AN OFFICIAL JOURNAL OF THE AMERICAN COLLEGE OF RHEUMATOLOGY

Arthritis & Rheumatism

VOLUME 44, NUMBER 1

JANUARY 2001

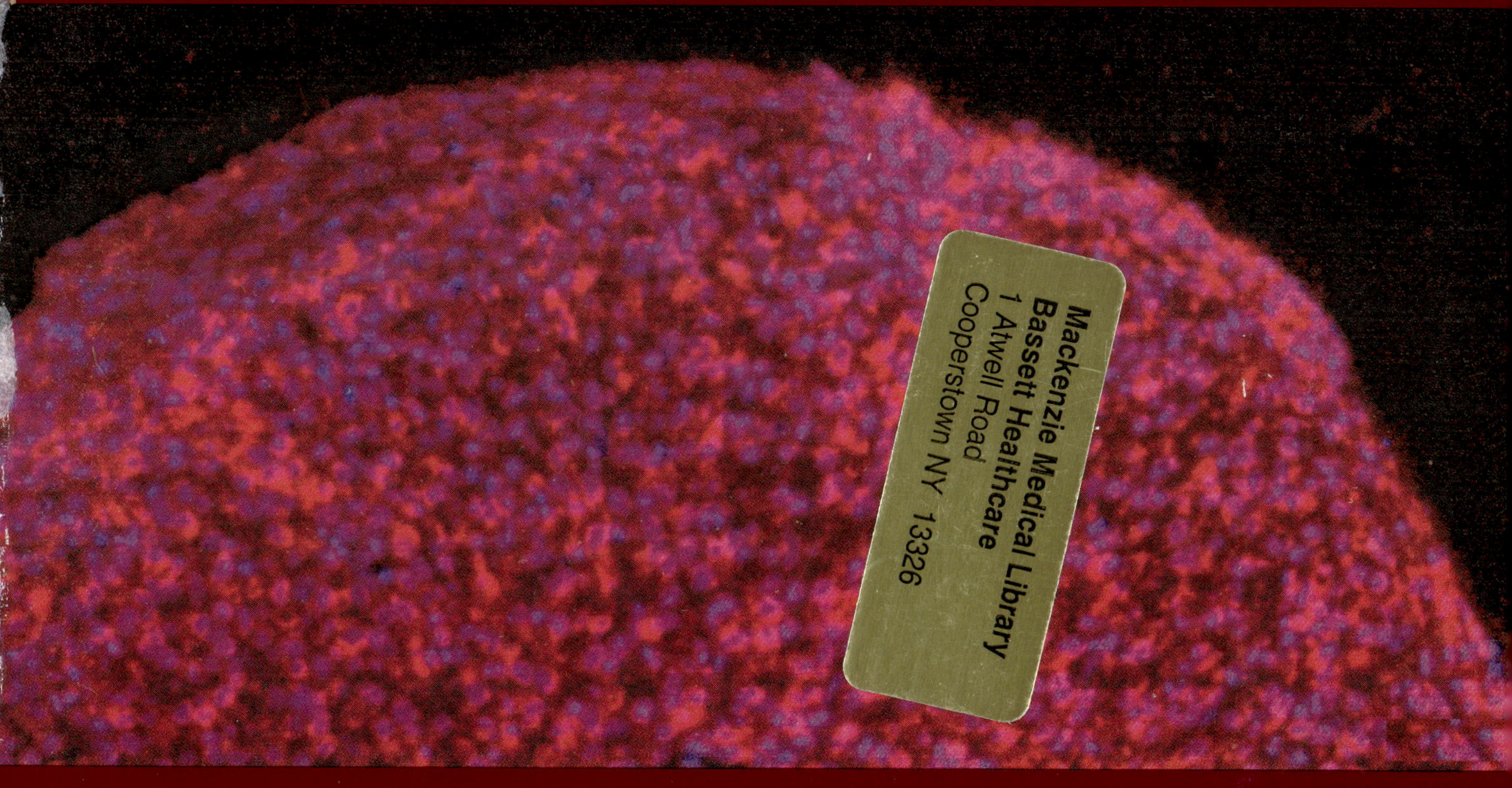

EDUCATION TREATMENT RESEARCH

AMERICAN COLLEGE OF RHEUMATOLOGY

www.arthritisrheum.org

WILEY InterScience®

www.interscience.wiley.com

She's got RA.

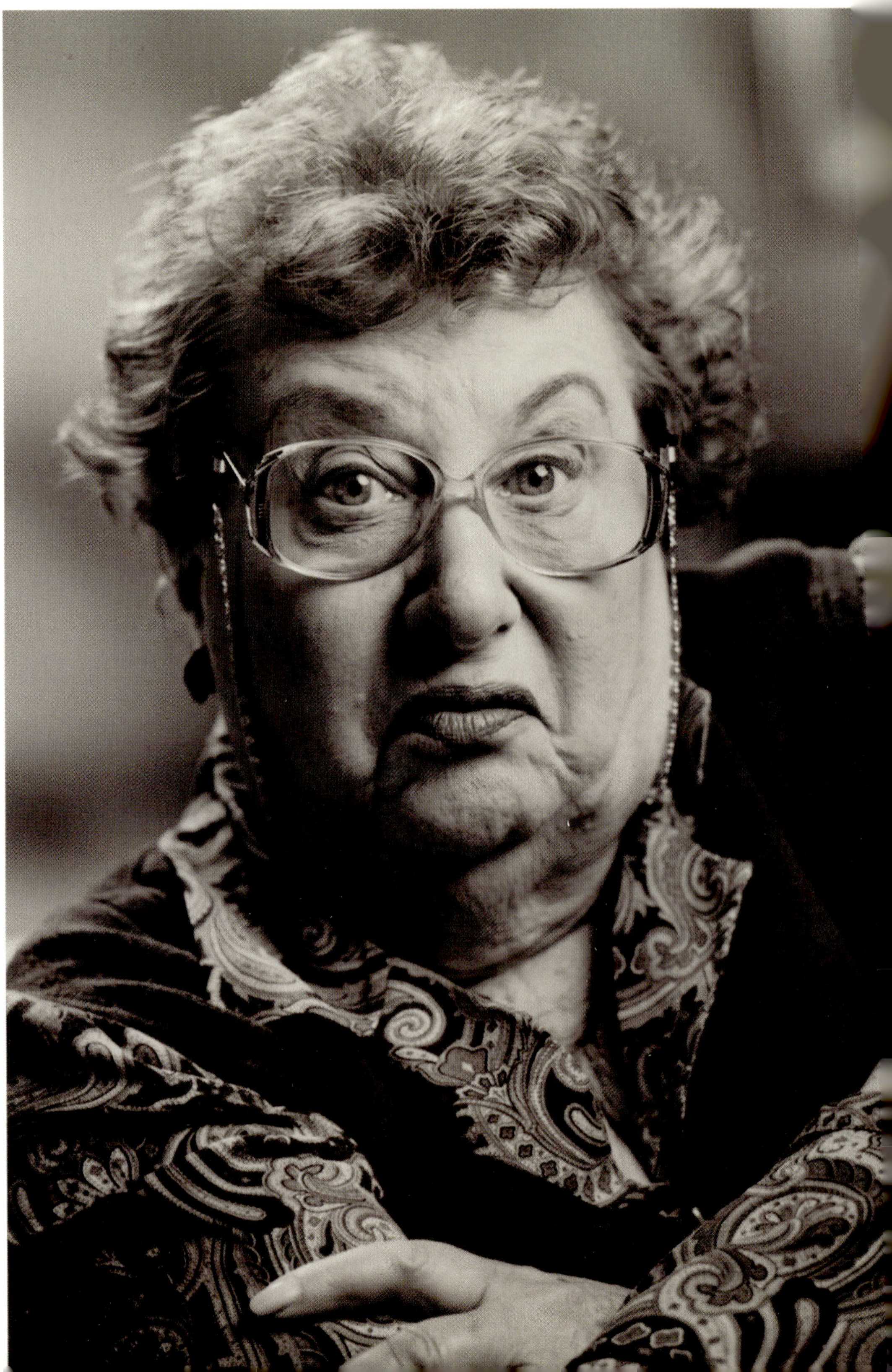

Arthritis & Rheumatism

Official Journal of the American College of Rheumatology
www.arthritisrheum.org and www.interscience.wiley.com

ARTHRITIS AND RHEUMATISM (Print ISSN 0004-3591; Online ISSN 1529-0131 at Wiley InterScience, www.interscience.wiley.com) is published monthly, except semi-monthly in February, April, June, August, October, and December by Wiley-Liss, Inc., a division of John Wiley & Sons, Inc., 605 Third Avenue, New York, NY 10158-0012. **Send subscription inquiries to:** John Wiley & Sons, Inc., Subscription Department, 9th Floor, 605 Third Avenue, New York, NY 10158-0012, (212) 850-6645. **Advertising sales contact:** Susan Tagliaferro, Accounts Representative, Pharmaceutical Media, Inc., 30 East 33rd Street, New York, NY 10016, phone (212) 685-5010. **Offprint sales and inquiries** should be directed to the Customer Service Department, John Wiley and Sons, 605 Third Avenue, New York, NY 10158-0012, (212) 850-8776. For 2001, Volumes 44 and 45; institutional rate in U.S., $560; outside U.S., $720; personal subscription rate in U.S., $207; outside U.S., $249. (Subscriptions outside North America are sent by air.) Payment must be made in U.S. dollars drawn on a U.S. bank. **Change of Address:** Please forward to the subscriptions address listed above 6 weeks prior to move; enclose present mailing label with change of address. **Claims** for undelivered copies will be accepted only after the following issue has been received. Please enclose a copy of the mailing label or cite your subscriber reference number in order to expedite handling. Missing copies will be supplied when losses have been sustained in transit and where reserve stock permits. Send claims to John Wiley & Sons, Inc., Customer Service, 605 Third Avenue, New York, NY 10158-0012. If claims are not resolved satisfactorily, please write to Caroline Rothaug, Subscription Fulfillment and Sales, John Wiley & Sons, Inc., 605 Third Avenue, New York, NY 10158-0012. **Cancellations:** Subscription cancellations will not be accepted after the first issue has been mailed. Periodicals postage paid at New York, N.Y., and at additional mailing offices. Printed in U.S.A. Copyright © 2001 Wiley-Liss, Inc., POSTMASTER: Send address changes to Arthritis and Rheumatism, Subscription Systems and Distribution, John Wiley & Sons, Inc., 605 Third Avenue, New York, NY 10158-0012.

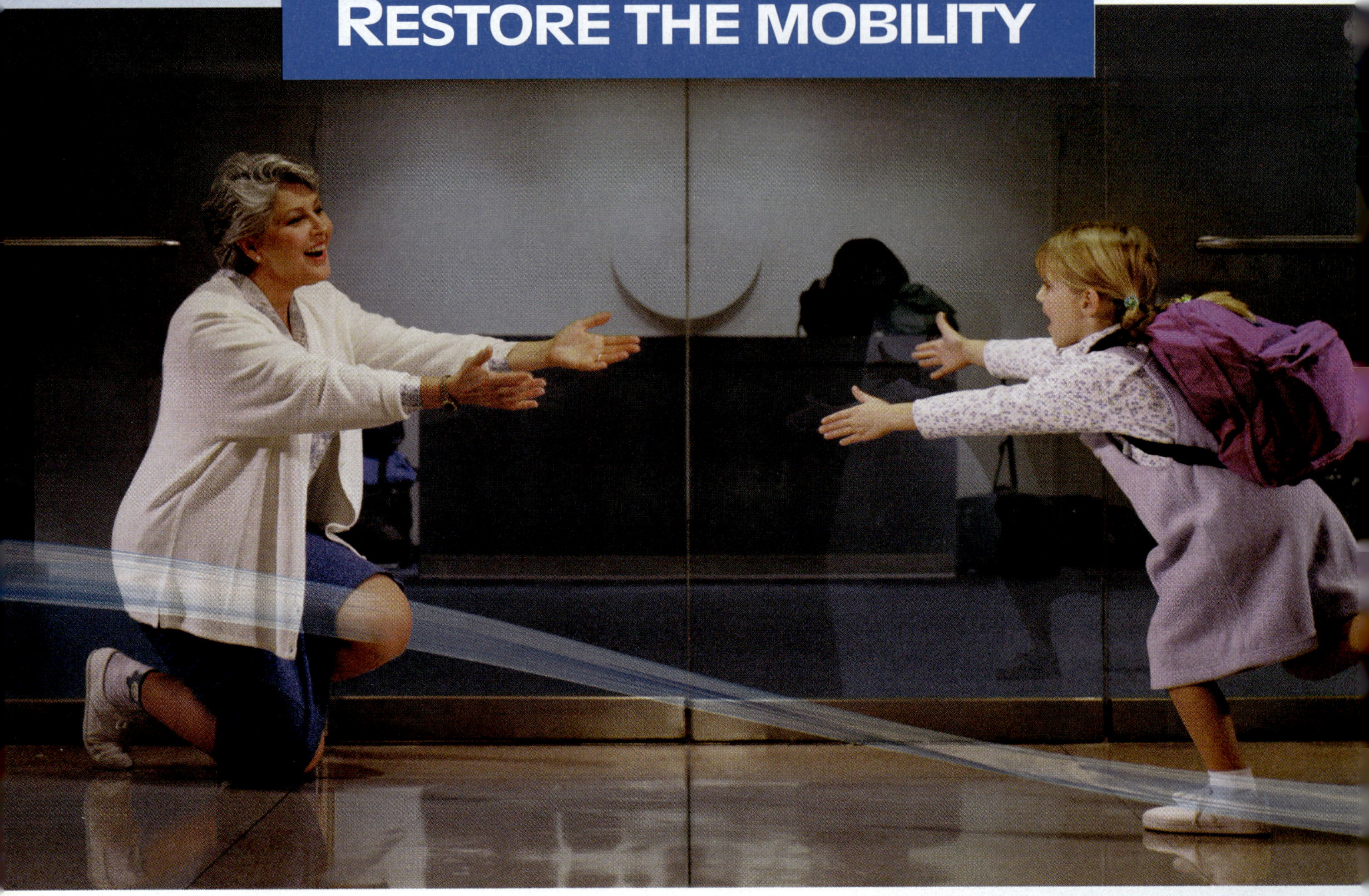

Arthritis & Rheumatism

Official Journal of the American College of Rheumatology
www.arthritisrheum.org and www.interscience.wiley.com

VOLUME 44 **JANUARY 2001** **NO. 1**

Special Articles

Editorial: The American College of Rheumatology Journals: New Directions for Y2K + 1
David S. Pisetsky 1

Review: Synergistic Activity of Interleukin-4 and Interleukin-10 in Suppression of Inflammation and Joint Destruction in Rheumatoid Arthritis
Joel A. G. van Roon, Floris P. J. G. Lafeber, and J. W. J. Bijlsma 3

Rheumatoid Arthritis

CD4+,CD28− T Cells in Rheumatoid Arthritis Patients Combine Features of the Innate and Adaptive Immune Systems
Kenneth J. Warrington, Seisuke Takemura, Jörg J. Goronzy, and Cornelia M. Weyand 13

Rheumatoid Arthritis Synovial Macrophages Express the Fas-Associated Death Domain–Like Interleukin-1β–Converting Enzyme–Inhibitory Protein and Are Refractory to Fas-Mediated Apoptosis
Harris Perlman, Lisa J. Pagliari, Hongtao Liu, Alisa E. Koch, G. Kenneth Haines, III, and Richard M. Pope 21

Regulation of Angiogenesis by the C-X-C Chemokines Interleukin-8 and Epithelial Neutrophil Activating Peptide 78 in the Rheumatoid Joint
Alisa E. Koch, Michael V. Volin, James M. Woods, Steven L. Kunkel, Matthew A. Connors, Lisa A. Harlow, Drew C. Woodruff, Marie D. Burdick, and Robert M. Strieter 31

Secretion of Anti–Citrulline-Containing Peptide Antibody by B Lymphocytes in Rheumatoid Arthritis
Carelle C. Reparon-Schuijt, Wim J. E. van Esch, Cees van Kooten, Gerard A. Schellekens, Ben A. W. de Jong, Walther J. van Venrooij, Ferdinand C. Breedveld, and Cornelis L. Verweij 41

The Influence of Synovial Fluid on Adenovirus-Mediated Gene Transfer to the Synovial Tissue
Paulien H. Goossens, Ronald Vogels, Elsbet Pieterman, Menzo J. E. Havenga, Abraham Bout, Ferdinand C. Breedveld, Dinko Valerio, and Tom W. J. Huizinga 48

Responsiveness of the Self-Assessed Rheumatoid Arthritis Disease Activity Index to a Flare of Disease Activity
Jaap Fransen, Hansjörg Häuselmann, Beat A. Michel, Miguel Caravatti, and Gerold Stucki 53

Association Between Rheumatoid Arthritis and Polymorphism of Tumor Necrosis Factor Receptor II, But Not Tumor Necrosis Factor Receptor I, in Caucasians
Anne Barton, Sally John, W. E. R. Ollier, Alan Silman, and Jane Worthington 61

The Clinical Significance of Amyloid Fat Deposits in Rheumatoid Arthritis: A Systematic Long-Term Followup Study using Abdominal Fat Aspiration
Emili Gómez-Casanovas, Raimon Sanmartí, Manel Solé, Juan D. Cañete, and José Muñoz-Gómez 66

Osteoarthritis and Cartilage

Hepatocyte Growth Factor Induction of Collagenase 3 Production in Human Osteoarthritic Cartilage: Involvement of the Stress-Activated Protein Kinase/c-Jun N-Terminal Kinase Pathway and a Sensitive p38 Mitogen-Activated Protein Kinase Inhibitor Cascade
Pascal Reboul, Jean-Pierre Pelletier, Ginette Tardif, Mohamed Benderdour, Pierre Ranger, Donald P. Bottaro, and Johanne Martel-Pelletier 73

Human Periosteum-Derived Cells Maintain Phenotypic Stability and Chondrogenic Potential throughout Expansion Regardless of Donor Age
Cosimo De Bari, Francesco Dell'Accio, and Frank P. Luyten 85

Nitric Oxide Regulates Mitochondrial Respiration and Functions of Articular Chondrocytes
Masuhiro Tomita, Eisuke F. Sato, Manabu Nishikawa, Yoshiki Yamano, and Masayasu Inoue 96

Mechanisms of Disease: Models and Genetics

Comparison of Differentiated Dendritic Cell Infiltration of Autoimmune and Osteoarthritis Synovial Tissue
Allison R. Pettit, Michael J. Ahern, Simone Zehntner, Malcolm D. Smith, and Ranjeny Thomas 105

Dependence of Interleukin-1–Induced Arthritis on Granulocyte–Macrophage Colony-Stimulating Factor
Yuan H. Yang and John A. Hamilton 111

Early Degradation of Type IX and Type II Collagen with the Onset of Experimental Inflammatory Arthritis
Toshihisa Kojima, Fackson Mwale, Tadashi Yasuda, Christiane Girard, A. Robin Poole, and Sheila Laverty 120
Disease-Modifying Activity of SB 273005, an Orally Active, Nonpeptide $\alpha_v\beta_3$ (Vitronectin Receptor) Antagonist, in Rat Adjuvant-Induced Arthritis
Alison M. Badger, Simon Blake, Rasesh Kapadia, Susanta Sarkar, Joshua Levin, Barbara A. Swift, Sandy J. Hoffman, George B. Stroup, William H. Miller, Maxine Gowen, and Michael W. Lark 128
Induction of Endothelial Cell Decay-Accelerating Factor by Vascular Endothelial Growth Factor: A Mechanism for Cytoprotection Against Complement-Mediated Injury during Inflammatory Angiogenesis
Justin C. Mason, Elaine A. Lidington, Helen Yarwood, Douglas M. Lublin, and Dorian O. Haskard 138
Insights from a Novel Three-Dimensional In Vitro Model of Lyme Arthritis: Standardized Analysis of Cellular and Molecular Interactions Between *Borrelia burgdorferi* and Synovial Explants and Fibroblasts
Juliane K. Franz, Olaf Fritze, Michael Rittig, Gernot Keyßer, Susanne Priem, Josef Zacher, Gerd-R. Burmester, and Andreas Krause 151
The MICA Region Determines the First Modifier Locus in Familial Mediterranean Fever
Isabelle Touitou, Marie-Christine Picot, Cécile Domingo, Cécile Notarnicola, Daniel Cattan, Jacques Demaille, and Isabelle Koné-Paut 163

Systemic Lupus Erythematosus and Autoimmunity

Treatment of Lupus-Induced Thrombocytopenia with Recombinant Human Interleukin-11
Shamiram Feinglass and Atul Deodhar 170
Genetic Association Between Interleukin-10 Promoter Region Polymorphisms and Primary Sjögren's Syndrome
Janne Hulkkonen, Marja Pertovaara, Jaakko Antonen, Nina Lahdenpohja, Amos Pasternack, and Mikko Hurme 176

Spondylarthropathy

Efficacy of Celecoxib, a Cyclooxygenase 2–Specific Inhibitor, in the Treatment of Ankylosing Spondylitis: A Six-Week Controlled Study with Comparison Against Placebo and Against a Conventional Nonsteroidal Antiinflammatory Drug
Maxime Dougados, Jehan-Michel Béhier, Irène Jolchine, Andrei Calin, Désirée van der Heijde, Ignazio Olivieri, Henning Zeidler, and Hélène Herman 180
Immunomodulatory Effects of Anti–Tumor Necrosis Factor α Therapy on Synovium in Spondylarthropathy: Histologic Findings in Eight Patients from an Open-Label Pilot Study
Dominique Baeten, Elli Kruithof, Filip Van den Bosch, Pieter Demetter, Nancy Van Damme, Claude Cuvelier, Martine De Vos, Herman Mielants, Eric M. Veys, and Filip De Keyser 186

Osteoporosis and Bone

A Functional Polymorphic Variant in the Interleukin-6 Gene Promoter Associated with Low Bone Resorption in Postmenopausal Women
S. L. Ferrari, P. Garnero, S. Emond, H. Montgomery, S. E. Humphries, and S. L. Greenspan 196
Two-Year Effects of Alendronate on Bone Mineral Density and Vertebral Fracture in Patients Receiving Glucocorticoids: A Randomized, Double-Blind, Placebo-Controlled Extension Trial
Jonathan D. Adachi, Kenneth G. Saag, Pierre D. Delmas, Uri A. Liberman, Ronald D. Emkey, Ego Seeman, Nancy E. Lane, Jean-Marc Kaufman, Patrice E. E. Poubelle, Federico Hawkins, Ricardo Correa-Rotter, Charles-Joel Menkes, Jose A. Rodriguez-Portales, Thomas J. Schnitzer, Joel A. Block, Jeffrey Wing, Harris H. McIlwain, Rene Westhovens, Jacques Brown, Jose A. Melo-Gomes, Barry L. Gruber, Melissa J. Yanover, Maria Odette R. Leite, Kerry G. Siminoski, Michael C. Nevitt, John T. Sharp, Marie-Pierre Malice, Thomas Dumortier, Michelle Czachur, Wendy Carofano, and Anastasia Daifotis 202

Epidemiology, Outcomes, and Treatment

Arthritis Prevalence and Activity Limitations in Older Adults
Dorothy D. Dunlop, Larry M. Manheim, Jing Song, and Rowland W. Chang 212
Alpha Sleep Characteristics in Fibromyalgia
Suely Roizenblatt, Harvey Moldofsky, Ana Amelia Benedito-Silva, and Sergio Tufik 222
Efficacy and Safety of Desensitization to Allopurinol following Cutaneous Reactions
Adel G. Fam, Shelly M. Dunne, John Iazzetta, and Thomas W. Paton 231

Concise Communications

Evidence for Linkage of the HLA–B Locus in Behçet's Disease, Obtained using the Transmission Disequilibrium Test
Ahmet Gül, Ali H. Hajeer, Jane Worthington, Jennifer H. Barrett, William E. R. Ollier, and Alan J. Silman 239

Beneficial Effect of Etanercept on Rheumatoid Lymphedema
Barbara E. Ostrov ... 240

Letters

Increase in the Heart Rate–Corrected QT Interval in Children of Anti-Ro–Positive Mothers, with a Further Increase in Those with Siblings with Congenital Heart Block: Comment on the Article by Cimaz et al
Patrick A. Gordon, Munther A. Khamashta, Graham R. V. Hughes, and Eric Rosenthal ... 242

Reply
Rolando Cimaz, Antonio Brucato, Marco Stramba-Badiale, Luca Catelli, and Pier Luigi Meroni ... 243

Shrinking Lung Syndrome in Patients without Systemic Lupus Erythematosus: Comment on the Concise Communication by Tavoni et al
Shahbaz Ahmed, Ariane Herrick, and B. Ronan O'Driscoll ... 243

Reply
A. Tavoni and S. Bombardieri ... 245

Similar Effects of Pulse Corticosteroid and Tumor Necrosis Factor α Blockade in Rheumatoid Arthritis: Comment on the Article by Taylor et al
Malcolm D. Smith, Michael J. Ahern, Peter J. Roberts-Thomson, and Peter P. Youssef ... 245

Reply
Peter C. Taylor, Ewa Paleolog, and Ravinder N. Maini ... 245

Clinical Images

Lupus Erythematosus Cells in the Kidney and Synovial Fluid
B. M. Atiquzzaman, Daniel D. Ricciardi, Yusuf Yazici, and Allan Gibofsky ... 169

Cervical Spinal Cord Compression
Kari Laiho, Markku Kauppi, and Irma Soini ... 241

ACR Announcements ... 43A

Cover image: The figure on the cover (from De Bari et al, page 92) shows immunofluorescence staining for type II collagen in transforming growth factor β1–treated micromasses derived from human periosteum-derived cells (PDC). The demonstration of type II collagen in these micromasses is evidence that PDC have chondrogenic potential and can develop into cartilage. The chondrogenic potential of PDC may provide the basis for tissue engineering to regenerate or resurface cartilage.

Erosion in rheumatoid arthritis

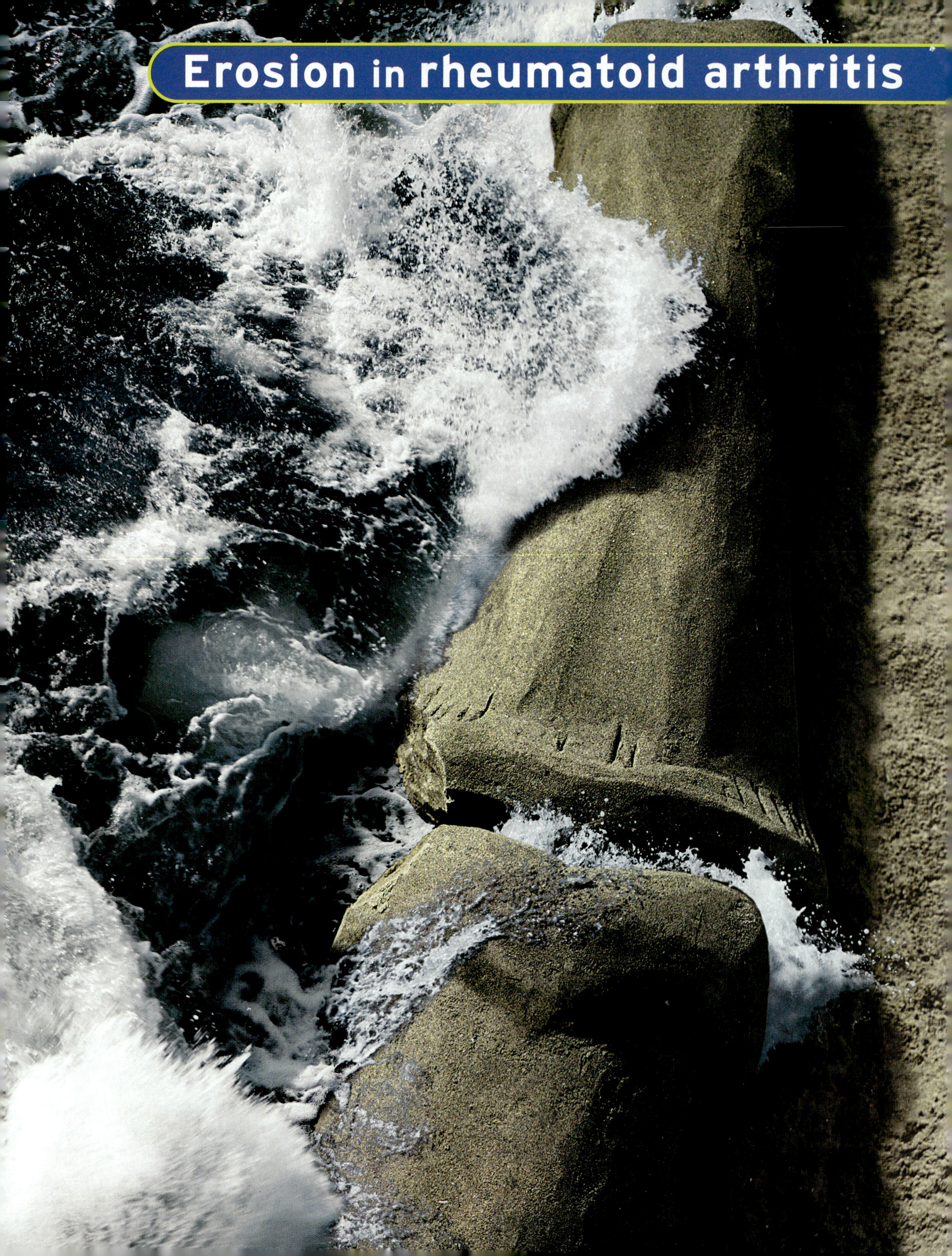

The critical role of IL-1

The pathogenesis of RA is a complex process that leads to joint inflammation and bone erosion. It's known to include several interdependent and variable interactions between pro-inflammatory and anti-inflammatory mechanisms.[1,2] Cytokines have been found to play a key role in promoting this disease process. The two pivotal cytokines in the pathogenesis of RA are interleukin-1 (IL-1) and tumor necrosis factor-alpha (TNF-α).[3,4]

IL-1 has been implicated in a destructive tide of events

In the RA disease process, IL-1 and TNF-α act synergistically to induce other cytokines and COX-2. Moreover, TNF-α induces IL-1,[5] IL-1 induces TNF-α,[6] and IL-1 induces IL-1.[7] This activity increases the production of PGE_2 and other arachidonic acid metabolites from synoviocytes[8,9] and accounts for much of the pain and swelling associated with RA.[10]

IL-1 is involved in many facets of the RA disease process. Pro-inflammatory cytokines cause neutrophils, monocytes, and lymphocytes to migrate to the synovium. In immunohistologic studies of macrophages accumulating in the synovial tissue, IL-1 production has been demonstrated in the cartilage-pannus junction as well as in the lining and sublining layers.[11,12]

Once in the synovium, neutrophils are activated and release mediators that stimulate mononuclear leukocytes, synoviocytes, and chondrocytes. These cells release IL-1 (more specifically, IL-1β) and other pro- and anti-inflammatory cytokines.[3,8,10]

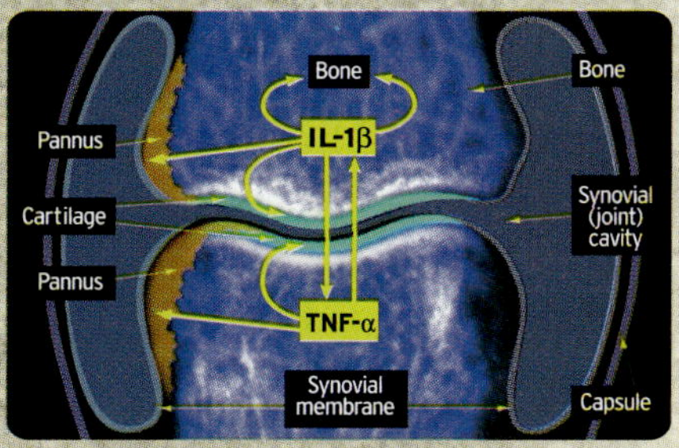

Then, once IL-1 and TNF-α are present, other interleukins (IL-6, IL-8, and IL-10) stimulate local fibroblast proliferation and recruit leukocytes. Although inflamed synovial cells express TNF-α, it is secreted to a far lesser extent than IL-1.[4,13] Early in the RA disease process, IL-1 causes cartilage degradation by inducing rapid loss of proteoglycans and stimulating the production of neutral proteinases in chondrocytes.[1,14] Since IL-1 also stimulates osteoclasts, bone resorption occurs.[15]

Higher levels of IL-1 seen with bone erosion

Animal studies, preclinical research, and early clinical studies all support the dominant role that IL-1 plays in cartilage damage and bone resorption, and suggest that TNF-α is more responsible for the inflammation in RA.[4,14,15]

In animal studies, joint swelling and cartilage damage are still present in TNF-α knockout mice (which cannot produce TNF-α), while there is an impressive reduction of cartilage damage, bone erosion, and chronic synovial infiltration in IL-1–deficient mice.[4]

These findings are supported by clinical evidence that patients with RA who have bone erosions also have higher IL-1 levels in their synovial fluid than RA patients who do not have bone erosions. Together, these findings point to the primary role of IL-1 in the bone and cartilage erosion seen in RA.[16]

The IL-1 gene family consists of IL-1α, IL-1β, and IL-1 receptor antagonist (IL-1Ra), which is the naturally occurring cytokine antagonist that normally balances the destructive effects of IL-1α and IL-1β in rheumatoid arthritis.[17] However, in RA, production of IL-1 cannot be sufficiently countered by endogenous IL-1Ra alone; this leads to the damaging bone and cartilage effects seen in rheumatoid joints.[17]

Amgen is conducting research in the area of rheumatology to develop new and important therapies.

AMGEN®

Advancing the science of rheumatology

References

1. Cush JJ, Lipsky PE. Cellular basis for rheumatoid inflammation. *Clin Orthop.* 1991;265:9-22.
2. Arend WP. Interleukin-1 receptor antagonist. *Adv Immunol.* 1993;54:167-227.
3. Buchan G, Barrett K, Turner M, Chantry D, Maini RN, Feldmann M. Interleukin-1 and tumour necrosis factor mRNA expression in rheumatoid arthritis: prolonged production of IL-1α. *Clin Exp Immunol.* 1998; 73:449-455.
4. van den Berg WB. Joint inflammation and cartilage destruction may occur uncoupled. *Springer Semin Immunopathol.* 1998;20:149-164.
5. Dinarello CA, Cannon JG, Wolff SM, et al. Tumor necrosis factor (cachectin) is an endogenous pyrogen and induces production of interleukin 1. *J Exp Med.* 1986; 163(6): 1433-1450.
6. Philip R, Epstein LB. Tumour necrosis factor as immuno-modulator and mediator of monocyte cytotoxicity induced by itself, γ-interferon and interleukin-1. *Nature.* 1986;323(6083):86-89.
7. Dinarello CA, Ikejima T, Warner SJC, et al. Interleukin 1 induces interleukin 1, I: induction of circulating interleukin 1 in rabbits in vivo and in human mononuclear cells in vitro. *J Immunol.* 1987;139(6):1902-1910.
8. Koch AE, Kunkel SL, Strieter RM. Cytokines in rheumatoid arthritis. *J Invest Med.* 1995;43:28-38.
9. Crofford LJ, Wilder RL, Ristimake AP. Cyclooxygenase-1 and -2 expression in rheumatoid synovial tissues: effects of interleukin-1β, phorbol ester, and corticosteroids. *J Clin Invest.* 1994;93(3):1095-1101.
10. Harris ED Jr. Rheumatoid arthritis: pathophysiology and implications for therapy. *New Engl J Med.* 1990;322:1277-1289.
11. Chu CQ, Field M, Allard S, Abney E, Feldmann M, Maini RN. Detection of cytokines at the cartilage/pannus junction in patients with rheumatoid arthritis: implications for the role of cytokines in cartilage destruction and repair. *Br J Rheumatol.* 1992;31(10):653-661.
12. Wood NC, Dickens E, Symons JA, Duff GW. In situ hybridization of interleukin-1 in CD14-positive cells in rheumatoid arthritis. *Clin Immunol Immunopathol.* 1992; 62(3):295-300.
13. van den Berg WB, Joosten LAB, van de Loo FAJ. TNFα and IL-1β are separate targets in chronic arthritis. *Clin Exp Rheumatol.* 1999;17(suppl 18):S105-S114.
14. van Lent PLEM, van de Loo FAJ, Astrid EM, et al. Major role for interleukin 1 but not for tumor necrosis factor in early cartilage damage in immune complex arthritis in mice. *J Rheumatol.* 1995;22:2250-2258.
15. Dinarello CA, Moldawer LL. *Proinflammatory and Anti-inflammatory Cytokines in Rheumatoid Arthritis: A Primer for Clinicians.* Thousand Oaks, Calif: Amgen Inc.; 1999:34.
16. Eastgate JA, Symons JA, Wood NC, Grinlinton FM, di Giovine FS, Duff GW. Correlation of plasma interleukin 1 levels with disease activity in rheumatoid arthritis. *Lancet.* 1988;2:706-709.
17. Arend WP, Malyak M, Guthridge CJ, Gabay C. Interleukin-1 receptor antagonist: role in biology. *Annu Rev Immunol.* 1998;16:27-55.

Notes to Contributors

(Note: the information that follows is also available online at www.arthritisrheum.org and www.interscience.wiley.com)

Manuscripts for publication, letters, news, and notes should be sent to:
David S. Pisetsky, MD, PhD, Editor, *Arthritis & Rheumatism*
2400 Pratt Street, Room 0311 Terrace Level
Duke University Medical Center Box 3806
Durham, NC 27710
phone (919) 668-0488, fax (919) 668-0744, e-mail jennifer.deyton@duke.edu

Articles are accepted for publication on the condition that they are submitted to this journal only. Articles should definitely pertain to the field of rheumatic disease.

Manuscripts not in compliance with the following instructions may be subject to a delay in the review process.

Format and organization

_____ Submit 5 copies of the manuscript, including tables and figures. For figures that are charts, graphs, or other line art that retains its readability when photocopied, the figures should be sent in the form of 1 photocopy attached to each copy of the manuscript, plus 1 high-quality original that will be used for printing if the manuscript is accepted. For radiographs, micrographs, and other halftone photographs, 5 high-quality glossy prints (not photocopies) should be sent (see Illustrations section below).

_____ A cover letter with the corresponding author's signature should accompany the manuscript. Note in cover letter what type of manuscript is enclosed (Full-Length Article, Brief Report, Case Report, Concise Communication, or Letter to the Editor). Confirm that the manuscript has not been submitted or is not simultaneously being submitted elsewhere for either print or electronic publication, and that no portion of the data has been or will be published, in print or electronic form, in proceedings or transactions of meetings or symposium volumes. The publication of data in abstracts, and presentation in oral or poster sessions at meetings, do not constitute previous publication. Indicate any financial support or other benefits from commercial sources for the work reported on in the manuscript, or any other financial interests that any of the authors may have, which could create a potential conflict of interest or the appearance of a conflict of interest with regard to the work. Corresponding author should include address, telephone number, fax number, and E-mail address if applicable.

_____ Type the manuscript in standard 12-point type on 8½ × 11″ paper with 1″ margins, double spaced throughout, including references, tables, and figure legends.

_____ Number all sheets in succession, including references, tables, and figure legends. Title page is page 1.

_____ On the first page, type the title, name(s) of the author(s) and their major degrees, grant supporter(s), address for reprint requests, and corresponding author's telephone and fax numbers and E-mail address.

Full-Length Articles and Brief Reports

Definition: Full-Length Articles are descriptions of original research that add to the body of knowledge in arthritis and the rheumatic diseases. Brief Reports are short papers of investigations into disease mechanisms, reports of clinical experience, therapeutic trials, or research and/or clinical contributions to diagnosis, treatment, etiopathology, and epidemiology of rheumatic diseases.

_____ On the second page of Full-Length Articles and Brief Reports, include an abstract of less than 250 words. The abstract should be divided into the following sections: Objective, Methods, Results, and Conclusion.

_____ On the third page, begin the introduction (no heading is necessary).

_____ Follow this plan of organization: Materials and Methods (or Patients and Methods), Results, Discussion, References, Tables, and Figure Legends.

_____ Full-Length Articles should not exceed 15 typed manuscript pages from introduction through discussion (not including references, tables, and figure legends).

_____ Brief Reports should not exceed 9 manuscript pages from introduction through references, and should contain no more than 3 tables and/or figures and no more than 15 references.

Case Reports

Definition: Case Reports are reports of single cases that contribute to the body of knowledge of rheumatic diseases by reporting in-depth observations and/or laboratory investigations that may reveal etiopathogenetic mechanisms of a broader significance, or by presenting a concise discussion of an infrequently encountered problem that emphasizes a particular clinical point not generally available in the literature. Emphasis will be placed on the scholarship of discussion.

_____ On the second page of Case Reports, include an abstract of less than 150 words. The abstract should not be divided into sections as required for Full-Length Articles and Brief Reports.

_____ On the third page, begin the introduction (no heading is necessary).

_____ After the introduction, include a description of the case, followed by a general discussion.

_____ Case Reports should not exceed 9 manuscript pages from introduction through references, and should contain no more than 3 tables and/or figures and no more than 15 references.

Radiologic/Dermatologic Vignettes and Clinical Images

_____ Radiologic Vignettes are short articles describing cases with interesting and significant radiologic features. The Vignette should present a case description with clinical findings, radiologic findings, differential diagnosis, final diagnosis, and discussion. No abstract is necessary. Page length should be less than that for a Brief Report or Case Report; up to 3 figures may be included. Dermatologic Vignettes describe cases with interesting and significant dermatologic features and should have a format similar to that of Radiologic Vignettes.

_____ Clinical Images are photographic depictions (clinical, radiologic, or pathologic) of interesting rheumatologic phenomena. The image and accompanying caption should be short enough to fit on half a page of the journal (i.e., no more than one half page of double-spaced typewritten text, with the image preferably oriented horizontally). All images must be in black and white. There is no page charge for Clinical Images.

Letters to the Editor/Concise Communications

Definitions: Letters to the Editor should be limited to commentaries on previous articles published in *Arthritis & Rheumatism* and issues affecting rheumatology and the American College of Rheumatology. Concise Communications should be very short reports of cases or research findings, with no abstract, subheads, or acknowledgments section.

_____ Letters to the Editor and Concise Communications should be double spaced throughout.

_____ Length of Letters to the Editor and Concise Communications should be no more than 4 pages, including references.

_____ Only 1 table or figure may accompany a Letter to the Editor or Concise Communication.

Content

_____ Do not use new technical words, laboratory slang, words not defined in dictionaries, or abbreviations or terminology not consistent with internationally accepted guidelines.

_____ Define any abbreviations the first time they are used. A list of standard abbreviations appears on pages 1903–1905 of the November 1998 issue.

______ In order to make the description of patients as clear as possible and to facilitate comparisons with other studies, the Methods section should include, whenever possible, a short paragraph detailing the proportion of patients who satisfy the ACR classification criteria for the particular disease described.

Compliance with research ethics standards

______ For articles reporting prospective research involving human or animal subjects, note in the Methods section that the study has been approved by the appropriate institutional review board or, if there is not an institutional review board or comparable formal ethics review committee, that the Declaration of Helsinki principles have been followed.

Illustrations

______ For illustrations that are photographs (as opposed to line art), send 5 packaged sets in labeled envelopes. For line art that reproduces well on a photocopier, include 1 copy with each copy of the manuscript, and also send 1 high-quality original to be used for printing.

______ Do not write on the back of any figure, but attach a label to each with the figure number and first author's name. Include on the label an arrow indicating which end is the top of the figure.

______ Lettering and symbols on figures should be large enough, and shading distinct enough, to remain readable after figure size is reduced to one column width.

______ Do not attach illustrations to the manuscript with a paperclip.

______ Obtain releases from any patients whose pictures will be printed in the journal. Blinders on the eyes are not a substitute for patient's permission.

______ Radiographs, micrographs, other halftones, and linecuts should be no more than 3¼″ square.

______ **Color figures:** Authors are entitled to one free page of color. Additional are billed to the author at the special reduced rate of $500 per page. All color figures will be reproduced in full color in the online edition of the journal at no cost to authors. Authors are encouraged to submit color illustrations that highlight the text and convey essential scientific information. For best reproduction, bright, clear colors should be used. Dark colors against a dark background do not reproduce well; please place your color images against a white background whenever possible. Please contact Jennifer Nowak at [jnowak@wiley.com] for further information.

Tables

______ Refer to current issues of the Journal for table style.

______ Provide each table with an explanatory title so that it is intelligible without specific reference to the text.

______ Provide each table column with an appropriate heading.

______ Indicate clearly any units of measure on a table.

References

______ Limit the length of the reference list by using only key references.

______ Double space references.

______ Compile references numerically according to the order of the citation.

______ Use abbreviations for titles of medical periodicals that conform to those in *Index Medicus*.

______ In 1997, the Journal changed its reference style to conform to the style suggested in the Uniform Requirements for Manuscripts Submitted to Biomedical Journals. All new submissions should use the new reference style, which can be found in the article "Uniform Requirements for Manuscripts Submitted to Biomedical Journals" (N Engl J Med, January 23, 1997, pp 309–15).

Assignment of reviewers

______ Authors are asked to suggest potential reviewers of their manuscript. If there are individuals they would prefer not to review their manuscript, they may also so indicate.

Related manuscripts/Duplicate publication

______ If the authors are aware of any related manuscript that has been or will be published by or submitted to another journal or to *Arthritis & Rheumatism* (e.g., another manuscript resulting from the same study), a copy of the other manuscript should be sent along with the one that is being submitted for publication in *Arthritis & Rheumatism*.

______ Articles are received only for exclusive publication in *Arthritis & Rheumatism* with the understanding that they have not been published elsewhere (in part or in full, in other words or in the same words, in letter or article form, in print or electronic form, or otherwise), are not at the time of submission under consideration by another journal or other publication, and will not be submitted elsewhere unless rejected by *Arthritis & Rheumatism.* If an author violates this requirement or engages in other similar misconduct, the Editor may, in addition to rejecting the manuscript, impose a moratorium on the acceptance of new manuscripts from the author and, if the misconduct is deemed sufficiently serious, may refer the matter to the author's academic institution or hospital and/or the appropriate state or local disciplinary body.

Disclosure of interest

______ The American College of Rheumatology's Board of Directors officially adopted Conflict of Interest Guidelines for *Arthritis & Rheumatism* on July 7, 1995. These guidelines, as they relate to authors, are as follows.

______ A cover letter to the Editor accompanying a submitted manuscript must disclose information about financial support and consulting activities, for *all* authors, that might be interpreted as constituting a possible conflict of interest for the described studies.

______ *All* authors of manuscripts (basic or clinical research, case reports, letters, reviews, editorials or commentary) accepted for publication will be asked to sign a full disclosure form regarding possible conflicts of interest for that individual, any member of his/her immediate family, or any other individual or entity with whom the author has a significant relationship, including: (a) ownership or control of stock in a company developing or distributing a product studied or discussed in the manuscript, or a competing product; (b) service as a consultant or advisor to a company developing or distributing a product studied or discussed in the manuscript, or a competing product; (c) the existence of any patent/license/royalty arrangements for any material studied or discussed in the manuscript; (d) any other possible financial benefit, such as derived income from a diagnostic test or product described or discussed in the manuscript, or frequent legal work as an expert witness or consultant in cases related to the content of the manuscript.

______ The Editor and Associate Editors will decide whether any of this information constitutes a possible conflict of interest, or the appearance thereof, and should be divulged in a footnote.

Publication procedures

______ In accordance with the 1978 Copyright Law, authors are requested to sign a provisional copyright transfer statement at the time manuscript revisions are requested.

______ Contributors are provided with page proofs and asked to check for errors and for editorial queries. Although the correction of editorial and typographical errors will be made without charge, the cost of excessive additional alterations may be charged to the author.

______ Authors are requested to return one set of proofs, the original manuscript and illustrations, and the reprint order within 48 hours. Publication of the article may be delayed if the proofs are not sent back on time.

Page charge

______ A $70 per page charge will be assessed for publication in *Arthritis & Rheumatism*. Instructions for payment will be sent to authors along with the proofs. In extreme cases of inability to pay, the page charge may be reduced or waived. There is no page charge for solicited articles, letters to the editor, or book reviews. Questions regarding the page charge should be directed to the Managing Editor, *Arthritis & Rheumatism*, 1800 Century Place, Suite 250, Atlanta, GA 30345-4300.

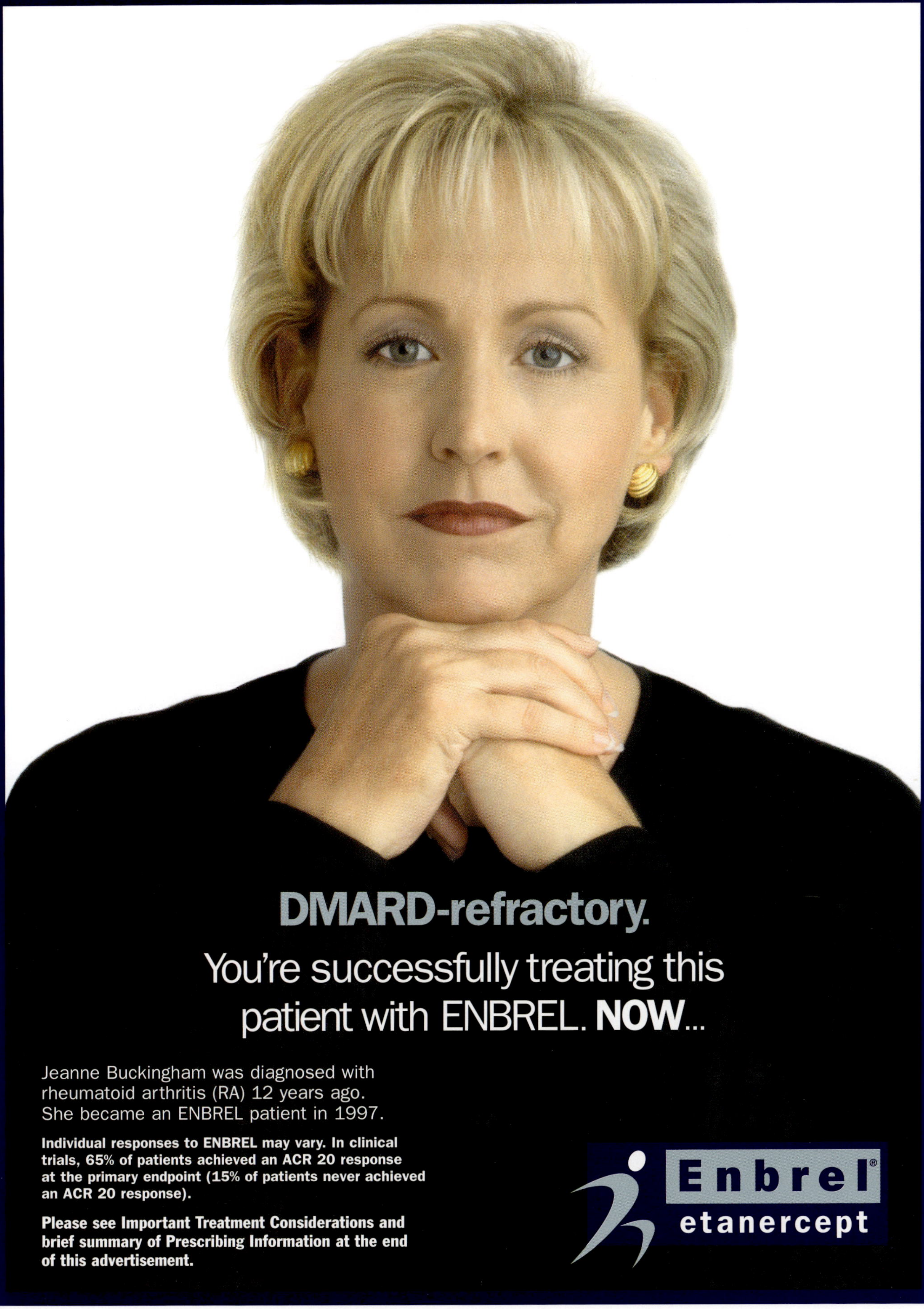
DMARD-refractory.
You're successfully treating this patient with ENBREL. NOW...
Jeanne Buckingham was diagnosed with rheumatoid arthritis (RA) 12 years ago. She became an ENBREL patient in 1997.
Individual responses to ENBREL may vary. In clinical trials, 65% of patients achieved an ACR 20 response at the primary endpoint (15% of patients never achieved an ACR 20 response).
Please see Important Treatment Considerations and brief summary of Prescribing Information at the end of this advertisement.
Enbrel®
etanercept

Important Treatment Considerations

IN POSTMARKETING USE, SERIOUS INFECTIONS AND SEPSIS, INCLUDING FATALITIES, HAVE BEEN REPORTED. MANY OF THESE EVENTS OCCURRED IN PATIENTS PREDISPOSED TO INFECTIONS, SUCH AS THOSE WITH ADVANCED OR POORLY CONTROLLED DIABETES. DISCONTINUE ENBREL IN PATIENTS WITH SERIOUS INFECTIONS OR SEPSIS. DO NOT START ENBREL IN THE PRESENCE OF SEPSIS, INFECTION (INCLUDING CHRONIC OR LOCALIZED), OR ALLERGY TO ENBREL OR ITS COMPONENTS. USE CAUTION IN PATIENTS PREDISPOSED TO INFECTION.

Rare cases of CNS demyelinating disorders have been reported, although the causal relationship to ENBREL remains unclear. Exercise caution when considering ENBREL for patients with these disorders. Rare cases of pancytopenia, including aplastic anemia, some fatal, have been reported in RA patients. Exercise caution in patients who have a previous history of significant hematologic abnormalities. Although the causal relationship to ENBREL remains unclear, advise patients to seek immediate medical attention if they develop signs or symptoms of blood dyscrasias or infection. If significant hematologic abnormalities are confirmed, consider discontinuing ENBREL.

The most frequent adverse events in placebo-controlled clinical trials (n=349) were injection site reactions (ISR) (37%), infections (35%), and headache (17%). Only the rate of ISR was higher than that of placebo. The most frequent adverse events in the methotrexate-controlled trial (n=415) were infections (64%), ISR (34%), and headache (24%). Only the rate of ISR was higher than that of MTX. In all RA patients treated in clinical trials (n=1,197), malignancies were rare (1%).

References: 1. ENBREL Prescribing Information, Immunex Corporation, Seattle, Wash. **2.** Data on file, Immunex Corporation, Seattle, Wash.

Enbrel®
etanercept

FREEDOM TO MOVE ON™

Please see brief summary of Prescribing Information at the end of this advertisement.

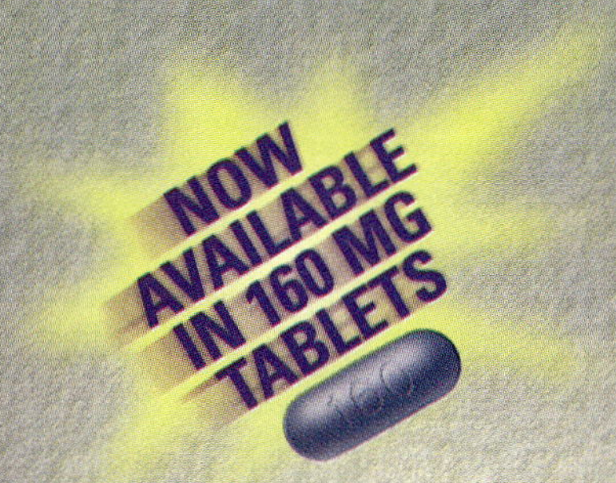

OxyContin 160 mg Tablets for use only in opioid-tolerant patients

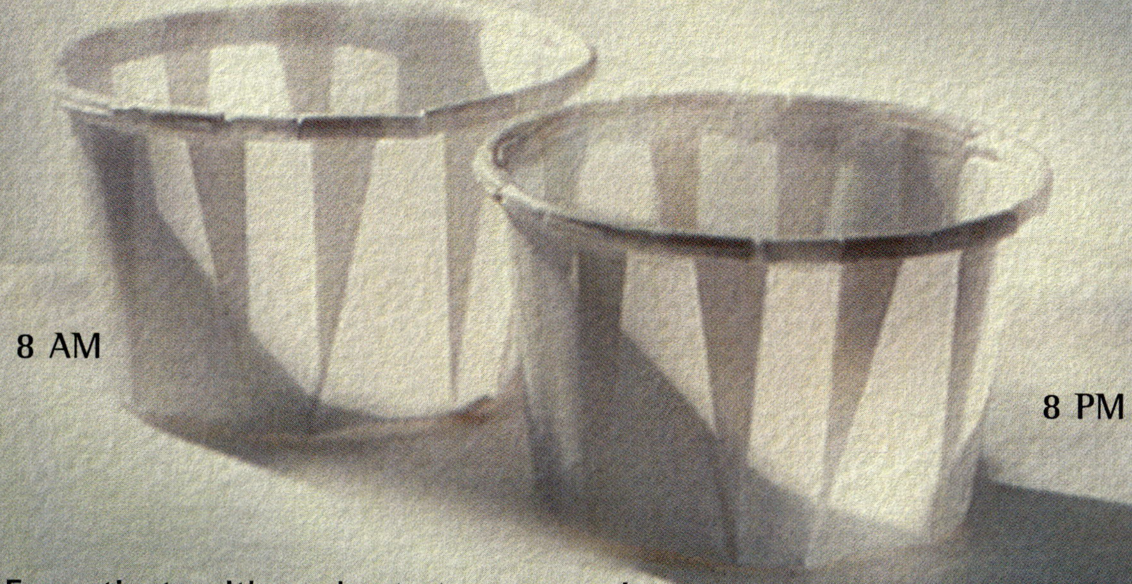

For patients with moderate to severe pain requiring opioid therapy for more than a few days

Q12h

OxyContin® CII

(OXYCODONE HCl CONTROLLED-RELEASE) TABLETS

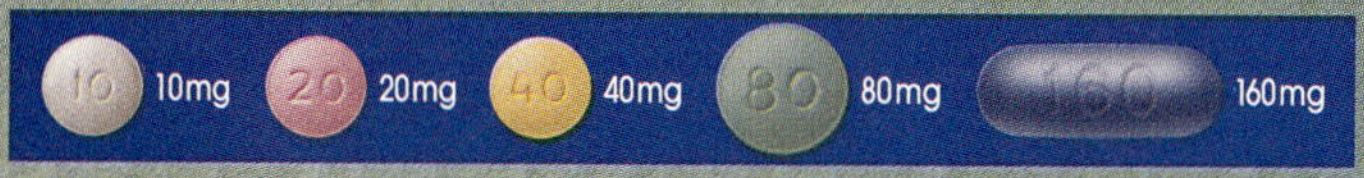

Small, color coded tablets (actual size)

OxyContin 80 and 160 mg Tablets for use only in opioid-tolerant patients requiring daily oxycodone equivalent dosages of 160 mg and 320 mg respectively.

OxyContin® Tablets are to be swallowed whole, and are not to be broken, chewed or crushed. Taking broken, chewed or crushed OxyContin Tablets could lead to the rapid release and absorption of a potentially toxic dose of oxycodone.

One OxyContin 160 mg Tablet is comparable to two 80 mg tablets when taken on an empty stomach. With a high fat meal, however, there is a 25% greater peak plasma concentration following one 160 mg tablet. Dietary caution should be taken when patients are initially titrated to 160 mg tablets.

The most serious risk associated with opioids, including OxyContin, is respiratory depression.

Common opioid side effects are constipation, nausea, sedation, dizziness, vomiting, pruritus, headache, dry mouth, sweating and weakness.

OxyContin is contraindicated in patients with known hypersensitivity to oxycodone, or in any situation where opioids are contraindicated. **(Please see Contraindications section in package insert.)**

For more information about pain management and prevention, visit our Web site: **www.partnersagainstpain.com**

Please read attached professional prescribing information.

Co-promoted by Purdue Pharma L.P. and Abbott Laboratories

PURDUE

A6571

PUR-4000665

OXYCONTIN® CII

(OXYCODONE HCl CONTROLLED-RELEASE) TABLETS

10 mg 20 mg 40 mg 80 mg* 160 mg*

*80 mg and 160 mg For use in opioid tolerant patients only.

Brief Summary on OxyContin® (oxycodone hydrochloride controlled-release) Tablets.

Before prescribing, see complete prescribing information, including DOSAGE AND ADMINISTRATION

INDICATIONS AND USAGE:

For the management of moderate to severe pain where use of an opioid analgesic is appropriate for more than a few days.

CONTRAINDICATIONS:

OxyContin® is contraindicated in patients with known hypersensitivity to oxycodone, or in any situation where opioids are contraindicated. This includes patients with significant respiratory depression (in unmonitored settings or the absence of resuscitative equipment), and patients with acute or severe bronchial asthma or hypercarbia. OxyContin is contraindicated in any patient who has or is suspected of having paralytic ileus.

WARNINGS:

OxyContin® TABLETS ARE TO BE SWALLOWED WHOLE, AND ARE NOT TO BE BROKEN, CHEWED OR CRUSHED. TAKING BROKEN, CHEWED OR CRUSHED OxyContin TABLETS COULD LEAD TO THE RAPID RELEASE AND ABSORPTION OF A POTENTIALLY TOXIC DOSE OF OXYCODONE.

Respiratory Depression

Respiratory depression, the chief hazard from all opioid agonist preparations, occurs most frequently in elderly or debilitated patients, usually following large initial doses in non-tolerant patients, or when opioids are given in conjunction with other agents that depress respiration.

Oxycodone should be used with extreme caution in patients with significant chronic obstructive pulmonary disease or cor pulmonale, and in patients having a substantially decreased respiratory reserve, hypoxia, hypercapnia, or preexisting respiratory depression. In such patients, even usual therapeutic doses of oxycodone may decrease respiratory drive to the point of apnea. In these patients alternative non-opioid analgesics should be considered, and opioids should be employed only under careful medical supervision at the lowest effective dose.

Head Injury

The respiratory depressant effects of opioids include carbon dioxide retention and secondary elevation of cerebrospinal fluid pressure, and may be markedly exaggerated in the presence of head injury, intracranial lesions, or other sources of preexisting increased intracranial pressure. Oxycodone produces effects which may obscure neurologic signs of further increases in intracranial pressure in patients with head injuries.

Hypotensive Effect

OxyContin®, like all opioid analgesics, may cause severe hypotension in an individual whose ability to maintain blood pressure has been compromised by a depleted blood volume, or after concurrent administration with drugs such as phenothiazines or other agents which compromise vasomotor tone. OxyContin may produce orthostatic hypotension in ambulatory patients. OxyContin, like all opioid analgesics, should be administered with caution to patients in circulatory shock, since vasodilation produced by the drug may further reduce cardiac output and blood pressure.

PRECAUTIONS:

Special precautions regarding OxyContin® 80 mg and 160 mg Tablets

OxyContin® 80 mg and 160 mg Tablets are for use only in opioid tolerant patients requiring daily oxycodone equivalent dosages of 160 mg or more for the 80 mg tablet and 320 mg or more for the 160 mg tablet. Care should be taken in the prescription of this tablet strength. Patients should be instructed against use by individuals other than the patient for whom it was prescribed, as such inappropriate use may have severe medical consequences.

One OxyContin® 160 mg tablet is comparable to two 80 mg tablets when taken on an empty stomach. With a high fat meal, however, there is a 25% greater peak plasma concentration following one 160 mg tablet. Dietary caution should be taken when patients are initially titrated to 160 mg tablets.

General — OxyContin® tablets are intended for use in patients who require oral pain therapy with an opioid agonist of more than a few days duration. As with any opioid analgesic, it is critical to adjust the dosing regimen individually for each patient.

Selection of patients for treatment with OxyContin should be governed by the same principles that apply to the use of similar controlled-release opioid analgesics. Opioid analgesics given on a fixed-dosage schedule have a narrow therapeutic index in certain patient populations, especially when combined with other drugs, and should be reserved for cases where the benefits of opioid analgesia outweigh the known risks of respiratory depression, altered mental state, and postural hypotension. Physicians should individualize treatment in every case, using non-opioid analgesics, prn opioids and/or combination products, and chronic opioid therapy with drugs such as OxyContin in a progressive plan of pain management such as outlined by the World Health Organization, the Agency for Health Care Policy and Research, and the American Pain Society.

Use of OxyContin is associated with increased potential risks and should be used only with caution in the following conditions: acute alcoholism; adrenocortical insufficiency (e.g., Addison's disease); CNS depression or coma; delirium tremens; debilitated patients; kyphoscoliosis associated with respiratory depression; myxedema or hypothyroidism; prostatic hypertrophy or urethral stricture; severe impairment of hepatic, pulmonary or renal function; and toxic psychosis.

The administration of oxycodone, like all opioid analgesics, may obscure the diagnosis or clinical course in patients with acute abdominal conditions. Oxycodone may aggravate convulsions in patients with convulsive disorders, and all opioids may induce or aggravate seizures in some clinical settings.

Interactions with other CNS Depressants

OxyContin, like all opioid analgesics, should be used with caution and started in a reduced dosage (1/3 to 1/2 of the usual dosage) in patients who are concurrently receiving other central nervous system depressants including sedatives or hypnotics, general anesthetics, phenothiazines, other tranquilizers, and alcohol. Interactive effects resulting in respiratory depression, hypotension, profound sedation, or coma may result if these drugs are taken in combination with the usual doses of OxyContin.

Interactions with Mixed Agonist/Antagonist Opioid Analgesics

Agonist/antagonist analgesics (i.e., pentazocine, nalbuphine, butorphanol, and buprenorphine) should be administered with caution to a patient who has received or is receiving a course of therapy with a pure opioid agonist analgesic such as oxycodone. In this situation, mixed agonist/antagonist analgesics may reduce the analgesic effect of oxycodone and/or may precipitate withdrawal symptoms in these patients.

Ambulatory Surgery

OxyContin is not recommended pre-operatively (preemptive analgesia) or for the management of pain in the immediate post-operative period (the first 12 to 24 hours following surgery) for patients not previously taking the drug, because its safety in this setting has not been established.

Patients who are already receiving OxyContin tablets as part of ongoing analgesic therapy may be safely continued on the drug if appropriate dosage adjustments are made considering the procedure, other drugs given and the temporary changes in physiology caused by the surgical intervention (see **PRECAUTIONS**; *Drug-Drug Interactions*).

Post-Operative Use

Morphine and other opioids have been shown to decrease bowel motility. Ileus is a common post-operative complication, especially after intra-abdominal surgery with opioid analgesia. Caution should be taken to monitor for decreased bowel motility in post-operative patients receiving opioids. Standard supportive therapy should be implemented.

Use in Pancreatic/Biliary Tract Disease

Oxycodone may cause spasm of the sphincter of Oddi and should be used with caution in patients with biliary tract disease, including acute pancreatitis. Opioids like oxycodone may cause increases in the serum amylase level.

Tolerance and Physical Dependence

Tolerance is the need for increasing doses of opioids to maintain a defined effect such as analgesia (in the absence of disease progression or other external factors). Physical dependence is the occurrence of withdrawal symptoms after abrupt discontinuation of a drug or upon administration of an antagonist. Physical dependence and tolerance are not unusual during chronic opioid therapy.

Significant tolerance should not occur in most of the patients treated with the lowest doses of oxycodone. It should be expected, however, that a fraction of cancer patients will develop some degree of tolerance and require progressively higher dosages of OxyContin to maintain pain control during chronic treatment. Regardless of whether this occurs as a result of increased pain secondary to disease progression or pharmacological tolerance, dosages can usually be increased safely by adjusting the patient's dose to maintain an acceptable balance between pain relief and side effects. The dosage should be selected according to the patient's individual analgesic response and ability to tolerate side effects. Tolerance to the analgesic effect of opioids is usually paralleled by tolerance to side effects, except for constipation.

Physical dependence results in withdrawal symptoms in patients who abruptly discontinue the drug or may be precipitated through the administration of drugs with opioid antagonist activity (see **OVERDOSAGE**). If OxyContin is abruptly discontinued in a physically dependent patient, an abstinence syndrome may occur. This is characterized by some or all of the following: restlessness, lacrimation, rhinorrhea, yawning, perspiration, chills, myalgia, and mydriasis. Other symptoms also may develop, including: irritability, anxiety, backache, joint pain, weakness, abdominal cramps, insomnia, nausea, anorexia, vomiting, diarrhea, or increased blood pressure, respiratory rate, or heart rate. If signs and symptoms of withdrawal occur, patients should be treated by reinstitution of opioid therapy followed by a gradual, tapered dose reduction of OxyContin combined with symptomatic support.

Information for Patients/Caregivers

If clinically advisable, patients receiving OxyContin should be given the following information by the physician:

1. OxyContin tablets were designed to work properly only if swallowed whole. They may release all their contents at once if broken, chewed or crushed, resulting in a risk of overdose.
2. Report episodes of breakthrough pain and adverse experiences occurring during therapy. Individualization of dosage is essential to make optimal use of this medication.
3. Do not adjust the dose of OxyContin without consulting the prescribing professional.
4. OxyContin may impair mental and/or physical ability required for the performance of potentially hazardous tasks (e.g., driving, operating heavy machinery).
5. Do not combine OxyContin with alcohol or other central nervous system depressants (sleep aids, tranquilizers) except by the orders of the prescribing physician, because additive effects may occur.
6. Women of childbearing potential who become, or are planning to become, pregnant should consult their physician regarding the effects of analgesics and other drug use during pregnancy on themselves and their unborn child.
7. OxyContin is a potential drug of abuse. Patients should protect it from theft, and it should never be given to anyone other than the individual for whom it was prescribed.
8. Patients may pass empty matrix "ghosts" (tablets) via colostomy or in the stool; this is of no concern since the active medication has already been absorbed.
9. If patients have been receiving treatment with OxyContin for more than a few weeks and cessation of therapy is indicated, it may be appropriate to taper the OxyContin dose, rather than abruptly discontinue it, due to the risk of precipitating withdrawal symptoms. Their physician can provide a dose schedule to accomplish a gradual discontinuation of the medication.

Laboratory Monitoring

Due to the broad range of plasma concentrations seen in clinical populations, the varying degrees of pain, and the development of tolerance, plasma oxycodone measurements are usually not helpful in clinical management. Plasma concentrations of the active drug substance may be of value in selected, unusual or complex cases.

Interactions with Alcohol and Drugs of Abuse

Oxycodone may be expected to have additive effects when used in conjunction with alcohol, other opioids or illicit drugs which cause central nervous system depression.

Use in Drug and Alcohol Addiction

OxyContin is an opioid with no approved use in the management of addictive disorders. Its proper usage in individuals with drug or alcohol dependence, either active or in remission, is for the management of pain requiring opioid analgesia.

Drug-Drug Interactions

Opioid analgesics, including OxyContin, may enhance the neuromuscular blocking action of skeletal muscle relaxants and produce an increased degree of respiratory depression.

Oxycodone is metabolized in part to oxymorphone via CYP2D6. While this pathway may be blocked by a variety of drugs (e.g., certain cardiovascular drugs and antidepressants), such blockade has not yet been shown to be of clinical significance with this agent. Clinicians should be aware of this possible interaction, however.

Use with CNS Depressants

OxyContin, like all opioid analgesics, should be started at 1/3 to 1/2 of the usual dosage in patients who are concurrently receiving other central nervous system depressants including sedatives or hypnotics, general anesthetics, phenothiazines, centrally acting anti-emetics, tranquilizers, and alcohol because respiratory depression, hypotension, and profound sedation or coma may result. No specific interaction between oxycodone and monoamine oxidase inhibitors has been observed, but caution in the use of any opioid in patients taking this class of drugs is appropriate.

Mutagenicity/Carcinogenicity

Oxycodone was not mutagenic in the following assays: Ames Salmonella and E. Coli test with and without metabolic activation at doses of up to 5000 μg, chromosomal aberration test in human lymphocytes in the absence of metabolic activation at doses of up to 1500 μg/ml and with activation 48 hours after exposure at doses of up to 5000 μg/ml, and in the in vivo bone marrow micronucleus test in mice (at plasma levels of up to 48 μg/ml). Mutagenic results occurred in the presence of metabolic activation in the human chromosomal aberration test (at greater than or equal to 1250 μg/ml) at 24 but not 48 hours of exposure and in the mouse lymphoma assay at doses of 50 μg/ml or greater with metabolic activation and at 400 μg/ml or greater without metabolic activation. The data from these tests indicate that the genotoxic risk to humans may be considered low.

Studies of oxycodone in animals to evaluate its carcinogenic potential have not been conducted owing to the length of clinical experience with the drug substance.

Pregnancy

Teratogenic Effects—Category B: Reproduction studies have been performed in rats and rabbits by oral administration at doses up to 8 mg/kg (48 mg/m^2) and 125 mg/kg (1375 mg/m^2), respectively. These doses are 3 and 47 times a human dose of 160 mg/day (90 mg/m^2), based on mg/kg of a 60 kg adult (0.5 and 15 times this human dose based upon mg/m^2). The results did not reveal evidence of harm to the fetus due to oxycodone. There are, however, no adequate and well-controlled studies in pregnant women. Because animal reproduction studies are not always predictive of human response, this drug should be used during pregnancy only if clearly needed.

Nonteratogenic Effects—Neonates whose mothers have been taking oxycodone chronically may exhibit respiratory depression and/or withdrawal symptoms, either at birth and/or in the nursery.

Labor and Delivery

OxyContin is not recommended for use in women during and immediately prior to labor and delivery because oral opioids may cause respiratory depression in the newborn.

Nursing Mothers

Low concentrations of oxycodone have been detected in breast milk. Withdrawal symptoms can occur in breast-feeding infants when maternal administration of an opioid analgesic is stopped. Ordinarily, nursing should not be undertaken while a patient is receiving OxyContin since oxycodone may be excreted in the milk.

Pediatric Use

Safety and effectiveness in pediatric patients below the age of 18 have not been established with this dosage form of oxycodone. However, oxycodone has been used extensively in the pediatric population in other dosage forms, as have the excipients used in this formulation. No specific increased risk is expected from the use of this form of oxycodone in pediatric patients old enough to safely take tablets if dosing is adjusted for the patient's weight. **It must be remembered that OxyContin tablets cannot be crushed or divided for administration.**

Geriatric Use

In controlled pharmacokinetic studies in elderly subjects (greater than 65 years) the clearance of oxycodone appeared to be slightly reduced. Compared to young adults, the plasma concentrations of oxycodone were increased approximately 15%. In clinical trials with appropriate initiation of therapy and dose titration, no untoward or unexpected side effects were seen based on age, and the usual doses and dosing intervals are appropriate for the geriatric patient. As with all opioids, the starting dose should be reduced to 1/3 to 1/2 of the usual dosage in debilitated, non-tolerant patients.

Hepatic Impairment

A study of OxyContin in patients with hepatic impairment indicates greater plasma concentrations than those with normal function. The initiation of therapy at 1/3 to 1/2 the usual doses and careful dose titration is warranted.

Renal Impairment

In patients with renal impairment, as evidenced by decreased creatinine clearance (<60 mL/min.), the concentrations of oxycodone in the plasma are approximately 50% higher than in subjects with normal renal function. Dose initiation should follow a conservative approach. Dosages should be adjusted according to the clinical situation.

Gender Differences

In pharmacokinetic studies, opioid-naive females demonstrate up to 25% higher average plasma concentrations and greater frequency of typical opioid adverse events than males, even after adjustment for body weight. The clinical relevance of a difference of this magnitude is low for a drug intended for chronic usage at individualized dosages, and there was no male/female difference detected for efficacy or adverse events in clinical trials.

Rectal Administration

OxyContin Tablets are not recommended for administration per rectum. A study in normal volunteers showed a significantly greater AUC and higher C_{max} during this route of administration.

ADVERSE REACTIONS:

Serious adverse reactions which may be associated with OxyContin® tablet therapy in clinical use are those observed with other opioid analgesics, including: respiratory depression, apnea, respiratory arrest, and (to an even lesser degree) circulatory depression, hypotension, or shock (see **OVERDOSAGE**).

The non-serious adverse events seen on initiation of therapy with OxyContin are typical opioid side effects. These events are dose-dependent, and their frequency depends upon the dose, the clinical setting, the patient's level of opioid tolerance, and host factors specific to the individual. They should be expected and managed as a part of opioid analgesia. The most frequent (>5%) include constipation, nausea, somnolence, dizziness, vomiting, pruritus, headache, dry mouth, sweating, and asthenia.

In many cases the frequency of these events during initiation of therapy may be minimized by careful individualization of starting dosage, slow titration, and the avoidance of large swings in the plasma concentrations of the opioid. Many of these adverse events will cease or decrease in intensity as OxyContin therapy is continued and some degree of tolerance is developed.

In clinical trials comparing OxyContin with immediate-release oxycodone and placebo, the most common adverse events (>5%) reported by patients (pts) at least once during therapy were:

	OxyContin (n=227)		Immediate-Release (n=225)		Placebo (n=45)	
	# Pts	(%)	# Pts	(%)	# Pts	(%)
Constipation	52	(23)	58	(26)	3	(7)
Nausea	52	(23)	60	(27)	5	(11)
Somnolence	52	(23)	55	(24)	2	(4)
Dizziness	29	(13)	35	(16)	4	(9)
Pruritus	29	(13)	28	(12)	1	(2)
Vomiting	27	(12)	31	(14)	3	(7)
Headache	17	(7)	19	(8)	3	(7)
Dry Mouth	13	(6)	15	(7)	1	(2)
Asthenia	13	(6)	16	(7)	—	—
Sweating	12	(5)	13	(6)	1	(2)

The following adverse experiences were reported in OxyContin treated patients with an incidence between 1% and 5%. In descending order of frequency they were anorexia, nervousness, insomnia, fever, confusion, diarrhea, abdominal pain, dyspepsia, rash, anxiety, euphoria, dyspnea, postural hypotension, chills, twitching, gastritis, abnormal dreams, thought abnormalities, and hiccups.

The following adverse reactions occurred in less than 1% of patients involved in clinical trials:

General: accidental injury, chest pain, facial edema, malaise, neck pain, pain

Cardiovascular: migraine, syncope, vasodilation, ST depression

Digestive: dysphagia, eructation, flatulence, gastrointestinal disorder, increased appetite, nausea and vomiting, stomatitis, ileus

Hemic and Lymphatic: lymphadenopathy

Metabolic and Nutritional: dehydration, edema, hyponatremia, peripheral edema, syndrome of inappropriate antidiuretic hormone secretion, thirst

Nervous: abnormal gait, agitation, amnesia, depersonalization, depression, emotional lability, hallucination, hyperkinesia, hypesthesia, hypotonia, malaise, paresthesia, seizures, speech disorder, stupor, tinnitus, tremor, vertigo, withdrawal syndrome with or without seizures

Respiratory: cough increased, pharyngitis, voice alteration

Skin: dry skin, exfoliative dermatitis, urticaria

Special Senses: abnormal vision, taste perversion

Urogenital: dysuria, hematuria, impotence, polyuria, urinary retention, urination impaired

DRUG ABUSE AND DEPENDENCE (Addiction):

OxyContin® is a mu-agonist opioid with an abuse liability similar to morphine and is a Schedule **II** controlled substance. Oxycodone products are common targets for both drug abusers and drug addicts. Delayed absorption, as provided by OxyContin tablets, is believed to reduce the abuse liability of a drug.

Drug addiction (drug dependence, psychological dependence) is characterized by a preoccupation with the procurement, hoarding, and abuse of drugs for non-medicinal purposes. Drug dependence is treatable, utilizing a multi-disciplinary approach, but relapse is common. Iatrogenic "addiction" to opioids legitimately used in the management of pain is very rare.

OxyContin consists of a dual-polymer matrix, intended for oral use only. Parenteral venous injection of the tablet constituents, especially talc, can be expected to result in local tissue necrosis and pulmonary granulomas.

OVERDOSAGE:

Acute overdosage with oxycodone can be manifested by respiratory depression, somnolence progressing to stupor or coma, skeletal muscle flaccidity, cold and clammy skin, constricted pupils, bradycardia, hypotension, and death.

In the treatment of oxycodone overdosage, primary attention should be given to the re-establishment of a patent airway and institution of assisted or controlled ventilation. Supportive measures (including oxygen and vasopressors) should be employed in the management of circulatory shock and pulmonary edema accompanying overdose as indicated. Cardiac arrest or arrhythmias may require cardiac massage or defibrillation.

The pure opioid antagonists such as naloxone or nalmefene are specific antidotes against respiratory depression from opioid overdose. Opioid antagonists should not be administered in the absence of clinically significant respiratory or circulatory depression secondary to oxycodone overdose. They should be administered cautiously to persons who are known, or suspected to be, physically dependent on any opioid agonist including OxyContin®. In such cases, an abrupt or complete reversal of opioid effects may precipitate an acute abstinence syndrome. The severity of the withdrawal syndrome produced will depend on the degree of physical dependence and the dose of the antagonist administered. Please see the prescribing information for the specific opioid antagonist for details of their proper use.

SAFETY AND HANDLING:

OxyContin® tablets are solid dosage forms that pose no known health risk to health-care providers beyond that of any controlled substance. As with all such drugs, care should be taken to prevent diversion or abuse by proper handling.

STORAGE: Store at 25°C (77°F); excursions permitted between 15°-30°C (59°-86°F).

CAUTION: DEA Order Form Required.

Manufactured by The PF Laboratories, Inc., Totowa, N.J. 07512

Distributed by Purdue Pharma L.P., Stamford, CT 06901-3431

U.S. Patent Numbers 4,861,598; 4,970,075; 5,266,331; 5,508,042; 5,549,912; and 5,656,295

March 17, 2000 L4909-BS

ARTHRITIS & RHEUMATISM
Vol. 44, No. 1, January 2001, pp 1–2

Arthritis & Rheumatism

Official Journal of the American College of Rheumatology
www.arthritisrheum.org and www.interscience.wiley.com

EDITORIAL

The American College of Rheumatology Journals: New Directions for Y2K + 1

David S. Pisetsky

Although I began my tenure as Editor of *Arthritis & Rheumatism* (*A&R*) on July 1, 2000, I have waited until the first issue of the year 2001 for this introductory editorial. This timing is motivated in part by my desire to settle in as Editor, learn the position better, and get a first-hand sense of the journal activities before this communication. With 6 months of the job, I have a clearer view of the current position of the journal and the prospects for the future. From this perspective, I can say the journal is very strong. It is an exciting, vibrant, and eclectic publication that encompasses the field of rheumatology remarkably well. It is preeminent among rheumatology journals and attracts and publishes outstanding articles from around the world. My predecessors, including Dr. William Arend who just finished his tenure as Editor, have set a high standard for the journal and worked hard to make *A&R* a publication of exceptional quality and relevance to both practitioner and scientist.

Another reason to wait until this issue is to welcome our new publisher, John Wiley & Sons. Wiley is a distinguished publisher in the field of science and medicine and was selected as the new publisher after a year-long search process led masterfully by Dr. Gary Hoffman, Chair of the Journal Publications Committee of the American College of Rheumatology (ACR). The world of science publishing is in a state of enormous flux, reflecting new electronic technologies, an increasingly crowded marketplace, and the desire by authors and readers alike for speed in everything—submission, review, and publication. In choosing Wiley as our publisher, the ACR wanted an organization that, while modern in its ability to navigate in today's publishing world, was traditional in its commitment to the excellence that a publication like *A&R* represents.

With both a new editor and a new publisher starting almost simultaneously, there is a spirit of adventure at the journal as we have recognized both the opportunities and the necessity for change. Indeed, we have already made changes at the journal. Whereas the Associate Editors of *A&R* previously have been centered at one institution or one city, the current members are now dispersed throughout the country. In assembling this group, I made the decision to recruit the best talent in editing that I could, on the belief that modern communications will keep us cohesive and interactive. Hence, we are now a bicoastal organization. In addition, I have recruited two deputy editors, Dr. Gary Firestein of the University of California at San Diego and Dr. Bill St. Clair of Duke University, to assist me with my editorial responsibilities. Both Dr. Firestein and Dr. St. Clair are outstanding individuals with strong records of accomplishment in basic and clinical research in rheumatology. With a team of exceptional advisory editors, the editorial group has breadth, experience, and judgment.

Other changes have already been made, and more will follow shortly. We have reorganized the table of contents. In place of sections on clinical and basic research, we have divided the articles by subject and disease group; we are now grouping articles on rheumatoid arthritis, for example, irrespective of methodology used. This format emphasizes the focus on important disease mechanisms and outcomes and not the approaches used to generate the data. In this way, we are trying to make the presentation of articles more accessible and allow the reader to discover better what's new and important in a specific area.

With our new publisher, we will also be changing the appearance of the journal, as is apparent in our new

---

David S. Pisetsky, MD, PhD: Editor, *Arthritis & Rheumatism*, Durham, North Carolina.
Submitted for publication October 20, 2000; accepted October 20, 2000.

cover, which includes an image to focus attention on a significant new concept or result. In the pages of the journal, we will also be seeing more and more color. The use of color is especially important because some of the best and most novel work in cell and molecular biology is in fact "colorful," with new techniques of microscopy producing images of great interest and beauty. The changes in the appearance of the journal will be evolutionary, and as we gain experience with our partners at Wiley we will be experimenting with other ways to improve the presentation of articles and showcase data. In addition, we are taking steps to implement electronic submission and review and are contemplating how best to use online publishing.

Perhaps the biggest change in the journal has been the creation of *Arthritis Care & Research* (*AC&R*) as a section of *A&R*. As a section, *AC&R* will retain an independent editorial board under the leadership of Dr. Gene Hunder of the Mayo Clinic and will continue to emphasize the clinical aspects of rheumatology, including rehabilitation, physical and occupational therapy, and outcomes research. A section designation, however, allows *AC&R* to bear an *A&R* volume number and share with *A&R* listing in the Index Medicus and the impact factor. The impact factor is a calculated number reflecting the number of times an article is cited in other publications and, as such, is a benchmark for importance in the field. This move is a major step for the ACR and signifies a commitment to publish top-flight articles on clinical topics and encourage even greater quality and diversity in this realm of our field.

The relationship between *AC&R* and *A&R* is evolving. Clearly, there are many manuscripts that could be published in either journal, and we have begun a process of acquainting authors with the new status of *AC&R* and, for certain manuscripts, suggesting that authors submit their report there as opposed to other rheumatology and specialty journals. I am in close communication with Dr. Hunder on how best to increase clinical submissions for both *AC&R* and *A&R* and develop a procedure for keeping the best clinical papers "within the family." I think that *AC&R* will be an outstanding journal with a distinct character, even in areas of overlap with *A&R*. From my perspective, I do not see any changes in the scope of *A&R*. The journal will remain diverse and comprehensive, covering the full gamut of basic and clinical investigation relevant to the field of rheumatology.

While 6 months on the job is really just a beginning, I already would like to offer my thanks to many people. First of all, I thank Bill Arend, who did a spectacular job as Editor, assuring the position of the journal as tops in the field. He made the transition from Denver to Durham as painless and seamless as possible. I want to thank my assistant editors, Jennifer Deyton and Julie Nash, for getting us off to a strong start. I also want to thank the officers and Board of Directors of the ACR for entrusting me with the editorship of the journal and bestowing upon me what is probably the best job in academic rheumatology. It is a great privilege and honor to discover and nurture important articles and help set the direction for the future of rheumatology.

Finally, I want to thank you, the members of the ACR, be you readers, authors, or reviewers. I thank you for submitting your work to us, providing detailed and scholarly reviews, and giving us your opinions through your letters and comments. I want the journal to be the product of the entire ACR and worldwide community of rheumatology. If you would like to serve as a reviewer, please let me know. You can send an e-mail with your name, contact information, and areas of expertise and interest. For those who have already been reviewers, we would appreciate updates on your interests and addresses. We receive more than 1,200 submissions each year, with subjects of dizzying diversity from the most basic molecular studies to the most applied social science. This science is then topped off with case reports, radiology features, and images. To assure quality of review, we need scores of reviewers at any time. My goal is to make the review process as fair and fast as possible. I thank you in advance for your thorough, thoughtful, and, hopefully, prompt reviews.

Rheumatology is one of the most vibrant specialties in medicine today, reflecting the advance of science and the extraordinary developments in new treatments. I want the journal to reflect this spirit and publish the best articles from around the world. The future of our specialty is very bright. I look forward to working with you over the coming years to improve the care of patients with arthritis by our dedication to research, scholarship, and scientific publication.

ARTHRITIS & RHEUMATISM
Vol. 44, No. 1, January 2001, pp 3–12

REVIEW

Synergistic Activity of Interleukin-4 and Interleukin-10 in Suppression of Inflammation and Joint Destruction in Rheumatoid Arthritis

Joel A. G. van Roon, Floris P. J. G. Lafeber, and J. W. J. Bijlsma

Introduction

Rheumatoid arthritis (RA) is a disease dominated by joint inflammation, accompanied by several peripheral inflammatory manifestations (1). Although the etiology of RA is still not fully understood, the pathogenesis is known to involve chronic synovitis leading to destruction of joint tissues (in particular, cartilage and bone) and consequently, serious impairment of joint function (2). Patients also exhibit features of systemic inflammation (such as marked acute-phase responses), and the disease is associated with autoimmune responses, the latter being most clearly displayed in the production of autoantibodies against the IgG Fc regions (rheumatoid factor) (3).

The important role of T helper cells, macrophages, dendritic cells (DC), and B cells in local tissue destruction in RA has been described extensively (4–7) (summarized in Figure 1). Macrophages and DC in the RA joint contribute strongly to inflammation by the production of proinflammatory mediators, uptake of (auto-)antigen, and presentation of peptides of processed antigen to T helper cells by class II major histocompatibility complex (MHC) molecules (HLA–DR1 and HLA–DR4, which are linked to RA) together with costimulatory molecules.

In addition to the cell–cell contact of T helper cells with macrophages and DC, there are a number of factors that cause costimulation of T helper cells (e.g., interleukin-7 [IL-7], IL-12, IL-15, and IL-18) in the joints of RA patients (8–11). A predominance of Th1 cell activity (defined by interferon-γ [IFNγ] production) and low Th2 cell activity (defined by IL-4 production) have been demonstrated in RA joints (12–14). This Th1/Th2 imbalance has been shown to strongly enhance activation of macrophages, DC, and B cells by cell–cell contact and secretion of cytokines (15–17). B cells are stimulated to differentiate and produce antigen-specific immunoglobulins, in particular, IgG (3,5). IgG interacts with antigen to form immune complexes, and its Fc constant region binds to Fcγ receptors (FcγR), causing activation of macrophages and DC by receptor crosslinkage (18). Apart from activation, this leads to increased and very efficient uptake of antigen, presentation of arthritogenic epitopes, and an increase or persistence of activation of inflammatory cells, and consequently, maintenance or stimulation of the inflammatory cascade. In addition, several other cell types, such as synovial fibroblasts and neutrophils, have been shown to increase joint inflammation and joint destruction (19,20).

As a consequence of the above inflammatory response, different cell types in the synovial tissue (ST), articular cartilage, and bone are transformed and destroyed by several mediators, such as cytokines (IL-1β, tumor necrosis factor α [TNFα], IL-15, IL-17), metalloproteinases (matrix metalloproteinase 1 [MMP-1] and MMP-3), and oxygen radicals (10,21–25). This ultimately results in serious impairment of joint function.

Several antiinflammatory mechanisms in response to the proinflammatory activity are activated in the RA joint in an attempt to control the dysregulated (auto)immune reactivity. These include the production of cytokines with antiinflammatory properties, such as IL-10, IL-13, and transforming growth factor β, present

Supported by the Nationaal Reumafonds (the Dutch League against Rheumatism).

Joel A. G. van Roon, PhD, Floris P. J. G. Lafeber, PhD, J. W. J. Bijlsma, PhD, MD: University Medical Center Utrecht, Utrecht, The Netherlands.

Address correspondence and reprint requests to Joel A. G. van Roon, PhD, Department of Rheumatology and Clinical Immunology (F01.127), University Medical Center Utrecht, PO Box 85500, 3508 GA Utrecht, The Netherlands.

Submitted for publication May 11, 2000; accepted in revised form August 26, 2000.

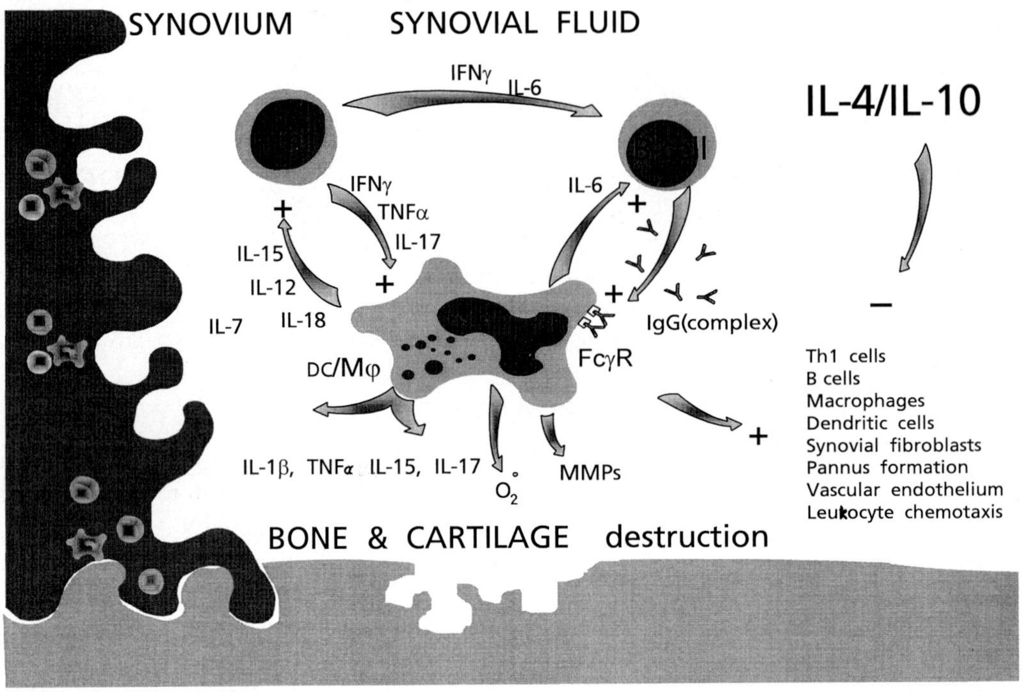

Figure 1. Prominence of the role of macrophages (Mφ), dendritic cells (DC), Th1 cells, and B cells and their products in the induction of rheumatoid arthritis. The synergistic down-regulation by interleukin-4 (IL-4)/IL-10, originally defined as Th2 cytokines, is also depicted. Macrophages and DC in the rheumatoid joint contribute strongly to inflammation by the production of proinflammatory mediators, uptake of (auto-)antigen, and presentation of peptides of processed antigen to Th. In addition, a number of factors, e.g., IL-7, IL-12, IL-15, and IL-18, cause costimulation of T helper cells. Induced Th1 cells in turn activate macrophages, DC, and B cells by cell–cell contact and secretion of interferon-γ (IFNγ), tumor necrosis factor α (TNFα), and IL-17. B cells are also stimulated to differentiate and produce antigen-specific immunoglobulins, in particular, IgG. IgG binds antigen to form immune complexes and interacts with Fcγ receptors (FcγR), causing activation of macrophages and DC by receptor crosslinkage. This leads to increased uptake of antigen, presentation of arthritogenic epitopes, and an increase or persistence of activation of T cells, B cells, macrophages, and DC. The final consequence of the above inflammatory response is the transformation and destruction of several cell types in the synovial tissue, articular cartilage, and bone by various mediators, such as cytokines (IL-1β, TNFα, IL-15, IL-17), metalloproteinases (matrix metalloproteinase 1 [MMP-1] and MMP-3), and oxygen radicals, resulting in impairment of joint function.

in significant amounts in the RA joint (26–28), as well as production of antagonists of inflammatory mediators, such as IL-1 receptor antagonist (IL-1Ra) and soluble TNF receptor (sTNFR) (29,30). These antiinflammatory mediators fall short of mitigating joint inflammation, and several groups have searched for causes of this and for possibilities of treatment with (other) immunosuppressive mediators.

Two mediators, IL-4 and IL-10, originally defined as specific Th2 cell products in mice, can affect Th2 cell activity (31) and have been tested for their antiarthritic properties. In particular, these cytokines can suppress and counterbalance Th1-driven proinflammatory responses in many different disorders (15). The ability of IL-4 to mimic Th2 cell activity, thus inhibiting Th1 cell activity and inflammation in RA and restoring the disturbed Th1/Th2 balance in this disease, has been investigated (16). IL-10 has been studied for similar purposes, although this cytokine cannot be considered a specific Th2 product since, in humans, it is also produced by B cells, monocyte/macrophages, and Th1-like cells (32). Studies in which the function of IL-4 or IL-10 in RA or experimental arthritis were investigated are listed in Table 1. The present report highlights the capacity of IL-4 and IL-10 to inhibit inflammation and joint destruction in RA and experimental arthritis (Table 2). The potential of IL-4 and IL-10 to act synergistically in suppressing in vitro inflammatory responses and ar-

Table 1. Regulation of inflammation in rheumatoid arthritis and experimental arthritis by IL-4 and IL-10*

Site and function studied	IL-4	IL-10	Refs.
T cells, isolated			
Th1 activity	–	0	45, 46
Th2 activity	+	0	45, 46
+ B cells	ND	+	63
IgG, IgM			
Monocyte/macrophages (synovial fluid)			
IL-1β, TNFα	0, –	–	39, 41, 43
IL-6, IL-10	–	–	56
IL-1Ra	+	+	43
Soluble TNFR-p75	–	+	59
Antigen presentation	+	–	60
GM-CSF	–	ND	57
HLA–DR	–	ND	57
FcγRI, FcγRIII	–	+	26, 57
FcγRIIb	+	ND	49
Dendritic cells (synovial fluid)			
Antigen presentation	ND	0	62
HLA–DR, CD86	ND	0	62
Monocyte/macrophages (peripheral blood)			
IL-1β, IL-6, TNFα, IL-12, IL-10	–	–	39, 41, 56
Soluble TNFR-p75	–	+	59
Antigen presentation	+	–	62
HLA–DR, CD86	+	–	62
Mononuclear cells (synovial fluid)			
Antigen presentation	–, +	–	17, 57, 62
MHC class I/II	+	–	57, 58
Th1, T cytotoxic 1 activity	–	–	17, 42, 47, 48
Th2, T cytotoxic 2 activity	+	0	47
IL-1β, TNFα, IL-8	–	–	17, 26, 40, 42
IL-1Ra	+	0	58
IL-12	–	ND	41
IL-10	0	ND	41
Mononuclear cells (peripheral blood)			
Th1 activity	–	–	17, 42, 48
Th2 activity	+	0	47, 48
IL-1β, TNFα	–	–	17, 42
IgM	–	0, +	65, 100
IgG	–	ND	100, 102
Soluble CD23	+	ND	100
Synovial tissue explants/synovial cells			
IL-1β, IL-6	–	–, +	27, 36, 43, 56
TNFα	–	–	27, 36
IL-8	–	–	27, 37
IL-1Ra	+	–, +	43
IgG, IgM	–	+	36, 64
Experimental arthritis			
Collagen-induced (mice)	–, 0	–	51–53, 68, 69
Collagen-induced (rats)	ND	–	66
Aggrecan-induced (mice)	–	–	50
SCW-induced mice (rats)	0, –	–	70

* IL-4 = interleukin-4; – = inhibition, down-regulation, or suppression; 0 = no effect; + = induction or up-regulation; ND = not done; TNFα = tumor necrosis factor α; IL-1Ra = IL-1 receptor antagonist; TNFR = TNF receptor; GM-CSF = granulocyte–macrophage colony-stimulating factor; FcγRI = Fcγ receptor I; MHC = major histocompatibility complex; SCW = streptococcal cell wall.

thritic responses in experimental models is reviewed, and the potential benefits of combined application in RA are discussed.

Regulation of inflammation in RA and experimental arthritis by IL-4

IL-4 is a specific and major defining product of Th2 cells (31,33), with the capacity to modulate the activity of many different cell types in RA. Inhibitory and stimulatory activities of IL-4 on T cells, B cells, and monocyte/macrophages from RA patients have been studied, in experiments with isolated as well as mixed cell populations, such as synovial fluid (SF) mononuclear cells and peripheral blood mononuclear cells (PBMC), and ST (Table 1).

In contrast to IL-4, which is virtually absent in the joints of RA patients, IL-13, considered to be a Th2-like cytokine, has been detected (26,28). IL-13 is strongly homologous with, and shares many functions with, IL-4. Similar to IL-4, it can act directly on monocyte/macro-

Table 2. Prevention of joint destruction by IL-4 and IL-10*

Site and function studied	IL-4	IL-10	Refs.
MMP (non-RA) monocytes			
MMP-1	–	–	72, 73
MMP-2	–	–	72, 73
TIMP-1	0	+	72, 73
TIMP-2	0	0	72
Cartilage			
Human explants			
Proteoglycan synthesis	0	+	42
Proteoglycan release	0	–	42
Human explants + SFMC/PBMC			
Proteoglycan synthesis	+	+	42
Proteoglycan release	–, 0	–	42
Chondrocyte death	–	ND	75
Isolated chondrocytes			
MMP-3	–	ND	71
TIMP-1	+	ND	71
Proteoglycan release	–	ND	71
Bone			
IL-6, LIF	–	ND	76
Osteoclasts	–	ND	76
Synovial fibroblasts (synoviocytes)			
MMP-1, MMP-3	–	ND	22, 81
IL-6	+, –	–	38, 74, 79
LIF, GM-CSF, PGE_2 (spont)	–	0	74, 79
PGE_2 (induced), COX-2	–	–	22, 74, 78
Proliferation	–	ND	77
TNF (by CD40 ligation)	+	–	104
Membrane TNFR	+	–	78
Soluble TNFR-p55, p75	+	+	78, 81
Experimental arthritis			
Collagen-induced (mice)	–	–	51–53, 67, 68
Aggrecan-induced (mice)	–	–	50
SCW-induced mice (rats)	0, –	–	70

* MMP = matrix metalloproteinase; RA = rheumatoid arthritis; TIMP-1 = tissue inhibitor of metalloproteinases 1; SFMC = synovial fluid mononuclear cells; PBMC = peripheral blood mononuclear cells; LIF = leukemia inhibitory factor; PGE_2 = prostaglandin E_2; spont = spontaneous; COX-2 = cyclooxygenase 2 (see Table 1 for other definitions).

phages and B cells, but not on T cells (34). Despite the fact that IL-13 seems to replace IL-4 in some immunoregulatory functions, inflammation and destruction persists in RA joints. Since the immunosuppressive potential of IL-4 has been demonstrated in many human conditions, as well as in several experimental in vivo and in vitro conditions in animals (35), it has been suggested that RA patients might benefit from treatment with this cytokine. Indeed, many in vitro experiments have demonstrated that IL-4 can inhibit arthritogenic activities. IL-4 has been shown to inhibit IL-1β, IL-6, and TNFα as well as IgM and IgG production by human ST cultures, and IL-1β, IL-6, and IL-8 by freshly isolated adherent synovial cells (36–38). Similarly, it inhibits IL-1β, IL-6, IL-8, and TNFα production by rheumatoid SF and PBMC, as well as by monocytes isolated from RA PB and ST (26,39–42). Furthermore, it has been found to induce the production of IL-1Ra by RA synovium (43).

An important regulatory activity of IL-4 is the stimulation of the antigen-presenting capacity of monocyte/macrophages from SF and PB of RA patients. Increased antigen presentation by macrophages is associated with up-regulation of class II MHC expression and of costimulatory molecules (B7-1 and B7-2), endocytosis, and fluid-phase pinocytosis, resulting in stimulation of T cell reactivity (44). This regulatory activity of IL-4 is associated with its ability to shift naive and memory CD4+ T cells toward the suppressive Th2 phenotype in patients with RA and to maintain memory Th2 cell activity, both in the absence and in the presence of antigen-presenting cells (APC) (17,42,45–47). In contrast to the stimulation of Th2 cell responses, IL-4 inhibits secretion of IFNγ and proliferation of Th1 and CD8+ T cytotoxic 1 cells in rheumatoid SF and PB (17,42,47,48). This can be mediated directly and indirectly through inhibition of Th1-stimulatory cytokines, such as IL-12, produced by monocytes and macrophages from the PB and SF of these patients (41).

In contrast to the stimulation by IL-4 of the above-mentioned antigen-presenting capacities, the expression of immune stimulatory Fcγ receptors FcγRI and FcγRIII on RA macrophages, both involved in antigen uptake and IgG immune complex–triggered responses in the RA joint, is down-regulated by this Th2-defining cytokine (18,26). Conversely, IL-4 has been shown to up-regulate the expression of the inhibitory receptor FcγRIIb2 (49). Taken together, these in vitro findings indicate that IL-4 has beneficial effects in counteracting joint inflammation in RA, by stimulation of suppressive cellular responses and inhibition of proinflammatory responses.

Data from studies of experimental arthritis in mice reveal similar responses to IL-4. Proteoglycan-induced arthritis, a Th1-mediated arthritis, in BALB/c mice is significantly suppressed by administration of IL-4, accompanied by inhibition of the Th1 response and of IL-1 and IL-6 production in the joints (50). Likewise, suppression of Th1-driven collagen-induced arthritis (CIA) in DBA/1 mice has been demonstrated (51). The delayed onset of arthritis and decrease in clinical scores was associated with a decrease in TNFα production and Th1-associated anticollagen IgG2a production (51). Treatment with vector cells engineered to secrete IL-4 also suppressed CIA in these mice (52).

In contrast to these findings, another study showed a lack of suppression of CIA in mice (DBA/1 LacJ) by IL-4 (53). Discrepancies in results may be due to the use of different dosages and forms of application. Whereas higher doses of IL-4 (3–5 μg/day; 10^9 units/mg) were sufficient to suppress both CIA and aggrecan-induced arthritis (50,51), IL-4 in lower doses (0.2 μg/day; 10^7 units/mg) was not able to suppress CIA (53). This implies that there may be certain dosage and administration requirements in patients with RA, which may be a major drawback in clinical trials (see below). Although the dosage of IL-4 and the route of administration seem to play a role in the final outcome of treatment, the overall assessment of these studies indicates that IL-4 is therapeutically beneficial in experimental arthritis.

Regulation of inflammation in RA and experimental arthritis by IL-10

In RA, IL-10 is produced by Th2 cells (as originally found in mice), but also by a variety of other cell types, including Th1 cells, B cells, and, in particular, monocytes and macrophages (31,54,55). Like IL-4, IL-10 has a broad range of activities on T cells, monocyte/macrophages, B cells, and other cell types in patients with RA. As with IL-4, the effects of IL-10 have been studied on isolated cell populations as well as mixed cell populations such as SF and PBMC, and ST explants (Table 1).

Although IL-10 is produced in substantial amounts in the RA joint, these levels are clearly insufficient to control inflammation (27). Notwithstanding this, studies involving neutralization of IL-10 demonstrated a suppressive role of endogenous IL-10, since this process led to an increase in levels of IL-1β, TNFα, and granulocyte–macrophage colony-stimulating factor (GM-CSF) (27). Administration of IL-10 to RA synovium cultures was shown to (further) suppress production of TNFα, IL-1β, and IL-6 (27,43), although stimulation of IL-1β and IL-6 production by IL-10 has also been reported (43,56). Production of these proinflammatory cytokines in unstimulated, Th1-activated, or lipopolysaccharide-stimulated rheumatoid SF mononuclear cells and PBMC was inhibited by IL-10 as well (42,57). Moreover, IL-10 induces sTNFR production by rheumatoid SF and PB monocyte/macrophages and has been found to have a limited stimulatory effect on IL-1Ra production (43,58,59).

The effect of IL-10 on monocyte/macrophages is achieved primarily by modulation of antigen presentation, which leads to inhibition of T cytotoxic cell and Th1 cell responses and thus indirectly to stimulation of Th2 cell activity (60). An important mechanism by which IL-10 achieves this effect is through inhibition of the production of IL-12 by RA monocyte/macrophages, which strongly induces Th1 activity (61). IL-10 also inhibits antigen presentation by macrophages from rheumatoid SF and PB, by inhibition of HLA–DR and B7 expression (57,60,62), which results in inhibition of spontaneous or Th1-induced lymphocyte activation (17).

IgM and IgG production by isolated B cells from RA patients in the presence of T cells or synovial fibroblasts (synoviocytes) is stimulated by IL-10 (63,64). However, a lack of stimulation of total IgM by IL-10 in the presence of other mononuclear cells (in particular, monocytes) has been reported, whereas specific production of IgM rheumatoid factor is stimulated (65).

In addition to the data on in vitro effects on RA inflammatory activity, results of studies on experimental models of arthritis demonstrate the beneficial effects of IL-10. Aggrecan-induced arthritis in BALB/c mice was down-regulated by IL-10, in association with inhibition of the Th1 response and of TNFα and IL-6 production in the joints and stimulation of peripheral Th2 activity (IL-4 and IL-10 production) (50). Administration of IL-10 to DBA/1 Lac/J mice as well as to DA rats led to a similar suppression of CIA (53,66–69). Also, injection of mice intravenously and intraarticularly with adenoviral vectors expressing viral IL-10 prevented induction of CIA and caused suppression of established CIA. This decrease in arthritis activity was associated with a reduction of collagen-specific lymphocyte activity, IL-2 messenger RNA (mRNA), Th1-associated IgG2a production, and IL-1β mRNA (67,68). Furthermore, inhibitory effects on streptococcal cell wall–induced arthritis have been observed (70). Together, these data and the in vitro data on RA inflammatory activity in general show that IL-10 has a clear suppressive effect on joint inflammation.

Prevention and reversal of joint destruction by IL-4 and IL-10

Both IL-4 and IL-10, in addition to controlling inflammation in RA, have effects on integrity of cartilage and subchondral bone as well as other joint tissues (Table 2). Both cytokines have been shown to directly inhibit MMP production by monocytes (MMP-1, MMP-2, and MMP-3, representing collagenase 1, gelatinase A/collagenase 4, and stromelysin 1, respectively) (71,72). Furthermore, IL-10 induces the expression of tissue inhibitor of metalloproteinases 1 (TIMP-1) by monocytes (72), an effect not found with IL-4. Both IL-4 and IL-10 have been demonstrated to have no effect on TIMP-2 expression by monocytes (73). As a consequence of their effects on joint production of destructive enzymes (74), directly on monocyte/macrophages and indirectly via suppression of IL-1β and TNFα production, IL-4 and IL-10 are capable of preventing cartilage degradation induced by stimulated rheumatoid SF and PBMC. This was demonstrated by the recovery of proteoglycan synthesis and inhibition of proteoglycan release (17,42). Likewise, irreversible joint damage induced by destructive hydroxyl radicals is prevented by IL-10. This type of joint damage as a consequence of chondrocyte apoptosis is induced by erythrocyte-activated mononuclear cells and monocytes (75).

In human chondrocytes, MMP production can also be inhibited directly by IL-4 and TIMP-1 production stimulated by IL-4 (71). Cartilage matrix synthesis (proteoglycans) can be stimulated by IL-10, whereas IL-4 has no such effect (42). IL-4, in contrast, inhibits bone resorption by a direct effect on bone osteoclasts and indirectly by inhibition of proinflammatory cytokine production (76).

Fibroblasts from the ST (synoviocytes) contribute to destruction of cartilage and bone. IL-4 has been shown to inhibit both MMP-1 and MMP-3 production by synovial fibroblasts and proliferation of these cells (22,77). In addition, IL-4 reduces production of leukemia inhibitory factor (LIF), prostaglandin E_2 (PGE_2), and GM-CSF by synovial fibroblasts, while inducing production of sTNFR (22,74,78–80). Addition of IL-10 to synovial fibroblasts did not alter spontaneous production of LIF, GM-CSF, or PGE_2 (74,78,80). The lack of expression of IL-10 receptor has been suggested as an explanation for this nonresponsiveness (80). However, production of PGE_2 by synovial fibroblasts, which is stimulated by TNFα, is inhibited by IL-10 (78,81). In addition, IL-10 induces the production of sTNFR-p75 by cytokine-stimulated synovial fibroblasts (78,81).

Whether the IL-10 receptor is up-regulated under these conditions remains to be determined.

Data from studies of experimental arthritis support the reported beneficial role of IL-4 and IL-10 in prevention of joint destruction. Cartilage destruction and subchondral bone erosion as a result of CIA were significantly reduced by administration of IL-4 as well as by administration of adenovirus-expressed IL-10 (51,67). Despite the fact that intraarticular injection of adenoviral vector expressing IL-4 did not inhibit joint inflammation, it prevented cartilage destruction. This was associated with reduced IL-1β production in the synovium, reduced MMP-3/TIMP-1 mRNA balance, and decreased granulocyte adherence to cartilage (82). Finally, joint abnormalities of CIA were prevented by the combined administration of IL-4 and IL-10 (see below) (53). Together, the beneficial effects of IL-4 and of IL-10 on several cell types in human and mouse RA joints indicate that these cytokines may prevent tissue damage in RA patients via several distinct and additive mechanisms.

Treatment of RA patients with IL-4 or IL-10

Despite the clear in vitro antiinflammatory effects of IL-4 and IL-10 in RA, confirmed by in vivo studies in several experimental animal models, clinical trials with either human IL-4 or IL-10 in RA patients show rather diverse responses, with limited disease suppression. Treatment of RA patients with recombinant human IL-4 (subcutaneous administration, up to 2 μg/kg 3 times per week for 6 weeks) in a multicenter, randomized, double-blind, placebo-controlled, dose-escalating phase I study ($n = 31$) did not result in significant improvement of disease activity, although the IL-4 was well tolerated (83).

In a similar clinical phase I study of treatment of RA patients ($n = 72$) with IL-10 (subcutaneous administration, up to 20 μg/kg daily for 4 weeks), IL-10 was also well tolerated but did not produce significant improvement in the disease, although a trend toward improvement (exceeding the American College of Rheumatology [ACR] 20% response criteria) was observed at 4 weeks with a 5-μg/kg daily dosage. Interestingly, circulating levels of sTNFR and IL-1Ra were significantly increased in patients who received IL-10 at the highest dose (84). Although not demonstrated in RA patients, IL-4 administration (10 μg/kg 3 times/day for a total of 10 days) to cancer patients resulted in a significant increase in circulating levels of IL-1Ra, whereas IgG, IgA, and IgM decreased (85). Furthermore, levels of soluble CD23 (type II IgE receptor) were increased with this IL-4 treatment and were accompanied by a decrease in IgE levels, without allergic manifestations (85). In particular, the absence of allergic manifestations is of importance since this has been considered as a potential side effect of IL-4 treatment. In addition, IL-10 given to healthy individuals resulted in suppression of IL-1β and TNFα production by whole blood cultures (86).

The above-described clinical responses in RA patients may be explained by the fact that both IL-4 and IL-10 not only down-regulate immune responses, but also up-regulate several immune functions (see Table 1). It has been found that IL-4 up-regulates soluble CD23 levels in human serum, and IL-10 has been shown to increase FcγR expression on monocyte/macrophages in the PB of patients with RA (van Roon JAG et al: unpublished results). Extrapolating from these findings, adjuvant therapy along with IL-4 and IL-10 treatment in RA may be indicated to enhance the immunosuppressive potential of both cytokines. This assumption is underscored by the results of a clinical study in which IL-10 treatment was accompanied by administration of methotrexate (MTX). Significant disease suppression (ACR 20% response criteria) was found in 65% of the patients who received IL-10 plus MTX, versus 10% of those who received placebo plus MTX (87). Since IL-4 and IL-10 have overlapping and also unique cross-regulatory activities, combination therapy may result in suppression of disease not accomplished with monotherapy with either of the 2 cytokines. Several of these unique features are discussed below.

Complementary effects of IL-4 and IL-10

The potential of IL-4 and IL-10 to mitigate RA will depend on the net result from immunoregulatory effects and interaction of the 2 cytokines. Individual effects of IL-4 and IL-10 on T and B cells, monocyte/macrophages, and synovial fibroblasts in arthritis have been tested (Tables 1 and 2).

Both *synergistic (additive)* and *antagonistic* immunoregulatory capacities of IL-4 and IL-10 may lead to a superior suppression of RA by the combination of cytokines than by either cytokine alone. Synergistic antiinflammatory mechanisms include the suppression of Th1 cell activity and the inhibition of proinflammatory cytokines in RA patients. The down-regulation of cytokine production illustrates that additive suppression may result from the interaction with different intracellular pathways: IL-4 increases degradation of proinflammatory cytokine mRNA, whereas IL-10 primarily inhibits its transcription by inhibition of nuclear factor κB generation (88). Proinflammatory cytokine production by isolated Th1-activated SF mononuclear cells and adherent cells from the ST and PBMC of RA patients has been shown to be inhibited synergistically (37,42). This consequently resulted in an additive prevention and reversal of cartilage degradation as determined in vitro (42). Combined treatment of CIA in mice with IL-4 and IL-10 similarly resulted in synergistic suppression of arthritic activity, cytokine production, and joint destruction, in contrast to the limited effects of either cytokine alone (53).

Several other synergistic antiinflammatory effects of the combination of IL-4 and IL-10 on various pathogenetic mechanisms have been documented in nonarthritic conditions. IL-4 and IL-10 act synergistically to inhibit T cell cytotoxicity (together with Th1 cell activity and stimulated Th2 cell activity), nitric oxide production by monocytes, neutrophil activity (cyclooxygenase 2 and PGE_2 production), and mast cell activity (Kit expression) (89–92). Furthermore, they have a synergistic effect on the induction of IL-1Ra production by neutrophils (93). Both neutrophils and, to a lesser extent, mast cells have been implicated in the pathogenesis of RA.

The value of IL-4 and IL-10 combination therapy in RA may also be mediated by antagonistic activities of both cytokines, by which adverse proinflammatory effects during down-regulation of inflammation, induced by one cytokine, are counteracted by the other. Several examples have been documented in RA and other conditions: 1) IL-10 up-regulates expression of FcγR on monocytes and stimulates IgG-mediated phagocytosis, endocytosis, and antibody-dependent cell-mediated cytotoxicity, whereas IL-4 suppresses these proinflammatory activities (94). 2) IL-4 may stimulate antigen-specific T cell responses, which can be down-regulated by IL-10 in the presence of autologous non–T cells (33,57,95), and leads to synergistic induction of Th2 cell activity in the context of mononuclear cells (47). 3) In the presence of GM-CSF, IL-4 can differentiate monocytes from the PB into pathogenic DC (7,96), whereas IL-10 can prevent this differentiation and leads to APC that skew T cells toward the Th2 phenotype (96–98). 4) IL-4 may induce IgE production by B cells (although no allergic reactions have been observed upon treatment of RA patients with IL-4), which, in the presence of APC such as monocytes, is suppressed by IL-10 (99). 5) IL-4 increases expression of FcεRII, which may facilitate inflammatory activities, whereas IL-10 down-regulates this expression (100,101). 6) IL-10 induces IgG and IgM production by B cells, stimulated by activated RA synovial fibroblasts (synoviocytes); IL-4 has been shown to down-regulate IgG and IgM production by ST explants as well as by PBMC (36,64,102). 7) IL-4 inhibits antiinflammatory sTNFR-p75 production by monocytes, whereas IL-10 stimulates this production (103); the opposite has been described for IL-1Ra production by ST explants (43). 8) IL-6 and TNFα production by cytokine-stimulated synoviocytes (stimulated with IL-1β, IL-17, and TNFα) is up-regulated by IL-4, but down-regulated by IL-10 (79,104). 9) IL-5 production by natural killer cells, encouraging allergic phenomena, is stimulated by IL-4 but inhibited by IL-10 (105).

In some cases, IL-4 has been shown to inhibit IL-10 production, and vice versa (95,106). Therefore, combined administration of IL-4 and IL-10 to RA patients may circumvent a shortage caused by down-regulation of endogenous IL-4, and, in particular, endogenous IL-10 production, since the latter is produced in considerable amounts in patients with RA.

Conclusion

Although both IL-4 and IL-10 separately inhibit inflammatory responses in vitro in patients with RA and in vivo in experimental arthritis models, the clinical benefit of either cytokine in the treatment of RA is limited. This may be because IL-4 and IL-10 have not only antiinflammatory, but also proinflammatory properties. In studies that take advantage of the distinct synergistic and antagonistic characteristics of both cytokines, significant suppression of inflammatory responses is found, to a level not reached by administration of either cytokine alone. This has been reported both for inflammatory cells of RA patients and in experimental arthritis. These data, along with the cartilage repair capacity of the combination of IL-4 and IL-10 (42,70), suggest that simultaneous administration of IL-4 and IL-10 to RA patients may lead to synergistic suppression of joint inflammation and reversal of joint destruction. Similar suppression may occur in other Th1-driven autoimmune diseases as well.

REFERENCES

1. Feldmann M, Brennan FM, Maini RN. Rheumatoid arthritis. Cell 1996;85:307–10.
2. Harris ED Jr. Rheumatoid arthritis: pathophysiology and implications for therapy. N Engl J Med 1990;322:1277–89.
3. Carson DA, Chen PP, Kipps TJ. New roles for rheumatoid factor. J Clin Invest 1991;87:379–83.
4. Burmester GR, Stuhlmüller B, Keyszer G, Kinne RW. Mononu-

clear phagocytes and rheumatoid synovitis: mastermind or workhorse in arthritis? Arthritis Rheum 1997;40:5–18.
5. Edwards JC, Cambridge G, Abrahams VM. Do self-perpetuating B lymphocytes drive human autoimmune disease? Immunology 1999;97:188–96.
6. Panayi GS, Lanchbury JS, Kingsley GH. The importance of the T cell in initiating and maintaining the chronic synovitis of rheumatoid arthritis. Arthritis Rheum 1992;35:729–35.
7. Thomas R, Lipsky PE. Could endogenous self-peptides presented by dendritic cells initiate rheumatoid arthritis? Immunol Today 1996;17:559–64.
8. Gracie JA, Forsey RJ, Chan WL, Gilmour A, Leung BP, Greer MR, et al. A proinflammatory role for IL-18 in rheumatoid arthritis. J Clin Invest 1999;104:1393–401.
9. Morita Y, Yamamura M, Nishida K, Harada S, Okamoto H, Inoue H, et al. Expression of interleukin-12 in synovial tissue from patients with rheumatoid arthritis. Arthritis Rheum 1998; 41:306–14.
10. McInnes IB, Liew FY. Interleukin 15: a proinflammatory role in rheumatoid arthritis synovitis. Immunol Today 1998;19:75–9.
11. Harada S, Yamamura M, Okamoto H, Morita Y, Kawashima M, Aita T, et al. Production of interleukin-7 and interleukin-15 by fibroblast-like synoviocytes from patients with rheumatoid arthritis. Arthritis Rheum 1999;42:1508–16.
12. Dolhain RJEM, van der Heiden AN, ter Haar NT, Breedveld FC, Miltenburg AMM. Shift toward T lymphocytes with a T helper 1 cytokine-secretion profile in the joints of patients with rheumatoid arthritis. Arthritis Rheum 1996;39:1961–9.
13. Morita Y, Yamamura M, Kawashima M, Harada S, Tsuji K, Shibuya K, et al. Flow cytometric single-cell analysis of cytokine production by CD4+ T cells in synovial tissue and peripheral blood from patients with rheumatoid arthritis. Arthritis Rheum 1998;41:1669–76.
14. Simon AK, Seipelt E, Sieper J. Divergent T-cell cytokine patterns in inflammatory arthritis. Proc Natl Acad Sci U S A 1994;91: 8562–6.
15. Abbas AK, Murphy KM, Sher A. Functional diversity of helper T lymphocytes. Nature 1996;383:787–93.
16. Miossec P, van den Berg W. Th1/Th2 cytokine balance in arthritis. Arthritis Rheum 1997;40:2105–15.
17. Van Roon JA, van Roy JL, Duits A, Lafeber FP, Bijlsma JW. Proinflammatory cytokine production and cartilage damage due to rheumatoid synovial T helper-1 activation is inhibited by interleukin-4. Ann Rheum Dis 1995;54:836–40.
18. Kimberly RP, Salmon JE, Edberg JC. Receptors for immunoglobulin G: molecular diversity and implications for disease. Arthritis Rheum 1995;38:306–14.
19. Firestein GS. Invasive fibroblast-like synoviocytes in rheumatoid arthritis: passive responders or transformed aggressors? Arthritis Rheum 1996;39:1781–90.
20. Chatham WW, Swaim R, Frohsin H Jr, Heck LW, Miller EJ, Blackburn WD Jr. Degradation of human articular cartilage by neutrophils in synovial fluid. Arthritis Rheum 1993;36:51–8.
21. Biemond P, Swaak AJG, Koster JF. Protective factors against oxygen free radicals and hydrogen peroxide in rheumatoid arthritis synovial fluid. Arthritis Rheum 1984;27:760–5.
22. Borghaei RC, Rawlings PL Jr, Mochan E. Interleukin-4 suppression of interleukin-1–induced transcription of collagenase (MMP-1) and stromelysin 1 (MMP-3) in human synovial fibroblasts. Arthritis Rheum 1998;41:1398–406.
23. Jovanovic DV, Martel-Pelletier J, di Battista JA, Mineau F, Jolicoeur FC, Benderdour M, et al. Stimulation of 92-kd gelatinase (matrix metalloproteinase 9) production by interleukin-17 in human monocyte/macrophages: a possible role in rheumatoid arthritis. Arthritis Rheum 2000;43:1134–44.
24. Kotake S, Udagawa N, Takahashi N, Matsuzaki K, Itoh K, Ishiyama S, et al. IL-17 in synovial fluids from patients with rheumatoid arthritis is a potent stimulator of osteoclastogenesis. J Clin Invest 1999;103:1345–52.
25. Wilbrink B, Nietfeld JJ, den Otter W, van Roy JL, Bijlsma JW, Huber-Bruning O. Role of TNF alpha, in relation to IL-1 and IL-6 in the proteoglycan turnover of human articular cartilage. Br J Rheumatol 1991;30:265–71.
26. Isomäki P, Luukkainen R, Toivanen P, Punnonen J. The presence of interleukin-13 in rheumatoid synovium and its antiinflammatory effects on synovial fluid macrophages from patients with rheumatoid arthritis. Arthritis Rheum 1996;39:1693–702.
27. Katsikis PD, Chu CQ, Brennan FM, Maini RN, Feldmann M. Immunoregulatory role of interleukin 10 in rheumatoid arthritis. J Exp Med 1994;179:1517–27.
28. Miossec P, Naviliat M, Dupuy d'Angeac A, Sany J, Banchereau J. Low levels of interleukin-4 and high levels of transforming growth factor β in rheumatoid synovitis. Arthritis Rheum 1990;33: 1180–7.
29. Cope AP, Maini RN. Soluble tumor necrosis factor receptors in arthritis. J Rheumatol 1995;22:382–4.
30. Firestein GS, Berger AE, Tracey DE, Chosay JG, Chapman DL, Paine MM, et al. IL-1 receptor antagonist protein production and gene expression in rheumatoid arthritis and osteoarthritis synovium. J Immunol 1992;149:1054–62.
31. Mosmann TR, Cherwinski H, Bond MW, Giedlin MA, Coffman RL. Two types of murine helper T cell clone. I. Definition according to profiles of lymphokine activities and secreted proteins. J Immunol 1986;136:2348–57.
32. Moore KW, O'Garra A, de Waal MR, Vieira P, Mosmann TR. Interleukin-10. Annu Rev Immunol 1993;11:165–90.
33. Del Prete GF, de Carli M, Mastromauro C, Biagiotti R, Macchia D, Falagiani P, et al. Purified protein derivative of Mycobacterium tuberculosis and excretory-secretory antigen(s) of Toxocara canis expand in vitro in human T cells with stable and opposite (type 1 T helper or type 2 T helper) profile of cytokine production. J Clin Invest 1991;88:346–50.
34. Zurawski G, de Vries JE. Interleukin 13, an interleukin 4-like cytokine that acts on monocytes and B cells, but not on T cells. Immunol Today 1994;15:19–26.
35. Chomarat P, Banchereau J. An update on interleukin-4 and its receptor. Eur Cytokine Netw 1997;8:333–44.
36. Miossec P, Briolay J, Dechanet J, Wijdenes J, Martinez-Valdez H, Banchereau J. Inhibition of the production of proinflammatory cytokines and immunoglobulins by interleukin-4 in an ex vivo model of rheumatoid synovitis. Arthritis Rheum 1992;35:874–83.
37. Sugiyama E, Kuroda A, Taki H, Ikemoto M, Hori T, Yamashita N, et al. Interleukin 10 cooperates with interleukin 4 to suppress inflammatory cytokine production by freshly prepared adherent rheumatoid synovial cells. J Rheumatol 1995;22:2020–6.
38. Suzuki H, Sugiyama E, Tunru IS, Yamashita N, Matsuno H, Hamazaki T, et al. Suppressive effect of interleukin-4 (IL-4) on IL-6 production by adherent rheumatoid synovial cells. Clin Immunol Immunopathol 1993;66:67–72.
39. Hart PH, Ahern MJ, Jones CA, Jones KL, Smith MD, Finlay-Jones JJ. Synovial fluid macrophages and blood monocytes differ in their response to IL-4. J Immunol 1993;151:3370–80.
40. Deleuran B, Iversen L, Kristensen M, Field M, Kragballe K, Thestrup-Pedersen K, et al. Interleukin-8 secretion and 15-lipoxygenase activity in rheumatoid arthritis: in vitro anti-inflammatory effects by interleukin-4 and interleukin-10, but not by interleukin-1 receptor antagonist protein. Br J Rheumatol 1994;33:520–5.
41. Bonder CS, Finlay-Jones JJ, Hart PH. Interleukin-4 regulation of human monocyte and macrophage interleukin-10 and interleukin-12 production: role of a functional interleukin-2 receptor gamma-chain. Immunology 1999;96:529–36.
42. Van Roon JAG, van Roy JLAM, Gmelig-Meyling FHJ, Lafeber FPJG, Bijlsma JWJ. Prevention and reversal of cartilage degra-

dation in rheumatoid arthritis by interleukin-10 and interleukin-4. Arthritis Rheum 1996;39:829–35.
43. Chomarat P, Vannier E, Dechanet J, Rissoan MC, Banchereau J, Dinarello CA, et al. Balance of IL-1 receptor antagonist/IL-1 beta in rheumatoid synovium and its regulation by IL-4 and IL-10. J Immunol 1995;154:1432–9.
44. Montaner LJ, da Silva RP, Sun J, Sutterwala S, Hollinshead M, Vaux D, et al. Type 1 and type 2 cytokine regulation of macrophage endocytosis: differential activation by IL-4/IL-13 as opposed to IFN-gamma or IL-10. J Immunol 1999;162:4606–13.
45. Skapenko A, Wendler J, Lipsky PE, Kalden JR, Schulze-Koops H. Altered memory T cell differentiation in patients with early rheumatoid arthritis. J Immunol 1999;163:491–9.
46. Van Roon JAG, Glaudemans CAFM, Lafeber FPJG, Bijlsma JWJ. Generation of suppressive Th2 cells from naive peripheral CD4+ T cells from rheumatoid arthritis patients using IL-7 and IL-4 [abstract]. Arthritis Rheum 1999;42 Suppl 9:S94.
47. Yin Z, Siegert S, Neure L, Grolms M, Liu L, Eggens U, et al. The elevated ratio of interferon gamma-/interleukin-4–positive T cells found in synovial fluid and synovial membrane of rheumatoid arthritis patients can be changed by interleukin-4 but not by interleukin-10 or transforming growth factor beta. Rheumatology (Oxford) 1999;38:1058–67.
48. Isomaki P, Luukkainen R, Lassila O, Toivanen P, Punnonen J. Synovial fluid T cells from patients with rheumatoid arthritis are refractory to the T helper type 2 differentiation-inducing effects of interleukin-4. Immunology 1999;96:358–64.
49. Pricop L, Redecha PB, Teillaud J-L, Fridman WH, Sautes-Fridman C, Salmon JE. Evidence for the presence of an inhibitory Fcγ receptor, FcγRIIb2, on human monocytes and neutrophils [abstract]. Arthritis Rheum 1999;42 Suppl 9:S274.
50. Finnegan A, Mikecz K, Tao P, Glant TT. Proteoglycan (aggrecan)-induced arthritis in BALB/c mice is a Th1-type disease regulated by Th2 cytokines. J Immunol 1999;163:5383–90.
51. Horsfall AC, Butler DM, Marinova L, Warden PJ, Williams RO, Maini RN, et al. Suppression of collagen-induced arthritis by continuous administration of IL-4. J Immunol 1997;159:5687–96.
52. Bessis N, Boissier MC, Ferrara P, Blankenstein T, Fradelizi D, Fournier C. Attenuation of collagen-induced arthritis in mice by treatment with vector cells engineered to secrete interleukin-13. Eur J Immunol 1996;26:2399–403.
53. Joosten LAB, Lubberts E, Durez P, Helsen MMA, Jacobs MJM, Goldman M, et al. Role of interleukin-4 and interleukin-10 in murine collagen-induced arthritis: protective effect of interleukin-4 and interleukin-10 treatment on cartilage destruction. Arthritis Rheum 1997;40:249–60.
54. Llorente L, Richaud-Patin Y, Fior R, Alcocer-Varela J, Wijdenes J, Fourrier BM, et al. In vivo production of interleukin-10 by non-T cells in rheumatoid arthritis, Sjögren's syndrome, and systemic lupus erythematosus: a potential mechanism of B lymphocyte hyperactivity and autoimmunity. Arthritis Rheum 1994; 37:1647–55.
55. Yudoh K, Matsuno H, Nakazawa F, Yonezawa T, Kimura T. Reduced expression of the regulatory CD4+ T cell subset is related to Th1/Th2 balance and disease severity in rheumatoid arthritis. Arthritis Rheum 2000;43:617–27.
56. Chomarat P, Banchereau J, Miossec P. Differential effects of interleukins 10 and 4 on the production of interleukin-6 by blood and synovium monocytes in rheumatoid arthritis. Arthritis Rheum 1995;38:1046–54.
57. Isomäki P, Luukkainen R, Saario R, Toivanen P, Punnonen J. Interleukin-10 functions as an antiinflammatory cytokine in rheumatoid synovium. Arthritis Rheum 1996;39:386–95.
58. Hart PH, Ahern MJ, Smith MD, Finlay-Jones JJ. Comparison of the suppressive effects of interleukin-10 and interleukin-4 on synovial fluid macrophages and blood monocytes from patients with inflammatory arthritis. Immunology 1995;84:536–42.
59. Hart PH, Hunt EK, Bonder CS, Watson CJ, Finlay-Jones JJ. Regulation of surface and soluble TNF receptor expression on human monocytes and synovial fluid macrophages by IL-4 and IL-10. J Immunol 1996;157:3672–80.
60. Mottonen M, Isomaki P, Saario R, Toivanen P, Punnonen J, Lassila O. Interleukin-10 inhibits the capacity of synovial macrophages to function as antigen-presenting cells. Br J Rheumatol 1998;37:1207–14.
61. Seder RA, Gazzinelli R, Sher A, Paul WE. Interleukin 12 acts directly on CD4+ T cells to enhance priming for interferon gamma production and diminishes interleukin 4 inhibition of such priming. Proc Natl Acad Sci U S A 1993;90:10188–92.
62. MacDonald KP, Pettit AR, Quinn C, Thomas GJ, Thomas R. Resistance of rheumatoid synovial dendritic cells to the immunosuppressive effects of IL-10. J Immunol 1999;163:5599–607.
63. Al Janadi M, al Dalaan A, al Balla S, al Humaidi M, Raziuddin S. Interleukin-10 (IL-10) secretion in systemic lupus erythematosus and rheumatoid arthritis: IL-10–dependent CD4+CD45RO+ T cell-B cell antibody synthesis. J Clin Immunol 1996;16:198–207.
64. Dechanet J, Merville P, Durand I, Banchereau J, Miossec P. The ability of synoviocytes to support terminal differentiation of activated B cells may explain plasma cell accumulation in rheumatoid synovium. J Clin Invest 1995;95:456–63.
65. Perez L, Orte J, Brieva JA. Terminal differentiation of spontaneous rheumatoid factor–secreting B cells from rheumatoid arthritis patients depends on endogenous interleukin-10. Arthritis Rheum 1995;38:1771–6.
66. Persson S, Mikulowska A, Narula S, O'Garra A, Holmdahl R. Interleukin-10 suppresses the development of collagen type II-induced arthritis and ameliorates sustained arthritis in rats. Scand J Immunol 1996;44:607–14.
67. Apparailly F, Verwaerde C, Jacquet C, Auriault C, Sany J, Jorgensen C. Adenovirus-mediated transfer of viral IL-10 gene inhibits murine collagen-induced arthritis. J Immunol 1998;160: 5213–20.
68. Ma Y, Thornton S, Duwel LE, Boivin GP, Giannini EH, Leiden JM, et al. Inhibition of collagen-induced arthritis in mice by viral IL-10 gene transfer. J Immunol 1998;161:1516–24.
69. Walmsley M, Katsikis PD, Abney E, Parry S, Williams RO, Maini RN, et al. Interleukin-10 inhibition of the progression of established collagen-induced arthritis. Arthritis Rheum 1996;39: 495–503.
70. Lubberts E, Joosten LA, Helsen MM, van den Berg WB. Regulatory role of interleukin 10 in joint inflammation and cartilage destruction in murine streptococcal cell wall (SCW) arthritis: more therapeutic benefit with IL-4/IL-10 combination therapy than with IL-10 treatment alone. Cytokine 1998;10: 361–9.
71. Shingu M, Miyauchi S, Nagai Y, Yasutake C, Horie K. The role of IL-4 and IL-6 in IL-1–dependent cartilage matrix degradation. Br J Rheumatol 1995;34:101–6.
72. Lacraz S, Nicod LP, Chicheportiche R, Welgus HG, Dayer JM. IL-10 inhibits metalloproteinase and stimulates TIMP-1 production in human mononuclear phagocytes. J Clin Invest 1995;96: 2304–10.
73. Lacraz S, Nicod L, Galve-de Rochemonteix B, Baumberger C, Dayer JM, Welgus HG. Suppression of metalloproteinase biosynthesis in human alveolar macrophages by interleukin-4. J Clin Invest 1992;90:382–8.
74. Dechanet J, Rissoan MC, Banchereau J, Miossec P. Interleukin 4, but not interleukin 10, regulates the production of inflammation mediators by rheumatoid synoviocytes. Cytokine 1995;7: 176–83.
75. Hooiveld MJJ, Roosendaal G, van Roon JAG, van den Berg HM, Lafeber FPJG, Bijlsma JWJ. Irreversible joint damage after joint bleeding can be prevented by IL-10 [abstract]. Arthritis Rheum 1999;42 Suppl 9:S254.

76. Miossec P, Chomarat P, Dechanet J, Moreau J-F, Roux J-P, Delmas P, et al. Interleukin-4 inhibits bone resorption through an effect on osteoclasts and proinflammatory cytokines in an ex vivo model of bone resorption in rheumatoid arthritis. Arthritis Rheum 1994;37:1715–22.
77. Dechanet J, Briolay J, Rissoan MC, Chomarat P, Galizzi JP, Banchereau J, et al. IL-4 inhibits growth factor-stimulated rheumatoid synoviocyte proliferation by blocking the early phases of the cell cycle. J Immunol 1993;151:4908–17.
78. Alaaeddine N, di Battista JA, Pelletier J-P, Kiansa K, Cloutier J-M, Martel-Pelletier J. Inhibition of tumor necrosis factor α–induced prostaglandin E_2 production by the antiinflammatory cytokines interleukin-4, interleukin-10, and interleukin-13 in osteoarthritic synovial fibroblasts: distinct targeting in the signaling pathways. Arthritis Rheum 1999;42:710–8.
79. Chabaud M, Fossiez F, Taupin JL, Miossec P. Enhancing effect of IL-17 on IL-1–induced IL-6 and leukemia inhibitory factor production by rheumatoid arthritis synoviocytes and its regulation by Th2 cytokines. J Immunol 1998;161:409–14.
80. Dechanet J, Taupin JL, Chomarat P, Rissoan MC, Moreau JF, Banchereau J, et al. Interleukin-4 but not interleukin-10 inhibits the production of leukemia inhibitory factor by rheumatoid synovium and synoviocytes. Eur J Immunol 1994;24:3222–8.
81. Taylor DJ. Interleukin-4 (IL-4) induces down-modulation and shedding of the p55 tumour necrosis factor receptor and inhibits TNF alpha's effect on rheumatoid synovial fibroblasts. Rheumatol Int 1994;14:21–5.
82. Lubberts E, Joosten LA, van Den BL, Helsen MM, Bakker AC, van Meurs JB, et al. Adenoviral vector-mediated overexpression of IL-4 in the knee joint of mice with collagen-induced arthritis prevents cartilage destruction. J Immunol 1999;163:4546–56.
83. Van den Bosch F, Russell A, Keystone EC, Moreland LW, St Clair EW, Weinblatt M, et al. rHuIL-4 in subjects with active rheumatoid arthritis: a phase I dose escalating safety study [abstract]. Arthritis Rheum 1998;41 Suppl 9:S56.
84. Maini RN, Paulus H, Breedveld FC, Moreland LW, St Clair EW, Russell AS, et al. rHuIL-10 in subjects with active rheumatoid arthritis: a phase I and cytokine response study [abstract]. Arthritis Rheum 1997;40 Suppl 9:S224.
85. Atkins MB, Vachino G, Tilg HJ, Karp DD, Robert NJ, Kappler K, et al. Phase I evaluation of thrice-daily intravenous bolus interleukin-4 in patients with refractory malignancy. J Clin Oncol 1992;10:1802–9.
86. Chernoff AE, Granowitz EV, Shapiro L, Vannier E, Lonnemann G, Angel JB, et al. A randomized, controlled trial of IL-10 in humans: inhibition of inflammatory cytokine production and immune responses. J Immunol 1995;154:5492–9.
87. Weinblatt ME, St Clair EW, Breedveld FC, Moreland LW, Keystone EC, Lee SH, et al. rHuIL-10 (TENOVIL) plus methotrexate (MTX) in active rheumatoid arthritis: a phase I/II study [abstract]. Arthritis Rheum 1999;42 Suppl 9:S170.
88. Wang P, Wu P, Siegel MI, Egan RW, Billah MM. Interleukin (IL)-10 inhibits nuclear factor kappa B (NF kappa B) activation in human monocytes: IL-10 and IL-4 suppress cytokine synthesis by different mechanisms. J Biol Chem 1995;270:9558–63.
89. Powrie F, Menon S, Coffman RL. Interleukin-4 and interleukin-10 synergize to inhibit cell-mediated immunity in vivo. Eur J Immunol 1993;23:3043–9.
90. Vouldoukis I, Becherel PA, Riveros-Moreno V, Arock M, da Silva O, Debre P, et al. Interleukin-10 and interleukin-4 inhibit intracellular killing of Leishmania infantum and Leishmania major by human macrophages by decreasing nitric oxide generation. Eur J Immunol 1997;27:860–5.
91. Niiro H, Otsuka T, Izuhara K, Yamaoka K, Ohshima K, Tanabe T, et al. Regulation by interleukin-10 and interleukin-4 of cyclooxygenase-2 expression in human neutrophils. Blood 1997;89: 1621–8.
92. Mirmonsef P, Shelburne CP, Yeatman CF II, Chong HJ, Ryan JJ. Inhibition of Kit expression by IL-4 and IL-10 in murine mast cells: role of STAT6 and phosphatidylinositol 3′-kinase. J Immunol 1999;163:2530–9.
93. Marie C, Pitton C, Fitting C, Cavaillon JM. IL-10 and IL-4 synergize with TNF-alpha to induce IL-1ra production by human neutrophils. Cytokine 1996;8:147–51.
94. Te Velde AA, de Waal MR, Huijbens RJ, de Vries JE, Figdor CG. IL-10 stimulates monocyte Fc gamma R surface expression and cytotoxic activity: distinct regulation of antibody-dependent cellular cytotoxicity by IFN-gamma, IL-4, and IL-10. J Immunol 1992;149:4048–52.
95. Del Prete G, de Carli M, Almerigogna F, Giudizi MG, Biagiotti R, Romagnani S. Human IL-10 is produced by both type 1 helper (Th1) and type 2 helper (Th2) T cell clones and inhibits their antigen-specific proliferation and cytokine production. J Immunol 1993;150:353–60.
96. Buelens C, Verhasselt V, de Groote D, Thielemans K, Goldman M, Willems F. Interleukin-10 prevents the generation of dendritic cells from human peripheral blood mononuclear cells cultured with interleukin-4 and granulocyte/macrophage-colony–stimulating factor. Eur J Immunol 1997;27:756–62.
97. De Smedt T, van Mechelen M, de Becker G, Urbain J, Leo O, Moser M. Effect of interleukin-10 on dendritic cell maturation and function. Eur J Immunol 1997;27:1229–35.
98. Thomas R, MacDonald KP, Pettit AR, Cavanagh LL, Padmanabha J, Zehntner S. Dendritic cells and the pathogenesis of rheumatoid arthritis. J Leukoc Biol 1999;66:286–92.
99. Punnonen J, de Waal MR, van Vlasselaer P, Gauchat JF, de Vries JE. IL-10 and viral IL-10 prevent IL-4-induced IgE synthesis by inhibiting the accessory cell function of monocytes. J Immunol 1993;151:1280–9.
100. Chomarat P, Briolay J, Banchereau J, Miossec P. Increased production of soluble CD23 in rheumatoid arthritis, and its regulation by interleukin-4. Arthritis Rheum 1993;36:234–42.
101. Morinobu A, Kumagai S, Yanagida H, Ota H, Ishida H, Matsui M, et al. IL-10 suppresses cell surface CD23/Fc epsilon RII expression, not by enhancing soluble CD23 release, but by reducing CD23 mRNA expression in human monocytes. J Clin Immunol 1996;16:326–33.
102. Briolay J, Dechanet J, Blanchard D, Banchereau J, Miossec P. Interleukin 4 inhibits polyclonal immunoglobulin secretion and cytokine production by peripheral blood mononuclear cells from rheumatoid arthritis patients. J Clin Immunol 1992;12:36–44.
103. Joyce DA, Gibbons DP, Green P, Steer JH, Feldmann M, Brennan FM. Two inhibitors of pro-inflammatory cytokine release, interleukin-10 and interleukin-4, have contrasting effects on release of soluble p75 tumor necrosis factor receptor by cultured monocytes. Eur J Immunol 1994;24:2699–705.
104. Harigai M, Hara M, Nakazawa S, Fukasawa C, Ohta S, Sugiura T, et al. Ligation of CD40 induced tumor necrosis factor-alpha in rheumatoid arthritis: a novel mechanism of activation of synoviocytes. J Rheumatol 1999;26:1035–43.
105. Warren HS, Kinnear BF, Phillips JH, Lanier LL. Production of IL-5 by human NK cells and regulation of IL-5 secretion by IL-4, IL-10, and IL-12. J Immunol 1995;154:5144–52.
106. De Waal MR, Abrams J, Bennett B, Figdor CG, de Vries JE. Interleukin 10 (IL-10) inhibits cytokine synthesis by human monocytes: an autoregulatory role of IL-10 produced by monocytes. J Exp Med 1991;174:1209–20.

ARTHRITIS & RHEUMATISM
Vol. 44, No. 1, January 2001, pp 13–20

CD4+,CD28− T Cells in Rheumatoid Arthritis Patients Combine Features of the Innate and Adaptive Immune Systems

Kenneth J. Warrington, Seisuke Takemura, Jörg J. Goronzy, and Cornelia M. Weyand

Objective. **To determine whether CD4+,CD28− T cells, which are expanded in patients with rheumatoid arthritis (RA), express receptors that typically regulate the function of natural killer (NK) cells.**

Methods. **Expression of the NK cell surface molecules CD158, p70, CD94, CD161, and CD8α on T cell subsets was determined by multicolor flow cytometric analysis of peripheral blood mononuclear cells from 36 RA patients. Expression of CD161 on tissue-infiltrating CD4 T cells was determined by 2-color immunohistochemistry analysis of synovial tissue samples.**

Results. **Killer cell–inhibitory receptors (KIR) and killer cell–activating receptors (KAR) were exclusively expressed on CD4+,CD28− T cells, with the CD158b molecule being the most frequently detected isoform. A coordinated mechanism inducing KIR/KAR expression was suggested by similarities in the expression of CD158b on CD4 and CD8 T cells. CD4+,CD28− T cells were also positive for CD8-αα homodimers, another characteristic shared with NK cells. Of the C-type lectin NK cell receptors (NK receptors), CD94 was consistently absent, but CD161 was found on a CD4 T cell population that is significantly expanded in RA patients (P = 0.01). Involvement in disease of NK receptor–expressing CD4 T cells was suggested by the presence of CD4+,CD161+ T cells in follicular microstructures typical of rheumatoid synovitis.**

Conclusion. **Patients with RA have an expanded and unusual subset of CD4 T cells that infiltrates the tissue lesions and is characterized by a deficiency of CD28, the expression of CD8-αα homodimers, and the expression of several types of HLA class I–recognizing NK receptors. CD4 T cells bearing NK receptors can bridge functions of the innate and adaptive immune systems, such as responsiveness to specific antigen, rapid release of interferon-γ, cytotoxicity, independence from classic costimulatory pathways, and integration of multiple activating and inhibitory signals to control effector functions.**

T lymphocytes are involved at multiple checkpoints in the immunopathogenesis of rheumatoid arthritis (RA) (1,2). T helper and regulatory cells play a key role in the formation and maintenance of chronic inflammatory lesions in the synovial membrane, and the depletion of tissue-infiltrating T cells promptly disrupts the production of proinflammatory cytokines as well as tissue-injurious metalloproteinases (3–7). Information on additional properties of synovial T cells derives from analysis of the lymphoid microstructures formed in the inflamed synovial membrane. In contrast to other inflammatory infiltrates, synovial lesions acquire a structured microarchitecture. Most notably, tissue-infiltrating T cells and B cells are arranged in follicles that support germinal center reactions, indicating that rheumatoid synovitis is associated with the formation of tertiary lymphoid tissues (8,9).

Additional aspects of abnormal T cell immunity in RA have recently come into focus. Besides the accumulation of activated T cells, B cells, macrophages, and dendritic cells in rheumatoid synovium, mechanisms of T cell homeostasis affecting the entire pool of T lymphocytes are also abnormal in patients with RA (10). While normal individuals have a highly diverse compartment of T cells, T cell diversity is contracted in RA patients and is accompanied by the emergence of grossly expanded clonotypes.

Expanded CD4 clonotypes are phenotypically

Supported by the Mayo Foundation and by NIH grants R01-AR-41974 and R01-AR-42527. Dr. Warrington's work was supported by a Clinical Investigator Fellowship from the General Mills Foundation.

Kenneth J. Warrington, MD, Seisuke Takemura, MD, Jörg J. Goronzy, MD, Cornelia M. Weyand, MD: Mayo Clinic, Rochester, Minnesota.

Address correspondence and reprint requests to Cornelia M. Weyand, MD, Mayo Clinic, 401 Guggenheim Building, 200 First Street SW, Rochester, MN 55905.

Submitted for publication May 2, 2000; accepted in revised form September 6, 2000.

and functionally distinct from classic T helper cells (11). Due to a transcriptional block of the *CD28* gene, clonally expanded CD4 T cells lack surface expression of the major costimulatory molecule CD28 (12). CD4+, CD28− T cells release large amounts of interferon-γ (IFNγ) (13) and contain intracellular perforin and granzyme B, providing them with the ability to lyse target cells (3). Their outgrowth into large clonal populations may be partially attributed to a defect in down-regulating Bcl-2 when deprived of T cell growth factors (14). In the absence of the CD28 molecule, these unusual CD4 T cells use alternate costimulatory pathways (13). Several of these functional features in CD4+,CD28− T cells are reminiscent of natural killer (NK) cells. Like NK cells, CD4+,CD28− T cells are cytotoxic and can express the CD57 marker (11,15). However, unlike previously described NK T cells, CD4+,CD28− T cells from RA patients are not biased toward using the T cell receptor BV11 and AV24 segments (16,17).

It is now clear that the function of NK cells is closely regulated by a family of polymorphic receptors that interact with polymorphic major histocompatibility complex (MHC) class I molecules, resulting in signals that control NK-mediated cytotoxicity and cytokine production (18–20). MHC class I–mediated triggering of the full-length NK cell receptors (NK receptors) transduces a dominant inhibitory signal that blocks the cytolytic activity and cytokine release of NK cells. Interestingly, both families also contain highly homologous members that have truncated cytoplasmic domains and transmit activating signals. MHC class I–recognizing receptors fall into two families: the C-type lectins, which consist of CD94/NKG2 and CD161; and the Ig superfamily, which includes CD158 and p70. CD158 includes both killer cell–inhibitory and killer cell–activating receptors (KIR and KAR, respectively), and p70 is only inhibitory.

The current project explored whether CD4+,CD28− T cells in patients with RA have features of NK cells, in particular the expression of MHC class I–recognizing receptors. The results demonstrate that multiple types of NK receptors are expressed on CD28-deficient CD4 T cells, suggesting that these unusual T cells represent hybrid cells that combine T cell receptor–mediated antigen recognition with signals derived from MHC class I–recognizing receptors.

PATIENTS AND METHODS

Study population. Samples were obtained with Mayo Foundation Internal Review Board approval and informed consent from all participants. Thirty-six patients with seropositive RA (16 men and 20 women, mean ± SD age 57 ± 12 years) were recruited from the rheumatology outpatient clinic at the Mayo Clinic. All study participants fulfilled the American College of Rheumatology (formerly, the American Rheumatism Association) 1987 revised diagnostic criteria for RA (21). Normal control samples were obtained from 40 healthy, age-matched donors (20 men and 20 women, mean ± SD age 51 ± 11 years).

Flow cytometry. Heparinized venous blood was collected, and peripheral blood mononuclear cells (PBMC) were isolated by density gradient centrifugation over Ficoll-Hypaque (Amersham Pharmacia Biotech, Piscataway, NJ). Cell surface staining was performed using combinations of the following antibodies: CD4–peridinin chlorophyll protein (CD4-PerCP), CD8-PerCP, CD28–fluorescein isothiocyanate (CD28-FITC), CD161-phycoerythrin (CD161-PE), CD158a-PE, DX9-PE, CD94-FITC, and CD8 β-chain–PE (all from Becton Dickinson, San Jose, CA), as well as CD158b-PE (BeckmanCoulter, Miami, FL). Samples were analyzed on a FACSCalibur flow cytometer (Becton Dickinson), and the frequencies of T cell subsets were calculated using WinMDI software (Joseph Trotter, Scripps Research Institute, La Jolla, CA). In selected experiments, CD4+ T cells were sorted into CD4+,CD28− and CD4+,CD28+ subsets on a FACSVantage flow cytometer (Becton Dickinson). Sorted populations were >99% pure as determined by flow cytometric analysis of the sorted samples.

Immunohistochemistry. Synovial tissue specimens obtained from RA patients undergoing joint surgery were embedded in OCT compound (Sakura Finetek USA, Torrance, CA). Cryostat sections (5 μm thick) were fixed in acetone for 10 minutes. Sections were incubated with mouse anti-CD161 monoclonal antibody (mAb) (1:200; PharMingen, San Diego, CA) for 30 minutes at room temperature. Thoroughly washed sections were treated for 30 minutes with a ready-to-use EnVision$^+$ reaction system (Dako, Carpinteria, CA) and developed with 3′,3′-diaminobenzidine tetrahydrochloride (DAB). The DAB-stained slides were washed in 0.5% Triton X-100/phosphate buffered saline for 10 minutes. Nonspecific binding was blocked for 15 minutes with 5% rabbit serum, and sections were stained with mouse anti-CD4 mAb (1:50; Dako) for 60 minutes at room temperature. After incubation with biotinylated rabbit anti-mouse Ig antibody (1:300; Dako), the slides were incubated with the VectaStain ABC-AP kit (Vector, Burlingame, CA) for 30 minutes and then developed with Vector Red substrate kit (Vector) for 3 minutes. Slides were counterstained with hematoxylin for 5 seconds and permanently mounted in Cytoseal-60 (Stephens Scientific, Riverdale, NJ). Negative controls consisted of slides stained without the primary antibodies.

Statistical analysis. All statistical analysis comparing cell populations was performed using the Mann-Whitney rank sum test (SigmaStat; SPSS, Chicago, IL).

RESULTS

Expression of Ig superfamily NK receptors on CD4+,CD28− T cells. Thirty-six patients with seropositive RA were enrolled in this study. Patients were

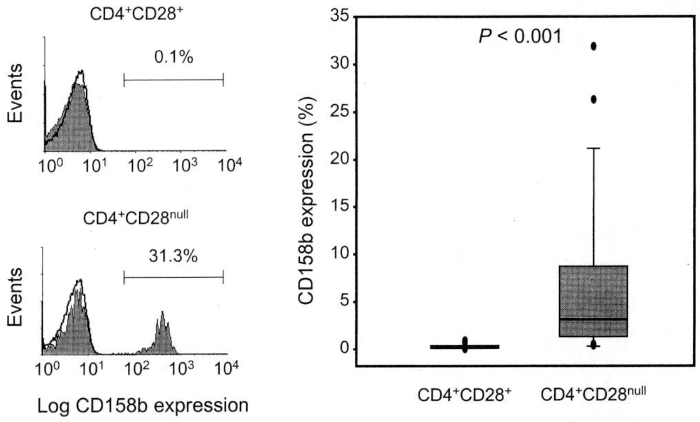

Figure 1. Expression of natural killer cell receptors (NK receptors) of the Ig superfamily by $CD4^+CD28^{null}$ T cells. Samples from rheumatoid arthritis patients with a $CD28^{null}$ compartment representing >1% of $CD4^+$ T cells were analyzed for expression of major histocompatibility complex class I–recognizing NK receptors (CD158a, CD158b, and p70) on $CD4^+$ T cells by 3-color flow cytometry. CD158b was the most common Ig-type NK receptor expressed on $CD4^+$ T cells. The frequency of CD158b-expressing T cells is shown as a box plot (right panel). CD158b expression was significantly increased on the T cells in the $CD4^+CD28^{null}$ subset ($P < 0.001$). Histograms representing CD158b expression on $CD4^+CD28^{null}$ T cells (lower left) and $CD4^+CD28^+$ T cells (upper left) are shown. Shaded areas represent staining with anti-CD158b; unshaded areas represent staining with an isotype-matched control antibody.

compared with age-matched normal individuals. In accordance with previous findings (22), CD28− T cells within the CD4 T cell population were significantly expanded in RA patients compared with normal control subjects ($P < 0.001$).

Antibodies specific for CD158a, CD158b, and p70 were used to stain receptors of the KIR/KAR families. As expected, CD158b was expressed by CD16+ NK cells and a small population of CD8 T cells. More interestingly, CD158b was also found on CD4 T cells. Among CD4 T cells, surface expression of CD158b was strictly limited to CD28-deficient T cells (Figure 1). CD4+,CD28+ T cells were consistently negative for CD158b molecules, but 0.4–31.9% (median 3.15%) of the CD4+,CD28− T cells expressed CD158b ($P < 0.001$). Of the RA patients with expansions of CD4+,CD28− T cells of >1%, 79% had CD158b-expressing CD4 T cells.

CD4+,CD158a+ and CD4+,p70+ T cells were less frequently represented. Again, CD158a and p70 receptors appeared exclusively on CD28-deficient T cells. Seven RA patients had CD158a+ T cells ranging between 1.3% and 6.1% of the CD4+,CD28− subset. In 5 patients, 1.0–11.6% of the CD4+,CD28− T cells expressed p70 (data not shown).

It is not currently understood how receptor expression on NK cells is regulated. An array of different receptors is usually found on a single cell, and there is marked variation in the number and combination of receptors on individual cells (23). There is no evidence that the repertoire of NK receptors expressed by NK cells is influenced by the host's MHC class I polymorphisms. Rather, it is believed that the repertoire of NK receptors is created by a stochastic process. In contrast, CD4+,CD28− T cells from RA patients appeared to preferentially express CD158b. To examine whether CD158b expression was random or selected, the frequencies of CD158b+ cells in the CD4, CD8, and NK compartments were compared. CD158b expression on CD4 T cells correlated with expression on CD8 T cells, but not on NK cells. RA patients with low CD4+, CD28−,CD158b+ frequencies (below the 50th percentile) also had low numbers of CD8+,CD28−,CD158b+ cells (median 4.8%), while the subset of patients with high expression of CD158b on CD4+,CD28− T cells (above the 50th percentile) also had significantly higher numbers of CD8+,CD28−,CD158b+ cells (median 10.95%) ($P = 0.03$). In contrast, the frequencies of CD158b+ NK cells did not differ in these two groups of patients ($P = 0.40$).

Expression of C-type lectin NK receptors on CD4 T cells. PBMC from patients and control subjects were analyzed for the expression of CD94 and CD161. CD94 dimerizes with the C-type lectin members of the NKG2 family; C94/NKG2 is the dominant MHC class I–recognizing receptor on NK cells, with the majority of cells expressing this molecule on the surface (23). However, CD94 could not be detected on CD4 T cells, again indicating that the emergence of NK receptors on T cells is a selective process. The second member of the C-type lectin family, CD161, was present on CD4 T cells. All patients and control subjects had CD4+,CD161+ cells with a wide range of expression (5.0–27.0% and 5.6–25.6%, respectively). In contrast to receptors of the Ig superfamily that displayed strict preference for CD28− T cells, CD161 was also encountered on a subset of CD4+,CD28+ T cells (Figure 2). However, expression of CD161 was typical for the majority of CD4+,CD28− T cells, but only occurred on a small fraction of CD4+,CD28+ T cells. Consequently, because CD4+, CD28− cells are more common in RA, CD161 frequencies were higher in the patients than in healthy individuals (15.8% versus 12.5%; $P = 0.01$).

Expression of CD8-$\alpha\alpha$ homodimers on CD4 T cells. In addition to expressing MHC class I–recognizing receptors, NK cells can also express low amounts of CD8

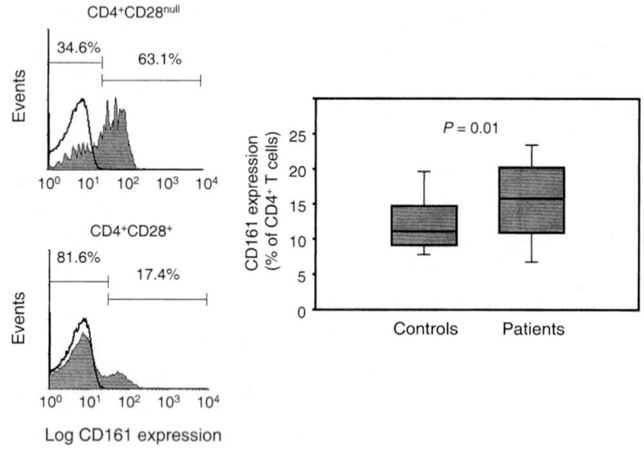

Figure 2. Expansion of $CD4^+CD161^+$ natural killer (NK) T cells in patients with seropositive rheumatoid arthritis (RA). The expression of CD161 on $CD4^+CD28^+$ and $CD4^+CD28^{null}$ T cells was determined by 3-color flow cytometry. Shown are representative histograms demonstrating surface expression of the C-type lectin receptor CD161 mostly on $CD4^+CD28^{null}$ T cells (left upper panel), but also on a subset of $CD4^+CD28^+$ T cells (left lower panel). The box plots in the right panel show that the number of $CD4^+CD161^+$ NK T cells was significantly increased in RA patients compared with age-matched control subjects ($P = 0.01$).

on the cell surface (24). The molecular correlate to the dim expression of CD8 consists of homodimers of CD8 α-chains, as opposed to CD8-$\alpha\beta$ heterodimers found on CD8 T cells (25). In cells with homodimerization of CD8 α-chains, the CD8 β-chain gene is transcriptionally blocked. By 3-color flow cytometry, CD4+,CD28+ and CD4+,CD28− T cells were analyzed for the presence of $CD8^{dim}$ cells. Among CD4+,CD28+ T cells, CD8 surface expression was extremely rare. All CD4+,$CD8^{dim}$ cells could be assigned to the CD4+,CD28− subset (Figure 3A). To confirm that $CD8^{dim}$ expression identified T cells with CD8 α-chain homodimers, T cells from RA patients were stained with antibodies specific for α- and β-chain epitopes. CD4+,CD28+ T cells included a very small population of CD8-$\alpha\beta^{bright}$ T cells, representing CD4+,CD8+ double-positive cells. CD4 T cells positive for CD8 α-chain binding but negative for CD8 β-chain binding were restricted to the subset of CD4+,CD28− T cells (Figure 3B).

Contribution of NK receptor–expressing CD4+ T cells to synovial lymphoid follicles. NK receptors have been implicated in regulating cytotoxic NK cells because they transduce either inhibitory or activating signals (20). Their functional role on T cells is much less understood. The expansion of CD4+ T cells with surface expression of NK receptors in RA raised the question of whether these unusual T cells influence pathogenic events in the synovium. CD161, the most common NK receptor, was chosen as a marker to detect and localize NK receptor–expressing CD4+ T cells in synovial lesions. Imaging with 2-color immunohistochemistry revealed the accumulation of CD4+,CD161+ T cells in the tissue infiltrates. Patients forming lymphoid follicles had higher frequencies of tissue-invading CD4+, CD161+ T cells than patients with diffuse synovitis lacking organized lymphoid architecture. CD4+ T cells expressing CD161 preferentially accumulated within the lymphoid follicles, which were composed of CD4+ T cells and CD20+ B cells (Figures 4A and C). In samples from some patients, CD4+,CD161+ T cells were also found at the outer edge of the lymphoid aggregates. Neither interfollicular zones nor the synovial lining was seeded by CD4+,CD161+ T cells. Also, the diffuse mononuclear infiltrate in the synovial tissue of a patient with connective tissue disease did not contain CD4+,CD161+ T cells (Figures 4B and D).

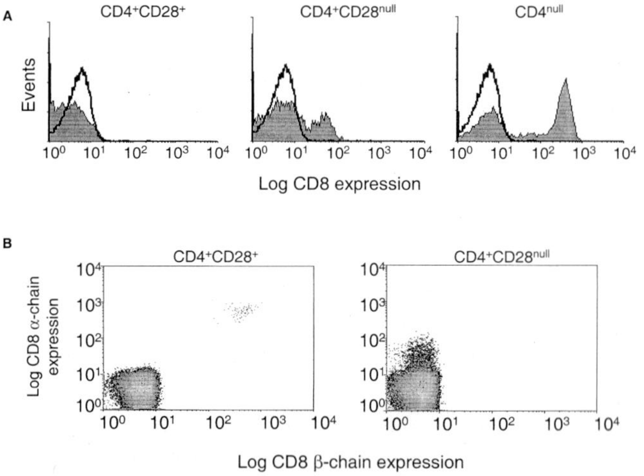

Figure 3. Expression of CD8-$\alpha\alpha$ homodimers by $CD4^+CD28^{null}$ T cells. **A,** CD8 surface expression of peripheral blood mononuclear cells was analyzed by 3-color flow cytometry. Gating on $CD4^+CD28^+$ (left panel) and $CD4^+CD28^{null}$ (center panel) subsets demonstrates that a double-positive ($CD4^+CD8^{dim}$) population is limited to the $CD28^{null}$ compartment. The right panel demonstrates $CD8^{bright}$ expression on typical $CD8^+CD4^{null}$ T cells for comparison. **B,** $CD4^+$ T cells were sorted into $CD4^+CD28^{null}$ and $CD4^+CD28^+$ subsets on a FACSVantage flow cytometer. Each subset was then analyzed for CD4, CD8 α-chain, and CD8 β-chain expression. $CD4^+CD8^{dim}CD28^{null}$ T cells expressed CD8 α-chain but not CD8 β-chain (right panel), indicating that the CD8 molecule in this subset was composed of $\alpha\alpha$ homodimers. Within the $CD28^+$ subset, <2% were double positive. These cells were all $CD4^+CD8^{bright}$ and were CD8 $\alpha\beta$-chain positive (left panel).

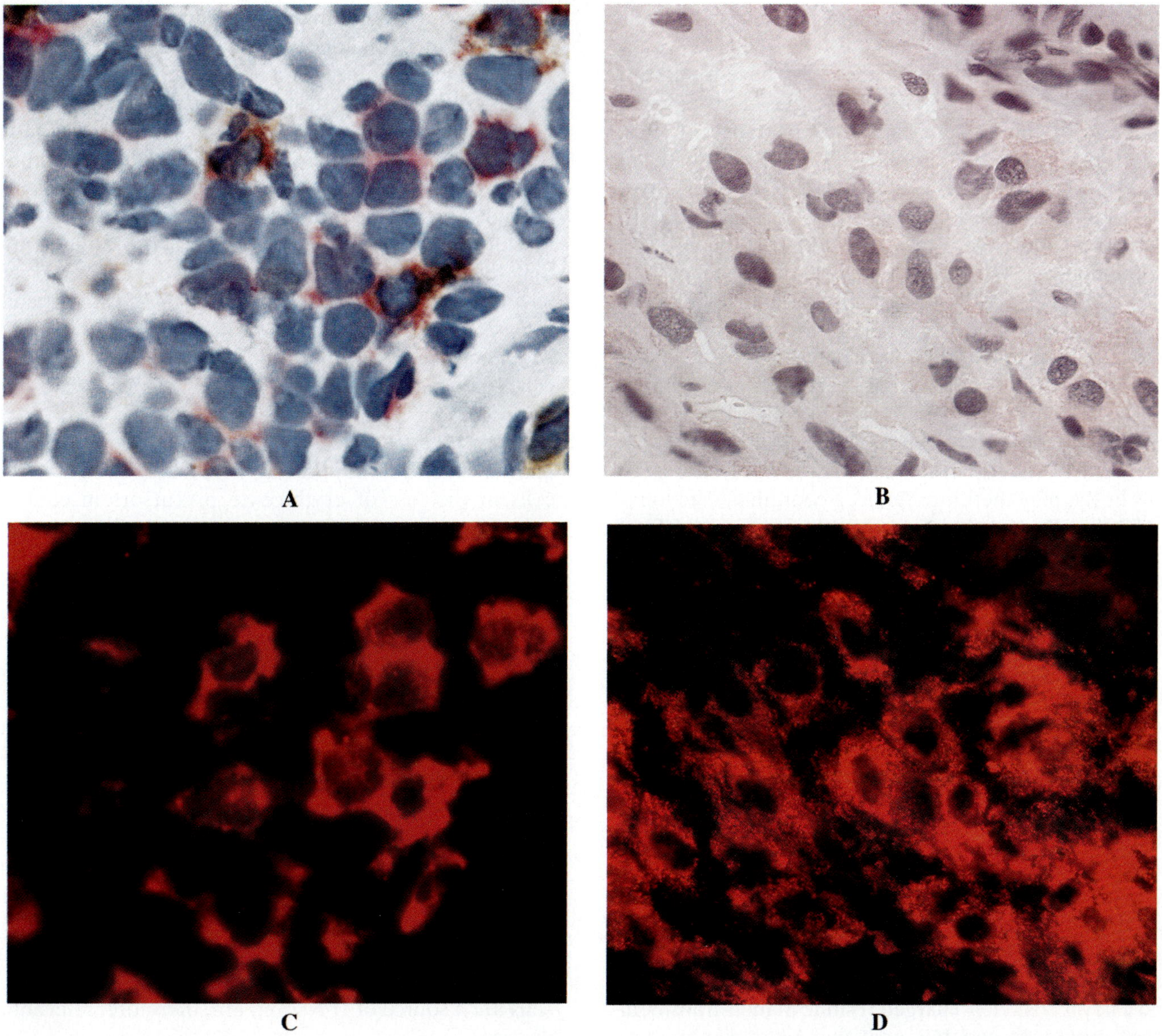

Figure 4. Contribution to synovial lymphoid follicles by natural killer cell receptor–expressing CD4+ T cells. **A,** Cryosections from synovial tissue specimens obtained from rheumatoid arthritis patients were analyzed by 2-color immunohistochemistry with anti-CD4 (red) and anti-CD161 (brown) antibodies. CD4+,CD161+ cells can be seen within synovial lymphoid follicles. **C,** Analysis of the identical tissue section by immunofluorescence shows CD4 staining on the surface of T cells. Most CD161+ cells in the tissue coexpressed CD4. **B,** Synovial tissue from a patient with connective tissue disease, which did not contain any CD161+ cells. **D,** CD4 stain corresponding to tissue section in **B**. (Original magnification × 1,000.)

DISCUSSION

The total number of lymphocytes circulating in the blood and their subset distribution is under strict homeostatic control (26). In patients with RA, there is a profound change in the representation of functionally and phenotypically distinct subsets of CD4 T cells. Best examined is the expansion of an unusual subpopulation of CD4 T cells characterized by clonal proliferation, loss of CD28 on the cell surface, production of large amounts of IFNγ, and intracellular storage of the cytolytic proteins, perforin and granzyme B. The basic mechanisms causing replacement of other CD4 T cells by CD4+,CD28− clonotypes are incompletely understood, but phenotypic and functional analysis of CD4+,CD28−

T cells has suggested that they are related to NK cells and represent a hybrid lineage of NK T cells (27).

In support of this hypothesis, we have found that CD4+,CD28− T cells express MHC class I–recognizing receptors of the Ig superfamily. Appearance of these receptors was strictly limited to CD4+ T cells with the CD28− phenotype. Selected members of the C-type lectin family were also expressed on CD4 T cells, with preference (but not exclusively so) for the CD28− subpopulation. Our data support the concept that CD4+,CD28− T cells share multiple features with NK cells and may combine functional properties relevant to innate and adaptive immunity. The presence of CD8-$\alpha\alpha$ homodimers and KIR/KAR receptors on CD4+, CD28− T cells suggests that the functional properties of these unusual T cells are under the control of MHC class I molecules. The expansion and activation of CD4 NK T cells in RA may therefore reflect a coordinated action of MHC class II– and class I–mediated stimulation of T cell receptors and KIR, respectively. The accumulation of NK receptor–expressing CD4 T cells in synovial follicles is compatible with a direct contribution of these unusual T cells to the tissue lesion.

How could functions mediated by the different NK receptors in T cells have relevance to the disease process of RA? KIR receptors on NK cells function as trans-acting inhibitors of cellular activation by recruiting phosphatases through an immunoreceptor tyrosine-based inhibition motif (ITIM) (20). While a detailed picture is emerging of how inhibitory NK receptors can prevent unwanted effector functions, such as cytolysis and cytokine production, much less is known about the biologic function and immunoregulatory consequences of activating NK receptors. Activating isoforms (KAR) use a different cytoplasmic tail lacking an ITIM motif and carry a positively charged residue in their transmembrane region. In general, activating NK receptors have been implicated in stimulating cytotoxicity and IFNγ production by NK cells and T cells and proliferation of MHC class I–restricted T cells (28). Such activating receptor forms are obvious candidates for costimulating CD4+ T cells in RA. They might be implicated in the outgrowth of the clonotypes and contribute fundamentally to the defect in T cell homeostasis in RA patients.

CD161 is a C-type lectin receptor with functions clearly different from those of the KIR/KAR or the CD94/NKG2 receptors (29). The ligand of CD161 is unknown and is not likely to be an MHC class I molecule. Human CD161 lacks a clear ITIM or immunoreceptor tyrosine-based activation motif in the cytoplasmic tail. However, CD161 has been shown to facilitate transendothelial migration, suggesting that it may play a role in T cell adhesion and tissue invasion (30,31).

So far, evidence for a possible contribution of NK T cells in RA pathogenesis has come from the observation that large granular lymphocytes express NK and T cell markers (32). Expansion of large granular lymphocytes is usually a feature of RA with extraarticular manifestations (i.e., Felty's syndrome or rheumatoid vasculitis) (33,34). In this context, it is interesting to note that the highest frequencies of CD4+,CD28− T cells have been described for RA patients with extraarticular disease (22). It is not known whether large granular lymphocytes have a direct contribution to leukopenia, which is used to establish the diagnosis of Felty's syndrome. Their cytolytic capability may be involved in injuring precursor cells, in a manner analogous to a pathomechanism implicating NK receptor–expressing cells in the loss of erythrocyte precursors in cases of aplastic anemia (35,36).

Results of this study provide direct evidence that CD4+ NK T cells can also be involved in the tissue-destructive lesions in the synovial membrane. It was surprising that CD4+,CD161+ T cells preferentially homed to follicular structures. Such follicular structures can form classic germinal centers and, as such, provide a microenvironment for antigen trapping, B cell hypermutation, and B cell memory generation. A cytolytic function of CD4+,CD161+ T cells is unlikely in this setting, because it should lead to cell death and destruction of the follicles. Instead, cytokine production by CD4+, CD161+ T cells may be more relevant (37). In vitro, CD4+,CD28− T cells resemble NK cells in the sense that they can rapidly release large amounts of IFNγ (13). IFNγ has been demonstrated to be critical in sustaining rheumatoid synovitis, suggesting that CD4+,CD161+ T cells are a source of IFNγ and are, therefore, relevant to disease.

Data presented here raise the question of whether CD4+,CD28− T cells are primarily derived from CD28− precursors and represent a special type of NK cells. CD4+,CD28− T cells in RA patients are different from NK T cells described previously, because they are not restricted in the use of T cell receptor AV segments. However, they can express the CD57 marker that is typically encountered on NK cells (11,15). Additionally, we report that CD4+,CD28− T cells have dim expression of CD8 on their surface. Phenotyping of CD8^{dim} T cells confirmed the expression of CD8-$\alpha\alpha$ homodimers. This homodimeric form of CD8 has been associated with extrathymic T cell development, particularly in the fetal intestine (38). CD4+ intestinal intraepithelial lymphocytes have been found in jejunal locations with high concentrations of recombinase, which supports the notion that these tissue sites are prone to extrathymic T cell generation (39).

An extrathymic origin of CD4+,CD8^{dim} T cells with CD8-$\alpha\alpha$ homodimers has also been suggested because of the expansion of such cells in clinical conditions associated with defective thymic function. CD4+, CD8^{dim} T cells are increased in frequency in patients who have been treated for Hodgkin's disease by mediastinal irradiation, and it has been proposed that extrathymic T cell differentiation is necessary to compensate for the loss of thymus-derived T cells (25). A similar scenario could explain the increased frequencies of CD4+,CD8^{dim} T cells in human immunodeficiency virus–related disease, in which virally induced destruction of the thymus is suspected (40–43). In RA, the increased frequency of CD4+,CD28− T cells could also reflect increased extrathymic T cell generation to compensate for decreased thymic function. Difficulties with T cell replenishment have been encountered in RA patients treated with T cell–depleting mAb. These patients developed longstanding lymphopenia with selectivity for T cells (44,45). More direct evidence for thymic dysfunction in RA has come from recent studies that show a decrease in recent thymic emigrants and a contracted peripheral repertoire (46).

The shared features of CD4+,CD28− T cells and NK cells cannot definitively settle the question of how these cells emerge. The lack of CD28 expression on CD4+,CD28− T cells is caused by a transcriptional block of the *CD28* gene due to the lack of two gene-specific nuclear proteins controlling the initiation of CD28 transcription (47). Principally, this cell type could also be derived from CD28+,CD4+ T cells that have down-regulated this costimulatory pathway, possibly as a result of chronic antigenic stimulation in the attempt to shut down T cell activation. In this scenario, CD4+, CD28+,CD161+ cells are the precursor cells that proceed to lose CD28 and to acquire the expression of KIR/KAR. In support of this model, we have recently found that CD28 expression can be reinduced by exposing CD28− T cells to interleukin-12 (Warrington KJ et al: unpublished observation).

In summary, RA patients carry CD4+ T cells that have several characteristics of NK cells, including the cell surface expression of regulatory killer cell–activating and –inhibitory receptors and CD8-$\alpha\alpha$ homodimers. Because these cells lack the expression of the costimulatory molecule CD28, activation of these cells may be regulated through MHC class I molecules and not through CD80/CD86. In contrast to classic T helper cells, CD4+,CD28− T cells are specialized in potentially tissue-injurious functions such as cytotoxicity and IFNγ production. The expression of CD161 enhances their ability to infiltrate inflamed, and possibly also noninflamed, tissues. We propose that individuals carrying such cell populations respond differently when exposed to exogenous as well as self antigens, predisposing them to chronic, smoldering immune responses in the synovial membrane.

ACKNOWLEDGMENTS

We gratefully acknowledge the support of our colleagues in the Division of Rheumatology and thank Tammy J. Dahl and James W. Fulbright for editorial assistance and manuscript preparation.

REFERENCES

1. Weyand CM, Goronzy JJ. HLA polymorphisms and T cells in rheumatoid arthritis. Int Rev Immunol 1999;18:37–59.
2. Panayi GS. T-cell-dependent pathways in rheumatoid arthritis. Curr Opin Rheumatol 1997;9:236–40.
3. Namekawa T, Wagner UG, Goronzy JJ, Weyand CM. Functional subsets of CD4 T cells in rheumatoid synovitis. Arthritis Rheum 1998;41:2108–16.
4. Rittner HL, Zettl A, Jendro MC, Bartz-Bazzanella P, Goronzy JJ, Weyand CM. Multiple mechanisms support oligoclonal T cell expansion in rheumatoid synovitis. Mol Med 1997;3:452–65.
5. Thomas R, McIlraith M, Davis LS, Lipsky PE. Rheumatoid synovium is enriched in CD45RB^{dim} mature memory T cells that are potent helpers for B cell differentiation. Arthritis Rheum 1992;35:1455–65.
6. Kohem CL, Brezinschek RI, Wisbey H, Tortorella C, Lipsky PE, Oppenheimer-Marks N. Enrichment of differentiated CD45RB^{dim}, CD27− memory T cells in the peripheral blood, synovial fluid, and synovial tissue of patients with rheumatoid arthritis. Arthritis Rheum 1996;39:844–54.
7. Klimiuk PA, Yang H, Goronzy JJ, Weyand CM. Production of cytokines and metalloproteinases in rheumatoid synovitis is T cell dependent. Clin Immunol 1999;90:65–78.
8. Berek C, Kim HJ. B-cell activation and development within chronically inflamed synovium in rheumatoid and reactive arthritis. Semin Immunol 1997;9:261–8.
9. Wagner UG, Kurtin PJ, Wahner A, Brackertz M, Berry DJ, Goronzy JJ, et al. The role of CD8+ CD40L+ T cells in the formation of germinal centers in rheumatoid synovitis. J Immunol 1998;161:6390–7.
10. Wagner UG, Koetz K, Weyand CM, Goronzy JJ. Perturbation of the T cell repertoire in rheumatoid arthritis. Proc Natl Acad Sci U S A 1998;95:14447–52.
11. Schmidt D, Goronzy JJ, Weyand CM. CD4+ CD7− CD28− T cells are expanded in rheumatoid arthritis and are characterized by autoreactivity. J Clin Invest 1996;97:2027–37.
12. Vallejo AN, Brandes JC, Weyand CM, Goronzy JJ. Modulation of CD28 expression: distinct regulatory pathways during activation and replicative senescence. J Immunol 1999;162:6572–9.
13. Park W, Weyand CM, Schmidt D, Goronzy JJ. Co-stimulatory pathways controlling activation and peripheral tolerance of human CD4+CD28− T cells. Eur J Immunol 1997;27:1082–90.
14. Schirmer M, Vallejo AN, Weyand CM, Goronzy JJ. Resistance to

apoptosis and elevated expression of Bcl-2 in clonally expanded CD4+CD28− T cells from rheumatoid arthritis patients. J Immunol 1998;161:1018–25.
15. Imberti L, Sottini A, Signorini S, Gorla R, Primi D. Oligoclonal CD4+ CD57+ T-cell expansions contribute to the imbalanced T-cell receptor repertoire of rheumatoid arthritis patients. Blood 1997;89:2822–32.
16. Schmidt D, Martens PB, Weyand CM, Goronzy JJ. The repertoire of CD4+ CD28− T cells in rheumatoid arthritis. Mol Med 1996;2:608–18.
17. Namekawa T, Snyder MR, Yen JH, Goehring BE, Leibson PJ, Weyand CM, et al. Killer cell activating receptors function as costimulatory molecules on CD4+CD28null T cells clonally expanded in rheumatoid arthritis. J Immunol 2000;165:1138–45.
18. Lopez-Botet M, Bellon T. Natural killer cell activation and inhibition by receptors for MHC class I. Curr Opin Immunol 1999;11:301–7.
19. Yokoyama WM. Natural killer cell receptors. Curr Opin Immunol 1998;10:298–305.
20. Lanier LL. NK cell receptors. Annu Rev Immunol 1998;16:359–93.
21. Arnett FC, Edworthy SM, Bloch DA, McShane DJ, Fries JF, Cooper NS, et al. The American Rheumatism Association 1987 revised criteria for the classification of rheumatoid arthritis. Arthritis Rheum 1988;31:315–24.
22. Martens PB, Goronzy JJ, Schaid D, Weyand CM. Expansion of unusual CD4+ T cells in severe rheumatoid arthritis. Arthritis Rheum 1997;40:1106–14.
23. Valiante NM, Uhrberg M, Shilling HG, Lienert-Weidenbach K, Arnett KL, D'Andrea A, et al. Functionally and structurally distinct NK cell receptor repertoires in the peripheral blood of two human donors. Immunity 1997;7:739–51.
24. Baume DM, Caligiuri MA, Manley TJ, Daley JF, Ritz J. Differential expression of CD8 alpha and CD8 beta associated with MHC-restricted and non-MHC-restricted cytolytic effector cells. Cell Immunol 1990;131:352–65.
25. Watanabe N, de Rosa SC, Cmelak A, Hoppe R, Herzenberg LA, Roederer M. Long-term depletion of naive T cells in patients treated for Hodgkin's disease. Blood 1997;90:3662–72.
26. Roederer M, De Rosa SC, Watanabe N, Herzenberg LA. Dynamics of fine T-cell subsets during HIV disease and after thymic ablation by mediastinal irradiation. Semin Immunol 1997;9:389–96.
27. Bix M, Locksley RM. Natural T cells: cells that co-express NKRP-1 and TCR. J Immunol 1995;155:1020–2.
28. Bottino C, Sivori S, Vitale M, Cantoni C, Falco M, Pende D, et al. A novel surface molecule homologous to the p58/p50 family of receptors is selectively expressed on a subset of human natural killer cells and induces both triggering of cell functions and proliferation. Eur J Immunol 1996;26:1816–24.
29. Lanier LL, Chang C, Phillips JH. Human NKR-P1A: a disulfide-linked homodimer of the C-type lectin superfamily expressed by a subset of NK and T lymphocytes. J Immunol 1994;153:2417–28.
30. Poggi A, Costa P, Zocchi MR, Moretta L. Phenotypic and functional analysis of CD4+ NKRP1A+ human T lymphocytes: direct evidence that the NKRP1A molecule is involved in transendothelial migration. Eur J Immunol 1997;27:2345–50.
31. Poggi A, Zocchi MR, Costa P, Ferrero E, Borsellino G, Placido R, et al. IL-12-mediated NKRP1A up-regulation and consequent enhancement of endothelial transmigration of V delta 2+ TCR gamma delta+ T lymphocytes from healthy donors and multiple sclerosis patients. J Immunol 1999;162:4349–54.
32. Kingreen D, Siegert W. Chronic lymphatic leukemias of T and NK cell type. Leukemia 1997;11 Suppl 2:S46–9.
33. Bowman SJ, Geddes GC, Corrigall V, Panayi GS, Lanchbury JS. Large granular lymphocyte expansions in Felty's syndrome have an unusual phenotype of activated CD45RA+ cells. Br J Rheumatol 1996;35:1252–5.
34. Starkebaum G, Loughran TP Jr, Gaur LK, Davis P, Nepom BS. Immunogenetic similarities between patients with Felty's syndrome and those with clonal expansions of large granular lymphocytes in rheumatoid arthritis. Arthritis Rheum 1997;40:624–6.
35. Tefferi A, Li CY, Witzig TE, Dhodapkar MV, Okuno SH, Phyliky RL. Chronic natural killer cell lymphocytosis: a descriptive clinical study. Blood 1994;84:2721–5.
36. Handgretinger R, Geiselhart A, Moris A, Grau R, Teuffel O, Bethge W, et al. Pure red-cell aplasia associated with clonal expansion of granular lymphocytes expressing killer-cell inhibitory receptors. N Engl J Med 1999;340:278–84.
37. Arase H, Arase N, Saito T. Interferon gamma production by natural killer (NK) cells and NK1.1+ T cells upon NKR-P1 cross-linking. J Exp Med 1996;183:2391–6.
38. Latthe M, Terry L, MacDonald TT. High frequency of CD8 alpha alpha homodimer-bearing T cells in human fetal intestine. Eur J Immunol 1994;24:1703–5.
39. Lundqvist C, Baranov V, Hammarstrom S, Athlin L, Hammarstrom ML. Intra-epithelial lymphocytes: evidence for regional specialization and extrathymic T cell maturation in the human gut epithelium. Int Immunol 1995;7:1473–87.
40. Gupta S. Abnormality of Leu 2+7+ cells in acquired immune deficiency syndrome (AIDS), AIDS-related complex, and asymptomatic homosexuals. J Clin Immunol 1986;6:502–9.
41. Su L, Kaneshima H, Bonyhadi M, Salimi S, Kraft D, Rabin L, et al. HIV-1-induced thymocyte depletion is associated with indirect cytopathogenicity and infection of progenitor cells in vivo. Immunity 1995;2:25–36.
42. Jamieson BD, Uittenbogaart CH, Schmid I, Zack JA. High viral burden and rapid CD4+ cell depletion in human immunodeficiency virus type 1-infected SCID-hu mice suggest direct viral killing of thymocytes in vivo. J Virol 1997;71:8245–53.
43. McCune JM, Loftus R, Schmidt DK, Carroll P, Webster D, Swor-Yim LB, et al. High prevalence of thymic tissue in adults with human immunodeficiency virus-1 infection. J Clin Invest 1998;101:2301–8.
44. Brett S, Baxter G, Cooper H, Johnston JM, Tite J, Rapson N. Repopulation of blood lymphocyte sub-populations in rheumatoid arthritis patients treated with the depleting humanized monoclonal antibody, CAMPATH-1H. Immunology 1996;88:13–9.
45. Jendro MC, Ganten T, Matteson EL, Weyand CM, Goronzy JJ. Emergence of oligoclonal T cell populations following therapeutic T cell depletion in rheumatoid arthritis. Arthritis Rheum 1995;38:1242–51.
46. Koetz K, Bryl E, Spickschen K, O'Fallon WM, Goronzy JJ, Weyand CM. T cell homeostasis in patients with rheumatoid arthritis. Proc Natl Acad Sci U S A 2000;97:9203–8.
47. Vallejo AN, Nestel AR, Schirmer M, Weyand CM, Goronzy JJ. Aging-related deficiency of CD28 expression in CD4+ T cells is associated with the loss of gene-specific nuclear factor binding activity. J Biol Chem 1998;273:8119–29.

ARTHRITIS & RHEUMATISM
Vol. 44, No. 1, January 2001, pp 21–30

Rheumatoid Arthritis Synovial Macrophages Express the Fas-Associated Death Domain–Like Interleukin-1β–Converting Enzyme–Inhibitory Protein and Are Refractory to Fas-Mediated Apoptosis

Harris Perlman,[1] Lisa J. Pagliari,[1] Hongtao Liu,[1] Alisa E. Koch,[1] G. Kenneth Haines, III,[2] and Richard M. Pope[1]

Objective. **The chronic inflammation and progressive joint destruction observed in rheumatoid arthritis (RA) are mediated in part by macrophages. A paucity of apoptosis has been observed in RA synovial tissues, yet the mechanism remains unknown. The present study sought to characterize the expression of Fas, Fas ligand (FasL), and Fas-associated death domain–like interleukin-1β–converting enzyme–inhibitory protein (FLIP), and to quantify the apoptosis induced by agonistic anti-Fas antibody, using mononuclear cells (MNC) isolated from the peripheral blood (PB) and synovial fluid (SF) of RA patients.**

Methods. **The expression of Fas, FasL, and FLIP and apoptosis induced by agonistic anti-Fas antibody in MNC from the PB and SF of RA patients were determined by flow cytometry. Immunohistochemistry employing a monospecific anti-FLIP antibody was performed on RA and osteoarthritis (OA) synovial tissue.**

Results. **CD14-positive monocyte/macrophages from normal and RA PB and from RA SF expressed equivalent levels of Fas and FasL. Furthermore, unlike the CD14-positive PB monocytes, RA SF monocyte/macrophages were resistant to the addition of agonistic anti-Fas antibody. In contrast, both CD14-positive PB and SF monocyte/macrophages were sensitive to apoptosis mediated by a phosphatidylinositol 3-kinase inhibitor. Intracellular staining of the caspase 8 inhibitor, FLIP, in CD14-positive SF monocyte/macrophages revealed a significant up-regulation of FLIP compared with normal and RA PB monocytes. Immunohistochemical analysis of synovial tissue from RA and OA patients revealed increased FLIP expression in the RA synovial lining compared with the OA synovial lining. Furthermore, FLIP expression was observed in the CD68-positive population in the RA synovial lining. Forced reduction of FLIP by a chemical inhibitor resulted in RA SF macrophage apoptosis that was enhanced by agonistic anti-Fas antibody, indicating that FLIP is necessary for SF macrophage survival.**

Conclusion. **These data suggest that up-regulation of FLIP in RA macrophages may account for their persistence in the disease. Thus, the targeted suppression of FLIP may be a potential therapeutic strategy for the amelioration of RA.**

Rheumatoid arthritis (RA) is an autoimmune disease characterized by infiltration of lymphocytes and macrophages into the synovium, hyperplasia of the synovial lining, and destruction of cartilage and bone. Macrophage-like and fibroblast-like synoviocytes comprise the normal synovial lining, which consists of 1–2 cell layers but increases to as much as 10 or more cell layers in active RA (1). Synovial macrophages express high levels of collagenase, stromelysin, interleukin-1β (IL-1β), tumor necrosis factor α (TNFα), granulocyte–

Dr. Perlman's work was supported by grants from the Northwestern Memorial Foundation and the NIH (AR-02147). Dr. Pope's work was supported by grants from the NIH (AR-43642 and AR-30692) and the Arthritis Foundation. Dr. Koch's work was supported by grants from the NIH (AR-41492 and AI-40987), funds from the VA Research Service, and a Gallagher Professorship for Arthritis Research.

[1]Harris Perlman, PhD, Lisa J. Pagliari, BS, Hongtao Liu, MD, PhD, Alisa E. Koch, MD, Richard M. Pope, MD: Northwestern University Medical School, and the Veterans Administration Chicago Healthcare System, Lakeside Division, Chicago, Illinois; [2]G. Kenneth Haines, III, MD: Northwestern University Medical School, Chicago, Illinois.

Address correspondence and reprint requests to Richard M. Pope, MD, Northwestern University Medical School, Department of Medicine, Division of Rheumatology, 303 East Chicago Avenue, Ward 3-315, Chicago, IL 60611.

Submitted for publication July 18, 2000; accepted in revised form September 6, 2000.

macrophage colony-stimulating factor, IL-6, IL-8, macrophage inhibitory protein 1α, and monocyte chemoattractant protein 1, all of which are mediators of inflammation and joint destruction (2,3). Thus, synovial macrophages contribute to the increase in synovial lining thickening, inflammation, and destruction of cartilage and bone.

Fas ligand (FasL), a type II membrane protein, is expressed on cells in immune privileged areas, cytotoxic lymphocytes, monocyte/macrophages, and certain tumor cells (4,5), while its cognate receptor Fas, a type I membrane receptor protein, is ubiquitously expressed (6). The Fas–FasL pathway is vital for maintaining immune homeostasis; mice and humans deficient for either Fas or FasL develop autoimmune disease (7). Ligation of Fas by FasL induces the oligomerization of Fas, resulting in the recruitment of Fas-associated death domain (FADD) and the zymogen form of the cysteine protease procaspase 8 to the cytoplasmic tail of Fas (8). Activation of caspase 8 following Fas–FasL interactions mediates the induction of the proteolytic cascade of apoptosis (9).

FLIP (FADD-like IL-1β–converting enzyme [FLICE]–inhibitory protein) (also called Casper [caspase 8–related protein], CLARP [caspase-like apoptosis-regulatory protein], FLAME-1 [FADD-like antiapoptotic molecule 1], I-FLICE [inhibitor of FLICE], CASH [caspase homolog], MRIT [MACH (MORT-associated CED-3 homolog)–related inducer of toxicity], and Usurpin), which exists as 2 splice variants, a short and a long isoform, inhibits the activation of caspase 8 (10). We recently identified FLIP to be essential for macrophage survival in culture (11). Normal macrophages express Fas and FasL, but apoptosis does not occur because of high expression of FLIP. In contrast to macrophages, peripheral blood (PB)–derived monocytes also express Fas and FasL, but lack detectable FLIP and readily undergo spontaneous apoptosis mediated by Fas–FasL interactions. Little is known about the in vivo expression of Fas, FasL, or FLIP by macrophages, including those obtained from an autoimmune disease such as RA.

Herein, we demonstrated that CD14-positive mononuclear cells (MNC) isolated from RA PB and synovial fluid (SF) express comparable levels of surface Fas and FasL, similar to normal monocytes and macrophages (11). Addition of agonistic anti-Fas antibody to cultured RA SF MNC revealed that the CD14-positive monocyte/macrophages were resistant to Fas-mediated apoptosis, while CD14-positive PB monocytes underwent cell death, suggesting that an inhibitory molecule involved in the Fas pathway is expressed in CD14-positive SF cells. In contrast, suppression of the phosphatidylinositol 3-kinase (PI 3-kinase) pathway by a pharmacologic inhibitor induced apoptosis in the CD14-positive monocyte/macrophages from both PB and SF. Flow cytometric analysis of intracellular FLIP in the CD14-positive SF monocyte/macrophages revealed a significant increase in FLIP expression compared with normal and with RA CD14-positive PB monocytes.

Analysis of RA and osteoarthritis (OA) synovial tissue demonstrated increased FLIP expression in RA synovial lining compared with OA synovial lining, which correlated with synovial lining thickening and inflammation. Furthermore, 2-color immunofluorescence showed that RA synovial lining CD68-positive macrophages were FLIP positive. Inhibition of FLIP resulted in macrophage apoptosis, which was enhanced by agonistic anti-Fas antibody, indicating that FLIP is necessary for macrophage survival. These data suggest that FLIP may be involved in preventing the removal of deleterious macrophages from the RA joint.

PATIENTS AND METHODS

Patients and cell and tissue preparation. Synovial fluid (n = 16) and synovial tissue (n = 15) were obtained at the time of arthroplasty from patients diagnosed as having RA or OA. All the patients met the American College of Rheumatology classification criteria for RA and OA, respectively (12,13). PB was obtained from 6 RA patients and 4 normal volunteer donors who were not matched for sex and age. MNC from the PB of normal subjects and RA patients and from the SF of RA patients were isolated by Histopaque (Sigma, St. Louis, MO) gradient centrifugation. All experiments on human cells and tissues were approved by the Institutional Review Board at Northwestern University.

Flow cytometric analysis. Immediately following isolation, MNC were blocked for 1 hour at room temperature in 50% human serum. Following blocking, MNC were stained with phycoerythrin (PE)–conjugated anti-CD14 (Beckman Coulter, Miami, FL) or control PE-labeled IgM (Beckman Coulter). Cells were then incubated with fluorescein isothiocyanate (FITC)–labeled $F(ab')_2$ anti-Fas antibody (clone UB2; Beckman Coulter) or with FITC-labeled $F(ab')_2$ IgG1 isotype control (Jackson ImmunoResearch, West Grove, PA). For surface FasL staining, CD14-stained RA MNC were incubated in 33% human serum/33% goat serum with either IgG rabbit anti-FasL (clone C-20; Santa Cruz Biotechnology, Santa Cruz, CA) or normal control rabbit IgG (Sigma). Cells were then incubated with FITC-labeled goat anti-rabbit antibody (Jackson ImmunoResearch).

Positive staining was determined by flow cytometry using a Beckman Coulter Epics XL flow cytometer and System 2 software, and gating on the CD14-positive population. For intracellular FLIP staining, CD14-labeled MNC were fixed in 4% neutral buffered formalin, permeabilized with 0.1% Nonidet P-40 (NP-40), blocked overnight at 4°C in 90% goat serum, and incubated at 4°C for 3–4 hours with rabbit anti-FLIP antibody (gift from Ken Walsh [11,14,15]) or control rabbit IgG (Sigma). Cells were then incubated with FITC-labeled goat anti-rabbit antibody (Jackson ImmunoResearch) at 4°C for 1–2 hours. FLIP expression was determined in the CD14-positive MNC by flow cytometry, and intracellular FLIP was quantified by the mean fluorescence intensity.

Apoptosis induction in SF macrophages. Isolated RA SF MNC were cultured in RPMI containing 20% heat-inactivated fetal bovine serum (FBS) plus 1 μg/ml of polymyxin B sulfate (Sigma) (16,17) in 24-well plates (Costar, Cambridge, MA). MNC were incubated with either agonistic anti-Fas antibody (clone CH11; Beckman Coulter), isotype control IgM (Dako, Carpinteria, CA), a PI 3-kinase inhibitor LY294002 (Sigma), or DMSO control for 24 hours. Triplicate cultures were harvested, incubated with annexin V as specified by the manufacturer (Beckman Coulter), and analyzed by flow cytometry. Prior to flow cytometric analysis for annexin V, non-treated MNC were stained with PE-labeled anti-CD14 antibody to identify the monocyte/macrophage population. Backgating on the CD14-positive population was then performed to quantitate the annexin V positivity.

Additionally, 9-day–adherent SF macrophages (<5% CD3 staining) were incubated with anti-Fas antibody or control IgM in the presence or absence of 50 n*M* bisindolylmaleimide I (GF 109203X; Sigma) for 24 hours. Cultures were then harvested by 0.02% EDTA, fixed overnight in 70% ethanol (18–20), stained with propidium iodide (Roche Molecular Biochemicals, Indianapolis, IN) (21), and the subdiploid peak, immediately adjacent to the G_0/G_1 peak (2N), was determined by flow cytometry using a Beckman Coulter Epics XL flow cytometer and System 2 software. Objects with minimal light scatter, which may represent debris, were excluded because they would have inappropriately enhanced our estimate of the subdiploid population (20).

Immunohistochemical analysis. Sections (5 μm) of synovial tissues fixed in 10% neutral buffered formalin were deparaffinized and blocked in 10% goat serum. Sections were incubated with rabbit anti-FLIP antibody (15) or normal rabbit IgG (Sigma). A biotinylated goat anti-rabbit secondary antibody (BioGenex, San Ramon, CA), followed by alkaline phosphatase (BioGenex) conjugated to streptavidin, was used to detect primary antibody complexes. Visualization was accomplished using the fast red–alkaline phosphatase substrate kit (BioGenex) and counterstained with hematoxylin.

The synovial lining thickness (median cell number), inflammation score (0–5 scale), which was estimated by the degree of sublining inflammatory cell infiltrate composed of macrophages, lymphocytes, and neutrophils, and the percentage of cells positive for FLIP were scored by a pathologist (GKH) who was blinded to the elements of the study (22–25).

Two-color immunofluorescence staining was performed with mouse anti-CD68 (Dako) and rabbit anti-FLIP antibodies or with control mouse and rabbit IgG. Slides were washed and incubated with FITC-conjugated goat anti-mouse antibody and rhodamine-conjugated donkey anti-rabbit antibody (Jackson ImmunoResearch). Nuclei were counterstained with Hoechst 33258. Slides were mounted with glass coverslips, using mounting medium for fluorescence (Kirkegaard & Perry, Gaithersburg, MD). Specimens were examined and photographed with a Nikon ES400 microscope (Nikon, Melville, NY) equipped for phase-contrast and epifluorescence visualization.

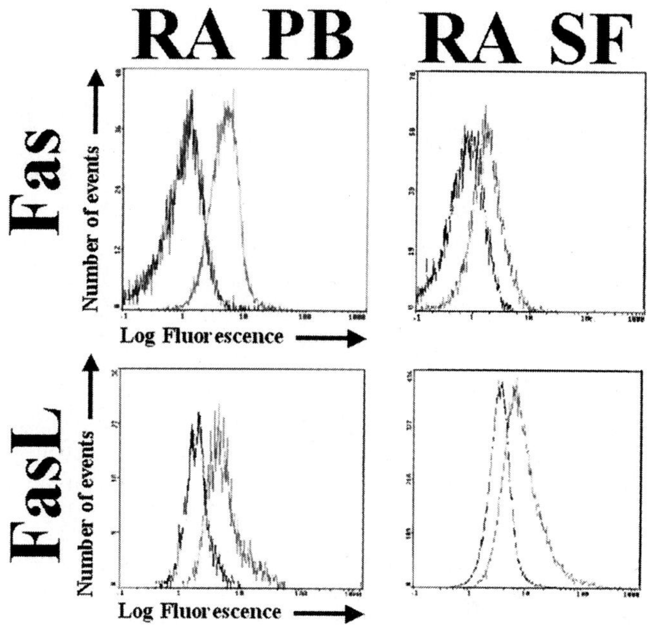

Figure 1. Expression of Fas and Fas ligand (FasL) on CD14-positive monocyte/macrophages. Rheumatoid arthritis (RA) peripheral blood (PB; n = 2) and synovial fluid (SF; n = 8) mononuclear cells (MNC) were blocked in human serum and stained with phycoerythrin-labeled anti-CD14 antibody. Cells were then stained with fluorescein isothiocyanate (FITC)–labeled anti-Fas antibody or isotype control. Additional CD14-labeled cells were stained with anti-FasL antibody or normal rabbit IgG and then with FITC-labeled goat anti-rabbit antibody. All cells were then analyzed by flow cytometry and gated for CD14 positivity. Darker lines are control Ig; lighter lines are experimental antibodies (anti-Fas, or anti-FasL).

Statistical analysis. Results are expressed as the mean plus or minus SEM. Differences between groups were analyzed using a Student's unpaired 2-tailed *t*-test. Correlations were determined by regression analysis.

RESULTS

Normal PB-derived monocytes and in vitro–differentiated macrophages express Fas and FasL (11,16,17,26). Although 1 investigation analyzed Fas and FasL messenger RNA (mRNA) expression in synovial tissue (27), no previous study has focused on the expression of surface Fas and FasL on macrophages obtained from the joints of patients with RA. Isolated MNC from RA SF and PB were analyzed for Fas and FasL expression by flow cytometry. The monocyte/macrophage population was identified by PE-labeled murine anti-CD14 antibody and by scatter properties as determined by flow

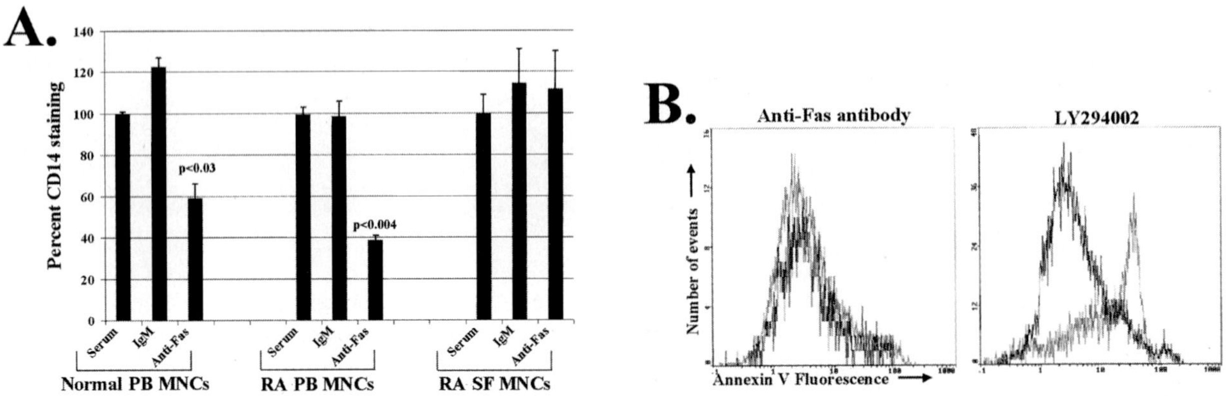

Figure 2. Fas-induced cell death of CD14-positive RA SF monocyte/macrophages. **A,** Susceptibility of normal and RA PB CD14-positive monocyte/macrophages to Fas-mediated cell death. Immediately after isolation, MNC from normal and RA PB and RA SF were cultured in duplicate for 24 hours, in the presence of serum alone or with agonistic anti-Fas antibody (1 μg/ml) or IgM control. The percentage of CD14 staining was determined as the ratio of serum-treated cultures to experimental cultures. Values are the mean and SEM of 2 independent experiments, which were compared for statistical significance by Student's unpaired 2-tailed *t*-test. $P < 0.03$ versus serum and versus IgM-treated MNC. **B,** Resistance of CD14-positive RA SF monocyte/macrophages to agonistic anti-Fas antibody. Following isolation, MNC from RA SF were cultured in triplicate for 24 hours in the presence of agonistic anti-Fas antibody (1 μg/ml), isotype control IgM, the phosphatidylinositol 3-kinase inhibitor LY294002 (50 μM), or DMSO. MNC were examined by annexin V staining to determine the amount of apoptosis and then analyzed by flow cytometry. Prior to analysis for apoptosis, the monocyte/macrophage population was predetermined by CD14 staining and scatter properties. Darker lines are control IgG or DMSO; lighter lines are anti-Fas antibody or LY294002. Histograms represent 1 of 3 replicate samples from 3 representative experiments. See Figure 1 for definitions.

cytometry. The gated CD14-positive RA SF (n = 8) and PB (n = 2) monocyte/macrophages expressed equivalent levels of Fas and FasL (Figure 1). The observed expression of Fas and FasL was similar to that in normal PB-derived monocytes and macrophages (11,16,17). These data demonstrate that the CD14-positive monocyte/macrophages from RA PB and SF express Fas and FasL.

PB monocytes undergo Fas-mediated apoptosis (11,16,17,26). Therefore, to examine the functional significance of Fas expression, MNC isolated from PB (n = 3) and SF (n = 3) were cultured for 24 hours in the presence of agonistic anti-Fas antibody or control IgM. A PI 3-kinase inhibitor, LY294002, was used as a positive control, since it was previously shown to induce macrophage apoptosis (28). Flow cytometric analysis of normal and RA PB monocytes revealed a decrease in the number of CD14-positive cells (Figure 2A) treated with anti-Fas antibody, suggesting that these cells were undergoing apoptotic cell death, as previously described (29,30). In contrast, no reduction in CD14-positive SF monocyte/macrophages was observed following incubation with anti-Fas antibody or control IgM.

To confirm that the RA SF monocyte/macrophages were viable and not undergoing apoptosis, annexin V staining was performed on anti-Fas antibody–treated MNC. Based on scatter properties and backgating on the CD14-positive cells in the anti-Fas antibody–treated or IgM-treated SF MNC, little or no annexin V staining was detected in the SF monocyte/macrophage population (Figure 2B). However, the SF monocyte/macrophages incubated with the PI 3-kinase inhibitor underwent apoptosis as compared with the control cultures (Figure 2B). These data suggest that there is an up-regulation of an inhibitory molecule that blocks the Fas death signal in RA SF monocyte/macrophages.

SF CD14-positive monocyte/macrophages expressed Fas and FasL, but were not susceptible to Fas-mediated apoptosis; therefore, studies were performed to define a potential mechanism responsible for this resistance. The expression of the antiapoptotic protein, FLIP, in the CD14-positive MNC from normal (n = 4) and RA (n = 8) PB and from RA SF (n = 10) was characterized by flow cytometry. Gated CD14-positive RA SF monocyte/macrophages displayed enhanced FLIP expression (Figure 3A) compared with CD14-positive normal and RA PB monocytes. Quantitative analysis of FLIP expression in the CD14-positive monocyte/macrophages revealed a mean ± SEM increase of 4.7 ± 0.8 fold (Figure 3B) compared with the rabbit IgG control. Staining of normal and RA CD14-positive PB monocytes showed only a 2.1 ± 0.2–fold and 2.3 ± 0.4–fold increase, respectively, compared with control rabbit IgG.

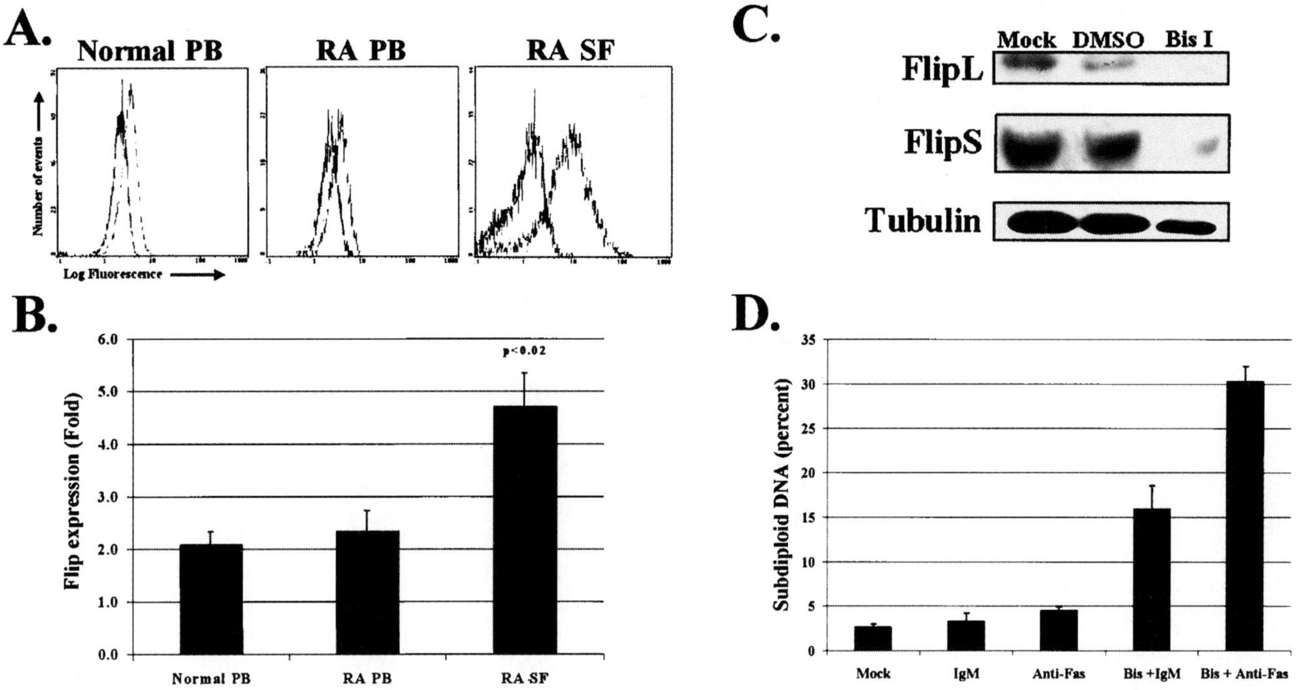

Figure 3. RA SF macrophages require FLIP (Fas-associated death domain–like interleukin-1β–converting enzyme–inhibitory protein). **A,** Intracellular FLIP expression in CD14-gated monocyte/macrophages. A representative fluorescence-activated cell sorter histogram showing control IgG (darker lines) and FLIP (lighter lines). Immediately after isolation, MNC from normal (n = 4) and RA (n = 8) PB and from RA SF (n = 10) were stained for CD14 and FLIP as described in Patients and Methods. **B,** Increased FLIP expression in SF monocyte/macrophages compared with normal and RA PB monocytes. The magnitude of increase in FLIP expression, as determined by the mean fluorescence intensity of FLIP-positive CD14-gated MNC divided by the isotype control, is shown. Values are the mean and SEM, and were compared for statistical significance by Student's unpaired 2-tailed *t*-test. $P < 0.02$ versus normal and RA PB CD14-positive MNC. **C,** Reduction of FLIP expression in macrophages by bisindolylmaleimide I (Bis I). Whole cell extracts (25 μg) were prepared from PB-derived monocyte-differentiated macrophages cultured in 20% fetal bovine serum/RPMI/1 μg/ml of polymyxin B, then treated with Bis I, DMSO, or serum only (Mock). Extracts were subjected to sodium dodecyl sulfate–polyacrylamide gel electrophoresis and probed with anti-FLIP antibody. The long (FlipL) and short (FlipS) forms are shown. **D,** FLIP inhibition and SF macrophage apoptosis. Triplicate cultures of 9-day–adherent SF macrophages were cultured for 24 hours with serum alone (mock), IgM, or anti-Fas antibody, in the presence or absence of 50 n*M* bisindolylmaleimide I (Bis) and analyzed by flow cytometry. Histograms were formed in the linear scale to identify subdiploid DNA (<2N), which is characteristic of apoptosis. Values are the mean and SEM of a representative experiment, which were compared for statistical significance by Student's unpaired 2-tailed *t*-test. See Figure 1 for other definitions.

To verify the positive FLIP expression found by flow cytometry, RT-PCR for *flip* mRNA was also performed on RA SF MNC isolated by sorting the CD14-positive cells. Both $FLIP_L$ (the long form) and $FLIP_S$ (the short form) were expressed at similar levels in the CD14-positive cells compared with the 3-day–differentiated macrophages from normal subjects (11) (data not shown). Thus, RA SF monocyte/macrophages displayed enhanced FLIP compared with normal or RA PB CD14-positive cells.

To demonstrate that FLIP is essential for SF macrophage survival, adherent SF macrophages were cultured with a selective protein kinase C (PKC) inhibitor, bisindolylmaleimide I (31), in the presence or absence of anti-Fas antibody or control IgM. Normal macrophages treated with bisindolylmaleimide I displayed a reduction in FLIP expression compared with untreated and DMSO-treated macrophages (Figure 3C). Furthermore, SF macrophages treated with bisindolylmaleimide plus IgM underwent apoptosis (mean ± SEM 16.0 ± 2.5%), which was enhanced by agonistic anti-Fas antibody (30.3 ± 1.7%) ($P < 0.01$), indicating that FLIP prevents Fas-mediated apoptosis in SF macrophages (Figure 3D).

Since FLIP was highly expressed in SF CD14-positive MNC, immunohistochemical analysis was performed to determine if FLIP is expressed in RA (n = 7) and OA (n = 8) synovial tissue. A previous investigation using rabbit anti-FLIP antibody revealed immunostaining specific for the FLIP antigen (15). Enhanced FLIP

Table 1. Correlation of FLIP expression with disease activity in RA and OA patients*

	RA patients (n = 7)	Correlation with % FLIP staining in RA				OA patients (n = 8)	Correlation with % FLIP staining in OA			
		Synovial lining		Sublining			Synovial lining		Sublining	
		r	*P*	r	*P*		r	*P*	r	*P*
Median synovial lining thickness, median cell number	2.1 ± 0.5	0.786	<0.008	0.28	NS	2.4 ± 0.2	0.003	NS	0.18	NS
Inflammation score, 0–5 scale	2.1 ± 0.4	0.64	<0.03	0.20	NS	1.7 ± 0.3	0.12	NS	0.02	NS
Vessel score, 1–4 scale	2.0 ± 0.2	0.19	NS	0.09	NS	2.2 ± 0.3	0.04	NS	0.04	NS
FLIP staining, % positive										
Synovial lining	63.6 ± 7.5	–	–	0.09	NS	9.6 ± 5.4	–	–	0.02	NS
Sublining	24.3 ± 7.1	0.41	NS	–	–	1.5 ± 0.6	0.03	NS	–	–

* Values are the mean ± SEM. *P* values were determined by regression analysis (NS = not significant). FLIP = Fas-associated death domain–like interleukin-1β–converting enzyme–inhibitory protein; RA = rheumatoid arthritis; OA = osteoarthritis.

expression was detected in RA synovial lining cells compared with OA synovial lining cells (mean ± SEM 63.6 ± 7.5% versus 9.6 ± 5.4%; $P < 0.00002$) (Table 1). Additionally, increased FLIP expression was observed in RA sublining cells compared with OA sublining cells (24.3 ± 7.1% versus 1.5 ± 0.6%; $P < 0.004$).

The percentage of FLIP-positive cells in the synovial lining correlated with the synovial lining thickness (r = 0.786, $P < 0.008$) and with the sublining inflammation score (r = 0.64, $P < 0.03$). In contrast, the percentage of FLIP-positive cells in the sublining region did not correlate significantly with the inflammation score (r = 0.20) or with the synovial lining thickness (r = 0.28). Furthermore, the percentage of FLIP-positive cells in the OA synovial lining or sublining did not correlate significantly with the lining thickness, inflammation score, or vessel score (Table 1). These observations suggest a relationship between FLIP expression and both synovial lining thickness and degree of inflammation.

Two-color immunofluorescence was utilized to identify which cell types in the synovial lining were FLIP positive; an anti-CD68 antibody was used to detect macrophages. The vast majority of CD68-positive RA synovial lining cells were FLIP positive (Figure 4B), indicating that synovial lining macrophages strongly express FLIP. However, CD68-negative/FLIP-positive cells were also detected in the lining and sublining, suggesting that a portion of synovial fibroblasts was also positive for FLIP (Figure 4B). Consistent with this possibility, immunoblot analysis of isolated RA synovial fibroblasts revealed weak FLIP expression compared with normal macrophages (results not shown). These studies support the potential role of FLIP in protecting against macrophage apoptosis mediated by Fas–FasL interactions in the rheumatoid joint.

DISCUSSION

Macrophage infiltration and activation leading to cartilage and bone destruction and enhanced cytokine production are characteristic of RA (32). One of the potential mechanisms of macrophage elimination is through the Fas–FasL pathway. Mice carrying functional mutations of Fas displayed elevated macrophage cell numbers (33) and developed autoimmune disease, supporting a role for Fas–FasL in regulating macrophage homeostasis. Numerous investigations have focused on the Fas–FasL pathway in RA synovial fibroblasts (24,34–36), but no previous report has described the expression of Fas and FasL on monocyte/macrophages obtained from the joints of RA patients.

In the present studies, we demonstrated the expression of Fas and FasL on the surfaces of normal and RA PB-derived monocytes and on monocyte/macrophages from RA SF. In contrast to normal and RA PB-derived monocytes, SF monocyte/macrophages were resistant to Fas-mediated apoptosis. Furthermore, FLIP was up-regulated in SF monocyte/macrophages compared with normal or RA PB-derived monocytes. We demonstrated that FLIP overexpression in monocytes inhibits Fas-mediated apoptosis (11), suggesting that the enhanced expression of FLIP observed in RA synovial macrophages compared with normal or RA PB monocytes may lead to their increased survival in RA. Moreover, FLIP expression was suppressed by a PKC inhibitor, which led to an increase in Fas-mediated apoptosis. The induction of PKC was shown to inhibit Fas-induced cell death through an unknown mechanism (37,38). Recently, bisindolylmaleimide inhibition of PKC ameliorated experimental arthritis through the facilitation of Fas-mediated apoptosis (39), presumably by down-regulating FLIP. A reduction in FLIP mediated by

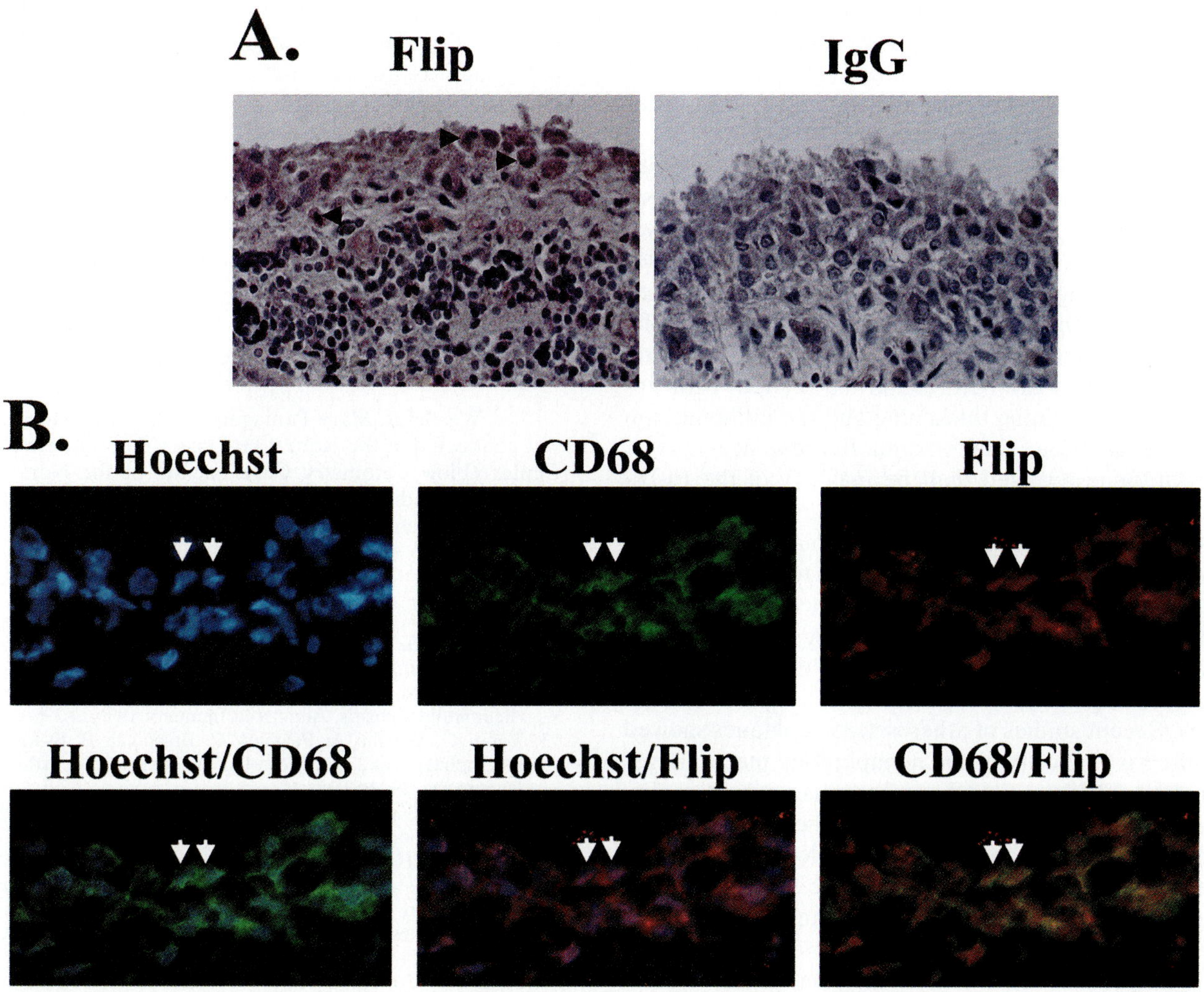

Figure 4. Expression of FLIP (Fas-associated death domain–like interleukin-1β–converting enzyme–inhibitory protein) in RA synovial tissues. **A,** Higher expression of FLIP in the synovial lining than in the sublining. Representative photomicrographs of RA synovial tissues (n = 7) were stained for FLIP (red) and counterstained with hematoxylin (blue). Sections were incubated with rabbit anti-FLIP antibody or isotype control IgG, followed by incubation with biotinylated anti-rabbit antibody. Streptavidin-conjugated alkaline phosphatase and a fast red–alkaline phosphatase substrate kit were used to visualize anti-FLIP complexes. **Arrowheads** show representative FLIP-positive cells. **B,** Predominant expression of FLIP in CD68-positive synovial lining cells. RA synovial tissue sections were analyzed by immunofluorescence following incubation with anti-FLIP and anti-CD68 antibodies. FLIP and CD68-positive complexes were identified by FITC- or rhodamine-conjugated secondary antibodies and nuclei stained with Hoechst 33258. CD68-positive, FLIP-positive, and CD68-positive/FLIP-positive cells were observed. **Arrowheads** show representative cells with colocalization of CD68 and FLIP. See Figure 1 for other definitions.

bisindolylmaleimide was confirmed in dendritic cells, allowing for the death signal induced by Fas–FasL interactions to proceed (40). Thus, the up-regulation of FLIP in synovial macrophages may lead to their enhanced survival in the RA joint.

FLIP expression in synovial macrophages may be responsible for the resistance to Fas-mediated apoptosis, as we have previously reported for normal in vitro–differentiated macrophages (11). In contrast, inhibition of the PI 3-kinase pathway resulted in macrophage apoptosis similar to that found in a previous study using peritoneal macrophages (28). These data suggest that FLIP expression has no inhibitory effect on apoptosis induced by suppression of the PI 3-kinase pathway, consistent with recent evidence that FLIP overexpression fails to prevent apoptosis induced by chemotherapeutic drugs or gamma irradiation (41). Collectively, our data (11) and those of others (42) indicate that FLIP may function to interrupt the death signal mediated by Fas–FasL ligation, while having a limited role in other apoptotic pathways.

A lack of macrophage apoptosis has been observed in the synovium of RA patients (22–25), suggesting that either enhanced expression of pro-survival proteins or a down-regulation of pro-death molecules may occur during disease progression. We demonstrated that FLIP was highly expressed in the RA synovial lining compared with the OA synovial lining. Furthermore, synovial lining FLIP expression correlated with increased synovial lining thickening and the inflammation score. In addition, dual immunofluorescence of RA synovial tissue revealed that the majority of the FLIP-positive cells were CD68-positive, suggesting that these cells were indeed macrophages. Since macrophage numbers and infiltration have been shown to correlate with articular destruction in RA (43) and since synovial lining thickness correlates with radiographic outcome (43), these data suggest that increased FLIP expression in the synovial lining may be associated with a worse outcome in RA. Recent studies of atherosclerotic plaques showed that the vast majority of the nonapoptotic macrophages expressed FLIP, while the macrophages undergoing apoptosis were FLIP negative (44). These data suggest that FLIP may be an important molecule in disease development, since macrophages are critical to the pathogenesis of both RA (43) and atherosclerosis (45–47).

Expression of FasL in the eye, testis, uterus, placenta, vessel wall, and in a number of solid tumors has raised the possibility that FasL expression renders these sites immune privileged (48,49). FLIP expression has also been localized to areas that are considered immune privileged, including the brain (50), vessel wall (14), and in solid tumors (10). These data are highlighted by the fact that tumors that overexpress FLIP in vivo displayed enhanced survival and growth (51,52), presumably through immune evasion. Thus, FLIP expression in RA monocyte/macrophages may enhance their survival by inhibiting apoptosis and subsequently increasing the numbers of RA synovial macrophages, similar to the effects of immune escape of cancer cells during tumor development (51,52). We recently demonstrated that TNFα induces FLIP expression in monocytic cells (data not shown), suggesting that the milieu of the joint may influence the survival of monocyte/macrophages.

Although the factors that regulate FLIP expression remain unidentified, it is possible that inhibition of transcription factors that are highly expressed in RA (53), such as nuclear factor κB (NF-κB) (54,55), may lead to a down-regulation of FLIP expression and subsequent increased apoptosis. This is exemplified in 2 recent studies demonstrating that inhibition of NF-κB led to increased apoptosis and amelioration of experimental arthritis (56,57). Thus, the inhibition or suppression of FLIP may lead to a decrease in macrophage number and activity, resulting in amelioration of RA.

ACKNOWLEDGMENTS

We thank Mary Paniagua for the flow cytometry that was conducted at the Robert H. Lurie Comprehensive Cancer Center (Flow Cytometry Core Facility of the Northwestern University Medical School, Chicago, IL) and Kathleen Carrigan for her technical assistance.

REFERENCES

1. Firestein GS. Invasive fibroblast-like synoviocytes in rheumatoid arthritis. Arthritis Rheum 1996;39:1781–90.
2. Feldmann M, Brennan FM, Maini RN. Role of cytokines in rheumatoid arthritis. Annu Rev Immunol 1996;14:397–440.
3. Yanni G, Whelan A, Feighery C, Bresnihan B. Synovial tissue macrophages and joint erosion in rheumatoid arthritis. Ann Rheum Dis 1994;53:39–44.
4. Peter ME, Krammer PH. Mechanisms of CD95 (APO-1/Fas)-mediated apoptosis. Curr Opin Immunol 1998;10:545–51.
5. French LE, Hahne M, Viard I, Radlgruber G, Zanone R, Becker K, et al. Fas and Fas ligand in embryos and adult mice: ligand expression in several immune-privileged tissues and coexpression in adult tissues characterized by apoptotic cell turnover. J Cell Biol 1996;133:335–43.
6. Nagata S, Golstein P. The Fas death factor. Science 1995;267:1449–56.
7. Cohen PL, Eisenberg RA. Lpr and gld: single gene models of systemic autoimmunity and lymphoproliferative disease. Annu Rev Immunol 1991;9:243–69.
8. Schulze-Osthoff K, Ferrari D, Los M, Wesselborg S, Peter ME. Apoptosis signaling by death receptors. Eur J Biochem 1998;254:439–59.
9. Thornberry NA, Lazebnik Y. Caspases: enemies within. Science 1998;281:1312–6.
10. Irmler M, Thome M, Hahne M, Schneider P, Hofmann K, Steiner V, et al. Inhibition of death receptor signals by cellular FLIP. Nature 1997;388:190–5.
11. Perlman H, Pagliari LJ, Georganas C, Mano T, Walsh K, Pope RM. FLICE inhibitory protein expression during macrophage differentiation confers resistance to Fas-mediated apoptosis. J Exp Med 1999;190:1679–88.
12. Arnett FC, Edworthy SM, Bloch DA, McShane DJ, Fries JF, Cooper NS, et al. The American Rheumatism Association 1987 revised criteria for the classification of rheumatoid arthritis. Arthritis Rheum 1988;31:315–24.
13. Altman R, Alarcón G, Appelrouth D, Bloch D, Borenstein D, Brandt K, et al. The American College of Rheumatology criteria for the classification and reporting of osteoarthritis of the hip. Arthritis Rheum 1991;34:505–14.
14. Sata M, Walsh K. Endothelial cell apoptosis induced by oxidized

LDL is associated with the down-regulation of the cellular caspase inhibitor FLIP. J Biol Chem 1998;273:33103–6.
15. Cheema ZF, Wade SB, Sata M, Walsh K, Sohrabji F, Miranda RC. Fas/Apo [apoptosis]-1 and associated proteins in the differentiating cerebral cortex: induction of caspase-dependent cell death and activation of NF-κB. J Neurosci 1999;19:1754–70.
16. Kiener PA, Davis PM, Starling GC, Mehlin C, Klebanoff SJ, Ledbetter JA, et al. Differential induction of apoptosis by Fas-Fas ligand interactions in human monocytes and macrophages. J Exp Med 1997;185:1511–6.
17. Kiener PA, Davis PM, Rankin BM, Klebanoff SJ, Ledbetter JA, Starling GC, et al. Human monocytic cells contain high levels of intracellular Fas ligand: rapid release following cellular activation. J Immunol 1997;159:1594–8.
18. Telford WG, King LE, Fraker PJ. Comparative evaluation of several DNA binding dyes in the detection of apoptosis-associated chromatin degradation by flow cytometry. Cytometry 1992;13: 137–43.
19. Fraker PJ, King LE, Lill-Elghanian D, Telford WG. Quantification of apoptotic events in pure and heterogeneous populations of cells using the flow cytometer. Methods Cell Biol 1995;46:57–76.
20. Darzynkiewicz Z, Juan G, Li X, Gorczyca W, Murakami T, Traganos F. Cytometry in cell necrobiology: analysis of apoptosis and accidental cell death (necrosis). Cytometry 1997;27:1–20.
21. Perlman H, Sata M, Le Roux A, Sedlak T, Branellec D, Walsh K. Bax-mediated cell death by the Gax homeoprotein requires mitogen-activation but is independent of cell cycle activity. EMBO J 1998:17:3576–86.
22. Ceponis A, Hietanen J, Tamulaitiene M, Partsch G, Patiala H, Konttinen YT. A comparative quantitative morphometric study of cell apoptosis in synovial membranes in psoriatic, reactive and rheumatoid arthritis. Rheumatology (Oxford) 1999;38:431–40.
23. Sugiyama M, Tsukazaki T, Yonekura A, Matsuzaki S, Yamashita S, Iwasaki K. Localization of apoptosis and expression of apoptosis related proteins in the synovium of patients with rheumatoid arthritis. Ann Rheum Dis 1995;55:442–9.
24. Nakajima T, Aono H, Hasunuma T, Yamamoto K, Shirai T, Hirohata K, et al. Apoptosis and functional Fas antigen in rheumatoid arthritis synoviocytes. Arthritis Rheum 1995;38: 485–91.
25. Matsumoto S, Muller-Ladner U, Gay RE, Nishioka K, Gay S. Ultrastructural demonstration of apoptosis, Fas and Bcl-2 expression of rheumatoid synovial fibroblasts. J Rheum 1996;23:1345–52.
26. Brown SB, Savill J. Phagocytosis triggers macrophage release of Fas ligand and induces apoptosis in bystander leukocytes. J Immunol 1999;162:480–5.
27. Asahara H, Hasunuma T, Kobata T, Inoue H, Muller-Ladner U, Gay S, et al. In situ expression of protooncogenes and Fas/Fas ligand in rheumatoid arthritis synovium. J Rheumatol 1997;24:430–5.
28. Koh JS, Lieberthal W, Heydrick S, Levine JS. Lysophosphatidic acid is a major serum noncytokine survival factor for murine macrophages which acts via the phosphatidylinositol 3-kinase signaling pathway. J Clin Invest 1998;102:716–27.
29. Heidenreich S, Schmidt M, August C, Cullen P, Rademaekers A, Pauels H-G. Regulation of human monocyte apoptosis by the CD14 molecule. J Immunol 1997;159:3178–88.
30. Heidenreich S. Monocyte CD14: a multifunctional receptor engaged in apoptosis from both sides. J Leukoc Biol 1999;65:737–43.
31. Toullec D, Pianetti P, Coste H, Bellevergue P, Grand-Perret T, Ajakane M, et al. The bisindolylmaleimide GF 109203X is a potent and selective inhibitor of protein kinase C. J Biol Chem 1991;266: 15771–81.
32. Van den Berg WB, van Lent PLEM. The role of macrophages in chronic arthritis. Immunobiol 1996;195:614–23.
33. Dang-Vu AP, Pisetsky DS, Weinberg JB. Functional alterations of macrophages in autoimmune MRL-lpr/lpr mice. J Immunol 1987; 138:1757–61.
34. Wakisaka S, Suzuki N, Takeba Y, Shimoyama Y, Nagafuchi H, Takeno M, et al. Modulation by proinflammatory cytokines of Fas/Fas ligand-mediated apoptotic cell death of synovial cells in patients with rheumatoid arthritis. Clin Exp Immunol 1998;114: 119–28.
35. Kawakami A, Eguchi K, Matsuoka N, Tsuboi M, Kawabe Y, Aoyagi T, et al. Inhibition of Fas antigen–mediated apoptosis of rheumatoid synovial cells in vitro by transforming growth factor β1. Arthritis Rheum 1996;39:1267–76.
36. Hashimoto H, Tanaka M, Suda T, Tomita T, Hayashida K, Takeuchi E, et al. Soluble Fas ligand in the joints of patients with rheumatoid arthritis and osteoarthritis. Arthritis Rheum 1998;41: 657–62.
37. Gomez-Angelats M, Bortner CD, Cidlowski JA. Protein kinase C (PKC) inhibits Fas receptor-induced apoptosis through modulation of the loss of K+ and cell shrinkage: a role for PKC upstream of Caspases. J Biol Chem 2000;275:19609–19.
38. Ruiz-Ruiz MC, Izquierdo M, de Murcia G, Lopez-Rivas A. Activation of protein kinase C attenuates early signals in Fas-mediated apoptosis. Eur J Immunol 1997;27:1442–50.
39. Zhou T, Song L, Yang P, Wang Z, Lui D, Jope RS. Bisindolylmaleimide VIII facilitates Fas-mediated apoptosis and inhibits T cell-mediated autoimmune diseases. Nat Med 1999;5:42–8.
40. Willems F, Amraoui Z, Vanderheyde N, Verhasselt V, Aksoy E, Scaffidi C, et al. Expression of c-FLIP(L) and resistance to CD95-mediated apoptosis of monocyte-derived dendritic cells: inhibition by bisindolylmaleimide. Blood 2000;95:3478–82.
41. Kataoka T, Schroter M, Hahne M, Schneider P, Irmler M, Thome M, et al. FLIP prevents apoptosis induced by death receptors but not by perforin/granzyme B, chemotherapeutic drugs, and gamma irradiation. J Immunol 1998;161:3936–42.
42. Tschopp J, Irmler M, Thome M. Inhibition of Fas death signals by FLIPs. Curr Opin Immunol 1998;10:552–8.
43. Mulherin D, FitzGerald O, Bresnihan B. Synovial tissue macrophage populations and articular damage in rheumatoid arthritis. Arthritis Rheum 1996;39:115–24.
44. Imanishi T, McBride J, Ho Q, O'Brien KD, Schwartz SM, Han DK. Expression of cellular FLICE-inhibitory protein in human coronary arteries and in a rat vascular injury model. Am J Pathol 2000;156:125–37.
45. Smith JD, Trogan E, Ginsberg M, Grigaux C, Tian J, Miyata M. Decreased atherosclerosis in mice deficient in both macrophage colony-stimulating factor (op) and apolipoprotein E. Proc Natl Acad Sci U S A 1995;92:8264–8.
46. Gu L, Okada Y, Clinton SK, Gerard C, Sukhova GK, Libby P, et al. Absence of monocyte chemoattractant protein-1 reduces atherosclerosis in low density lipoprotein receptor-deficient mice. Mol Cell 1998;2:275–81.
47. Gosling J, Slaymaker S, Gu L, Tseng S, Zlot CH, Young SG, et al. MCP-1 deficiency reduces susceptibility to atherosclerosis in mice that overexpress human apolipoprotein B. J Clin Invest 1999;103: 773–8.
48. Walker PR, Saas P, Dietrich PY. Tumor expression of Fas ligand (CD95L) and the consequences. Curr Opin Immunol 1998;10: 564–72.
49. Sata M, Walsh M. TNFα regulation of Fas ligand expression on vascular endothelium modulates leukocyte extravasation. Nature Med 1998;4:415–20.
50. Raoul C, Henderson CE, Pettmann B. Programmed cell death of embryonic motor neurons triggered through the fas death receptor. J Cell Biol 1999;147:1049–62.
51. Medema JP, de Jong J, van Hall T, Melief CJ, Offringa R. Immune escape of tumors in vivo by expression of cellular FLICE-inhibitory protein. J Exp Med 1999;190:1033–8.
52. Djerbi M, Screpanti V, Catrina AI, Bogen B, Biberfeld P, Gran-

dien A. The inhibitor of death receptor signaling, FLICE-inhibitory protein defines a new class of tumor progression factors. J Exp Med 1999;190:1025–32.
53. Roivainen A, Soderstrom KO, Pirila L, Aro H, Kortekangas P, Merilahti-Palo R, et al. Oncoprotein expression in human synovial tissue: an immunohistochemical study of different types of arthritis. Br J Rheumatol 1996;35:933–42.
54. Marok R, Winyard PG, Coumbe A, Kus ML, Gaffney K, Blades S, et al. Activation of the transcription factor nuclear factor–κB in human inflamed synovial tissue. Arthritis Rheum 1996;39: 583–91.
55. Handel ML, McMorrow LB, Gravallese EM. Nuclear factor–κB in rheumatoid synovium. Arthritis Rheum 1995;38:1762–70.
56. Tomita T, Takeuchi E, Tomita N, Morishita R, Kaneko M, Yamamoto K, et al. Suppressed severity of collagen-induced arthritis by in vivo transfection of nuclear factor κB decoy oligodeoxynucleotides as a gene therapy. Arthritis Rheum 1999;42: 2532–42.
57. Miagkov AV, Kovalenko DV, Brown CE, Didsbury JR, Cogswell JP, Stimpson SA, et al. NF-κB activation provides the potential link between inflammation and hyperplasia in the arthritic joint. Proc Natl Acad Sci U S A 1998;95:13859–64.

ARTHRITIS & RHEUMATISM
Vol. 44, No. 1, January 2001, pp 31–40

Regulation of Angiogenesis by the C-X-C Chemokines Interleukin-8 and Epithelial Neutrophil Activating Peptide 78 in the Rheumatoid Joint

Alisa E. Koch,[1] Michael V. Volin,[2] James M. Woods,[2] Steven L. Kunkel,[3] Matthew A. Connors,[2] Lisa A. Harlow,[2] Drew C. Woodruff,[2] Marie D. Burdick,[4] and Robert M. Strieter[4]

Objective. **Angiogenesis, the growth of new blood vessels, is vital to the ingress of inflammatory leukocytes in rheumatoid arthritis (RA) synovial tissue and to the growth and proliferation of RA pannus. The factors that mediate the growth of new blood vessels have not been completely defined. This study examined the ability of Glu-Leu-Arg (ELR)–containing chemokines to induce angiogenesis in the RA joint.**

Methods. **To reflect angiogenic activity in vivo, we selected a model using whole human synovial tissue rather than isolated cells. Tissues were examined by immunohistochemistry and enzyme-linked immunosorbent assay, and tissue homogenates were immunoneutralized and assayed for their ability to induce endothelial cell chemotaxis and rat corneal neovascularization.**

Results. **Cells expressing interleukin-8 (IL-8) and epithelial neutrophil activating peptide 78 (ENA-78) were located in proximity to factor VIII–related antigen–immunopositive endothelial cells. RA homogenates produced more IL-8 and ENA-78 compared with normal synovial tissue homogenates. Moreover, homogenates from RA synovial tissue produced significantly more chemotactic activity for endothelial cells in vitro and angiogenic activity in the rat cornea in vivo than did normal synovial tissue homogenates. The effects of IL-8 and ENA-78 accounted for a significant proportion of the chemotactic activity of endothelial cells and angiogenic activity found in RA synovial tissue homogenates.**

Conclusion. **These results indicate that the ELR-containing chemokines IL-8 and ENA-78 are important contributors to the angiogenic activity found in the inflamed RA joint. It is possible that efforts aimed at down-regulating these chemokines offer a novel targeted therapy for the treatment of RA.**

Rheumatoid arthritis (RA) is a chronic inflammatory disorder characterized by the infiltration of monocytes/macrophages, lymphocytes, and inflammatory cells into the hypertrophic synovial tissue (1–4). Interspersed in this chronic inflammatory infiltrate are a myriad of new blood vessels, the formation of which is termed angiogenesis. The growth of new synovial blood vessels is important in the pathogenesis of RA, primarily for two reasons: 1) the growth of new blood vessels facilitates the ingress of inflammatory leukocytes into the synovial tissue, and 2) the fibroproliferative state of the synovium culminates in synovial invasion of bone and cartilage, which characterizes RA (4,5).

There are a number of proangiogenic cytokines, growth factors, and adhesion molecules that may participate in the angiogenic activity found in the RA joint. These include vascular endothelial growth factor (VEGF), tumor necrosis factor α (TNFα), hepatocyte

Dr. Koch's work was supported by NIH grants AR-41492 and AI-40987, funds from the Veterans Administration Research Service, a grant from the American Heart Association, and funds from the Gallagher Research Professorship of Medicine. Dr. Kunkel's work was supported by NIH grant HL-46487. Dr. Strieter's work was supported by NIH grants HL-02401, HL-50057, CA-87879, and HL-66027.

[1]Alisa E. Koch, MD: Northwestern University Medical School and Veterans Administration Chicago Health Care System, Lakeside Division, Chicago, Illinois; [2]Michael V. Volin, PhD, James M. Woods, PhD, Matthew A. Connors, Lisa A. Harlow, MS, Drew C. Woodruff: Northwestern University Medical School, Chicago, Illinois; [3]Steven L. Kunkel, PhD: University of Michigan Medical School, Ann Arbor; [4]Marie D. Burdick, MS, Robert M. Strieter, MD: University of California at Los Angeles School of Medicine.

Address correspondence and reprint requests to Alisa E. Koch, MD, Gallagher Research Professor of Medicine, Northwestern University Medical School, Department of Medicine, Rheumatology Section, 303 East Chicago Avenue, Ward 3-315, Chicago, IL 60611.

Submitted for publication March 13, 2000; accepted in revised form August 21, 2000.

growth factor (HGF), platelet-derived growth factor, soluble vascular cell adhesion molecule 1 (sVCAM-1), and soluble E-selectin (sE-selectin) (6–19). Among the most potent angiogenic factors that may be involved in rheumatoid synovitis are the C-X-C chemokines.

The C-X-C chemokine family, so named for containing the first two cysteines separated by a nonconserved amino acid residue, is composed of a number of polypeptides with molecular weights of ~10 kd. These chemokines have been associated with mediating recruitment of polymorphonuclear neutrophils (PMNs). The C-X-C motif distinguishes this family from the C-C chemokines. The NH_2 terminus of the majority of the C-X-C chemokines contains the ELR motif (Glu-Leu-Arg), which confers the ability of these chemokines to bind and activate PMNs as well as to mediate angiogenesis (20–22). We have shown previously that interleukin-8 (IL-8) is up-regulated in RA compared with osteoarthritis synovial fluid, and that RA synovial tissue macrophages are potent producers of this angiogenic chemokine (9,23). We have also shown that the related ELR-containing C-X-C chemokines, epithelial neutrophil activating peptide 78 (ENA-78) and IL-8, contribute to the chemotactic activity of neutrophils found in the RA joint (24). To address the relative importance of the C-X-C chemokines in inducing angiogenesis in the RA synovium, we utilized a model of whole synovial tissue extracts. In this report, we demonstrate that IL-8 and ENA-78 are potent angiogenic factors in the RA synovium.

PATIENTS AND METHODS

Patient population. Synovial tissue was obtained from patients (70% female, 30% male) who were undergoing total joint replacement and who met the American College of Rheumatology (formerly, the American Rheumatism Association) criteria for RA (25). Sixteen of the 20 RA patients for whom additional data were obtained ranged in age from 21 years to 81 years, with a mean age of 56 years. While the majority of tissue was obtained from knee replacements (53%), tissue from hip (27%), hand (13%), and elbow (7%) surgeries was also included. Normal synovial tissue was obtained fresh from patients at the time of amputation for diabetes or other etiologies. These subjects were 78% female and 22% male and ranged in age from 41 years to 76 years, with a mean age of 66 years. All normal synovia were obtained from the knee. All procedures involving patients were performed with Institutional Review Board approval.

Reagents. Polyclonal anti-human IL-8 and anti–ENA-78 were produced by the immunization of rabbits with their respective recombinant proteins (R&D Systems, Minneapolis, MN) in multiple intradermal sites, with Freund's complete adjuvant (23,24,26). The specificity of each of these antibodies was assessed by Western blot analysis against a panel of other human recombinant cytokines. The antibodies were specific, without cross-reactivity to a panel of human interleukins including the IL-1 receptor antagonist protein, IL-1, IL-2, IL-4, IL-6, TNFα, interferon-γ, and other members of the C-X-C and C-C chemokine families. The anti–IL-8, anti–ENA-78, and anti-VEGF antibodies used to neutralize RA homogenates, as depicted in Figure 5, were purchased from R&D Systems. Control IgG antibody was purchased from Coulter (Hialeah, FL).

Antibodies used for dual fluorescence staining included mouse anti-human CD68 (Signet, Dedham, MA), mouse anti-human ENA-78 (R&D Systems), rhodamine isothiocyanate (RITC)–conjugated goat anti-mouse IgG (Jackson ImmunoResearch, West Grove, PA), fluorescein isothiocyanate (FITC)–conjugated anti-CD14 (BD-PharMingen, San Diego, CA), rabbit anti-human IL-8 (prepared as described above), RITC-conjugated goat anti-rabbit IgG (Jackson ImmunoResearch), FITC-conjugated donkey anti-mouse IgG (Jackson ImmunoResearch), and FITC-conjugated mouse anti-human proliferating cell nuclear antigen (PCNA; BD-PharMingen). The "anti-protease" buffer for tissue homogenization consisted of phosphate buffered saline (PBS) containing pronase (0.005 mg/ml), thermolysin (0.0005 mg/ml), pancrease extract (0.02 mg/ml), chymotrypsin (0.0015 mg/ml), and papain (0.33 mg/ml) (Complete; Boehringer Mannheim, Indianapolis, IN). Anti–factor VIII–related antigen was purchased from Dakopatts (Carpinteria, CA). Basic fibroblast growth factor (bFGF) was purchased from R&D Systems.

Synovial tissue homogenization. Synovial tissue specimens were homogenized in 1 ml of an "anti-protease" buffer as described (27). Samples were sonicated, centrifuged at 900*g* for 15 minutes, and filtered through a 1.2-μm pore size Sterile Acrodisk (Gelman Sciences, Ann Arbor, MI), and frozen at −70°C until thawed for assay. The specimens were lyophilized (SpeedVac; Savant, Farmingdale, NY), normalized to an equal amount of total protein, and used for chemotaxis assays for human dermal microvascular endothelial cells (HMVECs), or in the corneal bioassay for angiogenesis.

Enzyme-linked immunosorbent assay (ELISA) for chemokines. Homogenates were assayed for the chemokines IL-8 and ENA-78 using commercially available ELISA systems purchased from R&D Systems. Alternatively, ELISAs were performed as detailed previously (23,28). After assay, the samples whose values fell in the detectable range of the assay were normalized for total protein and the results expressed as pg/mg protein. All assays were specific for reactivity with their respective recombinant proteins.

Chemotaxis of HMVECs. HMVECs were purchased from BioWhittaker (Charlotte, NC). HMVEC chemotaxis was performed in 48-well blind-well chemotaxis chambers with polycarbonate membranes of 8-μm pore size (Neuroprobe, Cabinjohn, MD) (26). HMVECs (2.5×10^4 cells/well) in 25 μl RPMI media plus 0.1% fetal calf serum were added to the bottom wells of the chambers. Inverted chambers were incubated at 37°C for 2 hours, allowing endothelial cell attachment. Test substances were added to the top half of the reinverted chambers. Synovial tissue homogenates from 6 patients with RA and 6 normal controls were adjusted for total protein. RA as well as normal samples were pooled. In some cases, homogenates were incubated with a 1:500 dilution of either anti–IL-8 or anti–ENA-78 for 1 hour at 37°C. Alternatively, RA tissue homogenates were incubated with normal rabbit serum (1:500). In the experiments represented in Figure 5, RA homogenates were incubated with 10 μg/ml anti–IL-8, anti–ENA-78, anti-VEGF, or an equivalent concentration of isotype control antibody for 1 hour at 37°C. Controls for the chemotaxis assay included bFGF (60 n*M*) and PBS. Chemotaxis chambers were incubated for 2 hours, and the membranes were removed, fixed in methanol, and stained with Diff-Quik (Baxter Diagnostics, Chicago, IL). Each test group was assayed in quadruplicate. Three high-power microscope fields were counted in each replicate well, and results were expressed as cells per well.

Rat corneal assay for neovascularization. Angiogenic activity of pooled RA or normal synovial tissue homogenates was assayed in vivo in the avascular cornea of hooded Long-Evans rat eyes, as previously described (9,27). In brief, 1 μl of synovial tissue homogenate was combined with 4 μl of Hydron (Interferon Sciences, New Brunswick, NJ). The 5-μl pellets were allowed to polymerize and were then implanted in the normally avascular cornea of the rat at a distance of several millimeters from the limbus. Corneas were examined daily, and a permanent record was obtained by perfusion with colloidal carbon 6 days after implantation. No inflammatory response was observed in the corneas when data were obtained in this manner. Positive neovascular responses were recorded only if sustained directional growth of capillary sprouts and hairpin loops toward the implant were observed. Negative responses were recorded when either no growth was observed or only an occasional sprout or hairpin loop displaying no evidence of sustained growth was detected. All animal studies were performed with institutional Animal Care and Use Committee approval.

Immunoperoxidase staining. Fresh synovial tissues were frozen and 4-μm sections were cut and immunoperoxidase stained using an avidin–biotin technique (Vector Laboratories, Burlingame, CA) (29–32). Slides, air dried for 2–16 hours, were fixed in cold acetone for 20 minutes. All subsequent incubations were performed for 15 minutes at 37°C in a moist chamber. Synovial tissues were pretreated with 50 μl of diluted normal horse serum (150 μl of horse serum in 10 ml of PBS) and then incubated with antibodies, isotype-matched control monoclonal antibodies, or normal rabbit serum. Slides were washed twice and then incubated with a 1:400 dilution of anti-rabbit or anti-mouse biotinylated antibody in PBS, washed twice in PBS, and incubated with avidin-conjugated horseradish peroxidase complex. Slides were washed twice and then stained with diaminobenzidine tetrahydrochloride substrate for 5 minutes at room temperature, rinsed in tap water for 2 minutes, counterstained with Harris' hematoxylin, and dipped in saturated lithium carbonate solution for blue staining. Serial tissue sections were examined and cell types identified by morphology.

Dual immunofluorescence staining. RA synovial tissue sections were fixed in cold acetone for 20 minutes, blocked with 5% goat serum for 1 hour at room temperature, and incubated with primary antibodies overnight at 4°C. Antibodies included 1) rabbit anti-human IL-8 and mouse anti-human CD68 as primary antibodies, followed by RITC-conjugated goat anti-rabbit IgG and FITC-conjugated donkey anti-mouse IgG, 2) mouse anti-human ENA-78 and FITC-conjugated anti-human CD14 as primary antibodies, followed by RITC-conjugated goat anti-mouse IgG, or 3) rabbit anti-human IL-8 and FITC-conjugated mouse anti-human PCNA as primary antibodies, followed by RITC-conjugated goat anti-rabbit IgG. After 3 washes in PBS, secondary antibodies as described above were added for 45 minutes at room temperature in the dark. Immunofluorescence mounting media (Kirkegaard & Perry, Gaithersburg, MD) was used to mount slides after several additional washes.

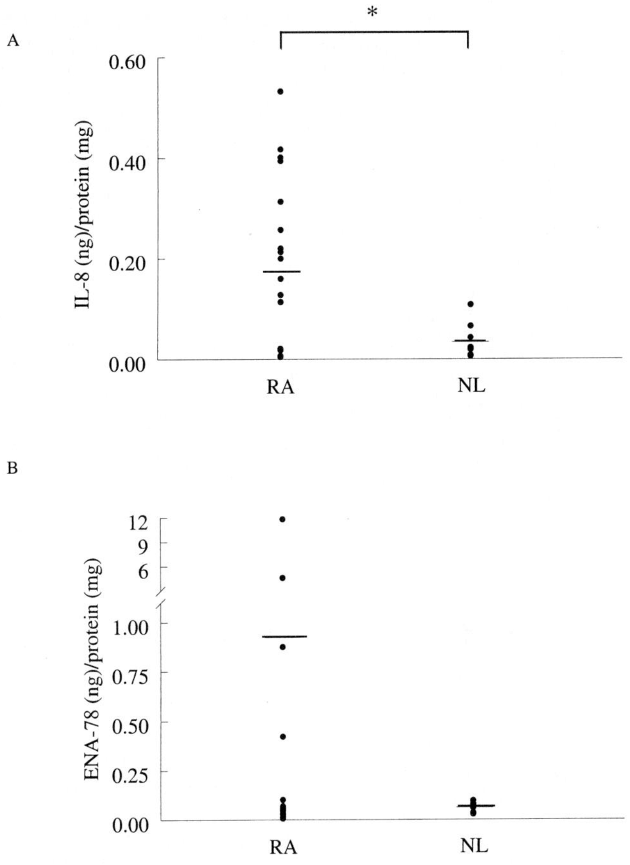

Figure 1. Enzyme-linked immunosorbent assays of rheumatoid arthritis (RA) and normal (NL) synovial tissue homogenates for interleukin-8 (IL-8) (**A**) and epithelial neutrophil activating peptide 78 (ENA-78) (**B**). Solid circles indicate individual values and the horizontal line indicates the mean. Results for samples falling within the detectable assay range were normalized for total protein. * = $P < 0.05$.

Statistical analysis. Statistical analysis was performed using Student's unpaired *t*-test. *P* values of less than 0.05 were considered significant.

RESULTS

Levels of angiogenic chemokines in RA and normal synovial tissue homogenates. Synovial tissue was obtained from RA patients and normal patients and homogenized in 1 ml "anti-protease" buffer. These

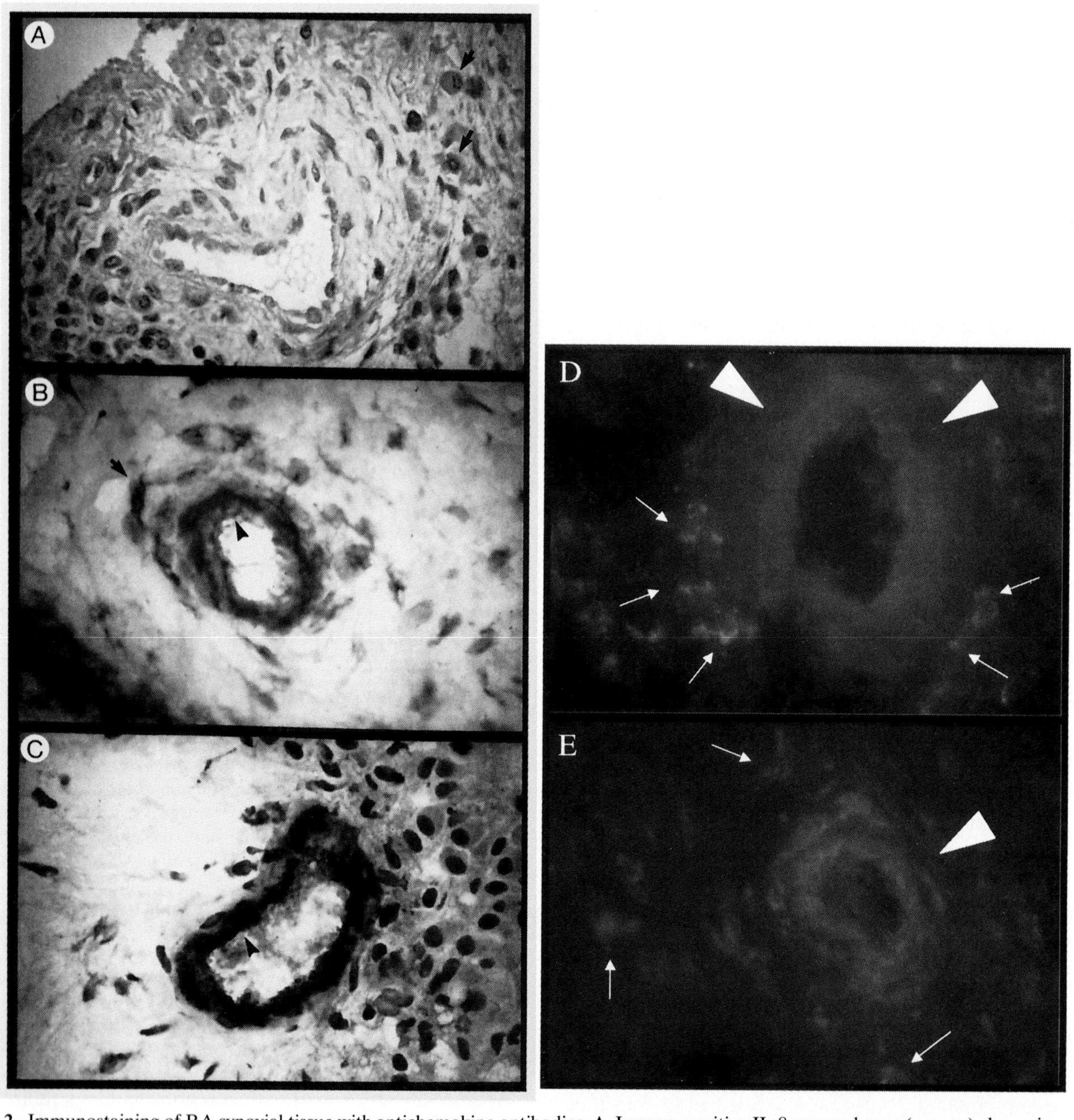

Figure 2. Immunostaining of RA synovial tissue with antichemokine antibodies. **A,** Immunopositive IL-8 macrophages **(arrows)** shown in proximity to a blood vessel. **B,** ENA-78–immunopositive macrophages **(arrow)** shown adjacent to an ENA-78–immunopositive blood vessel **(arrowhead). C,** Factor VIII–related antigen–immunopositive blood vessel in RA synovial tissue **(arrowhead). D,** Yellow staining **(arrows)** represents dual-colored ENA-78–positive (rhodamine isothiocyanate–conjugated [RITC]; red stained) and CD14-positive (fluorescein isothiocyanate–conjugated [FITC]; green stained) macrophages. **Arrowheads** indicate the close proximity of the ENA-78–producing macrophages to a blood vessel. **E,** IL-8 production **(arrows)** (RITC; red stained) adjacent to a blood vessel **(arrowhead),** where component cells are undergoing proliferation. The yellow color of the blood vessel indicates the dual staining of IL-8 (red stained) and proliferating cell nuclear antigen (FITC; green stained). (Original magnification × 576 in **A**, **B**, and **C**; × 457 in **D** and **E**.) See Figure 1 for other definitions.

homogenates were then assayed for the presence of chemokines using ELISA systems. Samples falling within the detectable range of the assay were normalized for total protein (Figure 1). The mean level of IL-8 in the homogenates was greater in RA compared with normal tissue homogenates ($P < 0.05$) (Figure 1A).

RA samples contained a mean (±SEM) of 0.173 ± 0.037 ng IL-8/mg protein compared with 0.033 ± 0.011 ng IL-8/mg protein in normal subjects. Likewise, mean ENA-78 levels in RA synovial tissue homogenates were higher than those found in normal synovial tissue homogenates (0.921 ± 0.617 ng/mg protein for RA compared with 0.055 ± 0.008 ng/mg protein for normal subjects) (Figure 1B). The RA values shown in Figure 1B were not normally distributed, as determined by a Shapiro-Wilk test of normality. Despite the difference in mean values, nonparametric analysis using a Wilcoxon rank sum test did not detect a significant difference between the groups.

Identification of cells immunopositive for angiogenic chemokines adjacent to blood vessels. We hypothesized that the angiogenic chemokines IL-8 and ENA-78 might be produced in vivo in areas adjacent to endothelial cells. To localize these chemokines, we utilized immunohistochemistry using anti–IL-8 and anti–ENA-78. The results are shown in Figure 2. Figure 2A shows a rheumatoid synovial biopsy specimen immunostained for IL-8. IL-8 immunoreactivity was present in the macrophages, as indicated by the arrows. Figure 2B shows ENA-78–immunopositive cells similarly located adjacent to blood vessels, with evidence of ENA-78–immunopositive vascular smooth muscle cells and endothelial cells (indicated by the arrowhead) and adjacent immunopositive macrophages (indicated by the arrow). Also of note is the presence of ENA-78–positive endothelial and smooth muscle cells.

Figure 2C shows vascular immunoreactivity with the endothelial marker, factor VIII–related antigen (indicated by the arrowhead). Figure 2D shows dual-labeled (stained yellow) macrophages that were CD14 positive and were producing ENA-78 in close proximity to a blood vessel. Similarly, we have seen dual staining of CD68-positive macrophages for IL-8 adjacent to blood vessels (results not shown), likewise indicating that chemokine-producing macrophages are prominent near blood vessels. Figure 2E shows that IL-8–positive cells (RITC-conjugated and stained red) were located near the blood vessels, where cells were undergoing proliferation. Since IL-8 can be produced by endothelial cells (33,34), the blood vessels appear yellow, indicating dual staining of IL-8 and PCNA. PCNA is a subunit of DNA polymerase delta, which is associated with DNA replication. Thus, chemokine-immunopositive cells were often located in the inflamed synovial tissues in close proximity to blood vessels.

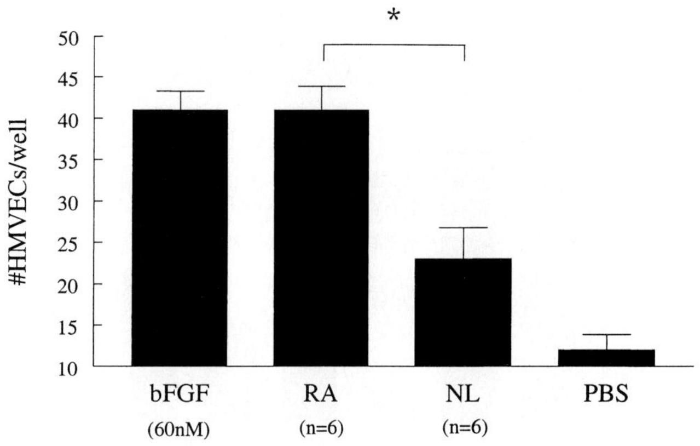

Figure 3. Human dermal microvascular endothelial cell (HMVEC) chemotaxis in response to rheumatoid arthritis (RA) compared with normal (NL) synovial tissue homogenates. Twelve high-power fields were assayed per sample and the results expressed as number of cells migrated per well. Bars show the mean and SEM of 4 separate experiments using homogenates from 6 patients with RA and 6 NL patients. * = $P < 0.05$. bFGF = basic fibroblast growth factor; PBS = phosphate buffered saline.

Chemotactic activity of HMVECs in RA synovial homogenates. Since one of the hallmarks of RA synovial tissue is its increased vascularity compared with that in normal synovial tissue, we next determined whether synovial tissue homogenates from RA patients contained more angiogenic activity than did normal synovial tissue homogenates. Synovial tissue homogenates from RA and normal patients were assayed for chemotactic activity of HMVECs, as shown in Figure 3. RA tissue possessed almost double the chemotactic activity in endothelial cells than did normal synovial tissue ($P < 0.05$).

Effects of immunodepletion of chemokines IL-8 or ENA-78 on the chemotactic activity of endothelial cells in RA homogenates. To determine whether the increased chemotactic activity of endothelial cells found in RA synovial tissue homogenate was due to the angiogenic chemokines, immunodepletion experiments were performed. RA synovial tissue homogenates were incubated with an antibody excess of anti–IL-8 or anti–ENA-78. Alternatively, RA synovial tissue homogenates were incubated with normal rabbit serum. Chemotaxis assays were performed and the results are shown in Figure 4 and Table 1. Incubation of RA homogenates with anti–IL-8 resulted in a 42% decrease in the chemotactic activity of HMVECs ($P < 0.05$). Similarly, incubation with anti–ENA-78 resulted in a 44% decrease in chemotactic activity ($P < 0.05$). The results presented represent 1 of 4 separate experiments.

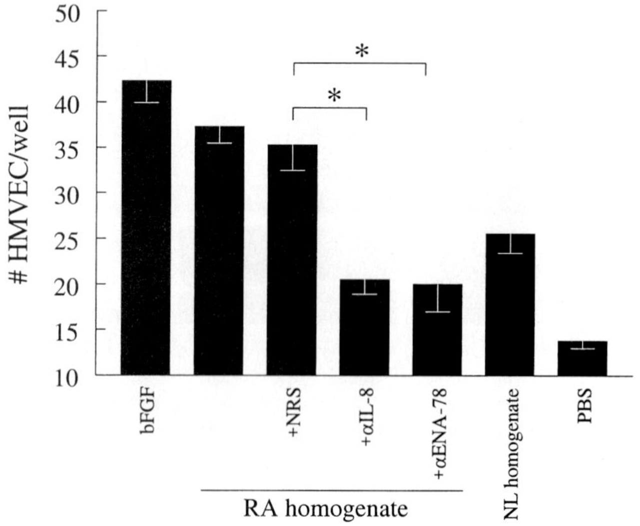

Figure 4. HMVEC chemotaxis in response to RA synovial tissue homogenates in the presence or absence of immunodepletion of IL-8 or ENA-78. Bars show the mean and SEM of each assay well. Twelve high-power fields were assayed per sample and the results expressed as the number of cells migrated per well. Results represent 1 of 4 experiments using synovial tissue from 6 patients with RA and 6 NL controls. * = $P < 0.05$. NRS = normal rabbit serum (see Figures 1 and 3 for other definitions).

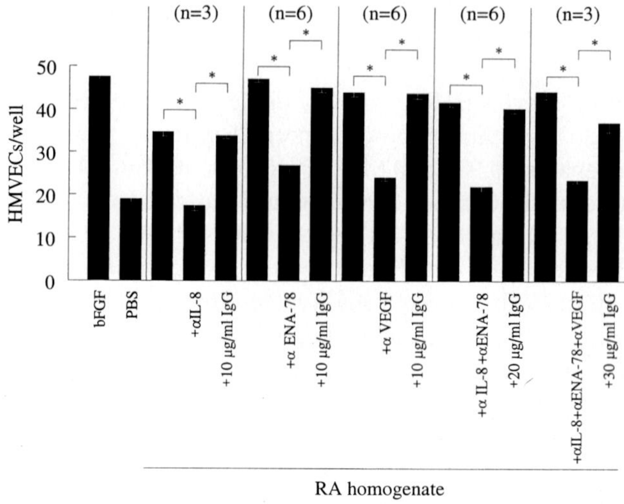

Figure 5. HMVEC chemotaxis in response to RA synovial tissue homogenate alone, in the presence of antibodies to IL-8, ENA-78, vascular endothelial growth factor (VEGF), or combinations thereof, or control IgG antibodies. The RA homogenate for the experiments shown was derived from a common pool of the same 3 RA patients. Bars show the mean and SEM of multiple combined assays, and the number of samples is reported above each condition. Twelve high-power fields were assayed per sample and the results expressed as the number of cells migrated per well. * = $P < 0.05$. See Figures 1 and 3 for other definitions.

A separate set of experiments, performed on a common pool of RA synovial tissue homogenate, used antibodies from a separate source to demonstrate similar results (Figure 5). A comparison of the assay results with anti–IL-8 and that with its IgG control demonstrated a 49% reduction in RA homogenate–induced chemotaxis. Similarly, anti–ENA-78 reduced chemotaxis by 40% and anti-VEGF reduced chemotaxis by 45%. The combination of anti–IL-8 and anti–ENA-78 reduced chemotaxis by 46%, and including anti-VEGF with these antibodies reduced chemotaxis by 36%. While use of multiple antibodies did not have additive effects, it is interesting to note that the single use of these antibodies reduced chemotaxis to near the levels found in assays with PBS.

Table 1. Suppression of RA synovial tissue homogenate–induced HMVEC migration in the presence versus absence of anti–IL-8 or anti–ENA-78*

Test group	No. HMVECs migrated/well (mean ± SEM)	% suppression	P†
RA + normal rabbit serum	36 ± 2.8		
RA + anti–IL-8	21 ± 1.6	42	<0.05
RA + anti–ENA-78	20 ± 3.0	44	<0.05

* RA = rheumatoid arthritis; HMVEC = human dermal microvascular endothelial cell; IL-8 = interleukin-8; ENA-78 = epithelial neutrophil activating peptide 78.
† Compared with RA + normal rabbit serum.

In vivo angiogenic activity of RA homogenates in response to IL-8 and ENA-78. To determine whether the effects seen on endothelial cells in vitro were also present in an angiogenic assay in vivo, the rat corneal bioassay was performed and the results are shown in Table 2 and Figure 6. Normal synovial tissue extracts did not elicit a neovascular response. In contrast, RA synovial tissue extracts elicited a positive corneal neovascular response in 6 of 6 corneas tested (Figure 6A). RA synovial tissue extracts incubated in the presence of normal rat serum were angiogenic in 88% of the assays. In contrast, incubation of RA synovial tissue extracts with anti–IL-8 resulted in a corneal response in only 20% of corneas assayed (Figure 6B). Incubation of RA synovial tissue extracts with anti–ENA-78 likewise did not result in a neovascular response (Figure 6C). These results suggest that the angiogenic activity present in RA synovial extracts is, in large part, due to ENA-78 and IL-8.

DISCUSSION

We and others have directly implicated several proangiogenic factors in the neovascular activity associ-

Table 2. Synovial tissue angiogenic activity*

Condition	Number positive/ total corneas	% positive corneal response
Normal synovial tissue	0/6	0
RA synovial tissue	6/6	100
RA + normal rabbit serum	7/8	88
RA + anti–IL-8	1/5	20
RA + anti–ENA-78	0/5	0

* See Table 1 for definitions.

ated with the pathogenesis of RA. These factors include VEGF, IL-8, TNFα, HGF, platelet-activating factor, sVCAM-1, and sE-selectin (6–9,35–37). Some proangiogenic factors such as transforming growth factor β have been described in the joint, but their role in joint angiogenesis has not been elucidated (38–43). Other proangiogenic factors, such as bFGF, have been localized to the RA joint by immunohistochemistry, yet little or no detectable amounts have been found in RA synovial fluid, and their role in mediating synovial angiogenesis remains unclear (44–47).

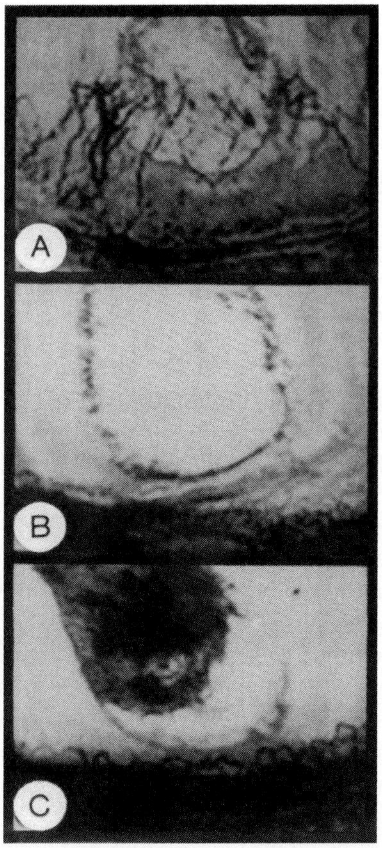

Figure 6. A, RA homogenate and normal rabbit serum implanted in a rat cornea. A brisk angiogenic response is seen. **B,** RA homogenate and anti–IL-8 implanted in a rat cornea. No angiogenic response is observed. **C,** RA homogenate and anti–ENA-78 implanted in a rat cornea. No angiogenesis is present. See Figure 1 for definitions.

To date, previous studies have been performed mainly using RA synovial fluid or supernatants from cells such as isolated RA synovial tissue macrophages. In the current study, to better determine the role of angiogenic chemokines in vivo, we used homogenates of whole RA synovial tissue. With this model we found that these tissues produced more IL-8 and ENA-78 compared with normal synovial tissues.

Since these chemokines were overproduced in RA compared with normal synovial tissues, we next determined whether cells producing these chemokines were located adjacent to blood vessels, and thus might directly mediate angiogenesis via production of chemokines. Indeed, IL-8– and ENA-78–immunopositive macrophages were often located in direct proximity to RA synovial blood vessels. Therefore, we hypothesized that these chemokines might mediate angiogenesis in the RA synovium.

To test this hypothesis, we performed assays for chemotaxis of endothelial cells, a facet of the angiogenic response. These assays indicated that RA synovial tissues produce significantly more chemotactic activity in endothelial cells than do normal tissues. In this system, not only IL-8, but also ENA-78 mediates a large portion of the chemotactic activity of endothelial cells found in the RA synovial tissue. Each of these chemokines accounted for between 42% and 44% of the chemotactic activity of HMVECs found in the RA synovial tissue homogenates. Chemokines use a complex and promiscuous set of receptors. Endothelial cells express the C-X-C chemokine receptors CXCR1, CXCR2, and CXCR4 (48,49). While CXCR1 is specific for IL-8, CXCR2, for instance, binds multiple ELR-containing chemokines. Therefore, it is likely that many ELR-containing chemokines may be binding to the same receptor on HMVECs, both in vitro and in vivo, to induce angiogenesis.

Since the in vitro chemotactic activity of endothelial cells is not always representative of conditions found in vivo, we utilized the rat corneal model of angiogenesis to analyze the in vivo angiogenic activity. Results using this model were similar to those found in vitro. IL-8 and ENA-78 contributed to the angiogenic activity found in the RA joint.

The issue of the contribution of chemokines in the RA angiogenic cascade relative to other angiogenic mediators is a difficult one to address. As with most biologic systems, it is unlikely that any one factor or family of factors accounts for all of the angiogenic bioactivity found in the RA joint. Other mediators may play a role. For instance, we found that a significant portion of the RA synovial fluid angiogenic activity was due to VEGF (6). The angiogenic activity found in synovial fluid would likely be derived from synovial tissue and cartilage. In contrast, in the current study, we found that the chemokines IL-8 and ENA-78 accounted for a large portion of the angiogenic activity found in the synovial tissue per se. However, since we demonstrated (in Figure 2B) ENA-78–positive macrophages near an ENA-78–positive blood vessel, it is possible that this chemokine may play a role in driving the proliferative phase of angiogenesis as opposed to establishing a gradient that guides the direction of neovascularization. Nonetheless, it is likely that these chemokines play a prominent role in angiogenic activity directly attributable to the RA inflammatory synovial pannus.

The net result of a chemokine–receptor interaction depends on a complex cascade determined by the cell type, ligand, structure, and configuration of the receptor, the G proteins present, and the available enzymes that can be activated. It is not clear why neutralization of a single chemoattractant within the complex RA homogenate reduces chemotaxis to the levels attained with PBS. A possible explanation could lie in receptor desensitization. Receptors for C-X-C chemokines are 7 transmembrane domain–containing G protein–coupled receptors. Receptor desensitization is a relatively transient event that can occur when receptors are exposed to a high concentration of ligand (50). Perhaps this phenomenon explains why chemotaxis concentration curves in response to various substances taper off at high concentrations. Heterologous desensitization of receptors is a reversible loss of responsiveness to multiple ligands. Such desensitization of chemokine receptors may involve protein kinase A (PKA) and PKC phosphorylation of multiple ligand-specific receptors, which uncouple them from association with their related G protein (50). Since IL-8 and ENA-78 are reported to share common C-X-C receptor–binding sites (51), it is possible that neutralization of IL-8 may overexpose the receptor to ENA-78 (and vice versa), thereby resulting in heterologous desensitization of multiple receptors.

In the current study, we have addressed the proangiogenic factors in the inflamed RA joint. Balancing the proangiogenic factors are the angiostatic factors. These factors are often cartilage-derived (52–58). In general, there appears to be a paucity of endogenous angiostatic factors in the joint. We have recently shown that the cytokine IL-4 is a potent inhibitor of angiogenesis, yet IL-4 is minimally detectable or absent in the RA joint (59–61).

Recent evidence suggests that in a number of disease states, there appears to be a balance between angiogenic and angiostatic chemokines as well. For example, we have shown previously that the ELR-containing chemokines IL-8 and ENA-78 contribute to tumorigenesis and concomitant angiogenesis of human non–small cell lung cancer in SCID mice (62,63). Similarly, the balance between ELR-containing proangiogenic chemokine IL-8 and the ELR-deficient angiostatic chemokine IP-10 appears to regulate the angiogenic activity found in human idiopathic pulmonary fibrosis (27). Thus, angiogenesis may predominate in disease states when the physiologic balance is weighted in favor of proangiogenic, compared with angiostatic, chemokines.

Modulation of cytokines may have a great impact on the course of RA in patients. Clinical trials have shown that measures aimed at decreasing TNFα in RA patients, such as the use of anti-TNFα, results in marked amelioration of disease with improvement in clinical parameters (64–72). This improvement in clinical disease may, in part, be due to the effects on angiogenesis from TNFα inhibition. Recent work has indicated that TNFα may mediate its angiogenic effect via IL-8 and VEGF (73). In fact, treatment strategies aimed at decreasing TNFα using RA synovial tissue mononuclear cells in vitro resulted in decreased angiogenic IL-8 production by these cells (74). Moreover, treatment of RA patients with therapies directed against TNFα also resulted in "vascular deactivation," with decreased serum levels of angiogenic VEGF and decreased levels of sE-selectin (18,75). Future therapies for RA may include direct augmentation of angiostatic cytokines, such as IL-4, or of angiostatic, non–ELR-containing chemokines. Alternative therapies may include methods aimed at down-regulating proangiogenic, ELR-containing C-X-C chemokines.

In summary, in this study we have shown that RA synovium produces more angiogenic activity than does normal synovium. RA synovial tissue, compared with normal synovial tissue, produces greater amounts of the angiogenic chemokines IL-8 and ENA-78. Angiogenic chemokines are often located in the synovial tissue in proximity to blood vessels. Moreover, the ELR-containing angiogenic chemokines IL-8 and ENA-78 contribute to the chemotactic activity of endothelial cells in vitro and the angiogenic activity in vivo found in the RA synovium. Dissecting the role of angiogenesis-promoting cytokines in the RA joint may help us design better therapies to benefit patients with RA.

REFERENCES

1. Harris ED. Pathogenesis of rheumatoid arthritis: a disorder associated with dysfunctional immunoregulation. In: Gallin JI, Goldstein IM, Snyderman R, editors. Inflammation: basic principles and clinical correlates. New York: Raven Press; 1988. p. 751–73.
2. Harris ED Jr. Rheumatoid arthritis: pathophysiology and implications for therapy. N Engl J Med 1990;332:1277–87.
3. Harris ED Jr. Rheumatoid arthritis. Curr Opin Rheumatol 1994; 6:287–9.
4. Szekanecz Z, Szegedi G, Koch AE. Angiogenesis in rheumatoid arthritis: pathogenic and clinical significance. J Investig Med 1998;46:27–41.
5. Koch AE. Angiogenesis: implications for rheumatoid arthritis. Arthritis Rheum 1998;41:951–62.
6. Koch AE, Harlow LA, Haines GK, Amento EP, Unemori EN, Wong WL, et al. Vascular endothelial growth factor: a cytokine modulating endothelial function in rheumatoid arthritis. J Immunol 1994;152:4149–56.
7. Koch AE, Halloran MM, Haskell CJ, Shah MR, Polverini PJ. Angiogenesis mediated by soluble forms of E-selectin and vascular cell adhesion molecule-1. Nature 1995;376:517–9.
8. Koch AE, Halloran MM, Hosaka S, Shah MR, Haskell CJ, Baker SK, et al. Hepatocyte growth factor: a cytokine mediating endothelial migration in inflammatory arthritis. Arthritis Rheum 1996; 39:1566–75.
9. Koch AE, Polverini PJ, Kunkel SL, Harlow LA, DiPietro LA, Elner VM, et al. Interleukin-8 as a macrophage-derived mediator of angiogenesis. Science 1992;258:1798–801.
10. Bottomley MJ, Webb NJ, Watson CJ, Holt PJ, Freemont AJ, Brenchley PE. Peripheral blood mononuclear cells from patients with rheumatoid arthritis spontaneously secrete vascular endothelial growth factor (VEGF): specific up-regulation by tumour necrosis factor-alpha (TNF-alpha) in synovial fluid. Clin Exp Immunol 1999;117:171–6.
11. Maeno N, Takei S, Imanaka H, Takasaki I, Kitajima I, Maruyama I, et al. Increased circulating vascular endothelial growth factor is correlated with disease activity in polyarticular juvenile rheumatoid arthritis. J Rheumatol 1999;26:2244–8.
12. Oppenheimer-Marks N, Lipsky PE. Adhesion molecules in rheumatoid arthritis. Springer Semin Immunopathol 1998;20:95–114.
13. Fox DA. Cytokine blockade as a new strategy to treat rheumatoid arthritis: inhibition of tumor necrosis factor. Arch Intern Med 2000;160:437–44.
14. Feldmann M, Maini RN. The role of cytokines in the pathogenesis of rheumatoid arthritis. Rheumatology 1999;38 Suppl 2:3–7.
15. Yukioka K, Inaba M, Furumitsu Y, Yukioka M, Nishino T, Goto H, et al. Levels of hepatocyte growth factor in synovial fluid and serum of patients with rheumatoid arthritis and release of hepatocyte growth factor by rheumatoid synovial fluid cells. J Rheumatol 1994;21:2184–9.
16. Remmers EF, Sano H, Lafyatis R, Case JP, Kumkumian GK, Hla T, et al. Production of platelet derived growth factor B chain (PDGF-B/c-sis) mRNA and immunoreactive PDGF B-like polypeptide by rheumatoid synovium: coexpression with heparin binding acidic fibroblast growth factor-1. J Rheumatol 1991;18:7–13.
17. Littler AJ, Buckley CD, Wordsworth P, Collins I, Martinson J, Simmons DL. A distinct profile of six soluble adhesion molecules (ICAM-1, ICAM-3, VCAM-1, E-selectin, L-selectin and P-selectin) in rheumatoid arthritis. Br J Rheumatol 1997;36:164–9.
18. Paleolog EM, Young S, Stark AC, McCloskey RV, Feldmann M, Maini RN. Modulation of angiogenic vascular endothelial growth factor by tumor necrosis factor α and interleukin-1 in rheumatoid arthritis. Arthritis Rheum 1998;41:1258–65.
19. Oliver SJ, Cheng TP, Banquerigo ML, Brahn E. Suppression of collagen-induced arthritis by an angiogenesis inhibitor, AGM-1470, in combination with cyclosporin: reduction of vascular endothelial growth factor (VEGF). Cell Immunol 1995;166:196–206.
20. Hebert CA, Vitangcol RV, Baker JB. Scanning mutagenesis of interleukin-8 identifies a cluster of residues required for receptor binding. J Biol Chem 1991;266:18989–94.
21. Clark-Lewis I, Dewald B, Geiser T, Moser B, Baggiolini M. Platelet factor 4 binds to interleukin 8 receptors and activates neutrophils when its N terminus is modified with Glu-Leu-Arg. Proc Natl Acad Sci U S A 1993;90:3574–7.
22. Strieter RM, Polverini PJ, Kunkel SL, Arenberg DA, Burdick MD, Kasper J, et al. The functional role of the ELR motif in CXC chemokine-mediated angiogenesis. J Biol Chem 1995;270: 27348–57.
23. Koch AE, Kunkel SL, Burrows JC, Evanoff HL, Haines GK, Pope RM, et al. Synovial tissue macrophage as a source of the chemotactic cytokine IL-8. J Immunol 1991;147:2187–95.
24. Koch AE, Kunkel SL, Harlow LA, Mazarakis DD, Haines GK, Burdick MD, et al. Epithelial neutrophil activating peptide-78: a novel chemotactic cytokine for neutrophils in arthritis. J Clin Invest 1994;94:1012–8.
25. Arnett FC, Edworthy SM, Bloch DA, McShane DJ, Fries JF, Cooper NS, et al. The American Rheumatism Association 1987 revised criteria for the classification of rheumatoid arthritis. Arthritis Rheum 1988;31:315–24.
26. Koch AE, Kunkel SL, Shah MR, Hosaka S, Halloran MM, Haines GK, et al. Growth-related gene product alpha: a chemotactic cytokine for neutrophils in rheumatoid arthritis. J Immunol 1995; 155:3660–6.
27. Keane MP, Arenberg DA, Lynch JP III, Whyte RI, Iannettoni MD, Burdick MD, et al. The CXC chemokines, IL-8 and IP-10, regulate angiogenic activity in idiopathic pulmonary fibrosis. J Immunol 1997;159:1437–43.
28. Halloran MM, Woods JM, Strieter RM, Szekanecz Z, Volin MV, Hosaka S, et al. The role of an epithelial neutrophil-activating peptide-78–like protein in rat adjuvant-induced arthritis. J Immunol 1999;65:7492–500.
29. Koch AE, Kunkel SL, Chensue SW, Haines GK, Strieter RM. Expression of interleukin-1 and interleukin-1 receptor antagonist by human rheumatoid synovial tissue macrophages. Clin Immunol Immunopathol 1992;65:23–9.
30. Koch AE, Burrows JC, Domer PH, Ashmun RA, Look TA, Leibovich SJ. Monoclonal antibodies defining shared human macrophage-endothelial antigens. Pathobiology 1992;60:59–67.
31. Koch AE, Kunkel SL, Harlow LA, Johnson B, Evanoff HL, Haines GK, et al. Enhanced production of monocyte chemoattractant protein-1 in rheumatoid arthritis. J Clin Invest 1992;90:772–9.
32. Koch AE, Kunkel SL, Harlow LA, Mazarakis DD, Haines GK, Burdick MD, et al. Macrophage inflammatory protein-1 alpha: a novel chemotactic cytokine for macrophages in rheumatoid arthritis. J Clin Invest 1994;93:921–8.
33. Nilsen EM, Johansen FE, Jahnsen FL, Lundin KE, Scholz T, Brandtzaeg P, et al. Cytokine profiles of cultured microvascular endothelial cells from the human intestine. Gut 1998;42:635–42.
34. Krishnaswamy G, Smith JK, Mukkamala R, Hall K, Joyner W, Yerra L, et al. Multifunctional cytokine expression by human coronary endothelium and regulation by monokines and glucocorticoids. Microvasc Res 1998;55:189–200.
35. Lupia E, Montrucchio G, Battaglia E, Modena V, Camussi G. Role of tumor necrosis factor-alpha and platelet-activating factor in neoangiogenesis induced by synovial fluids of patients with rheumatoid arthritis. Eur J Immunol 1996;26:1690–4.
36. Fava RA, Olsen NJ, Spencer-Green G, Yeo KT, Yeo TK, Berse B, et al. Vascular permeability factor/endothelial growth factor (VPF/VEGF): accumulation and expression in human synovial fluids and rheumatoid synovial tissue. J Exp Med 1994;180:341–6.
37. Paleolog EM. Angiogenesis: a critical process in the pathogenesis of RA—a role for VEGF? Br J Rheumatol 1996;35:917–9.

38. Szekanecz Z, Haines GK, Harlow LA, Shah MR, Fong TW, Fu R, et al. Increased synovial expression of TGF-β receptor endoglin and TGF-β1 in rheumatoid arthritis. Clin Immunol Immunopathol 1995;76:187–94.
39. Fava R, Olsen N, Keski-Oja J, Moses H, Pincus T. Active and latent forms of transforming growth factor β activity in synovial effusions. J Exp Med 1989;169:291–6.
40. Fava RA, Broadley KN, Davidson JM, Nanney LB, Cooper WO, Townes AS. Intra-articular injection of transforming growth factor β1 (TGF/β1) in rat knee joints mimics events associated with early stages of arthritis. In: Dinarello CA, editor. The physiological and pathological effects of cytokines. New York: Wiley-Liss; 1990. p. 99–104.
41. Fava RA, Olsen NJ, Postlethwaite AE, Broadley KN, Davidson JM, Nanney LB, et al. Transforming growth factor β1 (TGF-β1) induced neutrophil recruitment to synovial tissues: implications for TGF-β–driven synovial inflammation and hyperplasia. J Exp Med 1991;173:1121–32.
42. Wilder RL, Lafyatis R, Roberts AB, Case JP, Kumkumian GK, Sano H, et al. Transforming growth factor-β in rheumatoid arthritis. Ann N Y Acad Sci 1990;593:197–207.
43. Chu CQ, Field M, Abney E, Zheng RQH, Allard S, Feldmann M, et al. Transforming growth factor-β1 in rheumatoid synovial membrane and cartilage/pannus junction. Clin Exp Immunol 1991;86:380–6.
44. Hosaka S, Shah MR, Barquin N, Haines GK, Koch AE. Expression of basic fibroblast growth factor and angiogenin in arthritis. Pathobiology 1995;63:249–56.
45. Qu Z, Huang XN, Ahmadi P, Andresevic J, Planck SR, Hart CE, et al. Expression of basic fibroblast growth factor in synovial tissue from patients with rheumatoid arthritis and degenerative joint disease. Lab Invest 1995;73:339–46.
46. Remmers EF, Sano H, Wilder RL. Platelet-derived growth factors and heparin-binding (fibroblast) growth factors in the synovial tissue pathology of rheumatoid arthritis. Semin Arthritis Rheum 1991;21:191–9.
47. Nakashima M, Eguchi K, Aoyagi T, Yamashita I, Ida H, Sakai M, et al. Expression of basic fibroblast growth factor in synovial tissues from patients with rheumatoid arthritis: detection by immunohistological staining and in situ hybridisation. Ann Rheum Dis 1994;53:45–50.
48. Gupta SK, Lysko PG, Pillarisetti K, Ohlstein E, Stadel JM. Chemokine receptors in human endothelial cells: functional expression of CXCR4 and its transcriptional regulation by inflammatory cytokines. J Biol Chem 1998;273:4282–7.
49. Schonbeck U, Brandt E, Petersen F, Flad HD, Loppnow H. IL-8 specifically binds to endothelial but not to smooth muscle cells. J Immunol 1995;154:2375–83.
50. Ben-Baruch A, Michiel DF, Oppenheim JJ. Signals and receptors involved in recruitment of inflammatory cells. J Biol Chem 1995;270:11703–6.
51. Wuyts A, Proost P, Lenaerts JP, Ben-Baruch A, Van DJ, Wang JM. Differential usage of the CXC chemokine receptors 1 and 2 by interleukin-8, granulocyte chemotactic protein-2 and epithelial-cell-derived neutrophil attractant-78. Eur J Biochem 1998;255: 67–73.
52. Kuettner KE, Hiti J, Eisenstein R, Harper E. Collagenase inhibition by cationic proteins derived from cartilage and aorta. Biochem Biophys Res Commun 1976;72:40–6.
53. Brem H, Folkman J. Inhibition of tumor angiogenesis mediated by cartilage. J Exp Med 1975;141:427–39.
54. Langer R, Brem H, Falterman K, Klein M, Folkman J. Isolation of a cartilage factor that inhibits tumor neovascularization. Science 1976;193:70–2.
55. Kuettner KE, Pauli BU. Inhibition of neovascularization by a cartilage factor. Ciba Found Symp 1983;100:163–73.
56. Lee A, Langer R. Shark cartilage contains inhibitors of tumor angiogenesis. Science 1983;221:1185–7.
57. Langer R, Conn H, Vacanti J, Haudenschild C, Folkman J. Control of tumor growth in animals by infusion of an angiogenesis inhibitor. Proc Natl Acad Sci U S A 1980;77:4331–5.
58. Moses MA. A cartilage-derived inhibitor of neovascularization and metalloproteinases. Clin Exp Rheumatol 1993;11:S67–9.
59. Firestein GS. Cytokines in autoimmune diseases. In: Cruise JM, Lewis RE, editors. Clinical and molecular aspects of autoimmune diseases. New York: Karger; 1992. p. 129–60.
60. Firestein GS, Alvaro-Gracia JM, Maki R. Quantitative analysis of cytokine gene expression in rheumatoid arthritis. J Immunol 1990;144:3347–53.
61. Volpert OV, Fong T, Koch AE, Peterson JD, Waltenbaugh C, Tepper RI, et al. Inhibition of angiogenesis by interleukin 4. J Exp Med 1998;188:1039–46.
62. Smith DR, Polverini PJ, Kunkel SL, Orringer MB, Whyte RI, Burdick MD, et al. Inhibition of interleukin 8 attenuates angiogenesis in bronchogenic carcinoma. J Exp Med 1994;179:1409–15.
63. Arenberg DA, Kunkel SL, Polverini PJ, Glass M, Burdick MD, Strieter RM. Inhibition of interleukin-8 reduces tumorigenesis of human non-small cell lung cancer in SCID mice. J Clin Invest 1996;97:2792–802.
64. Maini RN, Brennan FM, Williams R, Chu CQ, Cope AP, Gibbons D, et al. TNF-α in rheumatoid arthritis and prospects of anti-TNF therapy. Clin Exp Rheumatol 1993;11 Suppl 8:S173–5.
65. Maini RN, Elliott M, Brennan FM, Williams RO, Feldmann M. Targeting TNF alpha for the therapy of rheumatoid arthritis. Clin Exp Rheumatol 1994;12 Suppl 11:S63–6.
66. Maini RN, Elliott M, Brennan FM, Williams RO, Feldmann M. TNF blockade in rheumatoid arthritis: implications for therapy and pathogenesis. APMIS 1997;105:257–63.
67. Elliott MJ, Maini RN, Feldmann M, Long-Fox A, Charles P, Katsikis P, et al. Treatment of rheumatoid arthritis with chimeric monoclonal antibodies to tumor necrosis factor α. Arthritis Rheum 1993;36:1681–90.
68. Elliott MJ, Maini RN, Feldmann M, Kalden JR, Antoni C, Smolen JS, et al. Randomised double-blind comparison of chimeric monoclonal antibody to tumour necrosis factor alpha (cA2) versus placebo in rheumatoid arthritis. Lancet 1994;344:1105–10.
69. Elliott MJ, Maini RN. New directions for biological therapy in rheumatoid arthritis. Int Arch Allergy Immunol 1994;104:112–25.
70. Feldmann M, Brennan FM, Elliott MJ, Williams RO, Maini RN. TNF alpha is an effective therapeutic target for rheumatoid arthritis. Ann N Y Acad Sci 1995;766:272–8.
71. Moreland LW, Margolies G, Heck LW Jr, Saway A, Blosch C, Hanna R, et al. Recombinant soluble tumor necrosis factor receptor (p80) fusion protein: toxicity and dose finding trial in refractory rheumatoid arthritis. J Rheumatol 1996;23:1849–55.
72. Moreland LW, Baumgartner SW, Schiff MH, Tindall EA, Fleischmann RM, Weaver AL, et al. Treatment of rheumatoid arthritis with a recombinant human tumor necrosis factor receptor (p75)-Fc fusion protein. N Engl J Med 1997;337:141–7.
73. Yoshida S, Ono M, Shono T, Izumi H, Ishibashi T, Suzuki H, et al. Involvement of interleukin-8, vascular endothelial growth factor, and basic fibroblast growth factor in tumor necrosis factor alpha-dependent angiogenesis. Mol Cell Biol 1997;17:4015–23.
74. Butler DM, Maini RN, Feldmann M, Brennan FM. Modulation of proinflammatory cytokine release in rheumatoid synovial membrane cell cultures: comparison of monoclonal anti TNF-alpha antibody with the interleukin-1 receptor antagonist. Eur Cytokine Netw 1995;6:225–30.
75. Paleolog EM, Hunt M, Elliott MJ, Feldmann M, Maini RN, Woody JN. Deactivation of vascular endothelium by monoclonal anti-tumor necrosis factor α antibody in rheumatoid arthritis. Arthritis Rheum 1996;39:1082–91.

VIOXX® (rofecoxib tablets and oral suspension)

Brief Summary of Prescribing Information

INDICATIONS AND USAGE: VIOXX is indicated for: relief of the signs and symptoms of osteoarthritis (OA); management of acute pain in adults; treatment of primary dysmenorrhea.

CONTRAINDICATIONS: VIOXX is contraindicated in patients with known hypersensitivity to rofecoxib or any other component of VIOXX.

VIOXX should not be given to patients who have experienced asthma, urticaria, or allergic-type reactions after taking aspirin or other nonsteroidal anti-inflammatory drugs (NSAIDs). Severe, rarely fatal, anaphylactic-like reactions to NSAIDs have been reported in such patients (see WARNINGS, *Anaphylactoid Reactions* and PRECAUTIONS, *Preexisting Asthma*).

WARNINGS: *Gastrointestinal (GI) Effects—Risk of GI Ulceration, Bleeding, and Perforation:* Serious GI toxicity, such as bleeding, ulceration, and perforation of the stomach, small intestine, or large intestine, can occur at any time, with or without warning symptoms, in patients treated with NSAIDs. Minor upper GI problems, such as dyspepsia, are common and may also occur at any time during NSAID therapy. Therefore, physicians and patients should remain alert for ulceration and bleeding, even in the absence of previous GI tract symptoms. Patients should be informed about the signs and/or symptoms of serious GI toxicity and the steps to take if they occur. The utility of periodic laboratory monitoring has not been demonstrated, nor has it been adequately assessed. Only 1 in 5 patients who develop a serious upper GI adverse event on NSAID therapy is symptomatic. It has been demonstrated that upper GI ulcers, gross bleeding, or perforation caused by NSAIDs, appear to occur in approximately 1% of patients treated for 3–6 months, and in about 2%–4% of patients treated for 1 year. These trends continue thus, increasing the likelihood of developing a serious GI event at some time during the course of therapy. However, even short-term therapy is not without risk.

It is unclear, at the present time, how the above rates apply to VIOXX. Among 3,357 patients who received VIOXX in controlled clinical trials of 6 weeks to 1 year in duration (most were enrolled in 6-month or longer studies) at a daily dose of 12.5 mg to 50 mg, a total of 4 patients experienced a serious upper GI event, using protocol-derived criteria. Two patients experienced an upper GI bleed within 3 months (at Days 62 and 87, respectively) (0.06%). One additional patient experienced an obstruction within 6 months (Day 130) and the remaining patient developed an upper GI bleed within 12 months (Day 322) (0.12%). Approximately 23% of these 3,357 patients were in studies that required them to be ulcer free at study entry. It is unclear if this study population is representative of the general population. Prospective, long-term studies required to compare the incidence of serious, clinically significant upper GI adverse events in patients taking VIOXX vs comparator NSAID products have not been performed.

NSAIDs should be prescribed with extreme caution in patients with a prior history of ulcer disease or GI bleeding. Most spontaneous reports of fatal GI events are in elderly or debilitated patients and therefore special care should be taken in treating this population. **To minimize the potential risk for an adverse GI event, the lowest effective dose should be used for the shortest possible duration.** For high-risk patients, alternate therapies that do not involve NSAIDs should be considered.

Studies have shown that patients with a *prior history of peptic ulcer disease and/or GI bleeding* and who use NSAIDs, have a greater than 10-fold higher risk for developing a GI bleed than patients with neither of these risk factors. In addition to a past history of ulcer disease, pharmacoepidemiologic studies have identified several other cotherapies or comorbid conditions that may increase the risk for GI bleeding, such as: treatment with oral corticosteroids, treatment with anticoagulants, longer duration of NSAID therapy, smoking, alcoholism, older age, and poor general health status.

Anaphylactoid Reactions: As with NSAIDs in general, anaphylactoid reactions have occurred in patients without known prior exposure to VIOXX. In postmarketing experience, rare cases of anaphylactoid reactions and angioedema have been reported in patients receiving VIOXX. VIOXX should not be given to patients with the aspirin triad. This symptom complex typically occurs in asthmatic patients who experience rhinitis with or without nasal polyps, or who exhibit severe, potentially fatal bronchospasm after taking aspirin or other NSAIDs (see CONTRAINDICATIONS and PRECAUTIONS, *Preexisting Asthma*). Emergency help should be sought in cases where an anaphylactoid reaction occurs.

Advanced Renal Disease: No safety information is available regarding the use of VIOXX in patients with advanced kidney disease. Therefore, treatment with VIOXX is not recommended in these patients. If VIOXX therapy must be initiated, close monitoring of the patient's kidney function is advisable (see PRECAUTIONS, *Renal Effects*).

Pregnancy: In late pregnancy, VIOXX should be avoided because it may cause premature closure of the ductus arteriosus.

PRECAUTIONS: *General:* VIOXX cannot be expected to substitute for corticosteroids or to treat corticosteroid insufficiency. Abrupt discontinuation of corticosteroids may lead to exacerbation of corticosteroid-responsive illness. Patients on prolonged corticosteroid therapy should have their therapy tapered slowly if a decision is made to discontinue corticosteroids.

The pharmacologic activity of VIOXX in reducing inflammation, and possibly fever, may diminish the utility of these diagnostic signs in detecting infectious complications of presumed noninfectious, painful conditions.

Hepatic Effects: Borderline elevations of 1 or more liver tests may occur in up to 15% of patients taking NSAIDs, and notable elevations of ALT or AST (~3 or more times the upper limit of normal) have been reported in approximately 1% of patients in clinical trials with NSAIDs. These laboratory abnormalities may progress, may remain unchanged, or may be transient with continuing therapy. Rare cases of severe hepatic reactions, including jaundice and fatal fulminant hepatitis, liver necrosis, and hepatic failure (some with fatal outcome) have been reported with NSAIDs. In controlled clinical trials of VIOXX, the incidence of borderline elevations of liver tests at doses of 12.5 mg and 25 mg daily was comparable to the incidence observed with ibuprofen and lower than that observed with diclofenac. In placebo-controlled trials, approximately 0.5% of patients taking rofecoxib (12.5 mg or 25 mg q.d.) and 0.1% of patients taking placebo had notable elevations of ALT or AST.

A patient with symptoms and/or signs suggesting liver dysfunction, or in whom an abnormal liver test has occurred, should be monitored carefully for evidence of the development of a more severe hepatic reaction while on therapy with VIOXX. Use of VIOXX is not recommended in patients with moderate or severe hepatic insufficiency. If clinical signs and symptoms consistent with liver disease develop, or if systemic manifestations occur (e.g., eosinophilia, rash, etc.), VIOXX should be discontinued.

Renal Effects: Long-term administration of NSAIDs has resulted in renal papillary necrosis and other renal injury. Renal toxicity has also been seen in patients in whom renal prostaglandins have a compensatory role in the maintenance of renal perfusion. In these patients, administration of an NSAID may cause a dose-dependent reduction in prostaglandin formation and, secondarily, in renal blood flow, which may precipitate overt renal decompensation. Patients at greatest risk of this reaction are those with impaired renal function, heart failure, liver dysfunction, those taking diuretics and angiotensin-converting enzyme (ACE) inhibitors, and the elderly. Discontinuation of NSAID therapy is usually followed by recovery to the pretreatment state. Clinical trials with VIOXX at daily doses of 12.5 mg and 25 mg have shown renal effects (e.g., hypertension, edema) similar to those observed with comparator NSAIDs; these occur with an increased frequency with chronic use of VIOXX at doses above the 12.5-mg to 25-mg range (see ADVERSE REACTIONS). Caution should be used when initiating treatment with VIOXX in patients with considerable dehydration. It is advisable to rehydrate patients first and then start therapy with VIOXX. Caution is also recommended in patients with preexisting kidney disease (see WARNINGS, *Advanced Renal Disease*).

Hematologic Effects: Anemia is sometimes seen in patients receiving VIOXX. In placebo-controlled trials, there were no significant differences observed between VIOXX and placebo in clinical reports of anemia. Patients on long-term treatment with VIOXX should have their hemoglobin or hematocrit checked if they exhibit any signs or symptoms of anemia or blood loss. VIOXX does not generally affect platelet counts, prothrombin time, or partial thromboplastin time, and does not inhibit platelet aggregation at indicated dosages.

Fluid Retention and Edema: Fluid retention and edema have been observed in some patients taking VIOXX® (rofecoxib tablets and oral suspension) (see ADVERSE REACTIONS). VIOXX should be used with caution and should be introduced at the lowest recommended dose in patients with fluid retention, hypertension, or heart failure.

Preexisting Asthma: Patients with asthma may have aspirin-sensitive asthma. The use of aspirin in patients with aspirin-sensitive asthma has been associated with severe bronchospasm, which can be fatal. Since cross-reactivity, including bronchospasm, between aspirin and other NSAIDs has been reported in such aspirin-sensitive patients, VIOXX should not be administered to patients with this form of aspirin sensitivity and should be used with caution in patients with preexisting asthma.

Information for Patients: VIOXX can cause discomfort and, rarely, more serious side effects, such as GI bleeding, which may result in hospitalization and even fatal outcomes. Although serious GI tract ulcerations and bleeding can occur without warning symptoms, patients should be alert for the signs and symptoms of ulcerations and bleeding, and should ask for medical advice when observing any indicative signs or symptoms. Patients should be apprised of the importance of this follow-up (see WARNINGS, *Gastrointestinal (GI) Effects—Risk of GI Ulceration, Bleeding, and Perforation)*.

Patients should promptly report signs or symptoms of GI ulceration or bleeding, skin rash, unexplained weight gain, or edema to their physicians.

Patients should be informed of the warning signs and symptoms of hepatotoxicity (e.g., nausea, fatigue, lethargy, pruritus, jaundice, right upper quadrant tenderness, and "flu-like" symptoms). If these occur, patients should be instructed to stop therapy and seek immediate medical therapy.

Patients should also be instructed to seek immediate emergency help in the case of an anaphylactoid reaction (see WARNINGS).

In late pregnancy, VIOXX should be avoided because it may cause premature closure of the ductus arteriosus.

Laboratory Tests: Because serious GI tract ulcerations and bleeding can occur without warning symptoms, physicians should monitor for signs or symptoms of GI bleeding.

Drug Interactions: ACE Inhibitors: Reports suggest that NSAIDs may diminish the antihypertensive effect of ACE inhibitors. In patients with mild to moderate hypertension, administration of 25 mg daily of VIOXX with the ACE inhibitor benazepril, 10 to 40 mg for 4 weeks, was associated with an average increase in mean arterial pressure of about 3 mmHg compared to ACE inhibitor alone. This interaction should be given consideration in patients taking VIOXX concomitantly with ACE inhibitors. *Aspirin:* Concomitant administration of low-dose aspirin with VIOXX may result in an increased rate of GI ulceration or other complications, compared to use of VIOXX alone. At steady state, VIOXX 50 mg once daily had no effect on the antiplatelet activity of low-dose (81 mg once daily) aspirin, as assessed by ex vivo platelet aggregation and serum TXB_2 generation in clotting blood. VIOXX is not a substitute for aspirin for cardiovascular prophylaxis. *Cimetidine:* Coadministration with high doses of cimetidine (800 mg twice daily) increased the C_{max} of rofecoxib by 21%, the $AUC_{0\text{-}120hr}$ by 23%, and the $t_{1/2}$ by 15%. These small changes are not clinically significant and no dose adjustment is necessary. *Digoxin:* Rofecoxib 75 mg once daily for 11 days does not alter the plasma concentration profile or renal elimination of digoxin after a single 0.5-mg oral dose. *Furosemide:* Clinical studies, as well as postmarketing observations, have shown that NSAIDs can reduce the natriuretic effect of furosemide and thiazides in some patients. This response has been attributed to inhibition of renal prostaglandin synthesis. *Ketoconazole:* Ketoconazole 400 mg daily did not have any clinically important effect on the pharmacokinetics of rofecoxib. *Lithium:* NSAIDs have produced an elevation of plasma lithium levels and a reduction in renal lithium clearance. In postmarketing experience, there have been reports of increases in plasma lithium levels. Thus, when VIOXX and lithium are administered concurrently, subjects should be observed carefully for signs of lithium toxicity. *Methotrexate:* VIOXX 75 mg administered once daily for 10 days increased plasma concentrations by 23%, as measured by $AUC_{0\text{-}24hr}$ in patients receiving methotrexate 7.5 mg to 15 mg/week for rheumatoid arthritis. An equivalent magnitude of reduction in methotrexate renal clearance was observed. At 24 hours postdose, a similar proportion of patients treated with methotrexate alone (94%) and subsequently treated with methotrexate coadministered with 75 mg of rofecoxib (88%) had methotrexate plasma concentrations below the measurable limit (5 ng/mL). The effects of the recommended doses for OA (12.5 mg and 25 mg) of VIOXX on plasma methotrexate levels are unknown. Standard monitoring of methotrexate-related toxicity should be continued if VIOXX and methotrexate are administered concomitantly. *Oral Contraceptives:* Rofecoxib did not have any clinically important effect on the pharmacokinetics of ethinyl estradiol and norethindrone. *Prednisone/Prednisolone:* Rofecoxib did not have any clinically important effect on the pharmacokinetics of prednisone or prednisolone. *Rifampin:* Coadministration of VIOXX with rifampin 600 mg daily, a potent inducer of hepatic metabolism, produced an approximate 50% decrease in rofecoxib plasma concentrations. Therefore, a starting daily dose of 25 mg of VIOXX should be considered for the treatment of OA when VIOXX is coadministered with potent inducers of hepatic metabolism. *Warfarin:* Anticoagulant activity should be monitored, particularly in the first few days after initiating or changing VIOXX therapy in patients receiving warfarin or similar agents, since these patients are at an increased risk of bleeding complications. In single- and multiple-dose studies in healthy subjects receiving both warfarin and rofecoxib, prothrombin time (measured as INR) was increased by approximately 8% to 11%. In postmarketing experience, bleeding events have been reported, predominantly in the elderly, in association with increases in prothrombin time in patients receiving VIOXX concurrently with warfarin.

Carcinogenesis, Mutagenesis, Impairment of Fertility: Rofecoxib was not carcinogenic in mice given oral doses up to 30 mg/kg (male) and 60 mg/kg (female) (~5- and 2-fold the human exposure at 25 mg and 50 mg daily based on $AUC_{0\text{-}24}$) and in male and female rats given oral doses up to 8 mg/kg (~6- and 2-fold the human exposure at 25 mg and 50 mg daily based on $AUC_{0\text{-}24}$) for 2 years. Rofecoxib was not mutagenic in an Ames test or in a V-79 mammalian cell mutagenesis assay, nor clastogenic in a chromosome aberration assay in Chinese hamster ovary (CHO) cells, in an in vitro and an in vivo alkaline elution assay, or in an in vivo chromosomal aberration test in mouse bone marrow. Rofecoxib did not impair male fertility in rats at oral doses up to 100 mg/kg (~20- and 7-fold human exposure at 25 mg and 50 mg daily based on $AUC_{0\text{-}24}$) and rofecoxib had no effect on fertility in female rats at doses up to 30 mg/kg (~19- and 7-fold human exposure at 25 mg and 50 mg daily based on $AUC_{0\text{-}24}$).

Pregnancy: Teratogenic Effects: Pregnancy Category C. Rofecoxib was not teratogenic in rats at dosages up to 50 mg/kg/day (~28- and 10-fold human exposure at 25 mg and 50 mg daily based on $AUC_{0\text{-}24}$). There was a slight, nonstatistically significant increase in the overall incidence of vertebral malformations only in the rabbit at doses of 50 mg/kg/day (~1- or <1-fold human exposure at 25 mg and 50 mg daily based on $AUC_{0\text{-}24}$). There are no studies in pregnant women. VIOXX should be used during pregnancy only if the potential benefit justifies the potential risk to the fetus.

Nonteratogenic Effects: Rofecoxib produced periimplantation and postimplantation losses and reduced embryo/fetal survival in rats and rabbits at oral doses ≥10 and ≥75 mg/kg/day, respectively (~9- and 3-fold [rats] and 2- and <1-fold [rabbits] human exposure based on $AUC_{0\text{-}24}$ at 25 mg and 50 mg daily). These changes are expected with inhibition of prostaglandin synthesis and are not the result of permanent alteration of female reproductive function. There was an increase in the incidence of postnatal pup mortality in rats at ≥5 mg/kg/day (~5- and 2-fold human exposure at 25 mg and 50 mg daily based on $AUC_{0\text{-}24}$). In studies in pregnant rats administered single doses of rofecoxib, there was a treatment-related decrease in the diameter of the ductus arteriosus at all doses used (3–300 mg/kg: 3 mg/kg is ~2- and <1-fold human exposure at 25 mg or 50 mg daily based on $AUC_{0\text{-}24}$). As with other drugs known to inhibit prostaglandin synthesis, use of VIOXX during the third trimester of pregnancy should be avoided.

Labor and Delivery: Rofecoxib produced no evidence of significantly delayed labor or parturition in females at doses 15 mg/kg in rats (~10- and 3-fold human exposure as measured by the $AUC_{0\text{-}24}$ at 25 mg and 50 mg). The effects of VIOXX on labor and delivery in pregnant women are unknown. Merck & Co., Inc., maintains a registry to monitor the pregnancy outcomes of women exposed to VIOXX while pregnant. Healthcare providers are encouraged to report any prenatal exposure to VIOXX by calling the Pregnancy Registry at 1-800-986-8999.

Nursing Mothers: Rofecoxib is excreted in the milk of lactating rats at concentrations similar to those in plasma. There was an increase in pup mortality and a decrease in pup body weight following exposure of pups to milk from dams administered VIOXX® (rofecoxib tablets and oral suspension) during lactation. The dose tested represents an approximate 18- and 6-fold human exposure at 25 mg and 50 mg daily based on $AUC_{0\text{-}24}$. It is not known whether this drug is excreted in human milk. Because many drugs are excreted in human milk and because of the potential for serious adverse reactions in nursing infants from VIOXX, a decision should be made whether to discontinue nursing or to discontinue the drug, taking into account the importance of the drug to the mother.

Pediatric Use: Safety and effectiveness in pediatric patients below the age of 18 years have not been evaluated.

Geriatric Use: Of the patients who received VIOXX in OA clinical trials, 1,455 were 65 years of age or older (this included 460 who were 75 years or older). No substantial differences in safety and effectiveness were observed between these subjects and younger subjects. Greater sensitivity of some older individuals cannot be ruled out. Dosage adjustment in the elderly is not necessary; however, therapy with VIOXX should be initiated at the lowest recommended dose. In 1 of these studies (a 6-week, double-blind, randomized clinical trial), VIOXX 12.5 mg or 25 mg once daily was administered to 174 OA patients ≥80 years of age. The safety profile in this elderly population was similar to that of younger patients treated with VIOXX.

ADVERSE REACTIONS: *OA:* Approximately 3,600 patients with OA were treated with VIOXX; approximately 1,400 patients received VIOXX for 6 months or longer, and approximately 800 patients for 1 year or longer. The following paragraph lists all adverse events, regardless of causality, occurring in at least 2% of patients receiving VIOXX in 9 controlled studies of 6 weeks' to 6 months' duration conducted in patients with OA at the therapeutically recommended doses (12.5 mg and 25 mg), which included a placebo and/or positive control group.

Clinical adverse experiences occurring in ≥2.0% of patients treated with VIOXX vs placebo, ibuprofen 2400 mg, or diclofenac 150 mg: *Body as a Whole/Site Unspecified:* abdominal pain, 3.4% (vs 4.1%, placebo; 4.6%, ibuprofen; 5.8%, diclofenac); asthenia/fatigue, 2.2% (vs 1.0%; 2.0%; 2.6%); dizziness, 3.0% (vs 2.2%; 2.7%; 3.4%); influenza-like disease, 2.9% (vs 3.1%; 1.5%; 3.2%); lower extremity edema, 3.7% (vs 1.1%; 3.8%; 3.4%); upper respiratory infection, 8.5% (vs 7.8%; 5.8%; 8.2%). *Cardiovascular System:* hypertension, 3.5% (vs 1.3%; 3.0%; 1.6%). *Digestive System:* diarrhea, 6.5% (vs 6.8%; 7.1%; 10.6%); dyspepsia, 3.5% (vs 2.7%; 4.7%; 4.0%); epigastric discomfort, 3.8% (vs 2.8%; 9.2%; 5.4%); heartburn, 4.2% (vs 3.6%; 5.2%; 4.6%); nausea, 5.2% (vs 2.9%; 7.1%; 7.4%). *Eyes, Ears, Nose, and Throat:* sinusitis, 2.7% (vs 2.0%; 1.8%; 2.4%). *Musculoskeletal System:* back pain, 2.5% (vs 1.9%; 1.4%; 2.8%). *Nervous System:* headache, 4.7% (vs 7.5%; 6.1%; 8.0%). *Respiratory System:* bronchitis, 2.0% (vs 0.8%; 1.4%; 3.2%). *Urogenital System:* urinary tract infection, 2.8% (vs 2.7%; 2.5%; 3.6%).

The general safety profile of VIOXX 50 mg q.d. in OA clinical trials of up to 6 months (476 patients) was similar to that of VIOXX at the recommended OA doses of 12.5 mg and 25 mg q.d., except for a higher incidence of GI symptoms (abdominal pain, epigastric pain, heartburn, nausea, and vomiting), lower extremity edema (6.3%), and hypertension (8.2%).

In the OA studies, the following spontaneous adverse events occurred in >0.1% to 1.9% of patients treated with VIOXX, regardless of causality:

Body as a Whole: abdominal distension, abdominal tenderness, abscess, chest pain, chills, contusion, cyst, diaphragmatic hernia, fever, fluid retention, flushing, fungal infection, infection, laceration, pain, pelvic pain, peripheral edema, postoperative pain, syncope, trauma, upper extremity edema, viral syndrome. *Cardiovascular System:* angina pectoris, atrial fibrillation, bradycardia, hematoma, irregular heartbeat, palpitation, premature ventricular contraction, tachycardia, venous insufficiency. *Digestive System:* acid reflux, aphthous stomatitis, constipation, dental caries, dental pain, digestive gas symptoms, dry mouth, duodenal disorder, dysgeusia, esophagitis, flatulence, gastric disorder, gastritis, gastroenteritis, hematochezia, hemorrhoids, infectious gastroenteritis, oral infection, oral lesion, oral ulcer, vomiting. *Eyes, Ears, Nose, and Throat:* allergic rhinitis, blurred vision, cerumen impaction, conjunctivitis, dry throat, epistaxis, laryngitis, nasal congestion, nasal secretion, ophthalmic injection, otic pain, otitis, otitis media, pharyngitis, tinnitus, tonsillitis. *Immune System:* allergy, hypersensitivity, insect bite reaction. *Metabolism and Nutrition:* appetite change, hypercholesterolemia, weight gain. *Musculoskeletal System:* ankle sprain, arm pain, arthralgia, back strain, bursitis, cartilage trauma, joint swelling, muscular cramp, muscular disorder, muscular weakness, musculoskeletal pain, musculoskeletal stiffness, myalgia, osteoarthritis, tendinitis, traumatic arthropathy, wrist fracture. *Nervous System:* hypesthesia, insomnia, median nerve neuropathy, migraine, muscular spasm, paresthesia, sciatica, somnolence, vertigo. *Psychiatric:* anxiety, depression, mental acuity decreased. *Respiratory System:* asthma, cough, dyspnea, pneumonia, pulmonary congestion, respiratory infection. *Skin and Skin Appendages:* abrasion, alopecia, atopic dermatitis, basal cell carcinoma, blister, cellulitis, contact dermatitis, herpes simplex, herpes zoster, nail unit disorder, perspiration, pruritus, rash, skin erythema, urticaria, xerosis. *Urogenital System:* breast mass, cystitis, dysuria, menopausal symptoms, menstrual disorder, nocturia, urinary retention, vaginitis.

The following serious adverse events have been reported rarely (estimated <0.1%) in patients taking VIOXX, regardless of causality. Cases reported only in the postmarketing experience are indicated in italics.

Cardiovascular: cerebrovascular accident, congestive heart failure, deep venous thrombosis, myocardial infarction, pulmonary embolism, transient ischemic attack, unstable angina. *GI:* cholecystitis, colitis, colonic malignant neoplasm, *duodenal perforation*, duodenal ulcer, *esophageal ulcer*, *gastric perforation, gastric ulcer*, GI bleeding, *hepatitis,* intestinal obstruction, *jaundice,* pancreatitis. *Hemic and Lymphatic: agranulocytosis, leukopenia,* lymphoma, *thrombocytopenia. Immune System: anaphylactoid reaction, angioedema. Nervous System: aseptic meningitis. Psychiatric: confusion, hallucinations. Skin and Skin Appendages: severe skin reactions, including Stevens-Johnson syndrome. Urogenital System: acute renal failure,* breast malignant neoplasm, *interstitial nepphritis*, prostatic malignant neoplasm, urolithiasis, *worsening chronic renal failure.*

In 1-year controlled clinical trials and in extension studies for up to 86 weeks (~800 patients treated with VIOXX for 1 year or longer), the adverse-experience profile was qualitatively similar to that observed in studies of shorter duration.

Analgesia, Including Primary Dysmenorrhea: Approximately 1,000 patients were treated with VIOXX in analgesia studies. All patients in postdental surgery pain studies received only a single dose of study medication. Patients in primary dysmenorrhea studies may have taken up to 3 daily doses of VIOXX, and those in the postorthopedic surgery pain study were prescribed 5 daily doses of VIOXX.

The adverse-experience profile in the analgesia studies was generally similar to those reported in the OA studies. The following additional adverse experience, which occurred at an incidence of ≥2% of patients treated with VIOXX, was observed in the postdental pain surgery studies: postdental extraction alveolitis (dry socket).

In 110 patients treated with VIOXX (average age ~65 years) in the postorthopedic surgery pain study, the most commonly reported adverse experiences were constipation, fever, and nausea.

DOSAGE AND ADMINISTRATION: VIOXX is administered orally. The lowest dose of VIOXX should be sought for each patient.

OA: The recommended starting dose of VIOXX is 12.5 mg once daily. Some patients may receive additional benefit by increasing the dose to 25 mg once daily. The maximum recommended daily dose is 25 mg.

Management of Acute Pain and Treatment of Primary Dysmenorrhea: The recommended initial dose of VIOXX is 50 mg once daily. Subsequent doses should be 50 mg once daily as needed. Use of VIOXX for more than 5 days in management of pain has not been studied.

VIOXX Tablets may be taken with or without food.

Oral Suspension: VIOXX Oral Suspension 12.5 mg/5 mL or 25 mg/5 mL may be substituted for VIOXX Tablets 12.5 mg or 25 mg, respectively, in any of the above indications. Shake before using.

For more detailed information, consult your Merck representative and read the full Prescribing Information.

MERCK

ARTHRITIS & RHEUMATISM
Vol. 44, No. 1, January 2001, pp 41–47

Secretion of Anti–Citrulline-Containing Peptide Antibody by B Lymphocytes in Rheumatoid Arthritis

Carelle C. Reparon-Schuijt,[1] Wim J. E. van Esch,[1] Cees van Kooten,[1]
Gerard A. Schellekens,[2] Ben A. W. de Jong,[2] Walther J. van Venrooij,[2]
Ferdinand C. Breedveld,[1] and Cornelis L. Verweij[1]

Objective. **To understand the regulation of anti–citrulline-containing peptide antibody (anti-CCP) production in rheumatoid arthritis (RA), production of anti-CCP by B cells derived from peripheral blood (PB), bone marrow (BM), and synovial fluid (SF) was examined.**

Methods. **Purified PB and SF B cells were isolated by negative selection and then cultured in the absence or presence of L–CD40 ligand cells and interleukin-10 or anti-CD3–activated T cells. Total IgM and IgM–anti-CCP were detected after 14 days of culture by enzyme-linked immunosorbent assay. Enzyme-linked immunospot assays were performed to analyze the frequency of cells that spontaneously produced IgM–anti-CCP in BM and SF B cells.**

Results. **IgM–anti-CCP autoantibodies were induced in PB B cells from healthy controls and RA patients following coculture with activated T cells or application of the CD40 activation system, whereas no production could be detected when PB B cells were cultured in the absence of a stimulus. SF and BM B cells from anti-CCP–seropositive RA patients, but not anti-CCP–seronegative patients, actively produced IgM–anti-CCP without stimulation. The frequency of spontaneous production of IgM–anti-CCP among the IgM-secreting cells ranged from 2.2% to 25%.**

Conclusion. **These results indicate the presence of B cell precursors for anti-CCP autoantibodies that are able to produce antibodies upon stimulation in the PB B cell repertoire of healthy controls and patients with RA. In contrast, B cells that actively secreted anti-CCP were specifically present in the BM and SF compartment of anti-CCP–seropositive RA patients. The local presence of anti-CCP–secreting cells in the inflamed joints provides evidence for an antigen-driven maturation of CCP-specific B cells at the site of inflammation in RA.**

Rheumatoid arthritis (RA) is a systemic disease characterized by chronic inflammation of multiple joints (1), which may lead to destruction of cartilage and bone and thus cause permanent disability. Based on evidence of the accumulation of T and B cells, association with HLA class II alleles (2), and presence of (auto)antibodies (3–5), both cellular and humoral autoimmune mechanisms have been implicated in the pathogenesis of RA. The presence of rheumatoid factor (RF), a type of antibody directed to the constant region of IgG, is one of the characteristics of RA (6). In addition to RF, other autoantibodies have been described in the serum of patients with RA, such as antiperinuclear factor (APF) (3), antikeratin (AKA) (4), anticollagen (5), and antinuclear proteins (7). Among these, 2 closely related autoantibodies, APF and AKA, have been demonstrated to be the most specific for RA. The presence of these autoantibodies before disease presentation is suggestive of a role in disease pathogenesis.

The nature of the antigen recognized by both APF and AKA has recently been identified (8). Both APF and AKA, which are reactive toward filaggrin (filament-aggregating protein) extracted from human epidermis, were shown to bind synthetic peptides containing the amino acid citrulline (9), a posttranslational modified arginine residue (10,11). Application of the citrulline-containing peptide (CCP) in enzyme-linked

[1]Carelle C. Reparon-Schuijt, PhD, Wim J. E. van Esch, MSc, Cees van Kooten, PhD, Ferdinand C. Breedveld, MD, Cornelis L. Verweij, PhD: Leiden University Medical Center, Leiden, The Netherlands; [2]Gerard A. Schellekens, PhD, Ben A. W. de Jong, Walther J. van Venrooij, PhD: University of Nijmegen, Nijmegen, The Netherlands.

Address correspondence and reprint requests to Cornelis L. Verweij, PhD, Leiden University Medical Center, Department of Rheumatology, C4-R, PO Box 9600, 2300 RC Leiden, The Netherlands.

Submitted for publication February 11, 2000; accepted in revised form September 5, 2000.

immunosorbent assay (ELISA) revealed the presence of anti-CCP autoantibodies in 76% of RA sera, with a specificity of 95–100% (9,12). This high specificity combined with their presence early in the disease, even before the disease is manifest, suggests a role for these autoantibodies in the pathogenesis of RA. Therefore, exploration of the regulation of anti-CCP production might lead to insight into the pathogenesis of RA.

In this study, the anti-CCP–producing capacity of highly purified B cells from the synovial fluid (SF) and peripheral blood (PB) of patients with RA and from the PB B cells of healthy controls was analyzed. It was demonstrated that healthy control subjects and RA patients have a pool of precursor B cells in the circulation that are capable of producing anti-CCP upon activation. SF and bone marrow (BM) B cells from patients with RA contain a population of B cells that spontaneously produce anti-CCP antibodies. These spontaneously producing B cells are specific for anti-CCP–positive patients with RA. These data confirm the local presence of anti-CCP–producing cells at the site of inflammation. The high frequency of these cells in the SF B cell population supports the notion of a local mechanism of activation.

PATIENTS AND METHODS

Patient material. Peripheral blood mononuclear cells (PBMC), synovial fluid mononuclear cells (SFMC), and bone marrow mononuclear cells (BMMC) were obtained from patients with RA who fulfilled the American College of Rheumatology (formerly, the American Rheumatism Association) criteria for RA (13).

Antibodies. The enrichment cocktail for human B cells and magnetic colloid were obtained from Stemcell Technologies (Vancouver, British Columbia, Canada) and monoclonal antibodies against CD3, CD14, CD19, CD20, and CD38 were obtained from Becton Dickinson (Mountain View, CA). The peptides cfc1-cyc2-biotin and cfc1-cyc2, in which arginine residues were substituted with citrulline (9), were used for measurement of IgM–anti-CCP by ELISA. The antibodies used for detection of IgM and IgM–anti-CCP were purchased from the following sources: anti-IgM (HB57) from American Type Culture Collection (Rockville, MD), horseradish peroxidase (HRP)–conjugated and alkaline phosphatase (AP)–conjugated anti-IgM from Dako (Glostrup, Denmark), and biotinylated goat (Fab_2)–anti-IgM from Tago Immunologicals (Burlingame, CA).

Cells and culture conditions. PBMC, SFMC, and BMMC were obtained by separation on Ficoll-Hypaque density gradient centrifugation (ρ = 1.077 gm/ml; Pharmacia Biotech, Uppsala, Sweden) and frozen in liquid nitrogen until used. PBMC and SFMC were thawed and incubated with the Stemsep enrichment cocktail for human B cells, followed by incubation with magnetic colloid (using standard Stemcell Technologies procedures). B cells were negatively selected using the gravity feed Stemsep column system (Stemcell Technologies), and the cells obtained contained >95% B cells, <1% CD3+ cells, and <3% CD14+ cells, as determined by fluorescence-activated cell sorter analysis (results not shown).

The mouse fibroblast L cells, stable-transfected with CD40 ligand (L-CD40L cells), were described before (14) and were cultured in Iscove's modified Dulbecco's medium with glutamax (IMDM; Gibco, Breda, The Netherlands) supplemented with 10% (volume/volume) heat-inactivated fetal calf serum (FCS; Bodinco, Alkmaar, The Netherlands), 100 IU/ml penicillin, and 100 μg/ml streptomycin (Boehringer Mannheim, Mannheim, Germany). Ten thousand purified B cells were cultured on a layer of 5,000 70-Gy γ-irradiated L-CD40L cells in 96-well flat-bottom tissue culture plates, in the presence of cytokines in a total volume of 200 μl IMDM/10% FCS with penicillin/streptomycin at 37°C, 5% CO_2. Culture supernatants were harvested after 14 days and analyzed for IgM and IgM–anti-CCP by ELISA.

Autoreactive T cell clone K15. The SF autoreactive CD4+ T cell clone was derived from a T cell line of a patient with RA that responded to autologous SF in vitro as described previously in detail (15). To maintain the T cell clone, T cells (3×10^5/ml) were stimulated weekly with 1 μg/ml phytohemagglutinin (Murex Diagnostics, Dartford, England) and cultured in the presence of irradiated allogeneic PBMC (10^6/well, 30 Gy) and a B lymphoblastoid cell line (10^5/well, 50 Gy) in 24-well tissue culture plates (Greiner, Alphen a/d Rijn, The Netherlands) at 37°C, 5% CO_2. Culture medium (IMDM) was supplemented with 10% (v/v) FCS (Bodinco), 100 IU/ml penicillin, 100 μg/ml streptomycin (Boehringer Mannheim), and 10 units/ml interleukin-2 (IL-2; Cetus, Gouda, The Netherlands). Rested T cells were frozen in liquid nitrogen until further use.

Quantitation of Ig. Total IgM concentrations in the culture supernatants were determined by ELISA as described previously (16). The detection limit was 1 ng/ml.

IgM–anti-CCP was measured in a modified version of the previously described peptide-based anti-CCP ELISA (9). Peptides were covalently coupled to 96-well assay plates (Costar, Cambridge, MA) at 1 μg/ml, pH 9.0, at 4°C overnight. Wells were blocked with 2% bovine serum albumin (BSA; Sigma, St. Louis, MO) for 1 hour at room temperature. Further incubations were also performed at room temperature and wells were washed between incubations with phosphate buffered saline (PBS)/0.05% (v/v) Tween 20 (PBS/Tw20). Supernatants were diluted 4-fold in 1% BSA, 350 m*M* NaCl, 10 m*M* Tris HCl, pH 7.6, 1% (v/v) Triton X-100, 0.1% sodium dodecyl sulfate, and incubated for 1.5 hours. A control serum was used to monitor plate-to-plate variation, with the results expressed in arbitrary units.

For detection of background staining, culture medium was used. After washing, the wells were successively incubated with 100 μl of biotinylated goat (Fab_2)–anti-IgM (10 μg/ml), streptavidin-HRP (Zymed Laboratories, San Francisco, CA), biotin-tyramine (Sigma), and again streptavidin-HRP. Finally, the bound antibody was detected using 3,3′-5,5′-methylbenzidine (Sigma) as a substrate. The color reaction was stopped after 10 minutes by adding 10% (v/v) H_2SO_4 and read in the ELISA reader at 450 nm.

Enzyme-linked immunospot assay (ELISpot) analysis. The frequency of IgM- and IgM–anti-CCP–producing cells was determined by ELISpot. Nitrocellulose plates (Millipore, Bedford, MA) were coated overnight at 4°C with 100 μl anti-IgM (10 μg/ml) or streptavidin (1 μg/ml) diluted in PBS. For the IgM–anti-CCP ELISpot, plates were washed and incubated for 3 hours with cfc1-cyc2-biotin. After washing the plates with PBS and blocking with IMDM/10% FCS, the wells were incubated overnight with B cells in IMDM/10% FCS. The cells were removed the next day and the plates were washed with PBS and PBS/Tw20 followed by incubation with biotinylated antibody, goat (Fab_2)-anti-IgM (10 μg/ml) for IgM in PBS/Tw20/BSA (1%), and AP-conjugated anti-IgM for IgM–anti-CCP for 1 hour at 37°C. After extensively washing with PBS/Tw20, IgM plates were incubated with ExtrAvidin-alkaline for 1 hour at room temperature, followed by washing with PBS/Tw20 and PBS. The color reaction was initiated with BCIP–nitroblue tetrazolium (Sigma). The color reaction was terminated with tap water. Spots were counted using a binocular microscope (M3Z; Wild, Heerbrugg, Switzerland).

Statistical analysis. Differences in IgM and IgM–anti-CCP levels between patients with RA and healthy control subjects were tested by a Mann-Whitney U test.

RESULTS

In vitro generation of anti-CCP antibodies by PB B cells. In vitro production of anti-CCP antibodies by B cells derived from the circulation of 8 patients with RA was examined. For that purpose, highly purified PB B cells were cultured in the presence or absence of L-CD40L cells and IL-10 or anti-CD3–activated T cells. After 14 days of culture, Ig production was determined by ELISA. No detectable levels of IgM–anti-CCP could be found in PB B cells cultured in the absence of fibroblasts or T cells, and production of IgM remained low or not detectable (results not shown). Coculture of PB B cells with L-CD40L cells and IL-10 resulted in production of IgM and IgM–anti-CCP (Figure 1A). Similar results were obtained when PB B cells were cultured with anti-CD3–activated T cells.

To determine whether the IgM–anti-CCP–producing capacity of RA PB B cells differed from that of the PB B cells derived from healthy controls, the same conditions as above were applied to the control B cells (n = 9) and supernatants were analyzed for Ig production (Figure 1B). These experiments revealed essentially similar results as found for RA PB B cells. However, PB B cell cultures from patients with RA showed higher levels of IgM–anti-CCP compared with that in control B cell cultures (2.6-fold higher [$P = 0.016$] and 1.5-fold higher [$P = 0.897$] in the CD40 and T cell activation systems, respectively), whereas the amount of total IgM was lower in B cell cultures from patients with RA

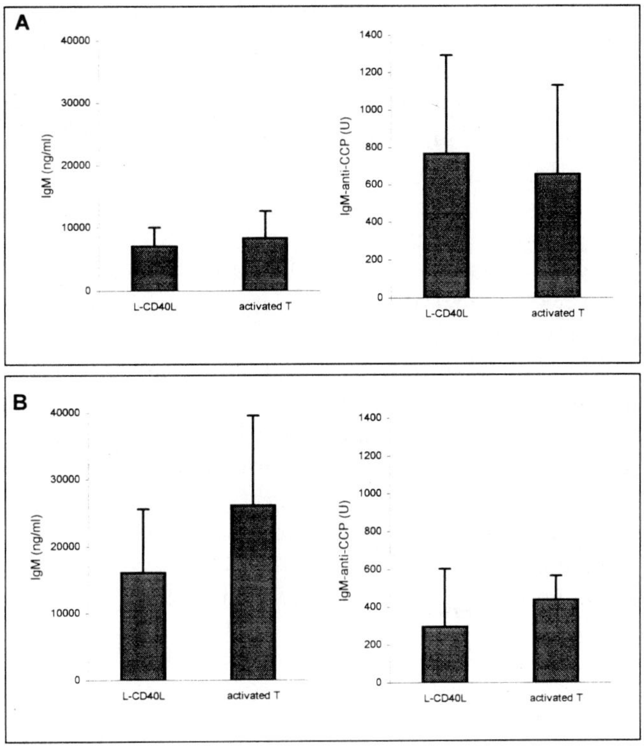

Figure 1. In vitro generation of anti–citrulline-containing peptide (anti-CCP) antibodies. Ten thousand peripheral blood B cells derived from **A,** patients with rheumatoid arthritis (RA) or **B,** healthy controls were cultured either with 5×10^3 irradiated L cells stable-transfected with CD40 ligand (L-CD40L) plus interleukin-10 (50 ng/ml) or with 1×10^5 anti-CD3 (50 μg/ml)–activated T cells for 14 days. IgM and IgM–anti-CCP production was measured by enzyme-linked immunosorbent assay. Bars show the mean and SD of 8 patients with RA and 9 healthy controls.

compared with that in control subjects (2.3-fold lower [$P = 0.043$] in the CD40 activation system and 3-fold lower [$P = 0.020$] with activated T cells) (Figure 1B). These results do not provide evidence for the presence of constitutive production of anti-CCP by B cells in the circulation of patients with RA, but do show that precursor B cells with the potential to produce anti-CCP are present in the PB B cell compartment of both patients with RA and healthy controls.

Anti-CCP antibody production by SF B cells. We next studied anti-CCP production by paired PB and SF B cells from 7 anti-CCP–seropositive and 4 anti-CCP–seronegative patients with RA. For this analysis, purified B cells were cultured in the absence or presence of L-CD40L and IL-10. Similar to the findings in PB B cells (Figure 2A), SF B cells from both anti-CCP–seropositive and anti-CCP–seronegative patients produced IgM

(2,450 ± 1,393 ng/ml and 1,846 ± 193 ng/ml, respectively) and IgM–anti-CCP (980 ± 654 units and 354 ± 136 units, respectively) when cultured with L-CD40L and IL-10 (Figure 2B). In contrast to PB B cells, SF B cells derived from seropositive patients with RA produced IgM–anti-CCP after 14 days of culture in the absence of a stimulus (24 ± 20 units in PB versus 314 ± 160 units in SF). Culture supernatants of SF B cells from anti-CCP–seronegative patients did not contain detectable IgM–anti-CCP after culture without additional stimuli (22 ± 3 units). This suggests that B cells with the potential to produce anti-CCP antibodies are present in the SF of patients who are either seropositive or seronegative for anti-CCP antibodies, but that spontaneous production of anti-CCP by B cells is restricted to the SF of anti-CCP–seropositive patients.

Frequency of spontaneous IgM–anti-CCP–secreting cells in SF and BM. To further investigate spontaneous production of IgM–anti-CCP in SF B cells,

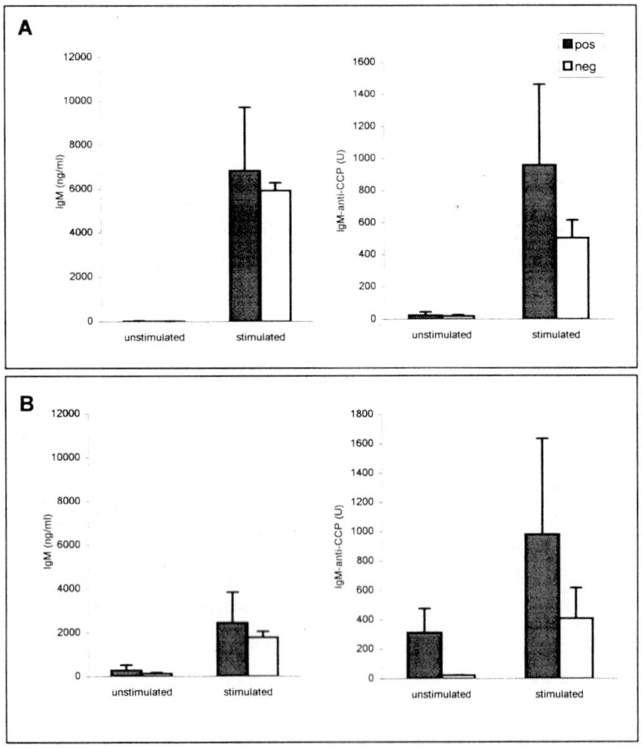

Figure 2. Ig production by peripheral blood (PB) B cells and synovial fluid (SF) B cells. Ten thousand PB B cells (**A**) and SF B cells (**B**) from 7 seropositive (pos) patients with rheumatoid arthritis and 4 seronegative (neg) patients were cultured with or without 5×10^3 irradiated L cells stable-transfected with CD40 ligand plus interleukin-10 (50 ng/ml). IgM and IgM–anti–citrulline-containing peptide (anti-CCP) antibody production were measured by enzyme-linked immunosorbent assay. Bars show the mean and SD.

Table 1. Frequencies of IgM-producing synovial fluid cells with anti–citrulline-containing peptide antibody (anti-CCP) activity*

Patient	Disease	Medication	Serum	Anti-CCP frequency
1	RA	N + D	+	1:8
2	RA	N + D	+	1:4
3	RA	D	+	1:41
4	RA	N + D	+	1:8
5	RA	N	+	1:7
6	RA	N + D	+	1:9
7	RA	D	+	1:12
8	RA	N + D	+	1:27
9	RA	N + D	–	–
10	RA	N	–	–
11	RA	–	–	–
12	RA	N + D	–	–
13	RA	N	+	1:34

* RA = rheumatoid arthritis; N = nonsteroidal antiinflammatory drug; D = disease-modifying antirheumatic drug (no corticosteroids or cytotoxic drugs).

ELISpot analysis was performed. Purified SF B cells were serially diluted and incubated on CCP-coated nitrocellulose. After 16 hours of incubation, the ELISpot was developed. IgM and IgM–anti-CCP–positive spots were counted and frequencies of citrulline-specific cells were calculated. SF B cells from 9 RA patients seropositive for anti-CCP antibodies (patients 1–8 and 13 in Table 1) and 4 anti-CCP–seronegative patients (patients 9–12) were tested. SF B cells derived from anti-CCP–seropositive patients were capable of secreting IgM–anti-CCP, and the frequency of anti-CCP–producing cells ranged from 1:4 to 1:41 of IgM-producing cells. Although SF B cells from anti-CCP–seronegative patients actively produced IgM antibodies, cells with anti-CCP specificity were not detected (<1:150, 1:178, 1:266, and 1:50 of IgM-producing cells). The results from the ELISpot analysis 1) confirm the results on the selective presence of spontaneous anti-CCP–producing B cells in the SF B cell cultures of anti-CCP–seropositive patients with RA, and 2) reveal that the percentage of anti-CCP–producing cells may range from 2.4% to 25% of the IgM-producing cells.

We next studied whether the BM of anti-CCP–seropositive RA patients contained plasma cells that actively secreted anti-CCP antibodies. Similar to the findings in SF B cells, we determined the presence of spontaneous IgM- and IgM–anti-CCP–producing BM cells by ELISpot. BM cells from 4 patients with anti-CCP–seropositive RA (patients 15–18 in Table 2) and, as negative controls, BM cells from 3 patients with anti-CCP–seronegative RA (patients 14, 21, and 22), from 1 patient with scleroderma (patient 19), and from 1 patient with undifferentiated arthritis (patient 20)

Table 2. Frequencies of IgM-producing bone marrow cells with anti-CCP activity*

Patient	Disease	Medication	Serum	Anti-CCP frequency
14	RA	N + D	–	–
15	RA	N + D	+	1:5
16	RA	N + D	+	1:6
17	RA	D	+	1:46
18	RA	N + D	+	1:39
19	Scleroderma	N	–	–
20	Undifferentiated arthritis	–	–	–
21	RA	N	–	–
22	RA	N + D	–	–

* See Table 1 for definitions.

were analyzed. The results revealed that the anti-CCP–seropositive patients with RA contained actively secreting IgM–anti-CCP cells. The frequencies of the anti-CCP–secreting BM cells ranged from 1:5 to 1:46 of IgM-secreting cells. As anticipated, actively producing anti-CCP–positive B cells were not detected in the BM samples of the anti-CCP–seronegative patients.

Together, these results demonstrate the presence of active secretion of anti-CCP by both SF and BM plasma cells in anti-CCP–seropositive patients with RA.

DISCUSSION

One of the characteristics of RA is the presence of autoantibodies in the circulation. These autoantibodies might directly contribute to the inflammatory response (6). In addition to RF, autoantibodies directed against citrullinated peptides are of diagnostic and predictive value in RA (9,17). These autoantibodies are strongly associated with RA, with a published specificity of 95–100% (9). Despite the correlation of these autoantibodies with RA, our data demonstrate that anti-CCP precursors are present not only in the circulation of patients with RA, but also in the B cell repertoire of healthy subjects. PB B cells only produce detectable anti-CCP antibodies upon activation. In contrast, the SF and BM compartments of anti-CCP–seropositive RA patients contain a population of B cells that actively produce anti-CCP antibodies in the absence of a stimulus. By means of ELISpot we were able to determine that 2.2–25% of the IgM-producing cells in both SF and BM are active anti-CCP–secreting B cells.

The systems we have used allow evaluation of the PB B cell repertoire under conditions of non–antigen-specific activation. No production of anti-CCP antibodies could be detected in any of the PB B cells tested in the absence of stimulation. Both coculture of B cells with anti-CD3–activated T cells and application of the CD40 activation system induced anti-CCP antibody production when using PB B cells. B cells from RA patients as well as healthy controls can be induced in vitro to produce anti-CCP antibodies in these systems. This observation supports the notion that the presence of anti-CCP precursors among each healthy control subject and each patient with RA tested is a normal component of the B cell repertoire. The capacity of PB B cells to produce increased anti-CCP antibody levels in patients with RA compared with healthy controls suggests a higher frequency of precursor cells or the presence of anti-CCP cells that respond more strongly following stimulation. The PB B cell compartment likely consists of self-reactive anti-CCP B cell precursors that circulate in a nonresponsive state which can be altered in vitro by T cell help. Clearly, the in vitro capacity of the PB B cells to produce anti-CCP does not correlate with the presence of circulating antibodies in the sera of the individuals tested, indicative that PB B cells are not directly involved in the production of circulating anti-CCP.

In contrast to the requirements for anti-CCP antibody production, RF production required coculture with activated T cells, but no detectable RF production occurred in the CD40 activation system (18). This indicates that anti-CCP and RF precursor B cells are probably in a different state of tolerance and require different activation conditions.

Differences in the conditions required to break tolerance in autoreactive B cells have been described for anti-DNA and anti-hen-egg lysozyme autoantibody–producing cells in transgenic mouse models (19). It appeared that the nature of the antigens for which these B cells were specific determined their responsiveness. This difference could be based on the capacity of antigens to interact with other proteins, thereby facilitating T cell help through T cell recognition against the interacting protein. Both anti-DNA (anti-DNA/DNA/exogenous binding proteins) and RF (anti-IgG/IgG/foreign antigen) fall in this bridging category.

Recently, we gained preliminary evidence that optimal T cell help for RF production is provided by T cells in a specific activation status (van Esch WJE, Reparon-Schuijt CC, and Verweij CL: unpublished observations). The anti-CCP response has requirements similar to that of the total Ig response, whereas the requirements for the RF response are different. Because of the difference in disease specificity between anti-CCP (95–100%) and RF (91%) (9,20), it is tempting to speculate that this is a reflection of functionally distinct precursor B cells that are regulated differentially.

The rheumatoid synovial compartment is known as an active site for the production of Ig and autoantibodies. The synovial tissue of RA patients contains germinal center (GC)–like structures that are thought to contribute to the local generation of antigen-specific memory B cells (CD20+,CD38−) and terminally differentiated plasma cells (CD20−,CD38+) (18,21), which constitute the predominant B lymphocyte subsets in the inflamed joint (mean ± SD 46.0 ± 24.0% and 45.8 ± 19.6%, respectively).

The results revealed that the BM compartment of anti-CCP–seropositive patients also contained active anti-CCP–secreting cells. These findings suggest that both the BM and the synovial compartment contain a population of B cells that actively contribute to circulating anti-CCP antibodies. These cells may have originated from precursor B cells present in the normal B cell repertoire. It is tempting to speculate that the SF B cells have locally matured into terminally differentiated antibody-secreting cells in the inflamed joint. Evidence exists that processes of clonal expansion, somatic mutation, and affinity selection take place in the ectopic synovial GC-like structures (22). Consequently, the relatively high proportion of anti-CCP–secreting cells in the synovial B cell compartment favors the local maturation of these cells as a consequence of an antigen-specific immune response. Memory B cells formed at the site of inflammation locally differentiate into anti-CCP antibody–producing plasma cells and/or enter the circulation and migrate into the BM, where they differentiate into anti-CCP–secreting plasma cells. Both the inflamed synovium and BM provide an ideal environment for high-level production and B cell survival (23).

Although anti-CCP autoantibodies were first identified as antifilaggrin antibodies, deiminated epidermal filaggrin (24) is not likely to be the autoantigen that drives the anti-CCP response in the RA synovium, since epidermis is not a target of rheumatoid inflammation. Knowing that peptidylarginine deiminase, the enzyme responsible for deimination of arginine, is expressed in a broad range of tissues and cell types (25,26), it is tempting to speculate that unknown deiminated antigens formed in the inflamed synovium drive the local antibody response. Insight into the local immune response that drives the maturation of anti-CCP–secreting B cells is essential for understanding the significance of the presence of anti-CCP and might provide insight into the etiology of RA.

REFERENCES

1. McCarthy DJ, Koopman WJ. Arthritis and allied conditions: a textbook of rheumatology. 12th ed. Philadelphia: Lea & Febiger; 1993.
2. Gregersen PK, Silver J, Winchester RJ. The shared epitope hypothesis: an approach to understanding the molecular genetics of susceptibility to rheumatoid arthritis. Arthritis Rheum 1987;30: 1205–13.
3. Nienhuis RLF, Mandema EA. A new serum factor in patients with rheumatoid arthritis. Ann Rheum Dis 1964;23:302–5.
4. Young BJJ, Mallya RK, Leslie RDJ, Clark CJM, Hamblin TJ. Anti-keratin antibodies in rheumatoid arthritis. BMJ 1979;2:97–9.
5. Bang H, Mollenhauer J, Schulmeister A, Nager C, van Eden W, Wand-Württenberger A, et al. Isolation and characterization of a cartilage-specific membrane antigen (CH65): comparison with cytokeratins and heat-shock proteins. Immunology 1994;81:322–9.
6. Carson DA, Chen PP, Fox RI, Kipps TJ, Jirik F, Goldfien RD, et al. Rheumatoid factor and immune networks. Annu Rev Immunol 1987;5:109–26.
7. Steiner G, Harmuth K, Skriner K, Maurer-Fogy I, Skinski A, Thalmann E, et al. Purification and partial sequencing of the nuclear autoantigen RA33 shows that it is indistinguishable from the A2 protein of the heterogeneous nuclear ribonucleoprotein complex. J Clin Invest 1992;90:1061–6.
8. Simon M, Girbal E, Sebbag M, Gomés-Daudrix V, Vincent C, Salema G, et al. Serre G. The cytokeratin filament-aggregating protein filaggrin is the target of the so called "antikeratin antibodies," autoantibodies specific for rheumatoid arthritis. J Clin Invest 1993;92:1387–93.
9. Schellekens GA, de Jong BAW, van den Hoogen FHJ, van de Putte LBA, van Venrooij WJ. Citrulline is an essential constituent of antigenic determinants recognized by rheumatoid arthritis-specific autoantibodies. J Clin Invest 1998;101:273–81.
10. Tarcsa E, Marekov LN, Mei G, Melino G, Lee SC, Steinert PM. Protein unfolding by peptidylarginine deiminase: substrate specificity and structural relationship of the natural substrates trichohyalin and filaggrin. J Biol Chem 1996;271:30709–17.
11. Girbal-Neuhauser E, Durieux JJ, Arnaud M, Dalbon P, Sebbag M, Vincent C, et al. The epitopes targeted by the rheumatoid arthritis-associated antifilaggrin autoantibodies are post-translationally generated on various sites of (pro)filaggrin by deimination of arginine residues. J Immunol 1999;162:585–94.
12. Vincent C, Simon M, Sebbag M, Girbal-Neuhauser E, Durieux JJ, Cantagrel A, et al. Immunoblotting detection of autoantibodies to human epidermis filaggrin: a new diagnostic test for rheumatoid arthritis. J Rheumatol 1998;25:838–46.
13. Arnett FC, Edworthy SM, Bloch DA, McShane DJ, Fries JF, Cooper NS, et al. The American Rheumatism Association 1987 revised criteria for the classification of rheumatoid arthritis. Arthritis Rheum 1988;31:315–24.
14. Garrone P, Neidhardt E-M, Garcia E, Galibert L, van Kooten C, Banchereau J. Fas ligation induces apoptosis of CD40-activated human B lymphocytes. J Exp Med 1995;182:1265–73.
15. Maurice MM, Res PCM, Leow A, van Hall T, Daha MR, Struijk P, et al. Joint-derived T cells in rheumatoid arthritis proliferate to antigens present in autologous synovial fluid. Scand J Rheumatol 1995;24:169–77.
16. Otten HG, Daha MR, Dolhain RJEM, de Rooy HH, Breedveld FC. Rheumatoid factor production by mononuclear cells derived from different sites of patients with rheumatoid arthritis. Clin Exp Immunol 1993;94:236–40.
17. Schellekens GA, Visser H, de Jong BAW, van den Hoogen FHJ,

Hazes JMW, Breedveld FC, et al. The diagnostic properties of rheumatoid arthritis antibodies recognizing a cyclic citrullinated peptide. Arthritis Rheum 2000;43:155–63.
18. Reparon-Schuijt CC, van Esch WJE, van Kooten C, Levarht EWN, Breedveld FC, Verweij CL. Functional analysis of rheumatoid factor–producing B cells from the synovial fluid of rheumatoid arthritis patients. Arthritis Rheum 1998;41:2211–20.
19. Goodnow CC, Brink R, Adams E. Breakdown of self-tolerance in anergic B lymphocytes. Nature 1991;352:532–6.
20. Hoet RM, van Venrooij WJ. The antiperinuclear factor and antikeratin antibodies in rheumatoid arthritis. In: Smolen JS, Kalden JR, Maini RN, editors. Rheumatoid arthritis. Berlin: Springer-Verlag; 1992. p. 299–318.
21. Reparon-Schuijt CC, van Esch WJE, van Kooten C, Rozier BCD, Levarht EWN, Breedveld FC, et al. Regulation of synovial B cell survival in rheumatoid arthritis by vascular cell adhesion molecule 1 (CD106) expressed on fibroblast-like synoviocytes. Arthritis Rheum 2000;43:1115–21.
22. Schröder AE, Greiner A, Seyfert C, Berek C. Differentiation of B cells in the nonlymphoid tissue of the synovial membrane of patients with rheumatoid arthritis. Proc Natl Acad Sci U S A 1996;93:221–5.
23. Merville P, Dechanet J, Desmouliere A, Durand I, de Bouteiller O, Garrone P, et al. Bcl-2^+ tonsillar plasma cells are rescued from apoptosis by bone marrow fibroblasts. J Exp Med 1996;183: 227–36.
24. Senshu T, Kan S, Ogawa H, Manabe M, Asaga H. Preferential deimination of keratin K1 and filaggrin during the terminal differentiation of human epidermis. Biochem Biophys Res Commun 1996;225:712–9.
25. Sugawara K, Oikawa Y, Ouchi T. Identification and properties of peptidylarginine deiminase from rabbit skeletal muscle. J Biol Chem 1982;91:1065–71.
26. Lamensa JWE, Moscarello MA. Deimination of human myelin basic protein by a peptidylarginine deiminase from bovine brain. J Neurochem 1993;61:987–96.

ARTHRITIS & RHEUMATISM
Vol. 44, No. 1, January 2001, pp 48–52

The Influence of Synovial Fluid on Adenovirus-Mediated Gene Transfer to the Synovial Tissue

Paulien H. Goossens,[1] Ronald Vogels,[2] Elsbet Pieterman,[1] Menzo J. E. Havenga,[2] Abraham Bout,[2] Ferdinand C. Breedveld,[1] Dinko Valerio,[2] and Tom W. J. Huizinga[1]

Objective. To determine the effect of synovial fluid (SF) from rheumatoid arthritis (RA) patients on adenovirus type 5 (Ad5)–mediated gene transfer to synoviocytes, and to explore new strategies for vector development based on the neutralization data obtained.

Methods. SF was derived from 63 randomly selected RA patients. Ten samples were used to study the effect of SF on Ad5-mediated gene transfer in synoviocytes. IgG and <100-kd fractions were purified from these 10 SF, and their effect on gene transfer was determined. Neutralizing activity against wild-type Ad5 (wt-Ad5), wt-Ad26, wt-Ad34, wt-Ad35, and wt-Ad48 was tested in the SF from the remaining 53 patients.

Results. Seven of 10 SF samples inhibited Ad5-mediated gene transfer. Purified antibodies exhibited inhibition patterns similar to those seen with unfractionated SF. In 5 of 10 SF samples, low molecular weight fractions inhibited gene transfer at low dilutions. Neutralization of wt-Ad35 by SF from RA patients was less frequent than neutralization of other wt-Ad tested (4% versus 42–72%; n = 53).

Conclusion. SF from 70% of the RA patients contained neutralizing antibodies that hamper Ad5-mediated gene transfer to synoviocytes. The activity of neutralizing antibodies may be circumvented in the majority of RA patients when vectors based on an Ad35 backbone are used.

Supported in part by the Dutch Organization for Scientific Research (project 940-37-001).

[1]Paulien H. Goossens, MD, Elsbet Pieterman, PhD, Ferdinand C. Breedveld, MD, Tom W. J. Huizinga, MD: Leiden University Medical Center, Leiden, The Netherlands; [2]Ronald Vogels, MD, Menzo J. E. Havenga, PhD, Abraham Bout, PhD, Dinko Valerio, PhD: Crucell BV, Leiden, The Netherlands.

Address correspondence and reprint requests to Tom W. J. Huizinga, MD, Department of Rheumatology, Leiden University Medical Center, C4-R, PO Box 9600, 2300 RC Leiden, The Netherlands.

Submitted for publication June 5, 2000; accepted in revised form September 6, 2000.

It has been demonstrated that adenovirus serotype 5 (Ad5)–based vectors can deliver genes to the synovial tissue after intraarticular administration in various animal models for rheumatoid arthritis (RA), such as mouse, guinea pig, rabbit, and nonhuman primate models (1–4). However, there are several problems with the use of the current-generation adenovirus vectors. There is considerable concern that high doses of these vectors can induce inflammation. Data from mouse studies indicate that systemic in vivo gene transfer with adenoviral vectors is successful only in the absence of antibodies against the adenovirus used (5). On the other hand, adenoviral vectors have advantages over other therapeutic vectors, including efficient delivery of genes to both dividing and nondividing target cells, and high levels of gene expression. The ideal adenoviral vector for gene transfer to the synovium is one that can efficiently infect the synovial tissue, is not immunogenic, does not induce inflammation in the synovium, and can be administered repeatedly.

Many different strategies to improve adenoviral vectors or methods of delivery are under investigation. The present study focused on the effect of synovial fluid (SF) on efficiency of gene transfer. The results indicated that 70% of patients with RA had neutralizing antibodies against Ad5 in their SF. Thus, only in 30% of the patients was Ad5-mediated gene transfer not hampered by the antibody response. This highlights the need for new strategies for vector development. It may be possible to circumvent the neutralizing activity of the SF by using an adenovirus derived from an alternative serotype that is not associated with high neutralizing activity. We therefore analyzed the neutralizing activity of the RA patients' SF against different serotypes of wild-type adenovirus (wt-Ad).

PATIENTS AND METHODS

Patients, SF samples, and serum samples. SF samples were obtained from 63 selected patients with RA according to the criteria of the American College of Rheumatology (formerly, the American Rheumatism Association) (6). Serum was collected simultaneously with the SF in 39 of the 63 patients. The RA patients were classified according to disease severity. Severe disease was defined as erosive, rheumatoid factor (RF)–positive disease for which at least 2 disease-modifying antirheumatic drugs (DMARDs) had been taken. Mild disease was defined as nonerosive, RF-negative disease for which ≤1 DMARD had been taken. If a patient's RA did not fulfill the criteria for severe or mild disease, the disease activity was defined as intermediate.

Ten SF samples (from 6 women and 4 men, mean age 56 years, 50% RF positive, mean disease duration 12 years) were used to study inhibition of gene transfer. Samples from the remaining 53 patients (38 women and 15 men, mean age 61 years, 75% RF positive, mean disease duration 13 years) were used to study inhibition of different wt-Ad in SF. Sterile SF was collected in 50-ml tubes containing 100 μl heparin (5,000 IU/ml; Leo Pharmaceutical, Weesp, The Netherlands). Serum was collected in heparin tubes (150 USH per tube; Becton Dickinson, Plymouth, UK). The tubes were centrifuged at 1,500 revolutions per minute for 20 minutes at 4°C. The supernatant was collected and stored at –20°C until use.

Synoviocytes. Synovial tissue was obtained from RA patients at the time of joint replacement surgery and was collected in sterile phosphate buffered saline (PBS). Synovial tissue was digested with 1 mg/ml collagenase IA (Sigma, St. Louis, MO) at 37°C for 2 hours. Cells were cultured in Iscove's modified Dulbecco's medium (IMDM) supplemented with glutamine (Life Technologies, Paisley, Scotland) and 10% fetal calf serum (FCS) at 37°C in a 5% CO_2 incubator.

Adenoviral vectors. The recombinant Ad5 vector used in this study contains the luciferase gene inserted into the E1 region, thereby rendering it replication defective. The vector IG.Ad5.clip.luc contains the nucleotides −601 to −14 of the wild-type cytomegalovirus promoter sequence and the SV40 intron/polyA from pcDNA1/amp (*Hha* I–*Avr* II fragment; Invitrogen, Carlsbad, CA). The vectors were generated and produced in PER.C6 cells (7), thereby avoiding the formation of replication-competent adenovirus. The production yield, as determined by high-performance liquid chromatography (8), was 1.6×10^{12} virus particles (VP)/ml. The concentration of infective units, as determined by end point titration on 911 cells, was 2.4×10^{11} infective units/ml (9).

Gene transfer experiments. The day prior to infection, synovial cells were plated at a density of 15,000 per well (12-well plate; Cellstar Greiner, Alphen a/d Rijn, The Netherlands) in 1 ml of IMDM–10% FCS. At infection, the medium was replaced by SF in concentrations ranging from 1:4 to 1:2,048, mixed with 5,000 VP of IG.Ad5.clip.luc per synoviocyte in IMDM–10% FCS. After 24 hours, the cells were washed twice and incubated in IMDM–10% FCS. Three days postinfection, the synoviocytes were lysed with 100 μl of lysis buffer (Promega, Madison, WI). Luciferase counts in 20 μl of the lysate were determined by luminometric methods, as described by the supplier (Promega). Experiments were repeated 2 additional times. The average SF concentration that resulted in ≥50% inhibition of gene expression was calculated.

Purification of immunoglobulins. SF was centrifuged at 7,000 rpm for 20 minutes at 4°C. The supernatant was filtered through a 0.45-μm filter (Schleicher & Schuell, Dassel, Germany) and the remnant was centrifuged again after precipitation with 50% $(NH_4)_2SO_4$. The pellet was dissolved in H_2O and dialyzed against PBS (pH 7.0) twice for at least 4 hours at 4°C. The dialyzed SF was supplemented to a quantity of 5 ml with PBS and put on a Hi Trap protein–G Sepharose column (Pharmacia LKB, Erlangen, Germany). The column was washed with 5 ml 20 m*M* $NaPO_4$ (pH 7.0). IgG was washed off the column using 9 ml of 0.1*M* glycine-HCl (pH 2.7). One-milliliter fractions of the eluate were collected in tubes containing 60 μl of 1*M* Tris (pH 9.0). All fractions were measured with a photospectrometer at 280 nm, and the elution fractions with the highest optical density (OD) were dialyzed overnight against PBS at 4°C. The fractions were sterilized using a 0.22-μm filter and reconstituted to initial SF volumes with PBS. All fractions were stored at –20°C until analysis. Inhibition of gene transfer by the IgG fraction was studied similarly to the study of inhibition by complete SF. The purity of the IgG fraction was confirmed by sodium dodecyl sulfate–polyacrylamide gel electrophoresis (SDS-PAGE). A 10% nondenaturing gel (Bio-Rad, Hercules, CA) was used to avoid disintegration of the immunoglobulin chains. Ten-microgram samples were placed on the gel for 1 hour (50 mA) and stained with Coomassie brilliant blue (Mallickrodt Baker, Phillipsburg, NJ).

Purification of low molecular weight fractions. SF was centrifuged at 7,000 rpm for 20 minutes at 4°C. Four milliliters of the supernatant was placed on an Amicon-100 filter (Amicon, Beverly, MA) and spun for 3 hours at 1,000*g* at 4°C. The fractions obtained were sterilized using a 0.22-μm filter. The <100-kd concentration that resulted in ≥50% inhibition of gene expression as compared with medium was determined.

Wild-type adenoviruses. The inhibition of wt-Ad was tested in a replicating system. Replication of wt-Ad on cells leads to a cytopathic effect and cell death (10). When the SF neutralizes the wt-Ad, the Ad can no longer infect the cells and no cytopathic effect is seen. In this study, wt-Ad in a quantity that gives a cytopathic effect on PER.C6 cells in 5 days was preincubated for 30 minutes in diluted SF from RA patients. After preincubation, 5×10^4 PER.C6 cells were added. Final dilutions of SF ranged from 1:4 to 1:64. Five days later, cell viability was measured with the MTT assay (Promega). The minimum concentration of SF (expressed as percentage SF) causing ≥50% inhibition of cytopathic effect or cell death was calculated.

RESULTS

Effect of SF on adenovirus-mediated gene transfer. The effect of SF on Ad5-mediated gene transfer to synoviocytes was tested in SF from 10 different RA

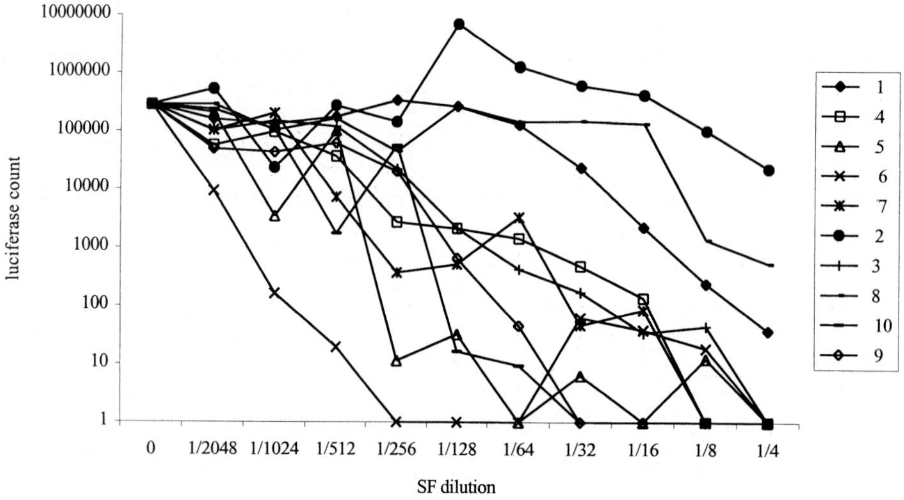

Figure 1. Influence of synovial fluid (SF) on gene transfer. Synoviocytes were incubated overnight with 5,000 virus particles of IG.Ad5.clip.luc per cell in SF diluted in Iscove's modified Dulbecco's medium–10% fetal calf serum. Three days postinfection, luciferase activity was measured. Each line represents SF from 1 rheumatoid arthritis patient; patient numbers correspond to those in Table 1.

patients (Figure 1), and the concentration of SF that induced ≥50% inhibition of gene expression was determined (Table 1). SF from at least 7 patients showed inhibition of gene transfer as compared with incubation of the vectors in medium. In 6 of 7 SF samples, inhibition of Ad5-mediated gene transfer was seen at high dilutions (≥1:1,024).

Effect of immunoglobulin fractions on gene transfer. To determine the effect of the IgG fraction, IgG fractions were purified from the SF with a protein G–Sepharose column. Eluted fractions with highest OD at 280 nm (mean ± SD OD_{280} after 10× sample dilution 2.3 ± 0.4) were collected and reconstituted to initial volumes. Purity of the IgG fractions was confirmed by SDS-PAGE (results not shown). Purified IgG fractions inhibited gene transfer to synoviocytes in a pattern that showed a high resemblance to the inhibition pattern of the complete SF (Table 1). As a control, the neutralizing effect of the SF that did not stick to the column was determined. Figure 2 shows a representative example of this experiment (patient 5). The IgG-depleted SF inhibited gene transgene expres-

Table 1. Neutralization of IG.Ad5.clip.luc*

Patient	SF	IgG Fraction	<100-kd Fraction
1	1:64	1:256	–
2	1:4	1:16	–
3	1:2,048	1:1,024	1:4
4	1:1,024	1:1,024	1:4
5	1:2,048	1:1,024	1:4
6	1:2,048	1:2,048	1:16
7	1:1,024	1:1,024	–
8	1:16	1:64	1:4
9	1:256	1:128	–
10	1:2,048	1:1,024	–

* Synoviocytes were incubated overnight with 5,000 virus particles of IG.Ad5.clip.luc per cell in synovial fluid (SF) or in the IgG or <100-kd fraction of SF, diluted in Iscove's modified Dulbecco's medium–10% fetal calf serum. Three days postinfection, the dilution that resulted in ≥50% inhibition of luciferase gene expression was determined.

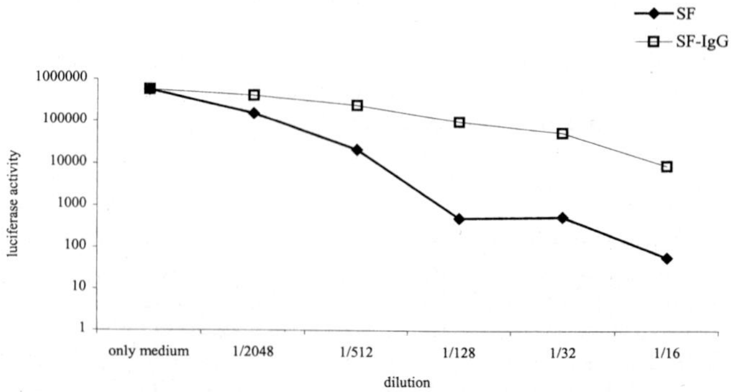

Figure 2. Effect of IgG-depleted synovial fluid (SF-IgG) versus whole SF on adenovirus 5–mediated gene transfer. Results shown are from a representative patient (patient 5).

sion far less than the initial SF. The remaining inhibition can probably be explained by the incomplete removal of the IgG and possible other inhibiting fractions in the SF.

Effect of low molecular weight fractions on gene transfer. In order to obtain a fraction that contains proteases but no immunoglobulin, a <100-kd fraction was purified from the SF. Low molecular weight fractions inhibited gene transfer at concentrations of up to 1:16 in 5 of 10 patients (Table 1).

Influence of the SF on wt-Ad5. The same 10 samples of SF that were used to test the effect on gene transfer were used to test the effect of SF on infection by wt-Ad5. The 6 SF samples that inhibited gene transfer at dilution of ≥1:1,024 also neutralized the wt-Ad5 at the highest dilution. The 2 samples of SF with the lowest titer of inhibition of gene transfer (patients 2 and 8) did not neutralize wt-Ad. The 2 samples of SF with intermediate titers of inhibition of gene transfer (patients 1 and 9) also neutralized wt-Ad5 at intermediate titers.

Relationship of neutralizing activity against wt-Ad5 in the SF and that in the serum. The correlation between neutralizing activity against Ad5 in SF and serum was studied in 39 RA patients. Twenty-nine patients (74%) exhibited neutralizing activity against wt-Ad5 in both SF and serum. SF and serum of 9 patients (23%) did not neutralize wt-Ad5. In 1 patient, the serum neutralized wt-Ad5 whereas the SF did not. These results indicate that it is possible to predict the Ad5-neutralizing activity of the SF by testing the patient's serum.

To investigate a possible correlation between disease severity and antibody titer, RA patients were classified according to disease severity. No differences in neutralizing activity between any of the disease severity groups were observed (Table 2).

Influence of the SF on different wild-type adenoviruses. To explore new strategies for the development of gene therapy vectors, the neutralization of different wt-Ad was determined in SF samples from 53 RA patients (Table 3). Strikingly, in the vast majority of the SF samples, wt-Ad35 was not neutralized. For the other wild-type viruses that were tested, a significant percentage of the SF samples showed neutralizing activity.

Table 2. Neutralizing activity against wild-type adenovirus 5 in the synovial fluid, by severity of rheumatoid arthritis*

Disease severity	No neutralizing activity (n = 15)	Neutralizing activity (n = 38)
Mild	1 (6.7)	4 (10.5)
Intermediate	6 (40)	11 (28.9)
Severe	5 (33.3)	16 (42.1)
Unknown	3 (20)	7 (18.4)

* Values are the number of patients (% of total no-neutralizing-activity or neutralizing-activity group).

Table 3. Inhibition of various wild-type adenoviruses (Ad) by synovial fluid*

Adenovirus	No inhibition	1:4–1:16	1:16–1:64	>1:64
Ad5	15	3	4	31
Ad26	18	11	6	18
Ad34	29	6	8	10
Ad35	51	1	1	0
Ad48	31	18	2	2

* Values are the number of patients in whom a dilution resulted in ≥50% inhibition of cytopathic effect or cell death.

DISCUSSION

This study focused on the effect of SF on gene transfer to synoviocytes. The commonly used adenoviral vector for gene therapy protocols is based on adenovirus type 5 (11). Our results show that neutralizing antibodies in the SF are responsible for blocking Ad5-mediated gene transfer to synoviocytes. Furthermore, we found that SF from 72% of the RA patients contained neutralizing antibodies against Ad5. In contrast, SF from only 4% of the RA patients contained neutralizing antibodies against Ad35, and these were found in low titer. Therefore, it may be possible to overcome neutralization when Ad35-based vectors are used.

The effect of SF on Ad5-mediated gene transfer was tested in samples from 10 randomly selected RA patients. It was found that SF from 7 patients inhibited gene transfer at low SF concentrations, whereas all SF inhibited gene transfer to some extent at higher SF concentrations. Experiments with wt-Ad5 in a replication system (see Patients and Methods) confirmed the neutralization of Ad5 by SF. In this assay no neutralization was detected in the SF of 2 patients, whereas in the luciferase inhibition assay low neutralizing titers were found. Since the recombinant adenoviral vector and the wild-type adenoviral vector do not differ in protein shell, we would not expect differences in neutralization between the replicating virus and the recombinant adenovirus. Thus, it appears that the test used to estimate the neutralization of wild-type adenovirus, which depends on cytopathic effect and cell death, is less sensitive than the luciferase activity assay.

In order to determine the cause of inhibition, an

IgG fraction and a <100-kd fraction were separated from the SF. The IgG fractions inhibited gene transfer with inhibition patterns similar to those observed with the complete SF. It was concluded that IgG directed against Ad5 plays a major role in the inhibitory effect of SF. However, other SF components besides immunoglobulin, such as proteases, may also play a role in the inhibition of gene transfer. Because the fallthrough of proteinase G columns may contain some overload IgG, we purified a fraction from the SF with a molecular weight of <100 kd, thus containing the proteases (<100 kd) but not the immunoglobulin (~150 kd). The low molecular weight fractions inhibited gene transfer only at high concentrations in 50% of the patients. In addition, high molecular weight fractions, such as macromolecules or fibrin, may inhibit in vivo gene transfer. We suggest that lavage of the joint prior to injection of the vector may increase infection efficiency by removal of proteases and other inhibitory molecules in the SF.

The neutralizing antibodies in the SF pose a problem because it is likely that they will hamper in vivo Ad5-mediated gene transfer to the human synovium. It does not appear that joint lavage would effectively remove all neutralizing antibodies, since gene transfer is inhibited even at low SF concentrations (≤1:1,024). Our study shows that the presence of antibodies against Ad5 in the serum of the patient can accurately predict the presence of antibodies in the SF. Therefore, we suggest that patients with antibodies to Ad5 found in the serum should be excluded from studies which aim at Ad5-mediated transfer of genes to the synovial tissue.

One might hypothesize that the titer of antibodies against Ad5 depends on the severity of the RA. However, the percentage of RA patients with neutralizing antibodies in their serum is comparable with that in the general population. Furthermore, we found no correlation between Ad5-neutralizing activity and disease severity. These results indicate that Ad5-neutralizing activity in SF will also pose problems in diseases other than RA. Based on the findings in this study, one would predict that Ad5-mediated gene transfer would be successful in only ~30% of patients with RA. Therefore, new strategies for vector development need to be explored. We found that neutralizing activity against wt-Ad35 in the SF was less frequent (4% of RA patients) than that against other wt-Ad tested (42–72% of RA patients). Furthermore, we demonstrated that neutralization of wt-Ad5 correlates well with neutralization of Ad5-based vectors. This indicates that use of Ad35-based vectors can circumvent the problem of neutralization by the SF.

In conclusion, optimal gene transfer to synoviocytes with current adenoviral vectors seems possible only in patients who lack antibodies to Ad5. Lavage of the joints of RA patients without antibodies prior to injection of the vector may enhance efficiency of gene transfer. In order to circumvent the effect of neutralizing antibodies in the SF, we suggest that vectors based on an Ad35 backbone are the most suitable tool for gene transfer to human synovial tissue.

ACKNOWLEDGMENTS

We wish to thank Rob Nelissen and Prof. Dr. P. M. Rozing (Department of Orthopedics, Leiden University Medical Center) and Annekoos Huidekooper for collecting synovial tissue.

REFERENCES

1. Sawchuk SJ, Boivin GP, Duwel LE, Ball W, Bove K, Trapnell B, et al. Anti-T cell receptor monoclonal antibody prolongs transgene expression following adenovirus-mediated in vivo gene transfer to mouse synovium. Hum Gene Ther 1996;7:499–506.
2. Roessler BJ, Allen ED, Wilson JM, Hartman JW, Davidson BL. Adenoviral mediated gene transfer to rabbit synovium in vivo. J Clin Invest 1993;92:1085–92.
3. Ikeda T, Kubo T, Arai Y, Nakanishi T, Kobayashi K, Takahashi K, et al. Adenovirus mediated gene delivery to the joints of guinea pigs. J Rheumatol 1998;25:1666–73.
4. Goossens PH, Schouten GJ, 'tHart BA, Bout A, Brok HPM, Kluin PM, et al. Feasibility of adenovirus-mediated non-surgical synovectomy in CIA affected Rhesus monkeys (M. mulatta). Hum Gene Ther 1999;10:1139–49.
5. Ilan Y, Sauter B, Chowdury NR, Reddy BV, Thumalla NR, Droguett G, et al. Oral tolerization to adenoviral proteins permits repeated adenovirus-mediated gene therapy in rats with pre-existing immunity to adenoviruses. Hepatology 1998;27:1368–74.
6. Arnett FC, Edworthy SM, Bloch DA, McShane DJ, Fries JF, Cooper NS, et al. The American Rheumatism Association 1987 revised criteria for the classification of rheumatoid arthritis. Arthritis Rheum 1988;31:315–24.
7. Fallaux FJ, Bout A, van der Velde I, van den Wollenberg DJ, Hehir KM, Keegan J, et al. New helper cells and matched early-region 1-deleted adenovirus vectors prevent generation of replication competent adenoviruses. Hum Gene Ther 1998;9: 1909–17.
8. Shabram PW, Giroux DD, Goudreau AM, Gregory RJ, Horn MT, Huyghe BG, et al. Analytical anion-exchange HPLC of recombinant type-5 adenoviral particles. Hum Gene Ther 1997;8:453–65.
9. Fallaux FJ, Kranenburg O, Cramer SJ, Houweling A, van Ormondt H, Hoeben RC, et al. Characterization of 911: a new helper cell line for the titration and propagation of early region 1-deleted adenoviral vectors. Hum Gene Ther 1996;7:215–22.
10. Wigand R, Schulz R. Laboratory procedures in adenoviruses. II. Sensitivity of various cell cultures as determined by endpoint titration. Zentralbl Bakteriol 1975;231:31–41.
11. Smith AE. Gene therapy: where are we? Lancet 1999;354 Suppl 1:1–4.

ARTHRITIS & RHEUMATISM
Vol. 44, No. 1, January 2001, pp 53–60

Responsiveness of the Self-Assessed Rheumatoid Arthritis Disease Activity Index to a Flare of Disease Activity

Jaap Fransen,[1] Hansjörg Häuselmann,[2] Beat A. Michel,[1] Miguel Caravatti,[1] and Gerold Stucki[3]

Objective. **To assess the responsiveness of the Rheumatoid Arthritis Disease Activity Index (RADAI) to increases in disease activity, using the occurrence of a flare of disease activity as an external standard.**

Methods. **A post hoc analysis was performed on data from a randomized, double-blind, controlled trial of methotrexate versus type II collagen in 92 patients with rheumatoid arthritis (RA). Responsiveness was analyzed by 1) correlating change in the RADAI score with change in the Disease Activity Score (DAS28), 2) determining the RADAI's ability to detect a disease flare by plotting a receiver operating characteristic (ROC) curve, and 3) using a responsiveness statistic, the standardized effect size (SES). The contribution of the single RADAI items to the change in total RADAI score was analyzed by the item score change in absolute value, the item responsiveness by the standardized response mean, and the correlation of item score change with total RADAI score change by Cronbach's alpha.**

Results. **Changes in the RADAI score correlated strongly with changes in the DAS28 (R^2 = 0.70, $P <$ 0.0001). The area under the ROC curve for the RADAI was 0.88 (95% confidence interval 0.78–0.95), which was similar to that for the DAS28. The SES for the RADAI was 1.56, which was also similar to that for the DAS28. The RADAI items of past global disease activity and morning stiffness contributed least to the total score change.**

Conclusion. **This study provides evidence that the RADAI is sensitive to relevant increases in disease activity in RA patients. The RADAI may complement clinical measures in clinical studies, or may be used as a proxy for disease activity in epidemiologic studies.**

[1]Jaap Fransen, MSc, Beat A. Michel, MD, Miguel Caravatti, MD: University Hospital Zurich, Zurich, Switzerland; [2]Hansjörg Häuselmann, MD: Center for Rheumatology and Bone Disease, Klinik im Park, Zurich, Switzerland; [3]Gerold Stucki, MD, MS: University of Munich, Munich, Germany.

Address correspondence and reprint requests to Jaap Fransen, MSc, Department of Rheumatology and Institute of Physical Medicine, University Hospital Zurich, Gloriastrasse 25, 8091 Zurich, Switzerland.

Submitted for publication November 24, 1999; accepted in revised form August 25, 2000.

Because there is no "gold standard" of disease activity in rheumatoid arthritis (RA), multiple measures are used and needed in clinical studies (1), as well as for monitoring individual patients in clinical practice for disease management (2). Progress has been made in rheumatology by the adoption of a core set of measures to be used in trials of antirheumatic drugs (3), and by the use of index measures (4). With both core set and index measures, the comparability between studies is enhanced.

The main advantages of indices over single measures are the avoidance of duplication and increased sensitivity to change (4). The avoidance of duplication reduces the risk of making a Type I error when performing multiple statistical testing and eliminates the difficulties that arise in attempting to interpret different changes in multiple measures simultaneously. Increased sensitivity to change is a result of reduction in measurement error (5,6). Combining items to increase validity and reliability is a common practice in creating questionnaires. The main disadvantages of indices are concerns about validity as well as practical problems such as interpretation and computational difficulties (4). The validity of an index depends on the validity of the measures that are included and their appropriate weighting. Interpretation of an index becomes easier when more information from validity (e.g., discriminative or predictive validity) studies is available and when there is growing familiarity with an index.

The Disease Activity Score (DAS28) combines the erythrocyte sedimentation rate (ESR), a swollen joint count, a tender joint count, and, sometimes, a general health assessment into a single index (7). An example of a self-administered index is the Rheumatoid Arthritis Disease Activity Index (RADAI), a short questionnaire that combines the following 5 items into a single index: current and past global disease activity, pain, morning stiffness, and a joint count (8,9). The RADAI was developed to complement clinical measures in clinical studies and to serve as a proxy for disease activity in epidemiologic studies (9).

While the RADAI has been shown to be a valid measure of disease activity cross-sectionally (9,10), its responsiveness has not been studied. However, a major objective of the RADAI is the measurement of change. Measures that are cross-sectionally valid are not necessarily responsive (11). Responsiveness is the ability of a measure to capture clinically important changes (11–13).

Until now, most attention concerning responsiveness in RA has implicitly been given to changes in direction of improvement; however, in a fluctuating chronic disease such as RA, patients also show worsening of disease (14). A measure that shows adequate responsiveness in the direction of improvement need not show the same responsiveness in the opposite direction. For constructed measurement instruments such as the RADAI, this may depend on the scaling properties (i.e., unidimensionality of the scale [15], item spacing [16], and relative scale length [ceiling or floor effects] [17]).

The objective of this study was to assess the responsiveness, or sensitivity to change, of the RADAI to increases in disease activity in RA patients. The occurrence of a flare of disease activity was used as an external standard of change. To assess concurrent validity, the RADAI was compared with the DAS28. In addition, to assess content validity, the relative contribution of the individual RADAI items to the amount of change in the RADAI score was determined.

PATIENTS AND METHODS

Patients. We made use of the data from a randomized, placebo-controlled trial of methotrexate (MTX) versus type II collagen that had examined whether type II collagen could sustain an MTX-induced treatment effect. The study sample and design were described in detail by Häuselmann et al (18). Informed consent was obtained from all patients before inclusion.

Included were patients diagnosed as having RA according to the 1987 revised criteria of the American College of Rheumatology (ACR; formerly, the American Rheumatism Association) (19) and having a functional status of class I–III (20). The patients had to have been treated with an unchanged regimen of MTX monotherapy for at least 8 weeks. Concurrent treatment with glucocorticoids or nonsteroidal antiinflammatory drugs (NSAIDs) was allowed, provided that the dosage was unchanged for the previous 2 weeks (and provided that the dosage was $\leq$12.5 mg/day in the case of glucocorticoids). Excluded were patients of age $<$18 years, as well as patients who had received intraarticular glucocorticoid injections within 3 weeks of the beginning of the study.

Ninety-two patients were randomly assigned to receive either type II collagen with MTX placebo or MTX with type II collagen placebo for 3 months in a blinded manner. If patients were being treated concurrently with NSAIDs or glucocorticoids, the dosages were kept constant for the entire trial period. The study protocol was approved by the ethics committee of the University Hospital Zurich.

Measurements. The patients were assessed by the same clinician (who was blinded to group assignment) at baseline, 30 days, and 90 days. At baseline, sociodemographic data were obtained, and radiographs of the hands and feet were obtained and scored according to the Larsen method (21,22). Laboratory testing was performed for rheumatoid factor and antinuclear antibodies (ANA), and included HLA class II typing (23,24) with subsequent classification according to RA severity (25).

The following disease parameters were measured at all visits: ESR (Westergren method) and C-reactive protein level, number of swollen joints (28-joint count), number of tender joints (28-joint count), physician's global assessment of disease activity (scale of 0–10), pain assessed by the patient (scale of 0–10), and patient's global assessment of disease activity (scale of 0–10).

The DAS28 (DAS28 swollen + tender) was calculated from the results of the joint counts and the ESR (26). A German version of the Stanford Health Assessment Questionnaire (HAQ) (27,28) and a German version of the RADAI (9) were used.

The RADAI is a 5-item questionnaire. The items ask the patient about 1) global disease activity during the last 6 months, 2) today's disease activity in terms of swollen and tender joints, 3) today's amount of arthritis pain, 4) today's duration of morning stiffness, and 5) today's amount of pain in each of several joint areas (tender joints). The first 3 items are all rated on an anchored numerical scale from 0 to 10, where higher scores indicate more disease activity. The scores on items 4 and 5 range from 0 to 6 and from 0 to 48, respectively, but are transformed into the same scale of 0–10 used for the first 3 items. The patient is required to answer all items. The scores are then added and divided by the number of items to provide a single index of patient-assessed disease activity.

The duration of participation in the study protocol was recorded as either termination at the end of the study or discontinuation prior to the end (with subsequent recording, in the latter instance, of the exact length of participation in the study and the specific reason for dropping out). For patients who dropped out, clinical and laboratory assessments, as described above, were performed immediately after dropout.

A dropout due to a flare of disease activity was defined as a patient-perceived increase in disease activity leading to the patient's wish to quit the study protocol and/or the requirement for a change in medication that caused a protocol violation.

Statistical analysis. We analyzed patients' reasons for dropping out of the study. Patients with reasons other than a flare of disease activity (e.g., adverse effects) were excluded from the analysis. There were therefore 2 groups of patients: those who discontinued (flare group) and those who stayed in the study (nonflare group). The groups were not further classified according to study medication, because splitting the sample into 4 groups would have induced a significant loss of power. To our knowledge, in the case of a flare of disease, no differential effects of MTX and type II collagen should be expected regarding the clinical parameters most relevant to this study (ESR, numbers of swollen and tender joints, and patient perception of disease activity). For data with an approximately normal distribution (according to the histogram, normal probability plot, median and mean, skewness and kurtosis), parametric statistics were applied and means and SDs are presented. For data with a skewed distribution, nonparametric statistics were applied and medians and interquartile ranges are presented. The flare and nonflare groups were analyzed for comparability at baseline. Between-group analysis was performed with the chi-square test, Fisher's exact test, the 2-sample *t*-test, or the 2-sample Wilcoxon test, as appropriate.

The flare and nonflare groups were compared with regard to changes from baseline to study termination in RADAI and DAS28 scores, as well as in other indicators of disease activity. The 1-sample *t*-test was used for analyzing within-group differences, while the 2-sample *t*-test and 2-sample Wilcoxon test were used for between-group differences. Linear regression was used to study change in disease activity (change in the DAS28) as a function of disease activity at baseline.

Responsiveness was analyzed by 1) correlating change in the RADAI score with change in the DAS28 score (using R^2), 2) determining the RADAI's ability to detect a disease flare by plotting a receiver operating characteristic (ROC) curve (29) representing the sensitivity and specificity of a decision (flare or nonflare) for all possible cutoff points of an underlying variable (change in RADAI score) and calculating the discriminative ability (area under the curve [AUC]), and 3) using a responsiveness statistic, the standardized effect size (SES) (29). The SES was calculated as the difference of the within-group changes of the flare and nonflare groups divided by the pooled SDs of change. The SES values for the RADAI and DAS28 were compared approximately using a Z statistic (30).

We preferred to use the DAS28 to test for concurrent validity across the various individual indicators of disease activity for the following reasons: 1) the DAS28 has been shown to be a valid estimator of disease activity (26) and is responsive to improvements in disease activity (31), 2) an index combining 3 items may be a better estimator than 3 separate items, 3) the statistical problem of multiple testing is avoided and interpretation is facilitated (3), and, especially important, 4) for the correlational method, there is no need to develop an a priori expectation of the degrees of correlation of the various individual indicators of disease activity.

The contribution of the single RADAI items to the change in total RADAI score of the flare group was analyzed by the item score change in absolute value, the item responsiveness by the standardized response mean (SRM) (32), and the correlation of item score change with total RADAI score change by Cronbach's alpha. The SRM is calculated as the ratio of the mean change to the SD of change. Higher values indicate a better responsiveness. SRMs are most easily interpreted relative to each other within the same study.

It is unclear whether different responsiveness statistics, such as SRM (32), effect size (the ratio of the mean change to the SD at baseline) (33), or the responsiveness statistic proposed by Guyatt et al (the ratio of a clinically important difference to the variability in stable subjects) (11), will lead to comparable results (34), as has been suggested (35). Therefore, we preferred to use the SES and the SRM, because they represent change and the same population in both numerator and denominator.

The level of statistical significance was set at $P = 0.05$ (2-sided). Data were stored in a MedLog database (Information Analysis, Incline Village, NV) and analyzed with the SAS 6.11 statistical software package (SAS Institute, Cary, NC).

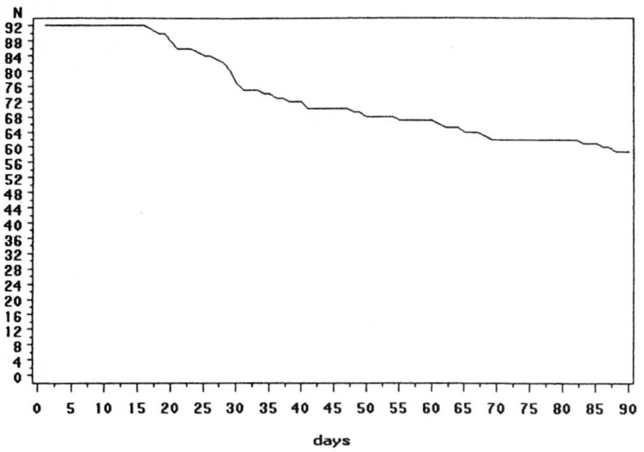

Figure 1. Dropouts (n = 33 patients) due to flares of disease activity during the 90 days of the study (see ref. 18).

RESULTS

Flare and nonflare groups. Within the 90-day study duration, 26 of the 46 patients (57%) who were receiving type II collagen dropped out. Of the 46 patients receiving MTX, only 7 (15%) dropped out. No reasons were noted for leaving the study protocol other than flares of disease activity. The median time-to-flare was 31 days (range 17–88 days) (Figure 1). At baseline, patients in the flare group did not differ significantly in demographic or disease variables from those who continued the study successfully, except in disease duration and ANA positivity (Table 1). The sex distribution did not differ significantly between the groups. In addition, there were no statistically significant differences in demographic or disease variables between women and men. Regarding the clinical parameters at baseline (Table 2), the only significant difference between the groups was in the pain rating. The DAS28 score reflects the range from remission to high levels of disease activity (31). A high level of DAS28 (31) at baseline was not associated with the later development of a flare ($P =$ 0.69, by Fisher's exact test).

Table 1. Baseline population characteristics and differences between nonflare and flare groups*

	Nonflare (n = 59)	Flare (n = 33)	*P*	Total (n = 92)
Men, no. (%)	8 (14)	8 (24)	0.20†	16 (17)
Women, no. (%)	51 (86)	25 (76)		76 (83)
Age, years, mean ± SD	51 ± 12	53 ± 13	0.37	52 ± 13
Disease duration, years, median (IQR)	7 (3–11)	13 (6–16)	0.0014	9 (4–14)
BMI, kg/m², median (IQR)	23 (21–25)	23 (21–26)	0.89	23 (21–25)
Taking steroids, no. (%)	23 (39)	18 (55)	0.17	41 (45)
Taking NSAIDs, no. (%)	49 (83)	24 (73)	0.26	73 (79)
ANA positive, no. (%)	39 (66)	30 (91)	0.011	69 (75)
RF positive, no. (%)	49 (83)	31 (94)	0.32	80 (87)
HLA–DRB1 A–D positive, no. (%)‡	31 (62)	19 (66)	0.35	50 (63)
Larsen radiographic score, 0–5 points, median (IQR)	2.3 (2.0–3.1)	2.5 (2.1–3.1)	0.27	2.3 (2.1–3.1)
ACR functional class, no. (%)				
I	13 (22)	3 (9)		16 (17)
II	16 (27)	12 (36)	0.26§	28 (30)
III	30 (51)	18 (55)		48 (52)
IV	–	–		0

* IQR = interquartile range; BMI = body mass index; NSAIDs = nonsteroidal antiinflammatory drugs; ANA = antinuclear antibody; RF = rheumatoid factor; ACR = American College of Rheumatology.
† For flare status in men versus women.
‡ HLA–DRB1 A–D allele classification according to disease severity (see ref. 25). Numbers of patients were lower for this measure due to missing values (nonflare group n = 50, flare group n = 29).
§ For flare status across functional classes.

Changes within and between groups. At study termination, the nonflare group showed no statistically significant changes from baseline in any indicator of disease activity, although all disease activity indicators were significantly increased in the flare group ($P < 0.0001$, by 1-sample *t*-test). The changes in the flare

Table 2. Changes in measures of disease activity for nonflare and flare groups from baseline to study termination*

		Baseline, median (IQR)†			Change from baseline, median (IQR)‡		Change from baseline, mean ± SD‡		Responsiveness§		
Measure	Range	Nonflare	Flare	*P*	Nonflare	Flare	Nonflare	Flare	R^2	AUC	SES
CRP, mg/liter	–	12 (5–29)	11 (4–25)	0.62	−1 (−5–6)	18 (7–75)	−1.1 ± 35	39 ± 46	0.34	0.84	1.03
ESR, mm/hour	–	16 (8–33)	18 (12–25)	0.91	0 (−4–6)	10 (4–31)	0 ± 13	19 ± 20	0.38	0.81	1.18
Swollen joints, no.	0–28	5 (2–9)	5 (3–10)	0.46	0 (−2–1)	3 (0–6)	−0.3 ± 3.0	3.4 ± 3.8	0.41	0.78	1.14
Tender joints, no.	0–28	5 (2–8)	6 (2–9)	0.54	0 (−2–1)	3 (2–8)	−0.6 ± 4.5	4.4 ± 4.8	0.61	0.80	1.08
Pain scale	0–10	3 (2–5)	4 (3–6)	0.032	0 (−1–1)	3 (2–5)	−0.2 ± 2.0	3.3 ± 2.4	0.79¶	0.89	1.67
Patient's global assessment scale	0–10	3 (2–5)	4 (3–6)	0.32	0 (−1–1)	3 (2–5)	−0.3 ± 2.3	3.1 ± 2.3	0.84¶	0.87	1.51
Physician's global assessment scale	0–10	3 (2–4)	3 (3–5)	0.23	0 (−1–1)	3 (2–5)	0 ± 1.3	2.0 ± 1.6	0.61	0.84	1.46
HAQ score	0–3	1.0 (0.4–1.5)	1.3 (0.5–1.8)	0.38	0 (−0.4–0.1)	0.4 (0.2–0.7)	−0.1 ± 0.5	0.47 ± 0.5	0.77	0.80	1.16
RADAI score	0–10	2.0 (0.8–3.7)	2.8 (1.5–4.7)	0.082	−0.3 (−0.9–0.6)	2.7 (1.1–4.5)	−0.3 ± 1.7	2.6 ± 2.0	1.00	0.88	1.56
DAS28	0–9	4.3 ± 1.4	4.3 ± 1.3	0.89	–	–	−0.1 ± 0.8	1.2 ± 0.8	0.70	0.87	1.58

* IQR = interquartile range; CRP = C-reactive protein; ESR = erythrocyte sedimentation rate; HAQ = Health Assessment Questionnaire; RADAI = Rheumatoid Arthritis Disease Activity Index; DAS28 = Disease Activity Score.
† DAS28 values are the mean ± SD.
‡ All non-negative values indicate higher disease activity levels, all negative values indicate reductions in disease activity. $P \leq 0.0001$ for between-group differences, for changes in medians or means (by 2-sample *t*-test).
§ R^2 = correlation of change with change in RADAI; AUC = area under the curve; SES = standardized effect size. All R^2 were significantly different from 0 ($P < 0.001$), and all AUC were significantly different from 0.5 ($P < 0.05$).
¶ Item correlation with the RADAI after deletion of that item from the RADAI.

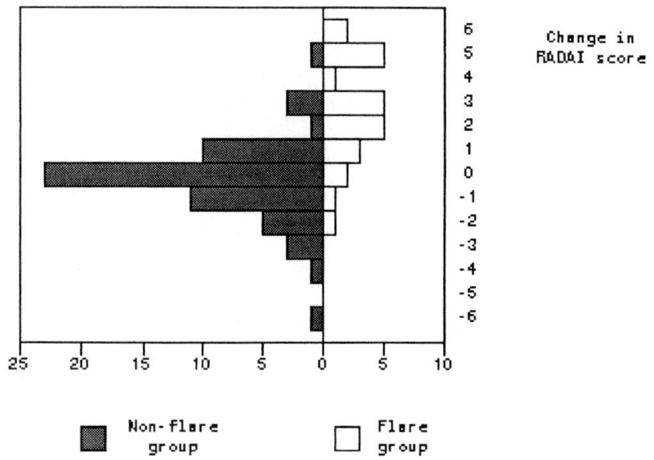

Figure 2. Frequency distribution of the change in Rheumatoid Arthritis Disease Activity Index (RADAI) score in the non-flare group (n = 59) and the flare group (n = 33). Numbers of patients are shown on the x-axis.

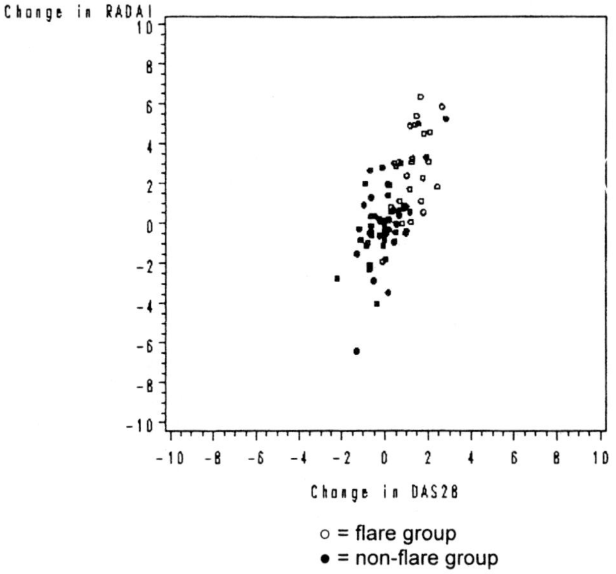

Figure 3. Scatterplot of change in Rheumatoid Arthritis Disease Activity Index (RADAI) score versus concurrent change in Disease Activity Score (DAS28) in the non-flare group (n = 59) and the flare group (n = 33).

group were significantly greater than those in the non-flare group ($P < 0.0001$, by 2-sample *t*-test) (Table 2). The RADAI and DAS28 scores in the flare group were also significantly increased from baseline compared with those in the nonflare group. The changes from baseline had normal or near-normal distributions. To interpret the changes from baseline in relation to the median values at baseline, both median and mean changes are presented. In the flare group, DAS28 scores at baseline explained 7% of the variance of change in DAS28 scores ($P = 0.012$, by F test). The distribution of score changes in the RADAI is shown in Figure 2. There was some overlap in score changes between the flare and nonflare groups, which means that some of the patients in both groups shared the same amount of change in RADAI score.

Responsiveness. The RADAI and DAS28 scores were correlated at baseline (Spearman's rank correlation [r_s] = 0.58, $P < 0.0001$). As can be seen in the scatterplot (Figure 3), the changes in RADAI score were strongly correlated with changes in the DAS28 score ($R^2 = 0.70$, $P < 0.0001$).

The discriminative ability (AUC) of the RADAI for detecting a relevant change (a flare) was 0.88 (95% confidence interval [95% CI] 0.78–0.95). This is also illustrated by the form of the ROC curve extending toward the upper left corner of the graph in Figure 4. The discriminative ability of the DAS28 for detecting the occurrence of a flare was similar (AUC 0.87 [95% CI 0.81–0.95]). The SES for the RADAI of 1.56 (i.e., [2.61 − −0.27]/1.85) was not significantly different ($P =$ 0.95) from the SES for the DAS28 of (1.58, i.e., [1.19 − −0.07]/0.80). The responsiveness statistics for the several indicators of disease activity are shown in Table 2. It should be noted that pain and patient's global assessment are included in the RADAI, while ESR and the joint counts are included in the DAS28.

Contribution of single items. The SRMs of the single RADAI items were lower than the SRM of the

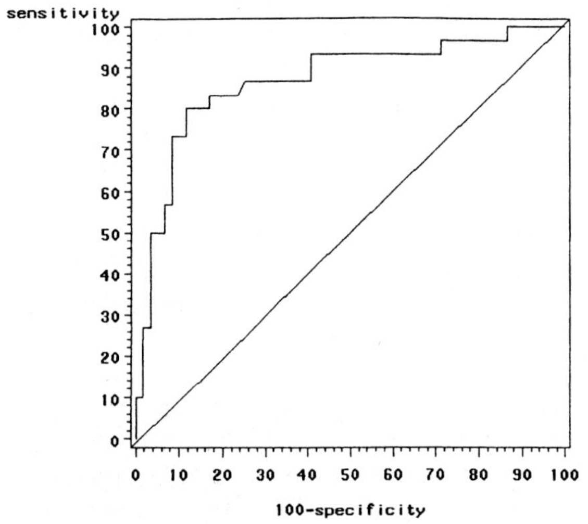

Figure 4. Receiver operating characteristic curve for the detection of a flare on the basis of a change in the Rheumatoid Arthritis Disease Activity Index score (n = 92).

Table 3. Contribution to change in score of single items on the Rheumatic Arthritis Disease Activity Index (RADAI)*

RADAI item	Change, mean ± SD	SRM	α	R^2
1. In general, how active has your arthritis been over the past 6 months?	2.5 ± 3.2	0.78	0.84	0.43
2. In terms of joint tenderness and swelling, how active is your arthritis today?	2.9 ± 2.6	1.12	0.72	0.84
3. How much arthritis pain do you feel today?	3.5 ± 3.0	1.17	0.73	0.79
4. Were your joints stiff when you woke up today? If yes, how long did this stiffness last? (no = 0, <30 minutes = 1, 30 minutes–1 hour = 2, 1–2 hours = 3, 2–4 hours = 4, >4 hours = 5, all day = 6)	2.2 ± 2.7	0.81	0.83	0.47
5. Please indicate the amount of pain you are having today in each of the joint areas listed below. (none = 0, mild = 1, moderate = 2, severe = 3; shoulders, elbows, wrists, fingers, hips, knees, ankles, toes)	1.9 ± 1.6	1.19	0.79	0.58
Total RADAI score	2.6 ± 2.0	1.31	0.82†	–

* Shown are the changes in scores for the flare group (n = 33). SRM = standardized response mean; α = Cronbach's alpha of the RADAI without the item; R^2 = correlation of change in the item with change in all other items.
† For the total RADAI score, the Cronbach's alpha is on all items.

total score (Table 3). In absolute values, items 2 and 3 contributed most to the overall change in RADAI score. Items 1 and 4 had the lowest SRMs and the lowest correlations with change in all other items. Further, the Cronbach's alpha of the RADAI score was raised most by leaving out one of these items.

DISCUSSION

The results of this post hoc analysis of data from a randomized, double-blind, clinical trial of MTX versus type II collagen provide evidence that the RADAI is sensitive to relevant increases in disease activity in patients with RA. The occurrence of a flare of disease activity was used as an external standard of change and was associated with raised values in all disease activity indicators used. In addition to the DAS28 and the RADAI, these were measures included in the World Health Organization/International League Against Rheumatism core set of end points for RA clinical trials (3).

The responsiveness of the RADAI was confirmed in several ways. First, the changes in the RADAI were well correlated with changes in the DAS28. Second, the discriminative ability of the RADAI and of the DAS28, reflected by the AUC, were virtually the same. The area was significantly different from 0.5, where 0.5 indicates that no information is provided (13). Finally, the SES values of the RADAI and the DAS28 were approximately the same and were >1. Interpretation guidelines were not available, but the SES values we found were quite high compared with values found elsewhere. Buchbinder et al (30) reported SES values for clinical measures ranging from 0.70 (physician's global assessment) to 0.07 (ESR). Vliet Vlieland et al (36) reported SES values ranging from 0.98 (Ritchie Articular Index) to 0.30 (duration of morning stiffness).

Of the single RADAI items, the first item (global disease activity in the past 6 months) and the fourth item (duration of morning stiffness) appeared to be the least responsive. However, with an SRM of ~0.80 or higher, these measures can be considered very sensitive (32). Given the subjective nature of the question, the item about the level of disease activity in the past 6 months cannot be expected to be very responsive, even if the patient's impression of the level of past disease activity may be influenced by the disease activity currently experienced.

There may be some practical and economic reasons to replace physician assessments with patient questionnaires. However, the fact that the RADAI and the DAS28 perform similarly well does not mean one can automatically replace the DAS28 with the RADAI (10). The DAS28 and the RADAI both aim to measure the same underlying construct—arthritis inflammatory activity—from two different perspectives (10). The patient's perspective is formed by perceptions of symptoms and signs, while that of the physician is formed by judgments of joint swelling, joint tenderness, and ESR.

One of the reasons the RADAI performed comparably with the DAS28 may have been the use of a disease flare as an external standard of change. The RADAI may measure this unpleasant experience more directly than the DAS28. However, the DAS28 may more directly reflect the underlying arthritis inflammatory activity (37).

A limitation of this study is that a flare of disease activity is a large change for an RA patient. It is possible that, for example, morning stiffness may not be very responsive to smaller but relevant changes in disease activity. However, the correlation and scatterplot of RADAI and DAS28 changes show that the RADAI may also be sensitive to smaller changes. In future studies, the sensitivity of the RADAI for small but clinically relevant changes in disease activity has to be assessed together with its smallest detectable difference.

To avoid the loss of statistical power, we chose not to stratify our sample into subsamples according to medication. We found no strong indication that patients who had disease flares while receiving MTX differed from those who had disease flares while receiving type II collagen, either at baseline or in their responses (data not shown). It appears that no important bias was introduced. The criterion of a disease flare was based on the assumption that patients had stable disease activity at baseline and that improvements were not expected by patients or physicians. Indeed, the flare group showed significant increases in all indicators of disease activity, while the nonflare group showed no changes. A high DAS28 score at baseline did not predict development of a flare later on. Further, the amount of change in DAS28 score was largely independent of the baseline DAS28 score in the flare group. Thus, it is unlikely that patients dropped out due to persistently high levels of disease activity instead of a flare, or that patients with high levels of disease activity at baseline could not "express" their flare on the DAS28.

In contrast to our study, most studies of responsiveness of measures in RA concentrate on treatment effects, and an improvement of disease activity is expected. Few studies have examined the responsiveness of questions (such as those on the RADAI) concerning patient perceptions of signs and symptoms. In a trial of multidisciplinary treatment in RA, the visual analog scale (VAS) for severity of morning stiffness was more responsive than the VAS for morning stiffness duration (36). Moreover, the morning stiffness severity measure was the most responsive of all (core set) end point measures used. In a randomized controlled trial comparing low-dose cyclosporine with placebo, morning stiffness (in minutes) and pain (VAS and Likert scale) were among the least responsive measures. However, the combination of 4 arthritis pain–related questions (from the Arthritis Impact Measurement Scales [38], specifically, the AIMS-2) appeared to be the only measure more responsive than the standard tender joint count (30). In a trial of several antirheumatic drug treatment strategies, the physical discomfort measures, pain and well being, were the most responsive for treatment effect at 3 months (39).

In two other responsiveness studies in RA (8,40), no external standard of change was used. Although it was likely that some worsening of the disease occurred, this was not clearly addressed in the reports of the results. A questionnaire with a format similar to that of the RADAI was tested for agreement on change by computing the intraclass correlation coefficients between patients and clinicians for changes in scores across a mean interval of 6 months. However, the changes in questionnaire scores were not compared with external indicators of change in disease activity, rendering uncertain the extent of clinically relevant changes (8). In an observational 60-week study of 24 RA patients, it was found that physician and patient global assessments, pain scores, and the HAQ were more sensitive to change than other clinical measures, while laboratory measures were generally less sensitive to change (40).

Thus, it appears that the responsiveness of questions about patient perceptions of signs and symptoms may at least equal the responsiveness of clinical measures. The different findings for morning stiffness may illustrate the importance of the design of the question and the scaling. To further increase the responsiveness of the RADAI, the morning stiffness item could be changed to measure severity instead of duration (36). The RADAI item on past disease activity could be replaced by a question regarding general well being in the context of the arthritis (41).

In summary, this study provides evidence that the RADAI, a self-administered rheumatoid arthritis disease activity index, is sensitive to relevant increases in disease activity in RA patients. Future studies must assess the sensitivity of the RADAI to small but clinically relevant increases and decreases in disease activity. The RADAI may complement clinical measures in clinical studies, or may be used as a proxy for disease activity in epidemiologic studies.

ACKNOWLEDGMENTS

We are grateful for the critical reading of the manuscript by Anke van Gestel, MSc, Department of Rheumatology, University Hospital, Nijmegen, The Netherlands. We thank Leanne Pobjoy for her assistance in the preparation of the manuscript.

REFERENCES

1. Kirwan JR. A theoretical framework for process, outcome and prognosis in rheumatoid arthritis. J Rheumatol 1992;19:333–6.

2. Stucki G, Langenegger T. Management of rheumatoid arthritis. Curr Opin Rheumatol 1997;9:229–35.
3. Boers M, Tugwell P, Felson DT, van Riel PLCM, Kirwan JR, Edmonds JP, et al. World Health Organisation and International League of Associations for Rheumatology core endpoints for symptom modifying antirheumatic drugs in rheumatoid arthritis clinical trials. J Rheumatol 1994;41 Suppl:86–9.
4. Boers M, Tugwell P. The validity of pooled outcome measures (indices) in rheumatoid arthritis clinical trials. J Rheumatol 1993; 20:568–74.
5. Roberts RS. Pooled outcome measures in arthritis: the pros and cons. J Rheumatol 1993;20:566–7.
6. Goldsmith CH, Smythe HA, Helewa A. Interpretation and power of a pooled index. J Rheumatol 1993;20:575–8.
7. Van der Heijde DM, Van 't Hof MA, van Riel PLCM, Theunisse LA, Lubberts EW, van Leeuwen MA, et al. Judging disease activity in clinical practice in rheumatoid arthritis: first step in the development of a disease activity score. Ann Rheum Dis 1990;49: 916–20.
8. Mason JH, Anderson JJ, Meenan RF, Haralson KM, Lewis-Stevens D, Kaine JL. The Rapid Assessment of Disease Activity in Rheumatology (RADAR) questionnaire: validity and sensitivity to change of a patient self-report measure of joint count and clinical status. Arthritis Rheum 1992;35:156–62.
9. Stucki G, Liang MH, Stucki S, Brühlmann P, Michel BA. A self-administered Rheumatoid Arthritis Disease Activity Index (RADAI) for epidemiologic research: psychometric properties and correlation with parameters of disease activity. Arthritis Rheum 1995;38:795–8.
10. Fransen J, Langenegger T, Michel BA, Stucki G. Feasibility and validity of the RADAI, a self-administered rheumatoid arthritis disease activity index. Rheumatology (Oxford) 2000;39:321–7.
11. Guyatt G, Walter S, Norman G. Measuring change over time: assessing the usefulness of evaluative instruments. J Chronic Disease 1987;40:171–8.
12. Kirshner B, Guyatt G. A methodological framework for assessing health indices. J Chronic Disease 1985;38:27–36.
13. Deyo RA, Diehr P, Patrick DL. Reproducibility and responsiveness of health status measures: statistics and strategies for evaluation. Control Clin Trials 1991;12 Suppl 4:142S–58S.
14. Fortin PR, Stucki G, Katz JN. Measuring relevant change: an emerging challenge in rheumatologic clinical trials. Arthritis Rheum 1995;38:1027–30.
15. Silverstein B, Kilgore KM, Fisher WP, Harley P, Harvey RF. Applying psychometric criteria to functional assessment in medical rehabilitation. I. Exploring unidimensionality. Arch Phys Med Rehabil 1991;72:631–7.
16. Silverstein B, Fisher WP, Kilgore KM, Harley P, Harvey RF. Applying psychometric criteria to functional assessment in medical rehabilitation. II. Defining interval measures. Arch Phys Med Rehabil 1992;73:507–18.
17. Nunnally JC, Bernstein IH. Psychometric theory. 3rd ed. New York: McGraw-Hill; 1994.
18. Häuselmann HJ, Caravatti M, Seifert B, Wang K, Bruckner P, Stucki G, et al. Can collagen type II sustain a methotrexate-induced therapeutic effect in patients with long-standing rheumatoid arthritis? A double-blind, randomized trial. Br J Rheumatol 1998;37:1110–7.
19. Arnett FC, Edworthy SM, Bloch DA, McShane DJ, Fries JF, Cooper NS, et al. The American Rheumatism Association 1987 revised criteria for the classification of rheumatoid arthritis. Arthritis Rheum 1988;31:315–24.
20. Hochberg MC, Chang RW, Dwosh I, Lindsey S, Pincus T, Wolfe F. The American College of Rheumatology 1991 revised criteria for the classification of global functional status in rheumatoid arthritis. Arthritis Rheum 1992;35:498–502.
21. Larsen A, Dale K, Eek M. Standard radiographs of rheumatoid arthritis. Oslo: Department of Radiology, Sanitatsforenings Rheumatism Hospital; 1975.
22. Larsen A. How to apply Larsen score in evaluating radiographs of rheumatoid arthritis in longterm studies. J Rheumatol 1995;22:1974–5.
23. Olerup O, Zetterquist H. HLA–DR typing by PCR amplification with sequence-specific primers (PCR–SSP) in 2 hours: an alternative to serological DR typing in clinical practice including donor-recipient matching in cadaveric transplantation. Tissue Antigens 1992;39:225–35.
24. Blasczyk R, van Lessen A, Schwella N, Huhn D, Salama A. A novel HLA–DR13 allele (DRB1*1314) identified by single-strand conformation polymorphism analysis and confirmed by direct sequencing. Hum Immunol 1995;43:309–12.
25. Weyand CM, Hicok KC, Conn DL, Goronzy JJ. The influence of HLA–DRB1 genes on disease severity in rheumatoid arthritis. Ann Intern Med 1992;117:801–6.
26. Prevoo MLL, Van 't Hof MA, Kuper HH, van Leeuwen MA, van de Putte LBA, van Riel PLCM. Modified disease activity scores that include twenty-eight–joint counts: development and validation in a prospective longitudinal study of patients with rheumatoid arthritis. Arthritis Rheum 1995;38:44–8.
27. Fries JF, Spitz P, Kraines RG, Holman HR. Measurement of patient outcome in arthritis. Arthritis Rheum 1980;23:137–45.
28. Bruhlmann P, Stucki G, Michel BA. Evaluation of a German version of the physical dimensions of the Health Assessment Questionnaire in patients with rheumatoid arthritis. J Rheumatol 1994;21:1245–9.
29. Deyo RA, Centor RM. Assessing the responsiveness of functional scales to clinical change: an analogy to diagnostic test performance. J Chronic Disease 1986;39:897–906.
30. Buchbinder R, Bombardier C, Yeung M, Tugwell P. Which outcome measures should be used in rheumatoid arthritis clinical trials? Clinical and quality-of-life measures' responsiveness to treatment in a randomized controlled trial. Arthritis Rheum 1995;38:1568–80.
31. Van Gestel AM, Haagsma CJ, van Riel PLCM. Validation of rheumatoid arthritis improvement criteria that include simplified joint counts. Arthritis Rheum 1998;41:1845–50.
32. Liang MH, Fossel AH, Larson MG. Comparisons of five health status instruments for orthopedic evaluation. Med Care 1990;28:632–42.
33. Kazis LE, Anderson JJ, Meenan RF. Effect sizes for interpreting changes in health status. Med Care 1989;27 Suppl 3:S178–89.
34. Wright JG, Young NL. A comparison of different indices of responsiveness. J Clin Epidemiol 1997;50:239–46.
35. Stucki G, Liang MH, Fossel AH, Katz JN. Relative responsiveness of condition-specific and generic health status measures in degenerative lumbar spinal stenosis. J Clin Epidemiol 1995;48:1369–78.
36. Vliet Vlieland TPM, Zwinderman AH, Breedveld FC, Hazes JMW. Measurement of morning stiffness in rheumatoid arthritis clinical trials. J Clin Epidemiol 1997;50:757–63.
37. Van der Heijde DMFM, van 't Hof MA, van Riel PLCM, van Leeuwen MA, van Rijswijk MH, van de Putte LBA. Validity of single variables and composite indices for measuring disease activity in rheumatoid arthritis. Ann Rheum Dis 1992;51:177–81.
38. Meenan RF, Gertman PM, Mason JH. Measuring health status in arthritis: the Arthritis Impact Measurement Scales. Arthritis Rheum 1980;23:146–52.
39. Van der Heide A, Jacobs JWG, Schenk Y, Bijlsma JWJ. Endpoint measures in rheumatoid arthritis clinical trials: group summary and individual patient analysis. J Rheumatol 1994;21:2195–9.
40. Ward MW. Clinical measures in rheumatoid arthritis: which are most useful in assessing patients? J Rheumatol 1994;21:17–27.
41. Hanly JG, Mosher D, Sutton E, Weerasinghe S, Theriault D. Self-assessment of disease activity by patients with rheumatoid arthritis. J Rheumatol 1996;23:1531–8.

ARTHRITIS & RHEUMATISM
Vol. 44, No. 1, January 2001, pp 61–65

Association Between Rheumatoid Arthritis and Polymorphism of Tumor Necrosis Factor Receptor II, But Not Tumor Necrosis Factor Receptor I, in Caucasians

Anne Barton, Sally John, W. E. R. Ollier, Alan Silman, and Jane Worthington

Objective. **Tumor necrosis factor (TNF) is a powerful mediator of inflammation in rheumatoid arthritis (RA). In vivo, its acute effects are limited by binding to soluble receptors (TNFR), suggesting that TNFR genes could be important candidate risk factors. The present study was undertaken to investigate association of polymorphisms of TNFRI and TNFRII with RA in subjects in the UK.**

Methods. **Unrelated Caucasian RA patients (n = 291) and healthy Caucasian controls (n = 143) were genotyped for A/G polymorphism in exon 1 of TNFRI. From this sample, 240 of the patients and 137 controls were also typed for a single-nucleotide polymorphism (SNP) in exon 6 of the TNFRII gene. In followup studies, DNA samples from UK Caucasian RA patients with a positive family history (n = 149) and UK Caucasian patients with sporadic RA (n = 208) were also typed for the exon 6 TNFRII polymorphism.**

Results. **TNFRI polymorphism was not associated with RA (odds ratio [OR] for GG genotype 0.93, 95% confidence interval [95% CI] 0.54–1.60). For TNFRII, in the initial study group, patients with RA were significantly more likely to be positive for both the G allele and GG genotype than were controls (OR for GG genotype 2.55, 95% CI 1.11–5.86). The association appeared to be confined to those with a family history of RA. This finding was replicated in an independent cohort of patients with familial RA.**

Conclusion. **The results of this study provide evidence of association between an SNP in the TNFRII gene and RA, the strongest association being observed in patients with a family history. No evidence of association between RA and TNFRI was demonstrated.**

Supported by the Arthritis and Rheumatism Campaign, UK. Dr. Barton's work was supported by the Medical Research Council, UK.

Anne Barton, MBChB, Sally John, PhD, W. E. R. Ollier, PhD, Alan Silman, MD, Jane Worthington, PhD: University of Manchester, Manchester, UK.

Address correspondence and reprint requests to Anne Barton, MBChB, ARC-EU, Stopford Building, University of Manchester, Manchester M13 9PT, UK.

Submitted for publication July 19, 2000; accepted in revised form September 27, 2000.

Rheumatoid arthritis (RA) is a chronic inflammatory disease. Excess concordance in monozygotic compared with dizygotic twins suggests a genetic component to RA susceptibility (1). The genetic component in RA is 50–60% as calculated using Falconer's estimate of heritability (2). Although HLA is the only major locus that has been consistently identified to date, a single-locus model for RA has been rejected. HLA is estimated to contribute 20–50% of the total genetic component of disease susceptibility, and it is likely that there are a number of other genes involved, each making a smaller contribution (3). A better understanding of the genetic susceptibility factors contributing to RA may lead to the identification of novel therapeutic targets.

In a complex disease like RA, the detection of weak genetic effects can be complicated by the fact that genetic heterogeneity exists, i.e., different genes will contribute to disease susceptibility in different people. In families in which more than 1 individual has the disease, it is likely that the genetic component of disease susceptibility is stronger. Previous studies have shown this to be the case with the major RA genetic susceptibility locus, HLA. Probands with a family history of RA are more likely to be DR4 positive and have a younger age at disease onset (4,5). Studying such multicase RA families may facilitate identification of weak genetic effects.

Inflammation in RA is mediated by a number of cytokines, but tumor necrosis factor α (TNFα) appears to be particularly important. TNFα acts via binding to cell surface receptors I and II (TNFRI and TNFRII). The extracellular portions of both receptors can be shed and the soluble forms still retain the ability to bind to

TNFα, thus limiting its acute effects. Soluble TNFR (sTNFR) have a higher affinity for TNFα than membrane-bound TNFR. In inflammation, levels of both TNFα and TNFR are increased, but the levels of TNFR are inadequate for complete neutralization of TNFα. Animal studies using the collagen-induced arthritis (CIA) model of inflammatory arthritis have shown that mice deficient in TNFR have a more severe early inflammatory response (6). Furthermore, a modified TNFRI gene has been used to suppress CIA in rats (7). Recent clinical studies in which administration of sTNFRII was used to treat disease in patients with RA have highlighted its importance in the inflammatory process (8).

The TNFRI gene maps to 12p13 and the TNFRII gene to 1p36. Whole genome screens (WGS) in rats with adjuvant-induced arthritis (9) and mice with CIA (10) have revealed linkage to regions syntenic to 12p13. Linkage to this region was also detected in a WGS of European RA affected sibpair (ASP) families (11). Two genome-wide linkage scans in RA have shown linkage to markers mapping to 1p36 (11,12), and linkage has been replicated in a second cohort of European HLA-identical RA ASP families (13). One approach to following up linkage data is to investigate association between polymorphism in candidate genes mapping within regions of linkage and RA. Association studies provide a powerful approach to detecting genes with small effect. Demonstration of an association of RA either with specific alleles of a marker (resulting from linkage disequilibrium with a potential functional polymorphism within the gene) or with the functional polymorphism itself would provide evidence of a role in the pathogenesis of RA. TNFRI and TNFRII are strong candidate RA genes based on their known biologic function and on findings in animal models of inflammatory disease. The aim of the current study was to directly test for association between RA and the TNFRI and TNFRII genes.

PATIENTS AND METHODS

Study design. A case–control (association) study was performed to investigate the association of TNFRI and TNFRII with RA in patients in the UK. Cases with RA were compared with population controls for both phenotype and genotype at the 2 loci. Cases were stratified according to the presence of a family history in a first-degree relative. The study included 2 cohorts of patients: a test group and a verification group.

RA cases. Cases with RA were obtained from 2 main sources: from the Arthritis Research Council (ARC) National Repository of patients and families and from local clinics. Patients identified through the National Repository were examined by a metrologist using a standardized questionnaire and examination protocol, including completion of a questionnaire on family history. In the case of any relatives reported by probands to have RA, the RA was verified using the same approach. For clinic patients, there was no information available regarding presence or absence of a family history. Based on previous estimates, it can be assumed that up to 4% of patients will have a first-degree relative with RA. All RA cases had disease that satisfied the American College of Rheumatology (formerly, the American Rheumatism Association) 1987 criteria (14) modified for genetic studies of prevalent cases (15), and all were of UK caucasoid origin. The RA cases were divided into a test group and a replication group. In the test group, 80% of patients had a family history of RA in a first-degree relative, while the verification group comprised 149 probands with a family history of RA (41.7%) and 208 without (58.3%).

Controls. As controls, healthy subjects with no history of inflammatory joint disease were recruited from general practice (n = 67) or from among blood donors (n = 76). All controls were of UK caucasoid ethnic origin.

Power calculation. Sample sizes were calculated based on published allele frequencies so that each of the association studies had 80% power to detect a gene conferring a genotypic relative risk of 2.0 at the 5% significance level.

TNFRI restriction fragment length polymorphism (RFLP). A single-nucleotide polymorphism (SNP) at position 36 in exon 1 of the TNFRI gene (A/G), which creates a recognition site for the restriction enzyme *Msp* AII (New England Biolabs, Hertfordshire, UK) when the G allele is present but not when the A allele is present (16), has recently been identified. The primer sequences and reaction conditions have been described (16).

TNFRII RFLP. There is a T/G polymorphism at position 196 in exon 6 of the TNFRII gene, which creates a recognition site for the restriction enzyme *Nla* III (New England Biolabs) when the T allele is present but not when the G allele is present (17). This polymorphism results in an amino acid substitution (methionine to arginine), although the effect of this change on the function of the TNFRII gene is unknown. The primer sequences and reaction conditions are described elsewhere (17).

Statistical analysis. Allele and genotype frequencies in patient and control groups were calculated by direct counting. The association of the rarer G allele with RA for both SNPs was assessed by calculating the odds ratio (OR) and 95% confidence intervals (95% CI) for the G phenotype and the GG genotype. *P* values less than 0.05 were considered significant.

RESULTS

TNFRI polymorphism in patients and controls. DNA was available from 291 RA probands from the ARC National Repository (the test group). Seventy-nine percent were female, 80% had a family history of RA in a first-degree relative, 78% were rheumatoid factor (RF) positive, and 58% had erosive disease. There was

Table 1. Frequencies of the TNFRI position 36 polymorphism in UK RA patients and controls*

	AA	AG	GG
RA (n = 291)	95 (32.6)	152 (52.3)	44 (15)
Controls (n = 143)	44 (30.8)	76 (53.1)	23 (16.1)

* Values are the number (%) of patients. Odds ratio (OR) for the GG genotype 0.93 (95% confidence interval [95% CI] 0.54–1.60, $P = 0.79$); OR for the G phenotype 0.92 (95% CI 0.60–1.41, $P = 0.69$). For the overall distribution between the 2 groups, χ^2 (2 degrees of freedom) = 0.178, $P = 0.915$). TNFRI = tumor necrosis factor receptor I; RA = rheumatoid arthritis.

no significant difference in the frequency of the G allele between patients and controls (OR for GG genotype 0.93, 95% CI 0.54–1.60, $P = 0.79$; OR for G phenotype 0.92, 95% CI 0.60–1.41, $P = 0.69$) (Table 1). Allele frequencies were similar to those reported previously (16). Since RA is a heterogeneous disease, associations may be found in subgroups of patients. No association with subgroups stratified for sex, RF positivity, presence of erosions, family history, or age at onset of disease was identified. HLA data were available from 137 cases. Stratifying for the presence of the shared epitope did not affect the results.

TNFRII polymorphism in patients and controls. *Test cohort.* Based on published allele frequencies, we calculated that genotyping would have to be performed on 220 RA patients and 110 controls in order to achieve 80% power for detection of a gene conferring a genotypic relative risk of 2.0 at the 5% significance level. Of the 291 patients and 143 controls in the test group who were genotyped in the TNFRI study, 240 patients and 137 controls were also genotyped for the TNFRII exon 6 T/G polymorphism. Positivity for both the G allele and the GG genotype was significantly more frequent in patients with RA than in controls (OR for GG genotype 2.55, 95% CI 1.11–5.86, $P = 0.03$; OR for G phenotype 1.54, 95% CI 1.01–2.34, $P = 0.046$) (Table 2). When the test group was stratified according to presence or absence of a family history of RA, however, the RA cases without a family history showed allele and genotype frequencies that were similar to control frequencies. The differences in GG genotype and G phenotype frequencies were confined to those with a family history of RA (OR for GG genotype 2.89, 95% CI 1.24–6.72, $P = 0.013$; OR for G phenotype 1.81, 95% CI 1.16–2.81, $P = 0.009$).

Verification cohort. DNA was available from 149 RA probands from the ARC National Repository who had a family history of RA in a first-degree relative. Seventy-five percent were female, 84.8% were RF positive, and 75% had erosive disease. DNA was available from an additional 208 individuals with sporadic RA, of whom 74% were female, 72% were RF positive, and 68% had erosive disease. All were typed for the exon 6 TNFRII polymorphism. In this group, too, the frequency of both the G allele and GG genotype was statistically significantly different in RA cases with a family history of RA compared with controls (OR for GG genotype 3.05, 95% CI 1.28–7.24, $P = 0.011$ [Table 2]; OR for G phenotype 1.65, 95% CI 1.03–2.63, $P = 0.036$).

Combined test and verification groups. When data from the groups were combined, there was a highly

Table 2. Frequencies of the TNFRII exon 6 polymorphism in UK RA patients and controls*

	TT	TG	GG	OR, GG genotype (95% CI)	*P*
Initial study					
Combined RA	104 (43.3)	107 (44.6)	29 (12.1)	2.55 (1.1–5.9)	0.032
Familial RA	76 (39.4)	91 (47.1)	26 (13.5)	2.89 (1.2–6.7)	0.013
Nonfamilial	28 (59.6)	16 (34.0)	3 (6.4)	1.26 (0.3–4.7)	0.74
Controls	74 (54.0)	56 (40.9)	7 (5.1)		
Replication study					
Combined RA	168 (47.1)	152 (42.6)	37 (10.3)	2.15 (0.9–4.8)	0.066
Familial RA	62 (41.6)	66 (44.3)	21 (14.1)	3.05 (1.3–7.2)	0.01
Nonfamilial	106 (51.0)	86 (41.3)	16 (7.7)	1.55 (0.6–3.8)	0.35
Controls	74 (54.0)	56 (40.9)	7 (5.1)		
Combined groups					
Combined RA	272 (45.6)	259 (43.4)	66 (11.0)	2.30 (1.1–5.1)	0.04
Familial RA	138 (40.4)	157 (45.9)	47 (13.7)	2.96 (1.3–6.6)	0.007
Nonfamilial RA	134 (52.5)	102 (40.0)	19 (7.5)	1.50 (0.6–3.6)	0.37
Controls	74 (54.0)	56 (40.9)	7 (5.1)		

* Values are the number (%) of patients. TNFRII = tumor necrosis factor receptor II; RA = rheumatoid arthritis; OR = odds ratio; 95% CI = 95% confidence interval.

significant difference in the frequency of the G allele and GG genotype between familial RA cases and controls (OR for GG genotype 2.96, 95% CI 1.33–6.58, P = 0.007 [Table 2]; OR for G phenotype 1.74, 95% CI 1.17–2.59, P = 0.007).

DISCUSSION

The results of this study provide evidence of association between TNFRII and familial RA. This work extends from previous findings of linkage analysis in RA ASP families. Two genome-wide scans in RA ASP families have shown linkage to markers mapping to 1p36, close to the TNFRII locus (11,12), and linkage for one of these markers has been replicated in a group of HLA-concordant European RA ASPs (13). The results of the association study presented here suggest that a true RA susceptibility locus may lie within the TNFRII gene itself or may be in linkage disequilibrium with the exon 6 polymorphism. No evidence of an association with an exon 1 TNFRI polymorphism was detected.

The TNFRII association results could be a false-positive finding, but this is unlikely because 1) there was a significant increase in the OR for both the GG genotype and the G phenotype in familial RA cases compared with controls, 2) the association has been replicated in independent cohorts of familial RA cases, and 3) the controls were found to be in Hardy-Weinberg equilibrium, with allele frequencies that closely reflect those reported elsewhere (18).

The difference in association of familial RA versus sporadic RA with the TNFRII polymorphism is not unexpected. When considering a complex disease that exhibits genetic heterogeneity, families in which more than 1 individual have the disease are likely to have a greater genetic susceptibility. In effect, multicase families are likely to concentrate genetic susceptibility factors, and probands from such families are an ideal group to study since there will be a greater chance of detecting even weak genetic effects. Differences between familial and nonfamilial RA have been reported previously. Sanders et al found that the frequency of HLA–DR4 was significantly higher in familial RA cases compared with RA probands without familial RA (4), and this finding has recently been replicated by another group (5).

It may be speculated that polymorphism within the TNFR genes could alter binding of ligands such as TNFα or cleavage enzymes, thereby leading to an inappropriate inflammatory response due to excessive circulating TNFα, and hence contributing to RA susceptibility. One might therefore expect an association with both TNFRI and TNFRII. However, no difference in allele or genotype frequencies between RA cases and controls was detected in studies using an A/G polymorphism in exon 1 of the TNFRI gene. The lack of association between TNFRI and RA may be a false-negative result. The polymorphism examined was nonfunctional, but it would be expected to be in linkage disequilibrium with any nearby functional polymorphism. Results reported by Kruglyak suggest that such an assumption may not always be valid (19). However, another study has failed to demonstrate an association with 2 TNFRI SNPs in a population of Dutch RA patients (20). The difference in association of TNFRI with RA versus that of TNFRII with RA may therefore be real. The receptors are expressed on different cells, and several lines of evidence suggest that they may have differing functions in addition to the common function of binding and neutralizing free TNFα (21).

The T/G SNP in exon 6 of the TNFRII gene results in an amino acid substitution (methionine to arginine), but the effect of this substitution on the function of the TNFRII gene is not known. The polymorphic site lies in the membrane-proximal extracellular domain of the TNFRII protein and may therefore affect binding of ligands.

We have found evidence of an association between familial RA and TNFRII, but we have not demonstrated an association between RA and TNFRI. Further work will be needed to attempt to replicate these findings in other populations. Interestingly, a recent study in a Japanese population failed to demonstrate an association between the exon 6 TNFRII polymorphism and RA (22). Functional studies to define the effect of the methionine-to-arginine amino acid substitution in the TNFRII protein are also needed. Information on the effect of genotype upon response to treatment with sTNFRII would also be of interest since RA does not respond to this expensive therapy in all patients.

REFERENCES

1. Silman AJ, MacGregor AJ, Thomson W, Holligan S, Carthy D, Farhan A, et al. Twin concordance rates for rheumatoid arthritis: results from a nationwide study. Br J Rheumatol 1993;32:903–7.
2. MacGregor AJ, Snieder H, Rigby AS, Koskenvuo M, Kaprio J, Aho K, et al. Characterizing the quantitative genetic contribution to rheumatoid arthritis using data from twins. Arthritis Rheum 2000;43:30–7.
3. Deighton CM, Walker DJ, Griffiths ID, Roberts DF. The contribution of HLA to rheumatoid arthritis. Clin Genet 1989;36: 178–82.
4. Sanders PA, Grennan DM, Dyer PA, Thomson W, deLange GG.

A comparison of clinical and immunogenetic features in familial and sporadic rheumatoid arthritis. J Rheumatol 1987;14:718–22.
5. Laivoranta-Nyman S, Möttönen T, Luukkainen R, Hakala M, Yli-Kerttula U, Hannonen P, et al. Immunogenetic differences between patients with familial and non-familial rheumatoid arthritis. Ann Rheum Dis 2000;59:173–7.
6. Mori L, Iselin S, de Libero G, Lesslauer W. Attenuation of collagen-induced arthritis in 55kDa TNF receptor type 1 (TNFR1)-IgG1-treated and TNFR1-deficient mice. J Immunol 1996;157:3178–82.
7. Le CH, Nicolson G, Morales A, Sewell KL. Suppression of collagen-induced arthritis through adenovirus-mediated transfer of a modified tumor necrosis factor α receptor gene. Arthritis Rheum 1997;40:1662–9.
8. Moreland LW, Schiff MH, Baumgartner SW, Tindall EA, Fleischmann RM, Bulpitt KJ, et al. Etanercept therapy in rheumatoid arthritis: a randomized, controlled trial. Ann Intern Med 1999;130: 478–86.
9. Lorentzen JC, Glaser A, Jacobsson L, Galli J, Fakhrai-rad H, Klareskog L, et al. Identification of rat susceptibility loci for adjuvant-oil-induced arthritis. Proc Natl Acad Sci U S A 1998;95: 6383–7.
10. McIndoe RA, Bohlman B, Chi E, Schuster E, Lindhardt M, Hood L. Localization of non-MHC collagen-induced arthritis susceptibility loci in DBA/1j mice. Proc Natl Acad Sci U S A 1999;96: 2210–4.
11. Cornelis F, Faure S, Martinez M, Prud'homme JF, Fritz P, Dib C, et al. New susceptibility locus for rheumatoid arthritis suggested by a genome-wide linkage study. Proc Natl Acad Sci U S A 1998;95: 10746–50.
12. Shiozawa S, Hayashi S, Tsukamoto Y, Goko H, Kawasaki H, Wada T, et al. Identification of the gene loci that predispose to rheumatoid arthritis. Int Immunol 1998;10:1891–5.
13. Cornélis F, for ECRAF, the European Consortium on RA Families. New susceptibility locus on chromosome 1 for rheumatoid arthritis [abstract]. Arthritis Rheum 1998;41 Suppl 9:S242.
14. Arnett FC, Edworthy SM, Bloch DA, McShane DJ, Fries JF, Cooper NS, et al. The American Rheumatism Association 1987 revised criteria for the classification of rheumatoid arthritis. Arthritis Rheum 1988;31:315–24.
15. MacGregor AJ, Bamber S, Silman AJ. A comparison of the performance of different methods of disease classification for rheumatoid arthritis: results from an analysis from a nationwide twin study. J Rheumatol 1994;21:1420–6.
16. Pitts SA, Olomolaiye OO, Elson CJ, Westacoll CI, Bidwell JL. An MspA1 I polymorphism in exon 1 of the human TNF receptor type 1 (p55) gene. Eur J Immunogenet 1998;25:269–70.
17. Al-Ansari AS, Ollier WE, Villarreal J, Ordi J, Teh LS, Hajeer AH. Tumor necrosis factor receptor II (TNFRII) exon 6 polymorphism in systemic lupus erythematosus. Tissue Antigens 2000;55:97–9.
18. Pantelidis P, Lympany PA, Foley PJ, Fanning GC, Welsh KI, du Bois RM, et al. Polymorphic analysis of the high-affinity tumour necrosis factor receptor 2. Tissue Antigens 1999;54:585–91.
19. Kruglyak L. Prospects for whole-genome linkage disequilibrium mapping of common disease genes. Nat Genet 1999;22:139–44.
20. Kaijzel EL, Bakker AM, van Krugten MV, Huizinga TWJ, Breedveld FC, Verweij CL. Polymorphisms of tumor necrosis factor receptor I and II in patients with rheumatoid arthritis. Arthritis Rheum 1999;42 Suppl 9:S194.
21. Santee SM, Owen-Schaub LB. Human tumor necrosis factor receptor p75/80 (CD120b) gene structure and promoter characterization. J Biol Chem 1996;271:21151–9.
22. Shibue T, Tsuchiya N, Komata T, Matsushita M, Shiota M, Ohashi J, et al. Tumor necrosis factor α 5′-flanking region, tumor necrosis factor receptor II, and HLA–DRB1 polymorphisms in Japanese patients with rheumatoid arthritis. Arthritis Rheum 2000;43: 753–7.

ARTHRITIS & RHEUMATISM
Vol. 44, No. 1, January 2001, pp 66–72

The Clinical Significance of Amyloid Fat Deposits in Rheumatoid Arthritis

A Systematic Long-Term Followup Study using Abdominal Fat Aspiration

Emili Gómez-Casanovas,[1] Raimon Sanmartí,[1] Manel Solé,[2] Juan D. Cañete,[1] and José Muñoz-Gómez[1]

Objective. **To analyze the prevalence of subclinical amyloid fat deposits in patients with rheumatoid arthritis (RA) and to evaluate its clinical significance.**

Methods. **A cohort of 313 adult RA patients were included in this prospective observational study. Systematic abdominal subcutaneous fat aspiration (ASFA) was performed on all patients at study entry. The prevalence of visceral amyloidosis at study entry and at the end of followup was analyzed for patients with a positive ASFA test result. Followup ranged from 1 to 14 years (mean ± SD 6.7 ± 4.1 years). Patients with clinical and subclinical amyloidosis were compared with regard to clinical characteristics and the degree of amyloid deposits in abdominal fat.**

Results. **The first ASFA test found amyloid in the abdominal fat of 51 patients (16.3%), and subsequent ASFA tests found amyloid in the abdominal fat of 10 additional patients. At the time of the ASFA test, amyloidosis was subclinical in 45 of these 61 patients, 41 of whom were followed up. During followup, 11 of these 41 patients developed renal involvement, 5 due to amyloid nephropathy. Thus, amyloidosis remained subclinical in at least 30 of 41 patients (73%) throughout followup. Marked amyloid fat deposits were found more frequently in patients with clinical amyloidosis than in those whose amyloidosis remained subclinical at the end of followup (57% versus 22%; *P* = 0.04).**

Conclusion. **Amyloid fat deposits are not uncommon in adult RA. In the majority of patients, the deposits do not indicate clinically evident organic dysfunction, even after several years of followup. Patients with more extensive fat deposits may have a higher risk of developing clinical amyloidosis.**

Rheumatoid arthritis (RA) constitutes the most frequent cause of reactive (secondary), or type AA, amyloidosis in first-world countries. The development of clinical visceral amyloid involvement in RA, generally as nephropathy and less commonly as digestive disease, is associated with a poor prognosis and is the direct cause of death in 2–9% of patients (1,2).

The definitive diagnosis of amyloidosis is usually based on the typical histopathologic findings of amyloid deposits in affected tissues. Abdominal subcutaneous fat aspiration (ASFA) is a nonaggressive technique with good sensitivity that is widely used as a screening test in the diagnosis of systemic amyloidosis (3–6). This technique has been used in our rheumatology service since 1983 on a nonselection basis in patients with chronic inflammatory arthritis. In some of these patients, most of whom had RA, amyloid deposits were detected unambiguously in the absence of symptoms suggesting visceral amyloid involvement. The exact clinical significance of these subclinical amyloid deposits is not known. The aims of this study were to analyze the prevalence of amyloid fat deposits in a large cohort of patients with unselected adult RA and to determine whether a positive ASFA test result predicts the development of clinical amyloidosis throughout a long-term followup.

[1]Emili Gómez-Casanovas, MD, Raimon Sanmartí, MD, Juan D. Cañete, MD, PhD, José Muñoz-Gómez, MD, FRCP(Ed): Institut Clínic de l'Aparell Locomotor (ICAL) and Institut d'Investigacions Biomèdiques August Pi i Sunyer (IDIBAPS), Hospital Clínic, Barcelona, Spain; [2]Manel Solé, MD: Hospital Clínic, Barcelona, Spain.

Address correspondence and reprint requests to Raimon Sanmartí, MD, Servicio de Reumatologia, Hospital Clínic, Villarroel 170, 08036 Barcelona, Spain.

Submitted for publication March 31, 2000; accepted in revised form September 27, 2000.

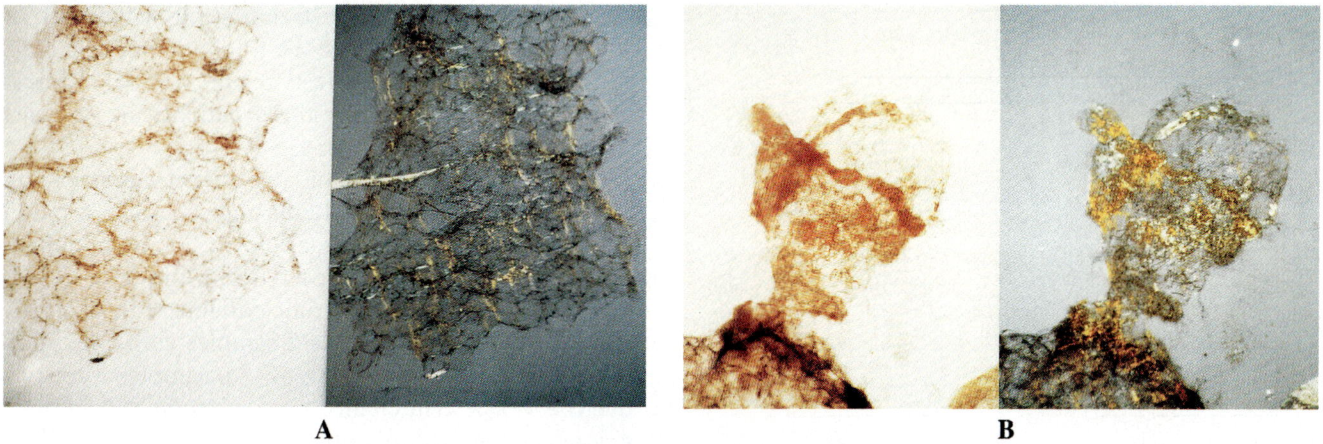

Figure 1. Specimens obtained by abdominal subcutaneous fat aspiration from patients with rheumatoid arthritis. **A,** Amyloid deposition in adipose tissue showing linear pattern under normal (left) and polarized (right) light. **B,** Massive amyloid deposition under normal (left) and polarized (right) light. (Congo red stained; original magnification × 40.)

PATIENTS AND METHODS

Patients. During a 15-year period (September 1983 to December 1998), all patients with chronic inflammatory arthritis of >5 years' duration treated at our rheumatology service were routinely screened for amyloidosis. A total of 313 patients fulfilled, either at present or in the past, the American College of Rheumatology (formerly, the American Rheumatism Association) diagnostic criteria for RA (7). Patients were excluded who met the criteria for juvenile chronic arthritis (disease onset at <16 years of age).

Procedures and followup. Abdominal subcutaneous fine-needle aspiration using standard procedures (6) was performed on RA patients, regardless of clinical symptoms or laboratory data suggestive of systemic amyloidosis. Congo red–stained smears were examined with polarizing light microscopy. The presence of amyloid deposits was confirmed when the typical apple-green birefringence was observed (positive ASFA test result). Positive specimens were reevaluated by the same pathologist (MS) in a blinded manner and classified as +++ (marked), ++ (moderate), and + (mild) according to the amount of amyloid deposits. Marked refers to massive amyloid deposition in >25% of the tissue fragments sampled and/or linear deposits in >75% of fragments, moderate refers to massive amyloid deposits in <25% of fragments or linear deposition in >25% of fragments, and mild refers to linear deposits in <25% of fragments (Figure 1). Very small and isolated Congo red–positive deposits were considered inconclusive and, for purposes of this study, were classified as negative.

In the case of 15 patients with a positive ASFA test result, part of the aspiration specimen was fixed in formalin and processed as a cell block for immunohistochemical analysis, which was performed using antibodies against protein A, κ and λ light chains, and prealbumin (transthyretin) (Dako, Glostrup, Denmark).

The following variables were recorded at the time of fat aspiration in patients who were diagnosed as having adult RA and who had a positive ASFA test result: age, sex, age at disease onset, years of disease evolution, number of swollen joints, C-reactive protein and hemoglobin levels, the presence of rheumatoid factor (by nephelometry; positive >30 IU/liter), the presence of joint erosions on radiographs of the hands and/or feet, and previous arthroplasties. At the time of fat aspiration, as well as during followup (every 3–6 months), we also assessed patients for clinical amyloidosis, defined as the presence of symptoms or laboratory findings suggestive of visceral amyloid involvement, mainly proteinuria (>0.3 gm/24-hour urine sample) or renal insufficiency (serum creatinine >1.4 mg/dl). Other tissue biopsy samples were obtained from some patients according to clinical or laboratory data. A new ASFA test was performed after 2–5 years of followup in patients with a negative ASFA test result at study entry.

RA patients with a positive ASFA test result and previous histopathologic diagnosis of amyloidosis or with renal involvement consistent with amyloid nephropathy at the time of the ASFA test were classified as having "visceral or clinical amyloidosis at entry." Only those patients with a positive ASFA test result and no evidence of visceral amyloid involvement, coupled with a minimum of 1 year of followup, were considered to belong to the true subclinical amyloidosis population (or asymptomatic population with a positive ASFA test result).

Statistical methods. For statistical analysis, patients with a positive ASFA test result were initially classified into 2 groups: those with visceral amyloidosis at entry and those with subclinical amyloidosis at entry. In the latter group, patients who remained asymptomatic at the end of followup and those who developed clinical manifestations during the evolution of the study were analyzed separately; patients with kidney disease other than amyloidosis or those who were not sufficiently studied, as well as patients with subclinical amyloidosis who were followed up for <1 year, were excluded from the statistical analyses. Descriptive analyses (arithmetic mean, standard deviation, minimum and maximum values for continuous variables, percentages for categorical variables) were performed on the different variables present at the time of the

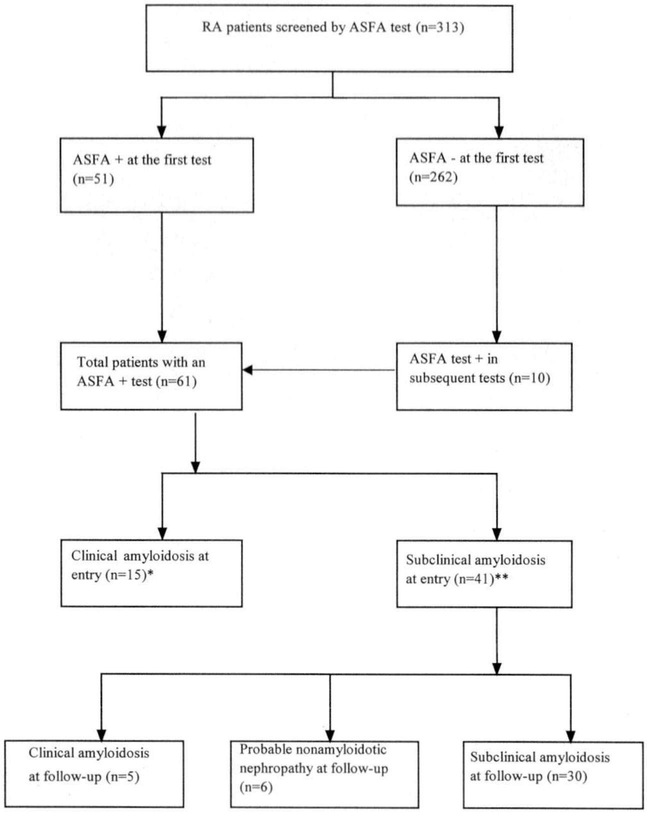

Figure 2. Flow diagram showing derivation of the study groups and subgroups. *One patient with mild renal insufficiency without proteinuria, unrelated to amyloidosis, was excluded from this subgroup (see Results). **Four patients with subclinical amyloidosis who were followed up for <1 year were excluded from this subgroup (see Results). RA = rheumatoid arthritis; ASFA = abdominal subcutaneous fat aspiration.

positive ASFA test result, together with univariate logistic regression analysis among the different groups of patients. The results are expressed as odds ratios (ORs) and 95% confidence intervals (95% CIs). *P* values <0.05 were considered significant. Stata software (8) was used for the analyses.

RESULTS

Amyloid deposits in subcutaneous abdominal fat were observed at study entry in 51 of 313 RA patients (16.3%) (Figure 2). The deposits in 4 other patients were inconclusive and considered negative. Of the 262 patients with a negative ASFA test result at study entry, 74 were retested (33 of them had ≥2 retests); amyloid deposits were observed in 10 of the retested patients after 2–12 years of followup. The remaining patients were not eligible for retest because they were lost to followup, there was insufficient followup time, or (in the case of 58 patients) the treating physician did not consider it necessary. Thus, the total number of patients with a positive ASFA test result was 61. Clinical and demographic data for these patients are shown in Table 1.

The degree of amyloid deposition was assessed in biopsy samples from 51 patients and classified as mild in 12, moderate in 19, and marked in 20. Immunohistochemical analysis found type AA amyloid deposit in all but 2 of the 15 samples from patients with a positive ASFA test result; the other 2 samples contained insufficient material for the analysis. No samples were positive for κ or λ light chains or prealbumin. No causes of secondary amyloidosis, other than RA, could be found in these patients with positive ASFA test results.

Clinical manifestations or laboratory findings consistent with amyloidosis were present in 15 patients at the time of the ASFA test, with histopathologic confirmation in other tissues in 10 patients (total of 13 biopsies: kidney 8, rectum 3, small bowel 1, and esophagus 1). An initial ASFA test result was negative in 1 of these patients. We excluded 1 additional patient with a positive ASFA test result who presented with mild renal insufficiency without proteinuria, unrelated to amyloidosis.

No evidence of renal or other visceral amyloid involvement was found in the remaining 45 patients with positive ASFA test results. In this population, the group with true subclinical amyloidosis, 41 patients were followed up for >1 year; those followed up for <1 year were excluded from the analysis. After a followup of 1–14 years (mean ± SD 6.7 ± 4.1 years), 11 of these 41 patients (26.8%) developed some type of renal involvement. In only 5 of these patients (12.2% of 41 patients) did the renal involvement prove to be due to amyloid nephropathy; in all 5 of these patients, the presence of amyloid deposits was confirmed in other organs or tissues. The latency period between the positive ASFA test result and the first clinical manifestation of systemic amyloidosis was 62 months (range 18–164 months). The clinical evolution of these 5 patients is shown in Table 2.

The existence of amyloid nephropathy could not be confirmed in the remaining 6 patients with renal disease. In 3 of these patients, kidney involvement was attributed to other causes (arterial hypertension and hepatitis C virus–associated mixed cryoglobulinemia in 1 patient, diabetes and chrysotherapy in 1 patient, and sepsis plus treatment with aminoglycosides in 1 patient). The fourth patient developed mild renal insufficiency, and the remaining 2 patients presented with discrete

Table 1. Demographic, clinical, and biologic features of the different groups of ASFA-positive patients at the time of the ASFA test*

			Subclinical amyloidosis at entry		
	All patients (n = 61)	Clinical amyloidosis at entry (n = 15)	Total (n = 41)	Clinical amyloidosis at followup (n = 5)	Subclinical amyloidosis at end of followup (n = 30)
Age, mean ± SD years	61.4 ± 13.7	60.6 ± 15.2	61.5 ± 13.4	56.2 ± 10.9	61.4 ± 14.6
No. of men/no. of women	3/58	0/15	1/40	1/4	0/30
Age at disease onset, mean ± SD (range) years	44.9 ± 14.4 (17–74)	40.6 ± 13.8 (17–68)	45.9 ± 14.2 (17–71)	41 ± 17.2 (20–56)	46.7 ± 14.3 (17–71)
Disease duration, mean ± SD (range) years	16.8 ± 10.5 (5–49)	18.4 ± 11.7 (7–41)	16.5 ± 10.5 (5–49)	17.4 ± 12.1 (7–38)	15.6 ± 8.8 (5–42)
Followup, mean ± SD (range) months	69.7 ± 53.3 (0–175)	62.7 ± 54.6 (0–168)	80.8 ± 49.7 (14–175)	115.6 ± 45 (70–171)	79.5 ± 51.7 (14–175)
RF positive, no. (%)	46 (75)	11 (73)	34 (83)	3 (60)	25 (83)
Erosive disease, no. (%)	57 (93)	14 (93)	41 (100)	5 (100)	30 (100)
CRP level, mean ± SD mg/dl	2.9 ± 2.9	2.6 ± 2.2	2.7 ± 2.6	ND	2.9 ± 2.7
Hemoglobin, gm/dl, mean ± SD	11.5 ± 1.7	10.7 ± 1.6†	11.8 ± 1.6	11.6 ± 1	11.8 ± 1.5
No. of swollen joints, mean ± SD	5.5 ± 4.2	6.1 ± 4.1	5.7 ± 4.2	5.8 ± 5.2	5 ± 4
Arthroplasty, no. (%)	8 (13)	1 (7)	7 (17)	2 (40)	6 (20)
Renal insufficiency, no. (%)	9 (15)	9 (60)	0 (0)	0 (0)	0 (0)
Proteinuria, no. (%)	8 (13)	8 (53)	0 (0)	0 (0)	0 (0)
Fat deposit analysis, no. (%)‡	51 (84)	14 (93)	32 (78)	5 (100)	23 (77)
+	12 (24)	1 (7)	9 (28)	1 (20)	7 (30)
++	19 (37)	5 (36)	13 (41)	2 (40)	11 (48)
+++	20 (39)	8 (57)§	10 (31)	2 (40)	5 (22)
Receiving DMARDs, no. (%)	57 (93)	14 (93)	40 (98)	5 (100)	29 (97)
IM gold	17 (30)	5 (36)	11 (28)	2 (40)	7 (24)
Chloroquine	25 (44)	2 (14)	22 (55)	2 (40)	16 (55)
Methotrexate	4 (7)	1 (7)	3 (8)	0 (0)	3 (10)
Others	11 (19)	6 (43)	4 (10)	1 (20)	3 (10)

* ASFA = abdominal subcutaneous fat aspiration; RF =rheumatoid factor; CRP = C-reactive protein; ND = not done; DMARDs = disease-modifying antirheumatic drugs; IM = intramuscular.
† Odds ratio (OR) 0.63 (95% confidence interval [95% CI] 0.39–0.99), *P* = 0.04 versus the 41 patients with subclinical amyloidosis at entry.
‡ + = mild; ++ = moderate; +++ = marked (see Patients and Methods for further details).
§ OR 11.2 (95% CI 1–120), *P* = 0.04 versus the 30 patients with subclinical amyloidosis at the end of followup.

Table 2. Evolution of disease in the 5 patients with a positive ASFA test result and subclinical amyloidosis at study entry who developed visceral involvement during followup*

Patient/age/sex	Disease duration, years	RF	Erosions	Arthroplasty	Degree of amyloid fat deposits	Latency period, months†	Type of visceral involvement	Other tissues with positive biopsy result	Treatment	Evolution	Followup period, months‡
1/37/F	17	+	Yes	Yes	+++	51	Renal insufficiency, proteinuria	Kidney	Cyclophosphamide	Improvement	120
2/59/F	14	+	Yes	No	+	35	Renal insufficiency, proteinuria	Kidney	Cyclophosphamide, colchicine	Improvement	54
3/59/F	11	–	Yes	No	++	164	Renal insufficiency, malabsorption	Rectum	Cyclophosphamide	Worsening	6
4/63/M	38	+	Yes	No	++	18	Renal insufficiency, malabsorption	Rectum	–	Death	60
5/63/F	7	–	Yes	Yes	+++	43	Renal insufficiency, proteinuria	Urinary bladder, small bowel	Cyclophosphamide	Death	27

* See Table 1 for definitions and other explanations.
† Interval between positive ASFA test result and first clinical manifestation of visceral amyloid involvement.
‡ Interval between first clinical manifestation of visceral amyloid involvement and last followup visit.

Table 3. Life-table analysis of the 35 patients with subclinical amyloidosis and a positive ASFA test result at study entry*

Interval, months	No. of patients with a positive ASFA test result	No. of patients with clinical amyloidosis	No. of patients lost to followup
1–12	35	0	0
13–24	35	1	8
25–36	26	1	1
37–48	24	1	0
49–60	23	1	2
61–72	20	0	4
73–84	16	0	2
85–96	14	0	1
97–108	13	0	1
109–120	12	0	1
121–132	11	0	4
133–144	7	0	2
145–156	5	0	3
157–168	2	1	0
169–180	1	0	1

*Six patients with a positive abdominal subcutaneous fat aspiration (ASFA) test result and nephropathy that was probably unrelated to amyloidosis at the end of followup were excluded.

proteinuria (<500 mg/24 hours) which could not be studied, since they were lost to followup.

Thus, at least 30 of the 41 patients (73%) had no evidence of clinical visceral involvement at the end of the study; in 10 of these patients, the followup period was >10 years (Table 3). Twelve of these patients underwent a second ASFA test 0.5–9 years after the first, and the existence of amyloid deposits in the abdominal fat was again confirmed. In 6 of these 30 patients, biopsy samples were obtained from other tissues, and in 3 of these 6 patients, amyloid deposits were found (rectum, stomach, and gum).

At the time of the positive ASFA test result, no significant differences were observed between the 15 patients with visceral amyloidosis and the 41 patients with subclinical amyloidosis in clinical, laboratory, and radiologic parameters, except for the expected existence of proteinuria and/or renal insufficiency, together with lower hemoglobin levels (mean ± SD 10.7 ± 1.6 versus 11.8 ± 1.6 gm/dl; $P = 0.04$) in the first group. Marked amyloid fat deposits were observed in 57% of patients with visceral amyloidosis at entry and in 31% of those with subclinical amyloidosis; in the group of patients who remained asymptomatic at the end of followup, the prevalence of marked deposits at entry was only 22%. The risk of marked amyloid fat deposits for those with visceral amyloidosis at entry was significantly greater than for those who remained asymptomatic at the end of followup (OR 11.2 [95% CI 1–120], $P = 0.04$). In the group with subclinical amyloidosis at study entry, no differences were observed between the 5 patients who developed visceral amyloidosis with nephropathy and the 30 patients whose amyloidosis remained subclinical at the end of followup. All of these results are shown in Table 1.

DISCUSSION

Different studies have evaluated the prevalence of reactive, or type AA, amyloidosis in RA with varying results, depending on the type of population, geographic area studied, and diagnostic methods used (9–16). At least 6 systematic studies (other than at autopsy) have been conducted using abdominal fat, rectal, or gastroduodenal biopsy samples obtained from RA patients (10–15). The first series showed a relatively low prevalence of type AA amyloidosis (~5% using rectal biopsy material [10] and 4.3% using subcutaneous fat aspiration biopsy material [11]). Recent studies using abdominal fat biopsy material as a screening method with relatively small samples of RA patients have shown higher prevalences of ~8% (12) and even 23% (13) or 78% (14). The largest series is that of Kobayashi et al (15), which demonstrated the presence of amyloid in 13.3% of gastroduodenal mucosa samples in a group of 407 Japanese RA patients.

In our study, the largest published series in nonselected Caucasian RA patients (and using subcutaneous fat biopsy as a screening method), we found a slightly higher prevalence than that in the Japanese series (16%). This may be because we did not include patients with RA of <5 years' duration, and amyloidosis is known to be a late complication of RA. As in other series, our patients had longstanding active and erosive disease, and some of our patients with destructive arthritis required arthroplasty. Previous analysis of a subgroup of patients included in the present study showed no differences between patients with positive or negative ASFA test results, except for the tendency toward a longer duration of arthritis and a significantly increased prevalence of destructive arthropathy in the first group (17).

It is well established that the presence of clinical manifestations due to amyloidosis is associated with a poor prognosis and a lower survival rate, particularly if renal insufficiency is present (18,19). However, our study and other systematic studies (10,12,15) included patients with histopathologic evidence of amyloidosis but without clinical manifestations of visceral involvement. In fact, most of our patients with amyloid deposits in abdominal fat had no symptoms of (and no laboratory findings confirming) amyloidosis at the time of the ASFA test. The true significance and prognostic value of this finding are unknown, and the present study is the first to attempt to answer this question with the long-term followup of these patients.

Our data show that although some patients develop visceral amyloidosis with evident nephropathy and even die, the majority of those with a positive ASFA test result continue to show no evidence of kidney disease or other clinical findings due to amyloidosis throughout a followup of up to 14 years, although a much longer followup period is required to definitively ascertain the prognostic significance of subclinical amyloidosis. The majority of these patients were treated with disease-modifying antirheumatic drugs, but none were treated with alkylating cytostatic drugs just because amyloid deposits were observed in abdominal fat. This circumstance is observed not only in RA patients, but also in patients with other chronic inflammatory rheumatic diseases, such as ankylosing spondylitis (AS). Using the same methods, investigators in our group have observed that although the prevalence of amyloid in the abdominal fat of AS patients is significantly lower (7%) than that in RA patients, amyloid deposition also remains subclinical in the majority of patients after several years of followup (20).

We observed no significant differences at the time of the ASFA test between the 5 patients who developed systemic amyloidosis with nephropathy and the patients whose amyloidosis remained subclinical at the end of followup, although the number of patients was too low for conclusions to be drawn. Kobayashi et al (15) found an association between clinical manifestations of systemic amyloidosis and a greater degree of amyloid deposition in gastroduodenal mucosa. In our study as well, the frequency of marked deposits was significantly higher in the group of patients with visceral amyloidosis at the time of the ASFA test than in those whose amyloidosis remained subclinical at the end of followup (57% versus 22%). It would be logical to think that a larger deposit in the abdominal fat testifies to a greater accumulation of amyloid substance in other organs, with consequent organic dysfunction. Nevertheless, 3 of the 5 patients who initially had subclinical deposits and who later developed visceral amyloidosis had no marked deposits at study entry, and some patients with marked deposits had not developed clinical amyloidosis by the end of followup.

Systematic biopsies of other organs were not considered on ethical grounds; in this respect, the use of a noninvasive, highly sensitive and specific imaging technique such as serum amyloid P scintigraphy (21) might be of great interest for ascertaining the extent and evolution of amyloid deposition in these patients. Unfortunately, this technique is not currently available at our hospital. However, the possibility of quantitatively analyzing the protein A of the amyloid in abdominal fat aspirate by enzyme-linked immunosorbent assay methods, such as those described recently, could help to determine definitively whether the degree of amyloid deposition in fat has prognostic value (22).

Aspiration biopsy of subcutaneous fat is a nonaggressive technique used in recent years to diagnose amyloidosis. Its sensitivity is somewhat inferior to that of rectal biopsy, ranging from 54% to 84% in some reports (3,5,6,23). Although all patients with clinical amyloidosis in the present series had a positive ASFA test result at the time of symptomatic involvement, a negative test result does not necessarily indicate the absence of systemic amyloidosis. On the other hand, Congo red is a highly specific stain for amyloid, and false-positive results are therefore unlikely (23). Caution should be exercised, however, to avoid overstaining, since yellowish birefringence of collagen can be confused with amyloid, particularly by inexperienced observers and especially when seeking very small amyloid deposits (24). Moreover, several fixatives, including alcohol, are responsible for nonspecific green birefringence in normal tissues (25). In our study, all specimens were air-dried and the process of the technique was strictly controlled; therefore, it is highly unlikely that the deposits represent false-positive results. Furthermore, when the ASFA test was repeated after several years of followup in 12 of the 30 patients whose amyloidosis remained subclinical at the end of followup, the presence of amyloid substance was again demonstrated in all patients. Thus, although only 15 specimens were processed for immunohistochemical analysis, the presence of type AA amyloid was confirmed in all evaluable specimens.

In conclusion, we found that 16.3% of patients with RA of >5 years' evolution have amyloid deposits in their abdominal fat; these patients usually have longstanding and erosive disease and, in some cases, destructive arthritis. Nevertheless, this finding is not associated with clinical amyloid disease in the majority of patients. This is true not only at the time of the ASFA test, but also after a long followup period. However, these patients must be periodically monitored for clinical symptoms or laboratory findings suggestive of amyloidosis, since they may develop symptomatic involvement after a variable period of time. In no case does aggressive treatment with cytostatic drugs appear justified if the amyloid deposition remains subclinical. Whether patients with more extensive deposits in their abdominal fat aspirate have a greater risk of developing clinical amyloidosis, as suggested by our findings, requires confirmation by subsequent studies.

ACKNOWLEDGMENTS

The authors are greatly indebted to Dr. Rosa Roselló and Dr. Jaume Rotés-Querol, who first introduced the ASFA test to our hospital. We are grateful to the rheumatologists (Dr. Antonio Collado, Dr. Jordi Gratacós, Dr. Núria Guañabens, Dr. José A. del Olmo, Dr. Miquel Sala) at the Hospital Clínic for their enthusiastic cooperation. We also thank Llorenç Quintó for advice with statistics and Dr. Josep Maria Campistol and Dr. Pilar Peris for cogent manuscript review.

REFERENCES

1. Mitchell DM, Spitz PW, Young DY, Bloch DA, McShane DJ, Fries JF. Survival, prognosis, and causes of death in rheumatoid arthritis. Arthritis Rheum 1986;29:706–14.
2. Mutru O, Laakso M, Isomaki H, Koota K. Ten year mortality and causes of death in patients with rheumatoid arthritis. BMJ 1985; 290:1197–9.
3. Duston MA, Skinner M, Shirahama T, Cohen AS. Diagnosis of amyloidosis by abdominal fat aspiration: analysis of four years' experience. Am J Med 1987;82:412–4.
4. Rosselló R, Solé M. La biopsia de la grasa subcutánea abdominal en el diagnóstico de amiloidosis. Med Clin (Barc) 1985;85:691–4.
5. Klemi PJ, Sorsa S, Happonen RP. Fine-needle aspiration biopsy from subcutaneous fat: an easy way to diagnose secondary amyloidosis. Scand J Rheumatol 1987;16:429–31.
6. Breedveld FC, Markusse HM, MacFarlane JD. Subcutaneous fat biopsy in the diagnosis of amyloidosis secondary to chronic arthritis. Clin Exp Rheumatol 1989;7:407–10.
7. Arnett FC, Edworthy SM, Bloch DA, McShane DJ, Fries JF, Cooper NS, et al. The American Rheumatism Association 1987 revised criteria for the classification of rheumatoid arthritis. Arthritis Rheum 1988;31:315–24.
8. Stata Corporation. Stata statistical software: release 6.0. College Station (TX): Stata Corporation; 1999.
9. Husby RA. Amyloidosis and rheumatoid arthritis. Clin Exp Rheumatol 1985;3:173–80.
10. Arakapis G, Tribe CR. Amyloidosis in rheumatoid arthritis investigated by means of rectal biopsy. Ann Rheum Dis 1963;22: 256–62.
11. Stenkvist B, Westermark P, Wibell L. Simple method of diagnostic screening for amyloidosis. Ann Rheum Dis 1974;33:75–6.
12. Tiitinen S, Kaarela K, Helin H, Kautiainen H, Isomäki H. Amyloidosis-incidence and early risk factors in patients with rheumatoid arthritis. Scand J Rheumatol 1993;22:158–61.
13. Päi S, Helin H, Isomäki H. Frequency of amyloidosis in Estonian patients with rheumatoid arthritis. Scand J Rheumatol 1993;22: 248–9.
14. Barile L, Ariza R, Muci H, Pizarro S, Fraga A, Lavalle C, et al. Tru-cut needle biopsy of subcutaneous fat in the diagnosis of secondary amyloidosis in rheumatoid arthritis. Arch Med Res 1993;24:189–92.
15. Kobayashi H, Tada S, Fuchigami T, Okuda Y, Takagusi K, Matsumoto T, et al. Secondary amyloidosis in patients with rheumatoid arthritis: diagnostic and prognostic value of gastroduodenal biopsy. Br J Rheumatol 1996;35:44–9.
16. Boers M, Croonen AM, Dijkmans BAC, Breedveld FC, Eulderink F, Cats A, et al. Renal findings in rheumatoid arthritis; clinical aspects of 132 necropsies. Ann Rheum Dis 1987;46:658–63.
17. Roselló R, Solé M. Incidencia de amiloidosis secundaria en los reumatismos inflamatorios crónicos. Med Clin (Barc) 1986;87: 525–8.
18. Gertz MA, Kyle RA. Secondary systemic amyloidosis: response and survival in 64 patients. Medicine (Baltimore) 1991;70:246–56.
19. Hazenberg BPC, van Rijswijk MH. Clinical and therapeutic aspects of AA amyloidosis. Baillieres Clin Rheumatol 1994;8: 661–90.
20. Gratacós J, Orellana C, Sanmartí R, Solé M, Collado A, Gómez-Casanovas E, et al. Secondary amyloidosis in ankylosing spondylitis: a systematic survey of 137 patients using abdominal fat aspiration. J Rheumatol 1997;24:912–5.
21. Hawkins PN, Lavender JP, Pepys MB. Evaluation of systemic amyloidosis by scintigraphy with 123 I-labeled serum amyloid P component. N Engl J Med 1990;323:508–13.
22. Hazenberg BPC, Limburg PC, Bijzet J, van Rijswijk MH. A quantitative method for detecting deposits of amyloid A protein in aspirated tissue of patients with arthritis. Ann Rheum Dis 1999; 58:96–102.
23. Duston MA, Skinner M, Meenan RF, Cohen AS. Sensitivity, specificity, and predictive value of abdominal fat aspiration for the diagnosis of amyloidosis. Arthritis Rheum 1989;32:82–5.
24. Blumenfeld W, Hildebrandt RH. Fine-needle aspiration of abdominal fat for the diagnosis of amyloidosis. Acta Cytol 1993;37: 170–4.
25. Klatskin G. Nonspecific green birefringence in Congo red-stained tissues. Am J Pathol 1969;56:1–12.

Please see brief summary of prescribing information on the adjacent page.

SALAGEN® Tablets
(pilocarpine hydrochloride)

Brief Summary

Consult package insert for full prescribing information

INDICATIONS AND USAGE: SALAGEN® Tablets are indicated for 1) the treatment of symptoms of dry mouth from salivary gland hypofunction caused by radiotherapy for cancer of the head and neck; and 2) the treatment of symptoms of dry mouth in patients with Sjogren's syndrome.

CONTRAINDICATIONS: SALAGEN® Tablets are contraindicated in patients with uncontrolled asthma, known hypersensitivity to pilocarpine, and when miosis is undesirable, e.g., in acute iritis and in narrow-angle (angle closure) glaucoma.

WARNINGS:

Cardiovascular Disease: Patients with significant cardiovascular disease may be unable to compensate for transient changes in hemodynamics or rhythm induced by pilocarpine. Pulmonary edema has been reported as a complication of pilocarpine toxicity from high ocular doses given for acute angle-closure glaucoma. Pilocarpine should be administered with caution in and under close medical supervision of patients with significant cardiovascular disease.

Ocular: Ocular formulations of pilocarpine have been reported to cause visual blurring which may result in decreased visual acuity, especially at night and in patients with central lens changes, and to cause impairment of depth perception. Caution should be advised while driving at night or performing hazardous activities in reduced lighting.

Pulmonary Disease: Pilocarpine has been reported to increase airway resistance, bronchial smooth muscle tone, and bronchial secretions. Pilocarpine hydrochloride should be administered with caution to and under close medical supervision in patients with controlled asthma, chronic bronchitis, or chronic obstructive pulmonary disease requiring pharmacotherapy.

PRECAUTIONS:

General: Pilocarpine toxicity is characterized by an exaggeration of its parasympathomimetic effects. These may include: headache, visual disturbance, lacrimation, sweating, respiratory distress, gastrointestinal spasm, nausea, vomiting, diarrhea, atrioventricular block, tachycardia, bradycardia, hypotension, hypertension, shock, mental confusion, cardiac arrhythmia, and tremors.

The dose-related cardiovascular pharmacologic effects of pilocarpine include hypotension, hypertension, bradycardia, and tachycardia.

Pilocarpine should be administered with caution to patients with known or suspected cholelithiasis or biliary tract disease. Contractions of the gallbladder or biliary smooth muscle could precipitate complications including cholecystitis, cholangitis, and biliary obstruction.

Pilocarpine may increase ureteral smooth muscle tone and could theoretically precipitate renal colic (or "ureteral reflux"), particularly in patients with nephrolithiasis.

Cholinergic agonists may have dose-related central nervous system effects. This should be considered when treating patients with underlying cognitive or psychiatric disturbances.

Renal Insufficiency: The pharmacokinetics of orally administered pilocarpine in patients with renal and hepatic disease is not known.

Information for Patients: Patients should be informed that pilocarpine may cause visual disturbances, especially at night, that could impair their ability to drive safely.

If a patient sweats excessively while taking pilocarpine hydrochloride and cannot drink enough liquid, the patient should consult a physician. Dehydration may develop.

Drug Interactions: Pilocarpine should be administered with caution to patients taking beta adrenergic antagonists because of the possibility of conduction disturbances. Drugs with parasympathomimetic effects administered concurrently with pilocarpine would be expected to result in additive pharmacologic effects. Pilocarpine might antagonize the anticholinergic effects of drugs used concomitantly. These effects should be considered when anticholinergic properties may be contributing to the therapeutic effect of concomitant medication (e.g., atropine, inhaled ipratropium).

While no formal drug interaction studies have been performed, the following concomitant drugs were used in at least 10% of patients in either or both Sjogren's efficacy studies: acetylsalicylic acid, artificial tears, calcium, conjugated estrogens, hydroxychloroquine sulfate, ibuprofen, levothyroxine sodium, medroxyprogesterone acetate, methotrexate, multivitamins, naproxen, omeprazole, paracetamol, and prednisone.

Carcinogenesis, Mutagenesis, Impairment of Fertility: No definitive long term animal studies have evaluated the carcinogenic potential of pilocarpine. No evidence that pilocarpine has the potential to cause genetic toxicity was obtained in a series of studies that included: 1) bacterial assays (Salmonella and E. coli) for reverse gene mutations; 2) an *in vitro* chromosome aberration assay in a Chinese hamster ovary cell line; 3) an *in vivo* chromosome aberration assay (micronucleus test) in mice; and 4) a primary DNA damage assay (unscheduled DNA synthesis) in rat hepatocyte primary cultures.

Oral administration of pilocarpine to male and female rats at a dosage of 18 mg/kg/day (approximately 5 times the maximum recommended dose for a 50 kg human when compared on the basis of body surface area (mg/m^2) estimates) resulted in impaired reproductive function, including reduced fertility, decreased sperm motility, and morphologic evidence of abnormal sperm. It is unclear whether the reduction in fertility was due to effects on male animals, female animals, or both males and females. In dogs, exposure to pilocarpine at a dosage of 3 mg/kg/day (approximately 3 times the maximum recommended dose for a 50 kg human when compared on the basis of body surface area (mg/m^2) estimates) for six months resulted in evidence of impaired spermatogenesis. The data obtained in these studies suggest that pilocarpine may impair the fertility of male and female humans.

SALAGEN® Tablets should be administered to individuals who are attempting to conceive a child only if the potential benefit justifies potential impairment of fertility.

Pregnancy: Teratogenic effects.

Pregnancy Category C: Pilocarpine was associated with a reduction in the mean fetal body weight and an increase in the incidence of skeletal variations when given to pregnant rats at a dosage of 90 mg/kg/day (approximately 26 times the maximum recommended dose for a 50 kg human when compared on the basis of body surface area (mg/m^2) estimates). These effects may have been secondary to maternal toxicity. In another study, oral administration of pilocarpine to female rats during gestation and lactation at a dosage of 36 mg/kg/day (approximately 10 times the maximum recommended dose for a 50 kg human when compared on the basis of body surface area (mg/m^2) estimates) resulted in an increased incidence of stillbirths; decreased neonatal survival and reduced mean body weight of pups were observed at dosages of 18 mg/kg/day (approximately 5 times the maximum recommended dose for a 50 kg human when compared on the basis of body surface area (mg/m^2) estimates) and above. There are no adequate and well-controlled studies in pregnant women. SALAGEN® Tablets should be used during pregnancy only if the potential benefit justifies the potential risk to the fetus.

Nursing Mothers: It is not known whether this drug is excreted in human milk. Because many drugs are excreted in human milk and because of the potential for serious adverse reactions in nursing infants from SALAGEN® Tablets, a decision should be made whether to discontinue nursing or to discontinue the drug, taking into account the importance of the drug to the mother.

Pediatric Use: Safety and effectiveness in pediatric patients have not been established.

Geriatric Use: Head and Neck Cancer Patients: In the placebo-controlled clinical trials (see Clinical Studies section in full prescribing information) the mean age of patients was approximately 58 years (range 19 to 80). Of these patients, 97/369 (61/217 receiving pilocarpine) were over the age of 65 years. In the healthy volunteer studies, 15/150 subjects were over the age of 65 years. In both study populations, the adverse events reported by those over 65 years and those 65 years and younger were comparable. Of the 15 elderly volunteers (5 women, 10 men), the 5 women had higher C_{max}'s and AUC's than the men.

Sjogren's Syndrome Patients: In the placebo-controlled clinical trials, the mean age of patients was approximately 55 years (range 21 to 85). The adverse events reported by those over 65 years and those 65 years and younger were comparable except for notable trends for urinary frequency, diarrhea, and dizziness (see **ADVERSE REACTIONS** section).

ADVERSE REACTIONS: Head & Neck Cancer Patients: In controlled studies, 217 patients received pilocarpine, of whom 68% were men and 32% were women. Race distribution was 91% Caucasian, 8% Black, and 1% of other origin. Mean age was approximately 58 years. The majority of patients were between 50 and 64 years (51%), 33% were 65 years and older and 16% were younger than 50 years of age.

The most frequent adverse experiences associated with SALAGEN® Tablets were a consequence of the expected pharmacologic effects of pilocarpine.

Adverse Event	10 mg t.i.d. (30mg/day) n=121	5 mg t.i.d. (15mg/day) n=141	placebo (t.i.d.) n=152
Sweating	68%	29%	9%
Nausea	15	6	4
Rhinitis	14	5	7
Diarrhea	7	4	5
Chills	15	3	<1
Flushing	13	8	3
Urinary Frequency	12	9	7
Dizziness	12	5	4
Asthenia	12	6	3

In addition, the following adverse events (≥3% incidence) were reported at dosages of 15-30 mg/day in the controlled clinical trials: Headache (11%), dyspepsia (7%), lacrimation (6%), edema (5%), abdominal pain (4%), amblyopia (4%), vomiting (4%), pharyngitis (3%), hypertension (3%).

The following events were reported with treated head and neck cancer patients at incidences of 1% to 2% at dosages of 7.5 to 30 mg/day: abnormal vision, conjunctivitis, dysphagia, epistaxis, myalgias, pruritus, rash, sinusitis, tachycardia, taste perversion, tremor, voice alteration.

The following events were reported rarely in treated head and neck cancer patients (<1%): Causal relation is unknown.

Body odor, hypothermia, mucous membrane abnormality, bradycardia, ECG abnormality, palpitations, syncope, anorexia, increased appetite, esophagitis, gastrointestinal disorder, tongue disorder, leukopenia, lymphadenopathy, anxiety, confusion, depression, abnormal dreams, hyperkinesia, hypoesthesia, nervousness, paresthesias, speech disorder, twitching, increased sputum, stridor, yawning, seborrhea, deafness, eye pain, glaucoma, dysuria, metrorrhagia, urinary impairment.

In long-term treatment were two patients with underlying cardiovascular disease of whom one experienced a myocardial infarct and another an episode of syncope. The association with drug is uncertain.

Sjogren's Syndrome Patients: In controlled studies, 376 patients received pilocarpine, of whom 5% were men and 95% were women. Race distribution was 84% Caucasian, 9% Oriental, 3% Black, and 4% of other origin. Mean age was 55 years. The majority of patients were between 40 and 69 years (70%), 16% were 70 years and older and 14% were younger than 40 years of age. Of these patients, 161/629 (89/376 receiving pilocarpine) were over the age of 65 years. The adverse events reported by those over 65 years and those 65 years and younger were comparable except for notable trends for urinary frequency, diarrhea, and dizziness. The incidences of urinary frequency and diarrhea in the elderly were about double those in the non-elderly. The incidence of dizziness was about three times as high in the elderly as in the non-elderly. These adverse experiences were not considered to be serious. In the 2 placebo-controlled studies, the most common adverse events related to drug use were sweating, urinary frequency, chills, and vasodilatation (flushing). The most commonly reported reason for patient discontinuation of treatment was sweating. Expected pharmacologic effects of pilocarpine include the following adverse experiences associated with SALAGEN® Tablets:

Adverse Event	5 mg q.i.d. (20 mg/day) n=255	Placebo (q.i.d.) n=253
Sweating	40%	7%
Urinary Frequency	10	4
Nausea	9	9
Flushing	9	2
Rhinitis	7	8
Diarrhea	6	7
Chills	4	2
Increased Salivation	3	0
Asthenia	2	2

In addition, the following adverse events (≥3% incidence) were reported at dosing of 20 mg/day in the controlled clinical trials: Headache (13%), flu syndrome (9%), dyspepsia (7%), dizziness (6%), pain (4%), sinusitis (4%), abdominal pain (3%), pharyngitis (2%), rash (2%), infection (2%).

The following events were reported in Sjögren's patients at incidences of 1% to 2% at dosing of 20 mg/day: accidental injury, allergic reaction, back pain, blurred vision, constipation, increased cough, edema, epistaxis, face edema, fever, flatulence, glossitis, lab test abnormalities including chemistry, hematology, and urinalysis, myalgia, palpitation, pruritus, somnolence, stomatitis, tachycardia, tinnitus, urinary incontinence, urinary tract infection, vaginitis, vomiting.

The following events were reported rarely in treated Sjogren's patients (<1%): Causal relation is unknown.

Chest pain, cyst, death, moniliasis, neck pain, neck rigidity, photosensitivity reaction, angina pectoris, arrhythmia, ECG abnormality, hypotension, hypertension, intracranial hemorrhage, migraine, myocardial infarction, anorexia, bilirubinemia, cholelithiasis, colitis, dry mouth, eructation, gastritis, gastroenteritis, gastrointestinal disorder, gingivitis, hepatitis, abnormal liver function tests, melena, nausea & vomiting, pancreatitis, parotid gland enlargement, salivary gland enlargement, sputum increased, taste loss, tongue disorder, tooth disorder, hematuria, lymphadenopathy, abnormal platelets, thrombocythemia, thrombocytopenia, thrombosis, abnormal WBC, peripheral edema, hypoglycemia, arthralgia, arthritis, bone disorder, spontaneous bone fracture, pathological fracture, myasthenia, tendon disorder, tenosynovitis, aphasia, confusion, depression, abnormal dreams, emotional lability, hyperkinesia, hypesthesia, insomnia, leg cramps, nervousness, paresthesias, abnormal thinking, tremor, bronchitis, dyspnea, hiccup, laryngismus, laryngitis, pneumonia, viral infection, voice alteration, alopecia, contact dermatitis, dry skin, eczema, erythema nodosum, exfoliative dermatitis, herpes simplex, skin ulcer, vesiculobullous rash, cataract, conjunctivitis, dry eyes, ear disorder, ear pain, eye disorder, eye hemorrhage, glaucoma, lacrimation disorder, retinal disorder, taste perversion, abnormal vision, breast pain, dysuria, mastitis, menorrhagia, metrorrhagia, ovarian disorder, pyuria, salpingitis, urethral pain, urinary urgency, vaginal hemorrhage, vaginal moniliasis.

The following adverse experiences have been reported rarely with ocular pilocarpine: A-V block, agitation, ciliary congestion, confusion, delusion, depression, dermatitis, middle ear disturbance, eyelid twitching, malignant glaucoma, iris cysts, macular hole, shock, and visual hallucination.

MANAGEMENT OF OVERDOSE: Fatal overdosage with pilocarpine has been reported in the scientific literature at doses presumed to be greater than 100 mg in two hospitalized patients. 100 mg of pilocarpine is considered potentially fatal. Overdosage should be treated with atropine titration (0.5 mg to 1.0 mg given subcutaneously or intravenously) and supportive measures to maintain respiration and circulation. Epinephrine (0.3 mg to 1.0 mg, subcutaneously or intramuscularly) may also be of value in the presence of severe cardiovascular depression or bronchoconstriction. It is not known if pilocarpine is dialyzable.

DOSAGE AND ADMINISTRATION:

Head & Neck Cancer Patients:

The recommended initial dose of SALAGEN® Tablets is one tablet (5 mg) taken three times a day. Dosage should be titrated according to therapeutic response and tolerance. The usual dosage range is up to 3-6 tablets or 15-30 mg per day. (Not to exceed 2 tablets per dose.) Although early improvement may be realized, at least 12 weeks of uninterrupted therapy with SALAGEN® Tablets may be necessary to assess whether a beneficial response will be achieved. The incidence of the most common adverse events increases with dose. The lowest dose that is tolerated and effective should be used for maintenance.

Sjögren's Syndrome Patients:

The recommended dose of SALAGEN® Tablets is one tablet (5 mg) taken four times a day. Efficacy was established by 6 weeks of use.

Manufactured by Boehringer Ingelheim Pharmaceuticals, Inc., Ridgefield, CT 06877

For MGI PHARMA, INC., Bloomington, MN 55438-2318

MGI® and Salagen® are registered trademarks of MGI PHARMA, INC.

MGI PHARMA
MGI PHARMA, INC.
Bloomington, MN 55438-2318

ARTHRITIS & RHEUMATISM
Vol. 44, No. 1, January 2001, pp 73–84

Hepatocyte Growth Factor Induction of Collagenase 3 Production in Human Osteoarthritic Cartilage

Involvement of the Stress-Activated Protein Kinase/c-Jun N-Terminal Kinase Pathway and a Sensitive p38 Mitogen-Activated Protein Kinase Inhibitor Cascade

Pascal Reboul,[1] Jean-Pierre Pelletier,[1] Ginette Tardif,[1] Mohamed Benderdour,[1] Pierre Ranger,[2] Donald P. Bottaro,[3] and Johanne Martel-Pelletier[1]

Objective. **Osteoarthritis (OA) involves both a decreased reparative process and an increased degradative phenomenon. Several cytokines and growth factors are known to facilitate the repair of articular cartilage defects. The hepatocyte growth factor (HGF) present in OA cartilage is suggested to be involved in the cartilage repair process as well as in matrix remodeling and chondrocyte migration, leading to partial reconstruction of articular cartilage. Since cell migration is often correlated with metalloprotease activity, the effect of HGF on collagenase 3 production was studied because of its possible implication in OA cartilage remodeling.**

Methods. **We examined HGF-stimulated collagenase 3 production in human OA chondrocytes by Western and Northern blotting. Furthermore, we explored the intracellular signaling pathways through which HGF induced collagenase 3 production.**

Results. **This study showed that HGF stimulated collagenase 3 production in human OA chondrocytes at the transcriptional level, and this induction was mediated by activation of the stress-activated protein kinase (SAPK)/c-Jun N-terminal kinase (JNK) pathway, but not the p38 mitogen-activated protein kinase (MAPK). The p44/42 MAPKs were also phosphorylated and the use of their specific inhibitor (PD 98059) did not affect HGF-induced collagenase 3 production in OA chondrocytes. Induced collagenase 3 production via the SAPK/JNK pathway was mediated, at least in part, by the TRE site in the promoter, and in the activator protein 1 complex, c-Jun, JunD, and Fra-1 were activated. Surprisingly, further experiments revealed that the specific p38 MAPK inhibitor SB 202190 also inhibited collagenase 3 production early in the HGF-induced process. The 50% inhibitory concentration was as low as 50 n*M*, which is unlikely to be related to p38 MAPK inhibition (which is usually in the μM range), suggesting the involvement of another kinase sensitive to SB 202190.**

Conclusion. **This is the first study to show that HGF has the ability to induce both the expression and synthesis of collagenase 3 in OA chondrocytes. The effect is mediated by kinase cascades involving SAPK/JNK and another, unidentified kinase. This study provides novel information implicating a role for HGF in the pathophysiology of OA through its effect on the production of collagenase 3, which is an enzyme that is possibly involved in OA cartilage remodeling.**

[1]Pascal Reboul, PhD, Jean-Pierre Pelletier, MD, Ginette Tardif, PhD, Mohamed Benderdour, PhD, Johanne Martel-Pelletier, PhD: Hôpital Notre-Dame, Centre Hospitalier de l'Université de Montreal, Montreal, Quebec, Canada; [2]Pierre Ranger, MD: Hôpital Sacré-Coeur, Montreal, Quebec, Canada; [3]Donald P. Bottaro, PhD: National Cancer Institute, Bethesda, Maryland.

Address correspondence and reprint requests to Pascal Reboul, PhD, Unité de Recherche en Arthrose, Hôpital Notre-Dame, Centre Hospitalier de l'Université de Montréal, 1560 rue Sherbrooke est, Montreal, Quebec H2L 4M1, Canada.

Submitted for publication May 5, 2000; accepted in revised form September 6, 2000.

Cartilage is composed of a highly organized extracellular matrix, mainly type II collagen and aggrecan, as well as other minor collagen types and proteoglycans that play an important role in maintaining matrix organization. Although chondrocytes represent <5% of cartilage weight, this unique cell type controls cartilage homeostasis (1,2).

Age-related pathologic processes occur at a high frequency in cartilage, and osteoarthritis (OA) is one of the most prevalent diseases in older individuals. OA involves both a decreased reparative process and an increased degradative phenomenon (3,4), thereby limiting the capacity for articular cartilage repair (5,6). Isolated chondrocyte transplantation seems promising, and has been attempted clinically (7); however, this method could benefit from an improved knowledge of the cartilage repair process. Several cytokines and growth factors are known to facilitate the repair of defects in the articular cartilage of animals, but not in histologically complete hyaline cartilage (8,9). Some growth factors, however, such as transforming growth factor β (TGFβ) and basic fibroblast growth factor (bFGF), have been found in vitro to be involved in the cartilage repair process (8,9). In contrast with these latter findings, TGFβ may also be involved in vivo in the degradation of proteoglycans and the formation of osteophytes (10), and bFGF has also been found to induce catabolic processes, including up-regulation of some matrix metalloproteases (MMPs) (11). Recently, hepatocyte growth factor (HGF) has been suggested as having a role in the processes of cartilage repair, matrix remodeling, and chondrocyte migration (12–14).

HGF, also known as a scatter factor, was first isolated from the serum of rats after partial hepatectomy, and has been shown to be a potent hepatocyte mitogenic molecule. This factor consists of both heavy and light chains held together by a disulfide bond, with molecular weights of 70 kd and 35 kd, respectively. HGF is structurally related to the family of serine proteases, but lacks 2 amino acids found in the catalytic triad required for proteolytic function (15–18). HGF stimulates proliferation of various cell types, including epithelial cells, keratinocytes, and melanocytes, promotes motility of keratinocytes and endothelial cells, induces branching tubule formation of canine kidney cells, and plays a key role in organ regeneration in various adult animals (19–22). In brief, HGF is a multifunctional factor and has properties that allow it to induce proliferation, motility, and morphogenesis. HGF binds to the protooncogene c-Met, a receptor belonging to the transmembrane tyrosine kinase cell surface receptor (23).

By immunohistochemistry, HGF was found at slight-to-moderate levels in chondrocyte cytosol, but also in the territorial matrix surrounding the OA chondrocytes of calcified cartilage and within the deep zone of normal cartilage (24,25). Although the exact role of HGF in the joint remains unknown, this factor is suggested to play a role in cartilage homeostasis and repair in early OA.

In the early stages of OA, mechanical erosion involves mainly the upper layers of cartilage (superficial zone), with the majority of chondrocytes of the deep zone remaining metabolically active. A suggested way to retard the OA process is to impede inflammation while stimulating chondrocytes to migrate from the deep zone to the upper zone, consequently facilitating cartilage reparation. Motility and extracellular matrix remodeling are important components in the repair process. It has been demonstrated in vitro, using a Boyden chamber system, that chondrocytes are able to migrate (12,13) and that molecules such as fibronectin and types I and II collagen could promote the haptotactic and chemotactic migration of chondrocytes. Recently, Wakitani et al have also shown in vivo that HGF has chemotactic properties in growth plate–isolated chondrocytes and chondrocytes isolated from adolescent (6-month-old) rabbits (14). Another interesting finding is that cell migration appeared to be accompanied by an increased level of MMP activity. In cartilage, it is well known that members of the MMP family are involved in the homeostatic process, as well as being etiopathologically associated with the progression of joint destruction in OA.

Recently, a new collagenase, collagenase 3 (or MMP-13), has been discovered, and studies have demonstrated its possible role in cartilage remodeling. Briefly, collagenase 3 has a high level of activity on type II collagen in OA and is localized predominantly in the lower intermediate and deep layers (deep zone) of cartilage (26,27). This is important because in this cartilage zone, type II collagen fibers are of the largest size and chondrocytes are most efficient in reconstituting qualitative as well as quantitative extracellular matrix (28).

To better understand the cartilage repair process, and since both HGF and collagenase 3 are produced preferentially in the deep zone of the cartilage (25–27) and appear to be implicated in cartilage remodeling, we first studied the effect of HGF on the production of collagenase 3. We then explored the major intracellular signaling pathways involved in HGF-induced collagenase 3 production.

PATIENTS AND METHODS

Specimen selection and cell culture. Human chondrocytes from articular cartilage (femoral condyles and tibial plateaus) were obtained from 12 OA patients (mean ± SD age 69 ± 9 years) who had undergone total knee arthroplasty. All OA patients were evaluated by a certified rheumatologist and were diagnosed as having OA based on the criteria developed by the American College of Rheumatology Diagnostic Subcommittee for OA (29). Chondrocytes were released from the articular cartilage by sequential enzymatic digestion at 37°C, as previously described (30), and cultured in Dulbecco's modified Eagle's medium (DMEM; Gibco BRL, Burlington, Ontario, Canada) supplemented with 10% fetal bovine serum (FBS; Gibco BRL) and an antibiotic mixture (100 units/ml penicillin base, 100 μg/ml streptomycin base; Gibco BRL) at 37°C in a humidified atmosphere of 5% CO_2/95% air.

Effect of HGF on collagenase 3 production. *Protein level.* First-passage cultured OA chondrocytes were seeded at 2×10^5 cells in 24-well plates in DMEM containing 10% FBS for 48 hours, and then the medium was replaced for 24 hours by DMEM containing 0.5% FBS. After this period, cells were incubated for 24 hours in fresh media containing 0.5% FBS, in the presence or absence of recombinant human HGF (rHuHGF) (10 ng/ml; R&D Systems, Minneapolis, MN) or recombinant human interleukin-1β (rHuIL-1β) (100 pg/ml; R&D Systems) as a positive control. Further experiments examining the effect of the putative endogenous production of IL-1β by OA chondrocytes on HGF-induced collagenase 3 production involved the addition of IL-1 receptor antagonist (IL-1Ra) at 0.5 ng/ml and 10 ng/ml (Amgen, Boulder, CO).

Determination of collagenase 3 synthesis was carried out using Western immunoblot as previously described (30). Briefly, culture media were recovered and electrophoresed in discontinuous 4–12% sodium dodecyl sulfate–polyacrylamide gel electrophoresis (SDS-PAGE) gels and transferred to nitrocellulose membranes (Bio-Rad, Mississauga, Ontario, Canada) according to the method of Towbin et al (31). The membranes were immersed overnight at 4°C in a blocking buffer (Superblock blocking buffer; Pierce, Rockford, IL), followed by a 2-hour incubation at room temperature in a blocking buffer containing 0.1% Tween 20 and anti-human collagenase 3 (mouse monoclonal IgG F17-1C2, diluted 1:10,000; generously provided by Pfizer Central Research, Groton, CT) (30). Membranes were then washed with TTBS (Tris 20 m*M*, NaCl 150 m*M*, Tween 20 0.05%, pH 7.4) and incubated for 1 hour with the secondary antibody (anti-mouse IgG–horseradish peroxidase conjugate, diluted 1:25,000; Pierce). Detection was performed by chemiluminescence analysis with SuperSignal Ultra Chemiluminescent Substrate (Pierce), diluted 1:10 in TTBS according to the manufacturer's recommendations.

Messenger RNA (mRNA) level. First-passage cultured OA chondrocytes were seeded at 8×10^5 cells in 6-well plates in DMEM containing 10% FBS for 48 hours, and then the medium was replaced for 24 hours with DMEM containing 0.5% FBS. After this period, cells were preincubated for 30 minutes with either actinomycin D (2 μg/ml; Sigma-Aldrich, Oakville, Ontario, Canada) or cycloheximide (2 μg/ml; Sigma-Aldrich) in fresh DMEM containing 0.5% FBS, before adding rHuHGF (10 ng/ml). Cells were then incubated for 8 hours.

Collagenase 3 expression was determined by Northern blotting as previously described (32). Briefly, total RNA was extracted using TRIzol reagent (Gibco BRL) as previously described (32), and the RNA was quantitated by RiboGreen RNA quantitation reagent (Molecular Probes, Eugene, OR). Five micrograms of total RNA was resolved on 1.2% formaldehyde–agarose gel and transferred electrophoretically overnight at 4°C to nylon membranes (Hybond-N; Amersham Pharmacia Biotech, Baie d'Urfé, Quebec, Canada) in a 10 m*M* sodium acetate buffer (pH 7.8), containing 20 m*M* Tris and 0.5 m*M* EDTA. RNA was cross-linked to the membranes by exposure to ultraviolet light. The collagenase 3 RNA probe sequences were as previously described (32). The RNA probes were transcribed and labeled with digoxigenin-11-UTP and revealed using CDP-Star (Roche Molecular Biochemicals, Laval, Quebec, Canada) as the chemiluminescence reagent. Films were subjected to an image analyzer for densitometry (ChemiImager 4000; Alpha Innotech, San Leandro, CA), and the mRNA values were calculated according to the relative expression of collagenase 3 normalized to 28S RNA. The results were expressed as a percentage of the control, which was assigned a value of 100.

Protein kinase phosphorylation. First-passage cultured OA chondrocytes were processed as described above. Chondrocytes were then treated in the presence or absence of 10 ng/ml HGF for different periods of time (0–24 hours), or with 100 pg/ml rHuIL-1β for 1 hour as a positive control. Levels of phosphorylation were detected for the stress-activated protein kinase (SAPK)/c-Jun N-terminal kinase (JNK) kinases, and the p44/42 and p38 mitogen-activated protein kinases (MAPKs) from chondrocyte lysates using specific PhosphoPlus kits with a Phototope-HRP Western detection system (New England Biolabs, Mississauga, Ontario, Canada) as previously described (33). After washing cells with ice-cold phosphate buffered saline (PBS), chondrocytes were lysed directly in 1× Laemmli buffer to avoid modification of phosphorylation during cell recovery. Ten micrograms of lysate protein was loaded on a discontinuous 4–12% SDS-PAGE gel. Detection was performed with the SuperSignal Ultra Chemiluminescent Substrate.

SAPK/JNK involvement in HGF-stimulated collagenase 3 production. *Chondrocyte transfections.* OA chondrocyte transfections were performed using the −133 chloramphenicol acetyltransferase (CAT) construct of the collagenase 3 promoter (34). The latter retained the TATA box as well as the activator protein 1 (AP-1) and polyoma virus enhancer 3 (PEA-3) sites. Transfections were carried out according to the calcium phosphate coprecipitation method (35), with a glycerol shock to improve DNA uptake (36). Briefly, first-passage OA chondrocytes were seeded at 6×10^5 cells in 6-well plates in DMEM containing 10% FBS for 24 hours. These cells were then transfected with a DNA–calcium phosphate preparation consisting of 125 m*M* $CaCl_2$, 10 μg −133 CAT collagenase 3 promoter construct, and 5 μg plasmid pSV-β-galactosidase (Promega, Madison, WI). The β-galactosidase plasmid was used as a positive transfection control. Following overnight incubation, chondrocytes were further incubated for 48 hours with or without 10 ng/ml rHuHGF. Cells were then washed and lysed in Triton X-100/MOPS buffered saline. Cellular extracts were evaluated for CAT, β-galactosidase, and total protein determinations. CAT and β-galactosidase were measured using enzyme-linked immunosorbent assay (ELISA) kits (Roche Molecular Biochemicals), and total proteins were assessed with the bicinchoninic acid method (Pierce). Transfections were performed in 5 independent experiments. Results were normalized according to the level of total protein and expressed as a percentage of the stimulation relative to that of non–HGF-treated cells.

Comparative effect of HGF and HGF/N-terminal hairpin and first two kringle domains (NK2) on SAPK/JNK pathway activation in chondrocytes. We performed Western blotting of nuclear extracts (10 μg) from first-passage OA chondrocytes untreated or treated with rHuHGF (10 ng/ml) or HGF/NK2 (10 ng/ml) for different periods of time. HGF/NK2 was produced in a bacterial expression system, purified, and refolded as previously described (37). This factor is a naturally truncated isoform of HGF that binds to the HGF receptor with an affinity similar to that of HGF, but induces the phosphorylation of p44/42 as well as phosphatidylinositol 3-kinase (PI 3-K), but not SAPK/JNK, in 184B5 cells (38). Detection was achieved by subsequently using a specific phospho c-Jun antibody (dilution 1:2,500; New England Biolabs), an anti-rabbit IgG horseradish peroxidase conjugate (dilution 1:10,000), and the SuperSignal Ultra Chemiluminescent Substrate (Pierce).

Comparative effect of HGF and HGF/NK2 on collagenase 3 production. First-passage cultured OA chondrocytes were seeded at 2×10^5 cells in 24-well plates in DMEM containing 10% FBS for 48 hours, and then the medium was replaced by DMEM containing 0.5% FBS. After 24 hours, cells were incubated for another 24 hours in fresh media containing 0.5% FBS, in the presence or absence of rHuHGF (10 ng/ml) or HGF/NK2 (10 ng/ml). Following incubation, collagenase 3 levels were determined on the culture medium with a specific collagenase 3 ELISA (Amersham Pharmacia Biotech).

Transcription factors. The AP-1 and PEA-3 transcription factor activity was determined using the DNA-binding electrophoretic mobility shift assay (EMSA). Nuclear extractions were performed as previously described (39). Chondrocytes were incubated with 10 ng/ml rHuHGF, then lysed in ice-cold hypotonic buffer containing 10 m*M* HEPES–KOH (pH 7.9), 10 m*M* KCl, 1.5 m*M* $MgCl_2$, 0.5 m*M* dithiothreitol (DTT), 1% Nonidet P40, 10 μg/ml each of aprotinin, leupeptin, and pepstatin, 1 m*M* orthovanadate, and 1 m*M* phenylmethylsulfonyl fluoride (PMSF). Nuclei were recovered by a brief centrifugation, washed once, and subjected to extraction with a high-salt buffer containing 20 m*M* HEPES–KOH (pH 7.9), 420 m*M* NaCl, 1.5 m*M* $MgCl_2$, 0.5 m*M* DTT, 0.2 mM EDTA, 25% glycerol, 10 μg/ml each of aprotinin, leupeptin, and pepstatin, 1 m*M* orthovanadate, and 0.5 m*M* PMSF as previously described (39). Nuclear extracts were recovered by centrifugation at 16,000*g* for 10 minutes at 4°C.

DNA probes and competitors were complementary oligonucleotides: AP-1 sense TAA-GTG-ATG-ACT-CAC-CAT-TGC, mutated AP-1 sense CCT-ATC-CAT-AAG-TGA-TCC-CTC-ACC-ATT-GCA-GGC-C, PEA-3 sense AGT-GAC-TAG-GAA-GTG-GAA-ACC, and GA sense GAG-GGA-AAA-GAA-AAA-GTC-GCC. Oligonucleotides were annealed and labeled with γ^{32}P–ATP by T4 polynucleotide kinase. Nuclear extracts (2 μg) were preincubated at room temperature for 10 minutes with or without competitor oligonucleotides in a binding buffer (Promega). The 20-minute binding reaction was initiated through the addition of 1 μl (80 fmol) of a ^{32}P-labeled probe at room temperature. The amount of unlabeled competitor DNA added was 400 fmoles. Samples were electrophoresed on prerun 6% polyacrylamide gels containing 2.5% glycerol in 0.5× TBE (Tris 22 m*M*, borate 22 m*M*, EDTA 0.5 m*M*) at 200 volts for 150 minutes at 4°C. Gels were then fixed with 7% acetic acid, dried, and subjected to autoradiography.

We further examined the different nuclear factors binding to the AP-1 probe using supershift EMSA experiments as previously described (39). The binding reaction was processed as described above, and then specific antibodies against Fra-1, Fra-2, FosB, c-Jun, and JunD (Santa Cruz Biotechnology, Santa Cruz, CA) in a 1:10 dilution were added and an immunogenic reaction was performed overnight at 4°C before electrophoresis.

Protein kinase inhibition. To define the pathways involved in activating HGF-induced collagenase 3 production, chondrocytes were preincubated for 30 minutes with inhibitors of several kinases, such as PD 98059 (50 μM) (MEK-1 inhibitor; New England Biolabs), wortmannin (100 n*M*) (PI 3-K inhibitor; Calbiochem-Novabiochem, San Diego, CA), and SB 202190 (2 μM) (p38 MAPK inhibitor; Upstate Biotechnology, Lake Placid, NY) followed by the addition of 10 ng/ml rHuHGF for 24 hours. Following incubation, collagenase 3 levels were determined on the culture medium with a specific ELISA (Amersham Pharmacia Biotech). Further experiments were carried out with SB 202190 wherein the inhibitory concentrations and time-dependent response were examined. In concentration studies, SB 202190 was preincubated for 30 minutes before adding 10 ng/ml rHuHGF, and cells were incubated for 24 hours. In kinetic experiments, 10 ng/ml rHuHGF was added for different time periods, followed by the addition of SB 202190 (2 μM) for 18 hours. Collagenase 3 levels were determined as above.

Determination of p38 MAPK activity. First-passage chondrocytes were incubated for 30 minutes with 10 ng/ml rHuHGF as described above. After washing cells with ice-cold PBS, they were recovered using a cell scraper in an ice-cold assay dilution buffer (20 m*M* MOPS, pH 7.2, 25 m*M* β-glycerol phosphate, 5 m*M* EGTA, 1 m*M* DTT, and 1 m*M* sodium orthovanadate). Cells were frozen and then thawed on ice, sonicated in a water bath containing melting ice water for 2 minutes, and centrifuged at 12,000*g* at 4°C for 10 minutes. The activity of p38 MAPK was measured on the supernatant according to the manufacturer's protocol (Upstate Biotechnology), which consists of activating recombinant MAPK-activated protein kinase 2 (MAPKAPK-2), which then phosphorylates a peptide. The p38 MAPK activity was expressed as counts per minute/μg protein. Results were expressed as a percentage of untreated cells (control), which was assigned a value of 100.

Statistical analysis. Data are expressed as the mean ± SEM. Student's 2-tailed *t*-tests were performed to assess differences between groups. *P* values less than 0.05 were considered significant.

RESULTS

HGF-induced collagenase 3 production. We evaluated the effect of HGF on collagenase 3 synthesis and expression in human OA chondrocytes. As illustrated in

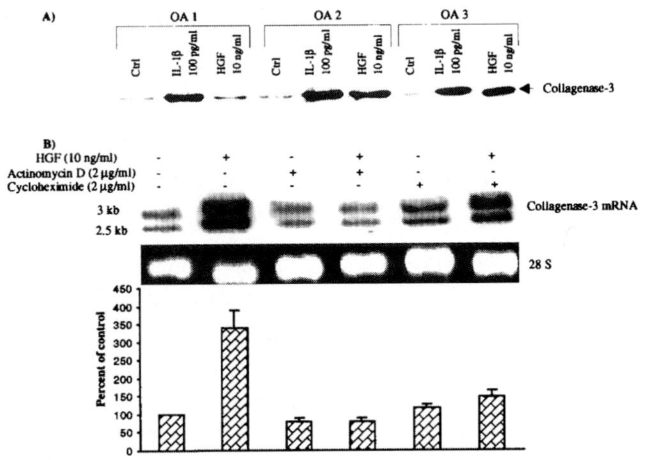

Figure 1. Stimulation of chondrocyte-synthesized collagenase 3 with hepatocyte growth factor (HGF). **A,** Three samples of human osteoarthritic (OA) chondrocytes (OA 1–OA 3) were treated with recombinant human interleukin-1β (IL-1β) (100 pg/ml) or recombinant human HGF (10 ng/ml) for 24 hours. Twenty micrograms of media proteins were blotted and immunodetection was performed with a monoclonal anti–collagenase 3 antibody. Ctrl = control. **B,** OA chondrocytes were preincubated with or without actinomycin D (2 μg/ml) or cycloheximide (2 μg/ml) for 30 minutes, followed by the addition of 10 ng/ml recombinant human HGF. Five micrograms of total RNA was transferred onto a nylon membrane. Collagenase 3 mRNA expression was normalized to the 28S ribosomal subunit (staining with ethidium bromide), and results are expressed as a percentage of the untreated cells (control). Bars show the mean and SEM of 3 independent experiments.

Figure 1A, 10 ng/ml of rHuHGF stimulated collagenase 3 synthesis (n = 3), but not to the same extent as did IL-1β in all human OA specimens. HGF was also proven capable of up-regulating the collagenase 3 mRNA level (n = 3) (Figure 1B). This stimulation was prevented by coincubation with actinomycin D (2 μg/ml) (an inhibitor of RNA transcription), suggesting that it did not occur through the HGF-stabilizing collagenase 3 transcripts. However, cycloheximide (2 μg/ml) (an inhibitor of mRNA translation) also partially inhibited the HGF-induced collagenase 3 mRNA level, suggesting that both endogenous and newly synthesized factors are necessary for complete stimulation by this factor.

To evaluate whether this response was specific for OA chondrocytes (versus normal chondrocytes), experiments were carried out with normal chondrocytes from humans (n = 2) and rabbits (n = 2). The rabbit was chosen because, unlike the mouse or rat, it expresses both collagenase 1 and collagenase 3, and HGF binds to rabbit HGF receptors with an affinity similar to that observed in humans (40). The results indicated that HGF also stimulated collagenase 3 production in normal chondrocytes (data not shown).

To further determine whether HGF-induced collagenase 3 production can be ascribed to an autocrine loop involving IL-1β, the OA chondrocytes were coincubated with HGF (10 ng/ml) and IL-1Ra (at 0.5 ng/ml and 10 ng/ml). The results indicate that blocking IL-1β activity had no effect on HGF-induced collagenase 3 production, since cotreatment with IL-1Ra produced similar levels of collagenase 3 as did treatment with HGF (mean ± SEM ng of collagenase 3/mg of protein [n = 5] 58.6 ± 23.9 in controls compared with 133.2 ± 31.1 with HGF, 135.6 ± 38.8 with HGF plus 0.5 ng/ml IL-1Ra, and 142.8 ± 41.4 with HGF plus 10 ng/ml IL-1Ra).

HGF signaling pathways in chondrocytes. To delineate the signaling pathway activated by HGF in human OA chondrocytes, we initially examined the HGF-induced phosphorylation patterns of MAPK over increasing periods of time. Results (n = 3) indicate that the SAPK/JNK kinases, as well as the p44/42 kinases, were phosphorylated within minutes of stimulation; however, there was no change in the p38 MAPK (Figure 2). Activation peaked at ~15 minutes for the p44/42 kinases and 30 minutes for SAPK/JNK, and phosphorylation levels returned to basal conditions after 2 hours of incubation. Interestingly, and in contrast with the effects of IL-1β, HGF stimulated the phosphorylation of only the p46 kinase, and not the p54.

The promoter regions of human collagenase 3 genes harbor *cis*-acting enhancer elements that are recognized, among others, by the *trans*-acting transcription factor AP-1. Because HGF stimulates SAPK/JNK

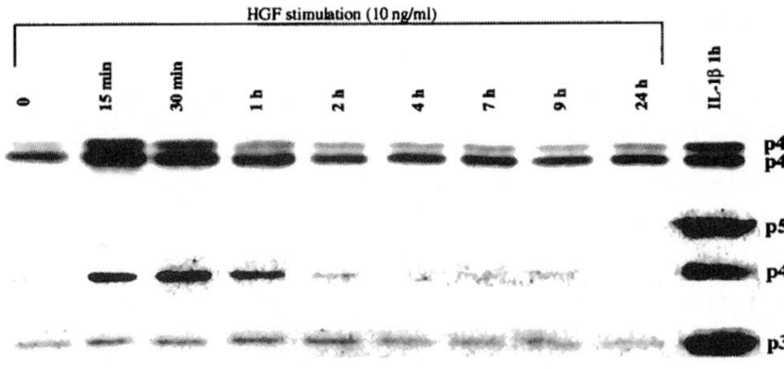

Figure 2. Kinetics of HGF-dependent phosphorylation of mitogen-activated protein kinase (MAPK). Immunoblots of HGF-stimulated OA chondrocyte protein lysates (10 μg) were reacted with phospho-specific p44/42 antibody, phospho-specific stress-activated protein kinase/c-Jun N-terminal kinase (p54/p46) antibody, or phospho-specific p38 MAPK. A protein lysate from OA chondrocytes stimulated with 100 pg/ml recombinant human IL-1β for 1 hour was used as positive control. Each blot is representative of 3 independent experiments. See Figure 1 for other definitions.

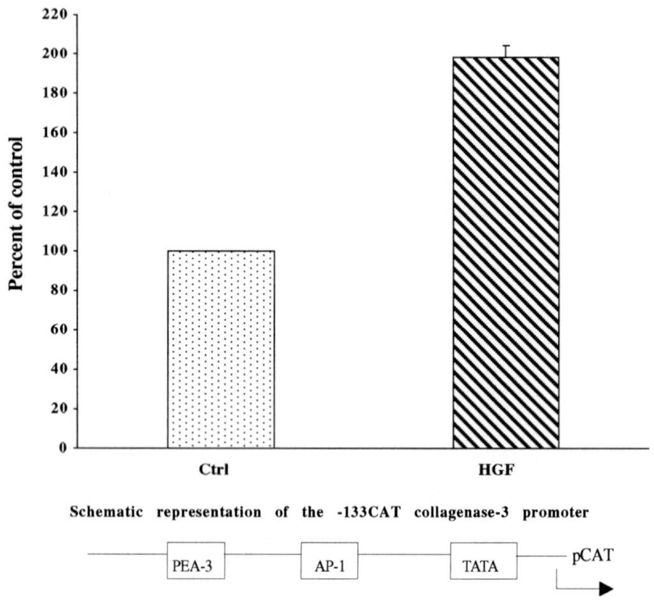

Figure 3. OA chondrocyte transfection with the −133 chloramphenicol acetyltransferase collagenase 3 promoter construct (−133CAT). OA chondrocytes were treated for 48 hours with or without recombinant human HGF (10 ng/ml). The expression of pCAT was measured with an enzyme-linked immunosorbent assay and reported as pg of pCAT/μg cell proteins. Results are expressed as the mean and SEM percentage (n = 5) of untreated cells (Ctrl), assigned a value of 100. PEA-3 = polyoma virus enhancer 3; AP-1 = activator protein 1; see Figure 1 for other definitions.

phosphorylation in OA chondrocytes, we further studied the effect of HGF on the collagenase 3 AP-1 site. To this end, we transfected the OA chondrocytes with a collagenase 3 promoter construct (−133 CAT) containing only the PEA-3 and AP-1 sites (34), and cells were left untreated or treated for 48 hours with HGF (10 ng/ml) (n = 5). Compared with the untreated transfected cells (control), HGF induced a 2-fold increase in expression of CAT (Figure 3). For comparison purposes, experiments were also performed with rHuIL-1β (100 pg/ml). The results showed a 2.2-fold increment of increase (data not shown). When chondrocytes were transfected with the empty vector, no CAT stimulation was found.

Further experiments were aimed at elucidating the role of the SAPK/JNK pathway in HGF-induced collagenase 3 production in OA chondrocytes. To this end, OA chondrocytes were treated with HGF/NK2, which is a truncated isoform of HGF that is able to induce the phosphorylation of p44/42 and PI 3-K, but not SAPK/JNK, in 184B5 cells (37,38). The presence of collagenase 3 was determined in the culture medium. In addition, in order to verify the absence of SAPK/JNK pathway activation, we looked at the phosphorylation of one of its target transcription factors, the c-Jun. The results showed that unlike HGF, HGF/NK2 was unable to activate c-Jun phosphorylation, demonstrating that this pathway is not induced when OA chondrocytes are incubated with HGF/NK2 (Figure 4A). Figure 4B illustrates the effect of HGF and HGF/NK2 on collagenase 3 production. The results (n = 11) showed that in contrast to HGF, HGF/NK2 slightly induced collagenase 3 production, but no statistically significant increase was reached. Additional experiments were carried out with increasing concentrations of HGF/NK2 (up to 40 ng/ml) and the findings revealed expression levels of collagenase 3 similar to those achieved with 10 ng/ml (results not shown). Taken together, these results, as well as those of the chondrocyte transfection experiments, indicate that the SAPK/JNK kinase pathway is a key factor in HGF-stimulated collagenase 3 production.

To more accurately identify whether the AP-1 or PEA-3 sequences were involved in HGF-induced collagenase 3 production, we evaluated the effects on HGF-induced nuclear DNA–binding proteins. HGF-stimulated the level of nuclear DNA–binding proteins,

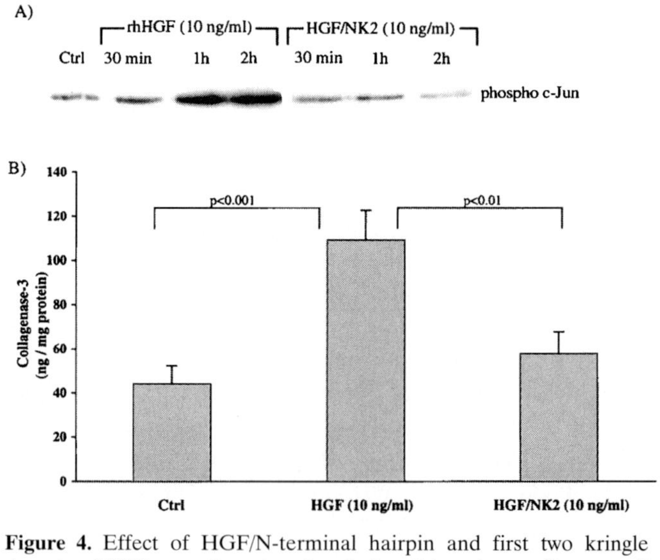

Figure 4. Effect of HGF/N-terminal hairpin and first two kringle domains (NK2) on c-Jun phosphorylation (**A**) and on collagenase 3 production (**B**) in OA chondrocytes. **A,** Phosphorylation of c-Jun was studied with OA chondrocytes left untreated or treated with recombinant human HGF (rhHGF) (10 ng/ml) and HGF/NK2 (10 ng/ml) for different periods of time. Nuclear proteins were extracted and 10 μg of protein was used for immunoblotting. **B,** OA chondrocytes were stimulated with either rhHGF (10 ng/ml) or HGF/NK2 for 24 hours, and collagenase 3 production was measured with a specific enzyme-linked immunosorbent assay. Bars show the mean and SEM (n = 11). See Figure 1 for other definitions.

in that the ^{32}P-labeled AP-1 oligonucleotide, but not the PEA-3, was recognized in OA chondrocytes treated with HGF (n = 3) (Figure 5A). Binding to the AP-1 sequence was specific, since it was displaced with a 5-fold excess of the probe and abrogated when using a mutant AP-1 probe. Moreover, a 5-fold excess of an unrelated probe (GA probe, a sequence in the 5′ end of the collagenase 3 −133 CAT construct) did not compete (Figure 5A). We then identified proteins that could constitute the AP-1 complex using supershift assay. Results (n = 2) showed that the binding of c-Jun, JunD, and Fra-1 was enhanced when chondrocytes were incubated with HGF (10 ng/ml) for 2 hours (Figure 5B). Neither FosB and Fra-2 (Figure 5B) nor JunB and cFos (results not shown) were implicated in this complex.

To better delineate the HGF signaling cascades involved in collagenase 3 production, we used cell-permeable chemical inhibitors of the intracellular process (n = 4) (Figure 6). The MEK-1 inhibitor PD 98059 (50 μM) had no effect on HGF-induced collagenase 3 synthesis, suggesting that MAPKs p44/42 are not implicated in this process. The wortmannin at 100 nM appeared to potentiate (stimulation of 60%) the effect of HGF on expression of collagenase 3, underlying a modulator effect generated by PI 3-K, although the difference did not reach statistical significance (Figure 6). Surprisingly, OA chondrocytes treated with the p38 MAPK inhibitor SB 202190 (2 μM) significantly decreased ($P < 0.02$) HGF-induced collagenase 3 synthesis by 60%.

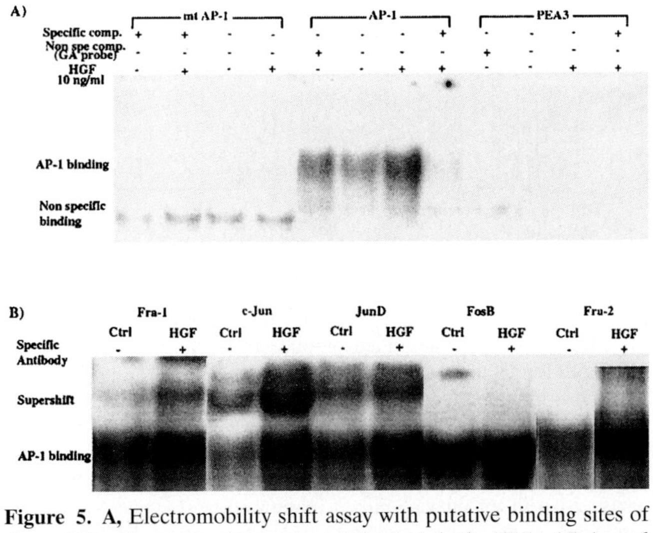

Figure 5. A, Electromobility shift assay with putative binding sites of the −133 collagenase 3 construct. Mutated (mt) AP-1, AP-1, and PEA3 probes were used in these assays. Stronger binding of AP-1 occurred when OA chondrocytes were treated with recombinant human HGF (10 ng/ml) for 2 hours. The specificity of binding is demonstrated with both the mt AP-1 probe and competition with either specific or unrelated (Non spe) competitors (comp.) (GA probe). No binding was demonstrated with the PEA3 probe. The gel is representative of 3 independent experiments. **B,** Analysis of the protein constituting AP-1 binding with HGF-stimulated chondrocytes. Binding assays were performed with nuclear extracts of unstimulated (Ctrl) or HGF-stimulated (10 ng/ml) OA chondrocytes for 2 hours. Supershifts were done using specific antibodies as described in Patients and Methods. The gel is representative of 2 independent experiments. See Figures 1 and 3 for other definitions.

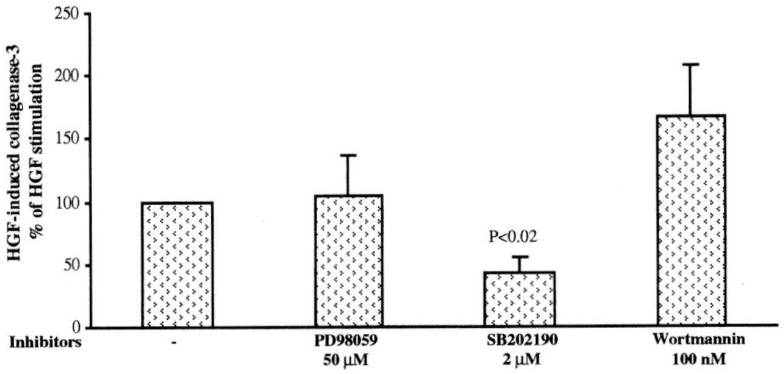

Figure 6. Effects of protein kinase inhibitors PD98059 (inhibitor of p44/42 MAPK), SB 202190 (inhibitor of p38 MAPK), and wortmannin (inhibitor of phosphatidylinositol 3-kinase) on HGF-induced collagenase 3 production. Cells were preincubated for 30 minutes with these different inhibitors followed by 24 hours' incubation in the presence of 10 ng/ml recombinant human HGF. Values are expressed as the mean and SEM percentage (n = 4) of the HGF control (-), assigned the value of 100. P value is versus control. See Figures 1 and 2 for definitions.

Since the above experiment suggested that a p38 MAPK inhibitor strongly inhibited HGF-induced collagenase 3 production, but that p38 was not phosphorylated by this factor (Figure 2), we further looked at the p38 MAPK activation via an assay kit using MAPKAPK-2 as substrate (Figure 7). The justification for this experiment is supported by a recent study that demonstrated, in another cell system, that HGF can phosphorylate another intracellular signaling cascade, the Smad-2, at a site other than the classic one induced by TGFβ (41). Therefore, if p38 MAPK is involved in HGF signaling in chondrocytes, a phosphorylation site different from the one recognized by the antibody may explain the negative findings that we (Figure 2) and others (42) have obtained using immunoblotting. By assessing the p38 MAPK activity using the assay kit (n = 4), the results showed that, after 30 minutes of treatment, HGF induced MAPKAPK-2 activation by 58% ($P < 0.03$) in OA chondrocytes (Figure 7). Moreover, IL-1β, used as a positive control, showed a 3-fold increase in stimulation. Interestingly, and although the IL-1β–induced activation of MAPKAPK-2 was partially

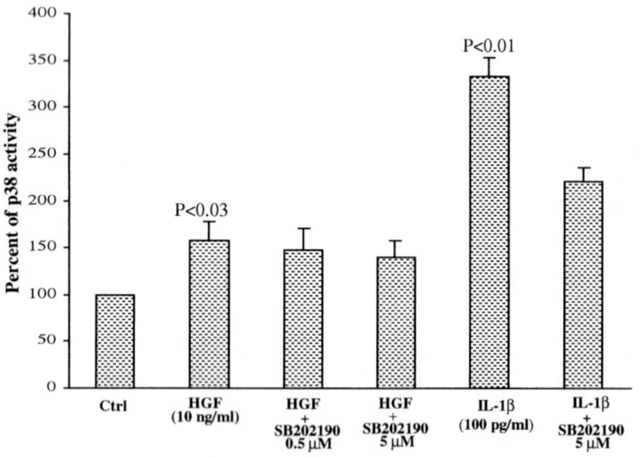

Figure 7. Effect of HGF on p38 MAPK activity. OA chondrocytes were treated with or without 10 ng/ml recombinant human HGF or 100 pg/ml recombinant human IL-1β for 30 minutes. Cells were lysed in an ice-cold assay dilution buffer and p38 activity was assayed as recommended by the manufacturer (Upstate Biotechnology) in the presence or absence of different concentrations of SB 202190. *P* values are versus control. Bars show the mean and SEM (n = 4). See Figures 1 and 2 for definitions.

inhibited by SB 202190 (5 μM), no inhibitory effect was noted in HGF-stimulated chondrocytes, suggesting that the HGF-induced MAPKAPK-2 activation did not occur through the p38 MAPK. This strongly suggests that SB 202190 may act on another kinase involved in the regulation of collagenase 3 expression.

To better characterize the p38 MAPK inhibitor effect, we performed a time-course study (n = 4) (Figure 8A) to assess the impact of the addition of SB 202190 during the early events of the HGF signaling cascades. OA chondrocytes were stimulated for different periods of time by 10 ng/ml of HGF, and then 2 μM of SB 202190 was added and incubation was maintained for 18 hours. During the first 30 minutes of HGF stimulation, SB 202190 decreased collagenase 3 production by 60% compared with the control level, followed by a dramatic time-dependent rise which reached the HGF control level at 2 hours of incubation, with no change thereafter. In light of this result and our finding that MAPKAPK-2 activity was not inhibited by 5 μM SB 202190 (Figure 7), suggesting that p38 MAPK was not implicated, we hypothesized that another kinase might be susceptible to this compound. We therefore performed dose-response studies (n = 3) (Figure 8B) with SB 202190 on HGF-induced collagenase 3 production. Interestingly, HGF-induced collagenase 3 production was inhibited in a dose-dependent manner, but with very low concentrations of SB 202190. Indeed, ~20% inhibition ($P <$

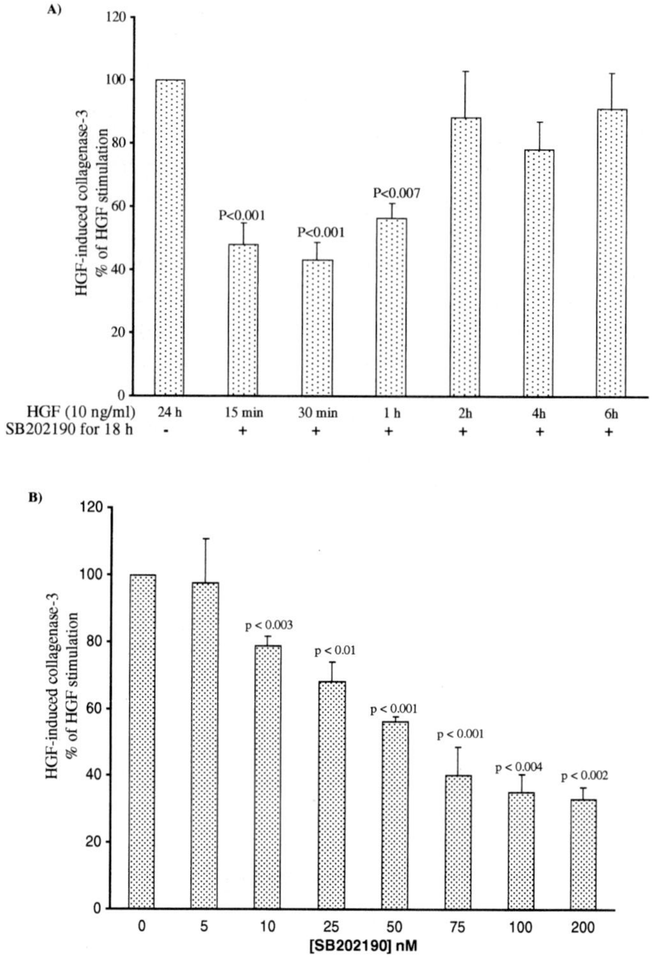

Figure 8. HGF-dependent collagenase 3 activation in the presence of SB 202190. **A,** OA chondrocytes (n = 4) were incubated for different periods of time with 10 ng/ml recombinant human HGF. Subsequently, SB 202190 (2 μM) was added at once in all wells and cells were incubated for 18 hours (h). **B,** Dose curve of SB 202190 and inhibition of HGF-stimulated collagenase 3 production. Chondrocytes were incubated for 30 minutes (min) with increasing concentrations of SB 202190, then 10 ng/ml recombinant human HGF was added and cells were incubated for 24 hours (n = 3). Collagenase 3 production was measured with an enzyme-linked immunosorbent assay. Values are expressed as the mean and SEM percentage of the HGF control, assigned a value of 100. *P* values are versus control. See Figure 1 for other definitions.

0.003) was obtained with 10 nM, and the maximum inhibition of ~66% was reached at 200 nM ($P < 0.002$), which is as potent as using 2 μM SB 202190.

DISCUSSION

In recent literature, interesting anabolic effects of the growth factor HGF on articular joint tissue suggest the possibility of this molecule's involvement in the cartilage repair process. One of its effects is that it stimulates chondrocyte migration, allowing partial reconstitution of hyaline cartilage in rabbits with experimentally induced cartilage defects (14). Since migration and repair processes have previously been coupled with MMP activities in other systems (42–44), and collagenase 3 is suggested to be implicated in the remodeling process of articular cartilage (45), we investigated the effect of HGF on collagenase 3 production and further examined the relevant intracellular signaling pathways. In this study, we showed that HGF stimulates collagenase 3 production in OA human chondrocytes. This occurs at the transcriptional level and requires a new synthesis of factors to fulfill its plenary potential. This effect is mediated by AP-1 via kinase cascades involving SAPK/JNK and another, unidentified kinase. Further data on HGF induction of collagenase 3 levels in human and rabbit normal chondrocytes suggested a general chondrocyte response mechanism. Moreover, the inability of IL-1Ra to inhibit the effects of HGF supports the involvement of a specific mechanism, rather than an endogenous IL-1β activation.

HGF binds to the c-Met, or HGF, receptor, which is a 190-kd protein tyrosine kinase formed by 2 polypeptide chains of 50 kd and 145 kd linked by disulfide bonds (23). Multiple signaling pathways have been identified that originate from this receptor on various cell systems. The cytoplasmic region of c-Met contains docking sites for PI 3-K (46–49) and MAPK through the Gab1/Grb2–Sos–Ras pathway (46), as well as other signaling molecules (46–49). However, the mechanism of signal transmission to target collagenase 3 following HGF stimulation has never been characterized. Because HGF can induce cell migration, division, and metabolic response, these events must be highly coordinated. Seeding chondrocytes at high density (100,000 cell/cm^2) simplifies our model, since experiments were conducted at confluence, where cells reach a stationary phase. Indeed, cell interactions between chondrocytes have been shown to inhibit cell proliferation.

Using specific antiphosphorylated protein antibodies, we found that the p44/42 MAPKs and the SAPK/JNK kinases, but not p38 MAPK, were phosphorylated in response to HGF. Previous reports (50,51) indicate that sustained activation of the MEK p42/44 signaling cascade results in the induction of cellular differentiation, while transient activation is associated with cell proliferation. As shown by our data, HGF induced a sustained activation of this pathway, suggesting that proliferation was not involved in our cultured chondrocytes. Moreover, HGF has recently been found in the matrix surrounding the chondrocytes of calcified cartilage in OA, suggesting its involvement in this particular stage of chondrocyte differentiation (25); this indicates that the effects of HGF in cartilage were more likely to be related to a differentiated cell state rather than to cell division in vivo. By using specific kinase inhibitors, our findings revealed that the p44/42 inhibitor (PD 98059) did not affect HGF-induced collagenase 3 production in OA chondrocytes. This is consistent with the findings of Johansson et al, who also showed that in TGFβ- or tumor necrosis factor α–stimulated transformed human epidermal keratinocytes, collagenase 3 was not regulated by p44/42 kinases (52). However, this statement cannot be extrapolated to all MMPs, because these same authors (52), as well as Zeigler et al (42), have demonstrated that p44/42 kinases play a role in regulating MMP-9 production in growth factor–stimulated human keratinocytes.

Our data also showed that wortmannin, a well-known PI 3-K inhibitor, had no major effect on collagenase 3 production. However, further experiments showed that this compound reduced HGF-induced OA chondrocyte migration (Reboul et al: personal observations), suggesting that PI 3-K is functional in these disease cells.

Herein we showed that HGF induced SAPK/JNK phosphorylation, and that the TRE site in the collagenase 3 promoter was also involved. In fact, the SAPK/JNK pathway appears to be crucial for HGF-induced collagenase 3 production, since HGF/NK2, a factor unable to activate SAPK/JNK kinases, demonstrated no true effect on the enzyme level. In OA chondrocytes, we showed that the AP-1 complex, which was able to bind on this site, consisted of c-Jun, JunD, and Fra-1, but not c-Fos, FosB, Fra-2, or JunB, which is in accordance with the observations on hepatocytes (53). It has recently been suggested that HGF is able to intracellularly generate reactive oxygen species (ROS) in sarcoma 180 (54). These molecules are produced during many physiologic intracellular reactions and generated in response to external stimuli such as ultraviolet radiation, which can activate SAPK/JNK. The ROS are generally considered to be cytotoxic, but several lines of evidence indicate that regulation of the intracellular redox status is a versatile control mechanism in gene expression and signal transduction (55,56). Using *N*-acetylcysteine (1–10 m*M*), which is a ROS inhibitor by its properties of intracellular free scavengers as well as a precursor of glutathione, we were not able to counteract the HGF-stimulated collagenase 3 production, suggesting that ROS are not implicated (results not shown).

In contrast to the kinase activation experiments, our data suggested that another factor, in addition to the SAPK/JNK, might also be involved in HGF-induced collagenase 3 production in OA chondrocytes. Indeed, experiments performed with a specific p38 MAPK inhibitor, SB 202190, induced a marked inhibition of HGF-induced collagenase 3 production. This inhibition was not related to cytotoxicity, since the stimulation of collagenase 3 was recovered when chondrocytes were treated for 2 hours with HGF followed by an 18-hour incubation with 2 μM of SB 202190. This experiment also demonstrated that the regulation of newly synthesized factors necessary for the production of collagenase 3 is no longer sensitive to the SB 202190 inhibitor after 2 hours of incubation with HGF. However, Clerk and Sugden (57) have shown that SB 203580, an analog of SB 202190 having less efficacy against p38 MAPK, is able to inhibit in vitro the activity of the purified p54, but not the p46, isoform of JNK-1, at a concentration of 3 μM. We showed that HGF activated only the phosphorylated p46 isoform. Therefore, the SB 202190 down-regulation of collagenase 3 expression in OA chondrocytes is not likely to be related to a direct inhibition of JNK-1.

Moreover, SB 202190 inhibits HGF-stimulated collagenase 3 production at a very low concentration (50% inhibitory concentration of 50 n*M*). This concentration is 40–200-fold lower than that usually used in cell culture systems (33,58,59). Such efficacy at this low concentration is indicative of high specificity. However, by using a p38 MAPK substrate, MAPKAPK-2, to determine p38 activity, HGF demonstrated its ability to activate this substrate in vitro, but unlike the effects following stimulation with IL-β, this activation was not reversed by SB 202190, even at a concentration of 5 μM and even after a longer period of chondrocyte stimulation with HGF (results not shown). The peptide substrate used to measure MAPKAPK-2 is also a substrate for other enzymes (Upstate Biotechnology), leading to background activity stimulation by HGF. Therefore, it would be reasonable to assume that the MAPKAPK-2 activation measured in HGF-treated chondrocytes was not due to p38 MAPK activity, and that SB 202190 may act on another, as-yet-unidentified kinase. The latter would be very sensitive to the inhibitor and involved in the regulation of collagenase 3 expression. It has been shown that SB 202190 inhibits p38α and β, but other isoforms, γ and δ, have been discovered (60,61). So far, these latter isoforms have not been described in chondrocytes. However, the p38δ isoform is not inhibited by SB 202190 (60) and the γ isoform is as sensitive as the α and β isoforms to this inhibitor (61), suggesting that the concentration of 50 n*M* SB 202190 would not be sufficient to inhibit the γ isoform.

In summary, this study shows for the first time that HGF has the ability to induce collagenase 3 expression and synthesis in OA chondrocytes. This appears to be mediated by the kinase cascades involving SAPK/JNK and another, as-yet-unidentified kinase, which are blocked at low concentrations and in the first 2 hours of HGF incubation by a p38 MAPK inhibitor, SB 202190. We are currently investigating the nature of this intermediary factor(s). Although the SAPK/JNK pathway is crucial, the p38 MAPK inhibitor-sensitive pathway also appears necessary. One could suggest that the SAPK/JNK pathway resembles an "on/off switch" which is needed for the stimulation of diverse MMPs, whereas the other pathway seems to be a fine regulation system more directed to collagenase 3. This phenomenon is of great significance, and may explain the diversity of HGF effects. Moreover, since HGF could be involved in the remodeling of cartilage, as well as in chondrocyte migration, use of this factor could prove to be an interesting approach in therapeutic strategies for the treatment of OA.

ACKNOWLEDGMENTS

The authors thank Mélanie Guèvremont and Kayghobad Kiansa for their technical expertise, and Shirley McCarthy for her assistance in manuscript preparation.

REFERENCES

1. Kuettner KE. Biochemistry of articular cartilage in health and disease. Clin Biochem 1992;25:155–63.
2. Von der Mark K, Kirsch T, Aigner T, Reichenberger E, Nerlich A, Weseloh G, et al. The fate of chondrocytes in osteoarthritic cartilage: regeneration, dedifferentiation, or hypertrophy? In: Kuettner K, Schleyerbach R, Peyron JG, Hascall VC; editors. Articular cartilage and osteoarthritis. New York: Raven Press; 1992. p. 221–34.
3. Dean DD, Martel-Pelletier J, Pelletier JP, Howell DS, Woessner JF Jr. Evidence for metalloproteinase and metalloproteinase inhibitor imbalance in human osteoarthritic cartilage. J Clin Invest 1989;84:678–85.
4. Poole AR. Cartilage in health and disease. In: Koopman WJ, editor. Arthritis and allied conditions: a textbook of rheumatology. 13th ed. Baltimore: Williams & Wilkins; 1997. p. 255–308.
5. Campbell CJ. The healing of cartilage defects. Clin Orthop 1969;64:45–63.
6. Kim HK, Moran ME, Salter RB. The potential for regeneration of articular cartilage in defects created by chondral shaving and subchondral abrasion: an experimental investigation in rabbits. J Bone Joint Surg Am 1991;73:1301–15.
7. Brittberg M, Lindahl A, Nilsson A, Ohlsson C, Isaksson O, Peterson L. Treatment of deep cartilage defects in the knee with

autologous chondrocyte transplantation. N Engl J Med 1994;331: 889–95.
8. Cuevas P, Burgos J, Baird A. Basic fibroblast growth factor (FGF) promotes cartilage repair in vivo. Biochem Biophys Res Commun 1988;156:611–8.
9. Hunziker EB, Schenk RK. A differential treatment protocol for inducing cartilage and bone repair in full-thickness articular cartilage defects [abstract]. Trans Orthop Res Soc 1995;20:170.
10. Van Beuningen HM, van der Kraan PM, Arntz OJ, van den Berg WB. Transforming growth factor-beta 1 stimulates articular chondrocyte proteoglycan synthesis and induces osteophyte formation in the murine knee joint. Lab Invest 1994;71:279–90.
11. Phadke K. Fibroblast growth factor enhances the interleukin-1–mediated chondrocytic protease release. Biochem Biophys Res Commun 1987;142:448–53.
12. Grumbles RM, Howell DS, Wenger L, Altman RD, Howard GA, Roos BA. Hepatocyte growth factor and its actions in growth plate chondrocytes. Bone 1996;19:255–61.
13. Takebayashi T, Iwamoto M, Jikko A, Matsumura T, Enomoto-Iwamoto M, Myoukai F, et al. Hepatocyte growth factor/scatter factor modulates cell motility, proliferation, and proteoglycan synthesis of chondrocytes. J Cell Biol 1995;129:1411–9.
14. Wakitani S, Imoto K, Kimura T, Ochi T, Matsumoto K, Nakamura T. Hepatocyte growth factor facilitates cartilage repair: full thickness articular cartilage defect studied in rabbit knees. Acta Orthop Scand 1997;68:474–80.
15. Nakamura T, Nawa K, Ichihara A, Kaise N, Nishino T. Purification and subunit structure of hepatocyte growth factor from rat platelets. FEBS Lett 1987;224:311–6.
16. Zarnegar R, Michalopoulos G. Purification and biological characterization of human hepatopoietin A, a polypeptide growth factor for hepatocytes. Cancer Res 1989;49:3314–20.
17. Rubin JS, Chan AM, Bottaro DP, Burgess WH, Taylor WG, Cech AC, et al. A broad-spectrum human lung fibroblast-derived mitogen is a variant of hepatocyte growth factor. Proc Natl Acad Sci U S A 1991;88:415–9.
18. Bottaro DP, Rubin JS, Faletto DL, Chan AM, Kmiecik TE, Vande Woude GF, et al. Identification of the hepatocyte growth factor receptor as the c-met proto-oncogene product. Science 1991;251: 802–4.
19. Matsumoto K, Hashimoto K, Yoshikawa K, Nakamura T. Marked stimulation of growth and motility of human keratinocytes by hepatocyte growth factor. Exp Cell Res 1991;196:114–20.
20. Nusrat A, Parkos CA, Bacarra AE, Godowski PJ, Delp-Archer C, Rosen EM, et al. Hepatocyte growth factor/scatter factor effects on epithelia: regulation of intercellular junctions in transformed and nontransformed cell lines, basolateral polarization of c-met receptor in transformed and natural intestinal epithelia, and induction of rapid wound repair in a transformed model epithelium. J Clin Invest 1994;93:2056–65.
21. Shiota G, Wang TC, Nakamura T, Schmidt EV. Hepatocyte growth factor in transgenic mice: effects on hepatocyte growth, liver regeneration and gene expression. Hepatology 1994;19: 962–72.
22. Inoue T, Nabeshima K, Shimao Y, Koono M. Hepatocyte growth factor/scatter factor (HGF/SF) is a regulator of fibronectin splicing in MDCK cells: comparison between the effects of HGF/SF and TGF-beta1 on fibronectin splicing at the EDA region. Biochem Biophys Res Commun 1999;260:225–31.
23. Naldini L, Vigna E, Narsimhan RP, Gaudino G, Zarnegar R, Michalopoulos GK, et al. Hepatocyte growth factor (HGF) stimulates the tyrosine kinase activity of the receptor encoded by the proto-oncogene c-MET. Oncogene 1991;6:501–4.
24. Wolf HK, Zarnegar R, Michalopoulos GK. Localization of hepatocyte growth factor in human and rat tissues: an immunohistochemical study. Hepatology 1991;14:488–94.
25. Pfander D, Cramer T, Weseloh G, Pullig O, Schuppan D, Bauer M, et al. Hepatocyte growth factor in human osteoarthritic cartilage. Osteoarthritis Cartilage 1999;7:548–59.
26. Moldovan F, Pelletier J-P, Hambor J, Cloutier J-M, Martel-Pelletier J. Collagenase-3 (matrix metalloprotease 13) is preferentially localized in the deep layer of human arthritic cartilage in situ: in vitro mimicking effect by transforming growth factor β. Arthritis Rheum 1997;40:1653–61.
27. Fernandes JC, Martel-Pelletier J, Lascau-Coman V, Moldovan F, Jovanovic D, Raynauld JP, et al. Collagenase-1 and collagenase-3 synthesis in early experimental osteoarthritic canine cartilage: an immunohistochemical study. J Rheumatol 1998;8:1585–94.
28. Aydelotte MB, Kuettner KE. Differences between sub-populations of cultured bovine articular chondrocytes. I. Morphology and cartilage matrix production. Connect Tissue Res 1988;18:205–22.
29. Altman R, Asch E, Bloch D, Bole G, Borenstein D, Brandt KD, et al. Development of criteria for the classification and reporting of osteoarthritis: classification of osteoarthritis of the knee. Arthritis Rheum 1986;29:1039–49.
30. Tardif G, Pelletier J-P, Dupuis M, Geng C, Cloutier J-M, Martel-Pelletier J. Collagenase 3 production by human osteoarthritic chondrocytes in response to growth factors and cytokines is a function of the physiological state of the cells. Arthritis Rheum 1999;42:1147–58.
31. Towbin H, Staehelin T, Gordon J. Electrophoretic transfer of proteins from polyacrylamide gels to nitrocellulose sheets: procedure and some applications. Proc Natl Acad Sci U S A 1979;76: 4350–4.
32. Reboul P, Pelletier JP, Tardif G, Cloutier JM, Martel-Pelletier J. The new collagenase, collagenase-3, is expressed and synthesized by human chondrocytes but not by synoviocytes: a role in osteoarthritis. J Clin Invest 1996;97:2011–9.
33. Martel-Pelletier J, Mineau F, Jovanovic D, Di Battista JA, Pelletier J-P. Mitogen-activated protein kinase and nuclear factor κB together regulate interleukin-17–induced nitric oxide production in human osteoarthritic chondrocytes: possible role of transactivating factor mitogen-activated protein kinase–activated protein kinase (MAPKAPK). Arthritis Rheum 1999;42:2399–409.
34. Tardif G, Pelletier JP, Dupuis M, Hambor JE, Martel-Pelletier J. Cloning, sequencing and characterization of the 5′-flanking region of the human collagenase-3 gene. Biochem J 1997;323:13–6.
35. Graham FL, van der Eb AJ. A new technique for the assay of infectivity of human adenovirus 5 DNA. Virology 1973;52:456–67.
36. Sambrook JF, Fritsch EF, Maniatis T. Molecular cloning: a laboratory manual. 2nd ed. New York: Cold Spring Harbor Laboratory Press; 1989.
37. Stahl SJ, Wingfield PT, Kaufman JD, Pannell LK, Cioce V, Sakata H, et al. Functional and biophysical characterization of recombinant human hepatocyte growth factor isoforms produced in Escherichia coli. Biochem J 1997;326:763–72.
38. Day RM, Cioce V, Breckenridge D, Castagnino P, Bottaro DP. Differential signaling by alternative HGF isoforms through c-Met: activation of both MAP kinase and PI 3-kinase pathways is insufficient for mitogenesis. Oncogene 1999;18:3399–406.
39. Miller C, Zhang M, He Y, Zhao J, Pelletier JP, Martel-Pelletier J, et al. Transcriptional induction of cyclooxygenase-2 gene by okadaic acid inhibition of phosphatase activity in human chondrocytes: co-stimulation of AP-1 and CRE nuclear binding proteins. J Cell Biochem 1998;69:392–413.
40. Matsumoto K, Nakamura T. Hepatocyte growth factor: molecular structure, roles in liver regeneration, and other biological functions. Crit Rev Oncog 1992;3:27–54.
41. Brown JD, DiChiara MR, Anderson KR, Gimbrone MA Jr, Topper JN. MEKK-1, a component of the stress (stress-activated protein kinase/c-Jun N-terminal kinase) pathway, can selectively activate Smad2-mediated transcriptional activation in endothelial cells. J Biol Chem 1999;274:8797–805.
42. Zeigler ME, Chi Y, Schmidt T, Varani J. Role of ERK and JNK

pathways in regulating cell motility and matrix metalloproteinase 9 production in growth factor-stimulated human epidermal keratinocytes. J Cell Physiol 1999;180:271–84.
43. Makela M, Larjava H, Pirila E, Maisi P, Salo T, Sorsa T, et al. Matrix metalloproteinase 2 (gelatinase A) is related to migration of keratinocytes. Exp Cell Res 1999;251:67–78.
44. Pilcher BK, Dumin JA, Sudbeck BD, Krane SM, Welgus HG, Parks WC. The activity of collagenase-1 is required for keratinocyte migration on a type I collagen matrix. J Cell Biol 1997;137: 1445–57.
45. Jimenez MJ, Balbin M, Lopez JM, Alvarez J, Komori T, Lopez-Otin C. Collagenase 3 is a target of Cbfa1, a transcription factor of the runt gene family involved in bone formation. Mol Cell Biol 1999;19:4431–42.
46. Ponzetto C, Bardelli A, Zhen Z, Maina F, dalla Zonca P, Giordano S, et al. A multifunctional docking site mediates signaling and transformation by the hepatocyte growth factor/scatter factor receptor family. Cell 1994;77:261–71.
47. Weidner KM, Di Cesare S, Sachs M, Brinkmann V, Behrens J, Birchmeier W. Interaction between Gab1 and the c-Met receptor tyrosine kinase is responsible for epithelial morphogenesis. Nature 1996;384:173–6.
48. Fournier TM, Kamikura D, Teng K, Park M. Branching tubulogenesis but not scatter of madin-darby canine kidney cells requires a functional Grb2 binding site in the Met receptor tyrosine kinase. J Biol Chem 1996;271:22211–7.
49. Nguyen L, Holgado-Madruga M, Maroun C, Fixman ED, Kamikura D, Fournier T, et al. Association of the multisubstrate docking protein Gab1 with the hepatocyte growth factor receptor requires a functional Grb2 binding site involving tyrosine 1356. J Biol Chem 1997;272:20811–9.
50. Schramek H, Schumacher M, Pfaller W. Sustained ERK-2 activation in rat glomerular mesangial cells: differential regulation by protein phosphatases. Am J Physiol 1996;271:F423–32.
51. Traverse S, Gomez N, Paterson H, Marshall C, Cohen P. Sustained activation of the mitogen-activated protein (MAP) kinase cascade may be required for differentiation of PC12 cells: comparison of the effects of nerve growth factor and epidermal growth factor. Biochem J 1992;288:351–5.
52. Johansson N, Ala-aho R, Uitto V, Grenman R, Fusenig NE, Lopez-Otin C, et al. Expression of collagenase-3 (MMP-13) and collagenase-1 (MMP-1) by transformed keratinocytes is dependent on the activity of p38 mitogen-activated protein kinase. J Cell Sci 2000;113:227–35.
53. Rahmani M, Nadori F, Durand-Schneider AM, Lardeux B, Bernuau D. Hepatocyte growth factor activates the AP-1 complex: a comparison between normal and transformed rat hepatocytes. J Hepatol 1999;30:916–25.
54. Arakaki N, Kajihara T, Arakaki R, Ohnishi T, Kazi JA, Nakashima H, et al. Involvement of oxidative stress in tumor cytotoxic activity of hepatocyte growth factor/scatter factor. J Biol Chem 1999;274: 13541–6.
55. Dean RT, Gieseg S, Davies MJ. Reactive species and their accumulation on radical-damaged proteins. Trends Biochem Sci 1993;18:437–41.
56. Buttke TM, Sandstrom PA. Oxidative stress as a mediator of apoptosis. Immunol Today 1994;15:7–10.
57. Clerk A, Sugden PH. The p38-MAPK inhibitor, SB203580, inhibits cardiac stress-activated protein kinases/c-Jun N-terminal kinases (SAPKs/JNKs). FEBS Lett 1998;426:93–6.
58. Singh RP, Dhawan P, Golden C, Kapoor GS, Mehta KD. One-way cross-talk between p38(MAPK) and p42/44(MAPK): inhibition of p38(MAPK) induces low density lipoprotein receptor expression through activation of the p42/44(MAPK) cascade. J Biol Chem 1999;274:19593–600.
59. Chen N, Ma W-Y, Huang C, Dong Z. Translocation of protein kinase Cϵ and protein kinase Cδ to membrane is required for ultraviolet B-induced activation of mitogen-activated protein kinases and apoptosis. J Biol Chem 1999;274:15389–94.
60. Jiang Y, Gram H, Zhao M, New L, Gu J, Feng L, et al. Characterization of the structure and function of the fourth member of p38 group mitogen-activated protein kinases, p38delta. J Biol Chem 1997;272:30122–8.
61. Li Z, Jiang Y, Ulevitch RJ, Han J. The primary structure of p38 gamma: a new member of p38 group of MAP kinases. Biochem Biophys Res Commun 1996;228:334–40.

ARTHRITIS & RHEUMATISM
Vol. 44, No. 1, January 2001, pp 85–95

Human Periosteum-Derived Cells Maintain Phenotypic Stability and Chondrogenic Potential throughout Expansion Regardless of Donor Age

Cosimo De Bari, Francesco Dell'Accio, and Frank P. Luyten

Objective. **To assess the in vitro chondrogenic potential of adult human periosteum-derived cells (PDCs) with regard to the number of cell passages and the age of the donor.**

Methods. **Cells were enzymatically released from the periosteum of the proximal tibia obtained from adult human donors and expanded in monolayer. PDCs were harvested at multiple passages for total RNA extraction and semiquantitative reverse transcription–polymerase chain reaction (RT-PCR) gene expression analysis. For the chondrogenesis assay, cells were plated in micromass and treated with transforming growth factor β1 (TGFβ1) in a chemically defined medium. At different time points, micromasses were either harvested for RT-PCR analysis for cartilage and bone markers or fixed, paraffin-embedded, and stained for cartilage matrix, and immunostained for type II collagen.**

Results. **At the first 2 passages, human PDCs from young donors formed chondrogenic nodules. This spontaneous chondrogenic activity was lost upon passaging, and it was not observed in donors older than 30 years. Using a panel of marker genes, PDCs were shown to be phenotypically stable during cell expansion. Regardless of donor age or cell passage, chondrogenesis could be induced consistently by combining micromass culture and TGFβ1 treatment. Histochemical and immunohistochemical analyses demonstrated the hyaline-like cartilage phenotype of the tissue generated in vitro. Other TGFβ superfamily members, such as growth differentiation factor 5/cartilage-derived morphogenetic protein 1, and bone morphogenetic proteins 2, 4, and 7, were poorly chondrogenic under the same culture conditions.**

Conclusion. **Adult human PDCs have the potential to differentiate toward the chondrocytic lineage in vitro, retaining this property even after extensive subculture. Human PDCs are easily accessible, expandable, and maintain their chondrogenic potential, and are therefore promising progenitor cells for use in the repair of joint surface defects.**

Supported by FWO grant G.0192.99.

Cosimo De Bari, MD, Francesco Dell'Accio, MD, Frank P. Luyten, MD, PhD: University Hospitals, Katholieke Universiteit Leuven, Leuven, Belgium.

Address correspondence and reprint requests to Frank P. Luyten, MD, PhD, Laboratory for Skeletal Development and Joint Disorders, Onderwijs & Navorsing, Herestraat 49, 3000 Leuven, Belgium. E-mail: frank.luyten@uz.kuleuven.ac.be.

Submitted for publication June 26, 2000; accepted in revised form September 20, 2000.

Articular cartilage has a limited capacity for repair. Whatever their etiology—whether acute or chronic processes—joint surface defects rarely heal completely. Most commonly, fibrocartilage or scar tissue forms. Eventually, the clinical picture can evolve into osteoarthritis and functional disability. For end-stage osteoarthritis, the usual treatment is prosthetic joint replacement, which is satisfactory for pain relief, but carries significant morbidity and a limited lifespan of the prosthesis. This poses a challenge in younger individuals. Therefore, joint surface defects represent a major health and social problem, which has spurred the search for techniques by which articular cartilage can be regenerated.

Repair of joint surface defects by transplantation of autologous chondrocytes has been described (1). Major drawbacks of this procedure are the source of the cells and the in vitro expansion of the chondrocytes. The donor tissue consists of articular cartilage specimens obtained from an "uninvolved" and minor load-bearing area of the same joint. This, however, results in additional injury to the joint surface, creating a potential *locus minoris resistentiae* and increased risk for developing osteoarthritis, especially in genetically predisposed individuals. Moreover, in some cases, there may be very little unaffected articular cartilage tissue available.

Chondrocyte expansion is essential for obtaining a sufficient number of cells. Unfortunately, the in vitro cell culture results in chondrocyte dedifferentiation (2), i.e., chondrocytes lose their phenotype and, potentially, are no longer able to organize and produce appropriate matrix, as in normal articular hyaline cartilage. The use of progenitor cells may circumvent these problems.

Studies of limb development indicate that the perichondrium may be embryologically related to the joint interzone and may contribute to the process of formation and differentiation of the joint-associated tissues, including articular cartilage (3–7). In addition, in postnatal fracture healing, mesenchymal progenitor cells in the periosteum form hyaline cartilage during endochondral ossification (8). Therefore, the periosteum can be a source of chondroprogenitor cells.

The in vitro and in vivo chondrogenic potential of periosteum-derived cells (PDCs) as reported in the literature appears to be dependent on the age of the donor and the number of cell passages (9–18). In most of the in vitro studies, cells are released from the periosteum of very young animals, in which the probability of obtaining progenitor cells is higher than in adult and elderly donors (11,19,20), and tested in chondrogenesis assays only at very early passages, when the cells have an inherent chondrogenic potential (12–14). The differentiation toward a chondrocyte phenotype is achieved in high-density culture and occurs spontaneously (12,13,15). The addition of growth factors seems to accelerate chondrogenesis, rather than induce it de novo (14,15).

In the present study, we confirmed the existence of a spontaneous chondrogenic activity at very early passages in PDCs from young donors. We then characterized the PDCs obtained from adult donors of various ages. We show that the PDCs can be expanded in vitro over at least 15 passages without loss of their phenotypic traits. We provide data demonstrating that adult human PDCs can be induced consistently into the chondrogenic differentiation pathway in vitro, regardless of donor age or cell passage number.

SUBJECTS AND METHODS

Harvest of periosteum and isolation of PDCs. A sample of periosteum measuring 1 cm^2 was harvested aseptically from the proximal medial tibia of human donors of various ages (mean 57 years, range 24–95 years); samples were obtained either postmortem (within 12 hours after death) or at the time of surgical knee replacement. Periosteum samples were rinsed twice with Hanks' balanced salt solution (Life Technologies, Merelbeke, Belgium) supplemented with antibiotic–antimycotic solution (100 units/ml penicillin, 100 μg/ml of streptomycin, and 0.25 μg/ml of amphotericin B; Life Technologies), minced finely, and digested with 0.2% collagenase (Life Technologies) in high-glucose Dulbecco's modified Eagle's medium (DMEM; Life Technologies) containing 10% fetal bovine serum (FBS; BioWhittaker, Verviers, Belgium) and antibiotics.

Following overnight incubation at 37°C, periosteal cells were collected by centrifugation, washed twice, resuspended in high-glucose DMEM supplemented with 10% FBS and antibiotics (growth medium), plated in a T25 culture flask, and allowed to attach for 4 days. Nonadherent cells were removed by changing the medium.

Cell expansion and cryopreservation. For expansion, cells were cultured in monolayer in growth medium at 37°C in a humidified atmosphere of 5% CO_2. The medium was replaced every 3 days. After 10–20 days of primary culture, when the sparsely attached cells reached confluence, they were washed twice with calcium- and magnesium-free phosphate buffered saline (PBS), harvested by treatment with trypsin–EDTA (0.25% trypsin, 1 m*M* EDTA; Life Technologies), and replated at a 1:4 dilution for the first subculture. Cell passages were continued in the same way with a 1:4 dilution every 6–12 days when cells reached confluence.

At passage 3 (P3), aliquots of trypsin-released primary PDC cultures in DMEM with 20% FBS and 10% DMSO (Sigma, Bornem, Belgium) were cryopreserved in liquid nitrogen, thawed after various times (range 1–18 months), replated, and expanded for the in vitro chondrogenesis assay.

Treatment with growth factors. Recombinant human bone morphogenetic protein 2 (BMP-2) and BMP-4 were obtained from Genetics Institute (Cambridge, MA); recombinant human BMP-7 and growth differentiation factor 5 (GDF-5)/cartilage-derived morphogenetic protein 1 (CDMP-1) were from Creative BioMolecules (Hopkinton, MA). These proteins were dissolved in 45% acetonitrile, 0.1% trifluoroacetic acid and added to the culture medium at final concentrations of 100–300 ng/ml. For all experiments, vehicle controls were performed in parallel cultures. The induction of alkaline phosphatase activity in ATDC5 and C2C12 cells was used to assess the biologic activity of the growth factors.

Recombinant human transforming growth factor β1 (TGFβ1; R&D Systems, Abingdon, UK) was dissolved in 4 m*M* HCl containing 1 mg/ml of bovine serum albumin (BSA; Serva, Heidelberg, Germany) and added to the culture medium at a final concentration of 10 ng/ml. Identical amounts of 4 m*M* HCl containing 1 mg/ml of BSA were added to parallel cultures as treatment controls.

Treatments were carried out in triplicate or quadruplicate for at least 6 days, both in growth medium and in a chemically defined serum-free medium (21).

In vitro chondrogenesis assay. Micromass cultures were performed as described elsewhere (22). Briefly, expanded PDCs were released by trypsin treatment, counted, tested for viability by trypan blue exclusion, and resuspended in growth medium at a density of 2.0×10^7 viable cells/ml. Micromass cultures were obtained by pipetting 20-μl droplets of cell suspension into individual wells of 24-well plates. After cells were allowed to attach without medium for 3 hours, the chemically defined serum-free medium was added. The day of plating in micromass culture was designated as day 0.

Table 1. Primers used for RT-PCR analysis and expected sizes of PCR products*

Gene	Sense primer	Antisense primer	Product
β-actin	5′-TGACGGGGTCACCCACACTGTGCCCATCTA-3′	5′-CTAGAAGCATTTGCGGTGGACGATGGAGGG-3′	661 bp
α1(II) collagen	5′-CCCTGAGTGGAAGAGTGGAG-3′	5′-GAGGCGTGAGGTCTTCTGTG-3′	511 bp
Sox9	5′-GAACGCACATCAAGACGGAG-3′	5′-TCTCGTTGATTTCGCTGCTC-3′	631 bp
Link protein	5′-CCTATGATGAAGCGGTGC-3′	5′-TTGTGCTTGTGGAACCTG-3′	618 bp
β1 integrin	5′-AATGAAGGGCGTGTTGGTAG-3′	5′-ATCTGTCCGTTGCTGGCTTC-3′	344 bp
TGFβRI	5′-TTCAGCCACAGATACCATTG-3′	5′-TTTGATGCCTTCCTGTTGAC-3′	430 bp
α1(I) collagen	5′-CGTGGTGACAAGGGTGAGAC-3′	5′-TAGGTGATGTTCTGGGAGGC-3′	827 bp
Osteocalcin	5′-TCACACTCCTCGCCCTATTG-3′	5′-GAAGAGGAAAGAAGGGTGCC-3′	362 bp

* RT-PCR = reverse transcription–polymerase chain reaction; TGFβRI = transforming growth factor β receptor type I.

Starting on day 1, when the culture medium was changed, TGFβ1 was added to the culture medium every other day, at a final concentration of 10 ng/ml. As a negative control, human dermal fibroblasts (kindly provided by S. Tejpar, Centrum Menselijke Erfelijkheid [CME], Leuven, Belgium) were kept under identical conditions. Micromass cultures were harvested after 6 days for Alcian blue staining and reverse transcription–polymerase chain reaction (RT-PCR) gene expression analysis.

Alcian blue staining in vitro. Cultures were rinsed twice with PBS, fixed with methanol for 30 minutes at −20°C, washed with distilled water, and covered with Alcian blue at pH 0.2 (0.5% Alcian blue 8 GS [Carl Roth, Karlsruhe, Germany] in 1*N* HCl). After overnight staining, cultures were washed extensively with distilled water. For quantitative analyses, Alcian blue–stained cultures were extracted with 200 μl of 6*M* guanidine HCl in Milli-Q water for 6 hours at room temperature. The optical density of the extracted dye was measured at 630 nm using a Spectronic 2000 spectrophotometer (Bausch & Lomb, Rochester, NY).

The specificity of Alcian blue staining at pH 0.2 in vitro and its correlation with the expression of type II collagen are described elsewhere (manuscript in preparation).

Total RNA extraction and semiquantitative RT-PCR analysis. Total RNA was extracted using a commercially available kit (SNAP kit; Invitrogen, Groningen, The Netherlands), according to the manufacturer's instructions. Complementary DNA (cDNA) was obtained by RT of 1 μg of total RNA (Thermoscript; Life Technologies) with oligo$(dT)_{20}$ as primer. PCR was performed in a volume of 10 μl; cDNA samples were added to the following PCR mixture: 0.5 units of *Taq* polymerase (Eurogentec, Seraing, Belgium), 0.2 m*M* dNTPs, 0.5 μ*M* specific primers, and 1.5 m*M* $MgCl_2$. Negative controls were either RT without enzyme or PCR with Milli-Q water instead of cDNA.

PCR reactions were carried out in a Perkin Elmer Thermal Cycler 9600 (Applied Biosystems, Lennik, Belgium). After 1 minute of denaturation at 95°C, cycles (19 for β-actin, 33 for type II collagen, 34 for osteocalcin, and 30 for the other genes) were 10 seconds at 94°C, 10 seconds at the optimal annealing temperature, and 30 seconds at 72°C. Cycling was followed by 10 minutes of elongation at 72°C. Primer pairs were designed using Vector NTI software (InforMax, North Bethesda, MD). The sequences of the primers and the sizes of the PCR products are shown in Table 1.

Complementary DNA samples were equalized for the expression of the housekeeping gene β-actin. PCR products were electrophoresed in 1.5% agarose gel in Tris–borate–EDTA electrophoresis buffer, stained with ethidium bromide, visualized by ultraviolet transillumination, and analyzed by densitometry using the Image Master software (Amersham Pharmacia Biotech, Roosendaal, The Netherlands).

Senescence-associated β-galactosidase (β-gal) staining. Staining for senescence-associated β-gal was performed as described (23). Early-passage (before P6) and late-passage (after P10) PDCs from young and old donors were plated in chamber slides and allowed to attach in growth medium. Cells were washed in PBS, fixed for 5 minutes at room temperature in 3% formaldehyde, washed, and incubated overnight in a humid chamber at 37°C with fresh β-gal staining solution: 1 mg of X-Gal per ml (Duchefa, Haarlem, The Netherlands), 40 m*M* citric acid/sodium phosphate at pH 6, 5 m*M* potassium ferrocyanide, 5 m*M* potassium ferricyanide, 150 m*M* NaCl, and 2 m*M* $MgCl_2$. Senescent human dermal fibroblasts were used as a positive control.

Histology and immunohistochemistry. For histologic and immunohistochemical analyses, 100 μl of PDC suspension was plated in micromass in individual wells of a 12-well plate. Micromasses were treated with 10 ng/ml of TGFβ1 or with the same amount of TGFβ1 carrier solution in the chemically defined serum-free medium. After 7 and 15 days, micromasses were peeled off the wells, fixed with 10% formalin, embedded in paraffin, and sectioned at 5 μm.

For histologic evaluation, sections were deparaffinized and stained with toluidine blue or Alcian blue at pH 2.5, according to standard protocols. In the Alcian blue–stained sections, neutral red was used for counterstaining the nuclei.

For immunohistochemical analysis, sections were deparaffinized and predigested with chondroitinase ABC (Sigma) at 50 mU/ml at room temperature for 1 hour to facilitate antibody access. Nonspecific antibody binding was blocked by incubating the slides for 1 hour in 5% BSA in PBS. Sections were then incubated for 1 hour with a mouse anti-human type II collagen monoclonal antibody (Chemicon, Hofheim, Germany) diluted 1:5 in 0.5% BSA in PBS. Reactivity was detected with fluorescence microscopy after incubation for 1 hour with a Cy3-conjugated secondary antibody (goat anti-mouse IgG; Jackson ImmunoResearch, West Grove, PA) that had been diluted 1:500 in 0.5% BSA in PBS. Nuclei were counterstained

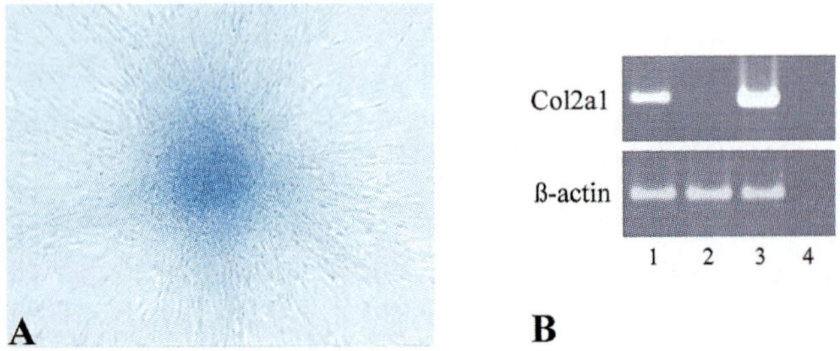

Figure 1. Spontaneous chondrogenic activity of periosteum-derived cells (PDCs) from young adult donors at very early passages. **A,** Nodule stained with Alcian blue. **B,** Semiquantitative reverse transcription–polymerase chain reaction (RT-PCR), showing the expression of α1(II) collagen (Col2a1) by PDCs at passage 1 (P1) (lane 1) but not at P4 (lane 2). Lane 3, Freshly isolated human articular chondrocytes (positive control); lane 4, RT-negative control of lane 1. Templates are equalized for the expression of β-actin.

with 4′,6-diamidino-2-phenylindole (ICN, Asse-Relegem, Belgium).

RESULTS

Loss of spontaneous chondrogenic activity on serial passaging and with increasing age of donor. At very early passages (P0 and P1), human PDCs from donors younger than 30 years formed densely packed nodules, with round or polygonal cells. The process of nodule formation from the adherent fibroblastic cell population was not uniform. Some cells appeared to give rise to nodules soon after adherence to the culture plate, whereas other cells did not contribute to nodule formation until they reached confluence.

A substantial number of nodules stained with Alcian blue, indicating the presence of proteoglycans (Figure 1A). Fibroblast-like cells were spreading between the nodules. The focal chondrogenic differentiation was confirmed by the detection of type II collagen messenger RNA (mRNA) in P0 and P1 monolayer cultures (Figure 1B). With the subsequent subculturing, PDCs lost the potential to form Alcian blue–positive nodules and appeared microscopically to be a relatively homogeneous population of fibroblast-like cells. PDCs from donors older than 30 years never formed chondrogenic nodules nor expressed type II collagen, having a fibroblast-like morphology from the beginning of the culture.

Phenotypic stability of PDCs through serial passaging and cryopreservation, independent of donor age. To define the effects of donor age and in vitro cell expansion on the molecular phenotype of PDCs, cells from donors of various ages were passaged serially. At multiple passages, gene expression analysis was performed by semiquantitative RT-PCR. The marker analysis included genes known to have a role in skeletal development and maintenance (3). The first 2 passages (P0 and P1) of PDCs obtained from donors younger than 30 years were not included in this experiment. The expression of 40 selected genes was analyzed (results not shown). Figure 2 shows a representative panel of the genes tested. The molecular profile of the cells was stable during serial passaging and independent of the age of the donors. No phenotypic differences were observed between samples obtained postmortem and samples obtained during surgical knee replacement (Figure 2).

To test whether cryopreservation could affect the phenotype of PDCs, the same panel of markers was tested for expression by cells that had been cryopreserved compared with passage-matched cells that had never been frozen. No phenotypic differences were detected between cryopreserved and noncryopreserved cells (results not shown).

Cell senescence during PDC expansion. Cell senescence, a common phenomenon occurring to various degrees in many somatic cells during in vitro culture expansion, is known to induce phenotypic and functional changes (24). Therefore, we analyzed senescence-associated β-gal activity in early-passage and late-passage PDCs from donors of different ages. Senescence-associated β-gal activity was not detected in PDCs (expanded up to P15) from donors younger than 30 years. PDCs from donors older than 60 years were largely β-gal negative at early passages, whereas weak-

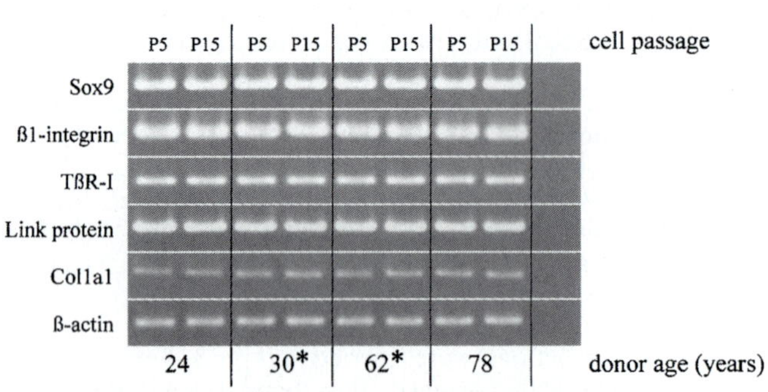

Figure 2. Stability of PDC phenotype independent of cell passage number or donor age. PDCs at P5 and P15 from 4 donors of different ages show a comparable molecular profile, as assessed by semiquantitative RT-PCR. A representative panel of the genes tested is shown here. In the last lane is Milli-Q water (negative control). Templates are equalized for β-actin expression. Col1a1 = α1(I) collagen. Asterisk indicates samples obtained postmortem. TβR-I = transforming growth factor β receptor type I (see Figure 1 for other definitions).

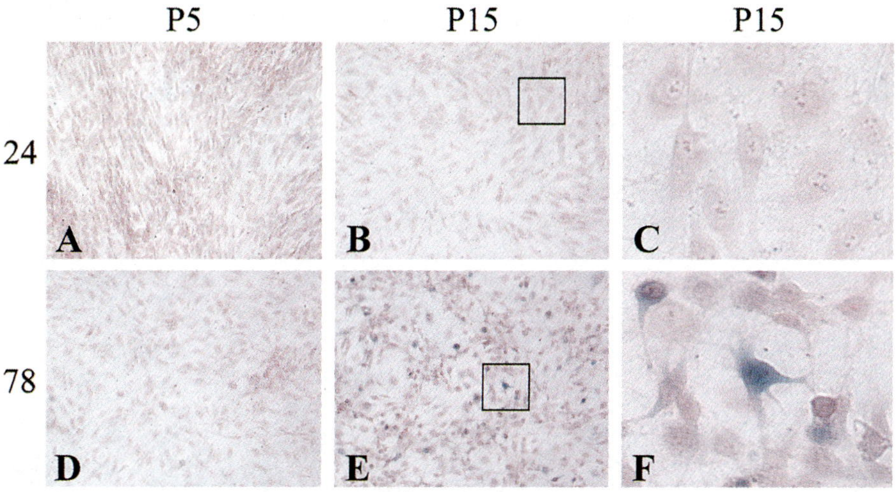

Figure 3. Senescence-associated β-galactosidase staining. PDCs at P5 and P15 from a 24-year-old donor (**A–C**) and from a 78-year-old donor (**D–F**) are shown. **C,** High-magnification view of the boxed area in **B**. **F,** High-magnification view of the boxed area in **E**, showing the detail of a senescent cell. PDCs from younger donors could be expanded for many passages without senescence. Few positive cells are visible in PDCs at P15 from the 78-year-old donor. (Neutral red counterstained; original magnification × 100 in **A**, **B**, **D**, and **E**; × 630 in **C** and **F**.) See Figure 1 for definitions.

to-moderate β-gal staining of a few scattered cells (5–10%) was observed at late passages (Figure 3).

Requirement for both micromass culture and TGFβ1 treatment for induction of chondrogenesis in vitro. We wished to determine whether it was possible to induce chondrogenesis in late-passage PDCs and in PDCs from older donors by using different culture systems and treatments. Supplementing the medium with growth factors, members of the TGFβ superfamily (TGFβ1, GDF-5/CDMP-1, and BMPs 2, 4, and 7), failed to induce chondrogenesis in confluent monolayer PDCs, as evaluated by Alcian blue staining and RT-PCR for

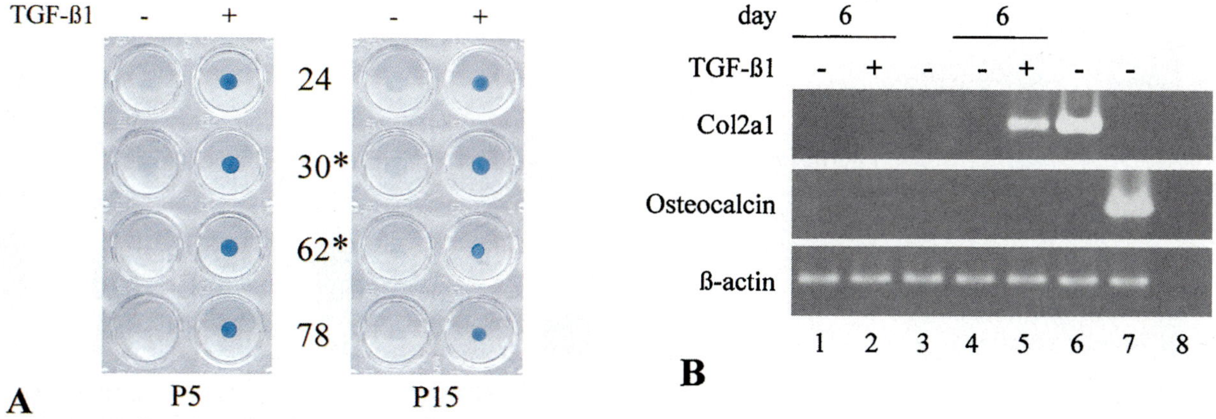

Figure 4. Stability of the chondrogenic potential of adult human PDCs over many passages and lack of impairment in older donors. **A,** PDCs at P5 and P15 from donors of different ages were plated in micromass culture and either treated or not treated with transforming growth factor β1 (TGF-β1). After 6 days, micromasses were fixed and stained with Alcian blue. The ages of the donors are shown in between the culture plates; asterisk indicates periosteum samples obtained postmortem. **B,** Semiquantitative RT-PCR for type II collagen and osteocalcin. Lanes 1 and 2, Human dermal fibroblasts in micromass; lane 3, PDCs at P16 in monolayer; lanes 4 and 5, PDCs at P16 in micromass; lane 6, freshly isolated human articular chondrocytes; lane 7, human trabecular osteoblasts; lane 8, RT-negative control of lane 5. All cDNA samples are equalized for β-actin expression. See Figure 1 for other definitions.

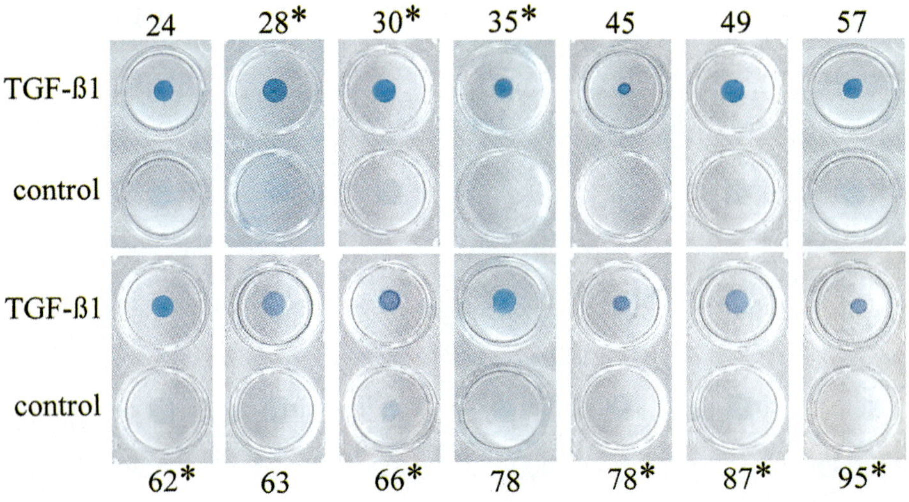

Figure 5. Induction of chondrogenesis in periosteum-derived cells (PDCs) from adult donors of various ages. PDCs were plated in micromass, treated or not treated with transforming growth factor β1 (TGF-β1) for 6 days, fixed, and stained with Alcian blue. The ages of the donors are shown across the top and the bottom; asterisk indicates periosteum samples obtained postmortem. For each donor, the chondrogenesis assay was carried out in triplicate.

type II collagen (results not shown). In contrast, differentiation toward the chondrocyte phenotype could be elicited reproducibly and consistently by combining the micromass culture system with TGFβ1 treatment. This treatment induced chondrogenesis regardless of the number of cell passages or the age of the donors. No difference was observed between samples obtained postmortem and samples obtained during surgical knee replacement (Figure 4). The expression of type I collagen remained unchanged during chondrogenic differentiation at all time points examined up to 21 days (results not shown). Human dermal fibroblasts under the same

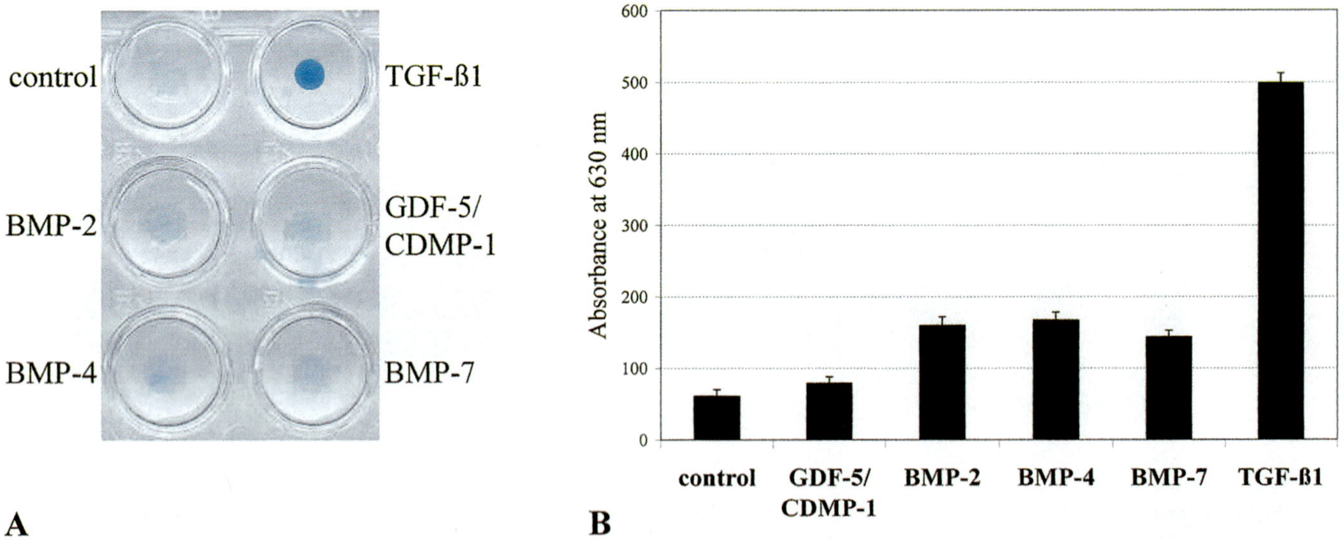

Figure 6. Chondrogenic potential of bone morphogenetic proteins (BMPs) compared with transforming growth factor β1 (TGF-β1). **A,** Periosteum-derived cells at passage 5 were plated in micromass culture and treated with growth factors, members of the TGFβ superfamily. Final concentrations were 10 ng/ml for TGF-β1 and 300 ng/ml for growth differentiation factor 5 (GDF-5)/cartilage-derived morphogenetic protein 1 (CDMP-1) and the BMPs. After 6 days, cultures were fixed and stained with Alcian blue. **B,** Stained micromasses were extracted with 6*M* guanidine HCl. The absorbance of the extracted dye was measured at 630 nm. Values are the mean and SD of 4 wells.

culture conditions and treatments failed to undergo chondrogenesis (Figure 4).

The chondrogenic differentiation could be reproduced in all donors tested (Figure 5). Importantly, no apparent impairment of the chondrogenic potential of PDCs was evident after cryopreservation. Under the same culture conditions, GDF-5/CDMP-1, BMP-2, BMP-4, and BMP-7 at concentrations of 100 or 300 ng/ml were poorly chondrogenic in comparison with TGFβ1 (Figure 6). The cell number was not affected by the treatments (results not shown). As proven by RT-PCR, PDCs expressed BMP receptors (results not shown). In the absence of TGFβ1, chondrogenesis did not take place even after 20 days of micromass culture, either in growth medium or in chemically defined serum-free medium (results not shown). As opposed to serially passaged PDCs, P0 and P1 cells in micromass cultures from donors younger than 30 years underwent chondrogenesis independent of TGFβ1 treatment (results not shown).

Histochemical and immunohistochemical characterization of periosteum-derived TGFβ1-induced neocartilage. Histochemical analysis of the micromass cultures treated with TGFβ1 displayed cartilage-specific metachromasia with toluidine blue dye and intense staining with Alcian blue, features which are highly suggestive of chondrogenic differentiation. Positive staining was evident only after 2 weeks. Untreated micromass cultures were all negative (Figures 7A–F). The detection of type II collagen protein by immunostaining further confirmed the cartilaginous nature of the tissue generated in vitro (Figures 7G and H). The extracellular matrix appeared to be homogeneous in all the histologic preparations. Hematoxylin and eosin staining as well as Masson's trichrome staining did not demonstrate the presence of dense fibrous bundles as in fibrocartilage tissue. This finding was confirmed by polarized light microscopy (results not shown). Alizarin red staining for calcium deposits (results not shown) and RT-PCR analysis for osteocalcin (Figure 4B) were negative at all time points examined up to 21 days.

The overall characteristics identified in the findings described above allow us to define the neocartilage as hyaline-like.

DISCUSSION

In the present study, we demonstrate that expanded adult human PDCs under appropriate culture conditions can be induced to form cartilage in vitro, independent of the number of cell passages or the age of the donors (within the ranges examined). We provide further characterization of a population of progenitor cells derived from human periosteum that possess high self-renewal capacity and retain their phenotype throughout expansion. We present additional data demonstrating full retention of the chondrogenic potential of this cell population following cryopreservation.

The chondrogenic potential of PDCs has been the subject of extensive investigation (9–18) and has been reported to be a phenomenon that is dependent on donor age and cell passage in culture (11). In most of the in vitro studies, PDCs were harvested from young animals, in which the probability of obtaining progenitor cells is very high (11,19,20), and were used in chondrogenesis assays at very early passages, when chondrogenesis seems to occur spontaneously (12–14).

Consistent with the results reported in the literature, we found that very early–passage PDCs from young adult human donors undergo spontaneous chondrogenesis in vitro. PDC cultures are initiated as primary cultures of fibroblast-like cells that grow out of PDC suspensions by selectively attaching to plastic tissue culture plates. In monolayer cultures, P0 and P1 PDCs from young donors express type II collagen and form nodules that stain with Alcian blue, indicating that at least a subpopulation of these cells has inherent chondrogenic potential. This phenomenon is rapidly lost upon cell passaging and is not observed in PDCs from donors older than 30 years.

The loss upon cell passaging of the spontaneous chondrogenic activity of PDCs from young donors may be due to factors related to the in vitro culture. Another possible explanation is that during the subculture period, a cell selection process takes place, so that PDCs responsible for the formation of chondrogenic nodules are overgrown by other cell subsets.

Not surprisingly, the decline in the in vitro chondrogenic potential of human PDCs is related to the age of the donor. In rabbit periosteum, it has been associated with a decrease in the size of the precursor pool in the cambium layer, where the progenitor cells reside (20). The observation that the in vitro chondrogenic potential of periosteum correlates directly with the thickness of the cambium layer and inversely with the age of the donor further supports this hypothesis (20,25). Alternatively, the age-related decline can also be attributable to a reduction in the inherent potential of the progenitor cells to undergo chondrogenic differentiation.

Regardless of the age, periosteum in vivo participates in bone remodeling and contributes to fracture healing by generating hyaline cartilage, which further

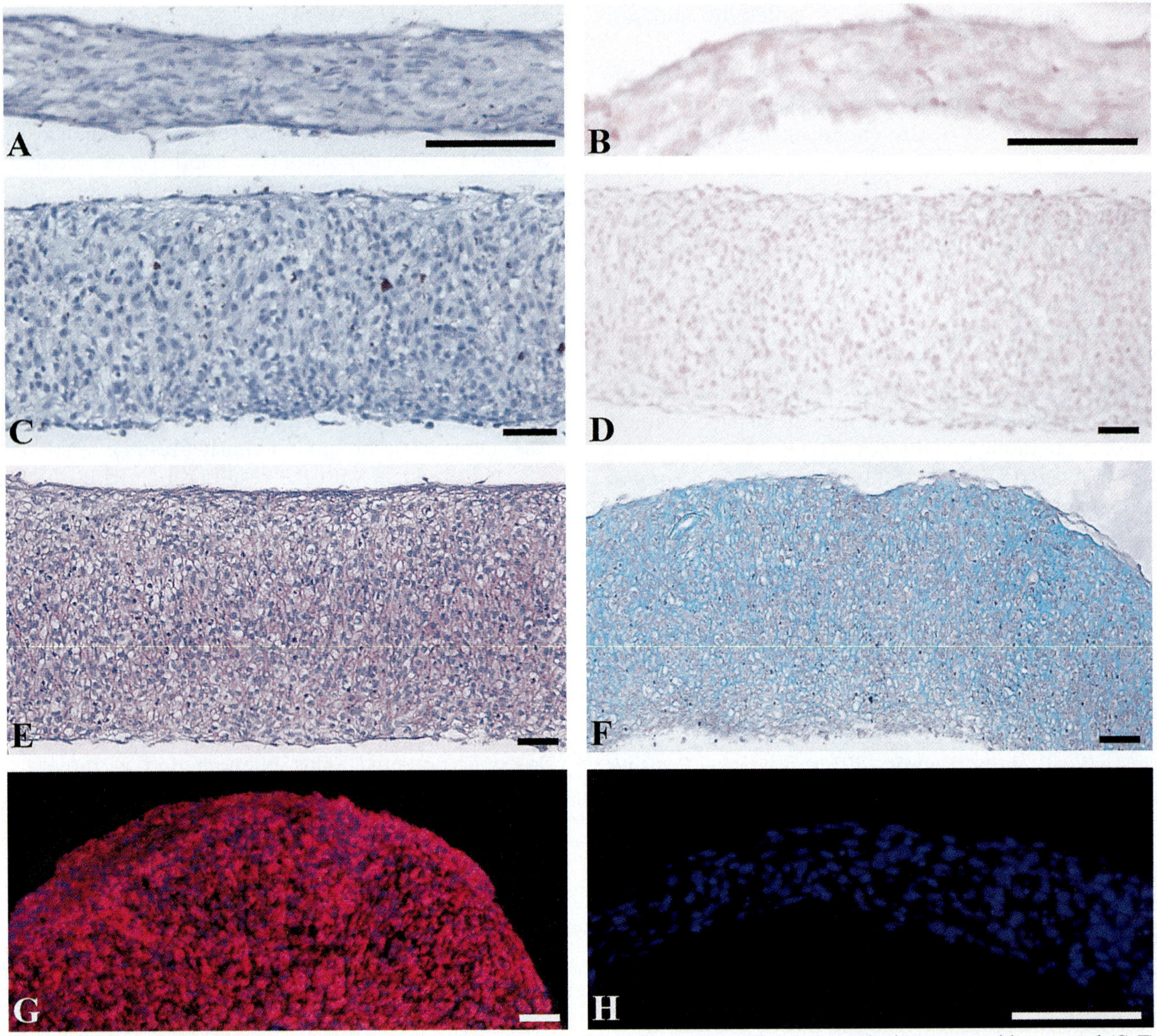

Figure 7. A–F, Toluidine blue (**A, C,** and **E**) and Alcian blue (**B, D,** and **F**) staining of paraffin sections of micromasses either treated (**C–F**) or not treated (**A** and **B**) with transforming growth factor β1 (TGFβ1) for 7 days (**C** and **D**) or 15 days (**A, B, E,** and **F**). **G** and **H,** Immunohistochemical analysis of paraffin sections with anti–type II collagen antibody. **G,** Micromass treated with TGFβ1 for 15 days. **H,** Untreated micromass. Nuclei were counterstained with 4′,6-diamidino-2-phenylindole (blue). Findings indicate the presence of cartilage differentiation in the micromasses treated with TGFβ1. Note the difference in scale between TGFβ1-treated and control micromasses. Bar = 50 μm.

undergoes endochondral ossification (26). With this observation in mind, we hypothesized that, independent of the age of the donor, an inducible chondrogenic potential of PDCs could be retained in vitro.

Treatments with growth factors, members of the TGFβ superfamily, which are known to be involved in morphogenesis, differentiation, and maintenance of cartilage (3–5,27), failed to induce chondrogenesis in confluent monolayer PDCs. Independent of the age of the donors or the number of cell passages, the differentiation toward the chondrocyte phenotype could be elicited reproducibly and consistently only when micromass culture and TGFβ1 treatment were combined. In contrast, neither untreated micromasses nor TGFβ1-treated monolayers could undergo chondrogenesis.

These results may appear to be at odds with the

previous literature reporting enhancement of in vitro chondrogenesis in PDCs using either the micromass culture system or TGFβ1 treatment alone (12–14). In those studies, however, PDCs were obtained from very young animals and assessed for chondrogenic potential at very early passages. Our data and data from previously published studies (14–16) demonstrate that in these settings, both culture conditions only enhance and accelerate an already spontaneous process.

We speculate that PDCs from young donors display spontaneous chondrogenesis that is lost with age or during in vitro cell expansion. Nevertheless, competence to respond to at least 1 chondrogenic signal is retained even in very elderly individuals or extensively passaged cells. The cytology, the presence of a metachromatic-staining matrix, and the detection of type II collagen mRNA and protein demonstrate the cartilage phenotype of the tissue generated in vitro. The positivity of the staining is evident only after 2 weeks, suggesting that, despite the early response to TGFβ1 treatment, time is required for the full maturation of PDCs to the cartilaginous phenotype.

The requirement for high cell density demonstrates the importance of cell–cell interactions for in vitro chondrogenic differentiation (28). In this respect, the micromass culture system reproduces cell interactions analogous to those occurring in precartilage mesenchymal condensation during limb development (3). However, in our system, this cell configuration alone was not sufficient for the induction of chondrogenesis; TGFβ1 treatment was also required. We hypothesize that PDCs in micromass culture would acquire competence to TGFβ1 signaling for chondrogenic differentiation.

Interestingly, under the same culture conditions, GDF-5/CDMP-1, BMP-2, BMP-4, and BMP-7 displayed a poor chondrogenic effect compared with TGFβ1. Our results are consistent with the observation that BMP-2 treatment does not affect chondrogenesis in high-density PDC cultures (16). However, BMPs have been shown to stimulate chondrogenesis in vitro (29–31). This discrepancy may be due to differences in the culture systems, BMP molecules, and concentrations used and/or the target cells. Specifically in human PDCs, the poor chondrogenic effect of BMPs as compared with that of TGFβ1 may depend on the relative levels of expression of TGFβ/BMP receptor subfamilies and related downstream factors or on distinctive regulation of their signaling pathways. These possibilities are currently under investigation.

For a potential use in tissue engineering protocols, PDCs should retain a stable phenotype as well as chondrogenic potential throughout extensive expansion and, possibly, after cryopreservation. Gene expression analysis by semiquantitative RT-PCR for a panel of genes known to be involved in skeletal development and maintenance (3) showed that, regardless of donor age, PDCs can be cryopreserved and largely expanded, retaining a stable phenotype and chondrogenic potential. Expanding further the number of marker genes, the analysis of PDC phenotype can lead to the identification of a set of molecular markers that is predictive of the chondrogenic potential of PDCs and other chondroprogenitor cell populations.

Cell senescence is known to alter the functional properties of somatic cells during in vitro expansion (23,24). We demonstrate that cell senescence is a limited event restricted to late-passage PDCs from elderly donors. Taking into consideration the high number of cells already obtainable after a few passages (about 1 billion cells after 6 passages, starting from a 1-cm^2 periosteum sample from the proximal medial tibia), senescence does not represent a significant factor limiting cell expansion.

A recent study showed a progressive decline in the chondrogenic potential of rabbit periosteum harvested postmortem (as soon as 4 hours after death) that was related to the viability of the tissue (32). In our study, no differences were observed in the molecular profile and chondrogenic potential of expanded cells obtained from periosteum harvested postmortem (within 12 hours) and at the time of surgical knee replacement. This apparent discrepancy can be explained by the different experimental settings. O'Driscoll et al (32) used an ex vivo organ culture of periosteum as a tissue. In our procedure, cells were first released and then selected based on their capacity to adhere to plastic. Adherent cells were a minority of the total pool of cells that were plated. The subsequent expansion of this selected cell subpopulation most probably corrected the possible differences in the number of viable chondroprogenitor cells present in the original tissue samples.

The characteristic poor capacity for repair of articular cartilage has prompted great interest in cartilage tissue engineering and regeneration. Autologous chondrocyte transplantation (1) is limited by the availability of cells, particularly in elderly individuals, and the well-known dedifferentiation events associated with chondrocyte expansion. In the selection of the optimal cells for repairing joint surface defects, the following criteria should be considered: the chondrogenic potential, the autologous source, the relative ease of access, the cell expandability, the phenotypic stability of the cells throughout the expansion procedures, and the least possible surgical morbidity. The potential use of human embryonic stem cells (33,34) for tissue regeneration therapy is very attractive, but ethical issues need to be resolved. Less controversial, but equally promising, is the perspective of using progenitor cells derived from adult tissues (35). These adult stem cells seem to retain a remarkable plasticity, since they have much wider differentiation potential than previously thought (36–43). This plasticity, however, presents the potential risk of cell differentiation toward an undesired direction(s) upon transplantation. It would be more reassuring, therefore, to use cells that have restricted differentiation potential.

We show that regardless of their age, adult human PDCs are easily accessible, expandable, and phenotypically stable. Moreover, they maintain their chondrogenic potential up to at least 15 passages and after cryopreservation. It has also been reported that human bone marrow–derived mesenchymal cells can be largely expanded in culture with retention of their chondrogenic potential, independent of donor age (44). However, in contrast to the broad plasticity of bone marrow–derived mesenchymal cells (37,41–43), PDCs are known to have bilineage potential, since they can give rise to cartilage and bone (11). At least in vitro, expanded PDCs can, under appropriate conditions, form a tissue close to that of hyaline cartilage, with no evidence of mineralization or bone differentiation. These characteristics make PDCs promising precursor cells for use in the repair of joint surface defects. If required in the in vivo environment, modern gene transfer technology and carrier systems can provide the means to deliver bioactive factors, such as TGFβ1, to prime chondrogenesis.

ACKNOWLEDGMENTS

We thank J. Bellemans (Department of Orthopedics, Katholieke Universiteit, Leuven, Belgium) for providing periosteum samples, S. Tejpar (CME, Katholieke Universiteit, Leuven, Belgium) for providing human dermal fibroblasts, and F. P. Cantatore (University of Bari, Bari, Italy) for providing human trabecular osteoblasts. Special thanks are also due to the people working in the mortuary of the Katholeike Universiteit Leuven. We are grateful to M. Moos and P. Tylzanowski for critical reading of the manuscript.

REFERENCES

1. Brittberg M, Lindahl A, Nilsson A, Ohlsson C, Isaksson O, Peterson L. Treatment of deep cartilage defects in the knee with autologous chondrocyte transplantation. N Engl J Med 1994;331: 889–95.
2. Benya PD, Shaffer JD. Dedifferentiated chondrocytes reexpress the differentiated collagen phenotype when cultured in agarose gels. Cell 1982;30:215–24.
3. Dell'Accio F, De Bari C, Luyten FP. Molecular basis of joint development. Jpn J Rheumatol 1999;9:17–29.
4. Thomas JT, Lin K, Nandedkar M, Camargo M, Cervenka J, Luyten FP. A human chondrodysplasia due to a mutation in a TGF-β superfamily member. Nat Genet 1996;12:315–7.
5. Thomas JT, Kilpatrick MW, Lin K, Erlacher L, Lembessis P, Costa T, et al. Disruption of human limb morphogenesis by a dominant negative mutation in CDMP1. Nat Genet 1997;17:58–64.
6. Tsumaki N, Tanaka K, Arikawa HE, Nakase T, Kimura T, Thomas JT, et al. Role of CDMP-1 in skeletal morphogenesis: promotion of mesenchymal cell recruitment and chondrocyte differentiation. J Cell Biol 1999;144:161–73.
7. Francis-West PH, Abdelfattah A, Chen P, Allen C, Parish J, Ladher R, et al. Mechanisms of GDF-5 action during skeletal development. Development 1999;126:1305–15.
8. Ham AW. A histological study of the early phases of bone repair. J Bone Joint Surg 1930;12:827–44.
9. Nakahara H, Bruder SP, Goldberg VM, Caplan AI. In vivo osteochondrogenic potential of cultured cells derived from the periosteum. Clin Orthop 1990;259:223–32.
10. Nakahara H, Bruder SP, Haynesworth SE, Holecek JJ, Baber MA, Goldberg VM, et al. Bone and cartilage formation in diffusion chambers by subcultured cells derived from the periosteum. Bone 1990;11:181–8.
11. Nakahara H, Goldberg VM, Caplan AI. Culture-expanded human periosteal-derived cells exhibit osteochondral potential in vivo. J Orthop Res 1991;9:465–76.
12. Nakahara H, Dennis JE, Bruder SP, Haynesworth SE, Lennon DP, Caplan AI. In vitro differentiation of bone and hypertrophic cartilage from periosteal-derived cells. Exp Cell Res 1991;195: 492–503.
13. Nakata K, Nakahara H, Kimura T, Kojima A, Iwasaki M, Caplan AI, et al. Collagen gene expression during chondrogenesis from chick periosteum-derived cells. FEBS Lett 1992;299:278–82.
14. Izumi T, Scully SP, Heydemann A, Bolander ME. Transforming growth factor beta 1 stimulates type II collagen expression in cultured periosteum-derived cells. J Bone Miner Res 1992;7: 115–21.
15. Iwasaki M, Nakata K, Nakahara H, Nakase T, Kimura T, Kimata K, et al. Transforming growth factor-beta 1 stimulates chondrogenesis and inhibits osteogenesis in high density culture of periosteum-derived cells. Endocrinology 1993;132:1603–8.
16. Iwasaki M, Nakahara H, Nakase T, Kimura T, Takaoka K, Caplan AI, et al. Bone morphogenetic protein 2 stimulates osteogenesis but does not affect chondrogenesis in osteochondrogenic differentiation of periosteum-derived cells. J Bone Miner Res 1994;9: 1195–204.
17. O'Driscoll SW, Recklies AD, Poole AR. Chondrogenesis in periosteal explants: an organ culture model for in vitro study. J Bone Joint Surg Am 1994;76:1042–51.
18. O'Driscoll SW. Articular cartilage regeneration using periosteum. Clin Orthop 1999;367 Suppl:186–203.
19. D'Ippolito G, Schiller PC, Ricordi C, Roos BA, Howard GA. Age-related osteogenic potential of mesenchymal stromal stem cells from human vertebral bone marrow. J Bone Miner Res 1999;14:1115–22.
20. O'Driscoll SW, Ito Y, Fitzsimmons JS. Age-related decrease in chondrogenic potential correlates with a decrease in chondrocyte precursor pool size [abstract]. Trans Orthop Res Soc 2000;25:935.
21. Harrison ET Jr, Luyten FP, Reddi AH. Osteogenin promotes reexpression of cartilage phenotype by dedifferentiated articular

chondrocytes in serum-free medium. Exp Cell Res 1991;192:340–5.
22. Chen P, Vukicevic S, Sampath K, Luyten FP. Bovine articular chondrocytes do not undergo hypertrophy when cultured in the presence of serum and osteogenic protein-1. Biochem Biophys Res Commun 1993;197:1253–9.
23. Dimri GP, Lee X, Basile G, Acosta M, Scott G, Roskelley C, et al. A biomarker that identifies senescent human cells in culture and in aging skin in vivo. Proc Natl Acad Sci U S A 1995;92:9363–7.
24. Goldstein S. Replicative senescence: the human fibroblast comes of age. Science 1990;249:1129–33.
25. Gallay SH, Miura Y, Commisso CN, Fitzsimmons JS, O'Driscoll SW. Relationship of donor site to chondrogenic potential of periosteum in vitro. J Orthop Res 1994;12:515–25.
26. Liu Z, Luyten FP, Lammens J, Dequeker J. Molecular signaling in bone fracture healing and distraction osteogenesis. Histol Histopathol 1999;14:587–95.
27. Erlacher L, Ng C-K, Ullrich R, Krieger S, Luyten FP. Presence of cartilage-derived morphogenetic proteins in articular cartilage and enhancement of matrix replacement in vitro. Arthritis Rheum 1998;41:263–73.
28. Solursh M. Formation of cartilage tissue in vitro. J Cell Biochem 1991;45:258–60.
29. Carrington JL, Chen P, Yanagishita M, Reddi AH. Osteogenin (bone morphogenetic protein-3) stimulates cartilage formation by chick limb bud cells in vitro. Dev Biol 1991;146:406–15.
30. Nakamura K, Shirai T, Morishita S, Uchida S, Saeki-Miura K, Makishima F. p38 mitogen-activated protein kinase functionally contributes to chondrogenesis induced by growth/differentiation factor-5 in ATDC5 cells. Exp Cell Res 1999;250:351–63.
31. Denker AE, Haas AR, Nicoll SB, Tuan RS. Chondrogenic differentiation of murine C3H10T1/2 multipotential mesenchymal cells. I. Stimulation by bone morphogenetic protein-2 in high-density micromass cultures. Differentiation 1999;64:67–76.
32. O'Driscoll SW, Meisami B, Miura Y, Fitzsimmons JS. Viability of periosteal tissue obtained postmortem. Cell Transplant 1999;8:611–6.
33. Thomson JA, Itskovitz-Eldor J, Shapiro SS, Waknitz MA, Swiergiel JJ, Marshall VS, et al. Embryonic stem cell lines derived from human blastocysts. Science 1998;282:1145–7.
34. Reubinoff BE, Pera MF, Fong CY, Trounson A, Bongso A. Embryonic stem cell lines from human blastocysts: somatic differentiation in vitro. Nat Biotechnol 2000;18:399–404.
35. Weissman IL. Translating stem and progenitor cell biology to the clinic: barriers and opportunities. Science 2000;287:1442–6.
36. Eglitis MA, Mezey E. Hematopoietic cells differentiate into both microglia and macroglia in the brains of adult mice. Proc Natl Acad Sci U S A 1997;94:4080–5.
37. Ferrari G, Cusella-De Angelis G, Coletta M, Paolucci E, Stornaiuolo A, Cossu G, et al. Muscle regeneration by bone marrow-derived myogenic progenitors. Science 1998;279:1528–30.
38. Bjornson CR, Rietze RL, Reynolds BA, Magli MC, Vescovi AL. Turning brain into blood: a hematopoietic fate adopted by adult neural stem cells in vivo. Science 1999;283:534–7.
39. Jackson KA, Mi T, Goodell MA. Hematopoietic potential of stem cells isolated from murine skeletal muscle. Proc Natl Acad Sci U S A 1999;96:14482–6.
40. Johansson CB, Momma S, Clarke DL, Risling M, Lendahl U, Frisen J. Identification of a neural stem cell in the adult mammalian central nervous system. Cell 1999;96:25–34.
41. Kopen GC, Prockop DJ, Phinney DG. Marrow stromal cells migrate throughout forebrain and cerebellum, and they differentiate into astrocytes after injection into neonatal mouse brains. Proc Natl Acad Sci U S A 1999;96:10711–6.
42. Petersen BE, Bowen WC, Patrene KD, Mars WM, Sullivan AK, Murase N, et al. Bone marrow as a potential source of hepatic oval cells. Science 1999;284:1168–70.
43. Pittenger MF, Mackay AM, Beck SC, Jaiswal RK, Douglas R, Mosca JD, et al. Multilineage potential of adult human mesenchymal stem cells. Science 1999;284:143–7.
44. Yoo JU, Barthel TS, Nishimura K, Solchaga L, Caplan AI, Goldberg VM, et al. The chondrogenic potential of human bone-marrow-derived mesenchymal progenitor cells. J Bone Joint Surg Am 1998;80:1745–57.

ARTHRITIS & RHEUMATISM
Vol. 44, No. 1, January 2001, pp 96–104

Nitric Oxide Regulates Mitochondrial Respiration and Functions of Articular Chondrocytes

Masuhiro Tomita, Eisuke F. Sato, Manabu Nishikawa, Yoshiki Yamano, and Masayasu Inoue

Objective. **Biologic effects of nitric oxide (NO) have been shown to increase under hypoxic conditions. Because the oxygen tension in joint cavities of patients with arthritis is fairly low, biologic effects of NO would be expected to be significantly large in these compartments. This study was undertaken to investigate the effects of NO on the energy metabolism and functions of articular chondrocytes under different oxygen tension conditions.**

Methods. **Articular chondrocytes from rabbits were cultured under various oxygen concentrations in the presence or absence of NO and NOC18, an NO donor. Cellular respiration was measured using a Clark-type oxygen electrode. Levels of ATP in the cells were determined according to the luciferin-luciferase method. Cellular synthesis of proteoglycans was determined by measuring the incorporation of radioactivity (derived from ^{35}S-labeled SO_4) into glycosaminoglycans. Expression of stress-related proteins was evaluated by Western blotting analysis using specific antibodies.**

Results. **Respiration and ATP synthesis of cultured chondrocytes were inhibited by NO, particularly under low oxygen concentrations. The presence of either NO or specific inhibitors of mitochondrial electron transport suppressed the synthesis of proteoglycans without affecting cell viability. When exposed to NO, cellular levels of heat-shock protein 70 (hsp70) and heme oxygenase 1 (HO-1) increased markedly. The presence of inhibitors of mitochondrial electron transport also increased cellular levels of hsp70 and HO-1.**

Conclusion. **These results suggest that NO generated in the joint might inhibit energy metabolism and the synthesis of proteoglycans of chondrocytes, thereby modulating pathophysiologic processes occurring in patients with arthritis.**

Nitric oxide (NO) is a multifunctional molecule that mediates various biologic processes, including relaxation of smooth muscles, host defense mechanisms against pathogens, and inflammation (1,2). Studies have revealed that both synovial cells and chondrocytes express the inducible type of NO synthase (iNOS) and that the synthesis of NO is enhanced in patients with rheumatoid arthritis (RA) or osteoarthritis (OA) (3–5). Inflammatory cytokines, such as interleukin-1 β and tumor necrosis factor α, increase the expression of iNOS in these cells (6). NO reversibly binds to mitochondrial cytochrome c oxidase and inhibits the respiration of various types of cells (7,8). Although the lifetime of NO has been postulated to be extremely short, and hence its biologic effects appear only transiently, recent studies revealed that NO exhibited strong effects for a fairly long time under conditions of low oxygen tension (9–12). Because oxygen concentrations in joint cavity and cartilage tissues, particularly those in patients with RA, are fairly low (13,14), effects of NO on chondrocyte metabolism might be stronger than those expected from in vitro experiments performed under air atmospheric conditions.

It is known that the amount of matrix in joint cartilage decreases in patients with arthritis, thereby causing dysfunction of their joints. Studies have shown that NO suppressed the synthesis of collagens and proteoglycans, thus destroying articular cartilage (15,16). Furthermore, plasma levels of nitrate, an oxidized metabolite of NO, were markedly increased in patients with RA (17). However, the possible involvement of NO in the pathogenesis of arthritis, and the nature of such possible involvement, remain to be elucidated. The present work demonstrates the effect of NO on the energy metabolism, proteoglycan synthesis,

Masuhiro Tomita, MD, Eisuke F. Sato, PhD, Manabu Nishikawa, MD, PhD, Yoshiki Yamano, MD, PhD, Masayasu Inoue, MD, PhD: Osaka City University Medical School, Osaka, Japan.

Address correspondence and reprint requests to Masuhiro Tomita, MD, Department of Biochemistry and Molecular Pathology, Osaka City University Medical School, 1-4-3 Asahimachi, Abeno, Osaka 545-8585, Japan.

Submitted for publication March 24, 2000; accepted in revised form September 18, 2000.

and viability of articular chondrocytes under different oxygen tension conditions.

MATERIALS AND METHODS

Reagents. NO and argon gas were obtained from Kinkisanki (Osaka, Japan). The NO donor 2,2′-(hydroxynitrosohydrazono)-bis-ethanamine (NOC18) was obtained from Dojindo Chemical (Kumamoto, Japan). ^{35}S-labeled sodium sulfate was from Amersham Pharmacia Biotech (Buckinghamshire, UK). Rotenone and antimycin A were from Wako Pure Chemical (Osaka, Japan) and Sigma (St. Louis, MO), respectively. All other reagents used were of analytical grade and were obtained from Wako Pure Chemical. Specific antibodies against type II collagen and aggrecan were purchased from Chemicon (Temecula, CA) and Biogenesis (Poole, UK), respectively. Antibodies against heat-shock protein 70 (hsp70), heme oxygenase 1 (HO-1), and Mn–superoxide dismutase (Mn-SOD) were obtained from Stress Gen (Victoria, BC, Canada), and those against Cu/Zn-SOD and Bcl-2 were from Calbiochem-Novabiochem (San Diego, CA) and Transduction Laboratory (Lexington, KY), respectively.

Preparation of NO solution. Saturated NO solution was prepared by bubbling NO gas through 50 m*M* HEPES-NaOH buffer (pH 7.4), as described previously (18). Briefly, 2 small tubes were fitted with an airtight septum with glass tubes inserted for delivery and escape of gases, with a first tube containing 5*M* KOH and a second tube containing 50 m*M* HEPES-NaOH buffer. Argon gas was delivered into the 2 tubes at a flow rate of 100 ml/minute. After 15 minutes, argon was replaced with NO at the same flow rate. The saturated NO solution (1.9 m*M*) was freshly prepared and used immediately for experiments.

Cell culture. Articular chondrocytes were isolated from the shoulder and knee joints of 4-week-old male rabbits, by the enzymatic digestion method of Green (19). Cartilage tissues from knee and shoulder joints were pooled, cut into small pieces, and digested with 0.2% trypsin and 0.2% collagenase for 0.5 hours and 3 hours, respectively. The isolated cells thus obtained were grown in Dulbecco's modified Eagle's medium (DMEM)/Ham's F-12 medium (Life Technologies, Grand Island, NY) supplemented with 10% fetal calf serum (FCS) and antibiotics, in 95% air and 5% CO_2. Confluent cells were washed with phosphate buffered saline, and the medium was replaced with DMEM/Ham's F-12 medium supplemented with 3% FCS and antibiotics. Skin fibroblasts were also obtained from rabbits, by the method of Touriol et al (20). AH-130 hepatoma cells were cultured as described previously (10). All animal experiments were approved by the Animal Care and Use Committee of Osaka City University Medical School.

Analysis of cell respiration. Respiration of chondrocytes was measured polarographically at 37°C, using a Clark-type oxygen electrode fitted to a 2-ml water-jacketed chamber (21). Cellular respiration was analyzed in Krebs-Ringer phosphate buffer (pH 7.4), consisting of 50 m*M* HEPES buffer, 100 m*M* NaCl, 5 m*M* KCl, 5 m*M* glucose, and 1 m*M* each of $MgCl_2$, NaH_2PO_4, and $CaCl_2$. The reaction was started by adding 10^7 cells to the assay mixture. During the experiments, aliquots of NO-saturated solution were added to the reaction mixture.

Determination of glucose, lactate, and ATP. Glucose concentration in the medium was measured with an assay kit, using glucose oxidase (Wako). Lactate concentration was determined spectrophotometrically, by the method of Goodall and Byers (22). Alanine aminotransferase was added to remove pyruvate in the medium to prevent the reverse reaction. ATP levels in chondrocytes were determined according to the luciferin-luciferase method, using an ATP bioluminescence assay kit (Roche Molecular Biochemicals, Mannheim, Germany).

Synthesis of proteoglycans. Synthesis of proteoglycans was determined by the method of Taskiran et al (23). Briefly, cells were labeled with ^{35}S-labeled sulfate (final concentration 20 μCi/ml) for 24 hours in the presence or absence of NOC18. After incubation, radioactive components in the cells were extracted at 4°C with 0.5*M* NaOH for 48 hours. Cell extracts and conditioned medium were subjected to column chromatography on Sephadex G-25M PD-10 columns (Amersham Pharmacia Biotech), using 50 m*M* Trizma buffer (pH 7.0) containing 4*M* guanidinium hydrochloride and 50 m*M* sodium sulfate. The radioactivity in de novo synthesized proteoglycans was determined by scintillation counting.

Analysis of DNA fragmentation. Cells (2×10^6) were incubated for 10 minutes in 100 μl ice-cold lysis buffer (10 m*M* Tris HCl [pH 7.4], 10 m*M* EDTA, 0.5% Triton X-100) at 4°C. After incubation for 20 minutes, the mixture was centrifuged at 10,000*g* for 20 minutes. The supernatant was incubated with 40 μg RNase A at 37°C for 1 hour, and then with 40 μg proteinase K for 1 hour. DNA was precipitated by incubating with 1 volume of isopropanol and 0.2 volumes of 5*M* NaCl at −20°C for 12 hours and centrifuging at 10,000*g* for 20 minutes. Pellets were air dried and dissolved in 10 μl of buffer consisting of 10 m*M* Tris HCl (pH 8.0) and 1 m*M* EDTA. The DNA samples thus obtained were subjected to 1.5% agarose gel electrophoresis at 100V using 40 m*M* Tris acetate (pH 8.0) and 1 m*M* EDTA as a running buffer. The gel was stained with 0.1 μg/ml of ethidium bromide and visualized under ultraviolet light.

Western blot and dot-blot analysis. Proteins (10 μg) from cell lysates were subjected to 10% and 15% sodium dodecyl sulfate–polyacrylamide gel electrophoresis and blotted onto a polyvinylidene difluoride membrane (Millipore, Bedford, MA) using a Bio-Rad (Richmond, CA) semidry blot system (15V for 1 hour in 192 m*M* Tris-glycine buffer). The sheets were incubated in Tris buffered saline–Tween (TBST) (150 m*M* NaCl, 50 m*M* Tris HCl [pH 7.2]) containing 0.05% Tween 20 and 5% lowfat milk powder, for 12 hours at 4°C. The sheets were then incubated with specific antibodies (1:1,000 in TBST with 5% lowfat milk powder) for 1 hour at 25°C. The incubated membranes were washed 3 times with TBST to eliminate nonspecific binding of the antibodies. After incubation with horseradish peroxidase–conjugated second antibody (1:1,000 in TBST with 5% lowfat milk powder) for 1 hour at 25°C, immunoreactive spots were analyzed by the enhanced chemiluminescence method (Amersham). The expression of specific proteins was determined using an imaging densitometer (model GS-700; Bio-Rad). Dot-blot analysis was carried out using 1-μg proteins of cell lysates from chondrocytes or fibroblasts, as described for Western blot analysis.

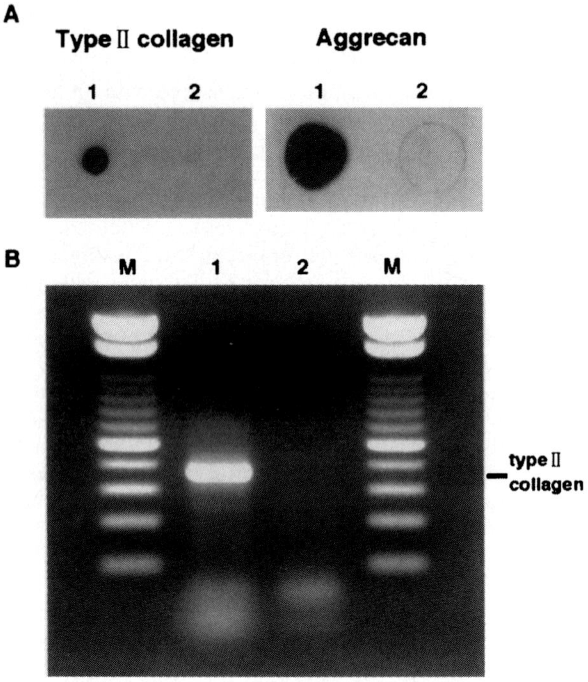

Figure 1. Expression of type II collagen and aggrecan in cultured chondrocytes. **A,** The expression of type II collagen and aggrecan in cultured articular chondrocytes (lane 1) and rabbit skin fibroblasts (lane 2) was determined by dot-blot analysis using specific antibodies against type II collagen and aggrecan. **B,** The expression of the type II collagen gene was also investigated by reverse transcriptase–polymerase chain reaction using 1 μg of total RNA from articular chondrocytes and fibroblasts, as described in the text.

Reverse transcriptase–polymerase chain reaction (RT-PCR) analysis. Total RNA was extracted from articular chondrocytes by the acid guanidium–phenol–chloroform method (24). Levels of messenger RNA for type II collagen were analyzed by RT-PCR (25). RT was carried out at 42°C for 15 minutes, and PCR was performed by 1 minute of denaturation at 95°C, 1 minute of hybridization at 57°C, and 2 minutes of extension at 72°C, for 35 cycles. The type II collagen primers used were 5′-ATGACAATCTGGCTCCCAACACTGC-3′ and 5′-GACCGGCCCTATGTCCACACCGAAT-3′ (26). PCR products were subjected to 1.5% agarose gel electrophoresis, stained with 0.1 μg/ml of ethidium bromide, and visualized under ultraviolet light.

Statistical analysis. All experiments were performed at least 3 times with similar results. Values were expressed as the mean ± SD. Statistical analysis was performed by analysis of variance and post hoc testing. *P* values less than 0.01 were considered significant.

RESULTS

Expression of type II collagen and aggrecan. To investigate the phenotypes of the cultured chondrocytes, dot-blot analysis of the expression of type II collagen and aggrecan was performed. The results clearly showed that both type II collagen and aggrecan were expressed in chondrocytes but not in fibroblasts (Figure 1A). We also found that the type II collagen gene was strongly expressed in cultured chondrocytes but not in fibroblasts, as analyzed by RT-PCR (Figure 1B). Thus, the phenotypes of primary cultured chondrocytes used for the present experiments were well maintained and not transformed to fibroblast-like cells. These chondrocytes were used for the subsequent experiments.

Effect of NO and O_2 on cellular respiration. Recent studies revealed that NO inhibited the respiration of isolated mitochondria and various types of cells (27,28). Figure 2 shows the effect of NO on the respiration of articular chondrocytes under different oxygen concentrations. The rates of coupled and dinitrophenol-uncoupled respiration of articular chondrocytes were 1.2 and 1.9 nmoles/minute/10^6 cells, respectively. These rates of respiration were similar to those reported by Stefanovic-Racic et al (29). The respiration was reversibly inhibited by NO at a fairly low concentration. The inhibitory effect of NO was increased by decreasing the

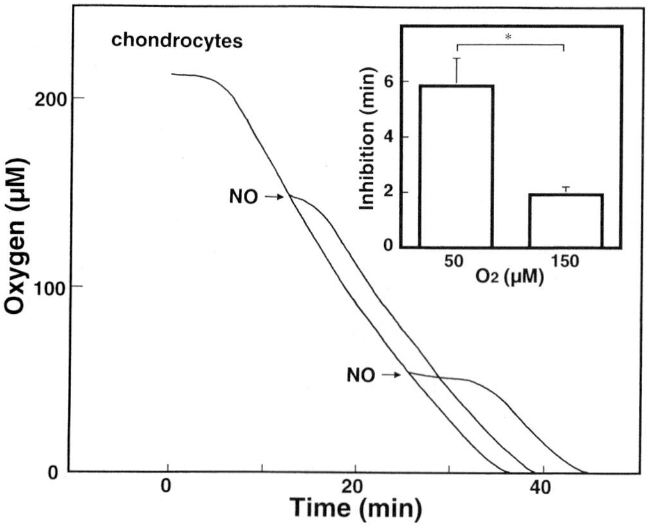

Figure 2. Effect of nitric oxide (NO) on oxygen consumption by chondrocytes. Chondrocytes (5 × 10^6/ml) were incubated in a closed chamber containing 2 ml of Krebs-Ringer phosphate buffer at 37°C in the presence of 5 m*M* glucose. At the indicated times (arrows), NO was added, to yield a final concentration of 2 μM. During the incubation, the oxygen concentration in the medium was monitored as described in the text. **Inset,** Effect of oxygen tension on the time required for disappearance of the inhibitory effect of NO. Values are the mean and SD. * = $P < 0.01$.

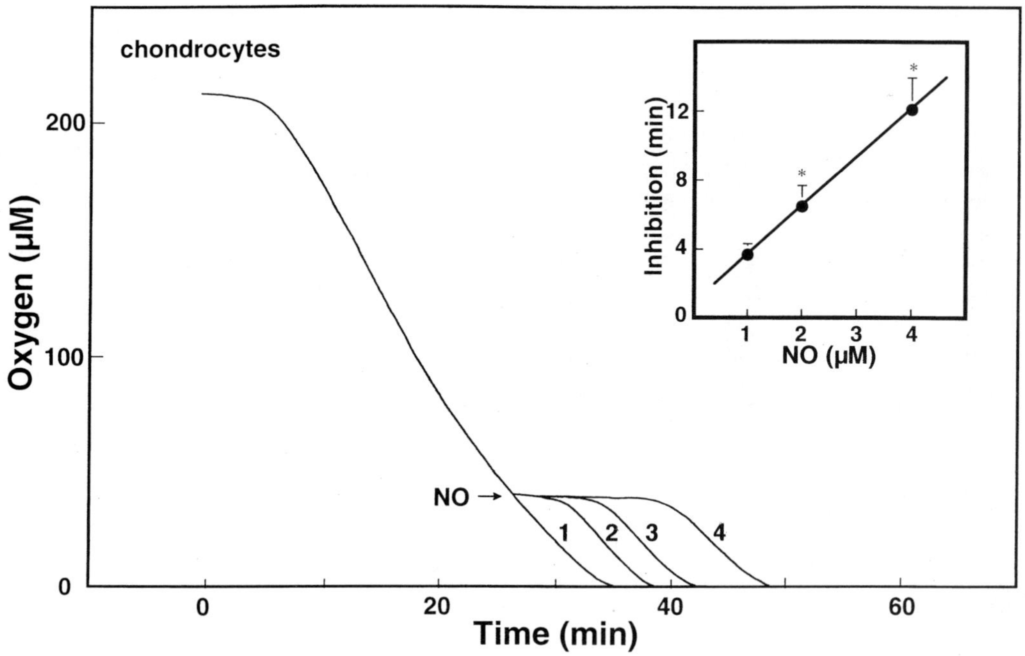

Figure 3. Effect of various doses of nitric oxide (NO) on oxygen consumption by chondrocytes. At the indicated times (arrows), NO was added to the reaction mixture to yield a final concentration of 0, 1, 2, or 4 μM (designated 1, 2, 3, and 4, respectively). **Inset,** Effect of various doses of NO on the time required for disappearance of the inhibitory effect of NO. Other conditions were as described in Figure 2. Values are the mean and SD. $* = P < 0.01$ versus control.

oxygen concentrations in the reaction mixture. NO inhibited the respiration of chondrocytes in a dose-dependent manner; the duration of the inhibition was proportional to the concentration of NO (Figure 3).

Effect of NO on cellular ATP levels. The effect of NO on cellular levels of ATP was studied with chondrocytes (Figure 4). The presence of NOC18, an NO donor, decreased the cellular levels of ATP in a dose-dependent manner. This inhibitory effect of NOC18 was stronger with an oxygen tension of 5% than with 20%. Using the trypan blue dye exclusion test (10), it was confirmed that the inhibitory effect of NO on cellular ATP levels was not due to a decrease in the viability of chondrocytes.

Effect of NO on glucose metabolism. Figure 5 shows the effect of NOC18 on glucose consumption and lactate production by chondrocytes. NOC18 increased the rate of glucose consumption, and this rate was higher at an oxygen tension of 5% than at 20%. NOC18 also increased the rate of lactate production; this rate, as well, was higher at the lower level of oxygen tension.

Effect of NO on the synthesis of proteoglycan by chondrocytes. Synthesis of proteoglycan is one of the important functions of articular chondrocytes. The synthesis of sulfated proteoglycans has been shown to be

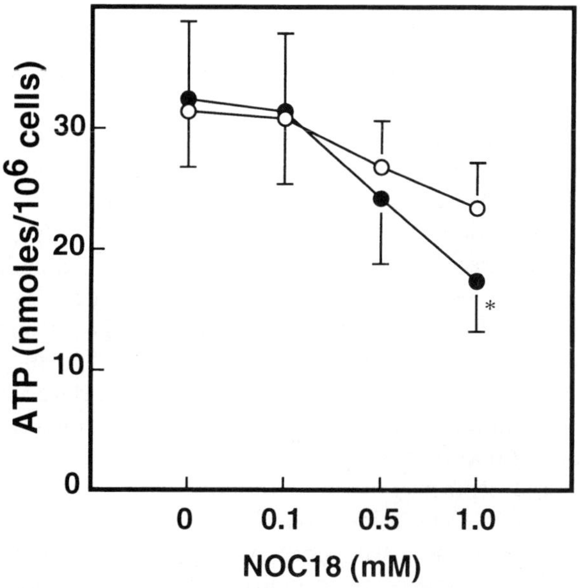

Figure 4. Effect of nitric oxide (NO) on cellular ATP levels. Chondrocytes were cultured for 24 hours in the presence of various concentrations of the NO donor NOC18, under oxygen concentrations of either 20% (open circles) or 5% (closed circles). After incubation for 24 hours, cellular ATP concentrations were measured as described in the text. Values are the mean and SD ($n = 6$). $* = P < 0.01$ versus oxygen concentration of 20%.

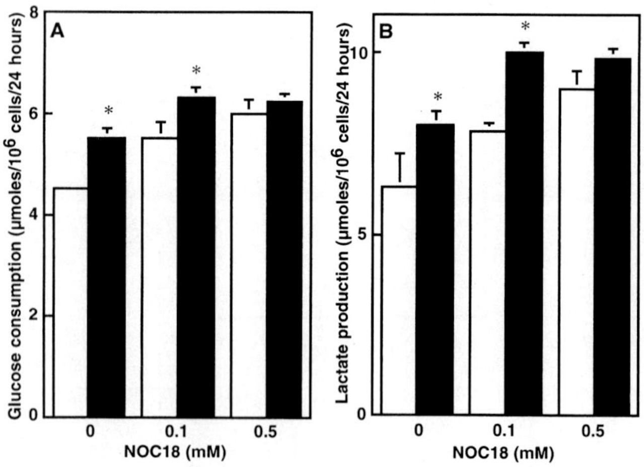

Figure 5. Effect of nitric oxide (NO) on the glucose metabolism of chondrocytes. Chondrocytes were cultured for 24 hours in the presence of various concentrations of the NO donor NOC18, under oxygen concentrations of either 20% (open columns) or 5% (closed columns). Concentrations of glucose (**A**) and lactate (**B**) in the medium were measured as described in the text. Values are the mean and SD (n = 6). * = $P < 0.01$ versus oxygen concentration of 20%.

regulated by cellular ATP (30). Thus, we studied the effect of NO on the incorporation of radioactive sulfate into proteoglycans of articular chondrocytes. The incorporation of radioactivity in cellular proteoglycans was inhibited by NOC18 in a dose-dependent manner (Figure 6).

Effect of NO on cellular DNA fragmentation. Fragmentation of internucleosomal DNA has been used as a marker of apoptosis of various types of cells. To test for the possible occurrence of apoptosis of NO-treated articular chondrocytes, DNA samples from the chondrocytes were isolated and analyzed by agarose gel electrophoresis. When cells were cultured for 24 hours under oxygen concentrations of either 20% or 5% in the presence or absence of 1 m*M* NOC18, no appreciable fragmentation of DNA was found to occur (Figure 7). When chondrocytes were cultured in the presence of 5 n*M* staurosporine, small amounts of cellular DNA underwent fragmentation. AH-130 cells, which easily undergo apoptosis (10), were also used, as a positive control. In contrast to chondrocytes, AH-130 cells cultured in the presence of NOC18 showed marked signs of DNA fragmentation.

Effect of specific mitochondrial electron transport inhibitors on cellular ATP and proteoglycan synthesis. NO has been shown to inhibit the electron transport system in mitochondria (8–12). Because rotenone and antimycin A specifically inhibit mitochondrial electron transport at complex I and complex III, respectively (31), we tested the effects of these 2 inhibitors on cellular functions (Table 1). Both inhibitors suppressed the ATP levels in articular chondrocytes during the first 2 hours. However, the inhibitory effect was no longer apparent after incubation for 12 hours. The effects of rotenone and antimycin A on the synthesis of proteoglycans were also investigated. Both inhibitors suppressed the cellular incorporation of radioactivity.

Effect of NO on cellular expression of various proteins. Recent studies have revealed that antioxidant enzymes, such as SOD isozymes, and heat-shock proteins protect various types of cells from cytotoxic effects of NO and its metabolites (32–34). To elucidate the mechanism by which articular chondrocytes showed strong resistance to NO despite the marked decrease in ATP levels and proteoglycans, effects of NOC18 on cellular levels of various proteins were investigated. Cellular levels of hsp70 and HO-1 were increased by

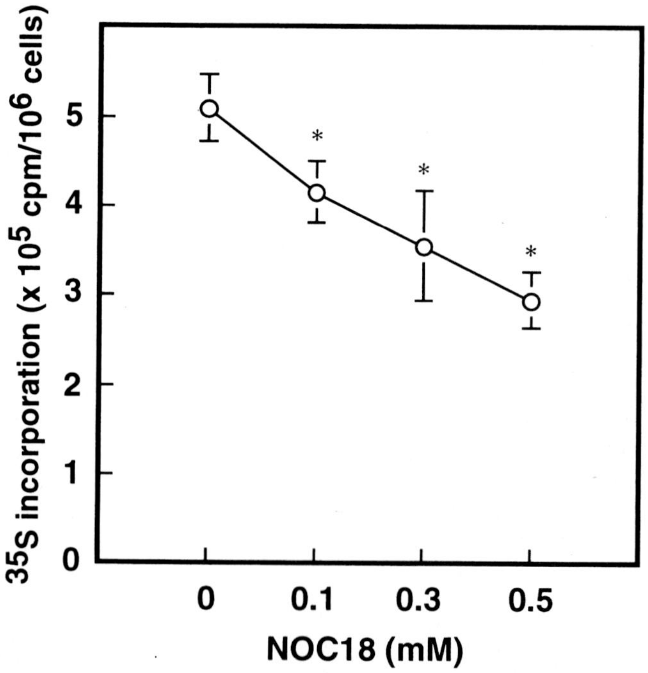

Figure 6. Effect of nitric oxide (NO) on the incorporation of ^{35}S in chondrocytes. Chondrocytes were cultured for 24 hours in the presence of various concentrations of the NO donor NOC18, under an oxygen concentration of 20%. After incubation for 24 hours, incorporation of ^{35}S was measured as described in the text. Values are the mean ± SD (n = 6). * = $P < 0.01$ versus control.

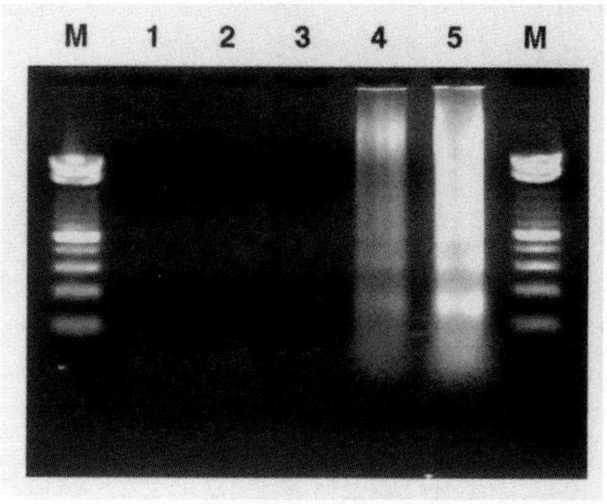

Figure 7. Effect of nitric oxide (NO) on DNA fragmentation. Chondrocytes (2×10^6) were cultured for 24 hours in the absence (lane 1) or presence (lanes 2 and 3) of 1 m*M* of the NO donor NOC18, under oxygen concentrations of either 20% (lane 2) or 5% (lane 3). Cells were also cultured for 5 days in the presence of 5 n*M* staurosporine, under an oxygen concentration of 20% (lane 4). AH-130 hepatoma cells (2×10^6), which easily undergo apoptosis, were also cultured for 24 hours in the presence of 1 m*M* NOC18, under an oxygen concentration of 20% (lane 5). DNA was extracted and subjected to agarose gel electrophoresis as described in the text. M = markers.

NOC18 in a dose-dependent manner (Figures 8 and 9). However, cellular levels of Mn-SOD, Cu/Zn-SOD, and Bcl-2 remained unaffected by NOC18 (Figure 10). The effect of NOC18 on hsp70 expression was greater at an oxygen tension of 5% than at 20%.

Effect of mitochondrial electron transport inhibitors on cellular levels of hsp70 and HO-1. Figure 11 shows the effect of rotenone and antimycin A on cellular levels of hsp70 and HO-1. Both rotenone and antimycin A increased the levels of hsp70 and HO-1 in chondrocytes.

Table 1. Effect of specific inhibitors of mitochondrial electron transport on cellular ATP levels and ^{35}S incorporation*

Experiment, incubation time	Control	Rotenone	Antimycin A
ATP			
2 hours	29.70 ± 4.92	22.73 ± 3.56	21.40 ± 2.56†
12 hours	31.03 ± 3.52	28.33 ± 3.21	27.42 ± 3.57
^{35}S incorporation			
12 hours	4.65 ± 0.26	4.19 ± 0.24†	3.33 ± 0.24†

* Chondrocytes were cultured in the presence or absence of either 2 μM rotenone or 1 μM antimycin A at an oxygen concentration of 20%. After incubation for 2 hours or 12 hours, cellular ATP (nmoles/10^6 cells) and incorporated ^{35}S (10^5 cpm/10^6 cells) were determined as described in the text. Values are the mean ± SD (n = 6).
† $P < 0.01$ versus control.

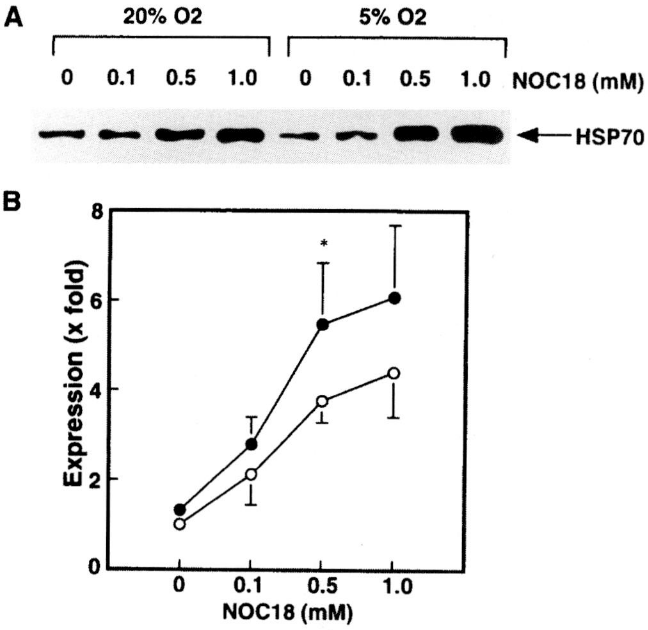

Figure 8. Effect of nitric oxide (NO) on cellular levels of heat-shock protein 70 (HSP70). Chondrocytes were cultured for 24 hours in the presence of various concentrations of the NO donor NOC18, under oxygen concentrations of either 20% (open circles) or 5% (closed circles). **A,** After 24 hours, cell lysates (10 μg protein) were electrophoresed and subjected to Western blot analysis using specific antibody against HSP70. **B,** Densitometric analysis of the findings shown in **A.** * = $P < 0.01$ versus oxygen concentration of 20%.

DISCUSSION

The present study demonstrates that NO reversibly inhibits mitochondrial respiration, ATP synthesis, and incorporation of ^{35}S into proteoglycans of chondrocytes without affecting cellular viability. Because the biologic effects of NO increase with concomitant decreases in oxygen tension (9–12), cellular respiration and ATP synthesis were inhibited strongly, particularly under conditions of low oxygen tensions. The concentrations of nitrite in synovial fluid from patients with RA and OA are reported to be ~0.91 and ~0.35 μM, respectively (3). This observation suggests the presence of NO in the articular space in these patients. Furthermore, oxygen tension in synovial fluid decreases in these patients, particularly those with RA (14). Thus, NO generated by inflammatory leukocytes and constituent cells in the joint might inhibit the respiration and ATP synthesis of articular chondrocytes, particularly in patients with RA.

When electron transport is blocked, mitochondria generate the superoxide radical which reacts with NO to form peroxynitrite (11). Cassina and Radi (9)

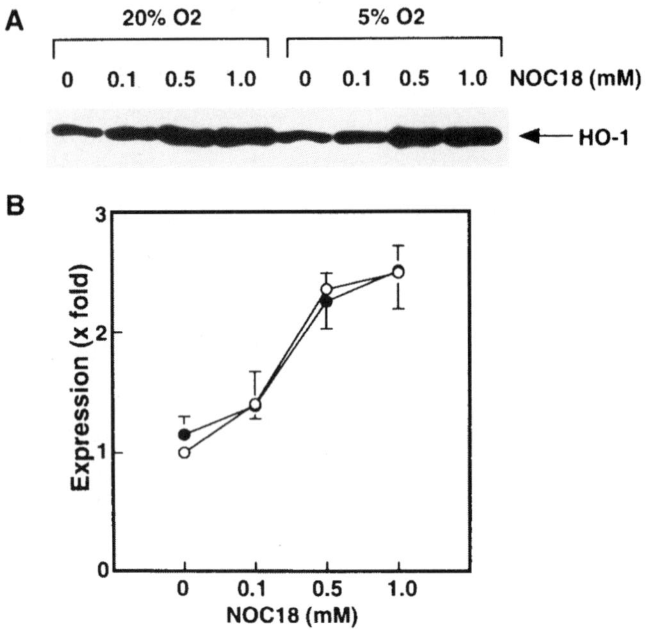

Figure 9. Effect of nitric oxide (NO) on cellular levels of heme oxygenase 1 (HO-1). Chondrocytes were cultured for 24 hours in the presence of various concentrations of the NO donor NOC18, under oxygen concentrations of either 20% (open circles) or 5% (closed circles). **A,** After 24 hours, cell lysates (10 μg protein) were electrophoresed and subjected to Western blot analysis using specific antibody against HO-1. **B,** Densitometric analysis of the findings shown in **A**.

reported that high concentrations of peroxynitrite (~1 m*M*) irreversibly inhibited respiration at complexes I and II without affecting the activity of cytochrome c oxidase. Because endogenously generated NO and related metabolites, including peroxynitrite, occur only in fairly low levels (9,11), we tested the effects of physiologically low levels of NO (~4 μM) in the present studies. Thus, hazardous metabolites, including peroxynitrite, may not be involved in the reversible inhibition of chondrocyte respiration by physiologically low levels of NO.

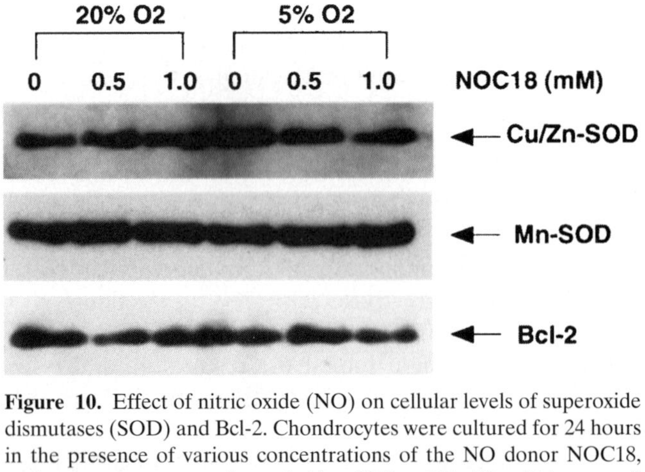

Figure 10. Effect of nitric oxide (NO) on cellular levels of superoxide dismutases (SOD) and Bcl-2. Chondrocytes were cultured for 24 hours in the presence of various concentrations of the NO donor NOC18, under oxygen concentrations of either 20% or 5%. After 24 hours, cell lysates (10 μg protein) were electrophoresed and subjected to Western blot analysis using specific antibodies against Mn-SOD, Cu/Zn-SOD, and Bcl-2.

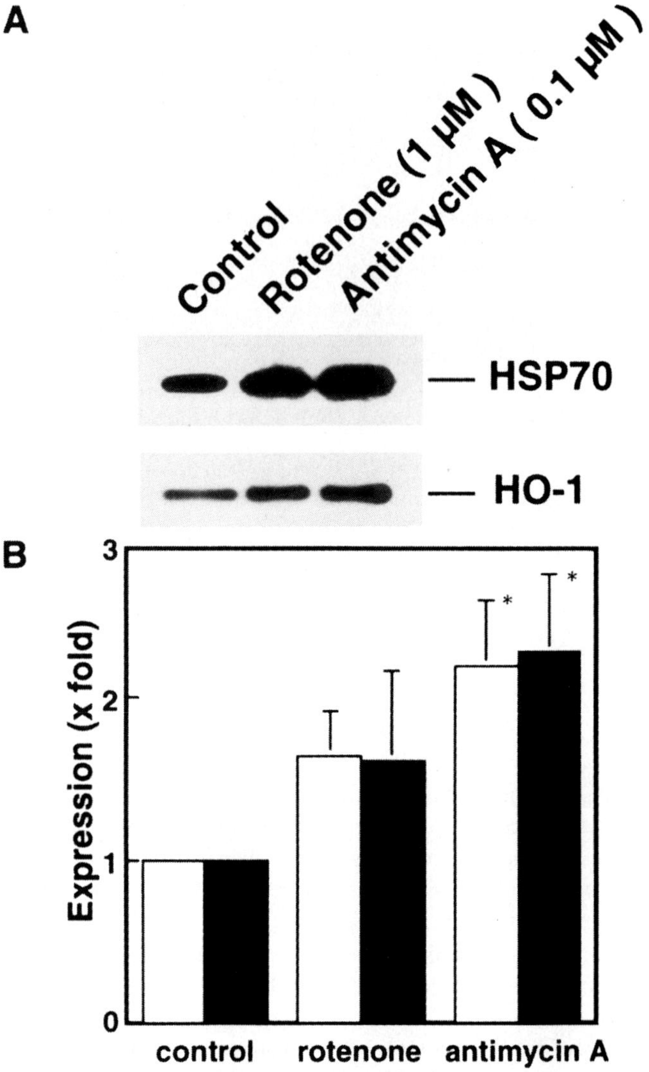

Figure 11. Effect of specific inhibitors of the mitochondrial electron transport system on cellular levels of heat-shock protein 70 (HSP70) and heme oxygenase 1 (HO-1). Chondrocytes were cultured for 24 hours in the presence or absence of either 1 μM rotenone or 0.1 μM antimycin A, under an oxygen concentration of 20%. After 24 hours, cell lysates (10 μg protein) were electrophoresed and subjected to Western blot analysis using specific antibodies against HSP70 and HO-1. * = $P < 0.01$ versus control.

Because NO inhibited the respiration of mitochondria, cellular glycolysis was enhanced significantly. Partly because of the increase in glycolysis, the effect on cellular ATP levels was rather mild, despite the inhibition of mitochondrial respiration by NO. Under standard experimental conditions, cultured chondrocytes consumed oxygen at a rate of 1.2 nmoles/minute/10^6 cells. Assuming 2.0 as the P:O ratio of the coupled respiration of mitochondria, ~4.8 nmoles of ATP/ minute could be synthesized aerobically by 10^6 cells. Under identical conditions, chondrocytes consumed glucose at a rate of 4.2 or 3.1 nmoles/minute/10^6 cells in the presence or absence, respectively, of 0.5 m*M* NOC18. Thus, the glycolytic activity of chondrocytes could theoretically cause synthesis of ATP at a rate of 8.4 or 6.2 nmoles/minute/10^6 cells in the presence or absence, respectively, of NOC18. The net increase in ATP synthesis by glycolysis of NOC18-treated chondrocytes would therefore be ~2.2 nmoles ATP/minute/10^6 cells. Thus, the enhanced glycolysis in NOC18-treated chondrocytes could theoretically compensate for the inhibited mitochondrial ATP synthesis by ~46%.

The present work also revealed that electron transport inhibitors decreased cellular ATP levels, particularly during the early period of incubation (~2 hours). Although cellular ATP levels in chondrocytes cultured in the presence of electron transport inhibitors returned to initial levels after long-term incubation (~12 hours), the total amount of ATP synthesized by cells would be significantly low as compared with that in the absence of the inhibitors. Thus, despite the enhanced glycolysis, the total amounts of ATP that could be utilized for the maintenance of cellular metabolism, including the synthesis of proteoglycans, would have been limited significantly in the presence of respiratory inhibitors.

ATP is the main energy source for cellular proliferation, differentiation, and apoptosis (35,36). Kanwar et al (30) demonstrated that depletion of cellular ATP markedly decreased the synthesis of sulfated proteoglycans, by a mechanism which was normalized by increasing cellular ATP levels. Because proteoglycans undergo significant posttranslational modifications, which require large amounts of ATP, their synthesis could readily be affected by ATP depletion.

The present work demonstrated that NO and specific inhibitors of electron transport of mitochondria significantly suppressed the synthesis of proteoglycans by chondrocytes. Because the sulfation of proteoglycans requires 3′-phosphoadenosine-5′-phosphosulfate, which is fueled by 2 moles of ATP, as a donor, an NO-induced decrease in ATP synthesis might result in the suppression of the de novo synthesis of ^{35}S-labeled proteoglycans. Such an inhibition of proteoglycan synthesis by NO, associated with increased levels of plasma nitrate, might underlie the pathogenesis of the destruction of joint cartilage in patients with RA. The fact that destruction of joint cartilage progresses more rapidly in RA than in OA is consistent with the above-described hypothesis.

NO has been found to induce apoptosis of various types of cells by decreasing mitochondrial membrane potential (due to increasing mitochondrial permeability transition), thereby releasing cytochrome c, which activates the caspase cascade (37,38). Blanco et al (39) showed that exogenously generated NO induced apoptosis of human articular chondrocytes, by glucose deprivation caused by the inhibition of aconitase. However, the present experiments clearly showed that low levels of NO did not induce apoptosis of chondrocytes, as measured by trypan blue dye exclusion and DNA fragmentation. Furthermore, glucose consumption was not enhanced sufficiently by NO to induce apoptosis. Thus, rabbit articular chondrocytes seem to be highly resistant to NO.

Western blot analysis revealed that both NO and specific inhibitors of mitochondrial electron transport increased the cellular expression of some proteins, such as hsp70 and HO-1. Heat-shock protein 70 functions as an important chaperone for denatured proteins, while HO-1 catalyzes the oxidative degradation of heme to generate carbon monoxide and bilirubin, a potent antioxidant (40–43). Thus, hsp70 and HO-1 play important roles in protecting cells against various types of biohazards (43,44). In fact, hsp70 has been shown to inhibit the apoptosis of ATP-depleted cells (45–47).

In conclusion, NO generated locally in the joints of patients with arthritis might enhance the expression of hsp70 and HO-1, thereby increasing the survival of chondrocytes despite the decrease of ATP and de novo synthesis of proteoglycans. Such effects of NO on the energy metabolism, proteoglycan synthesis, and upregulation of stress-induced proteins in chondrocytes might play important roles in the pathogenesis of cartilage destruction in patients with arthritis.

REFERENCES

1. Moncada S, Palmer RM, Higgs EA. Nitric oxide: physiology, pathophysiology, and pharmacology. Pharmacol Rev 1991;43: 109–42.
2. Nathan C. Nitric oxide as a secretory product of mammalian cells. FASEB J 1992;6:3051–64.
3. Farrell AJ, Blake DR, Palmer RM, Moncada S. Increased concentrations of nitrite in synovial fluid and serum samples suggest increased nitric oxide synthesis in rheumatic diseases. Ann Rheum Dis 1992;51:1219–22.
4. Kaur H, Halliwell B. Evidence for nitric oxide–mediated oxidative damage in chronic inflammation: nitrotyrosine in serum and synovial fluid from rheumatoid patients. FEBS Lett 1994;350:9–12.
5. Sakurai H, Kohsaka H, Liu MF, Higashiyama H, Hirata Y, Kanno K, et al. Nitric oxide production and inducible nitric oxide synthase expression in inflammatory arthritides. J Clin Invest 1995;96: 2357–63.
6. Stadler J, Stefanovic-Racic M, Billiar TR, Curran RD, McIntyre

LA, Georgescu HI, et al. Articular chondrocytes synthesize nitric oxide in response to cytokines and lipopolysaccharide. J Immunol 1991;147:3915–20.
7. Brookes PS, Bolanos JP, Heales SJ. The assumption that nitric oxide inhibits mitochondrial ATP synthesis is correct. FEBS Lett 1999;446:261–3.
8. Brown GC. Nitric oxide regulates mitochondrial respiration and cell functions by inhibiting cytochrome oxidase. FEBS Lett 1995; 369:136–9.
9. Cassina A, Radi R. Differential inhibitory action of nitric oxide and peroxynitrite on mitochondrial electron transport. Arch Biochem Biophys 1996;328:309–16.
10. Nishikawa M, Sato EF, Utsumi K, Inoue M. Oxygen-dependent regulation of energy metabolism in ascites tumor cells by nitric oxide. Cancer Res 1996;56:4535–40.
11. Brown GC. Nitric oxide and mitochondrial respiration. Biochim Biophys Acta 1999;1411:351–69.
12. Takehara Y, Kanno T, Yoshioka T, Inoue M, Utsumi K. Oxygen-dependent regulation of mitochondrial energy transfer reaction by nitric oxide. Arch Biochem Biophys 1995;323:27–32.
13. Mapp PI, Grootveld MC, Blake DR. Hypoxia, oxidative stress and rheumatoid arthritis. Br Med Bull 1995;51:419–36.
14. Richman AI, Su EY, Ho G Jr. Reciprocal relationship of synovial fluid volume and oxygen tension. Arthritis Rheum 1981;24:701–5.
15. Cao M, Westerhausen-Larson A, Niyibizi C, Kavalkovich K, Georgescu HI, Rizzo CF, et al. Nitric oxide inhibits the synthesis of type-II collagen without altering Col2A1 mRNA abundance: prolyl hydroxylase as a possible target. Biochem J 1997;324: 305–10.
16. Hauselmann HJ, Oppliger L, Michel BA, Stefanovic-Racic M, Evans CH. Nitric oxide and proteoglycan biosynthesis by human articular chondrocytes in alginate culture. FEBS Lett 1994;352: 361–4.
17. Ueki Y, Miyake S, Tominaga Y, Eguchi K. Increased nitric oxide levels in patients with rheumatoid arthritis. J Rheumatol 1996;23: 230–6.
18. Clancy RM, Miyazaki Y, Cannon PJ. Use of thionitrobenzoic acid to characterize the stability of nitric oxide in aqueous solutions and in porcine aortic endothelial cell suspensions. Anal Biochem 1990;191:138–43.
19. Green WT Jr. Behavior of articular chondrocytes in cell culture. Clin Orthop 1971;75:248–60.
20. Touriol C, Morillon A, Gensac MC, Prats H, Prats AC. Expression of human fibroblast growth factor 2 mRNA is post-transcriptionally controlled by a unique destabilizing element present in the 3′-untranslated region between alternative polyadenylation sites. J Biol Chem 1999;274:21402–8.
21. Packer L, Utsumi R, Mustafa MG. Oscillatory states of mitochondria. I. Electron and energy transfer pathways. Arch Biochem Biophys 1966;117:381–93.
22. Goodall SR, Byers FM. Automated micro method for enzymatic L (+) and D (−) lactic acid determinations in biological fluids containing cellular extracts. Anal Biochem 1978;89:80–6.
23. Taskiran D, Stefanovic-Racic M, Georgescu H, Evans CH. Nitric oxide mediates suppression of cartilage proteoglycan synthesis by interleukin-1. Biochem Biophys Res Commun 1994;200:142–8.
24. Chomczynski P, Sacchi N. Single-step method of RNA isolation by acid guanidinium thiocyanate-phenol-chloroform extraction. Anal Biochem 1987;162:156–9.
25. Frohman MA, Dush MK, Martin GR. Rapid production of full-length cDNAs from rare transcripts: amplification using a single gene-specific oligonucleotide primer. Proc Natl Acad Sci U S A 1988;85:8998–9002.
26. Nakanishi T, Nishida T, Shimo T, Kobayashi K, Kubo T, Tamatani T, et al. Effects of CTGF/Hcs24, a product of a hypertrophic chondrocyte-specific gene, on the proliferation and differentiation of chondrocytes in culture. Endocrinology 2000;141:264–73.
27. Nishikawa M, Takeda K, Sato EF, Kuroki T, Inoue M. Nitric oxide regulates energy metabolism and Bcl-2 expression in intestinal epithelial cells. Am J Physiol 1998;274:797–801.
28. Nishikawa M, Sato EF, Kuroki T, Inoue M. Role of glutathione and nitric oxide in the energy metabolism of rat liver mitochondria. FEBS Lett 1997;415:341–5.
29. Stefanovic-Racic M, Stadler J, Georgescu HI, Evans CH. Nitric oxide and energy production in articular chondrocytes. J Cell Physiol 1994;159:274–80.
30. Kanwar Y, Yoshinaga Y, Liu Z, Wallner E, Carone F. Biosynthetic regulation of proteoglycans by aldohexoses and ATP. Proc Natl Acad Sci U S A 1992;89:8621–5.
31. Kiningham KK, Oberley TD, Lin S, Mattingly CA, St. Clari DK. Overexpression of manganese superoxide dismutase protects against mitochondrial-initiated poly (ADP-ribose) polymerase-mediated cell death. FASEB J 1999;13:1601–10.
32. Ceneviva GD, Tzeng E, Hoyt DG, Yee E, Gallagher A, Engelhardt JF, et al. Nitric oxide inhibits lipopolysaccharide-induced apoptosis in pulmonary artery endothelial cells. Am J Physiol 1998;275:717–28.
33. Yabuki M, Kariya S, Ishisaka R, Yasuda T, Yoshioka T, Horton AA, et al. Resistance to nitric oxide-mediated apoptosis in HL-60 variant cells is associated with increased activities of Cu/Zn-superoxide dismutase and catalase. Free Radic Biol Med 1999;26:325–32.
34. Shimizu S, Eguchi Y, Kamiike W, Waguri S, Uchiyama Y, Matsuda H, et al. Bcl-2 blocks loss of mitochondrial membrane potential while ICE inhibitors act at a different step during inhibition of death induced by respiratory chain inhibitors. Oncogene 1996;13:21–9.
35. Hubbard SR. Structural analysis of receptor tyrosine kinases. Prog Biophys Mol Biol 1999;71:343–58.
36. Bernardi P, Scorrano L, Colonna R, Petronilli V, di Lisa F. Mitochondria and cell death: mechanistic aspects and methodological issues. Eur J Biochem 1999;264:687–701.
37. Crompton M. The mitochondrial permeability transition pore and its role in cell death. Biochem J 1999;341:233–49.
38. Paul A, Wilson S, Belham CM, Robinson CJ, Scott PH, Gould GW, et al. Stress-activated protein kinases: activation, regulation and function. Cell Signal 1997;9:403–10.
39. Blanco FJ, Ochs RL, Schwarz H, Lotz M. Chondrocyte apoptosis induced by nitric oxide. Am J Pathol 1995;146:75–85.
40. Hightower LE. Heat shock, stress proteins, chaperones, and proteotoxicity. Cell 1991;66:191–7.
41. Gething MJ, Sambrook J. Protein folding in the cell. Nature 1992;355:33–45.
42. Maines MD. The heme oxygenase system: a regulator of second messenger gases. Annu Rev Pharmacol Toxicol 1997;37:517–54.
43. Vile GF, Basu-Modak S, Waltner C, Tyrrell RM. Heme oxygenase 1 mediates an adaptive response to oxidative stress in human skin fibroblasts. Proc Natl Acad Sci U S A 1994;91:2607–10.
44. Kim YM, de Vera ME, Watkins SC, Billiar TR. Nitric oxide protects cultured rat hepatocytes from tumor necrosis factor-alpha-induced apoptosis by inducing heat shock protein 70 expression. J Biol Chem 1997;272:1402–11.
45. Van Why SK, Mann AS, Thulin G, Zhu XH, Kashgarian M, Siegel NJ. Activation of heat-shock transcription factor by graded reductions in renal ATP, in vivo, in the rat. J Clin Invest 1994;94: 1518–23.
46. Gabai VL, Kabakov AE. Rise in heat-shock protein level confers tolerance to energy deprivation. FEBS Lett 1993;327:247–50.
47. Kabakov AE, Gabai VL. Heat shock induced accumulation of 70-kDa stress protein (HSP70) can protect ATP-depleted tumor cells from necrosis. Exp Cell Res 1995;217:15–21.

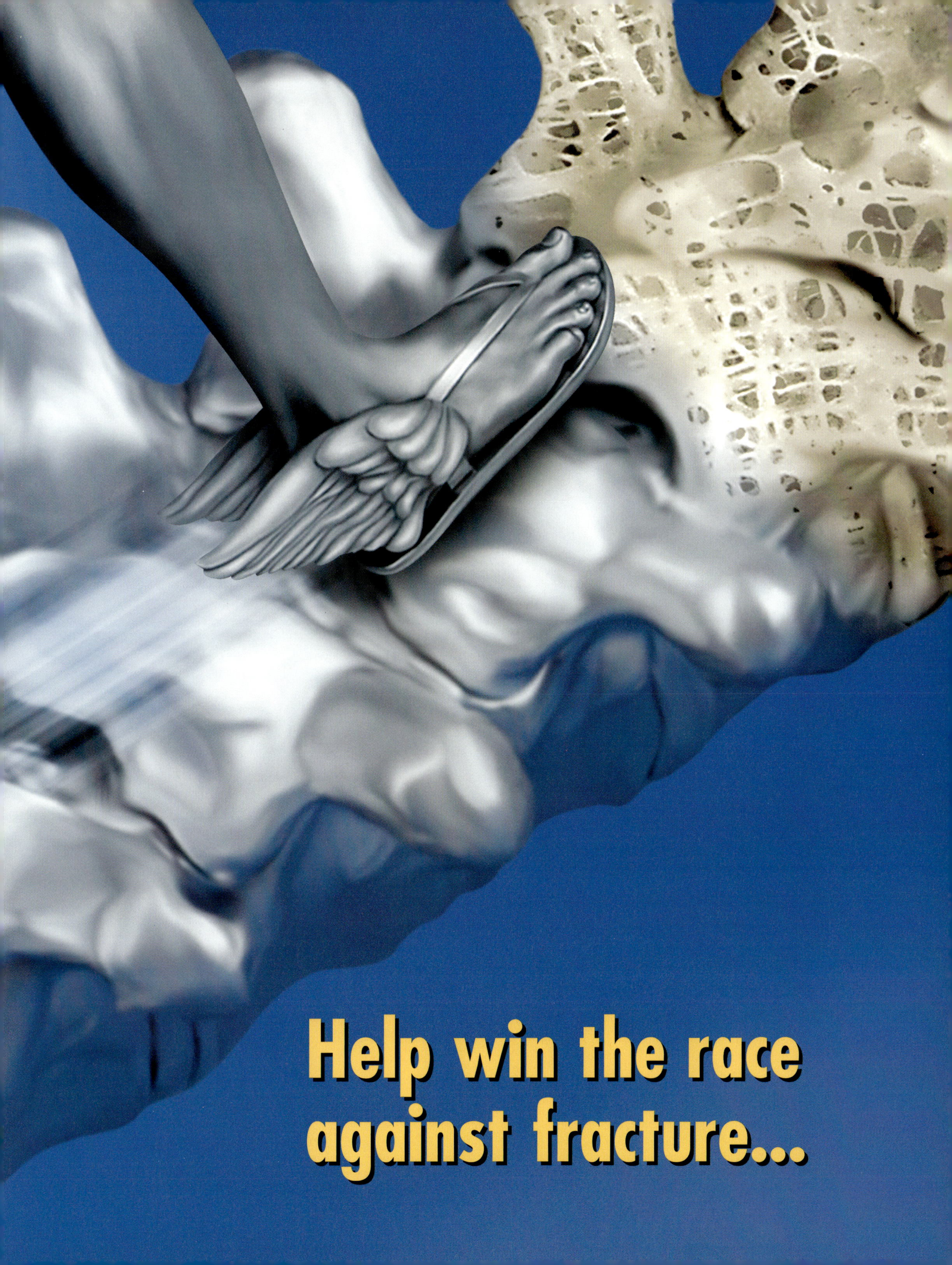
Help win the race
against fracture...

Tolerability you can trust.

Actonel is well tolerated, even in patients with active GI disease

Upper GI adverse events were comparable to placebo in over 5700 real world patients[4]

No GI exclusion criteria in any of the 7 Phase III clinical trials[4]

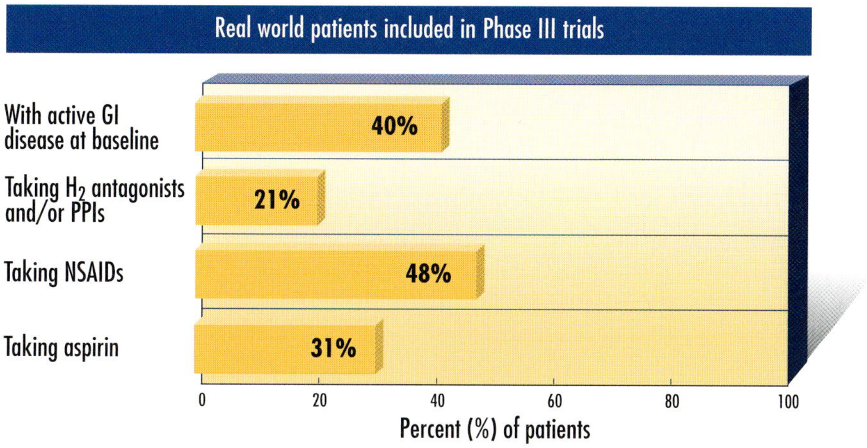

No increase in the incidence of upper GI adverse events vs placebo, even in patients with active GI disease at baseline or on NSAIDs, aspirin, H_2 antagonists, or PPIs[4]

Incidence of drug-related esophageal or gastric ulcers was comparable to placebo, even in patients with active GI disease at baseline[4]

Selected safety information

Patients should pay particular attention to the dosing instructions, as failure to take the drug according to instructions may compromise clinical benefits and may increase the risk of adverse events.

In clinical trials, Actonel was generally well tolerated. Actonel is contraindicated in patients with hypocalcemia, known hypersensitivity to any component of this product, or inability to stand or sit upright for at least 30 minutes. Hypocalcemia and other disturbances of bone and mineral metabolism should be effectively treated before starting Actonel therapy. Actonel is not recommended for use in patients with severe renal impairment (creatinine clearance <30 mL/min).

Bisphosphonates may cause upper gastrointestinal disorders such as dysphagia, esophagitis, and esophageal or gastric ulcer.

In clinical trials, the overall incidence of adverse events with Actonel was comparable to placebo. The most commonly reported adverse events regardless of causality were infection (primarily upper respiratory, placebo 29.7% vs Actonel 29.9%), back pain (23.6% vs 26.1%), and arthralgia (21.1% vs 23.7%).

Visit the Actonel Web site at http://www.actonel.com

Please see brief summary of prescribing information on the following page for more information about Actonel.

ACT NOW WITH

5 mg Actonel® (risedronate sodium tablets)

Rapid and Sustained

ACTONEL® (risedronate sodium tablets)
Brief Summary: See package insert for full prescribing information.

INDICATIONS AND USAGE

Postmenopausal Osteoporosis: ACTONEL is indicated for the treatment and prevention of osteoporosis in postmenopausal women.

Treatment of Osteoporosis: In postmenopausal women with osteoporosis, ACTONEL increases BMD and reduces the incidence of vertebral fractures and a composite endpoint of nonvertebral osteoporosis-related fractures (see CLINICAL STUDIES). Osteoporosis may be confirmed by the presence or history of osteoporotic fracture, or by the finding of low bone mass (for example, at least 2 SD below the premenopausal mean).

Prevention of Osteoporosis: ACTONEL may be considered in postmenopausal women who are at risk of developing osteoporosis and for whom the desired clinical outcome is to maintain bone mass and to reduce the risk of fracture.

Factors such as family history of osteoporosis, previous fracture, smoking, BMD (at least 1 SD below the premenopausal mean), high bone turnover, thin body frame, Caucasian or Asian race, and early menopause are associated with an increased risk of developing osteoporosis and fractures. The presence of these risk factors may be important when considering the use of ACTONEL for prevention of osteoporosis.

Glucocorticoid-Induced Osteoporosis: ACTONEL is indicated for the prevention and treatment of glucocorticoid-induced osteoporosis in men and women who are either initiating or continuing systemic glucocorticoid treatment (daily dosage equivalent to 7.5 mg or greater of prednisone) for chronic diseases. Patients treated with glucocorticoids should receive adequate amounts of calcium and vitamin D.

Paget's Disease: ACTONEL is indicated for treatment of Paget's disease of bone (osteitis deformans).

Treatment is indicated in patients with Paget's disease of bone (1) who have a level of serum alkaline phosphatase (SAP) at least two times the upper limit of normal, or (2) who are symptomatic, or (3) who are at risk for future complications from their disease, to induce remission (normalization of serum alkaline phosphatase).

CONTRAINDICATIONS

- Hypocalcemia (See PRECAUTIONS, General)
- Known hypersensitivity to any component of this product
- Inability to stand or sit upright for at least 30 minutes

WARNINGS: Bisphosphonates may cause upper gastrointestinal disorders such as dysphagia, esophagitis, and esophageal or gastric ulcer (see PRECAUTIONS).

PRECAUTIONS

General: Hypocalcemia and other disturbances of bone and mineral metabolism should be effectively treated before starting ACTONEL therapy. Adequate intake of calcium and vitamin D is important in all patients, especially in patients with Paget's disease in whom bone turnover is significantly elevated. ACTONEL is not recommended for use in patients with severe renal impairment (creatinine clearance < 30 mL/min).

Bisphosphonates have been associated with gastrointestinal disorders such as dysphagia, esophagitis, and esophageal or gastric ulcers. This association has been reported for bisphosphonates in postmarketing experience, but has not been found in most pre-approval clinical trials, including those conducted with ACTONEL. Patients should be advised that taking the medication according to the instructions is important to minimize the risk of these events. They should take ACTONEL with sufficient plain water (6 to 8 oz) to facilitate delivery to the stomach, and should not lie down for 30 minutes after taking the drug.

Glucocorticoid-Induced Osteoporosis: The risk versus benefit of ACTONEL for the prevention and treatment of glucocorticoid-induced osteoporosis at daily doses of glucocorticoids < 7.5 mg of prednisone or equivalent has not been established. Before initiating treatment, the hormonal status of both men and women should be ascertained and appropriate replacement considered.

The efficacy of ACTONEL has been established in studies of 1-year's duration. The efficacy of ACTONEL beyond 1 year has not been studied.

Information for Patients: The patient should be informed to pay particular attention to the dosing instructions as clinical benefits may be compromised by failure to take the drug according to instructions. Specifically, ACTONEL should be taken at least 30 minutes before the first food or drink of the day other than water.

To facilitate delivery to the stomach, and thus reduce the potential for esophageal irritation, patients should take ACTONEL while in an upright position (sitting or standing) with a full glass of plain water (6 to 8 oz). Patients should not lie down for 30 minutes after taking the medication (see PRECAUTIONS, General). Patients should not chew or suck on the tablet because of a potential for oropharyngeal irritation.

Patients should be instructed that if they develop symptoms of esophageal disease (such as difficulty or pain upon swallowing, retrosternal pain or severe persistent or worsening heartburn) they should consult their physician before continuing ACTONEL.

Patients should receive supplemental calcium and vitamin D if dietary intake is inadequate (see PRECAUTIONS, General). Calcium supplements or calcium-, aluminum-, and magnesium-containing medications may interfere with the absorption of ACTONEL and should be taken at a different time of the day, as with food.

Weight-bearing exercise should be considered along with the modification of certain behavioral factors, such as excessive cigarette smoking, and/or alcohol consumption, if these factors exist. Physicians should instruct their patients to read the Patient Information before starting therapy with ACTONEL 5 mg and to re-read it each time the prescription is renewed.

Drug Interactions: No specific drug-drug interaction studies were performed. Risedronate is not metabolized and does not induce or inhibit hepatic microsomal drug-metabolizing enzymes (Cytochrome P450).

Calcium Supplements/Antacids: Co-administration of ACTONEL and calcium, antacids, or oral medications containing divalent cations will interfere with the absorption of ACTONEL.

Hormone Replacement Therapy: One study of about 500 early postmenopausal women has been conducted to date in which treatment with ACTONEL (5 mg/day) plus estrogen replacement therapy was compared with estrogen replacement therapy alone. Exposure to study drugs was approximately 12 to 18 months and the primary endpoint was change in BMD. If considered appropriate, ACTONEL may be used concomitantly with hormone replacement therapy.

Aspirin/Nonsteroidal Anti-Inflammatory Drugs (NSAIDs): Of over 5700 patients enrolled in the ACTONEL Phase 3 osteoporosis studies, aspirin use was reported by 31% of patients, 24% of whom were regular users (3 or more days per week). Forty-eight percent of patients reported NSAID use, 21% of whom were regular users. Among regular aspirin or NSAID users, the incidence of upper gastrointestinal adverse experiences in ACTONEL-treated patients (24.5%) was similar to that in placebo-treated patients (24.8%).

H_2 Blockers and Proton Pump Inhibitors (PPIs): Of over 5700 patients enrolled in the ACTONEL Phase 3 osteoporosis studies, 21% used H_2 blockers and/or PPIs. Among these patients, the incidence of upper gastrointestinal adverse experiences in the ACTONEL-treated patients was similar to that in placebo-treated patients.

Drug/Laboratory Test Interactions: Bisphosphonates are known to interfere with the use of bone-imaging agents. Specific studies with ACTONEL have not been performed.

Carcinogenesis, Mutagenesis, Impairment of Fertility:

Carcinogenesis: In a 104-week carcinogenicity study, rats were administered daily oral doses up to 24 mg/kg/day (approximately 7.7 times the maximum recommended human daily dose of 30 mg based on surface area, mg/m^2). There were no significant drug-induced tumor findings in male or female rats. The high dose male group of 24 mg/kg/day was terminated early in the study (Week 93) due to excessive toxicity, and data from this group were not included in the statistical evaluation of the study results. In an 80-week carcinogenicity study, mice were administered daily oral doses up to 32 mg/kg/day (approximately 6.4 times the 30 mg/day human dose based on surface area, mg/m^2). There were no significant drug-induced tumor findings in male or female mice.

Mutagenesis: Risedronate did not exhibit genetic toxicity in the following assays: *In vitro* bacterial mutagenesis in *Salmonella* and *E. coli* (Ames assay), mammalian cell mutagenesis in CHO/HGPRT assay, unscheduled DNA synthesis in rat hepatocytes and an assessment of chromosomal aberrations *in vivo* in rat bone marrow. Risedronate was positive in a chromosomal aberration assay in CHO cells at highly cytotoxic concentrations (> 675 mcg/mL, survival of 6% to 7%). When the assay was repeated at doses exhibiting appropriate cell survival (29%), there was no evidence of chromosomal damage.

Impairment of Fertility: In female rats, ovulation was inhibited at an oral dose of 16 mg/kg/day (approximately 5.2 times the 30 mg/day human dose based on surface area, mg/m^2). Decreased implantation was noted in female rats treated with doses ≥ 7 mg/kg/day (approximately 2.3 times the 30 mg/day human dose based on surface area, mg/m^2). In male rats, testicular and epididymal atrophy and inflammation were noted at 40 mg/kg/day (approximately 13 times the 30 mg/day human dose based on surface area, mg/m^2). Testicular atrophy was also noted in male rats after 13 weeks of treatment at oral doses of 16 mg/kg/day (approximately 5.2 times the 30 mg/day human dose based on surface area, mg/m^2). There was moderate-to-severe spermatid maturation block after 13 weeks in male dogs at an oral dose of 8 mg/kg/day (approximately 8 times the 30 mg/day human dose based on surface area, mg/m^2). These findings tended to increase in severity with increased dose and exposure time.

Pregnancy: Pregnancy Category C: Survival of neonates was decreased in rats treated during gestation with oral doses ≥ 16 mg/kg/day (approximately 5.2 times the 30 mg/day human dose based on surface area, mg/m^2). Body weight was decreased in neonates from dams treated with 80 mg/kg (approximately 26 times the 30 mg/day human dose based on surface area, mg/m^2). In rats treated during gestation, the number of fetuses exhibiting incomplete ossification of sternebrae or skull was statistically significantly increased at 7.1 mg/kg/day (approximately 2.3 times the 30 mg/day human dose based on surface area, mg/m^2). Both incomplete ossification and unossified sternebrae were increased in rats treated with oral doses ≥ 16 mg/kg/day (approximately 5.2 times the 30 mg/day human dose based on surface area, mg/m^2). A low incidence of cleft palate was observed in fetuses from female rats treated with oral doses ≥ 3.2 mg/kg/day (approximately 1 time the 30 mg/day human dose based on surface area, mg/m^2). The relevance of this finding to human use of ACTONEL is unclear. No significant fetal ossification effects were seen in rabbits treated with oral doses up to 10 mg/kg/day during gestation (approximately 6.7 times the 30 mg/day human dose based on surface area, mg/m^2). However, in rabbits treated with 10 mg/kg/day, 1 of 14 litters were aborted and 1 of 14 litters were delivered prematurely.

Similar to other bisphosphonates, treatment during mating and gestation with doses as low as 3.2 mg/kg/day (approximately 1 time the 30 mg/day human dose based on surface area, mg/m^2) has resulted in periparturient hypocalcemia and mortality in pregnant rats allowed to deliver.

There are no adequate and well-controlled studies of ACTONEL in pregnant women. ACTONEL should be used during pregnancy only if the potential benefit justifies the potential risk to the mother and fetus.

Nursing Women: Risedronate was detected in feeding pups exposed to lactating rats for a 24-hour period post-dosing, indicating a small degree of lacteal transfer. It is not known whether risedronate is excreted in human milk. Because many drugs are excreted in human milk and because of the potential for serious adverse reactions in nursing infants from bisphosphonates, a decision should be made whether to discontinue nursing or to discontinue the drug, taking into account the importance of the drug to the mother.

Pediatric Use: Safety and effectiveness in pediatric patients have not been established.

Geriatric Use: Of the patients receiving ACTONEL in postmenopausal osteoporosis studies (see CLINICAL STUDIES), 43% were between 65 and 75 years of age, and 20% were over 75. The corresponding proportions were 26% and 11% in glucocorticoid-induced osteoporosis trials, and 40% and 26% in Paget's disease trials. No overall differences in efficacy or safety were observed between these patients and younger patients.

Use in Men: Safety and effectiveness have been demonstrated in clinical studies in men receiving ACTONEL both for Paget's disease and for treatment and prevention of glucocorticoid-induced osteoporosis. However, the safety and effectiveness in men for osteoporosis due to other causes have not been established.

ADVERSE REACTIONS

Osteoporosis: ACTONEL has been studied in over 5700 patients enrolled in the Phase 3 glucocorticoid-induced osteoporosis clinical trials and in postmenopausal osteoporosis trials of up to 3 years duration. The overall adverse event profile of ACTONEL 5 mg in these studies was similar to that of placebo. Most adverse events were either mild or moderate and did not lead to discontinuation from the study. The incidence of serious adverse events in the placebo group was 24.9% and in the ACTONEL 5 mg group was 26.3%. The percentage of patients who withdrew from the study due to adverse events was 14.4% and 13.5% for the placebo and ACTONEL 5 mg groups, respectively. Table 1 lists adverse events from the Phase 3 osteoporosis trials reported in ≥ 2% of patients and in more ACTONEL-treated patients than placebo-treated patients. Adverse events are shown without attribution of causality.

Table 5
Adverse Events Occurring at a Frequency ≥ 2% and in More ACTONEL-Treated Patients than Placebo-Treated Patients Combined Phase 3 Osteoporosis Trials

Body System	Placebo % (N = 1914)	ACTONEL 5 mg % (N = 1916)
Body as a Whole		
Infection	29.7	29.9
Back Pain	23.6	26.1
Pain	13.1	13.6
Abdominal Pain	9.4	11.6
Neck Pain	4.5	5.3
Asthenia	4.3	5.1
Chest Pain	4.9	5.0
Neoplasm	3.0	3.3
Hernia	2.5	2.9
Cardiovascular		
Hypertension	9.0	10.0
Cardiovascular Disorder	1.7	2.5
Angina Pectoris	2.4	2.5
Digestive		
Nausea	10.7	10.9
Diarrhea	9.6	10.6
Flatulence	4.2	4.6
Gastritis	2.3	2.5
Gastrointestinal Disorder	2.1	2.3
Rectal Disorder	1.9	2.2
Tooth Disorder	2.0	2.1
Hemic and Lymphatic		
Ecchymosis	4.0	4.3
Anemia	1.9	2.4
Musculoskeletal		
Arthralgia	21.1	23.7
Joint Disorder	5.4	6.8
Myalgia	6.3	6.6
Bone Pain	4.3	4.6
Bone Disorder	3.2	4.0
Leg Cramps	2.6	3.5
Bursitis	2.9	3.0
Tendon Disorder	2.5	3.0
Nervous		
Depression	6.2	6.8
Dizziness	5.4	6.4
Insomnia	4.5	4.7
Anxiety	3.0	4.3
Neuralgia	3.5	3.8
Vertigo	3.2	3.3
Hypertonia	2.1	2.2
Paresthesia	1.8	2.1
Respiratory		
Pharyngitis	5.0	5.8
Rhinitis	5.0	5.7
Dyspnea	3.2	3.8
Pneumonia	2.6	3.1
Skin and Appendages		
Rash	7.2	7.7
Pruritus	2.2	3.0
Skin Carcinoma	1.8	2.0
Special Senses		
Cataract	5.4	5.9
Conjunctivitis	2.8	3.1
Otitis Media	2.4	2.5
Urogenital		
Urinary Tract Infection	9.7	10.9
Cystitis	3.5	4.1

Duodenitis and glossitis have been reported uncommonly (0.1% to 1%). There have been rare reports (< 0.1%) of abnormal liver function tests.

Laboratory Test Findings: Asymptomatic and small decreases were observed in serum calcium and phosphorus levels. Overall, mean decreases of 0.8% in serum calcium and of 2.7% in phosphorus were observed at 6 months in patients receiving ACTONEL. Throughout the Phase 3 studies, serum calcium levels below 8 mg/dL were observed in 18 patients, 9 (0.5%) in each treatment arm (ACTONEL and placebo). Serum phosphorus levels below 2 mg/dL were observed in 14 patients, 11 (0.6%) treated with ACTONEL and 3 (0.2%) treated with placebo.

Endoscopic Findings: ACTONEL clinical studies enrolled over 5700 patients, many with pre-existing gastrointestinal disease and concomitant use of NSAIDs or aspirin. Investigators were encouraged to perform endoscopies in any patients with moderate-to-severe gastrointestinal complaints while maintaining the blind. These endoscopies were ultimately performed on equal numbers of patients between the treated and placebo groups [75 (14.5%) placebo; 75 (11.9%) ACTONEL]. Across treatment groups, the percentage of patients with normal esophageal, gastric, and duodenal mucosa on endoscopy was similar (20% placebo, 21% ACTONEL). The number of patients who withdrew from the studies due to the event prompting endoscopy was similar across treatment groups. Positive findings on endoscopy were also generally comparable across treatment groups. There was a higher number of reports of mild duodenitis in the ACTONEL group, however there were more duodenal ulcers in the placebo group. Clinically important findings (perforations, ulcers, or bleeding) among this symptomatic population were similar between groups (51% placebo; 39% ACTONEL).

Paget's Disease: ACTONEL has been studied in 392 patients with Paget's disease of bone. As in trials of ACTONEL for other indications, the adverse experiences reported in the Paget's disease trials have generally been mild or moderate, have not required discontinuation of treatment, and have not appeared to be related to patient age, gender, or race.

In a double-blind, active-controlled study, the adverse event profile was similar for ACTONEL and Didronel: 6.6% (4/61) of patients treated with ACTONEL 30 mg/day for 2 months discontinued treatment due to adverse events, compared with 8.2% (5/61) of patients treated with Didronel 400 mg/day for 6 months.

Table 6
Adverse Events Reported in ≥ 2% of ACTONEL-Treated Patients* in Phase 3 Paget's Disease Trials

Body System	30 mg/day x 2 months ACTONEL % (N = 61)	400 mg/day x 6 months Didronel % (N = 61)
Body as a Whole		
Flu Syndrome	9.8	1.6
Chest Pain	6.6	3.3
Asthenia	4.9	0
Neoplasm	3.3	1.6
Gastrointestinal		
Diarrhea	19.7	14.8
Abdominal Pain	11.5	8.2
Nausea	9.8	9.8
Constipation	6.6	8.2
Belching	3.3	1.6
Colitis	3.3	3.3
Metabolic & Nutritional		
Peripheral Edema	8.2	6.6
Musculoskeletal		
Arthralgia	32.8	29.5
Bone Pain	4.9	4.9
Leg Cramps	3.3	3.3
Myasthenia	3.3	0
Nervous		
Headache	18.0	16.4
Dizziness	6.6	4.9
Respiratory		
Bronchitis	3.3	4.9
Sinusitis	4.9	1.6
Skin		
Rash	11.5	8.2
Special Senses		
Amblyopia	3.3	3.3
Tinnitus	3.3	3.3
Dry Eye	3.3	0

*Considered to be possibly or probably causally related in at least one patient

Three patients that received ACTONEL 30 mg/day experienced acute iritis in one supportive study. All three patients recovered from their events; however, in one of these patients, the event recurred during ACTONEL treatment and again during treatment with pamidronate. All patients were effectively treated with topical steroids.

OVERDOSAGE

Decreases in serum calcium and phosphorus following substantial overdose may be expected in some patients. Signs and symptoms of hypocalcemia may also occur in some of these patients. Milk or antacids containing calcium should be given to bind ACTONEL and reduce absorption of the drug.

In cases of substantial overdose, gastric lavage may be considered to remove unabsorbed drug. Standard procedures that are effective for treating hypocalcemia, including the administration of calcium intravenously, would be expected to restore physiologic amounts of ionized calcium and to relieve signs and symptoms of hypocalcemia.

Lethality after single oral doses was seen in female rats at 903 mg/kg and male rats at 1703 mg/kg. The minimum lethal dose in mice and rabbits was 4000 mg/kg and 1000 mg/kg. These values represent 320 to 620 times the 30-mg human dose based on surface area (mg/m^2).

DOSAGE AND ADMINISTRATION

ACTONEL should be taken once per day at least 30 minutes before the first food or drink of the day other than water.

To facilitate delivery to the stomach, ACTONEL should be swallowed while the patient is in an upright position and with a full glass of plain water (6 to 8 oz). Patients should not lie down for 30 minutes after taking the medication (see PRECAUTIONS, General).

Patients should receive supplemental calcium and vitamin D if dietary intake is inadequate (see PRECAUTIONS, General). Calcium supplements and calcium-, aluminum-, and magnesium-containing medications may interfere with the absorption of ACTONEL and should be taken at a different time of the day. ACTONEL is not recommended for use in patients with severe renal impairment (creatinine clearance < 30 mL/min). No dosage adjustment is necessary in patients with a creatinine clearance ≥ 30 mL/min or in the elderly.

Treatment and Prevention of Postmenopausal Osteoporosis/Glucocorticoid-Induced Osteoporosis (see INDICATIONS AND USAGE): The recommended regimen is 5 mg orally daily.

Paget's Disease (see INDICATIONS AND USAGE): The recommended treatment regimen is 30 mg once daily for 2 months. Retreatment may be considered (following post-treatment observation of at least 2 months) if relapse occurs, or if treatment fails to normalize serum alkaline phosphatase. For retreatment, the dose and duration of therapy are the same as for initial treatment. No data are available on more than one course of retreatment.

Store at controlled room temperature 20°-25°C (68°-77°F) [See USP].

Mfg. and Dist. by:
Procter & Gamble Pharmaceuticals, TM Owner
Cincinnati, Ohio 45202
Mkt. with:
Aventis Pharmaceuticals Inc.
(formerly Hoechst Marion Roussel, Inc.)
Kansas City, Missouri 64137
AUGUST 2000

5 mg Actonel® (risedronate sodium tablets)

References: 1. Actonel [package insert]. Cincinnati, Ohio: Procter & Gamble; 2000. **2.** Harris ST, Watts NB, Genant HK, et al. Effects of risedronate treatment on vertebral and nonvertebral fractures in women with postmenopausal osteoporosis: a randomized controlled trial. *JAMA.* 1999;282(14):1344-1352. **3.** Reginster J-Y, Minne HW, Sorensen OH, et al. Randomised trial of the effects of risedronate on vertebral fractures in women with established postmenopausal osteoporosis. *Osteoporos Int.* 2000;11:83-91. **4**. Data on file, Procter & Gamble, Cincinnati, Ohio.

ARTHRITIS & RHEUMATISM
Vol. 44, No. 1, January 2001, pp 105–110

Comparison of Differentiated Dendritic Cell Infiltration of Autoimmune and Osteoarthritis Synovial Tissue

Allison R. Pettit,[1] Michael J. Ahern,[2] Simone Zehntner,[1] Malcolm D. Smith,[2] and Ranjeny Thomas[1]

Objective. **Infiltration of rheumatoid arthritis (RA) synovial tissue (ST) by differentiated dendritic cells (DC) is a consistent feature in patients with active disease. However, mononuclear cells (MNC), including DC, may be nonspecifically chemoattracted to inflammatory sites regardless of etiology. Therefore, to evaluate the specificity of ST infiltration by differentiated DC, synovial biopsies from patients with RA, spondylarthropathy (SpA), osteoarthritis (OA), and gout were examined.**

Methods. **Formalin-fixed ST sections were analyzed by double immunohistochemical staining for vascularity and infiltration by differentiated DC, lymphocytes, and macrophages.**

Results. **DC containing nuclear RelB were found in perivascular MNC aggregates from patients with all arthritides studied. Infiltration by differentiated DC was similar in RA and SpA ST, but reduced in OA ST. Differentiated DC were always observed in close association with lymphocytes, and the correlation between these variables suggested that the infiltration of inflammatory sites by DC and lymphocytes was associated.**

Conclusion. **Perivascular infiltration by DC, lymphocytes, and macrophages is nonspecifically related to inflammation, but signals present in RA and SpA ST lead to more intense cellular infiltration and accumulation.**

Supported by the National Health and Medical Research Council of Australia and the Arthritis Foundation of Australia. Dr. Thomas' work was supported by the Arthritis Foundation of Queensland.

[1]Allison R. Pettit, BSc (Hons), Simone Zehntner, PhD, Ranjeny Thomas, MBBS, MD: University of Queensland, Princess Alexandra Hospital, Brisbane, Queensland, Australia; [2]Michael J. Ahern, MD, Malcolm D. Smith, MD, PhD: Repatriation General Hospital, Adelaide, South Australia, Australia.

Address correspondence and reprint requests to Ranjeny Thomas, MBBS, MD, Center for Immunology and Cancer Research, University of Queensland, Princess Alexandra Hospital, Ipswich Road, Woolloongabba, Brisbane, Queensland 4102, Australia.

Submitted for publication May 2, 2000; accepted in revised form August 25, 2000.

Differentiated dendritic cells (DC) have been found within perivascular mononuclear cell (MNC) aggregates in synovial tissue (ST) from patients with active, untreated rheumatoid arthritis (RA) (1). We have previously demonstrated that differentiated DC can be identified in formalin-fixed tissue sections by nuclear expression of RelB, a member of the nuclear factor κB/Rel family, in the absence of B cell and monocyte/macrophage markers. Expression of nuclear RelB (nRelB) was associated with efficient antigen-presenting cell (APC) function (1,2).

The presentation of arthritogenic antigen by DC to CD4+ T cells is thought to be important in the disease process, and is reflected by the previous demonstration that nRelB+ differentiated DC, lymphocytes, and macrophages are closely associated within perivascular aggregates (1). Histopathologic studies of nonrheumatoid chronic inflammatory arthritides have demonstrated ST similar in appearance to RA ST, with some qualitative and quantitative differences that may result from differences in disease pathogenesis (3,4). While DC have been found in the synovial fluid and skin of psoriatic arthritis patients, their presence and phenotype in ST of spondylarthropathies (SpA) have not been previously investigated (2,5). The current studies were undertaken to examine the specificity of perivascular DC and MNC aggregation in RA ST. Therefore, ST from patients with SpA, osteoarthritis (OA; a disease with predominantly noninflammatory initiation), and gout, a nonautoimmune, crystal-induced inflammatory arthropathy, were obtained in order to examine DC infiltration associated with different levels of inflammation.

PATIENTS AND METHODS

Patients and tissue processing. Twenty-six ST biopsy samples were obtained at arthroscopy from 18 RA patients with active disease that fulfilled the American College of

Rheumatology (ACR; formerly, the American Rheumatism Association) 1987 revised criteria (6). Some of the samples were collected as part of a larger study of synovial immunopathology in response to treatment (Pettit AR, et al: unpublished observations). ST biopsy specimens were collected at the time of knee joint replacement from 10 patients with severe OA, 13 patients with SpA (at the time of knee arthroscopy), and 5 patients with gouty arthritis. All OA patients fulfilled the ACR criteria for OA of the knee (7).

The 18 RA patients included 10 women and 8 men with a mean ± SD age of 70 ± 10 years (range 56–86 years). Thirteen of the RA patients (72%) were positive for rheumatoid factor. At the time of biopsy, 12 patients were receiving no treatment. The others were taking methotrexate (n = 5), intramuscular gold (n = 4), D-penicillamine (n = 1), sulfasalazine (n = 5), and hydroxychloroquine (n = 3).

The SpA patients included 9 men and 4 women—5 with ankylosing spondylitis, 5 with psoriatic arthritis, 2 with reactive arthritis, and 1 with ulcerative colitis with associated joint inflammation (8). The mean ± SD age of these patients was 51 ± 19 years. Two patients were taking methotrexate and 3 were taking sulfasalazine. One patient was taking no disease-modifying antirheumatic drug (DMARD). All had active synovitis in at least 1 knee joint.

The OA patients included 5 women and 5 men with a mean ± SD age of 72 ± 8 years. These patients had no swollen joints and were taking no DMARD. ST biopsy samples were formalin fixed, embedded in paraffin, and 4-μm serial sections were cut.

Antibodies and immunohistochemical staining. The antibodies used included C-19 (directed against RelB) (Santa Cruz Biotechnology, Santa Cruz, CA), as well as TAL.1B5 (directed against HLA–DR), L26 (directed against CD20), polyclonal antibody (directed against CD3), and PG-M1 (directed against CD68) (all from Dako, Carpinteria, CA). Biotinylated *Ulex europaeus* agglutinin type I (*Ulex*), a lectin that binds endothelial cells, was purchased from Vector (Burlingame, CA). Control antibodies included isotype-matched mouse and rabbit control Ig (Dako). Immunohistochemical double staining used an immunoperoxidase–immunoalkaline phosphatase staining procedure with diaminobenzidine and fast red (Dako) as chromogens, and hematoxylin counterstaining, as described (1).

Analysis of DC and lymphocyte infiltration and vascularity. ST from 12 SpA and 8 OA biopsies were randomly selected for quantitative analysis. The same observers quantitatively analyzed all biopsies, including the 26 from RA patients. Biopsy sections were randomized and the clinical diagnosis coded prior to analysis by a blinded observer (ARP).

Biopsies from all disease groups were analyzed using the following methodology. To determine differentiated DC infiltration, the number of nRelB+ cells was counted in each tissue section at high power. For each biopsy, this number was corrected for the area of the section to obtain the number of nRelB+ cells/mm^2. The percentage of MNC aggregates (>10 cells) containing nRelB+ cells was determined by counting at high power. The number of vessels/mm^2 of tissue, or vascularity, was determined by counting vascular structures stained with *Ulex*. Lymphocytic infiltration was assessed by 2 independent observers (ARP and SZ) using a semiquantitative 10-point scoring system. Each high-power field in the whole section was scored, and the scores were averaged. The variability between scorers was minimal, with a mean difference in final score of 0.2, and 98% of all scores fell within half a point of each other. The gout sections could not be analyzed quantitatively due to incomplete adherence of sections to the slides after washing, resulting in a large degree of inconsistency through serial sections.

Statistical analysis. We compared histologic features of ST in 26 RA biopsy samples, 5 OA biopsy samples, and 6 SpA biopsy samples. Differences between ST sections from patients with different arthritides were determined using unpaired *t*-tests. Correlations between ST pathologic variables within each group of arthritis patients were determined using Spearman correlation coefficients (r_s). *P* values less than 0.05 were considered significant.

RESULTS

DC infiltration in OA, RA, and SpA ST. ST sections obtained from patients with OA, SpA, and gout were analyzed by immunohistochemical staining for infiltration by nRelB+ DC, lymphocytes, and macrophages, as well as for the degree of tissue vascularity. Cells infiltrating ST derived from each group of arthritis patients contained cytoplasmic RelB and nRelB (Figure 1). Approximately 85% of the nRelB+ cells could be identified as HLA–DR+,CD20−,CD68− differentiated DC, as previously defined (data not shown) (1). OA and SpA ST were compared with RA ST (Figures 1 and 2). Histologic analysis of RelB+ differentiated DC in RA ST has been published previously (1). In SpA ST, frequent perivascular cellular aggregates of varying sizes were observed, along with minimal lining layer hyperplasia and a high level of vascularity (Figure 1A) (4). Varying numbers of nRelB+ differentiated DC (Figure 1B), CD3+ T cells and CD20+ B cells (Figure 1C), and CD68+ macrophages (results not shown) infiltrated sublining perivascular regions. A mean ± SD of 44 ± 17% of perivascular aggregates (n = 5) contained nRelB+ differentiated DC. The percentage of perivascular aggregates that contained nRelB+ DC was significantly lower in SpA ST than that in RA ST (73 ± 15%, n = 4) (*P* = 0.035).

Although all of the biopsied SpA patients were taking DMARDs, only 8 of the 26 RA synovial biopsies were from patients treated with DMARDs. It is therefore possible that this treatment may have affected the immunopathology seen here. However, treated and untreated patients from both disease groups had active disease at the time of biopsy. In preliminary analysis of RA biopsy findings before and after treatment, we have found that clinical activity has a more significant impact than DMARD intervention on immunopathology (Pettit AR et al: unpublished observations).

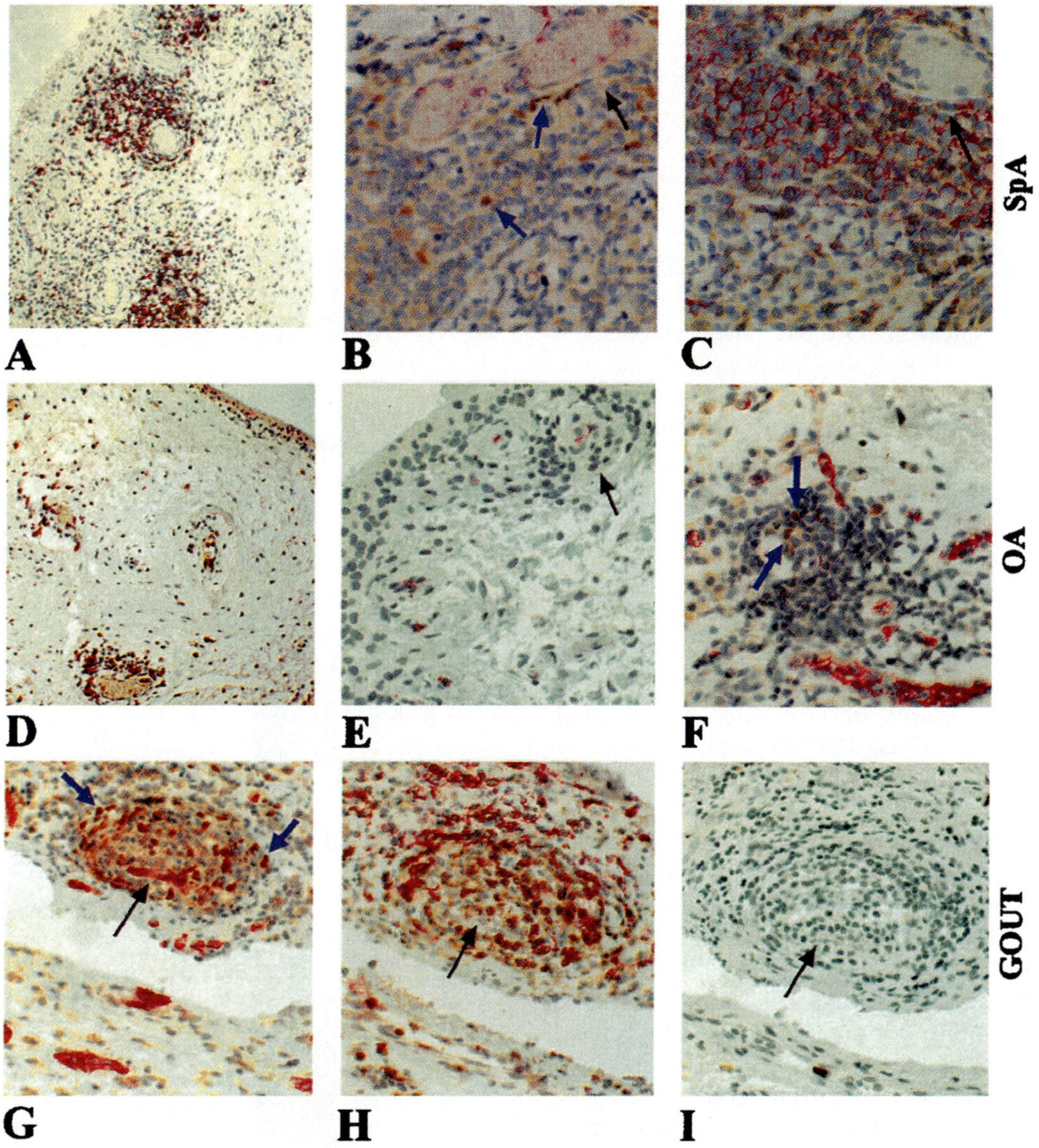

Figure 1. Nuclear RelB+ differentiated dendritic cells observed within perivascular mononuclear cell aggregates in synovial tissue (ST) from patients with spondylarthropathy (SpA), osteoarthritis (OA), and gout. Formalin-fixed tissue sections were stained as described in Patients and Methods, using an immunoperoxidase–immunoalkaline phosphatase technique with hematoxylin counterstaining (blue). Double staining of SpA ST is shown for CD3 (brown) and CD20 (red) (**A**), RelB (brown; **blue arrows** indicate examples of nRelB+ cells) and the endothelial cell marker biotinylated *Ulex europaeus* agglutinin type I (*Ulex*; red) (**B**), and CD3 (brown) and CD20 (red) of a serial section (**C**). **Black arrows** in **B** and **C** indicate the same blood vessel. Double staining of OA ST is shown for CD3 (brown) and CD20 (red) (**D**), as well as for RelB (brown; **blue arrows** indicate examples of nRelB+ cells) and *Ulex* (red) (**E** and **F**). **Black arrow** in **E** indicates a perivascular aggregate. Hematoxylin counterstaining was used to estimate lining layer hyperplasia and sublining cellularity. Double staining of gout ST is shown for RelB (brown; **blue arrows** indicate examples of nRelB+ cells) and *Ulex* (red) (**G**), CD3 (brown) and CD20 (red) in a serial section (**H**), and RelB control peptide–competed anti-RelB antibody in a serial section (**I**). **Black arrows** in **G–I** indicate the same blood vessel. Results are representative of 13 SpA, 10 OA, and 5 gout patients. (Original magnification × 32 in **A** and **D**; × 80 in **B**, **C**, and **E–I**.)

In contrast to SpA ST, sublining areas of OA ST were comparatively less cellular, with minimal-to-moderate lining layer hyperplasia (Figure 1D), as has been previously shown (5). Perivascular MNC aggregates were smaller and less frequent than those observed in RA or SpA ST (Figures 1D and F). Some perivascular aggregates contained nRelB+ differentiated DC (Figure 1F), CD20+ B cells, CD3+ T cells, and CD68+ macrophages (results not shown), but ~84% of perivascular MNC aggregates lacked nRelB+ differentiated DC (Figure 1E). The percentage of perivascular aggregates that contained nRelB+ cellular infiltration was significantly lower in OA ST than in RA ST ($P = 0.0005$) or SpA ST ($P = 0.02$). Therefore, just as in RA ST, differentiated DC, lymphocytes, and macrophages infiltrated perivascular regions of SpA and OA ST, but this infiltration was reduced in OA ST. Since lymphocytic infiltration was scored on a semiquantitative scale, the exact ratio of T cells to B cells in each lymphocytic aggregate was not quantitated. However, when examining multiple lymphocytic aggregates in biopsies from a number of individuals, there was no consistent predominance of either B cell or T cell infiltration in any disease subgroup analyzed.

Differentiated DC and blood vessels were quantitated per mm^2 of RA, SpA, or OA ST, and lymphocytic infiltration was scored on a semiquantitative scale in a proportion of biopsies. RA and SpA ST did not differ with regard to vascularity or infiltration by DC, but lymphocytic infiltration of RA ST was significantly greater (Figure 2). Infiltration by differentiated DC was significantly lower in OA ST than in RA and SpA ST (Figure 2B). Lymphocytic infiltration of RA ST, but not SpA ST, was significantly greater than that of OA ST (Figure 2C). While OA ST tended to be less vascular than SpA or RA ST, the differences were not significant (Figure 2A). Analysis of all biopsies (n = 37) from the 3 arthritis groups showed that DC infiltration correlated with lymphocytic infiltration ($r_s = 0.82$, $P < 0.0001$) and vascularity ($r_s = 0.33$, $P < 0.02$). Vascularity and lymphocytic infiltration were also correlated ($r_s = 0.29$, $P < 0.05$). Therefore, these histopathologic features represent associated events in synovial inflammation.

Nuclear RelB+ cell infiltration associated with lymphocytes in gout ST. ST collected from patients with gout displayed a complex phenotype, with variations in histology within sections. While large areas contained minimal lymphocytic or nRelB+ cell infiltration (results not shown), infrequent perivascular aggregates were present in other areas. Such aggregates contained nRelB+ cells (Figure 1G) and lymphocytes (Figure 1H). Other areas of gout ST contained scattered CD3+ T cells mixed with nRelB+ cells that were not clustered around blood vessels (results not shown). Finally, follicle-like structures containing CD20+ B cells and scattered nRelB+ cells were present (results not shown). The majority of the nRelB+ cells within these

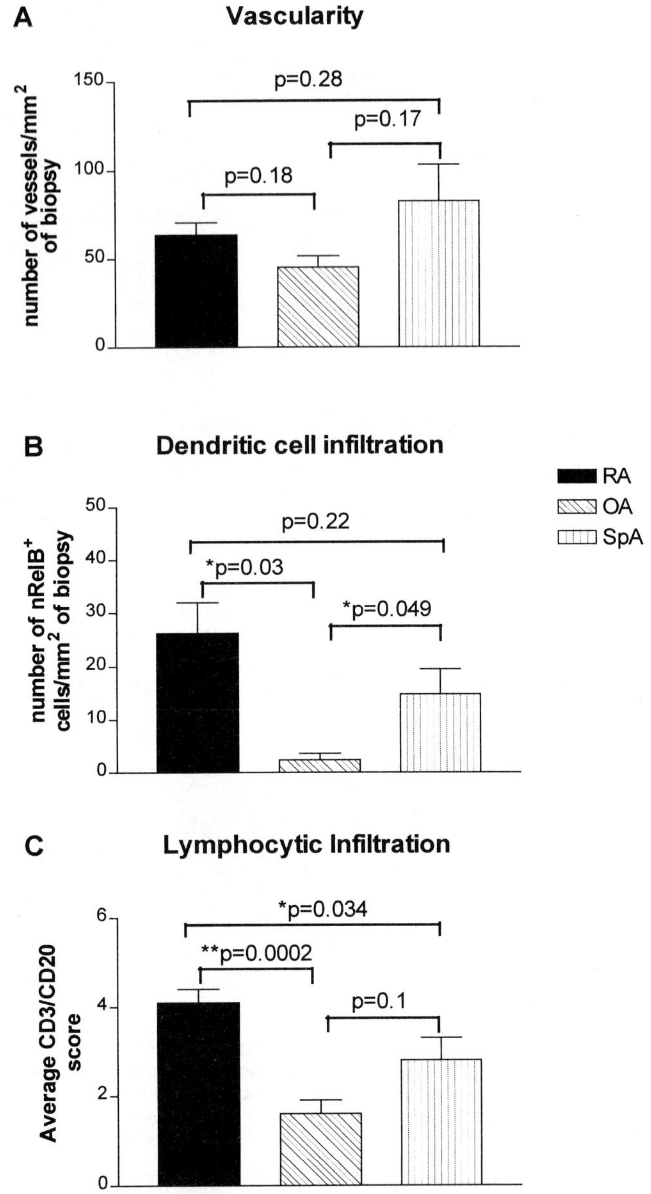

Figure 2. Comparison of vascularity (**A**), dendritic cell (DC) infiltration (**B**), and lymphocytic infiltration (**C**) in 26 biopsy samples from patients with active rheumatoid arthritis (RA), 6 samples from patients with active SpA, and 5 samples from patients with chronic OA. DC and lymphocytic infiltration were significantly higher in RA ST than in OA ST. The levels of nRelB+ DC and lymphocytic infiltration and tissue vascularity in ST were determined as described in Patients and Methods and compared using unpaired *t*-tests. See Figure 1 for other definitions.

follicle-like structures also expressed HLA–DR, suggesting that they were not follicular DC (1,2). However, specific stains for follicular DC could not be performed on these formalin-fixed tissues to confirm this. These structures resemble B cell follicles, similar to those observed in RA and SpA ST (4). The data indicate that infiltration of gout ST by nRelB+ cells also occurs in association with lymphocytes. Therefore, differentiated DC infiltration was observed in all arthritis tissues, but the extent of cellular infiltration varied for each type of arthritis.

DISCUSSION

Infiltration of perivascular MNC aggregates by nRelB+ differentiated DC is a consistent feature of the inflammatory response occurring in RA ST (1). The nuclear translocation of RelB by these DC implies that they are fully functional APC in situ (2). The close interaction of functional differentiated DC and lymphocytes in ST might reflect the local presentation of arthritogenic antigen by DC to CD4+ T cells (9). While DC infiltration is a consistent feature of RA ST, DC and other cells may be nonspecifically chemoattracted to inflammatory sites across activated endothelium regardless of etiology (10). Therefore, in the current studies we examined synovial biopsies from patients with 2 autoimmune arthropathies (RA and SpA), OA, and a crystal-induced arthropathy (gout) to evaluate the specificity of ST infiltration by differentiated DC in RA.

Biopsies from patients with SpA, OA, RA, and gout ST displayed perivascular MNC aggregates containing DC, lymphocytes, and macrophages. The extent of DC and lymphocytic infiltration was similar in SpA and RA ST, but lower in OA ST. This finding was supported by the reduced levels, compared with RA ST, of DC-containing lymphocytic aggregates and lymphocytic infiltration in OA ST. Recent evidence indicates that inflammation is common in OA ST, especially in later stages of disease, and is likely to be a consequence of bone and cartilage damage (3). In those studies, synovial inflammation in OA was also less intense than that in RA. It should be emphasized that OA ST was obtained in the current studies from patients with late-stage OA at joint replacement surgery. Urate crystal deposition in ST is likely to initiate synovial inflammation in gout (8). On qualitative examination, gout ST also contained fewer perivascular aggregates than RA ST. Finally, the current studies are the first to demonstrate quantitative differences between lymphocytic infiltration and DC-containing lymphocytic aggregates in SpA in a direct comparison with RA. The data suggest that perivascular infiltration by DC, lymphocytes, and macrophages is nonspecifically related to inflammation, but that the signals present, particularly in RA and, to a lesser extent, in SpA, lead to intense cellular infiltration and accumulation in the tissue.

The major histocompatibility complex (MHC) associations of RA and SpA, and the T cell reactivity demonstrable in these diseases, imply that presentation of self and/or bacterial or viral antigens to T cells by DC is integral to their perpetuation (4,11,12). Presentation of self antigen at inflammatory sites and draining lymph nodes of joints affected by gout or OA is a potential consequence of the infiltration by differentiated DC and T cells. However, it is probable that MHC haplotype, T cell repertoire, available antigen, and very likely other genes are critical contributors to the outcome of DC infiltration, such as perpetuation or resolution of inflammation as a result of antigen presentation. Therefore, the current studies imply that nonspecific stimuli of synovial inflammation may trigger a more intense and prolonged autoimmune response in susceptible individuals (13).

In all tissues examined, differentiated DC were always observed in close association with lymphocytes. Correlation between these variables suggested that they were associated with one another in inflammation. It is possible that differentiated DC in perivascular regions actively recruit and subsequently activate lymphocytes in ST through the secretion of chemokines and cytokines (14,15). In addition, lymphocytes may induce local DC accumulation and differentiation as a result of the secretion of cytokines or the engagement of surface molecules, including C-C chemokines and CD40 ligand (16). Monocyte secretion of tumor necrosis factor α plays a critical role in endothelial cell activation and DC differentiation. The correlations of DC and lymphocytic infiltration with vascularity suggest that the number of blood vessels influences the level of cellular recruitment into ST. Therefore, as a result of various proinflammatory stimuli, the formation of perivascular MNC aggregates is likely to be stimulated by interactions among DC, lymphocytes, and blood vessels (12). These perivascular aggregates, common to all inflammatory arthritides, therefore generate a microenvironment that may stimulate optimal effector cell function at inflammatory sites.

ACKNOWLEDGMENTS

The authors thank Dr. Geoff Strutton for assistance with pathologic sections, Dr. John Hay for advice with statistics, and Dr. Malcolm Handel for critical reading of the manuscript.

REFERENCES

1. Pettit AR, MacDonald KPA, O'Sullivan B, Thomas R. Differentiated dendritic cells expressing nuclear RelB are predominantly

located in rheumatoid synovial tissue perivascular mononuclear cell aggregates. Arthritis Rheum 2000;43:791–800.
2. Pettit AR, Quinn C, MacDonald KP, Cavanagh LL, Thomas G, Townsend W, et al. Nuclear localization of RelB is associated with effective antigen-presenting cell function. J Immunol 1997;159: 3681–91.
3. Smith MD, Triantafillou S, Parker A, Youssef PP, Coleman M. Synovial membrane inflammation and cytokine production in patients with early osteoarthritis. J Rheumatol 1997;24:365–71.
4. Cunnane G, Bresnihan B, FitzGerald O. Immunohistologic analysis of peripheral joint disease in ankylosing spondylitis. Arthritis Rheum 1998;41:180–2.
5. Goldenberg DL, Cohen AS. Synovial membrane histopathology in the differential diagnosis of rheumatoid arthritis, gout, pseudogout, systemic lupus erythematosus, infectious arthritis and degenerative joint disease. Medicine (Baltimore) 1978;57:239–52.
6. Arnett FC, Edworthy SM, Bloch DA, McShane DJ, Fries JF, Cooper NS, et al. The American Rheumatism Association 1987 revised criteria for the classification of rheumatoid arthritis. Arthritis Rheum 1988;31:315–24.
7. Altman R, Asch E, Bloch D, Bole G, Borenstein D, Brandt K, et al. Development of criteria for the classification and reporting of osteoarthritis: classification of osteoarthritis of the knee. Arthritis Rheum 1986;29:1039–49.
8. Klippel JH, Dieppe PA. Rheumatology. St. Louis (MO): Mosby; 1998.
9. Thomas R, Lipsky PE. Presentation of self peptides by dendritic cells: possible implications for the pathogenesis of rheumatoid arthritis. Arthritis Rheum 1996;39:183–90.
10. Sozzani S, Sallusto F, Luini W, Zhou D, Piemonti L, Allavena P, et al. Migration of dendritic cells in response to formyl peptides, C5a, and a distinct set of chemokines. J Immunol 1995;155:3292–5.
11. Veale D, Rogers S, Fitzgerald O. Immunolocalization of adhesion molecules in psoriatic arthritis, psoriatic and normal skin. Br J Dermatol 1995;132:32–8.
12. Winchester R. Psoriatic arthritis and the spectrum of syndromes related to the SAPHO (synovitis, acne, pustulosis, hyperostosis, and osteitis) syndrome. Curr Opin Rheumatol 1999;11:251–6.
13. Thomas R, Quinn C. Functional differentiation of dendritic cells in rheumatoid arthritis: role of CD86 in the synovium. J Immunol 1996;156:3074–86.
14. Ludewig B, Odermatt B, Landmann S, Hengartner H, Zinkernagel RM. Dendritic cells induce autoimmune diabetes and maintain disease via de novo formation of local lymphoid tissue. J Exp Med 1998;188:1493–501.
15. Tang HL, Cyster JG. Chemokine up-regulation and activated T cell attraction by maturing dendritic cells. Science 1999;284: 819–22.
16. MacDonald KPA, Nishioka N, Lipsky PE, Thomas R. Functional CD40-ligand is expressed by T cells in rheumatoid arthritis. J Clin Invest 1997;100:2404–14.

ARTHRITIS & RHEUMATISM
Vol. 44, No. 1, January 2001, pp 111–119

Dependence of Interleukin-1–Induced Arthritis on Granulocyte–Macrophage Colony-Stimulating Factor

Yuan H. Yang and John A. Hamilton

Objective. **To determine whether granulocyte–macrophage colony-stimulating factor (GM-CSF) and macrophage CSF (M-CSF or CSF-1) are involved in the methylated bovine serum albumin/interleukin-1 (mBSA/IL-1)–induced arthritis model.**

Methods. **Following systemic injection, IL-1 has been shown to augment a weak inflammatory response to mBSA in murine joints and to induce an acute erosive arthritis. GM-CSF and M-CSF have been implicated in inflammatory reactions, including those in joints, and have recently been shown to exacerbate murine arthritis. Since in vitro studies have found that IL-1 can enhance GM-CSF and M-CSF production, we reasoned that they might be playing a part in IL-1–mediated arthritis. GM-CSF–deficient (GM-CSF−/−) and M-CSF–deficient (*op/op*) mice were injected intraarticularly with mBSA and subcutaneously with IL-1. Arthritis was monitored histologically on day 7. Normal mice were also treated intraperitoneally with blocking monoclonal antibodies to GM-CSF and M-CSF, and to the M-CSF receptor. Numbers of macrophages (Mac-2 and F4/80 staining) were monitored, as was the number of cycling (bromodeoxyuridine-positive) cells.**

Results. **GM-CSF−/− mice and normal mice treated with anti–GM-CSF antibody did not show IL-1–induced arthritis progression. There was a dramatic reduction in synovial cellularity, including reduced numbers of macrophages and cycling cells. The *op/op* mice did not develop mBSA/IL-1–induced disease, but blocking antibody to M-CSF or to the M-CSF receptor failed to diminish disease in normal mice.**

Conclusion. **GM-CSF is involved in the IL-1–induced arthritis that follows mBSA injection; M-CSF involvement in the model is also suggested, since *op/op* mice did not develop arthritis. These studies provide the first in vivo evidence for a role of GM-CSF, and possibly M-CSF, in the proinflammatory actions of IL-1.**

There are data to support the concept that the colony-stimulating factors (CSFs), granulocyte–macrophage CSF (GM-CSF) and macrophage CSF (M-CSF or CSF-1), should be viewed as proinflammatory cytokines in addition to their traditional roles as hemopoietic growth factors (1–3). For example, they have been detected in the synovial fluids of patients with rheumatoid arthritis (RA) (4,5), and GM-CSF therapy for patients with Felty's syndrome can result in flares of RA (6).

Cytokines, such as interleukin-1 (IL-1) and tumor necrosis factor α (TNFα), can stimulate GM-CSF and M-CSF production in vitro by a number of cell types, including synovial fibroblasts and chondrocytes (7–10). IL-1 and TNFα are produced by macrophages at sites of inflammation, and macrophage numbers correlate with the degree of tissue damage, for example, in RA (11). It has therefore been proposed that GM-CSF and M-CSF form part of a "CSF network" at a site of inflammation in which they can act to promote macrophage survival and proliferation, leading to increased numbers of cells, and can therefore enhance inflammatory mediator levels (12); GM-CSF could also promote neutrophil function in lesions (13).

Investigators in our group recently obtained more direct evidence of a role for GM-CSF in inflammatory arthritis by demonstrating that GM-CSF can exacerbate disease symptoms when injected into mice with collagen-induced arthritis (CIA) (14), and by showing that GM-CSF–deficient (GM-CSF−/−) mice are

Supported by grants from the National Health and Medical Research Council of Australia.

Yuan H. Yang, PhD, John A. Hamilton, DSc, PhD: University of Melbourne, The Royal Melbourne Hospital, Parkville, Victoria, Australia.

Address correspondence and reprint requests to Yuan H. Yang, PhD, Arthritis and Inflammation Research Centre, Department of Medicine, University of Melbourne, The Royal Melbourne Hospital, Parkville, Victoria 3050, Australia.

Submitted for publication April 11, 2000; accepted in revised form September 27, 2000.

resistant to the induction of CIA (15). Although a previous study described exacerbation of disease in the *Streptococcus agalactiae* rat arthritis model by intravenous injection of M-CSF (16), it is not known whether M-CSF is required for arthritis development.

In a rapid-onset monarticular arthritis model with histopathologic features similar to those seen in RA, Staite et al (17) reported that subcutaneous (SC) injection of IL-1 exacerbated the arthritis in the knees of mice injected intraarticularly with methylated bovine serum albumin (mBSA). A prominent feature of this model is the rapid development of synovial hyperplasia, making it particularly suitable for studies of these changes in RA. In studies of experimental arthritis, there are some advantages of the mBSA model over other more traditional models, such as CIA. The most notable of these advantages are its acute onset, restriction to a specific joint, and dependence upon a defined cytokine which is strongly implicated in RA (18–21). The mechanism by which IL-1 transforms a mild inflammatory reaction to intraarticular mBSA into an acute destructive arthritis is unclear. It was suggested that IL-1 might stimulate local or systemic immunity to intraarticular mBSA or, alternatively, that it might induce other cytokines (17,22).

Investigators in our group recently found that SC injection of GM-CSF or M-CSF could replace IL-1 in this model (22). Since, as mentioned before, IL-1 can stimulate CSF formation in vitro by a number of cell types and tissues (7–10), we determined whether either or both of these CSFs might be critical for arthritis progression in this model. Using GM-CSF−/− mice and blocking antibody, we found that the arthritis-inducing capability of IL-1 was GM-CSF dependent; M-CSF–deficient mice did not develop disease.

MATERIALS AND METHODS

Reagents and antibodies. Methylated BSA was purchased from Sigma (St. Louis, MO). Recombinant human IL-1β (specific activity 5×10^8 units/mg) was a gift from Amgen (Thousand Oaks, CA). Endotoxin levels were routinely monitored by *Limulus* amebocyte cell lysate assays (CSL, Parkville, Victoria, Australia) with a minimum detectable level of 0.01 ng/ml.

The rat anti-mouse monoclonal antibodies (mAb) to Mac-2 (M3/38) and to F4/80 were obtained from the American Type Culture Collection (Rockville, MD), and a murine anti-bromodeoxyuridine (anti-BrdU) mAb was obtained from Boehringer (Mannheim, Germany). The rat anti-murine GM-CSF hybridoma, 22E9.11, was obtained from J. Abrams of the DNAX Research Institute (Palo Alto, CA), and the IgG was purified. This hybridoma produces a neutralizing mAb to murine GM-CSF of the IgG2a isotype (23). As an isotype-matched control, mAb from the rat anti-mouse β-galactosidase hybridoma, GL117.41 (DNAX Research Institute), was used. Rat mAb (IgG1) to M-CSF, 5A1, was a gift from F. Kull (Glaxo Wellcome, Research Triangle Park, NC). The neutralizing capacity of 5A1 was 7×10^5 units of M-CSF/mg of 5A1. The neutralizing anti-murine M-CSF receptor antibody, AFS-98 (24), was a gift from S.-I. Nishikawa, Kyoto, Japan. Antibodies were purified on a protein G–Sepharose column.

Animals. C57BL/6 mice were supplied by Monash University, Central Animal Services, (Clayton, Victoria, Australia). Mice heterozygous for a disrupted GM-CSF gene were provided by the Ludwig Institute for Cancer Research (Parkville, Victoria, Australia) (15). Germline transmitters of the mutated GM-CSF allele were crossed with C57BL/6 mice for 13 generations to yield the GM-CSF−/− mice used for the experiments. Animals used for all experiments, 8–12 weeks old and weighing 18–25 gm, were fed laboratory chow and tap water ad libitum and housed 5 to a cage. Osteopetrotic (*op*/*op*) mutant mice, as well as their littermate controls (+/+ or +/*op*), were obtained from the Ludwig Institute and maintained in microisolators within the Institute's animal house facility. Following weaning, the *op*/*op* mice, which lack incisors, were maintained on a diet of equal amounts of powdered chow and Ensure nutritional powder (VHA Trading, Mulgrave, Victoria, Australia) mixed in sterile water. All experiments were approved by the Royal Melbourne Hospital Research Foundation Animal Ethics Committee.

Induction of monarticular arthritis. Methylated BSA/IL-1–induced arthritis in mice was established as described previously (17,22). Briefly, 10 μl of mBSA at a concentration of 20 mg/ml in saline was injected into the knee joint. Twenty microliters of either IL-1β (250 ng) or saline was subcutaneously administered daily into the left rear footpad for 3 days (days 0–2). Contralateral control knee joints received vehicle (saline). To determine whether we could use more than 1 joint/mouse (thereby allowing us to use fewer mice), we examined what happened when mBSA was injected into both knees. We found with this protocol (and with IL-1 still administered subcutaneously into only 1 footpad) that the resulting arthritis was similar on both sides. For this reason, mBSA was often administered into both knees, leading to involvement of >1 joint. Animals were killed on day 7 following mBSA injection.

BrdU labeling in vivo. Mice were injected intraperitoneally with 250 μl of BrdU (8 mg/ml) 2 hours before they were killed (22). Control animals did not receive BrdU.

Histologic assessment of arthritis. Arthritis was assessed by histologic examination as described (22), but with some modifications. Knee joints were exposed by removal of the overlying skin and then excised. They were fixed in periodate–lysine–paraformaldehyde for 4 hours and decalcified in 10% EDTA (BDH Chemicals, Victoria, Australia) and 7.5% polyvinylpyrrolidone (Sigma) in Tris buffer (pH 6.95) for 7–10 days (25). A transverse cut was made when the bones were fully decalcified and processed to paraffin. Tissues were cut into 5-μm sections, placed on aminoalkylsilane-coated slides, and stained for routine histology with hematoxylin and eosin.

Five defined pathologic features were graded for severity from 0 (normal) to 5 (severe), according to Staite et al

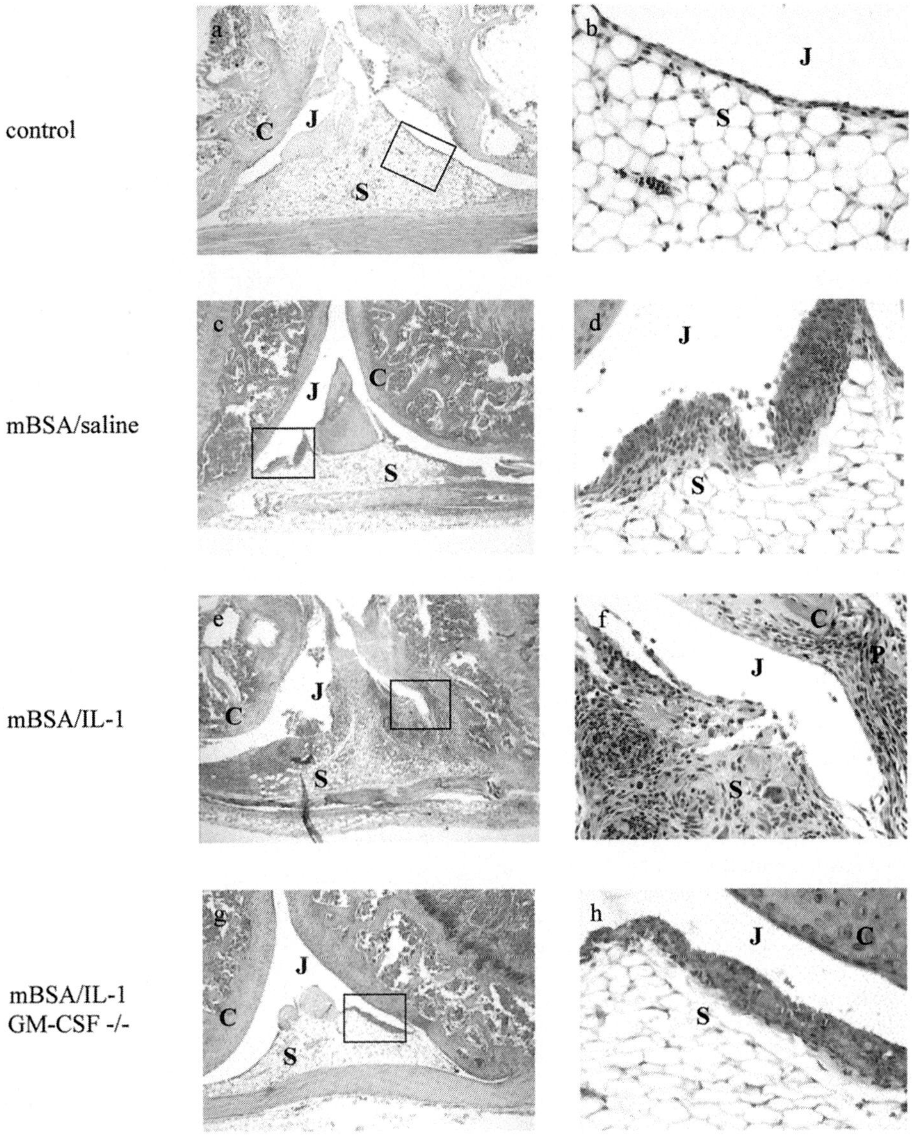

Figure 1. Histopathologic manifestations of the suppression of methylated bovine serum albumin/ interleukin-1 (mBSA/IL-1)–induced arthritis in granulocyte–macrophage colony-stimulating factor–deficient (GM-CSF−/−) mice. C57BL/6 or GM-CSF−/− mice were given intraarticular injections of either saline or mBSA (200 μg) on day 0 of the experiment; either saline or IL-1 (250 ng) was given subcutaneously on day 0 and for the following 2 days. Shown are sections of tissues from knee joints obtained on day 7 from C57BL/6 mice treated with saline/saline (**a** and **b**), mBSA/saline (**c** and **d**), and mBSA/IL-1 (**e** and **f**), as well as from GM-CSF−/− mice treated with mBSA/IL-1 (**g** and **h**). Panels at right correspond to boxed areas in the panels at left. **C** = articular cartilage; **J** = joint space; **S** = synovium; **P** = pannus formation. (Hematoxylin and eosin stained; original magnification × 100 in **a**, **c**, **e**, and **g**; × 400 in **b**, **d**, **f**, and **h**.)

(17), and in a blinded manner, as follows. *Soft tissue inflammation*, assessed in the infrapatellar fat pads, joint capsule, and the area adjacent to the periosteal sheath, was graded according to the extent of cellular infiltration and angiogenesis. *Joint space exudate* was identified as leukocytes scattered discretely or in aggregates in the joint space. *Synovitis* (synovial hyperplasia) was defined as hyperplasia of the synovium, but did not include pannus formation. *Pannus* was defined as hypertrophic synovial tissue forming a tight junction with the articular surface. Evaluation of *cartilage and bone damage* was based on loss of cartilage matrix, disruption and loss of cartilage surface, and the extent and depth of the subchondral bone erosion (22).

Antibody treatment. Mice were injected intraperitoneally with 100 μl of appropriate antibody at a concentration of 3 mg/ml.

Immunohistochemistry. For identification of synovial macrophages, deparaffinized sections were incubated with specific mAb against Mac-2 and F4/80, and subsequently stained for 1 hour using a peroxidase-conjugated rabbit anti-rat IgG (Dako, Carpinteria, CA). Endogenous peroxidase was blocked with 0.3% H_2O_2 (30% weight/volume; Sigma) in methanol. Peroxidase activity was demonstrated by incubation with 3,3′-diaminobenzidine tetrahydrochloride (DAB; Sigma)–H_2O_2 solution.

Local cell proliferation in the knee joint was examined by immunohistochemical staining using a specific anti-BrdU mAb. Briefly, knee joints were obtained 2 hours after intraperitoneal injection of BrdU. Deparaffinized sections were treated for 10 minutes at 60°C with 1*M* HCl. To enhance the immunohistochemical reactivity, the sections were further incubated with trypsin (1 mg/ml) for 40 minutes at room temperature prior to incubation with anti-BrdU mAb (5 μg/ml) overnight. Controls were sections from animals not given BrdU and sections from animals given BrdU but stained in the absence of anti-BrdU mAb. A peroxidase-conjugated rabbit anti-mouse IgG was incubated for 1 hour, and color was developed with DAB–H_2O_2 solution as described above.

For double staining, deparaffinized sections were incubated with anti–Mac-2, biotin-conjugated rabbit anti-rat IgG (Dako), and streptavidin–biotin–alkaline phosphatase (Dako). The color was developed by BCIP/nitroblue tetrazolium substrate detection kit (Zymed Laboratories, South San Francisco, CA). The sections were then incubated with anti-BrdU mAb following treatment with HCl and trypsin as described above. Immunoreactive cells were developed with DAB–H_2O_2 solution, and the counterstaining step was omitted. Macrophages appeared blue and BrdU+ cells appeared brown.

Statistical analysis. Data were analyzed using the Mann-Whitney 2-sample rank test to determine the significance of the difference between means of groups for histologic scores (22). Results are expressed as the mean ± SEM. For each test, *P* values less than 0.05 were considered significant.

RESULTS

Role of GM-CSF in the mBSA/IL-1 arthritis model. Arthritis was assessed by histologic examination 7 days after mBSA administration, i.e., at its peak (17,22). A weak, nonerosive synovitis was observed following an intraarticular mBSA injection alone, as previously reported (17,22). In comparison with normal joints (Figures 1a and b), mBSA-injected joints showed mild inflammation of soft tissue, synovial hyperplasia, and minimal leukocyte infiltration (Figures 1c and d). The additional SC administration of IL-1 resulted in a significant inflammatory response in the mBSA-injected knee joints (Figures 1e and f). The inflammatory reaction involved infiltration of inflammatory cells, hyperplasia of the synovial lining and sublining layer, pannus formation, and cartilage and subchondral bone damage that could be seen under the severe joint inflammation (17,22).

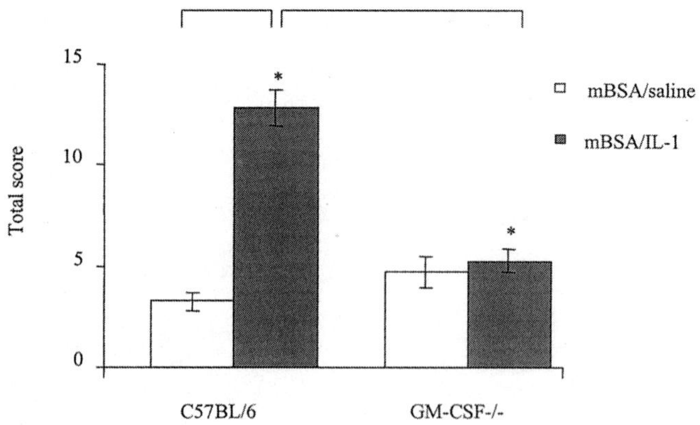

Figure 2. Suppression of mBSA/IL-1–induced arthritis in GM-CSF−/− mice. C57BL/6 and GM-CSF−/− mice were given intraarticular injections of mBSA (200 μg) on day 0 of the experiment; either saline or IL-1 (250 ng) was given subcutaneously on day 0 and for the following 2 days. Joint inflammation on day 7 was scored by histologic analysis on a scale of 0–5 for the 5 histopathologic features, as described (22) (see Materials and Methods). Values are the mean ± SEM total scores (maximum total score 25) obtained from groups of 12 GM-CSF−/− mice (n = 19 joints) and 28 C57BL/6 mice (n = 38 joints). * = $P < 0.001$ for mBSA/IL-1 treatment versus mBSA/saline treatment in C57BL/6 mice and for mBSA/IL-1 treatment in GM-CSF−/− mice versus C57BL/6 mice. See Figure 1 for definitions.

Investigators in our group recently showed that GM-CSF could substitute for IL-1 in the above model (22). Since IL-1 can stimulate GM-CSF in many cell types, including synovial fibroblasts and chondrocytes (7–10), we tested whether it might be involved in the establishment of the arthritis in this model. To evaluate the role of endogenous GM-CSF, we first used GM-CSF−/− mice. Although these mice have a characteristic pulmonary disease, they show little disturbance in resting hemopoiesis, with normal numbers of granulocytes and monocytes in the blood (26). Intraarticular injection of mBSA alone resulted in a weak inflammatory response in these mice (mean ± SEM total histologic score 4.7 ± 0.7, n = 7 joints) (Figure 2), similar to that observed in the C57BL/6 controls (3.3 ± 0.5, n = 21 joints). However, in contrast to the C57BL/6 group, in which the score increased to 13.2 ± 0.9 (n = 38 joints), the coadministration of mBSA and IL-1 in GM-CSF−/− mice did not significantly exacerbate the arthritis (5.4 ± 0.6; $P > 0.05$; n = 19 joints) (Figures 1g and h, Figure 2). We found no increased numbers of leukocytes in the circulation in either strain on days 3 and 7 in mice given mBSA/IL-1 (Figure 2 protocol). There was a suggestion of a slight increase in the percentage of polymorphonuclear cells on day 3 for both strains (n = 18 mice for each strain), but this was not statistically significant (data not shown).

As an additional approach to assessing the role of GM-CSF, a blocking anti–GM-CSF mAb was administered to normal mice. This treatment (300 μg/mouse/day) began 1 day prior to the injection of mBSA/IL-1 and was continued daily for an additional 5 days. Control animals received the same dosage of an isotype-matched control mAb. Evaluation of the diseased joints of anti–GM-CSF mAb–treated animals by histologic analysis revealed a significant reduction in the severity of joint inflammation compared with the control group (mean ± SEM 6.3 ± 0.5 versus 11.1 ± 1.0 total histologic score; $P < 0.001$; n = 20 joints per group) (Figure 3a). The soft tissue inflammation, cell exudate, synovitis, and cartilage and bone destruction were all reduced.

It should be noted that the reduced histologic score in the anti–GM-CSF mAb–treated group was similar to that found in the GM-CSF−/− mice, and was similar to that found in normal (control) mice given only mBSA/saline. These mild synovial changes in the GM-CSF–depleted mice given mBSA/IL-1 could simply have been due to the response to mBSA.

Role of M-CSF in the mBSA/IL-1 arthritis model. Investigators in our group recently reported that M-CSF could also replace IL-1 in exacerbating the arthritis caused by intraarticular injection of mBSA (22). Since IL-1 can also stimulate M-CSF formation in many cell types, again including synovial fibroblasts and chondrocytes (9,10), we examined whether M-CSF might also be playing a role in this model.

In contrast to GM-CSF, M-CSF circulates normally, and the *op/op* (M-CSF–deficient) mouse shows that it controls macrophage development in the steady state (27). For these reasons, we considered that the *op/op* mouse might not develop arthritis in the mBSA/IL-1 arthritis model because of the reduced numbers of macrophages, including those in the synovium (27), while disease suppression might be difficult to demonstrate by antibody blockade of M-CSF action in a normal mouse. As can be seen in Figure 3b, *op/op* mice were strikingly resistant to mBSA/IL-1–induced arthritis compared with their non-*op/op* littermates (mean ± SEM 2.3 ± 0.4 versus 9.5 ± 1.0 total histologic score [$P < 0.001$]; n = 23 and 19 joints, respectively). However, administration of either anti–M-CSF mAb or anti–M-CSF receptor mAb (300 μg/mouse/day) for 6 days to mBSA/IL-1–treated

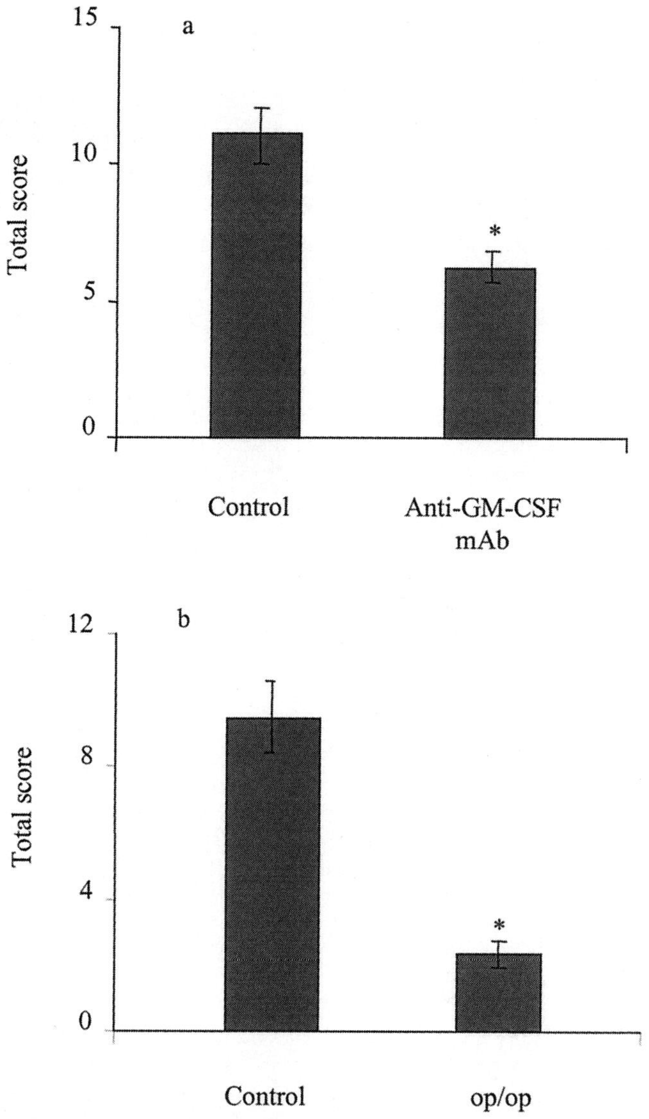

Figure 3. Suppression of mBSA/IL-1–induced arthritis by anti–GM-CSF monoclonal antibody (mAb) in C57BL/6 and in *op/op* mice. **A,** C57BL/6 mice were given mBSA/IL-1 using the same protocol as that for Figure 1; they were also treated with anti–GM-CSF or control mAb by intraperitoneal injection 1 day before the injections of mBSA/IL-1 and daily for the following 5 days. Clinical assessment was made on day 7 by histologic examination. Values are the mean ± SEM total scores obtained from each group of 13 mice (n = 20 joints per group). **B,** The *op/op* mice and their littermate controls (+/+ or +/*op* mice) were given mBSA/IL-1 using the same protocol as that for Figure 1. Clinical assessment was made on day 7 by histologic examination. Values are the mean ± SEM total scores from each group of 12 mice (n = 23 and 19 joints, respectively). * = $P < 0.001$ versus control group. See Figure 1 for other definitions.

C57BL/6 mice had no effect on the joint inflammation (9.9 ± 0.9 or 10.3 ± 1.6, respectively, versus score for controls of 9.1 ± 1.3; n = 19, 8, and 18 joints, respectively).

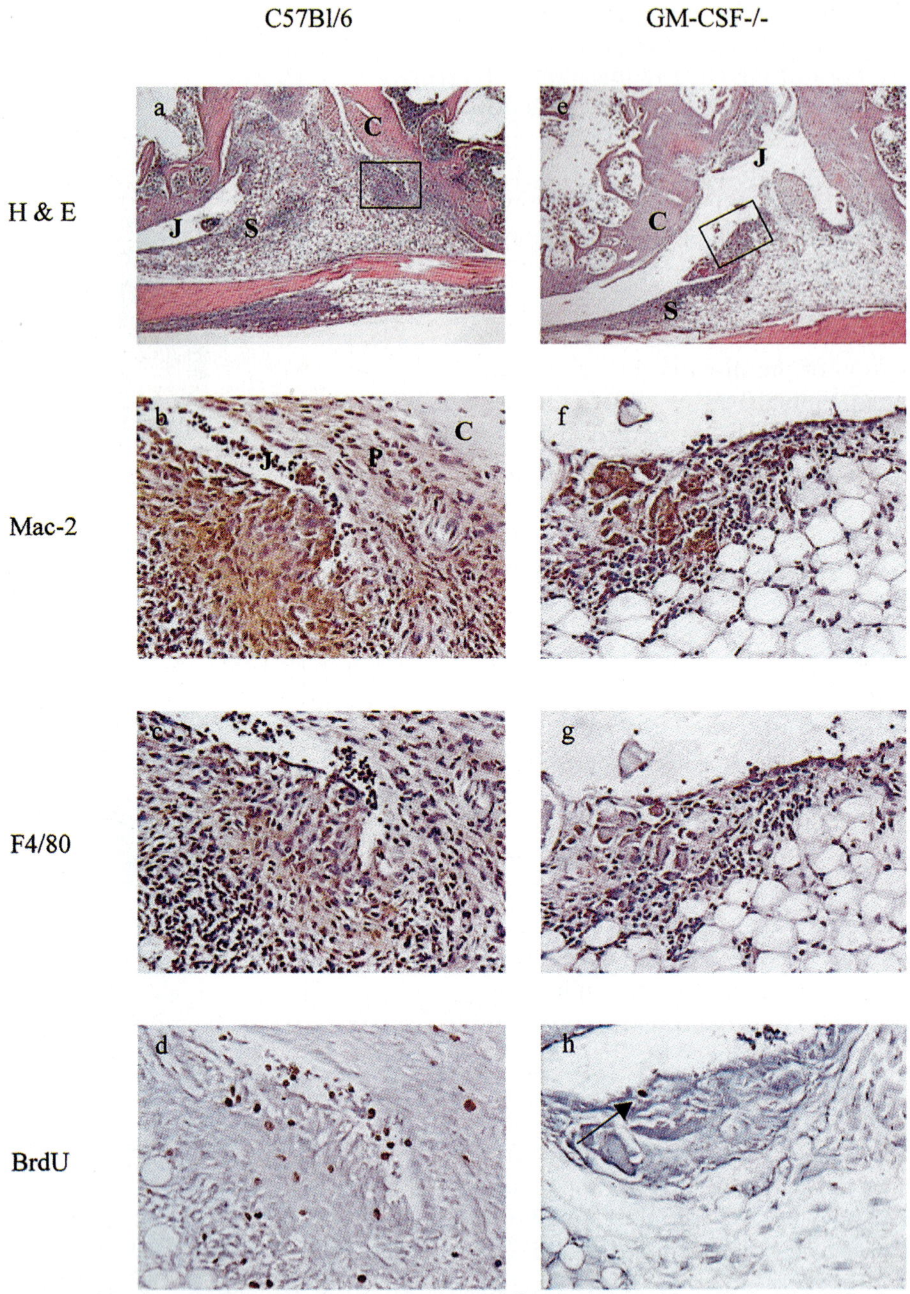

Figure 4. Numbers of macrophages and bromodeoxyuridine (BrdU)–positive cells in GM-CSF−/− mice following mBSA/IL-1 treatment. Knee joints were removed on day 7 from C57BL/6 and GM-CSF−/− mice after treatment with mBSA/IL-1 and were processed for histology and immunohistochemistry (see Materials and Methods). Joint sections were stained with hematoxylin and eosin (H&E) (**a** and **e**), anti–Mac-2 mAb (**b** and **f**), anti-F4/80 mAb (**c** and **g**), and anti-BrdU mAb (**d** and **h**) (**arrow** in **h** indicates a BrdU+ cell). Immunoreactive cells are stained brown; light counterstaining is with hematoxylin. **b–d** are from the inset in panel **a**; **f–h** are from the inset in panel **e**. (Original magnification × 100 in **a** and **e**; × 400 in **b–d** and **f–h**.) See Figures 1 and 3 for other definitions.

Numbers of macrophages. In the above results, it was noted that there was a marked reduction in overall cellularity in both mBSA/IL-1–treated GM-CSF−/− and *op*/*op* mice compared with the similarly treated wild-type controls. The macrophage is one cell type whose functions, including survival and proliferation, are enhanced by both GM-CSF and M-CSF (27,28). We therefore monitored numbers of macrophages in the joints of the GM-CSF−/− mice and *op/op* mice subjected to the arthritogenic protocol. We confirmed higher numbers of macrophages (by Mac-2 or F4/80 staining) in the synovial lining of the arthritic joints of mBSA/IL-1–treated C57BL/6 mice (Figures 4b and c), with cells intensely immunoreactive for Mac-2 localized around blood vessels in particular (22). We found fewer macrophages following treatment with mBSA/IL-1 in GM-CSF−/− mice than in control mice (Figures 4f and g). Similarly, anti–GM-CSF mAb significantly reduced the numbers of both Mac-2+ and F4/80+ cells in the arthritic joints of C57BL/6 mice (data not shown).

No macrophages could be seen in the synovium of 8-week-old *op/op* mice, as previously reported (27), although a few macrophages staining for Mac-2, but not for F4/80, did appear in the joints of these mice after treatment with mBSA/IL-1 (data not shown). However, treatment of arthritic C57BL/6 mice with anti–M-CSF mAb or anti–M-CSF receptor mAb failed to reduce the numbers of macrophages (data not shown).

Local cell proliferation. Local cell proliferation in arthritic joints was examined by immunohistochemistry following a 2-hour BrdU pulse in vivo. We confirmed by immunohistochemistry the significantly increased BrdU labeling of cells resembling macrophages, fibroblasts, or endothelial cells scattered within the inflamed synovium and neighboring tissue (Figure 4d), along with a small subpopulation of BrdU+,Mac-2+ macrophages (data not shown) (22). Since there was a marked reduction in cellularity in the GM-CSF−/− mice treated with mBSA/IL-1 (Figures 1g and h and 4a and e), it was not surprising that the vast majority of the BrdU+ cells were absent (Figure 4h; arrow indicates a BrdU+ cell). Likewise, for mBSA/IL-1–treated *op/op* mice, the dramatic reduction in cell numbers in the joint compared with the numbers observed in control (littermate) mice meant that the proliferating cells were virtually absent (data not shown).

DISCUSSION

It is not completely known how IL-1 functions as a critical inflammatory mediator, e.g., in inflammatory joint disease. The model described by Staite et al (17) was used since it allows us to monitor the IL-1–mediated progression from a mild inflammatory reaction to an acute destructive arthritis within an individual joint. Since two stimuli (mBSA and IL-1) are involved in the development of the model, the action of either or both may depend on CSF. For GM-CSF−/− mice and anti–GM-CSF antibody–treated C57BL/6 mice, addition of IL-1 did not potentiate the weak response to mBSA. Since GM-CSF can replace IL-1 in this model, and since IL-1 can induce GM-CSF in vitro in a number of cell types (7,8), our data indicate that GM-CSF is required for the arthritogenic action of IL-1 in this model; to our knowledge, this represents the first in vivo evidence for GM-CSF involvement in the proinflammatory actions of IL-1 (12). Since IL-1 is considered to be an important cytokine in RA (18–21), our findings support a possible role for GM-CSF in the human disease. For the *op/op* mice, the response to mBSA itself was diminished, presumably due to the reduced numbers of monocyte/macrophages in their synovium and blood (27). However, since IL-1 can also enhance M-CSF production in cells in vitro, and since M-CSF can replace IL-1 to some extent (see below), it is also possible that M-CSF is required for IL-1 action.

Investigators in our group have previously shown, using GM-CSF−/− mice, that GM-CSF is a critical mediator in CIA (15). We now demonstrate that this cytokine is also critical for the development of arthritis in another model. Regarding the function of GM-CSF in the promotion of the arthritis in the model under study, there was a marked reduction in the overall cellularity in the joints following IL-1 administration when GM-CSF was depleted. Since GM-CSF is a survival and developmental factor for both neutrophils and macrophages (28–31), reduced numbers of these cells could result from the local absence of GM-CSF in the inflamed joint—in this connection, fewer cycling cells were in the inflamed joint when GM-CSF was depleted (Figure 4h). In addition to its role in increasing numbers of inflammatory cells, there is both in vitro and in vivo evidence that GM-CSF is likely to prime or activate these cells to liberate inflammatory mediators such as cytokines or neutral proteinases (1,3). Since the mBSA/IL-1 model is T cell dependent (Campbell I: personal communication), a reduced T cell function could be contributing to the reduction in the severity of the arthritis, in addition to the loss of myeloid cell responses. Such reduced T cell function in these mice upon challenge with other antigens (32) has been reported and may reflect the ability of GM-CSF to participate in antigen-presenting cell development (33).

We suggest that the above data lend support to the CSF network hypothesis previously proposed (7,8,12), in which IL-1 can induce GM-CSF locally (for example, in joints), which in turn can feed back to act on myeloid cells (macrophages, granulocytes, and possibly precursors) to enhance the number of inflammatory cells. GM-CSF depletion could be interrupting the cytokine network proposed by this hypothesis.

The M-CSF–deficient (*op/op)* mouse is a unique tool for studying the role of M-CSF in disease models and the influence of macrophage depletion in vivo without the use of toxic agents. The *op/op* mice did not develop mBSA/IL-1–dependent arthritis, which is consistent with the hypothesis that M-CSF, acting by altering the number (or some property) of macrophage-lineage cells, influences arthritis susceptibility. If some of the M-CSF–dependent events happen to be downstream of the IL-1 action, then the findings would support another aspect of the CSF network hypothesis (9,10,12).

In contrast to GM-CSF−/− mice, in which myelopoiesis is intact (26), *op/op* mice are deficient in certain macrophage populations, although they appear to have normal T cell–dependent immune responses (27,34). The synovium is one tissue in *op/op* mice where the numbers of macrophages in the steady state are dramatically reduced (27). The inflammatory reaction to the mBSA injection alone was also very mild in the *op/op* mice (data not shown); also, synovial macrophage depletion by liposome-encapsulated clodronate reduces disease severity in murine arthritis models (35,36). Our data provide support for the importance of the resident macrophage type (type A) synovial lining cells in the model. Just as in the case of the foam cells in the atherosclerotic apoE−/− mouse (37), the use of *op/op* mice has also shown the dependence on M-CSF of the macrophage population(s) involved in the inflammatory reactions occurring in this arthritis model. Interestingly, numbers of granulocytes as well as macrophages were reduced compared with the response of the littermate controls, suggesting that M-CSF–dependent macrophage functions are somehow contributing to the granulocyte response in the synovium.

In contrast to the *op/op* data and the data derived from using antibody to GM-CSF, antibodies to either M-CSF or its receptor failed to suppress the arthritis. The reason for this failure could be that M-CSF, unlike GM-CSF, circulates normally, thereby controlling macrophage lineage development (27). Consistent with this difference, we recently found that exogenous M-CSF was not as potent as GM-CSF in exacerbating disease when either was used to replace IL-1, possibly because of the presence of the endogenous material (Yang YH, Hamilton JA: unpublished observations). It could be that the antibodies to the ligand or its receptor, at the levels administered, could not sufficiently block the action of the endogenous M-CSF. Also, in contrast to the case of the *op/op* mouse, in which numbers of macrophages are reduced at the outset, anti–M-CSF or anti–M-CSF receptor antibody treatment of a normal mouse has to block the function of and/or deplete existing cells in the short time available, and, presumably, also prevent development of new macrophages.

ACKNOWLEDGMENTS

We thank R. Sallay for typing of the manuscript and A. Cook for critical reading of the manuscript.

REFERENCES

1. Hamilton JA, Stanley ER, Burgess AW, Shadduck RK. Stimulation of macrophage plasminogen activator activity by colony-stimulating factors. J Cell Physiol 1980;103:435–45.
2. Alvaro-Gracia JM, Zvaifler NJ, Firestein GS. Cytokines in chronic inflammatory arthritis. IV. Granulocyte/macrophage colony-stimulating factor-mediated induction of class II MHC antigen on human monocytes: a possible role in rheumatoid arthritis. J Exp Med 1989;170:865–75.
3. Hamilton JA. Colony stimulating factors, cytokines and monocyte-macrophages—some controversies (a review). Immunol Today 1993;14:18–24.
4. Firestein GS, Xu WD, Townsend K, Broide D, Alvaro-Gracia J, Glasebrook A, et al. Cytokines in chronic inflammatory arthritis. I. Failure to detect T cell lymphokines (interleukin 2 and interleukin 3) and presence of macrophage colony-stimulating factor (CSF-1) and a novel mast cell growth factor in rheumatoid synovitis. J Exp Med 1988;168:1573–86.
5. Xu WD, Firestein GS, Taetle R, Kaushansky K, Zvaifler NJ. Cytokines in chronic inflammatory arthritis. II. Granulocyte-macrophage colony-stimulating factor in rheumatoid synovial effusions. J Clin Invest 1989;83:876–82.
6. De Vries EG, Willems PH, Biesma B, Stern AC, Limburg PC, Vellenga E. Flare-up of rheumatoid arthritis during GM-CSF treatment after chemotherapy. Lancet 1991;338:517–8.
7. Leizer T, Cebon J, Layton JE, Hamilton JA. Cytokine regulation of colony-stimulating factor production in cultured human synovial fibroblasts: I. Induction of GM-CSF and G-CSF production by interleukin-1 and tumor necrosis factor. Blood 1990;76:1989–96.
8. Campbell IK, Novak U, Cebon J, Layton JE, Hamilton JA. Human articular cartilage and chondrocytes produce hemopoietic colony-stimulating factors in culture in response to IL-1. J Immunol 1991;147:1238–46.
9. Hamilton JA, Filonzi EL, Ianches G. Regulation of macrophage colony-stimulating factor (M-CSF) production in cultured human synovial fibroblasts. Growth Factors 1993;9:157–65.
10. Campbell IK, Ianches G, Hamilton JA. Production of macrophage colony-stimulating factor (M-CSF) by human articular cartilage and chondrocytes: modulation by interleukin-1 and tumor necrosis factor alpha. Biochim Biophys Acta 1993;1182:57–63.
11. Firestein GS. Cytokine networks in rheumatoid arthritis: implications for therapy. Agents Actions Suppl 1995;47:37–51.
12. Hamilton JA. Rheumatoid arthritis: opposing actions of haemopoietic growth factors and slow-acting anti-rheumatic drugs [see comments]. Lancet 1993;342:536–9.
13. Coxon A, Tang T, Mayadas TN. Cytokine-activated endothelial cells delay neutrophil apoptosis in vitro and in vivo: a role for granulocyte/macrophage colony-stimulating factor. J Exp Med 1999;190:923–34.

14. Campbell IK, Bendele A, Smith DA, Hamilton JA. Granulocyte-macrophage colony stimulating factor exacerbates collagen induced arthritis in mice. Ann Rheum Dis 1997;56:364–8.
15. Campbell IK, Rich MJ, Bischof RJ, Dunn AR, Grail D, Hamilton JA. Protection from collagen-induced arthritis in granulocyte-macrophage colony-stimulating factor-deficient mice. J Immunol 1998;61:3639–44.
16. Abd AH, Savage NW, Halliday WJ, Hume DA. The role of macrophages in experimental arthritis induced by Streptococcus agalactiae sonicate: actions of macrophage colony-stimulating factor (CSF-1) and other macrophage-modulating agents. Lymphokine Cytokine Res 1991;10:43–50.
17. Staite ND, Richard KA, Aspar DG, Franz KA, Galinet LA, Dunn CJ. Induction of an acute erosive monarticular arthritis in mice by interleukin-1 and methylated bovine serum albumin. Arthritis Rheum 1990;33:253–60.
18. Feldmann M, Brennan FM, Maini RN. Role of cytokines in rheumatoid arthritis. Annu Rev Immunol 1996;14:397–440.
19. Jorgensen C, Apparailly F, Sany J. Immunological evaluation of cytokine and anticytokine immunotherapy in vivo: what have we learnt? Ann Rheum Dis 1999;58:136–41.
20. Van den Berg WB, Bresnihan B. Pathogenesis of joint damage in rheumatoid arthritis: evidence of a dominant role for interleukin-I. Baillieres Best Pract Res Clin Rheumatol 1999;13:577–97.
21. Cunnane G, Hummel KM, Muller-Ladner U, Gay RE, Gay S. Mechanism of joint destruction in rheumatoid arthritis. Arch Immunol Ther Exp (Warsz) 1998;46:1–7.
22. Bischof RJ, Zafiropoulos D, Hamilton JA, Campbell IK. Exacerbation of acute inflammatory arthritis by the colony-stimulating factors CSF-1 and granulocyte macrophage (GM)-CSF: evidence of macrophage infiltration and local proliferation. Clin Exp Immunol 2000;119:361–7.
23. O'Garra A, Barbis D, Wu J, Hodgkin PD, Abrams J, Howard M. The BCL1 B lymphoma responds to IL-4, IL-5, and GM-CSF. Cell Immunol 1989;123:189–200.
24. Sudo T, Nishikawa S-I, Ogawa M, Kataoka H, Ohno N, Izawa A, et al. Functional hierarchy of c-kit and c-fms in intramarrow production of CFU-M. Oncogene 1995;11:2469–76.
25. Leech M, Metz C, Santos L, Peng T, Holdsworth SR, Bucala R, et al. Involvement of macrophage migration inhibitory factor in the evolution of rat adjuvant arthritis. Arthritis Rheum 1998;41:910–7.
26. Stanley E, Lieschke GJ, Grail D, Metcalf D, Hodgson G, Gall JA, et al. Granulocyte/macrophage colony-stimulating factor-deficient mice show no major perturbation of hematopoiesis but develop a characteristic pulmonary pathology. Proc Natl Acad Sci U S A 1994;91:5592–6.
27. Cecchini MG, Dominguez MG, Mocci S, Wetterwald A, Felix R, Fleisch H, et al. Role of colony stimulating factor-1 in the establishment and regulation of tissue macrophages during postnatal development of the mouse. Development 1994;120:1357–72.
28. Metcalf D. The Florey Lecture, 1991. The colony-stimulating factors: discovery to clinical use. Philos Trans R Soc Lond B Biol Sci 1991;333:147–73.
29. Colotta F, Re F, Polentarutti N, Sozzani S, Mantovani A. Modulation of granulocyte survival and programmed cell death by cytokines and bacterial products. Blood 1992;80:2012–20.
30. Rossi AG, Cousin JM, Dransfield I, Lawson MF, Chilvers ER, Haslett C. Agents that elevate cAMP inhibit human neutrophil apoptosis. Biochem Biophys Res Commun 1995;217:892–9.
31. Brach MA, deVos S, Gruss HJ, Herrmann F. Prolongation of survival of human polymorphonuclear neutrophils by granulocyte-macrophage colony-stimulating factor is caused by inhibition of programmed cell death. Blood 1992;80:2920–4.
32. Wada H, Noguchi Y, Marino MW, Dunn AR, Old LJ. T cell functions in granulocyte/macrophage colony-stimulating factor deficient mice. Proc Natl Acad Sci U S A 1997;94:12557–61.
33. Inaba K, Inaba M, Romani N, Aya H, Deguchi M, Ikehara S, et al. Generation of large numbers of dendritic cells from mouse bone marrow cultures supplemented with granulocyte/macrophage colony-stimulating factor. J Exp Med 1992;176:1693–702.
34. Chang MD, Stanley ER, Khalili H, Chisholm O, Pollard JW. Osteopetrotic (op/op) mice deficient in macrophages have the ability to mount a normal T-cell-dependent immune response. Cell Immunol 1995;162:146–52.
35. Van Lent PL, van den Hoek AE, van den Bersselaar LA, Spanjaards MF, van Rooijen N, Dijkstra CD, et al. In vivo role of phagocytic synovial lining cells in onset of experimental arthritis. Am J Pathol 1993;143:1226–37.
36. Van Lent PLEM, Holthuysen AEM, van den Bersselaar LA, van Rooijen N, Joosten LAB, van de Loo FAJ, et al. Phagocytic lining cells determine local expression of inflammation in type II collagen–induced arthritis. Arthritis Rheum 1996;39:1545–55.
37. Smith JD, Trogan E, Ginsberg M, Grigaux C, Tian J, Miyata M. Decreased atherosclerosis in mice deficient in both macrophage colony-stimulating factor (op) and apolipoprotein E. Proc Natl Acad Sci U S A 1995;92:8264–8.

ARTHRITIS & RHEUMATISM
Vol. 44, No. 1, January 2001, pp 120–127

Early Degradation of Type IX and Type II Collagen with the Onset of Experimental Inflammatory Arthritis

Toshihisa Kojima,[1] Fackson Mwale,[1] Tadashi Yasuda,[1] Christiane Girard,[2] A. Robin Poole,[1] and Sheila Laverty[2]

Objective. **To determine whether following the onset of intraarticular inflammation, there is early damage to articular cartilage, specifically to types II and IX collagen, and the proteoglycan (PG) aggrecan, and whether measurement of the degradation products of these molecules in synovial fluid (SF) and serum may permit the detection of cartilage damage.**

Methods. **A rabbit model of rheumatoid arthritis, antigen (ovalbumin)–induced arthritis, was studied. Articular cartilage samples were analyzed by immunoassays for total type II collagen content, its denaturation and cleavage by collagenases, and for type IX collagen content. PG content was determined by colorimetric assay. In serum and SF, total PG content and collagenase-generated peptides of type II collagen were measured.**

Results. **After 6 days, both the PG content and the NC4 domain of type IX collagen were reduced in femoral and tibial cartilage, concomitant with the onset of arthritis. In only the tibial cartilage did this reduction in PG persist up to day 20. However, denatured type II collagen was increased in all cartilage samples, but only on day 20. In SF, the PG content was significantly reduced on day 20, and products of type II collagen cleavage by collagenase were significantly increased on both day 6 and day 20.**

Conclusion. **This study, which is the first of its kind examining changes in both types II and IX collagen and PG content, reveals early damage to both types of collagen as well as to PG in articular cartilage samples following induction of joint inflammation. SF analyses reveal this early damage and may be of value in the study and treatment of inflammatory arthritic diseases such as rheumatoid arthritis.**

Collagen fibrils of the cartilage matrix principally contain type II collagen, but types XI and IX collagen are present as well, the latter being found on the surface of the fibril (1). Aggrecan is the largest proteoglycan (PG) found in the interfibrillar matrix. The loss of PG and damage to type II collagen, because of its enhanced denaturation and cleavage by collagenase, are principle features of the articular cartilage matrix breakdown in both osteoarthritis (OA) and rheumatoid arthritis (RA) (1–5). Molecular abnormalities involving type IX collagen (6) and type II collagen (7) can each independently cause premature degeneration of human articular cartilage (e.g., in familial OA), demonstrating the importance of these collagens in the maintenance of the structure and function of the cartilage matrix.

It is important to examine both PG and these collagens in studies of early degradation of articular cartilage in arthritis. There is currently no information concerning the relative cleavage and degradation of types II and IX collagen in vitro or in vivo and how these features relate to PG degradation. It has been shown in culture that PG loss precedes cleavage and damage to type II collagen when cartilage degradation is induced by interleukin-1 (8–10). In studying the degradation of articular cartilage, it is important to use in vivo analyses, especially in the early stages of degradation, so that the relative attack on different matrix molecules can be more clearly understood.

We therefore selected a rabbit model of antigen-induced arthritis in which intraarticular inflammation can be induced in a single knee joint and compared with its contralateral control joint. Previous work has re-

Dr. Poole's work was supported by the Medical Council of Canada, Shriners Hospitals for Children, the Canadian Arthritis Network, and the National Institute on Aging, NIH. Dr. Laverty's work was supported by the Canadian Arthritis Network.

[1]Toshihisa Kojima, MD, PhD, Fackson Mwale, PhD, Tadashi Yasuda, MD, PhD, A. Robin Poole, PhD, DSc: McGill University, Montreal, Quebec, Canada; [2]Christiane Girard, DMV, Dipl ACVP, Sheila Laverty, MVB, Dipl ACVS: University of Montreal, St. Hyacinthe, Quebec, Canada.

Address correspondence and reprint requests to Sheila Laverty, MVB, Dipl ACVS, Department of Clinical Sciences, Faculty of Veterinary Medicine, University of Montreal, 3200 rue Sicotte, St. Hyacinthe, Quebec J2S 7C6, Canada.

Submitted for publication May 12, 2000; accepted in revised form August 25, 2000.

vealed that there is early damage to PG in articular cartilage in this model (11) which, in many ways, resembles the intraarticular inflammation seen in RA. Information gained from such studies may therefore be of value in the management of early and established RA. We selected a larger animal since analytic work on inflammatory arthritis in rats and mice (such as antigen-induced arthritis or type II collagen–induced arthritis) is restricted to immunohistochemical analyses of joint cartilage samples. In the rabbit, quantitative immunoanalyses of cartilage changes are possible in view of the increased joint size and therefore increased mass of the articular cartilage that is available for study.

Using immunoanalyses that we recently developed, we demonstrated that following induction of experimental intraarticular inflammation in rabbits, there is early damage to PG (principally aggrecan) and to the collagen fibril in the extracellular matrix of cartilage. This damage involves early increases in collagenase activity, which can be detected by analyses of SF.

MATERIALS AND METHODS

Animals. Male New Zealand white rabbits 16–18 weeks old were used. The experimental protocol was approved by the Animal Care Committee of the Faculty of Veterinary Medicine, University of Montreal.

Development of antigen-induced arthritis. Rabbits were earmarked and randomly assigned to experimental groups. The baseline animals ($n = 5$) were euthanized before immunization. All other rabbits ($n = 12$ per group) were sensitized with an emulsion of 4 mg of ovalbumin (OVA) (chicken egg albumin, grade VI; Sigma, St Louis, MO) in 0.5 ml of Freund's complete adjuvant (Sigma) and 0.5 ml of phosphate buffered saline. The emulsion was administered intradermally, in 100-μl volumes, at 5 intrascapular sites. A similar booster injection (OVA in Freund's incomplete adjuvant) was given 2 weeks later. Four days after the booster injection (day 0), knee joints were challenged with intraarticular (IA) injection of 1.5 mg of OVA in 0.5 ml of saline into the left knee and an equivalent volume of sterile saline alone into the right knee. In the control group, both joints were injected with 0.5 ml of sterile saline alone. Hypnorm, 0.2 ml/kg intramuscularly (fentanyl citrate; Janssen Animal Health, Janssen Pharmaceutica, Beerse, Belgium), was used for neuroleptanalgesia prior to IA injections.

The animals were examined daily for joint swelling. The diameter of the joint was measured at the same site (mediolateral measurement at the level of the proximal limit of the tibial crest) each day for 6 days using 15-cm dial calipers (General, Tool Canada, Pointe Claire, Quebec, Canada). Analgesia with buprenorphine HCl, 0.3 mg/kg subcutaneously (Temgesic; Reckitt & Coleman, Kingston-upon-Hull, UK), was provided for 6 days following IA injection. On day 6 and day 20 following IA injection of OVA, 6 rabbits from each group (OVA-treated and control) were euthanized.

Serum, SF, cartilage, and synovial membrane sampling. Blood samples were obtained on days −21, −11, −4, 3, 6, 10, 17, and 20 from the auricular artery of the ear. Lavage

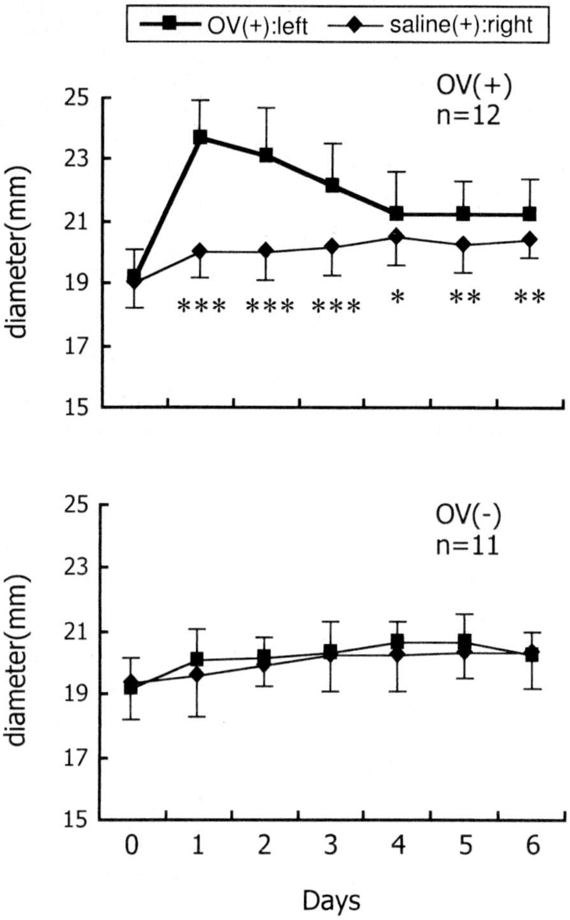

Figure 1. Joint swelling in ovalbumin (OV)–injected (+) and OV-uninjected (−) NZW rabbits. Values are the mean and SD. * = $P < 0.05$, ** = $P < 0.01$, and *** = $P \leq 0.0001$ for left knees versus right knees, by paired t-test.

synoviocentesis was performed immediately after euthanasia, by injecting 1.5 ml of sterile saline into the joint space, followed by 10 flexions and extensions, and immediate synoviocentesis. This was also performed following neuroleptanalgesia with an intramuscular injection of Hypnorm 1 week before IA challenge. Both serum and SF samples were centrifuged at 3,000 revolutions per minute for 20 minutes, and the supernatants were frozen at −70°C until analyzed.

The articular cartilage was harvested by shaving from the patellofemoral and femorotibial surfaces of the femoral condyles and the tibial plateau down to the subchondral bone. Samples were stored at −20°C until analyzed.

Synovial membrane histopathologic evaluation. A specimen of the synovial membrane was collected from each femorotibial joint, lateral to the patella, fixed in 10% buffered formalin, and embedded in paraffin. Six-micrometer–thick sections were stained with hematoxylin–phloxine–saffron. The presence of synoviocyte hyperplasia, synovial membrane erosion, fibrin, fibrosis, inflammatory cell infiltrates (polymorphonuclear cells, macrophages, lymphocytes, or plasma cells), and angiogen-

Table 1. Histopathologic scoring of synovial membranes in OVA-injected and control groups*

Evaluation point, study group	Synovial hyperplasia	Synovial erosions	Fibrin	Polymorpho-nuclear leukocytes	Macrophages	Lymphocytes	Plasma cells	Joint score
Day 6								
OVA-injected animals (n = 6)	1.83 ± 0.41†	1.17 ± 0.75	1.33 ± 0.52	1.33 ± 0.52	0	1.33 ± 0.52†	1.5 ± 0.83	8.5 ± 2.7†
Saline-injected controls (n = 6)	0	0	0	0	0	0	0	0
Day 20								
OVA-injected animals (n = 6)	1.0 ± 0.63	0	0	0.83 ± 0.75	0.33 ± 0.52	0.33 ± 0.52	0.83 ± 0.75	3.3 ± 2.7
Saline-injected controls (n = 5)	0	0	0	0	0	0	0	0

* Values are the mean ± SD. See Materials and Methods for explanation of scoring system.
† $P < 0.05$ versus ovalbumin (OVA)–injected group on day 20.

esis was evaluated and scored semiquantitatively on a scale of 0–3, where 0 = absent, 1 = mild, 2 = moderate, and 3 = severe. A total joint score was obtained by adding the individual scores for each parameter studied (maximum score 18).

Extraction and assay of cartilage for collagenase-cleaved, denatured, and total type II collagen content. The method used to extract Col2-3/4m (4) and Col2-3/4C_{short} (2) epitopes from cartilage was described previously (2,3). The α-chymotrypsin extracts were analyzed for both the collagenase-generated Col2-3/4C_{short} neoepitope and the intrachain hidden Col2-3/4m epitope. The undigested cartilage was incubated overnight at 56°C with proteinase K. The total collagen content in the cartilage was determined from the content of Col2-3/4m in both the α-chymotrypsin and proteinase K digests.

Determination of PG content. The hyaluronidase-digested SF and both the α-chymotrypsin and proteinase K cartilage digests were assayed for glycosaminoglycan, which represents primarily a measure of PG content, using a modification of the colorimetric 1,9-dimethylmethylene blue dye assay (12).

Determination of the NC4 domain of type IX collagen content in the cartilage. The NC4 domain of type IX collagen α1(IX) chain in the cartilage was measured from both the α-chymotrypsin and proteinase K digests using a new immunoassay recently developed in this laboratory (13).

Determination of DNA content in the cartilage. The DNA content of the articular cartilage was measured in the proteinase K digest as described previously (2,14). The contents of Col2-3/4C_{short}, Col2-3/4m, and NC4 epitopes were expressed as moles of peptide per microgram of cartilage DNA. PG content was expressed as micrograms per microgram of cartilage DNA.

Assays of SF and serum for collagen degradation products. SF was digested overnight at 37°C with 0.4 turbidity-reducing units/ml of *Streptomyces* hyaluronidase (Sigma) in 10 m*M* sodium acetate, pH 5.0, with proteinase inhibitors (1 m*M* EDTA, 1 m*M* phenylmethylsulfonyl fluoride, 1 m*M* iodoacetamide, and 5 μg/ml of pepstatin A) to decrease the viscosity of the fluid. This digest and serum were assayed for collagenase-generated neoepitope of type II collagen, Col2-3/4$C_{long\ mono}$ (C2C), using the immunoassay developed in this laboratory (15). The C2C antibody does not cross-react with collagenase-generated neoepitopes of type I collagen, which are also recognized by Col2-3/4C_{short} antibody. We could not use the C2C antibody to determine the collagenase-generated neoepitope of type II collagen in the cartilage because this epitope is digested by α-chymotrypsin. The epitope content recognized by Col2-3/4$C_{long\ mono}$ antibody was expressed as picomoles of peptide per milliliter of SF or serum.

Statistical analysis. The effect of OVA injection was analyzed by comparisons between saline-injected right knee joints and OVA-injected left knee joints by use of paired *t*-tests for analytic data. We also performed paired *t*-tests between the right and left joints in the baseline and control groups to detect possible differences. In serum samples, two-way repeated-measures analysis of variance was fitted with the factors of treatment and time. For histologic analyses, the Mann-Whitney U test was applied.

RESULTS

Findings of clinical evaluation of antigen-induced arthritis. Joint swelling resulted from IA injection of OVA and was clearly detectable up to day 6 and peaking on day 1, compared with saline-injected contralateral joints (Figure 1). No significant between-joint differences were detected in control rabbits. One rabbit in the control group was eliminated during the study because of acquired trauma to the knee during the experimental period.

Findings of histopathologic evaluation of antigen-induced arthritis. The changes observed in OVA-treated animals were characterized by mild-to-moderate synovial hyperplasia with mild-to-moderate inflammation. Polymorphonuclear and plasma cells predominated and were associated with lymphocytes and some macrophages. Mild-to-moderate erosions with exudation of fibrin were observed in 5 animals, 4 of which were noted on day 6. There was no evidence of fibrosis and neoangiogenesis.

The synovial membrane from the saline-injected

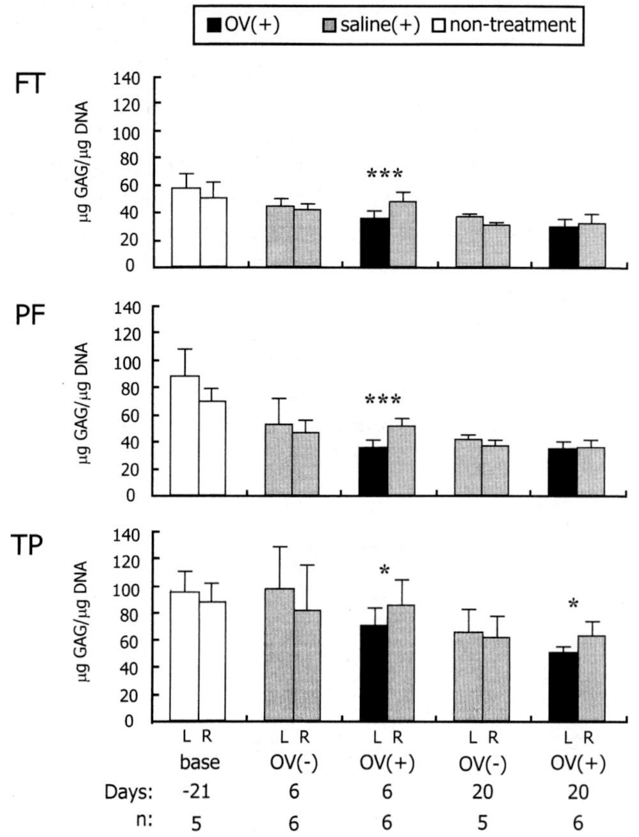

Figure 2. Proteoglycan (PG) content in cartilage from ovalbumin (OV)–injected (+) and OV-uninjected (−; non-treatment) NZW rabbits. PG content in α-chymotrypsin and proteinase K digests of cartilage were determined by dimethylmethylene blue assay. Values are the mean and SD. * = $P < 0.05$ and *** = $P < 0.001$ for left knees versus right knees, by paired *t*-test. FT = femorotibial surface of femoral condyles; PF = patellofemoral surface of femoral condyle; TP = tibial plateau; GAG = glycosaminoglycan; base = baseline group (see Materials and Methods for details); n = number of animals.

right knee joint was normal in all OVA-treated animals. No pathology was observed in the synovia from the left and right joints of the control rabbits (data not shown). The total joint scores in OVA-treated rabbits are shown in Table 1. Scores were higher on day 6 (acute phase) than on day 20 (chronic phase) for each histologic parameter except macrophages.

Findings of cartilage and SF analyses. Results of cartilage analyses were expressed in terms of DNA content since analyses of the DNA contents per wet weight (~1 μg/mg) revealed that there were no significant differences ($P \leq 0.05$) between the left and right knees in any experimental group. *P* values ranged from 0.11 to 0.82 in the femorotibial cartilage, from 0.08 to 0.53 in the patellofemoral cartilage from the femoral condyles, and from 0.11 to 0.49 in the tibial plateau cartilage. Dry weights could not be determined since the drying process causes denaturation of type II collagen.

Findings of PG degradation analyses. Since DNA contents were ~1 μg/mg wet weight, the PG content in control joints was similar to published results for bovine nasal cartilage (10). In uninjected baseline animals (−21 days), we detected no significant differences in cartilage PG content between joints. In OVA-treated rabbits, a reduction in cartilage PG content was detected on day 6 in all IA sites and on day 20 in the tibial plateau of only the OVA-injected joints. Control animals, which did not receive IA injections of OVA, showed no significant differences in cartilage PG content (Figure 2). The progressive decline in PG content with time is a reflection of growth-related changes, since these rabbits had not finished growing.

The release of PG into SF did not reflect the reduction in tissue content. The PG content in SF was significantly decreased in OVA-injected joints on day 20 compared with contralateral saline-injected joints, and although not significantly different, the PG content was also reduced on day 6. In baseline and control rabbits, there was no significant difference between right and left knee joints in terms of PG release into SF (Figure 3).

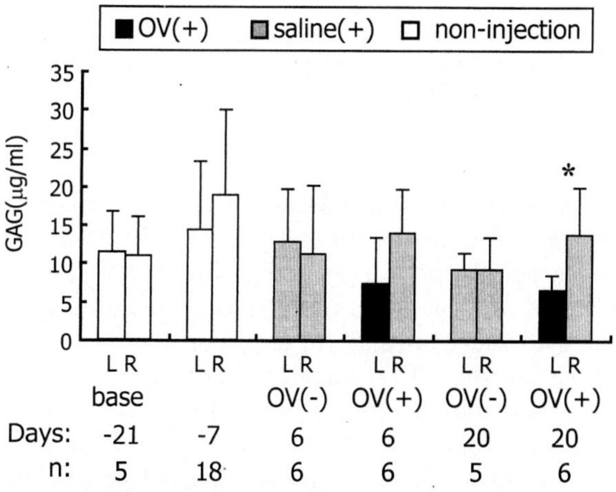

Figure 3. Proteoglycan (PG) content in synovial fluid from ovalbumin (OV)–injected (+) and OV-uninjected (−; non-injection) NZW rabbits. PG content in hyaluronidase digests was determined by dimethylmethylene blue assay. Values are the mean and SD. * = $P < 0.05$ for left knees versus right knees, by paired *t*-test. GAG = glycosaminoglycan; base = baseline group (see Materials and Methods for details); n = number of animals.

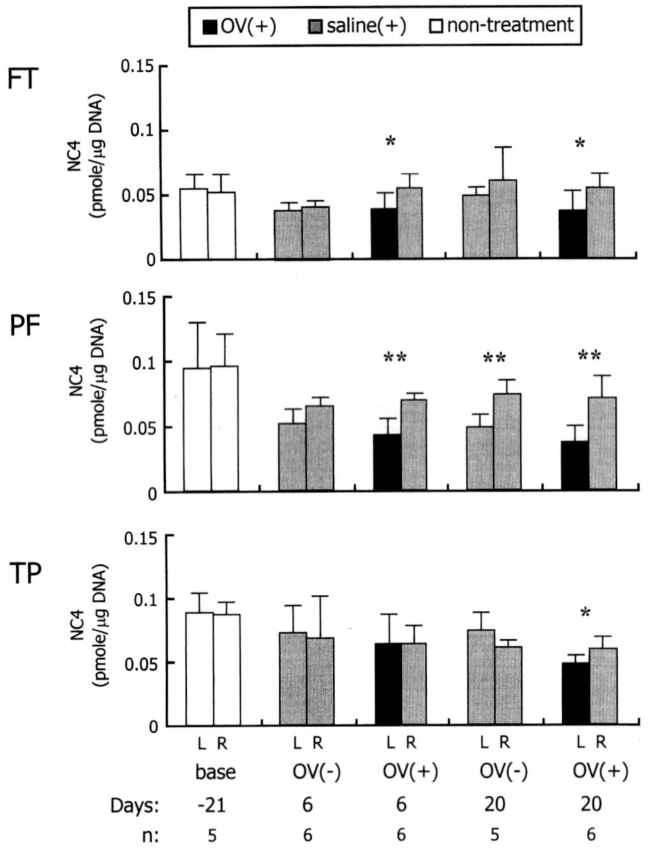

Figure 4. Content of the NC4 domain of type IX collagen in cartilage from ovalbumin (OV)–injected (+) and OV-uninjected (−; non-treatment) NZW rabbits. NC4 domain content in α-chymotrypsin and proteinase K digests was determined by immunoassay. Values are the mean and SD. * = $P < 0.05$ and ** = $P < 0.01$ for left knees versus right knees, by paired *t*-test. FT = femorotibial surface of femoral condyles; PF = patellofemoral surface of femoral condyle; TP = tibial plateau; base = baseline group (see Materials and Methods for details); n = number of animals.

Content and degradation of type IX collagen. In OVA-treated animals, the cartilage NC4 domain content was significantly decreased in the femorotibial and patellofemoral cartilage of OVA-injected joints compared with the contralateral joints on day 6 and in all sites within the OVA-injected joints on day 20. In baseline and control rabbits, no significant differences in the NC4 content were detected between right and left knees, except in the patellofemoral cartilage on day 20 (Figure 4).

Collagenase-cleaved, denatured, and total type II collagen content. No significant differences in the total type II collagen content of articular cartilage were observed between joints in the baseline, control, and OVA-treated groups during the experimental period (Figure 5). Cleavage of type II collagen by collagenase(s) in the cartilage was also not significantly different in either the baseline, control, or OVA-treated rabbits when comparing right and left knees (Figure 6). However, on day 20, an increase in denatured type II collagen was clearly detectable in all compartments of the OVA-treated injected joints compared with the contralateral saline-injected joints. No such differences were observed at any other time in the baseline, control, and OVA-treated rabbits (Figure 7).

The denatured collagen content represented ~2.5% of the total collagen in control cartilage samples. The content of denatured and type II collagen (4) and collagen cleavage products (2,10) in control cartilage was similar to published values for adult human and

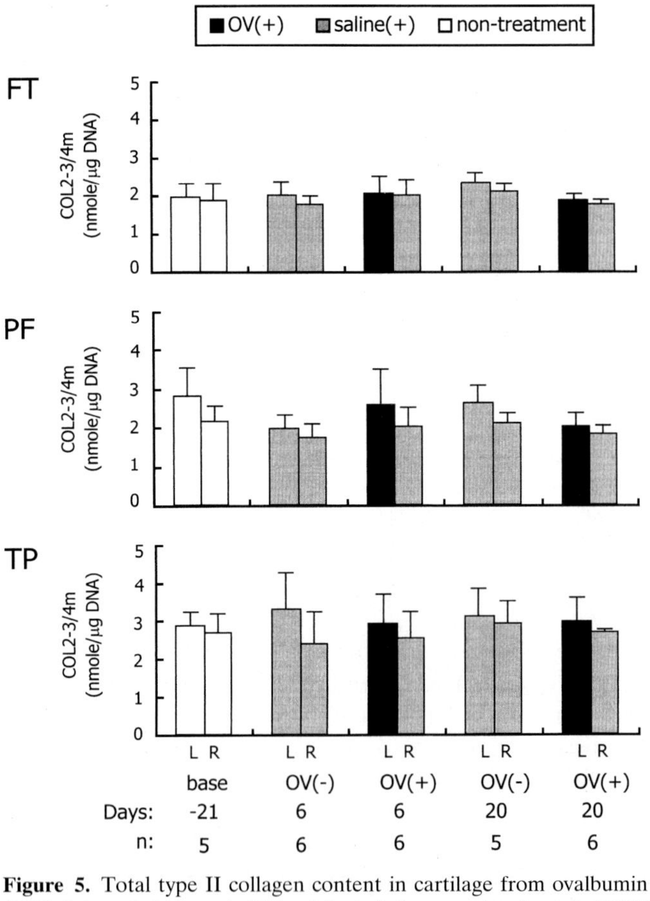

Figure 5. Total type II collagen content in cartilage from ovalbumin (OV)–injected (+) and OV-uninjected (−; non-treatment) NZW rabbits. The combined COL2-3/4m epitope content in α-chymotrypsin and proteinase K digests was determined by immunoassay. Values are the mean and SD. There were no significant differences between left and right knees in any group, by paired *t*-test. FT = femorotibial surface of femoral condyles; PF = patellofemoral surface of femoral condyle; TP = tibial plateau; base = baseline group (see Materials and Methods for details); n = number of animals.

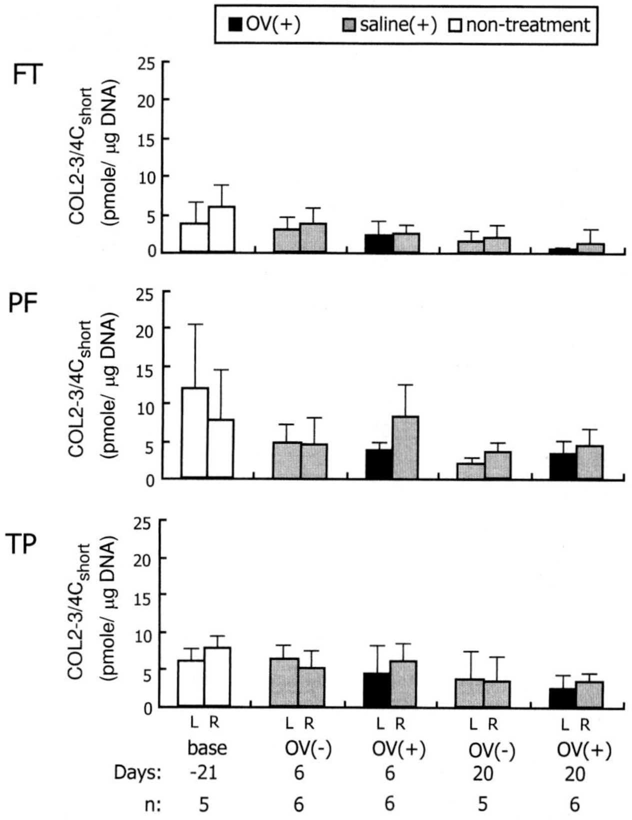

Figure 6. Content of cleaved type II collagen in cartilage from ovalbumin (OV)–injected (+) and OV-uninjected (−; non-treatment) NZW rabbits. The COL2-3/4C_{short} epitope content in α-chymotrypsin digests was determined by immunoassay. Values are the mean and SD. There were no significant differences between left and right knees in any group, by paired t-test. FT = femorotibial surface of femoral condyles; PF = patellofemoral surface of femoral condyle; TP = tibial plateau; base = baseline group (see Materials and Methods for details); n = number of animals.

bovine articular cartilage (4,10). In normal cartilage, the collagenase-cleaved collagen represented ~15% of the denatured collagen. This often decreased severalfold with cartilage damage, reflecting a selective loss of the cleavage neoepitope.

In SF, this loss from cartilage was reflected by a significant increase in the collagenase-generated neoepitope in OVA-injected joints compared with contralateral saline-injected joints on both day 6 and day 20 (Figure 8). There was no significant difference in the SF content of the neoepitope in the baseline and control groups. These changes were not reflected in serum.

DISCUSSION

Little is known about whether there is damage to collagen as well as to PGs in articular cartilage following the onset of inflammation such as that which occurs in inflammatory joint diseases such as RA. Recent analyses of human articular cartilage, however, have revealed that type II collagen is degraded within months after rupture of the anterior cruciate ligament, which can frequently result in the development of a posttraumatic OA (16). Early changes in articular cartilage can be conveniently studied in animal models.

Previous work has focused mainly on analyses of changes involving the PG aggrecan (11,17). In the present study, we determined how this inflammation affects not only this PG, but also types II and IX collagen of the collagen fibril. We elected to analyze changes on days 6 and 20 since those would likely reflect early damage to cartilage at the end of the initial acute phase of inflammation (days 0–4) and during the early chronic phase (days 4–20). In other studies of joint inflammation in

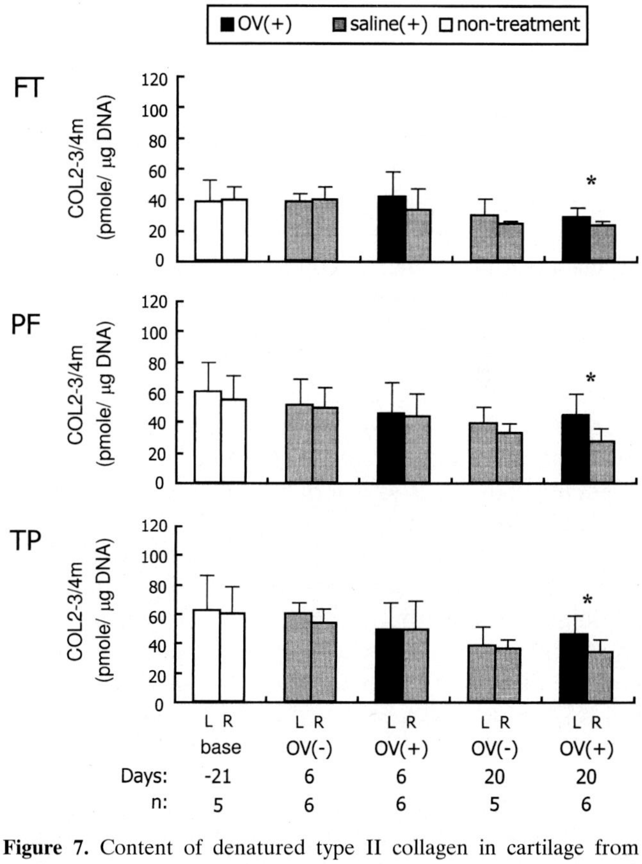

Figure 7. Content of denatured type II collagen in cartilage from ovalbumin (OV)–injected (+) and OV-uninjected (−; non-treatment) NZW rabbits. The COL2-3/4m epitope content in α-chymotrypsin digests was determined by immunoassay. Values are the mean and SD. * = $P < 0.05$ for left knees versus right knees, by paired t-test. FT = femorotibial surface of femoral condyles; PF = patellofemoral surface of femoral condyle; TP = tibial plateau; base = baseline group (see Materials and Methods for details); n = number of animals.

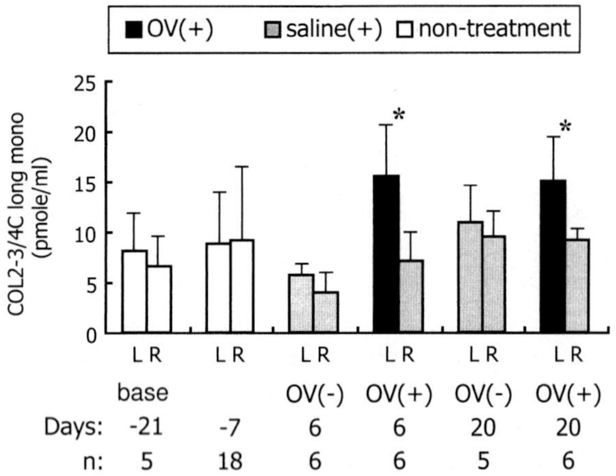

Figure 8. Collagenase-generated peptides of type II collagen in synovial fluid from ovalbumin (OV)–injected (+) and OV-uninjected (−; non-treatment) NZW rabbits. The COL2-3/4C$_{\text{long mono}}$ epitope in synovial fluid after hyaluronidase digestion was determined by immunoassay. Values are the mean and SD. * = $P < 0.05$ for left knees versus right knees, by paired *t*-test. base = baseline group (see Materials and Methods for details); n = number of animals.

rats, we have observed evidence of early damage to articular cartilage in the acute phase but more pronounced subsequent damage during the development of joint destruction (15). Moreover, recent studies of mice have revealed the importance of conducting longitudinal analyses to identify the progressive involvement of proteinases in the development of articular cartilage damage (17–19). Articular cartilage was analyzed to determine whether there are compartmental differences in the knee in response to IA inflammation, as has been observed by other investigators in murine studies (18,19). In addition, we examined body fluids to determine whether early changes are also reflected in these sites.

Only those joints injected intraarticularly with OVA showed inflammation and damage to articular cartilage. Animals that did not receive IA injections of OVA showed no differences between joints, except in the case of type IX collagen, where a reduced content of the NC4 domain was observed in the left knee joints of control animals on day 20. We have no explanation for this difference.

The NC4 domain of type IX collagen protrudes from the surface of the type II collagen fibril. It has been suggested that this collagen may provide a molecular link between the fibrils and other interfibrillar matrix components such as PG (20). The molar ratio of the NC4 domain to that of type II collagen is ~1:30–40 × 10^3. This very low level contrasts with a much higher content of this collagen as purified from nonarticular human hyaline cartilage samples, where a content of ~5% type IX and 90% type II collagen has been reported (21). This would translate into a molar ratio of type IX:type II of ~1:15. However, using the same methodology as we used here, we have determined that in cultured bovine growth plate cartilage, the minimal molar ratio of type IX collagen bearing the NC4 domain to type II collagen is ~1:50 (13), indicating that the content of the type IX collagen NC4 domain is much lower in rabbit articular cartilage than in other cartilages examined to date.

Our studies reveal that loss of the NC4 domain is an early event that accompanies PG loss in most compartments and precedes detectable damage to type II collagen within the cartilage. However, our SF analyses revealed that type II collagen cleavage by collagenase was indeed an early event, in that it occurred when type IX collagen and PG were first degraded and lost from the cartilage. However, this increased cleavage was never detectable in articular cartilage until day 20, when we observed increased denaturation, which results from collagen cleavage. The lack of detection of the cleavage product in cartilage likely results from rapid proteolysis of the denatured α chains of the three-quarter and one-quarter fragments, which are then susceptible to cleavage by proteinases such as matrix metalloproteinase 1 (MMP-1), MMP-2, MMP-3, MMP-9, and MMP-13.

In recent studies of the intraarticular degeneration of articular cartilage in the mouse, the induction of increased denaturation (18) and collagenase cleavage (18,19) of type II collagen were observed immunohistochemically as early events that accompanied cleavage of aggrecan by the metalloproteinase and aggrecanase(s) (19). These changes can vary according to the joint compartment (18), as was the case in our studies. The nature of the collagenase(s) involved in the cleavage of type II collagen in the present studies remains to be established. Recently, we have found evidence to indicate that chondrocytes utilize primarily collagenase 3 (MMP-13) in collagen cleavage of bovine (induced by interleukin-1α) (10) and human (22) OA articular cartilage. In rabbit inflammatory arthritis, collagenase 1 (MMP-1) and MMP-13 may also be contributed by activated synovial cells (23).

How type IX collagen is degraded is not known. But MMP-3, which is involved in PG degradation (19), has been reported to be capable of cleaving type IX collagen within its NC2 domain (24). A cleavage site produced by an unknown proteinase has also been identified close to or within the NC4 domain (13).

SF analyses of PG did not reflect the reduction

in PG content in articular cartilage. Only on day 20 were significant differences observed, and then, in contrast to earlier reports, PG was reduced. This could be explained if the inflammation resulted in the release of PG as a product of degradation of newly synthesized molecules. Inflammation has been shown to inhibit PG aggrecan synthesis via induction of interleukin-1 (17). Thus, it would reduce the substrate available for proteolysis. Similar observations of a reduction of PG aggrecan have been made in SF from patients with OA, where the PG content was inversely related to joint inflammation (25).

In conclusion, there is rapid and extensive extracellular matrix degradation involving both PG and collagens in articular cartilage that is caused by joint inflammation in the early phase of antigen-induced arthritis in rabbits. Degradation of both collagen fibrils and PG are also reflected in the SF, but collagen cleavage by collagenase is detected much earlier. Analyses of SF of humans with arthritis may provide an opportunity to study early damage to articular cartilage in diseases such as in RA.

REFERENCES

1. Poole AR. Cartilage in health and disease. In: Koopman W, editor. Arthritis and allied conditions. Baltimore (MD): Williams & Wilkins; 1997. p. 255–308.
2. Billinghurst RC, Dahlberg L, Ionescu M, Reiner A, Bourne R, Rorabeck C, et al. Enhanced cleavage of type II collagen by collagenases in osteoarthritic articular cartilage. J Clin Invest 1997;99:1534–45.
3. Dodge GR, Poole AR. Immunohistochemical detection and immunochemical analysis of type II collagen degradation in human normal, rheumatoid and osteoarthritic articular cartilages and in explants of bovine articular cartilage cultured with interleukin 1. J Clin Invest 1989;83:647–61.
4. Hollander AP, Heathfield TF, Webber C, Iwata Y, Bourne R, Rorabeck C, et al. Increased damage to type II collagen in osteoarthritic articular cartilage detected by a new immunoassay. J Clin Invest 1994;93:1722–32.
5. Hollander AP, Pidoux I, Reiner A, Rorabeck C, Bourne R, Poole AR. Damage to type II collagen in aging and osteoarthritis starts at the articular surface, originates around chondrocytes, and extends into the cartilage with progressive degeneration. J Clin Invest 1995;96:2859–69.
6. Paassilta P, Lohiniva J, Annunen S, Bonaventure J, Le Merrer M, Pai L. et al. Col 9A3: a third locus for multiple epiphyseal dysplasia. Am J Hum Genet 1999;64:1036–44.
7. Ala-Kokko L, Baldwin CT, Moskowitz RW, Prockop DJ. Single base mutation in the type II procollagen gene (COL2A1) as a cause of primary osteoarthritis associated with a mild chondrodysplasia. Proc Natl Acad Sci U S A 1990;87:6565–8.
8. Kozaci LD, Buttle DJ, Hollander AP. Degradation of type II collagen, but not proteoglycan, correlates with metalloproteinase activity in cartilage explant cultures. Arthritis Rheum 1997;40: 164–74.
9. Dingle JT, Horsfield P, Fell HB, Barratt MEJ. Breakdown of proteoglycan and collagen induced in pig articular cartilage in organ culture. Ann Rheum Dis 1995;34:303–11.
10. Billinghurst RC, Wu W, Ionescu M, Reiner A, Dahlberg L, Chen J, et al. Comparison of the degradation of type II collagen and proteoglycan in nasal and articular cartilages induced by interleukin-1 and the selective inhibition of type II collagen cleavage by collagenase. Arthritis Rheum 2000;43:664–72.
11. Pettipher ER, Henderson B, Hardingham T, Ratcliffe A. Cartilage proteoglycan depletion in acute and chronic antigen-induced arthritis. Arthritis Rheum 1989;32:601–7.
12. Farndale R, Buttle DJ, Barrett AJ. Improved quantitation and discrimination of sulphated glycosaminoglycans by use of dimethylmethylene blue. Biochim Biophys Acta 1986;883:173–7.
13. Mwale F, Billinghurst RC, Wu W, Alini M, Webber C, Reiner A, et al. Selective assembly and remodelling of collagens II and IX associated with expression of the chondrocyte hypertrophic phenotype. Dev Dyn 2000;218:648–62.
14. Labarca C, Paigen K. A simple, rapid, and sensitive DNA assay procedure. Anal Biochem 1980;102:344–52.
15. Song X-Y, Zeng L, Jin W, Thompson J, Mizel DE, Lei K-J, et al. Secretory leukocyte protease inhibitor suppresses the inflammation and joint damage of bacterial cell wall-induced arthritis. J Exp Med 1999;190:535–42.
16. Price JS, Till SH, Bickerstaff DR, Bayliss MT, Hollander AP. Degradation of cartilage type II collagen precedes the onset of osteoarthritis following anterior cruciate ligament rupture. Arthritis Rheum 1999;42:2390–8.
17. Van de Loo FA, Arntz OJ, Otterness IG, van den Berg WB. Protection against cartilage proteoglycan synthesis inhibition by antiinterleukin 1 antibodies in experimental arthritis. J Rheumatol 1992;19:348–56.
18. Stoop R, van der Kraan PM, Buma P, Hollander AP, Billinghurst CR, Poole AR, et al. Denaturation of type II collagen in articular cartilage in experimental murine arthritis: evidence for collagen degradation in both reversible and irreversible cartilage damage. J Pathol 1999;188:329–37.
19. Van Meurs J, van Lent P, Stoop R, Holthuysen A, Singer I, Bayne E, et al. Cleavage of aggrecan at the Asn^{341}–Phe^{342} site coincides with the initiation of collagen damage in murine antigen-induced arthritis. Arthritis Rheum 1999;42:2074–84.
20. Vasios G, Nishimura I, Konomi H, van der Rest M, Ninomiya Y, Olsen BR. Cartilage type IX collagen-proteoglycan contains a large amino-terminal globular domain encoded by multiple exons. J Biol Chem 1988;263:2324–9.
21. Diab M, Wu J-J, Shapiro F, Eyre D. Abnormality of type IX collagen in a patient with diastrophic dysplasia. Am J Med Gen 1994;49:402–9.
22. Dahlberg L, Billinghurst RC, Manner P, Nelson F, Webb G, Ionescu M, et al. Selective enhancement of collagenase-mediated cleavage of resident type II collagen in cultured osteoarthritic cartilage and arrest with a synthetic inhibitor that spares collagenase 1 (matrix metalloproteinase 1). Arthritis Rheum 2000;43: 673–82.
23. Vincenti MP, Coon CI, Mengshol JA, Yocum S, Mitchell P, Brinckerhoff CE. Cloning of the gene for interstitial collagenase-3 (matrix metalloproteinase-13) from rabbit synovial fibroblasts: differential expression with collagenase-1 (matrix metalloproteinase-1). Biochem J 1998;331:341–6.
24. Wu JJ, Lark MW, Chun LE, Eyre DR. Sites of stromelysin cleavage in collagen types II, IX, X, and XI of cartilage. J Biol Chem 1991;266:5625–8.
25. Poole AR, Ionescu M, Swan A, Dieppe PA. Changes in cartilage metabolism in arthritis are reflected by altered serum and synovial fluid levels of the cartilage proteoglycan aggrecan: implications for pathogenesis. J Clin Invest 1994;94:25–33.

ARTHRITIS & RHEUMATISM
Vol. 44, No. 1, January 2001, pp 128–137

Disease-Modifying Activity of SB 273005, an Orally Active, Nonpeptide $\alpha_v\beta_3$ (Vitronectin Receptor) Antagonist, in Rat Adjuvant-Induced Arthritis

Alison M. Badger, Simon Blake, Rasesh Kapadia, Susanta Sarkar, Joshua Levin, Barbara A. Swift, Sandy J. Hoffman, George B. Stroup, William H. Miller, Maxine Gowen, and Michael W. Lark

Objective. **To evaluate the effects of SB 273005, a potent, orally active nonpeptide antagonist of the integrin $\alpha_v\beta_3$ vitronectin receptor, on joint integrity in rats with adjuvant-induced arthritis (AIA).**

Methods. **Male Lewis rats with AIA were orally dosed either prophylactically (days 0–20) or therapeutically (days 10–20) with SB 273005. Efficacy was determined by measurement of paw inflammation, assessment of bone mineral density using dual-energy x-ray absorptiometry (DEXA), magnetic resonance imaging (MRI), and histologic evaluation.**

Results. **SB 273005 is a potent antagonist of the closely related integrins, $\alpha_v\beta_3$ (Ki = 1.2 n*M*) and $\alpha_v\beta_5$ (Ki = 0.3 n*M*). When SB 273005 was administered prophylactically to AIA rats twice per day, it inhibited paw edema at doses of 10, 30, and 60 mg/kg, by 40%, 50%, and 52%, respectively. Therapeutic administration twice daily was also effective, and a reduction in paw edema was observed at 30 mg/kg and 60 mg/kg of the antagonist (by 36% and 48%, respectively). SB 273005 was also effective when administered once per day, both prophylactically and therapeutically. Significant improvement in joint integrity in treated rats was shown using DEXA and MRI analyses. These findings were confirmed histologically, and significant protection of bone, cartilage, and soft tissue was observed within the joint.**

Conclusion. **Symptoms of AIA in rats were significantly reduced by either prophylactic or therapeutic treatment with the $\alpha_v\beta_3$ antagonist, SB 273005. Measurements of paw inflammation and of bone, cartilage, and soft tissue structure indicated that this compound exerts a protective effect on joint integrity and thus appears to have disease-modifying properties.**

Alison M. Badger, PhD, Simon Blake, PhD, Rasesh Kapadia, PhD (current address: Scanco USA, Inc., Wayne, Pennsylvania), Susanta Sarkar, PhD, Joshua Levin, PhD, Barbara A. Swift, BS, Sandy J. Hoffman, BS, George B. Stroup, MS, William H. Miller, PhD, Maxine Gowen, PhD, Michael W. Lark, PhD: SmithKline Beecham Pharmaceuticals, King of Prussia, Pennsylvania.

Address correspondence and reprint requests to Alison M. Badger, PhD, SmithKline Beecham Pharmaceuticals, 709 Swedeland Road, King of Prussia, PA 19406.

Submitted for publication May 31, 2000; accepted in revised form September 20, 2000.

Alpha$_v$beta$_3$ is a member of the integrin family of adhesion molecules. It is a 160/85-kd heterodimer that mediates cell adhesion to extracellular matrix and serum proteins by recognition of the arg-gly-asp (RGD) sequence. This integrin is expressed by proliferating and migrating endothelial cells (1) and has been proposed to play a role in angiogenesis and neovascularization (2,3). Alpha$_v$beta$_3$ is also expressed by malignant melanoma cells and its expression appears to correlate with tumor progression (4). Antagonists of this receptor have been shown to promote tumor regression by inducing apoptosis of angiogenic blood vessels (5–7), and antibodies generated against the receptor block human breast cancer growth and angiogenesis in human skin (8).

High-level expression of $\alpha_v\beta_3$ has also been shown on bone-resorbing osteoclasts, and this appears to play an essential role in mediating the attachment of these cells to bone matrix to allow active bone resorption (9–12). Antagonism of the receptor with neutralizing antibodies (13) or with small peptide inhibitors (14–16) has proven effective in inhibiting bone resorption in animal models of osteopenia. Unlike $\alpha_v\beta_3$, which is expressed on mature osteoclasts, $\alpha_v\beta_5$ is expressed on osteoclast precursors and has been proposed to play a role in osteoclast differentiation (17). It was recently reported that small nonpeptide $\alpha_v\beta_3/\alpha_v\beta_5$ inhibitors are effective in the ovariectomized (ovx) rat model of bone resorption (18,19). Several studies from our laboratories have demonstrated that orally available antagonists prevent bone loss in both in vitro and in vivo models of bone resorption (19–22), and these agents show great promise as therapeutic agents for the treatment of osteoporosis.

In the therapeutic area of rheumatoid arthritis (RA), compounds with the ability to inhibit osteoclast-mediated bone resorption as well as angiogenesis have shown high potential. An angiogenesis inhibitor, AGM-1470, has been shown to inhibit joint inflammation and disease severity in the adjuvant-induced arthritis (AIA) rat model (23) and in a rat model of collagen-induced arthritis, when used both alone and in combination with cyclosporin A (24). In addition, it has recently been shown that an $\alpha_v\beta_3$ antagonist has beneficial effects in a rabbit model of inflammatory arthritis (25). In these studies, intraarticular administration of a cyclic peptide antagonist of $\alpha_v\beta_3$ to rabbits with antigen-induced arthritis, early in disease, inhibited synovial angiogenesis and reduced inflammatory cell infiltration, pannus formation, and cartilage erosions. These results, along with the studies showing protection of bone in the ovx rat, suggested to us that these molecules might be effective in AIA in the rat. This animal model of RA displays an aggressive inflammatory component and destructive joint disease. In the studies reported herein we show that SB 273005, a potent antagonist of the $\alpha_v\beta_3$ and $\alpha_v\beta_5$ integrins, inhibits both paw edema and destruction of bone and cartilage in AIA.

MATERIALS AND METHODS

Animals. Male, inbred Lewis rats were obtained from Charles River Breeding Laboratories (Raleigh, NC). Within any given experiment, only animals of the same age were used. All experimental procedures were in accordance with protocols approved by the SmithKline Beecham Institutional Animal Care and Use Committee, and met or exceeded the standards of the American Association for the Accreditation of Laboratory Animal Care, the United States Department of Health and Human Services, and all local and federal animal welfare laws.

Materials. SB 273005 (Figure 1) was synthesized at SmithKline Beecham Pharmaceuticals (20). For in vivo experiments, SB 273005 was administered orally in 1% methyl cellulose, adjusted to pH 3.5 (Sigma, St. Louis, MO).

Induction of arthritis. AIA was induced by a single injection of 0.75 mg of *Mycobacterium butyricum* (Difco, Detroit, MI), suspended in paraffin oil, into the base of the tail of male Lewis rats, ages 6–8 weeks and weighing 160–180 gm. Hind-paw volumes were measured by a water displacement method on day 20 (26). Test compounds were homogenized in

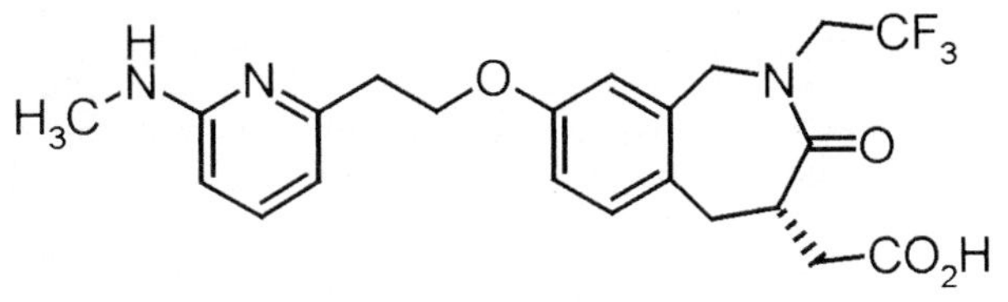

Figure 1. Structure of SB 273005.

1% methyl cellulose and administered orally in a volume of 10 ml/kg. Control animals were administered vehicle alone. Two dosing protocols were used: prophylactic dosing (1, 3, 10, 30, and 60 mg/kg/day either once or twice daily) initiated on the day of adjuvant injection, and therapeutic administration initiated on day 10 after injection.

Change in paw volume is presented as the mean and SEM percentage inhibition of hind-paw edema in 10–12 animals per group, which was calculated as follows:

$$\%\ \text{inhibition} = 1 - \left[\frac{\text{AIA (treated)} - \text{non-AIA control}}{\text{AIA (control)} - \text{non-AIA control}}\right] \times 100.$$

For statistical analysis, the paw volumes of AIA rats treated with SB 273005 were compared with those of the untreated controls (AIA and non-AIA) by Student's *t*-test.

Bone mineral density (BMD) measurement. Animals were killed on day 21 and the hind limbs were removed and fixed in 70% ethanol. The BMD of the distal tibia was determined by dual-energy x-ray absorptiometry (DEXA) using the Hologic QDR-1000 equipped with high-resolution scanning software. Quality control of the instrument was carried out each day prior to sample analysis by scanning both a human anthropomorphic spine phantom (low resolution) and the lumbar portion of a rat spine (high resolution), both of which were embedded in methylmethacrylate. All high-resolution scans were carried out with the sample placed on top of an acrylic block, 1.5 inches deep. The x-ray beam was collimated to a diameter of 1.27 mm and line spacing and point resolution were 0.25 mm and 0.127 mm, respectively.

Scans were made of the distal tibia region of bones that had been excised and stored in 70% ethanol in a square plastic container. The depth of the liquid was constant for all samples and was sufficient to cover the limbs by ~0.5 inches. BMD, as well as bone mineral content (BMC) and bone area, were determined for the distal tibia. The region of interest was defined as the area between a line drawn parallel to the proximal edge of the calcaneus and a second line drawn perpendicular to the long axis of the tibia, midway between the first line and the point where the tibia meets the fibula. The point of connection between the fibula and tibia had to be approximated in some samples with low BMD. The width of the region of interest was kept constant between samples.

Magnetic resonance imaging (MRI). All MRI studies were carried out on a 9.4-Tesla AMX spectrometer with microimaging accessories (Bruker Instruments, Billerica, MA). Coronal sections (250-μm thick) of rat tibiotarsal joints were imaged with an in-plane resolution of 70 × 70 μm. A repetition time of 1 second and an echo time of 7.5 ms were used, with a data matrix of 256 × 256. The morphologic changes in the joint architecture of the AIA rats were compared with those in the normal (non-AIA) controls and with those in the AIA rats treated with SB 273005. The joints were graded by a blinded observer (RK), and joint integrity was expressed as the percentage of joints with 1) no protection (i.e., severe disease similar to that in the AIA controls), 2) moderate protection, or 3) significant protection (i.e., similar to that in the non-AIA control animals).

Histology. Hind-limb tibiotalus joints from the following groups of rats were evaluated and scored for histologic changes: 4 normal rats, 11 rats with AIA, and 2 groups of 12 rats with AIA treated with SB 273005 at either 60 mg/kg or 30 mg/kg once per day. Rats were killed on day 21 by CO_2 administration, and the hind legs were fixed in formalin and decalcified in Cal-Rite (Richard-Allen Scientific, Kalamazoo, MI). The paws were then removed from the legs at the distal tibial diaphysis. After routine processing, the samples were embedded and coronal sections were cut in the plane midway through the tibiotalus and talartarsal joints. Sections were stained with Safranin O and counterstained with fast green.

The histologic characteristics of the bone and articular cartilage/periarticular soft tissue were scored separately by a blinded observer (SB). The bone was graded as follows: 0 = normal, 1 = subperiosteal fibrosis with periosteal woven bone formation, 2 = definite marrow inflammation, endosteal and trabecular bone resorption, and periosteal woven bone formation with osteophytes, 3 = extensive marrow inflammation with concomitant endosteal and trabecular bone resorption, and extensive periosteal woven bone formation with osteophytes, and 4 = marrow replaced by granulation tissue, little or no trabecular bone remaining, woven bone in marrow cavity, extensive obliteration of cortical contours by osteoclastic resorption, and cortex usually breached at the metaphysis. The cartilage/synovium was graded as follows: 0 = normal, 1 = mild lymphocytic infiltration of the synovium and surrounding tissues, 2 = synovial fibrosis and edema, partial lymphocytic infiltration of the joint space, and minor pannus erosion of the cartilage, and 3 = extensive infiltration of the joint space, fibrous ankylosis of the joints, peripheral and subchondral cartilage erosion, and extensive fibrosis of soft tissue with regional necrotic liquefaction.

RESULTS

Effect of prophylactic and therapeutic treatment with SB 273005 in AIA rats. *Paw inflammation.* The effect of SB 273005 was evaluated using the prophylactic dosing protocol, in which compound was administered to male Lewis rats starting on the day of adjuvant injection. SB 273005 was administered twice daily in acidified 1% methyl cellulose, and paw inflammation was measured on day 20 after adjuvant injection. Hind-paw inflammation was effectively inhibited at SB 273005 dose levels of 60 mg/kg (by 52%), 30 mg/kg (by 50%), and 10 mg/kg (by 40%) (all $P < 0.001$ versus controls) (Figure 2A). Although no clear dose-response curve was observed in this experiment, there was a statistically significant difference between the 52% inhibition in the group treated prophylactically with 60 mg/kg and the 40% inhibition achieved with 10 mg/kg ($P < 0.05$).

SB 273005 was also tested in the AIA rat using a therapeutic dosing protocol, which was used to more closely represent the clinical setting. In these experiments, rats were immunized with adjuvant on day 0 and treated with compound twice daily on days 10–20. Using this protocol, hind-paw inflammation was reduced at 60 mg/kg (by 48%) and 30 mg/kg (by 36%) of SB 273005 (both $P < 0.001$ versus controls), but not at 10 mg/kg (13% reduction) (P not significant versus controls) (Figure 2B).

Inhibition of hind-paw inflammation was also

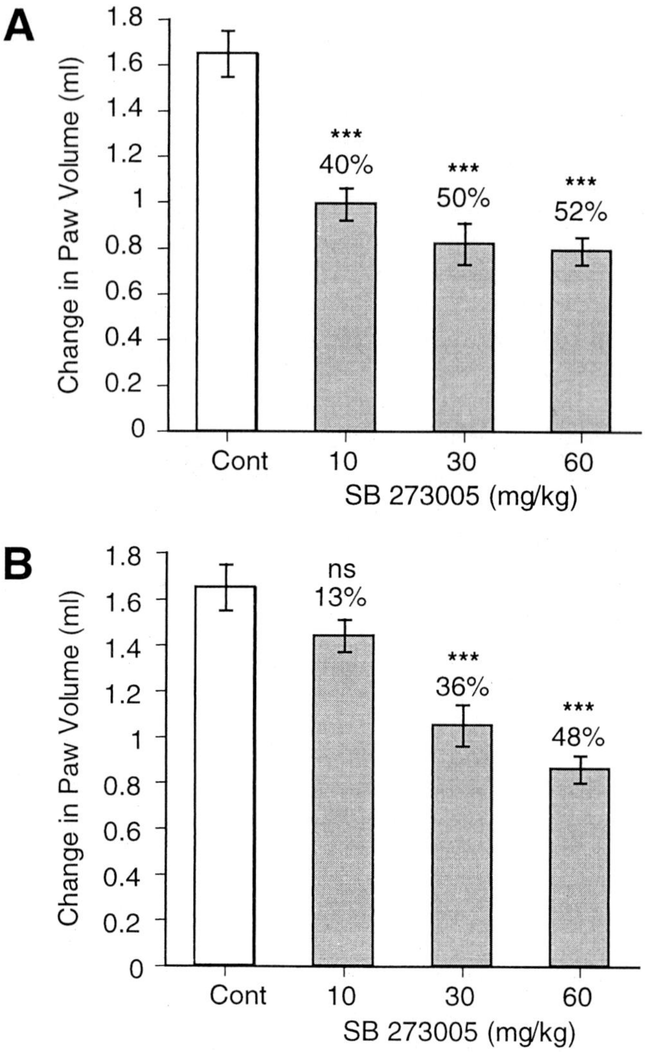

Figure 2. Inhibition of paw edema in Lewis rats with adjuvant-induced arthritis (AIA), in which rats were orally dosed with SB 273005 at 10, 30, and 60 mg/kg, twice daily, in 1% methyl cellulose, during days 0–20 in the prophylactic protocol (**A**) or days 10–20 in the therapeutic protocol (**B**). Bars show the mean and SEM of 12 rats per group. Treated groups were compared with the untreated AIA controls (Cont) by Student's t test. *** = $P < 0.001$. ns = not significant.

observed when SB 273005 was administered prophylactically and therapeutically only once per day, although this was somewhat less effective than the twice-daily administration. With the prophylactic protocol, inhibition was observed at 60 mg/kg (by 40%), 30 mg/kg (by 28%), 10 mg/kg (by 30%) (all $P < 0.001$ versus controls), and 3 mg/kg (by 18%) ($P < 0.01$ versus controls) (Figure 3A). Inhibition following therapeutic administration was observed at 60 mg/kg (by 22%), 30 mg/kg (by 24%) (both $P < 0.001$ versus controls), and 10 mg/kg (by 19%) ($P < 0.05$ versus controls) (Figure 3B).

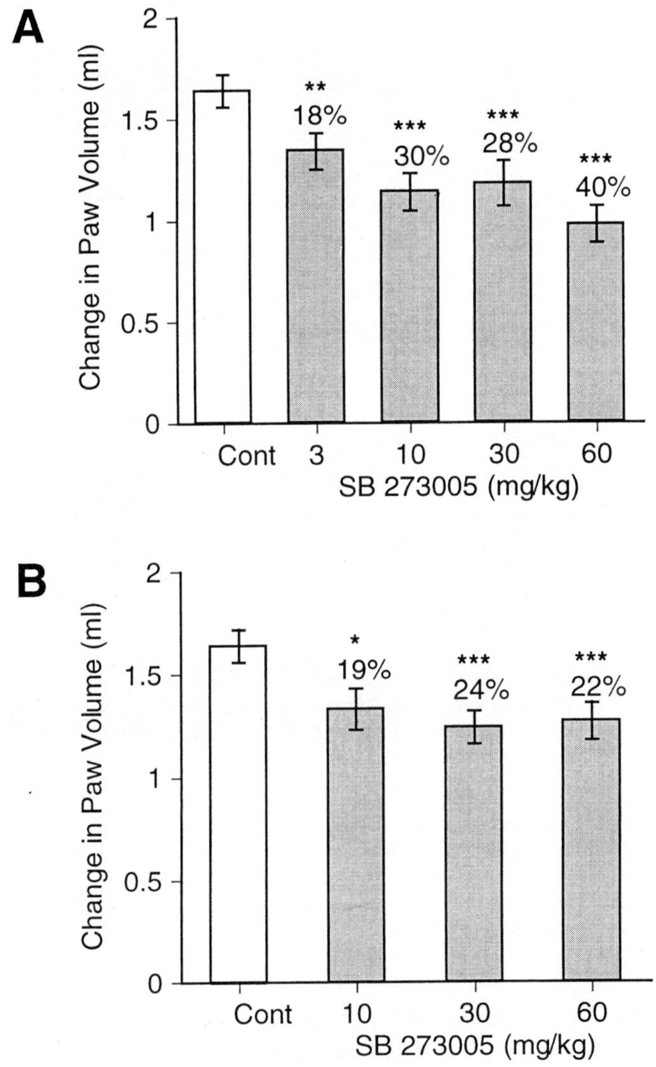

Figure 3. Inhibition of paw edema in Lewis rats with adjuvant-induced arthritis (AIA) using a prophylactic dosing protocol once per day. Rats were treated with SB 273005 at 3, 10, 30, and 60 mg/kg orally in 1% methyl cellulose, during days 0–20 in the prophylactic protocol (**A**) or days 10–20 in the therapeutic protocol (**B**). Bars show the mean and SEM of 12 rats per group. Treated groups were compared with the untreated AIA controls (Cont) by Student's t-test. $* = P < 0.05$; $** = P < 0.01$; $*** = P < 0.001$.

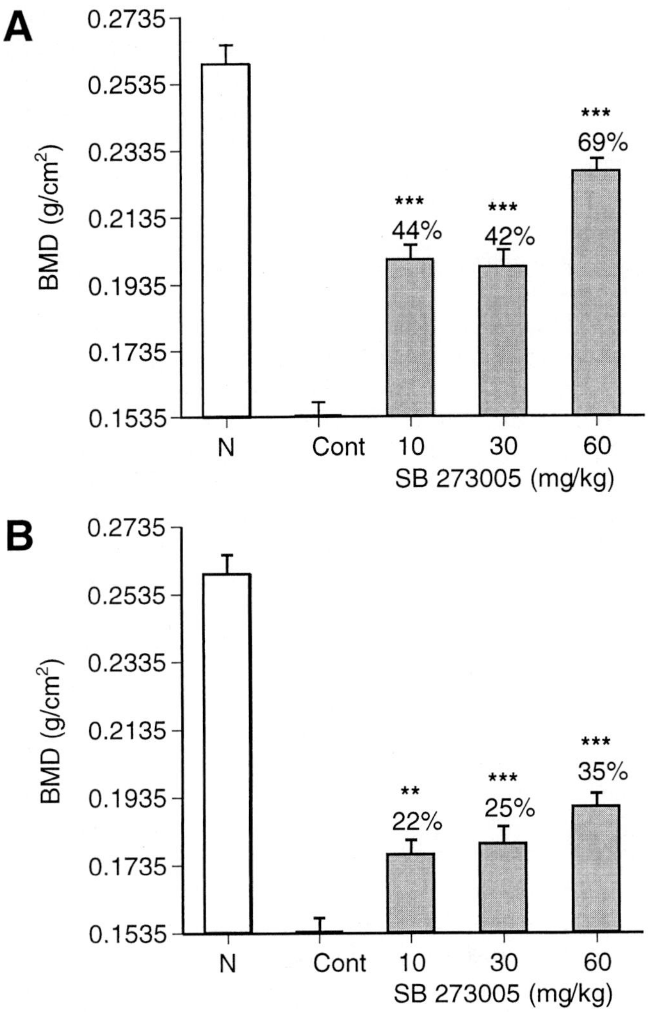

Figure 4. Bone densitometry evaluation of the distal tibia in adjuvant-induced arthritis (AIA) rats treated with SB 273005. Rats were treated with various doses of compound twice daily during days 0–20 (prophylactic) (**A**) or days 10–20 (therapeutic) (**B**). Values are the percentage change in bone mineral density (BMD) relative to the BMD in non-AIA normal controls (N; assigned a value of 100%). Bars show the mean and SEM of 12 animals per group. Treated groups were compared with the untreated AIA controls (Cont) by Student's t-test. $** = P < 0.01$; $*** = P < 0.001$.

BMD changes. BMD was monitored by DEXA using the Hologic QDR-1000 equipped with high-resolution scanning software. Scans were made of the distal tibia obtained from the animals on day 21. The BMD, as well as the BMC and bone area, were determined. However, because the improvements in the BMC values were identical to those in the BMD, we have chosen to report only the BMD data. The bone integrity of normal control rats was assigned a value of 100%, and that of AIA rats, a value of 0%. Compared with the AIA control rats, animals treated prophylactically with SB 273005 at 60, 30, and 10 mg/kg twice daily showed a significant normalization of BMD. There was 69%, 42%, and 44% normalization of BMD (all $P < 0.001$ versus controls) at 60, 30, and 10 mg/kg twice daily, respectively (Figure 4A).

Following therapeutic treatment, in which animals were dosed starting on day 10 following adjuvant injection and then dosed daily until day 20, there was also a significant normalization of BMD. There was 35%, 25% (both $P < 0.001$ versus controls), and 22% ($P < 0.01$ versus controls) normalization of BMD at 60, 30, and 10 mg/kg twice daily, respectively (Figure 4B). Following the single daily dose of SB 273005, the only significant improvement in BMD was observed when SB 273005 was administered prophylactically at 60 mg/kg (24% normalization; $P < 0.05$ versus controls) (results not shown).

MRI findings. Using MRI, the morphologic changes in the joint architecture of AIA rats were compared with those in normal (non-AIA) control rats and with those in AIA rats treated twice daily prophylactically or therapeutically with 60, 30, and 10 mg/kg SB 273005. Ex vivo MR images were obtained on day 21 from the intact left and right tibiotalar joints, and a total of 21–24 joints per group were evaluated. The images from AIA control rats (Figure 5A) were interpreted as demonstrating no protection against AIA, in which significant damage as well as swelling and marked loss in cortical as well as trabecular bone were observed. In comparison, in treated AIA rats, either moderate protection (Figure 5B) or significant protection (Figure 5C) was evident, in which the distal tibia, fibula, and talus were well defined and edema was minor (similar to that in a non-AIA normal rat). Following prophylactic treatment, 80% of the joints showed significant protection at the 60 mg/kg twice-daily dose, whereas ~40% of the joints from the animals dosed with either 30 or 10 mg/kg twice daily showed significant protection (Figure 6A). In the rats treated therapeutically with SB 273005, there was significant protection in 65% of the joints from the 60 mg/kg group and in 20% of the joints from the 30 mg/kg group (Figure 6B).

Histologic features. The histologic changes occurring in the bone and soft tissue compartments of AIA rats treated with SB 273005 at 60, 30, and 10 mg/kg (once daily) were compared with those in the vehicle-treated AIA controls. Histologic changes to the bone (the tibia and the talus) were scored 0–4 (normal to severely affected), whereas cartilage/soft tissue changes were scored on a scale of 0–3 depending on the severity, as described in Materials and Methods. Normal, non-AIA rats were scored 0 for all components. The mean severity scores for the lesions in the tibia, talus, and cartilage/soft tissue in AIA rats were determined separately, and the mean histologic scores for these regions are shown in Figure 7.

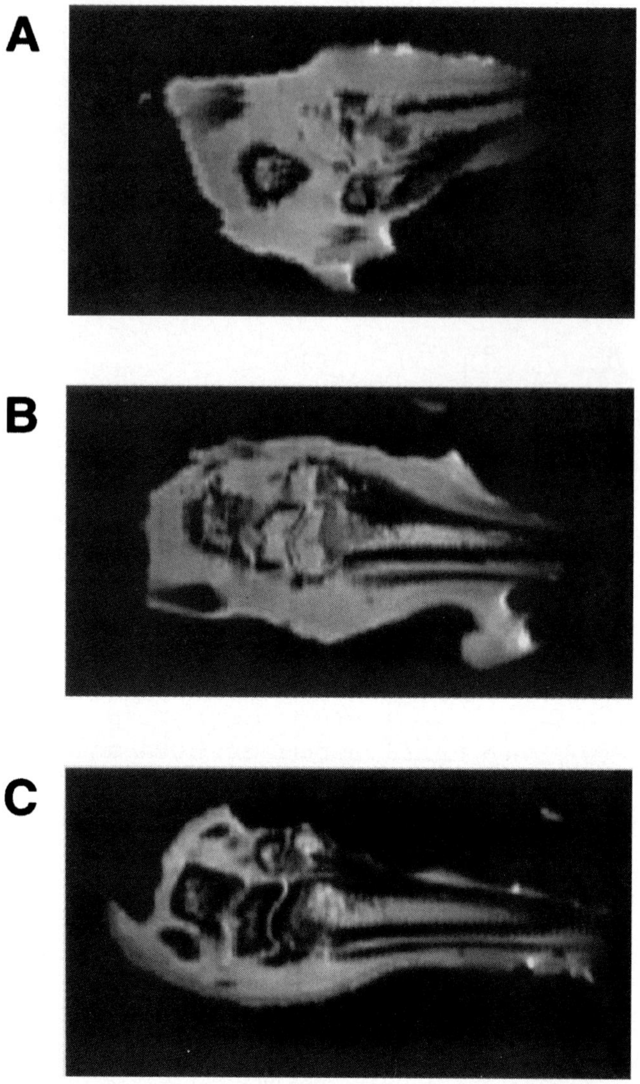

Figure 5. Representative magnetic resonance images on day 21 of a joint from an untreated rat with adjuvant-induced arthritis (AIA), in which no protection of joint integrity is evident (**A**), a joint from an AIA rat treated with SB 273005, showing moderate protection (**B**), or a joint from a treated AIA rat, showing significant protection (**C**). White areas indicate soft tissue and inflammation and the black areas indicate the bone.

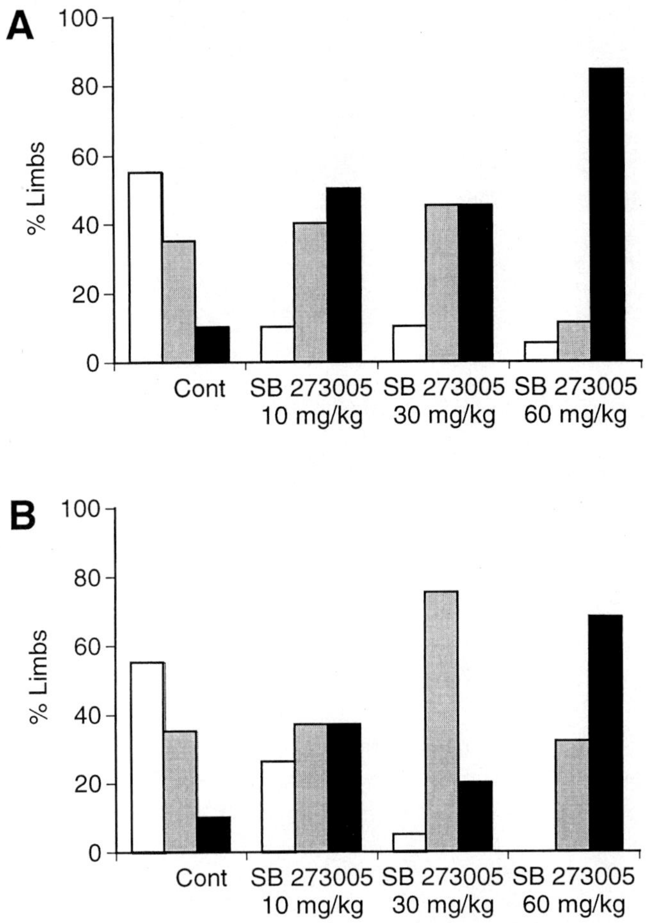

Figure 6. Evaluation of treatment effects based on magnetic resonance imaging of the tibiotarsal joints of adjuvant-induced arthritis (AIA) rats treated prophylactically (**A**) or therapeutically (**B**) with SB 273005 (twice daily). Values are expressed as the percentage of joints showing no protection (open bars), moderate protection (shaded bars), or significant protection (black bars). There were 20–24 limbs imaged in each group. Cont = untreated AIA control rats.

Of the 24 vehicle-treated AIA rat joints evaluated, all but 2 showed moderate-to–extremely severe changes in the tibia, talus, and cartilage/soft tissue components. The mean scores for the vehicle-treated groups were 2.6 for the tibia, 2.2 for the talus region, and 2.5 for the soft tissue. Administration of 60 mg/kg SB 273005 to AIA rats resulted in significant protection in both the bone and cartilage/soft tissue. None of these compound-treated animals was scored extremely severe for any component, and only 2 animals were scored severe (3.0) for bone lesions and 1 animal was scored 3.0 for cartilage/soft tissue damage. The mean scores for the tibia, talus, and cartilage for the 60 mg/kg group were 1.6, 1.3, and 1.5, respectively. In AIA rats treated with 30

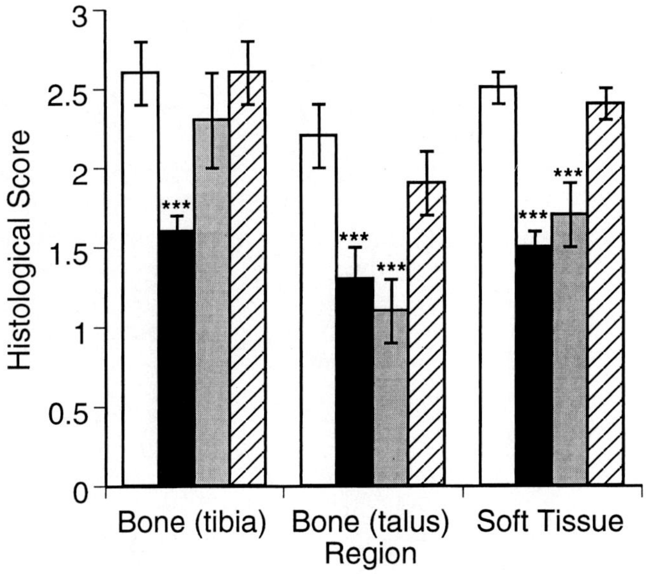

Figure 7. Histologic evaluation of the tibiotalus joints of adjuvant-induced arthritis (AIA) rats treated with SB 273005 once per day. Open bars = control AIA rats; black bars = AIA rats treated with 60 mg/kg; shaded bars = AIA rats treated with 30 mg/kg; hatched bars = AIA rats treated with 10 mg/kg. Bars show the mean ± SEM histologic score of 22–24 limbs for each group. Treated groups were compared with the untreated AIA controls by Mann-Whitney U test. *** = $P <$ 0.001 versus controls.

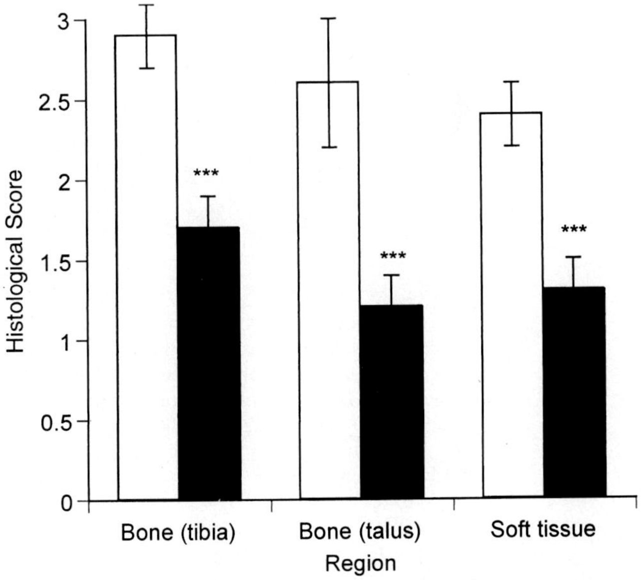

Figure 8. Histologic evaluation of the tibiotalus joints of rats treated with SB 273005 twice per day. Open bars = control adjuvant-induced arthritis (AIA) rats; black bars = AIA rats treated with 10 mg/kg twice daily. Bars show the mean ± SEM histologic score of 22–24 limbs for each group. The treated group was compared with the untreated AIA controls by Mann-Whitney U test. *** = $P < 0.001$ versus controls.

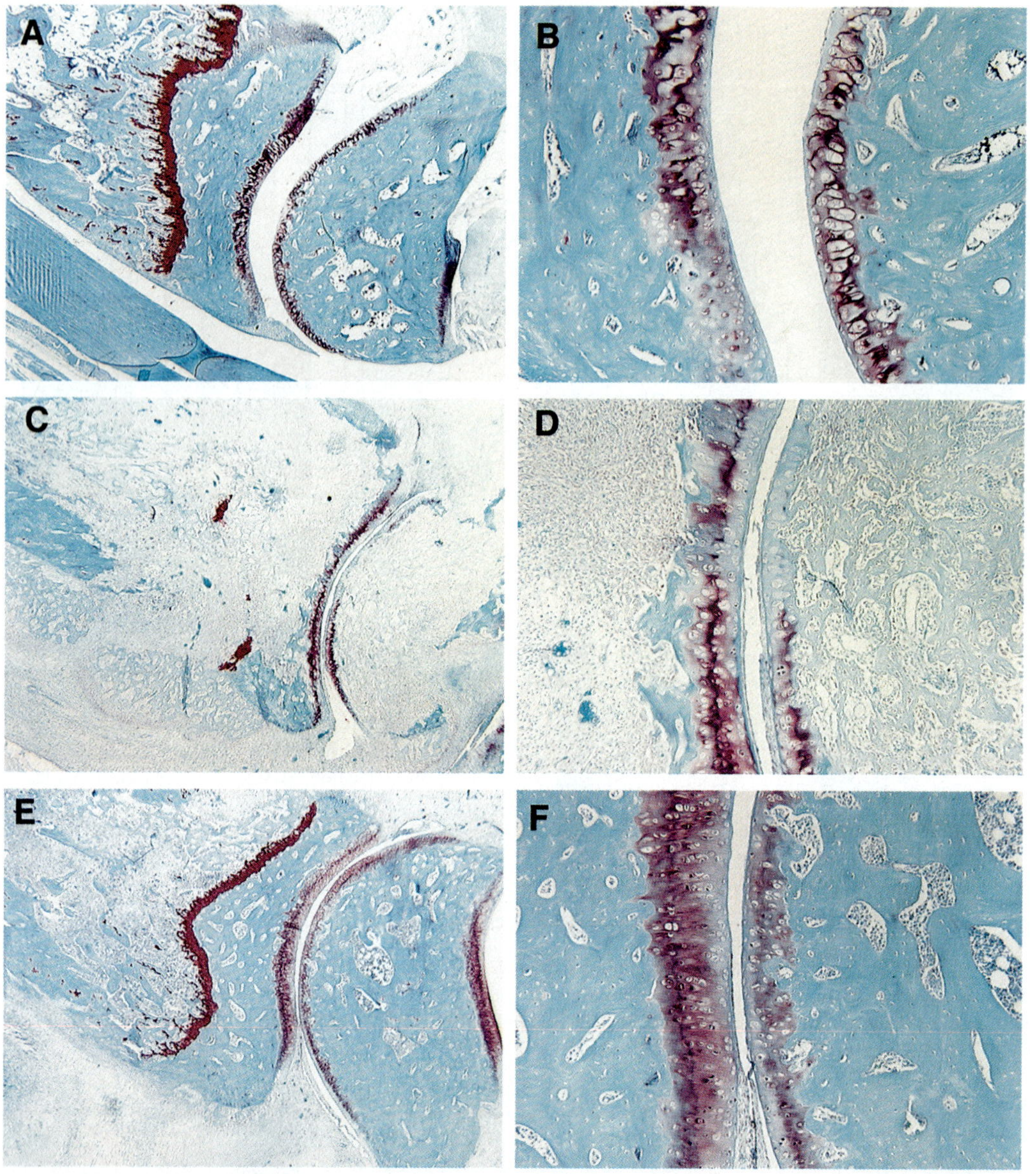

Figure 9. Photomicrographs of coronal sections of rat tibiotalus joints. **A** and **B,** normal tibiotalus joints from a normal, non–adjuvant-induced arthritis (AIA) rat. Articular cartilage is stained with Safranin O (pink), and other tissues are stained blue/green. The articulation of the distal tibia and proximal talus runs vertically through the image. **C** and **D,** Section of a tibiotalus joint from a vehicle-treated AIA rat. **E** and **F,** Tibiotalus joint from an AIA rat administered 60 mg/kg SB 273005 once per day on days 0–20. Note that compared with the joint from the AIA control rat, joint integrity has been significantly maintained with SB 273005. (Original magnification × 5 in **A**, **C**, and **E**; × 25 in **B**, **D**, and **F**.)

mg/kg SB 273005, the lesions in the talus and the cartilage, but not the tibia, were protected, with mean scores being 1.1, 1.7, and 2.3, respectively (Figure 7).

There was no significant protection observed on any parameter at the 10 mg/kg dose administered once per day. To determine whether a 10 mg/kg dose of SB 273005 administered twice daily would protect the joint integrity of AIA rats, joints from these animals were examined histologically and compared with those of vehicle-treated controls. The mean scores for the vehicle-treated groups were 2.9 for the tibia, 2.6 for the talus region, and 2.4 for the soft tissue. Administration of 10 mg/kg SB 273005 twice daily resulted in significant protection in all tissues. The mean scores for these groups were 1.7 for the tibia, 1.2 for the talus, and 1.3 for the soft tissue (Figure 8).

Representative photomicrographs of the joints from a normal rat, a vehicle-treated rat with AIA, and a rat with AIA treated prophylactically with 60 mg/kg SB 273005 once per day are shown in Figure 9. The joint architecture of the normal, non-AIA joint (Figures 9A and B) was scored 0 for all 3 components. In the AIA animals dosed with vehicle, inflammation was both extensive and severe (Figures 9C and D). The majority of the original bone in both the tibia and talus was lost. The marrow cavities were replaced with granulation tissue and reactive woven bone. As a result, a score of 3.0 was given for both of these bone components. Articular cartilage showed full-depth loss of proteoglycan (as indicated by reduced Safranin O staining) and the joint space had been infiltrated with granulation tissue. There was also extensive fibrosis of the surrounding soft tissues (not shown in this photomicrograph) and as a result, a score of 3.0 was given for this component. Compared with the joint from the vehicle-treated control rat, inflammation was markedly attenuated in the joints of animals treated with SB 273005 at 60 mg/kg once daily (Figures 9E and F). Although some inflammation was apparent in the marrow of the tibia, the talus appeared histologically normal. Therefore, the tibia and talus components were scored 1.0 and 0, respectively. The articular cartilage demonstrated some surface loss of proteoglycan, and the surrounding soft tissue contained a lymphocytic infiltrate and was edematous. This resulted in a score of 2.0 being assigned to the treated joints.

DISCUSSION

SB 273005 is an orally active, nonpeptide, RGD-mimetic $\alpha_v\beta_3$ antagonist. This compound binds $\alpha_v\beta_3$ and the closely related integrin, $\alpha_v\beta_5$, with low n*M* affinity, but binds only weakly to the related integrins $\alpha_{IIb}\beta_3$ and $\alpha_5\beta_1$ (20). The compound also inhibits $\alpha_v\beta_3$-mediated cell adhesion (at a 50% inhibition concentration [IC_{50}] of 3 n*M*) (20), endothelial cell migration (IC_{50} 1.8 n*M*), and osteoclast-mediated bone resorption in vitro (IC_{50} 11 n*M*). Studies in animal models of bone resorption have shown that this compound, as well as other small-molecule nonpeptide vitronectin receptor antagonists, inhibit bone loss in the thyroparathyroidectomized and chronic ovx rat models of bone resorption in vivo (18–20).

In addition to the effects observed with vitronectin receptor antagonists in animal models of bone resorption, a cyclic peptide $\alpha_v\beta_3$ antagonist was shown to decrease synovial vascularity and swelling in antigen-induced arthritis in rabbits (25). Angiogenesis is one of the earliest histopathologic findings in RA and appears to play a significant role in pannus formation. Suppression of angiogenesis, therefore, may impact disease progression and this has been observed in animal models of both adjuvant- and collagen-induced arthritis (23,24). In the rabbit model of antigen-induced arthritis, the angiogenic basic fibroblast growth factor was utilized to increase angiogenesis and this, in turn, increased the arthritic response to antigen in the animals (25). Treatment with the cyclic-peptide $\alpha_v\beta_3$ antagonist inhibited synovial angiogenesis, and reduced synovial cell infiltrate, pannus formation, and cartilage erosions.

The beneficial effects of antagonizing $\alpha_v\beta_3$ that were observed in the rabbit model of arthritis (25) and in the bone resorption models (18–20) encouraged us to examine the effects of SB 273005 in the rat AIA model. Inhibition of paw edema was observed in AIA in Lewis rats when SB 273005 was administered orally either twice or once per day. The lowest effective dose following prophylactic twice-daily dosing was 10 mg/kg, in which a 40% inhibition of inflammation was observed; lower doses were not tested in this experiment. However, in another experiment, 3 mg/kg twice daily was shown to be inactive (Badger AM: unpublished observations). The minimum effective dose using therapeutic twice-daily dosing was 30 mg/kg. Using a once-per-day dosing protocol, prophylactic dosing was clearly superior to therapeutic dosing. The effect of SB 273005 on paw edema is unlikely to be a direct antiinflammatory effect, which would resemble that of a nonsteroidal antiinflammatory drug, since studies in a classic model of carrageenan-induced inflammation, in which indomethacin showed strong activity, demonstrated that SB 273005 was inactive at 30 mg/kg and showed only 25% inhibition of inflammation at 60 mg/kg (Griswold D: unpublished observations).

It has previously been reported that SB 273005 potently inhibits both human endothelial cell migration and osteoclast-mediated bone resorption (19–22). The compound could have beneficial effects in inflammatory arthritis by preventing new vessel formation in the inflamed synovium as well as osteoclast-mediated bone resorption. It is possible that in adjuvant-driven disease, there is significant release of proinflammatory factors due to the significant destruction of bone and cartilage. Degraded matrix components may drive the inflammatory response and once this matrix degradation is blocked, inflammation subsides. In addition, the combination of inhibition of angiogenesis and proinflammatory products released from the bone could result in a significant reduction in pannus formation. An additional potential mechanism for the efficacy of SB 273005 in the AIA rat is that of inhibiting leukocyte migration to the joints. For example, CD31/platelet endothelial cell adhesion molecule 1 is a ligand for $\alpha_v\beta_3$ that is involved in the adhesion of leukocytes to endothelium (27,28), and interference with this interaction by the vitronectin receptor antagonist could reduce cell trafficking into the joint.

Evidence of the protection of bone integrity by SB 273005 was provided by DEXA, in which there was a remarkable 69% normalization of BMD at the 60 mg/kg twice-daily dose. Additional evidence of the disease-modifying activity of the compound was provided by the obvious improvement observed in the MR images, in which 80% of the joints were significantly protected by prophylactic treatment at the 60 mg/kg twice daily dose, and >60% of the joints were protected at this dose administered therapeutically. Of particular interest was the finding that in the groups treated therapeutically, the MR images indicated better protection than would have been suggested by the effect on inflammation. Histologic evaluation of the joints also showed that treatment with SB 273005 resulted in significant protective effects on both the bone and cartilage/soft tissue. Again, these data are consistent with those generated for the $\alpha_v\beta_3$ antagonist cyclic peptide (25), which prevented cartilage erosions in the rabbit model of inflammatory arthritis.

The profile of activity described here for SB 273005 suggests strongly that orally active, small-molecule vitronectin receptor antagonists could provide significant benefit in the treatment of inflammatory diseases such as RA. These compounds may prevent not only the swelling associated with this disease, but also the loss of bone, cartilage, and soft tissue structure within articulating joints.

ACKNOWLEDGMENTS

The authors would like to acknowledge the contribution of Don Griswold for providing assistance in developing the inflammation model, and the secretarial assistance of Nancy Cosgrove.

REFERENCES

1. Brooks PC, Clark RAF, Cheresh DA. Requirement of vascular integrin $\alpha_v\beta_3$ for angiogenesis. Science 1994;264:569–71.
2. Horton AH. The $\alpha_v\beta_3$ integrin "vitronectin receptor." Int J Biochem Cell Biol 1997;29:721–5.
3. Eliceiri BP, Cheresh DA. The role of α_v integrins during angiogenesis: insights into potential mechanisms of action and clinical development. J Clin Invest 1999;103:1227–30.
4. Albelda SM, Mett SA, Elder DE, Stewart R, Damjanovich L, Herlyn M, et al. Integrin distribution in malignant melanoma: association of β3 subunit with tumor progression. Cancer Res 1990;50:6757–64.
5. Brooks PC, Montgomery AMP, Rosenfeld M, Reisfeld RA, Hu T, Klier G, et al. Integrin $\alpha_v\beta_3$ antagonists promote tumor regression by inducing apoptosis of angiogenic blood vessels. Cell 1994;79: 1157–64.
6. Carron CP, Meyer DM, Pegg JA, Engleman VW, Nickols MA, Settle SL, et al. A peptidomimetic antagonist of the integrin $\alpha_v\beta_3$ inhibits Leydig cell tumor growth and the development of hypercalcemia of malignancy. Cancer Res 1998;58:1930–5.
7. Kerr JS, Wexler RS, Mousa SA, Robinson CS, Wexler EJ, Mohamed S, et al. Novel small molecule α_v integrin antagonists: comparative anti-cancer efficacy with known angiogenesis inhibitors. Anticancer Res 1999;19:959–68.
8. Brooks PC, Stromblad S, Klemke R, Visscher D, Sarkar FH, Cheresh DA. Antiintegrin $\alpha_v\beta_3$ blocks human breast cancer growth and angiogenesis in human skin. J Clin Invest 1995;96: 1815–22.
9. Clover J, Dodds RA, Gowen M. Integrin subunit expression by human osteoblasts and osteoclasts in situ and in culture. J Cell Sci 1992;103:267–71.
10. Helfrich MH, Nesbitt SA, Horton MA. Integrins on rat osteoclasts: characterization of two monoclonal antibodies (F4 and F11) to rat beta 3. J Bone Miner Res 1992;7:345–51.
11. Nesbitt S, Nesbit A, Helfrich M, Horton M. Biochemical characterization of human osteoclast integrins: osteoclasts express alpha v beta 3, alpha 2 beta 1, and alpha v beta 1 integrins. J Biol Chem 1993;268:16737–45.
12. Shinar DM, Schmidt A, Halperin D, Rodan GA, Weinreb M. Expression of alpha v and beta 3 integrin subunits in rat osteoclasts in situ. J Bone Miner Res 1993;8:403–14.
13. Crippes BA, Engleman VW, Settle SL, Delarco J, Ornberg RL, Helfrich MH, et al. Antibody to β_3 integrin inhibits osteoclast-mediated bone resorption in the thyroparathyroidectomized rat. Endocrinology 1996;137:918–24.
14. Fisher JE, Caalfield MP, Sato M, Quartuccio HA, Gould RJ, Garsky VM, et al. Inhibition of osteoclastic bone resorption in vivo by echistatin, an "arginyl–glycyl–aspartyl" (RGD)–containing protein. Endocrinology 1993;132:1411–3.
15. Yamamoto M, Balena R, Markatos A, Gentile M, Garsky VM, Rodan GA. Direct demonstration of inhibitory effect of echistatin on PTH-induced bone resorption in vivo in mice [abstract]. J Bone Miner Res 1993;8:123a.
16. Yamamoto M, Fisher JE, Gentile M, Seedor JG, Leu C-T, Rodan SB, et al. The integrin ligand echistatin prevents bone loss in ovariectomized mice and rats. Endocrinology 1998;139:1411–9.
17. Sago K, Teitelbaum SL, Venstrom K, Reichardt LF, Ross FP. The integrin $\alpha_v\beta_5$ is expressed on avian osteoclast precursors and regulated by retinoic acid. J Bone Miner Res 1999;14:32–8.
18. Engleman VW, Nickols GA, Ross FP, Horton MA, Griggs DW, Settle SL, et al. A peptidomimetic antagonist of the $\alpha_v\beta_3$ integrin inhibits bone resorption in vitro and prevents osteoporosis in vivo. J Clin Invest 1997;99:2284–92.
19. Lark MW, Stroup GB, Hwang SM, James IE, Rieman DJ, Drake FH, et al. Design and characterization of orally active Arg–Gly–Asp peptidomimetic vitronectin receptor antagonist SB 265123 for prevention of bone loss in osteoporosis. J Pharmacol Exp Ther 1999;291:612–7.

20. Lark MW, Stroup GB, Dodds RA, Kapadia R, Hoffman SJ, Hwang SM, et al. Antagonism of the osteoclast vitronectin receptor with an orally active non-peptide inhibitor prevents cancellous bone loss in the ovariectomized rat. J Bone Miner Res; in press.
21. Miller WH, Bondinell WE, Cousins RD, Erhard KF, Jakas DR, Keenan RM, et al. Highly orally bioavailable nonpeptide vitronectin receptor antagonists with efficacy in an osteoporosis model. Bioorg Med Chem Lett 1999;9:1807–12.
22. Miller WH, Alberts DP, Bhatnagar PK, Bondinell WE, Callahan JF, Calvo RR, et al. Discovery of orally active non-peptide vitronectin receptor antagonists based on a 2-benzazapine gly–asp mimetic. J Med Chem 2000;43:22–6.
23. Peacock DJ, Banquerigo ML, Brahn E. A novel angiogenesis inhibitor suppresses rat adjuvant arthritis. Cell Immunol 1995;160: 178–84.
24. Oliver SJ, Cheng TP, Banquerigo ML, Brahn E. Suppression of collagen-induced arthritis by an angiogenesis inhibitor, AGM-1470, in combination with cyclosporin: reduction of vascular endothelial growth factor (VEGF). Cell Immunol 1995;166: 196–206.
25. Storgard CM, Stupack DG, Jonczyk A, Goodman SL, Fox RI, Cheresh DA. Decreased angiogenesis and arthritic disease in rabbits treated with an $\alpha_v\beta_3$ antagonist. J Clin Invest 1999;103: 47–54.
26. Webb EF, Griswold DE. Microprocessor-assisted plethysmograph for the measurement of mouse paw volume. J Pharmacol Methods 1984;12:149–53.
27. Piali L, Hammel P, Uherek C, Bachmann F, Gisler RH, Dunon D, et al. CD31/PECAM-1 is a ligand for $\alpha_v\beta_3$ integrin involved in adhesion of leukocytes to endothelium. J Cell Biol 1995;130: 451–60.
28. Wakelin MW, Sanz MJ, Dewar A, Albelda SM, Larkin SW, Boughton-Smith N, et al. An anti-platelet-endothelial molecule-1 antibody inhibits leukocyte extravasation from mesenteric microvessels in vivo by blocking the passage through the basement membrane. J Exp Med 1996;184:229–39.

ARTHRITIS & RHEUMATISM
Vol. 44, No. 1, January 2001, pp 138–150

Induction of Endothelial Cell Decay-Accelerating Factor by Vascular Endothelial Growth Factor

A Mechanism for Cytoprotection Against Complement-Mediated Injury during Inflammatory Angiogenesis

Justin C. Mason,[1] Elaine A. Lidington,[1] Helen Yarwood,[1] Douglas M. Lublin,[2] and Dorian O. Haskard[1]

Objective. **Decay-accelerating factor (DAF) is a widely expressed, multifunctional cell surface protein involved in complement regulation and cell signaling. Previous studies have demonstrated that endothelial cell (EC) DAF is up-regulated by tumor necrosis factor α and inhibits complement binding. Because vascular endothelial growth factor (VEGF) is cytoprotective to endothelium and is expressed at sites of chronic inflammation, we hypothesized that VEGF may induce DAF expression during inflammatory angiogenesis.**

Methods. **Human umbilical vein and dermal microvascular EC were isolated using routine procedures, and the regulation and function of DAF, as well as other complement-regulatory proteins (membrane cofactor protein and CD59), were analyzed following stimulation with VEGF.**

Results. **Incubation of large- or small-vessel EC with VEGF led to increased expression of DAF, with maximal expression after 48–72 hours of stimulation. This effect depended on the activation of protein kinase C (PKC) and required increased steady-state messenger RNA levels and de novo protein synthesis. Although VEGF-induced EC proliferation was inhibited by both p38 and p42/44 mitogen-activated protein kinase (MAPK) antagonists, DAF up-regulation in response to VEGF was only sensitive to inhibition of p38 MAPK. VEGF-stimulated EC showed a 60% reduction in C3 deposition following complement activation, and this resulted in a marked reduction in complement-mediated EC lysis. These protective effects were abolished by anti-DAF monoclonal antibody 1H4.**

Conclusion. **This study confirms the importance of PKC for the regulation of DAF expression by EC and reveals VEGF to be a physiologic agonist for this pathway. The up-regulation of DAF expression by VEGF may represent an important mechanism for the protection of EC from complement-mediated injury during angiogenesis in inflammatory rheumatic diseases.**

Complement plays a critical role in the host defense against microorganisms and in the modulation of inflammatory responses. However, by the nature of its cytolytic effects, the complement cascade also has the potential to injure host tissues (1) and has been implicated in a variety of autoimmune disease states, including rheumatoid arthritis (RA), systemic lupus erythematosus (SLE), and Behçet's syndrome (2–4). The membrane-bound complement–regulatory proteins decay-accelerating factor (DAF; CD55), protectin (CD59), and membrane cofactor protein (MCP; CD46) are thought to protect cells against the constant low-level activity of the complement cascade (5,6). These factors utilize distinct mechanisms for the regulation of complement and may act cooperatively. DAF, which prevents the formation of and accelerates the decay of C3 and C5 convertases (5,7), and MCP, which binds C3b and C4b and facilitates their

Supported by a discretionary professorial award from the British Heart Foundation. Dr. Mason's work was supported by Arthritis Research Campaign grant M0572.

[1]Justin C. Mason, PhD, MRCP, Elaine A. Lidington, PhD, Helen Yarwood, PhD, Dorian O. Haskard, DM, FRCP: Imperial College School of Science, Technology, and Medicine, Hammersmith Hospital, London, UK; [2]Douglas M. Lublin, MD, PhD: Washington University School of Medicine, St. Louis, Missouri.

Address correspondence and reprint requests to Justin C. Mason, PhD, MRCP, The BHF Cardiovascular Medicine Unit, Imperial College School of Science, Technology, and Medicine, Hammersmith Hospital, Du Cane Road, London W12 ONN, UK.

Submitted for publication June 6, 2000; accepted in revised form August 26, 2000.

degradation by factor I (8), operate at the proximal end of the cascade. In contrast, CD59 serves to inhibit the membrane attack complex (C5b–9) by inhibiting the incorporation of C9 (9).

Although DAF, CD59, and MCP are each expressed by endothelial cells (EC) and contribute to the control of complement activation on the cell surface (6,10,11), the specific contributions made by these different molecules to the protection of the endothelium remain to be determined (12). In our previous work, we have shown that expression of DAF, but not that of MCP or CD59, is inducible on EC in response to the proinflammatory mediators tumor necrosis factor α (TNFα) and interferon-γ (IFNγ), as well as by the C5b–9 membrane attack complex (13). Furthermore, the up-regulation of DAF expression by these mediators was shown to protect EC from complement activation by reducing the binding of C3 to the EC surface, suggesting that DAF up-regulation may be important for maintaining the integrity of the microvasculature during subacute and chronic inflammatory responses involving complement activation (13).

There is increasing awareness of the importance of angiogenesis, the multistage process by which new blood vessels develop from the established vasculature, in the tissue remodeling that occurs in chronic inflammatory diseases such as RA (14) and psoriasis (15). Since vascular endothelium in chronic inflammatory tissues may be continuously exposed to sublytic levels of activated complement components (1,2,16,17), new blood vessels are at risk of complement-mediated injury and complement-induced cellular activation (1,18–21). We therefore postulated that the maintenance of vascular integrity during angiogenesis in the presence of low-grade complement activation might be facilitated by the induction of one or more of the complement-regulatory proteins DAF, CD59, and MCP.

Whereas the effects of TNFα, IFNγ, and C5b–9 on DAF expression are not affected by a pharmacologic inhibitor of protein kinase C (PKC) (13), the broadly active PKC agonist phorbol-12,-13-dibutyrate (PBu) is known to increase DAF expression by EC (22), suggesting that stimuli acting through PKC-dependent pathways may also stimulate expression of this complement regulator. One such candidate stimulus is vascular endothelial growth factor (VEGF), which is known to utilize PKC for stimulating EC proliferation and increased endothelial permeability to proteins (23,24). In this study, we show that VEGF does indeed stimulate DAF expression by a PKC-dependent pathway and that this leads to a reduction in the binding of complement C3 to the EC surface, thus conferring protection against subsequent cell lysis.

MATERIALS AND METHODS

Monoclonal antibodies (mAb) and other reagents. The mAb A35 (IgG1) against CD59 and the TRA-2-10 mAb (IgG1) against MCP were kind gifts from Professor B. P. Morgan (University of Wales, Cardiff, UK) and Professor J. P. Atkinson (Washington University School of Medicine, St. Louis, MO), respectively. The anti-DAF mAb used included mAb 1H4 (IgG1) and 5B2 (IgG1), which were a kind gift from Dr. T. Fujita (University of Tsukuba, Tsukuba, Japan). The anti-endoglin (CD105) mAb RMAC8 (IgG2a) was a kind gift from Dr. A. d'Apice (St. Vincent's Hospital, Victoria, Australia). IgG1 and IgG2a control mAb were obtained from the adhesion panel of the Fifth CD Workshop, and the EC-specific mAb EN4 (IgG1) was from Sanbio (Uden, The Netherlands). Recombinant human VEGF 165 was purchased from PeproTech (London, UK). Placental growth factor (PlGF) was purchased from R&D Systems (Abingdon, UK). The PKC agonist PBu, bovine serum albumin (BSA), nonenzymatic cell dissociation solution, and cycloheximide were purchased from Sigma (Poole, UK). The PKC antagonists RO 31-8220 and RO 32-0432 (25), the cell-permeable selective mitogen-activated protein kinase (MAPK) kinase 1 (MEK-1) inhibitor PD 98059, which inhibits activation of p42/44 MAPK (26), and the p38 MAPK inhibitor SB 202190 (27) were purchased from Calbiochem (Nottingham, UK).

Normal human serum (NHS) was obtained from samples of blood taken from healthy volunteers. The NHS was collected under sterile conditions into glass tubes and allowed to clot at 37°C, prior to further incubation at 4°C for 2 hours to induce clot retraction. Following centrifugation at 1,800*g*, the NHS was collected, pooled, and stored at −70°C.

Cell isolation and culture. Human umbilical vein endothelial cells (HUVEC) were isolated from umbilical cords by digestion with type II collagenase (Boehringer Mannheim, Lewes, UK) as described previously (28), and cultured in 1% gelatin-coated tissue culture flasks (Costar, Cambridge, MA) in medium 199 (M199; ICN Biomedicals, Costa Mesa, CA) supplemented with 20% fetal bovine serum (FBS; Hyclone Laboratories, Logan, UT), 100 IU/ml penicillin, 0.1 mg/ml streptomycin, 2 m*M* L-glutamine (all from Gibco Life Technologies, Paisley, UK), 10 units/ml heparin (Leo Laboratories, Prince Risborough, UK), and 30 μg/ml EC growth factor (ECGF; Sigma). Human dermal microvascular EC (DMEC) were isolated from human foreskins and cultured in fibronectin-coated flasks in M199 supplemented with 20% heat-inactivated human serum, 100 IU/ml penicillin, 0.1 mg/ml streptomycin, 2 m*M* L-glutamine, 10 units/ml heparin, and 60 μg/ml ECGF, as previously described in detail (29).

Flow cytometry. Following stimulation with test factors, monolayers of EC were harvested by exposure to trypsin/EDTA (ICN Biomedicals) for 1 minute at 37°C. EC were then stained with the appropriate primary mAb for 30 minutes at 4°C. After washing twice in phosphate buffered saline (PBS)/2.5% FBS, EC were resuspended in fluorescein isothiocyanate (FITC)–labeled rabbit anti-mouse Ig (Dako, Glostrup, Denmark) for 30 minutes at 4°C, followed by washing as above and fixation in 1% paraformaldehyde. Samples were analyzed on an Epics XL-MCL flow cytometer (Coulter, Hialeah, FL) by counting 10,000 cells per sample. In experiments involving RO 31-8220, RO 32-0432, PD 98059, SB 202190, and cycloheximide, each inhibitor was added 60 minutes prior to the addition of VEGF. In some experiments, the results are expressed as the relative fluorescence intensity (RFI), which represents the mean fluorescence intensity (MFI) with test mAb divided by the MFI with an isotype-matched irrelevant mAb. In all experiments, prior to staining, cell viability was assessed by examination of EC monolayers with the use of phase-contrast microscopy, cell counting, and estimation of trypan blue exclusion.

Northern blot analysis. VEGF-stimulated or unstimulated EC were lysed in guanidium isothiocyanate (Sigma) and RNA was extracted as described by Chomczynski and Sacchi (30). Purified RNA was resuspended in 20 μl RNase-free water and stored at −70°C before use. The probe for DAF was obtained from a plasmid vector (31) (kindly provided by Professor B. P. Morgan), and the DAF insert was released by incubation for 2 hours at 37°C with the *Sal* I and *Xba* I restriction enzymes. The technique used for Northern blotting was as previously described in detail (13). Northern blots were quantified by the Appligene Image Analysis system (Appligene, Durham, UK) and densitometry was performed using the National Institutes of Health Image program, version 1.52 (Bethesda, MD). Values were corrected with respect to ethidium bromide–stained ribosomal RNA loading patterns, and an arbitrary value of 1 was assigned to unstimulated EC.

Cell proliferation and bromodeoxyuridine (BrdU) double-staining assays. HUVEC (5×10^3 cells per well) were added to gelatin-coated 96-well plates (Costar) in M199 containing 10% FBS, 100 IU/ml penicillin, 0.1 mg/ml streptomycin, and 2 m*M* L-glutamine (plain medium). Following culture for 24 hours in the absence of growth factors, the medium was aspirated and replaced with plain medium alone or with plain medium containing 25 ng/ml VEGF. The cells were then incubated for a further 48–72 hours, with the addition of ^{3}H-thymidine (1 μCi/ml; Amersham Pharmacia Biotech, Buckinghamshire, UK) 16 hours before the end of the assay. The EC were then harvested using an automated Betaplate 96-well harvester (Wallac, Turku, Finland) and transferred to filtermats (Wallac) that were counted on a Betaplate liquid scintillation counter (Wallac), with the results expressed in counts per minute.

In the BrdU incorporation experiments, subconfluent EC were treated with 25 ng/ml VEGF for 48 hours, with the addition of BrdU (final concentration 20 μ*M*) 16 hours prior to the end of the assay. Following harvesting with trypsin/EDTA, the cells were resuspended in ice-cold PBS and fixed by adding slowly to 70% ethanol at 4°C and incubating on ice for 30 minutes. Following centrifugation at 500*g* and washing in PBS/1% BSA, 0.2*M* HCl was slowly added to the EC while maintaining a vortex. After 10 minutes and centrifugation at 500*g*, 1 ml of 0.1*M* $Na_2B_4O_7 \cdot 10\ H_2O$, pH 8.5, was added to neutralize the acid. Following centrifugation as described above and washing in PBS/1% BSA/0.5% Tween 20, the cells were transferred to 96-well V-bottom plates and primary antibodies were added for 30 minutes at 4°C. After 2 washes in PBS/1% BSA, biotinylated F(ab′)$_2$ rabbit anti-mouse Ig was added for 30 minutes at 4°C. After 2 washes, the cells were incubated with streptavidin–phycoerythrin (Vector Laboratories, Burlingame, CA) and FITC-conjugated anti-BrdU mAb (Becton Dickinson, Mountain View, CA) with 10% mouse serum for 30 minutes at 4°C, and expression of VEGF-induced DAF was then analyzed on a Becton Dickinson FACScan flow cytometer.

C3 binding and cell lysis assays. EC were plated in 35-mm petri dishes (3×10^5 cells per dish) and cultured overnight at 37°C in HUVEC media without ECGF (plain medium). The next day EC monolayers were washed once in Hanks' balanced salt solution (HBSS) and fresh plain medium was added, with or without VEGF (25 ng/ml). Following incubation for 48 hours, EC were harvested, pelleted in 96-well V-bottom plates, and incubated with anti-endoglin mAb RMAC8 for 30 minutes at 4°C. After washing with HBSS/1% BSA, EC were incubated with 100 μl of 20% NHS in M199 for 3 hours at 37°C prior to washing with HBSS/1% BSA and addition of FITC-conjugated rabbit anti-human C3c (Dako) at 1:40 dilution for 30 minutes at 4°C. After washing twice with HBSS/1% BSA, the presence of C3c was estimated using flow cytometric analysis. Controls included the omission of NHS and the addition of 10 m*M* EDTA to the NHS to inhibit complement activation. In the inhibition studies, blocking mAb were added to the assay with RMAC8 to achieve a concentration of 25 μg/ml.

In the cell lysis experiments, EC were cultured overnight in 24-well plates at 37°C prior to the addition of VEGF or plain medium alone for 48 hours. EC were then incubated for 30 minutes at 37°C in M199 with 10% FBS containing 7 μ*M* calcein–acetoxymethyl ester (calcein-AM; Molecular Probes, Leiden, The Netherlands). Following washing in M199/1% BSA, EC monolayers were opsonized with mAb RMAC8 for 30 minutes at 37°C. After washing with HBSS/1% BSA, EC were incubated with 5–20% baby rabbit complement (Serotec, Oxford, UK) in M199 for 30 minutes at 37°C. The supernatant from each well was then transferred to a 96-well microtiter plate (Costar), and after washing in M199/1% BSA, the calcein remaining in the cells was released by incubation with 250 μl M199/1% BSA/0.1% Triton X-100 (Sigma). The lysate was then transferred to a 96-well plate, and the calcein released by complement and detergent was estimated using a CytoFluor 2300 fluorescence plate reader (Millipore, Bedford, MA). The percentage of specific lysis in triplicate wells was calculated as

$$\frac{\text{Complement-mediated release} - \text{spontaneous release}}{\text{Maximal release} - \text{spontaneous release}} \times 100\%$$

where maximal release is the complement-mediated release plus detergent-mediated release of calcein. Spontaneous release was <20% in all experiments.

Statistical analysis. Differences between the results of experimental treatments were evaluated by the Mann-Whitney U test. Differences were considered significant at *P* values of less than 0.05.

RESULTS

VEGF induction of DAF expression on HUVEC and DMEC. Although DAF is known to be abundantly expressed on the surface of HUVEC and DMEC in culture (10,13), our preliminary immunohistologic stud-

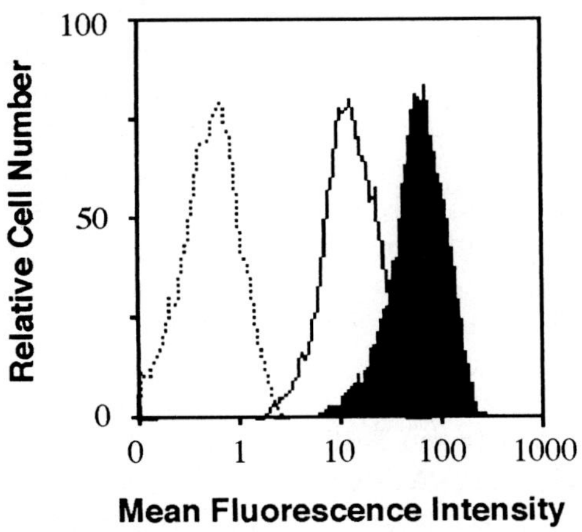

Figure 1. Up-regulation of decay-accelerating factor (DAF) expression by vascular endothelial growth factor (VEGF) on human umbilical vein endothelial cells (HUVEC). The expression of DAF on HUVEC was assessed by flow cytometry using monoclonal antibody (mAb) 5B2. DAF expression on HUVEC is shown in the absence of growth factors (mean fluorescence intensity [MFI] 12.5) (open histogram with solid line) and following 48 hours of stimulation with VEGF (20 ng/ml; MFI 56.4) (shaded histogram). Background fluorescence (irrelevant mAb and fluorescein isothiocyanate–labeled rabbit anti-mouse Ig) is also shown (open histogram with dotted line).

ies of normal human skin showed only minimal DAF expression by vascular EC (32). This suggested to us that DAF expression on cultured EC might be a consequence of cell proliferation and that the molecule might be regulated by growth factors. To test this hypothesis, HUVEC were cultured without growth factor for 24 hours and then stimulated with VEGF for 48 hours.

A low level of constitutive DAF expression was detected in growth factor–deprived cells, whereas culture with VEGF led to a significant unimodal increase in the expression of cell surface DAF (MFI 12.5 without VEGF compared with 56.4 with VEGF for 48 hours) (Figure 1). This up-regulation was dose dependent, with maximal expression occurring with 25 ng/ml of VEGF (Figure 2A). In 20 separate experiments, VEGF up-regulated the level of DAF up to 4-fold above the basal level on unstimulated EC (RFI ± SD 23.5 ± 5.5 in unstimulated EC versus 65.3 ± 13.0 in VEGF-stimulated EC; $P < 0.01$). In contrast, in parallel cultures, VEGF did not increase the expression of either MCP or CD59 (Figures 2B and C).

To determine the kinetics of DAF induction by VEGF, HUVEC monolayers were stimulated for up to 72 hours with VEGF, and DAF expression was then analyzed by flow cytometry. As seen in Figure 3A, up-regulation was detectable following 8 hours of stim-

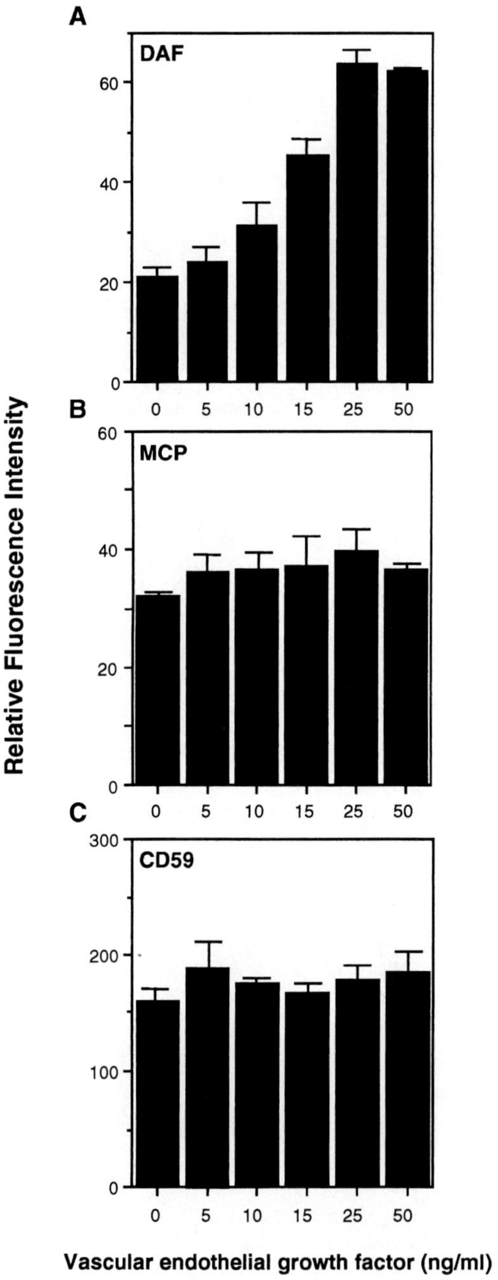

Figure 2. Analysis of DAF, CD59, and membrane cofactor protein (MCP) expression on HUVEC following stimulation with VEGF. HUVEC monolayers were incubated for 48 hours in the presence of varying concentrations of VEGF before harvesting and analysis by flow cytometry. DAF, CD59, and MCP were detected using mAb 1H4, A35, and TRA-2-10, respectively. The results are expressed as the relative fluorescence intensity (MFI of test sample divided by MFI of irrelevant isotype-matched negative control) for **A,** DAF, **B,** CD59, and **C,** MCP. Bars show the mean and SD of 3 separate experiments performed on different HUVEC cultures. See Figure 1 for other definitions.

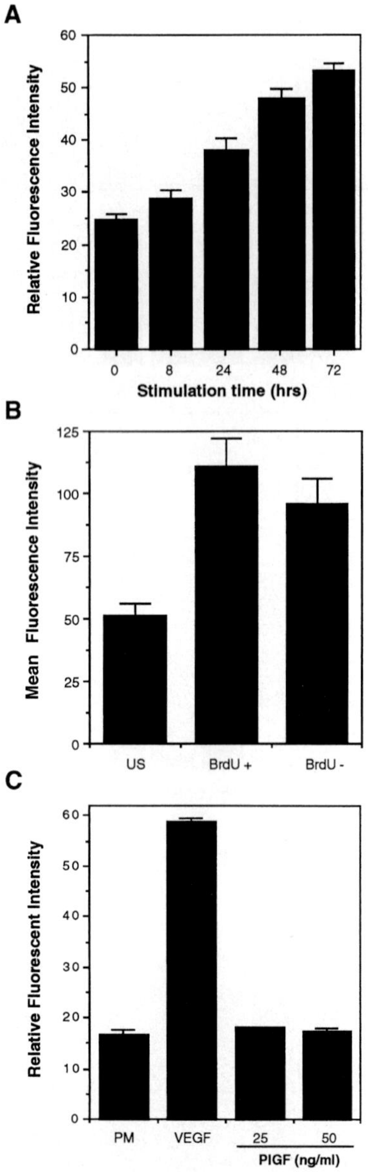

Figure 3. **A,** Time course for the regulation of DAF by VEGF. HUVEC were stimulated for up to 72 hours with VEGF (25 ng/ml). Following harvesting, single cell suspensions were analyzed by flow cytometry for the expression of DAF using mAb 1H4. **B,** HUVEC plated at subconfluence were stimulated for 48 hours with VEGF (25 ng/ml) and bromodeoxyuridine (BrdU; 20 μM) was added for the final 16 hours of incubation. Following harvesting, fixation, and permeabilization of EC, BrdU incorporation and DAF expression were assessed by flow cytometry. Bars show the mean and SEM (n = 3). **C,** HUVEC were stimulated for 48 hours with VEGF (25 ng/ml), placental growth factor (PlGF; 25 and 50 ng/ml), or plain medium (PM) alone prior to harvesting and analysis by flow cytometry for the expression of DAF using mAb 1H4. Bars show the mean and SD (n = 3). Results are representative of 3 similar experiments performed on different HUVEC cultures. US = unstimulated cells (see Figure 1 for other definitions).

ulation and was maximal after 48–72 hours. Parallel experiments performed on the same cells at these time points demonstrated no change in the levels of MCP or CD59 (results not shown). In order to determine whether an increase in DAF expression was confined to EC that were actively proliferating in response to VEGF, subconfluent cultures were treated with VEGF for 48 hours and then pulsed with BrdU for the final 16 hours. The cells were then double-stained for DAF and BrdU and examined by flow cytometry. In 3 separate experiments, there was no significant difference in DAF expression between BrdU-positive cells (MFI ± SEM 111 ± 11) and BrdU-negative cells (MFI ± SEM 96 ± 10) (Figure 3B), suggesting that DAF expression in this context is not dependent on the stage of the cell cycle.

Further experiments comparing the ability of VEGF and PlGF to induce DAF expression suggested that VEGF-induced DAF up-regulation was mediated through ligation of VEGF receptor 2 (VEGFR-2/kinase domain region). As seen in Figure 3C, VEGF, which can bind to and activate VEGFR-1 (flt-1) and VEGFR-2 (33), induced DAF expression, whereas PlGF, which only activates VEGFR-1 (33), had no effect. However, since HUVEC are large-vessel EC of fetal origin and may not accurately represent the EC of the microvasculature, which are involved in angiogenesis, we isolated EC from human dermis and performed experiments with these cells in a manner similar to that described for HUVEC.

As shown in Figure 4A, DMEC also showed an increase in DAF expression after stimulation with VEGF for 48 hours, whereas no change in MCP or CD59 expression was observed. Failure to demonstrate an increase in expression of MCP and CD59 was not due to the proteolytic effects of trypsin, since identical results were obtained when DAF, MCP, and CD59 were measured on EC harvested with a nonenzymatic cell dissociation solution (results not shown). As seen in Figure 4B, the up-regulation of DAF by VEGF on DMEC was also mediated by ligation of VEGFR-2, since PlGF had no effect on DAF expression.

PKC involvement in VEGF-induced DAF on HUVEC. In a previous study we demonstrated that DAF expression by EC can be stimulated by both PKC-dependent and -independent pathways (13). To investigate whether PKC is involved in the VEGF-mediated stimulation of DAF expression, we used the PKC antagonists RO 31-8220 and RO 32-0432 (25), which we have previously found to be effective and nontoxic inhibitors of EC PKC (29,34). The concentration of PKC antagonists used was based on levels established in our previous

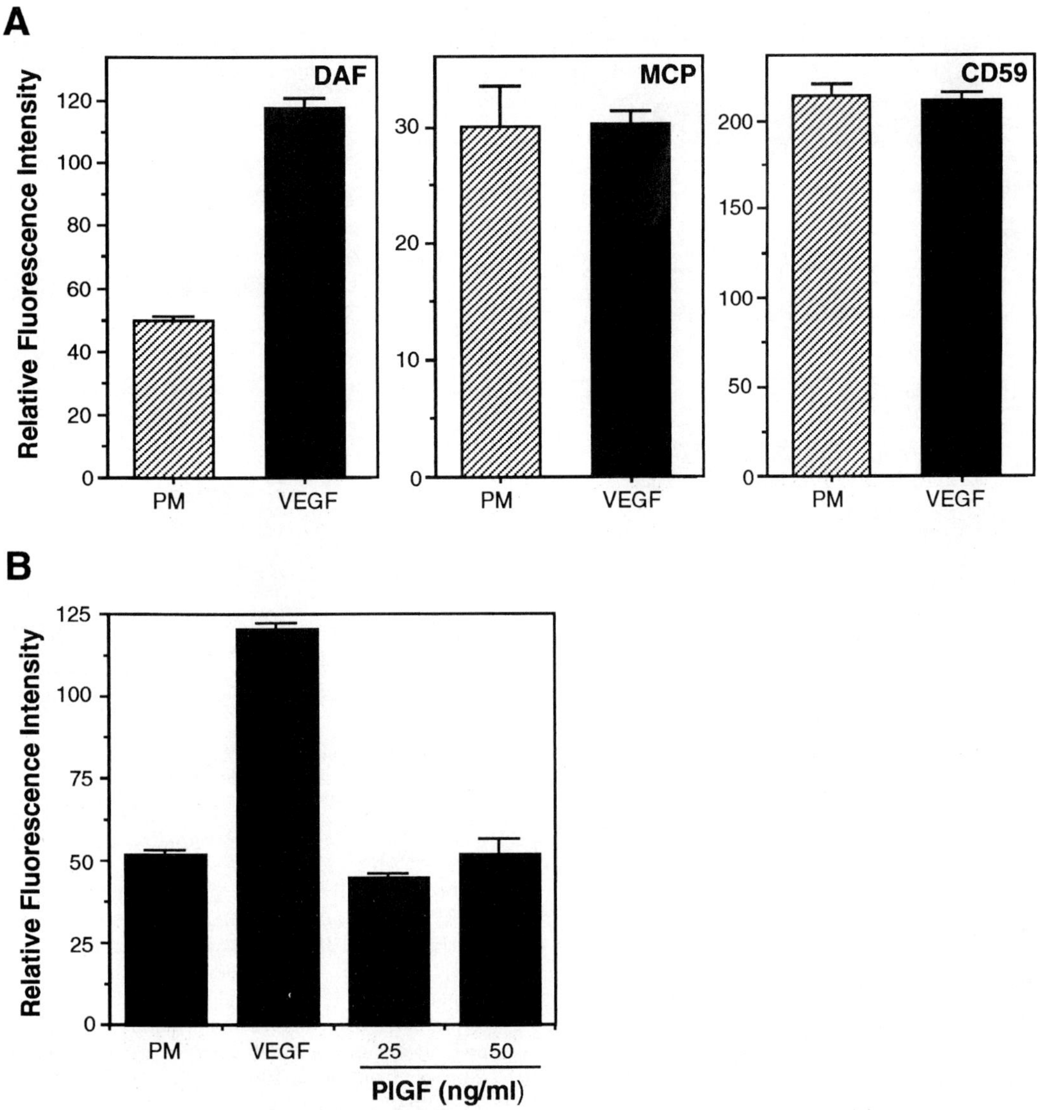

Figure 4. **A,** VEGF up-regulation of DAF, but not MCP or CD59, expression by human dermal microvascular endothelial cells (DMEC). Monolayers of DMEC were stimulated for 48 hours with VEGF (25 ng/ml) or PM alone and then analyzed by flow cytometry for expression of DAF, CD59, and MCP using mAb 1H4, A35, and TRA-2-10, respectively. **B,** DMEC were stimulated for 48 hours with VEGF (25 ng/ml), PlGF (25 and 50 ng/ml), or plain medium alone (PM) prior to harvesting and analysis by flow cytometry for the expression of DAF using mAb 1H4. Bars show the mean and SD (n = 3). Results are representative of 3 similar experiments performed on different DMEC cultures. See Figures 1–3 for other definitions.

work in which we observed complete inhibition of phorbol ester–induced effects on EC (13). As shown in Figure 5, pretreatment of EC (13) for 30 minutes with RO 31-8220 (0.75 μM) prior to stimulation with VEGF led to significant inhibition of EC proliferation (Figure 5A) and also of DAF expression (Figure 5B). Similar results were obtained when PKC was inhibited with RO 32-0432 (3 μM) (results not shown). These observations demonstrate that PKC activation is required to stimulate the effect of VEGF on EC DAF expression, just as previously observed for EC proliferation (23).

Role of p38 MAPK in VEGF-induced DAF on HUVEC. To further define the signaling pathways involved in the regulation of DAF expression by VEGF,

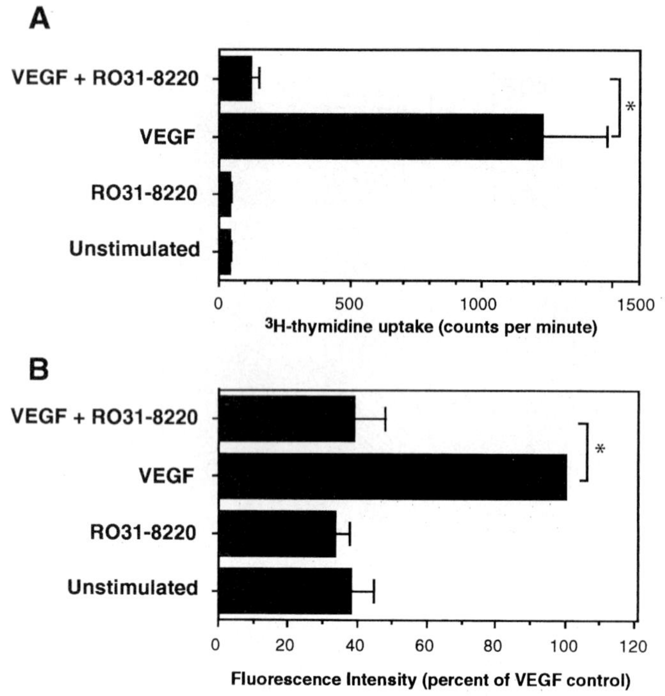

Figure 5. Effect of the protein kinase C antagonist RO31-8220 on VEGF-induced EC proliferation and DAF up-regulation. **A,** HUVEC were cultured in 96-well microtiter plates (5×10^3 EC per well) in medium 199 with 10% fetal bovine serum and no endothelial cell growth factor for 24 hours prior to the addition of VEGF (25 ng/ml). They were then cultured for a further 72 hours before harvesting. Following the addition of ^{3}H-thymidine (1 μCi/ml) 16 hours before the end of the assay, the plates were read on an automated plate reader. In test wells, EC were preincubated with RO31-8220 (0.75 μM) for 30 minutes prior to the addition of VEGF. Bars show the mean and SD uptake of ^{3}H-thymidine (n = 4). **B,** HUVEC monolayers were treated with RO31-8220 (0.75 μM) or plain medium alone for 30 minutes prior to the addition of VEGF (25 ng/ml) and cultured for a further 48 hours. Following harvesting, EC were analyzed by flow cytometry for the expression of DAF using mAb 1H4. The mean ($\pm$SEM) fluorescence intensity of DAF on VEGF-stimulated cells was 46.2 $\pm$ 7.4. The data are expressed as a percentage of the DAF expression on VEGF-treated cells and are presented as the mean and SEM from 4 experiments on separate HUVEC lines. * = $P < 0.02$. See Figure 1 for definitions.

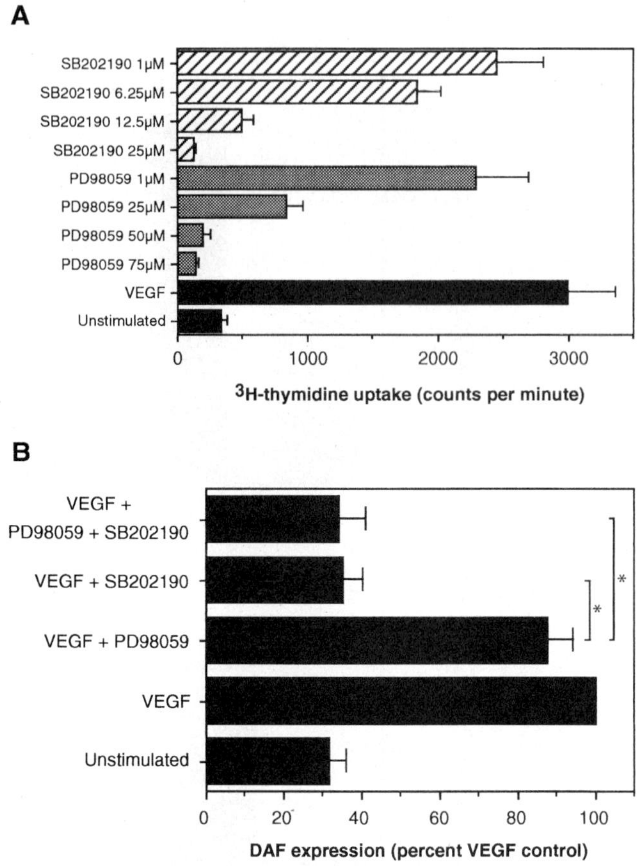

Figure 6. Involvement of p38 mitogen-activated protein kinase (MAPK), but not p42/44 MAPK, in VEGF-induced DAF expression by HUVEC. **A,** HUVEC were cultured in 96-well microtiter plates (5×10^3 cells per well) in medium 199 with 10% fetal bovine serum for 24 hours prior to the addition of VEGF (25 ng/ml). They were then cultured for a further 72 hours before harvesting. ^{3}H-thymidine (1 μCi/ml) was added 16 hours before the end of the assay and the plates were read on an automated plate reader. In test wells, EC were preincubated with inhibitors of p38 MAPK (SB202190) or MAPK kinase 1 (PD98059), at the concentrations shown, for 60 minutes prior to the addition of VEGF. Bars show the mean and SD uptake of ^{3}H-thymidine (n = 4). **B,** HUVEC were plated at confluence in 35-mm petri dishes (5×10^5 cells/dish) and cultured overnight at 37°C. The EC were then preincubated with the inhibitors SB202190 (25 μM) or PD98059 (75 μM) for 60 minutes prior to the addition of VEGF (25 ng/ml). Cells were then cultured for a further 48 hours. Following harvesting, DAF expression was measured by flow cytometry using mAb 1H4. The mean ($\pm$SEM) fluorescence intensity of DAF on VEGF-stimulated cells was 36.4 $\pm$ 5.5. The data are expressed as a percentage of the DAF expression on VEGF-treated cells and are presented as the mean and SEM from 3 experiments on separate EC lines. * = $P < 0.05$. See Figure 1 for other definitions.

we used PD 98059, a specific inhibitor of MEK-1 that prevents p42/44 MAPK phosphorylation (26), and SB 202190, which inhibits p38 MAPK (27). As shown in Figure 6A, pretreatment of EC for 60 minutes with either PD 98059 or SB 202190 prior to stimulation with VEGF led to dose-dependent inhibition of EC proliferation.

Similar experiments were subsequently performed to assess the role of MAPK in VEGF-induced DAF up-regulation. Following preliminary dose-titration studies to determine the optimal inhibitor concentrations, HUVEC were preincubated with SB 202190 (25 μM) for 1 hour prior to the addition of VEGF. As shown in Figure 6B, this led to significant inhibition of

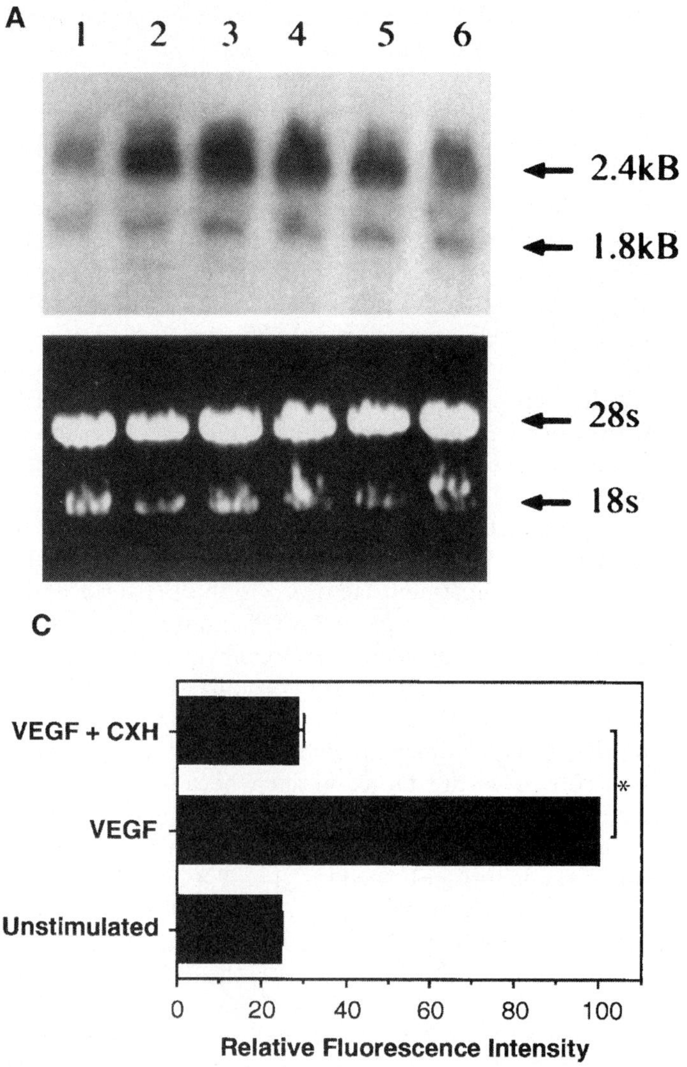

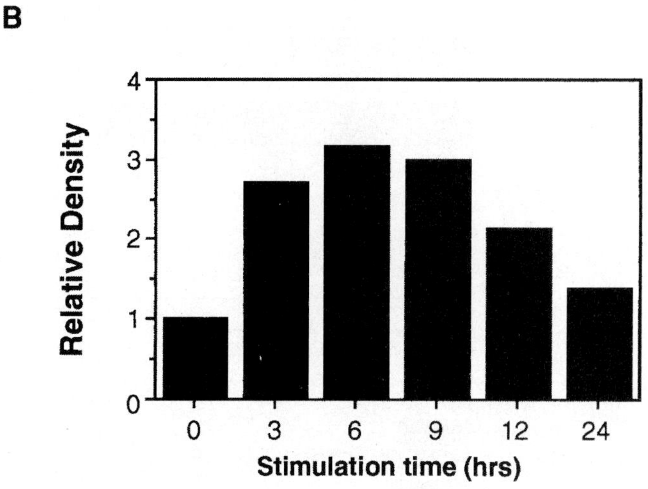

Figure 7. Involvement of increased steady-state DAF mRNA and de novo protein synthesis in VEGF-induced surface expression of DAF. **A** and **B,** HUVEC were cultured for up to 24 hours in plain medium alone or in medium supplemented with VEGF (25 ng/ml). **A,** Total RNA was isolated and Northern blots were prepared for detection of mRNA in cultures containing unstimulated EC (lane 1), VEGF for 3 hours (lane 2), VEGF for 6 hours (lane 3), VEGF for 9 hours (lane 4), VEGF for 12 hours (lane 5), and VEGF for 24 hours (lane 6). **B,** Levels of mRNA in resting and VEGF-stimulated EC were quantified using densitometric scanning. **C,** To determine whether VEGF-induced DAF expression was dependent on de novo protein synthesis, HUVEC were plated at confluence in 35-mm petri dishes (5×10^5 cells/dish) and cultured overnight at 37°C. They were then pretreated with cycloheximide (CXH; 3 μg/ml) for 30 minutes prior to the addition of VEGF (25 ng/ml) for a further 48 hours. Following harvesting, DAF expression was measured by flow cytometry using mAb 1H4. The data are expressed as a percentage of the DAF expression on VEGF-treated cells. Bars show the mean and SEM from 3 experiments performed on separate EC lines. $* = P < 0.02$. See Figure 1 for other definitions.

DAF up-regulation, as detected after 48 hours of culture ($P < 0.05$). In contrast, in parallel experiments, PD 98059 had no significant effect at concentrations up to 100 μM. These 2 agents, and particularly SB 202190, induced EC shape change but did not lead to any demonstrable cytotoxicity at the concentrations used, with EC remaining >90% viable as assessed by cell counting and trypan blue exclusion on the EC populations and also by flow cytometric analysis of CD31 expression (results not shown). These data therefore suggest that VEGF-induced DAF expression on EC is dependent on a signaling cascade that requires activation of p38 MAPK, but, unlike EC proliferation, probably does not require activation of p42/44 MAPK.

Association of VEGF-induced DAF expression with increased steady-state mRNA levels and de novo protein synthesis. Northern blot analysis was performed using mRNA extracted from unstimulated HUVEC and from cells stimulated with VEGF for up to 24 hours. As shown in Figure 7A, DAF mRNA was detectable at a low level in unstimulated EC. Following VEGF stimulation, an increase in DAF mRNA was first detectable at 3 hours, reached maximal levels at 6–9 hours, and declined to basal levels by 24 hours poststimulation. Two DAF mRNA transcripts (2.4 kb and 1.8 kb) were detected, as previously reported (31,35). Quantification of mRNA levels in resting and VEGF-stimulated EC using densitometric scanning of the 2.4-kb band demon-

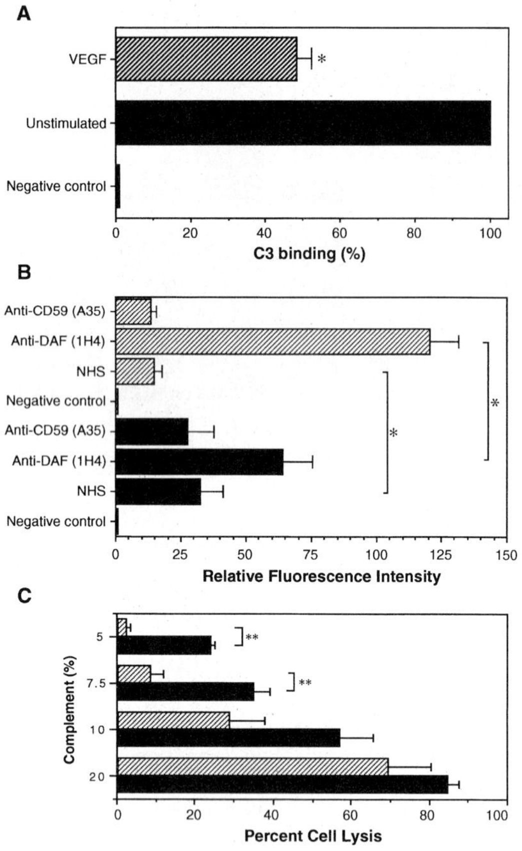

Figure 8. Reduction of binding of C3 to opsonized HUVEC by VEGF-induced DAF expression. HUVEC were plated at confluence in 35-mm petri dishes (5×10^5 cells/dish) and cultured overnight at 37°C prior to stimulation with VEGF (25 ng/ml) for 48 hours. Following harvesting, EC were incubated with the anti-endoglin mAb RMAC8 or plain medium alone for 30 minutes at 4°C. The EC were then washed in Hanks' balanced salt solution (HBSS)/1% bovine serum albumin (BSA) prior to addition of up to 20% normal human serum (NHS) for 3 hours at 37°C. Binding of C3 was detected by flow cytometry using fluorescein isothiocyanate–conjugated rabbit anti-human C3c. **A,** Percentage of C3 binding (mean and SD; n = 3) to unstimulated EC (solid bars) and VEGF-stimulated HUVEC (hatched bars), with binding to unstimulated EC (relative fluorescence intensity [RFI] ± SD 20.3 ± 5.0) shown as 100%. The negative control represents C3 binding in the presence of heat-inactivated human serum (HIHS) without preincubation with RMAC8. **B,** C3 binding (RFI and SD; n = 3) on unstimulated (solid bars) and VEGF-stimulated (hatched bars) HUVEC in the presence of inhibitory mAb 1H4 (anti-DAF) and A35 (anti-CD59). The negative control represents C3 binding in the presence of HIHS without preincubation with RMAC8. **C,** HUVEC plated at confluence (1.5×10^5 cells/well) in 24-well plates were cultured overnight prior to stimulation with VEGF (25 ng/ml) (hatched bars) or plain medium alone (solid bars) for 24 hours. Following loading with calcein–acetoxymethyl ester, EC were incubated with mAb RMAC8 for 30 minutes at 37°C. The EC were then washed in HBSS/1% BSA prior to the addition of baby rabbit complement or HIHS for 45 minutes at 37°C. Calcein release was measured and the percentage of cell lysis (mean and SD; n = 3) was calculated as described in Materials and Methods. Results are representative of 3 similar experiments performed on different EC cultures. * = $P < 0.05$; ** = $P < 0.01$. See Figure 1 for other definitions.

strated a 3-fold increase above baseline levels at 6 hours after stimulation (Figure 7B).

In order to determine whether the up-regulation of DAF that was observed following VEGF stimulation was dependent on de novo protein synthesis, HUVEC were pretreated with cycloheximide (3 μg/ml) prior to the addition of VEGF. We have previously shown that this concentration of cycloheximide is capable of inhibiting protein synthesis in EC (13,29). As shown in Figure 7C, cycloheximide led to a complete abrogation of the increased DAF expression seen in response to VEGF ($P < 0.02$). Thus, the up-regulation of DAF expression on the cell surface following stimulation of HUVEC with VEGF is associated with a transient increase in steady-state DAF mRNA levels and de novo protein synthesis.

Reduction of complement-mediated injury to HUVEC by VEGF-induced expression of DAF. The binding of complement factor C3 to the EC surface was used to investigate whether VEGF-induced DAF could afford increased protection to EC against complement-mediated injury. HUVEC were opsonized with an IgG2a anti-endoglin mAb, RMAC8 (36). IgG2a is the optimal murine isotype for complement fixation, and endoglin was chosen as the target antigen because it is highly expressed on the EC surface and was found to be not influenced by incubation of HUVEC with VEGF for 48 hours (endoglin RFI ± SD 92.1 ± 8.8 in unstimulated EC compared with 98.3 ± 5.7 in VEGF-treated EC). HUVEC were then incubated with 20% NHS for 3 hours, after which C3 binding to the cell surface was quantified by flow cytometry using an FITC-labeled antibody against C3. In a control experiment, addition of 10 m*M* EDTA to the NHS completely inhibited C3 binding, consistent with the response being dependent on complement activation (results not shown).

Stimulation of EC with VEGF for 48 hours prior to performing the C3 binding assay led to a reduction in C3 deposition on the cell surface by up to 60% compared with that in unstimulated cells ($P = 0.02$) (Figure 8A). To confirm the role of DAF in the reduction of C3 binding following VEGF stimulation, the anti-DAF mAb 1H4, which inhibits DAF function but does not fix complement, was included in the assay. The non–complement-fixing inhibitory mAb against CD59 (A35), which would not be expected to inhibit C3 binding, was also studied. As seen in Figure 8B, the addition of 1H4, but not A35, markedly increased the binding of C3 to unstimulated, opsonized EC exposed to 20% NHS. Furthermore, adding anti-DAF mAb 1H4 to HUVEC that had been preincubated for 48 hours with VEGF reversed the protective effect of VEGF and led to a marked increase in C3 binding, such that it significantly exceeded that observed in unstimulated cultures ($P < 0.05$).

To assess further the physiologic relevance of these data, we sought to determine whether a reduction of 60% in C3 binding resulted in reduced complement-mediated EC lysis. HUVEC were loaded with calcein-AM and opsonized with mAb RMAC8 and then exposed to baby rabbit complement. Endothelial lysis was subsequently measured by estimation of calcein release. As seen in Figure 8C, pretreatment of EC with VEGF for 48 hours was cytoprotective, significantly reducing cell lysis following the addition of 5–10% baby rabbit complement. At complement concentrations of 20% or higher, the cytoprotective effect of VEGF was overcome. These observations suggest that the increased levels of cell surface DAF seen in response to VEGF provide additional protection to EC against complement-mediated injury.

DISCUSSION

The fact that DAF is expressed on a wide variety of cell types suggests that it plays an important role in protecting against the deleterious effects of autologous complement activation (12). Furthermore, it is now recognized that the surface expression of DAF may be regulated during physiologic and pathophysiologic events (37,38). Despite this, our understanding of the regulation of DAF and its functional significance in vivo remains incomplete (5,39). On vascular endothelium, the constitutive expression of complement-regulatory proteins is thought to protect EC against the constant low-level activity of the complement cascade (5,6). However, the potential for local endothelial injury is greatly increased following activation of the alternative or classical pathways, and under these circumstances, up-regulation of complement-regulatory gene expression might be expected to enhance the protection of host tissues. To this end, we have previously demonstrated that the proinflammatory mediators TNFα, IFNγ, and C5b–9 upregulate the expression of DAF on EC (13).

This led us to consider the role of DAF, CD59, and MCP in the maintenance of vascular integrity during inflammatory angiogenesis, and to hypothesize that the expression of these proteins may be increased on the developing neovasculature. This hypothesis was further advanced by the observation that whereas the expression of DAF on resting endothelium in situ is often low (32,40,41), there is increased expression on large- and small-vessel EC in vitro (10,13) and in vivo on the microvasculature of the rheumatoid synovium and on the glomerulus in renal disease (17,40).

We initially tested the effect of VEGF on the expression of DAF on EC, since activation of PKC is known to be involved in VEGF-induced endothelial proliferation and permeability to proteins in vitro (23,24) and DAF has been shown to be inducible by a PKC-dependent pathway (22). We duly found that DAF expression was stimulated by VEGF and that this was PKC dependent, as demonstrated by complete inhibition of the effect by the PKC antagonists RO 31-8220 and RO 32-0432. The relatively delayed time course of DAF protein expression on EC is not unique and is comparable with that seen in response to cytokines (13) and other molecules, including Thy-1 (29). Furthermore, the prolonged expression of DAF on the EC surface suggests that DAF expression in vivo is likely to be persistent, rather than transient, in the face of chronic VEGF exposure. Thus, VEGF and thrombin (42) represent the first reported physiologic agonists for the known PKC-dependent pathway of DAF regulation (22).

It is of interest that in addition to up-regulating surface expression of DAF, activation of PKC by phorbol esters also results in deposition of the molecule into the subendothelial matrix, a response that is not seen following activation of the PKC-independent pathway (43). Previous studies have suggested that TNFα (44), and possibly VEGF (45), alter the morphology of EC monolayers in vitro, thus exposing the underlying basement membrane, which may fix complement. It is therefore possible that the PKC-dependent pathway of DAF regulation is important for regulating complement during angiogenesis in 2 ways: first, by acting to prevent complement deposition on the EC lumenal surface, and second, by reducing complement activation on exposed subendothelial matrix (44).

The MAPK cascade has been implicated in the downstream signaling pathway following PKC activation (46,47). Although the precise role of MAPK in VEGF-mediated EC functions remains unclear, it has been demonstrated that VEGF can activate both p42/44 and p38 MAPK in EC (48,49). The interaction between these pathways is of particular interest, and indeed, a recent study demonstrated cross-talk in which p38 MAPK negatively regulated the p42/44 MAPK cascade (50). In our experiments, EC proliferation could be inhibited by pharmacologic blockade of either p38 or p42/44 MAPK, whereas DAF expression was inhibited by suppression of p38 only. This suggests that DAF might be a useful cell surface reporter of a restricted aspect of VEGF-mediated signaling. However, endothelial MAPK signaling pathways remain to be fully elucidated and caution is required in interpreting results obtained using pharmacologic inhibitors. PD 98059 is the most specific inhibitor of MEK-1 available and has been extensively tested against 18 different kinases to confirm its specificity (26). Although the specificity of the pyridinyl imidazole inhibitors of p38 MAPK (SB 202190 and SB 203580 [27]) has varied between studies, they have been shown to inhibit other kinases, including c-Jun N-terminal kinase β1 (JNKβ1) and cRaf-1, in addition to p38 MAPK (51). Therefore, a role for both JNKβ1 and cRaf-1 in the VEGF-induced up-regulation of DAF cannot be excluded.

DAF exerts its actions at the proximal end of the complement cascade by accelerating the decay of the C3 and C5 convertases (12). Therefore, to confirm the beneficial functional role of VEGF-induced DAF, we used a flow cytometric assay that allows the detection of surface-bound C3 on opsonized EC exposed to normal human serum. Initial experiments demonstrated the cytoprotective potential of VEGF treatment, which resulted in a 60% reduction in C3 binding to the EC surface following complement activation, as compared with that in untreated control cells. The role of DAF in mediating this effect was confirmed by inclusion of the inhibitory anti-DAF mAb 1H4, which resulted in a significant increase in specific C3 binding to VEGF-stimulated EC, as compared with that in untreated cells. The reason that C3 binding to VEGF-treated EC was significantly greater than that to unstimulated EC following mAb 1H4 inhibition of DAF is unclear, but on the basis of preliminary further observations, this may be due to the induction of apoptosis by the anti-DAF mAb with exposure of phosphatidylserine (52) and increased cell surface binding of C1q (53) and C3 (54). The inhibition of C3 binding by VEGF is especially relevant in view of the relative inefficiency of C5 activation, which is critically dependent on an absolute excess of activated C3 (55). Thus, reduced C3 binding was translated into a significant reduction in complement-mediated lysis in EC pretreated with VEGF.

The complement system has been implicated in the pathogenesis of rheumatic diseases, including RA, SLE, and dermatomyositis (2,4,16,56). However, despite the deposition of C5b–9 on the endothelial surface (2,17), significant EC lysis is rarely seen. This is due, at least in part, to the effects of membrane regulators of complement activation, including DAF, that may be induced on the microvasculature of the rheumatoid synovium (17). We recently described a PKC-independent pathway for this response, activated by the cytokines TNFα and IFNγ and the C5b–9 complex, which results in a feedback loop of vascular protection through the up-regulation of DAF on the EC surface (13). The induction of DAF by VEGF through a PKC-dependent pathway provides an alternative mechanism for DAF induction on EC. The demonstration of distinct pathways regulating DAF expression raises the question of whether DAF may have functions beyond decay-accelerating activity, and this possibility is supported by the identification of the 7-span transmembrane molecule CD97 as an adhesive ligand for DAF (57). Since CD97 is expressed on peripheral blood leukocytes (58), the CD97/DAF ligand receptor pair may be involved in leukocyte–EC adhesive and/or signaling interactions (59).

There is now considerable evidence in support of a role for VEGF as a survival factor for the developing neovasculature during angiogenesis, and withdrawal of VEGF may induce vessel regression and EC death by apoptosis (60,61). VEGF is readily detectable at inflammatory sites (62–64) and has recently been reported to mediate vascular cytoprotection and endothelial repair in glomerulonephritis (65). These actions of VEGF are dependent on VEGFR-2 and phosphatidylinositol 3′-kinase/Akt signal transduction pathways (66), and on the induction of the antiapoptotic proteins Bcl-2 and A1 (67). We believe that DAF should now be added to this emerging list of cytoprotective genes induced by VEGF. Furthermore, an improved understanding of the mechanisms underlying vascular cytoprotection, including expression of the membrane regulators of complement, will facilitate the development of future therapeutic approaches by which the endothelium can be conditioned for the prevention and treatment of local or systemic inflammatory rheumatic diseases.

ACKNOWLEDGMENTS

We thank P. Kiely, P. Singh, and M. McNamara for their collection of foreskins, and the maternity unit of Hammersmith Hospital in London for the provision of umbilical cords. We would also like to thank M. Walport, K. Davies, B. Morley, M. Botto, B. P. Morgan, A. d'Apice, and J. Atkinson for their help with this study.

REFERENCES

1. Morgan BP. Complement membrane attack on nucleated cells: resistance, recovery and non-lethal effects. Biochem J 1989;264: 1–14.
2. Biesecker G, Katz S, Koffler D. Renal localization of the membrane attack complex in systemic lupus erythematosus nephritis. J Exp Med 1981;154:1779–94.
3. Rumfeld WR, Morgan BP, Campbell AK. The ninth complement component in rheumatoid arthritis, Behcet's disease and other rheumatic diseases. Br J Rheumatol 1986;25:266–70.
4. Morgan BP, Daniels RH, Williams BD. Measurement of terminal complement complexes in rheumatoid arthritis. Clin Exp Immunol 1988;73:473–8.

5. Lublin DM, Atkinson JP. Decay-accelerating factor: biochemistry, molecular biology and function. Annu Rev Immunol 1989;7:35–58.
6. Brooimans RA, van Wieringen PAM, van Es LA, Daha MR. Relative roles of decay-accelerating factor, membrane cofactor protein, and CD59 in the protection of human endothelial cells against complement mediated lysis. Eur J Immunol 1992;22: 3135–40.
7. Nicholson-Weller A, Burge J, Fearon DT, Weller PF, Austen KF. Isolation of a human erythrocyte membrane glycoprotein with decay-accelerating activity for C3 convertases of the complement system. J Immunol 1982;129:184–9.
8. Liszewski MK, Post TW, Atkinson JP. Membrane cofactor protein (MCP or CD46): newest member of the regulators of the complement activation gene cluster. Annu Rev Immunol 1991;9:431–55.
9. Davies A, Simmons DL, Hale G, Harrison RA, Tighe H, Lachmann PJ, et al. CD59, an LY-6–like protein expressed in human lymphoid cells, regulates the action of the complement membrane attack complex on homologous cells. J Exp Med 1989;170:637–54.
10. Asch AS, Kinoshita T, Jaffe EA, Nussenzweig V. Decay-accelerating factor is present on cultured human umbilical vein endothelial cells. J Exp Med 1986;163:221–6.
11. McNearney T, Ballard L, Seya T, Atkinson JP. Membrane cofactor protein of complement is present on human fibroblast, epithelial, and endothelial cells. J Clin Invest 1989;84:538–45.
12. Liszewski MK, Farries TC, Lublin DM, Rooney IA, Atkinson JP. Control of the complement system. Adv Immunol 1996;61:201–83.
13. Mason JC, Yarwood H, Sugars K, Morgan BP, Davies KA, Haskard DO. Induction of decay-accelerating factor by cytokines or the membrane-attack complex protects vascular endothelial cells against complement deposition. Blood 1999;94:1673–82.
14. Koch AE. Angiogenesis: implications for rheumatoid arthritis. Arthritis Rheum 1998;41:951–62.
15. Nickoloff BJ, Mitra RS, Varani J, Dixit VM, Polverini PJ. Aberrant production of interleukin-8 and thrombospondin-1 by psoriatic keratinocytes mediates angiogenesis. Am J Pathol 1994;144: 820–8.
16. Kissel JT, Mendell JR, Rammohan KW. Microvascular deposition of complement membrane attack complex in dermatomyositis. N Engl J Med 1986;314:329–34.
17. Tarkowski A, Trollmo C, Seifert PS, Hansson GK. Expression of decay-accelerating factor on synovial lining cells in inflammatory and degenerative arthritides. Rheumatol Int 1992;12:201–5.
18. Hattori R, Hamilton KK, McEver RP, Sims PJ. Complement proteins C5b-9 induce secretion of high molecular weight multimers of endothelial von Willebrand factor and translocation of granule membrane protein GMP-140 to the cell surface. J Biol Chem 1989;264:9053–60.
19. Kilgore KS, Shen JP, Miller BF, Ward PA, Warren JS. Enhancement by the complement membrane attack complex of tumor necrosis factor-alpha–induced endothelial cell expression of E-selectin and ICAM-1. J Immunol 1995;155:1434–41.
20. Saadi S, Holzknecht RA, Patte CP, Stern DM, Platt JL. Complement-mediated regulation of tissue factor activity in endothelium. J Exp Med 1995;182:1807–14.
21. Tedesco F, Pausa M, Nardon E, Introna M, Mantovani A, Dobrina A. The cytolytically inactive terminal complement complex activates endothelial cells to express adhesion molecules and tissue factor procoagulant activity. J Exp Med 1997;185:1619–27.
22. Bryant RW, Granzow CA, Siegel MI, Egan RW, Billah MM. Phorbol esters increase synthesis of decay-accelerating factor, a phosphatidylinositol-anchored surface protein, in human endothelial cells. J Immunol 1990;144:593–8.
23. Xia P, Aiello LP, Ishii H, Jiang ZY, Park DJ, Robinson GS, et al. Characterization of vascular endothelial cell growth factor's effect on the activation of protein kinase C, its isoforms, and endothelial cell growth. J Clin Invest 1996;98:2018–26.
24. Nagpala PG, Malik AB, Vuong PT, Lum H. Protein kinase C β1 overexpression augments phorbol ester-induced increase in endothelial permeability. J Cell Physiol 1996;166:249–55.
25. Davis PD, Hill CH, Keech E, Lawton G, Nixon JS, Sedgwick AD, et al. Potent selective inhibitors of protein kinase C. FEBS lett 1989;259:61–3.
26. Alessi DR, Cuenda A, Cohen P, Dudley DT, Saltiel AR. PD 098059 is a specific inhibitor of the activation of mitogen-activated protein kinase kinase in vitro and in vivo. J Biol Chem 1995;270: 27489–94.
27. Lee JC, Laydon JT, McDonnell PC, Gallagher TF, Kumar S, Green D, et al. A protein kinase involved in the regulation of inflammatory cytokine biosynthesis. Nature 1994;372:739–46.
28. Wellicome SM, Thornhill MH, Pitzalis C, Thomas DS, Lanchbury JS, Panayi GS, et al. A monoclonal antibody that detects a novel antigen on endothelial cells that is induced by tumor necrosis factor, IL-1, or lipopolysaccharide. J Immunol 1990;144:2558–65.
29. Mason JC, Yarwood H, Tárnok A, Sugars K, Harrison AA, Robinson PJ, et al. Human Thy-1 is cytokine inducible on vascular endothelial cells and is a signaling molecule regulated by protein kinase C. J Immunol 1996;157:874–83.
30. Chomczynski P, Sacchi N. Single-step method of RNA isolation by acid guanidinium thiocyanate-phenol-chloroform extraction. Anal Biochem 1987;162:156–9.
31. Medof ME, Lublin DM, Holers VM, Ayers DJ, Getty RR, Leykam JF, et al. Cloning and characterization of cDNAs encoding the complete sequence of decay-accelerating factor of human complement. Proc Natl Acad Sci U S A 1987;84:2007–11.
32. Mason JC, Yarwood H, Harrison AA, Davies KAA, Haskard DO. Expression and regulation of complement regulatory proteins CD59 and decay-accelerating factor (DAF) on endothelial cells [abstract]. Arthritis Rheum 1997;40:S77.
33. Veikkola T, Alitalo K. VEGFs, receptors and angiogenesis. Cancer Biol 1999;9:211–20.
34. Mason JC, Yarwood H, Sugars K, Haskard DO. Human umbilical vein and dermal microvascular endothelial cells show heterogeneity in response to activation of protein kinase C. Am J Physiol 1997;273:C1233–40.
35. Caras IW, Davitz MA, Rhee L, Weddell G, Martin DW Jr, Nussenzweig V. Cloning of decay-accelerating factor suggests novel use of splicing to generate two proteins. Nature 1987;325: 545–9.
36. O'Connell PJ, McKenzie A, Fisicaro N, Rockman SP, Pearse MJ, d'Apice AJ. Endoglin: a 180-kD endothelial cell and macrophage restricted differentiation molecule. Clin Exp Immunol 1992;90:154–9.
37. Uesu T, Mizuno M, Inoue H, Tomoda J, Tsuji T. Enhanced expression of decay accelerating factor and CD59/homologous restriction factor 20 on the colonic epithelium of ulcerative colitis. Lab Invest 1995;72:587–91.
38. Sasaki M, Joh T, Tada T, Okada N, Yokoyama Y, Itoh M. Altered expression of membrane inhibitors of complement in human gastric epithelium during Helicobacter-associated gastritis. Histopathology 1998;33:554–60.
39. Nicholson-Weller A, Wang CE. Structure and function of decay accelerating factor CD55. J Lab Clin Med 1994;123:485–91.
40. Cosio FG, Sedmak DD, Mahan JD, Nahman NS Jr. Localization of decay accelerating factor in normal and diseased kidneys. Kidney Int 1989;36:100–7.
41. Asghar SS. Membrane regulators of complement activation and their aberrant expression in disease. Lab Invest 1995;72:254–71.
42. Lidington EA, Haskard DO, Mason JC. Induction of decay-accelerating factor by thrombin through a protease-activated receptor 1 and protein kinase C-dependent pathway protects vascular endothelial cells from complement-mediated injury. Blood 2000;96:2784–92.
43. Hindmarsh EJ, Marks RM. Decay-accelerating factor is a component of subendothelial extracellular matrix in vitro and is aug-

mented by activation of protein kinase C. Eur J Immunol 1998; 28:1052–62.
44. Hindmarsh EJ, Marks RM. Complement activation occurs on subendothelial extracellular matrix. J Immunol 1998;160:6128–36.
45. Kevil CG, Payne DK, Mire E, Alexander JS. Vascular permeability factor/vascular endothelial cell growth factor-mediated permeability occurs through disorganization of endothelial junctional proteins. J Biol Chem 1998;273:15099–103.
46. Schönwasser DC, Marais RM, Marshall CJ, Parker PJ. Activation of the mitogen-activated protein kinase/extracellular signal-regulated kinase pathway by conventional, novel, and atypical protein kinase C isotypes. Mol Cell Biol 1998;18:790–8.
47. Dana A, Skarli M, Papakrivopoulou J, Yellon DM. Adenosine A1 receptor induced delayed preconditioning in rabbits: induction of p38 mitogen-activated protein kinase activation and Hsp27 phosphorylation via a tyrosine kinase– and protein kinase C–dependent mechanism. Circ Res 2000;89:989–97.
48. D'Angelo G, Struman I, Martial J, Weiner RI. Activation of mitogen-activated protein kinases by vascular endothelial growth factor and basic fibroblast growth factor in capillary endothelial cells is inhibited by the antiangiogenic factor 16-kDa N-terminal fragment of prolactin. Proc Natl Acad Sci U S A 1995;92:6374–8.
49. Rousseau S, Houle F, Landry J, Huot J. p38 MAP kinase activation by vascular endothelial growth factor mediates actin reorganization and cell migration in human endothelial cells. Oncogene 1997;15:2169–77.
50. Singh RP, Dhawan P, Golden C, Kapoor GS, Mehta KD. One-way cross-talk between p38(MAPK) and p42/44(MAPK): inhibition of p38(MAPK) induces low density lipoprotein receptor expression through activation of the p42/44(MAPK) cascade. J Biol Chem 1999;274:19593–600.
51. Badger AM, Griswold DE, Kapadia R, Blake S, Swift BA, Hoffman SJ, et al. Disease-modifying activity of SB 242235, a selective inhibitor of p38 mitogen-activated protein kinase, in rat adjuvant-induced arthritis. Arthritis Rheum 2000;43:175–83.
52. Mevorach D, Frolekis I, Shapira I. Stereo-specific activation of the complement system by phosphatidylserine appearing on apoptotic cells [abstract]. Arthritis Rheum 1999;42:S406.
53. Navratil JS, Wisnieski JJ, Ahearn JM. The globular heads of C1q bind specifically to surface blebs of apoptotic human endothelial cells: implications for immune tolerance [abstract]. Mol Immunol (supplement) 1998;35:398.
54. Tsuji S, Kaji K, Nagasawa S. Activation of the alternative pathway of human complement by apoptotic human umbilical vein endothelial cells. J Biochem (Tokyo) 1994;116:794–800.
55. Bhakdi S, Fassbender W, Hugo F, Carreno MP, Berstecher C, Malasit P, et al. Relative inefficiency of terminal complement activation. J Immunol 1988;141:3117–22.
56. Brodeur JP, Ruddy S, Schwartz LB, Moxley G. Synovial fluid levels of complement SC5b–9 and fragment Bb are elevated in patients with rheumatoid arthritis. Arthritis Rheum 1991;34:1531–7.
57. Hamann J, Vogel B, van Schijndel GMW, van Lier RAW. The seven-span transmembrane receptor CD97 has a cellular ligand (CD55 DAF). J Exp Med 1996;184:1185–9.
58. Eichler W, Hamann J, Aust G. Expression characteristics of the human CD97 antigen. Tissue Antigens 1997;50:429–38.
59. Hamann J, Wishaupt JO, van Lier RAW, Smeets TJM, Breedveld FC, Tak PP. Expression of the activation antigen CD97 and its ligand CD55 in rheumatoid synovial tissue. Arthritis Rheum 1999;42:650–8.
60. Alon T, Hemo I, Itin A, Peer J, Stone J, Keshet E. Vascular endothelial growth factor acts as a survival factor for newly formed retinal vessels and has implications for retinopathy of prematurity. Nat Med 1995;1:1024–8.
61. Yuan F, Chen Y, Dellian M, Safabakhsh N, Ferrara N, Jain RK. Time-dependent vascular regression and permeability changes in established human tumor xenografts induced by an anti-vascular endothelial growth factor/vascular permeability factor antibody. Proc Natl Acad Sci U S A 1996;93:14765–70.
62. Koch AE, Harlow LA, Haines GK, Amento EP, Unemori EN, Wong WL, et al. Vascular endothelial growth factor: a cytokine modulating endothelial function in rheumatoid arthritis. J Immunol 1994;152:4149–56.
63. Fava RA, Olsen NJ, Spencer-Green G, Yeo K-T, Yeo T-K, Berse B, et al. Vascular permeability factor/endothelial growth factor (VPF/VEGF): accumulation and expression in human synovial fluids and rheumatoid synovial tissue. J Exp Med 1994;180:341–6.
64. Palelog EM. Angiogenesis: a critical process in the pathogenesis of RA—a role for VEGF? Br J Rheumatol 1996;35:917–20.
65. Ostendorf T, Kunter U, Eitner F, Loos A, Regele H, Kerjaschki D, et al. VEGF(165) mediates glomerular endothelial repair. J Clin Invest 1999;104:913–23.
66. Gerber HP, McMurtrey A, Kowalski J, Yan M, Keyt BA, Dixit V, et al. Vascular endothelial growth factor regulates endothelial cell survival through the phosphatidylinositol 3′-kinase/Akt signal transduction pathway: requirement for Flk/KDR activation. J Biol Chem 1998;273:30336–43.
67. Gerber HP, Dixit V, Ferrara N. Vascular endothelial growth factor induces expression of the antiapoptotic proteins Bcl-2 and A1 in vascular endothelial cells. J Biol Chem 1998;273:13313–6.

Cassette Order Form

ACR / ARHP 2000 ANNUAL SCIENTIFIC MEETING

ACR COURSES

____ #1 (3 Tapes, $33) **CLINICAL UPDATE ON NEW THERAPIES IN RHEUMATIC DISEASES**
- Perspectives on Anti-TNF Therapy in RA — *Larry G. Anderson, MD*
- New Treatments in Development for Rheumatoid Arthritis — *Edward C. Keystone, MD*
- Osteoarthritis: Neutraceuticals, Viscosupplementation, and Other New Therapies — *David T. Felson, MD, MPH*
- New Approaches to the Treatment of SLE: An Overview — *Ellen M. Ginzler, MD, MPH*
- Pharmacoeconimic Analysis in the Rheumatic Diseases — *Sherine E. Gabriel, MD, MSc*

____ #2 (5 Tapes, $55) **ACR REVIEW COURSE**
- Hepatitis C Infection and the Silent Epidemic: Immunologic Complications — *Leonard H. Calabrese, DO*
- Novel Treatments for Rheumatoid Arthritis: Beyond Monotherapy with Disease-Modifying Anti-Rheumatic Drugs — *James R. O'Dell, MD*
- Magnetic Resonance Imaging of the Shoulder and Knee — *Clyde Helms, MD*
- Systemic Sclerosis: Insights into Pathogenesis and Treatment — *Joseph H. Korn, MD*
- Medical Management of Low Back Pain: Challenges and Pitfalls — *Alexander Vaccaro, MD*
- Neonatal Lupus: Bedside to Bench and Back — *Jill P. Buyon, MD*

____ #3 (3 Tapes, $33) **ACR FRONTIERS IN BASIC RESEARCH COURSE – Frontiers in Molecular Medicine**
- Genetic Medicine in the New Millennium – From Linkage Mapping to Finding Genes — *Matthew Brown, MB, BS, MD*
- Homocysteine and Connective Tissue Disease: To Treat or Not to Treat — *David Cole, MD*
- Pharmacogenetics: The Future of Individualized Therapy — *Mary Relling, PharmD*
- The Human Genome Project in the New Millennium — *Daniel L. Kastner, MD, PhD*
- The Future of Genetic Testing for Common, Complex Diseases — *Neil A. Holtzman, MD*

____ #4 **OPENING LECTURE: PAUL KLEMPERER, MD MEMORIAL LECTURESHIP – Innate Immunity: New Roles in Host Defense and Rheumatic Disease** — *John P. Atkinson, MD*

____ #5 (2 Tapes, $22) **PLENARY SESSION I**

____ #6 **MEDICAL ASPECTS OF RHEUMATIC DISEASES LECTURE – Evolving Concepts in the Diagnosis, Pathogenesis, and Management of Autoimmune Hepatitis** — *Albert J. Czaja, MD*

____ #7 **STATE-OF-THE-ART LECTURE – Steroid-Induced Osteoporosis** — *Kenneth G. Saag, MD*

____ #8 **CLINICAL SCIENCE SYMPOSIUM – Skin Manifestations of Rheumatic Diseases**
- Pathogenic Mechanisms Involved in Cutaneous Lupus Erythematosus — *Daniel P. McCauliffe, MD*
- Mechanisms Involved in Psoriasis — *Kevin D. Cooper, MD*
- Cutaneous Side Effects of Immunomodulatory Agents — *Victoria P. Werth, MD*

____ #9 **MINI SYMPOSIUM – Gene Expression Patterns, Genetic Polymporphisms in Sceroderma and Gene Regulation in Scleroderma** — *Sergio Jimenez, MD*

PHILADELPHIA 2000

CME Unlimited is proud to be the official recording and marketing company for the **American College of Rheumatology and Association of Rheumatology Health Professionals 2000 Annual Scientific Meeting**, held Oct. 28 – Nov. 2, in Philadelphia.

Audiocassette copies of sessions listed are available via **TELEPHONE, FAX, MAIL** or **ONLINE ORDERS.** All orders will be shipped within five business days.

To order immediately, have your credit card ready and call toll-free **1-800-776-5454** from 8:00 AM to 5:00 PM (PST), Monday-Friday.

Or visit the **Online Tape Store** via **www.rheumatology.org/products/other/audio.html.**

For mail or fax orders, please mark your selections, complete the coupon on the opposite side, include full payment, and send this entire order form to CME Unlimited. For your convenience, we accept VISA, MasterCard, American Express, as well as checks. Thank you!

ACR / ARHP TAPE SPECIALS

Product Description	Price
Individual Audio Tapes	$ 11.00
Any 8 Audio Tapes ($10.50/Each)	$ 84.00
Any 16 Audio Tapes with Free Album ($10.00/Each)	$ 160.00
Any 32 Audio Tapes with Free Albums ($9.50/Each)	$ 304.00
Full Set of 114 Audio Tapes with Free Albums	$ 899.00

____ #10 **MINI SYMPOSIUM – Epidemiology of Rheumatology** — *Deborah Symmons, MD*

____ #11 **SPECIAL LECTURE – ADVANCES IN RHEUMATIC DISEASE RESEARCH: Presentations of ACR's Distinguished Award Recipients**

____ #12 **ABSTRACT CONCURRENT SESSION – Organ Involvement in SLE**

____ #13 **ABSTRACT CONCURRENT SESSION – Cell-cell, Cell-matrix Interactions**

____ #14 **ABSTRACT CONCURRENT SESSION – Novel Findings in Chondrocyte/ Synoviocyte Biology in OA**

____ #15 **ABSTRACT CONCURRENT SESSION – Vasculitis: Diagnosis and Management**

____ #16 **ABSTRACT CONCURRENT SESSION – Assessment of Functional Disability in Musculoskeletal Disease**

____ #17 **CLINICAL SCIENCE SYMPOSIUM – Inflammation and Atherosclerotic Cardiovascular Disease**
- Inflammation and Atherosclerotic Risk — *Paul Ridker, MD*
- Techniques for the Detection of Preclinical ASCVD and their Application in SLE — *Mary Roman, MD*
- Risk Factors for Cardiovascular Mortality and Morbidity — *John Esdaile, MD*

____ #18 **SPECIAL LECTURE – Marshall J. Schiff, MD, Memorial Lectureship**
- The Bone and Joint Decade 2000 - 2010 – An Update — *Lars Lidgren, MD*
- Beyond Prosthetic Joint Replacement: The Repair and Regeneration of Skeletal Tissues — *Thomas Einhorn, MD*

____ #19 **MINI-SYMPOSIUM – RA Animal Models** — *Marie Griffiths, MD*

____ #20 **MINI-SYMPOSIUM – New Insight Antibody** — *John Harley, MD, PhD*

____ #21 **CONCURRENT SESSION – Late-breaking Abstracts**

____ #22 **CONCURRENT SESSION – Potpourri in Pediatric Rheumatology**

____ #23 **CONCURRENT SESSION – Infection-related Rheumatic Disease**

____ #24 **CONCURRENT SESSION – Sjögren's/Myositis**

____ #25 **CONCURRENT SESSION – Gene Therapy**

____ #26 **CONCURRENT SESSION – Epidemiology of Osteoarthritis**

____ #27 (2 Tapes, $22) **CONCURRENT SESSION – Potential Mechanisms in Fibromyalgia**

____ #28 **STUDY GROUP – Non-Articular Rheumatism**

____ #29 **STUDY GROUP – Pediatrics**

____ #30 (2 Tapes, $22) **STUDY GROUP – Scleroderma**

____ #31 **STUDY GROUP – Systemic Lupus Erthematosus**

____ #32 (2 Tapes, $22) **PLENARY SESSION II**

____ #33 **MEDICAL ASPECTS OF RHEUMATIC DISEASE LECTURE – Ocular Manifestations** — *James T. Rosenbaum, MD*

____ #34 **ACR/ARHP COMBINED CLINCAL SYMPOSIUM – Meeting Unmet Drug Needs: Development of Disease Therapies** — *James P. Witter, MD, PhD; John F. Beary, III, MD; Cheryl H. Yarboro, RN, BSPA*

____ #35 **MINI-SYMPOSIUM – Cytokines in Inflammatory Rheumatic Diseases** — *Lain McInnes, MD*

____ #36 **MINI-SYMPOSIUM – Gene Expression and Myositis** — *Salvestere Di Mauro, MD*

____ #37 **MINI-SYMPOSIUM – Phagocytes and Inflammation** — *Steven Abramson, MD*

____ #38 **ABSTRACT CONCURRENT SESSION – RA Therapy: Long-term Observations with New Therapies**

____ #39 **ABSTRACT CONCURRENT SESSION – Novel Therapeutic Agents for SLE**

____ #40 **ABSTRACT CONCURRENT SESSION – Tolerance Abrogation in Lupus**

____ #41 **ABSTRACT CONCURRENT SESSION – Markers and Protective Agents for Osteoarthritis**

____ #42 **ABSTRACT CONCURRENT SESSION – RA Genetics**

____ #43 **STATE-OF-THE-ART LECTURE – Fibromyalgia: Advances in Understanding and Improvements in Management** — *Daniel J. Clauw, MD*

____ #44 **CLINICAL SCIENCE SYMPOSIUM – New Drug Targets: Signal Transduction and Matrix Metalloproteinases**
- NF-KB and MAP Kinase Pathways: New Targets for DMARDs? — *Anthony Manning, PhD*
- MMP — *Randall M. Stevens, MD*

____ #45 **MINI-SYMPOSIUM – Crystal and Metabolic Arthropathies (Klinenberg Memorial Lecture)** — *Herbert Diamond, MD*

____ #46 **MINI-SYMPOSIUM – Clinical Aspects of APL Syndrome** — *Roger Levy, MD*

____ #47 **ABSTRACT CONCURRENT SESSION – Regulation Gene Expression**

____ #48 **ABSTRACT CONCURRENT SESSION – Genetics of Lupus**

____ #49 **ABSTRACT CONCURRENT SESSION – Chemokines & Cytokines**

____ #50 **SPECIAL LECTURE – Rheumatoid Arthritis and Atherosclerotic Cardiovascular Disease: Shared Disease Mechanisms** — *Cornelia M. Weyand, MD*

Continued on Opposite Side

Proven Results

Patients With Sjögren's Syndrome

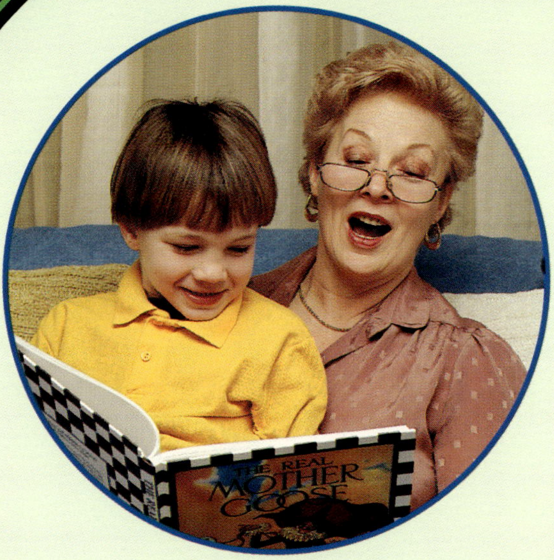

Evoxac™
(cevimeline HCl) 30 mg Capsules TID

Proven Relief...
Proven Results

- Cevimeline can potentially alter cardiovascular function. Consult the brief summary of prescribing information concerning these potential effects
- Caution should be advised while driving at night or performing hazardous activities in reduced lighting

* At study endpoint in 3 placebo-controlled trials at 30 mg TID.
† Patients self-reported overall feeling of dry mouth compared with before the study as "better," "no change," or "worse" at study endpoint.
‡ Significant improvement in the symptoms of dry mouth was observed in 2 of 3 trials versus placebo. However, there was a higher placebo response rate in one 12-week study versus the study arm.
§ Change from predose to postdose at final visit and week 6 in placebo-controlled trials.

Evoxac™ ('ē vō zak)

(cevimeline HCl) 30 mg Capsules

EVOXAC™ Capsules
(cevimeline hydrochloride)

Brief Summary
Consult package insert for full prescribing information.

INDICATIONS AND USAGE: Cevimeline is indicated for the treatment of symptoms of dry mouth in patients with Sjögren's Syndrome.

CONTRAINDICATIONS: Cevimeline is contraindicated in patients with uncontrolled asthma, known hypersensitivity to cevimeline, and when miosis is undesirable, e.g., in acute iritis and in narrow-angle (angle-closure) glaucoma.

WARNINGS:

Cardiovascular Disease: Cevimeline can potentially alter cardiac conduction and/or heart rate. Patients with significant cardiovascular disease may potentially be unable to compensate for transient changes in hemodynamics or rhythm induced by EVOXAC™. EVOXAC™ should be used with caution and under close medical supervision in patients with a history of cardiovascular disease evidenced by angina pectoris or myocardial infarction.

Pulmonary Disease: Cevimeline can potentially increase airway resistance, bronchial smooth muscle tone, and bronchial secretions. Cevimeline should be administered with caution and with close medical supervision to patients with controlled asthma, chronic bronchitis, or chronic obstructive pulmonary disease.

Ocular: Ophthalmic formulations of muscarinic agonists have been reported to cause visual blurring which may result in decreased visual acuity, especially at night and in patients with central lens changes, and to cause impairment of depth perception. Caution should be advised while driving at night or performing hazardous activities in reduced lighting.

PRECAUTIONS:

General: Cevimeline toxicity is characterized by an exaggeration of its parasympathomimetic effects. These may include: headache, visual disturbance, lacrimation, sweating, respiratory distress, gastrointestinal spasm, nausea, vomiting, diarrhea, atrioventricular block, tachycardia, bradycardia, hypotension, hypertension, shock, mental confusion, cardiac arrhythmia, and tremors.

Cevimeline should be administered with caution to patients with a history of nephrolithiasis or cholelithiasis. Contractions of the gallbladder or biliary smooth muscle could precipitate complications such as cholecystitis, cholangitis and biliary obstruction. An increase in the ureteral smooth muscle tone could theoretically precipitate renal colic or ureteral reflux in patients with nephrolithiasis.

Information for Patients: Patients should be informed that cevimeline may cause visual disturbances, especially at night, that could impair their ability to drive safely.

If a patient sweats excessively while taking cevimeline, dehydration may develop. The patient should drink extra water and consult a health care provider.

Drug Interactions: Cevimeline should be administered with caution to patients taking beta adrenergic antagonists, because of the possibility of conduction disturbances. Drugs with parasympathomimetic effects administered concurrently with cevimeline can be expected to have additive effects. Cevimeline might interfere with desirable antimuscarinic effects of drugs used concomitantly.

Drugs which inhibit CYP2D6 and CYP3A3/4 also inhibit the metabolism of cevimeline. Cevimeline should be used with caution in individuals known or suspected to be deficient in CYP2D6 activity, based on previous experience, as they may be at a higher risk of adverse events. In an *in vitro* study, cytochrome P450 isozymes 1A2, 2A6, 2C9, 2C19, 2D6, 2E1, and 3A4 were not inhibited by exposure to cevimeline.

Carcinogenesis, Mutagenesis and Impairment of Fertility: Lifetime carcinogenicity studies were conducted in CD-1 mice and F-344 rats. A statistically significant increase in the incidence of adenocarcinomas of the uterus was observed in female rats that received cevimeline at a dosage of 100 mg/kg/day (approximately 8 times the maximum human exposure based on comparison of AUC data). No other significant differences in tumor incidence were observed in either mice or rats.

Cevimeline exhibited no evidence of mutagenicity or clastogenicity in a battery of assays that included an Ames test, an *in vitro* chromosomal aberration study in mammalian cells, a mouse lymphoma study in L5178Y cells, or a micronucleus assay conducted *in vivo* in ICR mice.

Cevimeline did not adversely affect the reproductive performance or fertility of male Sprague-Dawley rats when administered for 63 days prior to mating and throughout the period of mating at dosages up to 45 mg/kg/day (approximately 5 times the maximum recommended dose for a 60 kg human following normalization of the data on the basis of body surface area estimates). Females that were treated with cevimeline at dosages up to 45 mg/kg/day from 14 days prior to mating through day seven of gestation exhibited a statistically significantly smaller number of implantations than did control animals.

Pregnancy: Pregnancy Category C.

Cevimeline was associated with a reduction in the mean number of implantations when given to pregnant Sprague-Dawley rats from 14 days prior to mating through day seven of gestation at a dosage of 45 mg/kg/day (approximately 5 times the maximum recommended dose for a 60 kg human when compared on the basis of body surface area estimates). This effect may have been secondary to maternal toxicity. There are no adequate and well-controlled studies in pregnant women. Cevimeline should be used during pregnancy only if the potential benefit justifies the potential risk to the fetus.

Nursing Mothers: It is not known whether this drug is secreted in human milk. Because many drugs are excreted in human milk, and because of the potential for serious adverse reactions in nursing infants from EVOXAC™, a decision should be made whether to discontinue nursing or discontinue the drug, taking into account the importance of the drug to the mother.

Pediatric Use: Safety and effectiveness in pediatric patients have not been established.

Geriatric Use: Although clinical studies of cevimeline included subjects over the age of 65, the numbers were not sufficient to determine whether they respond differently from younger subjects. Special care should be exercised when cevimeline treatment is initiated in an elderly patient, considering the greater frequency of decreased hepatic, renal, or cardiac function, and of concomitant disease or other drug therapy in the elderly.

ADVERSE REACTIONS: Cevimeline was administered to 1777 patients during clinical trials worldwide, including Sjögren's patients and patients with other conditions. In placebo-controlled Sjögren's studies in the U.S., 320 patients received cevimeline doses ranging from 15 mg tid to 60 mg tid, of whom 93% were women and 7% were men. Demographic distribution was 90% Caucasian, 5% Hispanic, 3% Black, and 2% of other origin. In these studies, 14.6% of patients discontinued treatment with cevimeline due to adverse events.

The following adverse events associated with muscarinic agonism were observed in the clinical trials of cevimeline in Sjögren's syndrome patients:

Adverse Event	Cevimeline 30 mg (tid) n* = 533	Placebo (tid) n = 164	Adverse Event	Cevimeline 30 mg (tid) n* = 533	Placebo (tid) n = 164
Excessive Sweating	18.7%	2.4%	Urinary Frequency	0.9%	1.8%
Nausea	13.8%	7.9%	Asthenia	0.5%	0.0%
Rhinitis	11.2%	5.4%	Flushing	0.3%	0.6%
Diarrhea	10.3%	10.3%	Polyuria	0.1%	0.6%
Excessive Salivation	2.2%	0.6%			

*n is the total number of patients exposed to the dose at any time during the study

EVOXAC™ Capsules
(cevimeline hydrochloride)

In addition, the following adverse events (≥3% incidence) were reported in the Sjögren's clinical trials:

Adverse Event	Cevimeline 30 mg (tid) n* = 533	Placebo (tid) n = 164	Adverse Event	Cevimeline 30 mg (tid) n* = 533	Placebo (tid) n = 164
Headache	14.4%	20.1%	Conjunctivitis	4.3%	3.6%
Sinusitis	12.3%	10.9%	Dizziness	4.1%	7.3%
Upper Respiratory Tract Infection	11.4%	9.1%	Bronchitis	4.1%	1.2%
			Arthralgia	3.7%	1.8%
Dyspepsia	7.8%	8.5%	Surgical Intervention	3.3%	3.0%
Abdominal Pain	7.6%	6.7%	Fatigue	3.3%	1.2%
Urinary Tract Infection	6.1%	3.0%	Pain	3.3%	3.0%
Coughing	6.1%	3.0%	Skeletal Pain	2.8%	1.8%
Pharyngitis	5.2%	5.4%	Insomnia	2.4%	1.2%
Vomiting	4.6%	2.4%	Hot Flushes	2.4%	0.0%
Injury	4.5%	2.4%	Rigors	1.3%	1.2%
Back Pain	4.5%	4.2%	Anxiety	1.3%	1.2%
Rash	4.3%	6.0%			

*n is the total number of patients exposed to the dose at any time during the study

The following events were reported in Sjögren's patients at incidences of <3% and ≥1%: constipation, tremor, abnormal vision, hypertonia, peripheral edema, chest pain, myalgia, fever, anorexia, eye pain, earache, dry mouth, vertigo, salivary gland pain, pruritus, influenza-like symptoms, eye infection, post-operative pain, vaginitis, skin disorder, depression, hiccup, hyporeflexia, infection, fungal infection, sialoadenitis, otitis media, erythematous rash, pneumonia, edema, salivary gland enlargement, allergy, gastroesophageal reflux, eye abnormality, migraine, tooth disorder, epistaxis, flatulence, toothache, ulcerative stomatitis, anemia, hypoesthesia, cystitis, leg cramps, abscess, eructation, moniliasis, palpitation, increased amylase, xerophthalmia, allergic reaction.

The following events were reported rarely in treated Sjögren's patients (<1%): Causal relation is unknown:

Body as a Whole Disorders: aggravated allergy, precordial chest pain, abnormal crying, hematoma, leg pain, edema, periorbital edema, activated pain trauma, pallor, changed sensation to temperature, weight decrease, weight increase, choking, mouth edema, syncope, malaise, face edema, substernal chest pain

Cardiovascular Disorders: abnormal ECG, heart disorder, heart murmur, aggravated hypertension, hypotension, arrhythmia, extrasystoles, t wave inversion, tachycardia, supraventricular tachycardia, angina pectoris, myocardial infarction, pericarditis, pulmonary embolism, peripheral ischemia, superficial phlebitis, purpura, deep thrombophlebitis, vascular disorder, vasculitis, hypertension

Digestive Disorders: appendicitis, increased appetite, ulcerative colitis, diverticulitis, duodenitis, dysphagia, enterocolitis, gastric ulcer, gastritis, gastroenteritis, gastrointestinal hemorrhage, gingivitis, glossitis, rectum hemorrhage, hemorrhoids, ileus, irritable bowel syndrome, melena, mucositis, esophageal stricture, esophagitis, oral hemorrhage, peptic ulcer, periodontal destruction, rectal disorder, stomatitis, tenesmus, tongue discoloration, tongue disorder, geographic tongue, tongue ulceration, dental caries

Endocrine Disorders: increased glucocorticoids, goiter, hypothyroidism

Hematologic Disorders: thrombocytopenic purpura, thrombocythemia, thrombocytopenia, hypochromic anemia, eosinophilia, granulocytopenia, leucopenia, leukocytosis, cervical lymphadenopathy, lymphadenopathy

Liver and Biliary System Disorders: cholelithiasis, increased gamma-glutamyl transferase, increased hepatic enzymes, abnormal hepatic function, viral hepatitis, increased serum glutamate oxaloacetic transaminase (SGOT)(also called AST-aspartate aminotransferase), increased serum glutamate pyruvate transaminase (SGPT)(also called ALT-alanine aminotransferase)

Metabolic and Nutritional Disorders: dehydration, diabetes mellitus, hypercalcemia, hypercholesterolemia, hyperglycemia, hyperlipemia, hypertriglyceridemia, hyperuricemia, hypoglycemia, hypokalemia, hyponatremia, thirst

Musculoskeletal Disorders: arthritis, aggravated arthritis, arthropathy, femoral head avascular necrosis, bone disorder, bursitis, costochondritis, plantar fasciitis, muscle weakness, osteomyelitis, osteoporosis, synovitis, tendinitis, tenosynovitis

Neoplasms: basal cell carcinoma, squamous carcinoma

Nervous Disorders: carpal tunnel syndrome, coma, abnormal coordination, dysesthesia, dyskinesia, dysphonia, aggravated multiple sclerosis, involuntary muscle contractions, neuralgia, neuropathy, paresthesia, speech disorder, agitation, confusion, depersonalization, aggravated depression, abnormal dreaming, emotional lability, manic reaction, paroniria, somnolence, abnormal thinking, hyperkinesia, hallucination

Miscellaneous Disorders: fall, food poisoning, heat stroke, joint dislocation, post-operative hemorrhage

Resistance Mechanism Disorders: cellulitis, herpes simplex, herpes zoster, bacterial infection, viral infection, genital moniliasis, sepsis

Respiratory Disorders: asthma, bronchospasm, chronic obstructive airway disease, dyspnea, hemoptysis, laryngitis, nasal ulcer, pleural effusion, pleurisy, pulmonary congestion, pulmonary fibrosis, respiratory disorder

Rheumatologic Disorders: aggravated rheumatoid arthritis, lupus erythematosus rash, lupus erythematosus syndrome

Skin and Appendages Disorders: acne, alopecia, burn, dermatitis, contact dermatitis, lichenoid dermatitis, eczema, furunculosis, hyperkeratosis, lichen planus, nail discoloration, nail disorder, onychia, onychomycosis, paronychia, photosensitivity reaction, rosacea, scleroderma, seborrhea, skin discoloration, dry skin, skin exfoliation, skin hypertrophy, skin ulceration, urticaria, verruca, bullous eruption, cold clammy skin

Special Senses Disorders: deafness, decreased hearing, motion sickness, parosmia, taste perversion, blepharitis, cataract, corneal opacity, corneal ulceration, diplopia, glaucoma, anterior chamber eye hemorrhage, keratitis, keratoconjunctivitis, mydriasis, myopia, photopsia, retinal deposits, retinal disorder, scleritis, vitreous detachment, tinnitus

Urogenital Disorders: epididymitis, prostatic disorder, abnormal sexual function, amenorrhea, female breast neoplasm, malignant female breast neoplasm, female breast pain, positive cervical smear test, dysmenorrhea, endometrial disorder, intermenstrual bleeding, leukorrhea, menorrhagia, menstrual disorder, ovarian cyst, ovarian disorder, genital pruritus, uterine hemorrhage, vaginal hemorrhage, atrophic vaginitis, albuminuria, bladder discomfort, increased blood urea nitrogen, dysuria, hematuria, micturition disorder, nephrosis, nocturia, increased nonprotein nitrogen, pyelonephritis, renal calculus, abnormal renal function, renal pain, strangury, urethral disorder, abnormal urine, urinary incontinence, decreased urine flow, pyuria

In one subject with lupus erythematosus receiving concomitant multiple drug therapy, a highly elevated ALT level was noted after the fourth week of cevimeline therapy. In two other subjects receiving cevimeline in the clinical trials, very high AST levels were noted. The significance of these findings is unknown.

Additional adverse events (relationship unknown) which occurred in other clinical studies (patient population different from Sjögren's patients) are as follows:

cholinergic syndrome, blood pressure fluctuation, cardiomegaly, postural hypotension, aphasia, convulsions, abnormal gait, hyperesthesia, paralysis, abnormal sexual function, enlarged abdomen, change in bowel habits, gum hyperplasia, intestinal obstruction, bundle branch block, increased creatine phosphokinase, electrolyte abnormality, glycosuria, gout, hyperkalemia, hyperproteinemia, increased lactic dehydrogenase (LDH), increased alkaline phosphatase, failure to thrive, abnormal platelets, aggressive reaction, amnesia, apathy, delirium, delusion, dementia, illusion, impotence, neurosis, paranoid reaction, personality disorder, hyperhemoglobinemia, apnea, atelectasis, yawning, oliguria, urinary retention, distended vein, lymphocytosis

MANAGEMENT OF OVERDOSE: Management of the signs and symptoms of acute overdosage should be handled in a manner consistent with that indicated for other muscarinic agonists: general supportive measures should be instituted. If medically indicated, atropine, an anti-cholinergic agent may be of value as an antidote for emergency use in patients who have had an overdose of cevimeline. If medically indicated, epinephrine may also be of value in the presence of severe cardiovascular depression or bronchoconstriction. It is not known if cevimeline is dialyzable.

DOSAGE AND ADMINISTRATION: The recommended dose of cevimeline is 30 mg taken three times a day. There is insufficient safety information to support doses greater than 30 mg tid. There is also insufficient evidence for additional efficacy of cevimeline at doses greater than 30 mg tid.

Rx Only

Manufactured by:
YAMANOUCHI PHARMA TECHNOLOGIES, INC., Palo Alto, CA 94304

for:
SnowBrand Pharmaceuticals, Inc., Rockville, MD 20850

Distributed and Marketed by:
Daiichi Pharmaceutical Corporation, Montvale, NJ 07645

02/2000 Printed in U.S.A.

DAIICHI
Daiichi Pharmaceutical Corporation

www.daiichius.com

For additional information please call toll free:
1-877-DAIICHI 1-877-324-4244

Reference: 1. Data on file, Daiichi Pharmaceutical Corporation.

ARTHRITIS & RHEUMATISM
Vol. 44, No. 1, January 2001, pp 151–162

Insights from a Novel Three-Dimensional In Vitro Model of Lyme Arthritis

Standardized Analysis of Cellular and Molecular Interactions Between *Borrelia burgdorferi* and Synovial Explants and Fibroblasts

Juliane K. Franz,[1] Olaf Fritze,[1] Michael Rittig,[2] Gernot Keyßer,[3] Susanne Priem,[1] Josef Zacher,[4] Gerd-R. Burmester,[1] and Andreas Krause[1]

Objective. **To develop a novel 3-dimensional (3-D) in vitro model of Lyme arthritis to use in the study of the interactions between *Borrelia burgdorferi* (Bb) and human synovial host cells with respect to phagocytosis and potential persistence of Bb as well as the induction of proinflammatory cytokines and chemokines.**

Methods. **Two distinct culture systems, consisting of synovial membrane explants or interactive synovial cells embedded in 3-D fibrin matrices, were chosen. Both systems were artificially infected with Bb, and the interactions between Bb and synovial tissue/cells were studied by histology, immunohistochemistry, and electron microscopy. Functional analyses included the induction/secretion of cytokines by Bb in the model system.**

Results. **Both culture systems proved to be stable and reproducible. The host cells and spirochetes showed high levels of viability and maintained their physiologic shape for >3 weeks. Bb invaded the synovial tissue and the artifical matrix in a time-dependent manner. Host cells were activated by Bb, as indicated by the induction of interleukin-1β and tumor necrosis factor α. Electron microscopic analysis revealed Bb intracellularly within macrophages as well as synovial fibroblasts, suggesting that not only professional phagocytes, but also resident synovial cells are capable of phagocytosing Bb. Most interestingly, the uptake of the spirochetes appeared to cause severe damage of the synovial fibroblasts, since the majority of these cells displayed ultrastructural features of disintegration.**

Conclusion. **A novel 3-D in vitro model has been established that allows the study of distinct aspects of Lyme arthritis under conditions that resemble the pathologic condition in humans. This reproducible, standardized model supplements animal studies and conventional 2-D cultures. The disintegration of synovial fibroblasts containing Bb or Bb fragments challenges the concept of an intracellular persistence of Bb and may instead reflect a mechanism that contributes to the inflammatory processes characteristic of Lyme arthritis.**

Lyme arthritis is one of the most common clinical manifestations of Lyme borreliosis. Early in the disease, migratory arthralgias and transient arthritides may occur. In chronic Lyme disease, arthritis typically manifests as an intermittent or chronic monarticular or oligoarticular arthritis that usually involves the larger joints, especially the knee.

Although the etiology of Lyme arthritis is known, the pathogenesis has not yet been fully elucidated. Most cases appear to be associated with the presence of spirochetes in the affected joints. The isolation and cultivation of *Borrelia burgdorferi* (Bb) from synovial fluid has rarely been successful (1), but novel molecular

Presented in part at the 63rd Annual Scientific Meeting of the American College of Rheumatology, Boston, MA, November 1999.
Supported by BMFT grant 01 KI 9503 and by DFG grant KR 997/2-1.
[1]Juliane K. Franz, MD, Olaf Fritze, Susanne Priem, MD, Gerd-R. Burmester, MD, Andreas Krause, MD: Charité University Hospital, Berlin, Germany; [2]Michael Rittig, MD: University of Montpellier, Montpellier, France; [3]Gernot Keyßer, MD: University Hospital Kröllwitz, Halle, and Charité University Hospital, Berlin, Germany; [4]Josef Zacher, MD: Orthopedic Clinic, Berlin-Buch, Germany.
Address correspondence and reprint requests to Andreas Krause, MD, Professor of Rheumatology, Department of Medicine, Rheumatology and Clinical Immunology, Charité University Hospital, Schumannstrasse 20/21, 10098 Berlin, Germany.
Submitted for publication February 22, 2000; accepted in revised form July 28, 2000.

techniques, such as polymerase chain reaction, have allowed the detection of Bb DNA in synovial fluids and synovial tissues in >80% of untreated patients with Lyme arthritis (2).

However, ~10% of patients do not respond to antibiotic therapy and develop chronic Lyme disease. Two not-mutually-exclusive pathogenetic concepts of chronic Lyme arthritis are currently being explored: persistent infection and infection-induced immunopathology. Intraarticular persistence of Bb is suspected because Bb DNA could be demonstrated in synovial tissue but not in synovial fluid from European patients with treatment-resistant Lyme arthritis (2). Therefore, the spirochetes are thought to persist *within* the synovial tissue. Ultrastructural studies suggest that they may be found not only extracellularly, but also within the cytoplasm of synovial cells (3). However, a recent study by Carlson et al (4) was unable to detect Bb DNA in patients with treatment-resistant Lyme arthritis in the United States, illustrating that in addition to the persistence of the spirochetes, other mechanisms, such as autoimmunity, might also be responsible for chronic Lyme arthritis (5).

Another riddle in the pathogenesis of Lyme arthritis is the paucity of spirochetes at lesional sites; this contrasts with the clinical and histologic signs of a strong local inflammatory reaction, signs which are often indistinguishable from those found in patients with rheumatoid arthritis (RA). Bb appears to induce mechanisms that sufficiently amplify the local inflammatory response. Thus, it has been shown that Bb strongly activates monocytes, resulting in the induction of proinflammatory cytokines, such as interleukin-1β (IL-1β) and tumor necrosis factor α (TNFα) (6). Of note, not only infiltrating inflammatory cells, such as monocytes and lymphocytes, but also resident fibroblasts can be activated by Bb to produce various cytokines, chemokines, and adhesion molecules (7), which indicates their involvement in the pathogenesis of Lyme arthritis.

The establishment of an experimental model system to study the cellular and molecular interactions of Bb and synovial tissue and cells is difficult to achieve. Although animal systems have revealed important aspects of the disease, they are difficult to standardize and are not fully representative of the conditions in humans. Most in vitro studies were performed on monolayer cell cultures in which cells show a different morphology and function as compared with the conditions in vivo. Apart from the fact that adherence of cells to the plastic surface of culture dishes causes an activation of cells (e.g., the induction of cytokines), monolayer cultures do not provide a 3-dimensional (3-D) extracellular matrix, which is of crucial importance for the invasion of spirochetes into human tissue (8). To overcome these shortcomings, a novel 3-D in vitro model was developed to study the interactions of Bb and human synovial cells and tissue under reproducible and standardized conditions.

MATERIALS AND METHODS

Bb isolates. In pilot studies, the experiments were performed with the *Borrelia burgdorferi* sensu stricto strains N40 (passages 0–2) and ZS7 (passages 4–6) and the *Borrelia afzelii* strain Pko (passages 4–6), in parallel. The 3 different strains gave comparable results. For further experiments, strain N40 was used exclusively. This isolate was passaged through SCID mice and stored in aliquots at −70°C. For the experiments, aliquots were thawed and the Bb organisms were passaged for 2–8 passages prior to use. This Bb isolate was infectious at the time it was used for our experiments.

Synovial tissue and cells. Synovial tissue specimens were obtained from 6 osteoarthritis (OA) patients undergoing synovectomy or joint replacement surgery at the orthopedic department of the Charité University Hospital and from 4 patients during arthroscopy for nonarthritic diseases. Significant inflammation was excluded by microscopic evaluation of hematoxylin and eosin–stained cryosections. One part of the synovial tissue was used for explant cultures, the other part for isolation of synovial fibroblasts.

For cell isolation, synovial tissue was minced and enzymatically dispersed for 1 hour with a mixture of collagenase P (0.17 mg/ml; Boehringer, Mannheim, Germany) in RPMI 1640 medium (Biochrom, Berlin, Germany) supplemented with heat-inactivated 10% fetal calf serum (FCS), 25 m*M* HEPES, 100 units/ml of penicillin, and 100 μg/ml of streptomycin (Seromed, Berlin, Germany). Isolated cells were plated into culture dishes and cultured over 4–5 passages to obtain fibroblasts. Adherent cells were harvested by trypsin–EDTA digestion and used for interactive 3-D cultures.

Culture conditions for Bb and for synovial explants and synovial cells. Bb were cultured in BSK-H medium supplemented with 6% rabbit serum (Sigma, Steinheim, Germany) and 2 m*M* L-glutamine (Biochrom). Synovial cells were cultured in RPMI 1640 (Biochrom) supplemented with heat-inactivated 10% FCS, 25 m*M* HEPES, 100 units/ml of penicillin, and 100 μg/ml of streptomycin (Seromed). To coculture the borreliae and the synovial cells, a mixture of two-thirds supplemented BSK-H medium and one-third RPMI medium supplemented with heat-inactivated 10% FCS and 25 m*M* HEPES, but without antibiotics (see above), proved to be suitable for both the spirochetes and the human cells (coculture medium; see also the Results section).

Preparation of tissue explant cultures. Synovial membrane tissue was used immediately after surgery. Samples were cut into 2–4-mm pieces. After histologic analysis, synovial tissue explants were cultured in 48-well tissue culture plates (Nunc, Wiesbaden, Germany) in coculture medium (two-thirds supplemented BSK-H and one-third RPMI supplemented with heat-inactivated 10% FCS and 25 m*M* HEPES;

see above) for 24 hours to allow cells to adapt to the conditions for coculture with Bb.

The 3-D matrix. Among various artificial matrices tested for the 3-D culture, fibrin was the most suitable in terms of cell viability and morphology as well as for penetration by the spirochetes. Pure collagen did not form a solid matrix. The highly viscous gel did not allow the synovial cells to grow and to form their physiologic spatial shape. Agarose at different concentrations also inhibited normal cell morphology. In addition, Bb did not appear to actively invade the agarose gel. The ECM Gel (extracellular matrix gel; Sigma), which is composed of collagen, glycoproteins, and proteoglycans, provided a suitable 3-D matrix. Cells could form their physiologic structures, and the spirochetes were able to invade the matrix. However, the necessity of preparing the ECM Gel on ice under sterile conditions limits its application. Based on these limitations of the matrices, fibrin was selected for the 3-D cell cultures.

The best concentration of thrombin and fibrinogen had been determined in pilot studies. A 1:100 dilution of the thrombin provided in the Tissucol Duo-S1 Fibrin Glue system (55 IU/ml; Immuno, Heidelberg, Germany) was sufficient to induce polymerization of fibrinogen. Fibrinogen (70–110 mg/ml) was diluted 50%, 33%, 25%, 12.5%, 8.3%, 5%, and 2.3% in phosphate buffered saline (PBS). At a concentration of $<2\%$, no solid gel was obtained. A concentration of $>10\%$ appeared to reduce the motility of the spirochetes. However, up to a concentration of 25%, Bb were able to penetrate the matrix.

Preparation of 3-D cell cultures. Synovial fibroblasts were prepared as described above. The number of viable cells was determined by hemocytometer counting, using trypan blue exclusion staining. The Tissucol Duo-S1 Fibrin Glue system, consisting of a fibrinogen glue component and a thrombin component, were mixed to obtain a gel structure. The optimal thrombin concentration for polymerization was a 1:10 dilution in PBS. Fibrinogen was mixed with the synovial cell suspension (density 5–10 $\times$ 10^6 cells/ml) or with the spirochete suspension. Cryosections (6 μm) of 3-D cell cultures were stained with hematoxylin and eosin to assess the even distribution of synovial cells within the matrix of the specimens.

Mode of infection. The experiments were performed with the Bb sensu stricto strain N40 (see above) exclusively. For the tissue explant cultures, experiments were performed in 48-well tissue culture plates (Nunc). The specimens were allowed to adapt to the coculture medium for 24 hours. Thereafter, they were infected with 5 $\times$ 10^6 spirochetes/ml of medium. Two-thirds of the medium was changed daily, according to the generation time of the spirochetes, to keep the number of spirochetes constant throughout the culture period (see Results). For the 3-D cell cultures, a fibrin layer containing the spirochetes was overlaid with a second layer of fibrin containing isolated synovial cells embedded in the fibrin matrix (sandwich culture; see Results). In this setting, the medium was replaced completely every day. Cultures were maintained for up to 21 days.

The viability of the spirochetes was controlled by daily darkfield microscopy. Motile spirochetes were considered viable. The adherence of the spirochetes to synovial tissue and cells was checked daily during the culture period using an inverted light microscope and confirmed by immunohistochemistry (borreliae adjacent to synovial cells) and ultrastructural analysis (borreliae in close contact with or within synovial cells).

Culture supernatants and cryoconservation. At the end of the respective culture periods, culture supernatants were harvested and maintained at $-20°C$ until further use. The tissue explants as well as the 3-D interactive cultures were immediately embedded in Tissue-Tek OCT medium (Miles, Elkhart, IN), snap-frozen, and stored at $-80°C$.

Immunohistochemistry for Bb. Cryosections (6 μm) were mounted onto aminoalkylsilane-coated slides (Sigma) and fixed for 15 minutes with 4% formalin in PBS. All incubations were performed at room temperature. After blocking with 4% dry milk powder/2% goat serum in Tris–NaCl (pH 7.6), sections were incubated with the respective primary anti-Bb antibody for 1 hour. Among the different primary antibodies tested (monoclonal mouse anti-Bb IgG antibodies LA1, LA10, and LA21 ([target antigen flagellin; kind gift of Dr. M. G. Kramer, Heidelberg, Germany], polyclonal rabbit anti-Bb IgG [target antigen whole Bb organism; Seramun, Dolgenbrodt, Germany], and the polyclonal rabbit anti-Bb IgG [target antigens 83-kd, 41-kd, 34-kd, and 31-kd proteins of Bb; Quartett, New Fields, UK]), the polyclonal rabbit anti-Bb antibody (Seramun) was the most suitable with regard to specificity and signal intensity. This antibody was used in all further procedures at a concentration of 0.01 mg/ml in Tris–NaCl (pH 7.6). Rabbit IgG of the same concentration served as negative control.

For signal detection, various systems were compared: indirect immunofluorescence with fluorescein isothiocyanate–labeled secondary antibodies, alkaline phosphatase staining, and peroxidase staining. Although all systems worked, alkaline phosphatase staining (EnVision; Dako, Carpinteria, CA) was the most suitable because it allowed the simultaneous detection of specific messenger RNA (mRNA) by in situ hybridization and counterstaining of nuclei.

In situ hybridization. In situ hybridization was performed as previously described (9). Briefly, 6-μm cryostat sections were fixed in 3% paraformaldehyde in diethyl pyrocarbonate–PBS and hybridized with the digoxigenin-labeled riboprobes (either antisense or sense) specific for IL-16 or cyclooxygenase 2 (COX-2) for 16 hours at 50°C. For generation of the riboprobes, complementary DNA fragments specific for IL-16 (311 bp) or COX-2 (303 bp), which had been transcribed and amplified from synovial fibroblasts obtained from patients with RA, were inserted into a Bluescript II SK vector (Stratagene, La Jolla, CA). Digoxigenin-labeled sense and antisense riboprobes were transcribed using a commercially available transcription kit (Stratagene) and T3 or T7 polymerases (Boehringer). For immunologic detection, antidigoxigenin–alkaline phosphatase–conjugated Fab (Boehringer) and BCIP/NBT color substrate solution (Boehringer) containing 1 m*M* levamisole (Dako, Zug, Switzerland) were used.

Ultrastructural analysis. The specimens were trimmed to small cubes measuring $\sim$1 mm^3 and then processed for electron microscopy according to standard protocols. Briefly, the cubes were fixed in cacodylate-buffered cold 2.5% (volume/volume) glutaraldehyde for 8 hours at 4°C, postfixed in 1% (v/v) reduced ferricyanide–reduced osmium tetroxide, stained en bloc with a mixture of uranyl acetate and phospho-

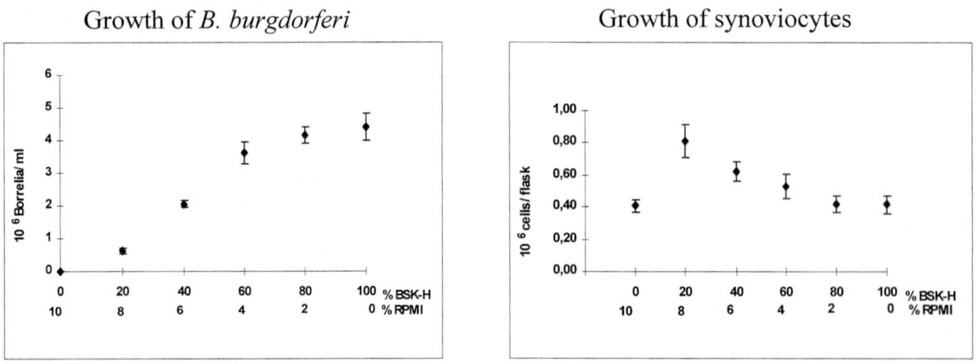

A B

Figure 1. Determination of the optimum coculture medium. To find a culture medium meeting the requirements of both the synovial cells and the spirochetes, RPMI 1640 medium and the *Borrelia*-specific medium BSK-H were mixed at various ratios. The growth rates of *Borrelia burgdorferi* (**A**) and synovial cells (**B**) in different dilutions of BSK-H/RPMI 1640 were determined separately. A reduction of the BSK-H medium to 40% resulted in a >50% decrease in the number of spirochetes (**A**). Synovial cells were less sensitive, showing a viability rate of 90–98% in all BSK-H/RPMI 1640 mixtures (**B**). For all further experiments, a coculture medium consisting of 2 parts BSK-H and 1 part RPMI 1640 was used. Small quantities of BSK-H appeared to have a stimulatory effect on synovial cells; this effect could not be observed at higher BSK-H concentrations (**B**).

tungstic acid in ethanol solution, dehydrated in a series of graded ethanol solutions ending with pure acetone, and finally embedded in Epon 812. Ultrathin sections were placed onto 200-mesh standard square copper grids, contrasted with uranyl acetate and lead citrate, and evaluated with a Zeiss 906 transmission electron microscope (Zeiss, Wetzlar, Germany). All chemicals were obtained from Roth, Karlsruhe, Germany.

Enzyme-linked immunosorbent assay (ELISA) for cytokines. Levels of the proinflammatory cytokines IL-1β and TNFα in the culture supernatants were determined by ELISA (Milenia-Assays; Diagnostic Products, Bad Nauheim, Germany) according to the manufacturer's protocol. The lower detection limits were 3 pg/ml for IL-1β and 6 pg/ml for TNFα.

RESULTS

Development of the 3-D model. *Coculture medium.* To find a culture medium suitable for both human synovial cells *and* Bb, cell medium RPMI 1640 and *Borrelia*-specific medium BSK-H were mixed at various ratios, and the growth rates of cells and the spirochetes were determined separately. As shown in Figure 1A, a reduction of the concentration of the BSK-H medium to 40% resulted in a >50% decrease in the number of spirochetes. Synovial cells were less sensitive, showing a viability rate of 90–98% in all RPMI 1640/BSK-H mixtures (Figure 1B). Small quantities of BSK-H appeared to have a stimulatory effect on synovial cells. This effect could not be observed at higher concentrations of the BSK-H medium (Figure 1B). For all further experiments, a coculture medium consisting of 2 parts BSK-H and 1 part RPMI 1640 was used.

We also assessed the influence of serum supplementation. Growth rates of the spirochetes and synovial cells in coculture medium supplemented with either 6% rabbit serum or 6% FCS were measured. Whereas

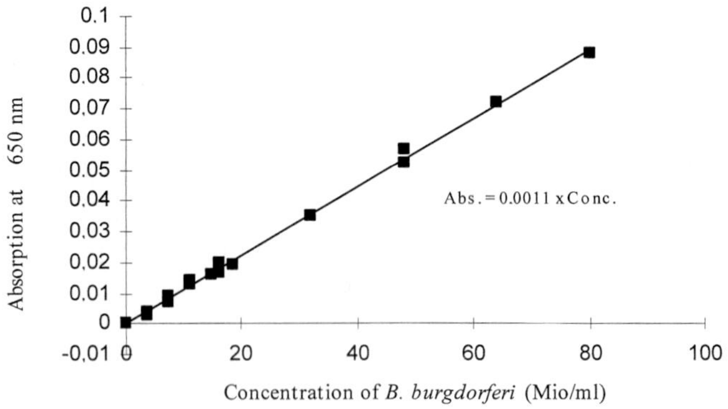

Figure 2. Densitometric determination of the concentration (Conc.) of *Borrelia burgdorferi*. To quantify the number of spirochetes used for infection in the model system, the optical density (OD) of suspensions of defined numbers of spirochetes was determined at an absorption (Abs.) level of 650 nm after equilibration of the pH of the culture medium with 1*M* HCl. Since the OD correlated with the number of spirochetes, the number of spirochetes can be extrapolated from the OD of a given suspension of spirochetes. Mio/ml = 10^6 infecting organisms/ml.

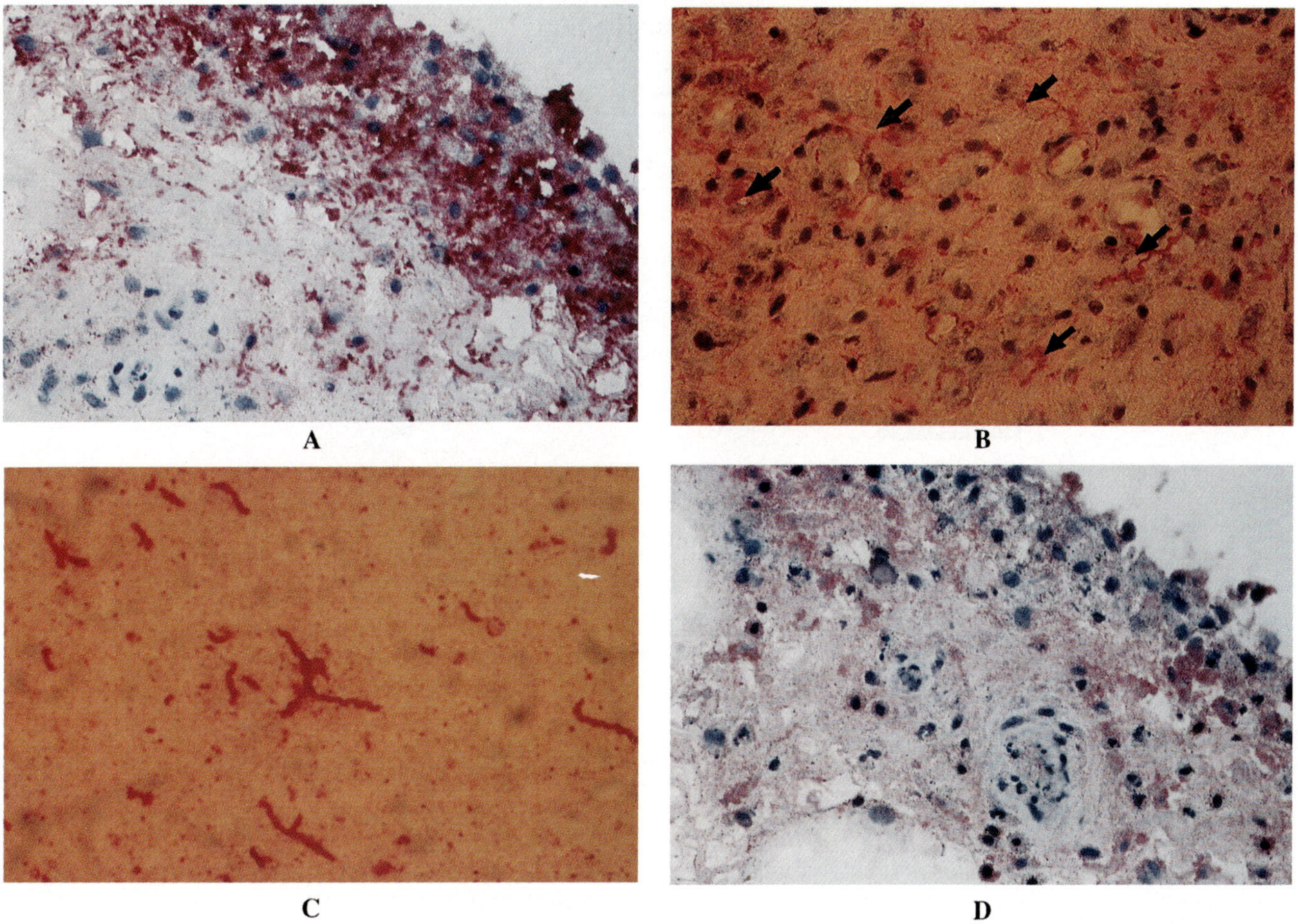

Figure 3. Immunohistochemistry for *Borrelia burgdorferi* (Bb). Specific staining of Bb (red; **arrows**) in the tissue explant culture (**A** and **C**) and in the fibrin gel of the 3-dimensional cell culture (**D**). The negative control, applying rabbit IgG instead of the rabbit anti-Bb antibody, is shown in **B**. In the tissue explants, spirochetes appeared to bind especially to the lining layer of synovium (**A**) but were also found in deeper areas (**C**). (Original magnification × 600 in **A**, **B**, and **C**; × 1,000 in **D**.)

synovial cells showed similar growth and viability in 6% rabbit serum and 6% FCS, the spirochetes survived only in 6% rabbit serum and not in 6% FCS.

Standardization of the Bb infective dose. To quantify the number of spirochetes used to infect tissue explant cultures and 3-D cell cultures, a novel densitometric technique was established. The optical densities (ODs) of suspensions of defined numbers of spirochetes were determined at 650 nm after equilibration of the pH of the medium with HCl to eliminate optical differences between fresh and used medium. As shown in Figure 2, the OD correlated with the number of spirochetes ($r = 0.99$). Therefore, the number of spirochetes can be extrapolated from the OD of a given suspension of spirochetes by applying the formula $N(t) = c \times a^t$, where N(t) is the time-dependent concentration, c is the initial concentration, and a is a growth coefficient specific for each strain of Bb.

Generation times of 14–18 hours were determined for all Bb strains used in this study. Based on this finding, two-thirds of the medium was replaced every day to keep the number of spirochetes constant during the culture period.

Immunohistochemistry for Bb. Bb could be detected within both the tissue explant cultures (Figures 3A and C) and the 3-D cell culture (Figure 3D). Because of the excellent ratio between strong specific staining and low background staining, the polyclonal rabbit anti-

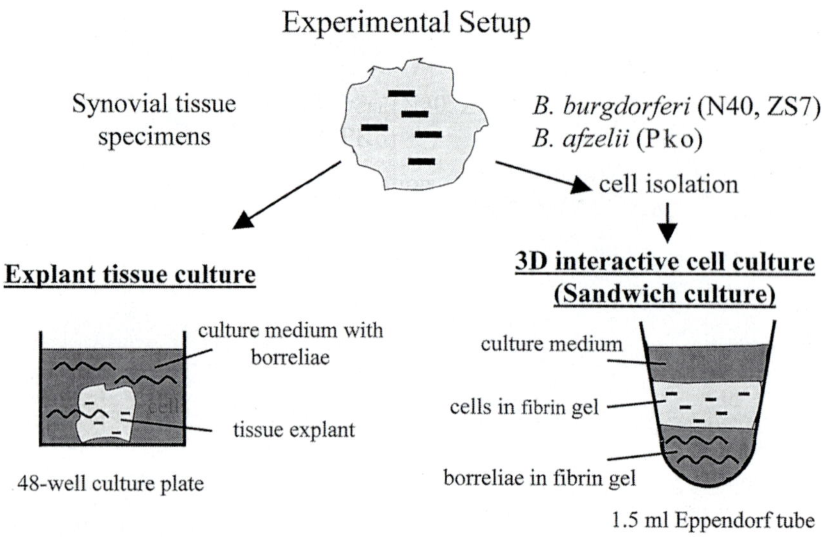

Figure 4. Experimental setup/"sandwich" culture. For the tissue explant cultures, tissue specimens were placed into 48-well culture plates and infected with the spirochetes **(left)**. For the 3-dimensional (3D) cell culture, a fibrin layer containing the spirochetes was overlaid with a matrix/cell suspension. After solidification of the gel, coculture medium was added, and cultures were incubated for up to 21 days. Since the nutrition medium was placed on top of the culture, the spirochetes penetrated the cell layer, following the nutrition gradient.

Bb antibody (Seramun) was used for further experiments. Staining with isotype-specific IgG did not result in any staining (negative control) (Figure 3B).

Infection of the 3-D cell culture/novel sandwich culture. For the 3-D cell culture, several settings were tested. The incubation of synovial cells within the fibrin matrix with Bb in a liquid medium phase did not result in a migration of the spirochetes into the gel. In another system, a central cylinder of synovial cells in fibrin was surrounded by Bb embedded in fibrin. This approach allowed only an incomplete penetration into the cell compartment by the spirochetes.

A novel sandwich culture was therefore developed (Figure 4). A fibrin layer containing the spiro-

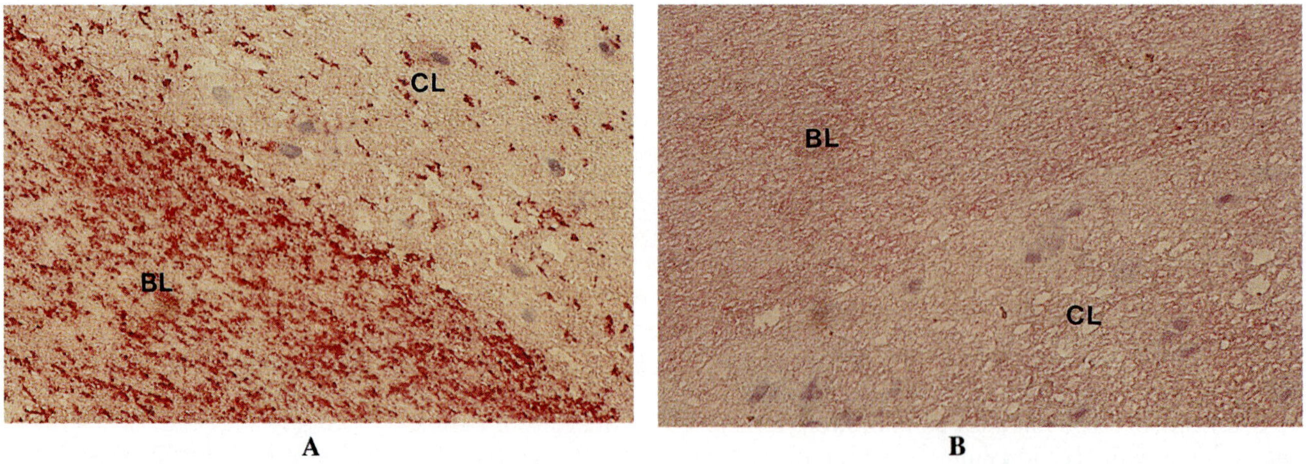

Figure 5. Kinetics of invasion by *Borrelia burgdorferi* (Bb). To assess the time course of invasion of the matrix by Bb, the 3-dimensional cell culture was analyzed by immunohistochemistry at daily intervals. After 24 hours, the first spirochetes were already detectable within the cell layer (red). After 5 days, the spirochetes were distributed homogenously. **A,** Invasion of the cell layer after an incubation period of 62 hours. **B,** Immunohistochemistry with isotype-specific IgG did not result in any staining. CL = cell layer; BL = Bb-containing layer. (Original magnification × 400.)

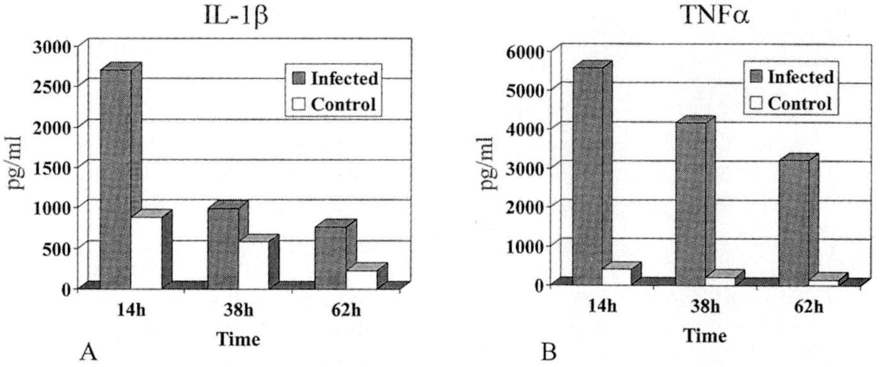

Figure 6. Increase in proinflammatory cytokines induced by *Borrelia burgdorferi*. Infection of the 3-dimensional cell culture system resulted in an increase in **A,** interleukin-1β (IL-1β) and **B,** tumor necrosis factor α (TNFα) in the culture supernatants, as determined by enzyme-linked immunosorbent assay. The highest levels were reached within 24 hours after infection.

chetes (20–50 $\times$ 10^6 spirochetes/ml of gel) was overlaid with a matrix/cell suspension (5–10 $\times$ 10^6 cells/ml of gel). For this purpose, 10 μl of a 1:10 dilution of thrombin was placed at the bottom of an Eppendorf tube, mixed with 0.2 ml of the suspension of spirochetes in 10% fibrinogen, and allowed to polymerize for 10 minutes at 37°C. Thereafter, another 10 μl of a 1:10 dilution of thrombin was put on the Bb-containing layer and mixed with the synovial cell/fibrinogen suspension. After solidification, coculture medium was added, and cultures were incubated at 37°C for up to 21 days.

Infection of tissue explant culture. For the tissue explant cultures, tissue specimens were used immediately after surgery. After a 24-hour period of adaptation to the coculture medium, the tissue explants were infected with the spirochetes (infective dose 5 $\times$ 10^6 spirochetes/ml of medium). As shown in Figure 3A, Bb adhered preferentially to the synovial lining layer, but also penetrated into deeper areas.

Time course of invasion. All 3 strains of Bb tested were able to invade both the tissue explants and the 3-D matrix (Figures 3A–C). There was no difference between the synovial cells/synovial tissue from OA patients and the synovial cells/synovial tissue from patients without an inflammatory joint disease. To characterize the time course of invasion, sandwich cultures were analyzed at daily intervals by cell culture microscopy, darkfield microscopy of the supernatants, and immunohistochemistry.

After 24 hours, some viable spirochetes were already visible within the culture supernatant of the 3-D interactive cultures, as detected by darkfield microscopy. Immunohistochemical analysis revealed that after 24 hours, only some spirochetes had invaded the cell layer of the sandwich cultures (Figure 5A). The number of invading spirochetes increased daily. Of interest, the borreliae invaded the cell layer with different velocities and did not move together as a "front of invasion." After an incubation period of 5 days, about one-third of the spirochetes from the lower layer (Bb-containing layer in Figure 5A) had invaded the upper cell layer and were homogenously distributed within the cell layer.

Applications of the 3-D model. *Cytokines in Bb-infected cultures.* To test the model with respect to the induction of cytokines, the synovial tissue explants and the 3-D cell cultures were incubated with Bb. After 24 hours, the concentrations of TNFα and IL-1β were measured within the culture supernatants. Despite the variations in individual levels of TNFα and IL-1β among the cultures (both basal and peak level), both cytokines were significantly elevated in the supernatants of infected explant cultures ($n = 3$) as compared with noninfected cultures (Figures 6A and B). The highest levels for both IL-1β and TNFα were reached within 24 hours after infection. Since at this time, only a few, single spirochetes had invaded the tissue, soluble factors of Bb are assumed to be involved in the activation of host cells.

In the interactive cell cultures, only a slight increase of both cytokines could be observed (data not shown). The controls (coculture medium) showed no elevation in the cytokine levels.

Induction of mRNA for IL-16 and COX-2. The induction of cytokines by Bb on the mRNA level was assessed by in situ hybridization. We focused on IL-16, since it is known to induce chemoattraction to CD4+ cells and because the infiltration of the synovial membrane with CD4+ cells is characteristic of Lyme arthritis. Expression of COX-2 was assessed since COX-2 is up-regulated in other inflammatory arthritides, such as

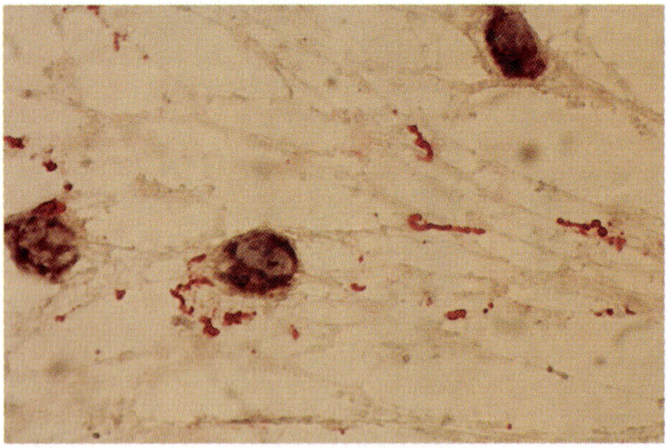

Figure 7. In situ hybridization for assessment of the induction of interleukin-16 (IL-16) mRNA by *Borrelia burgdorferi*. In the 3-dimensional cell culture system, ~80% of synovial cells expressed IL-16 mRNA (brown), whereas only a few, single cells showed positive signals in uninfected cultures. After hybridization, immunohistochemical double-labeling of the spirochetes (red) and counterstaining (hematoxylin) for nuclei was performed. (Original magnification × 1,000.)

RA. Interactive cultures infected with Bb showed a strong expression of IL-16 mRNA in ~80% of synovial cells (Figure 7), whereas only a few, single cells expressed IL-16 mRNA in uninfected cultures. Comparable results were obtained for COX-2 mRNA (data not shown).

Electron microscopic analysis of Bb. The tissue explant cultures and the 3-D cell cultures were analyzed by electron microscopy. Bb were present throughout the tissue explant cultures and the 3-D cell cultures, both within the extracellular matrix and within synovial cells. Within the extracellular matrix of the biopsy material, the spirochetes were typically situated in the loose connective tissue separating bundles of horizontally striped thick collagen fibers (Figure 8A). Most interestingly, a spirochete was also seen *within* such a fiber bundle (Figure 8B). In most cases, the borreliae were oriented parallel to the longitudinal axis of the adjacent fibers. The spirochetes were often located adjacent to synovial cells such as fibroblasts, mast cells, and macrophages, but without obvious preference for any cell population.

Bb could also be detected intracellularly, within macrophages and synovial fibroblasts (Figures 8C and D). Although the process of uptake itself was not witnessed, intact synovial fibroblasts contained internalized spirochetes inside a spacious vacuole (Figures 8C and D). The loose-fitting wall of the vacuole, the additional presence of fluffy material in the vacuolar space, and the fact that the intravacuolar borreliae displayed ultrastructural features of beginning disintegration (e.g., swelling of the periplasmic space, rupture of the outer and protoplasmic membranes, or clumping of the protoplasm) all indicated that the spirochete-bearing vacuole was a phagolysosome provided with antimicrobial mechanisms. Of special interest, the majority of synovial fibroblasts containing spirochetes or fragments of spirochetes exhibited signs of severe damage, such as massive swelling of the cytoplasm and rupture of membrane-bound intracellular compartments (Figures 8E and F), most likely indicating that the uptake of the spirochetes causes cell lysis of synovial fibroblasts.

DISCUSSION

In vivo studies addressing the pathogenesis of Lyme arthritis are difficult to perform because of the paucity of spirochetes within infected tissues (1). Several animal models of Lyme disease (10–13) have allowed the analysis of distinct aspects of the disease. However, these experimental approaches are limited by ethical considerations as well as the fact that not all data can be applied to the situation in humans. Most in vitro studies are based on findings in monolayer cell cultures (14–19). The major shortcoming of these experimental settings is the loss of the physiologic 3-D arrangement of the cells, which leads to changes in morphology and function.

In the present study, a 3-D system was developed which allowed cells to keep a spatial orientation similar to that in vivo. Two different approaches were chosen: explants of synovial tissue containing the natural mixture of cells and the physiologic extracellular matrix, and isolated synovial fibroblasts embedded into an artificial matrix were infected with Bb. These two settings were used based on their specific advantages. In the tissue explant culture, the natural 3-D structure of synovial tissue remains intact throughout the incubation period, and the in vivo mixture of cells allows interactions between different cell types but excludes systemic, blood-derived factors, such as complement, blood cells, and antibodies. In the 3-D cell culture, the specific cellular and molecular interactions between Bb and distinct cell populations can be studied separately. For example, it appears to be of crucial importance to analyze whether resident synovial cells are able to phagocytize Bb and whether they thereby contribute to the elimination or the potential persistence of Bb. Moreover, the 3-D cell culture can easily be manipulated, and therefore allows us to standardize the model

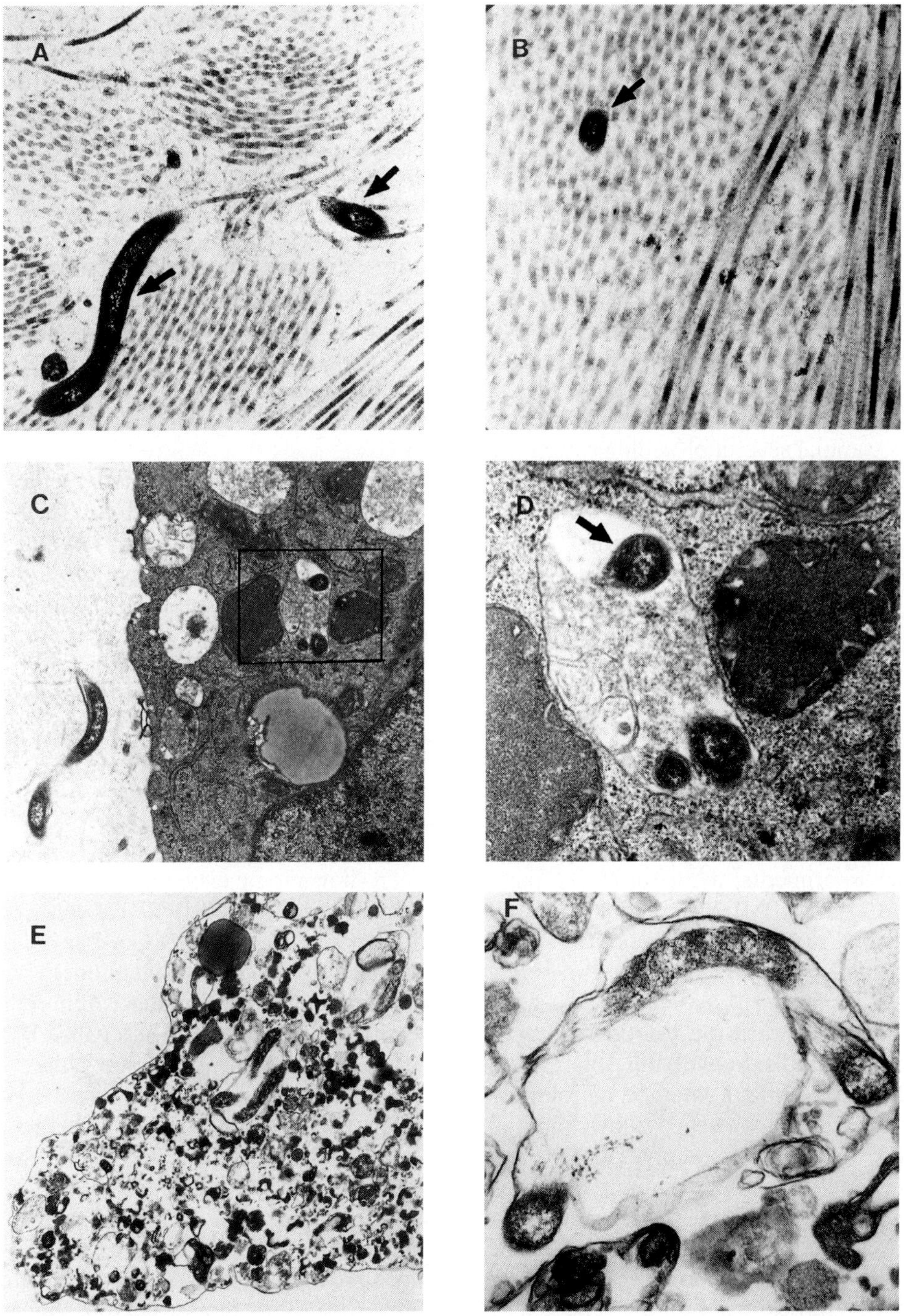

Figure 8. Ultrastructural analysis of *Borrelia burgdorferi* (Bb). Bb could be detected by electron microscopy within the tissue explant cultures and the 3-dimensional cell cultures, both within the extracellular matrix and within synovial cells. **A,** Within the extracellular matrix of the tissue explants, Bb was typically found in the loose connective tissue separating bundles of collagen fibers **(arrows)**. **B,** A spirochete was also seen *within* such a fiber bundle **(arrow)**. **C,** Bb was also detectable intracellularly, within synovial fibroblasts. **D,** Higher magnification view of the boxed area shown in **C,** demonstrating an intact synovial fibroblast containing internalized spirochetes inside a spacious vacuole **(arrow)**. The loose-fitting wall of the vacuole, the presence of fluffy material, and the beginning disintegration of the spirochete indicate an ongoing antimicrobial mechanism. **E** and **F,** The majority of synovial fibroblasts containing spirochetes displayed features of severe damage. (Original magnification × 29,000 in **A**; × 21,560 in **B**; × 19,000 in **C**; × 71,000 in **D** and **F**; × 15,000 in **E**.)

with regard to cell density, infective dose, and a defined extracellular matrix. The matrix produced by fibroblasts in vitro (20,21) can be saved in this setting, in contrast to the monolayer system, where it is discharged at the changes of the medium.

The extracellular matrix, a complex network of collagens, glycoproteins, proteoglycans, and glucosaminoglycans, allows cells to adhere, to form their 3-D arrangement, and to interact. For the spirochetes, binding to matrix components of the host is one virulence factor, since they are able to activate host plasminogen leading to fibrinolysis, and thereby, to invade host tissues (22). For our purpose, the artificial extracellular matrix had to meet the requirements for both the synovial cells and the spirochetes. Among several physiologic matrices tested, such as collagen, fibrin, ECM Gel, and agarose, fibrin turned out to be the most suitable matrix. The only problem was the variable pore size of the fibrin network, most likely caused by matrix-degrading proteases produced by synovial fibroblasts.

In vitro culture of Bb has been considered to be difficult, since the spirochetes require special culture media and conditions (23,24). With the use of BSK-H medium supplemented with 6% rabbit serum, we did observe very good viability or growth rate of the spirochetes (number doubled every 15 hours) over a period of at least 8 weeks. For coculture of the spirochetes with mammalian cells, a special medium had to be established (25). In our experiments, a mixture of 2 parts BSK-H medium and 1 part RPMI 1640 medium allowed both the spirochetes and the fibroblasts to survive and to keep their characteristic morphologic and functional properties.

An important step toward the reproducibility of the model was the standardization of the counting of spirochetes. Since the conventional method of counting the spirochetes at darkfield microscopy allows only an estimation of their number, we supplemented this method with a novel densitometric technique. Based on the generation time of 14–18 hours, as determined for the 3 *Borrelia* strains used in our study, 75% of the coculture medium was changed every second day to keep the number of spirochetes at the same range throughout culture period.

Immunohistochemical analysis revealed that the spirochetes were concentrated at the outer layer of the synovium (lining layer) but were also found to have penetrated into the deeper areas of the synovial tissue explants. In the 3-D cell cultures, Bb invaded the artificial matrix homogenously and were often found adjacent to synovial cells.

The involvement of proinflammatory cytokines in the pathophysiology of Lyme arthritis has been well established. Thus, levels of TNFα, interferon-γ, and IL-1 have been reported to be elevated in patients with Lyme disease (26,27). To test our model, we exposed both the synovial tissue explants and the interactive cell cultures to Bb for 24 hours and measured the production of TNFα and IL-1β in the culture supernatants. Levels of both cytokines were significantly elevated in the supernatants of infected explant cultures as compared with noninfected cultures. The highest levels of both IL-1β and TNFα were reached within 24 hours. The increase in proinflammatory cytokines in our test system demonstrates that the model reflects interactions that occur in vivo.

We further examined the expression of IL-16 based on the fact that IL-16 displays a chemoattractant activity toward CD4+ cells (28) and that inflammatory infiltrates of CD4+ lymphocytes within the synovial membrane are an important hallmark of Lyme arthritis (1). Applying in situ hybridization with IL-16–specific riboprobes, we found a strong expression of IL-16 in ~80% of synovial cells after infection with Bb. In contrast, uninfected cultures showed only a weak staining in some single cells. Therefore, Bb appears to strongly induce IL-16 mRNA. Comparable results were obtained for the expression of COX-2, the key enzyme for the synthesis of inflammatory prostaglandins that has been shown to be elevated in RA synovium (29). Further studies are required to assess the pathophysiologic significance of IL-16 and COX-2 in Lyme disease. From a technical point of view, the model is suited for advanced double-labeling techniques (immunohistochemistry and in situ hybridization) to colocalize Bb and the molecule of interest to the same tissue slide.

In favor of the potential persistence of Bb as a mechanism of chronic Lyme arthritis, several groups have tried to discover escape mechanisms of Bb into immunologically privileged sites, such as intracellular compartments or tissues with low turnover rates and the paucity of immune effector cells. The present study is the first to show internalized Bb within intact synovial fibroblasts, thus demonstrating that in addition to professional phagocytes (neutrophils, monocytes, and macrophages), other cells, such as synovial cells, are able to phagocytize spirochetes (3,30–32). These morphologic findings cannot answer the questions of whether the intracellularly detectable Bb are viable or degraded spirochetes, whether the nonprofessional phagocytes are able to kill the internalized spirochetes, or whether the nonprofessional phagocytes act as a "Trojan horse."

Data supporting the notion of intracellular survival have been obtained from some coculture studies (32–34). However, the significance of those observations appears to be limited, since in our experience, it is hardly possible to definitely remove all extracellular spirochetes from the coculture system. Other studies describing the light microscopic colocalization of Bb and either human umbilical vein endothelial cells (HUVEC) (18), fibroblasts (33), or fibroblast-like cells (L929) (35) cannot be equated with an intracellular persistence of the spirochetes because of the restricted resolution of light microscopy. Ultrastructural studies have shown borreliae invaginating into HUVEC (36), tendocytes (37), and synovial cells (32), and/or located in tunnel-like vacuoles near the surface of these cells. However, such interaction of Bb with the cell surface of mammalian cells is not evidence of subsequent internalization.

In the current study, the internalized spirochetes were attached to a host cell–derived membrane and displayed ultrastructural features of beginning disintegration, indicating that the intravacuolar pathogens were killed in the phagolysosome. Thus, the uptake of spirochetes by synovial fibroblasts is unlikely to provide a protective niche, but rather, to contribute to the clearance of the Bb cells from infected joints. Moreover, in our study, the majority of synovial fibroblasts containing spirochetes or fragments of spirochetes displayed features of severe damage. Comparable findings were obtained by 2 other electron microscopic studies that also demonstrated spirochetes inside damaged fibroblast-like synovial cells (3,32). Taking previous and current data together, we hypothesize that the uptake of Bb by resident synovial fibroblasts does not lead to intracellular survival of the spirochetes, but provokes the disintegration and lysis of these cells, and thereby contributes to the local inflammation in Lyme arthritis. The present study does not rule out a potential extracellular persistence of Bb, since an association of the spirochetes with collagen fiber bundles could be demonstrated, which is consistent with previous reports (37,38).

The preferential localization in the loose connective tissue spaces between the collagen fiber bundles may reflect the well-known binding affinity of the spirochetes to components of the extracellular matrix, especially proteoglycans (39–41). It is tempting to speculate that the low tissue turnover of collagenous connective tissue coupled with the paucity of immune effector cells may contribute to the persistence of Bb in this immunologically privileged site. Further applications of the novel 3-D model will contribute to the resolution of this issue.

In summary, our 3-D model of Lyme arthritis provides a reproducible and standardized system for analyzing the interactions of Bb and host cells or tissues. The setting is suited for the application of advanced histologic techniques to the colocalization of Bb and molecules of interest. The exclusive use of human tissues and the avoidance of animal experiments are further advantages of the model. The first applications of the model have demonstrated its great potential for unraveling distinct pathophysiologic mechanisms that might be operative in chronic Lyme arthritis.

ACKNOWLEDGMENT

We would like to acknowledge the kind support of Steffen Gay, MD, in whose laboratory the in situ hybridization technique for IL-16 and COX-2 was developed.

REFERENCES

1. Steere AC, Duray PH, Butcher EC. Spirochetal antigens and lymphoid cell surface markers in Lyme synovitis: comparison with rheumatoid synovium and tonsillar lymphoid tissue. Arthritis Rheum 1988;31:487–95.
2. Priem S, Burmester GR, Kamradt T, Wolbart K, Rittig MG, Krause A. Detection of Borrelia burgdorferi by polymerase chain reaction in synovial membrane, but not in synovial fluid from patients with persisting Lyme arthritis after antibiotic treatment. Ann Rheum Dis 1998;57:18–121.
3. Chary-Valckenaere I, Jaulhac B, Champigneulle J, Piemont Y, Mainard D, Pourel J. Ultrastructural demonstration of intracellular localization of Borrelia burgdorferi in Lyme arthritis [letter]. Br J Rheumatol 1998;37:468–70.
4. Carlson D, Hernandez J, Bloom BJ, Coburn J, Aversa JM, Steere AC. Lack of Borrelia burgdorferi DNA in synovial samples from patients with antibiotic treatment-resistant Lyme arthritis. Arthritis Rheum 1999;42:2705–9.
5. Gross DM, Forsthuber T, Tary-Lehmann M, Etling C, Ito K, Nagy ZA, et al. Identification of LFA-1 as a candidate autoantigen in treatment-resistant Lyme arthritis. Science 1998;281:703–6.
6. Radolf JD, Arndt LL, Akins DR, Curetty LL, Levi ME, Shen Y, et al. Treponema pallidum and Borrelia burgdorferi lipoproteins and synthetic lipopeptides activate monocytes/macrophages. J Immunol 1995;154:2866–77.
7. Ebnet K, Brown KD, Siebenlist UK, Simon MM, Shaw S. Borrelia burgdorferi activates nuclear factor-kappa B and is a potent inducer of chemokine and adhesion molecule gene expression in endothelial cells and fibroblasts. J Immunol 1997;158:3285–92.
8. Kimsey RB, Spielman A. Motility of Lyme disease spirochetes in fluids as viscous as the extracellular matrix. J Infect Dis 1990;162:1205–8.
9. Kriegsmann J, Keyszer GM, Geiler T, Bräuer R, Gay RE, Gay S. Expression of vascular cell adhesion molecule-1 mRNA and protein in rheumatoid synovium demonstrated by in situ hybridization and immunohistochemistry. Lab Invest 1995;72:209–14.
10. Keane-Myers A, Nickell SP. Role of IL-4 and IFN-γ in modulation of immunity to Borrelia burgdorferi in mice. J Immunol 1995;155:2020–8.
11. Appel MJG, Allen S, Jacobson RH, Lauderdale T-L, Chang Y-F, Shin SJ, et al. Experimental Lyme disease in dogs produces arthritis and persistent infection. J Infect Dis 1993;167:651–64.
12. Barthold SW, Beck DS, Hansen GM, Terwilliger GA, Moody KD.

Lyme borreliosis in selected strains and ages of laboratory mice. J Infect Dis 1990;162:133–8.
13. Galbe JL, Guy E, Zapatero JM, Peerschke EI, Benach JL. Vascular clearance of Borrelia burgdorferi in rats. Microb Pathog 1993;14:187–201.
14. Fuchs H, Simon MM, Wallich R, Bechtel R, Kramer MG. Borrelia burgdorferi induces secretion of pro-urokinase-type plasminogen activator by human monocytes. Infect Immun 1996;64:4307–12.
15. Sprenger H, Krause A, Kaufmann A, Priem S, Fabian D, Burmester GR, et al. Borrelia burgdorferi induces chemokines in human monocytes. Infect Immun 1997;65:4384–8.
16. Georgilis K, Peacocke M, Klempner MS. Fibroblasts protect the Lyme disease spirochete, Borrelia burgdorferi, from ceftriaxone in vitro. J Infect Dis 1992;166:440–4.
17. Montgomery RR, Nathanson MH, Malawista SE. The fate of Borrelia burgdorferi, the agent for Lyme disease, in mouse macrophages: destruction, survival, recovery. J Immunol 1993;150: 909–15.
18. Ma Y, Sturrock A, Weis JJ. Intracellular localization of Borrelia burgdorferi within human endothelial cells. Infect Immun 1991; 59:671–8.
19. Leong JM, Wang H, Magoun L, Field JA, Morrissey PE, Robbins D, et al. Different classes of proteoglycans contribute to the attachment of Borrelia burgdorferi to cultured endothelial and brain cells. Infect Immun 1998;66:994–9.
20. Sittinger M, Bujia J, Rotter N, Reitzel D, Minuth WW, Burmester GR. Tissue engineering and autologous transplant formation: practical approaches with resorbable biomaterials and new cell culture techniques. Biomaterials 1996;17:237–42.
21. Ishukawa O, Kondo A, Okada K, Miyachi Y, Furumura M. Morphological and biochemical analyses on fibroblasts and self-produced collagens in a novel three-dimensional culture. Br J Dermatol 1997;136:6–11.
22. Fuchs H, Wallich R, Simon MM, Kramer MD. The outer surface protein A of the spirochete Borrelia burgdorferi is a plasmino-(gen) receptor. Proc Natl Acad Sci U S A 1994;91:12594–8.
23. Pollack RJ, Telford SR III, Spielman A. Standardization of medium for culturing Lyme disease spirochetes. J Clin Microbiol 1993;131:1251–5.
24. Straubinger RK, Straubinger AF, Summers BA, Erb HN, Härter L, Appel MJ. Borrelia burgdorferi induces the production and release of proinflammatory cytokines in canine synovial explant cultures. Infect Immun 1998;66:247–58.
25. Guner E. Retention of Borrelia burgdorferi pathogenicity and infectivity after multiple passages in a co-culture system. Experientia 1994;50:54–9.
26. Yin Z, Braun J, Neure L, Wu P, Eggens U, Krause A, et al. T cell cytokine pattern in the joints of patients with Lyme arthritis and its regulation by cytokines and anticytokines. Arthritis Rheum 1997; 40:69–79.
27. Gross DM, Steere AC, Huber BT. T helper 1 response is dominant and localized to the synovial fluid in patients with Lyme arthritis. J Immunol 1998;160:1022–8.
28. Cruikshank WW, Center DM, Nisar N, Natke B, Theodore A, Kornfeld H. Molecular and functional analysis of a lymphocyte chemoattractant factor: association of biological function with CD4 expression. Proc Natl Acad Sci U S A 1994;91:5109–13.
29. Crofford LJ, Tan B, McCarthy CJ, Hla T. Involvement of nuclear factor κB in the regulation of cyclooxygenase-2 expression by interleukin-1 in rheumatoid synoviocytes. Arthritis Rheum 1997; 40:226–36.
30. Dorward DW, Fischer ER, Brooks DM. Invasion and cytopathic killing of human lymphocytes by spirochetes causing Lyme disease. Clin Infect Dis 1997;25:S2–8.
31. Nanagara R, Duray PH, Schumacher HR Jr. Ultrastructural demonstration of spirochetal antigens in synovial fluid and synovial membrane in chronic Lyme disease: possible factors contributing to persistence of organisms. Hum Pathol 1996;27:1025–34.
32. Girschick HJ, Huppertz HI, Russmann H, Krenn V, Karch H. Intracellular persistence of Borrelia burgdorferi in human synovial cells. Rheumatol Int 1996;16:125–32.
33. Klempner MS, Noring R, Rogers RA. Invasion of human skin fibroblasts by the Lyme disease spirochete, Borrelia burgdorferi. J Infect Dis 1993;167:1074–81.
34. Brouqui P, Badiaga S, Raoult D. Eucaryotic cells protect Borrelia burgdorferi from the action of penicillin and ceftriaxone but not from the action of doxycycline and erythromycin. Antimicrob Agents Chemother 1996;40:1552–4.
35. Tylewska-Wierzbanowska S, Chmielewski T. The isolation of Borrelia burgdorferi spirochetes from clinical material in cell line cultures. Zentralbl Bakteriol 1997;286:363–70.
36. Szczepanski A, Furie MB, Benach JL, Lane BP, et al. Interaction between Borrelia burgdorferi and endothelium in vitro. J Clin Invest 1990;85:1637–47.
37. Häupl T, Hahn G, Rittig M, Krause A, Schoerner C, Schönherr U, et al. Persistence of Borrelia burgdorferi in ligamentous tissue from a patient with chronic Lyme borreliosis. Arthritis Rheum 1993;36:1621–6.
38. Pachner AR, Basta J, Delaney E, Hulinska D. Localization of Borrelia burgdorferi in murine Lyme borreliosis by electron microscopy. Am J Trop Med Hyg 1995;52:128–33.
39. Isaacs RD. Borrelia burgdorferi bind to epithelial cell proteoglycans. J Clin Invest 1994;93:809–19.
40. Guo BP, Norris SJ, Rosenberg LC, Hook M. Adherence of Borrelia burgdorferi to the proteoglycan decorin. Infect Immun 1995;63:3467–72.
41. Leong JM, Robbins D, Rosenfeld L, Lahiri B, Parveen N. Structural requirements for glycosaminoglycan recognition by the Lyme disease spirochete, Borrelia burgdorferi. Infect Immun 1998;66: 6045–8.

ARTHRITIS & RHEUMATISM
Vol. 44, No. 1, January 2001, pp 163–169

The MICA Region Determines the First Modifier Locus in Familial Mediterranean Fever

Isabelle Touitou,[1] Marie-Christine Picot,[1] Cécile Domingo,[2] Cécile Notarnicola,[1] Daniel Cattan,[3] Jacques Demaille,[1] and Isabelle Koné-Paut[4]

Objective. **Familial Mediterranean fever (FMF) is a genetically recessive inflammatory disease caused by mutations in the MEFV gene. Most patients of non-Ashkenazi Jewish ancestry or those who are homozygous for M694V manifest a severe disease course, but some express a mild form of the disease. We therefore searched for other genes which could possibly be implicated in the disease phenotype. We tested MICA (major histocompatibility complex class I chain–related gene A) because it has been associated with a number of other inflammatory disorders.**

Methods. **One hundred fifty FMF probands and their family members were evaluated. The MEFV gene was screened by a combination of denaturing gradient-gel electrophoresis, restriction fragment length polymorphism, and amplification refractory mutation system. The MICA transmembrane polymorphism in exon 5 was analyzed after biotin-labeled polymerase chain reaction products were loaded onto sequencing gels and subjected to autoradiography.**

Results. **The contribution of MICA to the FMF phenotype was confirmed after adjustment for the patient's ancestry and for the MEFV genotype. MEFV was individually the most important prognostic factor for the disease. However, the impact of M694V homozygosity on the age at disease onset (OR 2.3) was aggravated if patients also inherited MICA-A9 (OR 6.3). In contrast, the frequency of attacks was found to be dramatically reduced (OR 0.16) in patients with MICA-A4.**

Conclusion. **We have identified the first FMF modifier locus, MICA. FMF is the first model of a Mendelian disease associated with MICA. These results clarify, at least partly, the inconsistent phenotype–MEFV correlation in FMF.**

Familial Mediterranean fever (FMF) is an inflammatory disorder with symptoms that include recurrent febrile attacks, synovitis, and cutaneous signs. It mainly affects populations of Mediterranean ancestry (1) and is especially severe in non-Ashkenazi Jews (NAJs) (2). To date, more than 20 mutations have been detected in the gene responsible for FMF (MEFV) (3–8). The role of the corresponding protein (marenostrin/pyrin) is still unknown.

The discovery of MEFV has provided the first specific biologic tool for the diagnosis of FMF. Indeed, FMF can be accurately pinpointed among various inflammatory disorders through MEFV mutation screening. However, screening alone cannot be used as a prognostic test because of the lack of complete correlation between the clinical features of the disease and the MEFV mutations (6–9). Currently, the clearest available data concerning phenotype–genotype relate to M694V, the most frequent FMF mutation. M694V accounts for 70–90% of the FMF chromosomes in NAJs and for 30–60% of those in other populations. Homozygosity for M694V has been reproducibly demonstrated to be associated with a severe disease course in NAJs and Armenians (2,8,10–13), but not in Turks (9). This genotype is practically fully penetrant. The greater disease severity in NAJs has therefore been attributed to the higher M694V frequency in this population. M694V-homozygous patients may nevertheless display a wide array of clinical features, ranging from rare isolated bouts of fever to severe renal amyloidosis with dramatic

Supported by the Regional Hospital Center of Montpellier, France.

[1]Isabelle Touitou, MD, PhD, Marie-Christine Picot, MD, Cécile Notarnicola, MS, Jacques Demaille, MD, PhD: Arnaud de Villeneuve Hospital, Montpellier, France; [2]Cécile Domingo, MS: Visible Genetics, Evry, France; [3]Daniel Cattan, MD: Villeneuve St. Georges Hospital, Villeneuve St. Georges, France; [4]Isabelle Koné-Paut, MD, PhD: correspondence and Nord Hospital, Marseilles, France.

Address correspondence and reprint requests to Isabelle Touitou, MD, PhD, Laboratory of Genetics, Arnaud de Villeneuve Hospital, 34295 Montpellier, France.

Submitted for publication June 19, 2000; accepted in revised form August 26, 2000.

attacks of inflammatory pain. Differences in disease severity occur not only between ethnic groups, but also between siblings (11,14,15).

The existence of intrafamilial phenotype variations suggests that, apart from likely environmental factors, genes other than MEFV are also involved in FMF expression. The major histocompatibility complex (MHC), comprising most notably the HLA genes, is a relevant candidate as a modifier locus for FMF because it has been clearly associated with numerous other inflammatory diseases, for example, Behçet's disease, rheumatoid arthritis, and inflammatory bowel diseases (16–19). Nevertheless, findings of previous association and linkage studies did not support the involvement of HLA in FMF (20–22). Other MHC genes, such as MICA (MHC class I chain–related gene A), have also been shown to be involved in inflammatory diseases.

MICA was first associated with Behçet's disease: both the A6 allele of the microsatellite polymorphism in the transmembrane region (exon 5) and the A009 allele in exons 2–4 were found to be more frequent in patients than in healthy controls (16,17). More recently, MICA was further found to be associated with acute anterior uveitis (23), psoriatic arthritis (24), Addison's disease (25), and diabetes (26,27).

Since the known MEFV mutations do not explain all FMF phenotype subtypes, we conducted a study aimed at identifying modifier genes in this disease. Considering that FMF and other inflammatory diseases are sometimes difficult to differentiate clinically and can occasionally be identified in a single patient (28–30), we hypothesized that the MICA locus might be a common genetic factor for inflammation. We therefore designed a molecular study to test for its possible involvement in FMF, taking into account the ancestry and MEFV genotype of patients. Our study revealed that at least 3 factors are involved in the clinical expression of FMF: MEFV, MICA or a tightly linked gene, and one (or more) still unknown population-specific epigenetic or genetic factor(s).

PATIENTS AND METHODS

Patients. One hundred fifty unrelated FMF patients were genotyped. Seventy-nine patients were NAJs, 22 were Turks, 15 were Armenians, 14 were Arabs, and 20 were southern Europeans who did not have any of these ancestries. Patients were included in the present study if 2 MEFV mutations were detected or if they had a definitive clinical diagnosis according to established criteria (31).

The control group consisted of the parents' chromosomes that were not inherited by the patients, as previously described (22). The allele frequency in the untransmitted chromosomes gives a good estimate of the allele frequency in the general population and is advantageously ethnically matched (32). In controls, the MICA phenotype distribution was deduced from the phenotype frequency, which was calculated from the observed MICA allele frequency as follows: phenotype frequency = 2 × allele frequency − (allele frequency)^2.

All participants gave their informed consent and were assigned a code number for blind analysis. We used the same questionnaire and computer files as previously described (10). Data were available for >84% patients. The symptoms studied were those that were manifested by the patients prior to colchicine treatment.

MEFV mutations. Denaturing gradient-gel electrophoresis (DGGE) was performed to screen for mutations in exon 10. A complementary method was systematically used for the most frequent mutations amplification-refractory mutation system (ARMS) for M694V and M694I and restriction fragment length polymorphism (RFLP) for R761H, V726A, and M680I. If a rare or unknown DGGE band shift was detected, the variants were identified by sequencing or ARMS. Mutations in exon 2 (E148Q, E167D, and T267I) were examined by RFLP. All these approaches have been described in detail elsewhere (3,6). The known mutations in exons 3 and 5 (6–8) were not systematically searched for because they were too rare.

MICA alleles. DNA samples were amplified using the primers described previously (16). One of the 2 primers (MICA5F) was 5′ biotinylated. The polymerase chain reaction (PCR) conditions were as follows: 2 minutes of denaturation at 94°C, then 27 cycles of denaturation at 94°C for 30 seconds, annealing at 58°C for 30 seconds, and extension at 72°C for 1 minute. PCR fragments were directly loaded onto a sequencing gel. The gels were transferred to an N+ membrane (Appligene, Illkirch, France) for 2 hours and fixed for 3 minutes under ultraviolet light. The membranes were washed at 42°C for at least 1 hour in standard hybridization buffer (Boehringer, Meylan, France), then incubated at 37°C for 30 minutes with 30 ml of a solution containing 1.5 units of streptavidin coupled with peroxidase in 1% blocking reagent (Boehringer), 0.1*M* maleic acid, 0.15*M* NaCl, pH 7.5.

The membranes were washed twice with 2× saline–sodium citrate, 0.1% sodium dodecyl sulfate, once with phosphate buffered saline, and then subjected for 1 minute to enhanced chemiluminescence (Amersham, Les Ulis, France) before exposure to Kodak X-Omat AR film. Alleles were blindly and independently read by 2 different investigators (IT and CD).

Statistical analysis. The distribution of alleles between the patient and the control group, as well as between FMF patients, was compared by chi-square analysis, or by Fisher's exact test if chi-square was not a valid test. When necessary, a correction for multiple tests (Bonferroni) was made. *P* values less than or equal to 0.05 were considered significant. Odds ratios (ORs) and their 95% confidence intervals (95% CIs) were calculated. The more relevant cutoff values in our sample were determined to be 10 for the age at onset, and 1/month for the frequency of attacks (data not shown).

Table 1. Effect of MEFV genotype on the age at onset of familial Mediterranean fever, according to the MICA phenotype*

	Age at onset			
	≤10 years	>10 years	P	OR (95% CI)
All patients				
M694V homozygous	54 (82)	12 (18)		
Not M694V homozygous	36 (51)	35 (49)	0.001	4.4 (2–9.5)
Patients with the following MICA phenotype				
With the A9 allele				
M694V homozygous	21 (95)	1 (5)		
Not M694V homozygous	9 (60)	6 (40)	0.01	14 (1.5–134)
Without the A9 allele				
M694V homozygous	33 (75)	11 (25)		
Not M694V homozygous	27 (48)	29 (52)	0.007	3.2 (1.4–7.6)

* Values are the number (%) of patients. OR = odds ratio; 95% CI = 95% confidence interval.

The relative importance of the predictive variables of severity was assessed through a multivariate analysis consisting of a stepwise logistic regression (33). The dependent variables were the patient's clinical features. SAS software, version 6.12/UNIX, was used for statistical analysis (SAS Institute, Cary, NC).

RESULTS

MEFV and MICA distribution in FMF patients and controls. Two MEFV mutations were detected in 121 of the 150 patients (81%), including 71 (47%) homozygous for the M694V mutation. The prevalence of the M694V homozygous genotype differed dramatically between NAJs (52 of 79, or 66%) and the other patients (19 of 71, or 27%), $P < 0.0001$. Of the 150 patients, 18 (12%) had 1 unknown mutation and 11 (7%) had 2 unknown mutations.

The 5 common alleles (A9, A6, A5.1, A5, and A4) of the MICA microsatellite in the transmembrane region were found in our patient sample. The MICA phenotype, defined as the presence of at least 1 of the MICA alleles of interest, was determined in patients and controls. In controls, the prevalence of the MICA-A5 phenotype was lower in NAJs (8 of 79, or 10%) than in non-NAJs (22 of 71, or 31%) (corrected P [P_{corr}] = 0.05). In FMF patients, the prevalence of the A5.1 phenotype was higher in NAJs (33 of 79, or 42%) than in non-NAJs (16 of 71, or 23%) (P_{corr} = 0.05). In addition, MICA-A5.1 was less frequent in patients that did not have a high-risk ancestry for FMF than in controls (2 of 20, 10% versus 13 of 20, 65%) (P_{corr} = 0.002). No other significant differences in MICA phenotype were detected between ethnic groups or between FMF patients and controls.

Effect of MEFV, MICA, and ancestry on the course of FMF. We evaluated the patients for the occurrence of fever, peritonitis, arthritis, pleuritis, erysipelas, splenomegaly, frequency of attacks, age at onset of FMF, and response to colchicine treatment. Renal complications were too rare in our patient sample to accurately test this parameter. The association of MEFV, MICA, and patient ancestry with these clinical features was examined.

The known association of M694V homozygosity with a severe form of FMF was confirmed in relation to 3 clinical features. Patients with this MEFV genotype displayed an earlier age at onset (P = 0.001, OR 4.4, 95% CI 2–9.5) (Table 1) and more frequent attacks (P = 0.001, OR 4, 95% CI 1.7–10) (Table 2). The incidence of arthritis was also more frequent (78% versus 59%; P = 0.02, OR 2.5, 95% CI 1.2–5.2). We focused the rest of the study on these 3 clinical parameters because the others were not more frequent or were only slightly more frequent in M694V-homozygous patients (data not shown).

A possible individual MICA effect was also investigated. Two features differed according to the MICA phenotype. Early onset of disease tended to be more frequent in patients bearing the A9 allele (81% versus 60%; P = 0.02, P_{corr} = 0.1, OR 2.9, 95% CI 1.1–7). The attacks tended to be less frequent in patients with the A4 allele (59% versus 73%; P = 0.03, P_{corr} = 0.15, OR 0.4, 95% CI 0.2–0.9).

Detection of this second possible prognostic factor prompted us to investigate whether MEFV and MICA interacted. We sought the effect of MEFV according to the MICA background of the patients. The

Table 2. Effect of MEFV genotype on the frequency of attacks of familial Mediterranean fever, according to the MICA phenotype*

	Frequency of attacks			
	≥1/month	<1/month	*P*	OR (95% CI)
All patients				
M694V homozygous	53 (87)	8 (13)		
Not M694V homozygous	40 (62)	25 (38)	0.001	4 (1.7–10)
Patients with the following MICA phenotype				
With the A4 allele				
M694V homozygous	10 (67)	5 (33)		
Not M694V homozygous	9 (53)	8 (47)	NS	1.8 (0.4–7.5)
Without the A4 allele				
M694V homozygous	43 (93)	3 (7)		
Not M694V homozygous	31 (65)	17 (35)	0.001	8 (2–29)

* Values are the number (%) of patients. OR = odds ratio; 95% CI = 95% confidence interval; NS = not significant.

impact of M694V homozygosity on age at disease onset was more severe in patients with MICA-A9 than in those without MICA-A9, as shown by the gain in odd ratios in these patients (OR 14 with A9 and 3.2 without A9) (Table 1). In contrast, the effect of MEFV on the frequency of attacks was enhanced in patients without MICA-A4 (OR 1.8 with A4 and 8 without A4) (Table 2). We also searched for a MICA effect according to the MEFV genotype; there was no significant difference.

Patient ancestry was found to be a third prognostic factor in our study groups. NAJ patients more often had >1 attack/month (85% versus 60%; $P = 0.008$, OR 2.7, 95% CI 1.3–5.5) and more often manifested the disease before the age of 10 (76% versus 54%; $P = 0.001$, OR 3.4, 95% CI 1.6–7.3) than patients of other ancestries. The other ethnic groups were too small to be tested individually.

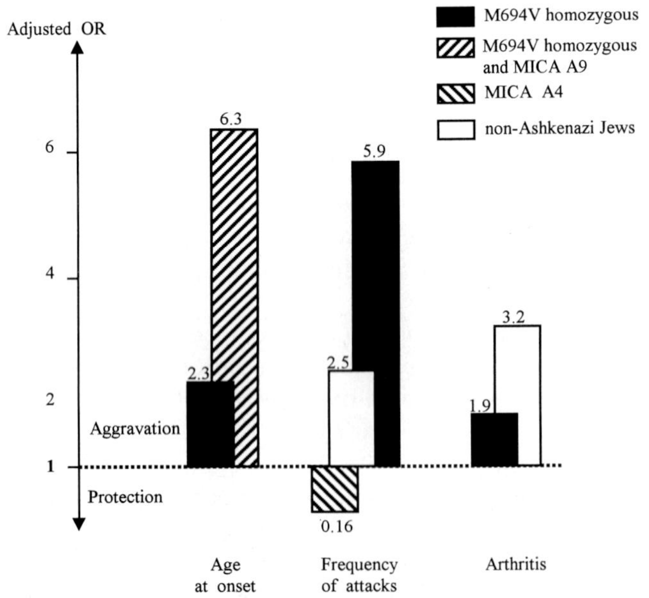

Figure 1. Relative contributions of MEFV, MICA, and ancestry to familial Mediterranean fever. Numbers above and below the bars show the adjusted odds ratios (OR), as determined by multivariate analysis. See text for *P* values and 95% confidence intervals. Combining ancestry with either MEFV or MICA yielded no significant results.

Relative contribution of MEFV, MICA, and ancestry in FMF. Each of the 3 variables were adjusted for each other using a multivariate analysis (Figure 1). The most robust prognostic factor was MEFV. After adjustment, M694V homozygosity remained an aggravating factor for the 3 clinical features tested (for age at onset $P = 0.0001$, adjusted OR [OR_{adj}] 2.3, 95% CI 1–5.8; for frequency of attacks $P = 0.001$, OR_{adj} 5.9, 95% CI 1.7–27; for arthritis $P = 0.02$, OR_{adj} 1.9, 95% CI 1.1–4.6).

Association of the MICA locus with the FMF phenotype was also confirmed after adjustment. Although MICA-A9 no longer showed a significant individual impact on disease onset, patients homozygous for M694V who also inherited MICA-A9 had an almost 3-fold higher risk of early onset of the disease ($P = 0.04$, OR_{adj} 6.3, 95% CI 1–119). It is noteworthy that the only patient with both an M694V homozygous genotype and MICA-A9 had a disease onset between the ages of 10 and 15, an age very close to the cutoff value of ≤10 (data not shown). Patients with MICA-A4 were still protected and experienced less frequent attacks ($P = 0.05$, OR_{adj} 0.16, 95% CI 0–0.8).

Finally, other genetic or environmental factors in NAJs remained a prognostic factor for the frequency of attacks ($P = 0.03$, OR_{adj} 2.5, 95% CI 1–6.5) and for arthritis ($P = 0.01$, OR_{adj} 3.4, 95% CI 1.4–8).

DISCUSSION

Our most important finding is the demonstration that some alleles in the MHC are prognostic factors for FMF. The MICA gene exhibits a microsatellite in its transmembrane domain that could easily be used in an extensive association analysis.

The case–control study disclosed no significant overrepresentation of a particular MICA allele in the patient group as a whole and within the group of NAJs. Larger samples are needed, however, to extend this result to other ethnic groups, especially those not commonly affected by FMF. Nevertheless, our results prove that MICA is not an important gene for the FMF outbreak in itself, at least in commonly affected patients. These data fit well with the Mendelian inheritance of the disease.

Reasoning that MICA could still modify the FMF phenotype, we stratified our sample according to patients' symptoms. Since both M694V homozygosity and the ancestry of the NAJs were confirmed to be associated with a severe form of the disease in our sample, these 2 variables had to be taken into account as possible confounding factors for MICA. We therefore adjusted step-by-step each of the 3 variables in relation to the others. This procedure eliminated any bias due to population admixture and gave the specific contribution of the 3 prognostic factors, each independently of the others (33).

These 3 prognostic factors were all valid, but only MEFV remained significant for all 3 clinical features. Patient ancestry remained a significant prognostic factor for the frequency of attacks and for arthritis. This finding shows that either a third gene, presumably deriving from a founder effect, or some population-specific epigenetic factors are yet to be identified. Recent studies by Mimouni et al (2), who used the same statistical approach, yielded results that were consistent with our findings.

The case of MICA is more puzzling. It remained a significant modifying locus, but the 2 alleles that were involved produced different effects. A9 increased the MEFV-associated severity, while A4 itself appeared to be protective. Unfortunately, we had too few A4 and A9 homozygotes to determine whether the 2 alleles produced an additive effect. For the same reason, we could not test each of the 15 possible MICA genotypes.

How can the MICA gene modulate the course of FMF? MICA is believed to serve as a sentinel for the detection of damaged, infected, or transformed cells. Owing to the presence of an Hsp70-like heat-shock element in its promoter (34), MICA behaves as a stress-inducible self-antigen. Before the identification of MEFV, FMF was long thought to be an autoimmune disease, and it is well known that fatigue, emotion, and infections favor attacks of FMF. Accordingly, the modifying effect of MICA on FMF appeared to be restricted to the course of the disease (age at onset and frequency of attacks) and did not seem to influence the location of manifestations (e.g., arthritis). We cannot exclude the possibility that each of the MICA alleles could have a modifying effect on the other clinical features in different or larger series of patients.

Recent studies showed that, interestingly, each single MICA allele may be overrepresented in inflammatory diseases, namely, A9 in psoriatic arthritis and diabetes (24,26), A6 in Behçet's disease (16), A5.1 in Addison's disease (25), A5 in human papillomavirus 18 seropositivity (35), and A4 in acute anterior uveitis (23). In contrast, MICA-A6 was protective in diabetes (27), and MICA-A4 was protective in Kawasaki disease (36). In relation to Behçet's disease, Yakubi and colleagues (37) suggested 2 hypotheses: either the MICA-A6 allele activates γ/δ T cells more efficiently than do the other alleles or some bacterial components may specifically induce MICA-A6 expression. Another hypothesis could be the existence of tissue-specific MICA-regulating factors.

FMF is the first model of a Mendelian disease associated with MICA. While in the polyfactorial diseases described above, it acts as a susceptibility factor, with 1 allele being more frequent in patients than in controls, in FMF, MICA acts as a modifier of the disease course. Hence, the FMF model provides new insights into MICA-association studies. First, it shows that phenotype–genotype correlations within patients, even in the absence of significant case–control differences, would be worth examining. Second, it suggests that the MICA locus may function by interacting with the disease-causing gene (e.g., MICA-A9 and age at onset). Third, it points to the necessity to take into account other prognostic factors, such as ethnicity.

None of the MICA studies, including ours, rules out the possibility that another gene in tight linkage disequilibrium with MICA could be the true disease-associated gene. For example, tumor necrosis factor, a gene closely linked to MICA that is located in the MHC, is associated with uveitis in Behçet's disease (38).

In conclusion, we have identified the first FMF modifier locus, MICA, which modulates the course of the disease but not the subset of its symptoms. Clinical expression of FMF, therefore, appears to be modulated by at least 3 factors: MEFV, MICA, and another as-yet-unidentified population-specific factor(s). These results may explain, at least in part, the lack of full phenotype–genotype correlation between severe FMF and M694V homozygosity.

ACKNOWLEDGMENTS

We thank Dr. J. Weissenbach, Dr. J. F. Eliaou, Dr. M. Dupont, and N. Molinari for helpful discussions.

REFERENCES

1. Sohar E, Gafni J, Pras M, Heller H. Familial Mediterranean fever: a survey of 470 cases and review of the literature. Am J Med 1967;43:227–53.
2. Mimouni A, Magal N, Stoffman N, Shohat T, Minasian A, Krasnov M, et al. Familial Mediterranean fever: effects of genotype and ethnicity on inflammatory attacks and amyloidosis. Pediatrics [article online]. 2000;105:E70. Accessed May 19, 2000. URL: http://www.pediatrics.org.
3. The French FMF Consortium. A candidate gene for familial Mediterranean fever. Nat Genet 1997;17:25–31.
4. The International FMF Consortium. Ancient missense mutations in a new member of the RoRet gene family are likely to cause familial Mediterranean fever. Cell 1997;90:797–807.
5. Booth DR, Gillmore JD, Booth MB, Pepys MB, Hawkins PN. Pyrin/marenostrin mutations in familial Mediterranean fever. QJM 1998;91:603–6.
6. Bernot A, da Silva C, Petit JL, Cruaud C, Caloustian C, Castet V, et al. Non-founder mutations in the MEFV gene establish this gene as the cause of familial Mediterranean fever (FMF). Hum Mol Genet 1998;7:1317–25.
7. Aksentijevich I, Torosyan Y, Samuels J, Centola M, Pras E, Chae JJ, et al. Mutation and haplotype studies in familial Mediterranean fever reveal new ancestral relationships and evidence for a high carrier frequency with reduced penetrance in the Ashkenazi Jewish population. Am J Hum Genet 1999;64:949–62.
8. Cazeneuve C, Sarkisian T, Pêcheux C, Dervichian M, Nédelec B, Reinert P, et al. MEFV gene analysis in Armenian patients with familial Mediterranean fever: diagnostic value, unfavorable renal prognosis of the M694V homozygous genotype, genetic and therapeutic implications. Am J Hum Genet 1999;65:88–97.
9. Yalcinkaya F, Cakar N, Misirlio M, Tumer N, Akar N, Tekin M, et al. Genotype-phenotype correlation in a large group of Turkish patients with familial Mediterranean fever: evidence for mutation-independent amyloidosis. Rheumatology 2000;39:67–72.
10. Dewalle M, Domingo C, Rozenbaum M, Ben-Chetrit E, Cattan D, Bernot A, et al. Phenotype-genotype correlation in Jewish patients suffering from familial Mediterranean fever (FMF). Eur J Hum Genet 1998;6:95–7.
11. Shohat M, Magal N, Shohat T, Chen X, Dagan T, Mimouni A, et al. Phenotype-genotype correlation in familial Mediterranean fever: evidence for an association between Met694Val and amyloidosis. Eur J Hum Genet 1999;7:287–92.
12. Livneh A, Langevitz P, Shinar Y, Zaks N, Kastner DL, Pras M, et al. MEFV mutation analysis in patients suffering from amyloidosis of familial Mediterranean fever. Amyloid 1999;6:1–6.
13. Brik R, Shinawi M, Kepten I, Berant M, Gershoni-Baruch R. Familial Mediterranean fever: clinical and genetic characterization in a mixed pediatric population of Jewish and Arab patients. Pediatrics [article online]. 1999;103:E70. Accessed May 19, 2000. URL: http://www.pediatrics.org.
14. Dupont M, Dross C, Smaoui N, Nedelec B, Grateau G, Clepet C, et al. Genotypic diagnosis of familial Mediterranean fever (FMF) using new microsatellite markers: example of two extensive non-Ashkenazi Jewish pedigrees. J Med Genet 1997;34:375–81.
15. Pras E, Langevitz P, Livneh A, Zemer D, Mal A, Padeh S, et al. Genotype-phenotype correlation in familial Mediterranean fever (a preliminary report). In: Sohar E, Gafni J, Pras M, editors. Familial Mediterranean fever. Tel Aviv: Freund Publishing House; 1997; p. 260–4.
16. Mizuki N, Ota M, Kimura M, Ohno S, Ando H, Katsuyama Y, et al. Triplet repeat polymorphism in the transmembrane region of the MICA gene: a strong association of six GCT repetitions with Behçet disease. Proc Natl Acad Sci U S A 1997;94:1298–303.
17. Wallace GR, Verity DH, Delemaine LJ, Ohno S, Inoko H, Ota M, et al. MIC-A allele profiles and HLA class I associations in Behçet's disease. Immunogenetics 1999;49:613–7.
18. McCurdy D. Genetic susceptibility to connective tissue diseases. Curr Opin Rheumatol 1999;11:329–407.
19. Stokkers PC, Reitsma PH, Tytgat GN, van Deventer SJ. HLA-DR and DQ phenotypes in inflammatory bowel disease: a meta-analysis. Gut 1999;45:395–401.
20. Chaouat Y, Tormen JP, Godeau P, Camus JP, Kahn MF, Ryckewaert A, et al. HLA markers and periodic disease (familial Mediterranean fever, FMF). Nouv Presse Med 1977;6: 2949–53.
21. Fradkin A, Zemer D, Pras M, Gazit E. Familial Mediterranean fever: no association of HLA with amyloidosis or colchicine treatment response. Isr J Med Sci 1985;21:757–8.
22. Shohat T, Shohat M, Tyan DB, Wang SJ, Sparkes AD, Swabe J, et al. Familial Mediterranean fever-linkage studies with genetic markers on chromosome 6. Tissue Antigens 1990;36:103–7.
23. Goto K, Ota M, Ando H, Mizuki N, Nakamura S, Inoue K, et al. MICA gene polymorphisms and HLA-B27 subtypes in Japanese patients with HLA-B27 associated acute anterior uveitis. Invest Ophthalmol Vis Sci 1998;39:634–7.
24. Gonzalez S, Martinez-Borra J, Torre-Alonso JC, Gonzalez-Roces S, Sanchez del Río J, Rodriguez Pérez A, et al. The MICA-A9 triplet repeat polymorphism in the transmembrane region confers additional susceptibility to the development of psoriatic arthritis and is independent of the association of Cw*0602 in psoriasis. Arthritis Rheum 1999;42:1010–6.
25. Gambelunghe G, Falorni A, Ghaderi M, Laureti S, Tortoioli C, Santeusanio F, et al. Microsatellite polymorphism of the MHC class I chain-related (MICA-A and MICA-B) genes marks the risk for autoimmune Addison's disease. J Clin Endocrinol Metab 1999;84:3701–7.
26. Lee YJ, Huang FY, Wang CH, Lo FS, Tsan KW, Hsu CH, et al. Polymorphism in the transmembrane region of the MICA gene and type 1 diabetes. J Pediatr Endocrinol Metab 2000;13: 489–96.
27. Kawabata Y, Ikegami H, Kawaguchi Y, Fujisawa T, Hotta M, Ueda H, et al. Age-related association of MHC class I chain-related gene A (MICA) with type 1 (insulin-dependent) diabetes mellitus. Hum Immunol 2000;61:624–9.
28. Schwartz T, Langevitz P, Zemer D, Pras M, Livneh A. Increased incidence of Behçet's disease in familial Mediterranean fever. In: Sohar E, Gafni J, Pras M, editors. Familial Mediterranean fever. Tel Aviv: Freund Publishing House; 1997. p. 148–50.
29. Birlik M, Tunca M, Hizli N, Soyturk M, Yenicerioglu Y, Ozcan MA, et al. Coexistence of familial Mediterranean fever with sacroiliitis and Behçet's disease: a rare occurrence. Clin Rheumatol 1998;17:397–99.
30. Cattan D, Notarnicola C, Molinari N, Touitou I. Inflammatory bowel disease in patients with familial Mediterranean fever. Lancet 2000;355:378–9.
31. Livneh A, Langevitz P, Zemer D, Zaks N, Kees S, Lidar T, et al. Criteria for the diagnosis of familial Mediterranean fever. Arthritis Rheum 1997;40:1879–85.

32. Falk CT, Rubinstein P. Haplotype relative risks: an easy reliable way to construct a proper control sample for risk calculations. Ann Hum Genet 1987;51:227–33.
33. Hosmer DW, Lemeshow S. Applied logistic regression. New York: John Wiley; 1989.
34. Bauer S, Groh V, Wu J, Steinle A, Phillips JH, Lanier LL, et al. Activation of NKG2D, a receptor for stress-inducible MICA. Science 1999;285:727–9.
35. Ghaderi M, Hjelmstrom P, Hallmans G, Wiklund F, Lenner P, Dillner J, et al. MICA gene polymorphism and the risk to develop cervical intraepithelial neoplasia. Hum Immunol 1999;10:970–3.
36. Huang F, Lee Y, Chen M, Hsu C, Lin S, Sung T, et al. Polymorphism of transmembrane region of MICA gene and Kawasaki disease. Exp Clin Immunogenet 2000;17:130–7.
37. Yakubi K, Mizuki N, Ota M, Katsuyama Y, Palimeris G, Stavropoulos C, et al. Association of MICA gene and HLA-B*5101 with Behçet's disease in Greece. Invest Ophthalmol Vis Sci 1999;40:1921–6.
38. Verity DH, Wallace GR, Vaughan RW, Kondeatis E, Madanat W, Zureikat H, et al. HLA and tumour necrosis factor (TNF) polymorphisms in ocular Behçet's disease. Tissue Antigens 1999;54:264–72.

Clinical Images: Lupus erythematosus cells in the kidney and synovial fluid

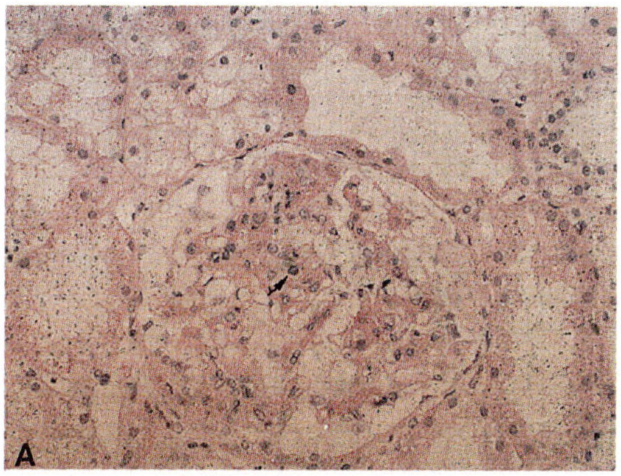

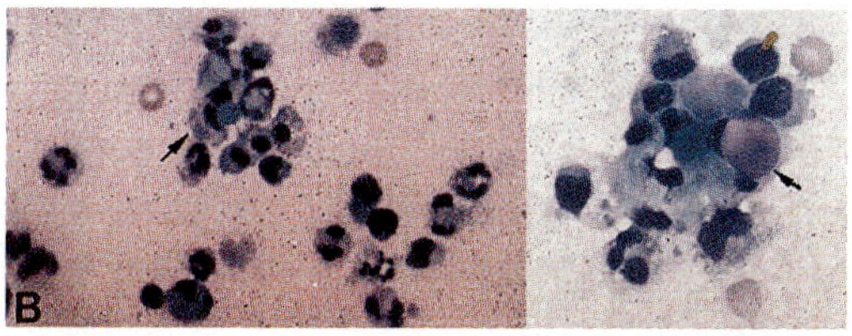

The patient, a 26-year-old woman with a 2-year history of systemic lupus erythematosus (SLE), presented with progressive swelling and pain in her knees, ankles, and right elbow of 10 days' duration. She had developed increasing fatigue, loss of appetite, and "puffiness" of her face over the last 2 months. Laboratory studies revealed the following: antinuclear antibody titer 1:1,280, anti–double-stranded DNA >300 IU/ml, C3 40 mg/dl, C4 <10 mg/dl, and 1,100 mg protein/24 hour urine collection. A kidney biopsy showed focal segmental glomerulonephritis and deposits of hematoxylin bodies in the glomeruli **(A; arrow).** Light microscopy of fluid aspirated from the right knee revealed numerous LE cells **(B; arrows).** The patient was treated with steroids and immunosuppressive agents and discharged after her symptoms resolved. LE cells, also referred to as hematoxylin bodies when seen in renal glomeruli, are very specific for SLE. Hematoxylin bodies are seen in ~2% of renal biopsy samples from patients with SLE; reports of LE cells in synovial fluid are few. This patient had both findings when she presented with a flare of her disease. Because immunologic tests are now commonly used for diagnosis of SLE, the recognition of these pathognomonic features by a new generation of physicians is unlikely.

B. M. Atiquzzaman, MD
Daniel D. Ricciardi, MD
Yusuf Yazici, MD
Allan Gibofsky, MD, JD
Long Island College Hospital
Brooklyn, NY

ARTHRITIS & RHEUMATISM
Vol. 44, No. 1, January 2001, pp 170–175

Treatment of Lupus-Induced Thrombocytopenia with Recombinant Human Interleukin-11

Shamiram Feinglass and Atul Deodhar

Autoimmune thrombocytopenia can be a serious manifestation of systemic lupus erythematosus (SLE) which necessitates treatment with immunosuppressive agents and platelet transfusions. Interleukin-11 (IL-11) is a unique thrombopoietic growth factor which causes proliferation of megakaryocyte progenitors as well as induces megakaryocytic maturation. To our knowledge, this agent has not been used in the treatment of autoimmune thrombocytopenia, since theoretically there is a danger of IL-11 stimulating the immune system by up-regulating the lymphoid stem cells. We describe a 36-year-old splenectomized woman with known SLE who presented with pulmonary hemorrhage, acute renal failure, change in mental status, and severe thrombocytopenia (platelet count 2,000/mm^3). Her pulmonary, renal, and central nervous system complications responded to intensive therapy with intravenous (IV) pulse methylprednisone and cyclophosphamide along with hemodialysis. The thrombocytopenia remained refractory to the above treatment plus daily multiple platelet transfusions and IV immunoglobulin. Treatment with recombinant human IL-11 (25 μg/kg/day subcutaneously) was initiated and continued for 5 days. Her platelet count improved to 25,000/mm^3 within 48 hours, and she experienced no adverse effects.

Autoimmune thrombocytopenia can be a life-threatening manifestation of systemic lupus erythematosus (SLE). The acute form necessitates treatment with immunosuppressive agents such as high-dose corticosteroids and cyclophosphamide (CYC) (1). In resistant cases, intravenous immunoglobulin (IVIG) infusion (2) and splenectomy (3,4) have been found to be useful. Platelet transfusions are used predominantly in bleeding-related emergencies, though the beneficial effects are only temporary because the circulating antibodies destroy the transfused platelets.

Interleukin 11 (IL-11), a cytokine produced by bone marrow stromal cells, is a unique thrombopoietic growth factor (5). Recombinant human IL-11 (rHuIL-11) (oprelvekin, Numega; Genetics Institute, Cambridge, MA) was approved in November 1997 for use in chemotherapy-induced thrombocytopenia, in a recommended dosage of 50 μg/kg subcutaneously daily for adults. The daily treatment is continued for 10–21 days until the postnadir platelet count is >50,000/mm^3; administration beyond 21 days is not recommended. In recent studies, rHuIL-11 has been shown to be safe and effective in reducing the need for platelet transfusions (6). It has not been used in the treatment of autoimmune thrombocytopenia, perhaps because of the possibility of stimulation of the immune system by up-regulation of lymphoid stem cells.

Herein we describe a case of systemic lupus erythematosus (SLE)–related severe refractory thrombocytopenia that responded to treatment with rHuIL-11. Use of this treatment in lupus-related thrombocytopenia has not previously been reported in the literature.

CASE REPORT

The patient, a 36-year-old woman with known SLE, presented to our hospital in January 1998 with abdominal pain and change in mental status of 1 week's duration. Her SLE had started in 1982 with a malar rash and deep venous thrombosis in the legs. Subsequent studies had revealed positive antinuclear antibody, positive anti–double-stranded DNA, and later, positive anticardiolipin antibody. Over the next 5 years she had 3 spontaneous abortions, autoimmune thrombocytopenia, a further episode of deep venous thrombosis with possible pulmonary embolism, arthritis of the small joints of

Shamiram Feinglass, MD, Atul Deodhar, MD, MRCP: Oregon Health Sciences University, Portland.

Address correspondence and reprint requests to Atul Deodhar, MD, MRCP, Division of Arthritis and Rheumatic Diseases (L329A), Oregon Health Sciences University, Portland, OR 97201.

Submitted for publication June 26, 2000; accepted in revised form September 6, 2000.

Table 1. Abnormal laboratory findings in the patient upon admission

Test	Result	Normal value
Hematocrit, %	18.7	37.0–46.0
White blood cell count, × 10^3/mm^3	20.6	3.4–10.0
Platelet count, × 10^3/mm^3	23	150.0–420.0
Blood urea nitrogen, mg/dl	69	6.0–23.0
Creatinine, mg/dl	4.7	0.7–1.2
Aspartate aminotransferase, units/liter	40	11.0–32.0
Alanine aminotransferase, units/liter	72	5.0–30.0
Alkaline phosphatase, units/liter	170	35–105
Lactate dehydrogenase, units/liter	420	110–205
Amylase, units/liter	459	28–100
Peripheral blood smear	Microcytic, normochromic, no schistocytes	
C3, mg/dl	61	8.8–203
C4, mg/dl	13.9	16.0–47.0
Anti–double-stranded DNA, units	25	0–34
Urinalysis	Large amount of blood, 30 mg protein, 8–12 red blood cells, no casts	
Hepatitis B surface antibody	Positive	
Hepatitis B core antibody	Positive	

the hands, discoid lupus skin changes, and "diffuse" glomerulonephritis (exact histopathology unknown). She underwent splenectomy for refractory thrombocytopenia and between 1993 and 1998 remained fairly asymptomatic, with platelet counts of ~70,000/mm^3.

The patient was in her usual state of health until approximately 2 weeks prior to admission, when she presented to her local hospital with abdominal pain. A presumptive diagnosis of acute cholecystitis and pancreatitis (amylase level 459 units/liter) was made. She underwent laparoscopic cholecystectomy, with some resolution of the pain. However, postoperatively her creatinine level rose from 1.3 mg/dl to 3.5 mg/dl, her hematocrit value and platelet count fell (25% and 23,000/mm^3, respectively), and schistocytes were noted in her blood smear. Additionally, chest radiography showed cardiomegaly and pulmonary vascular congestion. A nephrologist prescribed high-dose prednisone and furosemide, which resulted in improvement in the pulmonary congestion. However, her creatinine level remained unchanged, and she developed mild confusion. She was transferred to our hospital with a presumptive diagnosis of SLE flare with nephritis and cerebritis, or possibly thrombotic thrombocytopenic purpura (TTP). Upon arrival, she reported abdominal pain, nausea, and the presence of blood in her stool and urine for the last several days. She denied vomiting, shortness of breath, chest pain, dysuria, or diarrhea.

Physical examination revealed an ill-appearing woman with a blood pressure of 147/105 mm Hg, pulse rate of 109, and temperature of 36.9°C. In general, she was sleepy but arousable, and she said that she "felt confused," although findings of her mental status examination were normal. She had a malar rash and multiple discoid lupus lesions on her right arm. Her jugular venous pressure was increased at 9 cm, and she had crackles at the bottom one-third of the lung fields. Cardiovascular examination disclosed a grade II/VI ejection systolic flow murmur. On abdominal examination, she was tender in the right upper quadrant and mid-epigastrium, with healing laparoscopic surgery scars.

Laboratory studies (Table 1) showed microcytic anemia, leukocytosis, and a platelet count of 23,000/mm^3. Chemistry panel revealed increased levels of blood urea nitrogen and creatinine and abnormal liver enzyme values (Table 1). Chest radiography showed cardiomegaly and pulmonary vascular congestion, but no effusions or infiltrates. Echocardiography did not show Libman-Sack endocarditis. Abdominal ultrasound revealed mildly dilated intrahepatic veins.

The patient underwent a 4-day trial of plasma exchanges for presumed TTP based on the low platelet count and an increased lactate dehydrogenase level, despite negative findings on a peripheral blood smear. Hemodialysis was started, and she was also treated with a 500-mg IV CYC bolus and 100–120 mg IV methylprednisolone per day for 2 weeks, for lupus nephritis. When her platelet count worsened to 10,000/mm^3, leukocyte-depleted, single-donor platelet transfusions were instituted.

Six days after admission, she developed extreme

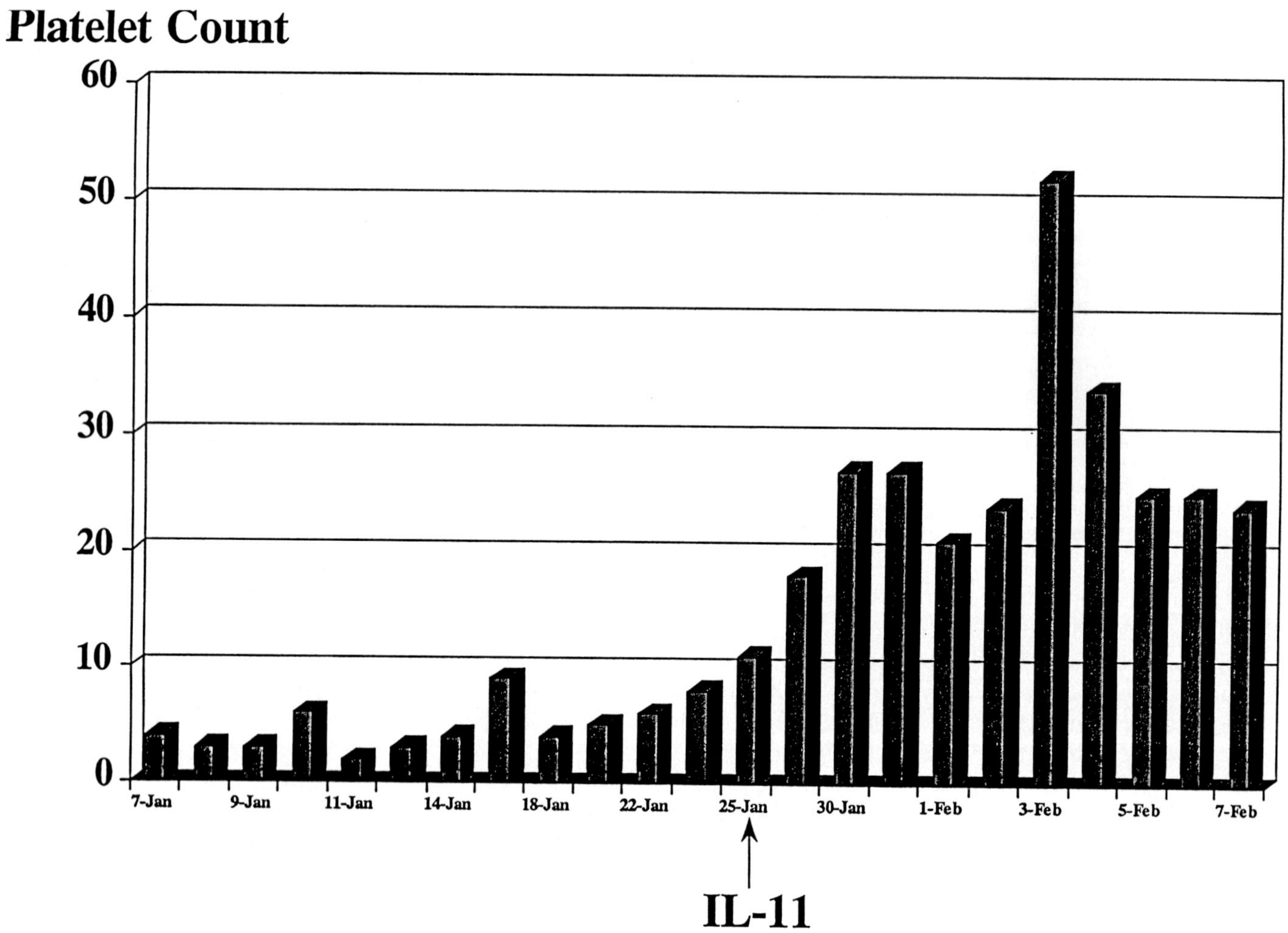

Figure 1. Platelet counts in the patient before and after treatment with recombinant human interleukin-11 (IL-11).

shortness of breath, frothy sputum, and decreasing oxygen saturation. She underwent bronchoscopy, which revealed intrabronchial hemorrhage with punctate lesions. Hemosiderin-laden macrophages seen on bronchoalveolar lavage confirmed the diagnosis of pulmonary alveolar hemorrhage. This was treated with a 3-day increase in the dosage of IV methylprednisolone.

After a brief stay in the intensive care unit, the patient was transferred to the medicine floor without further bleeding episodes. During the third week of her hospitalization, her overall condition started to improve. Her nephritis had stabilized upon treatment with methylprednisolone, CYC, and dialysis, and her pulmonary hemorrhage had resolved. Her mentation was normal. However, a severe, persistent thrombocytopenia (platelet counts of 2,000–5,000/mm^3) remained and was resistant to all of the treatments mentioned above, as well as IVIG (2 gm/kg over a 3-day period). A tagged red cell scan, to investigate for an accessory spleen, yielded negative results. She received another pulse of CYC (500 mg). However, her platelet count could be maintained only with daily platelet transfusions, with counts often falling to 2,000–3,000/mm^3 prior to transfusion and increasing only to 7,000–9,000/mm^3 post-transfusion.

The patient was then given rHuIL-11, 25 μg/kg/day subcutaneously for 5 days, an off-label use of this agent, for the refractory thrombocytopenia. Her platelet count improved to 25,000/mm^3 within 48 hours, eventually rising to 50,000/mm^3 (Figure 1). Treatment with rHuIL-11 did not result in a flare of the SLE, and she was discharged 10 days after completion of this treatment. Her platelet count at the time of discharge was 45,000/mm^3.

During the next 2 months, the patient had 1 more

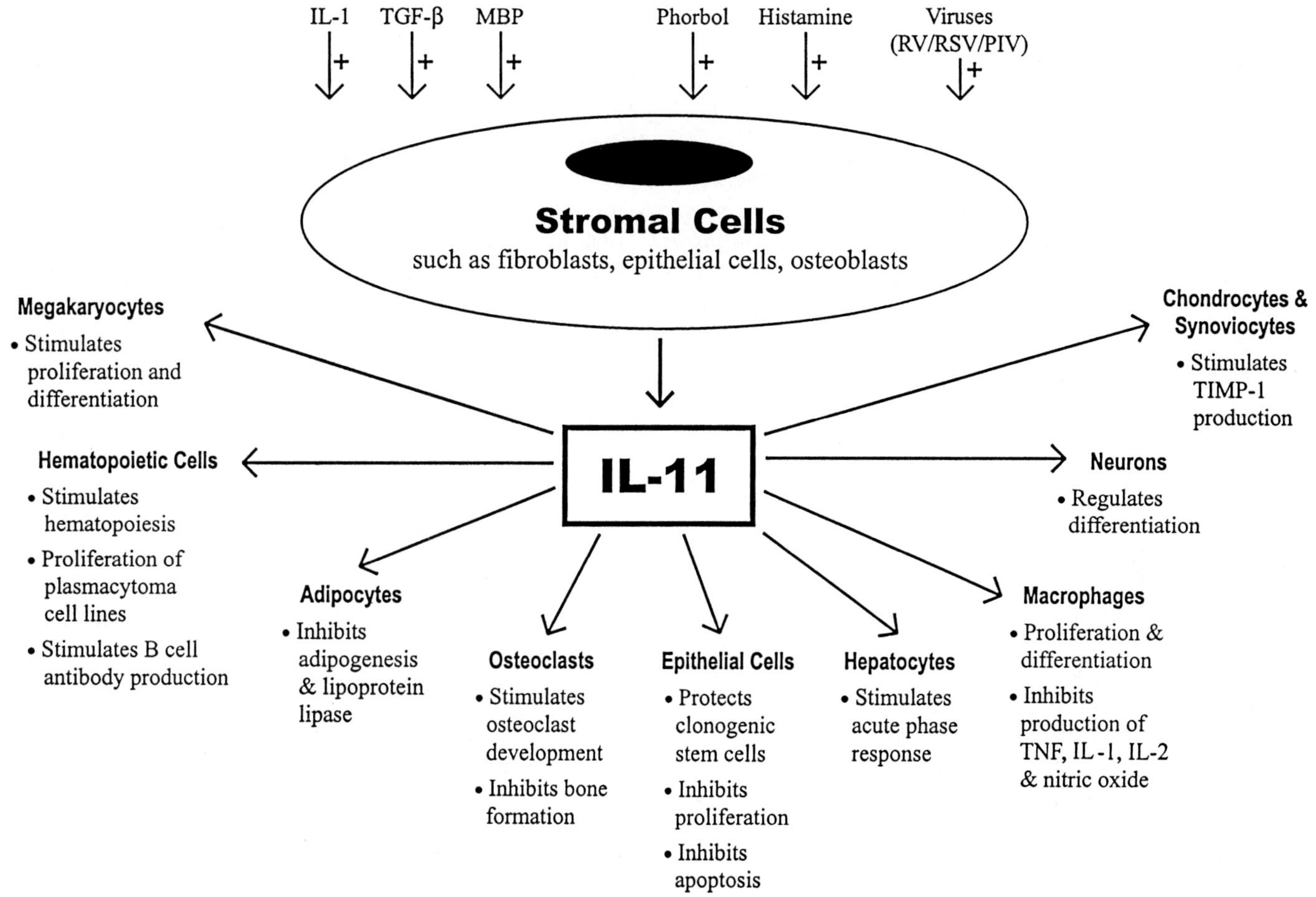

Figure 2. Biologic effects of interleukin-11 (IL-11). TGF-β = transforming growth factor β; MBP = myelin basic protein; RV = rhinovirus; RSV = respiratory syncytial virus; PIV = parainfluenza virus; TNF = tumor necrosis factor; TIMP-1 = tissue inhibitor of metalloproteinases 1. Reproduced, with permission, from ref. 5.

hospital admission, for acute pulmonary edema secondary to noncompliance with fluid restriction. This was treated with changes in her hemodialysis therapy. She was followed up by a private nephrologist and underwent hemodialysis 3 times per week. She was seen once in followup at our hospital when her platelet count was noted to be slightly higher than 25,000/mm^3. She continued to be noncompliant with her fluid intake restrictions and had 3 further episodes of pulmonary congestion noted by her nephrologist, who had assumed the role of her primary care provider. The episodes of pulmonary edema were treated with appropriate changes in the hemodialysis regimen.

Two months later, she was found dead at home. No autopsy was performed, and the cause of death, as certified by the nephrologist, was renal failure secondary to SLE and pulmonary edema.

DISCUSSION

To our knowledge, this is the first reported use of rHuIL-11 to treat immune-mediated severe thrombocytopenia. We were forced to try this approach in this splenectomized patient, given that the life-threatening thrombocytopenia was refractory to high-dose corticosteroids, pulse CYC, IVIG, plasma exchanges, and daily platelet transfusions.

Biologic features and effects of IL-11 are shown in Figure 2. IL-11 is produced by fibroblasts, epithelial cells, and osteoblasts, and it regulates various aspects of hematopoiesis (5). It stimulates all stages of megakaryocyte development independent of thrombopoietin, from the stem cell to the mature megakaryocyte (6). It also stimulates erythropoiesis and regulates macrophage proliferation and differentiation (5). The stimulatory effect of IL-11 on platelet production has been utilized clinically to accelerate recovery from thrombocytopenia induced by bone marrow transplantation or chemotherapy (7), but not in the setting of an autoimmune disease.

There were at least 3 possible causes of the severe thrombocytopenia in our patient. She had SLE and secondary antiphospholipid antibody syndrome, both of which are known causes of thrombocytopenia. She possibly could have had an episode of lupus-related TTP, although the peripheral smear did not clearly indicate this and the platelet count showed no response to plasma exchanges. A kidney biopsy to investigate for the presence or absence of microthrombi would have been helpful for the diagnosis of TTP, but the severely low platelet count made this investigation too risky. We instead elected to treat her aggressively with all of the conventional modalities available.

Thrombocytopenia in SLE is usually a chronic problem that persists for several years. Rarely, patients present with a devastating acute thrombocytopenia (counts $<20,000/mm^3$), leading to life-threatening bleeding manifestations. The underlying mechanism for both clinical types is the presence of antiplatelet antibodies that coat the platelets, causing them to be phagocytosed by splenic macrophages through their Fc receptors. The current treatment is therefore directed toward suppression of the peripheral destruction of platelets by suppressing the immune response.

High-dose oral and/or IV pulse corticosteroids are generally used in the initial stages of SLE-related acute thrombocytopenia. These agents inhibit macrophage ingestion of antibody-coated platelets and suppress antibody synthesis. If this fails, immunosuppression with agents such as azathioprine, vincristine, or CYC is used (1,2). There is a clear paradox in this treatment in that all of these agents may cause thrombocytopenia secondary to bone marrow suppression. However, in these circumstances, they suppress the antiplatelet antibody production and are often life saving. IVIG has been used for many years to treat childhood idiopathic thrombocytopenic purpura (ITP) (8). However, in the setting of lupus, it may have only a limited and transient effect (9). Splenectomy is effective in ~70–80% of patients with ITP (10). In a study of 13 patients with severe thrombocytopenia secondary to lupus and antiphospholipid antibody syndrome, complete remission of the thrombocytopenia was achieved with splenectomy in 9 (4). Danazol, a steroid-like molecule with weak androgenic properties and extracorporeal immunoadsorption using a staphylococcal A–silica column have also been shown to be effective in some cases (11,12). Platelet transfusions are reserved for prevention or control of acute bleeding in patients with dangerously low platelet counts.

Use of rHuIL-11 would be complementary to the immunosuppressive therapy in that it increases the platelet count by stimulating thrombopoiesis. However, there could be several problems associated with rHuIL-11 treatment in patients with SLE. Apart from its action on thrombopoiesis, IL-11 inhibits apoptosis, stimulates B cell immunoglobulin production, and in experimental models, causes proliferation of plasmacytoma cell lines (5), all of which could theoretically lead to a lupus flare. Additionally, it causes sodium and water retention, which in a patient such as ours, can lead to fluid overload. Thus, great precautions must be taken if this drug is to be used to treat SLE-induced thrombocytopenia.

Interleukins, such as IL-1, IL-2, IL-6, and IL-10, and tumor necrosis factor play a complex role in the pathogenesis of SLE (13–15). IL-6, a Th2-type cytokine, is associated with stimulating autoantibody-secreting B cells and could play a key role in SLE pathogenesis. Although the exact role of IL-11 in SLE is unknown, considering its similarities with IL-6, it could lead to a lupus flare. However, because of the cascade nature of cytokines, all components of the cytokine network need to be considered before any conclusions can be drawn.

This is the first report of the use of rHuIL-11 in the treatment of SLE-induced thrombocytopenia. Rheumatologists need to be aware that rHuIL-11 is commercially available for stimulating thrombopoiesis. In severe situations related to autoimmune thrombocytopenia, in which the main problem involves destruction, rather than reduced production, of platelets, it could still be used, but with great caution.

REFERENCES

1. Boumpas DT, Barez S, Klippel JH, Balow JE. Intermittent cyclophosphamide for the treatment of autoimmune thrombocytopenia in systemic lupus erythematosus. Ann Intern Med 1990;112:674–7.
2. Fessler BJ, Boumpas DT. Severe major organ involvement in systemic lupus erythematosus: diagnosis and management. Rheum Dis Clin North Am 1995;21:81–98.
3. Homan WP, Dineen P. The role of splenectomy in the treatment of thrombocytopenic purpura due to systemic lupus erythematosus. Ann Surg 1978;187:52–6.
4. Hakim AJ, Machin SJ, Isenberg DA. Autoimmune thrombocytopenia in primary antiphospholipid syndrome and systemic lupus erythematosus: the response to splenectomy. Semin Arthritis Rheum 1998;28:20–5.

5. Leng SX, Elias JA. Molecules in focus: interleukin 11. Int J Biochem Cell Biol 1997;29:1059–62.
6. Issacs C, Robert NJ, Bailey FA, Schuster MW, Overmoyer B, Graham M, et al. Randomized placebo-controlled study of recombinant human interleukin 11 to prevent chemotherapy induced thrombocytopenia in patients with breast cancer receiving dose intensive cyclophosphamide and doxorubicin. J Clin Oncol 1997; 15:3368–77.
7. Teramura M, Kobayashi S, Yoshinaga K, Iwabe K, Mizoguchi H. Effect of interleukin 11 on normal and pathological thrombopoiesis. Cancer Chemother Pharmacol 1996;38 Suppl:S99–102.
8. Imbach P, Barandun S, d'Apuzzo V, Baumgastner C, Hirt A, Morell A, et al. High dose intravenous gammaglobulin for idiopathic thrombocytopenic purpura in childhood. Lancet 1981; 1:1228–31.
9. Borg EJ, Kallenberg CG. Treatment of severe thrombocytopenia in systemic lupus erythematosus with intravenous gammaglobulin. Ann Rheum Dis 1992;51:1149–51.
10. Berchtold P, McMillan R. Therapy of chronic idiopathic thrombocytopenic purpura in adults. Blood 1989;74:2309–17.
11. West SG, Johnson SC. Danazol for the treatment of refractory autoimmune thrombocytopenia in systemic lupus erythematosus. Ann Intern Med 1988;108:703–6.
12. Muroi K, Sasaki R, Miura Y. The effect of immunoadsorption therapy by a protein A column on patients with thrombocytopenia. Semin Hematol 1989;26 Suppl 1:10–4.
13. Cross JT, Benton HP. The roles of interleukin 6 and interleukin 10 in B cell hyperactivity in systemic lupus erythematosus. Inflamm Res 1999;48:255–61.
14. Dayan M, Segal R, Mozes E. Cytokine manipulation by methotrexate treatment in murine experimental SLE. J Rheumatol 1997;24:1075–82.
15. Llorente L, Zou W, Levy Y, Richaud-Patin Y, Wijdenes J, Alcocer-Varela J, et al. Role of interleukin-10 in the B lymphocyte hyperactivity and autoantibody production of human systemic lupus erythematosus. J Exp Med 1995;181:839–44.

ARTHRITIS & RHEUMATISM
Vol. 44, No. 1, January 2001, pp 176–179

Genetic Association Between Interleukin-10 Promoter Region Polymorphisms and Primary Sjögren's Syndrome

Janne Hulkkonen,[1] Marja Pertovaara,[2] Jaakko Antonen,[3] Nina Lahdenpohja,[1] Amos Pasternack,[3] and Mikko Hurme[3]

Objective. **To determine whether the haplotypes formed on the basis of single-base–exchange polymorphisms at positions −1082, −819, or −592 of the interleukin-10 (IL-10) gene predispose subjects to primary Sjögren's syndrome (SS).**

Methods. **The frequency of IL-10 polymorphisms was analyzed in 62 patients with primary SS and in 400 healthy subjects. These data were assessed for correlations with the concentration of IL-10 in the plasma.**

Results. **The frequency of the IL-10 GCC haplotype (G at position −1082, C at position −819, and C at position −592 of the IL-10 gene) was increased (*P* < 0.05, odds ratio [OR] 1.90, 95% confidence interval [95% CI] 0.955–3.62) and the frequency of the ACC haplotype decreased (*P* < 0.05, OR 0.443, 95% CI 0.257–0.764) in primary SS patients compared with healthy controls. Moreover, the frequency of the ATA haplotype was similar in primary SS patients and healthy controls, but the incidence of the GCC/ATA genotype was elevated in the primary SS patients (*P* < 0.05, OR 2.19, 95% CI 1.19–4.03). The concentration of plasma IL-10 was significantly higher in patients carrying the GCC haplotype than in non-carriers of GCC.**

Conclusion. **These results suggest that the presence of the GCC haplotype or the GCC/ATA genotype and the absence of the ACC haplotype of the IL-10 gene are associated with an increased susceptibility to primary SS. This effect is probably mediated by the increased capability to produce IL-10 among carriers of the GCC haplotype.**

Supported by grants from the Medical Research Fund of Tampere University Hospital.

[1]Janne Hulkkonen, MD, Nina Lahdenpohja, PhD: University of Tampere Medical School and Institute of Medical Technology, Tampere, Finland; [2]Marja Pertovaara, MD: Tampere University Hospital, Tampere, Finland; [3]Jaakko Antonen, MD, PhD, Amos Pasternack, MD, PhD, Mikko Hurme, MD, PhD: University of Tampere Medical School and Tampere University Hospital, Tampere, Finland.

Address correspondence and reprint requests to Janne Hulkkonen, MD, Department of Microbiology and Immunology, Medical School, FIN-33014, University of Tampere, Finland.

Submitted for publication May 5, 2000; accepted in revised form September 6, 2000.

Primary Sjögren's syndrome (SS) is a systemic autoimmune disorder that primarily affects the salivary and lacrimal glands. The most important manifestations of the disease are keratoconjunctivitis sicca and oral dryness caused by diminished lacrimal and salivary gland secretory activity. Classically, this glandular dysfunction is associated with progressive lymphocytic infiltration, which leads to the destruction of acinar and ductal epithelial cells and loss of glandular parenchyma. Antibodies against ribonucleoproteins (SSA/Ro and SSB/La) are frequently present in the sera of SS patients. Recent studies also suggest that antibodies against muscarinic acetylcholine receptors may have a role in the development of glandular dysfunction (1). Moreover, B cell hyperreactivity and hypergammaglobulinemia are common in primary SS (2). Several cytokines, such as interleukin-10 (IL-10), IL-6, IL-1, tumor necrosis factor α, and interferon-γ, have been proposed to play a role in the pathogenesis of the disease (2–4).

IL-10 is a pleiotropic cytokine that is usually considered to have a role in the down-regulation of cell-mediated and cytotoxic inflammatory responses, thus being a potent antiinflammatory mediator. IL-10 also has some proinflammatory and hematologic functions. IL-10 promotes B cell activation and differentiation and induces immunoglobulin synthesis and autoantibody production (2). An increased frequency of IL-10–secreting mononuclear cells has been found in the peripheral blood of primary SS patients (2). Increased spontaneous IL-10 production has also been observed in cultures of mononuclear cells from primary SS patients (3). Moreover, the IL-10 messenger RNA (mRNA) expression is elevated in the salivary glands of SS patients (4).

Table 1. Demographic characteristics of primary Sjögren's syndrome patients (n = 62)

Variable	Value
Age, years (mean ± SD)	60 ± 11
Disease duration after diagnosis, years (mean ± SD)	9.1 ± 4.3
Sex, no. of women/no. of men	60/2

Twin studies and family studies have suggested that ~75% of the variation in IL-10 production is genetically determined (5). It seems that IL-10 production is mainly controlled at the transcriptional level (6). The 5′ flanking region of the IL-10 gene is polymorphic. Three single-base–exchange polymorphisms, sited at positions −1082 (G to A), −819 (C to T), and −592 (C to A), form haplotypes, of which only 3 forms (GCC, ACC, and ATA) have been described in Caucasian populations (6). The GCC haplotype has been associated with high IL-10 production in peripheral blood mononuclear cell cultures (6). The ATA haplotype, compared with the GCC haplotype, has been associated with lower transcriptional activity, and the ATA/ATA genotype has been associated with lower IL-10 production in whole blood cultures compared with other haplotypes (7). The presence of these different IL-10 haplotypes has been described to be associated with distinctive systemic lupus erythematosus (SLE) disease phenotypes (8).

In this study we analyzed IL-10 plasma levels and polymorphisms of the IL-10 gene in 62 primary SS patients, and compared the results with corresponding data from 400 healthy controls.

PATIENTS AND METHODS

Patients. All patients fulfilling 3 or more Californian criteria for primary SS (9), modified so that salivary flow determinations were not performed and histologic findings were graded on the Chisholm-Mason scale (10) (in which grades 3 and 4 were regarded as diagnostic), were selected from the records of patients with sicca symptoms. These patients were examined in the Department of Internal Medicine, Section of Rheumatology, at Tampere University Hospital in Finland during the years 1977 to 1992 (n = 111). Patients who were still alive were invited by letter to undergo cytokine and cytokine gene polymorphism determinations, and clinical specimens and samples were obtained for genotyping after informed consent was given by the 62 primary SS patients. Demographic characteristics of the patients at study entry are summarized in Table 1.

Normal controls. Blood samples (n = 400) from healthy blood donors (ages 18–60 years) were obtained from the Finnish Red Cross Blood Transfusion Centre in Tampere.

Clinical methods. A careful clinical examination with an in-depth interview with the primary SS patients, covering previous and concurrent diseases, duration of sicca symptoms, existence of recurrent parotid or submandibular gland swellings, and present sicca symptoms of the eyes and mouth, as well as extraglandular symptoms (dermatologic, endocrine, gastrointestinal, lymphoproliferative, musculoskeletal, neurologic, renal, respiratory, and vascular symptoms), was conducted (11).

Laboratory analyses. Antinuclear antibodies, antibodies against ribonuclear antigens SSA (Ro) and SSB (La), and serum concentrations of IgG were measured as previously described (11).

IL-10 determination. Plasma IL-10 concentrations in all primary SS patients and 202 healthy controls were determined by using commercially available enzyme-linked immunosorbent assays (Pelikine human IL-10 ELISA kit; Central Laboratory of The Netherlands Red Cross Blood Transfusion Service, Amsterdam) following the manufacturer's instructions. The assay contains reagents used to circumvent rheumatoid factor binding. The optical density of individual wells was determined with a Multiscan Bichromatic 348 spectrophotometer (Labsystems, Helsinki, Finland). The detection limit of the assay was 1.2 pg/ml.

Genotype analyses. DNA was isolated from blood samples and the G/A base-exchange polymorphism at −1082 of the IL-10 gene was analyzed by polymerase chain reaction (PCR) and cycle sequencing as previously described (12). The −819 C/T polymorphism and −592 C/A polymorphism of the IL-10 gene were analyzed by PCR and restriction fragment length polymorphism (RFLP) analysis (13,14). The validity of RFLP-based methodologies was confirmed by additionally analyzing 70 samples with direct sequencing.

Statistical analysis. Concentrations of IL-10 were compared using the Mann-Whitney U test and Kruskall-Wallis analysis of variance. Allelic frequencies were compared using chi-square test with Yates' correction when appropriate. Findings were considered statistically significant at P values less than 0.05.

RESULTS

IL-10 base-exchange polymorphisms. After determining the single-base–exchange polymorphism of −1082, −819, and −562 for each subject, the genotype distribution, the haplotype carrier rate, and the haplotype frequencies in primary SS patients and control subjects were analyzed (Table 2). In the haplotype analysis, the GCC haplotype frequency was significantly higher among primary SS patients (0.524) than among healthy controls (0.429) ($P < 0.05$). The ACC haplotype frequency was significantly lower in primary SS patients (0.258) than in healthy subjects (0.351) ($P < 0.05$). The ATA haplotype frequencies were similar in primary SS patients and in control subjects (0.218 and 0.220, respectively), but the proportion of the GCC/ATA genotype was higher in primary SS patients (29%) than in normal controls (16%) ($P < 0.05$). No correlation between

Table 2. Individual interleukin-10 genotypes, haplotype carrier rate, and haplotype carrier frequencies in healthy controls and in patients with primary Sjögren's syndrome (SS)

Genetic marker	Primary patients (n = 62)	Normal controls (n = 400)	Chi-square *P*
Genotype, n (%)			
GCC/ACC	15 (24)	126 (32)	0.245
GCC/GCC	16 (26)	77 (19)	0.231
GCC/ATA	18 (29)	63 (16)	0.011
ACC/ACC	5 (8)	46 (12)	0.558*
ACC/ATA	7 (11)	63 (16)	0.471*
ATA/ATA	1 (2)	25 (6)	0.239*
Haplotype carrier rate, n (%)			
GCC carriers	49 (79)	266 (67)	0.049
ACC carriers	27 (44)	235 (59)	0.025
ATA carriers	26 (42)	151 (38)	0.528
Haplotype frequency			
GCC	0.524	0.429	0.046
ACC	0.258	0.351	0.041
ATA	0.218	0.220	0.955

* Value with Yates' correction.

extraglandular symptoms and IL-10 haplotypes was found (results not shown).

IL-10 plasma levels. The IL-10 plasma levels were higher in the primary SS patients (mean ± SD 8.65 ± 23.6 pg/ml, n = 62) compared with those in the healthy controls (5.20 ± 15.8 pg/ml, n = 202), although this difference can only be considered a trend (P = 0.08). The patients were then classified according to their genotypes and haplotype-carrier state and the effects of these on the plasma IL-10 levels were analyzed (Figure 1). The plasma IL-10 levels were significantly higher among the primary SS patients who carried the GCC haplotype (10.4 ± 26.3 pg/ml) compared with the levels in GCC haplotype–negative patients (2.03 ± 3.26 pg/ml) ($P < 0.05$). The patients who were carriers of the ACC haplotype had slightly, but not significantly, lower IL-10 plasma levels (4.09 ± 6.08 pg/ml) than did ACC-negative patients (12.2 ± 30.7 pg/ml). The ATA-carrier status did not have any effect on plasma IL-10. No significant differences in the levels of plasma IL-10 among the healthy controls were seen when they were categorized on the basis of IL-10 haplotypes (results not shown).

DISCUSSION

In this study we analyzed polymorphisms of the IL-10 gene and found that the frequency of the GCC haplotype is increased and the frequency of the ACC haplotype is decreased in primary SS patients. Moreover, we measured the levels of circulating IL-10 and found that the GCC haplotype is associated with high plasma levels of IL-10 in primary SS, which is in agreement with the results observed by Turner et al in mononuclear cell cultures (6). Our findings concerning the IL-10 haplotypes may partly explain the results presented in a previous report by Llorente et al (2), in which the authors described elevated levels of IL-10 mRNA and IL-10 protein expression in peripheral blood mononuclear cell cultures in primary SS.

Abnormal frequencies of IL-10 haplotypes have been described in other autoimmune diseases; e.g., in SLE, the GCC haplotype has been shown to be associated with renal involvement in the disease (8). Moreover, the ATA haplotype of the IL-10 gene has been

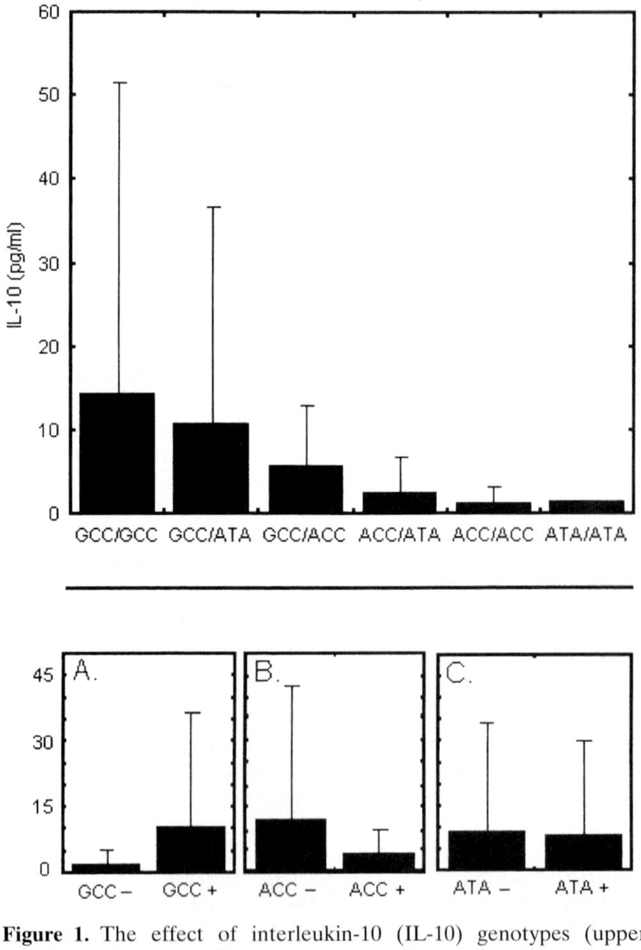

Figure 1. The effect of interleukin-10 (IL-10) genotypes (upper panel) on the plasma IL-10 concentration in primary Sjögren's syndrome patients. In the lower panel, IL-10 levels (mean and SD) are shown among the carriers and non-carriers of the IL-10 GCC haplotype (panel A), ACC haplotype (panel B), or ATA haplotype (panel C).

described to be related to the severity of juvenile chronic arthritis (7). Our study is the first one to demonstrate that the haplotypes formed on the basis of the IL-10 gene alleles (at the −1082, −819, and −592 locus) are related to the susceptibility to primary SS. Furthermore, for the first time, the IL-10 haplotypes have been found to regulate levels of circulating IL-10.

In the development of primary SS the pathologic features of glandular dysfunction are associated with a local and systemic increase of IL-6 and other proinflammatory cytokines (2–4). Polymorphic genetic loci with regulatory functions have been described in inflammatory as well as antiinflammatory cytokine genes. It could be possible that the combinations formed by these individual polymorphisms may also lead to an unfavorable cytokine imbalance and influence the disease outcome in subgroups of patients. The knowledge of these complex genetic factors and, especially, the understanding of their associations with autoimmune diseases are still in the very beginning stages.

Primary SS is characterized by B cell hyperactivity and hypergammaglobulinemia. IL-10 together with IL-6 plays a central role in the maturation of plasma cells and activation of immunoglobulin synthesis. No direct correlations of IL-10 haplotypes with total IgG, SSA or SSB antibodies, or antinuclear antibodies were found in our study (results not shown), but it is still probable that the increased levels of IL-10 contribute to the development of hypergammaglobulinemia and promote autoantibody production associated with primary SS. Potential mechanisms of hypergammaglobulinemia and B cell hyperreactivity have been comprehensively discussed in the recent study by Llorente et al (2). Moreover, it is known that patients with SS have an increased risk of developing lymphomas, and it is possible that persistently high levels of IL-10 may contribute to these conditions (15). In our cross-sectional study we did not observe any distinct associations with the IL-10 haplotypes and extraglandular manifestations of primary SS. Due to the subtle nature of allelic effects, it is quite probable that larger materials and longitudinal studies are needed to find these kinds of phenotypic differences. Moreover, the fact that the IL-10 haplotypes had no clear effect on circulating IL-10 in healthy controls suggests that the IL-10 polymorphism primarily regulates induced IL-10 responses, or that more sensitive methods are needed to detect the haplotype effect on basal IL-10 production.

In conclusion, we suggest that the abnormal distribution of IL-10 haplotypes may be a predisposing factor for primary SS. The increased proportion of the GCC, "IL-10 high producer" haplotype in primary SS may explain some of the cytokine findings observed in the disease.

REFERENCES

1. Fox RI, Törnwall J, Michelson P. Current issues in the diagnosis and treatment of Sjögren's syndrome. Curr Opin Rheumatol 1999;11:364–71.
2. Llorente L, Richaud-Patin Y, Fior R, Alcocer-Varela J, Wijdenes J, Fourrier BM, et al. In vivo production of interleukin-10 by non–T cells in rheumatoid arthritis, Sjögren's syndrome, and systemic lupus erythematosus: a potential mechanism of B lymphocyte hyperactivity and autoimmunity. Arthritis Rheum 1994; 37:1647–55.
3. Halse A, Tengner P, Wahren-Herlenius M, Haga H, Jonsson R. Increased frequency of cells secreting interleukin-6 and interleukin-10 in peripheral blood of patients with primary Sjögren's syndrome. Scand J Immunol 1999;49:533–8.
4. Fox RI, Kang HI, Ando D, Abrams J, Pisa E. Cytokine mRNA expression in salivary gland biopsies of Sjögren's syndrome. J Immunol 1994;152:5532–9.
5. Westendorp RG, Langermans JA, Huizinga TW, Elouali AH, Verweij CL, Boomsma DI, et al. Genetic influence on cytokine production and fatal meningococcal disease. Lancet 1997;349: 170–3.
6. Turner DM, Williams DM, Sankaran D, Lazarus M, Sinnott PJ, Hutchinson IV. An investigation of polymorphism in the interleukin-10 gene promoter. Eur J Immunogenet 1997;24:1–8.
7. Crawley E, Kay R, Sillibourne J, Patel P, Hutchinson I, Woo P. Polymorphic haplotypes of the interleukin-10 5′ flanking region determine variable interleukin-10 transcription and are associated with particular phenotypes of juvenile rheumatoid arthritis. Arthritis Rheum 1999;42:1101–8.
8. Lazarus M, Hajeer AH, Turner D, Sinnott P, Worthington J, Ollier WE, et al. Genetic variation in the interleukin 10 gene promoter and systemic lupus erythematosus. J Rheumatol 1997; 24:2314–7.
9. Fox RI, Robinson CA, Curd JG, Kozin F, Howell FV. Sjögren's syndrome: proposed criteria for classification. Arthritis Rheum 1986;29:577–85.
10. Chisholm DM, Mason DK. Labial salivary gland biopsy in Sjögren's disease. J Clin Pathol 1968;21:656–60.
11. Pertovaara M, Korpela M, Kouri T, Pasternack A. The occurrence of renal involvement in primary Sjögren's syndrome: a study of 78 patients. Rheumatology (Oxford) 1999;38:1113–20.
12. Helminen M, Lahdenpohja N, Hurme M. Polymorphism of the interleukin-10 gene is associated with susceptibility to Epstein-Barr virus infection. J Infect Dis 1999;180:496–9.
13. Mok CC, Lanchbury JS, Chan DW, Lau CS. Interleukin-10 promoter polymorphisms in Southern Chinese patients with systemic lupus erythematosus. Arthritis Rheum 1998;41:1090–5.
14. Edwards-Smith CJ, Jonsson JR, Purdie DM, Bansal A, Shorthouse C, Powell EE. Interleukin-10 promoter polymorphism predicts initial response of chronic hepatitis C to interferon alfa. Hepatology 1999;30:526–30.
15. Levy Y, Brouet JC. Interleukin-10 prevents spontaneous death of germinal center B cells by induction of the bcl-2 protein. J Clin Invest 1994;93:424–8.

ARTHRITIS & RHEUMATISM
Vol. 44, No. 1, January 2001, pp 180–185

Efficacy of Celecoxib, a Cyclooxygenase 2–Specific Inhibitor, in the Treatment of Ankylosing Spondylitis

A Six-Week Controlled Study with Comparison Against Placebo and Against a Conventional Nonsteroidal Antiinflammatory Drug

Maxime Dougados,[1] Jehan-Michel Béhier,[2] Irène Jolchine,[2] Andrei Calin,[3] Désirée van der Heijde,[4] Ignazio Olivieri,[5] Henning Zeidler,[6] and Hélène Herman[2]

Objective. **To evaluate the short-term efficacy of celecoxib, a cyclooxygenase 2–specific inhibitor, in the treatment of ankylosing spondylitis (AS).**

Methods. **The study was a 6-week randomized, double-blind, placebo-controlled trial with 3 treatment arms: placebo, ketoprofen 100 mg twice daily, and celecoxib 100 mg twice daily. Patients who had AS according to the modified New York criteria, without peripheral synovitis and with active disease (pain ≥40 mm on a 100-mm visual analog scale [VAS] and an increase in pain of at least 30% after nonsteroidal antiinflammatory drug withdrawal) were eligible for study. Primary outcome measures were change in pain intensity (VAS) and change in functional impairment (Bath Ankylosing Spondylitis Functional Index [BASFI]).**

Results. **Of the 246 randomized patients, 76 were allocated to receive placebo, 90 ketoprofen, and 80 celecoxib. There were no statistically significant differences between treatment groups at study entry. During the 6 weeks of the study, the decrease in pain and functional impairment was greater in the active treatment groups than in the placebo group, with a trend in favor of celecoxib when the 2 active treatments were compared. The mean changes were −13 mm, −21 mm, and −27 mm ($P = 0.006$) for pain and 1, −6, and −12 ($P = 0.0008$) for BASFI score in the placebo, ketoprofen, and celecoxib groups, respectively. During treatment, the number of patients reporting epigastric pain was 6 (8%), 13 (14%), and 10 (13%) in the placebo, ketoprofen, and celecoxib groups, respectively.**

Conclusion. **The results of this study confirm the clinically relevant antiinflammatory effect of celecoxib at a 200-mg daily dosage, with significant improvement of both pain and function in patients with AS.**

The group of diseases collectively labeled spondylarthropathies consists of several disorders: reactive arthritis, psoriatic arthritis, arthritis related to inflammatory bowel disease, a subgroup of juvenile chronic arthritis, and ankylosing spondylitis (AS), the latter being the prototype of this group of interrelated disorders (1). The rheumatic manifestations of these diseases include spinal symptoms, but also extraspinal joint disease and enthesopathic lesions (2). The monitoring and, to a lesser degree, the diagnosis and treatment of these diseases are related more to their clinical presentation than to the individual diagnosis (3). The objectives of treatment of the axial involvement of spondylarthropathy are to reduce and/or prevent the deleterious clinical effects of the 3 main clinical characteristics of the disease, i.e., inflammation, ankylosis, and abnormal postures.

Nonsteroidal antiinflammatory drugs (NSAIDs) are considered to be the cornerstone of drug therapy for such axial involvement. Most of the clinical trials evaluating NSAIDs clearly demonstrate substantial, quick

Supported in part by a grant from Searle Ltd.

[1]Maxime Dougados, MD: René Descartes University, Cochin Hospital, Paris, France; [2]Jehan-Michel Béhier, MD, Irène Jolchine, MD, Hélène Herman, MD: Searle Medical Department, Paris, France; [3]Andrei Calin, MD: Royal National Hospital for Rheumatic Diseases, Bath, UK; [4]Désirée van der Heijde, MD, PhD: University Hospital, Maastricht, The Netherlands; [5]Ignazio Olivieri, MD: Ospedale San Carlo, Potenza, Italy; [6]Henning Zeidler, MD: Medizinische Hochschule, Hannover, Germany.

Address correspondence and reprint requests to Maxime Dougados, MD, Université René Descartes, Hôpital Cochin—Rhumatologie B, 27, rue du Faubourg Saint Jacques, 75014 Paris, France.

Submitted for publication July 17, 2000; accepted in revised form September 5, 2000.

relief of symptoms. Because of the lack of knowledge of whether this symptomatic effect obtained in the short term will correlate with an improvement in the long-term prognosis, and due to the poor tolerability of conventional NSAIDs, the usual recommendation is to restrict the intake of NSAIDs to periods when the disease is causing pain (4).

Conventional NSAIDs inhibit the 2 isozymes cyclooxygenase 1 (COX-1) and COX-2. COX-1 is responsible for production of prostaglandins critical to the maintenance of gastric mucosal integrity and platelet function, and COX-2 is responsible for the biosynthesis of inflammatory prostaglandins (5).

Celecoxib has a high affinity for COX-2 enzyme at therapeutic doses (6). Experience in clinical trials conducted to date has consistently shown that treatment with celecoxib has been associated with improvement in the signs and symptoms of osteoarthritis and rheumatoid arthritis, with no appreciable effects on platelet function and no significantly increased rates of gastroduodenal ulcer as compared with placebo treatment (7–9). The effect of celecoxib on AS symptoms has not been evaluated previously. In the present study, we assessed the short-term efficacy of celecoxib 200 mg daily and ketoprofen (a widely used conventional NSAID) 200 mg daily, compared with placebo in the treatment of AS.

PATIENTS AND METHODS

Patient population. Outpatients fulfilling the modified New York criteria for AS (10) were recruited in 76 rheumatology centers, in France, after written informed consent was obtained. Other defined criteria for inclusion were 1) daily NSAID intake during the month preceding the screening visit; 2) NSAID washout period of 2–14 days before the baseline visit; and 3) a flare of the disease at baseline, defined both by pain scored as ≥40 mm on a 100-mm visual analog scale (VAS) and by an increase in pain of at least 30% between the screening and the baseline visits.

Patients with peripheral articular disease, defined by the presence of active (with swelling) peripheral arthritis (excluding hip and shoulder) at the screening visit and those with active inflammatory bowel disease were excluded, as were those with concomitant severe medical illness. Patients who had received corticosteroids during the previous 6 weeks and/or any disease-modifying antirheumatic drug with a change in dosage during the previous 6 months were excluded. Also excluded were patients with peptic ulcer confirmed by endoscopy within the year preceding the screening visit. At the screening visit, concomitant therapies with gastrointestinal (GI)–protective effects (misoprostol, proton pump inhibitors) were stopped when there was no history of gastroduodenal ulcers and were initiated and/or continued when there was a positive history of gastroduodenal ulcers.

Study design. The study was a multicenter, randomized, double-blind, placebo- and conventional NSAID–controlled trial of 6 weeks' duration. The design was approved by the Ethics Committee of Cochin Hospital.

Study drugs. After confirmation that the patient fulfilled the defined eligibility criteria, patients were randomly assigned to receive placebo, celecoxib 100 mg twice daily, or ketoprofen 100 mg twice daily. Patients took 4 capsules per day (2 at breakfast and 2 at dinner), every day during the 6 weeks of the trial, regardless of the level of symptoms. Compliance was evaluated by pill count at each visit. Acetaminophen (500-mg tablets, maximum of 6 tablets/day) was used as analgesic treatment during the study, when needed.

Assessment criteria. Clinical assessments were performed at baseline and after 1, 3, and 6 weeks, by the same investigator. The primary criteria were patient-reported global pain intensity over the 2 previous days (recorded using a 100-mm VAS) and patient-reported functional impairment (according to the Bath Ankylosing Spondylitis Functional Index [BASFI]) (11). The secondary criteria were patient's overall assessment of disease activity (100-mm VAS), patient-reported nocturnal pain intensity (100-mm VAS), and mobility (Schober test).

Other outcome measures included 1) degree of pain at physical examination, determined using a previously reported spinal articular index (12) that focuses on the cervical, thoracic, and lumbar spine as well as the sacroiliac joints (each area scored on a 0–4 scale; maximum possible score 16); 2) degree of clinical inflammation, assessed by the duration of morning stiffness; 3) degree of sleep impairment, measured using a 1–4 scale; 4) range of chest expansion in centimeters; and 5) overall assessment of the disease activity by the investigator. At each visit, the investigators checked for treatment compliance and tolerability. At the baseline visit and at week 6, blood samples were collected to evaluate hematologic, liver, and renal function and the C-reactive protein (CRP) level.

Sample size. The sample size needed in order to demonstrate a statistically significant difference between active NSAID and placebo in the change in pain intensity from baseline to 6 weeks was calculated. It was considered important to detect a difference of half a standard deviation (i.e., if the standard baseline deviation is 30 mm, then a difference of 15 is deemed clinically relevant). We calculated that a sample size of 80 patients per treatment group would allow demonstration of this difference with an α level of 0.05 and a power of at least 0.80 (2-tailed).

Statistical analysis. The efficacy analysis was conducted on the intent-to-treat (ITT) population, defined as all patients randomized in the study and receiving at least 1 dose of study drug, with the last-observation-carried-forward technique. For patients who withdrew without a treatment assessment, the baseline value was reported as the final value. For patients who withdrew after an intermediate visit, the last value recorded during treatment was reported as the final value.

The primary efficacy criteria (absolute changes in global pain intensity [VAS] and in functional impairment [BASFI]) were evaluated using a two-way analysis of covariance, with treatment and center as factors and baseline value as covariate. In cases of significant treatment effect, a pairwise comparison was conducted using the Hochberg procedure. For both primary variables, the ratio of celecoxib effect to ketoprofen effect was calculated and the 95% confidence interval (95% CI) of the ratio was estimated. The secondary criteria (overall assessment of disease activity by patient, nocturnal pain, Schober test) and the other outcome measures were analyzed in the same way as the primary criteria.

Responders were defined as patients in whom global

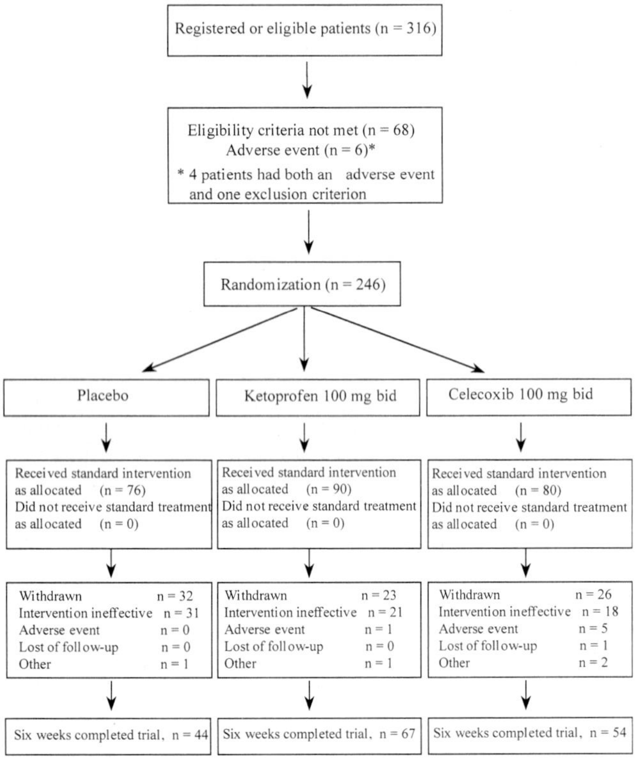

Figure 1. Patients and study course.

pain intensity decreased by at least 50% during the study period and who did not have to discontinue the drug because of lack of efficacy. Based on previous experiences (13–16), we anticipated a 20% placebo effect and a 50% active drug effect after 6 weeks of therapy. The number of responders was compared between treatment groups, by chi-square test.

An acceptable level of treatment compliance was defined a priori as an intake of capsules of at least 70% of the theoretical quantity expected to be taken. The safety analyses were performed on all randomized patients.

RESULTS

Patients and study course. Of the 316 patients screened, 246 were included in the trial (Figure 1). The most frequent reasons for noninclusion were a lack of flare after the NSAID washout period (68.6%) and a failure to achieve a washout of NSAIDs (11.4%).

Table 1 summarizes the patients' characteristics at the start of the trial. All 246 patients were included in the ITT analysis. There was no statistically significant difference in demographic data or clinical variables among the 3 treatment groups at baseline. The main reasons for discontinuation of the study drug were lack of efficacy in 23% of the patients in both active treatment groups and 41% of the patients in the placebo group. Compliance was good: the mean capsule intake was 97.5%, 100%, and 97.4% of the theoretical total in the celecoxib, ketoprofen, and placebo groups, respectively.

Assessment of efficacy. The mean ± SD changes in the global pain variable (VAS) were −13 ± 29 mm in the placebo group and −21 ± 26 mm in the ketoprofen group (P = 0.0512). The mean ± SD changes in the functional impairment variable (BASFI) were 1.3 ± 17.7 in the placebo group and −6.0 ± 20.8 in the ketoprofen group (P = 0.0436) (Table 2). Moreover, the percentage of patients in the placebo group who experienced an improvement in pain of at least 50% during the 6-week study (19.7%) was very close to that expected (20%). In the ketoprofen group, this percentage was 36% (P = 0.0024). The results obtained in the celecoxib group were also significantly different from those observed with placebo treatment (mean changes in pain and functional impairment were −27 ± 30 [P = 0.0068] and −12 ± 22 [P = 0.0006], respectively) (Table 2). The

Table 1. Baseline characteristics of the 246 randomized and treated ankylosing spondylitis patients, by treatment group*

	Treatment group		
Characteristic	Placebo (n = 76)	Ketoprofen 100 mg twice daily (n = 90)	Celecoxib 100 mg twice daily (n = 80)
Age, mean ± SD years	40 ± 11	38 ± 11	38 ± 11
% male	71	67	70
Body mass index, mean ± SD	24.6 ± 4.0	23.4 ± 3.3	24.1 ± 4.0
Disease duration, mean ± SD years	11 ± 9	11 ± 10	11 ± 9
History of peripheral articular disease, %	26.3	30.0	37.5
History of acute anterior uveitis, %	15.8	23.3	28.8
Family history of spondylarthropathy, %	34	31	38
HLA–B27 positive, %	84	89	84

* There were no statistically significant differences between groups for any of these baseline variables.

Table 2. Baseline values and mean changes in clinical and biologic variables during the 6 weeks of the study, by treatment group*

	Baseline†			Changes during the study			
Variable	Placebo (n = 76)	Ketoprofen 100 mg twice daily (n = 90)	Celecoxib 100 mg twice daily (n = 80)	Placebo (n = 76)	Ketoprofen 100 mg twice daily (n = 90)	Celecoxib 100 mg twice daily (n = 80)	*P*‡
Pain							
Global pain, VAS	70 ± 15	66 ± 15	70 ± 16	−13 ± 29	−21 ± 26§	−27 ± 30¶	0.0061
Spinal articular index	8.4 ± 2.7	7.9 ± 2.7	8.9 ± 2.9	−0.79 ± 2.38	−1.57 ± 2.78	−2.32 ± 3.16	0.0076
Function, BASFI	42 ± 25	39 ± 19	47 ± 23	1.3 ± 17.7	−6.0 ± 20.8#	−11.9 ± 22.0**	0.0008
Overall assessment, VAS							
Patient	66 ± 20	60 ± 24	67 ± 20	−8.8 ± 26.0	−16.7 ± 31.0	−24.5 ± 31.3	0.0028
Physician	59 ± 17	57 ± 18	59 ± 17	−5.6 ± 25.8	−16.6 ± 28.2	−18.6 ± 26.7	0.0025
Inflammation							
Night pain, VAS	54 ± 29	53 ± 28	56 ± 32	−0.2 ± 29.3	−16.0 ± 31.7	−17.7 ± 33.9	0.0002
Sleep disturbance, % yes††	67.1	67.8	61.3	59.2	34.4	38.8	0.003
Morning stiffness, minutes	86 ± 127	91 ± 149	83 ± 79	7 ± 128	−27 ± 154	−28 ± 74	NS
CRP, mg/liter	14.1 ± 16.0	14.5 ± 16.6	20.2 ± 28.5	−0.31 ± 9.13	−1.69 ± 8.15	−2.48 ± 11.32	NS
Range of motion							
Modified Schober test, mm	12.8 ± 1.5	12.8 ± 1.3	12.5 ± 1.4	0.16 ± 0.87	0.55 ± 1.07	0.48 ± 1.00	0.0314
Finger-to-floor distance, mm	23.1 ± 15.8	24.4 ± 16.4	27.2 ± 15.3	0.28 ± 9.75	−3.59 ± 12.16	−3.25 ± 9.0	NS
Chest expansion, cm	4.5 ± 2.0	4.8 ± 2.2	4.2 ± 2.1	−0.13 ± 0.99	0.24 ± 1.35	0.27 ± 1.54	NS

* Values are the mean ± SD. VAS = visual analog scale; BASFI = Bath Ankylosing Spondylitis Functional Index; CRP = C-reactive protein.
† There were no statistically significant differences at baseline for any of these variables.
‡ Determined by two-way analysis of covariance and, for the 2 main assessment criteria (pain and functional impairment), by pairwise comparison using the Hochberg procedure. NS = not significant.
§ *P* = 0.0512 versus placebo.
¶ *P* = 0.0068 versus placebo.
# *P* = 0.0436 versus placebo.
** *P* = 0.0006 versus placebo.
†† Score of 3 or 4 on a 1–4 scale.

trend in favor of the celecoxib group when compared with the ketoprofen group did not reach statistical significance for these variables. The ratio of the celecoxib effect to the ketoprofen effect was 1.30 (95% CI 0.98–1.62]) for pain intensity and 1.98 (95% CI 0.80–3.96) for functional impairment. The percentage of patients who experienced an improvement of at least 50% in the celecoxib group (48%) was very close to that expected (50%) and significantly different from placebo (20%) ($P = 0.001$).

The results observed for all of the other clinical variables and CRP levels are summarized in Table 2. All 3 secondary clinical assessments (patient global assessment, night pain, and Schober test) confirmed the efficacy of the active treatments. The remaining efficacy assessments yielded comparable results. The mean ± SD numbers of acetaminophen tablets used daily as analgesic rescue were similar in the celecoxib and ketoprofen groups (1.4 ± 1.6 and 1.3 ± 1.2, respectively) and lower than in the placebo group (1.8 ± 1.6) ($P = 0.09$).

A detailed analysis of the changes in pain and functional impairment over time (Figure 2) showed that the improvement in both the ketoprofen and the celecoxib groups was observed at the first treatment visit (which occurred after 7 days of treatment). The changes in the biologic variables (CRP) showed a trend in favor of the active treatment groups when compared with placebo (Table 2).

Assessment of tolerability. During the study, the incidence of any adverse event was statistically significantly higher in the 2 active treatment groups compared with the placebo group (42%, 60%, and 68% in the placebo, ketoprofen, and celecoxib groups, respectively) ($P = 0.005$). Moreover, the number of patients who had to withdraw from the study because of side effects was greater in the active treatment groups compared with the placebo group (0, 1, and 5 patients in the placebo, ketoprofen, and celecoxib groups, respectively). The patient in the ketoprofen group withdrew after 14 days of therapy because of abdominal symptoms (constipation, abdominal pain, and rectal bleeding). The 5 patients in the celecoxib group withdrew for various reasons, many of which were not considered to be drug related (renal colic in 1 patient, atrial fibrillation in 1, pruritus in 1, abdominal pain in 1, and heartburn in 1).

The adverse events with the highest incidence were upper GI symptoms (epigastric pain, heartburn, nausea, abdominal pain), diarrhea, headache, upper

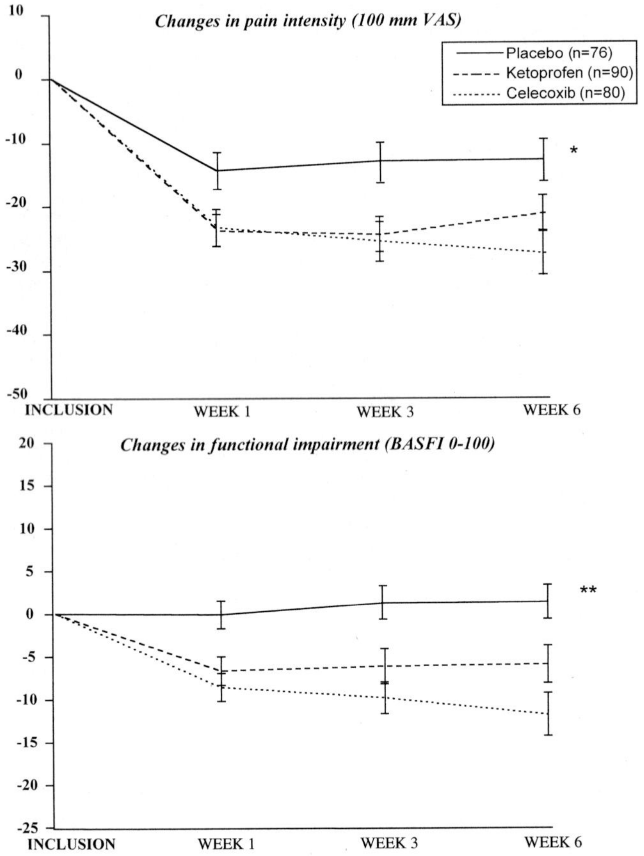

Figure 2. Changes over time in pain as assessed by visual analog scale (VAS) and in functional impairment as assessed by the Bath Ankylosing Spondylitis Functional Index (BASFI), by treatment group. * = $P = 0.0061$ for overall treatment effect on day 42 and $P = 0.0068$ for celecoxib versus placebo on day 42; ** = $P = 0.0008$ for overall treatment effect on day 42, $P = 0.0436$ for ketoprofen versus placebo on day 42, and $P = 0.0006$ for celecoxib versus placebo on day 42 (by two-way analysis of covariance and pairwise comparisons using the Hochberg procedure).

respiratory tract infection, and pruritus (Table 3). Epigastric pain occurred in 6 patients (7.9%), 13 patients (14.4%), and 10 patients (12.5%) in the placebo, ketoprofen, and celecoxib groups, respectively ($P = 0.42$).

One serious adverse event was reported in each active treatment group. In the celecoxib group, 1 patient died following discontinuation of treatment due to lack of efficacy. This event was considered unrelated to the drug. In the ketoprofen group, a gastric ulcer was diagnosed, with endoscopy performed, due to severe epigastric pain after 11 days of treatment.

One patient in the ketoprofen group had a significant decrease in the hemoglobin level, from 12.3 gm/dl to 8.8 gm/dl. There were no clinically significant changes in levels of creatinine or liver function enzymes in any of the 3 groups.

DISCUSSION

This study demonstrated that celecoxib 100 mg twice daily showed similar efficacy and safety to ketoprofen 100 mg twice daily during the 6-week period of treatment of AS; both celecoxib and ketoprofen demonstrated superior efficacy and safety when compared with placebo. The results obtained in the placebo group appear to mimic those observed in previous clinical trials (13–16). In addition, this trial confirmed the lack of placebo effect with the instruments used to evaluate the functional impairment of the patients, contrasting with a more relevant placebo effect in the instruments for evaluating patient global assessment and/or the level of pain (17,18).

In this study, celecoxib was compared with both an inactive control (placebo) and an active control (ketoprofen). Ketoprofen was chosen because of its well-known antiinflammatory effect (19) and because of a pharmacokinetic profile similar to that of celecoxib. A twice-daily dosage (once in the morning and once in the evening) was chosen for both drugs. The choice of the dosage of the active comparator is usually a concern when conducting clinical trials. The dosage of 100 mg twice daily for ketoprofen was considered to be the most appropriate since this is the dosage that is recommended and usually prescribed by rheumatologists in daily practice (20).

The present findings suggest that celecoxib at a daily dosage of 200 mg is sufficient to produce a substantial beneficial effect in 50% of patients with AS. The antiinflammatory effect is usually defined by an improvement in clinical variables that can be assessed by the patient, e.g., nocturnal pain, morning stiffness, general level of pain, and functional improvement. The

Table 3. Adverse events with an overall incidence of ≥5%, by treatment group*

Event	Placebo (n = 76)	Ketoprofen (n = 90)	Celecoxib (n = 80)
Epigastric pain	6 (7.9)	13 (14.4)	10 (12.5)
Diarrhea	1 (1.3)	6 (6.7)	6 (7.5)
Nausea	3 (3.9)	5 (5.6)	4 (5.0)
Heartburn	4 (5.3)	3 (3.3)	3 (3.8)
Abdominal pain	–	2 (2.2)	4 (5.0)
Headache	6 (7.9)	3 (3.3)	6 (7.5)
Bronchitis	–	3 (3.3)	4 (5.0)
Pharyngitis	4 (5.3)	6 (6.7)	1 (1.3)
Pruritus	1 (1.3)	3 (3.3)	4 (5.0)

* Values are the no. (%) of patients.

ability of conventional NSAIDs to provide a beneficial effect on biologic parameters of inflammation is considered to be questionable or marginal. In AS, the CRP level has been found to be correlated with clinical parameters of disease severity (such as decreased chest expansion) and predictive of structural disease progression (21,22). In this study, there was a trend in favor of an NSAID effect on the CRP level, with mean decreases of 0.3, 1.7, and 2.5 mg/liter in the placebo, ketoprofen, and celecoxib groups, respectively (see Table 2).

The beneficial antiinflammatory effect of celecoxib, which can be considered at least comparable with that of conventional NSAIDs, must be analyzed with respect to its safety profile. The evaluation of the safety profile of celecoxib was not the primary objective of the present study. It is important to note that treatment with GI-protective agents was maintained in select patients, in accordance with the study design. Nevertheless, our results confirm the acceptable short-term safety profile of celecoxib. One of the main concerns with the use of NSAIDs is the risk of occurrence of ulcers and their potential clinical complications, i.e., bleeding and perforation. Studies in other diseases have clearly demonstrated a better safety profile of celecoxib when compared with conventional NSAIDs (7–9). In those studies, the incidence of gastroduodenal ulcers in celecoxib-treated patients was similar to that in placebo-treated patients (8) and significantly lower than that observed with diclofenac (9) or naproxen (8). Regarding upper GI effects, the analysis of the present study has limited clinical relevance due to the relatively small sample size compared with the larger-scale trials performed with rheumatoid arthritis and osteoarthritis patients.

The results of this study strongly suggest that celecoxib 200 mg daily may be of benefit for patients with spondylitis with painful axial involvement. However, previous studies have suggested that a 6-week clinical trial is not of sufficient duration to detect the optimal dosage of NSAIDs to be used in AS (16). Therefore, further trials of longer duration and comparing different dosages are necessary to define the optimal dosage of celecoxib in these patients.

REFERENCES

1. Arnett FC. Seronegative spondylarthropathies. Bull Rheum Dis 1987;37:1–12.
2. Dougados M. Diagnostic features of ankylosing spondylitis. Br J Rheumatol 1995;34:301–5.
3. Dougados M. Diagnosis and monitoring of spondylarthropathy. Compr Ther 1990;16:52–6.
4. Toussirot E, Wendling D. Current guidelines for the drug treatment of ankylosing spondylitis. Drugs 1998;56:225–40.
5. Masferrer JL, Seibert K, Zweifel B, Needleman P. Endogenous glucocorticoids regulate an inducible cyclooxygenase enzyme. Proc Natl Acad Sci U S A 1992;89:3917–21.
6. Penning TD, Talley JJ, Bertenshaw SR, Carter JS, Collins PW, Docter S, et al. Synthesis and biological evaluation of the 1,5-diarypyrazole class of cyclooxygenase-2 inhibitors: identification of 4-[5-(4-methylphenyl)-3-(trifluoromethyl)-1H-pyrazol-1-yl] benzenesulfonamide (SC-58635, celecoxib). J Med Chem 1997;40: 1347–65.
7. Bensen WG, Fiechtner JJ, McMillen JI, Zhao WW, Yu SS, Woods EM, et al. Treatment of osteoarthritis with celecoxib, a cyclooxygenase-2 inhibitor: a randomized controlled trial. Mayo Clin Proc 1999;74:1095–105.
8. Simon LS, Weaver AL, Graham DY, Kivitz AJ, Lipsky PE, Hubbard RC, et al. Anti-inflammatory and upper gastrointestinal effects of celecoxib in rheumatoid arthritis: a randomized controlled trial. JAMA 1999;282:1921–8.
9. Emery P, Zeidler H, Kvien TK, Guslandi M, Naudin R, Stead H, et al. Celecoxib versus diclofenac in long-term management of rheumatoid arthritis: randomized double-blind comparison. Lancet 1999;354:2106–11.
10. Van der Linden S, Valkenburg HA, Cats A. Evaluation of diagnostic criteria for ankylosing spondylitis: a proposal for modification of the New York criteria. Arthritis Rheum 1984;27:361–8.
11. Calin A, Garrett S, Whitelock H, Kennedy LG, O'Hea J, Mallorie P, et al. A new approach to defining functional ability in ankylosing spondylitis: the development of the Bath Ankylosing Spondylitis Functional Index. J Rheumatol 1994;21:2281–5.
12. Dougados M. La Mesure: méthodes d'évaluation des affections rhumatismales. Paris: Expansion Scientifique; 1997.
13. Dougados M, Nguyen M, Nakache JP, Amor B. Spondylarthrite ankylosante et anti-inflammatoires. Concours Med 1987;30: 2780–6.
14. Dougados M, Caporal R, Doury P, Thiesce A, Pattin S, Laffez B, et al. A double blind crossover placebo controlled trial of ximoprofen in AS [letter]. J Rheumatol 1989;16:1167–9.
15. Dougados M, Nguyen M, Caporal R, Legeasi J, Bouxin-Sauzet A, Pellegri-Guegnault B, et al. Ximoprofen in ankylosing spondylitis: a double blind placebo controlled dose ranging study. Scand J Rheumatol 1994;23:243–8.
16. Dougados M, Gueguen A, Nakache J-P, Velicitat P, Veys EM, Zeidler H, et al. Ankylosing spondylitis: what is the optimum duration of a clinical study? A one year versus a 6 weeks nonsteroidal antiinflammatory drug trial. Br J Rheumatol 1999; 38:235–44.
17. Van der Heijde D, Bellamy N, Calin A, Dougados M, Khan MA, van der Linden S. Preliminary core sets for endpoints in ankylosing spondylitis. J Rheumatol 1997;24:2225–9.
18. Van der Heijde D, Calin A, Dougados M, Khan MA, van der Linden S, Bellamy N. Selection of instruments in the core set for DC-ART, SMARD, physical therapy, and clinical record keeping in ankylosing spondylitis: progress report of the ASAS Working Group. J Rheumatol 1999;26:951–4.
19. Brogden RN, Speight TM, Avery GS. Ketoprofen: a preliminary report of its pharmacological activity and therapeutic efficacy in rheumatic disorders. Drugs 1974;8:168–75.
20. Kantor TG. Ketoprofen: a review of its pharmacologic and clinical properties. Pharmacotherapy 1986;6:93–103.
21. Dougados M, Gueguen A, Nakache JP, Velicitat P, Zeidler H, Veys EM, et al. Clinical relevance of C-reactive protein in axial involvement of ankylosing spondylitis. J Rheumatol 1999;26: 971–4.
22. Taylor HG, Wardle T, Beswick EJ, Dawes PT. The relationship of clinical and laboratory measurements to radiological change in ankylosing spondylitis. Br J Rheumatol 1991;30:330–5.

ARTHRITIS & RHEUMATISM
Vol. 44, No. 1, January 2001, pp 186–195

Immunomodulatory Effects of Anti–Tumor Necrosis Factor α Therapy on Synovium in Spondylarthropathy

Histologic Findings in Eight Patients from an Open-Label Pilot Study

Dominique Baeten, Elli Kruithof, Filip Van den Bosch, Pieter Demetter, Nancy Van Damme, Claude Cuvelier, Martine De Vos, Herman Mielants, Eric M. Veys, and Filip De Keyser

Objective. **To assess the effects of treatment with anti–tumor necrosis factor α (anti-TNFα) on synovial histology in patients with spondylarthropathy (SpA) in order to confirm the effect on peripheral synovitis and to investigate the immunologic mechanisms involved in anti-TNFα therapy.**

Methods. **Patients with treatment-resistant SpA were treated with infliximab (5 mg/kg) at weeks 0, 2, and 6 in an open-label pilot study. In 8 patients, synovial biopsy tissues obtained at baseline, week 2, and week 12 were used for histologic and immunohistochemical evaluation.**

Results. **In all 8 patients (3 with ankylosing spondylitis, 1 with undifferentiated SpA, and 4 with psoriatic arthritis), there was a clear clinical improvement in the peripheral arthritis after anti-TNFα therapy. Histologic analysis of the synovial biopsy tissues indicated that the synovial lining layer thickness tended to decrease, with a significant reduction of CD55+ synoviocytes, at week 12. In the sublining layer, vascularity was reduced at week 12, with a decreased endothelial expression of vascular cell adhesion molecule 1 but not intercellular adhesion molecule 1, platelet endothelial cell adhesion molecule 1, and E-selectin. Although at week 2 and week 12, the number of neutrophils and CD68+ macrophages in the sublining layer was decreased, the overall degree of inflammatory infiltration remained unchanged. This could be related to the lymphocyte infiltration since at week 12, only CD4+ cells (but not CD3+, CD45RO+, and CD8+ cells) tended to decrease, while CD20+ lymphocytes and plasma cells were clearly increased.**

Conclusion. **The reduction in lining layer thickness, vascularity, and infiltration with neutrophils and macrophages paralleled the beneficial effect of anti-TNFα therapy on peripheral synovitis in 8 patients with different subtypes of SpA. The adhesion molecule expression, T cell infiltration, and, most important, B cell infiltration seemed to contrast with previous observations in RA. Although these preliminary data need to be confirmed in a larger cohort, they suggest distinct immunomodulatory mechanisms of anti-TNFα in SpA.**

Supported by a concerted action grant GOA96001 from the University of Ghent, Ghent, Belgium. Dr. Baeten is an FWO-Vlaanderen Research Assistant.

Dominique Baeten, MD, Elli Kruithof, MD, Filip Van den Bosch, MD, Pieter Demetter, MD, Nancy Van Damme, Claude Cuvelier, MD, PhD, Martine De Vos, MD, PhD, Herman Mielants, MD, PhD, Eric M. Veys, MD, PhD, Filip De Keyser, MD, PhD: Ghent University, Ghent, Belgium.

Address correspondence and reprint requests to Dominique Baeten, MD, Department of Rheumatology, 0K12IB, Ghent University Hospital, De Pintelaan 185, 9000 Ghent, Belgium.

Submitted for publication April 14, 2000; accepted in revised form September 6, 2000.

Tumor necrosis factor α (TNFα), a proinflammatory cytokine produced primarily by monocytes and macrophages, plays a central role in the pathophysiology of rheumatoid arthritis (RA), as suggested by the findings that mice transgenic for human TNFα develop a destructive arthritis (1), that TNFα is present in high concentrations in synovial tissue and synovial fluid of RA patients (2–6), and that blocking of TNFα in vitro interrupts the inflammatory cytokine cascade (7). The beneficial clinical effect of anti-TNFα in animal models of arthritis (8–10) and, most important, in human RA (11,12) provides further evidence that TNFα is a pivotal arthritogenic mediator and, thus, an important therapeutic target in RA. Studies evaluating the effect of anti-TNFα therapy on histologic features of the synovium in RA confirm the clinical improvement in joint inflammation and provide insights into the molecular and cellular mechanisms that are involved (13–16): reduction of synovial neovascularization and circulating levels of vascular endothelial growth factors; deactivation of the synovial endothelium by reduced expression of E-selectin, intercellular adhesion molecule 1 (ICAM-1), and vascular cell adhesion molecule 1 (VCAM-1); and reduction of the inflammatory infiltration of synovial tissue by neutrophils, macrophages, and lymphocytes.

Recent evidence indicates that anti-TNFα therapy could also have a therapeutic effect in the spondylarthropathies (SpA), a group of related, chronic autoimmune diseases of the joint with common clinical, radiologic, and genetic characteristics. The SpA encompass ankylosing spondylitis, reactive arthritis, psoriatic arthritis, inflammatory bowel disease, some forms of juvenile chronic arthritis, and acute anterior uveitis. Findings of several studies indicate an intriguing relationship between SpA and Crohn's disease: 20–30% of the patients with Crohn's disease have articular symptoms compatible with SpA (17), 40–60% of SpA patients have microscopic evidence of inflammation of the gut (18,19), and 6.5% of the SpA patients in a long-term followup study developed full-blown Crohn's disease (20). The relationship between these two diseases coupled with the beneficial effect of anti-TNFα treatment on the concomitant articular symptoms in therapy-resistant Crohn's disease (21) suggest a therapeutic potential for anti-TNFα therapy in SpA (22). The results of a recently performed open-label pilot study of anti-TNFα therapy in patients with SpA strengthen this concept, since treatment with infliximab had a convincing effect both on global disease parameters and on axial and peripheral joint inflammation (23).

The aim of the present study was to evaluate the effects of anti-TNFα treatment on histologic features of the synovium in patients with SpA in order to confirm a potential beneficial effect on peripheral synovitis and to investigate the immunologic mechanisms involved in anti-TNFα therapy.

PATIENTS AND METHODS

Patients. As described previously, 21 patients with SpA, according to the European Spondylarthropathy Study Group criteria (24), were treated in an open-label pilot study with anti-TNFα antibodies (23). All patients had active disease and were treated with intravenous infusions of 5 mg/kg of infliximab at baseline, week 2, and week 6. Synovial histology was performed on 8 of these patients (6 men and 2 women), who had been selected on the basis of active synovitis of the knee. All patients gave their informed consent, as approved by the Ethics Committee of the Ghent University Hospital.

All 8 study patients had active synovitis of the knee at baseline and had been diagnosed as having ankylosing spondylitis (n = 3), undifferentiated SpA (n = 1), or psoriatic arthritis (n = 4). The mean age of the patients was 48.8 years (range 39–58 years), and the mean disease duration was 19 years (range 2–43 years). HLA–B27 was positive in 4 patients, negative in 2 patients, and unknown in the 2 other patients. Treatment with disease-modifying antirheumatic drugs was stopped at least 4 weeks prior to the beginning of the study: 1 patient had been taking sulfasalazine, 3 had been taking methotrexate, and 1 had been taking methotrexate plus cyclosporine. Nonsteroidal antiinflammatory drugs and/or steroids were continued at stable dosages throughout the study: piroxicam in 5 patients (20–30 mg/day), phenylbutazone in 2 patients (200 and 400 mg/day, respectively), nimesulide in 1 patient (100 mg/day), and prednisolone in 2 patients (4 and 6 mg/day, respectively).

Global clinical evaluation of the patients at baseline, week 2, and week 12 included the patient's global assessment of disease activity (by 100-mm visual analog scale [VAS]), patient's assessment of pain (by 100-mm VAS), physician's global assessment of disease activity (by 100-mm VAS), erythrocyte sedimentation rate (ESR), and C-reactive protein (CRP) level. Evaluation of peripheral arthritis included estimations of pain (by 100-mm VAS) and duration of morning stiffness (in minutes) of the peripheral joints as assessed by the patient and counts of tender joints (of 68 joints) and swollen joints (of 66 joints) as assessed by the physician.

Synovial biopsies were performed at baseline (just before the first infusion with infliximab), week 2 (just before the second infusion), and week 12 by needle arthroscopy of the knee, as described previously (25). To provide a representative sample of the synovial membrane pathology that would allow for reliable semiquantitative scoring, 20 synovial biopsy samples (~3 × 3 × 3 mm) were obtained from the suprapatellar pouch and the medial gutter of each patient's affected knee (26,27). To avoid interference of the effect of the arthroscopy with the effect of the treatment on synovial inflammation, joint lavage was minimized (<150 ml of fluid), and no intraarticular steroids were injected.

Ten biopsy samples from each patient were stored in formaldehyde and embedded en bloc in paraffin. Sections (5 μm) were cut and stained with hematoxylin and eosin for histologic analysis. The remaining 10 biopsy samples were snap-frozen and mounted en bloc in Jung tissue freezing medium (Reichert-Jung, Nussloch, Germany). Frozen sections were mounted on Star Frost glass slides (Knittelgläser, Braunschweig, Germany) and used for immunohistochemistry.

Immunohistochemistry. Frozen sections were fixed for 10 minutes in acetone and incubated for 30 minutes with the following mouse monoclonal antibodies: anti-CD3 (clone UCHT-1; Dako, Glostrup, Denmark), anti-CD4 (clone MT310; Dako), anti-CD8 (clone DK25; Dako), anti-CD20 (clone L26; Dako), anti-CD45RO (clone OPD4; Dako), anti-CD55 (clone BRIC216; BioSource, Nivelles, Belgium), anti-

Table 1. Clinical evaluation of the effect of anti–tumor necrosis factor α in 8 spondylarthropathy patients at baseline, week 2, and week 12*

	Baseline	Week 2	Week 12
Patient's assessment of pain (by VAS)	59 (23–100)	27 (4–60)	13.5 (9–86)
Patient's global assessment (by VAS)	59 (45–100)	28 (3–50)	13.5 (7–73)
Physician's global assessment (by VAS)	49.5 (35–79)	22 (5–36)	22.5 (8–75)
Erythrocyte sedimentation rate (mm/h)	47 (17–92)	11.5 (2–30)	7.5 (2–59)
C-reactive protein (mg/dl)	4.8 (3.0–29.0)	0.3 (0.0–1.0)	0.6 (0.0–6.6)
Patient's assessment of pain in the peripheral joints (by VAS)	71.5 (31–99)	27 (1–49)	18 (0–84)
Duration of morning stiffness in the peripheral joints (minutes)	147.5 (10–300)	3.5 (0–150)	7.5 (0–60)
Tender joint score	7.5 (1–18)	1.5 (0–11)	0 (0–2)
Swollen joint score	8.5 (1–12)	2.5 (0–9)	2.5 (0–7)

* Values are the median (range). VAS = visual analog scale.

CD68 (clone PG-M1; Dako), anti–E-selectin (CD62E, clone 1.2B6; Dako), anti–ICAM-1 (CD54, clone 6.5B5; Dako), anti–VCAM-1 (CD106, clone 1.4C3; Dako), anti–platelet endothelial cell adhesion molecule 1 (anti–PECAM-1) (CD31, clone 9G11; R&D Systems, Minneapolis, MN), anti-IgA (clone 6E2C1; Dako), anti-IgD (polyclonal; Dako), anti-IgE (clone CIA-E-7.12; Dako), anti-IgG (clone A57H; Dako), and anti-IgM (clone R1/69; Dako).

Parallel sections were incubated with irrelevant isotype-matched monoclonal antibodies as negative controls. After rinsing, the endogenous peroxidase was blocked with 1% hydrogen peroxide. The sections were subsequently incubated for 15 minutes with a biotinylated anti-mouse secondary antibody, followed by incubation for 15 minutes with a streptavidin–peroxidase complex (LSAB+ kit; Dako). The color reaction was developed using 3-amino-9-ethylcarbazole substrate (Dako) as chromogen. Finally, the sections were counterstained with hematoxylin. All incubations were carried out at room temperature and the sections were washed with phosphate buffered saline between each step.

Microscopic analysis. Stained sections were coded and analyzed by 2 independent observers (DB and PD) who were blinded to the patients' data and time of biopsy sampling (baseline, week 2, or week 12). As previously described, both for histology and immunohistochemistry, 10 biopsy samples were mounted, cut, and stained en bloc. Based on validated semiquantitative scoring methods for synovial tissue (which appear to have sensitivity and reliability comparable to that of manual cell counting and digital image analysis), the analysis included all areas of the 10 biopsy samples, and a global semiquantitative score (0–3 scale, where 0 = lowest expression and 3 = highest expression) was given for each parameter (28–30). Because some histologic markers in synovial tissue are more abundant than others, the scoring system was calibrated separately for each marker by examining a representative number of synovial samples. This implies that a score of, for example, 2 can reflect a different absolute degree of abundance for 2 different markers and, thus, that this method doesn't allow the study of the relative expression of different markers in a single tissue sample. The scores obtained by the 2 observers were concordant for <90% of the samples. In cases of discordant scores, which differed by a maximum of 1 point, the mean of the 2 scores was used.

Histologic evaluation of the paraffin sections included the mean synovial lining layer thickness (0 = 1–2 cell layers, 1 = 3–4 cell layers, 2 = 5–6 cell layers, and 3 = ≥7 cell layers), degree of vascularity of the sublining layer, degree of infiltration of the sublining layer, number of lymphocytes, number of plasma cells, number of neutrophils, and number of lymphoid aggregates. Immunohistochemical evaluation of the synovial lining layer included CD55 (fibroblast-like synoviocytes) and CD68 (macrophage-like synoviocytes); sublining infiltration was assessed using CD3, CD4, CD8, CD20, CD45RO, and CD68. Expression of the adhesion molecules E-selectin, ICAM-1, VCAM-1, and PECAM-1 was scored in the synovial lining layer and endothelium of synovial blood vessels. Plasma cells present in the sublining layer were further characterized by evaluation of intracytoplasmic IgA, IgD, IgE, IgG, and IgM.

Statistical analysis. Scores obtained at week 2 and week 12 were compared with baseline scores using the paired Wilcoxon signed rank test. *P* values less than 0.05 were considered to be statistically significant. Since the analysis of each marker was considered as an individual comparison of paired scores before and after treatment, Bonferroni corrections for multiple comparisons were not applied in this exploratory study.

Table 2. Histologic evaluation of the effect of anti–tumor necrosis factor α in 8 spondylarthropathy patients at baseline, week 2, and week 12*

	Baseline	Week 2	Week 12
Synovial lining layer thickness	1 (1–2)	1 (1–2)	1 (1–1)
Sublining vascularity	2 (1–3)	2 (1–2.5)	1.25 (1–2)†
Degree of inflammatory cell infiltration	1.25 (0–3)	1 (0.5–3)	1 (0–2)
No. of lymphocytes	1.25 (0–3)	1 (0.5–3)	1 (0–2)
No. of plasma cells	0 (0–2.5)	0 (0–2.5)	0.75 (0–3)†
No. of neutrophils	1 (0–2)	0 (0–0)†	0 (0–0.5)†
No. of lymphoid aggregates	0 (0–1)	0 (0–0)	0 (0–0)

* Values are the median (range) of semiquantitative scores on a 0–3 scale.
† $P < 0.05$ versus baseline.

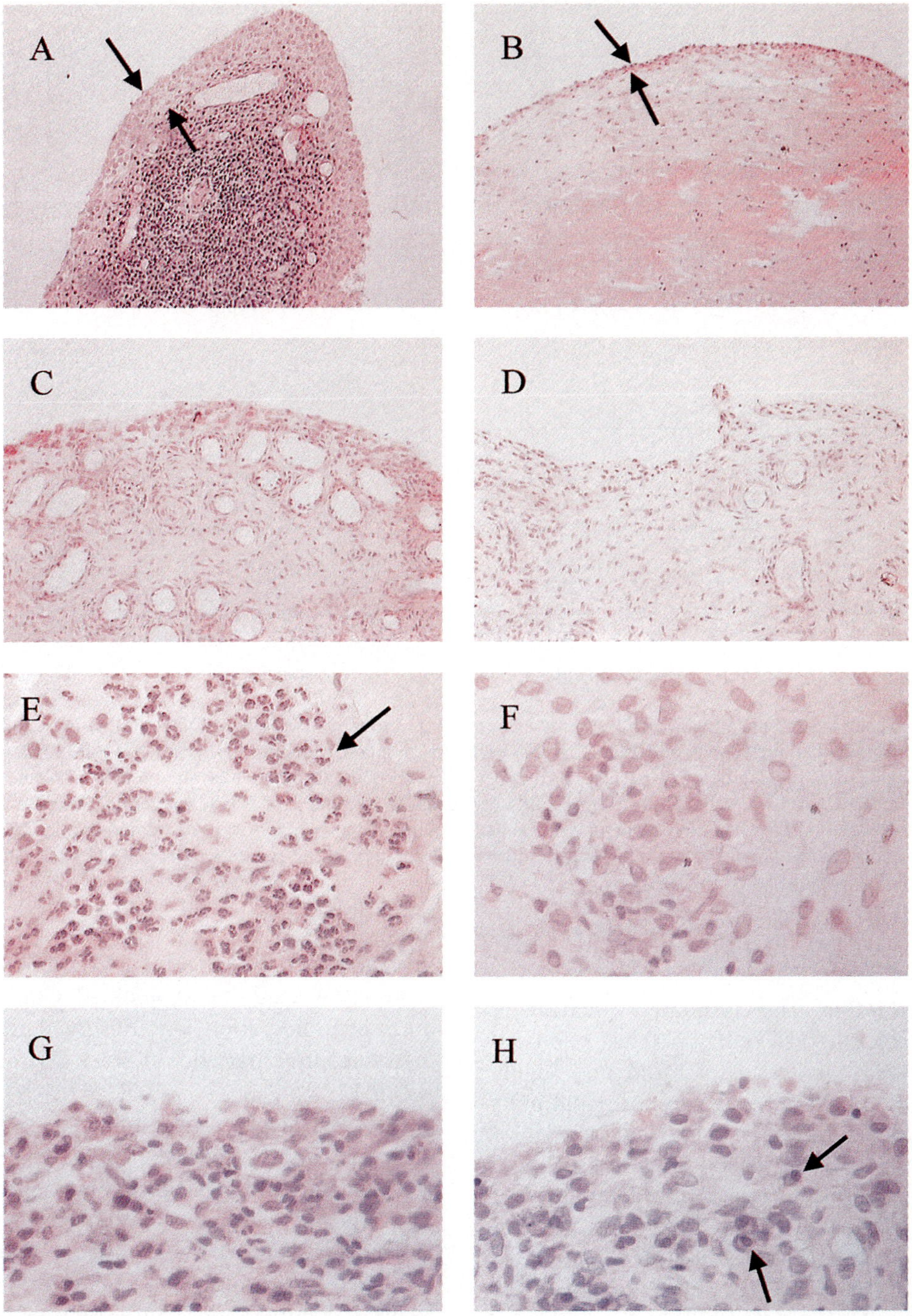

Figure 1. Effect of infliximab treatment (5 mg/kg intravenously at weeks 0, 2, and 6) on histologic features of the synovium in patients with spondylarthropathy. Representative sections from the evaluations done at baseline and at week 12 are shown, and the corresponding semiquantitative scores are indicated. All sections were obtained during clinical synovitis, except for the sections shown in **B** and **H**. The relevant histologic changes (hematoxylin and eosin staining) are as follows: **A,** synovial lining hyperplasia **(arrows)** (score 2) at baseline in patient 3; **B,** synovial lining hyperplasia **(arrows)** (score 1) at week 12 in patient 1; **C,** vascularity (score 2) at baseline in patient 6; **D,** vascularity (score 1) at week 12 in patient 6; **E,** neutrophil infiltration **(arrow)** (score 2) at baseline in patient 7; **F,** neutrophil infiltration (score 0) at week 12 in patient 7; **G,** plasma cell infiltration (score 0) at baseline in patient 3; and **H,** plasma cell infiltration **(arrows)** (score 3) at week 12 in patient 3. (Original magnification × 160 in **A–D**; × 640 in **E–H**.)

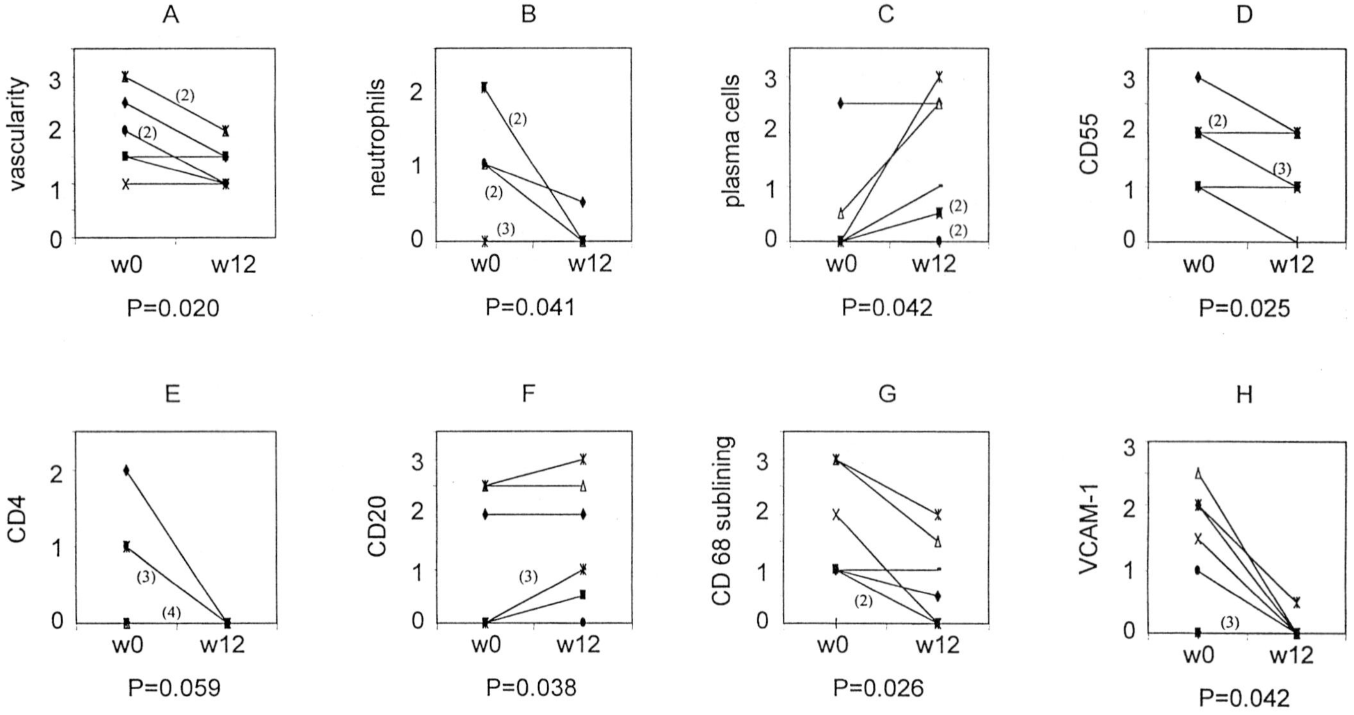

Figure 2. Effect of infliximab treatment (5 mg/kg intravenously at weeks 0, 2, and 6) on synovial histology in 8 patients with spondylarthropathy. Synovial biopsy samples obtained at week 0 (w0) and week 12 (w12) were scored on a semiquantitative scale of 0–3 by 2 independent observers. The evaluated parameters included **A,** the degree of vascularity, **B,** number of neutrophils, **C,** number of plasma cells, **D,** number of CD55+ synovial lining fibroblasts, **E,** number of CD4+ T cells, **F,** number of CD20+ B cells, **G,** number of CD68+ macrophages in the sublining layer, and **H,** vascular cell adhesion molecule 1 (VCAM-1) expression on synovial endothelium. All parameters were decreased at week 12 except for plasma cells and CD20+ B cells, which were increased. Numbers in parentheses indicate the number of patients represented by the data point. *P* values were calculated with the paired Wilcoxon signed rank test.

RESULTS

Clinical evaluation. The complete evaluation of the clinical effect of anti-TNFα in SpA has been reported previously (23), indicating a rapid and highly significant improvement in all parameters for patient's and physician's global assessments and assessment of peripheral arthritis. Both the baseline values and the improvement in the different clinical parameters after therapy were similar in the 8 patients of the present study, who were selected for histologic evaluation of peripheral synovitis, and in the entire group of 21 patients who were initially studied (23).

As indicated in Table 1, there was a clear improvement in all global clinical parameters (patient's assessment of pain, patient's global assessment of disease activity, physician's global assessment of disease activity, ESR, and CRP) at week 2 and at week 12 compared with baseline. A similar improvement in the peripheral arthritis (patient's assessment of pain in the peripheral joints, duration of morning stiffness in peripheral joints, and tender and swollen joint count) was noted at week 2 and at week 12. Clinical synovitis of the biopsied knee joint was observed in all 8 patients at baseline, in 3 patients at week 2, and in 4 patients at week 12.

Histologic evaluation. The histologic scores at baseline, week 2, and week 12 are summarized in Table 2. The thickness of the synovial lining layer was increased (3–5 cell layers compared with 1–2 cell layers in normal synovium) in 3 patients at baseline and had returned to normal (1–2 cell layers) in all patients at week 12 (*P* not significant) (Figures 1A and B). Vascularity, which was evaluated as the number of blood vessels in the sublining, was significantly reduced at week 12 compared with baseline ($P = 0.020$) (Figures 2A and 1C and D).

The overall degree of inflammatory cell infiltration of the sublining layer changed only slightly, whereas the number of neutrophils was reduced at week 2 and week 12 ($P = 0.038$ and $P = 0.041$, respectively) (Figures

Table 3. Immunohistochemical evaluation of the effect of anti–tumor necrosis factor α in 8 spondylarthropathy patients at baseline, week 2, and week 12*

	Baseline	Week 2	Week 12
Lining			
CD55	2 (1–3)	2 (1–3)	1 (0–2)†
CD68	0.5 (0–1)	0 (0–2)	1 (0–2)
Sublining			
CD3	1 (0–2.5)	1.25 (0–3)	1.5 (0–3)
CD45RO	0.5 (0–3)	0 (0–2)	1 (0–3)
CD4	0.5 (0–2)	0 (0–1)	0 (0–0)
CD8	1 (1–3)	1 (0–3)	1 (0–3)
CD20	0 (0–2.5)	0 (0–3)	1 (0–3)†
CD68	1 (0–3)	0 (0–2)†	0.25 (0–2)†
Endothelium			
E-selectin	0 (0–1)	0 (0–0)	0 (0–0)
ICAM-1	1 (1–2)	1 (0.5–2.5)	1.25 (1–2)
VCAM-1	1.25 (0–2.5)	0 (0–1)†	0 (0–0.5)†
PECAM-1	3 (2–3)	2.75 (2–3)	2.75 (2–3)

* Values are the median (range) of semiquantitative scores on a 0–3 scale. ICAM-1 = intercellular adhesion molecule 1; VCAM-1 = vascular cell adhesion molecule 1; PECAM-1 = platelet endothelial cell adhesion molecule 1.
† $P < 0.05$ versus baseline.

2B and 1E and F), and the number of lymphocytes tended to be decreased at week 12 (*P* not significant). In contrast, the number of plasma cells was significantly increased at week 12 ($P = 0.042$) (Figures 2C and 1G and H). This plasma cell infiltration was diffuse, without the formation of focal plasma cell aggregates. Lymphoid aggregates were seen in only 1 patient at baseline and in none of the patients at week 2 and week 12.

Immunohistochemical evaluation. The semiquantitative scores for the immunohistochemical evaluation are summarized in Table 3. In the synovial lining layer, the number of CD55+ type B synoviocytes, but not CD68+ type A synoviocytes, was reduced at week 12 ($P = 0.025$) (Figures 2D and 3A and B). In the sublining, the number of lymphocytes positive for CD3, CD45RO, and CD8 changed just slightly; only the number of CD4+ cells, which was already low at baseline, tended to diminish (*P* not significant) (Figure 2E). In contrast, CD20+ B cells increased at week 12 ($P = 0.038$) (Figure 2F); both at baseline and after therapy, B cells were present in foci around small blood vessels (Figures 3C and D). The number of CD68+ macrophages in the sublining layer was significantly decreased at both week 2 and week 12 ($P = 0.020$ and $P = 0.026$, respectively) (Figures 2G and 3E and F).

The expression of VCAM-1, but not E-selectin, ICAM-1, and PECAM-1, on the endothelium of synovial blood vessels and in the synovial lining layer was significantly reduced at week 2 and week 12 ($P = 0.042$ for both time points) (Figures 2H and 3G and H). It should be noted, however, that the expression of E-selectin was already minimal at baseline.

Immunohistochemical staining of Ig types indicated that the plasma cells present at week 12 were mainly IgG, while at baseline, intracellular IgG was nearly absent (Figures 3I and J); IgM+ cells were detected at a lower frequency, while IgD and IgE were only occasionally observed. Staining for IgA was negative.

DISCUSSION

Serial histologic evaluation of synovial tissue has previously been explored and validated in a number of trials evaluating anti-TNFα therapy (13–15), as well as other therapies (31–34), in RA. This approach turned out to be a powerful tool not only for confirming clinical effects on peripheral synovitis, but also for providing insights into the local immunomodulatory effects of the evaluated drug.

Our recent open-label study of infliximab (5 mg/kg intravenously at weeks 0, 2, and 6) was designed to evaluate the safety and the therapeutic potential of anti-TNFα therapy in SpA (23). The fact that anti-TNFα therapy has well-described immunomodulatory effects on synovial histologic features in RA (13,15) prompted us to include histologic evaluation of peripheral synovitis in this pilot study in SpA. Serial synovial biopsy samples (at baseline, week 2, and week 12) were obtained in 8 of the 21 patients of the original study (23); these 8 patients were selected on the basis of manifest clinical synovitis of the knee joint at baseline, since local disease activity has an important impact on synovial histologic features (28,35). As expected from previously reported data (23,36), anti-TNFα treatment induced a major clinical response, with a rapid improvement in both global and peripheral parameters of disease in these 8 patients, independently of the SpA subtype.

Histologic and immunohistochemical data at baseline were comparable with previous data on synovial histology and immunohistology in SpA (28). Likewise, there were no apparent differences between the SpA subgroups except for the presence of neutrophils, which were present in all 4 of the psoriatic arthritis patients but in only 1 of the other 4 SpA patients (28). Evaluation at week 2 showed a significant decrease in VCAM-1 expression on the synovial endothelium and of neutrophil and macrophage infiltration of the sublining layer, which was maintained throughout the study. This correlates well with previous observations in RA (13–15) and

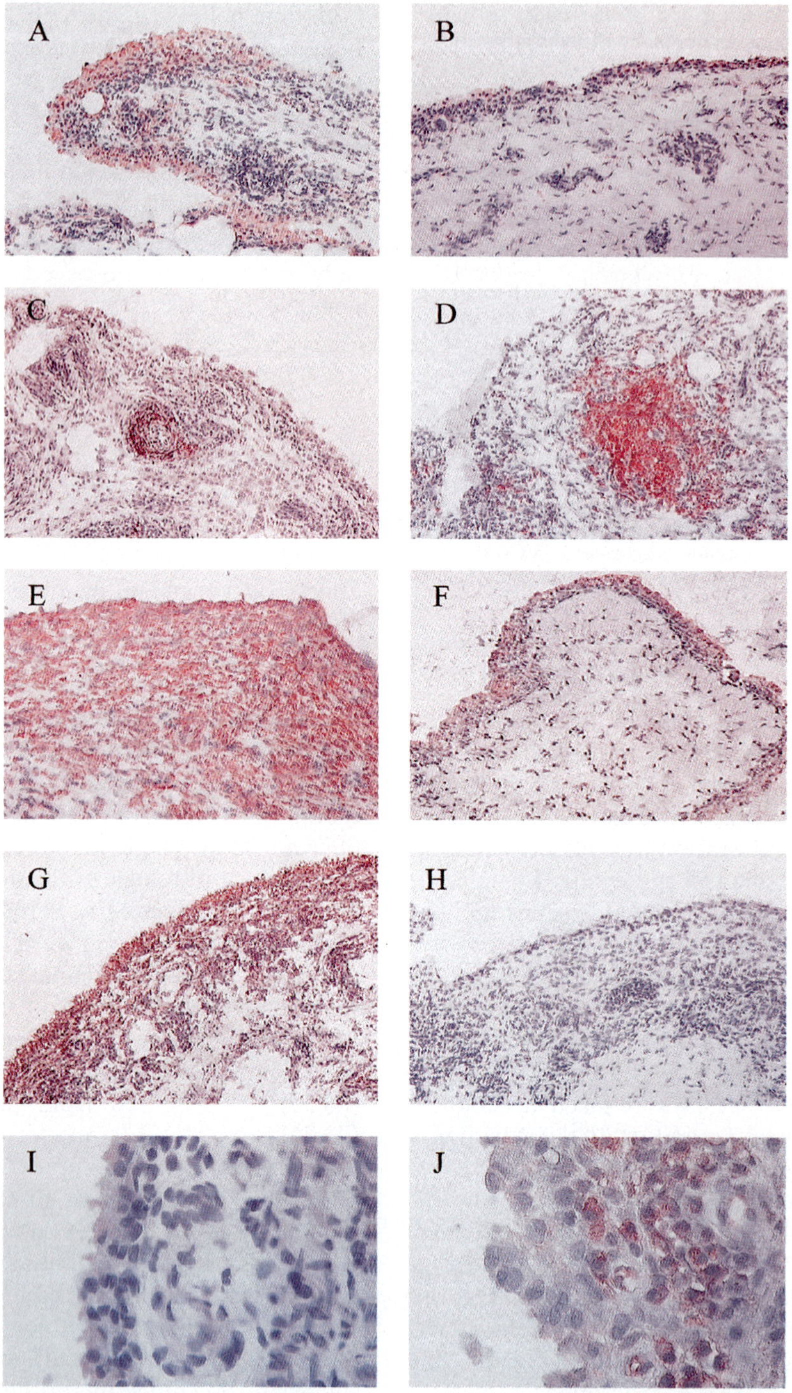

Figure 3. Effect of infliximab treatment (5 mg/kg intravenously at weeks 0, 2, and 6) on histologic features of the synovium in patients with spondylarthropathy. Representative sections from the evaluations done at baseline and at week 12 are shown, and the corresponding semiquantitative scores are indicated. All sections were obtained during clinical synovitis, except for the section shown in **J**. The relevant immunohistochemical changes (peroxidase staining) are as follows: **A,** CD55+ type B synoviocytes (score 2) at baseline in patient 3; **B,** CD55+ type B synoviocytes (score 1) at week 12 in patient 7; **C,** CD20+ B cells (score 2) at baseline in patient 1; **D,** CD20+ B cells (score 3) at week 12 in patient 1; **E,** CD68+ sublining macrophages (score 2) at baseline in patient 1; **F,** CD68+ sublining macrophages (score 0) at week 12 in patient 7; **G,** vascular cell adhesion molecule 1 (VCAM-1) expression (score 2) at baseline in patient 3; **H,** VCAM-1 expression (score 0) at week 12 in patient 1; **I,** absence of IgG+ plasma cells at baseline in patient 2; **J,** abundant intracellular IgG in plasma cells at week 12 in patient 2. (Original magnification × 160 in **A–F**; × 640 in **G–J**.)

suggests that one of the primary effects of anti-TNFα therapy is deactivation of the endothelium, which thereby reduces the migration and homing of inflammatory cells into the synovial tissue. Moreover, at week 12 there was a significant decrease in the vascularity of the synovium. This effect has also been observed in RA and could be related to a decrease in growth factors, such as vascular endothelial growth factor (16). Independently of the underlying mechanism, reduction of vascularity seems particularly relevant in SpA, since hypervascularity is one of the hallmarks of synovial inflammation in this disease (28,37,38).

Anti-TNFα treatment also had an effect on synovial hyperplasia. The thickness of the synovial lining was normalized at week 12. This effect is likely to be mediated by a reduction of TNF-induced proliferation and/or a restoration of Fas-mediated apoptotic cell death of synovial fibroblasts (39), since the number of CD55+ synovial lining fibroblasts was significantly reduced at week 12. It should be noted, however, that selective staining of synovial intimal fibroblasts remains difficult and that this possible effect should be confirmed by other methods. Alternatively, a decreased influx of macrophage-like synoviocytes could contribute to the reduction of hyperplasia, but in contrast to the sublining macrophages, the number of CD68+ cells in the synovial lining layer was not reduced in the present study. Preliminary stainings with the proliferation markers Ki-67 and proliferating cell nuclear antigen also did not show a significant reduction of proliferation in the lining layer (data not shown). However, these data should certainly be confirmed and extended in a larger number of patients before definite conclusions can be made about the mechanisms involved in the reduction of the synovial lining hyperplasia.

In summary, the deactivation of the endothelium, the reduced infiltration with neutrophils and macrophages, the decrease in vascularity, and the abrogation of lining hyperplasia found in the present study are concordant with previous observations in RA and parallel the beneficial effects of anti-TNFα therapy on synovial inflammation in SpA. Because of the relatively small number of patients and the fact that all patients responded well to the therapy, it was not possible to analyze correlations between single histologic parameters and clinical improvement.

Surprisingly, a number of histologic changes after anti-TNFα therapy in these SpA patients were clearly different from those observed in RA patients. Whereas the different lymphocyte subsets were reported to decrease after treatment in RA patients (13–16), only the CD4+ T lymphocyte subset tended to decrease in SpA patients. The fact that this decrease did not reach statistical significance could be related to the relatively low numbers of CD4+ cells at baseline. In contrast to the CD4+ T lymphocytes, the numbers of CD3+, CD45RO+, and CD8+ cells showed no trend toward diminution, but remained unchanged. Moreover, the numbers of CD20+ B cells and, even more clearly, plasma cells were significantly increased at week 12. The particularity of the increase of B cells and plasma cells is stressed by the fact that these cells are generally scarce in SpA synovium compared with RA synovium (28,29,40).

The plasma cells are probably polyclonal, as suggested by the production of different immunoglobulin isotypes, and seem not to be directly related to autoantibody production. All patients remained rheumatoid factor negative throughout the study, while 2 of the 8 patients became positive for antinuclear factor and anti-DNA antibodies. Those 2 patients, however, had no manifest increase in plasma cells in the synovial membrane and had no clinical symptoms of lupus. Further studies are needed to clarify the origin and reactivity (antigen-specific or not) of these plasma cells.

Possible explanations for the distinct immunomodulatory effect of anti-TNFα on specific lymphocyte subsets in SpA should consider at least two characteristics. First, anti-TNFα treatment is more likely to induce specific migration and homing of B cells into SpA synovial membrane, rather than local B cell proliferation, since B cells were absent in synovial samples from 5 of the 8 patients at baseline. A number of mediators of B cell migration, including adhesion molecules, such as VCAM-1, ICAM-1, and E-selectin (41,42), and specific chemokines and chemokine receptors (43–46), could be influenced by anti-TNFα treatment (13–15). Although there are no data on the expression of B cell–specific chemokines in the synovium, the present study provides preliminary arguments for a differential effect of anti-TNFα on the expression of ICAM-1 and E-selectin in SpA versus RA. Second, after homing to the synovial membrane, a large number of B cells seem to differentiate into IgG+ and IgM+ plasma cells. Since TNF has been reported to inhibit the differentiation of B cells through an effect on T helper cells (47,48), anti-TNFα therapy could possibly reverse this inhibition and lead to restored plasma cell maturation.

In conclusion, the present data confirm the impact of anti-TNFα therapy on peripheral synovitis in SpA and reveal immunomodulatory mechanisms involving adhesion molecule expression and lymphocyte infiltration that could be different from those observed previously in RA. Considering the few therapeutic alternatives in severe SpA, our findings warrant further evaluation of the clinical efficacy and the immunologic mechanisms of anti-TNFα in the treatment of SpA.

ACKNOWLEDGMENTS

We wish to thank Jenny Vermeersch and Annemie Herssens for their excellent technical contributions to this study.

REFERENCES

1. Keffer J, Probert L, Cazlaris H, Georgopoulos S, Kaslaris E, Kioussis D, et al. Transgenic mice expressing human tumor necrosis factor: a predictive genetic model of arthritis. EMBO J 1991;10:4025–31.
2. Husby G, Williams RC Jr. Synovial localization of tumor necrosis factor in patients with rheumatoid arthritis. J Autoimmun 1988;1: 363–71.
3. Feldmann M, Brennan FM, Maini RN. Role of cytokines in rheumatoid arthritis. Annu Rev Immunol 1996;14:397–440.
4. Chu CQ, Field M, Feldmann M, Maini RN. Localization of tumor necrosis factor α in synovial tissues and at the cartilage–pannus junction in patients with rheumatoid arthritis. Arthritis Rheum 1991;34:1125–32.
5. Tetta C, Camussi G, Modena V, Di Vittorio C, Baglioni C. Tumour necrosis factor in serum and synovial fluid of patients with active and severe rheumatoid arthritis. Ann Rheum Dis 1990;49: 665–7.
6. Saxne T, Palladino MA Jr, Heinegård D, Talal N, Wollheim FA. Detection of tumor necrosis factor α but not tumor necrosis factor β in rheumatoid arthritis synovial fluid and serum. Arthritis Rheum 1988;31:1041–5.
7. Brennan FM, Chantry D, Jackson A, Maini R, Feldmann M. Inhibitory effect of TNF α antibodies on synovial cell interleukin-1 production in rheumatoid arthritis. Lancet 1989;2:244–7.
8. Williams RO, Feldmann M, Maini R. Anti-tumor necrosis factor ameliorates joint disease in murine collagen-induced arthritis. Proc Natl Acad Sci U S A 1992;89:9784–8.
9. Piguet PF, Grau GE, Vesin C, Loetscher H, Gentz R, Lesslauer W. Evolution of collagen arthritis in mice is arrested by treatment with anti-tumor necrosis factor (TNF) antibody or a recombinant soluble TNF receptor. Immunology 1992;77:510–4.
10. Kuiper S, Joosten LA, Bendele AM, Edwards CK, Arntz OJ, Helsen MM, et al. Different roles of tumour necrosis factor alpha and interleukin 1 in murine streptococcal cell wall arthritis. Cytokine 1998;10:690–702.
11. Elliott MJ, Maini RN, Feldmann M, Long-Fox A, Charles P, Katsikis P, et al. Treatment of rheumatoid arthritis with chimeric monoclonal antibodies to tumor necrosis factor α. Arthritis Rheum 1993;36:1681–90.
12. Elliott MJ, Maini RN, Feldmann M, Kalden JR, Antoni C, Smolen J, et al. Randomised double blind comparison of a chimaeric monoclonal antibody to tumour necrosis factor α (cA2) versus placebo in rheumatoid arthritis. Lancet 1994;344:1105–10.
13. Tak PP, Taylor PC, Breedveld FC, Smeets TJM, Daha MR, Kluin PM, et al. Decrease in cellularity and expression of adhesion molecules by anti–tumor necrosis factor α monoclonal antibody treatment in patients with rheumatoid arthritis. Arthritis Rheum 1996;39:1077–81.
14. Paleolog EM, Hunt M, Elliott MJ, Feldmann M, Maini RN, Woody JN. Deactivation of vascular endothelium by monoclonal anti–tumor necrosis factor α antibody in rheumatoid arthritis. Arthritis Rheum 1996;39:1082–91.
15. Taylor PC, Peters AM, Paleolog E, Chapman PT, Elliott MJ, McCloskey R, et al. Reduction of chemokine levels and leukocyte traffic to joints by tumor necrosis factor α blockade in patients with rheumatoid arthritis. Arthritis Rheum 2000;43:38–47.
16. Maini RN, Taylor PC, Paleolog E, Charles P, Ballara S, Brennan FM, et al. Anti-tumour necrosis factor specific antibody (infliximab) treatment provides insights into the pathophysiology of rheumatoid arthritis. Ann Rheum Dis 1999;58 Suppl 1:156–60.
17. De Vlam K, De Vos M, Vandekerckhove K, Mielants H, Cesmeli E, De Keyser F, et al. Prevalence of clinical and subclinical spondyloarthropathy in patients with inflammatory bowel disease [abstract]. Arthritis Rheum 1998;41 Suppl 9:S113.
18. De Keyser F, Elewaut D, De Vos M, De Vlam K, Cuvelier C, Mielants H, et al. Bowel inflammation and the spondyloarthropathies. Rheum Dis Clin North Am 1998;24:785–813.
19. Mielants H, Veys EM, Goemaere S, Goethals K, Cuvelier C, De Vos M. Gut inflammation in the spondyloarthropathies: clinical, radiologic, biologic and genetic features in relation to the type of histology. A prospective study. J Rheumatol 1991;18:1542–51.
20. De Vos M, Mielants H, Cuvelier C, Elewaut A, Veys E. Long term evolution of gut inflammation in patients with spondyloarthropathy. Gastroenterology 1996;110:1696–1703.
21. Van den Bosch F, Kruithof E, De Vos M, De Keyser F, Veys EM, Mielants H. Crohn's disease associated with spondyloarthropathy: effect of TNF-α blockade (infliximab) on the articular symptoms. Lancet. In press.
22. De Keyser F, Van Damme N, De Vos M, Mielants H, Veys EM. Opportunities for immune modulation in the spondyloarthropathies with special reference to gut inflammation. Inflamm Res 2000;49:47–54.
23. Van den Bosch F, Kruithof E, Baeten D, De Keyser F, Mielants H, Veys EM. Effects of a loading dose regimen of 3 infusions of chimeric monoclonal antibody to tumor necrosis factor α (infliximab) in spondyloarthropathy: an open pilot study. Ann Rheum Dis 2000;59:428–33.
24. Dougados M, van der Linden S, Juhlin R, Huitfeldt B, Amor B, Calin A, et al. The European Spondylarthropathy Study Group preliminary criteria for the classification of spondylarthropathy. Arthritis Rheum 1991;34:1218–27.
25. Baeten D, Van Den Bosch F, Elewaut D, Stuer A, Veys EM, De Keyser F. Needle arthroscopy of the knee with synovial biopsy sampling: technical experience in 150 patients. Clin Rheumatol 1999;18:434–41.
26. Kirkham B, Portek I, Soon Lee C, Stavros B, Lenarczyk A, Lassere M, et al. Intraarticular variability of synovial membrane histology, immunohistology and cytokine mRNA expression in patients with rheumatoid arthritis. J Rheumatol 1999;26:777–84.
27. Dolhain RJEM, Ter Haar NT, De Kuiper R, Nieuwenhuis IG, Zwinderman AH, Breedveld FC, et al. Distribution of T cells and signs of T-cell activation in the rheumatoid joint: implications for semiquantitative comparative histology. Br J Rheumatol 1998;37: 324–30.
28. Baeten D, Demetter P, Cuvelier C, Van den Bosch F, Kruithof E, Van Damme N, et al. A comparative study of the synovial histology in rheumatoid arthritis, spondyloarthropathy and osteoarthritis: influence of disease duration and activity. Ann Rheum Dis. In press.
29. Smeets TJM, Dolhain RJEM, Breedveld FC, Tak PP. Analysis of the cellular infiltrates and expression of cytokines in synovial tissue from patients with rheumatoid arthritis and reactive arthritis. J Pathol 1998;186:75–81.
30. Kraan MC, Haringman JJ, Ahern MJ, Breedveld FC, Smith MD, Tak PP. Quantification of the cell infiltrate in synovial tissue by digital image analysis. Rheumatology (Oxford) 2000;40:43–9.
31. Tak PP, van der Lubbe PA, Cauli A, Daha MR, Smeets TJM,

Kluin PM, et al. Reduction of synovial inflammation after anti-CD4 monoclonal antibody treatment in early rheumatoid arthritis. Arthritis Rheum 1995;38:1457–65.
32. Veale DJ, Reece RJ, Parsons W, Radjenovic A, O'Connor PJ, Orgles CS, et al. Intra-articular primatised anti-CD4: efficacy in resistant rheumatoid knees: a study of combined arthroscopy, magnetic resonance imaging, and histology. Ann Rheum Dis 1999;58:342–9.
33. Youssef PP, Haynes DR, Triantafillou S, Parker A, Gamble JR, Roberts-Thomson PJ, et al. Effects of pulse methylprednisolone on inflammatory mediators in peripheral blood, synovial fluid, and synovial membrane in rheumatoid arthritis. Arthritis Rheum 1997; 40:1400–8.
34. Smeets TJM, Dayer JM, Kraan MC, Versendaal J, Chicheportiche R, Breedveld FC, et al. The effects of interferon-β treatment on synovial inflammation and expression of metalloproteinases in patients with rheumatoid arthritis. Arthritis Rheum 2000;43: 270–4.
35. Tak PP, Smeets TJM, Daha MR, Kluin PM, Meijers KAE, Brand R, et al. Analysis of the synovial cell infiltrate in early rheumatoid synovial tissue in relation to local disease activity. Arthritis Rheum 1997;40:217–25.
36. Brandt J, Haibel H, Cornely D, Golder W, Gonzalez J, Reddig J, et al. Successful treatment of active ankylosing spondylitis with the anti–tumor necrosis factor α monoclonal antibody infliximab. Arthritis Rheum 2000;43:1346–52.
37. Veale D, Yanni G, Rogers S, Barnes L, Bresnihan B, FitzGerald O. Reduced synovial membrane macrophage numbers, ELAM-1 expression, and lining layer hyperplasia in psoriatic arthritis as compared with rheumatoid arthritis. Arthritis Rheum 1993;36: 893–900.
38. Fearon U, Reece R, Smith J, Emery P, Veale DJ. Synovial cytokine and growth factor regulation of MMPs/TIMPs: implications for erosions and angiogenesis in early rheumatoid and psoriatic arthritis patients. Ann N Y Acad Sci 1999;878:619–21.
39. Ohshima S, Mima T, Sasai M, Nishioka K, Shimizu M, Murata N, et al. Tumour necrosis factor α (TNF-α) interferes with Fas-mediated apoptotic cell death on rheumatoid arthritis (RA) synovial cells: a possible mechanism of rheumatoid synovial hyperplasia and a clinical benefit of anti-TNF-α therapy for RA. Cytokine 2000;12:281–8.
40. Kraan MC, Haringman JJ, Post WJ, Versendaal J, Breedveld FC, Tak PP. Immunohistological analysis of synovial tissue for differential diagnosis in early arthritis. Rheumatology (Oxford) 1999;38: 1074–80.
41. Yago T, Tsukuda M, Tajima H, Nishi T, Kurata-Miura K, Ohkubo J, et al. Analysis of initial attachment of B cells to endothelial cells under flow conditions. J Immunol 1997;158:707–14.
42. Montoya MC, Holtmann K, Snapp KR, Borges E, Sanchez-Madrid F, Luscinkas FW, et al. Memory B lymphocytes from secondary lymphoid organs interact with E-selectin through a novel glycoprotein ligand. J Clin Invest 1999;103:1317–27.
43. Warnock RA, Campbell JJ, Dorf ME, Matsuzawa A, McEvoy LM, Butcher EC. The role of chemokines in the microenvironmental control of T versus B cell arrest in Peyer's patch high endothelial venules. J Exp Med 2000;191:77–88.
44. Bleul CC, Schultze JL, Springer TA. B lymphocyte chemotaxis regulated in association with microanatomic localization, differentiation state, and B cell receptor engagement. J Exp Med 1998; 187:753–62.
45. Legler DF, Loetscher M, Roos RS, Clark-Lewis I, Baggiolini M, Moser B. B cell-attracting chemokine 1, a human CXC chemokine expressed in lymphoid tissues, selectively attracts B lymphocytes via BLR1/CXCR5. J Exp Med 1998;187:655–60.
46. Forster R, Mattis AE, Kremmer E, Wolf E, Brem G, Lipp M. A putative chemokine receptor, BLR1, directs B cell migration to defined lymphoid organs and specific anatomic compartments of the spleen. Cell 1996;87:1037–47.
47. Kashiwa H, Wright SC, Bonavida B. Regulation of B cell maturation and differentiation: suppression of pokeweed mitogen-induced B cell differentiation by tumor necrosis factor (TNF). J Immunol 1987;138:1383–90.
48. Banchereau J, Briere F, Liu YJ, Rousset F. Molecular control of B lymphocyte growth and maturation. Stem Cells 1994;12:278–88.

ARTHRITIS & RHEUMATISM
Vol. 44, No. 1, January 2001, pp 196–201

A Functional Polymorphic Variant in the Interleukin-6 Gene Promoter Associated with Low Bone Resorption in Postmenopausal Women

S. L. Ferrari,[1] P. Garnero,[2] S. Emond,[1] H. Montgomery,[3] S. E. Humphries,[3] and S. L. Greenspan[4]

Objective. **To examine functional interleukin-6 (IL-6) −174 G→C allelic variants in relation to bone turnover and bone mineral density (BMD) in postmenopausal women.**

Methods. **Four hundred thirty-four healthy women living in the community (mean ± SD age 71.7 ± 5.7 years) were genotyped for the IL-6 −174 G→C polymorphism. Serum levels of C-telopeptide of type I collagen (CTx), a marker of bone resorption, and osteocalcin (OC), a marker of bone formation, were determined. BMD at the hip and forearm was measured by dual-energy x-ray absorptiometry.**

Results. **CTx levels differed significantly (P = 0.006) among IL-6 genotypes (mean ± SEM 0.275 ± 0.02 ng/ml, 0.325 ± 0.01 ng/ml, and 0.356 ± 0.02 ng/ml in women with the CC genotype [n = 68], the GC genotype [n = 204], and the GG genotype [n = 162], respectively). Compared with the GG group, age-adjusted odds ratios for high bone resorption were 0.65 (95% confidence interval [95% CI] 0.41–1.0, P = 0.06) and 0.37 (95% CI 0.18–0.73, P = 0.0047) in GC and CC subjects, respectively. In contrast, OC levels did not differ by genotype. BMD at the hip and forearm was 1.5–5% higher in CC subjects compared with GG subjects (P not significant). When the cohort was divided according to the median age (70.5 years), BMD was significantly decreased in older compared with younger postmenopausal women with the GG and GC genotypes (−9.6% on average; $P < 0.01$), but not in those with the CC genotype (−5.1% on average; P not significant).**

Conclusion. **Compared with the GC and GG IL-6 −174 G→C genotypes, the CC genotype is associated with lower bone resorption and lesser decrease in bone mass in older postmenopausal women. These results suggest that IL-6 −174 G→C alleles may be significant determinants of the risk for osteoporosis in elderly subjects.**

Primary osteoporosis is a major public health problem, particularly for women, who have a 40–50% lifetime risk of osteoporotic fractures (1–3). Moreover, systemic inflammatory disorders, such as rheumatoid arthritis, and long-term treatment with corticosteroids are frequently complicated by secondary osteoporosis (4,5). The occurrence of osteoporosis—defined as a bone mineral density (BMD) that is at least 2.5 standard deviations below the mean value in young adults (3)—depends on both the peak bone mass and the rate of bone loss. BMD can be easily and accurately assessed noninvasively by dual-energy x-ray absorptiometry (DXA) (3). In addition, specific and sensitive biochemical markers reflecting the overall rate of bone formation (such as osteocalcin [OC]) and resorption (such as serum C-telopeptide of type I collagen [CTx]) have improved the noninvasive assessment of bone turnover (6,7). However, DXA or biochemical markers of bone turnover, alone or in combination, are of limited value in predicting the long-term rate of bone loss or response to treatment in the individual patient (8–10).

Supported by grants from the NIH (R01-AG-13069) and the Harvard Thorndike General Clinical Research Center (M01-RR-01032). Drs. Montomery and Humphries' work was supported by the British Heart Foundation (RG95007 and SP96003).

[1]S. L. Ferrari, MD, S. Emond, BA: Beth Israel Deaconess Medical Center and Harvard Medical School, Boston, Massachusetts; [2]P. Garnero, PhD: Hôpital E. Herriot and Synarc, Lyon, France; [3]H. Montgomery, MD, S. E. Humphries, FRCPath, MRCP: Rayne Institute, Royal Free and University College, London Medical School, London, UK; [4]S. L. Greenspan, MD: Beth Israel Deaconess Medical Center and Harvard Medical School, Boston, Massachusetts, and University of Pittsburgh Medical Center, Pittsburgh, Pennsylvania.

Address correspondence and reprint requests to S. L. Ferrari, MD, Division of Bone and Mineral Metabolism, Beth Israel Deaconess Medical Center, 330 Brookline Avenue (HIM 944), Boston, MA 02215.

Submitted for publication May 24, 2000; accepted in revised form August 21, 2000.

Because both peak bone mass and age-related bone loss are under multiple environmental and genetic influences (11), attention has recently turned toward identifying polymorphic gene markers for osteoporosis (12,13). Identification of one or a few gene(s) associated with BMD, and particularly bone turnover, could greatly improve the evaluation and treatment of patients who are at increased risk of osteoporotic fractures. Among the multiple candidate genes investigated (13), vitamin D receptor, estrogen receptor, and type I collagen alleles have all shown some association with BMD and/or bone loss (12–16), but results have been inconsistent (17–19). One of the limitations pertinent to these candidate genes is the lack of demonstrated allele-mediated differences in gene and/or protein function.

The hallmark of osteoporosis is a reduction in skeletal mass caused by an imbalance between bone resorption and bone formation. Loss of gonadal function is the most important factor contributing to high bone resorption, and its effects appear to be dependent partly on increasing production of interleukin-6 (IL-6) by bone cells (20,21). Moreover, preliminary data from the European Vertebral Osteoporosis Study suggest that serum IL-6 concentrations predict femoral bone loss in postmenopausal women (22). Recently, a novel, functional G→C polymorphism at position −174 in the IL-6 gene promoter has been described (23). The in vitro transcriptional activity of the IL-6 −174 C allele was markedly lower compared with that of the G allele, and circulating IL-6 levels in healthy CC subjects were significantly lower than those in subjects with the other IL-6 genotypes (23). Moreover, the prevalence of the CC genotype was significantly lower than expected among patients with juvenile chronic arthritis (23), a disorder characterized by elevated IL-6 concentrations in the serum and synovial fluid of inflamed joints (24). These observations prompted us to investigate the relationship between the IL-6 −174 G→C allelic polymorphism, bone turnover, and BMD in a cohort of postmenopausal women.

PATIENTS AND METHODS

Subjects and bone mineral densitometry. Five hundred seventy healthy, ambulatory women living in the community (>94% Caucasians, the others being African Americans, Asians, and Asian Indians) over the age of 65 years were recruited from the greater Boston area to participate in a clinical trial on the prevention and treatment of postmenopausal osteoporosis. Entry criteria were not based on BMD, and 13% of the cohort had osteoporosis at the time of inclusion, as diagnosed by a T-score lower than −2.5 for BMD at the total hip (3). Potential subjects were excluded if they had been treated for osteoporosis with bisphosphonates, hormone replacement therapy, or calcitonin within 1 year of screening, or if they had significant disease of the digestive system or the kidney, had cancer in the last 5 years, unexplained weight loss in the past year, or uncontrolled high blood pressure, or a history of hyperparathyroidism, malabsorption, abnormal Pap smear, or thromboembolic disease. A food frequency questionnaire was utilized to estimate dietary calcium and vitamin D intakes (10). The study was approved by the Committee on Clinical Investigations, New Devices and New Forms of Therapy of the Beth Israel Deaconess Medical Center, where the study was led. All subjects participating in this study provided written informed consent.

BMD (gm/cm^2) was measured at baseline by DXA (QDR-4500A; Hologic, Waltham, MA). Measurements performed at the hip (total hip, femoral neck, and trochanter) and forearm (one-third distal, mid-distal, and ultradistal radius) were considered for analysis in the present study. The precision of this technique in our laboratory has previously been reported (10,25).

IL-6 genotyping. Whole blood samples from 461 women were available for DNA preparation. DNA was extracted according to standard methods and amplified by polymerase chain reaction (PCR) using forward primer 5′-TGACTTCAGCTTTACTCTTGT and reverse primer 5′-CTGATTGGAACCCTTATTAAG, as follows: 1 cycle of 95°C for 4 minutes, followed by 35 cycles of 95°C for 30 seconds, 50°C for 30 seconds, and 72°C for 90 seconds, followed by 1 cycle of 72°C for 5 minutes. The 190-bp PCR product was digested overnight at 37°C with *Nla* III. This enzyme recognizes a CATG sequence present in the C allele, leading to 2 DNA fragments of 143 bp and 47 bp, respectively, which were separated by 8% microliter array diagonal gel electrophoresis. Details of the procedure have been described previously (23).

Markers of bone turnover. After the subjects fasted overnight, serum samples were collected and frozen at −80°C until analysis. Serum type I collagen breakdown products were measured by a 2-site assay with an automatic analyzer (Elecsys, Roche Diagnostic, Nutley, NJ), using monoclonal antibodies raised against an 8–amino acid sequence from CTx. Intraassay variation is <3%, and interassay variation is <8% (7). The mean ± SD value in premenopausal women is 0.255 ± 0.12 ng/ml. Serum OC, a specific marker of bone formation, was measured by a 2-site assay measuring both intact and N-mid fragments, with an automatic system (Kryptor-Osteo; Cis-Biointernational, Gif/Yvette, France). Measuring the main proteolytic fragment of OC allows one to correct for the potential degradation of OC in vitro and obtain precise measurements. Intra- and interassay variations are <2.5% and <3%, respectively. The mean ± SD value in premenopausal women is 16.6 ± 4.5 ng/ml.

Statistical analysis. In order to avoid potential problems with outliers and non-normality, the association of IL-6 genotypes with markers of bone turnover and BMD was first assessed by Kruskal-Wallis test for differences between the 3 genotypes (26). These associations were further tested by analysis of variance (ANOVA) and by test for trend, used as standard linear regression with the number of G alleles (0, 1, or 2) as the independent variable.

Six clinical and dietary variables (age, weight, height,

Table 1. Characteristics of the study subjects*

Characteristic	IL-6 genotype GG	GC	CC	All
No. (% of total)	162 (37)	204 (47)	68 (16)	434
Age, years	71.4 ± 5.7	72.5 ± 6.0	71.1 ± 4.4	71.9 ± 5.6
Weight, kg	68.2 ± 14.5	69.7 ± 17.6	70.3 ± 14.3	69.2 ± 15.9
Height, cm	158.8 ± 6.4	158.4 ± 6.7	158.9 ± 5.7	158.6 ± 6.4
Body mass index, kg/m^2	27.0 ± 4.9	27.8 ± 6.4	27.8 ± 5.2	27.5 ± 5.6
Daily calcium intake, mg	871 ± 395	901 ± 450	832 ± 385	879 ± 419
Daily vitamin D intake, IU	244 ± 173	251 ± 190	256 ± 175	249 ± 181

* All subjects were postmenopausal women. Except where otherwise indicated, values are the mean ± SD. IL-6 = interleukin-6.

body mass index, and daily calcium and vitamin D intake) were evaluated as potential confounders of the association between IL-6 genotypes and outcome measurements, using the Kruskal-Wallis test for association with IL-6 genotypes and Spearman's rank correlation to test for association with BMD and bone marker measurements. P values less than 0.25 were required in both tests for a variable to be further considered as a potential confounder. Age was the only variable fulfilling this criterion ($P = 0.09$), and analyses of the association between IL-6 genotypes and outcome measurements were subsequently adjusted for age using the general linear model.

Logistic regression, using age as the continuous variable, was performed to calculate odds ratios and 95% confidence intervals (95% CI) for the risk of high bone turnover associated with the C allele, with the GG genotype used as the reference group.

The age-related decrease in BMD was estimated as the difference in BMD between older and younger postmenopausal women after dividing the cohort into 2 groups according to the median age (70.5 years). Planned orthogonal comparisons were performed within each genotype, using the t-test for independent groups with the Bonferroni adjustment for multiple comparisons (27). Accordingly, $P < 0.05$ was considered as the minimal level of significance for BMD differences between older and younger postmenopausal women in these groups (corresponding to $P < 0.003$ prior to adjustment for multiple comparisons).

RESULTS

From the original cohort of 461 postmenopausal women (mean ± SD age 71.7 ± 5.7 years) who completed screening and for whom DNA samples were available, genotypes for the IL-6 −174 G→C polymorphism could be determined in 434 subjects (Table 1). Genotype frequencies were as expected from Hardy-Weinberg proportions and were similar to those previously noted in Caucasian subjects from the United Kingdom (23). Age, weight, height, body mass index, and daily calcium and vitamin D intakes did not differ significantly among IL-6 genotypes (Table 1).

Levels of serum CTx, a marker of bone resorption, showed significant differences among IL-6 genotypes (mean ± SEM 0.275 ± 0.02 ng/ml, 0.325 ± 0.01 ng/ml, and 0.356 ± 0.02 ng/ml in women with the CC genotype [n = 68], the GC genotype [n = 204], and the GG genotype [n = 162], respectively) ($P = 0.014$ by Kruskal-Wallis test, $P = 0.021$ by ANOVA, and $P = 0.007$ and 0.006 by test for trend for the number of G alleles before and after adjustment for age, respectively) (Figure 1). In contrast, levels of serum OC, a marker of bone formation, did not differ significantly among IL-6 genotypes (Figure 1). High bone resorption, as defined by serum CTx values more than 1 SD above the mean in premenopausal women (0.375 ng/ml), was present in 42%, 33%, and 20% of GG, GC, and CC subjects, respectively ($P = 0.013$ by unadjusted chi-square analysis). Accordingly, odds ratios (adjusted for age) for the risk of high bone resorption decreased significantly with the number of C alleles (0.65 [95% CI 0.41–1.0, $P = 0.06$] and 0.37 [95% CI 0.18–0.73, $P = 0.0047$] in GC and CC subjects, respectively, as compared with GG subjects).

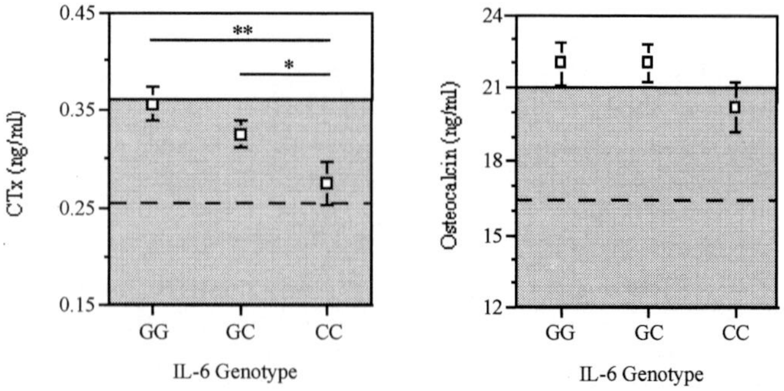

Figure 1. Mean ± SEM levels of serum C-telopeptide of type I collagen (CTx) and serum osteocalcin according to interleukin-6 (IL-6) −174 G→C genotype in postmenopausal women. Dashed lines indicate the mean value in premenopausal women; shaded areas indicate ±1 SD from this mean. ** = $P = 0.01$; * = $P = 0.02$.

Table 2. Bone mineral density by IL-6 genotype*

Region	IL-6 genotype			% difference, CC vs. GG		
	GG	GC	CC	All	Younger (age <70.5 years)	Older (age >70.5 years)
Total hip	0.786 ± 0.012	0.789 ± 0.010	0.806 ± 0.017	+2.5	+0.8	+5.6
Femoral neck	0.653 ± 0.009	0.659 ± 0.008	0.668 ± 0.014	+2.3	+0.3	+5.2
Trochanter	0.595 ± 0.010	0.601 ± 0.008	0.623 ± 0.014	+4.7	+3.5	+6.8
One-third distal radius	0.552 ± 0.007	0.552 ± 0.006	0.560 ± 0.010	+1.5	−0.1	+4.4
Mid-distal radius	0.479 ± 0.007	0.481 ± 0.005	0.486 ± 0.010	+1.5	−0.1	+5.3
Ultradistal radius	0.338 ± 0.006	0.342 ± 0.005	0.349 ± 0.009	+3.2	+2.8	+4.1

* Values are the mean ± SEM bone mineral density (gm/cm^2) and the percentage difference between interleukin-6 (IL-6) −174 CC and GG genotypes in younger and older postmenopausal women.

Age-adjusted differences in BMD by IL-6 genotype are shown in Table 2. In women with the CC genotype, there was a nonsignificant trend toward higher BMD in all subregions of the hip and forearm (distal radius) examined, compared with those with the GC or GG genotype. These differences were the largest in regions containing the highest amounts of trabecular bone, i.e., the trochanter and ultradistal radius ($P = 0.09$ for the trochanter, by test for trend), reaching 4.7% at the trochanter between alternate homozygotes CC and GG (Table 2).

To investigate whether BMD differences between IL-6 genotypes might increase with age (15), the cohort was further divided into 2 groups according to the median age (70.5 years); the mean ± SD age in the younger group was 67.5 ± 1.6 years, and that in the older group was 76.5 ± 4.8 years. Genotype distribution was similar in the 2 age groups (n = 31, 97, and 71 with CC, GC, and GG, respectively, in the older group; n = 29, 91, and 82, respectively, in the younger group). Consistent with the notion that IL-6 genotypes have a persistent influence on the level of bone resorption, differences in serum CTx levels between IL-6 genotypes were similar in the 2 age groups (data not shown), and no statistical interaction between genotype and age was found ($P = 0.023$ for genotypes, $P = 0.49$ for age, and $P = 0.86$ for genotype × age, by 2-factor ANOVA). In contrast, BMD differences between genotypes were more prominent among older than younger postmenopausal women ($P = 0.15$ for genotype × age). In the older group, BMD was as much as 6.8% higher in the women with CC compared with those with the GG genotype (Table 2), although none of the differences between genotypes achieved statistical significance (by test for trend).

To evaluate the influence of IL-6 genotypes on the age-related decrease in BMD, differences in BMD between older and younger postmenopausal women were calculated within each genotype. In older postmenopausal women, BMD was significantly decreased compared with that in younger postmenopausal women for most subregions of the hip and forearm among those with GG and GC, but not in those with CC (Figure 2).

DISCUSSION

The results of this study indicate that the level of bone resorption in healthy postmenopausal women living in the community, as evaluated by levels of serum CTx (6,7,9), is partly determined by allelic variation at the −174 G→C polymorphic locus of the IL-6 gene (23). Although these results must await confirmation in a second, independent population, the relatively large size of the present cohort, as well as the high prevalence of the IL-6 −174 C allelic variant (39%) and of the CC genotype (16%), make it unlikely that this observation is spurious.

This argument is strengthened by the large mag-

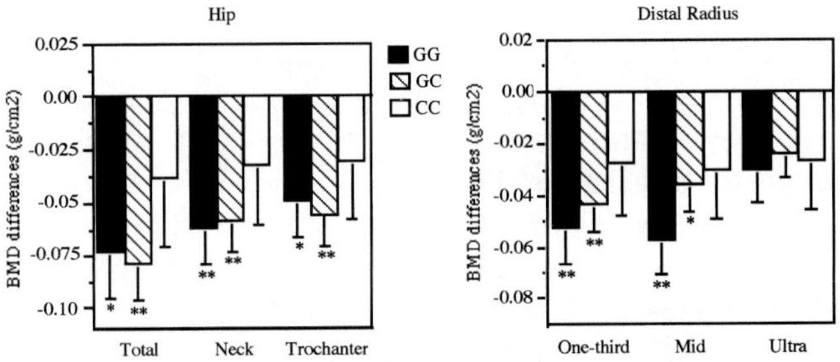

Figure 2. Mean and SEM differences in bone mineral density (BMD) at the hip (total hip, femoral neck, and trochanter) and forearm (one-third distal, mid-distal, and ultradistal radius) in older versus younger postmenopausal women according to interleukin-6 −174 G→C genotype. ** = $P = 0.01$; * = $P = 0.05$, older versus younger postmenopausal women, by *t*-test adjusted for multiple comparisons.

nitude of the differences in serum CTx levels (30%) between CC and GG homozygotes, as well as in the risk of high bone resorption, which decreases dramatically with the number of C alleles. The difference between mean CTx levels in the GG and CC women is biologically relevant and is about half as large as the previously reported difference between postmenopausal and premenopausal women (28). Our results thus suggest that the accelerated bone resorption normally caused by estrogen deprivation in postmenopausal women is being significantly slowed in the presence of the IL-6 −174 CC allele.

These findings are consistent with the previously demonstrated function of the −174 G→C IL-6 allelic variants in vitro and in vivo, as well as with the physiologic role of IL-6 in bone resorption. In vitro, the level of unstimulated IL-6 transcription associated with the C allele was 40% lower than with the G allele, and this difference was markedly exaggerated upon stimulation with proinflammatory mediators, such as IL-1 (23). Moreover, among 100 healthy men and women, serum IL-6 concentrations were ~40% lower in CC as compared with GG subjects (23). Most importantly, the IL-6 −174 C allele was identified less frequently than the G allele among patients with juvenile chronic arthritis, a condition in which IL-6 plays a prominent pathologic role (23). These findings, taken together with the facts that IL-6 is a major local factor in the mediation of bone resorption and that IL-6 transcription in osteoblastic cells increases dramatically in the absence of estrogens (20,21), make it plausible that postmenopausal women carrying the IL-6 −174 C allele have lower levels of bone resorption. For the same reasons, however, these results should not be extrapolated to premenopausal women or to men.

Due to the relatively large difference in bone resorption levels between IL-6 −174 G→C polymorphisms, it may appear surprising that BMD differences between IL-6 genotypes were not larger and/or statistically significant. Nevertheless, there was a consistent trend toward higher BMD in women with CC as compared with those with the GG genotype in all subregions of the hip and forearm examined, approaching 5% at skeletal sites containing mostly trabecular bone. In addition, BMD differences between IL-6 −174 G→C genotypes appeared to increase with age (Table 2), consistent with the notion that IL-6 genotypes have a persistent influence on the level of bone resorption. In accordance with these observations, it might take as much as 10 years before high versus low bone resorption, as evaluated by serum CTx levels, translates into a 5% difference in BMD in postmenopausal women (9).

Since our study was cross-sectional, a prospective evaluation of bone turnover markers and BMD changes in relation to IL-6 −174 G→C genotypes was not available. Nevertheless, the influence of IL-6 allelic polymorphisms on the rate of postmenopausal bone loss can be inferred from studies showing a significant positive correlation between bone resorption markers and bone loss (7–10), as well as between plasma IL-6 concentration and osteopenia (22,29). Consistent with these observations, BMD was significantly decreased in older compared with younger postmenopausal women carrying the GG and GC IL-6 genotypes (−9.6% on average; $P = 0.01$), but not significantly so in CC women (−5.1% on average). Accelerated bone loss is the primary consequence of estrogen deprivation and is mostly responsible for the age-related increase in the risk of osteoporotic fracture at the hip, wrist, and spine (30). Moreover, high rates of bone resorption are also associated with a disruption of the trabecular bone network, leading to a loss of connectivity that is not necessarily reflected in a measurable decrease of BMD but is an independent risk factor for fracture (31). Hence, dramatic differences in bone resorption rates associated with IL-6 −174 G→C genotypes could translate into differences in the risk of osteoporotic fractures well above those predicted by BMD measurements alone.

Recently, a common, functional polymorphism in the transforming growth factor β gene exon 1 (29T→C), another major regulator of bone metabolism acting downstream of estrogen, has been reported to be associated with the rate of bone loss in postmenopausal Japanese women (32). By comparison, the prevalence of the ss genotype at the collagen Iα1 Sp1 polymorphic locus, previously described to be associated with low BMD in the elderly, is ~3% among Caucasians (15). Identifying polymorphic genes with frequent allelic variants both improves the reliability of the association with any phenotypic trait and increases their predictive value for the general population. Thus, our results raise the possibility that prevention of postmenopausal bone loss by estrogens or bisphosphonates (33) could be modulated by IL-6 −174 allelic polymorphisms.

In conclusion, we have demonstrated that a common functional IL-6 genetic variant is related to bone resorption levels and possibly bone loss in postmenopausal women, with 1 in 6 Caucasian women having the protective CC genotype. Future studies should directly address the possibility that IL-6 −174 G→C allelic variants are associated with postmenopausal bone loss, osteoporosis, and, mostly, osteoporotic fractures in the elderly as well as in patients with systemic inflammatory disorders, such as rheumatoid arthritis (4,5).

ACKNOWLEDGMENTS

We thank Dr. R. Parker for directing the statistical analysis, Ms K. Staples and Mr. M. Halpern for preparing the DNA samples, Mr. Le Ahn-Luong for the genotyping, and the dietary, nursing, technical, and administrative staff of the General Clinical Research Center and the Osteoporosis Prevention and Treatment Center at Beth Israel Deaconess Medical Center.

REFERENCES

1. Melton LJ III, Chrischilles EA, Cooper C, Lane AW, Riggs BL. Perspective: how many women have osteoporosis? J Bone Miner Res 1992;7:1005–10.
2. Melton LJ III, Thamer M, Ray NF, Chan JK, Chesnut CH III, Einhorn TA, et al. Fractures attributable to osteoporosis: report from the National Osteoporosis Foundation. J Bone Miner Res 1997;12:16–23.
3. Kanis JA, Devogelaer JP, Gennari C. Practical guide for the use of bone mineral measurements in the assessment of treatment of osteoporosis: a position paper of the European Foundation for Osteoporosis and Bone Disease. Osteoporos Int 1996;6:256–61.
4. Laan RF, van Riel PL, van de Putte LB. Bone mass in patients with rheumatoid arthritis. Ann Rheum Dis 1992;51:826–32.
5. Laan RF, van Riel PL, van de Putte LB, van Erning LJ, van 't Hof MA, Lemmens JA. Low-dose prednisone induces rapid reversible axial bone loss in patients with rheumatoid arthritis. Ann Intern Med 1993;119:963–8.
6. Garnero P, Delmas PD. Biochemical markers of bone turnover: applications for osteoporosis. Endocrinol Metab Clin North Am 1998;27:303–23.
7. Rosenquist C, Fledelius C, Christgau S, Pedersen BJ, Bonde M, Qvist P, et al. Serum Crosslaps One Step ELISA: first application of monoclonal antibodies for measurement in serum of bone-related degradation products from C-terminal telopeptides of type I collagen. Clin Chem 1998;44:2281–9.
8. Marcus R, Holloway L, Wells B, Greendale G, James MK, Wasilauskas C, et al. The relationship of biochemical markers of bone turnover to bone density changes in postmenopausal women: results from the postmenopausal estrogen/progestin interventions (PEPI) trial. J Bone Miner Res 1999;14:1583–95.
9. Garnero P, Sornay-Rendu E, Duboeuf F, Delmas PD. Markers of bone turnover predict forearm bone loss over 4 years: the OFELY study. J Bone Miner Res 1999;14:1614–21.
10. Greenspan SL, Parker RA, Ferguson L, Rosen HN, Maitland-Ramsey L, Karpf DB. Early changes in biochemical markers of bone turnover predict the long-term response to alendronate therapy in representative elderly women: a randomized clinical trial. J Bone Miner Res 1998;13:1431–8.
11. Ferrari S, Rizzoli R, Bonjour JP. Heritable and nutritional influences on bone mineral mass. Aging (Milano) 1998:10:205–13.
12. Morrison NA, Qi JC, Tokita A, Kelly PJ, Crofts L, Nguyen TV, et al. Prediction of bone density from vitamin D receptor alleles. Nature 1994;367:284–7.
13. Ferrari S, Rizzoli R, Bonjour JP. Genetic aspects of osteoporosis. Curr Opin Rheumatol 1999;11:294–300.
14. Ferrari S, Rizzoli R, Chevalley T, Slosman D, Eisman JA, Bonjour JP. Vitamin-D-receptor-gene polymorphisms and change in lumbar-spine bone mineral density. Lancet 1995;345:423–4.
15. Uitterlinden AG, Burger H, Huang Q, Yue F, McGuigan FEA, Grant SFA, et al. Relation of alleles of the collagen type Iα1 gene to bone density and the risk of osteoporotic fractures in postmenopausal women. N Engl J Med 1998;338:1016–21.
16. Kobayashi S, Inoue S, Hosoi M, Ouchi Y, Shiraki M, Orimo H. Association of bone mineral density with polymorphism of the estrogen receptor gene. J Bone Miner Res 1996;11:306–11.
17. Ferrari SL, Rizzoli R, Slosman DO, Bonjour JP. Do dietary calcium and age explain the controversy surrounding the relation between bone mineral density and vitamin D receptor gene polymorphisms? J Bone Miner Res 1998;13:363–70.
18. Garnero P, Borel O, Grant SF, Ralston SH, Delmas PD. Collagen I-alpha-1 Sp1 polymorphism, bone mass and bone turnover in healthy French premenopausal women: the OFELY study. J Bone Miner Res 1998;13:813–7.
19. Salmen T, Heikkinen AM, Mahonen A, Kroger H, Komulainen M, Saarikoski S, et al. Early postmenopausal bone loss is associated with Pvu II estrogen receptor gene polymorphism in Finnish women: effect of hormone replacement therapy. J Bone Miner Res 2000;15:315–21.
20. Manolagas SC, Jilka RL. Bone marrow, cytokines and bone remodeling. N Engl J Med 1995;332:305–11.
21. Manolagas SC. Cellular and molecular mechanisms of osteoporosis. Aging Clin Exp Res 1998;10:182–90.
22. Scheidt-Nave CE, Bismar H, Leidig-Bruckner G, Seibel MJ, Ziegler R, Pfeilschifter J. Serum interleukin-6 is a major predictor of bone loss in women specific to the first decade past menopause [abstract]. J Bone Miner Res 1999;14 Suppl 1:S147.
23. Fishman D, Faulds G, Jeffery R, Mohamed-Ali V, Yudkin JS, Humphries S, et al. The effect of novel polymorphisms in the interleukin-6 (IL-6) gene on IL-6 transcription and plasma IL-6 levels, and an association with systemic-onset juvenile chronic arthritis. J Clin Invest 1998;102:1369–76.
24. De Benedetti F, Massa M, Robbioni P, Ravelli A, Burgio GR, Martini A. Correlation of serum interleukin-6 levels with joint involvement and thrombocytosis in systemic juvenile rheumatoid arthritis. Arthritis Rheum 1991;34:1158–63.
25. Bouxsein ML, Parker RA, Greenspan SL. Forearm bone mineral densitometry cannot be used to monitor response to alendronate therapy in postmenopausal women. Osteoporos Int 1999;10:505–9.
26. Daniel WW. Applied nonparametric analysis. Boston (MA): Houghton Mifflin; 1978.
27. Dawson-Saunders B, Trapp RG. Basic and clinical biostatistics. Norwalk (CT): Appleton & Lange; 1994.
28. Garnero P, Sornay-Rendu E, Chapuy MC, Delmas PD. Increased bone turnover in late postmenopausal women is a major determinant of osteoporosis. J Bone Miner Res 1996;11:337–49.
29. Pollak RD, Karmeli F, Eliakim R, Ackerman Z, Tabb K, Rachmilewitz D. Femoral neck osteopenia in patients with inflammatory bowel disease. Am J Gastroenterol 1998;93:1483–90.
30. Riggs BL, Khosla S, Melton LJ III. A unitary model for involutional osteoporosis: estrogen deficiency causes both type I and type II osteoporosis in postmenopausal women and contributes to bone loss in aging men. J Bone Miner Res 1998;13:763–73.
31. Parfitt AM. Age-related structural changes in trabecular and cortical bone: cellular mechanisms and biomechanical consequences. Calcif Tissue Int 1984;36 Suppl 1:S123–8.
32. Yamada Y, Harada A, Hosoi T, Miyauchi A, Ikeda K, Ohta H, et al. Association of transforming growth factor β1 genotype with therapeutic response to active vitamin D for postmenopausal osteoporosis. J Bone Miner Res 2000;15:415–20.
33. Eastell R. Treatment of postmenopausal osteoporosis. N Engl J Med 1998;338:736–46.

ARTHRITIS & RHEUMATISM
Vol. 44, No. 1, January 2001, pp 202–211

Two-Year Effects of Alendronate on Bone Mineral Density and Vertebral Fracture in Patients Receiving Glucocorticoids

A Randomized, Double-Blind, Placebo-Controlled Extension Trial

Jonathan D. Adachi,[1] Kenneth G. Saag,[2] Pierre D. Delmas,[3] Uri A. Liberman,[4] Ronald D. Emkey,[5] Ego Seeman,[6] Nancy E. Lane,[7] Jean-Marc Kaufman,[8] Patrice E. E. Poubelle,[9] Federico Hawkins,[10] Ricardo Correa-Rotter,[11] Charles-Joel Menkes,[12] Jose A. Rodriguez-Portales,[13] Thomas J. Schnitzer,[14] Joel A. Block,[14] Jeffrey Wing,[15] Harris H. McIlwain,[16] Rene Westhovens,[17] Jacques Brown,[9] Jose A. Melo-Gomes,[18] Barry L. Gruber,[19] Melissa J. Yanover,[20] Maria Odette R. Leite,[21] Kerry G. Siminoski,[22] Michael C. Nevitt,[23] John T. Sharp,[24] Marie-Pierre Malice,[25] Thomas Dumortier,[25] Michelle Czachur,[25] Wendy Carofano,[25] and Anastasia Daifotis[25]

Objective. **To evaluate the continued efficacy and safety of alendronate (ALN) for up to 2 years in patients receiving glucocorticoids.**

Methods. **This is a 12-month extension of a previously completed 1-year trial of daily ALN, performed to evaluate the effects of ALN over a total of 2 years in 66 men and 142 women continuing to receive at least 7.5 mg of prednisone or equivalent daily. All patients received supplemental calcium and vitamin D. The primary end point was the mean percentage change in lumbar spine bone mineral density (BMD) from baseline to 24 months. Other outcomes included changes in hip and total body BMD, biochemical markers of bone turnover, radiographic joint damage of the hands, and vertebral fracture incidence.**

Results. **The mean (±SEM) lumbar spine BMD increased by 2.8 ± 0.6%, 3.9 ± 0.7%, and 3.7 ± 0.6%, respectively, in the groups that received 5 mg, 10 mg, and 2.5/10 mg of ALN daily ($P \leq 0.001$) and decreased by −0.8 ± 0.6% in the placebo group (*P* not significant) over 24 months. In patients receiving any dose of ALN,**

Supported by grants from Merck & Co., Inc., the General Clinical Research Centers Programs, and the National Center for Research Resources, and NIH grant RR-00059.

[1]Jonathan D. Adachi, MD: McMaster University, Hamilton, Ontario, Canada; [2]Kenneth G. Saag, MD, MSc: University of Iowa College of Medicine, Iowa City; [3]Pierre D. Delmas, MD: Hospital Edouard Herriot, Lyon, France; [4]Uri A. Liberman, MD, PhD: Tel Aviv University, Petach Tikva, Israel; [5]Ronald D. Emkey, MD: Bone Research Center, West Reading, Pennsylvania; [6]Ego Seeman, MD: Austin and Repatriation Medical Center, Heidelberg, Australia; [7]Nancy E. Lane, MD: The Rosalind Russell Arthritis Research Laboratories, San Francisco, California; [8]Jean-Marc Kaufman, MD: Universitaire Ziekenhuizen Gent, Ghent, Belgium; [9]Patrice E. E. Poubelle, MD, Jacques Brown, MD: Le Centre Hospitalier Universitaire de Québec, Canada; [10]Federico Hawkins, MD: Hospital 12 de Octubre, Madrid, Spain; [11]Ricardo Correa-Rotter, MD: Instituto Nacional Nutrición Salvador Zubirán, Delegacion Tlalpan, Mexico; [12]Charles-Joel Menkes, MD: Hopital Cochin, Paris, France; [13]Jose A. Rodriguez-Portales, MD: Universidad Catolica De Chile, Santiago, Chile; [14]Thomas J. Schnitzer, MD, PhD, Joel A. Block, MD: Northwestern University, Chicago, Illinois; [15]Jeffrey Wing, MD: Johannesburg Hospital, Parktown, South Africa; [16]Harris H. McIlwain, MD: Tampa Medical Group, Tampa, Florida; [17]Rene Westhovens, MD, PhD: Universitaire Ziekenhuizen Leuven, Leuven, Belgium; [18]Jose A. Melo-Gomes, MD: Hospital Militar Principal, Lisbon, Portugal; [19]Barry L. Gruber, MD: University Hospital Medical Center, Stony Brook, New York; [20]Melissa J. Yanover, MD: Western Nephrology & Metabolic Bone Disease, PC, Lakewood, Colorado; [21]Maria Odette R. Leite, MD: Faculdade De Medicina Da Universidade De São Paulo, São Paulo, Brazil; [22]Kerry G. Siminoski, MD: Endocrine Centre of Edmonton, Edmonton, Alberta, Canada; [23]Michael C. Nevitt, PhD: University of California, San Francisco; [24]John T. Sharp, MD: Bainbridge Island, Washington; [25]Marie-Pierre Malice, PhD, Thomas Dumortier, MSc, Michelle Czachur, MPH, Wendy Carofano, RPh, Anastasia Daifotis, MD: Merck & Co., Inc., Rahway, NJ.

Address correspondence and reprint requests to Jonathan D. Adachi, MD, St. Joseph's Hospital, McMaster University, Department of Medicine, 25 Charlton Avenue East, Suite #501, Hamilton L8N1Y2, Ontario, Canada.

Submitted for publication November 11, 1999; accepted in revised form September 5, 2000.

BMD was increased at the trochanter ($P \leq 0.05$) and maintained at the femoral neck. Total body BMD was increased in patients receiving 5 or 10 mg ALN ($P \leq 0.01$). These 2 dose levels of ALN were more effective than placebo at all sites ($P \leq 0.05$). Bone turnover markers (N-telopeptides of type I collagen and bone-specific alkaline phosphatase) decreased 60% and 25%, respectively, during treatment with ALN ($P \leq 0.05$). There were fewer patients with new vertebral fractures in the ALN group versus the placebo group (0.7% versus 6.8%; $P = 0.026$). The safety profile was similar between treatment groups.

Conclusion. **Alendronate is an effective, well-tolerated therapy for the prevention and treatment of glucocorticoid-induced osteoporosis, with sustained treatment advantages for up to 2 years.**

Osteoporosis is a well-recognized complication of long-term glucocorticoid therapy, and ultimately leads to fractures in up to 50% of patients (1). There is a doubling of hip fracture risk compared with patients who have not received glucocorticoids (2). Estrogen (3), vitamin D and its active metabolites (4,5), and calcitonin (6) have been reported to be effective in preventing bone loss in some, but not all, patients treated with glucocorticoids. Bisphosphonates have been considered as a potential therapy for glucocorticoid-induced osteoporosis because of their ability to inhibit bone resorption and their relatively few side effects. In several studies of oral pamidronate (7), risedronate (8), and etidronate (9,10), spinal and hip bone mineral density (BMD) were increased or maintained in patients with glucocorticoid-induced osteoporosis. Greater therapeutic efficacy with bisphosphonate therapy than with either calcium, vitamin D, or calcitonin was reported in a recent meta-analysis (11).

Alendronate (ALN) is a potent bisphosphonate that has been reported to increase spine, hip, and total body BMD and reduce the incidence of spine and hip fractures (12–15) in osteoporotic postmenopausal women. ALN for 48 weeks has also been reported to increase spine, hip, and total body BMD in a heterogeneous population of glucocorticoid-treated patients (16) and to increase BMD in a study of sarcoid patients receiving glucocorticoids (17).

Herein we report the results of a 12-month extension of a previously reported 48-week trial (16). Our report summarizes 24 months of experience with continuous ALN treatment in both men and women undergoing long-term glucocorticoid therapy.

PATIENTS AND METHODS

Patients. The original 48-week study was a combined United States and multinational, randomized, double-blind, placebo-controlled trial of daily oral ALN at a dose of 2.5 mg (in the multinational study only), 5 mg, or 10 mg, in patients receiving at least 7.5 mg/day of prednisone or equivalent (16). The current study was a 12-month randomized, double-blind, placebo-controlled extension to the original trial. Patients who completed the first study and were still receiving at least 7.5 mg of oral prednisone or equivalent doses of other glucocorticoids daily for a variety of diseases were eligible for this extension study. The institutional review boards of the participating institutions approved the protocol, and all patients provided informed consent.

Treatment. Patients continued to receive the double-blind study medication to which they had been randomized at the beginning of year 1, except that patients in the multinational study who had been receiving 2.5 mg of ALN daily (a predicted suboptimal dose) were blindedly switched to a dose of 10 mg. Two patients receiving placebo and 1 patient receiving 2.5 mg ALN met the criteria for classification as fast bone losers (defined as >6% loss in spine BMD from baseline to 9 months) and were switched to open-label ALN at a dose of 10 mg in year 2. ALN sodium tablets and matching placebo were manufactured and supplied by Merck (Whitehouse Station, NJ). All patients continued to receive 800–1,000 mg of elemental calcium and 250–500 IU of vitamin D supplements daily. The patients' primary physicians managed their glucocorticoid therapy. The use of nonsteroidal antiinflammatory drugs (NSAIDs), including aspirin, was allowed.

Risk factor and outcome measurements. The patients were reevaluated at 18 and 24 months from the baseline time point of the original study. Glucocorticoid usage was recorded by the patients on diary cards, which were reviewed by the study staff at each visit. BMD of the lumbar spine, hip, and total body was measured by dual-energy x-ray absorptiometry with Hologic (Waltham, MA) or Lunar (Madison, WI) machines, and the results were centrally analyzed by Medical Data Management (Waltham, MA). A standard phantom was used at all sites for cross-calibration. Serum and urine samples, obtained for measurement of biochemical markers of bone turnover (serum bone-specific alkaline phosphatase [BSAP] and N-telopeptides of type I collagen [NTx] corrected for the creatinine concentration), were analyzed at a central reference laboratory (Mayo Medical Laboratories, Rochester, MN).

Followup radiographs of the lateral lumbar and thoracic spine were taken at baseline, 12, and 24 months or at the time of early discontinuation, according to current guidelines, and were evaluated at a central facility (University of California, San Francisco) by readers who were blinded to the treatment group. The measurement of changes in vertebral dimension by radiographic computerized digitization was the primary method of assessing incident vertebral fractures, defined as decreases of ≥20% and ≥4 mm in anterior, middle, or posterior vertebral body height (L1 to L5 and T4 to T12) between baseline and followup. Prevalent fractures were identified by binary (yes/no), semiquantitative (scale 0–3) visual assessment as those with a grade of 2 or higher (18).

Table 1. Baseline characteristics of the glucocorticoid-induced osteoporosis extension cohort*

	Placebo (n = 61)	ALN 5 mg (n = 63)	ALN 10 mg (n = 55)	ALN 2.5/10 mg (n = 29)
Age/years				
Mean ± SD	54 ± 15	53 ± 15	53 ± 15	56 ± 15
Range	23–76	22–76	21–78	30–79
Sex/menopausal status, no. (%)				
Men	19 (31)	18 (29)	15 (27)	14 (48)
Premenopausal women	17 (28)	16 (25)	14 (25)	5 (17)
Postmenopausal women				
Receiving estrogen (oral or transdermal)	7 (11)	10 (16)	8 (15)	2 (7)
Not receiving estrogen	18 (30)	19 (30)	18 (33)	8 (28)
Duration of prior glucocorticoid therapy, no. (%)				
<4 months	18 (30)	18 (29)	19 (35)	11 (38)
4–12 months	13 (21)	13 (21)	13 (24)	5 (17)
>12 months	30 (49)	32 (51)	23 (42)	13 (45)
Daily glucocorticoid dose, mg prednisone or equivalent				
Mean ± SD	20.4 ± 20.7	21.1 ± 21.6	17.4 ± 18.0	19.4 ± 21.5
Median	10.0	10.0	10.0	10.0
Range	7.5–120	7.5–135	7.5–95	5.3–100
Glucocorticoid-requiring illness, no. (%)				
Rheumatologic	42 (69)	45 (71)	37 (67)	21 (72)
Pulmonary	3 (5)	3 (5)	8 (15)	1 (3)
Dermatologic	5 (8)	8 (13)	5 (9)	4 (14)
Myasthenia and myasthenia gravis	9 (15)	1 (2)	0	1 (3)
Gastrointestinal†	1 (2)	2 (3)	0	0
Renal	1 (2)	4 (6)	5 (9)	2 (7)
Lumbar spine BMD, mean ± SD				
gm/cm^2‡	0.93 ± 0.15	0.92 ± 0.17	0.93 ± 0.15	0.89 ± 0.16
T-score§	−1.18 ± 1.31	−1.24 ± 1.59	−1.14 ± 1.41	−1.66 ± 1.43
Biochemical markers of bone turnover, mean ± SD				
Urine NTx/Cr, pmoles BCE/μmoles creatinine¶	42.5 ± 26.9	41.9 ± 25.1	45.2 ± 35.3	39.8 ± 25.7
Bone-specific alkaline phosphatase, ng/ml#	9.5 ± 4.7	9.7 ± 4.7	10.1 ± 3.9	10.0 ± 5.5
History of fractures, no. (%)				
Prior morphometric vertebral fracture	7 (11)	7 (11)	9 (16)	3 (10)
Prior nonvertebral fracture	16 (26)	16 (25)	17 (31)	8 (28)

* There were no significant differences between treatment groups. ALN = alendronate; BMD = bone mineral density; NTx = N-telopeptides of type I collagen; Cr = creatinine; BCE = bone collagen equivalent.
† Inflammatory bowel disease.
‡ Lunar values were converted to Hologic equivalents: Hologic = Lunar/1.1303.
§ T-score = standard deviations from the mean peak bone mass of sex-matched, healthy young adults. Normal ≥ −1; osteopenic ≥ −2 and < −1; osteoporotic <−2.
¶ Normal range 0.0–131.
# Normal range for men 4.4–17.2, for women 2.0–16.6.

Joint destruction at months 12 and 24 relative to baseline was assessed in rheumatoid arthritis patients (by JTS) according to previously described methods (19). Paired baseline and followup bilateral hand radiographs (blinded for treatment group and chronologic sequence) were scored for erosions, and joint space narrowing and a total radiographic score (erosion plus joint space narrowing) were calculated.

Statistical analysis. Data from all patients enrolled in the double-blind extension study were included in the BMD intention-to-treat analyses. The main efficacy measure was the percentage change in lumbar spine BMD from baseline (of the original study) to the last measurement obtained while the patients were receiving at least 7.5 mg of prednisone (or equivalent) per day. If no such measurement was available at month 24, the 18-month BMD measurement was used in the analysis. Other predefined efficacy end points included the percentage change in hip and total body BMD, biochemical markers of bone turnover, radiographic joint damage of the hands, and the incidence of fractures. Additional BMD analyses were performed in all patients, irrespective of glucocorticoid dose. The log-transformed fraction of the baseline value at month 24 was used to analyze biochemical markers. Data from patients identified as protocol violators were excluded from the biochemical marker analyses.

For the clinical and biochemical efficacy end points, comparisons of placebo with the 5-, 10-, and 2.5/10-mg doses of ALN were made with the step-down Tukey trend test adjusted for multiplicity (20,21). The difference in the percentage change in BMD between treatment groups was assessed using an analysis of variance (ANOVA) model including factors for treatment group, center, and duration of prestudy glucocorticoid therapy (0–4, 4–12, or >12 months). Possible differences in treatment response were assessed for patient subgroups that were defined by the previous and current dose of glucocorticoids, duration of glucocorticoid therapy, underlying disease, baseline spine BMD, sex/menopausal status, and estrogen use, by testing the interactions between subgroup and treatment group within the ANOVA model. All statistical tests were 2-sided. Subgroup analyses were performed only on the placebo and ALN 5- and 10-mg groups. Statistical comparisons within subgroups of patients were not preplanned and not performed since no treatment-by-subgroup interaction was detected. Moreover, sample sizes were too small to perform meaningful analyses within the various subgroups.

The presence of a treatment effect on the incidence of vertebral fractures was tested using Fisher's exact test after combining the ALN 5-, 10-, and 2.5/10-mg treatment groups.

Changes in radiographic scores of joint damage of the hands from baseline to followup were compared between the pooled 5-, 10-, and 2.5/10-mg ALN group and the placebo treatment group, using the Wilcoxon rank sum test. Patients were classified into the categories "Improvement/No change" or "Worsening," and logistic regression was performed on these data to adjust for any potentially significant differences in confounding variables.

The percentage of patients having 1 or more adverse experiences was compared between treatment groups by sequentially performing the Cochran-Armitage trend test, with no adjustment for multiplicity.

RESULTS

Patient characteristics. Of the 560 patients enrolled, 476 completed the original study. At the end of the first year, 389 were still receiving prednisone, 7.5 mg or equivalent, and were therefore eligible for the 1-year extension. This report presents the findings on the 208 patients who continued in the double-blind extension trial, of whom 166 (80%) completed 2 years. Of the remaining 181 patients who did not participate in the double-blind extension, 97 (54%) were at sites that closed (at the investigator's request due to concerns about continuing patients on masked treatment for an additional year or due to low patient enrollment), 75 (41%) did not provide consent, and 9 (5%) received 10 mg of open-label ALN in year 2.

Overall, the characteristics of the extension cohort were similar to those of the original study cohort, with a few exceptions. Because extension participants were required to be taking a minimum glucocorticoid dose of 7.5 mg/day of prednisone or equivalent, they had, as expected, a higher median daily glucocorticoid dose at 12 months compared with nonparticipants (10 mg versus 7.5 mg, respectively). Extension participants had a lower incidence of serious adverse experiences in year 1 compared with nonparticipants (13.6% versus 19.1%). Patients with underlying gastrointestinal (GI) and pulmonary diagnoses were less common in the extension cohort than in the original study cohort (1.4% versus 7.3% and 7.2% versus 14.6%, respectively), which

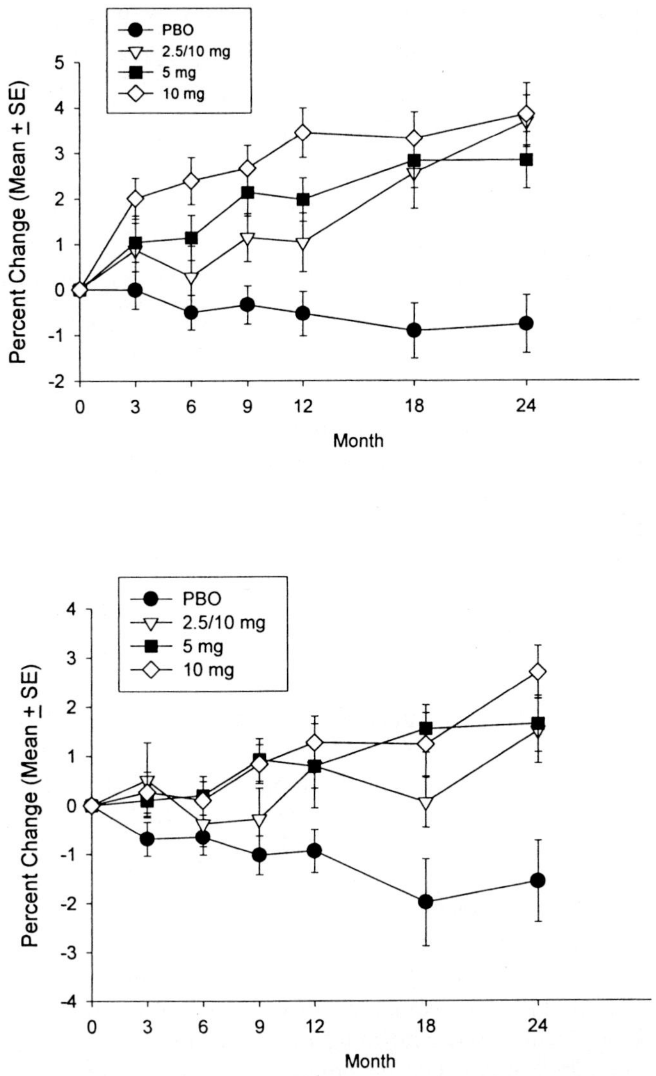

Figure 1. Two-year effects of alendronate (ALN) on bone mineral density (BMD) of the lumbar spine (upper panel) and total hip (lower panel) in patients receiving average daily doses of at least 7.5 mg of prednisone or equivalent. Bars show the mean ± SEM. Lumbar spine BMD increased significantly ($P \leq 0.001$) in all ALN-treated groups. PBO = placebo.

may be a reflection of the lower glucocorticoid doses used to treat these patients. There was no significant difference in the average (among the 3 ALN dose groups of 5, 10, and 2.5/10 mg) percentage gain in lumbar spine BMD observed at the end of year 1 between those who did and did not enter the extension (2.0% versus 2.2%, respectively; $P = 0.642$).

Baseline demographics of the extension cohort are presented in Table 1. There were no significant differences between treatment groups in terms of age,

Table 2. Percentage change in bone mineral density (BMD) from baseline to month 24*

	Lumbar spine		Femoral neck		Trochanter		Total hip		Total body	
Treatment	n	Mean ± SEM %	n	Mean ± SEM %	n	Mean ± SEM %	n	Mean ± SEM %	n	Mean ± SEM %
Placebo	53	−0.77 ± 0.64	53	−2.93 ± 0.86	53	−1.21 ± 0.85	45	−1.57 ± 0.83	40	−0.36 ± 0.45
5 mg ALN	59	2.84 ± 0.62	57	0.11 ± 0.64	57	2.16 ± 0.69	47	1.64 ± 0.57	44	0.77 ± 0.28
10 mg ALN	51	3.85 ± 0.68	51	0.61 ± 0.66	51	3.91 ± 0.71	40	2.69 ± 0.54	41	1.09 ± 0.33
2.5/10 mg ALN	27	3.69 ± 0.57	22	−0.43 ± 0.95	22	1.73 ± 0.73	19	1.50 ± 0.66	19	0.99 ± 0.61

* Patients were randomized to receive either placebo or different doses of alendronate (ALN). BMD at the hip was measured at sites only with Hologic densitometers. Total body BMD was not measured in patients with surgical implants. At any dose of ALN, BMD was increased at the trochanter ($P \leq 0.05$) and maintained at the femoral neck. Total body BMD was increased in patients receiving 5 or 10 mg of ALN ($P \leq 0.01$). These 2 dose levels of ALN were more effective than placebo at all sites ($P \leq 0.05$).

sex/menopausal status, duration of prior glucocorticoid use, daily baseline glucocorticoid dose, and underlying glucocorticoid-requiring illness. The average age of all patients was 54 years; 32% were male. The mean and median glucocorticoid doses at baseline were 20 mg and 10 mg, respectively. Thirty-two percent of patients were new steroid users (<4-month steroid use), 21% were intermediate steroid users (4–12-month history), and 47% were long-term steroid users (>12 months) at baseline. Approximately 70% of patients had underlying rheumatologic conditions, rheumatoid arthritis being the most common diagnosis (38.5%), 11% had dermatologic diagnoses, 7% had pulmonary diseases, and the remainder of patients had a variety of other glucocorticoid-requiring illnesses. Baseline lumbar spine BMD, biochemical markers of bone turnover, and history of morphometric vertebral and nonvertebral fractures were also comparable across treatment groups (Table 1). Approximately 45% of patients had spine BMD values in the normal range at baseline (T-score ≥ −1), 25% had a T-score between −2 and −1, and 30% had a T-score below −2.

The mean daily and cumulative prednisone-equivalent steroid doses at the end of 24 months were 10.1 mg and 9.16 gm, respectively, and there were no apparent differences between treatment groups. Approximately 36% of patients had a history of upper GI disease, including 10.6% with a history of gastric, duodenal, or peptic ulcer. Approximately 54% of patients were taking NSAIDs, including aspirin, and 28.8% received methotrexate during the study, with similar proportions of use in each treatment group.

BMD measurements. BMD of the lumbar spine, total hip (Figure 1 and Table 2), trochanter, and total body (Table 2) increased at 24 months following treatment with 5 or 10 mg ALN, relative both to the change values in the placebo group and to baseline values. The greatest increases occurred within the first year, with smaller increases occurring in the second year, which were significant at the spine and trochanter ($P \leq 0.05$). On average, 84% of patients treated with ALN gained spinal bone mass, compared with 45% receiving placebo. A significant effect on spine BMD relative to that at baseline and to that in the placebo group, which was seen as early as 3 months with 10 mg ALN and 6 months with 5 mg ALN, was sustained over 2 years.

At month 24, there was no significant difference in treatment effect between the 3 dosage regimens of ALN at any site except for the trochanter, in which the 10-mg ALN dose given for 24 months was significantly more effective (mean ± SEM 3.9 ± 0.7% change in BMD) than was the ALN 2.5-mg dose given for 1 year followed by 10 mg ALN in year 2 (1.7 ± 0.7%) ($P < 0.05$). Femoral neck BMD was increased, relative to the change in BMD in patients receiving placebo, in both the 5- and 10-mg ALN groups (Table 2), although there was a small, insignificant loss from year 1 to year 2. Patients receiving placebo continued to lose bone at all sites, most significantly at the femoral neck (average loss was −2.9 ± 0.9% over 2 years, and −1.6 ± 0.54% from year 1 to year 2) ($P \leq 0.01$) (Table 2). BMD results for patients receiving any dose of glucocorticoids were similar to those seen in patients receiving a minimum of 7.5 mg of prednisone or equivalent daily.

As shown in Table 3, in patients receiving 5 mg and 10 mg of ALN, spine BMD significantly increased from baseline, not only in patients receiving glucocorticoids over the long term, but also in patients who had recently started glucocorticoids (<4 months of use); trochanteric BMD also significantly increased (results not shown). In patients who recently started glucocorticoids and were receiving 10 mg ALN, substantial differences from the placebo group were seen in the change in BMD at the spine (6.8%), femoral neck (7.7%), trochanter (9.4%), and total body (2.4%). Smaller differences

Table 3. Subgroup analyses of the mean percentage change in lumbar spine bone mineral density (BMD) from baseline to month 24

	Placebo		Alendronate 5 mg		Alendronate 10 mg	
	n	Mean ± SEM %	n	Mean ± SEM %	n	Mean ± SEM %
Sex/menopausal status + estrogen use*						
Men	17	0.65 ± 1.27	17	4.29 ± 1.02	14	6.29 ± 1.15
Women	36	−1.43 ± 0.71	42	2.25 ± 0.76	37	2.92 ± 0.79
Premenopausal women	11	−0.96 ± 0.97	15	0.75 ± 1.10	12	2.34 ± 1.04
Postmenopausal women						
Receiving estrogen†	7	−3.98 ± 2.33	9	5.36 ± 1.40	7	1.40 ± 2.38
Not receiving estrogen	18	−0.73 ± 0.89	18	1.95 ± 1.24	18	3.91 ± 1.17
Duration of glucocorticoid therapy prior to study*						
Stratum I (<4 months)	16	−2.92 ± 1.16	18	2.01 ± 1.33	18	3.90 ± 1.30
Stratum II (4–12 months)	11	−1.39 ± 1.03	11	4.01 ± 1.42	13	1.97 ± 1.62
Stratum III (>12 months)	26	0.82 ± 0.91	30	2.91 ± 0.78	20	5.02 ± 0.70
Baseline BMD*						
T-score < −2 SD (osteoporotic)‡	13	0.41 ± 1.36	19	3.15 ± 1.33	14	5.02 ± 1.51
T-score ≥ −1 SD (normal)	24	−0.74 ± 0.75	22	2.63 ± 1.06	26	3.39 ± 0.98

* Subgroup-by-treatment interaction not significant.
† Oral or transdermal estrogen therapy used at least 50% of the time during study.
‡ T-score = standard deviations from the mean peak BMD value of sex-matched, healthy, young adults.

were seen with 5 mg ALN; however, no significant difference between the 2 doses was detected.

Increases in spine BMD from baseline were ~2% higher in men than in women ($P \leq 0.01$), but the treatment effect of ALN compared with placebo was similar in both sexes. Consistent with the year 1 findings, postmenopausal women not receiving estrogen and taking 10 mg ALN had a greater increase in spine BMD than did those taking 5 mg (Table 3), although this result was not significant in year 2. The number of postmenopausal women in the subgroup receiving estrogen was too small to draw any clinically meaningful conclusions. However, the data suggest that, overall, women receiving placebo continued to lose bone mass in year 2.

Biochemical markers of bone turnover. Markers of bone formation, i.e., BSAP, and bone resorption, i.e., NTx corrected for creatinine, decreased ~25% and ~60%, respectively ($P \leq 0.05$), on all doses of ALN during the first 48 weeks of therapy, to within the lower normal reference range for premenopausal women. These decreases persisted through 24 months (Figure 2). A small, significant decrease in NTx (−22%) ($P \leq 0.01$ versus baseline) was observed in the placebo group at 24 months, consistent with the 1-year results. No significant changes in BSAP were observed in placebo-treated patients in either year.

Fractures. Approximately 12.5% of patients had a prevalent morphometric vertebral fracture at baseline (Table 1). The incidence of vertebral fractures overall, by time, and by sex and hormonal status may be found in Table 4. The number of vertebral fractures in the study was small, and most occurred in the subgroup of postmenopausal women. By 2 years of followup, the incidence of morphometric vertebral fractures was decreased in the combined ALN 5-, 10-, and 2.5/10-mg treatment group (0.7%) compared with that in the placebo group (6.8%) ($P = 0.026$). No new vertebral fractures occurred in patients treated with any dose of ALN during the second year.

Six (9.8%) of 61 patients and 8 (5.4%) of 147 patients treated with placebo or any dose of ALN, respectively, experienced nonvertebral fractures over 24 months (no significant between-group difference). The incidence of nonvertebral fractures decreased in the combined ALN treatment group from 4.1% in year 1 to 1.4% in year 2, while the incidence in the placebo group remained constant (4.9%) during years 1 and 2. In patients receiving 10 mg ALN for 24 months, no new nonvertebral fractures occurred in the second year of therapy (results not shown).

Joint erosion scores. There were no significant differences between the placebo and ALN treatment groups with respect to the change from baseline in juxtaarticular erosion, joint space narrowing, total radiographic damage scores, or proportion of patients with newly involved areas of joint damage at either month 12

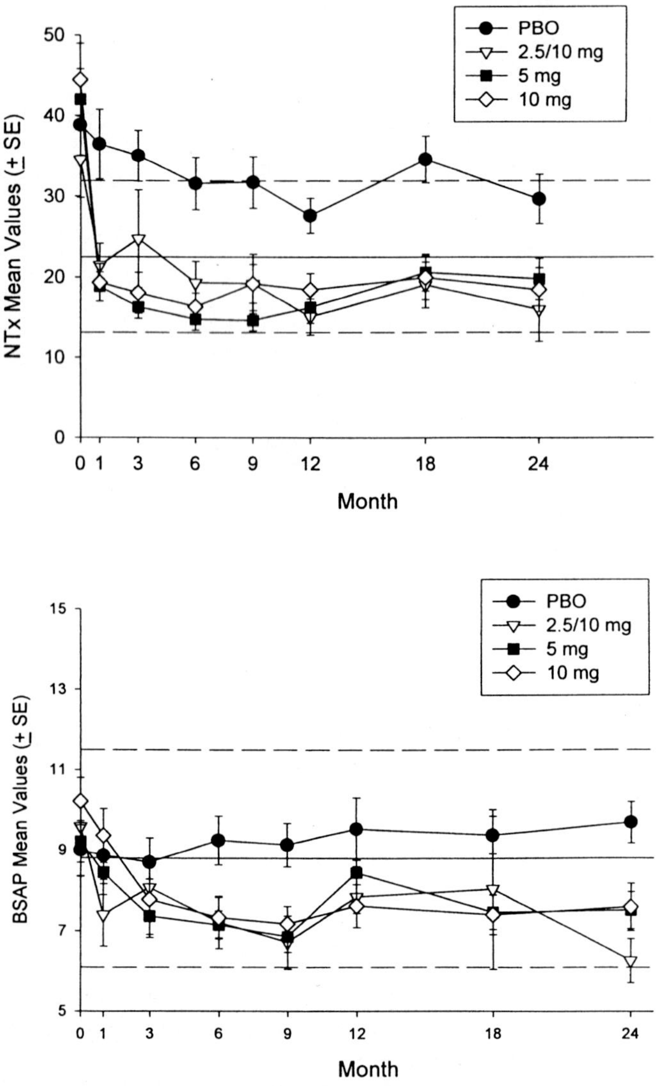

Figure 2. Two-year effects of alendronate on biochemical markers of bone resorption (urine N-telopeptides of type I collagen [NTx]/creatinine in pmoles bone collagen equivalent/μmoles creatinine [upper panel]) and bone formation (bone-specific alkaline phosphatase [BSAP] in ng/ml [lower panel]) in patients receiving average daily doses of at least 7.5 mg of prednisone or equivalent. Bars show the mean ± SEM. The solid horizontal lines indicate the mean reference values for premenopausal women, and the dotted horizontal lines are 1 SD above and below the mean (30–31). PBO = placebo.

or month 24. Similarly, there were no significant differences between groups in the proportions of patients showing a worsening in any of these end points at either time point (results not shown).

Adverse effects. The overall safety profile was similar between treatment groups. No meaningful differences were noted between treatment groups in the overall incidence of adverse experiences or in the incidence of adverse experiences that were considered serious or that led to withdrawal from the study (Table 5).

There was no difference between treatment groups in the extension cohort in the overall incidence of upper GI adverse experiences or in the incidence of upper GI adverse experiences considered serious or that led to withdrawal from the study (Table 5). Three patients treated with placebo experienced a serious upper GI adverse event (2 cases of abdominal pain and 1 case of gastroenteritis), and 1 patient receiving 10 mg ALN experienced a serious gastric ulcer; all events resolved, none were considered drug related, and none resulted in withdrawal from the study. No specific upper GI adverse experience increased in frequency in patients receiving ALN, except for clinical reflux esophagitis, which occurred in 4 (7.3%) of 55 patients receiving 10 mg ALN, compared with 0 of 61 placebo-treated patients. Two of these 4 patients did not have evidence of esophagitis on endoscopy. The other 2 patients, who were not evaluated by endoscopy, had a history of reflux disease or dysphagia. Three of the 4 cases occurred during the first year. None was serious and none resulted in discontinuation of treatment. The relative risk of developing an upper GI adverse experience was similar between patients treated with placebo and those treated with ALN, irrespective of concomitant NSAID/aspirin use.

DISCUSSION

In this randomized, prospective, double-blind, placebo-controlled extension trial, we examined the effect of continuous daily ALN treatment for up to 2 years in the prevention and treatment of bone loss in

Table 4. Incidence of morphometric vertebral fractures at 24 months*

	Placebo	Alendronate
Overall	4/59 (6.8)	1/143 (0.7)†
By time		
Year 1	1/59 (1.7)	1/143 (0.7)
Year 2	3/59 (5.1)	0/143 (0.0)
By sex and hormonal status		
Men	0/19 (0.0)	0/46 (0.0)
Women	4/40 (10.0)	1/97 (1.0)
Premenopausal	1/17 (5.9)	0/35 (0.0)
Postmenopausal	3/23 (13.0)	1/62 (1.6)

* Values are the number of patients with at least 1 morphometric vertebral fracture/number of patients with digitized spine radiographs (%) in the placebo and combined alendronate (5-, 10-, and 2.5/10-mg) groups.
† $P = 0.026$ by Fisher's exact test.

Table 5. Clinical adverse experience profile at 24 months*

	Placebo (n = 61)	ALN 5 mg (n = 63)	ALN 10 mg (n = 55)	ALN 2.5/10 mg (n = 29)
Adverse experience—all	55 (90.2)	59 (93.7)	51 (92.7)	26 (89.7)
Serious adverse experience†	19 (31.1)	14 (22.2)	9 (16.4)	5 (17.2)
Adverse experience leading to withdrawal	3 (4.9)	2 (3.2)	3 (5.5)	1 (3.4)
Upper GI adverse experience	19 (31.1)	13 (20.6)	17 (30.9)	5 (17.2)
Serious upper GI adverse experience†	3 (4.9)	0	1 (1.8)	0
Upper GI adverse experience leading to withdrawal	0	0	1 (1.8)	0
Specific upper GI adverse experiences‡				
Abdominal pain	9 (14.8)	6 (9.5)	4 (7.3)	3 (10.3)
Acid regurgitation	3 (4.9)	1 (1.6)	5 (9.1)	0
Gastritis	2 (3.3)	1 (1.6)	3 (5.5)	1 (3.4)
Nausea	3 (4.9)	3 (4.8)	3 (5.5)	0
Reflux esophagitis	0	0	4 (7.3)§	0

* Values are the no. (%) of patients with 1 or more experience. ALN = alendronate; GI = gastrointestinal.
† Defined as a condition that required or prolonged hospitalization, was fatal, was life threatening, or was diagnosed as cancer.
‡ Incidence of at least 5% in any treatment group.
§ Significant dose-response trend compared with placebo and lower doses of ALN.

patients receiving pharmacologic doses (≥7.5 mg/day) of glucocorticoids for a variety of diseases. A significant and clinically relevant increase in lumbar spine BMD was observed in all groups of patients treated with 5 mg and 10 mg of ALN, relative to baseline and placebo BMD values, after 24 months of treatment, and this was evident as early as 3 months after starting ALN. Trochanteric and total body BMD were also significantly increased during treatment with ALN, and BMD was maintained at the femoral neck. This was true of all groups studied, including men as well as premenopausal and postmenopausal women who were either taking or not taking estrogen replacement therapy. Increases in BMD were greatest within the first year of therapy and continued to increase, albeit at a lesser rate, over the second year. On average, patients who were given 2.5 mg ALN in year 1 showed significant increases in BMD following 10 mg in year 2, confirming the beneficial effects of initiating ALN therapy any time during the course of glucocorticoid treatment. In spite of supplementation with calcium and vitamin D as per the American College of Rheumatology guidelines (22), 70% of patients treated with placebo continued to lose bone (>2% at the spine or hip) over 24 months, suggesting that although this treatment alone is not adequate to maintain bone mass in the majority of patients, it may be effective in some patients.

Treatment with ALN for 2 years was associated with a significant reduction in the proportion of patients who sustained new vertebral fractures, although the number of events overall was small. This reduction was most notable in the subgroup of postmenopausal women, in whom the majority of new vertebral fractures occurred. This is consistent with the fact that the risk of fracture due to glucocorticoids was superimposed on the risk associated with postmenopausal bone loss. Furthermore, during the second year of treatment, no new vertebral fractures occurred in patients treated with any dose of ALN. Consistent with this finding, the incidence of nonvertebral fractures was also lower with ALN relative to placebo, although this difference was not statistically significant. The reduction in the incidence of vertebral and nonvertebral fractures documented in this study is consistent with the magnitude of fracture reductions previously seen after 3 years (12–15) and 1 year (23) of ALN treatment in postmenopausal women with osteoporosis. Of note, this is the first randomized, prospective study to show sustained positive effects (specifically at the spine and trochanter) on the prevention and treatment of glucocorticoid-induced osteoporosis, with a significant effect on prevention of spinal fracture through 2 years.

Although the study was not statistically powered for many of the subgroup analyses (especially for subgroups with small sample sizes), they were undertaken for clinical interest, and in fact, the results generally support what is known from the literature on glucocorticoid use (1,2,24–27). The treatment effect of ALN was consistent in both male and female patients receiving any glucocorticoid dose for any duration, and was also consistent in patients with normal, osteopenic, or osteoporotic baseline spine BMD. Over 2 years, placebo-treated patients recently starting glucocorticoids lost more bone than did placebo-treated patients who had been on a prolonged regimen of glucocorticoids. In contrast, ALN treatment resulted in not only prevention of bone loss, but also substantial increases from baseline in the spine, femoral neck, and trochanter BMD. In other bisphosphonate studies of patients starting glucocorticoids, bone mass was maintained but did not increase; however, these studies used lower doses of calcium (9).

In addition, ALN increased bone mass in postmenopausal women receiving estrogen therapy and in patients receiving adequate doses of supplemental calcium and vitamin D. The consistent effect of ALN in increasing spine and hip BMD relative to both baseline and placebo values in this heterogeneous group of patients, independent of glucocorticoid use, sex, menopausal status, estrogen use, baseline spine BMD, and underlying disease, supports the use of ALN in a wide range of patients who are receiving glucocorticoids.

Overall, ALN was well tolerated in this high-risk, diverse population of patients being treated concurrently with glucocorticoids and NSAIDs, including aspirin. There were no new clinically meaningful adverse experiences identified, and the number of patients who dropped out due to adverse events was similar between treatment groups. Although there was a small increase in upper GI events seen in the first year in the 10-mg group, during the 2 years that the extension cohort was followed up, the GI safety profile was similar between groups, with no significant difference in the incidence of events that were serious or resulted in withdrawal from the study. No specific upper GI adverse experiences were increased in frequency among patients receiving ALN, except for a small increase in clinical reflux esophagitis following treatment with 10 mg of ALN, but this did not result in discontinuation. No effect of ALN treatment on the progression of joint disease in patients with chronic rheumatoid arthritis was observed. These data are consistent with the lack of effect reported following treatment with pamidronate in a study by Eggelmeijer et al (28). It is not known if higher doses or earlier use of ALN would demonstrate an effect on the progression of joint disease in patients with rheumatoid arthritis.

A limitation of the investigation is that it was not originally designed as a 2-year study, but was a 1-year study with a subsequent extension. A second limitation is that 2-year outcomes were not available on patients whose glucocorticoid dose was dropped below 7.5 mg of daily prednisone. However, although there were small differences with regard to disease distribution and serious adverse events, the group of patients in the extension were similar to the original cohort with regard to the relevant baseline measurements of BMD and prevalent vertebral fracture.

In conclusion, within 3 to 6 months of initiating ALN therapy, there were significant increases in BMD at all sites measured, which was maintained over 2 years. Although patients had a relatively low background prevalence of vertebral fractures (12–15%), there was a reduction in the incidence of new vertebral fractures at the end of year 1, which became significant over 2 years in this randomized, double-blind, placebo-controlled extension trial of glucocorticoid-treated patients. Alendronate is therefore an effective and well-tolerated therapy for the prevention and treatment of glucocorticoid-induced osteoporosis.

REFERENCES

1. Lukert BP, Raisz LG. Glucocorticoid-induced osteoporosis: pathogenesis and management. Ann Intern Med 1990;112:352–64.
2. Cooper C, Coupland C, Mitchell M. Rheumatoid arthritis, corticosteroid therapy and hip fracture. Ann Rheum Dis 1995;54:49–52.
3. Hall GM, Daniels M, Doyle DV, Spector TD. Effect of hormone replacement therapy on bone mass in rheumatoid arthritis patients treated with and without steroids. Arthritis Rheum 1994;37:1499–505.
4. Buckley LM, Leib ES, Cartularo KS, Vacek PM, Cooper SM. Calcium and vitamin D3 supplementation prevents bone loss in the spine secondary to low-dose corticosteroids in patients with rheumatoid arthritis: a randomized, double-blind, placebo-controlled trial. Ann Intern Med 1996;125:961–8.
5. Sambrook P, Birmingham J, Kelly P, Kempler S, Nguyen T, Pocock N, et al. Prevention of corticosteroid osteoporosis: a comparison of calcium, calcitriol, and calcitonin. N Engl J Med 1993;328:1747–52.
6. Adachi JD, Bensen WG, Bell MJ, Bianchi FA, Cividino AA, Craig GL, et al. Salmon calcitonin nasal spray in the prevention of corticosteroid-induced osteoporosis. Br J Rheumatol 1997;36:255–9.
7. Reid JR, Alexander CJ, King AR, Ibbertson HK. Prevention of steroid-induced osteoporosis with (3-amino-1-hydroxypropylidene)-1, 1-bisphosphonate (APD). Lancet 1988;8578:143–6.
8. Cohen S, Levy RM, Keller M, Boling E, Emkey RD, Greenwald M, et al. Risedronate therapy prevents corticosteroid-induced bone loss. Arthritis Rheum 1999;42:2309–18.
9. Adachi JD, Bensen WG, Brown J, Hanley D, Hodsman A, Josse R, et al. Intermittent etidronate therapy to prevent corticosteroid-induced osteoporosis. N Engl J Med 1997;337:382–7.
10. Roux C, Oriente P, Laan R, Hughes RA, Ittner J, Goemaere S, et al. Randomized trial of effect of cyclical etidronate in the prevention of corticosteroid-induced bone loss. J Clin Endocrinol Metab 1998;83:1128–33.
11. Amin S, LaValley MP, Simms RW, Felson DT. A meta-analysis

ranking efficacy of treatments for corticosteroid-induced osteoporosis (CSOP) [abstract]. Arthritis Rheum 1998;41 Suppl 9:S137.
12. Liberman UA, Weiss SR, Broll J, Minne HW, Quan H, Bell NH, et al. Effect of oral alendronate on bone mineral density and the incidence of fractures in postmenopausal osteoporosis. N Engl J Med 1995;333:1437–43.
13. Black DM, Cummings SR, Karpf DB, Cauley JA, Thompson DE, Nevitt MC, et al. Randomised trial of effect of alendronate on risk of fracture in women with existing vertebral fractures. Lancet 1996;348:1535–41.
14. Karpf DB, Shapiro DR, Seeman E, Ensrud KE, Johnston CC Jr, Adami S, et al. Prevention of nonvertebral fractures by alendronate: a meta-analysis. JAMA 1997;277:1159–64.
15. Cummings SR, Black DM, Thompson DE, Applegate WB, Barrett-Connor E, Musliner TA, et al. Effect of alendronate on risk of fracture in women with low bone density but without vertebral fractures: results from the Fracture Intervention Trial. JAMA 1998;280:2077–82.
16. Saag KG, Emkey R, Schnitzer TJ, Brown JP, Hawkins F, Goemaere S, et al. Alendronate for the prevention and treatment of glucocorticoid-induced osteoporosis. N Engl J Med 1998;339: 292–9.
17. Gonnelli S, Rottoli P, Cepollaro C, Pondrelli C, Cappiello V, Vagliasindi M, et al. Prevention of corticosteroid-induced osteoporosis with alendronate in sarcoid patients. Calcif Tissue Int 1997;61:382–5.
18. Genant HK, Jergas M, Palermo L, Nevitt M, Valentin RS, Black D, et al. Comparison of semiquantitative visual and quantitative morphometric assessment of prevalent and incident vertebral fractures in osteoporosis. J Bone Miner Res 1996;11:984–96.
19. Sharp JT, Young DY, Bluhm GB, Brook A, Brower AC, Corbett M, et al. How many joints in the hands and wrists should be included in a score of radiologic abnormalities used to assess rheumatoid arthritis? Arthritis Rheum 1985;28:1326–35.
20. Tukey JW, Ciminera JL, Heyse JF. Testing the statistical certainty of a response to increasing doses of a drug. Biometrics 1985;41: 295–301.
21. Capizzi T, Survill TT, Heyse JF, Malani H. An empirical and simulated comparison of some tests for detecting progressiveness of response with increasing doses of a compound. Biometrical Journal 1992;34:275–89.
22. American College of Rheumatology Task Force on Osteoporosis Guidelines. Recommendations for the prevention and treatment of glucocorticoid-induced osteoporosis. Arthritis Rheum 1996;39: 1791–801.
23. Pols HAP, Felsenberg D, Hanley DA. Multinational, placebo-controlled, randomized trial of the effects of alendronate on bone density and fracture risk in postmenopausal women with low bone mass: results of the FOSIT study. Osteoporos Int 1999;9:461–8.
24. Krogsgaard MR, Thamsborg G, Lund B. Changes in bone mass during low dose corticosteroid treatment in patients with polymyalgia rheumatica: a double-blind, prospective comparison between prednisolone and deflazacort. Ann Rheum Dis 1996;55:143–6.
25. Walsh LJ, Wong CA, Pringle M, Tattersfield AE. Use of oral corticosteroids in the community and the prevention of secondary osteoporosis: a cross sectional study. BMJ 1996;313:344–6.
26. Boumpas DT, Chrousos GP, Wilder RL, Cupps TR, Balow JE. Glucocorticoid therapy for immune-mediated diseases: basic and clinical correlates. Ann Intern Med 1993;119:1198–208.
27. Saag KG, Koehnke R, Caldwell JR, Brasington R, Burmeister LF, Zimmerman B, et al. Low dose long-term corticosteroid therapy in rheumatoid arthritis: an analysis of serious adverse events. Am J Med 1994;96:115–23.
28. Eggelmeijer F, Papapoulos SE, van Paassen HC, Dijkmans BAC, Valkema R, Westedt ML, et al. Increased bone mass with pamidronate treatment in rheumatoid arthritis: results of a three-year randomized, double-blind trial. Arthritis Rheum 1996;39:396–402.

APPENDIX A

Members of the Glucocorticoid-Induced Osteoporosis Intervention Extension Study Group are as follows. For the US study, R. D. Emkey, P. Moyer, G. Nuss, D. Rohrbach (Bone Research Center, West Reading, PA); B. Gruber, L. Kaufman, L. Titus, L. Rannazi (University Hospital Medical Center, Stony Brook, NY); N. E. Lane, P. Mroczkowski, C. Merrifield, R. Montanti (The Rosalind Russell Arthritis Research Laboratories, San Francisco, CA); K. G. Saag, R. Koehnke, J. Torner, M. Tullis, R. Wallace (University of Iowa College of Medicine, Iowa City); T. J. Schnitzer, J. A. Block, R. Balius, D. Olejinczak (Northwestern University, Chicago, IL); M. J. Yanover, P. D. Miller, H. Hainault, J. Kennedy (Western Nephrology & Metabolic Bone Disease, P. C., Lakewood, CO); H. McIlwain, J. Silverfield, M. C. Burnette, B. F. Germain, R. Altemose, J. LaPorte, P. Kaufman (Tampa Medical Group, Tampa, FL). For the multinational study, M. O. R. Leite, A. Borelli, E. Arioli, P. H. Correa, L. Galina (Hospital Das Clinicas, Faculdade De Medicina Da Universidade De São Paulo, Brazil); P. D. Delmas, E. Confavreux, C. Hardouin, F. Duboeuf (Hopital Edouard Herriot, Lyon, France); J. M. Kaufman, S. Goemaere, K. Toye, M. De Schepper (Universitaire Ziekenhuizen Gent, Ghent, Belgium); J. Wing, F. J. Raal, C. M. Schnitzler, S. J. Goldburgh, L. Wane, A. Grisillo (Johannesburg Hospital, Parktown, South Africa); R. Correa-Rotter, S. Jasqui, M. Cortés (Instituto Nacional Nutrición Salvador Zubirán, Mexico); R. Westhovens, J. Dequeker, J. Joly, J. Nijs (Universitaire Ziekenhuizen Leuven, Department of Rheumatology, Leuven, Belgium); P. E. E. Poubelle, J. Brown, E. Lejeune, N. Gagné, L. Mailloux (Le Centre Hospitalier Universitaire de Québec, Pavillon CHUL, Quebec, Canada); J. A. Melo-Gomes, R. André-Santos, P. Mateus (Unidade de Reumatologia, Hospital Militar Principal, Lisbon, Portugal); A. Cividino, W. Bensen, M. Gordon, J. Zahavich, L. McMahon (St. Joseph Hospital, Hamilton, Ontario, Canada); K. Siminoski, L. Creasy, N. Gann (Endocrine Centre of Edmonton, Alberta, Canada); J. A. Rodriguez-Portales, V. Cervilla, A. Rojas (Universidad Catolica De Chile, Santiago, Chile); F. Hawkins, L. Morillas, J. M. Padrino, D. Puente (Hospital 12 de Octubre, Madrid, Spain); U. A. Liberman, R. Arie, M. David, N. Katzenelesson, H. Trau, Z. Libman (Tel Aviv University, Petach Tikva, Israel); C.-J. Menkes, C. Cormier, E. Gallimard (Hopital Cochin, Paris, France); E. Seeman, S. M. Mathews (Austin and Repatriation Medical Center, Heidelberg, Australia); M.-P. Malice, T. Dumortier, M. Czachur, W. Carofano, A. Daifotis (Merck & Co., Inc., Rahway, NJ).

ARTHRITIS & RHEUMATISM
Vol. 44, No. 1, January 2001, pp 212–221

Arthritis Prevalence and Activity Limitations in Older Adults

Dorothy D. Dunlop,[1] Larry M. Manheim,[1] Jing Song,[1] and Rowland W. Chang[2]

Objective. **To evaluate the prevalence of arthritis and activity limitations among older Americans by assessing their demographic, ethnic, and economic characteristics.**

Methods. **Data from the Asset and Health Dynamic Survey Among the Oldest Old (AHEAD), a national probability sample of community-dwelling adults born before 1924, were analyzed cross-sectionally. Arthritis that resulted in a physician's visit or a joint replacement not associated with a hip fracture was ascertained by self-report.**

Results. **The prevalence of arthritis in older adults ranged from 25% in non-Hispanic whites to 40% in non-Hispanic blacks to 44% in Hispanics. A higher prevalence of arthritis was associated with less education as well as lower income and less wealth. The prevalence of limitations in activities of daily living (ADL) among non-Hispanic white, non-Hispanic black, and Hispanic adults who reported arthritis only was 29%, 30%, and 37%, respectively, and increased to 48%, 57%, and 56%, respectively, among those reporting arthritis plus other chronic conditions, after adjustment for age and sex.**

Conclusion. **Non-Hispanic black and Hispanic older adults reported having arthritis at a substantially higher frequency than did non-Hispanic whites. In addition, Hispanics reported higher rates of ADL limitations than did non-Hispanic whites with comparable disease burden. Further study is needed to confirm and elucidate the reasons for these racial and economic disparities in older populations.**

Supported by a grant from the Arthritis Foundation and by Multipurpose Arthritis Center grant AM-30692.

[1]Dorothy D. Dunlop, PhD, Larry M. Manheim, PhD, Jing Song, MS: Northwestern University, Evanston, Illinois; [2]Rowland W. Chang, MD, MPH: Northwestern University, Evanston, Illinois, and Northwestern University Medical School, Chicago, Illinois.

Address correspondence and reprint requests to Dorothy D. Dunlop, PhD, Institute for Health Services Research and Policy Studies, Northwestern University, 629 Noyes Street, Evanston, IL 60208.

Submitted for publication May 18, 2000; accepted in revised form September 18, 2000.

This report presents characteristics of older adults with arthritis and rheumatic conditions, hereafter referred to simply as "arthritis," who saw a physician for this condition in the previous year. Data were based on the Asset and Health Dynamic Survey Among the Oldest Old (AHEAD), a national probability sample of older Americans living in the community.

Demographic trends related to the baby boomer generation's approaching the retirement age as well as a decline in the prevalence and severity of fatal conditions over several decades will expose increasing numbers of Americans to diseases of aging (1–4). In addition, major changes in the health care system have created concerns regarding the quality of life among older Americans living with chronic diseases (1,5,6). Arthritis is ranked among the most prevalent chronic conditions in persons ages 65 years and older (7,8). It is also the most prevalent condition for white, black, and Hispanic ethnic groups (9). Arthritis is a leading cause of functional and activity limitations (7,8,10–12). The number of people with arthritis in the US is projected to increase from 15.0% of the 1990 population (37.9 million) to 18.2% (59.4 million) by the year 2020. These projected increases are largely due to the high prevalence rate of arthritis among older persons.

There are socioeconomic and ethnic disparities associated with arthritis. In the general population, the rate of arthritis and associated limitations in activity is higher among persons with low education and income (13–16). Arthritis is also more common among working-age adults with less income and wealth (17). Activity limitations attributable to arthritis are more frequent among blacks compared with whites (13,14). However, there is conflicting information regarding ethnic differences in the prevalence of arthritis. In the general population, whites and blacks are reported to have similar rates of disease (7,8,13,14). In contrast, among adults ages 51–61 years, higher prevalence rates of arthritis are reported for non-Hispanic blacks compared with whites and people of other races (18). Among older adults, which is the group with the highest prevalence rates of arthritis, little is known about the influence of socioeconomic and ethnic characteristics related to this disease.

The AHEAD study provides self-reported information on arthritis in older adults who saw a physician for this condition in the last year. The AHEAD interview asked each participant, "During the last 12 months, have you seen a doctor specifically for arthritis or rheumatism?" This question is designed to identify people who had symptoms severe enough to merit a physician visit for arthritis. The nature of this question in the AHEAD, which focuses on symptomatic arthritis and rheumatic conditions, is designed to obtain highly valid self-report responses. Indeed, it has been shown that the most valid self-reports of arthritis are based on symptomatic conditions (19).

In this study, we obtained information on the prevalence of arthritis by evaluating the demographic, social, ethnic, and economic characteristics of older adults, and compared the activity limitation experience of people with arthritis with that in people reporting other chronic conditions. Understanding the characteristics of older adults with arthritis and the impact of this condition on functional abilities will help policy makers to better target prevention and intervention programs.

POPULATION AND METHODS

Data source. For this analysis, we used 1993 data from the AHEAD, a longitudinal study based on a national probability sample of noninstitutionalized adults ages 70 years and older (born in 1923 or earlier). The objectives of AHEAD include monitoring transitions in physical and functional health in advanced old age and relating changes in health to the use of economic resources (20). The survey collects information on demographics, physical health, functioning, income, earnings, and assets. Of those selected in the multistage sample, 8,222 people participated in the 1993 interviews (an 80.0% response rate), of whom 7,447 were born in 1923 or earlier and an additional 775 were younger spouses/partners. The overall AHEAD sample size is sufficiently large to provide analyses of the oldest old (85 years or older) and includes an oversample of blacks and Hispanics to provide sufficiently large numbers of participants to allow differential examination of the characteristics of these groups in the elderly (21). The present analyses focus on the 7,447 adults who were members of the 1923 or earlier birth cohorts.

Physical health data. At the AHEAD 1993 interview, self-reported information was obtained about each individual's health, including the presence of arthritis and rheumatic conditions and 7 other categories of chronic conditions. A person was considered to have arthritis if an affirmative response was given regarding seeing a doctor within 12 months for arthritis or rheumatism or if a person reported a joint replacement that was not associated with a hip fracture. Participants were also asked whether they currently had diabetes and if they ever had been told by a doctor that they had cancer, a stroke, hypertension, lung disease, or a heart condition (including coronary heart disease, angina, congestive heart failure, heart attack, or other heart disease) or if they had ever seen a doctor for psychiatric problems. This information was used to partition the respondents into 5 health groups based on the report of 1) no chronic conditions, 2) arthritis only, 3) arthritis plus other chronic conditions, 4) 1 chronic condition other than arthritis, or 5) 2 or more chronic conditions other than arthritis.

Demographic data. The AHEAD survey collected demographic information that included marital status (married, divorced, separated, widowed, never married), education (years completed), age, sex, and ethnicity (white/Caucasian, black/African American, Hispanic, other). Ethnicity was used to categorize race into non-Hispanic white, non-Hispanic black, Hispanic, and other.

Economic data. Family income was determined from the income received by the respondent and spouse/partner from the preceding year from all sources. (AHEAD asks respondents about all income received during the previous month from Social Security, Supplemental Security Income, private pensions, labor income, annuities, individual retirement accounts, stocks and bonds, veteran's benefits, food stamps, and other sources.) (22). For respondents who were unable or unwilling to provide exact amounts, the interviewer gave the opportunity to provide an amount within a bracketed category. This information was used to improve imputed income estimates (23). Net assets were evaluated using AHEAD's household net worth category, which summarized the household's tangible wealth in terms of housing equity and nonhousing equity (e.g., savings) (22). Similar procedures were used to impute net assets when a response was not given. The imputed values provided on the public use files were used for cases of missing income and missing net asset data. Health insurance information comprised coverage from Medicare, Medicaid, other government insurance, and private insurance.

Activity limitations. Activity limitations included self-reported functional limitations in basic activities of daily living (ADL) or instrumental activities of daily living (IADL) tasks, and physical activity limitations. ADL limitations included reports of having difficulty or receiving help in the tasks of dressing, toileting, bathing, or eating, and reports of using a device, having difficulty, or receiving help in the tasks of walking across a room or transferring in and out of bed. IADL limitations included reports of having difficulty or receiving help with tasks related to hot meal preparation, shopping, using the telephone, taking medication, or managing money. Functional limitations were further categorized as no limitations or limitations in only IADL, 1–2 ADL, or 3 or more ADL. Limitations related to physical activities included reports of having difficulty with the ability to walk several blocks, climb one flight of stairs, pull/push heavy objects, carry 10 pounds, or pick up a dime.

Statistical analysis. The AHEAD comprises data on a probability sample of the national population. To reflect this population, all analyses were weighted and adjusted for the complex sampling design using SUDAAN software (24), to apply Taylor series methods with between-cluster robust estimation and to provide appropriate statistical tests based on the

Table 1. Self-reported arthritis rates by demographic and economic characteristics in the 1993 Asset and Health Dynamic Survey Among the Oldest Old

Characteristic	Sample size	Estimated population (thousands)*	Unadjusted arthritis rate %	Unadjusted 95% confidence interval	Adjusted arthritis rate† %	Adjusted 95% confidence interval
Women by age group, years						
70–74‡	1,627	4,710	25.99	±2.35	–	
75–79	1,263	3,629	35.02	±3.26	–	
80–84	953	2,702	33.08	±2.51	–	
85+	691	2,015	35.46	±3.54	–	
Men by age group, years						
70–74§	1,170	3,372	20.37	±2.21	–	
75–79	819	2,410	24.47	±3.31	–	
80–84	572	1,381	24.89	±4.67	–	
85+	347	790	24.21	±5.27	–	
Race/ethnicity						
White, non-Hispanic	5,911	17,815	25.89	±1.24	31.89	±2.63
Black, non-Hispanic	1,015	2,114	40.10	±4.63	46.95	±5.33
Hispanic	418	811	44.25	±6.46	52.26	±6.74
Other	98	269	35.63	±12.97	43.40	±13.49
Education, years						
<9	2,088	5,362	34.48	±2.86	40.90	±3.77
9–11	1,270	3,597	30.22	±2.99	36.51	±4.13
12	2,169	6,391	25.76	±1.87	31.79	±3.05
13 or more	1,915	5,659	23.55	±2.23	29.82	±3.64
Health insurance						
Medicare only	1,155	2,924	29.23	±2.83	34.93	±3.86
Medicare + private/government	5,310	15,634	26.34	±1.30	32.44	±2.68
Medicare + Medicaid	742	1,827	43.53	±6.36	48.95	±7.09
Other	235	624	23.51	±5.74	29.40	±6.49
Annual family income						
Less than $7,500	1,471	3,833	35.05	±3.30	39.42	±4.46
$7,500–$14,999	2,106	5,872	30.49	±2.55	35.72	±3.67
$15,000–$29,999	2,324	6,738	25.63	±1.66	31.97	±3.01
$30,000 or more	1,541	4,567	23.08	±2.09	29.88	±3.16
Net assets						
Less than $25,000	1,947	5,139	35.37	±2.96	40.59	±4.13
$25,000–$84,999	1,828	4,950	29.20	±3.04	34.84	±4.00
$85,000 or more	3,667	10,920	24.28	±1.30	30.62	±2.64

* Numbers are rounded to nearest thousand; group totals vary slightly due to rounding error.
† Rates are adjusted for age (70–74, **75–79,** 80–84, 85 years or older) and sex (male, **female**) and are reported for the boldfaced reference categories.
‡ Includes 8 women in the 1923 cohort who were 69 years at the time of the baseline (1993) interview.
§ Includes 9 men in the 1923 cohort who were 69 years at the time of the baseline (1993) interview.

sample size (25). Logistic regression was used to calculate adjusted rates for selected population characteristics. Adjusted rates are given for the median category related to each characteristic. For example, age- and sex-adjusted rates are reported for women (the prevalent sex), and for the age group 75–79 years (the median 5-year age category). Similarly, rates adjusted for socioeconomic status are reported for the median category associated with education, income, and net assets. The estimated logit from these analyses, i.e., logit(p) = $\log_e(p/1 - p) = \underline{b}^T\underline{X}$, was used to obtain estimates of adjusted rates and proportions, i.e., $p = \exp(\underline{b}^T\underline{X})/(1 + \exp(b^T\underline{X})$ (where p is a proportion, $\underline{X}$ is a covariate vector, and $\underline{b}$ is the associated vector of coefficients). The standard error of the adjusted rate, used to calculate the associated confidence interval, was estimated by the delta method (26). Statistical testing was done at a nominal 5% alpha significance level.

RESULTS

Data from responses to the 1993 AHEAD survey were analyzed. A total of 7,442 respondents born in 1923 or earlier provided information regarding the presence or absence of arthritis, and those data were used in these analyses. This sample represented the noninstitutionalized US population of older adults. The population was estimated to have a mean age of 77 years and a median family income of $15,000, and was predominantly non-Hispanic white (84.8%) and female (62.1%) with at least a high school education (58.8%), and almost all had Medicare coverage (97.0%).

Table 1 provides prevalence rates of self-reported

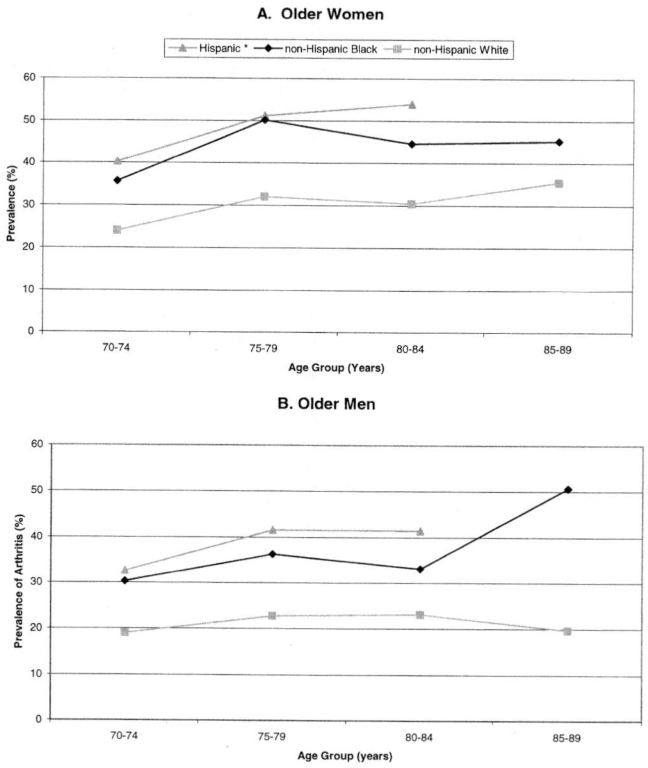

Figure 1. Unadjusted arthritis prevalence rates by age and sex (**A**, older women and **B**, older men) among 3 ethnic categories. * = insufficient sample size to estimate rate for the 85–89-year age group.

arthritis by demographic and economic characteristics. The prevalence of arthritis increased with age (from 24% for ages 70–74 years to 32% for ages 85 years or older) and was greater in women (31%) than in men (23%). The age/sex-adjusted arthritis prevalence rates indicated that non-Hispanic blacks and Hispanics reported higher rates of arthritis than did non-Hispanic white older adults. It is also evident from the age/sex-adjusted rates that arthritis was more prevalent among people with lower levels of education, lower levels of income, and lower net assets. In addition, the distribution of arthritis by health insurance coverage reflects the socioeconomic disparities in prevalence rates. Arthritis was more prevalent among people who received Medicaid plus Medicare coverage compared with people with only Medicare coverage or other supplemental coverage.

Figure 1 shows arthritis prevalence rates by age and sex for non-Hispanic white, non-Hispanic black, and Hispanic ethnic groups. Among women (Figure 1A), it is evident that the arthritis prevalence rates among non-Hispanic black and Hispanic women were more than 50% greater compared with the rates in non-Hispanic white women for the 70–74-year age group (i.e., non-Hispanic black 36% and Hispanic 40% versus non-Hispanic white 24%) and remained up to 25% higher for the over-80 age groups. Although prevalence rates of arthritis were lower among men compared with women of similar age, the same ethnic trends are evident among men. The arthritis prevalence rates for non-Hispanic black and Hispanic men (Figure 1B) were ~50% greater than the rates in non-Hispanic white men across all age groups.

Racial disparities in health related to differences in socioeconomic status are well known (27–29). Since racial disparities in disease rates can reflect socioeconomic differences between ethnic groups, we also estimated arthritis prevalence rates after adjusting for education, family income, and net assets, and the results are shown in Figure 2. Comparing the socioeconomic

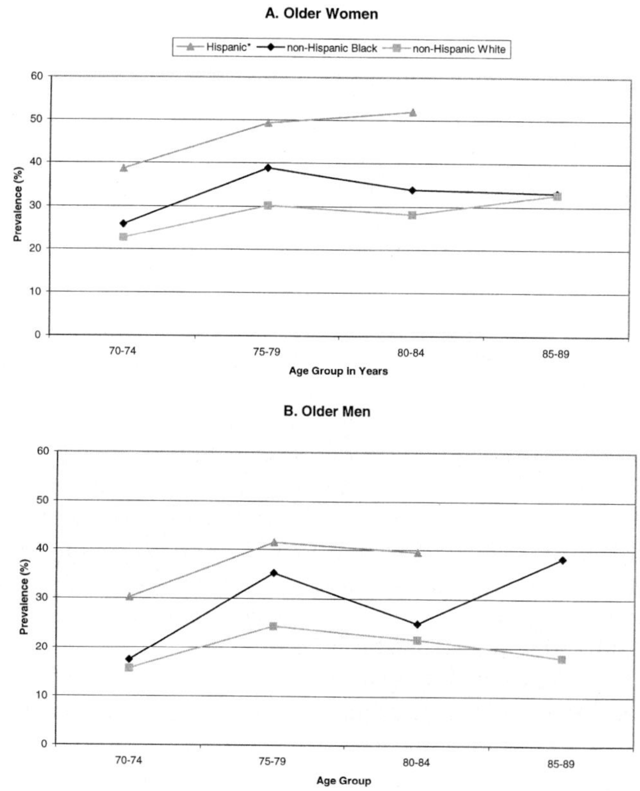

Figure 2. Arthritis prevalence rates by age and sex (**A**, older women and **B**, older men) among 3 ethnic categories adjusted for socioeconomic factors (education <9, 9–11, 12, and ≥13 years; family income <$7,500, $7,500–$14,999, $15,000–$29,999, and ≥$30,000; net assets <$25,000, $25,000–$84,000, and ≥$85,000). Data on the group with 12 years of education, family income between $7,500 and $14,999, and net assets between $25,000 and $84,999 are reported. * = insufficient sample size to estimate rate for the 85–89-year age group.

Table 2. Activity limitation rates by arthritis/chronic condition status*

	Self-reported arthritis							
	Arthritis only (N = 1,102,922) (n = 399)				Arthritis plus other chronic conditions (N = 4,811,697) (n = 1,752)			
	Mean age, years	% female	Unadjusted	Adjusted†	Mean age, years	% female	Unadjusted	Adjusted†
Demographic	78.06	69.62	–	–	78.03	69.32	–	–
Functional limitations								
None			54.01 (±5.87)	63.14 (±10.20)			41.89 (±2.85)	44.17 (±4.25)
IADL only			7.57 (±2.39)	6.61 (±4.70)			7.39 (±1.38)	5.80 (±1.90)
1–2 ADL			28.34 (±4.74)	22.69 (±9.80)			32.28 (±2.49)	32.42 (±4.00)
3+ ADL			10.07 (±3.06)	7.46 (±6.21)			18.44 (±1.85)	17.43 (±2.75)
Physical limitations								
Walk several blocks			43.14 (±5.34)	38.93 (±8.45)			61.32 (±2.60)	61.17 (±4.93)
Climb one flight of stairs			36.17 (±5.33)	35.74 (±8.92)			50.93 (±2.54)	53.60 (±4.84)
Pull/push heavy objects			40.83 (±5.67)	48.36 (±10.80)			58.93 (±1.94)	65.61 (±4.79)
Carry 10 pounds			39.85 (±5.63)	42.69 (±12.49)			55.67 (±2.69)	63.00 (±4.48)
Pick up dime			10.77 (±2.81)	11.90 (±7.18)			16.26 (±2.51)	13.64 (±3.08)

* Values for unadjusted and adjusted rates are the % of subjects (95% confidence interval). N = estimated population; n = sample size; IADL = instrumental activities of daily living; ADL = activities of daily living.
† Rates are adjusted for age (70–74, **75–79,** 80–84, 85 years or older) and sex (male, **female**) and are reported for the boldfaced reference categories.

status–adjusted rates in Figure 2 with the unadjusted rates in Figure 1, it is evident that the adjusted rates in the non-Hispanic black and non-Hispanic white populations are closer than are the unadjusted rates, for both women and men. These graphs indicate that the disparity in non-Hispanic black and non-Hispanic white arthritis prevalence rates is partly eliminated for older women (Figure 2A) and older men (Figure 2B) by adjusting for socioeconomic factors. However, as shown in Figure 2, even after accounting for socioeconomic factors, no moderating effect on the high prevalence rates among Hispanics compared with non-Hispanic whites is evident for either women or men. In additional analyses (data not shown), we found that arthritis prevalence rates in non-Hispanic black and Hispanic older adults were significantly higher than those in non-Hispanic white older adults even after adjustment for age, sex, and socioeconomic factors. These findings indicate that socioeconomic differences do not adequately account for the ethnic disparities found in the prevalence of arthritis among older adults.

Table 2 shows the distribution of the activity limitation characteristics of older adults with and without arthritis. People with arthritis were divided into 2 groups: those for whom arthritis was the only reported chronic condition and those reporting arthritis plus at least 1 other chronic condition. People without arthritis were divided into 3 groups based on the report of no chronic conditions, 1 chronic condition, and 2 or more chronic conditions. There were differences in the distribution of age and sex across the 5 chronic condition groups, with the highest proportions of women found in the 2 arthritis groups, while people reporting no chronic conditions were younger. For this reason, the age/sex-adjusted rates and the associated confidence intervals are provided to allow a comparison across the 5 chronic condition groups.

As seen in Table 2, activity limitations were much greater among people with arthritis than in people without arthritis. People with arthritis were more likely to report some functional limitation (arthritis only 37%, arthritis plus other conditions 56%) compared with people without arthritis who had similar chronic disease burden (1 other condition 22%, multiple other condi-

Table 2. *(Cont'd)*

Self-reported chronic conditions other than arthritis								No chronic conditions			
One condition (N = 5,496,515) (n = 1,922)				Multiple conditions (N = 5,778,888) (n = 2,031)				None reported (N = 3,818,952) (n = 1,338)			
Mean age, years	% female	Unadjusted	Adjusted†	Mean age, years	% female	Unadjusted	Adjusted†	Mean age, years	% female	Unadjusted	Adjusted†
77.29	58.99	–	–	77.29	58.39	–	–	77.20	61.17	–	–
		71.49	77.79			56.33	57.98			75.48	77.47
		(±2.46)	(±5.09)			(±1.87)	(±4.20)			(±2.66)	(±4.97)
		11.35	9.40			11.49	9.24			9.90	11.34
		(±1.63)	(±3.17)			(±1.54)	(±2.59)			(±2.05)	(±4.46)
		12.19	10.36			19.74	20.06			10.75	8.65
		(±1.40)	(±3.00)			(±1.61)	(±3.43)			(±2.00)	(±3.88)
		4.97	2.08			12.45	12.81			3.86	2.36
		(±0.98)	(±1.37)			(±1.55)	(±3.69)			(±1.10)	(±1.97)
		28.56	27.24			47.68	49.14			18.94	17.51
		(±1.91)	(±4.90)			(±2.47)	(±5.48)			(±2.11)	(±4.52)
		19.74	17.96			36.92	39.32			14.90	13.58
		(±2.23)	(±3.71)			(±1.93)	(±4.77)			(±2.22)	(±4.18)
		27.87	31.68			46.33	54.77			22.10	26.18
		(±2.43)	(±4.95)			(±2.88)	(±5.90)			(±2.26)	(±6.28)
		24.69	25.78			41.53	49.62			18.10	21.62
		(±1.99)	(±4.43)			(±1.88)	(±5.03)			(±1.50)	(±4.53)
		4.62	3.43			9.70	7.58			4.01	3.32
		(±1.10)	(±1.65)			(±1.33)	(±2.45)			(±1.18)	(±2.22)

tions 42%), based on the adjusted rates. This pattern of higher limitation rates among people with arthritis compared with those without is also evident among all the physical activities evaluated. The adjusted limitation rates for people with arthritis, in walking several blocks, climbing stairs, pulling/pushing heavy objects, carrying 10 pounds, or picking up a dime, were greater than the rates for similar people without arthritis. For example, older adults with arthritis were more likely to report limitation in walking several blocks (arthritis only 39%, arthritis plus other conditions 61%) than were people without arthritis who reported similar chronic disease burden (1 other condition 27%, multiple conditions 49%) or no chronic conditions (18%), based on the adjusted rates.

Recognizing that there were higher rates of arthritis among non-Hispanic blacks and Hispanics compared with non-Hispanic whites, and higher rates of ADL limitations among people with arthritis compared with people not reporting arthritis, it was of interest to see if there were differential rates of ADL limitations among ethnic groups within the 5 chronic disease categories. Figure 3A shows the percentages of ADL limitations by ethnicity for each of the 5 chronic disease groups, adjusted for age and sex. Percentages adjusted for age, sex, education, income, and net assets are shown in Figure 3B. Socioeconomic status had no appreciable impact on the ADL limitation differences across the chronic condition and ethnic groups.

Several features should be noted about the data shown in Figure 3. First, across all ethnic groups, the rates of ADL limitations increased with the presence of arthritis and the presence of chronic conditions, with the highest rates of ADL limitations being among older people with arthritis and other chronic conditions. Specifically, in Figure 3A, the rate of ADL limitations among non-Hispanic white, non-Hispanic black, and Hispanic adults reporting no arthritis or chronic conditions was 10%, 12%, and 17%, respectively, but among people reporting *only* arthritis, the corresponding rates increased to 29%, 30%, and 37%, respectively, and further increased among those reporting arthritis *plus* other chronic conditions, to 48%, 57%, and 56%, respectively, after adjustment for age and sex. Also, these rates among people with arthritis were higher compared with those in people with similar chronic disease burden but *not* reporting arthritis.

Second, Figure 3A shows that some of the ethnic differences in ADL limitation rates are related to arthritis/chronic condition status. Similar age/sex-adjusted rates of ADL limitations among persons reporting only arthritis were found for non-Hispanic

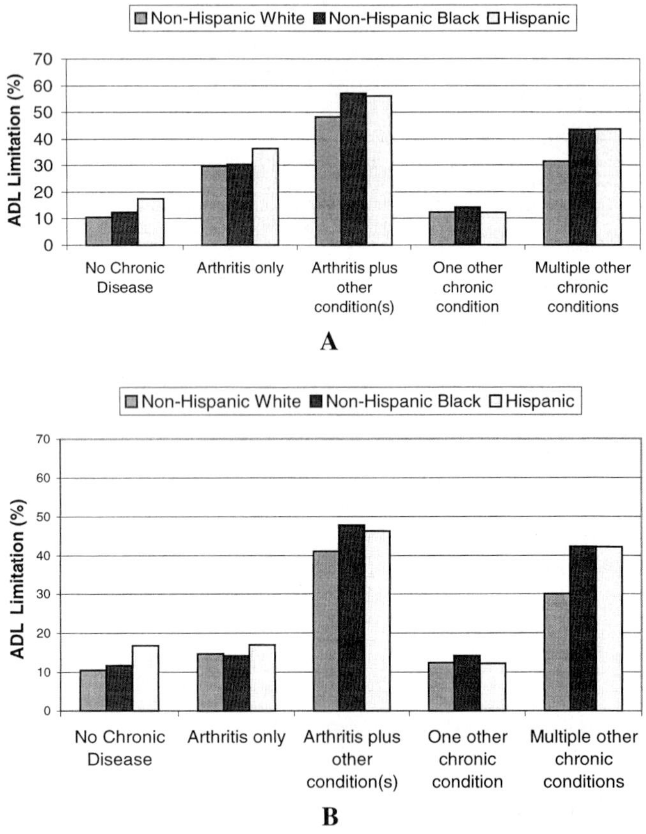

Figure 3. Rates of limitation in activities of daily living (ADL) by ethnicity and chronic condition status adjusted for **A,** age and sex, and **B,** age, sex, and socioeconomic factors. See Figures 1 and 2 for age and socioeconomic factor categories. Data on the 75–79-year female age group are reported in **A.** Data on the 75–79-year female age group with 12 years of education, family income between $7,500 and $14,999, and net assets between $25,000 and $84,999 are reported in **B.**

blacks (30%) and non-Hispanic whites (29%). In contrast, non-Hispanic blacks reported higher adjusted ADL limitation rates (57%) than did non-Hispanic whites (48%) among people reporting arthritis *plus* other chronic conditions. Likewise, among people with multiple chronic conditions but *not* reporting arthritis, non-Hispanic blacks had higher adjusted ADL limitation rates (44%) than did non-Hispanic whites (31%), but both ethnic groups had similar rates among people with only 1 chronic condition unrelated to arthritis (14% versus 12%, respectively). This suggests that the higher age/sex-adjusted rates of ADL limitations experienced by non-Hispanic blacks compared with non-Hispanic whites with arthritis are largely due to comorbidity.

Finally, it should be noted that ethnic differences remained after adjusting the ADL rates for socioeconomic status, age, and sex (Figure 3B). This indicates that socioeconomic factors do not explain the observed ethnic disparities found in the frequency of ADL limitations.

DISCUSSION

The purpose of this study was to evaluate the prevalence of arthritis among older Americans by assessing their demographic, social, ethnic, and economic characteristics, and to describe the activity limitation experience of older adults with and without arthritis. Our study is unique in that it uses data from the AHEAD cohort, which has sufficient numbers of non-Hispanic black and Hispanic older adults to compare these ethnic groups. In addition, AHEAD is based on a national probability sample, which allows findings to be generalized to the US population of older adults. This study shows ethnic differences in arthritis prevalence rates as well as ethnic differences in the frequency of ADL limitations among older people with arthritis and other chronic conditions.

Ethnic differences were found in the arthritis prevalence rates among older adults. Twenty-five percent of non-Hispanic white, 40% of non-Hispanic black, and 44% of Hispanic older adults reported seeing a doctor for arthritis in the previous year. After adjustment for age and sex, arthritis prevalence rates among non-Hispanic blacks and Hispanics in this study were more than 50% higher than among non-Hispanic whites. The finding of higher arthritis prevalence rates among non-Hispanic blacks compared with non-Hispanic whites based on the 1993 AHEAD data is in contrast to the findings of Lawrence and colleagues (14), which were based on the 1989–1991 National Health Interview Survey (NHIS). Their data showed almost identical age-adjusted arthritis prevalence rates for blacks compared with whites and lower rates among Hispanics compared with non-Hispanics.

There are a number of issues that may contribute to the differences in our findings of ethnic disparity from the AHEAD data compared with the findings in the NHIS data. First, the arthritis prevalence rates from AHEAD were based on adults older than 70 years of age, while the age-adjusted rates reported by Lawrence and colleagues were based on the general population over 15 years of age. However, age-specific rates for people over age 65 based on the 1991–1993 NHIS also showed a similar prevalence of arthritis for blacks and whites (7), which suggests that differences in the range of ages surveyed is an inadequate explanation. A second potential difference is the years of the survey: 1989–1991 for the NHIS versus 1993 for the AHEAD survey. However, since the 1991–1993 NHIS rates showed trends that were similar to the 1989–1991 NHIS rates (7,13), the year of the surveys does not seem to be a contributing factor.

A third issue is differences in defining the ethnic groups. The prevalence rates reported from the AHEAD data were based on 3 mutually exclusive groups: non-Hispanic whites, non-Hispanic blacks, and Hispanics. The study by Lawrence and colleagues gave NHIS rates for whites versus blacks, both of which include Hispanics, and also for Hispanics versus non-Hispanics. However, age/sex-adjusted arthritis prevalence rates from the 1989–1991 NHIS, which used mutually exclusive ethnic groups, showed lower arthritis prevalence rates for Hispanics (11.2%) compared with non-Hispanic whites (15.5%) and non-Hispanic blacks (15.4%) (30). These NHIS findings are in direct contrast to the much higher arthritis prevalence rates found among Hispanics and non-Hispanic blacks compared with non-Hispanic whites in AHEAD.

Fourth, the sampling frames of the studies are different. In particular, the NHIS oversampled blacks but not Hispanics, while AHEAD oversampled blacks and Hispanics. However, the major advantage of oversampling Hispanics is to have sufficient numbers for statistical comparisons. Since the variances in the age/sex-adjusted NHIS arthritis rates were small enough to detect statistical differences related to lower arthritis prevalence rates among Hispanics compared with other ethnic groups, the NHIS Hispanic sample size is not problematic for this question.

A more relevant issue related to the ethnic disparities between the populations in the AHEAD and NHIS surveys is the question used to solicit the self-report of arthritis. The AHEAD monitors self-reports of arthritis for which a person visited a physician in the past 12 months, while the NHIS collects self-reports of arthritis within the preceding 12 months. The difference in the questions is evident in the lower arthritis prevalence rates captured by the AHEAD (29% overall for adults ages 70 years or above) compared with the rates from the the NHIS (43% and 55% overall for adults ages 65–74 years and 75 years or above, respectively) (7). These lower arthritis prevalence rates in the AHEAD compared with the NHIS are consistent with the report that ~16% of Americans who report arthritis never see a doctor for the problem (31). Recall bias may be a contributing factor to lower rates of self-reported arthritis-related physician visits versus self-reported arthritis. Alternatively, the AHEAD report of arthritis that is associated with a physician visit may capture more severe arthritis than would the self-report of arthritis in the NHIS. If the prevalence of self-reported arthritis is similar in whites and blacks, as shown by the NHIS, but the severity of disease in blacks is greater, one would expect a larger proportion of black adults to report arthritis-related physician visits, which is consistent with the AHEAD data.

The finding of higher arthritis prevalence rates among non-Hispanic blacks compared with non-Hispanic whites is compatible with the findings of Kingston and Smith (18), who based their study on the 1992 Health and Retirement Survey (HRS) of older adults ages 51–61 years. Their results showed that non-Hispanic blacks were more likely to report arthritis than were non-Hispanic whites. Also, similar to our findings, they reported that controlling for socioeconomic factors reduced the disparity in arthritis prevalence rates between these 2 groups. However, in contrast to our AHEAD findings, the HRS data showed similar rates of arthritis reported among Hispanics and non-Hispanic whites. Our finding of higher rates of self-reported arthritis among Hispanics compared with non-Hispanic whites may reflect our evaluation of an older cohort (70 years or older). Alternatively, it may reflect differences related to the HRS instrument, which inquired if respondents *ever had* or were told by a doctor that they had arthritis. The AHEAD question, which solicits information on arthritis only if associated with a physician's visit, may capture more severe arthritis, as noted above.

Across all ethnic groups, the rates of ADL limitations increased with the presence of arthritis and the presence of other chronic conditions, with the highest rates of ADL limitations being among older people with arthritis and other chronic conditions. However, additional ethnic differences were found with regard to ADL limitation rates and chronic condition groups. Similar rates of ADL limitations were found for non-Hispanic blacks and non-Hispanic whites among persons reporting arthritis only. In contrast, non-Hispanic blacks reported higher ADL limitation rates than did non-Hispanic whites among people reporting arthritis *plus* other chronic conditions. Likewise, for people *not* reporting arthritis, non-Hispanic blacks reported higher ADL limitation rates than did non-Hispanic whites among people with multiple chronic conditions, but reported similar rates among people with only 1 chronic condition. This suggests that the higher rates of ADL limitations experienced by non-Hispanic blacks compared with non-Hispanic whites with arthritis are largely due to comorbidity. In addition, it is notable that adjusting for socioeconomic status resulted in *similar* ethnic differences within arthritis/chronic disease groups related to ADL limitations.

Findings from other studies that have shown higher rates of activity limitations for blacks versus whites attributable to arthritis do not provide related comorbidity information (3,14). Our findings indicate that ethnicity and other chronic conditions may interact in relation to the rate of functional limitations among older adults with arthritis. These results point to the importance of further investigation of ethnic differences in older adults and the role that arthritis may play in concert with other chronic conditions in relation to functional limitations.

Finally, the AHEAD data indicate that the prevalence rates of arthritis are associated with socioeconomic factors in older adults. The prevalence rates of arthritis increased among older adults with less education, less income, and fewer net assets. These findings are similar to other evaluations of socioeconomic factors in the general population (13–16). They are also compatible with the observations of Yelin (17), who showed that based on the HRS data, persons ages 51–61 years with musculoskeletal conditions and comorbidity reported lower family income and fewer assets than the average values for these factors. Recent reports based on national probability surveys show different socioeconomic effects on the relationship between race and arthritis prevalence. Findings from the 1992 HRS data showed a higher age/sex-adjusted prevalence of arthritis for blacks and a similar adjusted prevalence of arthritis for Hispanics compared with whites/others among adults ages 51–61 (18). Further adjustment for wealth, education, and income resulted in lower arthritis prevalence rates for both blacks and Hispanics compared with whites/others. A report based on the 1993 AHEAD data also showed higher arthritis prevalence rates for blacks compared with whites (22). However, consistent with our findings, controlling for socioeconomic status reduced, but did not eliminate, the higher arthritis prevalence rates reported among blacks compared with whites. Our findings and these reports indicate that differences in socioeconomic factors may attenuate, but do not entirely account for, the observed differences in arthritis prevalence among ethnic groups.

Several limitations of this study should be noted. First, this evaluation uses cross-sectional data. Longitudinal studies are needed to further evaluate the impact of ethnic and socioeconomic factors on the occurrence of arthritis in older adults. Second, attribution of activity limitations to particular chronic conditions was not ascertained by the AHEAD survey. Third, the AHEAD relies on self-reported as opposed to physician-confirmed diagnoses of arthritis and rheumatism. The presence of arthritis was defined on the basis of self-reported physician contacts for arthritis and rheumatic conditions. This approach assumes that individuals had symptoms of arthritis (e.g., pain, swelling, stiffness, limitation) severe enough to seek care for this problem from a physician. Prior studies indicate that the most reliable self-reports of arthritis are associated with symptomatic conditions (19). Furthermore, people who see a physician tend to have more activity limitations than those who do not see a physician (31). Whether or not one visits a physician can be related to one's level of income, education, and insurance coverage. In this population of people 70 years of age or older, essentially all had health insurance through Medicare, and we controlled for the remaining socioeconomic factors in assessing differences across ethnic groups. A relevant question is whether racial disparities are adequately represented using a definition of arthritis related to a physician visit, since other factors (e.g., a regular source of medical care, Medigap policy, social support) may influence seeing a physician. However, if an ethnic group receives sporadic health care due to access barriers, medical care is more likely to be pursued for acute, rather than chronic, problems, resulting in an under-report of arthritis. In this situation, further adjustment for such differences would show even greater ethnic disparity.

Despite these limitations, this study extends our understanding of arthritis in older adults in several ways. First, it indicates that there are ethnic disparities related to the prevalence of arthritis among older adults. The finding of higher rates of self-reported arthritis for which an older adult sees a physician among non-Hispanic blacks and Hispanics compared with non-Hispanic whites suggests that arthritis may be more severe in those ethnic groups. In addition this is the first study, to our knowledge, to use recent population-based data to report higher arthritis prevalence rates among Hispanics compared with non-Hispanic white older adults. Second, our findings show higher rates of ADL limitations among Hispanics compared with similar non-Hispanic white older adults who see a physician for arthritis. Third, this study indicates that ethnicity and comorbidity may interact in relation to the rate of functional limitations among older adults with arthritis. These findings point to the need for further study to confirm and elucidate the reasons for these racial disparities in elderly populations.

ACKNOWLEDGMENT

The authors thank Alan Dyer, PhD for his comments.

REFERENCES

1. Manton KG, Stallard E, Corder L. The dynamics of dimensions of age-related disability 1982 to 1994 in the U.S. elderly population. J Gerontol 1998;53a:B59–65.
2. Crimmins EM, Hayward MD, Saito Y. Changing mortality and morbidity rates and the health status and life expectancy of the older population. Demography 1994;31:159–75.
3. Crimmins EM, Saito Y, Reynolds SL. Further evidence on recent trends in the prevalence and incidence of disability among older Americans from two sources: the LSOA and the NHIS. J Gerontol B Psychol Sci Soc Sci 1997;52B:S59–71.
4. Manton KG, Corder L, Stallard E. Chronic disability trends in elderly United States populations: 1982–1994. Proc Nat Acad Sci U S A 1997;94:2593–8.
5. Manheim LM. Managed care and arthritis care: patients and providers under the new medical care organizations. Arthritis Care Res 1995;8:298–303.
6. Guralnik JM, Fried LP, Salive ME. Disability as a public health outcome in the aging population. Annu Rev Public Health 1996; 17:25–46.
7. Collins JG. Prevalence of selected chronic conditions. Vital Health Stat 10 1997;194:1–89.
8. Centers for Disease Control and Prevention. Prevalence and impact of arthritis by race and ethnicity, United States, 1996. MMWR 1996;45:373–8.
9. Centers for Disease Control and Prevention. Impact of arthritis and other rheumatic conditions on the health-care system. MMWR 1999;48:349–52.
10. Centers for Disease Control and Prevention. Prevalence and impact of chronic joint symptoms—seven states, United States, 1996. MMWR 1998;47:345–50.
11. Yelin E. Arthritis: the cumulative impact of a common chronic condition. Arthritis Rheum 1992;35:489–97.
12. Verbrugge LM, Lepkowski JM, Konkol LL. Comorbidity and its impact on disability. Milbank Q 1989;67:450–84.
13. Centers for Disease Control and Prevention. Arthritis prevalence and activity limitations, United States, 1990. MMWR 1994;43: 433–8.
14. Lawrence RC, Helmick CG, Arnett FC, Deyo RA, Felson DT, Giannini EH, et al. Estimates of the prevalence of arthritis and selected musculoskeletal disorders in the United States. Arthritis Rheum 1998;41:778–99.
15. Helmick CG, Lawrence RC, Pollard RA, Lloyd E, Heyse SP, for the National Arthritis Data Workgroup. Arthritis and other rheumatic conditions: who is affected now, who will be affected later? Arthritis Care Res 1995;8:203–11.
16. US Department of Health and Human Services. Arthritis, Osteoporosis, and Chronic Back Conditions. Healthy People 2010 (conference edition, vol. 1). Washington DC: US Department of Health and Human Services; 2000.
17. Yelin E. The earnings, income and assets of persons aged 51–61 with and without musculoskeletal conditions. J Rheumatol 1997; 24:2024–30.
18. Kingston RS, Smith JP. Socioeconomic status and racial and ethnic differences in functional status associated with chronic diseases. Am J Public Health 1997;87:805–10.
19. Hughes SL, Edelman P, Naughton B, Singer RH, Schuette P, Liang G, et al. Estimates and determinants of valid self-reports of musculoskeletal disease in the elderly. J Aging Health 1993;5: 244–63.
20. Herringa SG. Technical description of the Asset and Health Dynamics Among the Oldest Old (AHEAD) study sample design. Ann Arbor (MI): Population Studies Center; 1995. HRS Documentation Report DR-003.
21. Soldo BJ, Hurd MD, Rodgers WL, Wallace RB. Asset and Health Dynamics Among the Oldest Old: an overview of the AHEAD study. J Gerontol B Psychol Sci Soc Sci 1997;52B:1–20.
22. Schoenbaum M, Waidmann T. Race, socioeconomic status, and health: accounting for racial differences in health. J Gerontol B Psychol Sci Soc Sci 1997;52B:61–73.
23. Smith J. Wealth inequality among older Americans. J Gerontol B Psychol Sci Soc Sci 1997;52B:74–81.
24. Shah BV, Barnwell BG, Bieler GS. SUDAAN user's manual release 7.5. Research Triangle Park (NC): Research Triangle Institute; 1997.
25. Williams R. A note on variance estimation for cluster-correlated data. Biometrics 2000;56:218–9.
26. Tamhane AC, Dunlop DD. Statistics and data analysis. Upper Saddle River (NJ): Prentice-Hall; 2000.
27. Menchik PL. 1993. Economic status as a determinant of mortality among black and white older men: does poverty kill? Popul Stud 1993;47:427–36.
28. Furner SE. 1992. Chartbook on health data on older Americans: United States, 1992. Vital Health Stat 3 1992;29:37–56.
29. Manton KG, Patrick CH, Johnson KW. Health differentials between blacks and whites: recent trends in mortality and morbidity. Milbank Q 1987;87:129–99.
30. Centers for Disease Control and Prevention. Prevalence and impact of arthritis by race and ethnicity—United States 1989–1991. MMWR 1996;45:273–8.
31. Rao JK, Callahan LF, Helmick CG. Characteristics of persons with self-reported arthritis and other rheumatic conditions who do not see a doctor. J Rheumatol 1997;24:169–73.

ARTHRITIS & RHEUMATISM
Vol. 44, No. 1, January 2001, pp 222–230

Alpha Sleep Characteristics in Fibromyalgia

Suely Roizenblatt,[1] Harvey Moldofsky,[2] Ana Amelia Benedito-Silva,[1] and Sergio Tufik[1]

Objective. **To characterize the patterns of alpha electroencephalographic sleep and their associations with pain and sleep in patients with fibromyalgia.**

Methods. **Pain and sleep symptoms of 40 female patients with fibromyalgia and 43 healthy control subjects were studied before and after overnight polysomnography. Blinded analyses of alpha activity in non–rapid eye movement (non-REM) sleep were performed using time domain, frequency domain, and visual analysis techniques.**

Results. **Three distinct patterns of alpha sleep activity were detected in fibromyalgia: phasic alpha (simultaneous with delta activity) in 50% of patients, tonic alpha (continuous throughout non-REM sleep) in 20% of patients, and low alpha activity in the remaining 30% of patients. Low alpha activity was exhibited by 83.7% of control subjects ($P < 0.01$). All fibromyalgia patients who displayed phasic alpha sleep, activity reported worsening of pain after sleep, compared with 58.3% of patients with low alpha activity ($P < 0.01$) and 25.0% of patients with tonic alpha activity ($P < 0.01$). Postsleep increase in the number of tender points occurred in 90.0% of patients with phasic alpha activity, 41.7% of patients with low alpha activity, and 25.0% of patients with tonic alpha activity ($P < 0.01$). Self ratings of poor sleep were reported by all patients with phasic alpha activity, 58.3% of patients with low alpha activity ($P < 0.01$), and 12.5% of patients with tonic alpha activity ($P < 0.01$). Patients with phasic alpha activity reported longer duration of pain than patients in other subgroups ($P < 0.01$). Additionally, patients with phasic alpha sleep activity exhibited less total sleep time than patients in other subgroups ($P < 0.05$), as well as lower sleep efficiency ($P < 0.05$) and less slow wave sleep ($P < 0.05$) than patients with a tonic alpha sleep pattern.**

Conclusion. **Alpha intrusion during sleep can be of different patterns. Phasic alpha sleep activity was the pattern that correlated better with clinical manifestations of fibromyalgia.**

Supported by Fundação de Amparo à Pesquisa grants 95/09421-9 and 96/06940-8 and by Associação Fundo de Incentivo à Psicofarmacologia.

[1]Suely Roizenblatt, MD, PhD, Ana Amelia Benedito-Silva, PhD, Sergio Tufik, MD, PhD: São Paulo Federal University, São Paulo, Brazil; [2]Harvey Moldofsky, MD, FRCP(C): University of Toronto, Toronto, Ontario, Canada.

Address correspondence and reprint requests to Suely Roizenblatt, MD, PhD, Departamento de Psicobiologia, Universidade Federal de São Paulo, Rua Napoleão de Barros 925, CEP: 04024 – 002, São Paulo SP, Brazil.

Submitted for publication May 8, 2000; accepted in revised form September 27, 2000.

Nonrestorative sleep and fatigue are prominent features in patients with fibromyalgia. The unrefreshing sleep occurs in 76–90% of the patients with this condition (1–7), compared with 10–30% of normal subjects (8). Studies show that sleep disturbances per se may produce an overnight increase in pain and stiffness, particularly in painful musculoskeletal conditions (9–15). Investigators have not been able to draw a clear causal connection between pain severity and sleep disturbances in patients with chronic pain disorder and fibromyalgia, but psychological distress has been found to be associated with the poor sleep (9,16–19). Indeed, poor sleep occurs nonspecifically in various chronic musculoskeletal pain conditions (17,18,20–26). However, in fibromyalgia there is evidence for prolonged sleep latencies (27,28), low sleep efficiency (26,29), and an increased amount of stage 1 non–rapid eye movement (non-REM) sleep (7,16,28,30). In addition, these patients exhibit a reduction in slow wave sleep (27–29,31) and in REM sleep percentages (28), as well as an increased number of arousals (16,27–29,32–34) and restless leg movements (26,35). In particular, a number of reports describe the presence of alpha electroencephalographic (EEG) activity during non-REM sleep (7,11,28,31,36–38).

In studies that have used varying methodologies (27,37–42), the association of alpha EEG sleep with vigilance during sleep, drowsiness, and the subjective experience of nonrefreshing sleep has not been uniformly demonstrated. Initially, the alpha/delta sleep EEG was reported in a group of patients reported to have psychiatric disorders (43), and it was subsequently identified in patients with fibrositis or fibromyalgia who had chronic musculoskeletal complaints, fatigue, and negative mood (7,38,44,45). The association mentioned above has also been described in postinfectious and posttraumatic conditions (46), chronic fatigue syndrome (39), and even in normal individuals who submitted to experimental stimulation (13,14,47–49). Other studies have indicated the existence of different types of alpha activity (40,50,51), but the clinical implication of specific alpha sleep patterns still remains unclear.

The aim of this study was to evaluate the characteristics of the different alpha sleep patterns of activity in fibromyalgia patients. We hypothesized that there is an association between alpha EEG activity and the clinical symptoms in this musculoskeletal pain condition.

PATIENTS AND METHODS

Patients and control subjects. Forty Caucasian postmenopausal women <60 years of age with active fibromyalgia symptoms (3) were enrolled in this study. The patients were randomly drawn from a list of 185 available outpatients with fibromyalgia who attended the Rheumatology Clinic at Hospital São Paulo, Universidade Federal de São Paulo. The list of patients was arranged alphabetically and only contained information about age, sex, and address.

Forty-three healthy Caucasian women without chronic pain or sleep disturbance at the time of the study served as control subjects. They were matched 1:1 with the fibromyalgia patients with regard to age, postmenopausal condition, body mass index, and education level. These subjects were selected from healthy maintenance personnel at the university.

Criteria for exclusion from the study were the regular intake or abuse of medications that could interfere with sleep; the presence of neurologic, psychiatric, or other rheumatologic disorders (including, among others, rheumatoid arthritis and systemic lupus erythematosus); endocrine disorders (diabetes, thyroid disorders, obesity); or other inflammatory or infectious conditions.

All participants consented to the protocol that was previously approved by the Medical Ethics Committee of Universidade Federal de São Paulo.

Clinical assessment. All studied patients and control subjects completed an initial screening questionnaire to evaluate the characteristics and duration of pain (52) as well as the quality of sleep (53). Participants were instructed to score their sleep quality as well as their pain intensity before and after sleep recording in the laboratory. A numeric rating scale from 0 to 10 was used, where 0 corresponded to the lowest and 10 to the highest sleep quality or pain intensity. Sleep was considered poor when the self-rated sleep score was ≤ 4.

The Beck Inventory for depression was used, comprising 21 self-report questions. Scores of <20 were classified as low, 20–40 as moderate, and >40 as associated with a high likelihood of clinical depression (54).

All subjects underwent clinical evaluation and tender pnt count immediately before and after sleep recording (12). Using digital palpation, a trained investigator (SR) performed the examination of the tender points. According to accepted clinical criteria for fibromyalgia (3), only those patients or control subjects presenting with ≥ 11 positive tender points were included in the study.

Sleep recording. All medications that could interfere with sleep were discontinued for a minimum of 4 weeks before the recordings. Smoking and the use of alcohol or caffeine were not allowed for at least 24 hours prior to the polysomnography. After patients and control subjects underwent a first night of adaptation, overnight polysomnography, starting at their usual bedtime, was performed in the sleep laboratory. Sleep recordings of both nights were performed using the 9.2 Medilog Sleep Analyzer Computer (Oxford Medical, Oxon, UK) (11), with a sampling rate of 500 Hz and resolution of 12 bits. The signals were amplified and digitized by a 5.0V analog-to-digital converter and band-pass filters. The montage employed C3-A2, C4-A1, and Oz-Fz EEG derivations placed according to the International 10-20 System; bilateral electrooculography (EOG); submental electromyography (EMG); bilateral anterior tibial EMG; electrocardiography; nasal airflow thermistor; respiratory belts; and oxygen saturation recording (Ohmeda, Helsinki, Finland). The settings for the recording were 90 Hz for the high-pass filter, 0.3 Hz for the low-pass filter, time constant of 0.4 seconds, and sensitivity of 50 μV/cm. Adaptation and second-night sleep recordings were stored on optical disks.

Sleep scoring. Sleep stages were scored manually in a blinded manner for consecutive 30-second epochs according to standardized criteria (55), and successive non-REM–REM cycles were identified, taking into account the REM periods. Latency to sleep onset corresponded to the time elapsed from "lights out" to the first epoch in stage 2 non-REM sleep, and sleep efficiency expressed the percentage of time in bed that was actually spent sleeping. The percentages of sleep stages were considered in relation to total sleep time (time in minutes that the individual really spent sleeping at bedtime). Stages 3 and 4 of non-REM sleep were considered together as slow wave sleep (SWS). Arousals were considered as an abrupt shift in EEG frequencies, with activation of submental EMG or EOG, lasting for >3 seconds and preceded by 10 seconds of continuous sleep (56). The arousal index was obtained during the first and second sleep cycles and was expressed as the number of arousals per hour of sleep.

Hypopnea or apnea events were visually detected when the nasal air-flow thermistor recording slowed or stopped for >10 seconds, excluding stage 1 non-REM sleep, waking, or movement time epochs. Hypopnea was scored when ventilation was reduced by at least 50% of baseline and there was a drop of at least 4% in O_2 saturation; apnea was scored when there was no evidence of ventilation. Both hypopnea and apnea had to exceed 10 seconds to be scored. An apnea-plus-hypopnea index (AHI) value of >5 events/hour of sleep was considered pathologic.

To evaluate the reliability of the second-night analysis, the degree of agreement (weighted kappa [Kw]) of sleep parameters between the adaptation night and the second night was calculated from a sample comprising sleep recordings of 12 fibromyalgia patients and 12 control subjects. Substantial agreement was obtained with regard to the percentage of stage

2 non-REM sleep (Kw = 0.69) and SWS (Kw = 0.74), sleep efficiency (Kw = 0.79), arousals (Kw = 0.63), and AHI (Kw = 0.80). Moderate agreement was noted for sleep latency (Kw = 0.59) and total sleep time (Kw = 0.55).

Microstructure of sleep. Quantitative scoring of alpha and delta activities was analyzed from the stored digitized EEG data obtained throughout stages 2, 3, and 4 of non-REM sleep. Based on the fact that alpha intrusion in non-REM sleep is observed particularly during the first half of the night (28), we analyzed this event throughout the first 2 sleep cycles, both visually and by means of time domain (Polysmith; Neurotronics, Gainesville, FL) and power spectral analysis (fast Fourier transform [FFT]; Meditron, São Paulo, Brazil) softwares.

The time domain software for waveform analysis was based on the detection of each zero crossing of the digitized EEG signal (i.e., polarity changes from positive to negative and vice versa). Frequency bands were computed using the following bandwidths: alpha, in the range of 7.0–12.0 Hz, with minimum peak-to-peak amplitude of 5 μV; and delta, in frequencies of 0.5–2.0 Hz, with minimum amplitude of 30 μV. Averaged alpha and delta time values, expressed in seconds per epoch, were obtained for the visually scored stage 2 non-REM sleep and SWS during the first 2 sleep cycles.

Frequency domain analysis was estimated using the FFT (57), performed at each 1-Hz band. Consecutive 2-second samples were visually selected during stage 2 non-REM sleep and SWS, up to a maximum of 640 contiguous seconds. Arousals, baseline oscillations, and artifact segments of EEG were not included in the analysis. The frequency bands of interest were delta-1 (0.5–2.0 Hz) and alpha (7.0–12.0 Hz). The upper limit of 2.0 Hz for the delta band was chosen to avoid confusion with SWS breakthrough during non-REM apneas (58). The voltage amplitude and frequencies comprised in every 2-second segment were obtained, and spectral activity was expressed as a percentage of the total power. The data obtained from the selected samples of EEG were averaged.

Visual alpha scoring was performed according to the previously described method (59). Briefly, alpha activity was defined as frequencies in the range of 7.0–12.0 Hz, with minimum peak-to-peak amplitude of 5 μV, and rated according to the percentage of alpha events per epoch of stage 2 non-REM sleep and SWS. Arousal events and artifacts were eliminated from the analysis. After scoring each epoch, averaged percentage-of-alpha rating values were obtained for stage 2 non-REM sleep and for SWS during the first and second sleep cycles.

Statistical analysis. The intergroup differences in frequency distribution were assessed by chi-square test or Fisher's exact test, as appropriate. The modification in pain parameters, after sleeping at the laboratory, was established by the significance of change observed between postsleep and presleep pain score or tender point count (by Student's *t*-test) and by the percentage of this modification, expressed as $\Delta = [(\text{final value} - \text{initial value})/\text{initial value}] \times 100$. Descriptive data were expressed as mean ± SD. The level of significance was established at $P < 0.05$.

For comparisons among the 3 subgroups of fibromyalgia patients and control subjects, analysis of variance (ANOVA) was used, followed by Duncan's test for multiple comparisons. For comparison of alpha and delta activity values obtained by time domain analysis among fibromyalgia subgroups, the Kruskal-Wallis ANOVA was used, followed by the least significance of differences test for multivariate analysis.

The degree of correlation between clinical and sleep parameters (Spearman's rank correlation [r_s]) and the degrees of agreement (Kw) between first- and second-night polysomnography and between FFT and visual alpha scoring were classified as almost perfect (≥0.81), substantial (0.61–0.80), moderate (0.41–0.60), and mild (≤0.40).

RESULTS

As a result of the matching process, fibromyalgia patients did not differ in age from control subjects (mean ± SD 46 ± 4 versus 47 ± 7 years, respectively). The mean ± SD duration of fibromyalgia manifestations was 5 ± 3 years. There were significant differences between the groups in postsleep pain and sleep quality scores. Although worsening of pain symptoms after sleep was reported by 72% of the fibromyalgia patients, this was observed in only 12% of the control subjects ($P < 0.01$). The subjective assessment of worsening pain was accompanied by an increase in the number of tender points observed in 93% of these fibromyalgia patients after sleep. The self-rated sleep quality score was significantly lower in the fibromyalgia patients than in the control subjects (mean ± SD 3.8 ± 2.0 versus 8.4 ± 1.8; $P = 0.04$). Poor sleep quality (self-rated score of ≤4) was reported by 70% of the fibromyalgia patients and by none of the control subjects.

We compared the sleep structure in the groups. The fibromyalgia patients exhibited an increase in the percentage of stage 1 non-REM sleep (mean ± SD 13 ± 2.1% versus 8.9 ± 2.4%; $P = 0.04$) and an increase in alpha activity in both stage 2 non-REM sleep and SWS during the first 2 sleep cycles (70% versus 16%; $P < 0.01$).

Three distinct patterns of alpha activity were identified. Figure 1 illustrates a typical tracing of each pattern. The phasic alpha sleep pattern is characterized by an episodic alpha rhythm occurring simultaneously with delta activity. In the tonic alpha sleep pattern, alpha activity is continuously present throughout non-REM sleep, independent of delta activity. The third pattern is characterized by low alpha activity. The specific prevalence of each of these 3 patterns was quite distinct for the fibromyalgia patients and control subjects. Although the phasic alpha EEG pattern was the most common pattern in the fibromyalgia group (50% of patients), it was observed in only 7% of the control subjects. In the latter group, the low alpha EEG pattern was the most common, observed in 83.7% of control subjects versus 30% of fibromyalgia patients ($P < 0.01$). The tonic alpha

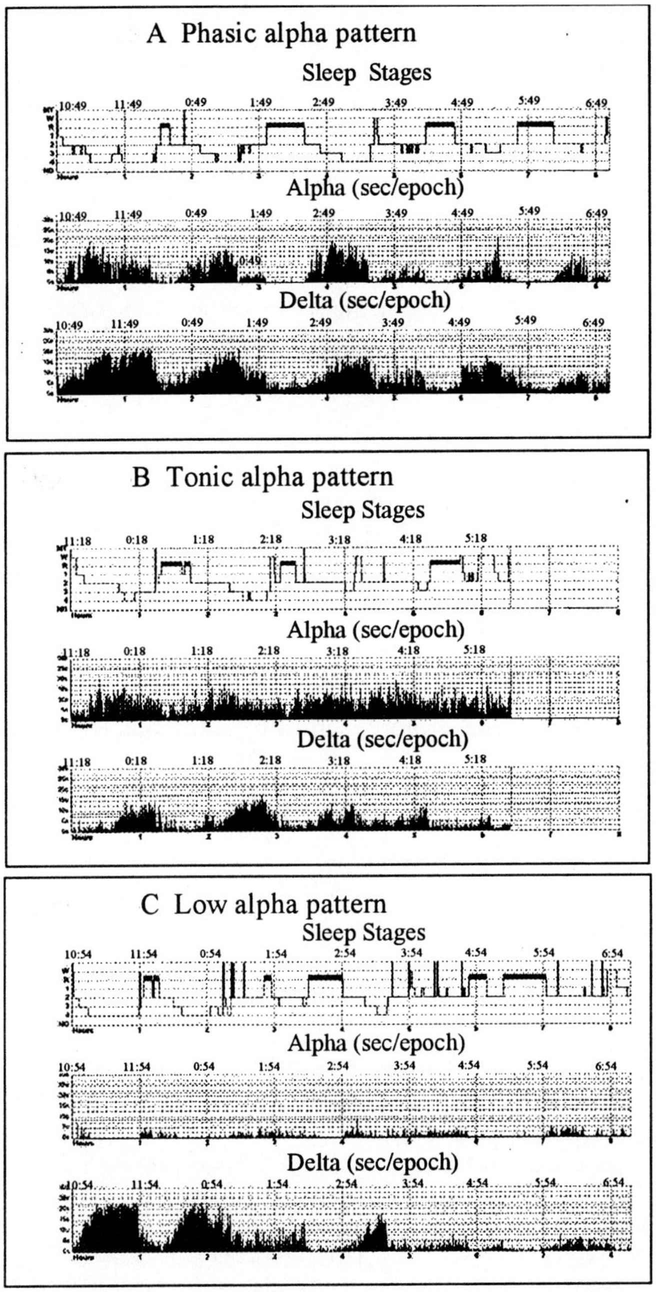

Figure 1. Different patterns of alpha activity during sleep recording. **A,** Phasic alpha pattern, **B,** Tonic alpha pattern, **C,** Low alpha pattern. Within each of the 3 patterns shown, the first plot (Sleep Stages) is a hypnogram, while the second and third plots show alpha and delta activity, respectively (in seconds/epoch), during sleep.

sleep pattern was observed in only 20% and 9% of the fibromyalgia patients and control subjects, respectively.

To further elucidate the clinical significance of the 3 alpha EEG sleep patterns, we evaluated their associations with parameters indicative of pain and sleep quality in the fibromyalgia patients. Among these patterns, the phasic alpha EEG was associated with longer-lasting pain symptoms as well as with poor sleep (Table 1). When self-rated sleep quality and postsleep pain scores were evaluated, the phasic alpha sleep pattern was associated with both subjective (pain score) and objective (tender point count) increases in morning pain, and with the lowest subjective sleep quality scores (Table 2). The majority of the 29 fibromyalgia patients who reported worsening of pain score after sleeping in the laboratory exhibited the phasic alpha sleep pattern rather than the low alpha and tonic alpha sleep patterns (69% versus 24% and 7%; $P < 0.01$). Further, all of the 20 fibromyalgia patients who displayed phasic alpha sleep activity reported worsening of self-rated pain scores after sleep, compared with 58.3% of those who displayed low alpha sleep, activity ($P < 0.01$) and 25.0% of those who displayed tonic alpha sleep activity ($P < 0.01$). Regarding postsleep number of tender points, the increase in the tender point count occurred in 90.0% of the patients with phasic alpha sleep activity, 41.7% of

Table 1. Characteristics of 40 fibromyalgia patients according to their alpha sleep patterns*

	Phasic alpha	Tonic alpha	Low alpha
Patients, no. (%)	20 (50)	8 (20)	12 (30)
Age in years, mean ± SD	46 ± 5	46 ± 4	45 ± 2
Duration of pain symptoms in years, mean ± SD	7 ± 2†	3 ± 1	3 ± 1
Patients with nonrefreshing sleep, %	100‡	25§	58
Patients with depression, %	30	37	33

* P values were calculated by analysis of variance followed by Duncan's test for multiple comparisons, chi-square test, or Fisher's exact test, as appropriate.
† $P < 0.01$ versus other alpha sleep patterns.
‡ $P < 0.05$ versus other alpha sleep patterns.
§ $P < 0.05$ versus low alpha sleep pattern.

Table 2. Clinical parameters of fibromyalgia according to the alpha sleep pattern*

Alpha sleep pattern	NRS pain score		Tender point count		NRS sleep quality score
	Presleep	Postsleep	Presleep	Postsleep	
Phasic	3.6 ± 0.5	5.8 ± 0.7†	12.4 ± 0.9	16.5 ± 1.3†	2.6 ± 0.7‡
Tonic	4.6 ± 1.3	4.9 ± 1.8§	13.8 ± 1.6	14.3 ± 2.2§	6.2 ± 1.2
Low	4.3 ± 1.5	4.7 ± 1.3§	14.1 ± 1.7	14.6 ± 1.6	6.3 ± 1.4

* Values are the mean ± SD. NRS = numeric rating scale.
† $P < 0.01$ versus presleep condition, by Student's t-test.
‡ $P < 0.01$ versus other alpha sleep patterns, by analysis of variance followed by Duncan's test for multiple comparisons.
§ $P < 0.05$ versus presleep condition, by Student's t-test.

Table 3. Polysomnographic parameters in fibromyalgia according to the alpha sleep pattern*

	Phasic alpha	Tonic alpha	Low alpha
Total sleep time, minutes	335 ± 45†	398 ± 23	383 ± 46
Sleep latency, minutes	12.8 ± 6.1	9.7 ± 1.6	12.1 ± 4.3
REM latency, minutes	94.6 ± 15.1	94.4 ± 8.4	102.1 ± 7.0
Sleep efficiency, %	87.0 ± 8.2‡	92.9 ± 4.6	89.9 ± 6
Stage 1 non-REM sleep, %	13.9 ± 4.2	12.0 ± 3.5	11.5 ± 5.7
Stage 2 non-REM sleep, %	51.3 ± 4.1	44.9 ± 12.1	50.4 ± 3.6
Slow wave sleep, %	12.9 ± 4.1‡	19.9 ± 2.6	14.4 ± 4.5
REM sleep, %	21.9 ± 3.9	23.1 ± 3.6	22.7 ± 3.3

* Values are the mean ± SD. *P* values were calculated by analysis of variance followed by Duncan's test for multiple comparisons. REM = rapid eye movement.
† $P < 0.05$ versus other alpha sleep patterns.
‡ $P < 0.05$ versus tonic alpha sleep pattern.

Table 4. Spearman's rank correlations (r_s) of clinical data with alpha sleep activity during slow wave sleep detected by means of different techniques*

	Phasic alpha activity		Tonic alpha activity	
	FFT	Visual	FFT	Visual
Sleep score	−0.74	−0.76	−0.52	−0.47
Postsleep pain score	0.67	0.89	0.21	0.40
Postsleep tender point count	0.52	0.85	NS	0.32

* No significant correlations were obtained for these variables in fibromyalgia patients with low alpha sleep activity. The level of significance was set at $P < 0.05$. FFT = fast Fourier transform; NS = not significant.

those with low alpha sleep activity, and 25.0% of those with tonic alpha sleep activity ($P < 0.01$).

In the fibromyalgia patients with the phasic alpha sleep pattern, the mean ± SD values for the percentage of modification (Δ) of self-rated pain score and of tender point count before and after sleep were 58.7 ± 17.4 and 33.3 ± 10.1, respectively. These values were significantly higher ($P < 0.01$) than the Δ of the self-rated pain score and the Δ of the tender point count observed in patients with the tonic alpha sleep pattern (13.3 ± 9.0 and 8.1 ± 4.7, respectively) or the low alpha sleep pattern (18.2 ± 13.9 and 19.9 ± 7.2, respectively).

With regard to the self-rated sleep quality score in the laboratory, poor sleep (score of ≤4) was reported by 28 of the fibromyalgia patients: by all of the 20 patients who displayed the phasic alpha sleep pattern, by 1 patient with tonic alpha activity ($P < 0.01$), and by 7 patients with low alpha activity ($P < 0.01$). The phasic alpha sleep pattern was not detected in any of the patients with better sleep quality scores, but was present in 2 of the 6 control subjects who reported poor quality of sleep.

Polysomnography parameters are listed in Table 3. Total sleep time, percentage of sleep efficiency, and percentage of SWS were significantly reduced in the fibromyalgia patients with the phasic alpha sleep pattern ($P < 0.05$). There was no significant association between AHI and a specific alpha EEG sleep pattern. None of the subgroups exhibited elevation of the arousal index beyond 9.1 arousals/hour, which corresponded to the maximum normal value as determined by the 95% confidence interval in the group of control subjects.

Significant correlations between self-rated sleep quality scores and objective parameters measured by polysomnography were observed in the fibromyalgia patients. These included total sleep time ($r_s = 0.49$, $P < 0.01$), sleep efficiency ($r_s = 0.37$, $P = 0.02$), percentage of SWS ($r_s = 0.48$, $P < 0.01$), and alpha EEG activity in SWS detected by FFT ($r_s = -0.43$, $P < 0.01$). Alpha EEG activity in the phasic alpha sleep pattern correlated with poor sleep and also with postsleep pain parameters (Table 4). Furthermore, self-rated sleep quality scores

Table 5. Techniques of alpha detection according to the alpha sleep pattern in fibromyalgia*

	Phasic alpha	Tonic alpha	Low alpha
Time domain, median (interquartile range/2)			
Stage 2 non-REM sleep			
Alpha, seconds/epoch	0.1 (0.02)	0.3 (0.03)†	0.02 (0.05)
Alpha:delta ratio	1.0 (0.22)	3.6 (1.8)†	0.2 (0.22)
SWS			
Alpha, seconds/epoch	0.5 (0.25)†	0.3 (0.14)†	0.04 (0.05)
Alpha:delta ratio	1.2 (0.95)†	0.9 (0.12)†	0.1 (0.10)
Frequency domain analysis using FFT, mean ± SD			
Stage 2 non-REM sleep			
Alpha, %	16.1 ± 1.6‡	22.4 ± 1.6§	4.6 ± 1.1
Alpha:delta ratio	0.6 ± 0.2‡	1.0 ± 0.1§	0.2 ± 0.06
SWS			
Alpha, %	44.2 ± 5.9‡§	27.3 ± 1.9§	5.4 ± 0.8
Alpha:delta ratio	0.9 ± 0.2‡§	0.5 ± 0.05†	0.09 ± 0.02
Visual scoring, mean ± SD			
Stage 2 non-REM sleep			
Alpha, score	2.1 ± 0.4‡	3.8 ± 0.5†	1.2 ± 0.4
SWS			
Alpha, score	4.3 ± 0.8‡§	3.2 ± 0.5†	1.3 ± 0.5

* *P* values were calculated by analysis of variance (ANOVA) followed by Duncan's test for multiple comparisons or by Kruskal-Wallis ANOVA, followed by the least significance of differences test for multivariate analysis, as appropriate. REM = rapid eye movement; SWS = slow wave sleep; FFT = fast Fourier transform.
† $P < 0.05$ versus low alpha sleep pattern.
‡ $P < 0.05$ versus tonic alpha sleep pattern.
§ $P < 0.01$ versus low alpha sleep pattern.

correlated with postsleep pain intensity scores (r_s = −0.83, $P < 0.01$).

To evaluate the accuracy of the two automated EEG interpretation methods, we compared the results of time domain and FFT techniques with those obtained by the visual inspection method. Using time domain analysis, in spite of the nonparametric distribution of the data (Table 5), it was possible to detect increases in alpha time (seconds/epoch) and alpha:delta ratio during stage 2 non-REM sleep in the tonic alpha sleep pattern compared with the other 2 alpha EEG patterns ($P <$ 0.05). During SWS, however, increases in alpha time and alpha:delta ratio were detected indistinctly in patients with phasic or tonic alpha sleep patterns compared with patients with low alpha activity ($P < 0.05$). Additionally, a negative correlation between the amount of alpha and delta time during SWS was found in fibromyalgia patients with phasic alpha ($r_s = -0.76$, $P < 0.01$) or tonic alpha ($r_s = -0.76$, $P = 0.02$) sleep patterns.

Regarding frequency analysis and visual scoring, both techniques were able to detect the highest alpha EEG power during stage 2 non-REM sleep ($P < 0.01$) in the tonic alpha sleep pattern and during SWS ($P < 0.01$) in the phasic alpha sleep pattern (Table 5). For alpha activity detection, the degree of agreement (Kw) between FFT and visual scoring was 0.49 (moderate) for stage 2 non-REM sleep and 0.61 (substantial) for SWS.

DISCUSSION

Poor sleep quality and morning musculoskeletal pain are commonly reported by fibromyalgia patients (7,14,16,26,27–33). In the present study, which was designed to evaluate these symptoms objectively, we were able to document worsening of pain after poor sleep in patients with fibromyalgia. Polysomnography and alpha activity analysis of patients with this condition provided additional and important information. The phasic alpha sleep pattern was associated with longer duration of pain symptoms and superficial sleep. The role of depression in the manifestations mentioned above is controversial (16,19,38,43) and could not be confirmed in the present study.

It has previously been reported that so-called alpha/delta sleep interferes with sleep function, resulting in nonrestorative sleep (7,16,26–35,46,50,60,61), daytime fatigue, and musculoskeletal pain rather than in behavioral changes or shortened sleep (44). Painful musculoskeletal conditions in humans (10,14,18–20,22,24–26,35,62–67) and even in animals (68) have been reported to be leading causes of nonrestorative sleep. Although normal individuals report less pain sensitivity during the morning (69), fibromyalgia patients experience a tendency toward a worsening of symptoms overnight, resulting in fatigue more intense in the morning than in the prior night, as well as in a diurnal variation in symptoms (14,44,64,67,70,71). Furthermore, it has also been suggested that fibromyalgia patients with alpha/delta sleep pattern are those with the best clinical response to amytriptyline (60). In this study, morning stiffness, diffuse pain, and discomfort after awakening were common in fibromyalgia patients with phasic alpha sleep. Although a cause–effect relationship between pain and sleep cannot be established, the data presented here suggest that the phasic alpha sleep pattern is associated with longer duration of pain symptoms, perception of poor sleep, and morning pain.

According to findings of previous studies, the association between alpha anomaly and nonrestorative sleep, pain, or fatigue (37,38,43–45) does not depend on the reduction in SWS (31,36,51). Disruptions in sleep continuity, although not sufficient to induce awakening (37,62), are postulated to be more detrimental to the restorative property of sleep (64–67) than SWS or total sleep deprivation (13–15). In experimental studies, external stimulation insufficient to wake the subjects induced changes in sleep architecture, including stage shift or alpha EEG intrusion, even in normal individuals (37,48). Studies of normal subjects (62,64–67,69) and subjects with sleep disorders (32,61,63,70–76) have shown nonrestorative sleep, daytime sleepiness, and pain symptoms secondary to multiple brief disruptions in sleep continuity without sleep deprivation (64–67).

Arousals may also result in fragmented sleep (14,16,29,34,50) rather than in behavioral awakening or shortened sleep (37,48,62), but in this study, EEG segments with arousal events were not included in alpha activity analysis, and the arousal index was not significantly increased among the fibromyalgia patients. The K-alpha phenomenon, described in association with periodic limb movements during sleep, fatigue, and musculoskeletal pain, should also be mentioned. It is defined as a K-complex followed immediately by a burst of alpha activity lasting <5 seconds. Although it also corresponds to a phasic event, it differs from phasic alpha sleep pattern in that it appears primarily in stage 2 non-REM sleep and, less frequently, in SWS (77).

Alpha activity in non-REM sleep has been reported in painful conditions by investigators using visual (43,59) or computerized (11,26–28,36,60) sleep analysis. Despite the current tendency toward the use of automated systems for sleep analysis, the importance of visual scoring methodologies is undeniable in light of the many elements involved in detecting a given waveform. In sleep laboratory analyses, computerized sleep EEG scoring systems often require manual correction. In this context, the ideal software for sleep analysis should allow a critical evaluation of the stage scoring, as well as of the detection of respiratory and motor events. With reference to alpha EEG sleep analysis, the ideal system should permit the recognition of superimposed wave frequencies and also offer flexibility in sample selection, to permit the exclusion of artifacts and arousal events.

The available automated methods that quantify alpha activity are based on frequency domain (28,50,60,78) or time domain (79–81) analyses, methodologies that are not equivalent in their practical applications and that do not provide concordant data (81), as could be confirmed in the present study. Spectral analysis, in which the FFT procedure (57) is the most common tool, provides independent measurements of frequency bands, even when these are hidden by superimposed frequencies (82). Time domain analysis is based on the detection of the number of zero crossings per second and on the evaluation of waveform amplitude. The zero-crossing techniques consider one frequency in a given period of time, and since low-amplitude fast waves are superimposed on high-amplitude slow waves in the alpha/delta phenomenon, there is a bias related to the detection of faster waveforms riding on a large-amplitude slow wave (81,83). This aspect could be verified in the present study, in spite of the use of frequency-selective band filters for time domain analysis. In the current study, the FFT data correlated better with visual scoring than with time domain analysis for the recognition of the different patterns of alpha EEG activity. Additionally, alpha activity obtained by visual scoring showed a closer correlation with pain and sleep symptoms than did automated sleep analysis.

For the study of data relative to sleep architecture (Table 3), and for the detection of alpha and delta activities (Figure 1), all sleep cycles were taken into account. Nevertheless, for comparison among the 3 distinct techniques of sleep microstructure analysis (visual scoring, FFT, and time domain), quantification of alpha and delta activities was restricted to the first 2 sleep cycles. Such restriction was necessary to avoid dealing with missing data, because 11 of 12 fibromyalgia patients exhibited SWS only in the first 2 non-REM–REM complete sleep cycles.

Despite the progressive reduction of delta EEG activity and of SWS over the sequence of non-REM–REM sleep cycles verified in this and other studies (28,84), the pattern of alpha activity was preserved throughout the sleep cycles during the entire night sleep recording: alpha activity concomitant with delta activity in the phasic pattern, independent of delta activity in the tonic pattern, and very low in the low pattern (Figure 1). Another reason for limiting this study to the first 2 sleep cycles was that the time domain method quantified alpha and delta activities not as percentages, as do visual scoring and FFT techniques, but as averaged alpha time and delta time values (seconds/epoch). Since alpha and delta sleep frequencies tend to be less prominent during the second half of the night, the detection of alpha and delta activities would become more difficult using the time domain technique if the entire sleep were to be analyzed numerically. Although the current practice is to study the alpha phenomenon during the entire non-REM sleep (26–28,36,59,60), our results suggest that the procedure of analyzing stage 2 non-REM sleep separately from SWS is valid for measuring the differentiation of alpha EEG sleep patterns (Table 5).

In conclusion, fibromyalgia patients show distinctive patterns of alpha intrusion in non-REM sleep. The current data suggest that sleep EEG evaluation may assist in the detection of the phasic alpha sleep pattern, which is found in patients with severe symptoms. This finding could be useful in selecting therapeutic modalities and in assessing the response to a specific treatment that might improve sleep quality, pain, and fatigue in fibromyalgia.

ACKNOWLEDGMENTS

We are grateful to Jaques Belik, MD, for the careful revision of the manuscript, and to engineer James Schubert for providing technical support to this study.

REFERENCES

1. Smythe HA, Moldofsky H. Two contributions to understanding "fibrositis" syndrome. Bull Rheum Dis 1977;28:928–31.
2. Yunus MB, Masi AT, Calabro JJ, Miller KA, Feigenbaum SI. Primary fibromyalgia (fibrositis): clinical study of 50 patients with matched normal controls. Semin Arthritis Rheum 1981;11:151–72.
3. Wolfe F, Smythe HA, Yunus MB, Bennett RM, Bombardier C, Goldenberg DL, et al. The American College of Rheumatology 1990 criteria for the classification of fibromyalgia: report of the multicenter criteria committee. Arthritis Rheum 1990;33:160–72.
4. Campbell SM, Clark S, Tindall EA, Forehand ME, Bennett RM. Clinical characteristics of fibrositis. I. A "blinded," controlled study of symptoms and tender points. Arthritis Rheum 1983;26: 817–24.
5. Wolfe F, Cathey MA. Prevalence of primary and secondary fibrositis. J Rheumatol 1983;10:965–8.
6. Schaefer KM. Sleep disturbance and fatigue in women with

fibromyalgia and chronic fatigue syndrome. J Obstet Gynecol Neonatal Nurs 1995;24:229–33.
7. Moldofsky H, Scarisbrick P, England R, Smythe H. Musculoskeletal symptoms and non-REM sleep disturbance in patients with 'fibrositis syndrome' and healthy subjects. Psychosom Med 1975; 37:341–51.
8. Lugaresi E, Cirignotta F, Zucconi M, Mondini S, Lenzi PL, Coccagna G. Good and poor sleepers: an epidemiological survey of the San Marino population. In: Guilleminault C, Lugaresi E, editors. Sleep/wake disorders: natural history. New York: Raven Press; 1981. p. 1–12.
9. Affleck G, Urrows S, Tennen H, Higgins P, Abeles M. Sequential daily relations of sleep, pain intensity, and attention to pain among women with fibromyalgia. Pain 1996;68:363–8.
10. Hemmeter U, Kocher R, Ladewig D, Hatzinger M, Seifritz E, Lauer CJ, et al. Sleep disorders in chronic pain and generalized tendomyopathy. Schweiz Med Wochenschr 1995;125:2391–7.
11. Roizenblatt S, Tufik S, Goldenberg J, Pinto LR, Feldman DP. Juvenile fibromyalgia: clinical and polysomnographic aspects. J Rheumatol 1997;24:579–85.
12. Croft P, Schollum J, Silman A. Population study of tender point counts and pain as evidence of fibromyalgia. BMJ 1994;309:696–9.
13. Moldofsky H, Scarisbrick P. Induction of neurasthenic musculoskeletal pain syndrome by selective sleep stage deprivation. Psychosom Med 1976;38:35–44.
14. Older SA, Battafarano DF, Danning CL, Ward JA, Grady EP, Derman S, et al. The effect of delta wave sleep interruption on pain thresholds and fibromyalgia-like symptoms in healthy subjects: correlations with insulin-like growth factor I. J Rheumatol 1998;25:1180–6.
15. Walsh JK, Hartman PG, Schweitzer PK. Slow wave sleep deprivation and waking function. J Sleep Res 1994;3:16–25.
16. Shaver JLF, Lentz M, Landis CA, Heitkemper NN, Buchwald DS, Woods NF. Sleep, psychological distress, and stress arousal in women with fibromyalgia. Res Nurs Health 1997;20:247–57.
17. Hyyppä MT, Kronholm E. Nocturnal motor activity in fibromyalgia patients with poor sleep quality. J Psychosom Res 1995;39: 85–91.
18. Pilowsky I, Crettenden I, Townly M. Sleep disturbance in pain clinic patients. Pain 1985;23:27–33.
19. Phillips GD, Cousins MJ. Neurological mechanisms of pain and the relationship of pain, anxiety, and sleep. In: Cousins MJ, Philips GD, editors. Acute pain management. New York: Churchill Livingstone; 1986. p. 21–48.
20. Mahowald MW, Mahowald ML, Bundlie SR, Ytterberg SR. Sleep fragmentation in rheumatoid arthritis. Arthritis Rheum 1989;32: 974–83.
21. Kryeger JM. Cytokines and sleep. Int Arch Allergy Immunol 1995;106:97–100.
22. Hirsch M, Carlander B, Vergé M, Tafti M, Anaya J-M, Billiard M, et al. Objective and subjective sleep disturbances in patients with rheumatoid arthritis: a reappraisal. Arthritis Rheum 1994;37:41–9.
23. Kryger M, Shapiro CM. Pain and distress at night. Sleep Solutions 1992;5:1–20.
24. Leigh TJ, Hindmarch I, Bird HA, Wright V. Comparison of sleep in osteoarthritic patients and age–sex matched healthy controls. Ann Rheum Dis 1988;47:40–2.
25. Greenberg HE, Ney G, Ravdin L, Scharf SM, Hilton E. Sleep quality in Lyme disease. Sleep 1995;18:912–6.
26. Wittig RM, Zorick FJ, Blumer D, Heilbronn M, Roth T. Disturbed sleep in patients complaining of chronic pain. J Nerv Ment Dis 1982;170:429–31.
27. Horne JA, Shackell BS. Alpha-like EEG activity in non-REM sleep and the fibromyalgia (fibrositis) syndrome. Electroencephalogr Clin Neurophysiol 1991;79:271–6.
28. Branco J, Atalaia A, Paiva T. Sleep cycles and alpha-delta sleep in fibromyalgia syndrome. J Rheumatol 1994;21:1113–7.
29. Touchon J, Besset A, Billiard M, Simon L, Herrison C, Cadihac J. Fibrositis syndrome: polysomnographic and psychological aspects. In: Koella WP, Obál F, Schulz H, Visser P, editors. Sleep '86. New York: Gustav Fischer Verlag; 1988, p. 445–7.
30. Anch AM, Lue FA, MacLean AW, Moldofsky H. Sleep physiology and psychological aspects of fibrositis (fibromyalgia) syndrome. Can J Exp Psychol 1991;45:179–84.
31. Drewes AM, Nielsen KD, Taagholt SJ, Bjerregard K, Svendsen L, Gade J. Sleep intensity in fibromyalgia: focus on the microstructure of the sleep process. Br J Rheumatol 1995;34:629–35.
32. Molony RR, MacPeek DM, Schiffman PL, Frank M, Neubauer JA, Schwartzberg M, et al. Sleep, sleep apnea, and fibromyalgia syndrome. J Rheumatol 1986;13:797–800.
33. Clauw D, Blank C, Hiltz R, Katz P, Potolicchio S. Polysomnography in fibromyalgia patients [abstract]. Arthritis Rheum 1994;37 Suppl 9:S348.
34. Staedt J, Windt H, Hajaki G, Soppe G, Rudolph G, Ensink FBM, et al. Cluster arousal analysis in chronic pain-disturbed sleep. J Sleep Res 1993;2:134–7.
35. Atkinson JH, Ancoli-Israel S, Slater MA, Garfin SR, Gillin JC. Subjective sleep disturbance in chronic back pain. Clin J Pain 1988;4:225–32.
36. Drewes AM, Gade J, Nielsen KD, Bjerrard K, Taagholt SJ, Svendsen L. Clustering of sleep electroencephalopathic patterns in patients with the fibromyalgia syndrome. Br J Rheumatol 1995;34: 1151–40.
37. Perlis ML, Giles DE, Bootzin RR, Dikman ZV, Fleming GM, Drummond SPA, et al. Alpha sleep and information processing, perception of sleep, pain, and arousability in fibromyalgia. Int J Neurosci 1997;89:265–80.
38. Ware JC, Russell IJ, Campos E. Alpha intrusions into the sleep of depression and fibromyalgia syndrome (fibrositis) patients [abstract]. Sleep Res 1986;15:210.
39. Manu P, Lane TJ, Matthews DA, Castriotta RJ, Watson RK, Abeles M. Alpha-delta sleep in patients with a chief complaint of chronic fatigue. South Med J 1994;87:465–70.
40. Scheuler W, Stinshoff D, Kubicki S. The alpha sleep pattern: different from other sleep patterns and effects of hypnotics. Neuropsychobiology 1983;10:183–9.
41. Broughton R, Hasan J, Dunham W. Anterior slow alpha of drowsiness: topography, source dipole analysis [abstract]. Sleep Res 1994;23:5.
42. Scheuler W, Kubicki S, Marquardt J, Scholz G, Wei KH, Henkes H, et al. The sleep pattern: quantitative analysis and functional aspects. In: Koella WP, Obál F, Schulz H, Visser P, editors. Sleep '86. New York: Gustav Fischer Verlag; 1988. p. 284–6.
43. Hauri P, Hawkins DR. Alpha-delta sleep. Electroencephalogr Clin Neurophysiol 1973;34:233–7.
44. Moldofsky H, Lue FA. The relationship of alpha and delta EEG frequencies to pain and mood in "fibrositis" patients treated with chlorpromazine and L-tryptophan. Electroencephalogr Clin Neurophysiol 1980;50:71–80.
45. Coté KA, Moldofsky H. Sleep, daytime symptoms, and cognitive performance in patients with fibromyalgia. J Rheumatol 1997;24: 2014–23.
46. Moldofsky H. Sleep-wake mechanisms in fibrositis. J Rheumatol 1989;16 Suppl 19:47–8.
47. Stepanski E, Lamphere J, Roehrs T, Zorick F, Roth T. Experimental sleep fragmentation in normal subjects. Int J Neurosci 1987;33:207–14.
48. Drewes AM, Nielsen KD, Arendt-Nielsen L, Birket-Smith L, Hansen LM. The effect of cutaneous and deep pain on the electroencephalogram during sleep: an experimental study. Sleep 1997;20:632–40.
49. Chediak AD, Demirozu MC, Nay KN. Alpha EEG sleep produced by balloon catheterization of the esophagus [letter]. Sleep 1990; 13:369–70.

50. Scheuler W, Rappelsberger P, Schmatz F, Pastelak-Price C, Petsche H, Kubicki S. Periodicity anaysis of sleep EEG in the second and minute ranges: example of application in different alpha activities in sleep. Electroencephalogr Clin Neurophysiol 1990;76:222–34.
51. Pivik RT, Harman K. A reconceptualization of EEG alpha activity as an index of arousal during sleep: all alpha activity is not equal. J Sleep Res 1995;4:131–7.
52. Braz S, Neumann BRG, Tufik S. Avaliação dos distúrbios do sono: elaboração e validação de um questionário. Rev Assoc Bras Psiquiatr 1987;9:9–14.
53. Bennett K, Cardiel MH, Ferraz MB, Riedemann P, Goldsmith CH, Tugwell P. Community screening for rheumatic disorder: cross cultural adaptation and screening characteristics of the COPCORD Core Questionnaire in Brazil, Chile, and Mexico. J Rheumatol 1997;24:160–8.
54. Gorenstein C, Andrade L. Validation of a Portuguese version of The Beck Inventory and State-Trait Inventory in Brazilian subjects. J Med Biol Res 1996;29:452–7.
55. Rechtschaffen A, Kales A, editors. A manual of standardized terminology, techniques and scoring systems for sleep stages of human subjects. Los Angeles: BIS/RRI, UCLA; 1968.
56. Bonnet M, Carley D, Carskadon M, Easton P, Guilleminault C, Harper R, et al. ASDA report. EEG arousals: scoring rules and examples. A preliminary report from the Sleep Disorders Atlas Task Force of the American Sleep Disorders Association. Sleep 1992;15:173–84.
57. Cooley WJ, Tukey JW. An algorithm for the machine calculation of complex Fourier series. Math Comput 1965;19:297–301.
58. Svanborg E, Guilleminault C. EEG frequency changes during sleep apneas. Sleep 1996;19:248–54.
59. MacLean AW, Lue F, Moldofsky H. The reliability of visual scoring of alpha EEG activity during sleep. Sleep 1995;18:565–9.
60. Carette S, Oakson G, Guimont C, Steriade M. Sleep electroencephalography and the clinical response to amytriptyline in patients with fibromyalgia. Arthritis Rheum 1995;38:1211–7.
61. Lavigne GJ, Vally-Miguel AM, Montplaisir J. Muscle pain, dyskinesia and sleep. Can J Physiol Pharmacol 1991;69:678–82.
62. Akerstedt T, Hume K, Minors D, Waterhouse J. The meaning of good sleep: a longitudinal study of polysomnography and subjective sleep quality. J Sleep Res 1994;3:152–8.
63. Carskadon MA, Dement WC, Mitler MM, Guilleminault C, Zarcone V, Speigel R. Self-reports versus sleep laboratory findings in 122 drug-free subjects with complaints of chronic insomnia. Am J Psychiatry 1976;133:1382–8.
64. Stepanski E, Lamphere J, Roehrs T, Zorick F, Roth T. Sleep fragmentation and daytime sleepiness. Sleep 1984;7:18–26.
65. Bonnet MH. Infrequent periodic sleep disruption: effects on sleep, performance and mood. Physiol Behav 1989;45:1049–55.
66. Levine B, Roehrs T, Stepanski E, Zorick F, Roth T. Fragmenting sleep diminishes its recuperative value. Sleep 1987;10:590–9.
67. Roehrs T, Merlotti L, Petrucelli N, Stepanski E, Roth T. Experimental sleep fragmentation. Sleep 1994;17:438–43.
68. Landis CA, Robinson CR, Helms C, Levine JD. Differential effects of acetylsalicylic acid and acetaminophen on sleep abnormalities in a rat chronic pain model. Brain Res 1989;488:195–201.
69. Procacci P. Methods for the study of pain thresholds in man. In: Bonica ER, editor. Advances in pain research and therapy. Vol. 3. New York: Raven Press; 1979. p. 781–90.
70. Moldofsky H. Sleep and fibrositis syndrome. Rheum Dis Clin North Am 1989;15:91–103.
71. Reilly PA, Littlejohn GO. Diurnal variation in symptoms and signs of the fibromyalgia syndrome (FS). J Musculoskeletal Pain 1993; 1:237–43.
72. Hench PK. Sleep and rheumatic diseases. Bull Rheum Dis 1996; 45:1–6.
73. Kempenaers C, Simenon G, Elst MV, Fransolet L, Mingard P, de Maertelaer V, et al. Effect of an antidiencephalon immune serum on pain and sleep in primary fibromyalgia. Neuropsychobiology 1994;30:66–72.
74. Haytornthwaite JA, Hegel MT, Kernz RD. Development of a sleep diary for chronic pain patients. J Pain Symptom Manage 1991;6:65–72.
75. Magni G, Moreschi C, Rigatti-Luchini S, Merskey H. Prospective study on the relationship between depressive symptoms and chronic musculoskeletal pain. Pain 1994;56:289–97.
76. Wilson KG, Watson ST, Currie SR. Daily diary and ambulatory activity monitoring of sleep in patients with insomnia associated with chronic musculoskeletal pain. Pain 1998;75:75–84.
77. MacFarlane JG, Shahal B, Mously C, Moldofsky H. Periodic K-alpha sleep EEG activity and periodic limb movements during sleep: comparisons of clinical features and sleep parameters. Sleep 1996;19:200–4.
78. Nielsen KD, Drewes AM, Svendsen L, Bjerregard K, Taagholt S. Ambulatory recording and power spectra analysis by autoregressive modeling of polygraphic sleep signals in patients suffering from chronic pain. Methods Inf Med 1994;33:76–8.
79. Hasan J. Automatic analysis of sleep recordings: a critical review. Ann Clin Res 1985;17:280–7.
80. Kuwahara H, Higashi H, Mizuki Y, Matsunari S, Tanaka M, Inanaga K. Automatic real time analysis of human sleep stages by an interval histogram method. Electroencephalogr Clin Neurophysiol 1988;70:220–9.
81. Geering BA, Achermann P, Eggimann F, Borbéry A. Period-amplitude analysis and power spectral analysis: a comparison based on all-night sleep EEG recordings. J Sleep Res 1993;2: 121–9.
82. Achermann P, Dijk DJ, Brunner DP, Borbély AA. A model of human sleep homeostasis based on EEG slow-wave activity: quantitative comparison of data and simulations. Brain Res Bull 1993;31:97–113.
83. Armitage R, Roffwarg HP, Rush AJ, Calhoun JS, Purdy DG, Giles DE. Digital period analysis of sleep EEG in depression. Biol Psychiatry 1992;31:52–68.
84. Steriade M. Brain electrical activity and sensory processing during waking and sleep stages. In: Kryger MH, Roth T, Dement WC, editors. Principles and practice of sleep medicine. 2nd ed. Philadelphia: WB Saunders; 1994. p.105–24.

FOSAMAX®(alendronate sodium tablets) **BRIEF SUMMARY OF PRESCRIBING INFORMATION**

CONTRAINDICATIONS

- Abnormalities of the esophagus which delay esophageal emptying such as stricture or achalasia
- Inability to stand or sit upright for at least 30 minutes
- Hypersensitivity to any component of this product
- Hypocalcemia (see PRECAUTIONS, *General*)

WARNINGS

FOSAMAX, like other bisphosphonates, may cause local irritation of the upper gastrointestinal mucosa. Esophageal adverse experiences, such as esophagitis, esophageal ulcers and esophageal erosions, occasionally with bleeding and rarely followed by esophageal stricture, have been reported in patients receiving treatment with FOSAMAX. In some cases these have been severe and required hospitalization. Physicians should therefore be alert to any signs or symptoms signaling a possible esophageal reaction and patients should be instructed to discontinue FOSAMAX and seek medical attention if they develop dysphagia, odynophagia, retrosternal pain, or new or worsening heartburn. The risk of severe esophageal adverse experiences appears to be greater in patients who lie down after taking FOSAMAX and/or who fail to swallow it with a full glass (6–8 oz) of water, and/or who continue to take FOSAMAX after developing symptoms suggestive of esophageal irritation. Therefore, it is very important that the full dosing instructions are provided to, and understood by, the patient (see DOSAGE AND ADMINISTRATION). In patients who cannot comply with dosing instructions due to mental disability, therapy with FOSAMAX should be used under appropriate supervision. Because of possible irritant effects of FOSAMAX on the upper gastrointestinal mucosa and a potential for worsening of the underlying disease, caution should be used when FOSAMAX is given to patients with active upper gastrointestinal problems (such as dysphagia, esophageal diseases, gastritis, duodenitis, or ulcers). There have been post-marketing reports of gastric and duodenal ulcers, some severe and with complications, although no increased risk was observed in controlled clinical trials.

PRECAUTIONS

General

Causes of osteoporosis other than estrogen deficiency, aging, and glucocorticoid use should be considered. Hypocalcemia must be corrected before initiating therapy with FOSAMAX (see CONTRAINDICATIONS). Other disturbances of mineral metabolism (such as vitamin D deficiency) should also be effectively treated. Presumably due to the effects of FOSAMAX on increasing bone mineral, small, asymptomatic decreases in serum calcium and phosphate may occur, especially in patients with Paget's disease, in whom the pretreatment rate of bone turnover may be greatly elevated and in patients receiving glucocorticoids, in whom calcium absorption may be decreased. Ensuring adequate calcium and vitamin D intake is especially important in patients with Paget's disease of bone and in patients receiving glucocorticoids.

Renal insufficiency

FOSAMAX is not recommended for patients with renal insufficiency (creatinine clearance <35 mL/min). (See DOSAGE AND ADMINISTRATION.)

Glucocorticoid-induced osteoporosis

The risk versus benefit of FOSAMAX for treatment at daily dosages of glucocorticoids less than 7.5 mg of prednisone or equivalent has not been established (see INDICATIONS AND USAGE). Before initiating treatment, the hormonal status of both men and women should be ascertained and appropriate replacement considered. A bone mineral density measurement should be made at the initiation of therapy and repeated after 6 to 12 months of combined FOSAMAX and glucocorticoid treatment. The efficacy of FOSAMAX for the treatment of glucocorticoid-induced osteoporosis has been shown in patients with a median bone mineral density which was 1.2 standard deviations below the mean for healthy young adults. The efficacy of FOSAMAX has been established in studies of two years' duration. The greatest increase in bone mineral density occurred in the first year with maintenance or smaller gains during the second year. Efficacy of FOSAMAX beyond two years has not been studied. The efficacy of FOSAMAX in respect to fracture prevention has been demonstrated for vertebral fractures. However, this finding was based on very few fractures that occurred primarily in postmenopausal women. The efficacy for prevention of non-vertebral fractures has not been demonstrated.

Information for Patients

General

Physicians should instruct their patients to read the patient package insert before starting therapy with FOSAMAX and to reread it each time the prescription is renewed. Patients should be instructed to take supplemental calcium and vitamin D, if daily dietary intake is inadequate. Weight-bearing exercise should be considered along with the modification of certain behavioral factors, such as cigarette smoking and/or excessive alcohol consumption, if these factors exist.

Dosing Instructions

Patients should be instructed that the expected benefits of FOSAMAX may only be obtained when each tablet is swallowed with plain water the first thing upon arising for the day at least 30 minutes before the first food, beverage, or medication of the day. Even dosing with orange juice or coffee has been shown to markedly reduce the absorption of FOSAMAX (see CLINICAL PHARMACOLOGY, *Pharmacokinetics, Absorption*). To facilitate delivery to the stomach and thus reduce the potential for esophageal irritation patients should be instructed to swallow FOSAMAX with a full glass of water (6–8 oz) and not to lie down for at least 30 minutes and until after their first food of the day. Patients should not chew or suck on the tablet because of a potential for oropharyngeal ulceration. Patients should be specifically instructed not to take FOSAMAX at bedtime or before arising for the day. Patients should be informed that failure to follow these instructions may increase their risk of esophageal problems. Patients should be instructed that if they develop symptoms of esophageal disease (such as difficulty or pain upon swallowing, retrosternal pain or new or worsening heartburn) they should stop taking FOSAMAX and consult their physician. Patients should be instructed that if they miss a dose of once weekly FOSAMAX, they should take one tablet on the morning after they remember. They should not take two tablets on the same day but should return to taking one tablet once a week, as originally scheduled on their chosen day.

Drug Interactions (also see CLINICAL PHARMACOLOGY, *Pharmacokinetics, Drug Interactions*)

Estrogen/hormone replacement therapy (HRT)

Concomitant use of HRT (estrogen ± progestin) and FOSAMAX was assessed in two clinical studies of one or two years' duration in postmenopausal osteoporotic women. In these studies, the safety and tolerability profile of the combination was consistent with those of the individual treatments; however, the degree of suppression of bone turnover (as assessed by mineralizing surface) was significantly greater with the combination than with either component alone. The long-term effects of combined FOSAMAX and HRT on fracture occurrence have not been studied (see CLINICAL PHARMACOLOGY, *Clinical Studies, Concomitant use with estrogen/hormone replacement therapy (HRT)* and ADVERSE REACTIONS, *Clinical Studies, Concomitant use with estrogen/hormone replacement therapy*).

Calcium Supplements/Antacids

It is likely that calcium supplements, antacids, and some oral medications will interfere with absorption of FOSAMAX. Therefore, patients must wait at least one-half hour after taking FOSAMAX before taking any other oral medications.

Aspirin

In clinical studies, the incidence of upper gastrointestinal adverse events was increased in patients receiving concomitant therapy with daily doses of FOSAMAX greater than 10 mg and aspirin-containing products.

Nonsteroidal Anti-inflammatory Drugs (NSAIDs)

FOSAMAX may be administered to patients taking NSAIDs. In a 3-year, controlled, clinical study (n=2027) during which a majority of patients received concomitant NSAIDs, the incidence of upper gastrointestinal adverse events was similar in patients taking FOSAMAX 5 or 10 mg/day compared to those taking placebo. However, since NSAID use is associated with gastrointestinal irritation, caution should be used during concomitant use with FOSAMAX.

Pregnancy

Pregnancy Category C:

Reproduction studies in rats showed decreased postimplantation survival at 2 mg/kg/day and decreased body weight gain in normal pups at 1 mg/kg/day. Sites of incomplete fetal ossification were statistically significantly increased in rats beginning at 10 mg/kg/day in vertebral (cervical, thoracic, and lumbar), skull, and sternebral bones. The above doses ranged from 0.26 times (1 mg/kg) to 2.6 times (10 mg/kg) a maximum recommended daily dose of 40 mg (Paget's disease) based on surface area, mg/m^2. No similar fetal effects were seen when pregnant rabbits were treated at doses up to 35 mg/kg/day (10.3 times a 40 mg human daily dose based on surface area, mg/m^2). Both total and ionized calcium decreased in pregnant rats at 15 mg/kg/day (3.9 times the 40 human daily dose based on surface area, mg/m^2) resulting in delays and failures of delivery. Protracted parturition due to maternal hypocalcemia occurred in rats at doses as low as 0.5 mg/kg/day (0.13 times a 40 mg human daily dose based on surface area, mg/m^2) when rats were treated from before mating through gestation. Maternotoxicity (late pregnancy deaths) occurred in the female rats treated with 15 mg/kg/day for varying periods of time ranging from treatment only during pre-mating to treatment only during early, middle, or late gestation; these deaths were lessened but not eliminated by cessation of treatment. Calcium supplementation either in the drinking water or by minipump could not ameliorate the hypocalcemia or prevent maternal and neonatal deaths due to delays in delivery; calcium supplementation IV prevented maternal, but not fetal deaths. There are no studies in pregnant women. FOSAMAX should be used during pregnancy only if the potential benefit justifies the potential risk to the mother and fetus.

Nursing Mothers

It is not known whether alendronate is excreted in human milk. Because many drugs are excreted in human milk, caution should be exercised when FOSAMAX is administered to nursing women.

Pediatric Use

Safety and effectiveness in pediatric patients have not been established.

Use in the Elderly

Of the patients receiving FOSAMAX in the United States and Multinational osteoporosis treatment studies in women, the osteoporosis study in men, glucocorticoid-induced osteoporosis studies, and Paget's disease studies (see CLINICAL PHARMACOLOGY, *Clinical Studies*), 45%, 50%, 37%, and 70%, respectively, were 65 years of age or over. No overall differences in efficacy or safety were observed between these patients and younger patients but greater sensitivity of some older individuals cannot be ruled out.

ADVERSE REACTIONS

Clinical Studies

In clinical studies of up to five years in duration adverse experiences associated with FOSAMAX usually were mild, and generally did not require discontinuation of therapy. FOSAMAX has been evaluated for safety in approximately 8000 postmenopausal women in clinical studies.

Treatment of osteoporosis

Postmenopausal women

In two identically designed, three-year, placebo-controlled, double-blind, multicenter studies (United States and Multinational; n=994), discontinuation of therapy due to any clinical adverse experience occurred in 4.1% of 196 patients treated with FOSAMAX 10 mg/day and 6.0% of 397 patients treated with placebo. In the Fracture Intervention Trial (n=6459), discontinuation of therapy due to any clinical adverse experience occurred in 9.1% of 3236 patients treated with FOSAMAX 5 mg/day for 2 years and 10 mg/day for either one or two additional years and 10.1% of 3223 patients treated with placebo. Discontinuations due to upper gastrointestinal adverse experiences were: FOSAMAX, 3.2%; placebo, 2.7%. In these study populations, 49-54% had a history of gastrointestinal disorders at baseline and 54-89% used nonsteroidal anti-inflammatory drugs or aspirin at some time during the studies. Adverse experiences from these studies considered by the investigators as possibly, probably, or definitely drug related in ≥1% of patients treated with either FOSAMAX or placebo are presented in the following table.

Osteoporosis Treatment Studies in Postmenopausal Women–Adverse Experiences Considered Possibly, Probably, or Definitely Drug Related by the Investigators and Reported in ≥1% of Patients

	United States/Multinational Studies		Fracture Intervention Trial	
	FOSAMAX* % (n=196)	Placebo % (n=397)	FOSAMAX** % (n=3236)	Placebo % (n=3223)
Gastrointestinal				
abdominal pain	6.6	4.8	1.5	1.5
nausea	3.6	4.0	1.1	1.5
dyspepsia	3.6	3.5	1.1	1.2
constipation	3.1	1.8	0.0	0.2
diarrhea	3.1	1.8	0.6	0.3
flatulence	2.6	0.5	0.2	0.3
acid regurgitation	2.0	4.3	1.1	0.9
esophageal ulcer	1.5	0.0	0.1	0.1
vomiting	1.0	1.5	0.2	0.3
dysphagia	1.0	0.0	0.1	0.1
abdominal distension	1.0	0.8	0.0	0.0
gastritis	0.5	1.3	0.6	0.7
Musculoskeletal				
musculoskeletal (bone, muscle or joint) pain	4.1	2.5	0.4	0.3
muscle cramp	0.0	1.0	0.2	0.1
Nervous System/Psychiatric				
headache	2.6	1.5	0.2	0.2
dizziness	0.0	1.0	0.0	0.1
Special Senses				
taste perversion	0.5	1.0	0.1	0.0

*10 mg/day for three years **5 mg/day for 2 years and 10 mg/day for either 1 or 2 additional years

Rarely, rash and erythema have occurred.

One patient treated with FOSAMAX (10 mg/day) who had a history of peptic ulcer disease and gastrectomy and who was taking concomitant aspirin developed an anastomotic ulcer with mild hemorrhage, which was considered drug related. Aspirin and FOSAMAX were discontinued and the patient recovered.

The adverse experience profile was similar for the 401 patients treated with either 5 or 20 mg doses of FOSAMAX in the United States and Multinational studies. The adverse experience profile for the 296 patients who received continued treatment with either 5 or 10 mg doses of FOSAMAX in the two-year extension of these studies (treatment years 4 and 5) was similar to that observed during the three-year placebo-controlled period. During the extension period, of the 151 patients treated with FOSAMAX 10 mg/day, the proportion of patients who discontinued therapy due to any clinical adverse experience was similar to that during the first three years of the study.

In a one-year, double-blind multicenter study, the overall safety and tolerability profiles of once weekly FOSAMAX 70 mg and FOSAMAX 10 mg daily were similar. The adverse experiences were considered by investigators as possibly, probably, or definitely drug related in ≥1% of patients treated with either FOSAMAX 70 mg once weekly (n=519), or FOSAMAX 10 mg daily (n=370), respectively, were: *Gastrointestinal:* abdominal pain (3.7%; 3.0%), dyspepsia (2.7%; 2.2%), acid regurgitation (1.9%; 2.4%), nausea (1.9%; 2.4%), abdominal distension (1.0%; 1.4%), constipation (0.8%; 1.6%), flatulence (0.4%; 1.6%), gastritis (0.2%; 1.1%), gastric ulcer (0.0%; 1.1%); *Musculoskeletal:* musculoskeletal (bone, muscle, joint) pain (2.9%; 3.2%), muscle cramp (0.2%; 1.1%).

Men

In a two-year, placebo-controlled, double-blind multicenter study, discontinuation of therapy due to any clinical adverse experience occurred in 2.7% of men treated with FOSAMAX 10 mg/day and 10.5% of men treated with placebo. The adverse experiences considered by investigators as possibly, probably, or definitely drug related in ≥2% of patients treated with either FOSAMAX 10 mg/day (n=146), or placebo (n=95), respectively, were: *Gastrointestinal:* acid regurgitation (4.1%; 3.2%), flatulence (4.1%; 1.1%), dyspepsia (3.4%; 0.0%), abdominal pain (2.1%; 1.1%), nausea (2.1%; 0.0%).

Prevention of osteoporosis in postmenopausal women

The safety of FOSAMAX 5 mg/day in postmenopausal women 40-60 years of age has been evaluated in three double-blind, placebo-controlled studies involving over 1,400 patients randomized to receive FOSAMAX for either two or three years. In these studies the overall safety profiles of FOSAMAX 5 mg/day and placebo were similar. Discontinuation of therapy due to any clinical adverse experience occurred in 7.5% of 642 patients treated with FOSAMAX 5 mg/day and 5.7% of 648 patients treated with placebo.

In a one-year, double-blind multicenter study, the overall safety and tolerability profiles of once weekly FOSAMAX 35 mg and FOSAMAX 5 mg daily were similar.

The adverse experiences from these studies considered by the investigators as possibly, probably, or definitely drug related in ≥1% of patients treated with either once weekly FOSAMAX 35 mg, FOSAMAX 5mg/day or placebo are presented in the following table.

Osteoporosis Prevention Studies in Postmenopausal Women–Adverse Experiences Considered Possibly, Probably, or Definitely Drug Related by the Investigators and Reported in ≥1% of Patients

	Two/Three-Year Studies		One-Year Study	
	FOSAMAX 5 mg/day % (n=642)	Placebo % (n=648)	FOSAMAX 5 mg/day % (n=361)	Once-Weekly FOSAMAX 35 mg % (n=362)
Gastrointestinal				
dyspepsia	1.9	1.4	2.2	1.7
abdominal pain	1.7	3.4	4.2	2.2
acid regurgitation	1.4	2.5	4.2	4.7
nausea	1.4	1.4	2.5	1.4
diarrhea	1.1	1.7	1.1	0.6
constipation	0.9	0.5	1.7	0.3
abdominal distension	0.2	0.3	1.4	1.1
Musculoskeletal				
musculoskeletal (bone, muscle or joint) pain	0.8	0.9	1.9	2.2

Concomitant use with estrogen/hormone replacement therapy

In two studies (of one and two years' duration) of postmenopausal osteoporotic women (total: n=853), the safety and tolerability profile of combined treatment with FOSAMAX 10 mg once daily and estrogen ± progestin (n=354) was consistent with those of the individual treatments.

Treatments of glucocorticoid-induced osteoporosis

In two one-year, placebo-controlled, double-blind multicenter studies, in patients receiving glucocorticoid treatment, the overall safety and tolerability profiles of FOSAMAX 5 and 10 mg/day were generally similar to that of placebo. The adverse experiences considered by the investigators as possibly, probably, or definitely drug related in ≥1% of patients treated with either FOSAMAX 10 mg/day (n=157), FOSAMAX 5 mg/day (n=161), or placebo (n=159), respectively, were: *Gastrointestinal:* abdominal pain (3.2%; 1.9%; 0.0%), acid regurgitation (2.5%; 1.9%; 1.3%), constipation (1.3%; 0.6%; 0.0%), melena (1.3%; 0.0%; 0.0%), nausea (0.6%; 1.2%; 0.6%), diarrhea (0.0%; 0.0%; 1.3%), *Nervous System/Psychiatric:* headache (0.6%; 0.0%; 1.3%).

The overall safety and tolerability profile in the glucocorticoid-induced osteoporosis population that continued therapy for the second year of the studies (FOSAMAX: n=147) was consistent with that observed in the first year.

Paget's disease of bone

In clinical studies (osteoporosis and Paget's disease), adverse experiences reported in 175 patients taking FOSAMAX 40 mg/day for 3-12 months were similar to those in postmenopausal women treated with FOSAMAX 10 mg/day. However, there was an apparent increased incidence of upper gastrointestinal adverse experiences in patients taking FOSAMAX 40 mg/day (17.7% FOSAMAX vs. 10.2% placebo). One case of esophagitis and two cases of gastritis resulted in discontinuation of treatment. Additionally, musculoskeletal (bone, muscle, or joint) pain, which has been described in patients with Paget's disease treated with other bisphosphonates, was considered by the investigators as possibly, probably, or definitely drug related in approximately 6% of patients treated with FOSAMAX 40 mg/day vs. approximately 1% of patients treated with placebo, but rarely resulted in discontinuation of therapy. Discontinuation of therapy due to any clinical adverse experience occurred in 6.4% of patients with Paget's disease treated with FOSAMAX 40 mg/day and 2.4% of patients treated with placebo.

Laboratory Test Findings

In double-blind, multicenter, controlled studies, asymptomatic, mild, and transient decreases in serum calcium and phosphate were observed in approximately 18% and 10%, respectively, of patients taking FOSAMAX versus approximately 12% and 3% of those taking placebo. However, the incidences of decreases in serum calcium to <8.0 mg/dL (2.0 mM) and serum phosphate to ≤2.0 mg/dL (0.65 mM) were similar in both treatment groups.

Post-Marketing Experience

The following adverse reactions have been reported in post-marketing use: *Body as a Whole:* hypersensitivity reactions including urticaria and rarely angioedema. *Gastrointestinal:* esophagitis, esophageal erosions, esophageal ulcers, rarely esophageal stricture, and oropharyngeal ulceration. Gastric or duodenal ulcers, some severe and with complications have also been reported (see WARNINGS, PRECAUTIONS, and *Information for Patients,* and DOSAGE AND ADMINISTRATION). *Skin:* rash (occasionally with photosensitivity). *Special Senses:* rarely uveitis.

For more detailed information, consult your Merck representative or see the full Prescribing Information.

ARTHRITIS & RHEUMATISM
Vol. 44, No. 1, January 2001, pp 231–238

Efficacy and Safety of Desensitization to Allopurinol following Cutaneous Reactions

Adel G. Fam,[1] Shelly M. Dunne,[2] John Iazzetta,[1] and Thomas W. Paton[1]

Objective. **To evaluate the long-term efficacy and safety of slow oral desensitization in the management of patients with hyperuricemia and allopurinol-induced maculopapular eruptions.**

Methods. **A retrospective evaluation of an oral desensitization regimen using gradual dosage-escalation of allopurinol in 32 patients (30 with gout and 2 with chronic lymphocytic leukemia) whose therapy was interrupted because of a pruritic cutaneous reaction to the drug.**

Results. **Twenty-one men and 11 women with a mean age of 63 years (range 17–83 years), a mean serum urate level of 618 μmoles/liter (range 495–750) (or, mean 10.4 mg/dl [range 8.3–12.6]), and a mean serum creatinine level of 249 μmoles/liter (range 75–753) (or, mean 2.8 mg/dl [range 0.8–8.5]) were studied. Desensitization failed in 4 patients because of unmanageable recurrent rash. Twenty-eight patients completed the desensitization procedure to a target allopurinol dosage of 50–100 mg/day, 21 without deviation from the protocol for a mean of 30.5 days (range 21–56 days) and 7 requiring dosage adjustments because of a recurrent rash over 53.8 days (range 40–189 days). Seven of these 28 patients developed late cutaneous reactions 1–20 months postdesensitization, 4 responding to dosage modification and 3 discontinuing the drug. Twenty-five of the 32 patients (78%) continued to take allopurinol; their mean duration of followup was 32.6 months (range 3–92 months) and the mean postdesensitization serum urate level was 318 μmoles/liter (range 187–452) (or, mean 5.3 mg/dl [range 3.0–7.5]).**

Conclusion. **The study confirms the long-term efficacy and safety of slow oral desensitization to allopurinol in patients with maculopapular eruptions, particularly in those with gout, who cannot be treated with uricosurics or other urate-lowering drugs. Although pruritic skin eruptions may recur both during and after desensitization, most of these cutaneous reactions can be managed by temporary withdrawal of allopurinol and dosage adjustment.**

Allopurinol is an effective urate-lowering drug which has been the mainstay of treatment of hyperuricemia and gout for the last 36 years (1). The drug is well tolerated by the majority of patients, and serious side effects are rare (1–4). However, an estimated 2% of patients receiving allopurinol therapy, particularly those with chronic renal insufficiency, may experience a pruritic maculopapular rash that precludes further administration (1–4). This poses an obstacle to the treatment of hyperuricemia, particularly in patients with gout and renal insufficiency, which renders uricosurics ineffective (5), and in patients receiving chemotherapy for myeloproliferative or lymphoproliferative diseases, in whom uricosurics are not recommended.

Desensitization procedures (6), including both true immunologic desensitization (e.g., to penicillin) and test-dosing or tolerance-induction protocols (e.g., "desensitization" to sulfasalazine [7], trimethoprim/sulfamethoxazole [8], and ciprofloxacin [9]), have been successfully used for the management of drug-induced cutaneous reactions. In 1992, we reported our experience with desensitization to allopurinol, using a schedule of graded dosages, in a group of 9 patients with gout and renal impairment who had their therapy interrupted because of a maculopapular eruption in response to the drug (10). Findings from the study indicated that slow oral desensitization to allopurinol is a feasible and

Presented at the 62nd Annual Scientific Meeting of the American College of Rheumatology, San Diego, CA, November 1998.

Supported in part by a grant from the Sunnybrook Trust for Medical Research.

[1]Adel G. Fam, MD, FRCP(C), John Iazzetta, PharmD, Thomas W. Paton, PharmD: University of Toronto, Toronto, Ontario, Canada; [2]Shelly M. Dunne, MD, FRCP(C): Toronto East General Hospital, Toronto, Ontario, Canada.

Address correspondence and reprint requests to Adel G. Fam, MD, Sunnybrook Health Science Centre, 2075 Bayview Avenue M-1402, Toronto, Ontario M4M 3M5, Canada.

Submitted for publication June 23, 2000; accepted in revised form August 26, 2000.

acceptably safe approach to therapy, particularly in patients who cannot be treated with other urate-lowering drugs (10). Other investigators have reported similar results with allopurinol desensitization (11–17), including rapid intravenous desensitization in 1 patient (18), re-desensitization after initial failure in 1 patient (19), and desensitization of 2 siblings with allopurinol-induced rash (20). Recently, desensitization to allopurinol-induced fixed drug eruptions has also been described (21–23). However, only a small number of patients have been studied, and there is limited information regarding the long-term outcome of allopurinol desensitization.

The present study (24) retrospectively evaluates the outcome, safety, and long-term clinical utility of allopurinol desensitization in a larger group of patients with hyperuricemic disorders (mainly gout) and cutaneous reactions who were desensitized during the period 1991–1998, with a further followup of the original 9 patients who underwent desensitization from 1980 to 1990 (10). A secondary objective of the investigation was to define the indications and dosing guidelines for allopurinol desensitization.

PATIENTS AND METHODS

Patient population. Sunnybrook Health Science Centre is a tertiary referral teaching hospital. Preparation of the allopurinol suspension and the protocol for desensitization were established by the Ambulatory Patient Pharmacy since our initial publication in 1980 (25) and the larger study in 1992 (10). Patients were either referred to our unit or the desensitization schedule was prescribed by their physicians and dispensed by the pharmacy at Sunnybrook. A computer printout generated by the Ambulatory Patient Pharmacy was used to identify all patients for whom allopurinol suspension was prescribed for desensitization during 1991–1998. Desensitization was the only indication for allopurinol suspension in this setting. No patient was inadvertently excluded, as verified by reviewing the pharmacy's computer records. A list was also compiled of the original 9 patients who had undergone desensitization from 1980 to 1990 (10). Study approval was granted by the Research Ethics Board of Sunnybrook Health Science Centre.

Patients received a consent form approved by the Research Ethics Board describing the nature of the study and requesting permission to review personal medical records and, if necessary, participate in a telephone interview. The study included patients with gouty arthritis or other hyperuricemic states requiring urate-lowering therapy with allopurinol who had a well-documented recent history of a pruritic, erythematous maculopapular or morbilliform eruption occurring following initiation of allopurinol, which resolved after discontinuation of the drug, and who subsequently underwent oral desensitization to allopurinol, as recorded in the pharmacy computer. In all patients, the rash was documented in the outpatient chart or hospital record by the examining physician and verified to be temporally related to allopurinol administration.

Based on data from the original study (10), patients did not undergo desensitization if their hemoglobin value was <90 gm/liter, total leukocyte count was $<4.0 \times 10^9$/liter, platelet count was $<100.0 \times 10^9$/liter, or findings of liver function tests were >2-fold elevated, or if they had experienced toxic epidermal necrolysis or other catastrophic reaction associated with allopurinol.

Clinical data included age, sex, indication for allopurinol therapy, presence of renal impairment, hypertension, alcoholism, heart failure, or history of nephrolithiasis, concomitant medications (including diuretics, low-dose aspirin, and cyclosporine), a description of the original cutaneous reaction to allopurinol and any history of inadvertent reexposure, and other therapies for acute and chronic gout.

Results of the following studies performed before, during, and after desensitization were recorded: complete blood cell count, urinalysis, serum creatinine (normal <120 μmoles/liter [or, <1.5 mg/dl]), serum urate (normal for men 180–450 μmoles/liter [or, 3–7 mg/dl] and for women 150–360 μmoles/liter [or, 2–6 mg/dl]), alanine aminotransferase, aspartate aminotransferase, gamma glutamyl transferase, bilirubin, and albumin, as well as a pretreatment 24-hour urinary urate excretion study while eating a regular diet (normal <4.76 mmoles/day [or, 800 mg/day]).

Desensitization procedure. Desensitization was performed as previously described (10). Briefly, a suspension of allopurinol was prepared by the outpatient pharmacy as follows: two 100-mg tablets of allopurinol were crushed in a mortar, and 33 ml of 1% methylcellulose solution was slowly added to make a slurry. Both 4 ml of cherry flavor and simple sugar were then added and mixed to a volume of 100 ml to yield a concentration of allopurinol of 10 mg/5 ml. Ten milliliters of this suspension was further diluted with the same ingredients to 100 ml, yielding a 1 mg/5 ml (200 μg/ml) concentration.

Using the high- and low-concentration suspensions, unit doses containing 10 μg, 25 μg, 50 μg, 100 μg, 200 μg, 500 μg, 1 mg, 5 mg, 10 mg, and 25 mg of allopurinol were prepared; 50-mg and 100-mg doses were then administered as one-half and whole 100-mg tablets, respectively. Predesensitization intradermal tests using a solution of allopurinol and oxypurinol were not performed. The desensitization procedure and its potential risks were discussed with each patient and after obtaining the patient's informed consent, the *standard protocol* was administered as follows (Table 1): an initial dosage of 50 μg of allopurinol/day, which was progressively and cautiously increased every 3 days to 100 μg, 200 μg, 500 μg, 1 mg, 5 mg, 10 mg, 25 mg, and finally to a target dosage of 50–100 mg of allopurinol/day. Further dosage increments were based upon the individual patient's serum urate and creatinine levels, aiming at reducing and maintaining serum urate levels at <300–350 μmoles/liter (or, <5–6 mg/dl), which is well below the levels at which urate saturates the extracellular fluid (~404 μmoles/liter [or, 6.8 mg/dl] at 37°C).

A *modified desensitization protocol*, with initial daily doses of allopurinol of 10 μg and 25 μg, and a dosage change every 5–10 days or longer, was initially prescribed for frail, elderly patients with multiple comorbid medical conditions,

Table 1. Standard allopurinol desensitization protocol*

Daily dose	Preparation†	Days (approximate)
50 μg	0.25-ml suspension (1 mg/5 ml)	1–3
100 μg	0.5-ml suspension (1 mg/5 ml)	4–6
200 μg	1-ml suspension (1 mg/5 ml)	7–9
500 μg	2.5-ml suspension (1 mg/5 ml)	10–12
1 mg	5-ml suspension (1 mg/5 ml)	13–15
5 mg	2.5-ml suspension (10 mg/5 ml)	16–18
10 mg	5-ml suspension (10 mg/5 ml)	19–21
25 mg	12.5-ml suspension (10 mg/5 ml)	22–24
50 mg	One-half a 100-mg tablet	25–27
100 mg	One 100-mg tablet	28+

* For high-risk patients, a modified desensitization protocol, with initial allopurinol doses of 10 μg and 25 μg (0.05 ml and 0.12 ml of 1 mg/5 ml suspension, respectively), and a dosage escalation every 5–10 days or longer, is recommended.
† Two concentrations of allopurinol suspension were used: 1 mg/5 ml and 10 mg/5 ml, depending on the dosage required.

including renal impairment, as well as for patients with more widespread, confluent, allopurinol-induced eruptions, particularly when associated with facial or tongue swelling, fever, stomatitis, or eosinophilia.

All patients undergoing desensitization were cautioned about possible severe reactions and were instructed to stop allopurinol and consult their physician if an adverse reaction, such as fever, pruritus, or skin eruption, occurred. In such an event, allopurinol was withheld until the reaction had resolved, reintroduced cautiously at one-half the previously tolerated dosage, and the rate of dosage escalation was slowed to every 5–10 days or longer.

Outcome assessment. Followup data were collected through active clinic assessments, chart review, and if necessary, by telephone interview. Short-term and long-term assessments of outcome were made. In the short-term outcome assessment, successful desensitization was defined as the ability to tolerate allopurinol at a dosage of 50–100 mg/day. The time taken to reach the target dosage and the occurrence of recurrent rash or other adverse events during desensitization were documented. In the long-term outcome assessment made after desensitization, we evaluated the control of hyperuricemia, the effects of treatment on the frequency of gouty attacks, as confirmed by interview with the patients and review of their medical records, and on the number and size of tophi, as documented by the treating physician, late cutaneous reactions, and discontinuation of allopurinol for any reason.

RESULTS

Patient population. The clinical characteristics of the 32 patients who had undergone desensitization to allopurinol are outlined in Table 2. This patient group consisted of 9 previously described patients who had been desensitized to the drug between 1980 and 1990 (10) and an additional 23 patients who were consecutively enrolled between 1991 and 1998.

Thirty patients had gout, and 2 had chronic lymphocytic leukemia. All patients with gout experienced recurrent gouty attacks, and 21 had tophi and disabling chronic tophaceous gouty arthritis. Eight of the patients with gout had a history of renal calculi. Indications for allopurinol desensitization in patients with gouty arthritis included renal insufficiency, which renders uricosurics ineffective, in 26 patients, intolerance to uricosurics in 3 patients, and contraindication to uricosuric therapy in 1 patient because of nephrolithiasis and hyperuricosuria of 5.6 mmoles/day.

Allopurinol therapy had been withdrawn in all patients because of a pruritic maculopapular or morbilliform eruption, which in the majority of patients (24 of 32, or 75%) developed within 3 months of initiating treatment. The rash was associated with fever in 6 patients, 3 of whom also had eosinophilia and facial swelling, and with stomatitis in 1 patient. None of these individuals had experienced a severe allopurinol hypersensitivity reaction (e.g., Stevens-Johnson syndrome, toxic epidermal necrolysis, acute hepatitis, or acute interstitial nephritis) or had previously failed desensitization to the drug. In 4 patients, inadvertent reexposure to allopurinol prior to desensitization resulted in recurrence of the rash, which resolved following withdrawal of the drug.

Twenty-two of the 32 patients undergoing desensitization had been referred to our unit; in the remaining 10 patients, desensitization was initiated by their physi-

Table 2. Clinical characteristics of 32 patients undergoing allopurinol desensitization for cutaneous reactions

Feature	Frequency
Age, mean (range) years	63 (17–83)
Sex, no. of men:no. of women	21:11
Indication for allopurinol desensitization, no. positive/total	
Gout and renal insufficiency	26/32
Gout and intolerance/contraindication to uricosurics	4/32
Chemotherapy for chronic lymphocytic leukemia	2/32
Serum urate, mean (range) μmoles/liter	618 (495–750)
Twenty-four–hour urinary urate, mean (range) mmoles/day*	2.3 (0.5–5.6)
Serum creatinine, mean (range) μmoles/liter	249 (75–753)
Patients with gout, no. (%)†	
Recurrent gouty arthritis	30/30 (100)
Tophi and chronic tophaceous gouty arthritis	21/30 (70)
Renal calculi	8/30 (27)

* Represents 13 of 32 patients.
† Represents 30 patients.

cians. Allopurinol dosages prior to the cutaneous reaction were not always appropriate for the degree of renal impairment: 21 of 26 patients with renal insufficiency were receiving 300 mg/day, and 4 were maintained on 200 mg/day. Only 1 patient with advanced renal disease was receiving 100 mg of allopurinol daily.

The mean serum urate concentration before desensitization was 618 μmoles/liter (range 495–750) (or, 10.4 mg/dl [range 8.3–12.6]), with a mean of 631 μmoles/liter (or, 10.6 mg/dl) in men and 594 μmoles/liter (or, 10.0 mg/dl) in women. The mean 24-hour urinary urate level in 13 of 32 patients was 2.3 mmoles/day (range 0.5–5.6) (or, 390 mg/day [range 80–940]). The mean predesensitization serum creatinine concentration was 249 μmoles/liter (range 75–753) (or, 2.8 mg/dl [range 0.8–8.5]).

Risk factors in the 30 patients with gout included renal insufficiency in 26 patients (88%), hypertension in 25 (83%), chronic diuretic therapy in 22 (73%), cardiac failure in 8 (25%), long-term low-dose aspirin in 8 (25%), cyclosporine following renal transplantation in 3 (10%), family history of gout in 3 (10%), and ethanol abuse in 2 (7%).

Drug therapies for acute gouty attacks included corticosteroids in 18 patients, colchicine in 13, and nonsteroidal antiinflammatory drugs (NSAIDs) in 8. None of the patients were receiving long-term NSAIDs. Twelve patients were treated with uricosurics (sulfinpyrazone in 8 and probenecid in 4) but with little benefit in 9 and intolerance in 3 patients. No data were available on individuals with cutaneous reactions to allopurinol who declined desensitization.

Desensitization and outcome of therapy. The immediate and long-term outcomes of allopurinol desensitization are summarized in Table 3. Twenty-three individuals underwent desensitization as outpatients, and in 9 patients, the desensitization procedure was initiated in the hospital.

Short-term outcome. The dosage of allopurinol was escalated every 3 days (standard protocol) in 23 patients and every 5–10 days or longer (modified protocol) in 9 patients. Four patients (12.5%) were unable to complete the desensitization procedure because of recurrent rashes (Table 3): 1 patient also had nausea and oral ulcers, 1 had nausea and facial swelling, 1 refused to continue with further desensitization, and 1 developed an unmanageable rash despite repeated dosage adjustments.

Twenty-eight patients (87.5%) completed the desensitization protocol to a target allopurinol dosage of 50–100 mg/day. Desensitization was achieved in 21 patients (75%) without any adverse reaction or deviation from the set protocol, with dosage escalation every 3 days in 19 patients and every 5 days in the other 2. The mean duration of desensitization in this group of patients was 30.5 days (range 21–56 days). The other 7 patients (25%) required single (6 patients) or repeated (1 patient) dosage modifications because of a transient recurrent rash. These cutaneous reactions occurred at allopurinol dosages of <5 mg/day in 5 patients, 50 mg/day in 1, and 100 mg/day in 1. These patients required a slower rate of desensitization, with dosage changes every 5–10 days or longer (*modified desensitization protocol*), with a mean duration of the desensitization procedure of 53.8 days (range 40–189 days).

Long-term outcome. Followup was complete through 1999, with an observation period of 902 patient-months, or a mean of 32.6 months per patient (median 24 months, range 3–92 months per patient). Seven of 28 patients (25%) developed late, postdesensitization, recurrent cutaneous eruptions, 2 of whom also had "early" rash occurring during the desensitization procedure. These late cutaneous reactions occurred at a mean of 6 months (range 1–20 months) following desensitization. Four of the 7 patients responded to dosage adjustment, but the other 3 discontinued allopurinol treatment because of either an unmanageable recurrent rash (1 patient) or an unwillingness to continue treatment (2 patients).

Table 3. Short-term and long-term outcome of allopurinol desensitization in 32 patients

	Number (%) of patients	
Outcome	Continued administration	Drug withdrawal
Short-term outcome (n = 32)*		
Reactions during desensitization (n = 11)		
Recurrent rash (n = 9)†	7	2
Rash, nausea, and oral ulcers (n = 1)	0	1
Rash, nausea, and facial swelling (n = 1)	0	1
Completion of desensitization protocol	28 (87.5)	4 (12.5)
Long-term outcome (n = 28)‡		
Postdesensitization reactions (n = 7)		
Recurrent rash (n = 7)†	4	3
Overall outcome (n = 32)	25 (78)	7 (22)

* Percentage success rate of desensitization and adverse events.
† Two patients had rashes both during and after desensitization.
‡ Postdesensitization long-term tolerance to allopurinol for 32.6 months (range 3–92 months).

Thus, the overall success rate of desensitization was 25 of 32 patients, or 78% (Table 3). In the remaining 7 patients (22%), failure of allopurinol desensitization was the result of unmanageable recurrent rashes that occurred during (4 patients) and after (3 patients) desensitization. No patient experienced any serious hypersensitivity reactions, significant abnormal laboratory findings, or required hospitalization, emergency department care, or medications other than diphenhydramine for recurrent pruritic rash.

Maintenance dosages of allopurinol following desensitization in the 25 patients who remained evaluable for long-term tolerance were notably lower than predesensitization dosages: 100 mg/day in 8 patients, 150 mg/day in another 8 patients, 200 mg/day in 6 patients, and 300 mg/day, 250 mg/day, and 50 mg/day in 1 patient each. Twenty-three patients with gout improved clinically, with complete (n = 14) or partial (n = 9) cessation of gouty attacks. The mean postdesensitization serum urate level in 20 of the 25 long-term–evaluable patients was 318 μmoles/liter (range 187–452) (or, 5.3 mg/dl [range 3.0–7.5]), with only 2 patients having levels above 350 μmoles/liter (or, 6.0 mg/dl). Resolution of tophi, which occurred in 16 of 18 patients, was complete in 4 patients and partial in 12.

Two patients inadvertently stopped taking allopurinol for about a week at 3 and 6 months following successful desensitization. In both patients, the drug was successfully reintroduced at one-half the previously tolerated dosage, followed by gradual escalation of the dosage to its previous level.

Reasons for late, postdesensitization withdrawals included death from unrelated causes in 11 patients (3–84 months postdesensitization due to heart failure in 2, myocardial infarction in 2, metastatic carcinoma in 3, chronic lymphocytic leukemia in 1, aplastic crisis secondary to systemic lupus erythematosus in 1, stroke in 1, and septic shock in 1), loss to followup in 4 patients (11–24 months postdesensitization), improvement of gout following renal transplantation in 1 patient (42 months postdesensitization), and improvement of gout with home hemodialysis in 1 patient (49 months following desensitization).

Eight patients were receiving allopurinol at 13–92 months postdesensitization (mean 44 months, median 36 months); the mean serum urate level in 7 of these patients was 353 μmoles/liter (range 267–412) (or, 5.9 mg/day [range 4.8–6.9]); only 1 patient had a serum urate level of 412 μmoles/liter (or, 6.9 mg/dl). Six patients reported complete cessation of gouty attacks, and 2 reported less frequent attacks. Five of these 8 patients had tophi, which resolved completely in 3 patients and partially in 2 patients.

DISCUSSION

An estimated 2% of patients receiving allopurinol experience a pruritic maculopapular rash, sometimes associated with fever, facial swelling, or eosinophilia (1–4). More severe reactions, including toxic epidermal necrolysis, erythema multiforme or exfoliative dermatitis with leukocytosis, acute hepatitis, and/or acute interstitial nephritis with renal failure (allopurinol hypersensitivity syndrome), are rare (~0.4% of patients) (26–28). The exact pathogenesis of these hypersensitivity events, whether immune-mediated and/or toxic in nature, are unclear. Accumulation of oxypurinol (principal metabolite of allopurinol) due to renal impairment or coadministration of thiazide diuretics (26–28), genetic factors (20,29), abnormal T lymphocyte–mediated immune responses to oxypurinol, and to a lesser extent, allopurinol (30,31), and formation of immune complexes (28,32) have been implicated. A recent study suggests that in vitro allopurinol-induced release of interferon-γ from peripheral blood T lymphocytes may be a useful test in the diagnosis of Stevens-Johnson syndrome and other sensitivity reactions to allopurinol (33). Skin testing with either allopurinol or oxypurinol is less specific and has yielded conflicting results (18,28,30).

Many of those who experience allopurinol hypersensitivity are elderly patients with renal impairment in whom the dosage of the drug has not been reduced appropriately (26–29). In the present study, 26 of the 32 patients (81%) who underwent desensitization had renal insufficiency; 18 of them (69%) were taking concomitant diuretics, and 21 (80%) were receiving 300 mg of allopurinol daily—an inappropriate dosage for their degree of renal insufficiency. Recent reports indicate that allopurinol, at a "standard" dosage of 300 mg/day, is the most frequently prescribed urate-lowering drug (34,35) and that not all physicians adjust the initial dosage according to the degree of renal insufficiency (35). In this study, daily allopurinol dosages following desensitization were considerably lower than the predesensitization dosages, further emphasizing the importance of dosage reduction in patients with renal impairment (26).

The occurrence of cutaneous reactions to allopurinol severely limits the ability to manage hyperuricemia, particularly in individuals who cannot be treated with an alternative, equally effective, urate-lowering

Table 4. Indications for desensitization in patients with allopurinol-induced pruritic maculopapular eruptions

Patients with gout and renal insufficiency, and those requiring concomitant cardioprotective low-dose aspirin, which renders uricosurics ineffective (5,36–38)
Patients with gout, "overproduction" hyperuricemia, hyperuricosuria, and nephrolithiasis in whom uricosurics can increase the risk of stone formation, renal colic, and renal failure (36–39)
Patients with gout and "underexcretion" hyperuricemia who are either allergic or intolerant to both probenecid and sulfinpyrazone
Patients with malignancy-associated hyperuricemia due to cytolytic therapy for myeloproliferative or lymphoproliferative disorders; the resulting massive uricosuria precludes the use of a uricosuric agent (40)

drug. Table 4 lists the indications for desensitization in patients with such reactions to allopurinol. In the present study, we evaluated allopurinol desensitization as a potential therapy for patients in whom long-term control of hyperuricemia has proved difficult to achieve because of a pruritic maculopapular reaction to the drug. Overall, desensitization was successful in 78% of the patients (95% confidence interval 63–93%), enabling them to tolerate long-term allopurinol therapy (up to 92 months) as effective treatment for hyperuricemia and gout. To our knowledge, this is the largest reported series of patients who have undergone allopurinol desensitization.

Although the present study was limited by its retrospective, uncontrolled, open-label design, a number of observations can be made. First, cautious reinstitution of allopurinol, through reexposure to graded oral doses (test dosing or tolerance induction strategy) is a viable, acceptably safe approach to therapy in patients with allopurinol-related rash in whom other urate-lowering drugs are ineffective, poorly tolerated, or contraindicated (Table 4). We were unable to identify any antecedent clinical or laboratory parameter(s) that was predictive of either the immediate or long-term outcome of desensitization. Second, while transient pruritic rashes may recur both during (about one-third of patients) and after desensitization (about one-fourth of patients), more than 60% of the cutaneous reactions in the present study were managed by temporary withdrawal of allopurinol until the rash had subsided, followed by cautious reintroduction of the drug at one-half the previously tolerated dosage, and a slower rate of incremental dosage change. Medication compliance is important, since it is unclear whether the loss of sensitivity in these individuals is temporary or permanent. In the present investigation, 2 patients inadvertently interrupted their allopurinol treatment for about a week, and it was possible to reintroduce the drug at one-half the previously tolerated dosage, followed by gradual dosage escalation. However, it is not known whether a longer lapse of therapy would require a full re-desensitization procedure. Third, while no severe cutaneous reaction, hepatitis, interstitial nephritis, or hematologic toxicity was encountered in any of the 32 patients who underwent allopurinol desensitization, the procedure can occasionally result in life-threatening reactions (15,19). To minimize such a risk, timely recognition of any sign of intolerance, such as pruritus, cutaneous erythema, fever, or oral ulcers, and prompt withdrawal of allopurinol are essential.

A major obstacle to the management of hyperuricemia in allopurinol-intolerant patients is the limited availability of suitable, equally effective, alternative urate-lowering drugs, particularly in patients who are refractory to treatment with or are intolerant of uricosuric drugs. Oxypurinol at a dosage of 100–600 mg/day has been used to treat allopurinol-sensitive individuals, but cross-hypersensitivity with allopurinol has been reported in up to 40% of these patients (41–43).

Urate oxidase, or uricase, is an enzyme that catalyzes the conversion of uric acid into allantoin, which is 10 times more soluble than uric acid and is more readily eliminated by the kidneys (40,44–48). Humans and certain primates lack this enzyme activity (48). When given parenterally, urate oxidase is a more potent and faster acting urate-lowering drug than is allopurinol (40,44–48). Uricozyme, a nonrecombinant urate oxidase derived from cultures of *Aspergillus flavus,* has been used in Europe since 1974 as a short-term adjunct to cytolytic therapy for childhood leukemia and other myeloproliferative and lymphoproliferative disorders (40,44,45). It is not available in the United States or Canada, and its use for prolonged therapy of gout is limited by the need for parenteral administration, its potential immunogenicity, and its side effects (allergic rash, anaphylaxis, bronchospasm, and hemolytic anemia) (40,44,45). Recently, recombinant urate oxidase, a complementary DNA clone derived from *Aspergillus flavus* and biosynthesized in the yeast strain *Saccharomyces cerevisiae* (Sanofi-Synthelabo, New York, NY) has been utilized in the prophylaxis and treatment of chemotherapy-associated hyperuricemia in patients with leukemia and lymphoma (47). However, its long-term parenteral use in allopurinol-sensitive patients with chronic gout and renal insufficiency has not been examined.

As renal function deteriorates, uricosurics lose their efficacy as urate-lowering drugs (5,36–38). Benzbromarone seems to be an exception; a number of studies suggest that at dosages of 25–150 mg/day, the drug retains its uricosuric properties in patients who have mild-to-moderate renal impairment with a creatinine clearance of >25 ml/minute (49–51). The risk of uric acid nephrolithiasis and hepatotoxicity in these patients requires further study (52). The drug is marketed in Europe, but is not available in Canada or the United States.

In summary, results from the present study confirm the long-term efficacy and safety of slow oral desensitization to the minor rashes induced by allopurinol. Although the mechanism underlying "desensitization" to allopurinol has not yet been established, the data presented indicate that this "graded reintroduction strategy" can restore tolerability to the drug in the majority of patients. The procedure can be carried out in an ambulatory setting under close supervision. Careful planning and detailed discussion of the desensitization protocol with each patient prior to initiating therapy are essential. Desensitization to allopurinol poses potential risks (15,19) and is not recommended as first-choice treatment for all patients with pruritic maculopapular eruptions to the drug. The procedure is beneficial in selected patients who cannot be treated with other urate-lowering drugs, particularly those with gout and renal insufficiency (Table 4). Continued monitoring of these patients, both during and following desensitization, is important because sensitivity to the drug may recur.

Given the potential morbidity and mortality from the allopurinol hypersensitivity syndrome, desensitization is not recommended in patients with previous Stevens-Johnson syndrome, toxic epidermal necrolysis, or other life-threatening reactions to the drug (10,53). A slower incremental dosing regimen, with dosage changes every 5–10 days or longer, increases the likelihood of successful desensitization and is recommended for the following high-risk patients: those who are frail and elderly and have multiple medical conditions; those who have had a confluent widespread allopurinol rash, especially when associated with fever, stomatitis, facial or tongue swelling, or eosinophilia (which have been associated with potentially more severe drug-induced cutaneous reactions [54]); and those who have experienced recurrent rashes during the desensitization procedure.

Additional prospective, long-term, dose-ranging studies are required to address the issues of optimal initial dosages and the duration and rate of desensitization to allopurinol. More work remains to be done to define the pathogenesis of allopurinol hypersensitivity events, elucidate the mechanisms underlying desensitization, and explore new xanthine oxidase inhibitors and other novel therapeutic interventions to treat hyperuricemia in patients who are refractory to both allopurinol and uricosuric drugs.

ACKNOWLEDGMENTS

The authors wish to gratefully acknowledge Dr. Donald Redelmeier for helpful suggestions, Ms Marilyn Bacher for generating the Ambulatory Pharmacy computer printout, and Ms Kathy Carey for secretarial assistance.

REFERENCES

1. Rundles RW. The development of allopurinol. Arch Intern Med 1985;145:1492–503.
2. Boston Collaborative Drug Surveillance Program. Excess of ampicillin rashes associated with allopurinol or hyperuricemia. N Engl J Med 1972;286:505–7.
3. McInnes GT, Lawson DH, Jick H. Acute adverse reactions attributed to allopurinol in hospitalized patients. Ann Rheum Dis 1981;40:245–9.
4. Rundles RW, Metz EN, Silberman HR. Allopurinol in the treatment of gout. Ann Intern Med 1966;64:229–58.
5. Wallace SL, Singer JZ. Therapy in gout. Rheum Dis Clin North Am 1988;14:441–57.
6. Greenberger PA. Drug challenge and desensitization protocols. Immun Allergy Clin North Am 1998;18:759–72.
7. Bax DE, Amos RS. Sulphasalazine in rheumatoid arthritis: desensitizing the patient with a skin rash. Ann Rheum Dis 1986;45: 139–40.
8. Rich JD, Sullivan T, Greineder D, Kazanjian PH. Trimethoprim/ sulphamethoxazole incremental dosage regimen in human immunodeficiency virus-infected persons. Ann Allergy Asthma Immunol 1997;79:409–14.
9. Lantner RR. Ciprofloxacin desensitization in a patient with cystic fibrosis. J Allergy Clin Immunol 1995;96:1001–2.
10. Fam AG, Lewtas J, Stein J, Paton TW. Desensitization to allopurinol in patients with gout and cutaneous reactions. Am J Med 1992;93:299–302.
11. Meyrier A. Desensitization in a patient with chronic renal disease and severe allergy to allopurinol [letter]. BMJ 1976;2:458.
12. Webster E, Panush RS. Allopurinol hypersensitivity in a patient with severe, chronic, tophaceous gout. Arthritis Rheum 1985;28: 707–9.
13. Northridge DB, Almack PM. Allopurinol desensitization. Br J Pharm Pract 1986;8:200.
14. Kelsey SM, Stuthers GR, Beswick T, Blake DR. Desensitization to allopurinol [letter]. Ann Rheum Dis 1987;46:84.
15. Unsworth J, Black DR, D'Assis Fonseca AE, Beswick DT. Desensitization to allopurinol: a cautionary tale [letter]. Ann Rheum Dis 1987;46:646.
16. Ridley MG, Mathews JA. Desensitization to allopurinol [letter]. Ann Rheum Dis 1987;46:875.
17. Gillott TJ, Whallett A, Zaphiropoulos G. Oral desensitization in patients with chronic tophaceous gout and allopurinol hypersensitivity [letter]. Rheumatology (Oxford) 1999;38:85–6.
18. Walz-LeBlanc BAE, Reynolds WJ, MacFadden DK. Allopurinol sensitivity in a patient with chronic tophaceous gout: success of intravenous desensitization after failure of oral desensitization. Arthritis Rheum 1991;34:1329–31.
19. Tanna SB, Barnes JF, Seth SK. Desensitization to allopurinol in a patient with previous failed desensitization. Ann Pharmacother 1999;33:1180–3.

20. Melson RD. Familial hypersensitivity to allopurinol with subsequent desensitization [letter]. Rheumatology 1999;38:1301.
21. Garces M, Alonso L, Perez R, Marcos L, Juste S, Blanco J, et al. Successful oral desensitization in a patient with fixed eruption from allopurinol [abstract]. Allergy 1995;50 Suppl:213.
22. Kelso JM, Keating RM. Successful desensitization for treatment of a fixed drug eruption to allopurinol. J Allergy Clin Immunol 1996;97:1171–2.
23. Umpierrez A, Cuesta-Herranz J, De Las Heras M, Lluch-Bernal M, Figueredo E, Sastre J. Successful desensitization of a fixed drug eruption caused by allopurinol. J Allergy Clin Immunol 1998;101: 286–7.
24. Fam AG, Paton TW, Chaiton A. Reinstitution of allopurinol therapy for gouty arthritis after cutaneous reactions. CMAJ 1980; 123:128–9.
25. Dunne SM, Fam AG, Iazzetta J, Paton TW. Efficacy and safety of desensitization to allopurinol following cutaneous reactions [abstract]. Arthritis Rheum 1998;41 Suppl 9:S151.
26. Hande KR, Noone RM, Stone WJ. Severe allopurinol toxicity: description and guidelines for prevention in patients with renal insufficiency. Am J Med 1984;76:47–56.
27. Singer JZ, Wallace SL. The allopurinol hypersensitivity syndrome: unnecessary morbidity and mortality. Arthritis Rheum 1986;29: 82–7.
28. Arellano F, Sacristan JA. Allopurinol hypersensitivity syndrome: a review. Ann Pharmacother 1993;27:337–43.
29. Chan SH, Tan T. HLA and allopurinol drug eruption. Dermatologica 1989;179:32–3.
30. Emmerson BT, Hazelton RA, Frazer IH. Some adverse reactions to allopurinol may be mediated by lymphocyte reactivity to oxypurinol. Arthritis Rheum 1988;31:436–40.
31. Braden GL, Warzynski MJ, Golightly M, Ballow M. Cell-mediated immunity in allopurinol-induced hypersensitivity. Clin Immunol Immunopathol 1994;70:145–51.
32. Morel D, Guez S, Merville P, Deminiere C, Tamisier JM, Potaux L. Recurrent renal failure associated with hypersensitivity to allopurinol. Nephrol Dial Transplant 1999;14:780–1.
33. Halevy S, Cohen AD, Livni E. The diagnostic role of the in vitro drug-induced interferon-γ release test in Stevens-Johnson syndrome. Int J Dermatol 1999;38:835–40.
34. Bellamy N, Gilbert JR, Brooks PM, Emmerson BT, Campbell J. A survey of current prescribing practices of antiinflammatory and urate lowering drugs in gouty arthritis in the Province of Ontario. J Rheumatol 1988;15:1841–7.
35. Zell SC, Carmichael JM. Evaluation of allopurinol use in patients with gout. Am J Hosp Pharm 1989;46:1813–6.
36. Fam AG. Strategies and controversies in the treatment of gout and hyperuricemia. Baillieres Clin Rheumatol 1990;42:177–92.
37. Emmerson BT. The management of gout. N Engl J Med 1996;334: 445–51.
38. Wortmann RL. Effective management of gout: an analogy. Am J Med 1998;105:513–4.
39. Kovalchik MT III. Sulfinpyrazone induced uric acid urolithiasis with renal failure. Conn Med 1981;45:423–4.
40. Jones DP, Mahmoud H, Chesney RW. Tumor lysis syndrome: pathogenesis and management. Pediatric Nephrol 1995;9:206–12.
41. Earll JM, Saavedra M. Oxypurinol therapy in allopurinol-allergic patients. Am Fam Physician 1983;28:147–8.
42. Lockard O Jr, Harmon C, Nolph K, Irvin W. Allergic reaction to allopurinol with cross-reactivity to oxypurinol. Ann Intern Med 1976;85:333–5.
43. O'Duffy JD. Oxipurinol therapy in allopurinol-sensitive patients. Arthritis Rheum 1993;36 Suppl 9:S159.
44. Masera G, Jankovic M, Zurlo MG, Locasciulli A, Rossi MR, Uderzo C, et al. Urate-oxidase prophylaxis of uric acid-induced renal damage in childhood leukemia. J Pediatr 1982;100:152–5.
45. Pui C-H, Relling MV, Lascombes F, Harrison PL, Struxiano A, Mondesir JM, et al. Urate oxidase in prevention and treatment of hyperuricemia associated with lymphoid malignancies. Leukemia 1997;11:1813–6.
46. Rozenberg S, Koeger A-C, Bougeois P. Urate oxydase for gouty arthritis in cardiac transplant recipients [letter]. J Rheumatol 1993;20:2171.
47. Mahmoud HH, Leverger G, Patte C, Harvey E, Lascombes F. Advances in the management of malignancy-associated hyperuricemia. Br J Cancer 1998;77 Suppl 4:18–20.
48. Lee CC, Wu XW, Gibbs RA, Cook RG, Muzny DM, Casky CT. Generation of cDNA probes directed by amino acid sequence: cloning of urate oxidase. Science 1988;239:1288–91.
49. Zurcher RM, Bock HA, Thiel G. Excellent uricosuric efficacy of benzbromarone in cyclosporine-A–treated renal transplant patients: a prospective study. Nephrol Dial Transplant 1994;9: 548–51.
50. Grahame R, Simmonds HA, McBride MB, Marsh FP. How should we treat tophaceous gout in patients with allopurinol hypersensitivity? Adv Exp Med Biol 1998;431:19–23.
51. Perez-Ruiz F, Calabozo M, Fernandez-Lopez MJ, Herrero-Beites A, Ruiz-Lucea E, Garcia-Erauskin G, et al. Treatment of chronic gout in patients with renal function impairment: an open, randomized, actively controlled study. J Clin Rheumatol 1999;5:49–55.
52. Perez-Ruiz F, Alonzo-Ruiz A, Calabozo M, Herrero-Beites A, Garcia-Erauskin G, Ruiz-Lucea E. Efficacy of allopurinol and benzbromarone for the control of hyperuricemia: a pathogenic approach to the treatment of primary chronic gout. Ann Rheum Dis 1998;57:545–9.
53. Roujeau J-C, Kelly JP, Naldi L, Rzany B, Stern RS, Anderson T. Medication use and the risk of Stevens-Johnson syndrome or toxic epidermal necrolysis. N Engl J Med 1995;333:1600–7.
54. Roujeau J-C, Stern RS. Severe adverse cutaneous reactions to drugs. N Engl J Med 1994;331:1272–85.

ARTHRITIS & RHEUMATISM
Vol. 44, No. 1, January 2001, pp 239–241

CONCISE COMMUNICATIONS

Evidence for linkage of the HLA–B locus in Behçet's disease, obtained using the transmission disequilibrium test

Behçet's disease is a systemic vasculitic disorder characterized mainly by recurrent oral and genital ulceration, skin lesions, and uveitis. The etiology of Behçet's disease is unknown, but available data support the possible involvement of some microbial agents in genetically susceptible individuals (1).

The majority of Behçet's disease patients have sporadic disease with no family history; however, the familial recurrence risk is probably increased. A recent study revealed a sibling recurrence risk of 4.2% and a λ_S value of 11.4–52.5 for Behçet's disease in Turkey (2). Association of HLA–B51 with Behçet's disease is regarded as being the strongest evidence of genetic contribution described to date (3). However, whether HLA–B51 is a Behçet's disease susceptibility gene itself or if this strong association reflects linkage disequilibrium with another gene has yet to be elucidated. Recent studies with polymorphic microsatellite DNA markers suggested that the disease susceptibility locus is probably located within a 46-kb segment between the major histocompatibility complex class I chain–related gene family A (MICA) and HLA–B genes (4,5).

Although the strong association of HLA–B51 with Behçet's disease has been confirmed in different ethnic groups, genetic linkage of this region to Behçet's disease has not yet been documented. Association studies are subject to error based on selection of cases and healthy controls, with population stratification rather than disease possibly explaining any differences observed. We have therefore ascertained whether there is genetic linkage between HLA–B and Behçet's disease using the transmission disequilibrium test (TDT), since it is a test for linkage in the presence of association and is not sensitive to a stratified population (6).

The study group consisted of 81 individuals from 12 multicase families of Turkish origin. Both of the parents were available in 9 families, and 1 parent was missing in 3. Thirty-three of the study subjects (22 male, 11 female) met the criteria of the International Study Group (ISG) for the diagnosis of Behçet's disease (7). There were 8 sib-pairs, 1 sib-trio, and 3 sib-quadruples; in 2 families, 1 of the parents was also affected. Ten individuals with isolated recurrent oral ulcers and/or other Behçet's disease–related manifestations who did not fulfill the ISG criteria were classified as "unknown" cases. Statistical analyses were carried out using the data only from 33 individuals who met the ISG criteria.

Data on HLA–B and HLA–A antigens, determined by standard serologic methods, were available in all but 1 family (72 individuals). To cover a region between HLA–A and HLA–DQ, 5 different polymorphic microsatellite markers, i.e., MICA5, tumor necrosis factor a (TNFa), TNFb, TNFd, and DQCAR, were analyzed by polymerase chain reaction amplification and electrophoresis on denaturing polyacrylamide gel using a 373A automated DNA sequencer (PE Applied Biosystems, Foster City, CA).

TDT was performed using the Extended TDT (ETDT) package, which is a version of TDT for markers with multiple alleles, which uses a logistic regression method (8). For evaluation of the empiric significance, we performed a Monte Carlo simulation of ETDT (9) with 1,000 replicates.

ETDT analysis revealed evidence of linkage to Behçet's disease only for HLA–B, with both allele-wise statistics and the Monte Carlo simulation (Table 1). Chi-square analysis of the individual alleles revealed a positive result only for HLA–B51 (Table 2) (P = 0.0003, P_{corr} = 0.0042). No significant results were found for the other markers.

Table 1. Allele-wise ETDT results for HLA–A, HLA–B, and 5 microsatellite markers in multicase Behçet's disease families*

Marker	χ^2	df	Asymptotic P	Empiric P (SE)†
HLA–A	12.5	9	0.18	0.25 (0.01)
HLA–B	28.4	14	0.01	0.02 (0.005)
MICA5	4.0	4	0.41	0.47 (0.02)
TNFb	9.0	5	0.11	0.20 (0.01)
TNFa	6.9	8	0.55	0.73 (0.01)
TNFd	4.3	4	0.37	0.49 (0.02)
DQCAR	15.3	8	0.054	0.11 (0.01)

* ETDT = Extended transmission disequilibrium test; df = degrees of freedom; MICA5 = microsatellite marker in exon 5 of the major histocompatibility complex class I chain–related gene family A; TNFb = tumor necrosis factor microsatellite marker b; SE = standard error.

† Results of a Monte Carlo simulation with 1,000 replicates.

We also estimated the contribution of HLA–B ($\lambda_{HLA–B}$) to the overall genetic susceptibility to Behçet's disease, using identity-by-descent (IBD) sharing of HLA–B alleles in these families (10). The frequencies of IBD-shared HLA–B alleles in Behçet's disease patients were found to be 15.4%, 50%, and 34.6% for 0-allele, 1-allele, and 2-allele sharing, respectively, using the SPLINK program (11). Based on the proportion of affected pairs sharing 0 alleles, we calculated $\lambda_{HLA–B}$ to be 1.6 (10). Thus, the highest contribution of HLA–B to the overall genetic susceptibility to Behçet's disease was estimated to be 19%, using the method of Risch (10) and assuming a multiplicative interaction between disease susceptibility loci (19% for λ_S = 11.4 and 12% for λ_S = 52.5).

A strong association between HLA–B51 and Behçet's disease has long been known, but this study is the first to demonstrate evidence for linkage of the HLA–B locus with Behçet's disease. Although the recent fine mapping study in Behçet's disease cases and controls, covering a 900-kb region surrounding the HLA–B locus, refined the critical region for Behçet's disease to a 46-kb segment between MICA and HLA–B, HLA–B51 showed the strongest association with Behçet's disease, and no other functioning gene could be identified by sequencing of this segment (4,5,12).

The contribution of the HLA–B locus to the overall genetic susceptibility to Behçet's disease is relatively small,

Table 2. Number of transmissions of individual HLA–B alleles from parents to the children with Behçet's disease

	HLA–B allele														
	7	8	13	18	27	35	38	44	50	51	52	55	57	60	62
Passed	0	1	1	2	0	3	0	2	1	23	1	2	0	3	2
Not passed	2	3	3	5	4	3	4	4	1	4	1	4	2	1	0

even with an assumption of multiplicative interaction between Behçet's disease susceptibility loci based on our observations in other extended families (2,10). Further studies are needed to map the susceptibility genes for Behçet's disease on the other chromosomal regions, with larger numbers of families as well as sporadic disease cases and matched controls.

Dr. Gül's work was supported by the European Science Exchange Programme (the Royal Society and Scientific and Technical Research Council of Turkey).

Ahmet Gül, MD
University of Istanbul
Istanbul, Turkey
Ali H. Hajeer, PhD
Jane Worthington, PhD
Jennifer H. Barrett, PhD
William E. R. Ollier, PhD
Alan J. Silman, MD
University of Manchester
Mancheter, UK

1. Sakane T, Takeno M, Suzuki N, Inaba G. Behçet's disease. N Engl J Med 1999;341:1284–91.
2. Gül A, Inanc M, Ocal L, Aral O, Konice M. Familial aggregation of Behçet's disease in Turkey. Ann Rheum Dis 2000;59:622–5.
3. Mizuki N, Inoko H, Ohno S. Pathogenic gene responsible for the predisposition of Behçet's disease. Int Rev Immunol 1997;14:33–48.
4. Ota M, Mizuki N, Katsuyama Y, Tamiya G, Shiina T, Oka A, et al. The critical region for Behçet's disease in the human major histocompatibility complex is reduced to a 46-kb segment centromeric of HLA-B, by association analysis using refined microsatellite mapping. Am J Hum Genet 1999;64:1406–10.
5. Mizuki N, Ota M, Katsuyama Y, Yabuki K, Ando H, Goto K, et al. Association analysis between the MIC-A and HLA–B alleles in Japanese patients with Behçet's disease. Arthritis Rheum 1999;42: 1961–6.
6. Schaid DJ. Transmission disequilibrium, family controls, and great expectations. Am J Hum Genet 1998;63:935–41.
7. International Study Group for Behçet's disease. Criteria for diagnosis of Behçet's disease. Lancet 1990;335:1078–80.
8. Sham PC, Curtis D. An extended transmission/disequilibrium test (TDT) for multi-allele marker loci. Ann Hum Genet 1995;59:323–36.
9. Zhao JH, Sham PC, Curtis D. A program for the Monte Carlo evaluation of significance of the extended transmission/disequilibrium test. Am J Hum Genet 1999;64:1484–5.
10. Risch N. Assessing the role of HLA-linked and unlinked determinants of disease. Am J Hum Genet 1987;40:1–14.
11. Holmans P, Clayton D. Efficiency of typing unaffected relatives in an affected-sib-pair linkage study with single-locus and multiple tightly linked markers. Am J Hum Genet 1995;57:1221–32.
12. Shiina T, Tamiya G, Oka A, Takishima N, Inoko H. Genome sequencing analysis of the 1.8 Mb entire human MHC class I region. Immunol Rev 1999;167:193–9.

Beneficial effect of etanercept on rheumatoid lymphedema

Since 1998, rheumatologists nationwide have been able to prescribe anti–tumor necrosis factor (anti-TNF) therapy for their patients with rheumatoid arthritis (RA), often with dramatic improvement in the arthropathy (1,2). There is little information, however, on the benefit of this therapy for the extraarticular manifestations of RA. Common extraarticular features include rheumatoid nodules, interstitial lung disease, vasculitis, neuropathy, and Sjögren's syndrome. A less common complication is rheumatoid lymphedema (3,4). Described herein is a patient with longstanding seropositive RA complicated by rheumatoid lymphedema, who was prescribed etanercept in March 2000 after failure to respond to other agents. She experienced a dramatic response of the arthritis as well as the lymphedema, for the first time in her disease course.

The patient presented in 1993 at 51 years of age, with rheumatoid factor–positive polyarthritis. Antinuclear antibody was negative, and her erythrocyte sedimentation rate (ESR) was 105 mm/hour. She was treated initially with nonsteroidal antiinflammatory drugs (NSAIDs) and low-dose prednisone; after 1 year, methotrexate (MTX) was instituted. She improved clinically, and the corticosteroids were discontinued in 1995. In May 1995, she developed diffuse right wrist and forearm swelling with no evidence of vascular compromise. She had no adenopathy, breast masses, or skin changes. The area was nontender, and there was no warmth or erythema. Her other joints appeared normal, although her ESR was 41 mm/hour. The MTX dosage was increased from 12.5 mg/week to 17.5 mg/week, without any change in the arm. Corticosteroids were reinstituted, again with no change noted. Her disease followed a fluctuating course over the next 4½ years, requiring 5–10 mg/day of prednisone in addition to the MTX and NSAIDs.

In March 2000, etanercept was instituted at 25 mg subcutaneously twice weekly. Within 8 weeks her synovitis improved, and by 12 weeks the lymphedema was dramatically reduced. Except for some residual tightness and swelling of the palm and dorsum of the hand, the swelling of the forearm up to the elbow had virtually resolved.

Rheumatoid lymphedema is an uncommon extraarticular feature of RA, which has been reported in <30 patients in the literature. It is thought to be due to complications of synovitis with the development of inflammation and possible fibrosis of the superficial lymph vessels, with subsequent obstruction of lymphatic flow (3–5). Treatment is usually symptomatic, with pressure stockings and, in rare instances, surgery. These approaches have been only partially successful. Previously, medical management of RA has not been of consistent benefit for the lymphedema, and in the majority of patients, it is a longstanding problem even with good control of the inflammatory joint disease. Anti-TNF therapy in this patient dramatically reduced the lymphedema after <4 months of therapy. The mechanism of action of etanercept in the treatment of lymphedema is speculative. Assuming synovitis causes adjacent lymphatic inflammation and ultimate fibrosis, maximal control of active rheumatoid synovitis could abrogate this reaction. Further reports of improvement and/or resolution of a variety of extraarticular features of RA, including rheumatoid lymphedema, with the use of anti-TNF agents will likely be forthcoming in the next few years.

Barbara E. Ostrov, MD
Milton S. Hershey Medical Center
Hershey, PA

1. Weinblatt ME, Kremer JM, Bankhurst AD, Bulpitt KJ, Fleischman RM, Fox RI, et al. A trial of etanercept, a recombinant tumor necrosis factor receptor:Fc fusion protein, in patients with rheumatoid arthritis receiving methotrexate. N Engl J Med 1999;340:253–9.
2. Maini RN, Breedveld FC, Kalden JR, Smolen JS, Davis D, Macfarlane JD, et al. Therapeutic efficacy of multiple intravenous infusions of anti–tumor necrosis factor α monoclonal antibody

combined with low-dose weekly methotrexate in rheumatoid arthritis. Arthritis Rheum 1998;41:1552–63.
3. Dacre JE, Scott DL, Huskisson EC. Lymphedema of the limbs as an extra-articular feature of RA. Ann Rheum Dis 1990;49:722–4.
4. Athreya BH, Ostrov BE, Eichenfeld AH, Goldsmith DP. Lymphedema associated with juvenile rheumatoid arthritis. J Rheumatol 1989;16:1338–40.
5. Mulherin DM, FitzGerald O, Bresnihan B. Lymphedema of the upper limb in patients with psoriatic arthritis. Semin Arthritis Rheum 1993;22:350–6.

Clinical Images: Cervical spinal cord compression

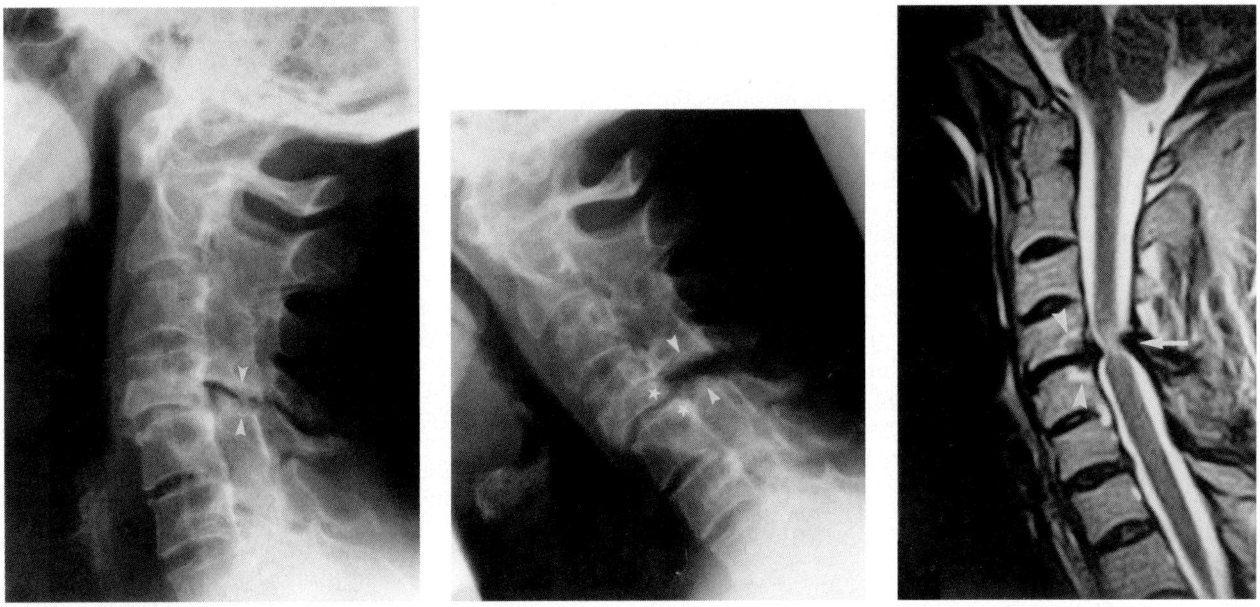

A B C

The patient, a 38-year-old woman, had had juvenile rheumatoid arthritis since 1973. On admission to the hospital in 1998, she reported having experienced numbness, tingling, and pain in her arms for several months, with no deterioration in arm function. She had felt minor symptoms in her neck. On clinical examination, the neck was stiff and the biceps tendon and patella reflexes hyperactive. Laboratory tests revealed an erythrocyte sedimentation rate of 42 mm/hour, a C-reactive protein level of 20 mg/liter, and a serum alkaline phosphatase level of 130 units/liter. Cervical spine radiographs taken at extension (**A**) and flexion (**B**) revealed apophyseal joint ankylosis at C2–4 and C5–6, and instability at C4–5. The joint surfaces of the C4–5 apophyseal joint were uneven and the joint space widened due to erosions (**A; arrowheads**). The width of the apophyseal joint space was increased in flexion (**B; arrowheads**), and there was mild anterior displacement of the C4 vertebral body (**B; asterisks**). T2-weighted sagittal magnetic resonance images of the cervical spine (fast spin echo, 4,000 ms/160 ms, 4.0 mm, 270 mm, 256 $\times$ 256) showed spinal canal stenosis, cord compression, and medullopathy (bright signal) at the C4–5 level (**C; arrow**). Further erosions were seen at the posterior portions of vertebral end plates (**C; arrowheads**). Spinal canal decompression and spondylodesis at C4–5 were performed. Postoperatively, numbness remained in the hands.

Kari Laiho, MD
Markku Kauppi, MD, PhD
Irma Soini, MD, PhD
Rheumatism Foundation Hospital
Heinola, Finland

ARTHRITIS & RHEUMATISM
Vol. 44, No. 1, January 2001, pp 242–246

LETTERS

Increase in the heart rate–corrected QT interval in children of anti-Ro–positive mothers, with a further increase in those with siblings with congenital heart block: comment on the article by Cimaz et al

To the Editor:

We read with great interest the article by Cimaz et al on prolongation of the QT interval in asymptomatic infants who are positive for anti-Ro but do not have congenital heart block (CHB) (1). These findings are consistent with our belief that CHB is only one end of a spectrum of anti-Ro antibody–associated cardiac abnormality.

In a minority (<5%) of pregnancies in which the mother is anti-Ro positive, the offspring is born with CHB (2,3). Thus, it appears that only a subset of anti-Ro–positive sera is pathogenic. However, even in the subset of anti-Ro–positive women who give birth to a child with CHB, the recurrence rate is only 16% (4). In addition, there are many reports in the literature of twins discordant for CHB (5–7).

Certainly lesser degrees of heart block have been reported to occur in children born to anti-Ro–positive mothers (8,9). In addition, there are reports of a prolonged heart rate–corrected QT interval (QTc) occurring in infants with CHB (10,11), and Cimaz et al found that the QTc was prolonged in children of anti-Ro–positive mothers.

To pursue our hypothesis that CHB is only one end of a spectrum of anti-Ro–associated congenital heart disease, we are currently assessing electrocardiographic findings in 3 groups of children: the children of anti-Ro–positive mothers attending our pregnancy clinic (children born since January 1997, and their siblings [mean age 27.8 months; n = 19]) (group 1), the children of anti-Ro–negative mothers with connective tissue disease (children born since March 1999 [mean age 1.8 months; n = 7]) (group 2), and the siblings of children with CHB born to anti-Ro–positive mothers (from 13 families with a total of 15 children with CHB and 1 child with second-degree heart block [mean age 103 months; n = 19]) (group 3). We are assessing the QTc (using Bazett's formula), PR interval, and QRS duration in these children. Because our study is ongoing, the number of subjects in group 2 is as yet small.

Our preliminary data showed no significant difference between the groups in PR interval or QRS duration. None of the children had CHB (group 3 by selection). However the QTc was significantly longer in the children of all anti-Ro–positive mothers (groups 1 and 3 combined, mean ± SD 379 ± 26 msec) compared with the children of Ro-negative mothers (group 2; 332 ± 20 msec) ($P < 0.0001$, 95% confidence interval 26.7–68.3). Furthermore, among children of anti-Ro–positive mothers, the QTc in the siblings of children with CHB (group 3; 395 ± 22 msec) was significantly longer than that in children from families without CHB (group 1; 365 ± 21 msec) ($P < 0.0001$, 95% confidence interval 15.9–43.5).

There is some evidence that the QTc varies with age not only in early life (12) but throughout life (13). This relationship was demonstrable in our study population, with linear regression demonstrating a significant association between age and QTc. To confirm that the difference in QTc between the groups was not merely secondary to the age differences, we further analyzed the data using multiple regression. When corrected for age by multiple regression, the differences in QTc between the groups remained significant. Therefore, although there is an association between QTc and age, our results demonstrate that both maternal anti-Ro antibody status and history of a sibling with CHB are also associated with the QTc.

None of the children had a QTc above the upper limit of normal (>440 msec). Notably, in 1 family in which a child had CHB, sudden infant death syndrome had occurred in a sibling.

It is tempting to speculate that there is a common pathologic link between prolongation of the QTc and conduction defects in anti-Ro antibody–associated CHB. However, there is no obvious mechanism to support such a theory. At a molecular level, prolonged QTc has been causally linked to Na^+ and K^+ channel defects (14) whereas CHB has been associated with the slow L-type $Ca2^+$ channels (15). Pseudo 2:1 atrioventricular (AV) block may occur in the long QTc syndrome secondary to prolonged ventricular refractoriness, but this is pathologically unrelated to the true AV block with AV nodal fibrosis, as found in CHB. Therefore, further research on this possible association is needed.

In conclusion, we were able to confirm that the QTc is longer in children of anti-Ro–positive mothers. However we could not confirm the presence of a prolonged QTc (>440 msec) in the children in our series. In addition, we showed that among children of anti-Ro–positive mothers, the QTc is significantly longer in the subset who have a sibling with CHB. This suggests that prolongation of the QTc is a part of the spectrum of anti-Ro–positive–associated congenital heart pathology. Surprisingly, we were unable to demonstrate a relationship between the PR interval or QRS interval and a history of CHB in a sibling or Ro positivity in the mother.

Supported by the British Heart Foundation.

Patrick A. Gordon, MRCP
Munther A. Khamashta, MD, MRCP, PhD
Graham R.V. Hughes, MD, FRCP
St. Thomas Hospital
London, UK
Eric Rosenthal, FRCP, MD, MRCPCH
Guy's Hospital
London, UK

1. Cimaz R, Stramba-Badiale M, Brucato A, Catelli L, Panzeri P, Meroni PL. QT interval prolongation in asymptomatic anti-SSA/Ro–positive infants without congenital heart block. Arthritis Rheum 2000;43:1049–53.
2. Lockshin MD, Bonfa E, Elkon K, Druzin ML. Neonatal lupus risk to newborns of mothers with systemic lupus erythematosus. Arthritis Rheum 1988;31:697–701.
3. Ramsey-Goldman R, Hom D, Deng J-S, Ziegler GC, Kahl LE, Steen VD, et al. Anti-SS-A antibodies and fetal outcome in maternal systemic lupus erythematosus. Arthritis Rheum 1986;29: 1269–73.
4. Buyon J, Hiebert R, Copel J, et al. Autoimmune-associated

congenital heart block: demographics, mortality, morbidity and recurrence rates obtained from a national neonatal lupus registry. J Am Coll Cardiol 1998;31:1658–66.

5. Cooley HM, Keech CL, Melny BJ, Menahem S, Morahan G, Kay TWH. Monozygotic twins discordant for congenital complete heart block. Arthritis Rheum 1997;40:381–4.
6. Watson RM, Scheel JN, Petri M, Kan JS, Provost TT, Ratric H III, et al. Neonatal lupus erythematosus: report of serological and immunogenetic studies in twins discordant for congenital heart block. Br J Dermatol. 1994;130:342–8.
7. Kaaja R, Julkunen H, Ammala P, Kurki P, Koskimies S. Congenital heart block in one of the HLA identical twins. Eur J Obstet Reprod Biol 1993;51:78–80.
8. Saleeb S, Copel J, Friedman D, Buyon JP. Comparison of treatment with fluorinated glucocorticoids to the natural history of autoantibody-associated congenital heart block: retrospective review of the Research Registry for Neonatal Lupus. Arthritis Rheum 1999;42:2335–45.
9. Uzun O, Gibbs JL. Progressive disease of the atrioventricular conduction axis in an infant of an anti-Ro positive mother. Cardiol Young. 1999;9:192–3.
10. Esscher E, Michaelsson M. Q-T interval in congenital complete heart block. Pediatr Cardiol 1983;4:121–4.
11. Esscher E. Congenital complete heart block. Acta Paediatr Scand 1981;70:131–6.
12. Schwartz PJ, Montemerlo M, Facchini M, Salice P, Rosti D, Poggio G, et al. The QT interval throughout the first 6 months of life: a prospective study. Circulation 1982;66:496–501.
13. Carter N, Snieder H, Jeffrey S, Saumarez R, Varma C, Antoniades L, et al. QT interval in twins. J Hum Hypertens 2000;14:389–90.
14. Vincent GM, Timothy K, Fox J, Zhang L. The inherited long QT syndromes: from ion channel to bedside. Cardiol Rev 1999;7:44–5.
15. Boutjdir M, Chen L, Zhang ZH, Tseng CE, DiDonato F, Rashbaum W, et al. Arrhythmogenicity of IgG and anti–52-kD SSA/Ro affinity purified antibodies from mothers of children with congenital heart block. Circ Res 1997;80:354–62.

Reply

To the Editor:

We thank Dr. Gordon and his coworkers for their interest in our article on QT interval prolongation in anti-Ro–positive infants without heart block, and for sharing the preliminary results of their study. As they state, their findings and ours are supportive of the same hypothesis, i.e., that the presence of anti-Ro antibodies can be related to cardiac disturbances other than CHB. In this respect we find it very interesting that, in a pair of siblings in their series, 1 had CHB and the other died of sudden infant death syndrome (SIDS). We wonder if an electrocardiogram (EKG) had ever been obtained in this latter baby prior to death. In fact, not only is a prolonged QT interval thought to be a risk factor for SIDS (Schwartz PJ, Stramba-Badiale M, Segantini A, Austoni P, Bosi G, Giorgetti R, et al. Prolongation of the QT interval and the sudden infant death syndrome. N Engl J Med 1998;338: 1709–14), but a recent report described an infant who nearly died of SIDS and in whom the long QT syndrome was diagnosed (Schwartz PJ, Priori SG, Dumaine R, Napolitano C, Antzelevitch C, Stramba-Badiale M, et al. A molecular link between the sudden infant death syndrome and the long-QT syndrome. N Engl J Med 2000;343:262–7).

We would like to comment on the fact that none of the children in Gordon et al's study had a prolonged QTc (>440 msec), in contrast to our findings. A possible reason for this might be related to the different ages of patients in the 2 series. The mean age in Gordon and colleagues' group 1, the group that most closely matches our study sample, was 27.8 months, and in the other children of anti-Ro–positive mothers (group 3), the mean age was 103 months, whereas the EKG was recorded during their first 6 months of life (median 75 days) in all of the children we studied. If the hypothesis is that anti-Ro interferes with ventricular repolarization, the EKG result is most likely to be abnormal when these antibodies are still present in the baby's serum. Since maternal autoantibodies are cleared from the baby's circulation by age 1 year at the latest, we cannot exclude the possibility that the QTc in Gordon et al's patients might have been prolonged during the first months of life. Followup of our anti-Ro–positive children with prolonged QTc is ongoing, so that we will be able to assess whether this is a transient phenomenon.

Rolando Cimaz, MD
Istituti Clinici di Perfezionamento
Milan, Italy
Antonio Brucato, MD
Ospedale Niguarda
Milan, Italy
Marco Stramba-Badiale, MD, PhD
Luca Catelli, MD
Pier Luigi Meroni, MD
Istituto Auxologico Italiano
Milan, Italy

Shrinking lung syndrome in patients without systemic lupus erythematosus: comment on the concise communication by Tavoni et al

To the Editor:

We read with interest the concise communication by Tavoni et al on shrinking lung syndrome in primary Sjögren's syndrome (1). We too have observed shrinking lung syndrome in systemic autoimmune disease other than systemic lupus erythematosus (SLE).

The first patient presented in July 1997 at the age of 46, with a cough, bilateral pleuritic chest pain, and shortness of breath. Seropositive erosive rheumatoid arthritis had been diagnosed in 1994. At the time of presentation in 1997, her rheumatoid factor (RF) titer was 1:1,024 by sheep cell agglutination test (SCAT). Her antinuclear antibody (ANA) titer was 1:100, and double-stranded DNA (dsDNA) antibodies and antibodies to extractable nuclear antigen (ENA) were absent. Chest radiography revealed elevated diaphragms, small bilateral pleural effusions, and basal atelectasis. Findings on ventilation-perfusion scan and echocardiogram were normal. Spirometry revealed a restrictive defect, with a forced expiratory volume in 1 second/forced vital capacity (FEV_1/FVC) of 1.12 liters/1.39 liters (predicted value 2.99 liters/3.47 liters) and normal gas transfer (Kco 97% of predicted). Findings on a

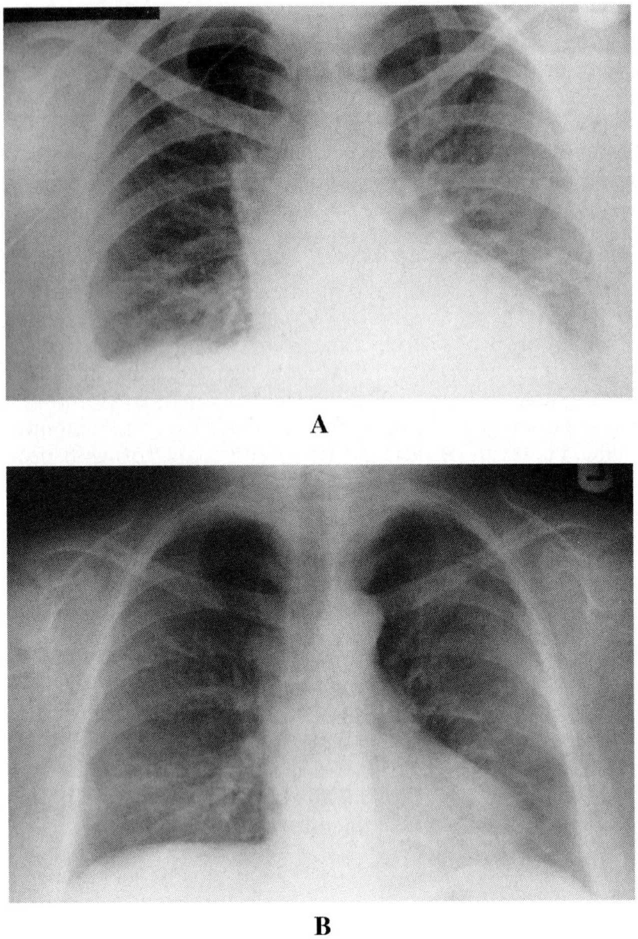

Figure 1. Chest radiographs of the second patient on presentation (A), showing elevated diaphragms, right basal consolidation, and basal atelectasis, and after steroid therapy (B).

high-resolution computed tomography (CT) scan of the chest excluded interstitial lung disease. Her maximum inspiratory mouth pressure (PImax) and maximum expiratory mouth pressure (PEmax) were 28 cm water (normal >70) and 44 cm water (normal >90), respectively.

Treatment with prednisolone 40 mg/day was started, and by November 1997 her PImax and PEmax had increased to 67 cm water and 54 cm water, respectively. In February 1998 the steroids were tapered and discontinued. Four weeks later, her breathing began to deteriorate. Prednisolone was restarted at 15 mg/day, and her breathing improved. In August 1999, steroids were again discontinued, and her FEV_1/FVC remained stable at 1.4 liters/1.74 liters.

The second patient presented in July 1997 at the age of 53, with dyspnea, right-sided pleuritic chest pain, cough, and pain and stiffness in her wrists and shoulder joints. Ten years previously, she had experienced proximal muscle pain and had been treated with corticosteroids. On examination in 1997, she was found to have a low-grade fever and tenderness at the wrists, shoulders, and thighs bilaterally, with restriction of movement. Her ANA titer was 1:1,000, dsDNA and ENA were absent, as was RF (by SCAT). Muscle enzyme levels were normal. Chest radiography (Figure 1A) revealed elevated diaphragms, right basal consolidation, and basal atelectasis. Ventilation-perfusion scan showed matched basal defects. Spirometry showed a restrictive defect, with an FEV_1/FVC of 1.1 liters/1.5 liters (predicted value 2.4 liters/2.8 liters) and normal gas transfer. A high-resolution CT scan of the chest excluded interstitial lung disease. Her PImax and PEmax were 36 cm water and 44 cm water, respectively.

There was no response to a course of antibiotics. The clinical features of her disease were not typical of SLE. In view of the arthralgias and positive ANA, her illness was categorized as undifferentiated connective tissue disease. Prednisolone 20 mg/day was started in August 1997. In November 1997, her PImax and PEmax had increased to 48 cm water and 77 cm water, respectively, and the steroid dosage was decreased to 10 mg/day. Her FVC had improved to 2.4 liters in June 1998. Chest radiographic findings (Figure 1B) had also improved. In November 1999, she was still experiencing shortness of breath and was still taking prednisolone 10 mg/day.

Tavoni et al describe shrinking lung syndrome occurring in a patient with primary Sjögren's syndrome. Herein we have reported 2 further cases of shrinking lung syndrome in patients with autoimmune disease other than SLE. The shrinking lung syndrome is a rare but well-recognized complication of SLE (2). We are not aware, however, of any previous reports of this syndrome in patients with rheumatoid arthritis. Our second patient was of interest because, although she had some features suggestive of connective tissue disease (positive ANA, arthralgias), she did not fulfill criteria for SLE (3).

Shrinking lung syndrome should be suspected when chest radiography shows small lung volumes (4). PImax and PEmax are invariably reduced (5). The response to corticosteroids is variable (6). Treatment with β_2-agonists and theophyllines has been tried, with varying success (1). Some patients experience relentless deterioration, while others show a slow or nonprogressive course.

The case reported by Tavoni et al and the 2 cases described here demonstrate that the diagnosis of shrinking lung syndrome should be considered in patients with multisystem inflammatory disease other than definite SLE who present with shortness of breath. This is especially important given that a proportion of patients respond well to treatment.

Shahbaz Ahmed, MRCP
Ariane Herrick, FRCP
B. Ronan O'Driscoll, MD
Hope Hospital
Salford, UK

1. Tavoni A, Vitali C, Cirigliano G, Frigelli S, Stampacchia G, Bombardieri S. Shrinking lung in primary Sjögren's syndrome. Arthritis Rheum 1999;42:2249–50.
2. Soubrier M, Dubost JJ, Piette JC, Urosevic Z, Rami S, Oualid T, et al. Shrinking lung syndrome in systemic lupus erythematosus: a report of three cases. Rev Rhum 1995;62:395–8.
3. Tan EM, Cohen AS, Fries JF, Masi AT, McShane DJ, Rothfield NF, et al. The 1982 revised criteria for the classification of systemic lupus erythematosus. Arthritis Rheum 1982;25:1271–7.
4. Laroche CM, Mulvey DA, Hawkins PA, Walport MJ, Strickland B,

Moxham J. Diaphragm strength in the shrinking lung syndrome of systemic lupus erythematosus. QJM 1989;71:429–39.
5. Bernstein RM, Ind PW, Elkon KB, Sewell JR, Gibson GJ, Hughes JMB, et al. Pulmonary function in SLE with a longitudinal study of the shrinking lungs syndrome [abstract]. Arthritis Rheum 1982;25 Suppl 4:S7.
6. Walz-Leblanc BAE, Urowitz MB, Gladman DD, Hanly PJ. The "shrinking lungs syndrome" in systemic lupus erythematosus: improvement with corticosteroid therapy. J Rheumatol 1992;19: 1970–2.

Reply

To the Editor:

We are grateful to Dr. Ahmed and colleagues for their observations, which are of great interest. They rightly point out that shrinking lung syndrome is a rare complication not only restricted to SLE but potentially occurring in all systemic autoimmune diseases. Most importantly, they note that if appropriate therapy is instituted early this potentially disabling condition might be controlled. With control of the condition, the most severe complications, such as lung infections, might be prevented.

Many aspects of this syndrome need to be better elucidated: we do not know, for instance, if the same pathogenetic mechanisms are responsible for the syndrome, either in patients with the same disease or in different clinical entities in which this complication has been observed. We are certainly aware that investigation of some of the mechanisms proposed to explain this syndrome, such as local myositis, vasculitis, or fibrosis of the diaphragm (Gibson GJ, Edmonds JP, Hughes GRV. Diaphragm function and lung involvement in systemic lupus erythematosus. Am J Med 1977;63:926–32), would require invasive procedures and would therefore be difficult to perform, but we would suggest that at least an electrophysiologic study of the phrenic nerve be included in the standard evaluation of these patients. This simple preliminary suggestion could improve our understanding whether shrinking lung syndrome involves a common pathogenetic mechanism in different autoimmune disorders, thus helping in the prediction and monitoring of the response to therapy.

A. Tavoni, MD
S. Bombardieri, MD
University of Pisa
Pisa, Italy

Similar effects of pulse corticosteroid and tumor necrosis factor α blockade in rheumatoid arthritis: comment on the article by Taylor et al

To the Editor:

We read with interest the article by Taylor et al (1) reporting the effects of tumor necrosis factor α (TNFα) blockade on synovial expression of interleukin-8 and monocyte chemotactic protein 1 and the reduction of inflammatory cell migration into joints in patients with rheumatoid arthritis. We commend the authors on their study.

It should be noted, however, that results very similar to those reported by Taylor et al were previously demonstrated to occur with high-dose intravenous (pulse) corticosteroid treatment, in a study using techniques very similar to theirs. Specifically, we have published extensively on the effects of pulse methylprednisolone therapy on neutrophil trafficking (2), cell subsets in synovial fluid (3), and chemokine and cytokine levels in serum, synovial fluid, and synovial membrane (4). Our results were very similar to Taylor et al's findings with TNFα blockade. It was somewhat surprising that the authors did not refer to our prior publications in their report (1).

Anti-TNFα therapy is expensive and is not readily available to patients in many countries at present. It is at least reassuring for those rheumatologists practicing in such countries to know that a relatively cheap and readily available therapeutic agent (intravenous pulse corticosteroids) has clinical and immunohistologic effects similar to those of one of the more expensive biologic therapies.

Malcolm D. Smith, MD
Michael J. Ahern, MD
Peter J. Roberts-Thomson, MD
Flinders Medical Centre and Repatriation General Hospital
Adelaide, Australia
Peter P. Youssef, MD
Rachel Forster Hospital
Sydney, Australia

1. Taylor PC, Peters AM, Paleolog E, Chapman PT, Elliott MJ, McCloskey R, et al. Reduction of chemokine levels and leukocyte traffic to joints by tumor necrosis factor α blockade in patients with rheumatoid arthritis. Arthritis Rheum 2000;43:38–47.
2. Youssef PP, Cormack J, Evill CA, Peter DT, Roberts-Thomson PJ, Ahern MJ, et al. Neutrophil trafficking into inflamed joints in patients with rheumatoid arthritis, and the effects of methylprednisolone. Arthritis Rheum 1996;39:216–25.
3. Youssef PP, Roberts-Thomson PJ, Ahern MJ, Smith MD. Pulse methylprednisolone in rheumatoid arthritis: effects on peripheral blood and synovial fluid neutrophil surface phenotype. J Rheumatol 1995;23:2065–71.
4. Youssef PP, Haynes DR, Triantafillou S, Parker A, Gamble JR, Roberts-Thomson PJ, et al. Effects of pulse methylprednisolone on inflammatory mediators in peripheral blood, synovial fluid, and synovial membrane in rheumatoid arthritis. Arthritis Rheum 1997; 40:1400–8.

Reply

To the Editor:

We have demonstrated that TNFα blockade in active rheumatoid arthritis (RA) results in reduced neutrophil traffic to synovial joints (1) and in diminished synovial inflammatory cell infiltration (2). This reduction is associated with decreases in the expression of synovial adhesion molecules (2), the serum concentration of soluble adhesion molecules (3), and the synovial expression of the chemokines interleukin-8 and monocyte chemotactic protein 1 (1). We agree that these findings are very similar to those observed following pulse methylprednisolone treatment in active RA, as demonstrated in an elegant series of studies by Dr. Smith and his colleagues (4–6). The similar biologic, immunohistologic, and clinical effects of a single intravenous administration of infliximab and an intravenous pulse of corticosteroid suggest a common mechanism of action through down-regulation of TNFα.

A single pulse of either infliximab or high-dose corticosteroid has a limited duration of clinical benefit. One potential indication for the use of such therapies is the treatment of RA flare. In disease that has been refractory to treatment with conventional disease-modifying antirheumatic drugs, however, the potential risks and benefits of repeated administration of any alternate therapy must be taken into account. In such patients, repeated administration of anti-TNFα agents has been shown to result in maintenance of good disease control with little toxicity in a randomized, placebo-controlled trial in which ~60% of patients had been receiving long-term treatment with prednisolone in doses of up to 10 mg daily (7). In contrast, there are no such trial data on extended and frequent treatment with high-dose corticosteroids, and this strategy is rarely used in patients with refractory RA, given the high level of associated toxicity. Therefore, in such situations, repeated administration of anti-TNF agents is preferable, despite the expense associated with currently available drugs.

Peter C. Taylor, PhD, FRCP
Ewa Paleolog, PhD
Ravinder N. Maini, MB, FRCP
Kennedy Institute of Rheumatology
London, UK

1. Taylor PC, Peters AM, Paleolog E, Chapman PT, Elliott MJ, McCloskey R, et al. Reduction of chemokine levels and leukocyte traffic to joints by tumor necrosis factor α blockade in patients with rheumatoid arthritis. Arthritis Rheum 2000;43:38–47.
2. Tak PP, Taylor PC, Breedveld FC, Smeets TJM, Daha MR, Kluin PM, et al. Decrease in cellularity and expression of adhesion molecules by anti–tumor necrosis factor α monoclonal antibody treatment in patients with rheumatoid arthritis. Arthritis Rheum 1996;39:1077–81.
3. Paleolog EM, Hunt M, Elliott MJ, Feldmann M, Maini RN, Woody JN. Deactivation of vascular endothelium by monoclonal anti–tumor necrosis factor α antibody in rheumatoid arthritis. Arthritis Rheum 1996;39:1082–91.
4. Youssef PP, Cormack J, Evill CA, Peter DT, Roberts-Thomson PJ, Ahern MJ, et al. Neutrophil trafficking into inflamed joints in patients with rheumatoid arthritis, and the effects of methylprednisolone. Arthritis Rheum 1996;39:216–25.
5. Youssef PP, Roberts-Thompson PJ, Ahern MJ, Smith MD. Pulse methylprednisolone in rheumatoid arthritis: effects on peripheral blood and synovial fluid neutrophil surface phenotype. J Rheumatol 1995;23:2065–71.
6. Youssef PP, Haynes DR, Triantafillou S, Parker A, Gamble JR, Roberts-Thomson PJ, et al. Effects of pulse methylprednisolone on inflammatory mediators in peripheral blood, synovial fluid, and synovial membrane in rheumatoid arthritis. Arthritis Rheum 1997; 40:1400–8.
7. Maini RN, St Clair EW, Breedveld FC, Furst D, Kalden JR, Weisman M, et al, and the ATTRACT study group. Randomised phase III trial of infliximab (Chimeric anti-TNFα monoclonal antibody) versus placebo in rheumatoid arthritis patients receiving concomitant methotrexate. Lancet 1999;354:1932–9.

REMICADE®

(infliximab)
for IV Injection
BRIEF SUMMARY
See package insert for full prescribing information.

INDICATIONS AND USAGE: Rheumatoid Arthritis REMICADE, in combination with methotrexate, is indicated for the reduction in signs and symptoms of rheumatoid arthritis in patients who have had an inadequate response to methotrexate. Crohn's Disease REMICADE is indicated for the reduction in signs and symptoms of Crohn's disease in patients with moderately to severely active Crohn's disease who have had an inadequate response to conventional therapy. **The safety and efficacy of therapy continued beyond a single dose have not been established.** REMICADE is indicated for the reduction in the number of draining enterocutaneous fistulae in patients with fistulizing Crohn's disease. **The safety and efficacy of therapy continued beyond three doses have not been studied.**
CONTRAINDICATIONS: REMICADE should not be administered to patients with known hypersensitivity to any murine proteins or other component of the product.

WARNINGS:

RISK OF INFECTIONS
SERIOUS INFECTIONS, INCLUDING SEPSIS AND FATAL INFECTIONS, HAVE BEEN REPORTED IN PATIENTS RECEIVING TNF-BLOCKING AGENTS. MANY OF THE SERIOUS INFECTIONS IN PATIENTS TREATED WITH REMICADE HAVE OCCURRED IN PATIENTS ON CONCOMITANT IMMUNOSUPPRESSIVE THERAPY THAT, IN ADDITION TO THEIR CROHN'S DISEASE OR RHEUMATOID ARTHRITIS, COULD PREDISPOSE THEM TO INFECTIONS. CAUTION SHOULD BE EXERCISED WHEN CONSIDERING THE USE OF REMICADE IN PATIENTS WITH A CHRONIC INFECTION OR A HISTORY OF RECURRENT INFECTION. REMICADE SHOULD NOT BE GIVEN TO PATIENTS WITH A CLINICALLY IMPORTANT, ACTIVE INFECTION. PATIENTS WHO DEVELOP A NEW INFECTION WHILE UNDERGOING TREATMENT WITH REMICADE SHOULD BE MONITORED CLOSELY. IF A PATIENT DEVELOPS A SERIOUS INFECTION OR SEPSIS, REMICADE THERAPY SHOULD BE DISCONTINUED (see *ADVERSE REACTIONS, Infections*).
Hypersensitivity REMICADE has been associated with hypersensitivity reactions that vary in their time of onset. Most hypersensitivity reactions, which include urticaria, dyspnea and/or hypotension, have occurred during or within 2 hours of infliximab infusion. However, in some cases, serum sickness-like reactions have been observed in Crohn's disease patients 3 to 12 days after REMICADE therapy was reinstituted following an extended period without REMICADE treatment. Symptoms associated with these reactions include fever, rash, headache, sore throat, myalgias, polyarthralgias, hand and facial edema and/or dysphagia. These reactions were associated with marked increase in antibodies to infliximab, loss of detectable serum concentrations of REMICADE, and possible loss of drug efficacy. REMICADE should be discontinued for severe reactions. Medications for the treatment of hypersensitivity reactions (e.g., acetaminophen, antihistamines, corticosteroids and/or epinephrine) should be available for immediate use in the event of a reaction (see *ADVERSE REACTIONS, Infusion-related Reactions*).

PRECAUTIONS: Autoimmunity Treatment with REMICADE may result in the formation of autoantibodies and, rarely, in the development of a lupus-like syndrome. If a patient develops symptoms suggestive of a lupus-like syndrome following treatment with REMICADE, treatment should be discontinued (see *ADVERSE REACTIONS, Autoantibodies/Lupus-like Syndrome*). **Malignancy** Patients with long duration of Crohn's disease or rheumatoid arthritis and chronic exposure to immunosuppressant therapies are more prone to develop lymphomas (see *ADVERSE REACTIONS, Malignancies/Lymphoproliferative Disease*). The impact of treatment with REMICADE on these phenomena is unknown. **Immunogenicity** Treatment with REMICADE can be associated with the development of antibodies to infliximab (also referred to as human antichimeric antibodies, HACA). One hundred thirty-four of the 199 Crohn's disease patients treated with REMICADE were evaluated for the development of infliximab-specific antibodies; 18 (13%) were antibody-positive (the majority at low titer, <1:20). Patients who were antibody-positive were more likely to experience an infusion reaction (see *ADVERSE REACTIONS, Infusion-related Reactions*). Antibody development was lower among rheumatoid arthritis and Crohn's disease patients receiving immunosuppressant therapies such as 6-MP, AZA or MTX. With repeated dosing of REMICADE, serum concentrations of infliximab were higher in rheumatoid arthritis patients who received concomitant MTX. There are limited data available on the development of antibodies to infliximab in patients receiving long-term treatment with REMICADE. Because immunogenicity analyses are product-specific, comparison of antibody rates to those from other products is not appropriate. **Vaccinations** No data are available on the response to vaccination or on the secondary transmission of infection by live vaccines in patients receiving anti-TNF therapy. It is recommended that live vaccines not be given concurrently. **Drug Interactions** Specific drug interaction studies, including interactions with MTX, have not been conducted. The majority of patients in rheumatoid arthritis or Crohn's disease clinical trials received one or more concomitant medications. In rheumatoid arthritis, concomitant medications besides MTX were nonsteroidal anti-inflammatory agents, folic acid, corticosteroids and/or narcotics. Concomitant Crohn's disease medications were antibiotics, antivirals, corticosteroids, 6-MP/AZA and aminosalicylates. Patients with Crohn's disease who received immunosuppressants tended to experience fewer infusion reactions compared to patients on no immunosuppressants (see *PRECAUTIONS, Immunogenicity* and *ADVERSE REACTIONS, Infusion-related Reactions*). **Carcinogenesis, Mutagenesis and Impairment of Fertility** Long-term studies in animals have not been performed to evaluate the carcinogenic potential. No clastogenic or mutagenic effects of infliximab were observed in the *in vivo* mouse micronucleus test or the *Salmonella-Escherichia coli* (Ames) assay, respectively. Chromosomal aberrations were not observed in an assay performed using human lymphocytes. It is not known whether infliximab can impair fertility in humans. No impairment of fertility was observed in a fertility and general reproduction toxicity study conducted in mice using an analogous antibody that selectively inhibits the functional activity of mouse TNFα. **Pregnancy Category C** Since infliximab does not cross-react with TNFα in species other than humans and chimpanzees, animal reproduction studies have not been conducted with REMICADE. It is not known whether REMICADE can cause fetal harm when administered to a pregnant woman or can affect reproduction capacity while infliximab is present in the serum. REMICADE should be given to a pregnant woman only if clearly needed. No evidence of maternal toxicity, embryotoxicity or teratogenicity was observed in a developmental toxicity study conducted in mice using an analogous antibody that selectively inhibits the functional activity of mouse TNFα. **Nursing Mothers** It is not known whether infliximab is excreted in human milk or absorbed systemically after ingestion. Because many drugs and immunoglobulins are excreted in human milk, and because of the potential for adverse reactions in nursing infants from REMICADE, a decision should be made whether to discontinue nursing or to discontinue the drug, taking into account the importance of the drug to the mother. **Pediatric Use** Safety and effectiveness of REMICADE in patients with juvenile rheumatoid arthritis and in pediatric patients with Crohn's disease have not been established. **Geriatric Use** In the ATTRACT study, no overall differences were observed in effectiveness or safety in the 72 patients aged 65 or older compared to younger patients. In Crohn's disease studies, there were insufficient numbers of patients aged 65 or older to determine whether they respond differently from patients aged 18 to 65. Because there is a higher incidence of infections in the elderly population in general, caution should be used in treating the elderly (see *ADVERSE REACTIONS, Infections*).

ADVERSE REACTIONS: A total of 771 patients were treated with REMICADE in clinical trials. In both rheumatoid arthritis and Crohn's disease trials, approximately 5% of patients discontinued REMICADE because of adverse experiences. The most common reasons for discontinuation of treatment were dyspnea, urticaria and headache. **Infusion-related Reactions** *Acute infusion reactions* An infusion reaction was defined as any adverse event occurring during the infusion or within 1 to 2 hours after the infusion. Seventeen percent of REMICADE-treated patients in all clinical trials experienced an infusion reaction compared to 7% of placebo-treated patients. Among the 3284 REMICADE infusions, 4% were accompanied by nonspecific symptoms such as fever or chills, 1% were accompanied by pruritus or urticaria, 1% were accompanied by cardiopulmonary reactions (primarily chest pain, hypotension, hypertension or dyspnea), and 0.1% were accompanied by combined symptoms of pruritus/urticaria and cardiopulmonary reactions. Less than 2% of patients discontinued REMICADE because of infusion reactions, and all patients recovered with treatment and/or discontinuation of infusion. REMICADE infusions beyond the initial infusion in rheumatoid arthritis patients were not associated with a higher incidence of reactions. Patients with Crohn's disease who became positive for antibodies to infliximab were more likely to develop infusion reactions than were those who were negative (36% vs. 11% respectively). Use of concomitant immunosuppressant agents appeared to reduce the frequency of antibodies to infliximab and infusion reactions (see *PRECAUTIONS, Immunogenicity* and *Drug Interactions*). *Reactions following readministration* In a clinical trial of forty patients with Crohn's disease retreated with infliximab following a 2 to 4 year period without infliximab treatment, 10 patients experienced adverse events manifesting 3 to 12 days following infusion of which 6 were considered serious. Signs and symptoms included myalgia and/or arthralgia with fever and/or rash, with some patients also experiencing pruritus, facial, hand or lip edema, dysphagia, urticaria, sore throat, and headache. Patients experiencing these adverse events had not experienced infusion-related adverse events associated with their initial infliximab therapy. Of the 40 patients enrolled, these adverse events occurred in 9 of 23 (39%) who had received liquid formulation which is no longer in use and 1 of 17 (6%) who received lyophilized formulation. The clinical data are not adequate to determine if occurrence of these reactions is due to differences in formulation. Patients' signs and symptoms improved substantially or resolved with treatment in all cases. There are insufficient data on the incidence of these events after drug-free intervals of less than 2 years. However, these events have been observed infrequently in clinical trials and post-marketing surveillance at intervals of less than 1 year. **Infections** In REMICADE (infliximab) clinical trials, infections were reported by 26% of REMICADE-treated patients (average of 27 weeks of follow-up) and by 16% of placebo-treated patients (average of 20 weeks of follow-up). The infections most frequently reported were upper respiratory tract infections (including, sinusitis, pharyngitis, and bronchitis) and urinary tract infections. No increased risk of serious infections or sepsis has been observed with Remicade compared to placebo. Among REMICADE-treated patients, these serious infections included pneumonia, cellulitis, pyelonephritis and sepsis. In the ATTRACT study, one patient died with disseminated tuberculosis and one died with disseminated coccidioidomycosis. The relationship to REMICADE is unknown (see *WARNINGS, Risk of Infections*). Twelve percent of patients with fistulizing Crohn's disease developed a new abscess 8 to 16 weeks after the last infusion of REMICADE. **Autoantibodies/Lupus-like Syndrome** Patients were tested for autoantibodies at multiple time points. In the rheumatoid arthritis ATTRACT study, 23% of REMICADE-treated patients developed antinuclear antibodies (ANA) between screening and last evaluation, compared to 6% of placebo-treated patients. Anti-dsDNA antibodies developed in approximately 4% of REMICADE-treated patients, compared to none of the placebo-treated patients. No association was seen between REMICADE dose/schedule and development of ANA or anti-dsDNA. Of Crohn's disease patients treated with REMICADE who were evaluated for antinuclear antibodies (ANA), 34% developed ANA between screening and last evaluation. Anti-dsDNA antibodies developed in approximately 9% of Crohn's disease patients treated with REMICADE. The development of anti-dsDNA antibodies was not related to either the dose or duration of REMICADE treatment. However, baseline therapy with an immunosuppressant in Crohn's disease patients was associated with reduced development of anti-dsDNA antibodies (3% compared to 21% in patients not receiving any immunosuppressant). Crohn's disease patients were approximately 2 times more likely to develop anti-dsDNA antibodies if they were ANA-positive at study entry. Three patients developed clinical symptoms consistent with a lupus-like syndrome, two with rheumatoid arthritis and one with Crohn's disease. All three patients improved following discontinuation of therapy and appropriate medical treatment (see *PRECAUTIONS, Autoimmunity*). **Malignancies/Lymphoproliferative Disease** Five new and 2 recurrent malignancies were observed in 6 of 771 patients treated with REMICADE for up to 36 weeks in clinical trials. These were non-Hodgkin's B-cell lymphoma, breast cancer, melanoma, squamous cell cancer of the skin, and basal cell cancer. There are insufficient data to determine whether REMICADE contributed to the development of these malignancies. The observed rates and incidences were similar to those expected for the populations studied[1,2] (see *PRECAUTIONS, Malignancy*). **Other Adverse Reactions** Adverse events occurring at a frequency of at least 5% in trials in patients with rheumatoid arthritis or Crohn's disease are shown in the table below. Patients with Crohn's disease who were treated with REMICADE were more likely than patients with rheumatoid arthritis to experience adverse events associated with gastrointestinal symptoms.

ADVERSE EVENTS IN RHEUMATOID ARTHRITIS AND CROHN'S DISEASE TRIALS

	RHEUMATOID ARTHRITIS		CROHN'S DISEASE	
	Placebo (n=133)	REMICADE (n= 555)	Placebo (n=56)	REMICADE (n=199)
Avg. weeks of follow-up	22.3	26.9	14.7	27.0
Respiratory				
Upper respiratory infection	13%	20%	9%	16%
Coughing	5%	10%	0%	5%
Sinusitis	3%	9%	2%	5%
Rhinitis	4%	8%	4%	6%
Pharyngitis	5%	8%	5%	9%
Bronchitis	2%	4%	2%	7%
Gastrointestinal				
Nausea	17%	14%	4%	17%
Abdominal Pain	7%	8%	4%	12%
Vomiting	10%	5%	0%	9%
Other				
Headache	10%	20%	21%	23%
Rash	4%	9%	5%	6%
Fatigue	5%	6%	5%	11%
Fever	4%	6%	7%	10%
Back pain	2%	6%	4%	5%
Pain	4%	6%	5%	9%
Urinary tract infection	3%	6%	4%	3%
Pruritus	0%	5%	2%	5%
Moniliasis	2%	3%	0%	5%

Serious adverse events by body system that occurred in all patients treated with REMICADE at frequencies <2% are as follows:
Body as a whole: abdominal hernia, chest pain, fall, pain *Blood:* splenic infarction, splenomegaly *Cardiovascular:* hypertension, hypotension, syncope *Central & Peripheral Nervous:* dizziness, headache, upper motor neuron lesion *Collagen:* lupus erythematosus syndrome, rheumatoid nodules *Ear and Hearing:* ceruminosis *Gastrointestinal:* abdominal pain, Crohn's disease, diarrhea, gastric ulcer, intestinal obstruction, intestinal perforation, intestinal stenosis, nausea, pancreatitis, proctalgia, vomiting *Heart Rate and Rhythm:* palpitation, tachycardia *Liver and Biliary:* cholecystitis *Metabolic and Nutritional:* dehydration, pancreatic insufficiency, weight decrease *Musculoskeletal:* arthropathy, back pain, bone fracture, myalgia, tendon disorder, tendon injury *Myo-, Endo-, Pericardial and Coronary Valve:* cardiac failure, myocardial ischemia *Neoplasms:* lymphoma *Platelet, Bleeding and Clotting:* thrombocytopenia *Psychiatric:* anxiety, confusion, delirium, depression, somnolence, suicide attempt *Red Blood Cell:* anemia *Resistance Mechanism:* abscess, cellulitis, fever, infection bacterial, sepsis *Respiratory:* adult respiratory distress syndrome, bronchitis, coughing, dyspnea, pleurisy, pneumonia, pulmonary infiltration, respiratory insufficiency *Skin and Appendages:* furunculosis, rash, increased sweating *Urinary:* azotemia, dysuria, hydronephrosis, kidney infarction, renal failure, ureteral obstruction *Vascular (Extracardiac):* brain infarction, pulmonary embolism, thrombophlebitis deep *White cell and Reticuloendothelial:* leukopenia, lymphadenopathy A greater proportion of patients enrolled into the ATTRACT trial who received REMICADE plus MTX experienced mild, transient elevations (<2 times the upper limit of normal) in AST or ALT (37% each) compared to patients treated with placebo plus MTX (AST: 24%, ALT: 29%). Five (1.5%) patients treated with REMICADE and MTX experienced more prolonged elevations in their ALT.

OVERDOSAGE: Single doses up to 20 mg/kg have been administered without any direct toxic effect. In case of overdosage, it is recommended that the patient be monitored for any signs or symptoms of adverse reactions or effects and appropriate symptomatic treatment instituted immediately.

Storage Store the lyophilized product under refrigeration at 2°C to 8°C (36°F to 46°F). Do not freeze. Do not use beyond the expiration date. This product contains no preservative.

HOW SUPPLIED: REMICADE lyophilized concentrate for IV injection is supplied in individually-boxed single-use vials in the following strength:
NDC 57894-030-01 100 mg infliximab in a 20-mL vial

REFERENCES:

1. Greenstein AJ, Mullin GE, Strauchen JA, Heimann T, et al. Lymphoma in inflammatory bowel disease. *Cancer* 1992;69:1119-21.
2. Jones M, Symmons D, Finn J, Wolfe F. Does exposure to immunosuppressive therapy increase the 10 year malignancy and mortality risks in rheumatoid arthritis? A matched cohort study. *Br J Rheum* 1996;35:738-45.

Centocor, Inc., Malvern, PA 19355, USA
1-800-457-6399

License #1242
9 November 1999

ACR ANNOUNCEMENTS

AMERICAN COLLEGE OF RHEUMATOLOGY
1800 Century Place, Suite 250, Atlanta, Georgia 30345-4300

ACR Meetings

Annual Meetings
November 10–15, 2001, San Francisco
October 24–29, 2002, New Orleans
October 23–28, 2003, Orlando
October 7–12, 2004, San Antonio
November 12–17, 2005, San Diego

Winter Rheumatology Symposium
January 27–February 2, 2001, Snowmass

Innovative Therapies in Autoimmune Diseases: Clinical Development Challenges
March 8–10, 2001, San Francisco

State-of-the-Art Clinical Symposium
April 20–22, 2001, Chicago

Summer Clinical Meeting
June 21–24, 2001, Santa Barbara

For additional information, contact the ACR office.

ACR State-of-the-Art Clinical Symposium

The American College of Rheumatology will hold the State-of-the-Art Clinical Symposium April 20–22, 2001, at the Fairmont Hotel in Chicago. The conference will update physicians on recent developments in the broad field of rheumatology, with a special focus on the clinical perspective of rheumatology practice. Topics will reflect the needs and interests of ACR members by providing a forum for the medical community to address issues of professional significance. Sessions in both clinical and basic research will be offered. Program lecturers will outline the direction of state-of-the-art research and detail future prospects in the management of conditions addressed by practicing rheumatologists. In addition, the format will include both pro/con presentations and discussion between faculty and participants.

Sessions on basic immunology for clinicians, sports medicine and regional musculoskeletal disorders, and state-of-the-art treatments will be offered. Topics will include shoulder, common running and other sports-related injuries, neck/cervicalgia, the American Pain Society evidence-based clinical practice guidelines for the management of pain in osteoarthritis and rheumatoid arthritis, tumor necrosis factor antagonists versus combination disease-modifying antirheumatic drug therapy, outcomes and treatment of juvenile rheumatoid arthritis, inflammatory myopathy, osteoporosis, systemic lupus erythematosus, matrix precursors, the risks and interactions of alternative medicine, and computers.

In addition to the State-of-the-Art Clinical Symposium, an optional Committee on Rheumatologic Care (CORC) Practice Management Symposium will be held on April 20, 2001. Issues relevant to practicing rheumatologists—including new documentation guidelines, using hand-held computers and personal digital assistants in rheumatology practice, and benchmarking in rheumatology—will be presented.

The registration and housing deadline for the State-of-the-Art Clinical Symposium is Friday, March 16, 2001. If received by that date, the registration fee is $250 for ACR members, $370 for nonmembers, $95 for member trainees, and $115 for nonmember trainees. The registration fee after March 16, 2001 is $325 for ACR members, $445 for nonmembers, $120 for member trainees, and $140 for nonmember trainees. Guest registration is free. Registration for the optional CORC Practice Management Symposium is $125. This fee is in addition to the State-of-the-Art Clinical Symposium registration fee and includes lunch. The ACR special housing rate at the Fairmont Hotel is $179 per night single/double, plus 14.5% tax. After March 16, 2001, this special group rate cannot be guaranteed.

Complete registration, housing, and course information can be obtained by calling the ACR Education Department at 404-633-3777. To register online or to obtain up-to-date information on this meeting, visit the ACR's Web site, http://www.rheumatology.org.

American Board of Internal Medicine Certification and Recertification Examinations

The ABIM 2001 Certification Examination in Rheumatology will be held November 7, 2001. The registration period is January 1–April 1, 2001; the late registration period is April 2–June 1, 2001. The ABIM's Recertification Program, which has been renamed the Program for Continuous Professional Development (CPD), consists of an at-home, open-book self-evaluation process and a proctored final examination which will be administered twice each year in May and November. To register for the examination, Diplomates must be enrolled in the CPD Program and be in at least year 6 of their certification cycle. For the 2001 Recertification Examinations in Internal Medicine, its Subspecialties, and Added Qualifications, the final examination will be administered May 1 (registration deadline March 1) and November 7 (registration deadline September 1). For additional information and registration forms, contact Registration Section, American Board of Internal Medicine, 510 Walnut Street, Suite 1700, Philadelphia, PA 19106-3699, phone 800-441-2246 or 215-446-3500, fax 215-446-3590, e-mail request@abim.org, or visit the ABIM's Web site at www.abim.org.

NIH/NIAMS Trial of Methotrexate Plus Infliximab Treatment in Early Rheumatoid Arthritis

The National Institute of Arthritis and Musculoskeletal and Skin Diseases is conducting a single-center trial of treatment of patients with early rheumatoid arthritis with methotrexate plus placebo versus methotrexate plus infliximab. After 6 months of double-blind administration, all patients will receive methotrexate plus infliximab for another 6 months. The trial is designed to assess the value of sensitive imaging modalities in detecting differences in erosion formation in the 2 treatment arms and to correlate serologic markers with imaging findings. Participation involves 13 monthly visits for infusions, clinical evaluation, specimen collections, and questionnaires. Patients who have rheumatoid arthritis of <2 years' duration, erosive disease, and an incomplete response to methotrexate at a minimum weekly dosage of 12.5 mg, and who have not received bisphosphonates in the past year, are being sought for the trial. For additional information, contact Raphaela Goldbach-Mansky, MD or Mildred Wilson, RN, NIAMS, NIH, Building 10, Room 9S205, 10 Center Drive, Bethesda, MD 20892, phone 301-496-3374 or 877-274-4981, e-mail goldbacr@mail.nih.gov or Wilsonl@mail.nih.gov.

Hopkins Cyclophosphamide Trial

The National Institute of Arthritis and Musculoskeletal and Skin Diseases is funding a randomized trial of high-dose immunoblative cyclophosphamide versus monthly (NIH) intravenous cyclophosphamide for patients with moderate-to-severe systemic lupus erythematosus who have not previously received cyclophosphamide. Patients randomized to receive high-dose immunoblative cyclophosphamide will need to stay in the Baltimore area for approximately 3–4 weeks. For information regarding patient referral, contact Michelle Petri, MD, MPH, The Johns Hopkins University Lupus Center, phone 410-955-3823, fax 410-614-0498.

Education Programs

20th Annual Scientific Meeting of the American Pain Society. April 19–22, 2001; Phoenix, AZ. For additional information, contact American Pain Society, 4700 West Lake Avenue, Glenview, IL 60025-1485, phone 847-375-4715, fax 888-508-7578, e-mail info@ampainsoc.org, or visit the Web site http://www.ampainsoc.org/meeting/.

First Joint Meeting of the International Bone and Mineral Society and the European Calcified Tissue Society. June 5–10, 2001, Madrid, Spain. For additional information, contact Lucia Calvo, IBMS/ECTS 2001, c/o Tilcsa OPC, SL, Londres 17, 28028 Madrid, Spain, phone 34-91-361-2600, fax 34-91-355-9208, e-mail ibms-ects2001@tilesa.es, or visit the Web site http://www.intercongres-2001.com.

20th International League of Associations for Rheumatology (ILAR) World Congress. August 26–31, 2001, Edmonton, Alberta. Canada. The theme of the congress will be Therapy for the 21st Century. For additional information, contact ILAR Secretariat, Health Care Communications, Suite 906, 50 Burnhamthorpe Road West, Mississauga, Ontario, L5B 3C2, Canada. phone 800-535-3330 (from within Canada) or 905-273-3080, fax 905-273-3611, e-mail healthcarecomm@sympatico.ca.

Controversies in Diagnosis, Management, and Costs of Osteoarticular Implications of Obesity. October 12–13, 2001, Brussels, Belgium. For additional information, contact Prof. Dr. M. Szpalski, Centre Hospitalier Molière Longchamps, Rue Marconi 142, 1180 Brussels, Belgium, fax 32-2-348-5694.

Third International Congress on Autoimmunity. February 20–24, 2002, Geneva, Switzerland. For additional information, contact Prof. Yehuda Shoenfeld, 3rd International Congress on Autoimmunity, PO Box 50006, Tel Aviv 61500, Israel, phone 972-3-5140018/9, fax 972-3-5175674 or 972-3-5172484, e-mail autoim02@kenes.com.

Arthritis & Rheumatism

Professional Opportunities

Reach the healthcare professionals of your needs - advertise in *Arthritis & Rheumatism* and get the results you want!

For advertising information contact:

Aileen Rivera • Pharmaceutical Media, Inc.
30 East 33rd St. • New York, NY 10016
Tel: (212) 685-5010 x111 • Fax: (212) 685-6126
Email: arivera@pminy.com

RHEUMATOLOGIST: Faculty position available for BC/BE Rheumatologist at the *University of North Texas Health Science Center.* Academic rank commensurate with experience. This is a 100% consultant practice that involves patient care, teaching of students and house staff, and clinical research. Base salary and incentive with excellent benefits. Please reply in confidence with CV and three references to: **Bernard Rubin, D.O., Professor of Medicine, Chief of Rheumatology, University of North Texas Health Science Center, 855 Montgomery, Fort Worth, TX 76107, Fax (817) 735-2673.**

The University of North Texas Health Science Center is an equal opportunity employer.

Busy 100% Rheumatology Practice For Sale in a large Western Canadian Centre. Send inquiries to:

Box# AR002
Pharmaceutical Media, Inc.
30 East 33rd Street
New York, NY 10016

BC/BE RHEUMATOLOGIST wanted to join busy solo physician's practice in northern Texas city with 200,000 population. Well-established practice, physician owned and directed. Exceptional opportunity to join a high-quality practice. Excellent environment for families, including outstanding schools and community involvement. Offering a competitive salary, attractive benefits, no state income tax and an opportunity for partnership. Send CV to:

Box AR#003 • Pharmaceutical Media, Inc.
30 East 33rd Street • New York, NY 10016

RHEUMATOLOGIST: *Bassett Healthcare,* a teaching affiliate of Columbia University of Physicians and Surgeons, is seeking a BC/BE Rheumatologist with a strong clinical background. Emphasis is on patient care and teaching, with Columbia faculty appointment. Bassett is a multi-specialty group practice, which provides primary and tertiary care services to a 10-county, predominantly rural region of Central New York. Cooperstown enjoys recreational facilities, excellent schools and a wide range of cultural activities. Please send CV and correspondence to: **Denise B. Harter, Medical Staff Affairs, One Atwell Road, Cooperstown, NY 13326, Fax: (607) 547-3844, email address: denise.harter@bassett.org, or for more information please call (607) 547-6982.**

FOR SALE:

Once in a life time opportunity to purchase in Southern California an exclusive 100% Rheumatologic Consultative Fee for Service 30 year old established solo practice. Situated in Santa Monica adjacent to West Los Angeles and Beverly Hills. Have no contracts with PPO's or HMO's. No General Internal Medicine. **Reply to: *Box AR#001 / Pharmaceutical Media, Inc. / 30 East 33rd Street / New York, NY 10016***

MAINE--A BETTER WAY OF LIFE:

We seek a third rheumatologist and partner for our very busy 100% rheumatology practice. Site of the Eastern Maine Medical Center, Bangor boasts its symphony orchestra, repertory theatre, and its location adjacent to the main campus of the University of Maine and its proximity to the Appalachian Trail and Acadia National Park. Earn as we do: your own receipts minus our shared overhead. You will do well and your family will thank you for choosing our practice and this area.

Contact: Sid Block or Geoff Gratwick
275 Union St. / Bangor, ME 04401
Fax (207) 942-5915 or email bjpa@acadia.net

RHEUMATOLOGIST

Opportunity for Rheumatologist to join progressive, successful solo practice. With the flexibility to work either full-time or part-time, you'll have access to the latest diagnostic equipment in two office locations, with on-site nurse practitioner. Contemporary practice offers its patients accepted alternative treatments. Affiliation with four hospitals, you will be within a short distance from both Yale-New Haven Hospital and UConn Medical Center. Great Central Connecticut location, with access to both country and city lifestyles. Enjoy theatre, ballet, fine restaurants, and professional sporting events, within easy commute to the amenities of the coast as well as New England skiing. ***To learn more about this opportunity, call 800-892-3846, or fax us your CV at 860-585-3086. Email address: cbourbeau@brishosp.chime.org***
EOE

UNIVERSITÉ DE GENÈVE
SWITZERLAND

FACULTY OF MEDICINE

Full or Associate Professor of Rhumatology

This position involves clinical responsibilities as chief of the Division of rhumatology in a University Hospital setting. Active involvement in pre and post-graduate teaching and continuing education in this field is also expected.

Candidates must have outstaning clinical skills, good teaching capabilities documented scientific experience in clinical and/or basic research rhumatology. Good knowledge of French is required.

Requirements: MD -- Certified Specialist in Rhumatology or equivalence.

This position is open for October 1st 2001 or at convenience.

Guidelines for application are available on request by Fax (004122 702.50.02) or E-mail (Dominique.Gehring@medecine.unige.ch)

Applications must be sent before March 20, 2001, to:

Doyen de la Faculté de médecine
Centre Médical Universitaire
-1, rue Michel-Servet
CH - 1211 Genève 4 SWITZERLAND

Women are encouraged to apply.

University of Iowa College of Medicine

The Department of Pediatrics, University of Iowa College of Medicine, seeks a pediatrician with fellowship training in pediatric rheumatology to serve as a consultant in pediatric rheumatology. The position may be filled at any rank on the tenure or non-tenure track: Associate, Assistant Professor, Associate Professor, or Professor. An enthusiasm for general pediatrics and for teaching medical students and residents as well as expertise in pediatric rheumatology, are essential. Candidates must be board certified/eligible in pediatrics and in pediatric rheumatology. Candidates for a tenure track position should possess research programs and skills. Candidates for the non-tenure track should have expectations for professional productivity.

Inquiries, including curriculum vitae, should be addressed to:

Frank H. Morriss, Jr., M.D.
Professor and Head
Department of Pediatrics
University of Iowa Hospital and Clinics
Iowa City, IA 52242
Please refer to F1936.

The University of Iowa is an Equal Employment Opportunity/ Affirmative Action Employer, and candidates who are women or members of minority groups are strongly encouraged to apply.

Division of Rheumatology

The Division of Rheumatology (www.med.ualberta.ca/medicine/rheumatology.htmweb), **Department of Medicine, University of Alberta** is seeking a clinician/basic scientist at the Assistant or Associate Professor level to develop a research program of relevance to the field of rheumatic disease. Preference will be given to candidates with proven expertise in cellular and molecular immunology. Applicants should have a PhD or MD with at least two years of postdoctoral training; MD's should be licensable to practice medicine in Alberta. Applicants will apply for personal support from the Medical Research Council of Canada and the Alberta Heritage Foundation for Medical Research (AHFMR) (http://www.AHFMR.ab.ca/). The divisional laboratory is housed in a state of the art facility (supported by the AHFMR) adjacent to the Department of Medical Microbiology and Immunology and has a well established program of research in immunogenetics, antigen processing, and advanced therapeutics. The Department of Medicine provides strong support for researchers including a mentoring program, internal reviews of grant applications and numerous collaborative opportunities in the Department and with other departments. The Department of Medicine has annual research funding of $14M. In accordance with Canadian Immigration requirements, priority will be given to Canadian citizens and permanent residents of Canada. If suitable Canadian citizens and permanent residents cannot be found, other individuals will be considered. Interested candidates should forward a curriculum vitae, a statement of interest and the names and addresses of three referees by January 31, 2001 to: Dr. A.S. Russell, Director, Division of Rheumatology, 562 HMRC, **University of Alberta**, Edmonton, Alberta, Canada, T6G 2R7. Tel: (780) 407-6296; Fax: (780) 407-6055; E-mail: asr@gpu.srv.ualberta.ca. The records arising from this competition will be managed in accordance with provisions of the Alberta Freedom of Information and Protection of Privacy Act (FOIPP). The University of Alberta hires on the basis of merit. We are committed to the principle of equity in employment. We welcome diversity and encourage applications from all qualified women and men, including persons with disabilities, members of visible minorities, and Aboriginal persons.

PHYSICIAN-RHEUMATOLOGY

The VA Medical Center in Louisville, Kentucky is seeking a part-time physician in the specialty of Rheumatology. Candidates must be board certified or board eligible in both Internal Medicine and Rheumatology. Experience with both an inpatient and outpatient population with a wide array of rheumatologic disorders is required. The successful candidate will also be expected to function as a primary care provider in an outpatient setting, as well as attend on one of the general internal medicine wards for part of the year. Applicants must have a background in participating in research initiatives and activities, and must demonstrate the ability to teach both internal medicine and rheumatology skills to housestaff that rotate through the teaching clinics at the medical center.

The Louisville VA Medical Center is an active, acute-care teaching center affiliated with the University of Louisville. This position is part-time, and candidates must be eligible for a faculty appointment at the University of Louisville. Salary and rank are commensurate with experience. *The Department of Veterans Affairs and the University of Louisville are equal opportunity employers.* Moving expenses are not authorized. Send C.V. and cover letter, to be received not later than February 2, 2001, to:

Angela Dutton
Personnel Staffing Specialist
VA Medical Center (05C)
800 Zorn Avenue / Louisville, KY 40206-1499
telephone (502) 894-6170

AN OFFICIAL JOURNAL OF THE AMERICAN COLLEGE OF RHEUMATOLOGY

Arthritis & Rheumatism

VOLUME 44, NUMBER 2

FEBRUARY 2001

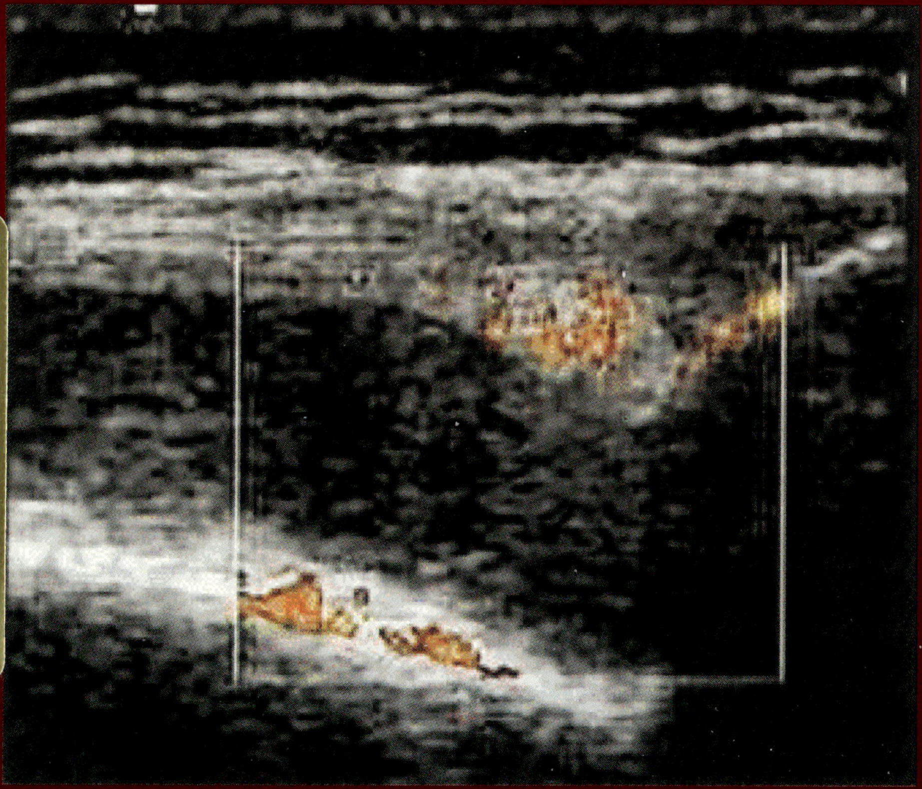

WILEY
InterScience®
www.interscience.wiley.com

AMERICAN COLLEGE OF RHEUMATOLOGY
www.arthritisrheum.org

ACTONEL® (risedronate sodium tablets)
Brief Summary: See package insert for full prescribing information.

INDICATIONS AND USAGE

Postmenopausal Osteoporosis: ACTONEL is indicated for the treatment and prevention of osteoporosis in postmenopausal women.

Treatment of Osteoporosis: In postmenopausal women with osteoporosis, ACTONEL increases BMD and reduces the incidence of vertebral fractures and a composite endpoint of nonvertebral osteoporosis-related fractures (see CLINICAL STUDIES). Osteoporosis may be confirmed by the presence or history of osteoporotic fracture, or by the finding of low bone mass (for example, at least 2 SD below the premenopausal mean).

Prevention of Osteoporosis: ACTONEL may be considered in postmenopausal women who are at risk of developing osteoporosis and for whom the desired clinical outcome is to maintain bone mass and to reduce the risk of fracture.

Factors such as family history of osteoporosis, previous fracture, smoking, BMD (at least 1 SD below the premenopausal mean), high bone turnover, thin body frame, Caucasian or Asian race, and early menopause are associated with an increased risk of developing osteoporosis and fractures. The presence of these risk factors may be important when considering the use of ACTONEL for prevention of osteoporosis.

Glucocorticoid-Induced Osteoporosis: ACTONEL is indicated for the prevention and treatment of glucocorticoid-induced osteoporosis in men and women who are either initiating or continuing systemic glucocorticoid treatment (daily dosage equivalent to 7.5 mg or greater of prednisone) for chronic diseases. Patients treated with glucocorticoids should receive adequate amounts of calcium and vitamin D.

Paget's Disease: ACTONEL is indicated for treatment of Paget's disease of bone (osteitis deformans).

Treatment is indicated in patients with Paget's disease of bone (1) who have a level of serum alkaline phosphatase (SAP) at least two times the upper limit of normal, or (2) who are symptomatic, or (3) who are at risk for future complications from their disease, to induce remission (normalization of serum alkaline phosphatase).

CONTRAINDICATIONS

- Hypocalcemia (See PRECAUTIONS, General)
- Known hypersensitivity to any component of this product
- Inability to stand or sit upright for at least 30 minutes

WARNINGS: Bisphosphonates may cause upper gastrointestinal disorders such as dysphagia, esophagitis, and esophageal or gastric ulcer (see PRECAUTIONS).

PRECAUTIONS

General: Hypocalcemia and other disturbances of bone and mineral metabolism should be effectively treated before starting ACTONEL therapy. Adequate intake of calcium and vitamin D is important in all patients, especially in patients with Paget's disease in whom bone turnover is significantly elevated. ACTONEL is not recommended for use in patients with severe renal impairment (creatinine clearance < 30 mL/min).

Bisphosphonates have been associated with gastrointestinal disorders such as dysphagia, esophagitis, and esophageal or gastric ulcers. This association has been reported for bisphosphonates in postmarketing experience, but has not been found in most pre-approval clinical trials, including those conducted with ACTONEL. Patients should be advised that taking the medication according to the instructions is important to minimize the risk of these events. They should take ACTONEL with sufficient plain water (6 to 8 oz) to facilitate delivery to the stomach, and should not lie down for 30 minutes after taking the drug.

Glucocorticoid-Induced Osteoporosis: The risk versus benefit of ACTONEL for the prevention and treatment of glucocorticoid-induced osteoporosis at daily doses of glucocorticoids < 7.5 mg of prednisone or equivalent has not been established. Before initiating treatment, the hormonal status of both men and women should be ascertained and appropriate replacement considered.

The efficacy of ACTONEL has been established in studies of 1-year's duration. The efficacy of ACTONEL beyond 1 year has not been studied.

Information for Patients: The patient should be informed to pay particular attention to the dosing instructions as clinical benefits may be compromised by failure to take the drug according to instructions. Specifically, ACTONEL should be taken at least 30 minutes before the first food or drink of the day other than water.

To facilitate delivery to the stomach, and thus reduce the potential for esophageal irritation, patients should take ACTONEL while in an upright position (sitting or standing) with a full glass of plain water (6 to 8 oz). Patients should not lie down for 30 minutes after taking the medication (see PRECAUTIONS, General). Patients should not chew or suck on the tablet because of a potential for oropharyngeal irritation.

Patients should be instructed that if they develop symptoms of esophageal disease (such as difficulty or pain upon swallowing, retrosternal pain or severe persistent or worsening heartburn) they should consult their physician before continuing ACTONEL.

Patients should receive supplemental calcium and vitamin D if dietary intake is inadequate (see PRECAUTIONS, General). Calcium supplements or calcium-, aluminum-, and magnesium-containing medications may interfere with the absorption of ACTONEL and should be taken at a different time of the day, as with food.

Weight-bearing exercise should be considered along with the modification of certain behavioral factors, such as excessive cigarette smoking, and/or alcohol consumption, if these factors exist.

Drug Interactions: No specific drug-drug interaction studies were performed. Risedronate is not metabolized and does not induce or inhibit hepatic microsomal drug-metabolizing enzymes (Cytochrome P450).

Calcium Supplements/Antacids: Co-administration of ACTONEL and calcium, antacids, or oral medications containing divalent cations will interfere with the absorption of ACTONEL.

Hormone Replacement Therapy: One study of about 500 early postmenopausal women has been conducted to date in which treatment with ACTONEL (5 mg/day) plus estrogen replacement therapy was compared with estrogen replacement therapy alone. Exposure to study drugs was approximately 12 to 18 months and the primary endpoint was change in BMD. If considered appropriate, ACTONEL may be used concomitantly with hormone replacement therapy.

Aspirin/Nonsteroidal Anti-Inflammatory Drugs (NSAIDs): Of over 5700 patients enrolled in the ACTONEL Phase 3 osteoporosis studies, aspirin use was reported by 31% of patients, 24% of whom were regular users (3 or more days per week). Forty-eight percent of patients reported NSAID use, 21% of whom were regular users. Among regular aspirin or NSAID users, the incidence of upper gastrointestinal adverse experiences in ACTONEL-treated patients (24.5%) was similar to that in placebo-treated patients (24.8%).

H_2 Blockers and Proton Pump Inhibitors (PPIs): Of over 5700 patients enrolled in the ACTONEL Phase 3 osteoporosis studies, 21% used H_2 blockers and/or PPIs. Among these patients, the incidence of upper gastrointestinal adverse experiences in the ACTONEL-treated patients was similar to that in placebo-treated patients.

Drug/Laboratory Test Interactions: Bisphosphonates are known to interfere with the use of bone-imaging agents. Specific studies with ACTONEL have not been performed.

Carcinogenesis, Mutagenesis, Impairment of Fertility:

Carcinogenesis: In a 104-week carcinogenicity study, rats were administered daily oral doses up to 24 mg/kg/day (approximately 7.7 times the maximum recommended human daily dose of 30 mg based on surface area, mg/m^2). There were no significant drug-induced tumor findings in male or female rats. The high dose male group of 24 mg/kg/day was terminated early in the study (Week 93) due to excessive toxicity, and data from this group were not included in the statistical evaluation of the study results. In an 80-week carcinogenicity study, mice were administered daily oral doses up to 32 mg/kg/day (approximately 6.4 times the 30 mg/day human dose based on surface area, mg/m^2). There were no significant drug-induced tumor findings in male or female mice.

Mutagenesis: Risedronate did not exhibit genetic toxicity in the following assays: *In vitro* bacterial mutagenesis in *Salmonella* and *E. coli* (Ames assay), mammalian cell mutagenesis in CHO/HGPRT assay, unscheduled DNA synthesis in rat hepatocytes and an assessment of chromosomal aberrations *in vivo* in rat bone marrow. Risedronate was positive in a chromosomal aberration assay in CHO cells at highly cytotoxic concentrations (> 675 mcg/mL, survival of 6% to 7%). When the assay was repeated at doses exhibiting appropriate cell survival (29%), there was no evidence of chromosomal damage.

Impairment of Fertility: In female rats, ovulation was inhibited at an oral dose of 16 mg/kg/day (approximately 5.2 times the 30 mg/day human dose based on surface area, mg/m^2). Decreased implantation was noted in female rats treated with doses ≥ 7 mg/kg/day (approximately 2.3 times the 30 mg/day human dose based on surface area, mg/m^2). In male rats, testicular and epididymal atrophy and inflammation were noted at 40 mg/kg/day (approximately 13 times the 30 mg/day human dose based on surface area, mg/m^2). Testicular atrophy was also noted in male rats after 13 weeks of treatment at oral doses of 16 mg/kg/day (approximately 5.2 times the 30 mg/day human dose based on surface area, mg/m^2). There was moderate-to-severe spermatid maturation block after 13 weeks in male dogs at an oral dose of 8 mg/kg/day (approximately 8 times the 30 mg/day human dose based on surface area, mg/m^2). These findings tended to increase in severity with increased dose and exposure time.

Pregnancy: Pregnancy Category C: Survival of neonates was decreased in rats treated during gestation with oral doses ≥ 16 mg/kg/day (approximately 5.2 times the 30 mg/day human dose based on surface area, mg/m^2). Body weight was decreased in neonates from dams treated with 80 mg/kg (approximately 26 times the 30 mg/day human dose based on surface area, mg/m^2). In rats treated during gestation, the number of fetuses exhibiting incomplete ossification of sternebrae or skull was statistically significantly increased at 7.1 mg/kg/day (approximately 2.3 times the 30 mg/day human dose based on surface area, mg/m^2). Both incomplete ossification and unossified sternebrae were increased in rats treated with oral doses ≥ 16 mg/kg/day (approximately 5.2 times the 30 mg/day human dose based on surface area, mg/m^2). A low incidence of cleft palate was observed in fetuses from female rats treated with oral doses ≥ 3.2 mg/kg/day (approximately 1 time the 30 mg/day human dose based on surface area, mg/m^2). The relevance of this finding to human use of ACTONEL is unclear. No significant fetal ossification effects were seen in rabbits treated with oral doses up to 10 mg/kg/day during gestation (approximately 6.7 times the 30 mg/day human dose based on surface area, mg/m^2). However, in rabbits treated with 10 mg/kg/day, 1 of 14 litters were aborted and 1 of 14 litters were delivered prematurely.

Similar to other bisphosphonates, treatment during mating and gestation with doses as low as 3.2 mg/kg/day (approximately 1 time the 30 mg/day human dose based on surface area, mg/m^2) has resulted in periparturient hypocalcemia and mortality in pregnant rats allowed to deliver.

There are no adequate and well-controlled studies of ACTONEL in pregnant women. ACTONEL should be used during pregnancy only if the potential benefit justifies the potential risk to the mother and fetus.

Nursing Women: Risedronate was detected in feeding pups exposed to lactating rats for a 24-hour period post-dosing, indicating a small degree of lacteal transfer. It is not known whether risedronate is excreted in human milk. Because many drugs are excreted in human milk and because of the potential for serious adverse reactions in nursing infants from bisphosphonates, a decision should be made whether to discontinue nursing or to discontinue the drug, taking into account the importance of the drug to the mother.

Pediatric Use: Safety and effectiveness in pediatric patients have not been established.

Geriatric Use: Of the patients receiving ACTONEL in postmenopausal osteoporosis studies (see CLINICAL STUDIES), 43% were between 65 and 75 years of age, and 20% were over 75. The corresponding proportions were 26% and 11% in glucocorticoid-induced osteoporosis trials, and 40% and 26% in Paget's disease trials. No overall differences in efficacy or safety were observed between these patients and younger patients.

Use in Men: Safety and effectiveness have been demonstrated in clinical studies in men receiving ACTONEL both for Paget's disease and for treatment and prevention of glucocorticoid-induced osteoporosis. However, the safety and effectiveness in men for osteoporosis due to other causes have not been established.

ADVERSE REACTIONS

Osteoporosis: ACTONEL has been studied in over 5700 patients enrolled in the Phase 3 glucocorticoid-induced osteoporosis clinical trials and in postmenopausal osteoporosis trials of up to 3 years duration. The overall adverse event profile of ACTONEL 5 mg in these studies was similar to that of placebo. Most adverse events were either mild or moderate and did not lead to discontinuation from the study. The incidence of serious adverse events in the placebo group was 24.9% and in the ACTONEL 5 mg group was 26.3%. The percentage of patients who withdrew from the study due to adverse events was 14.4% and 13.5% for the placebo and ACTONEL 5 mg groups, respectively. Table 1 lists adverse events from the Phase 3 osteoporosis trials reported in ≥ 2% of patients and in more ACTONEL-treated patients than placebo-treated patients. Adverse events are shown without attribution of causality.

Table 5
Adverse Events Occurring at a Frequency ≥ 2% and in More ACTONEL-Treated Patients than Placebo-Treated Patients Combined Phase 3 Osteoporosis Trials

Body System	Placebo % (N = 1914)	ACTONEL 5 mg % (N = 1916)
Body as a Whole		
Infection	29.7	29.9
Back Pain	23.6	26.1
Pain	13.1	13.6
Abdominal Pain	9.4	11.6
Neck Pain	4.5	5.3
Asthenia	4.3	5.1
Chest Pain	4.9	5.0
Neoplasm	3.0	3.3
Hernia	2.5	2.9
Cardiovascular		
Hypertension	9.0	10.0
Cardiovascular Disorder	1.7	2.5
Angina Pectoris	2.4	2.5
Digestive		
Nausea	10.7	10.9
Diarrhea	9.6	10.6
Flatulence	4.2	4.6
Gastritis	2.3	2.5
Gastrointestinal Disorder	2.1	2.3
Rectal Disorder	1.9	2.2
Tooth Disorder	2.0	2.1
Hemic and Lymphatic		
Ecchymosis	4.0	4.3
Anemia	1.9	2.4
Musculoskeletal		
Arthralgia	21.1	23.7
Joint Disorder	5.4	6.8
Myalgia	6.3	6.6
Bone Pain	4.3	4.6
Bone Disorder	3.2	4.0
Leg Cramps	2.6	3.5
Bursitis	2.9	3.0
Tendon Disorder	2.5	3.0
Nervous		
Depression	6.2	6.8
Dizziness	5.4	6.4
Insomnia	4.5	4.7
Anxiety	3.0	4.3
Neuralgia	3.5	3.8
Vertigo	3.2	3.3
Hypertonia	2.1	2.2
Paresthesia	1.8	2.1
Respiratory		
Pharyngitis	5.0	5.8
Rhinitis	5.0	5.7
Dyspnea	3.2	3.8
Pneumonia	2.6	3.1
Skin and Appendages		
Rash	7.2	7.7
Pruritus	2.2	3.0
Skin Carcinoma	1.8	2.0
Special Senses		
Cataract	5.4	5.9
Conjunctivitis	2.8	3.1
Otitis Media	2.4	2.5
Urogenital		
Urinary Tract Infection	9.7	10.9
Cystitis	3.5	4.1

Duodenitis and glossitis have been reported uncommonly (0.1% to 1%). There have been rare reports (< 0.1%) of abnormal liver function tests.

Laboratory Test Findings: Asymptomatic and small decreases were observed in serum calcium and phosphorus levels. Overall, mean decreases of 0.8% in serum calcium and of 2.7% in phosphorus were observed at 6 months in patients receiving ACTONEL. Throughout the Phase 3 studies, serum calcium levels below 8 mg/dL were observed in 18 patients, 9 (0.5%) in each treatment arm (ACTONEL and placebo). Serum phosphorus levels below 2 mg/dL were observed in 14 patients, 11 (0.6%) treated with ACTONEL and 3 (0.2%) treated with placebo.

Endoscopic Findings: ACTONEL clinical studies enrolled over 5700 patients, many with pre-existing gastrointestinal disease and concomitant use of NSAIDs or aspirin. Investigators were encouraged to perform endoscopies in any patients with moderate-to-severe gastrointestinal complaints while maintaining the blind. These endoscopies were ultimately performed on equal numbers of patients between the treated and placebo groups [75 (14.5%) placebo; 75 (11.9%) ACTONEL]. Across treatment groups, the percentage of patients with normal esophageal, gastric, and duodenal mucosa on endoscopy was similar (20% placebo, 21% ACTONEL). The number of patients who withdrew from the studies due to the event prompting endoscopy was similar across treatment groups. Positive findings on endoscopy were also generally comparable across treatment groups. There was a higher number of reports of mild duodenitis in the ACTONEL group, however there were more duodenal ulcers in the placebo group. Clinically important findings (perforations, ulcers, or bleeding) among this symptomatic population were similar between groups (51% placebo; 39% ACTONEL).

Paget's Disease: ACTONEL has been studied in 392 patients with Paget's disease of bone. As in trials of ACTONEL for other indications, the adverse experiences reported in the Paget's disease trials have generally been mild or moderate, have not required discontinuation of treatment, and have not appeared to be related to patient age, gender, or race.

In a double-blind, active-controlled study, the adverse event profile was similar for ACTONEL and Didronel: 6.6% (4/61) of patients treated with ACTONEL 30 mg/day for 2 months discontinued treatment due to adverse events, compared with 8.2% (5/61) of patients treated with Didronel 400 mg/day for 6 months.

Table 6
Adverse Events Reported in ≥ 2% of ACTONEL-Treated Patients* in Phase 3 Paget's Disease Trials

Body System	30 mg/day x 2 months ACTONEL % (N = 61)	400 mg/day x 6 months Didronel % (N = 61)
Body as a Whole		
Flu Syndrome	9.8	1.6
Chest Pain	6.6	3.3
Asthenia	4.9	0
Neoplasm	3.3	1.6
Gastrointestinal		
Diarrhea	19.7	14.8
Abdominal Pain	11.5	8.2
Nausea	9.8	9.8
Constipation	6.6	8.2
Belching	3.3	1.6
Colitis	3.3	3.3
Metabolic & Nutritional		
Peripheral Edema	8.2	6.6
Musculoskeletal		
Arthralgia	32.8	29.5
Bone Pain	4.9	4.9
Leg Cramps	3.3	3.3
Myasthenia	3.3	0
Nervous		
Headache	18.0	16.4
Dizziness	6.6	4.9
Respiratory		
Bronchitis	3.3	4.9
Sinusitis	4.9	1.6
Skin		
Rash	11.5	8.2
Special Senses		
Amblyopia	3.3	3.3
Tinnitus	3.3	3.3
Dry Eye	3.3	0

*Considered to be possibly or probably causally related in at least one patient

Three patients that received ACTONEL 30 mg/day experienced acute iritis in one supportive study. All three patients recovered from their events; however, in one of these patients, the event recurred during ACTONEL treatment and again during treatment with pamidronate. All patients were effectively treated with topical steroids.

OVERDOSAGE

Decreases in serum calcium and phosphorus following substantial overdose may be expected in some patients. Signs and symptoms of hypocalcemia may also occur in some of these patients. Milk or antacids containing calcium should be given to bind ACTONEL and reduce absorption of the drug.

In cases of substantial overdose, gastric lavage may be considered to remove unabsorbed drug. Standard procedures that are effective for treating hypocalcemia, including the administration of calcium intravenously, would be expected to restore physiologic amounts of ionized calcium and to relieve signs and symptoms of hypocalcemia.

Lethality after single oral doses was seen in female rats at 903 mg/kg and male rats at 1703 mg/kg. The minimum lethal dose in mice and rabbits was 4000 mg/kg and 1000 mg/kg. These values represent 320 to 620 times the 30-mg human dose based on surface area (mg/m^2).

DOSAGE AND ADMINISTRATION

ACTONEL should be taken once per day at least 30 minutes before the first food or drink of the day other than water.

To facilitate delivery to the stomach, ACTONEL should be swallowed while the patient is in an upright position and with a full glass of plain water (6 to 8 oz). Patients should not lie down for 30 minutes after taking the medication (see PRECAUTIONS, General).

Patients should receive supplemental calcium and vitamin D if dietary intake is inadequate (see PRECAUTIONS, General). Calcium supplements and calcium-, aluminum-, and magnesium-containing medications may interfere with the absorption of ACTONEL and should be taken at a different time of the day. ACTONEL is not recommended for use in patients with severe renal impairment (creatinine clearance < 30 mL/min). No dosage adjustment is necessary in patients with a creatinine clearance ≥ 30 mL/min or in the elderly.

Treatment and Prevention of Postmenopausal Osteoporosis/Glucocorticoid-Induced Osteoporosis (see INDICATIONS AND USAGE): The recommended regimen is 5 mg orally daily.

Paget's Disease (see INDICATIONS AND USAGE): The recommended treatment regimen is 30 mg once daily for 2 months. Retreatment may be considered (following post-treatment observation of at least 2 months) if relapse occurs, or if treatment fails to normalize serum alkaline phosphatase. For retreatment, the dose and duration of therapy are the same as for initial treatment. No data are available on more than one course of retreatment.

Store at controlled room temperature 20°-25°C (68°-77°F) [See USP].

Mfg. and Dist. by:
Procter & Gamble Pharmaceuticals, TM Owner
Cincinnati, Ohio 45202
Mkt. with:
Aventis Pharmaceuticals Inc.
(formerly Hoechst Marion Roussel, Inc.)
Kansas City, Missouri 64137
APRIL 2000

5 mg Actonel
(risedronate sodium tablets)

References: **1.** Actonel [package insert]. Cincinnati, Ohio: Procter & Gamble; 2000. **2.** Harris ST, Watts NB, Genant HK, et al. Effects of risedronate treatment on vertebral and nonvertebral fractures in women with postmenopausal osteoporosis: a randomized controlled trial. *JAMA.* 1999;282(14):1344-1352. **3.** Reginster J-Y, Minne HW, Sorensen OH, et al. Randomised trial of the effects of risedronate on vertebral fractures in women with established postmenopausal osteoporosis. *Osteoporos Int.* 2000;11:83-91. **4.** Data on file, Procter & Gamble, Cincinnati, Ohio.

Arthritis & Rheumatism

An Official Journal of the American College of Rheumatology
www.arthritisrheum.org and www.interscience.wiley.com

ARTHRITIS & RHEUMATISM (Print ISSN 0004-3591; Online ISSN 1529-0131 at Wiley InterScience, www.interscience.wiley.com) is published monthly, except semi-monthly in February, April, June, August, October, and December by Wiley-Liss, Inc., a division of John Wiley & Sons, Inc., 605 Third Avenue, New York, NY 10158-0012. **Send subscription inquiries to:** John Wiley & Sons, Inc., Subscription Department, 9th Floor, 605 Third Avenue, New York, NY 10158-0012, (212) 850-6645. **Advertising sales contact:** Susan Tagliaferro, Accounts Representative, Pharmaceutical Media, Inc., 30 East 33rd Street, New York, NY 10016, phone (212) 685-5010. **Offprint sales and inquiries** should be directed to the Customer Service Department, John Wiley and Sons, 605 Third Avenue, New York, NY 10158-0012, (212) 850-8776. For 2001, Volumes 44 and 45; institutional rate in U.S., $560; outside U.S., $720; personal subscription rate in U.S., $207; outside U.S., $249. (Subscriptions outside North America are sent by air.) Payment must be made in U.S. dollars drawn on a U.S. bank. **Change of Address:** Please forward to the subscriptions address listed above 6 weeks prior to move; enclose present mailing label with change of address. **Claims** for undelivered copies will be accepted only after the following issue has been received. Please enclose a copy of the mailing label or cite your subscriber reference number in order to expedite handling. Missing copies will be supplied when losses have been sustained in transit and where reserve stock permits. Send claims to John Wiley & Sons, Inc., Customer Service, 605 Third Avenue, New York, NY 10158-0012. If claims are not resolved satisfactorily, please write to Caroline Rothaug, Subscription Fulfillment and Sales, John Wiley & Sons, Inc., 605 Third Avenue, New York, NY 10158-0012. **Cancellations:** Subscription cancellations will not be accepted after the first issue has been mailed. Periodicals postage paid at New York, N.Y., and at additional mailing offices. Printed in U.S.A. Copyright © 2001 American College of Rheumatology. POSTMASTER: Send address changes to Arthritis & Rheumatism, Subscription Systems and Distribution, John Wiley & Sons, Inc., 605 Third Avenue, New York, NY 10158-0012.

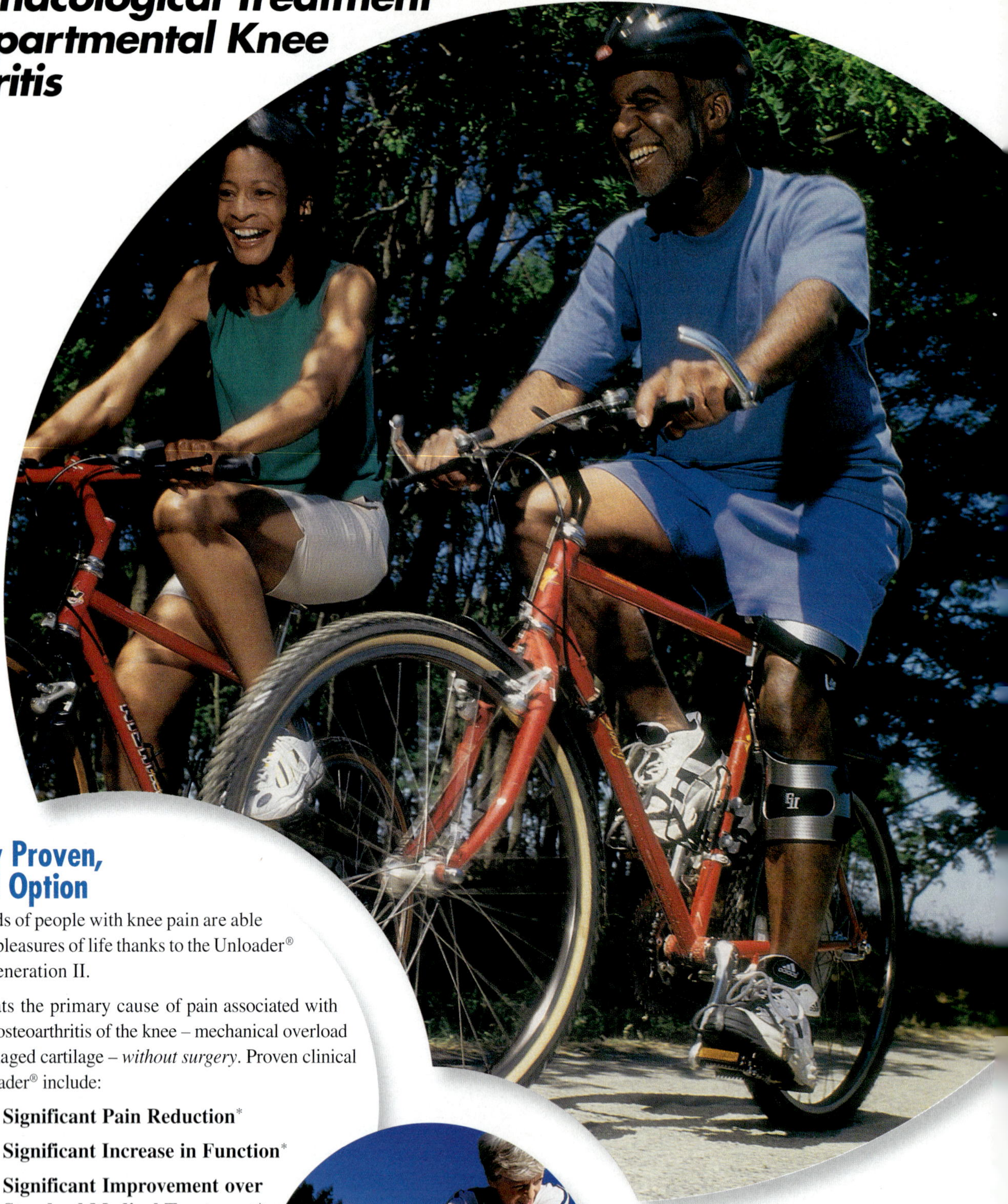

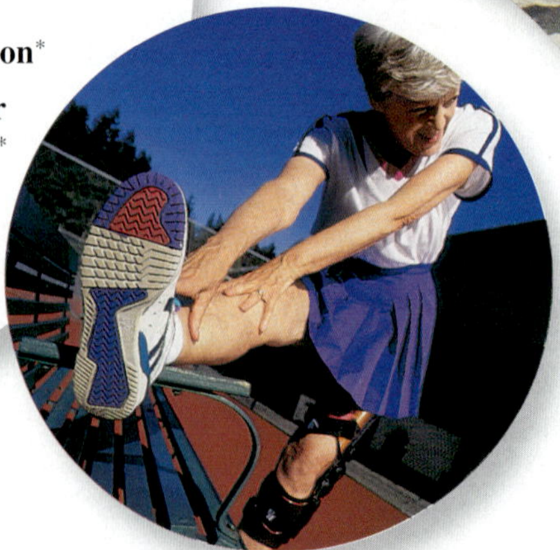

Arthritis & Rheumatism

An Official Journal of the American College of Rheumatology
www.arthritisrheum.org and www.interscience.wiley.com

VOLUME 44 **FEBRUARY 2001** **NO. 2**

Special Articles

ACR Presidential Address: The Future Is Now
Joseph D. Croft, Jr. 247

Review: The Role of Osteoprotegerin and Receptor Activator of Nuclear Factor κB Ligand in the Pathogenesis and Treatment of Rheumatoid Arthritis
Lorenz C. Hofbauer and Armin E. Heufelder 253

Rheumatoid Arthritis

Involvement of ErbB-2 in Rheumatoid Synovial Cell Growth
Koichiro Satoh, Shinichi Kikuchi, Masayuki Sekimata, Yukihito Kabuyama, Miwako K. Homma, and Yoshimi Homma 260

Overexpression of Transcription Factor Ets-1 in Rheumatoid Arthritis Synovial Membrane: Regulation of Expression and Activation by Interleukin-1 and Tumor Necrosis Factor α
Kurt Redlich, Hans P. Kiener, Georg Schett, Makiyeh Tohidast-Akrad, Edgar Selzer, Irene Radda, Georg H. Stummvoll, Carl W. Steiner, Marion Gröger, Peter Bitzan, Peter Zenz, Josef S. Smolen, and Günter Steiner 266

Interferon-γ–Inducing Activity of Interleukin-18 in the Joint With Rheumatoid Arthritis
Masahiro Yamamura, Masanori Kawashima, Madoka Taniai, Hiroshi Yamauchi, Tadao Tanimoto, Masashi Kurimoto, Yoshitaka Morita, Yasukazu Ohmoto, and Hirofumi Makino 275

Tumor Necrosis Factor Markers Show Sex-Influenced Association With Rheumatoid Arthritis
Joanne M. Meyer, Jinfeng Han, and George Moxley 286

Recognition of Cell Surface GD3 by Monoclonal Antibody Anti-6C2 in Rheumatoid Arthritis Synovial Fluid: Expression on Human T Cells With Transendothelial Migratory Activity
Toshio Homma, Osamu Hosono, Satoshi Iwata, Susumu Ando, Katsutoshi Sasaki, Tatsunari Nishi, Hiroshi Kawasaki, Hirotoshi Tanaka, and Chikao Morimoto 296

Rheumatoid Arthritis in Southern Spain: Toward Elucidation of a Unifying Role of the HLA Class II Region in Disease Predisposition
M. Pascual, A. Nieto, M. A. López-Nevot, L. Ramal, L. Matarán, A. Caballero, A. Alonso, J. Martín, and E. Zanelli 307

HLA Haplotype Analysis in Finnish Patients With Rheumatoid Arthritis
Juha Tuokko, Sergei Nejentsev, Reijo Luukkainen, Auli Toivanen, and Jorma Ilonen 315

The Association of Cigarette Smoking With Disease Outcome in Patients With Early Inflammatory Polyarthritis
Beverley J. Harrison, Alan J. Silman, Nicola J. Wiles, David G. I. Scott, and Deborah P. M. Symmons 323

Correlation of Power Doppler Sonography With Vascularity of the Synovial Tissue of the Knee Joint in Patients With Osteoarthritis and Rheumatoid Arthritis
Markus Walther, Harry Harms, Veit Krenn, Stephan Radke, Trutz-Peter Faehndrich, and Frank Gohlke 331

Development of Fulminant Hepatitis B (Precore Variant Mutant Type) After the Discontinuation of Low-Dose Methotrexate Therapy in a Rheumatoid Arthritis Patient
Satoshi Ito, Kiyoshi Nakazono, Akira Murasawa, Yusaku Mita, Kojiro Hata, Noriko Saito, Masatoshi Kikuchi, Kazukiyo Yoshida, Masaaki Nakano, and Fumitake Gejyo 339

Osteoarthritis and Cartilage

Effects of Intraarticular Glucocorticoids on Macrophage Infiltration and Mediators of Joint Damage in Osteoarthritis Synovial Membranes: Findings in a Double-Blind, Placebo-Controlled Study
Laurel Young, Amel Katrib, Carolyn Cuello, Ute Vollmer-Conna, James V. Bertouch, Peter J. Roberts-Thomson, Michael J. Ahern, Malcolm D. Smith, and Peter P. Youssef 343

Interleukin-1β Down-Regulates the Expression of Glucuronosyltransferase I, a Key Enzyme Priming Glycosaminoglycan Biosynthesis: Influence of Glucosamine on Interleukin-1β–Mediated Effects in Rat Chondrocytes
Jean-Noel Gouze, Karim Bordji, Sandrine Gulberti, Bernard Terlain, Patrick Netter, Jacques Magdalou, Sylvie Fournel-Gigleux, and Mohamed Ouzzine 351

Systemic Lupus Erythematosus and Autoimmunity

Low-Binding Alleles of Fcγ Receptor Types IIA and IIIA Are Inherited Independently and Are Associated With Systemic Lupus Erythematosus in Hispanic Patients
Ricardo Zuñiga, Sonia Ng, Margaret G. E. Peterson, John D. Reveille, Bruce A. Baethge, Graciela S. Alarcón, and Jane E. Salmon 361

The Appearance of U1 RNP Antibody Specificities in Sequential Autoimmune Human Antisera Follows a Characteristic Order That Implicates the U1–70 kd and B′/B Proteins as Predominant U1 RNP Immunogens
Eric L. Greidinger and Robert W. Hoffman 368

Anti–Topoisomerase I (Anti–Scl-70) Antibodies in Patients With Systemic Lupus Erythematosus
Hélène A. Elicha Gussin, Georghe P. Ignat, John Varga, and Marius Teodorescu 376

Detection of Autoantibodies to Killer Immunoglobulin-Like Receptors Using Recombinant Fusion Proteins for Two Killer Immunoglobulin-Like Receptors in Patients With Systemic Autoimmune Diseases
Toshihiro Matsui, Masataka Otsuka, Katsumi Maenaka, Hiroshi Furukawa, Toshio Yabe, Kazuhiko Yamamoto, Kusuki Nishioka, and Tomohiro Kato 384

The DNA Mismatch Repair Enzyme PMS1 Is a Myositis-Specific Autoantigen
Livia A. Casciola-Rosen, Ann F. Pluta, Paul H. Plotz, Amy E. Cox, Steven Morris, Fredrick M. Wigley, Michelle Petri, Allan C. Gelber, and Antony Rosen 389

Decreased Ras–Mitogen-Activated Protein Kinase Signaling May Cause DNA Hypomethylation in T Lymphocytes From Lupus Patients
Chun Deng, Mariana J. Kaplan, Jun Yang, Donna Ray, Zhiyong Zhang, W. Joseph McCune, Samir M. Hanash, and Bruce C. Richardson 397

"Lymphoid" Chemokine Messenger RNA Expression by Epithelial Cells in the Chronic Inflammatory Lesion of the Salivary Glands of Sjögren's Syndrome Patients: Possible Participation in Lymphoid Structure Formation
Georgina Xanthou, Mary Polihronis, Athanasios G. Tzioufas, Spyros Paikos, Paschalis Sideras, and Haralampos M. Moutsopoulos 408

Alteration of Peripheral Blood Dendritic Cells in Patients With Primary Sjögren's Syndrome
Yoshio Ozaki, Ryuichi Amakawa, Tomoki Ito, Hiroshi Iwai, Kenichirou Tajima, Kazutaka Uehira, Hideo Kagawa, Yoshiko Uemura, Toshio Yamashita, and Shirou Fukuhara 419

Mechanisms of Disease: Models and Genetics

Treatment With a Consensus Peptide Based on Amino Acid Sequences in Autoantibodies Prevents T Cell Activation by Autoantigens and Delays Disease Onset in Murine Lupus
Bevra H. Hahn, Ram R. Singh, Weng Kee Wong, Betty P. Tsao, Ken Bulpitt, and Fanny M. Ebling 432

Molecular and Cellular Mediators of Interleukin-1–Dependent Acute Inflammatory Arthritis
Kate E. Lawlor, Ian K. Campbell, Kristy O'Donnell, Li Wu, and Ian P. Wicks 442

Increased Production of Intracellular Interleukin-1 Receptor Antagonist Type I in the Synovium of Mice With Collagen-Induced Arthritis: A Possible Role in the Resolution of Arthritis
Cem Gabay, Liliana Marinova-Mutafchieva, Richard O. Williams, Jason P. Gigley, Debra M. Butler, Marc Feldmann, and William P. Arend 451

Vasculitis

Antineutrophil Cytoplasmic Antibodies Reacting With the Pro Form of Proteinase 3 and Disease Activity in Patients With Wegener's Granulomatosis and Microscopic Polyangiitis
Kimberly A. Russell, David N. Fass, and Ulrich Specks 463

Elevated Interleukin-4 and Interleukin-13 Production by T Cell Lines From Patients With Churg-Strauss Syndrome
M. Kiene, E. Csernok, A. Müller, C. Metzler, A. Trabandt, and W. L. Gross 469

Systemic Sclerosis

Blockade of Endogenous Transforming Growth Factor β Signaling Prevents Up-Regulated Collagen Synthesis in Scleroderma Fibroblasts: Association With Increased Expression of Transforming Growth Factor β Receptors
Hironobu Ihn, Kenichi Yamane, Masahide Kubo, and Kunihiko Tamaki 474

Epidemiology, Outcomes, and Treatment

Widespread Pain Among 11-Year-Old Finnish Twin Pairs
Marja Mikkelsson, Jaakko Kaprio, Jouko J. Salminen, Lea Pulkkinen, and Richard J. Rose 481

Concise Communications

Synovial Stimulatory Protein Fragments Copurify With Woodchuck Hepatitis Virus: Implications for the Etiology of Arthritis in Chronic Hepatitis B Virus Infection
Anand Mehta, Xuanyong Lu, Timothy Block, Anthony Willis, Raymond Dwek, Bud Tennant, and Baruch Blumberg 486

The Rate of Recurrence of Isolated Congenital Heart Block: A Population-Based Study
Heiki Julkunen and Marianne Eronen 487
Lupus Band Test Yields Negative Results in Primary Antiphospholipid Syndrome
Jean-Charles Piette, Eduardo Marinho, Du Le Thi Huong, Zahir Amoura, and Camille Francès 488
Letters
Monoclonal Expansion of B Cells in Sjögren's Syndrome: Comment on the Article by Martin et al
M. Voulgarelis, A. G. Tzioufas, and H. M. Moutsopoulos 490
Reply
Thierry Martin and Jean-Louis Pasquali 490
Is the Anti–Topoisomerase I Autoantibody Response Associated With a Distinct Amino Acid Sequence in the HLA–DQβ1 Domain?
Ayako Ueki, Yumika Isozaki, Akiko Tomokuni, Takemi Otsuki, Fuminori Hydoh, Haruko Sakaguchi, Shinichiro Tanaka, and Masayasu Kusaka 491
Clinical Image
Arthritis Induced by South American Blastomycosis 492
Morton A. Scheinberg and Moises Cohen
ACR Announcements 19A

Cover image: The figure on the cover (from Walther et al, page 333) illustrates the appearance of a knee joint of a patient with rheumatoid arthritis as visualized by power Doppler sonography (PDS). Vascularity of the synovium can be assessed from the extent of red and yellow coloration. PDS is one of the powerful new technologies to assess synovitis by noninvasive means.

Erosion in rheumatoid arthritis

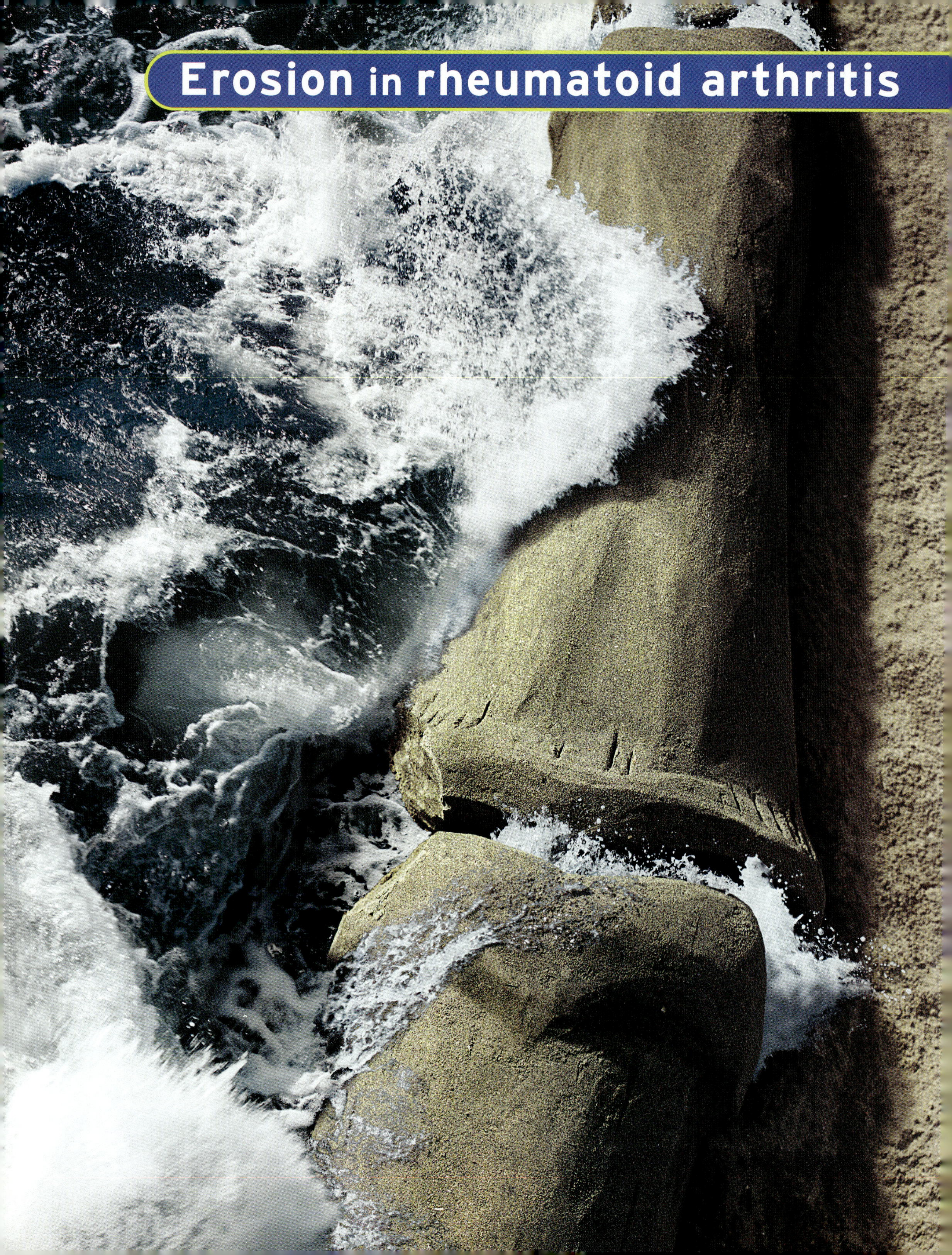

The critical role of IL-1

The pathogenesis of RA is a complex process that leads to joint inflammation and bone erosion. It's known to include several interdependent and variable interactions between pro-inflammatory and anti-inflammatory mechanisms.[1,2] Cytokines have been found to play a key role in promoting this disease process. The two pivotal cytokines in the pathogenesis of RA are interleukin-1 (IL-1) and tumor necrosis factor-alpha (TNF-α).[3,4]

IL-1 has been implicated in a destructive tide of events

In the RA disease process, IL-1 and TNF-α act synergistically to induce other cytokines and COX-2. Moreover, TNF-α induces IL-1,[5] IL-1 induces TNF-α,[6] and IL-1 induces IL-1.[7] This activity increases the production of PGE_2 and other arachidonic acid metabolites from synoviocytes[8,9] and accounts for much of the pain and swelling associated with RA.[10]

IL-1 is involved in many facets of the RA disease process. Pro-inflammatory cytokines cause neutrophils, monocytes, and lymphocytes to migrate to the synovium. In immunohistologic studies of macrophages accumulating in the synovial tissue, IL-1 production has been demonstrated in the cartilage-pannus junction as well as in the lining and sublining layers.[11,12]

Once in the synovium, neutrophils are activated and release mediators that stimulate mononuclear leukocytes, synoviocytes, and chondrocytes. These cells release IL-1 (more specifically, IL-1β) and other pro- and anti-inflammatory cytokines.[3,8,10]

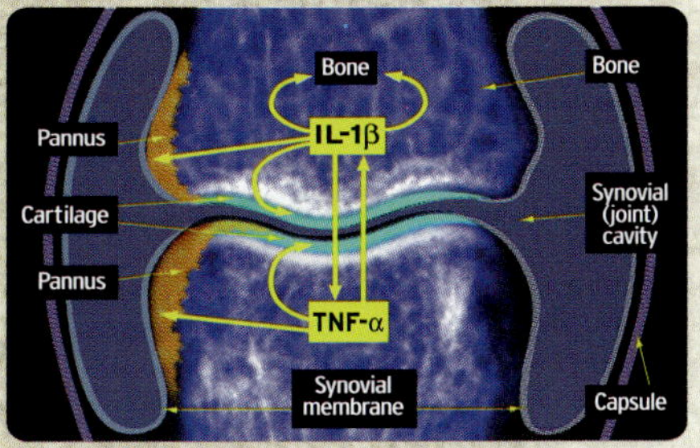

Then, once IL-1 and TNF-α are present, other interleukins (IL-6, IL-8, and IL-10) stimulate local fibroblast proliferation and recruit leukocytes. Although inflamed synovial cells express TNF-α, it is secreted to a far lesser extent than IL-1.[4,13] Early in the RA disease process, IL-1 causes cartilage degradation by inducing rapid loss of proteoglycans and stimulating the production of neutral proteinases in chondrocytes.[1,14] Since IL-1 also stimulates osteoclasts, bone resorption occurs.[15]

Higher levels of IL-1 seen with bone erosion

Animal studies, preclinical research, and early clinical studies all support the dominant role that IL-1 plays in cartilage damage and bone resorption, and suggest that TNF-α is more responsible for the inflammation in RA.[4,14,15]

In animal studies, joint swelling and cartilage damage are still present in TNF-α knockout mice (which cannot produce TNF-α), while there is an impressive reduction of cartilage damage, bone erosion, and chronic synovial infiltration in IL-1–deficient mice.[4]

These findings are supported by clinical evidence that patients with RA who have bone erosions also have higher IL-1 levels in their synovial fluid than RA patients who do not have bone erosions. Together, these findings point to the primary role of IL-1 in the bone and cartilage erosion seen in RA.[16]

The IL-1 gene family consists of IL-1α, IL-1β, and IL-1 receptor antagonist (IL-1Ra), which is the naturally occurring cytokine antagonist that normally balances the destructive effects of IL-1α and IL-1β in rheumatoid arthritis.[17] However, in RA, production of IL-1 cannot be sufficiently countered by endogenous IL-1Ra alone; this leads to the damaging bone and cartilage effects seen in rheumatoid joints.[17]

Amgen is conducting research in the area of rheumatology to develop new and important therapies.

AMGEN®

Advancing the science of rheumatology

References

1. Cush JJ, Lipsky PE. Cellular basis for rheumatoid inflammation. *Clin Orthop.* 1991;265:9-22.
2. Arend WP. Interleukin-1 receptor antagonist. *Adv Immunol.* 1993;54:167-227.
3. Buchan G, Barrett K, Turner M, Chantry D, Maini RN, Feldmann M. Interleukin-1 and tumour necrosis factor mRNA expression in rheumatoid arthritis: prolonged production of IL-1α. *Clin Exp Immunol.* 1998; 73:449-455.
4. van den Berg WB. Joint inflammation and cartilage destruction may occur uncoupled. *Springer Semin Immunopathol.* 1998;20:149-164.
5. Dinarello CA, Cannon JG, Wolff SM, et al. Tumor necrosis factor (cachectin) is an endogenous pyrogen and induces production of interleukin 1. *J Exp Med.* 1986; 163(6): 1433-1450.
6. Philip R, Epstein LB. Tumour necrosis factor as immuno-modulator and mediator of monocyte cytotoxicity induced by itself, γ-interferon and interleukin-1. *Nature.* 1986;323(6083):86-89.
7. Dinarello CA, Ikejima T, Warner SJC, et al. Interleukin 1 induces interleukin 1, I: induction of circulating interleukin 1 in rabbits in vivo and in human mononuclear cells in vitro. *J Immunol.* 1987;139(6):1902-1910.
8. Koch AE, Kunkel SL, Strieter RM. Cytokines in rheumatoid arthritis. *J Invest Med.* 1995;43:28-38.
9. Crofford LJ, Wilder RL, Ristimake AP. Cyclooxygenase-1 and -2 expression in rheumatoid synovial tissues: effects of interleukin-1β, phorbol ester, and corticosteroids. *J Clin Invest.* 1994;93(3):1095-1101.
10. Harris ED Jr. Rheumatoid arthritis: pathophysiology and implications for therapy. *New Engl J Med.* 1990;322:1277-1289.
11. Chu CQ, Field M, Allard S, Abney E, Feldmann M, Maini RN. Detection of cytokines at the cartilage/pannus junction in patients with rheumatoid arthritis: implications for the role of cytokines in cartilage destruction and repair. *Br J Rheumatol.* 1992;31(10):653-661.
12. Wood NC, Dickens E, Symons JA, Duff GW. In situ hybridization of interleukin-1 in CD14-positive cells in rheumatoid arthritis. *Clin Immunol Immunopathol.* 1992; 62(3):295-300.
13. van den Berg WB, Joosten LAB, van de Loo FAJ. TNFα and IL-1β are separate targets in chronic arthritis. *Clin Exp Rheumatol.* 1999;17(suppl 18):S105-S114.
14. van Lent PLEM, van de Loo FAJ, Astrid EM, et al. Major role for interleukin 1 but not for tumor necrosis factor in early cartilage damage in immune complex arthritis in mice. *J Rheumatol.* 1995;22:2250-2258.
15. Dinarello CA, Moldawer LL. *Proinflammatory and Anti-inflammatory Cytokines in Rheumatoid Arthritis: A Primer for Clinicians.* Thousand Oaks, Calif: Amgen Inc.; 1999:34.
16. Eastgate JA, Symons JA, Wood NC, Grinlinton FM, di Giovine FS, Duff GW. Correlation of plasma interleukin 1 levels with disease activity in rheumatoid arthritis. *Lancet.* 1988;2:706-709.
17. Arend WP, Malyak M, Guthridge CJ, Gabay C. Interleukin-1 receptor antagonist: role in biology. *Annu Rev Immunol.* 1998;16:27-55.

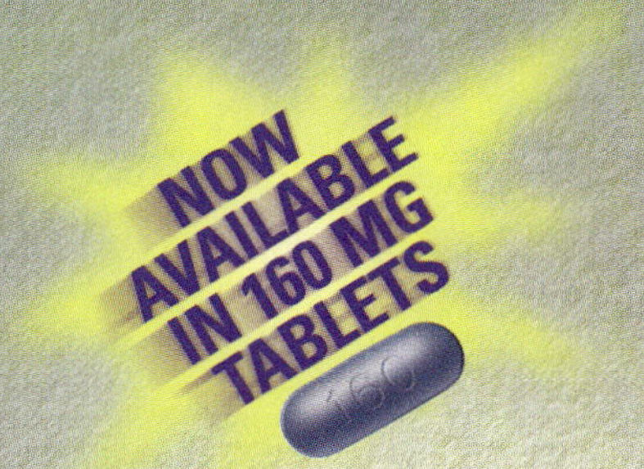

OxyContin 160 mg Tablets for use only in opioid-tolerant patients

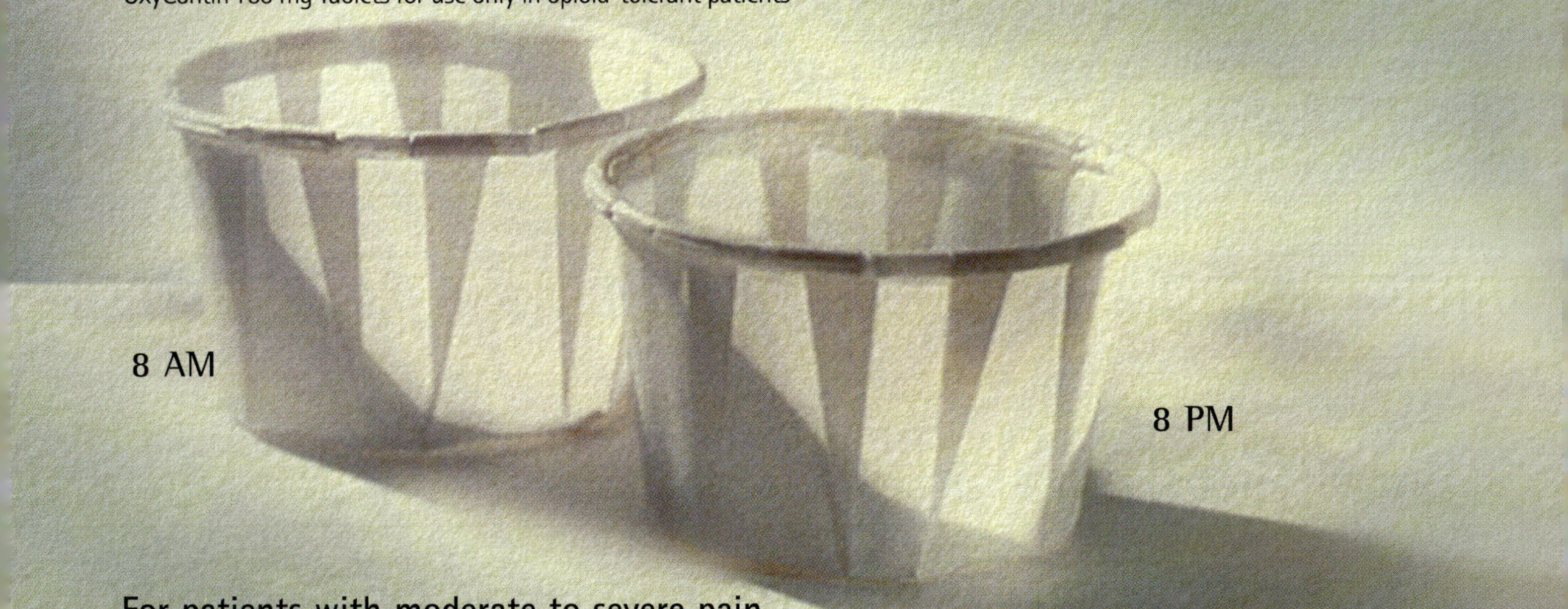

For patients with moderate to severe pain requiring opioid therapy for more than a few days

Q12h

OxyContin® CII

(OXYCODONE HCl CONTROLLED-RELEASE) TABLETS

10 10mg · 20 20mg · 40 40mg · 80 80mg · 160 160mg

Small, color coded tablets (actual size)

OxyContin 80 and 160 mg Tablets for use only in opioid-tolerant patients requiring daily oxycodone equivalent dosages of 160 mg and 320 mg respectively.

OxyContin® Tablets are to be swallowed whole, and are not to be broken, chewed or crushed. Taking broken, chewed or crushed OxyContin Tablets could lead to the rapid release and absorption of a potentially toxic dose of oxycodone.

One OxyContin 160 mg Tablet is comparable to two 80 mg tablets when taken on an empty stomach. With a high fat meal, however, there is a 25% greater peak plasma concentration following one 160 mg tablet. Dietary caution should be taken when patients are initially titrated to 160 mg tablets.

The most serious risk associated with opioids, including OxyContin, is respiratory depression.

Common opioid side effects are constipation, nausea, sedation, dizziness, vomiting, pruritus, headache, dry mouth, sweating and weakness.

OxyContin is contraindicated in patients with known hypersensitivity to oxycodone, or in any situation where opioids are contraindicated. **(Please see Contraindications section in package insert.)**

For more information about pain management and prevention, visit our Web site: **www.partnersagainstpain.com**

Please read attached professional prescribing information.

Co-promoted by Purdue Pharma L.P. and Abbott Laboratories

PURDUE

A6571

PUR-4000665

Notes to Contributors

(Note: the information that follows is also available online at www.arthritisrheum.org and www.interscience.wiley.com)

Manuscripts for publication, letters, news, and notes should be sent to:
David S. Pisetsky, MD, PhD, Editor, *Arthritis & Rheumatism*
2400 Pratt Street, Room 0311 Terrace Level
Duke University Medical Center Box 3806
Durham, NC 27710
phone (919) 668-0488, fax (919) 668-0744, e-mail jennifer.deyton@duke.edu

Articles are accepted for publication on the condition that they are submitted to this journal only. Articles should definitely pertain to the field of rheumatic disease.

Manuscripts not in compliance with the following instructions may be subject to a delay in the review process.

Format and organization

_____ Submit 5 copies of the manuscript, including tables and figures. For figures that are charts, graphs, or other line art that retains its readability when photocopied, the figures should be sent in the form of 1 photocopy attached to each copy of the manuscript, plus 1 high-quality original that will be used for printing if the manuscript is accepted. For radiographs, micrographs, and other halftone photographs, 5 high-quality glossy prints (not photocopies) should be sent (see Illustrations section below).

_____ A cover letter with the corresponding author's signature should accompany the manuscript. Note in cover letter what type of manuscript is enclosed (Full-Length Article, Brief Report, Case Report, Concise Communication, or Letter to the Editor). Confirm that the manuscript has not been submitted or is not simultaneously being submitted elsewhere for either print or electronic publication, and that no portion of the data has been or will be published, in print or electronic form, in proceedings or transactions of meetings or symposium volumes. The publication of data in abstracts, and presentation in oral or poster sessions at meetings, do not constitute previous publication. Indicate any financial support or other benefits from commercial sources for the work reported on in the manuscript, or any other financial interests that any of the authors may have, which could create a potential conflict of interest or the appearance of a conflict of interest with regard to the work. Corresponding author should include address, telephone number, fax number, and E-mail address if applicable.

_____ Type the manuscript in standard 12-point type on 8½ × 11″ paper with 1″ margins, double spaced throughout, including references, tables, and figure legends.

_____ Number all sheets in succession, including references, tables, and figure legends. Title page is page 1.

_____ On the first page, type the title, name(s) of the author(s) and their major degrees, grant supporter(s), address for reprint requests, and corresponding author's telephone and fax numbers and E-mail address.

Full-Length Articles and Brief Reports

Definition: Full-Length Articles are descriptions of original research that add to the body of knowledge in arthritis and the rheumatic diseases. Brief Reports are short papers of investigations into disease mechanisms, reports of clinical experience, therapeutic trials, or research and/or clinical contributions to diagnosis, treatment, etiopathology, and epidemiology of rheumatic diseases.

_____ On the second page of Full-Length Articles and Brief Reports, include an abstract of less than 250 words. The abstract should be divided into the following sections: Objective, Methods, Results, and Conclusion.

_____ On the third page, begin the introduction (no heading is necessary).

_____ Follow this plan of organization: Materials and Methods (or Patients and Methods), Results, Discussion, References, Tables, and Figure Legends.

_____ Full-Length Articles should not exceed 15 typed manuscript pages from introduction through discussion (not including references, tables, and figure legends).

_____ Brief Reports should not exceed 9 manuscript pages from introduction through references, and should contain no more than 3 tables and/or figures and no more than 15 references.

Case Reports

Definition: Case Reports are reports of single cases that contribute to the body of knowledge of rheumatic diseases by reporting in-depth observations and/or laboratory investigations that may reveal etiopathogenetic mechanisms of a broader significance, or by presenting a concise discussion of an infrequently encountered problem that emphasizes a particular clinical point not generally available in the literature. Emphasis will be placed on the scholarship of discussion.

_____ On the second page of Case Reports, include an abstract of less than 150 words. The abstract should not be divided into sections as required for Full-Length Articles and Brief Reports.

_____ On the third page, begin the introduction (no heading is necessary).

_____ After the introduction, include a description of the case, followed by a general discussion.

_____ Case Reports should not exceed 9 manuscript pages from introduction through references, and should contain no more than 3 tables and/or figures and no more than 15 references.

Radiologic/Dermatologic Vignettes and Clinical Images

_____ Radiologic Vignettes are short articles describing cases with interesting and significant radiologic features. The Vignette should present a case description with clinical findings, radiologic findings, differential diagnosis, final diagnosis, and discussion. No abstract is necessary. Page length should be less than that for a Brief Report or Case Report; up to 3 figures may be included. Dermatologic Vignettes describe cases with interesting and significant dermatologic features and should have a format similar to that of Radiologic Vignettes.

_____ Clinical Images are photographic depictions (clinical, radiologic, or pathologic) of interesting rheumatologic phenomena. The image and accompanying caption should be short enough to fit on half a page of the journal (i.e., no more than one half page of double-spaced typewritten text, with the image preferably oriented horizontally). All images must be in black and white. There is no page charge for Clinical Images.

Letters to the Editor/Concise Communications

Definitions: Letters to the Editor should be limited to commentaries on previous articles published in *Arthritis & Rheumatism* and issues affecting rheumatology and the American College of Rheumatology. Concise Communications should be very short reports of cases or research findings, with no abstract, subheads, or acknowledgments section.

_____ Letters to the Editor and Concise Communications should be double spaced throughout.

_____ Length of Letters to the Editor and Concise Communications should be no more than 4 pages, including references.

_____ Only 1 table or figure may accompany a Letter to the Editor or Concise Communication.

Content

_____ Do not use new technical words, laboratory slang, words not defined in dictionaries, or abbreviations or terminology not consistent with internationally accepted guidelines.

_____ Define any abbreviations the first time they are used. A list of standard abbreviations appears on pages 1903–1905 of the November 1998 issue.

______ In order to make the description of patients as clear as possible and to facilitate comparisons with other studies, the Methods section should include, whenever possible, a short paragraph detailing the proportion of patients who satisfy the ACR classification criteria for the particular disease described.

Compliance with research ethics standards

______ For articles reporting prospective research involving human or animal subjects, note in the Methods section that the study has been approved by the appropriate institutional review board or, if there is not an institutional review board or comparable formal ethics review committee, that the Declaration of Helsinki principles have been followed.

Illustrations

______ For illustrations that are photographs (as opposed to line art), send 5 packaged sets in labeled envelopes. For line art that reproduces well on a photocopier, include 1 copy with each copy of the manuscript, and also send 1 high-quality original to be used for printing.

______ Do not write on the back of any figure, but attach a label to each with the figure number and first author's name. Include on the label an arrow indicating which end is the top of the figure.

______ Lettering and symbols on figures should be large enough, and shading distinct enough, to remain readable after figure size is reduced to one column width.

______ Do not attach illustrations to the manuscript with a paperclip.

______ Obtain releases from any patients whose pictures will be printed in the journal. Blinders on the eyes are not a substitute for patient's permission.

______ Radiographs, micrographs, other halftones, and linecuts should be no more than 3¼″ square.

______ Color figures: Authors are entitled to one free page of color. Additional are billed to the author at the special reduced rate of $500 per page. All color figures will be reproduced in full color in the online edition of the journal at no cost to authors. Authors are encouraged to submit color illustrations that highlight the text and convey essential scientific information. For best reproduction, bright, clear colors should be used. Dark colors against a dark background do not reproduce well; please place your color images against a white background whenever possible. Please contact Jennifer Nowak at [jnowak@wiley.com] for further information.

Tables

______ Refer to current issues of the Journal for table style.

______ Provide each table with an explanatory title so that it is intelligible without specific reference to the text.

______ Provide each table column with an appropriate heading.

______ Indicate clearly any units of measure on a table.

References

______ Limit the length of the reference list by using only key references.

______ Double space references.

______ Compile references numerically according to the order of the citation.

______ Use abbreviations for titles of medical periodicals that conform to those in *Index Medicus*.

______ In 1997, the Journal changed its reference style to conform to the style suggested in the Uniform Requirements for Manuscripts Submitted to Biomedical Journals. All new submissions should use the new reference style, which can be found in the article "Uniform Requirements for Manuscripts Submitted to Biomedical Journals" (N Engl J Med, January 23, 1997, pp 309–15).

Assignment of reviewers

______ Authors are asked to suggest potential reviewers of their manuscript. If there are individuals they would prefer not to review their manuscript, they may also so indicate.

Related manuscripts/Duplicate publication

______ If the authors are aware of any related manuscript that has been or will be published by or submitted to another journal or to *Arthritis & Rheumatism* (e.g., another manuscript resulting from the same study), a copy of the other manuscript should be sent along with the one that is being submitted for publication in *Arthritis & Rheumatism*.

______ Articles are received only for exclusive publication in *Arthritis & Rheumatism* with the understanding that they have not been published elsewhere (in part or in full, in other words or in the same words, in letter or article form, in print or electronic form, or otherwise), are not at the time of submission under consideration by another journal or other publication, and will not be submitted elsewhere unless rejected by *Arthritis & Rheumatism.* If an author violates this requirement or engages in other similar misconduct, the Editor may, in addition to rejecting the manuscript, impose a moratorium on the acceptance of new manuscripts from the author and, if the misconduct is deemed sufficiently serious, may refer the matter to the author's academic institution or hospital and/or the appropriate state or local disciplinary body.

Disclosure of interest

______ The American College of Rheumatology's Board of Directors officially adopted Conflict of Interest Guidelines for *Arthritis & Rheumatism* on July 7, 1995. These guidelines, as they relate to authors, are as follows.

______ A cover letter to the Editor accompanying a submitted manuscript must disclose information about financial support and consulting activities, for *all* authors, that might be interpreted as constituting a possible conflict of interest for the described studies.

______ *All* authors of manuscripts (basic or clinical research, case reports, letters, reviews, editorials or commentary) accepted for publication will be asked to sign a full disclosure form regarding possible conflicts of interest for that individual, any member of his/her immediate family, or any other individual or entity with whom the author has a significant relationship, including: (a) ownership or control of stock in a company developing or distributing a product studied or discussed in the manuscript, or a competing product; (b) service as a consultant or advisor to a company developing or distributing a product studied or discussed in the manuscript, or a competing product; (c) the existence of any patent/license/royalty arrangements for any material studied or discussed in the manuscript; (d) any other possible financial benefit, such as derived income from a diagnostic test or product described or discussed in the manuscript, or frequent legal work as an expert witness or consultant in cases related to the content of the manuscript.

______ The Editor and Associate Editors will decide whether any of this information constitutes a possible conflict of interest, or the appearance thereof, and should be divulged in a footnote.

Publication procedures

______ In accordance with the 1978 Copyright Law, authors are requested to sign a provisional copyright transfer statement at the time manuscript revisions are requested.

______ Contributors are provided with page proofs and asked to check for errors and for editorial queries. Although the correction of editorial and typographical errors will be made without charge, the cost of excessive additional alterations may be charged to the author.

______ Authors are requested to return one set of proofs, the original manuscript and illustrations, and the reprint order within 48 hours. Publication of the article may be delayed if the proofs are not sent back on time.

Page charge

______ A $70 per page charge will be assessed for publication in *Arthritis & Rheumatism*. Instructions for payment will be sent to authors along with the proofs. In extreme cases of inability to pay, the page charge may be reduced or waived. There is no page charge for solicited articles, letters to the editor, or book reviews. Questions regarding the page charge should be directed to the Managing Editor, *Arthritis & Rheumatism*, 1800 Century Place, Suite 250, Atlanta, GA 30345-4300.

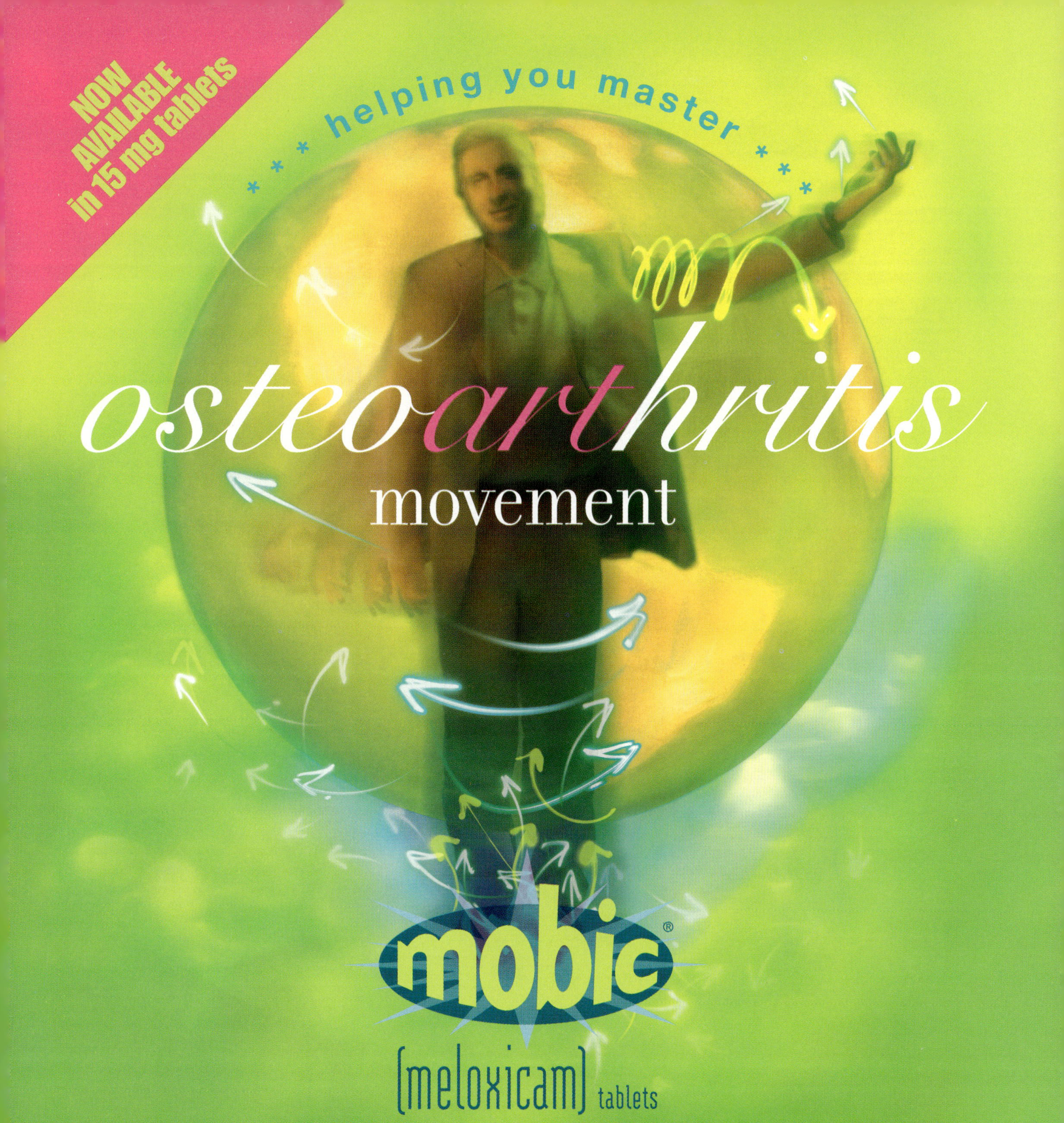

For relief of the signs and symptoms of osteoarthritis

7.5 mg once daily * Specially priced[1]

MOBIC is contraindicated in patients with known hypersensitivity to meloxicam. It should not be given to patients who have experienced asthma, urticaria, or allergic-type reactions after taking aspirin or other nonsteroidal anti-inflammatory drugs (NSAIDs). Severe, rarely fatal, anaphylactic-like reactions to NSAIDs have been reported in such patients.

Please see accompanying Brief Summary of Prescribing Information.

Reference: 1. Price Probe, FirstData Bank, March 2, 2000.

mobic®

(meloxicam) tablets

MOBIC® (meloxicam) Tablets 7.5 mg and 15 mg
Brief Summary of Prescribing Information

INDICATIONS AND USAGE

MOBIC is indicated for relief of the signs and symptoms of osteoarthritis.

CONTRAINDICATIONS

MOBIC is contraindicated in patients with known hypersensitivity to meloxicam. It should not be given to patients who have experienced asthma, urticaria, or allergic-type reactions after taking aspirin or other NSAIDs. Severe, rarely fatal, anaphylactic-like reactions to NSAIDs have been reported in such patients (see WARNINGS, Anaphylactoid Reactions, and PRECAUTIONS, Pre-existing Asthma).

WARNINGS

Gastrointestinal (GI) Effects - Risk of GI Ulceration, Bleeding, and Perforation:

Serious gastrointestinal toxicity, such as inflammation, bleeding, ulceration, and perforation of the stomach, small intestine or large intestine, can occur at any time, with or without warning symptoms, in patients treated with nonsteroidal anti-inflammatory drugs (NSAIDs). Minor upper gastrointestinal problems, such as dyspepsia, are common and may also occur at any time during NSAID therapy. Therefore, physicians and patients should remain alert for ulceration and bleeding, even in the absence of previous GI symptoms. Patients should be informed about the signs and/or symptoms of serious GI toxicity and the steps to take if they occur. The utility of periodic laboratory monitoring has not been demonstrated, nor has it been adequately assessed. Only one in five patients who develop a serious upper GI adverse event on NSAID therapy is symptomatic. It has been demonstrated that upper GI ulcers, gross bleeding or perforation, caused by NSAIDs, appear to occur in approximately 1% of the patients treated for 3-6 months, and in about 2-4% of patients treated for one year. These trends continue thus, increasing the likelihood of developing a serious GI event at some time during the course of therapy. However, even short-term therapy is not without risk.

NSAIDs should be prescribed with extreme caution in those with a prior history of ulcer disease or gastrointestinal bleeding. Most spontaneous reports of fatal GI events are in elderly or debilitated patients and therefore special care should be taken in treating this population. **To minimize the potential risk for an adverse GI event, the lowest effective dose should be used for the shortest possible duration.** For high-risk patients, alternate therapies that do not involve NSAIDs should be considered.

Studies have shown that patients with a *prior history of peptic ulcer disease and/or gastrointestinal bleeding* and who use NSAIDs, have a greater than 10-fold risk for developing a GI bleed than patients with neither of these risk factors. In addition to a past history of ulcer disease, pharmacoepidemiological studies have identified several other co-therapies or co-morbid conditions that may increase the risk for GI bleeding such as: treatment with oral corticosteroids, treatment with anticoagulants, longer duration of NSAID therapy, smoking, alcoholism, older age, and poor general health status.

Anaphylactoid Reactions

As with other NSAIDs, anaphylactoid reactions have occurred in patients without known prior exposure to MOBIC. MOBIC should not be given to patients with the aspirin triad. This symptom complex typically occurs in asthmatic patients who experience rhinitis with or without nasal polyps, or who exhibit severe, potentially fatal bronchospasm after taking aspirin or other NSAIDs (see CONTRAINDICATIONS and PRECAUTIONS, Pre-existing Asthma). Emergency help should be sought in cases where an anaphylactoid reaction occurs.

Advanced Renal Disease

In cases with advanced kidney disease, treatment with MOBIC is not recommended. If NSAID therapy must be initiated, close monitoring of the patient's kidney function is advisable (see PRECAUTIONS, Renal Effects).

Pregnancy

In late pregnancy, as with other NSAIDs, MOBIC should be avoided because it may cause premature closure of the ductus arteriosus.

PRECAUTIONS

General

MOBIC cannot be expected to substitute for corticosteroids or to treat corticosteroid insufficiency. Abrupt discontinuation of corticosteroids may lead to disease exacerbation. Patients on prolonged corticosteroid therapy should have their therapy tapered slowly if a decision is made to discontinue corticosteroids.

The pharmacological activity of MOBIC in reducing inflammation and possibly fever may diminish the utility of these diagnostic signs in detecting complications of presumed noninfectious, painful conditions.

Hepatic Effects

Borderline elevations of one or more liver tests may occur in up to 15% of patients taking NSAIDs, including MOBIC. These laboratory abnormalities may progress, may remain unchanged, or may be transient with continuing therapy. Notable elevations of ALT or AST (approximately three or more times the upper limit of normal) have been reported in approximately 1% of patients in clinical trials with NSAIDs. In addition, rare cases of severe hepatic reactions, including jaundice and fatal fulminant hepatitis, liver necrosis and hepatic failure, some of them with fatal outcomes, have been reported with NSAIDs.

Patients with signs and/or symptoms suggesting liver dysfunction, or in whom an abnormal liver test has occurred, should be evaluated for evidence of the development of a more severe hepatic reaction while on therapy with MOBIC. If clinical signs and symptoms consistent with liver disease develop, or if systemic manifestations occur (e.g., eosinophilia, rash, etc.), MOBIC should be discontinued.

Renal Effects

Caution should be used when initiating treatment with MOBIC in patients with considerable dehydration. It is advisable to rehydrate patients first and then start therapy with MOBIC. Caution is also recommended in patients with pre-existing kidney disease (see WARNINGS, Advanced Renal Disease).

Long-term administration of NSAIDs has resulted in renal papillary necrosis and other renal medullary changes. Renal toxicity has also been seen in patients in whom renal prostaglandins have a compensatory role in the maintenance of renal perfusion. In these patients, administration of NSAIDs may cause dose-dependent reduction in prostaglandin formation and, secondarily, in renal blood flow, which may precipitate overt renal decompensation. Patients at greatest risk of this reaction are those with impaired renal function, heart failure, liver dysfunction, those taking diuretics and ACE inhibitors, and the elderly. Discontinuation of NSAID therapy is usually followed by recovery to the pretreatment state.

The extent to which metabolites may accumulate in patients with renal failure has not been studied with MOBIC. Because some MOBIC metabolites are excreted by the kidney, patients with significantly impaired renal function should be more closely monitored.

Hematological Effects

Anemia is sometimes seen in patients receiving NSAIDs, including MOBIC. This may be due to fluid retention, GI blood loss, or an incompletely described effect upon erythropoiesis. Patients on long-term treatment with NSAIDs, including MOBIC, should have their hemoglobin or hematocrit checked if they exhibit any signs or symptoms of anemia.

Drugs which inhibit the biosynthesis of prostaglandins may interfere to some extent with platelet function and vascular responses to bleeding.

NSAIDs inhibit platelet aggregation and have been shown to prolong bleeding time in some patients. Unlike aspirin their effect on platelet function is quantitatively less, or of shorter duration, and reversible. MOBIC does not generally affect platelet counts, prothrombin time (PT), or partial thromboplastin time (PTT). Patients receiving MOBIC who may be adversely affected by alterations in platelet function, such as those with coagulation disorders or patients receiving anticoagulants, should be carefully monitored.

Fluid Retention and Edema

Fluid retention and edema have been observed in some patients taking NSAIDs, including MOBIC. Therefore, as with other NSAIDs, MOBIC should be used with caution in patients with fluid retention, hypertension, or heart failure.

Pre-existing Asthma

Patients with asthma may have aspirin-sensitive asthma. The use of aspirin in patients with aspirin-sensitive asthma has been associated with severe bronchospasm which can be fatal. Since cross reactivity, including bronchospasm, between aspirin and other nonsteroidal anti-inflammatory drugs has been reported in such aspirin-sensitive patients, MOBIC should not be administered to patients with this form of aspirin sensitivity and should be used with caution in patients with pre-existing asthma.

Information for Patients

MOBIC, like other drugs of its class, can cause discomfort and, rarely, more serious side effects, such as gastrointestinal bleeding, which may result in hospitalization and even fatal outcomes. Although serious GI tract ulcerations and bleeding can occur without warning symptoms, patients should be alert for the signs and symptoms of ulcerations and bleeding, and should ask for medical advice when observing any indicative signs or symptoms. Patients should be made aware of the importance of this follow-up (see WARNINGS, Gastrointestinal (GI) Effects - Risk of GI Ulceration, Bleeding and Perforation).

Patients should report to their physicians signs or symptoms of gastrointestinal ulceration or bleeding, skin rash, weight gain, or edema.

Patients should be informed of the warning signs and symptoms of hepatotoxicity (e.g., nausea, fatigue, lethargy, pruritus, jaundice, right upper quadrant tenderness, and "flu-like" symptoms). If these occur, patients should be instructed to stop therapy and seek immediate medical therapy.

Patients should also be instructed to seek immediate emergency help in the case of an anaphylactoid reaction (see WARNINGS, Anaphylactoid Reactions).

In late pregnancy, as with other NSAIDs, MOBIC should be avoided because it may cause premature closure of the ductus arteriosus.

Laboratory Tests

Patients on long-term treatment with NSAIDs should have their CBC and a chemistry profile checked periodically. If clinical signs and symptoms consistent with liver or renal disease develop, systemic manifestations occur (e.g., eosinophilia, rash, etc.) or if abnormal liver tests persist or worsen, MOBIC should be discontinued.

Drug Interactions

ACE inhibitors Reports suggest that NSAIDs may diminish the antihypertensive effect of angiotensin-converting enzyme (ACE) inhibitors. This interaction should be given consideration in patients taking NSAIDs concomitantly with ACE inhibitors.

Aspirin Concomitant administration of aspirin (1000 mg TID) to healthy volunteers tended to increase the AUC (10%) and C_{max} (24%) of meloxicam. The clinical significance of this interaction is not known; however, as with other NSAIDs, concomitant administration of meloxicam and aspirin is not generally recommended because of the potential for increased adverse effects. Concomitant administration of low-dose aspirin with MOBIC may result in an increased rate of GI ulceration or other complications, compared to use of MOBIC alone. MOBIC is not a substitute for aspirin for cardiovascular prophylaxis.

Cholestyramine Pretreatment for four days with cholestyramine significantly increased the clearance of meloxicam by 50%. This resulted in a decrease in $t_{1/2}$, from 19.2 hours to 12.5 hours, and a 35% reduction in AUC. This suggests the existence of a recirculation pathway for meloxicam in the gastrointestinal tract. The clinical relevance of this interaction has not been established.

Cimetidine Concomitant administration of 200 mg cimetidine QID did not alter the single-dose pharmacokinetics of 30 mg meloxicam.

Digoxin Meloxicam 15 mg once daily for 7 days did not alter the plasma concentration profile of digoxin after β-acetyldigoxin administration for 7 days at clinical doses. *In vitro* testing found no protein binding drug interaction between digoxin and meloxicam.

Furosemide Clinical studies, as well as post-marketing observations, have shown that NSAIDs can reduce the natriuretic effect of furosemide and thiazide diuretics in some patients. This effect has been attributed to inhibition of renal prostaglandin synthesis. Studies with furosemide agents and meloxicam have not demonstrated a reduction in natriuretic effect. Furosemide single and multiple dose pharmacodynamics and pharmacokinetics are not affected by multiple doses of meloxicam. Nevertheless, during concomitant therapy with furosemide and MOBIC, patients should be observed closely for signs of declining renal function (see PRECAUTIONS, Renal Effects), as well as to assure diuretic efficacy.

Lithium In clinical trials, NSAIDs have produced an elevation of plasma lithium levels and a reduction in renal lithium clearance. In a study conducted in healthy subjects, mean pre-dose lithium concentration and AUC were increased by 21% in subjects receiving lithium doses ranging from 804 to 1072 mg BID with meloxicam 15 mg QD as compared to subjects receiving lithium alone. These effects have been attributed to inhibition of renal prostaglandin synthesis by MOBIC. Patients on lithium treatment should be closely monitored when MOBIC is introduced or withdrawn.

Methotrexate A study in 13 rheumatoid arthritis (RA) patients evaluated the effects of multiple doses of meloxicam on the pharmacokinetics of methotrexate taken once weekly. Meloxicam did not have a significant effect on the pharmacokinetics of single doses of methotrexate. *In vitro,* methotrexate did not displace meloxicam from its human serum binding sites.

Warfarin Anticoagulant activity should be monitored, particularly in the first few days after initiating or changing MOBIC therapy in patients receiving warfarin or similar agents, since these patients are at an increased risk of bleeding. The effect of meloxicam on the anticoagulant effect of warfarin was studied in a group of healthy subjects receiving daily doses of warfarin that produced an INR (International Normalized Ratio) between 1.2 and 1.8. In these subjects, meloxicam did not alter warfarin pharmacokinetics and the average anticoagulant effect of warfarin as determined by prothrombin time. However, one subject showed an increase in INR from 1.5 to 2.1. Caution should be used when administering MOBIC with warfarin since patients on warfarin may experience changes in INR and an increased risk of bleeding complications when a new medication is introduced.

Carcinogenesis, Mutagenesis, Impairment of Fertility

No carcinogenic effect of meloxicam was observed in rats given oral doses up to 0.8 mg/kg/day (approximately 0.4-fold the human dose at 15 mg/day for a 50 kg adult based on body surface area conversion) for 104 weeks or in mice given oral doses up to 8.0 mg/kg/day (approximately 2.2-fold the human dose, as noted above) for 99 weeks.

Meloxicam was not mutagenic in an Ames assay, or clastogenic in a chromosome aberration assay with human lymphocytes and an *in vivo* micronucleus test in mouse bone marrow.

Meloxicam did not impair male and female fertility in rats at oral doses up to 9 and 5 mg/kg/day, respectively (4.9-fold and 2.5-fold the human dose, as noted above). However, an increased incidence of embryolethality at oral doses ≥ 1 mg/kg/day (0.5-fold the human dose, as noted above) was observed in rats when dams were given meloxicam 2 weeks prior to mating and during early embryonic development.

Pregnancy

Teratogenic Effects: Pregnancy Category C. Meloxicam caused an increased incidence of septal defect of the heart, a rare event, at an oral dose of 60 mg/kg/day (64.5-fold the human dose at 15 mg/day for a 50 kg adult based on body surface area conversion) and embryolethality at oral doses ≥ 5 mg/kg/day (5.4-fold the human dose, as noted above) when rabbits were treated throughout organogenesis. Meloxicam was not teratogenic in rats up to an oral dose of 4 mg/kg/day (approximately 2.2-fold the human dose, as noted above) throughout organogenesis. An increased incidence of stillbirths was observed when rats were given oral doses ≥1 mg/kg/day throughout organogenesis. Meloxicam crosses the placental barrier. There are no adequate and well-controlled studies in pregnant women. MOBIC should be used during pregnancy only if the potential benefit justifies the potential risk to the fetus.

Nonteratogenic Effects: Meloxicam caused a reduction in birth index, live births, and neonatal survival at oral doses ≥ 0.125 mg/kg/day (approximately 0.07-fold the human dose at 15 mg/day for a 50 kg adult based on body surface area conversion) when rats were treated during the late gestation and lactation period. No studies have been conducted to evaluate the effect of meloxicam on the closure of the ductus arteriosus in humans; use of meloxicam during the third trimester of pregnancy should be avoided.

Labor and Delivery

Studies in rats with meloxicam, as with other drugs known to inhibit prostaglandin synthesis, showed an increased incidence of stillbirths, increased length of delivery time, and delayed parturition at oral dosages ≥ 1 mg/kg/day (approximately 0.5-fold the human dose at 15 mg/day for a 50 kg adult based on body surface area conversion), and decreased pup survival at an oral dose of 4 mg/kg/day (approximately 2.1-fold the human dose, as noted above) throughout organogenesis. Similar findings were observed in rats receiving oral dosages ≥ 0.125 mg/kg/day (approximately 0.07-fold the human dose, as noted above) during late gestation and the lactation period.

Nursing Mothers

Studies of meloxicam excretion in human milk have not been conducted; however, meloxicam was excreted in the milk of lactating rats at concentrations higher than those in plasma. Because of the potential for serious adverse reactions in nursing infants from MOBIC, a decision should be made whether to discontinue nursing or to discontinue the drug, taking into account the importance of the drug to the mother.

Pediatric Use

Safety and effectiveness in pediatric patients under 18 years of age have not been established.

Geriatric Use

As with any NSAID, caution should be exercised in treating the elderly (65 years and older).

ADVERSE REACTIONS

The MOBIC phase 2/3 clinical trial database includes 10,122 patients treated with MOBIC 7.5 mg/day and 3,505 patients treated with MOBIC 15 mg/day. MOBIC at these doses was administered to 661 patients for at least 6 months and to 312 patients for at least one year. Approximately 10,500 of these patients were treated in ten placebo and/or active-controlled osteoarthritis trials. Gastrointestinal (GI) adverse events were the most frequently reported adverse events in all treatment groups across MOBIC trials.

A 12-week multicenter, double-blind, randomized trial was conducted in patients with osteoarthritis of the knee or hip to compare the efficacy and safety of MOBIC with placebo and with an active control.

The following adverse events (%) occurred in ≥ 2% of MOBIC 7.5 mg daily (n=154) and 15 mg daily (n=156) patients, respectively, in a 12-week osteoarthritis placebo- and active-controlled trial: abdominal pain, 1.9%, 2.6%; diarrhea, 7.8%, 3.2%; dyspepsia, 4.5%, 4.5%; flatulence, 3.2%, 3.2%; nausea, 3.9%, 3.8%; accident household, 4.5%, 3.2%; edema[1], 1.9%, 4.5%; fall, 2.6%, 0.0%; influenza-like symptoms, 4.5%, 5.8%; dizziness, 2.6%, 3.8%; headache, 7.8%, 8.3%; pharyngitis, 0.6%, 3.2%; upper respiratory tract infection, 3.2%, 1.9%; rash[2], 2.6%, 0.6%.

The following adverse events (%) occurred with MOBIC 7.5 mg daily in ≥ 2% of patients treated, respectively, in short-term (4-6 weeks) and long-term (6 months) active-controlled osteoarthritis trials: abdominal pain, 2.7%, 4.7%; constipation, 0.8%, 1.8%; diarrhea, 1.9%, 5.9%; dyspepsia, 3.8%, 8.9%; flatulence, 0.5%, 3.0%; nausea, 2.4%, 4.7%; vomiting, 0.6%, 1.8%; edema[1], 0.6%, 2.4%; pain, 0.9%, 3.6%; dizziness, 1.1%, 2.4%; headache, 2.4%, 3.6%; anemia, 0.1%, 4.1%; arthralgia, 0.5%, 5.3%; back pain, 0.5%, 3.0%; insomnia, 0.4%, 3.6%; coughing, 0.2%, 2.4%; upper respiratory tract infection, 0.2%, 8.3%; pruritus, 0.4%, 2.4%; rash[2], 0.3%, 3.0%; micturition frequency, 0.1%, 2.4%; urinary tract infection, 0.3%, 4.7%.

The following adverse events (%) occurred with MOBIC 15 mg daily in ≥ 2% of patients treated, respectively, in short-term (4-6 weeks) and long-term (6 months) active-controlled osteoarthritis trials: abdominal pain, 2.3%, 2.9%; constipation, 1.2%, 2.6%; diarrhea, 2.7%, 2.6%; dyspepsia, 7.4%, 9.5%; flatulence, 0.4%, 2.6%; nausea, 4.7%, 7.2%; vomiting, 0.8%, 2.6%; edema[1], 2.0%, 1.6%; pain, 2.0%, 5.2%; dizziness, 1.6%, 2.6%; headache, 2.7%, 2.6%; anemia, 0.0%, 2.9%; arthralgia, 0.0%, 1.3%; back pain, 0.4%, 0.7%; insomnia, 0.0%, 1.6%; coughing, 0.8%, 1.0%; upper respiratory tract infection, 0.0%, 7.5%; pruritus, 1.2%, 0.0%; rash[2], 1.2%, 1.3%; micturition frequency, 0.4%, 1.3%; urinary tract infection, 0.4%, 6.9%.

[1]WHO preferred terms edema, edema dependent, edema peripheral and edema legs combined

[2]WHO preferred terms rash, rash erythematous and rash maculo-papular combined

As with other NSAIDs, higher doses of MOBIC (e.g., chronic daily 30 mg dose) were associated with an increased risk of serious GI events, therefore the daily dose of MOBIC should not exceed 15 mg.

The following is a list of adverse drug reactions occurring in < 2% of patients receiving MOBIC in clinical trials involving approximately 15,400 patients. Adverse reactions reported only in worldwide post-marketing experience or the literature are shown in italics and are considered rare (< 0.1%).

Body as a Whole: allergic reaction, *anaphylactoid reactions including shock,* face edema, fatigue, fever, hot flushes, malaise, syncope, weight decrease, weight increase **Cardiovascular:** angina pectoris, cardiac failure, hypertension, hypotension, myocardial infarction, vasculitis **Central and Peripheral Nervous System:** convulsions, paresthesia, tremor, vertigo **Gastrointestinal:** colitis, dry mouth, duodenal ulcer, eructation, esophagitis, gastric ulcer, gastritis, gastroesophageal reflux, gastrointestinal hemorrhage, hematemesis, hemorrhagic duodenal ulcer, hemorrhagic gastric ulcer, intestinal perforation, melena, pancreatitis, perforated duodenal ulcer, perforated gastric ulcer, stomatitis ulcerative **Heart Rate and Rhythm:** arrhythmia, palpitation, tachycardia **Hematologic:** *agranulocytosis*, leukopenia, purpura, thrombocytopenia **Liver and Biliary System:** ALT increased, AST increased, bilirubinemia, GGT increased, hepatitis, *jaundice, liver failure* **Metabolic and Nutritional:** dehydration **Psychiatric Disorders:** abnormal dreaming, anxiety, appetite increased, confusion, depression, nervousness, somnolence **Respiratory:** asthma, bronchospasm, dyspnea **Skin and Appendages:** alopecia, angioedema, bullous eruption, *erythema multiforme,* photosensitivity reaction, pruritus, *Stevens-Johnson syndrome,* sweating increased, *toxic epidermal necrolysis,* urticaria **Special Senses:** abnormal vision, conjunctivitis, taste perversion, tinnitus **Urinary System:** albuminuria, BUN increased, creatinine increased, hematuria, *interstitial nephritis,* renal failure.

OVERDOSAGE

There is limited experience with meloxicam overdose. Four cases have taken 6 to 11 times the highest recommended dose; all recovered. Cholestyramine is known to accelerate the clearance of meloxicam.

Symptoms following acute NSAID overdose are usually limited to lethargy, drowsiness, nausea, vomiting, and epigastric pain, which are generally reversible with supportive care. Gastrointestinal bleeding can occur. Severe poisoning may result in hypertension, acute renal failure, hepatic dysfunction, respiratory depression, coma, convulsions, cardiovascular collapse, and cardiac arrest. Anaphylactoid reactions have been reported with therapeutic ingestion of NSAIDs, and may occur following an overdose.

Patients should be managed with symptomatic and supportive care following an NSAID overdose. In cases of acute overdose, gastric lavage followed by activated charcoal is recommended. Gastric lavage performed more than one hour after overdose has little benefit in the treatment of overdose. Administration of activated charcoal is recommended for patients who present 1-2 hours after overdose. For substantial overdose or severely symptomatic patients, activated charcoal may be administered repeatedly. Accelerated removal of meloxicam by 4 gm oral doses of cholestyramine given three times a day was demonstrated in a clinical trial. Administration of cholestyramine may be useful following an overdose. Forced diuresis, alkalinization of urine, hemodialysis, or hemoperfusion may not be useful due to high protein binding.

Rx only MB-BS-4058550/US/5(10/00)

Boehringer Ingelheim

ABBOTT LABORATORIES

MB-7681R

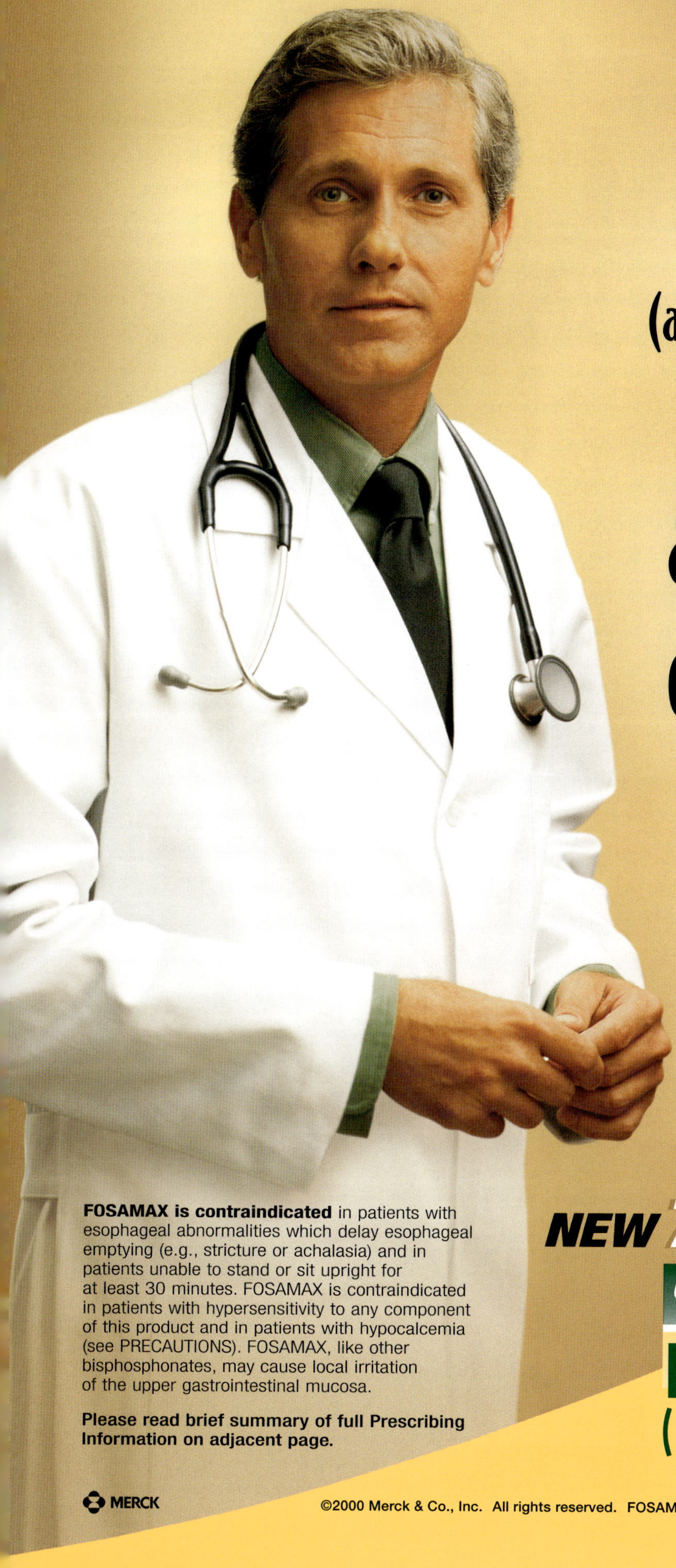

For the treatment of postmenopausal osteoporosis

"FOSAMAX® (alendronate sodium tablets) is now available in a once-weekly tablet?"

FOSAMAX is contraindicated in patients with esophageal abnormalities which delay esophageal emptying (e.g., stricture or achalasia) and in patients unable to stand or sit upright for at least 30 minutes. FOSAMAX is contraindicated in patients with hypersensitivity to any component of this product and in patients with hypocalcemia (see PRECAUTIONS). FOSAMAX, like other bisphosphonates, may cause local irritation of the upper gastrointestinal mucosa.

Please read brief summary of full Prescribing Information on adjacent page.

NEW 70 mg

ONCE WEEKLY

FOSAMAX®

(alendronate sodium tablets)

MERCK

FOSAMAX® (alendronate sodium tablets) BRIEF SUMMARY OF PRESCRIBING INFORMATION

CONTRAINDICATIONS

- Abnormalities of the esophagus which delay esophageal emptying such as stricture or achalasia
- Inability to stand or sit upright for at least 30 minutes
- Hypersensitivity to any component of this product
- Hypocalcemia (see PRECAUTIONS, *General*)

WARNINGS

FOSAMAX, like other bisphosphonates, may cause local irritation of the upper gastrointestinal mucosa. Esophageal adverse experiences, such as esophagitis, esophageal ulcers and esophageal erosions, occasionally with bleeding and rarely followed by esophageal stricture, have been reported in patients receiving treatment with FOSAMAX. In some cases these have been severe and required hospitalization. Physicians should therefore be alert to any signs or symptoms signaling a possible esophageal reaction and patients should be instructed to discontinue FOSAMAX and seek medical attention if they develop dysphagia, odynophagia, retrosternal pain, or new or worsening heartburn. The risk of severe esophageal adverse experiences appears to be greater in patients who lie down after taking FOSAMAX and/or who fail to swallow it with a full glass (6–8 oz) of water, and/or who continue to take FOSAMAX after developing symptoms suggestive of esophageal irritation. Therefore, it is very important that the full dosing instructions are provided to, and understood by, the patient (see DOSAGE AND ADMINISTRATION). In patients who cannot comply with dosing instructions due to mental disability, therapy with FOSAMAX should be used under appropriate supervision. Because of possible irritant effects of FOSAMAX on the upper gastrointestinal mucosa and a potential for worsening of the underlying disease, caution should be used when FOSAMAX is given to patients with active upper gastrointestinal problems (such as dysphagia, esophageal diseases, gastritis, duodenitis, or ulcers). There have been post-marketing reports of gastric and duodenal ulcers, some severe and with complications, although no increased risk was observed in controlled clinical trials.

PRECAUTIONS

General

Causes of osteoporosis other than estrogen deficiency, aging, and glucocorticoid use should be considered. Hypocalcemia must be corrected before initiating therapy with FOSAMAX (see CONTRAINDICATIONS). Other disturbances of mineral metabolism (such as vitamin D deficiency) should also be effectively treated. Presumably due to the effects of FOSAMAX on increasing bone mineral, small, asymptomatic decreases in serum calcium and phosphate may occur, especially in patients with Paget's disease, in whom the pretreatment rate of bone turnover may be greatly elevated and in patients receiving glucocorticoids, in whom calcium absorption may be decreased. Ensuring adequate calcium and vitamin D intake is especially important in patients with Paget's disease of bone and in patients receiving glucocorticoids.

Renal insufficiency

FOSAMAX is not recommended for patients with renal insufficiency (creatinine clearance <35 mL/min). (See DOSAGE AND ADMINISTRATION.)

Glucocorticoid-induced osteoporosis

The risk versus benefit of FOSAMAX for treatment at daily dosages of glucocorticoids less than 7.5 mg of prednisone or equivalent has not been established (see INDICATIONS AND USAGE). Before initiating treatment, the hormonal status of both men and women should be ascertained and appropriate replacement considered. A bone mineral density measurement should be made at the initiation of therapy and repeated after 6 to 12 months of combined FOSAMAX and glucocorticoid treatment. The efficacy of FOSAMAX for the treatment of glucocorticoid-induced osteoporosis has been shown in patients with a median bone mineral density which was 1.2 standard deviations below the mean for healthy young adults. The efficacy of FOSAMAX has been established in studies of two years' duration. The greatest increase in bone mineral density occurred in the first year with maintenance or smaller gains during the second year. Efficacy of FOSAMAX beyond two years has not been studied. The efficacy of FOSAMAX in respect to fracture prevention has been demonstrated for vertebral fractures. However, this finding was based on very few fractures that occurred primarily in postmenopausal women. The efficacy for prevention of non-vertebral fractures has not been demonstrated.

Information for Patients

General

Physicians should instruct their patients to read the patient package insert before starting therapy with FOSAMAX and to reread it each time the prescription is renewed. Patients should be instructed to take supplemental calcium and vitamin D, if daily dietary intake is inadequate. Weight-bearing exercise should be considered along with the modification of certain behavioral factors, such as cigarette smoking and/or excessive alcohol consumption, if these factors exist.

Dosing Instructions

Patients should be instructed that the expected benefits of FOSAMAX may only be obtained when each tablet is swallowed with plain water the first thing upon arising for the day at least 30 minutes before the first food, beverage, or medication of the day. Even dosing with orange juice or coffee has been shown to markedly reduce the absorption of FOSAMAX (see CLINICAL PHARMACOLOGY, *Pharmacokinetics, Absorption*). To facilitate delivery to the stomach and thus reduce the potential for esophageal irritation patients should be instructed to swallow FOSAMAX with a full glass of water (6–8 oz) and not to lie down for at least 30 minutes and until after their first food of the day. Patients should not chew or suck on the tablet because of a potential for oropharyngeal ulceration. Patients should be specifically instructed not to take FOSAMAX at bedtime or before arising for the day. Patients should be informed that failure to follow these instructions may increase their risk of esophageal problems. Patients should be instructed that if they develop symptoms of esophageal disease (such as difficulty or pain upon swallowing, retrosternal pain or new or worsening heartburn) they should stop taking FOSAMAX and consult their physician. Patients should be instructed that if they miss a dose of once weekly FOSAMAX, they should take one tablet on the morning after they remember. They should not take two tablets on the same day but should return to taking one tablet once a week, as originally scheduled on their chosen day.

Drug Interactions (also see CLINICAL PHARMACOLOGY, *Pharmacokinetics, Drug Interactions*)

Estrogen/hormone replacement therapy (HRT)

Concomitant use of HRT (estrogen ± progestin) and FOSAMAX was assessed in two clinical studies of one or two years' duration in postmenopausal osteoporotic women. In these studies, the safety and tolerability profile of the combination was consistent with those of the individual treatments; however, the degree of suppression of bone turnover (as assessed by mineralizing surface) was significantly greater with the combination than with either component alone. The long-term effects of combined FOSAMAX and HRT on fracture occurrence have not been studied (see CLINICAL PHARMACOLOGY, *Clinical Studies, Concomitant use with estrogen/hormone replacement therapy (HRT)* and ADVERSE REACTIONS, *Clinical Studies, Concomitant use with estrogen/hormone replacement therapy*).

Calcium Supplements/Antacids

It is likely that calcium supplements, antacids, and some oral medications will interfere with absorption of FOSAMAX. Therefore, patients must wait at least one-half hour after taking FOSAMAX before taking any other oral medications.

Aspirin

In clinical studies, the incidence of upper gastrointestinal adverse events was increased in patients receiving concomitant therapy with daily doses of FOSAMAX greater than 10 mg and aspirin-containing products.

Nonsteroidal Anti-inflammatory Drugs (NSAIDs)

FOSAMAX may be administered to patients taking NSAIDs. In a 3-year, controlled, clinical study (n=2027) during which a majority of patients received concomitant NSAIDs, the incidence of upper gastrointestinal adverse events was similar in patients taking FOSAMAX 5 or 10 mg/day compared to those taking placebo. However, since NSAID use is associated with gastrointestinal irritation, caution should be used during concomitant use with FOSAMAX.

Pregnancy

Pregnancy Category C:

Reproduction studies in rats showed decreased postimplantation survival at 2 mg/kg/day and decreased body weight gain in normal pups at 1 mg/kg/day. Sites of incomplete fetal ossification were statistically significantly increased in rats beginning at 10 mg/kg/day in vertebral (cervical, thoracic, and lumbar), skull, and sternebral bones. The above doses ranged from 0.26 times (1 mg/kg) to 2.6 times (10 mg/kg) a maximum recommended daily dose of 40 mg (Paget's disease) based on surface area, mg/m^2. No similar fetal effects were seen when pregnant rabbits were treated at doses up to 35 mg/kg/day (10.3 times a 40 mg human daily dose based on surface area, mg/m^2). Both total and ionized calcium decreased in pregnant rats at 15 mg/kg/day (3.9 times the 40 human daily dose based on surface area, mg/m^2) resulting in delays and failures of delivery. Protracted parturition due to maternal hypocalcemia occurred in rats at doses as low as 0.5 mg/kg/day (0.13 times a 40 mg human daily dose based on surface area, mg/m^2) when rats were treated from before mating through gestation. Maternotoxicity (late pregnancy deaths) occurred in the female rats treated with 15 mg/kg/day for varying periods of time ranging from treatment only during pre-mating to treatment only during early, middle, or late gestation; these deaths were lessened but not eliminated by cessation of treatment. Calcium supplementation either in the drinking water or by minipump could not ameliorate the hypocalcemia or prevent maternal and neonatal deaths due to delays in delivery; calcium supplementation IV prevented maternal, but not fetal deaths. There are no studies in pregnant women. FOSAMAX should be used during pregnancy only if the potential benefit justifies the potential risk to the mother and fetus.

Nursing Mothers

It is not known whether alendronate is excreted in human milk. Because many drugs are excreted in human milk, caution should be exercised when FOSAMAX is administered to nursing women.

Pediatric Use

Safety and effectiveness in pediatric patients have not been established.

Use in the Elderly

Of the patients receiving FOSAMAX in the United States and Multinational osteoporosis treatment studies in women, the osteoporosis study in men, glucocorticoid-induced osteoporosis studies, and Paget's disease studies (see CLINICAL PHARMACOLOGY, *Clinical Studies*), 45%, 50%, 37%, and 70%, respectively, were 65 years of age or over. No overall differences in efficacy or safety were observed between these patients and younger patients but greater sensitivity of some older individuals cannot be ruled out.

ADVERSE REACTIONS

Clinical Studies

In clinical studies of up to five years in duration adverse experiences associated with FOSAMAX usually were mild, and generally did not require discontinuation of therapy. FOSAMAX has been evaluated for safety in approximately 8000 postmenopausal women in clinical studies.

Treatment of osteoporosis

Postmenopausal women

In two identically designed, three-year, placebo-controlled, double-blind, multicenter studies (United States and Multinational; n=994), discontinuation of therapy due to any clinical adverse experience occurred in 4.1% of 196 patients treated with FOSAMAX 10 mg/day and 6.0% of 397 patients treated with placebo. In the Fracture Intervention Trial (n=6459), discontinuation of therapy due to any clinical adverse experience occurred in 9.1% of 3236 patients treated with FOSAMAX 5 mg/day for 2 years and 10 mg/day for either one or two additional years and 10.1% of 3223 patients treated with placebo. Discontinuations due to upper gastrointestinal adverse experiences were: FOSAMAX, 3.2%; placebo, 2.7%. In these study populations, 49-54% had a history of gastrointestinal disorders at baseline and 54-89% used nonsteroidal anti-inflammatory drugs or aspirin at some time during the studies. Adverse experiences from these studies considered by the investigators as possibly, probably, or definitely drug related in ≥1% of patients treated with either FOSAMAX or placebo are presented in the following table.

Osteoporosis Treatment Studies in Postmenopausal Women–Adverse Experiences Considered Possibly, Probably, or Definitely Drug Related by the Investigators and Reported in ≥1% of Patients

	United States/Multinational Studies		Fracture Intervention Trial	
	FOSAMAX* % (n=196)	Placebo % (n=397)	FOSAMAX** % (n=3236)	Placebo % (n=3223)
Gastrointestinal				
abdominal pain	6.6	4.8	1.5	1.5
nausea	3.6	4.0	1.1	1.5
dyspepsia	3.6	3.5	1.1	1.2
constipation	3.1	1.8	0.0	0.2
diarrhea	3.1	1.8	0.6	0.3
flatulence	2.6	0.5	0.2	0.3
acid regurgitation	2.0	4.3	1.1	0.9
esophageal ulcer	1.5	0.0	0.1	0.1
vomiting	1.0	1.5	0.2	0.3
dysphagia	1.0	0.0	0.1	0.1
abdominal distension	1.0	0.8	0.0	0.0
gastritis	0.5	1.3	0.6	0.7
Musculoskeletal				
musculoskeletal (bone, muscle or joint) pain	4.1	2.5	0.4	0.3
muscle cramp	0.0	1.0	0.2	0.1
Nervous System/Psychiatric				
headache	2.6	1.5	0.2	0.2
dizziness	0.0	1.0	0.0	0.1
Special Senses				
taste perversion	0.5	1.0	0.1	0.0

*10 mg/day for three years **5 mg/day for 2 years and 10 mg/day for either 1 or 2 additional years

Rarely, rash and erythema have occurred.

One patient treated with FOSAMAX (10 mg/day) who had a history of peptic ulcer disease and gastrectomy and who was taking concomitant aspirin developed an anastomotic ulcer with mild hemorrhage, which was considered drug related. Aspirin and FOSAMAX were discontinued and the patient recovered.

The adverse experience profile was similar for the 401 patients treated with either 5 or 20 mg doses of FOSAMAX in the United States and Multinational studies. The adverse experience profile for the 296 patients who received continued treatment with either 5 or 10 mg doses of FOSAMAX in the two-year extension of these studies (treatment years 4 and 5) was similar to that observed during the three-year placebo-controlled period. During the extension period, of the 151 patients treated with FOSAMAX 10 mg/day, the proportion of patients who discontinued therapy due to any clinical adverse experience was similar to that during the first three years of the study.

In a one-year, double-blind multicenter study, the overall safety and tolerability profiles of once weekly FOSAMAX 70 mg and FOSAMAX 10 mg daily were similar. The adverse experiences were considered by investigators as possibly, probably, or definitely drug related in ≥1% of patients treated with either FOSAMAX 70 mg once weekly (n=519), or FOSAMAX 10 mg daily (n=370), respectively, were: *Gastrointestinal*: abdominal pain (3.7%; 3.0%), dyspepsia (2.7%; 2.2%), acid regurgitation (1.9%; 2.4%), nausea (1.9%; 2.4%), abdominal distension (1.0%; 1.4%), constipation (0.8%; 1.6%), flatulence (0.4%; 1.6%), gastritis (0.2%; 1.1%), gastric ulcer (0.0%; 1.1%); *Musculoskeletal:* musculoskeletal (bone, muscle, joint) pain (2.9%; 3.2%), muscle cramp (0.2%; 1.1%).

Men

In a two-year, placebo-controlled, double-blind multicenter study, discontinuation of therapy due to any clinical adverse experience occurred in 2.7% of men treated with FOSAMAX 10 mg/day and 10.5% of men treated with placebo. The adverse experiences considered by investigators as possibly, probably, or definitely drug related in ≥2% of patients treated with either FOSAMAX 10 mg/day (n=146), or placebo (n=95), respectively, were: *Gastrointestinal:* acid regurgitation (4.1%; 3.2%), flatulence (4.1%; 1.1%), dyspepsia (3.4%; 0.0%), abdominal pain (2.1%; 1.1%), nausea (2.1%; 0.0%).

Prevention of osteoporosis in postmenopausal women

The safety of FOSAMAX 5 mg/day in postmenopausal women 40-60 years of age has been evaluated in three double-blind, placebo-controlled studies involving over 1,400 patients randomized to receive FOSAMAX for either two or three years. In these studies the overall safety profiles of FOSAMAX 5 mg/day and placebo were similar. Discontinuation of therapy due to any clinical adverse experience occurred in 7.5% of 642 patients treated with FOSAMAX 5 mg/day and 5.7% of 648 patients treated with placebo.

In a one-year, double-blind multicenter study, the overall safety and tolerability profiles of once weekly FOSAMAX 35 mg and FOSAMAX 5 mg daily were similar.

The adverse experiences from these studies considered by the investigators as possibly, probably, or definitely drug related in ≥1% of patients treated with either once weekly FOSAMAX 35 mg, FOSAMAX 5mg/day or placebo are presented in the following table.

Osteoporosis Prevention Studies in Postmenopausal Women–Adverse Experiences Considered Possibly, Probably, or Definitely Drug Related by the Investigators and Reported in ≥1% of Patients

	Two/Three-Year Studies		One-Year Study	
	FOSAMAX 5 mg/day % (n=642)	Placebo % (n=648)	FOSAMAX 5 mg/day % (n=361)	Once-Weekly FOSAMAX 35 mg % (n=362)
Gastrointestinal				
dyspepsia	1.9	1.4	2.2	1.7
abdominal pain	1.7	3.4	4.2	2.2
acid regurgitation	1.4	2.5	4.2	4.7
nausea	1.4	1.4	2.5	1.4
diarrhea	1.1	1.7	1.1	0.6
constipation	0.9	0.5	1.7	0.3
abdominal distension	0.2	0.3	1.4	1.1
Musculoskeletal				
musculoskeletal (bone, muscle or joint) pain	0.8	0.9	1.9	2.2

Concomitant use with estrogen/hormone replacement therapy

In two studies (of one and two years' duration) of postmenopausal osteoporotic women (total: n=853), the safety and tolerability profile of combined treatment with FOSAMAX 10 mg once daily and estrogen ± progestin (n=354) was consistent with those of the individual treatments.

Treatments of glucocorticoid-induced osteoporosis

In two one-year, placebo-controlled, double-blind multicenter studies, in patients receiving glucocorticoid treatment, the overall safety and tolerability profiles of FOSAMAX 5 and 10 mg/day were generally similar to that of placebo. The adverse experiences considered by the investigators as possibly, probably, or definitely drug related in ≥1% of patients treated with either FOSAMAX 10 mg/day (n=157), FOSAMAX 5 mg/day (n=161), or placebo (n=159), respectively, were: *Gastrointestinal:* abdominal pain (3.2%; 1.9%; 0.0%), acid regurgitation (2.5%; 1.9%; 1.3%), constipation (1.3%; 0.6%; 0.0%), melena (1.3%; 0.0%; 0.0%), nausea (0.6%; 1.2%; 0.6%), diarrhea (0.0%; 0.0%; 1.3%), *Nervous System/Psychiatric*: headache (0.6%; 0.0%; 1.3%).

The overall safety and tolerability profile in the glucocorticoid-induced osteoporosis population that continued therapy for the second year of the studies (FOSAMAX: n=147) was consistent with that observed in the first year.

Paget's disease of bone

In clinical studies (osteoporosis and Paget's disease), adverse experiences reported in 175 patients taking FOSAMAX 40 mg/day for 3-12 months were similar to those in postmenopausal women treated with FOSAMAX 10 mg/day. However, there was an apparent increased incidence of upper gastrointestinal adverse experiences in patients taking FOSAMAX 40 mg/day (17.7% FOSAMAX vs. 10.2% placebo). One case of esophagitis and two cases of gastritis resulted in discontinuation of treatment. Additionally, musculoskeletal (bone, muscle, or joint) pain, which has been described in patients with Paget's disease treated with other bisphosphonates, was considered by the investigators as possibly, probably, or definitely drug related in approximately 6% of patients treated with FOSAMAX 40 mg/day vs. approximately 1% of patients treated with placebo, but rarely resulted in discontinuation of therapy. Discontinuation of therapy due to any clinical adverse experience occurred in 6.4% of patients with Paget's disease treated with FOSAMAX 40 mg/day and 2.4% of patients treated with placebo.

Laboratory Test Findings

In double-blind, multicenter, controlled studies, asymptomatic, mild, and transient decreases in serum calcium and phosphate were observed in approximately 18% and 10%, respectively, of patients taking FOSAMAX versus approximately 12% and 3% of those taking placebo. However, the incidences of decreases in serum calcium to <8.0 mg/dL (2.0 mM) and serum phosphate to ≤2.0 mg/dL (0.65 mM) were similar in both treatment groups.

Post-Marketing Experience

The following adverse reactions have been reported in post-marketing use: *Body as a Whole*: hypersensitivity reactions including urticaria and rarely angioedema. *Gastrointestinal:* esophagitis, esophageal erosions, esophageal ulcers, rarely esophageal stricture, and oropharyngeal ulceration. Gastric or duodenal ulcers, some severe and with complications have also been reported (see WARNINGS, PRECAUTIONS, and *Information for Patients*, and DOSAGE AND ADMINISTRATION). *Skin:* rash (occasionally with photosensitivity). *Special Senses:* rarely uveitis.

For more detailed information, consult your Merck representative or see the full Prescribing Information.

007129(2)(017)-FOS Printed in USA Minimum 10% Recycled Paper

ACR ANNOUNCEMENTS

AMERICAN COLLEGE OF RHEUMATOLOGY
1800 Century Place, Suite 250, Atlanta, Georgia 30345-4300

ACR Meetings

Annual Meetings
- November 10–15, 2001, San Francisco
- October 24–29, 2002, New Orleans
- October 23–28, 2003, Orlando
- October 7–12, 2004, San Antonio
- November 12–17, 2005, San Diego

Innovative Therapies in Autoimmune Diseases: Clinical Development Challenges
- March 8–10, 2001, San Francisco

State-of-the-Art Clinical Symposium
- April 20–22, 2001, Chicago

Summer Clinical Meeting
- June 21–24, 2001, Santa Barbara

For additional information, contact the ACR office.

ACR Summer Clinical Symposium

The American College of Rheumatology will hold its First Annual Summer Clinical Symposium June 21–24, 2001, at Fess Parker's Doubletree Resort in Santa Barbara, California. The meeting, which will focus on rheumatology practice from a clinical perspective, will provide an update of current knowledge in the broad field of rheumatology, as well as a review of established concepts. Similar in format to the ACR State-of-the-Art Clinical Symposium held in the spring, the Summer Clinical Symposium will offer sessions in both clinical and basic research. Lecturers will outline the direction of state-of-the-art research and detail future prospects for the management of conditions treated by practicing rhematologists. In addition, the format will include both pro/con presentations and discussion between faculty and participants.

Session topics for the First Annual Summer Clinical Symposium are medical ethics in rheumatology practice, nonpharmacologic therapies for knee osteoarthritis, treatment of refractory rheumatoid arthritis, clinical issues in rheumatology, opioid dependency in the rheumatic disease patient, cyclooxygenase 2 inhibitors, refractory systemic lupus erythematosus, osteoarthritis, rheumatic diseases and sleep disorders, inflammatory myopathies, bone mass measurement for osteoporosis, metabolic myopathies, bone tumors, gout, pediatric rheumatology, bone marrow transplants, and sports medicine.

In addition to the educational courses, the Summer Clinical Symposium will feature family-oriented social activities at the end of each day. Activities will include a casual, family-friendly opening reception; a picnic on the beach complete with volleyball, Beach Boys music, and interactive games; and a Mexican Fiesta with a Mariachi band, piñata, paper flower makers, and great food.

The registration deadline for the meeting is Friday, May 18, 2001. If received by that date, the registration fee is $250 for ACR members, $370 for nonmembers, $95 for member trainees, and $115 for nonmember trainees. The registration fee after May 18 is $325 for ACR members, $445 for nonmembers, $120 for member trainees, and $140 for nonmember trainees. Guest registration is free. The ACR special housing rate at Fess Parker's Doubletree Resort is $209 per night single/double, plus tax. After May 18, this special group rate cannot be guaranteed.

Complete registration, housing, and course information can be obtained by calling the ACR Education Department at 404-633-3777. To register online or to obtain up-to-date information on this meeting, visit the ACR's Web site, http://www.rheumatology.org.

American Board of Internal Medicine Certification and Recertification Examinations

The ABIM 2001 Certification Examination in Rheumatology will be held November 7, 2001. The registration period is January 1–April 1, 2001; the late registration period is April 2–June 1, 2001. The ABIM's Recertification Program, which has been renamed the Program for Continuous Professional Development (CPD), consists of an at-home, open-book self-evaluation process and a proctored final examination which will be administered twice each year in May and November. To register for the examination, Diplomates must be enrolled in the CPD Program and be in at least year 6 of their certification cycle. For the 2001 Recertification Examinations in Internal Medicine, its Subspecialties, and Added Qualifications, the final examination will be administered May 1 (registration deadline March 1) and November 7 (registration deadline September 1). For additional information and registration forms, contact Registration Section, American Board of Internal Medicine, 510 Walnut Street, Suite 1700, Philadelphia, PA 19106-3699, phone 800-441-2246 or 215-446-3500, fax 215-446-3590, e-mail request@abim.org, or visit the ABIM's Web site at www.abim.org.

Education Programs

20th Annual Scientific Meeting of the American Pain Society. April 19–22, 2001; Phoenix, AZ. For additional information, contact American Pain Society, 4700 West Lake Avenue, Glenview, IL 60025-1485, phone 847-375-4715, fax 888-508-7578, e-mail info@ampainsoc.org, or visit the Web site http://www.ampainsoc.org/meeting/.

First Joint Meeting of the International Bone and Mineral Society and the European Calcified Tissue Society. June 5–10, 2001, Madrid, Spain. For additional information, contact Lucia Calvo, IBMS/ECTS 2001, c/o Tilcsa OPC, SL,

Londres 17, 28028 Madrid, Spain, phone 34-91-361-2600, fax 34-91-355-9208, e-mail ibms-ects2001@tilesa.es, or visit the Web site http://www.intercongres-2001.com.

20th International League of Associations for Rheumatology (ILAR) World Congress. August 26–31, 2001, Edmonton, Alberta. Canada. The theme of the congress will be Therapy for the 21st Century. For additional information, contact ILAR Secretariat, Health Care Communications, Suite 906, 50 Burnhamthorpe Road West, Mississauga, Ontario, L5B 3C2, Canada. phone 800-535-3330 (from within Canada) or 905-273-3080, fax 905-273-3611, e-mail healthcarecomm@sympatico.ca.

Controversies in Diagnosis, Management, and Costs of Osteoarticular Implications of Obesity. October 12–13, 2001, Brussels, Belgium. For additional information, contact Prof. Dr. M. Szpalski, Centre Hospitalier Molière Longchamps, Rue Marconi 142, 1180 Brussels, Belgium, fax 32-2-348-5694.

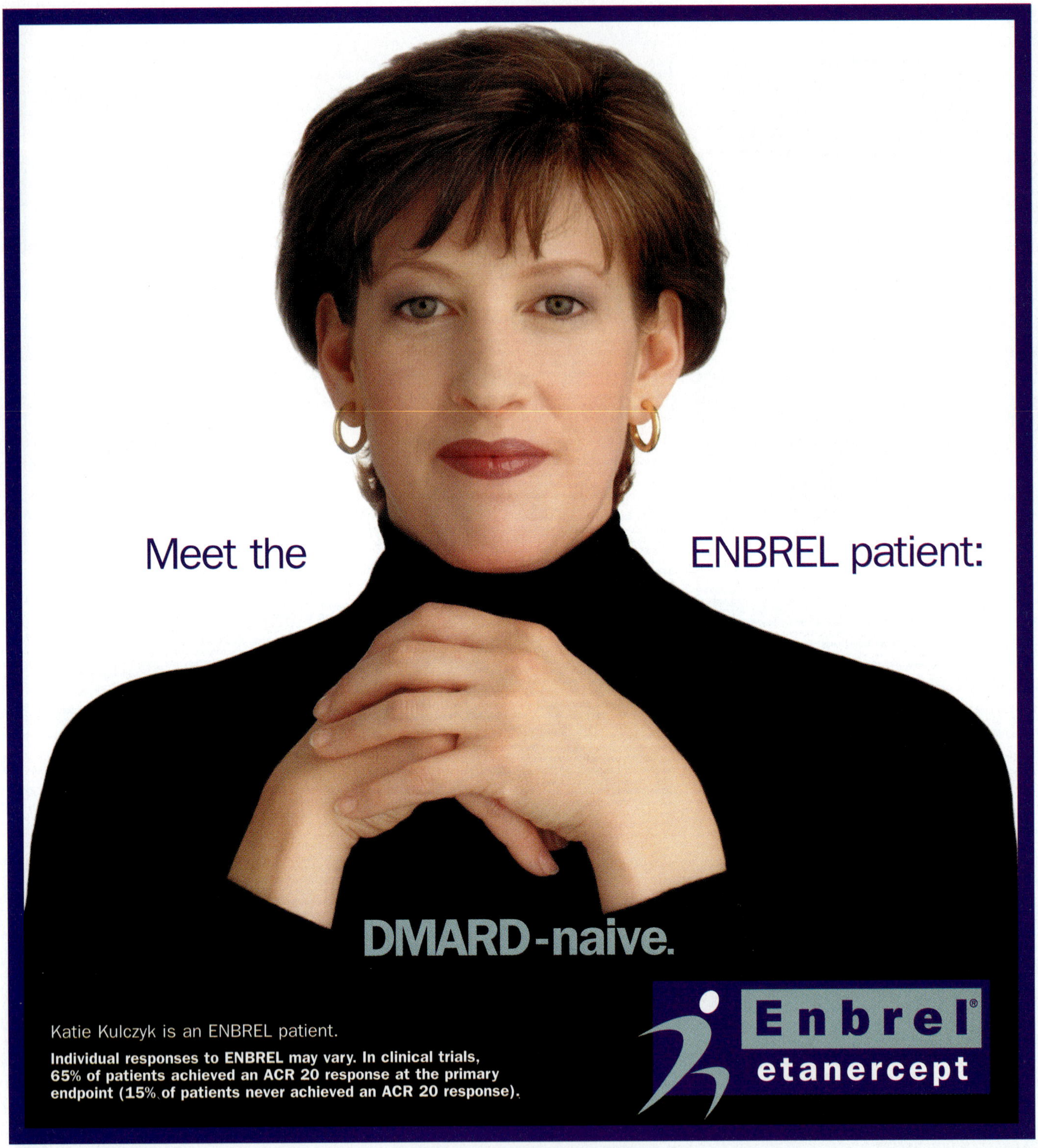
Meet the
ENBREL patient:
DMARD-naive.
Katie Kulczyk is an ENBREL patient.
Individual responses to ENBREL may vary. In clinical trials, 65% of patients achieved an ACR 20 response at the primary endpoint (15% of patients never achieved an ACR 20 response).
Enbrel®
etanercept

ARTHRITIS & RHEUMATISM
Vol. 44, No. 2, February 2001, pp 247–252

Arthritis & Rheumatism

An Official Journal of the American College of Rheumatology
www.arthritisrheum.org and www.interscience.wiley.com

ACR PRESIDENTIAL ADDRESS

The Future Is Now

Joseph D. Croft, Jr.

I am pleased to have this opportunity to review with you the state of the state of the American College of Rheumatology (ACR) and, more importantly, to expand upon the chronicles of our organizational advances and achievements that have transpired over the past year as well as the early years of the past 8 decades.

Before embarking upon this presentation I would like to depart from the traditional protocol that has characterized these presidential addresses. I wish to thank those special people who have encouraged me to serve, at the beginning of my reflections rather than at the end. This year has truly been an extraordinarily rewarding personal journey, and I have been blessed by having my wife, Jane Croft, who also happens to be my best friend, at my side. Our children, Joe Croft and Julia Croft Peterson, have provided encouragement to both Jane and me. Over the past 28 years I have been offered opportunities to serve the College in various capacities, and each of these individuals has been instrumental in sustaining my energy and enthusiasm for the ACR. Mark Andrejeski, our executive vice president, has justifiably been the recipient of multiple accolades, from this podium and elsewhere, for more than a decade. His devotion to the College, his comprehensive understanding of our organization, his commitment to detail and excellence, and his future vision have been inspirational. Sherrie Cathcart and all of the ACR staff and volunteers are examples of extraordinarily dedicated, energetic, and supportive individuals who have made major contributions to the success of our organization. My partners, John Melton, Bob Lloyd, and Jane Gilbert, and our office staff have soldiered through some of my absences with good spirit and reassuring support. To all of you I express my profound appreciation and gratitude.

Adlai Stevenson once said, "We can chart our future clearly and wisely only when we know the past which has led to the present." In order to better understand where we are and where we hope to go, I think it is imperative that we revisit some of those historical events that have served to shape our present and, I would submit, our future activities.

Our current venue, Philadelphia, has been the site of much of the development and success of rheumatology in America (1). Dr. Ralph Pemberton, who was a resident of this city, is regarded by many as the father of American rheumatology. He had a special interest in this field; he started the first arthritis clinic in Pennsylvania in 1926 at the Presbyterian Hospital and later moved to the Abington Hospital, where he limited his practice to rheumatic diseases. In 1927 he traveled to Europe, where he reviewed future needs and directions for the field of rheumatology with physicians who had similar interests, including Dr. van Breeman in Holland. He recognized that, in Europe, our field was represented by a group of professionals of high intellect, great visibility, and influence who had an unbridled commitment to an important cause. Upon his return to America he became an important figure in the establishment of the American Committee for the Control of Rheumatism, a forerunner of the American Rheumatism Association (ARA; now the ACR). He chaired the first scientific meeting of the Committee, held prior to the annual AMA meetings in New Orleans in 1932. Of note is the fact that one of the first papers presented at this meeting addressed the clinical and economic aspects of

---

Presented at the 64th Annual Scientific Meeting of the American College of Rheumatology, Philadelphia, PA, November 1, 2000.

Joseph D. Croft, Jr., MD, Chevy Chase, Maryland: President, American College of Rheumatology, 1999–2000.

Address correspondence and reprint requests to Joseph D. Croft, Jr., MD, 5454 Wisconsin Avenue, Suite 835, Chevy Chase, MD 20815.

Submitted for publication November 15, 2000; accepted November 15, 2000.

arthritis, topics which, of course, have been reviewed at the first plenary session of our 2000 Philadelphia meeting. He became the second President of the American Rheumatism Association (1938–1939), and he was the first American president of the International League of Associations for Rheumatology (ILAR) during the War years. The first International Committee on Rheumatism (the forerunner of ILAR) was founded in 1925, and I would like to take this moment to acknowledge the 75th anniversary of the formation of this important international body. Dr. Pemberton stimulated the interest of a number of Philadelphia physicians in rheumatology, including such notables as Drs. Bernard Comroe, John Lansbury, and Joseph Hollander, among others.

During the 1920s and 1930s there was a widespread campaign to combat rheumatism in the US. A number of new rheumatology units were established. The importance of these programs can hardly be overestimated, not only because of their teaching efforts, but also because of their focus on research and patient care. Some of the pre-1940 names associated with these programs that resonate in the archives of rheumatology include Walter Bauer, Ralph Boots, Joseph Bunim, Martin Dawson, Richard Freyberg, Philip Hench, Currier McEwen, Marian Ropes, Charles Short, Charley Smyth, and Louis Spear.

From an historical point of view, observations regarding notable events of the early twentieth century that served to promote the field of rheumatology certainly must include the initiatives of Philip S. Hench. As we have come to learn, when Dr. Hench was a resident physician at the Mayo Clinic, he developed an interest in rheumatology, and he was offered an opportunity to pursue further training in Germany. Upon his return in 1926, he developed what might be considered the first organized graduate training program in rheumatology in the US. His role in the development of such programs, as well as his efforts to define and treat various rheumatologic disorders, is legendary. He participated in the early US efforts to combat rheumatism on many fronts. As a member of the American Committee for the Control of Rheumatism, he participated in the first open meeting of this group in 1932 (Gallbladder Disease in Chronic Infectious Arthritis: Results of Cholecystectomy), and again at the second conference in 1933 (Analgesic Effect of Hepatitis and Jaundice on Arthritis and Rheumatic Pain). His presentation of the concept of palindromic rheumatism in 1940 is well known to all of us. He was the first chairman of *Rheumatism Reviews* (1934) and the third president of the American Rheumatism Association (1939–1940). He chaired the planning committee for the Seventh International Congress on Rheumatic Diseases which was held in New York in 1949, where he presented early observations on the effect of cortisone to a large group of US and international investigators and practitioners. This year marks the 50th anniversary of the Nobel Prize awarded to Drs. Edward Kendall and Philip Hench for the discovery and use of cortisone.

Clearly the advancement of rheumatology in the US between 1920 and 1940 was a consequence of contributions of a number of influential, experienced, respected, and committed physicians throughout the country. They played major roles in the development of knowledge, the training of students, and the care of patients with rheumatic diseases. A brief and incomplete roll call of these early pioneers might include such names as Russell Cecil, David Ghrist, Donald Hill, Paul Holbrook, Chester Keefer, Maxwell Lockie, H. M. Margolis, William Osler, Robert Stecher, LeRoy Steinberg, Otto Steinbrocker, and Hans Waine, among others. On a personal note, and departing from the pre-1940 focus of these reflections, I want to thank those individuals who have had a profound influence on my professional career, including Ralph Jacox, John Vaughan, and Darrell Crain.

Reflections on the American movement to combat rheumatic diseases certainly must include the efforts of the Arthritis Foundation (AF). Throughout the history of this campaign against rheumatism, there has been awareness on the part of the physician organizers that external financial support would be required in order to meet anticipated research and educational goals. In 1929 the American Committee for the Control of Rheumatism first sought financial support from laypersons. By 1947, members of the ARA, with input from a consultant and the National Research Council, were instrumental in the development and creation of a separate fundraising agency. This agency was incorporated in New York State in 1948 and became known as the American Rheumatism Foundation. It was later reorganized as the AF in 1964.

It was the hope and expectation of the organizing ARA members that the new foundation would develop financial resources that would be used to underwrite ARA programs. Over the intervening years, the AF has made significant financial contributions to research and educational activities in arthritis and rheumatic and musculoskeletal disorders. Between 1965 and 1985 the ARA was a section of the AF and, as you all know, we are now separate institutions. I am pleased to report that during the past year we have continued to interact frequently with the AF. Some of the areas of cooperation during 1999–2000 include expanding the matching research grant terms, presenting our collective interests to the Center for Scientific Review (CSR), the Arthritis Advocacy Partnership, and the National Arthritis Action Plan (NAAP). ACR members participate in various AF committees and leadership positions. Our executive groups continue to meet on a regular basis.

It is important to recognize that for many years there have been a number of additional extremely important supporters of ACR and ACR Research and Education Foundation (REF) activities, including our patients, 2 of whom have made substantial contributions within the past year, other members of the public, charitable organizations, and industry, to name a few.

I bring these matters to your attention not only because of their historical importance but also to point out that the growth and success of the American rheumatism movement has been multifactorial. The impact of committed, highly respected leaders in the medical profession who had a strong sense of volunteerism cannot be overestimated.

I would like to suggest that many current ACR activities bear a strong relationship to the goals and objectives of the original American Committee for the Control of Rheumatism. Early committee minutes, as well as an editorial in the *Journal of the American Medical Association* (July 7, 1928) (2), outline some of the plans, including the following:

1. Promotion of research
2. Improved education of medical students
3. Updating practicing physicians
4. Evaluation of therapies and measures of proven value
5. Establishment of databases and improvement of nomenclature
6. Timely delivery of information regarding existing therapies and measures of proven value

The American Committee became the American Association for the Control of Rheumatism in 1934. The name was changed to the American Rheumatism Association in 1937 and, of course, the ARA's name was changed to the ACR in 1988. Another notable moment in the history of the ACR was in 1994, when the Arthritis Health Professionals Association became a Division of the ACR as the Association of Rheumatology Health Professionals (ARHP).

In 1985, when the ARA became an independent organization, leadership convened and prepared a detailed plan for the future. The central focus of these deliberations was to identify those activities that were considered critical to the survival of this new association. Three principal survival issues were defined. One of the essential elements included attracting a committed membership which would represent many constituencies who would support the mission of the organization, namely research, education, and patient care. Additional, equally vital priorities included the need to conduct a successful annual meeting and the requirement to publish a financially sound journal of the highest scientific quality. Our commitment to these survival functions, combined with the efforts of the volunteers and staff, are vital to the success of our organization. An assessment of the College's activities during the past year confirms our ongoing commitment to these 3 activities:

1. The nucleus of our organization, the membership, continues to grow. Our current membership is over 7,200 (3,597 US Fellows). There are various categories of membership. The ARHP has over 850 members.
2. Attendance at our annual meeting has more than doubled over the past decade. The first annual meeting of the millennium has attracted over 7,100 physician attendees. The Committee on Continuing Medical Education, chaired by Maren Mahowald, has general oversight responsibilities for this annual meeting. The Professional Meetings Subcommittee, chaired by Len Calabrese, supervises interim meetings.
3. Abstract submissions for the annual meeting have increased approximately 50% since 1993. Peggy Crow, chair of the Annual Meeting Planning Subcommittee, Harvi Luthra, chair of the Abstract Selection Subcommittee, and their respective committee members have devoted an extraordinary level of energy and expertise in reviewing over 3,000 abstracts and preparing the scientific agenda for all phases of this meeting. Abstract submission rates remain high.
4. Journal submissions have increased over 60% from 1993. The Committee on Journal Publications, chaired by Gary Hoffman, has overseen important events that have transpired regarding our journals, *Arthritis & Rheumatism* (*A&R*) and *Arthritis Care and Research* (*AC&R*). David Pisetsky has been named the new editor of *A&R*, and Gene Hunder has accepted the editorship of *AC&R*. John Wiley and Sons will become the new publisher for both journals. *AC&R* has been designated as an official

journal of the College and will become a section of *A&R*. The Committee on Journal Publications has been reorganized to reflect this change. Both journals went online earlier this year. Submissions to both journals continue to increase, and their scientific quality remains highly acclaimed.

The past year has been very productive for the College in many areas, and I would like to update you on some of these activities and initiatives:

1. A new strategic plan has been developed that is designed to guide ACR activities over the next 3–5 years. This effort was chaired by Audrey Nelson. Part of our organizational culture has been to address anticipated future challenges *now*, with the expectation of setting a successful course and direction for future activities.
2. The Ethics Subcommittee, chaired by Rich Panush, has been charged with addressing a number of important issues, including establishing a code of conduct for many of our volunteers as well as revising our disclosure statement.
3. The High Impact Rheumatology program, under the auspices of Dr. Maren Mahowald and the Committee on Continuing Medical Education, was completed in March. This consisted of 120 programs for primary care physicians conducted by 34 groups in 84 cities, with a total attendance of over 3,900. The program was highly acclaimed by the attendees. Significant financial resources were allocated to the development of the curriculum as well as to the participating sites. The curriculum has been put on our Web site and on a CD-ROM and is intended for noncommercial educational purposes only. Exploratory discussions are under way with our international colleagues to present these materials to an international audience.
4. The Committee on Educational Products, chaired by Mike Maricic, continues to develop and produce interactive educational programs including placing the 1998 Core Curriculum Supplement Cases on CD-ROM (introduced at this meeting) and developing a Rheumatology Self-Assessment Program. The revision of the Core Curriculum is close to completion.
5. Our Board of Directors (BOD) has approved a report of the Blue Ribbon Committee on New Therapies. This Blue Ribbon Committee was chaired by David Wofsy. An ad hoc committee led by Mike Condit and Paul Katz has reviewed and prioritized the recommendations. Action plans and budget requests recommended by the ad hoc committee have been approved.
6. The ACR has accepted a seat on the International Steering Committee of the Decade of the Bone and Joint movement. The mission of the group is to (a) raise awareness of the growing burden of musculoskeletal disorders on society; (b) promote prevention of musculoskeletal disorders and empower patients through education campaigns; (c) advance research in prevention, diagnosis, and treatment of musculoskeletal disorders; and (d) improve diagnosis and treatment of musculoskeletal disorders. Ted Harris and Mark Hochberg have agreed to be our delegates to this group. The College plans to participate actively in furthering the efforts of the US National Action Committee.
7. The BOD has appointed an ad hoc Internet Technology Committee, chaired by Eric Schned, which is charged with the responsibility of defining our current capabilities as well as future technology needs of the College.
8. The Committee on Communications and Marketing, led by Eric Schned, will continue to be responsible for *ACR News* and *Hotline,* and it has forwarded recommendations for future media relations activities and membership surveys.
9. The Committee on Rheumatologic Care, chaired by Mark Robbins, has long been and will continue to be a valuable resource for practice management. The contributions of this group to improved practice reimbursement profiles are well known. They are planning to oversee the development of a practice analysis instrument, which will measure the financial and managerial health of clinical practices. The creation of a rheumatology-specific electronic medical template, as well as establishing benchmark data for academic rheumatology practices, are being considered.
10. The Committee on Government Affairs, chaired by Robert Yood, continues to advocate for full implementation of Resource-Based Practice Expense legislation. It has developed a Public Policy Plan, and it lobbies annually on Capitol Hill with Advocates for Arthritis (most recently advocating for increased federal funding for rheumatic disease research, patient protection in managed care, and increased funding for the NAAP). Additional coalitions have been formed, including the Arthritis Advocacy Partnership, and this committee continues to exhibit leadership in policy develop-

ment. There is ongoing monitoring of prescription drug coverage legislation, a very challenging issue.

11. The Committee on Rheumatology Training and Workforce Issues, chaired by Dennis Boulware, has been instrumental in establishing criteria for the Clinician Investigator and Clinician Scholar Educator awards. The fellowship program directors' retreats have been well received. The formation of a Fellowship Subcommittee with members from the trainee member category will foster development of future ACR leaders and give the Fellows a sense of identity with our organization.
12. The contributions of the Committee on Research, chaired by Mike Holers, include efforts to enhance the visibility of our specialty in the NIH scientific review process (CSR). The College will cosponsor a forthcoming NIAMS conference on the role of anti-TNF therapy in RA, and the Research Committee will serve as our liaison group. They are developing a strategy for immediate and ongoing review of new therapies. Over 500 individuals attended their Basic Research Conference just prior to our 2000 Annual Meeting.
13. The Committee on Nominations and Appointments, chaired by Bevra Hahn, set in place a new, detailed, and comprehensive process for appointing individuals to our very important volunteer corps, and this group, some of whom have been identified at this meeting, will play a critical role in the future success of the College. I am pleased to announce that this committee has suggested, and the BOD has recently recommended, the creation of an ACR Distinguished Service Award. This award will recognize an ACR member who, as an active volunteer, has provided outstanding service on behalf of the College.
14. The Committee on Finance, chaired by Betsy Tindall, has presided over a period of unprecedented prosperity and continues to be the important oversight body supervising the finances of the College. Our current total net assets of over 11 million dollars have more than doubled since 1997.

I also want to acknowledge the role of the ARHP, whose president this past year was Jill Noaker-Luck. Their contributions to this meeting, and to ACR activities in general, are greatly valued. They have worked diligently and with great expertise in preparing *AC&R* for the next century, and they are currently working to complete the second edition of *Clinical Care in the Rheumatic Diseases,* among other educational products. Several of their members currently participate in our new and very important Internet technology efforts.

The REF, whose current president is Stan Cohen, has expanded its very ambitious program. This group was established in 1986 to advance basic research in rheumatology. Its mission statement has recently been broadened to state a need to attract qualified physicians and other health care professionals into careers in rheumatology. It is anticipated that such a mission modification will provide a stimulus for the development and expansion of programs that are designed to address concerns regarding training and workforce challenges that confront our specialty.

In an effort to fund awards that will sustain the above mission, the REF has established an Industry Roundtable (IRT). Each of the 9 members, all of whom were recognized at our plenary session yesterday, has made a major 3-year financial commitment to the REF. The funds will be used to support current and expanded training, research, and educational programs sponsored by the REF. Such initiatives are vital to the success of the REF and the College. Long-term external financial support will be important in order to continue these scholarly activities. Instruments for creating a stable future financial environment for the support of these programs are being explored. Two weeks ago, one of our IRT partners announced a major gift to the REF, which will fund an endowment that will support our Pediatric Visiting Professor Program for many years to come. Our leadership and roundtable participants remain committed to the concept that the tone and agenda for such partnerships must reflect the high professional standards that have guided ACR actions over the years. Such a philosophy is consistent with membership expectations.

On a final note, I would like to emphasize that the ACR has been, and will continue to be, a global organization. We were an early contributor to ILAR (1934), a founding member of the Pan-American League Against Rheumatism (1944), and we have participated in and/or hosted a number of international meetings over the last 50 years. Our international friends make significant and very important contributions to the College. Over 70% of *A&R* journal submissions and over 60% of annual meeting abstract submissions come from the international community. Over half of our annual meeting attendees come from outside the US. I would anticipate that our international colleagues will continue to play an important role in our future successes. Our BOD has recently recommended that our most prestigious award, the Gold Medal, should be renamed the Presidential Gold Medal. Candidates for this award will include all US and international ACR members.

I have attempted to review past and present events that either have shaped or are likely to shape our future. The ACR is entering the new century on sound financial footing and with substantial financial commitments. We are fortunate in having a team of committed and talented volunteers. We must husband their time, talent, and skills with care. Our experienced professional staff will provide the structure and direction that will help us to prosper. Our well-constructed strategic plan provides an important template for a successful future.

These are challenging times for medicine. Managed care and Medicare changes have had a profound impact on our members who are engaged in research, education, and patient care. Recent critical commentary in the press and scientific journals reporting on ethical issues related to clinical research and patient care sends a sense of concern through the scientific community (3–7). The ACR mission, namely, to develop and deliver educational, research, and advocacy programs, is designed to foster excellence in the care of people with arthritis and rheumatic and musculoskeletal diseases. The College has been fortunate in having been served by a group of individuals of high integrity and high ethical standards. Our leadership will continue to serve as a "moral beacon," which will focus on the welfare of our patients. Such attention will serve to maintain our ethical integrity and, at the same time, maintain the sense of trust that has been bestowed upon us by the public. Our commitment to professionalism, as well as our tradition of "taking the moral high road," will serve us well. I am confident that, in light of the above organizational efforts and considerations, combined with our historical commitment to excellence, our launch into the 21st century will be highly successful.

REFERENCES

1. Smyth CJ, Freyberg RH, McEwen C. History of rheumatology. Atlanta: Arthritis Foundation; 1985.
2. Pemberton R. The control of rheumatism [editorial]. JAMA 1928; 91:30–1.
3. Companies' influence on medical studies is feared. Washington Post 2000 Aug 16; p. A8.
4. Pellegrino ED, Relman AS. Professional medical associations: ethical and practical guidelines. JAMA 1999;282:984–6.
5. Rothman DJ. Medical professionalism: focusing on the real issues. N Engl J Med 2000;342:1284–6.
6. Bodenheimer T. Uneasy alliance, clinical investigators and the pharmaceutical industry. N Engl J Med 2000;342:1539–44.
7. Angell M. Is academic medicine for sale? [editorial]. N Engl J Med 2000;342:1516.

ARTHRITIS & RHEUMATISM
Vol. 44, No. 2, February 2001, pp 253–259

REVIEW

The Role of Osteoprotegerin and Receptor Activator of Nuclear Factor κB Ligand in the Pathogenesis and Treatment of Rheumatoid Arthritis

Lorenz C. Hofbauer and Armin E. Heufelder

Introduction

The skeletal complications of rheumatoid arthritis (RA) include focal bone erosions and juxtaarticular osteopenia at sites of active inflammation, as well as systemic osteopenia, resulting in significant joint deformity, disability, and pain in addition to an increased risk of bone fractures (1,2). Several lines of evidence have clearly established that osteoclasts, multinucleated cells of the monocyte/macrophage lineage, are key mediators of bone loss in RA (2–4). Activated T cells, a proinflammatory cytokine milieu, and their interactions with cells of the bone microenvironment and the immune system have been suggested as potential mechanisms that promote the differentiation and activation of osteoclasts and lead to enhanced bone resorption (2).

The recent identification and characterization of receptor activator of nuclear factor κB ligand (RANKL), an essential cytokine for various osteoclast functions, its receptor, receptor activator of nuclear factor κB (RANK), and its decoy receptor, osteoprotegerin (OPG), have created a new molecular and cellular concept of osteoclast biology, bone resorption, and bone and cartilage homeostasis (5–7) (Table 1). The fact that RANK is expressed on osteoclasts and dendritic cells (DCs), that RANKL regulates important functions of osteoclasts, DCs, and T cells, and that bone marrow stromal cells and activated T cells produce RANKL suggests common paracrine pathways in the regulation of bone metabolism and immune functions. In this article, we highlight the potential roles of RANKL, RANK, and OPG in the pathogenesis and treatment of skeletal lesions in RA.

Dr. Hofbauer's work was supported by Deutsche Forschungsgemeinschaft grant Ho-1875/2-1.
Lorenz C. Hofbauer, MD, Armin E. Heufelder, MD: Philipps University, Marburg, Germany.
Address correspondence and reprint requests to Lorenz C. Hofbauer, MD, Division of Gastroenterology, Endocrinology, and Metabolism, Zentrum für Innere Medizin, Philipps University, Baldingerstrasse, D-35033 Marburg, Germany.
Submitted for publication July 26, 2000; accepted in revised form September 27, 2000.

Regulation of bone metabolism by RANKL, RANK, and OPG

RANKL (also called osteoprotegerin ligand [OPGL], osteoclast differentiation factor [ODF], tumor necrosis factor–related activation-induced cytokine [TRANCE]) is a membrane-bound peptide (317 amino acids) of the tumor necrosis factor (TNF) ligand superfamily (8–11). Posttranslational processing by TNFα-converting enzyme–like protease generates a soluble extracellular RANKL form of comparable biologic activity (12) (Figure 1). Rich sources of RANKL expression include T lymphocytes and osteoblastic lineage cells (marrow stromal cells and mature osteoblasts) (8–11). Of note, a squamous cell carcinoma cell line and activated T lymphocytes have been shown to express a secreted form of RANKL (13) (Figure 1).

In the presence of permissive concentrations of macrophage colony-stimulating factor (M-CSF), RANKL stimulates in vitro the differentiation, proliferation, fusion, and activation of osteoclastic lineage cells, and suppresses osteoclast apoptosis, resulting in an increased number of functionally active osteoclasts and enhanced bone resorption (14–17) (Figure 1). While RANKL and M-CSF are required and sufficient to stimulate osteoclast differentiation and activation, a recent report suggested that TNFα and interleukin-1 (IL-1) may regulate these processes in a RANKL-independent manner (18). In vivo, treatment of mice with RANKL activates osteoclasts, promotes bone loss, and causes severe hypercalcemia (8), whereas RANKL deletion results in the absence of mature osteoclasts and the subsequent development of osteopetrosis (generalized increased bone mass) (19).

Table 1. Glossary of abbreviations related to bone metabolism and immune function in rheumatoid arthritis

Abbreviation	Definition
DC	Dendritic cell
IL	Interleukin
M-CSF	Macrophage colony-stimulating factor
OPG	Osteoprotegerin
RA	Rheumatoid arthritis
RANK	Receptor activator of nuclear factor κB
RANKL	Receptor activator of nuclear factor κB ligand
TACE	Tumor necrosis factor α–converting enzyme–like protease
TNFα	Tumor necrosis factor α
TNFR	Tumor necrosis factor receptor
TRAF	Tumor necrosis factor receptor–associated factors
TRANCE	Tumor necrosis factor–related activation-induced cytokine

RANKL exerts its biologic effects upon binding to, and activating, RANK, a transmembrane receptor of the TNF receptor (TNFR) superfamily, which is mainly expressed by osteoclasts, DCs, and B and T lymphocytes (11,20,21). RANK signal transduction involves several TNFR-associated factors, including nuclear factor κB, c-Fos, c-Src, c-Jun N-terminal kinase, and the antiapoptotic serine/threonine kinase protein kinase B/Akt. Deletion of RANK in mice generates a phenotype identical to that of RANKL-deficient animals (22,23).

OPG is a soluble receptor that belongs to the TNFR superfamily and acts as a receptor antagonist (24,25). OPG is ubiquitously produced by a variety of tissues, cell types, and cell lines (7,24,25). OPG binds both the soluble and cell-bound forms of RANKL and, thus, prevents their interaction with, and stimulation of, RANK (14–17). Consistent with this, the in vitro effects of OPG include inhibition of osteoclast differentiation, survival, fusion, and activation of osteoclasts, as well as stimulation of osteoclast apoptosis, thereby reducing the pool of active osteoclasts that are capable of resorbing bone (14–17,24,25) (Figure 1). In vivo, overexpression of OPG in transgenic mice (24) or administration of OPG to normal rodents (24,25) substantially inhibits osteoclastogenesis, osteoclast activation, and bone resorption, resulting in an osteopetrotic phenotype. Moreover, OPG administration has been demonstrated to prevent ovariectomy-induced bone loss (24). In contrast, OPG deletion has been associated with enhanced osteoclastogenesis and osteoclast activation, increased bone resorption, and massive osteoporosis (26,27).

Modulation of the immune system by RANKL, RANK, and OPG

There is compelling experimental evidence that RANKL, RANK, and OPG are also critical determinants of DC functions and T cell–mediated immune responses (6). Before the search for the cognate ligand of OPG succeeded in identifying OPGL/ODF (8,9), 2 independent groups of investigators had identified RANKL or TRANCE as a T cell–derived immunomodulatory cytokine (10,11). DCs have the ability to present antigens to T cells and to activate a T cell response, highlighting their gatekeeping position in regulating cellular immune responses (6). Expression of RANK has been detected in DCs, and its activation by RANKL prevents apoptosis (by up-regulating Bcl-x_L expression) and increases survival of DCs, which results in enhanced DC-mediated T cell proliferation (11,12,28,29) (Figure 2).

All of these stimulatory effects of RANKL can be abrogated by OPG (6). DC-derived cytokines that are stimulated by RANKL–RANK interaction include proinflammatory cytokines, such as IL-6 and IL-11, as well as T cell growth and proliferation factors (IL-12,

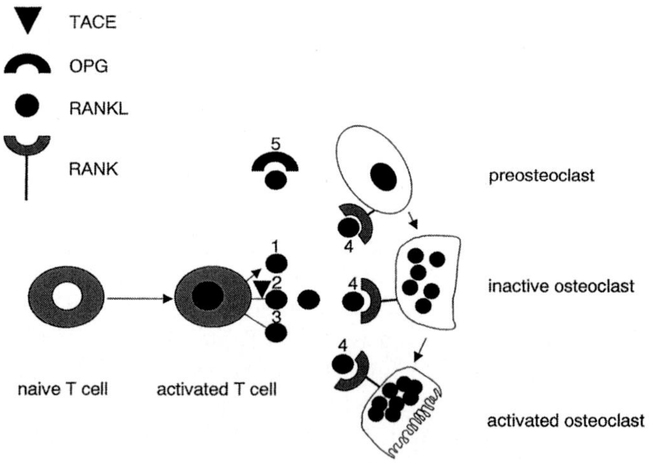

Figure 1. Roles of receptor activator of nuclear factor κB ligand (RANKL), receptor activator of nuclear factor κB (RANK), and osteoprotegerin (OPG) in T cell–osteoclast interactions. Activated T lymphocytes express a primary soluble form (**1**) and a cellular form (**3**) of RANKL, the latter of which is posttranslationally cleaved by the protease tumor necrosis factor α–converting enzyme–like protease (TACE) to give rise to a secondary soluble ectodomain form of RANKL (**2**). All 3 RANKL variants bind to and activate RANK, which is located on the surface of osteoclasts (**4**), induce osteoclast formation, survival, fusion, and activation, and inhibit osteoclast apoptosis, thus expanding the pool of osteoclasts that are capable of resorbing bone and cartilage. OPG represents a decoy receptor that blocks RANKL–RANK interactions (**5**).

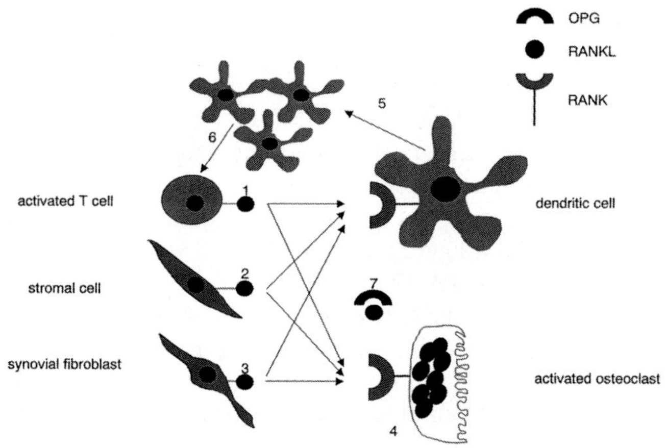

Figure 2. Link between bone metabolism and immune system in rheumatoid arthritis (RA) through RANKL, RANK, and OPG. In joint lesions affected by RA, RANKL is produced by activated T cells **(1)**, marrow stromal cells **(2)**, and synovial fibroblasts **(3)** (for clarity, only the cellular RANKL form is shown). RANKL activates its receptor RANK, which is located on osteoclasts and dendritic cells (DCs). Osteoclastic activation results in cartilage destruction and periarticular and systemic bone loss **(4)**, while RANK activation in DCs prolongs DC survival and inhibits their apoptosis **(5)**. Activated DCs may promote T cell activation through enhanced antigen presentation (and may facilitate the generation of autoreactive T cells) **(6)**. All these effects are antagonized by the decoy receptor OPG **(7)**. See Figure 1 for other definitions.

IL-15) (29). In addition, neutralization of RANKL by a soluble RANK prevented T helper cell activation following viral infection (30). Of note, a cell-bound form of OPG (which is up-regulated by CD40 ligand) has been exclusively demonstrated in a DC line (31) (Figure 2).

RANKL and RANK are also essential elements for the development of lymphoid tissues. Mice deficient in RANKL (19) or RANK (22,23) display severe immunologic defects, including abnormal thymocyte and B lymphocyte development as well as impaired DC-mediated T lymphocyte activation and cytokine production. Surprisingly, the phenotype of RANKL-deficient or RANK-deficient animals revealed (in addition to severe osteopetrosis) thymus and Peyer's patch hypoplasia, a complete lack of lymph nodes, and a normally structured, but enlarged spleen as a result of extramedullary hematopoiesis due to osteopetrosis (19,22,23).

Thus, RANKL–RANK interactions are critical for 2 pivotal functions of the immune system: 1) early development and maturation of pre–B cells and pre–T cells in the bone marrow and thymus; and 2) interactions between mature DCs and T cells. While the former function is required for the orderly formation and function of lymphoid structures, the latter function is critical in modulating immune responses and preventing inadequate activation of autoreactive T cells. The expression of RANK by osteoclasts and DCs, the production of RANKL by osteoblastic lineage cells and activated T cells, and the requirement of RANKL or RANK for the development of normal bone and lymphoid tissue (evident from the phenotypes of knockout mice) all support the concept that the pleiotropic RANKL–RANK–OPG system represents a central molecular link between bone metabolism and the immune system (Figure 2). This has obvious implications for the pathogenesis of RA, as discussed below.

Modulation of RANKL, RANK, and OPG by cytokines

Various proinflammatory and proresorptive cytokines (IL-1, IL-6, IL-11, IL-17, M-CSF, parathyroid hormone–related peptide, and TNFα) have been detected in inflamed synovial tissues and have been implicated as mediators of bone and cartilage loss through stimulation of osteoclastic bone resorption (2,32). Because of the essential roles of RANKL, RANK, and OPG in bone metabolism and immune function, it was hypothesized that these cytokines converge at the level of RANKL and OPG, and that proresorptive cytokines affect bone resorption through a modulation of the RANKL:OPG ratio (7). In fact, IL-1, IL-11, IL-17, oncostatin, TNFα, parathyroid hormone–related peptide, and prostaglandin E_2 have all been demonstrated to enhance RANKL messenger RNA (mRNA) levels, whereas parathyroid hormone–related peptide and prostaglandin E_2 concurrently inhibit OPG mRNA levels (5–7).

The net effect of IL-1 and TNFα on the RANKL:OPG ratio appears to be moderate, since these cytokines stimulate both RANKL and OPG mRNA to a similar extent (33). Both cytokines have also been shown to induce osteoclast activation through a RANKL-independent pathway (5–7). IL-6, a potent proresorptive cytokine, is capable of inducing RANKL mRNA in rodent marrow stromal cell systems, but not in human stromal cells (5–7,33).

Abnormalities of RANKL, RANK, and OPG in RA

In vitro studies. Activated T cells (which constitute a major population of immune cells in the inflamed synovium in RA), but not resting T cells, express RANKL and are capable of inducing functionally active osteoclasts (34,35) (Figure 1). Kong et al (34) used activated T cells (fixed with paraformaldehyde) or supernatant from activated T cells in a coculture model to generate osteoclasts. Of note, both the cell-bound and the soluble form of RANKL are produced by activated T cells and induce osteoclastogenesis to a similar extent, an effect which can be specifically blocked by OPG, but not by antibodies directed against other cytokines (34) (Figure 1). Horwood et al (35) used a coculture model of human activated T cells and murine splenocytes (which contain osteoclast precursor cells) to induce osteoclasts, and this process was enhanced by IL-1 and transforming growth factor β. It is important to note that many T cell–derived cytokines, such as interferon-γ, IL-4, and IL-10, inhibit osteoclast formation in vitro (36,37).

Thus, activated T cells are a potential source of RANKL and, provided that appropriate cell culture techniques are employed, may facilitate the formation and activation of osteoclasts. However, further studies are required to address the potency of T cell–derived RANKL (as compared with bone marrow stromal cells, osteoblasts, and synovial fibroblasts) on osteoclast biology and to dissect the role of secreted versus cell-bound RANKL.

Animal models. The concept that systemic activation of T cells promotes bone loss is supported by the severe osteoporosis in CTLA-4–deficient mice, in which T cells are spontaneously activated (34). In addition, transfer of bone marrow stromal cells derived from CTLA-4–deficient mice into RAG-1–deficient mice (which lack lymphocytes) or RANKL-deficient mice was also shown to cause osteoporosis associated with an increased number of osteoclasts, which could be prevented by daily administration of OPG. These results indicate that T cell–derived RANKL is sufficient to activate osteoclasts in vivo (34).

Using adjuvant-induced arthritis as an established rat model of RA (generated by subcutaneous injection of *Mycobacterium tuberculosis*), Kong et al (34) demonstrated that synovial fibroblasts and inflammatory cells express RANKL mRNA. Over the course of 7 days, rats developed a profound loss of cortical and trabecular bone, which was associated with an increased number of osteoclasts, extensive joint erosions with matrix degeneration, and signs and symptoms of crippling (34). In collagen-induced arthritis, an established murine model of RA (generated by intradermal injection of type II collagen), osteoclasts were detected at sites of active bone erosions and were found to be located adjacent to RANKL-producing, synovium-infiltrating mononuclear cells and chondrocytes (38). In this model, osteoclasts were found to produce RANKL, which suggests that this peptide may act as an autocrine factor for osteoclasts (38).

Human disease. Several studies in humans have indicated that RANKL and OPG may play key roles in mediating the bone and cartilage damage in RA (39–43). Immunohistochemical and in situ hybridization studies have localized RANKL expression to T cells within lymphoid aggregates of inflamed synovial tissues in patients with RA (35,39,40), but not in intact synovium (39) or in the synovium of patients with osteoarthritis (40). RANKL mRNA and protein were also detected in synovial fibroblasts and activated T lymphocytes cultured from these areas of inflamed synovium (39,40). Moreover, synovial fibroblasts derived from patients with RA promoted osteoclastogenesis when stimulated with 1,25-dihydroxyvitamin D_3, which was facilitated by an increase in RANKL and a decrease in OPG production, and could be abrogated by administration of OPG (40).

Consistent with these observations, immunohistochemical analyses in patients with RA demonstrated the presence of osteoclasts in areas of pannus invasion into bone and adjacent to sites where RANKL expression is highest, underscoring the concept that increased RANKL expression is biologically significant (39). In another study, synovial macrophages from patients with RA were capable of differentiating into osteoclasts in the presence of RANKL and M-CSF (43).

Of note, IL-17, a T cell–derived cytokine, may partly mediate T cell production of RANKL, since IL-17 was found in high concentrations in the synovial fluid and was shown to be a potent inducer of RANKL mRNA (41). Moreover, IL-17–stimulated osteoclast differentiation and activation was prevented by OPG, indicating that IL-17 may represent an up-stream signal that converges at RANKL to cause bone loss in RA (41). In addition to the increase in RANKL in the inflamed synovium of RA patients, OPG concentrations in the synovial fluid are lower in patients with RA (as compared with patients with other forms of arthritis), which results in an increased local and systemic RANKL:OPG ratio (42).

These data therefore suggest that RANKL is an important cytokine that mediates bone and joint destruction in human RA, and that OPG has a protective role in this condition.

Therapeutic potential of OPG

Based on the concept that an increased local or systemic ratio of RANKL to OPG may favor enhanced osteoclastic bone resorption in various metabolic bone diseases, exogenous administration of recombinant OPG has been successfully used in various animal models of bone diseases to control bone and mineral abnormalities resulting from inadequate osteoclast activity. These diseases include estrogen deficiency (24), humoral hypercalcemia of malignancy (44–46), hyperparathyroidism (46), metastatic bone tumors (47), and immobilization (48). OPG administration exerted a rapid and pronounced effect and had no adverse effects (24,44–48). A controlled clinical study has recently confirmed the antiresorptive effect of recombinant human OPG therapy in postmenopausal women (49). A single monthly injection of OPG decreased by 80% the concentrations of deoxypyridinoline, a biochemical marker of bone resorption, indicating that the data obtained in animals can be extrapolated to humans.

Because RANKL production by activated T cells and synovial fibroblasts is increased in inflamed joints in RA (38–41) and because OPG levels in the synovial fluid are inappropriately low to compensate for this (40,42), the RANKL:OPG ratio—a critical determinant of osteoclast differentiation and activation—is enhanced (40). In vitro administration of OPG prevented osteoclastogenesis by synovial fibroblasts derived from patients with RA, proving the principle that blocking RANKL through administration of OPG may provide a novel therapeutic strategy in RA (40). Kong and associates have convincingly demonstrated in vivo that neutralization of RANKL by daily injections of recombinant OPG completely prevents bone and joint abnormalities in rat adjuvant arthritis, without apparent adverse effects and without altering the inflammatory process (34).

These findings suggest that blockage of RANKL by OPG does not interfere with T cell–dependent effects on inflammation and immune response, and that the effects of RANKL on DC functions are not critical to the synovitis or inflammation in this model (34). Furthermore, the protective effects of OPG on cartilage matrix may involve other mechanisms in addition to blocking RANKL and inhibiting osteoclastic activity (34).

Moreover, suppression of synovial RANKL and IL-17 production by local overexpression of IL-4 in collagen-induced arthritis was found to prevent bone and joint erosions in a similar manner, suggesting that therapeutic strategies that enhance local IL-4 production may protect against cartilage and bone destruction in RA (50).

A recent study has suggested that combined neutralization of IL-1, TNFα, and RANKL by administration of either IL-1 receptor antagonist or soluble TNFR type I and OPG suppresses both inflammation and bone loss in rats with adjuvant arthritis (51). Taken together, these findings indicate that OPG treatment may evolve as a novel therapeutic modality for patients with severe RA once standard treatment regimens have failed.

Summary and integration of mechanisms

Activated autoreactive T cells and an increased number and activity of osteoclasts have long been implicated in the pathogenesis of bone and joint erosions in RA. Following identification of the novel TNF ligand and receptor triad, RANKL, RANK, and OPG, and their detailed characterization by in vitro, in vivo, and knockout studies, it has become evident that this cytokine system links the immune system to bone metabolism (Figure 2). RANKL is produced by bone marrow stromal cells and activated T cells, and is essential for the differentiation, activation, and survival of osteoclasts, the survival of DCs, and DC–T cell interactions, whereas OPG represents the endogenous decoy receptor with opposite effects.

Activation of osteoclasts through RANKL produced by activated T cells has been demonstrated by in vitro and in vivo systems, rodent models, and the pathologic features of RA in humans. The production of both the cell-bound and soluble forms of RANKL by activated T cells plausibly explains the entire spectrum of skeletal complications in RA, including bone and joint erosions (both forms), juxtaarticular osteoporosis (both forms), and systemic osteoporosis (soluble form). T cell–dependent activation of osteoclasts in RA may represent the prototype disease model for bone loss and osteoporosis associated with inflammatory, autoimmune, and lymphoproliferative diseases that are characterized by systemic activation of T cells, including chronic viral and bacterial infections, chronic inflammatory bowel diseases, and lymphoma or leukemia. Additional factors that may aggravate bone loss in RA include the systemic use of glucocorticoids and immobilization, both of which are associated with an increased RANKL:OPG ratio in bone (52,53) and can be prevented by exogenous administration of OPG (48).

Systemic parenteral administration of OPG has been shown to control the signs and symptoms of various metabolic bone diseases in animal models (44–48) and to prevent increased bone resorption in postmenopausal women (49). The beneficial effects of systemic administration of decoy receptors targeting other TNF ligands or lymphotoxins have been documented in animal models of autoimmune diseases, including systemic lupus erythematosus, inflammatory bowel disease, and graft-versus-host disease (54). Based on its molecular and cellular mode of action, its pleiotropic modulation of bone metabolism and immune function, and its compelling protective effects in animal models of RA, recombinant OPG will be a powerful and rational therapeutic approach that deserves careful evaluation in patients with RA.

REFERENCES

1. Gough AK, Lilley J, Eyre S, Holdin R, Emery P. Generalized bone loss in patients with rheumatoid arthritis. Lancet 1994;344:23–7.
2. Goldring SR, Gravallese EM. Pathogenesis of bone erosions in rheumatoid arthritis. Curr Opin Rheumatol 2000;12:195–9.
3. Bromley M, Woolley DE. Chondroclasts and osteoclasts at subchondral sites of erosion in the rheumatoid joint. Arthritis Rheum 1984;27:968–75.
4. Gravallese EM, Harada Y, Wang JT, Gorn AH, Thornhill TS, Goldring SR. Identification of cell types responsible for bone resorption in rheumatoid arthritis and juvenile rheumatoid arthritis. Am J Pathol 1998;152:943–51.
5. Suda T, Takahashi N, Udagawa N, Jimi E, Gillespie MT, Martin TJ. Modulation of osteoclast differentiation and function by the new members of the tumor necrosis factor receptor and ligand families. Endocr Rev 1999;20:345–57.
6. Wong BR, Josien R, Choi Y. TRANCE is a TNF family member that regulates dendritic cell and osteoclast function. J Leukoc Biol 1999;65:715–24.
7. Hofbauer LC, Khosla S, Lacey DL, Dunstan CR, Boyle WJ, Riggs BL. The roles of osteoprotegerin and osteoprotegerin ligand in the paracrine regulation of bone resorption. J Bone Miner Res 2000;15:2–12.
8. Lacey DL, Timms E, Tan H-L, Kelley MJ, Dunstan CR, Burgess T, et al. Osteoprotegerin (OPG) ligand is a cytokine that regulates osteoclast differentiation and activation. Cell 1998;93:165–76.
9. Yasuda H, Shima N, Nakagawa N, Yamaguchi K, Kinosaki M, Mochizuki S-I, et al. Osteoclast differentiation factor is a ligand for osteoprotegerin/osteoclastogenesis-inhibitory factor and is identical to TRANCE/RANKL. Proc Natl Acad Sci U S A 1998;95: 3597–602.
10. Wong BR, Rho J, Arron J, Robinson E, Orlinick J, Chao M, et al. TRANCE is a novel ligand of the tumor necrosis factor receptor family that activates c-jun N-terminal kinase in T cells. J Biol Chem 1997;272:25190–4.
11. Anderson MA, Maraskovsky E, Billingsley WL, Dougall WC, Tometsko ME, Roux ER, et al. A homologue of the TNF receptor and its ligand enhance T-cell growth and dendritic-cell function. Nature 1997;390:175–9.
12. Lum L, Wong BR, Josien R, Becherer JD, Erdjument-Bromage H, Schlöndorff J, et al. Evidence for a role of a tumor necrosis factor-α (TNF-α)-converting enzyme-like protease in shedding of TRANCE, a TNF family member involved in osteoclastogenesis and dendritic cell survival. J Biol Chem 1999;274:13613–8.
13. Nagai M, Kyakumoto S, Sato N. Cancer cells responsible for humoral hypercalcemia express mRNA encoding a secreted form of ODF/TRANCE that induces osteoclast formation. Biochem Biophys Res Commun 2000;269:532–6.
14. Quinn JMW, Elliott J, Gillespie MT, Martin TJ. A combination of osteoclast differentiation factor and macrophage-colony stimulating factor is sufficient for both human and mouse osteoclast formation in vitro. Endocrinology 1998;139:4424–7.
15. Fuller K, Wong B, Fox S, Choi Y, Chambers TJ. TRANCE is necessary and sufficient for osteoblast-mediated activation of bone resorption in osteoclasts. J Exp Med 1998;188:997–1001.
16. Burgess TL, Qian Y, Kaufman S, Ring BD, Van G, Capparelli C, et al. The ligand for osteoprotegerin (OPGL) directly activates mature osteoclasts. J Cell Biol 1999;145:527–38.
17. Jimi E, Akiyama S, Tsurukai T, Okahashi N, Kobayashi K, Udagawa N, et al. Osteoclast differentiation factor acts as a multifunctional regulator in murine osteoclast differentiation and function. J Immunol 1999;163:434–42.
18. Kobayashi K, Takahashi N, Jimi E, Udagawa N, Takami M, Kotake S, et al. Tumor necrosis factor alpha stimulates osteoclast differentiation by a mechanism independent of the ODF/RANKL-RANK interaction. J Exp Med 2000;191:275–86.
19. Kong Y-Y, Yoshida H, Sarosi I, Tan H-L, Timms E, Capparelli C, et al. OPGL is a key regulator of osteoclastogenesis, lymphocyte development and lymph-node organogenesis. Nature 1999;397: 315–23.
20. Hsu H, Lacey DL, Dunstan CR, Solovyev I, Colombero A, Timms E, et al. Tumor necrosis factor receptor family member RANK mediates osteoclast differentiation and activation induced by osteoprotegerin ligand. Proc Natl Acad Sci U S A 1999;96:3540–5.
21. Nakagawa N, Kinosaki M, Yamaguchi K, Shima N, Yasuda H, Yano K, et al. RANK is the essential signaling receptor for osteoclast differentiation factor in osteoclastogenesis. Biochem Biophys Res Commun 1998;253:395–400.
22. Dougall WC, Glaccum M, Charrier K, Rohrbach K, Brasel K, de Smedt T, et al. RANK is essential for osteoclast and lymph node development. Genes Dev 1999;13:2412–24.
23. Li J, Sarosi I, Yan X-Q, McCabe SM, Tan H-L, Capparelli C, et al. RANK is the intrinsic hematopoietic cell surface receptor that controls osteoclastogenesis and regulation of bone mass and calcium metabolism. Proc Natl Acad Sci U S A 2000;97:1566–71.
24. Simonet WS, Lacey DL, Dunstan CR, Kelley M, Chang M-S, Lüthy R, et al. Osteoprotegerin: a novel secreted protein involved in the regulation of bone density. Cell 1997;89:309–19.
25. Yasuda H, Shima N, Nakagawa N, Mochizuki S-I, Yano K, Fujise N, et al. Identity of osteoclastogenesis inhibitory factor (OCIF) and osteoprotegerin (OPG): a mechanism by which OPG/OCIF inhibits osteoclastogenesis in vitro. Endocrinology 1998;139: 1329–37.
26. Bucay N, Sarosi I, Dunstan CR, Morony S, Tarpley J, Capparelli C, et al. Osteoprotegerin-deficient mice develop early onset osteoporosis and arterial calcification. Genes Dev 1998;12:1260–8.
27. Mizuno A, Amizuka N, Irie K, Murakami A, Fujise N, Kanno T, et al. Severe osteoporosis in mice lacking osteoclastogenesis inhibitory factor/osteoprotegerin. Biochem Biophys Res Commun 1998;247:610–5.
28. Wong BR, Josien R, Lee SY, Sauter B, Li H-L, Steinman RM, et al. TRANCE (Tumor necrosis factor [TNF]-related activation-induced cytokine), a new TNF family member predominantly expressed in T cells, is a dendritic cell-specific survival factor. J Exp Med 1997:186:2075–80.
29. Josien R, Wong BR, Li H-L, Steinman RM, Choi Y. TRANCE, a TNF family member, is differentially expressed on T cell subsets and induces cytokine production in dendritic cells. J Immunol 1999;162:2562–8.
30. Bachmann MF, Wong BR, Josien R, Steinman RM, Oxenius A, Choi Y. TRANCE, a tumor necrosis factor family member critical for CD40 ligand-independent T helper cell activation. J Exp Med 1999;189:1025–31.
31. Yun TJ, Chaudhary PM, Shu GL, Frazer JK, Ewings MK, Schwartz SM, et al. OPG/FDCR-1, a TNF receptor family member, is expressed in lymphoid cells and is up-regulated by ligating CD40. J Immunol 1998;161:6113–21.

32. Feldmann M, Brennan FM, Maini RN. Role of cytokines in rheumatoid arthritis. Ann Rev Immunol 1996;14:397–440.
33. Hofbauer LC, Lacey DL, Dunstan CR, Spelsberg TC, Riggs BL, Khosla S. Interleukin-1β and tumor necrosis factor-α, but not interleukin-6 stimulate osteoprotegerin ligand gene expression in human osteoblastic cells. Bone 1999;25:255–9.
34. Kong Y-Y, Feige U, Sarosi I, Bolon B, Tafuri A, Morony S, et al. Activated T cells regulate bone loss and joint destruction in adjuvant arthritis through osteoprotegerin ligand. Nature 1999; 402:304–9.
35. Horwood NJ, Kartsogiannis V, Quinn JMW, Romas E, Martin TJ, Gillespie MT. Activated T cells support osteoclast formation in vitro. Biochem Biophys Res Commun 1999;265:144–50.
36. Hong MH, Williams H, Jin CH, Pike JW. The inhibitory effect of interleukin-10 on mouse osteoclast formation involves novel tyrosine-phosphorylated proteins. J Bone Miner Res 2000;15:911–8.
37. Lacey DL, Erdmann JM, Teitelbaum SL, Tan HL, Ohara J, Shioi A. Interleukin 4, interferon-γ, and prostaglandin E impact the osteoclastic cell-forming potential of murine bone marrow macrophages. Endocrinology 1995;136:2367–76.
38. Romas E, Bakharevski O, Hards DK, Kartsogiannis V, Quinn JMW, Ryan PFJ, et al. Expression of osteoclast differentiation factor at sites of bone erosion in collagen-induced arthritis. Arthritis Rheum 2000;43:821–6.
39. Gravallese EM, Manning C, Tsay A, Naito A, Pan C, Amento E, et al. Synovial tissue in rheumatoid arthritis is a source of osteoclast differentiation factor. Arthritis Rheum 2000;43:250–8.
40. Takayanagi H, Iizuka H, Juji T, Nakagawa T, Yamamoto A, Miyazaki T, et al. Involvement of receptor activator of nuclear factor κB ligand/osteoclast differentiation factor in osteoclastogenesis from synoviocytes in rheumatoid arthritis. Arthritis Rheum 2000;43:259–69.
41. Kotake S, Udagawa N, Takahashi N, Matsuzaki K, Itoh K, Ishiyama S, et al. IL-17 in synovial fluids from patients with rheumatoid arthritis is a potent stimulator of osteoclastogenesis. J Clin Invest 1999;103:1345–52.
42. Kotake S, Udagawa N, Takahashi N, Yano K, Tsuda E, Higashio K, et al. Presence of osteoclastogenesis inhibitory factor/osteoprotegerin in synovial fluids from patients with rheumatoid arthritis [abstract]. Arthritis Rheum 1998;41 Suppl 9:S320.
43. Itonaga I, Fujikawa Y, Sabokbar A, Murray DW, Athanasou NA. Rheumatoid arthritis synovial macrophage-osteoclast differentiation is osteoprotegerin ligand-dependent. J Pathol 2000;192: 97–104.
44. Akatsu T, Murakami T, Ono K, Nishikawa M, Tsuda E, Mochizuki S-I, et al. Osteoclastogenesis inhibitory factor exhibits hypocalcemic effects in normal mice and in hypercalcemic nude mice carrying tumors associated with humoral hypercalcemia of malignancy. Bone 1998;23:495–8.
45. Capparelli C, Kostenuik PJ, Morony S, Starnes C, Weimann B, Van G et al. Osteoprotegerin prevents and reverses hypercalcemia in a murine model of humoral hypercalcemia of malignancy. Cancer Res 2000;60:783–7.
46. Morony S, Capparelli C, Lee R, Shimamoto G, Boone T, Lacey DL, et al. A chimeric form of osteoprotegerin inhibits hypercalcemia and bone resorption induced by IL-1β, TNFα, PTH, PTHrP, and 1,25$(OH)_2D_3$. J Bone Miner Res 1999;14:1478–85.
47. Honore P, Luger NM, Sabino MAC, Schwei MJ, Rogers SD, Mach DB, et al. Osteoprotegerin blocks bone cancer-induced skeletal destruction, skeletal pain and pain-related neurochemical reorganization of the spinal cord. Nature Med 2000;5:521–8.
48. Bateman TA, Dunstan CR, Ferguson VL, Lacey DL, Ayers RA, Simske SJ. Osteoprotegerin mitigates tail suspension-induced osteopenia. Bone 2000;26:443–9.
49. Bekker PJ, Holloway D, Nakanishi A, Arrighi HM, Dunstan CR. Osteoprotegerin (OPG) has potent and sustained anti-resorptive activity in postmenopausal women [abstract]. J Bone Miner Res 1999;14 Suppl 1:1190.
50. Lubberts E, Joosten LAB, Chabaud M, van den Bersselaer L, Oppers B, Coenen-de Roo CJJ, et al. IL-4 gene therapy for collagen arthritis suppresses synovial IL-17 and osteoprotegerin ligand and prevents bone erosions. J Clin Invest 2000;105: 1697–710.
51. Bolon B, Campagnuolo G, Hu Y-L, Duryea D, Feige U. Arthritis patterns in rats with adjuvant-induced arthritis define distinct mechanisms of joint protection for IL-1ra, sTNF-RI, and OPG [abstract]. Ann Rheum Dis 2000;59 Suppl 1:355.
52. Hofbauer LC, Gori F, Riggs BL, Lacey DL, Dunstan CR, Spelsberg TC, et al. Stimulation of osteoprotegerin ligand and inhibition of osteoprotegerin production by glucocorticoids in human osteoblastic lineage cells: potential paracrine mechanisms of glucocorticoid-induced osteoporosis. Endocrinology 1999;140: 4382–9.
53. Rubin J, Murphy T, Nanes MS, Fan X. Mechanical strain inhibits expression of osteoclast differentiation factor by murine stromal cells. Am J Physiol Cell Physiol 2000;278:C1126–32.
54. Ware CF. Decoy receptors thwart B cells. Nature 2000;404: 949–50.

ARTHRITIS & RHEUMATISM
Vol. 44, No. 2, February 2001, pp 260–265

Involvement of ErbB-2 in Rheumatoid Synovial Cell Growth

Koichiro Satoh, Shinichi Kikuchi, Masayuki Sekimata, Yukihito Kabuyama, Miwako K. Homma, and Yoshimi Homma

Objective. The synovial tissue affected by rheumatoid arthritis (RA) is characterized by hyperproliferation of synovial cells. High amounts of epidermal growth factor (EGF) in the synovial fluid of RA patients contribute to the growth of rheumatoid synovial cells. To characterize the receptor for EGF in rheumatoid synovial cells, the expression and function of ErbB family members were examined.

Methods. Synovial tissues were obtained from surgical excisions. The expression of ErbB products was examined by immunohistochemistry and immunoblotting by using specific antibodies. Primary cultures were established from the surgical materials. Cell growth was measured using MTT. The levels and phosphorylation state of the ErbB-2 protein were analyzed by immunoprecipitation and immunoblotting.

Results. The expression of ErbB-2, but not other ErbB-related products, was detected in synovium with RA as compared with that with osteoarthritis (OA) and ligament injury. Growth of primary synovial cells with RA was inhibited by genistein, a tyrosine kinase inhibitor, and herceptin, a specific monoclonal antibody against ErbB-2. Herceptin showed a small effect on growth of primary synovial cells with OA. EGF stimulated the phosphorylation of ErbB-2 in primary synovial cells with RA. This EGF-stimulated phosphorylation was completely abrogated by genistein and herceptin.

Conclusion. ErbB-2 is expressed in rheumatoid synovial cells and may function as the receptor for EGF. Our data suggest that mitotic signals from EGF family members are transduced by ErbB-2 in these cells. Inhibition of ErbB-2 may provide a new approach to the effective treatment for RA.

Koichiro Satoh, MD, Shinichi Kikuchi, MD, PhD, Masayuki Sekimata, PhD, Yukihito Kabuyama, PhD, Miwako K. Homma, PhD, Yoshimi Homma, PhD: Fukushima Medical University School of Medicine, Fukushima, Japan.

Address correspondence and reprint requests to Koichiro Satoh, MD, Department of Orthopaedic Surgery, Fukushima Medical University, 1 Hikariga-oka, Fukushima 960-1295, Japan.

Submitted for publication May 22, 2000; accepted in revised form October 23, 2000.

Rheumatoid arthritis (RA) is a systemic, chronic, and inflammatory disease characterized by synovial proliferation and abnormal immune responses that ultimately lead to progressive destruction of tendons, cartilage, and bone (1). While there has been progress in defining the etiology and pathogenesis of RA, these are still incompletely understood. Overexpression of inflammatory cytokines is thought to play an important role in the pathogenesis of synovial hyperplasia and joint destruction. Synovial cells are the major source of these inflammatory cytokines; thus, it is important to control the growth and phenotype of synovial cells for the treatment of RA (2). Cytokines identified as major contributors in the hyperplasia of rheumatoid synovial cells include epidermal growth factor (EGF), platelet-derived growth factor (PDGF), and fibroblast growth factor (3). Histochemical studies have revealed enhanced expression levels of PDGF receptor on synovial cells and FGF receptor on lesional T cells.

Although the synovial fluid of RA tissue contains high concentrations of EGF (4), there is very little information about the receptor for EGF in this tissue. In addition to EGF receptor (EGFR), ErbB-2 (also designated c-neu or HER2), ErbB-3, and ErbB-4 (the products of the *erb* B-2, *erb* B-3, and *erb* B-4 genes, respectively) can also function as receptors for the EGF family of growth factors (5–8). EGFR, detected in various normal tissues at low levels (9), is overexpressed on epithelial cells in hyperplastic skin diseases. High levels of ErbB-2 are observed in 20–30% of carcinomas of the breast (10–13), stomach (14), ovary (15), and pancreas (16). These observations suggest that ErbB proteins may play important roles not only in the growth and differentiation, but also in the pathogenesis of hyperplastic diseases.

In this study, we attempted to identify the receptor for EGF on synovial cells and to examine EGFR and

Table 1. ErbB-2 expression in the patients with RA, OA, and ligament injury*

Diagnosis, patient/age/sex	ErbB-2 expression, densitometric units
RA	
1/67/F	0.10
2/42/F	0.51
3/42/F	0.31
4/45/F	0.36
5/78/F	0.12
6/71/M	0.26
OA	
1/54/F	0
2/76/F	0.08
3/51/M	0
4/49/F	0
Injury of ligament	
1/23/F	0
2/27/M	0

* RA = rheumatoid arthritis; OA = osteoarthritis.

ErbB proteins in rheumatoid synovium and synovial cells in primary cultures. We showed the expression of ErbB-2 in the synovium and cultured synovial cells from RA patients. The growth of synovial cells was inhibited by genistein, a tyrosine kinase inhibitor, and herceptin, an anti–ErbB-2 monoclonal antibody, suggesting that ErbB-2 plays an important role in RA synovial hyperproliferation.

PATIENTS AND METHODS

Patients. Synovial tissue samples were obtained, at the time of surgery, from 6 patients with RA (1 man and 5 women, mean age 57.5 years, range 42–78 years), 4 patients with osteoarthritis (OA) (1 man and 3 women, mean age 57.5 years, range 49–76 years), and 2 patients with knee ligament injury (1 man and 1 woman, mean age 25 years, range 23–27 years) (Table 1). The diagnosis was based on the clinical and radiologic findings.

Cell culture. Synovial cells were isolated from surgical samples as previously described (17). Briefly, synovial membranes prepared from surgical materials were minced and dissociated enzymatically with collagenase (4.0 mg/ml; Sigma, St. Louis, MO) in RPMI 1640 for 4 hours at 37°C. The cells thus obtained were cultured in a growth medium consisting of RPMI 1640 and 10% fetal bovine serum for several days at 37°C in 5% CO_2 in a humidified incubator. When the cells were grown to subconfluence, they were passaged at a ratio of 1:2 to 1:4. The medium was changed every 3–4 days, and the cells from passage 4–7 were used for the experiments.

Immunohistochemical detection. Synovial tissues obtained from patients with RA, OA, or ligament injury of the knees were fixed in buffered 4% paraformaldehyde. After embedding the tissues in paraffin, 4 μm–thick sections were made and enzymatically pretreated to enhance the immunoreactivity with 0.1% trypsin (Zymed, South San Francisco, CA) at 37°C for 10 minutes, and endogenous peroxidase activity was blocked by incubation with 0.3% H_2O_2. After blocking with 3% normal goat serum, samples were incubated with anti–EGFR, anti–c-neu, anti–ErbB-3 (Calbiochem, La Jolla, CA), or anti–ErbB-4 (Santa Cruz Biotechnology, Santa Cruz, CA) in a moist chamber. The samples were further incubated with the biotinylated second antibodies (Vector, Burlingame, CA), and then with avidin–peroxidase complex reagent (Vector). After washing thoroughly, positive signals were obtained by incubation with 3,3′-diaminobenzidine tetrahydrochloride (Wako, Osaka, Japan). Methyl green (Wako) was used to counterstain. All tissue sections were mounted with Canada balsam (Wako) and assessed by observers who were blinded as to the source.

Immunoblotting analysis. The tissue and cell lysates were prepared from surgical materials and confluent cultures of synovial cells. These tissue and cell samples were washed with ice-cold phosphate buffered saline and homogenized in a buffer consisting of 20 m*M* Tris HCl (pH 7.5), 1% Nonidet P40, 1 m*M* EDTA, 50 m*M* NaF, 50 m*M* β-glycerophosphate, 50 μM Na_3VO_4, 10 μg/ml of leupeptin, 10 μg/ml of aprotinin, and 100 μM phenylmethylsulfonyl fluoride. After centrifugation, the supernatant was incubated with anti–c-neu antibody. The immune complexes were collected by incubating the samples with 40 μl of protein G–Sepharose (50% slurry; Zymed) for 30 minutes at 4°C. After washing 5 times with Tris buffered saline (TBS), proteins were solubilized by heating at 90°C for 5 minutes in 20 μl sodium dodecyl sulfate (SDS) sample buffer (62.5 m*M* Tris HCl [pH 6.8], 10% glycerol, 2.3% SDS, 5% 2-mercaptoethanol) and subjected to SDS–polyacrylamide gel electrophoresis (SDS-PAGE).

Cellular proteins were transferred onto polyvinylidene difluoride filters. The filters were blocked with 5% nonfat dry milk in TBS containing 0.1% Tween 20 and incubated with anti–c-neu, followed by incubation with a second antibody, peroxidase-conjugated goat anti-mouse IgG (Dakopatts, Copenhagen, Denmark). A chemiluminescence-based detection system (Amersham International, Buckinghamshire, UK) was used to detect immunoreactivity. The intensity of each band was quantified by a densitometric analysis.

Phosphorylation analysis. Cultured cells were incubated with ^{32}P-orthophosphate and stimulated with various concentrations of EGF under the conditions indicated. The cell lysates obtained from these cells were treated with anti–c-neu antibody, and immune complexes were collected by incubating with 40 μl of protein G–Sepharose. After washing 5 times with TBS, proteins were solubilized by heating at 90°C for 5 minutes in 20 μl SDS sample buffer and analyzed by SDS-PAGE. The phosphorylated bands were visualized by autoradiography.

Measurement of cell growth. Cell growth was determined by an assay using MTT (Sigma) (18). Synovial cells were seeded in a 96-well microplate (5×10^3 cells/well) and incubated in the growth medium at 37°C overnight. The cells were washed and further incubated in the growth medium in the presence or absence of genistein or herceptin for 7 days, with the medium changed every 2 days. Two hours before the termination of culture, MTT (5 mg/ml) was added to each well. At the end of the incubation, 100 μl of dimethyl sulfoxide was added to each culture to solubilize the formazan complex. The optical density at 590 nm was measured using a 96-well

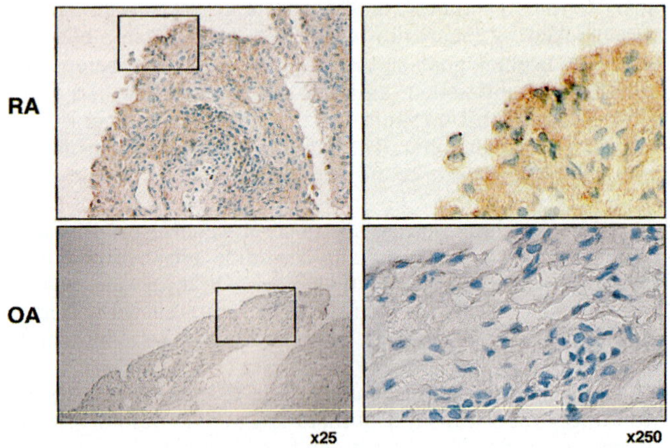

Figure 1. Immunohistochemical detection of ErbB-2 expression. Paraffin-embedded synovium sections derived from patients with rheumatoid arthritis (RA) and osteoarthritis (OA) were examined by staining with an anti–ErbB-2 antibody. A magnified view of the area indicated by the square in the left panel is shown in the right panel. Nuclei were stained with methyl green.

multiscanner (Immuno-Mini; Nihon Intermed, Tokyo, Japan). Each experiment was performed in quadruplicate.

RESULTS

Immunohistochemical detection of ErbB-2. Although normal synovium is histologically composed of 1–3 layers of synovial lining cells, synovial tissues from patients with RA are characterized by diffuse and nodular mononuclear cell infiltration and hyperplasia of synovial epithelial cells (Figure 1). In order to detect the EGFR and its related proteins in synovial tissues, we carried out immunohistochemical staining of samples from patients with RA, using specific antibodies against EGFR, ErbB-2, ErbB-3, and ErbB-4. Only anti–ErbB-2 antibody produced positive signals in samples from patients with RA (Figure 1). The expression of ErbB-2 was predominant in the plasma membrane and cytoplasm, which is similar to the cellular distribution of ErbB-2 in other ErbB-2–overexpressing cells, such as breast cancer cells. Neither anti-EGFR, anti–ErbB-3, nor anti–ErbB-4 detected significant levels of corresponding proteins.

Biochemical detection of ErbB-2. The expression levels of ErbB-2 in surgical samples were examined by Western blotting with anti–ErbB-2 antibody. This antibody recognized a specific component with an apparent molecular weight of 185 kd, which corresponds to ErbB-2 (Figure 2A). The expression of ErbB-2 was detected in all samples from 6 patients with RA, but not in samples from 4 patients with OA (Figures 2A and B and Table 1). The expression of ErbB-2 was observed in 1 sample with OA, but its level was quite low. The expression was not detected in surgical samples derived from ligament injury (Table 1). Primary cultures established from synovial tissue from RA patients and OA patients were also examined for the expression of ErbB-2. The expression was detected in all cultures derived from RA patients, but not in cultures from OA patients (Figure 2C). These results suggested that ErbB-2 plays an important role in growth of RA synovial cells.

Since ErbB-2 possesses an intrinsic protein tyrosine kinase domain, we next examined the phosphorylation of ErbB-2 of synovial cultures in response to extracellularly added EGF. When ^{32}P-labeled cells were stimulated with various concentrations of EGF for 10 minutes, ErbB-2 was phosphorylated in a dose-dependent manner (Figure 3A). These results indicate that ErbB-2 is activated in response to extracellularly added EGF.

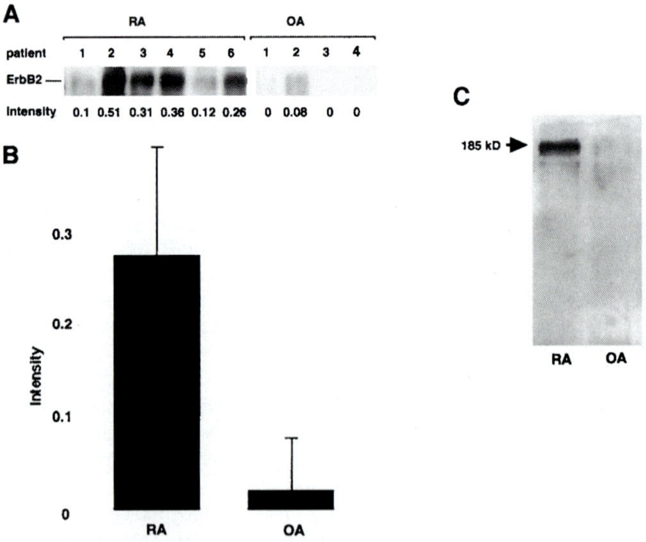

Figure 2. Biochemical detection of ErbB-2. **A,** Expression levels of ErbB-2 in surgical samples from 6 rheumatoid arthritis (RA) and 4 osteoarthritis (OA) patients were examined by Western blotting. The intensity of each band was quantified using Image Master (Pharmacia Biotech, Uppsala, Sweden). **B,** Expression levels (mean and SD) were compared in the RA and OA groups, and statistical analysis was performed using Student's t-test ($P < 0.05$). **C,** Expression levels of ErbB-2 in cultures of synovial cells from patients with RA or OA were analyzed by Western blotting. The position of 185 kD (corresponding to ErB-2) is indicated.

Effect of inhibitors on cell growth and tyrosine phosphorylation. In order to assess the involvement of ErbB-2 in growth of cultured synovial cells, we examined the effect on cell growth of genistein, a tyrosine kinase inhibitor, and herceptin, a specific inhibitor for ErbB-2 receptor. As shown in Figure 4A, genistein inhibited growth of synovial cells from RA and OA patients in a dose-dependent manner. The median infective dose (ID_{50}) was ~5 μg/ml. A cytotoxic effect was not observed with any concentration tested (up to 25 μg/ml). Herceptin also showed the cytostatic effect on RA cells in a dose-dependent manner without any cytotoxic effects. The ID_{50} was ~50 ng/ml. On the other hand, herceptin had a small effect on the growth of synovial cells from OA patients (Figure 4B).

Effects of these inhibitors on phosphorylation of ErbB-2 were also examined using ^{32}P-labeled RA cells. As shown in Figure 3B, the moderate level of ErbB-2 phosphorylation was detected under nonstimulating conditions. The phosphorylation was enhanced by EGF treatment. This enhancement was diminished by either genistein or herceptin. These results indicate a possible involvement of ErbB-2 in hyperproliferation of RA synovial cells through activation of intracellular signaling systems.

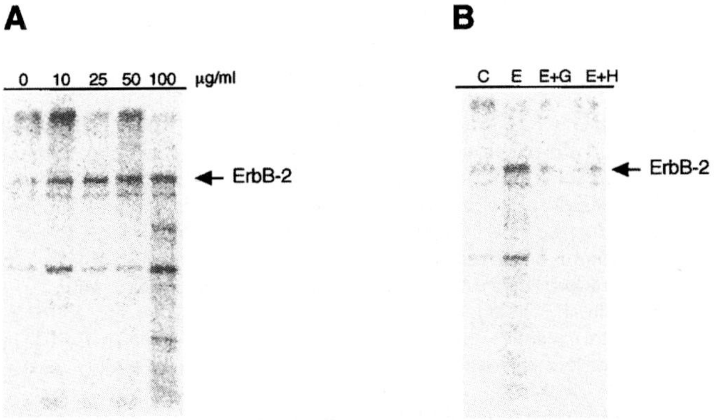

Figure 3. Detection of phosphorylation of ErbB-2. **A,** ^{32}P-labeled cells were stimulated with various concentrations of epidermal growth factor (EGF) for 10 minutes, and the cell lysates were treated with anti–ErbB-2 antibody. The resultant immunoprecipitates were analyzed by sodium dodecyl sulfate–polyacrylamide gel electrophoresis (SDS-PAGE). The phosphorylated bands were visualized by autoradiography. **B,** ^{32}P-labeled cells were pretreated with 20 μg/ml genistein (E+G) or 100 ng/ml herceptin (E+H) for 10 minutes. ^{32}P-labeled cells treated only with EGF (E) and untreated cells (control; C) were also prepared. Cell lysates obtained from these cells were treated with anti–ErbB-2 antibody, and the resultant immunoprecipitates were analyzed by SDS-PAGE. The phosphorylated bands were visualized by autoradiography.

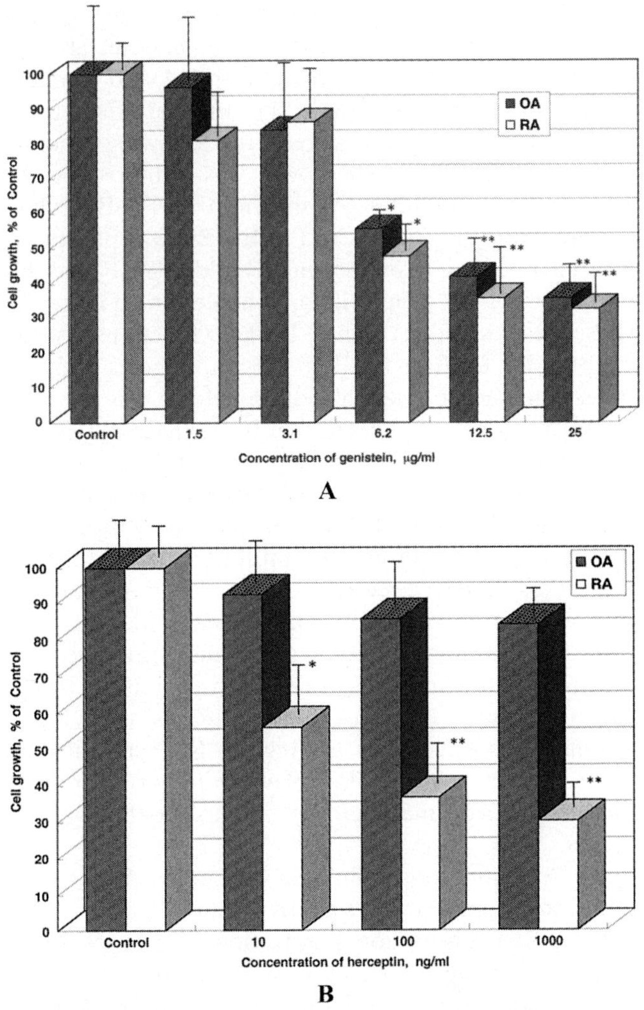

Figure 4. Effect of inhibitors on synovial cell growth. Cells from rheumatoid arthritis (RA) patients and osteoarthritis (OA) patients were cultured in fetal bovine serum–containing growth medium in the presence of the indicated amounts of **A,** genistein or **B,** herceptin for 7 days, and growth was determined using the MTT assay. Results (mean and SD; n = 4) are expressed as percentages of the values detected in cells in the absence of inhibitors. Statistical significance of the differences between control and treated groups was calculated by Student's *t*-test. $* = P < 0.05$; $** = P < 0.01$.

DISCUSSION

Synovial hyperplasia is one of the major characteristics observed in RA joints. Much evidence has accumulated concerning the hyperproliferation of synovial cells and infiltration of inflammatory cells, including the transformed appearance of synovium. In the present study, we examined the expression of ErbB-related products possibly serving as the receptor for EGF in synovial tissues, and found ErbB-2, but not other ErbB-related products including EGFR, expressed on synovial cells in RA synovium. ErbB-2 was undetectable in synovium obtained from patients with OA and ligament injury (Figure 1 and Table 1). Furthermore, using primary cultures of synovial cells, the following observations were made: 1) cell growth was inhibited by the tyrosine kinase inhibitor genistein and the ErbB-2 inhibitor herceptin (Figure 4); and 2) ErbB-2 was phosphorylated in response to extracellularly added EGF, and this was inhibited by genistein and herceptin (Figure 3). These results indicate that ErbB-2 functions as the receptor for EGF or EGF-like growth factors and mediates signaling to synovial cell growth.

It has been indicated that the activity of tyrosine kinases is important for hyperproliferation of synovial cells (19,20). Histochemical studies have revealed enhanced expression of PDGF receptor in synovial cells and FGF receptor in lesional infiltrates. In addition to these tyrosine kinase receptors, we now demonstrate the high expression of ErbB-2 in rheumatoid synovium. Moreover, results of our in vitro study revealed that ErbB-2 possibly functions as a growth-promoting receptor on synovial cells in RA. Since contents of EGF and its related growth factors are high in RA synovial fluid (4), it is certain that ErbB-2 plays an important role as the receptor for these growth factors in the synovial lesions.

A number of cellular components may be involved in the mechanism underlying the high expression of ErbB-2. Transcriptional activation may be one such mechanism. Considering previous findings that various transcription factors are induced by cytokines that are found at high levels in RA synovial fluid, the enhanced levels of transcription factors can be critical for the high expression of ErbB-2. In fact, AP-2, which is induced by inflammatory cytokines such as interleulin-6 and whose recognition sequence is contained in the upstream regulatory region of the ErbB-2 gene, was highly expressed in the RA lesions. On the other hand, we analyzed the upstream regulatory region of the ErbB-2 gene derived from RA and OA patients and could not detect any nucleotide substitutions specific to RA. Further studies should be undertaken to address this issue.

The results presented here suggest that ErbB-2 could be an important target for the growth inhibition of synovial cells in RA, which may provide a new approach to control RA. Genistein has an inhibitory effect on tyrosine kinases, with 50% inhibition at concentrations between 0.7 and 8.0 μg/ml (21).

In this study, we showed that genistein restricts the activities of ErbB-2 in a dose-dependent manner, and restricts the growth of synovial cells with 50% inhibition at 6.25 μg/ml. Herceptin is more specific for inhibition of ErbB-2. The murine monoclonal antibody (mAb) 4D5, directed against the extracellular domain of ErbB-2, is quite potent in inhibiting growth of human breast cancer cells that overexpress ErbB-2 (26). However, murine antibodies are limited for clinical use because they are immunogenic. For clinical application, mAb 4D5 was humanized by inserting the complementarity-determining regions of mAb 4D5 into the framework of a consensus human immunoglobulin, G1 (27). The resulting recombinant, humanized anti–ErbB-2 mAb (i.e., herceptin), has a higher affinity for ErbB-2 than the murine mAb 4D5 and a cytostatic growth inhibitory effect against breast cancer cells overexpressing ErbB-2 (27,28). Recent studies show that antibodies directed at ErbB-2 inhibit the growth of tumor xenografts and transform cells that express this protein at high levels (22–25). Here we demonstrate that herceptin results in concentration-dependent growth inhibitory effects on cultures of synovial cells from patients with RA. The half-maximal effect was observed at ~50 ng/ml, with no cytotoxic effects. Therefore, we suggest that herceptin may be useful in preventing pannus formation and irreversible joint destruction in RA, analogous to the therapeutic application of herceptin to cancers overexpressing ErbB-2.

REFERENCES

1. Gay S, Gay RE, Koopman WJ. Molecular and cellular mechanisms of joint destruction in rheumatoid arthritis: two cellular mechanisms explain joint destruction? Ann Rheum Dis 1993;52:S39–47.
2. Harris ED Jr. Rheumatoid arthritis: pathophysiology and implications for therapy. N Engl J Med 1990;322:1277–89.
3. Feldmann M, Brennan FM, Maini RN. Role of cytokines in rheumatoid arthritis. Annu Rev Immunol 1996;14:397–440.
4. Kusada J, Otsuka T, Matsui N, Hirano T, Asai K, Kato T. Immuno-reactive human epidermal growth factor (h-EGF) in rheumatoid synovial fluids. Nippon Seikeigeka Gakkai Zasshi 1993;67:859–65.
5. Wen D, Peles E, Cupples R, Suggs SV, Bacus SS, Luo Y, et al. Neu differentiation factor: a transmembrane glycoprotein containing an EGF domain and an immunoglobulin homology unit. Cell 1992;69:559–72.
6. Carraway KI III, Cantley LC. A neu acquaintance for erbB3 and erbB4: a role for receptor heterodimerization in growth signaling. Cell 1994;78:5–8.
7. Holmes WE, Sliwkowski MX, Akita RW, Henzel WJ, Lee J, Park JW, et al. Identification of heregulin, a specific activator of p185erbB2. Science 1992;256:1205–10.
8. Riese DJ II, van Raaij TM, Plowman GD, Andrews GC, Stern DF. The cellular response to neuregulins is governed by complex interactions of the erbB receptor family. Mol Cell Biol 1995;15: 5770–6.
9. Press MF, Cordon-Cardo C, Slamon DJ. Expression of the HER-

2/neu proto-oncogene in normal human adult and fetal tissues. Oncogene 1990;5:953–62.
10. Slamon DJ, Clark GM, Wong SG, Levin WJ, Ullrich A, McGuire WL. Human breast cancer: correlation of relapse and survival with amplification of the HER-2/neu oncogene. Science 1987;235: 177–82.
11. Borg A, Baldetorp B, Ferno M, Killander D, Olsson H, Ryden S, et al. ERBB2 amplification is associated with tamoxifen resistance in steroid-receptor positive breast cancer. Cancer Lett 1994;81: 137–44.
12. Tetu B, Brisson J. Prognostic significance of HER-2/neu oncoprotein expression in node-positive breast cancer. Cancer 1994;73: 2359–65.
13. King CR, Kraus MH, Aaronson SA. Amplification of a novel v-erbB-related gene in a human mammary carcinoma. Science 1985;229:974–6.
14. Kameda T, Yasui W, Yoshida K, Tsujino T, Nakayama H, Ito M, et al. Expression of ERBB2 in human gastric carcinomas: relationship between p185ERBB2 expression and the gene amplification. Cancer Res 1990;50:8002–9.
15. Slamon DJ, Godolphin W, Jones LA, Holt JA, Wong SG, Keith DE, et al. Studies of the HER-2/neu proto-oncogene in human breast and ovarian cancer. Science 1989;244:707–12.
16. Williams TM, Weiner DB, Greene MI, Maguire HC Jr. Expression of c-erbB-2 in human pancreatic adenocarcinomas. Pathobiology 1991;59:46–52.
17. Migita K, Eguchi K, Aoyagi T, Tsukada T, Tsuboi M, Kawabe Y, et al. The effects of the immunosuppressant rapamycin on the growth of rheumatoid arthritis (RA) synovial fibroblast. Clin Exp Immunol 1996;104:86–91.
18. Hansen MB, Nielsen SE, Berg K. Re-examination and further development of a precise and rapid dye method for measuring cell growth/cell kill. J Immunol Methods 1989;119:203–10.
19. Takeuchi T, Abe T. Tyrosine phosphorylated proteins in synovial cells of rheumatoid arthritis. Int Rev Immunol 1998;17:365–81.
20. Williams WV, VonFeldt JM, Ramanujam T, Weiner DB. Tyrosine kinase signal transduction in rheumatoid synovitis. Semin Arthritis Rheum 1992;21:317–29.
21. Akiyama T, Ishida J, Nakagawa S, Ogawara H, Watanabe S, Itoh N, et al. Genistein, a specific inhibitor of tyrosine-specific kinases. J Biol Chem 1987;262:5592–5.
22. Hancock MC, Langton BC, Chan T, Toy P, Monahan JJ, Mischak RP, et al. A monoclonal antibody against the c-erbB-2 protein enhances the cytotoxicity of cis-diaminedichloroplatinum against human breast and ovarian tumor cell lines. Cancer Res 1991;51: 4575–80.
23. Drebin JA, Link VC, Stern DF, Weinberg RA, Greene MI. Down-modulation of an oncogene protein product and reversion of the transformed phenotype by monoclonal antibodies. Cell 1985;41:697–706.
24. Stancovski I, Hurwitz E, Leitner D, Ullrich A, Yarden Y, Sela M. Mechanistic aspects of the opposing effects of monoclonal antibodies to the ERBB2 receptor on tumor growth. Proc Natl Acad Sci U S A 1991;88:8691–5.
25. McKenzie SJ, Marks PJ, Lam T, Morgan J, Panicali DL, Trimpe KL, et al. Generation and characterization of monoclonal antibodies specific for the human neu oncogene product, p185. Oncogene 1989;4:543–8.
26. Lewis GD, Figari I, Fendly B, Wong WL, Carter P, Gorman C, et al. Differential responses of human tumor cell lines to anti-p185HER2 monoclonal antibodies. Cancer Immunol Immunother 1993;37:255–63.
27. Carter P, Presta L, Gorman CM, Ridgway JB, Henner D, Wong WL, et al. Humanization of an anti-p185HER2 antibody for human cancer therapy. Proc Natl Acad Sci U S A 1992;89:4285–9.
28. Hudziak RM, Lewis GD, Winget M, Fendly BM, Shepard HM, Ullrich A. p185HER2 monoclonal antibody has antiproliferative effects in vitro and sensitizes human breast tumor cells to tumor necrosis factor. Mol Cell Biol 1989;9:1165–72.

ARTHRITIS & RHEUMATISM
Vol. 44, No. 2, February 2001, pp 266–274

Overexpression of Transcription Factor Ets-1 in Rheumatoid Arthritis Synovial Membrane

Regulation of Expression and Activation by Interleukin-1 and Tumor Necrosis Factor α

Kurt Redlich,[1] Hans P. Kiener,[1] Georg Schett,[1] Makiyeh Tohidast-Akrad,[2] Edgar Selzer,[1] Irene Radda,[1] Georg H. Stummvoll,[1] Carl W. Steiner,[1] Marion Gröger,[1] Peter Bitzan,[1] Peter Zenz,[3] Josef S. Smolen,[1] and Günter Steiner[1]

Objective. **To investigate the expression of the transcription factor Ets-1 in synovial tissue and cultured synovial fibroblasts from patients with rheumatoid arthritis (RA) and osteoarthritis (OA) and to study the regulation of Ets-1 expression and activation in synovial fibroblasts by proinflammatory cytokines.**

Methods. **In situ expression of Ets-1 in synovial tissue from RA and OA patients was examined by double immunohistochemistry. The effects of interleukin-1 (IL-1) or tumor necrosis factor α (TNFα) on Ets-1 expression and activation (DNA binding) in cultured synovial fibroblasts were analyzed by Western blotting and DNA gel shift assay, respectively. In addition, the intracellular location of Ets-1 in synovial fibroblasts was determined by immunofluorescence.**

Results. **Pronounced expression of Ets-1 was detected in synovial tissues from all RA patients evaluated, particularly in the synovial lining layer and the sublining areas. Ets-1 was expressed by both fibroblasts and macrophages as well as by endothelial cells, while only a few T cells stained positive for Ets-1. In synovial specimens from OA patients, Ets-1 expression was much less frequently observed and was largely restricted to vascular cells. Ets-1 was expressed to a similar degree in cultured synovial fibroblasts from RA and OA patients, as demonstrated by reverse transcriptase–polymerase chain reaction and Western blotting. Both IL-1 and TNFα induced pronounced up-regulation of Ets-1 in synovial fibroblasts. Moreover, binding of Ets-1 to its specific DNA binding site was induced by both cytokines, although with different time courses. Immunofluorescence staining revealed a dominant nuclear localization of Ets-1 in IL-1– or TNFα-stimulated synovial fibroblasts.**

Conclusion. **The overexpression of Ets-1 observed in RA synovial tissue appears to be caused by TNFα and IL-1, suggesting that Ets-1 may be an important factor in the cytokine-mediated inflammatory and destructive cascade characteristic of RA.**

Rheumatoid arthritis (RA) is a systemic autoimmune disorder of unknown etiology characterized by hyperplasia of the synovial membrane and degradation of articular cartilage and subchondral bone (1,2). The destructive invasion of cartilage and bone is accompanied by the appearance of proliferating fibroblast-like synoviocytes with pleomorphic nuclei which show elevated expression of protooncogenes and release large amounts of destructive metalloproteinases (MPs) (3,4). Furthermore, many proinflammatory cytokines and chemokines are overexpressed in the synovium of RA patients (5), among which tumor necrosis factor α (TNFα) and interleukin-1 (IL-1) are regarded as key players in the pathogenesis of RA (6,7), a concept

[1]Kurt Redlich, MD, Hans P. Kiener, MD, Georg Schett, MD, Edgar Selzer, MD, Irene Radda, Georg H. Stummvoll, MD, Carl W. Steiner, Marion Gröger, MD, Peter Bitzan, MD: Josef S. Smolen, MD, Günter Steiner, PhD: University of Vienna, Vienna, Austria; [2]Makiyeh Tohidast-Akrad, PhD: Ludwig Boltzmann Institute for Rheumatology, Vienna, Austria; [3]Peter Zenz, MD: Hospital Baumgartner Höhe, Vienna, Austria.

Address correspondence and reprint requests to Günter Steiner, PhD, Department of Internal Medicine III, Division of Rheumatology, University Hospital of Vienna, Währinger Gürtel 18-20, A-1090 Vienna, Austria.

Submitted for publication May 16, 2000; accepted in revised form October 23, 2000.

supported by the clinical efficacy of both TNFα and IL-1 blockade (8,9). However, blockade of cytokines, even though they constitute well-defined targets, is still a relatively nonspecific approach that interferes with all effects of the targeted cytokines rather than with those downstream events that may be of particular pathogenetic importance in RA.

Aberrant overproduction of cytokines by RA synoviocytes leads to persistent up-regulation of various molecules involved in the inflammatory and destructive processes, including adhesion molecules, heat-shock proteins (HSPs), and proteolytic enzymes. The expression of many of these molecules is regulated via specific transcription factors (10,11). For example, Hsp70 and its transcription factor heat-shock factor 1 have recently been demonstrated to be highly expressed in the rheumatoid synovium and to be inducible in cultured synovial fibroblasts by proinflammatory cytokines (12). However, HSP expression may be beneficial and protect cells from inflammatory damage (13). On the other hand, matrix metalloproteinases (MMPs) play a direct and crucial role in tissue destruction (14–16). Regulation of MMPs is complex and involves several transcription factors, although the details of this process are still not fully understood (17,18). One such transcription factor is Ets-1, which has been shown to be up-regulated by TNFα and IL-1 in human foreskin fibroblasts (19).

The Ets transcription factor, originally discovered as an oncogene (v-*ets*) within the genome of the avian leukemia virus (20), activates many viral and cellular genes, including those encoding growth factor genes, protooncogenes, and proteins important for immune functions (21–24). Furthermore, c-*ets* overexpression leads to transactivation of the stromelysin 1 promoter (25) and may contribute to transcriptional activation of the collagenase 1 gene (26).

In the present study, we investigated the expression of Ets-1 in synovial membrane tissue from patients with RA and osteoarthritis (OA) and studied the regulation of Ets-1 by cytokines in cultured synovial fibroblasts. The data obtained demonstrate that Ets-1 is highly overexpressed in RA, but not OA, synovial tissue and thus may be one of the factors downstream of the TNFα/IL-1 cascade involved in the pathogenetic events leading to the destructive processes characteristic of RA.

PATIENTS AND METHODS

Patients. Synovial tissue was obtained from 14 RA patients and 6 OA patients at the time of surgery for arthroplasty or synovectomy. In each case, informed consent was obtained before surgery. RA and OA patients fulfilled the respective classification criteria (27,28).

In situ staining experiments. Immunohistochemical analysis of Ets-1 expression was performed essentially as previously described (12,29). Briefly, 4–6-μm cryostat sections were prepared from synovial tissue of 6 RA patients and 6 OA patients and fixed in ice-cold acetone. For in situ detection of Ets-1, sections were incubated for 60 minutes with a monoclonal anti–Ets-1 antibody (Transduction Laboratories, Lexington, KY). After rinsing, endogenous peroxidase was blocked with 0.3% hydrogen peroxide in Tris buffered saline (10 m*M* Tris HCl, 140 m*M* NaCl, pH 7.4) for 10 minutes. This was followed by 30 minutes of incubation with a biotinylated horse anti-mouse IgG. Sections were then incubated with the Vectastain ABC reagent (Vector, Burlingame, CA) for another 30 minutes using diaminobenzidine (Sigma, St. Louis, MO) for the color reaction leading to brown staining of Ets-1–expressing cells. Finally, slides were counterstained with hematoxylin (Merck, Darmstadt, Germany).

Antibodies specific for fibroblasts (clone ASO2; Dianova, Hamburg, Germany), macrophages (anti-CD68; Dako, Glostrup, Denmark), T cells (anti-CD3; Becton Dickinson, Mountain View, CA), and endothelial cells (anti-CD34; Novocastra, Newcastle upon Tyne, UK) were used to characterize Ets-1–expressing cells in double-labeling experiments employing the alkaline phosphatase–anti–alkaline phosphatase detection system (Dako) for visualization of cell-specific antigens leading to blue staining of positive cells. Since diaminobenzidine (used for peroxidase staining) blocks the binding site on the first antibody (i.e., anti–Ets-1), false-positive results (due to binding of the alkaline phosphatase–labeled secondary antibody to the monoclonal anti–Ets-1 antibody) are avoided. Thus, under light microscopy, Ets-1–positive cells appeared brown or brown/blue. The percentage of positive cells was determined by counting all cells of a given section at 200× magnification. Isotype-matched monoclonal antibodies (Dako) served as controls.

Synovial fibroblast culture. Synovial fibroblasts were isolated by enzymatic digestion of synovectomy-derived tissue samples, essentially as described elsewhere (12). Cells were harvested after 3–4 passages. To investigate the induction of Ets-1, synovial fibroblasts were cultured in the presence of different concentrations of recombinant TNFα or recombinant human IL-1 (R&D Systems, Oxford, UK) in RPMI 1640 medium containing 10% fetal calf serum (Sera Lab, Crowley Down, UK) at 37°C for various periods of time.

Protein extraction and Western blot analysis. Total cellular protein extracts were obtained from synovial fibroblasts using radioimmunoprecipitation assay buffer (50 m*M* Tris HCl, 150 m*M* NaCl, 1% Triton X-100, 0.1% sodium dodecyl sulfate [SDS], pH 7.2). Extracted proteins (12.5 μg/lane) were resolved on 10% SDS-polyacrylamide gels and transferred onto nitrocellulose membranes (BA85; Schleicher & Schuell, Dassel, Germany). Membranes were probed with polyclonal rabbit anti-human Ets-1 antibody (Santa Cruz Biotechnology, Santa Cruz, CA) diluted 1:500 for 1 hour. The reaction was visualized using polyvalent horseradish peroxidase–conjugated goat anti-rabbit Ig second antibodies (Dako) and the ECL Western Blot Detection Kit (Amersham, Buckinghamshire, UK).

Reverse transcriptase–polymerase chain reaction (RT-PCR). Synovial fibroblasts from OA or RA patients were analyzed by RT-PCR essentially as described elsewhere (30). The complementary DNA (cDNA) was synthesized in a re-

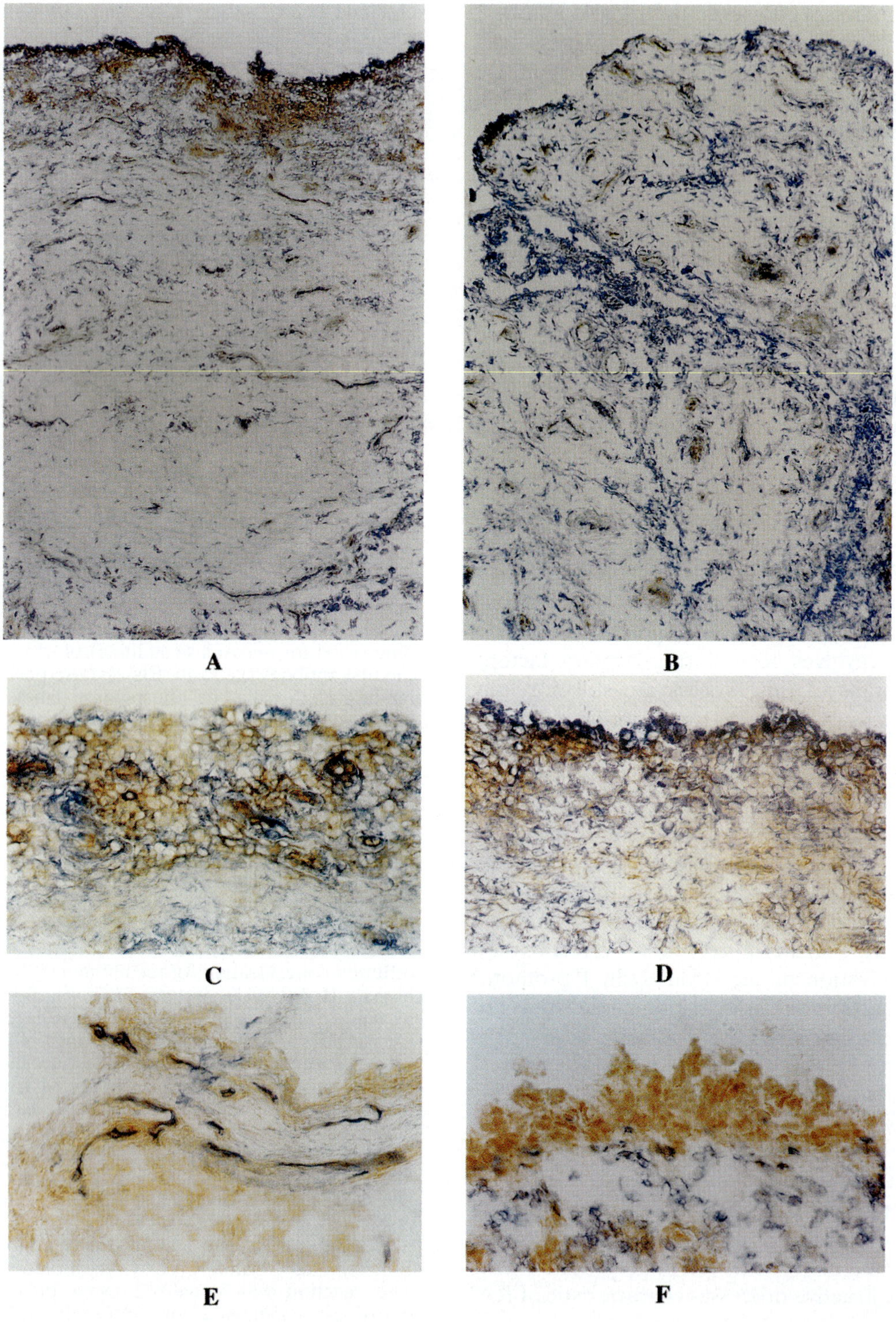

Figure 1. Immunohistochemical analysis of Ets-1 expression in synovial tissue from patients with rheumatoid arthritis (RA) and osteoarthritis (OA). Cryosections of synovial tissue from patients with RA (**A** and **C–F**) and OA (**B**) were stained with a monoclonal anti–Ets-1 antibody (brown staining) and cell type–specific antibodies (blue staining) such as the macrophage marker antibody CD68 (**A**, **B**, and **D**), the fibroblast marker ASO2 (**C**), the endothelial cell marker anti-CD34 (**E**), and the T cell marker anti-CD3 (**F**) to characterize the phenotype of Ets-1–expressing cells; or with an unrelated control antibody (not shown). (Original magnification × 100 in **A** and **B**; × 400 in **C–F**.)

verse transcription reaction mixture (First-Strand cDNA Synthesis kit; Pharmacia Biotech, Uppsala, Sweden) containing 4 μg total RNA from cultured synovial fibroblasts. Aliquots of the cDNA products (i.e., 2 μl for the constitutively expressed GAPDH as a positive internal control and 4 μl for Ets-1) were used for RT-PCR. A set of 4 primers was used (100 pmoles per reaction) that allowed us to distinguish among the following 4 alternative splice variants described for Ets-1 (31): Ets-1 exons III–V (5′-TAT-GGA-ATG-TGC-AGA-TGT-CC, 3′-TAA-TGA-AGT-AAT-CCG-AGG-T), Ets-1 exons VI–VIII (5′-GCA-GAA-TGA-CTA-CTT-TGC-TA, 3′-ATC-TCC-TGT-CCA-GCT-GAT-AA). GAPDH-specific primers were 5′-CCA-TGG-ACG-GTC-GGG-GTC-GCA-GTT-TC and 3′-GCA-GGG-GGG-AGC-CAA-AAG-GG. The various DNA fragments were amplified by 37 cycles at 94°C for 1 minute, 57°C for 2 minutes, and 72°C for 3 minutes after initial denaturation at 95°C for 1 minute. Aliquots of the PCR products were electrophoresed on a 2% agarose gel in 1× Tris–acetate–EDTA buffer, visualized by ethidium bromide staining, and photographed.

Gel mobility shift assays. For analysis of DNA binding of Ets-1, nuclear protein preparations from stimulated and unstimulated synovial fibroblasts were prepared. Subconfluent (80–90%) synovial fibroblasts were treated for various periods of time with TNFα or IL-1. Isolation of nuclear proteins and gel mobility shift assays were performed as previously described (12). The ETS-1 consensus double-stranded oligonucleotide (sequence 5′-GAT-CTC-GAG-CAG-GAA-GTT-CGA-3′) was purchased from Santa Cruz Biotechnology and 5′-end–labeled with γ^{32}P-ATP using polynucleotide kinase. To investigate DNA binding, 10 ng nuclear protein was incubated with 10 fmoles of the labeled oligonucleotide for 20 minutes on ice. Reaction buffer contained 20 m*M* HEPES (pH 7.6), 2 μg poly(dI-dC) (Pharmacia Biotech), 100 m*M* KCl, 1 m*M* $MgCl_2$, 0.1 m*M* EDTA, 0.1% Nonidet P40, and 1 m*M* spermidine. Samples were electrophoresed on 4% nondenaturing polyacrylamide gels in 0.5× Tris–borate–EDTA (TBE; 1× TBE consists of 89 m*M* Tris, 89 m*M* boric acid, 20 m*M* EDTA, pH 8.3), and gels were subsequently dried. The specific signal of Ets-1 binding was quantified on a Cyclone phosphorimager (Hewlett-Packard, Palo Alto, CA) using the 3-dimensional–image analysis software (Hewlett-Packard).

Immunofluorescence. Immunofluorescence studies were performed as described elsewhere (12), with slight modifications. Subconfluent synovial fibroblasts in 8-well chamber slides (Nunc, Naperville, IL) were treated with either TNFα (10 ng/ml) or IL-1 (5 ng/ml) for 3 hours, or left at 37°C. Cells were washed, permeabilized, and fixed with 4% paraformaldehyde for 30 minutes and absolute methanol for 5 minutes. Air-dried slides were then probed with a polyclonal rabbit anti-human Ets-1 antibody (Santa Cruz Biotechnology) diluted 1:20 for 1 hour at room temperature and subsequently with a fluorescein isothiocyanate–conjugated anti-rabbit Ig (Dako). Slides were analyzed in a confocal laser scanning microscope.

RESULTS

Expression of Ets-1 in RA and OA synovial tissue. To investigate the in situ expression of Ets-1 in synovial membranes, tissue sections from RA or OA patients were stained with a monoclonal antibody against Ets-1 and various cell lineage–specific antibodies, including anti-CD68 (macrophages), clone ASO2 (fibroblasts), anti-CD34 (endothelial cells), and anti-CD3 (T cells). Pronounced expression of Ets-1 was observed in sections from all 6 RA patients evaluated, particularly in the lining layer, the sublining area, at the site of blood vessels, and in areas of round-cell infiltrates (Figure 1A). In tissue sections from OA patients, Ets-1 expression was generally less abundant and appeared to be largely restricted to vascular sites (Figure 1B). In double-labeling studies, Ets-1 was detected in ASO2+ (fibroblasts) and CD68+ (macrophages) cells (Figures 1C and D, respectively).

Table 1. Quantitative analysis of Ets-1 expression in synovial tissue from 4 patients with rheumatoid arthritis*

Patient	No. of fibroblasts (% Ets-1+)†	No. of macrophages (% Ets-1+)‡
1	1,102 (5.9)	1,090 (7.0)
2	1,304 (5.1)	1,196 (5.7)
3	1,070 (6.4)	1,208 (6.6)
4	1,049 (6.9)	1,210 (6.3)

* Cells were double stained with a monoclonal antibody to Ets-1 and either the fibroblast-specific antibody ASO2 or the macrophage marker anti-CD68 (see Figures 1C and D, respectively). The percentage of Ets-1–expressing cells was determined by counting cells in 4–6 different areas at 400× magnification.
† A mean ± SD of 1,131 ± 117 fibroblasts were counted, of which 6.1 ± 0.8% were Ets-1 positive.
‡ A mean ± SD of 1,176 ± 58 macrophages were counted, of which 6.4 ± 0.5% were Ets-1 positive.

A detailed quantitative analysis revealed that 5.1–7% of RA synovial fibroblasts and macrophages expressed Ets-1 (Table 1), while <1% of these cells stained positive in OA specimens. Interestingly, however, CD34+ endothelial cells were commonly Ets-1–positive in sections from both RA (Figure 1E) and OA (not shown) patients. Expression in T cells was rarely seen, however, with the majority of T cell infiltrates staining negative (Figure 1F).

RT-PCR analysis of Ets-1 expression in cultured RA and OA synovial fibroblasts. Four related transcripts can be generated by alternative splicing of the 6.8-kb Ets-1 pre–messenger RNA (pre-mRNA), leading to skipping of exon IV and/or exon VII (31). To investigate expression of Ets-1 splice variants in cultured synovial fibroblasts from RA and OA patients, primer oligonucleotides complementary to sequences in exons III, V, VI, and VIII were used. Thus, 3 RT-PCR reactions were performed, encompassing exons III–V, III–VIII, and VI–VIII, respectively (Figure 2A). In all cases, only one single major PCR product was obtained (Figures 2B and C), demonstrating that the full-length mRNA containing exons IV and VII was the major isoform expressed. Thus, PCR products of 398 bp (exons III–V) and 994 bp (exons III–VIII) can be seen in Figure 2B, and a single PCR product of 421 bp (exons VI–VIII) can be seen in Figure 2C, which shows 5 RT-PCR reactions performed with mRNA from RA or OA patients. In this experiment, no major qualitative or quantitative difference in Ets-1 expression was seen between RA and OA synovial fibroblasts, since the intensity of the 421-bp band was similar in all reactions.

Up-regulation of Ets-1 protein by TNFα and IL-1 in cultured synovial fibroblasts. We next investigated semiquantitatively the expression of Ets-1 in cultured synovial fibroblasts from 10 RA and 6 OA patients at the

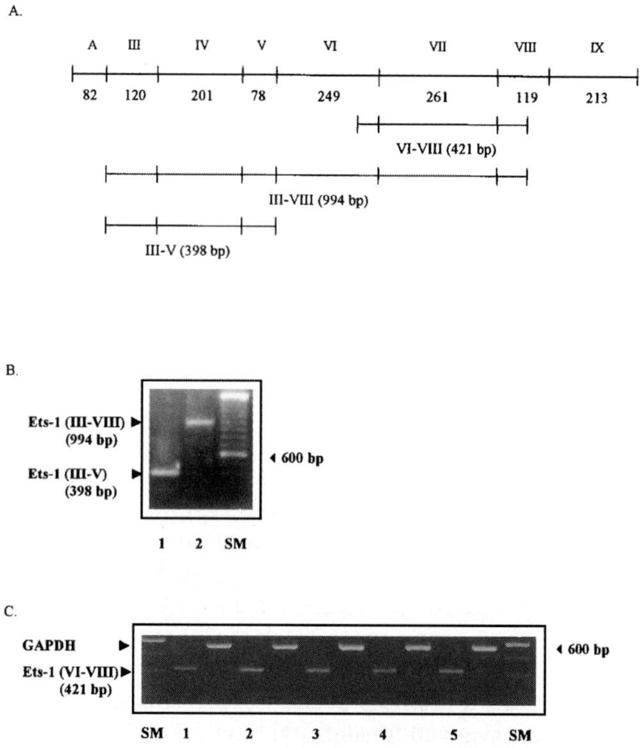

Figure 2. Reverse transcriptase–polymerase chain reaction (RT-PCR) analysis of Ets-1 expression in cultured synovial fibroblasts. **A,** Schematic representation of the exon structure of Ets-1 and of the RT-PCR reactions performed. Shown are sizes of exons and of the major PCR products obtained. **B,** RT-PCR analysis of Ets-1 expression in synovial fibroblasts from an RA patient, showing bands of 398 bp (lane 1) and 994 bp (lane 2) corresponding to exons III–V and III–VIII, respectively. SM indicates a 100-bp DNA ladder size marker with the 600-bp band indicated. **C,** RT-PCR analysis of Ets-1 expression in synovial fibroblasts from 2 RA patients (lanes 1 and 2) and 3 OA patients (lanes 3–5), showing a 421-bp band corresponding to exons VI–VIII. GAPDH served as a control, and the 600-bp band of the size marker is again indicated. See Figure 1 for other definitions.

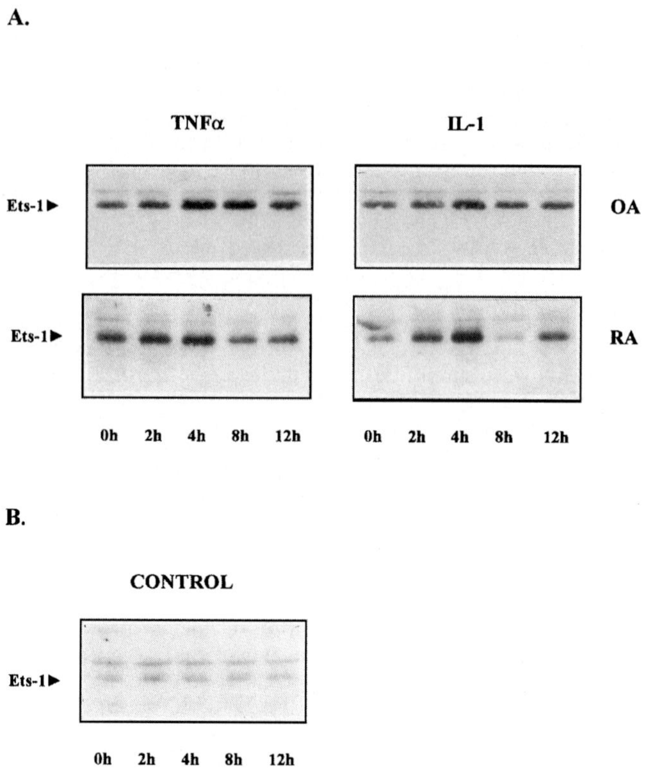

Figure 3. Regulation of Ets-1 expression by tumor necrosis factor α (TNFα) and interleukin-1 (IL-1) in RA and OA synovial fibroblasts analyzed by Western blotting. Synovial fibroblasts were incubated with TNFα (10 ng/ml) or IL-1 (5 ng/ml) for up to 12 hours (**A**) or cultured in medium alone (**B**). Whole cell extracts were separated on a 10% sodium dodecyl sulfate polyacrylamide gel (12.5 μg/lane), blotted onto nitrocellulose membranes, and probed with a polyclonal anti–Ets-1 antibody. See Figure 1 for other definitions.

protein level by Western blotting. Consistent with the RT-PCR data, only the full-length 51-kd Ets-1 protein was seen in all synovial fibroblasts investigated, confirming the results of the RT-PCR analysis (Figure 3). Both TNFα and IL-1 enhanced Ets-1 protein levels severalfold in a time-dependent manner, with maximum expression after 4 hours and a subsequent decline to basal levels after 8–12 hours (Figure 3A). The observed effects were similar for the two cytokines, with no significant quantitative differences detectable between individual patients, irrespective of their diagnoses. In contrast, Ets-1 expression remained constant when cells were cultured in medium alone (Figure 3B).

TNFα and IL-1 activation of DNA binding of Ets-1. To analyze DNA binding of Ets-1 (as an indicator of functional activation) in response to TNFα or IL-1, gel mobility shift assays were performed using a radiolabeled DNA containing the ETS-1–binding motif. Nu-

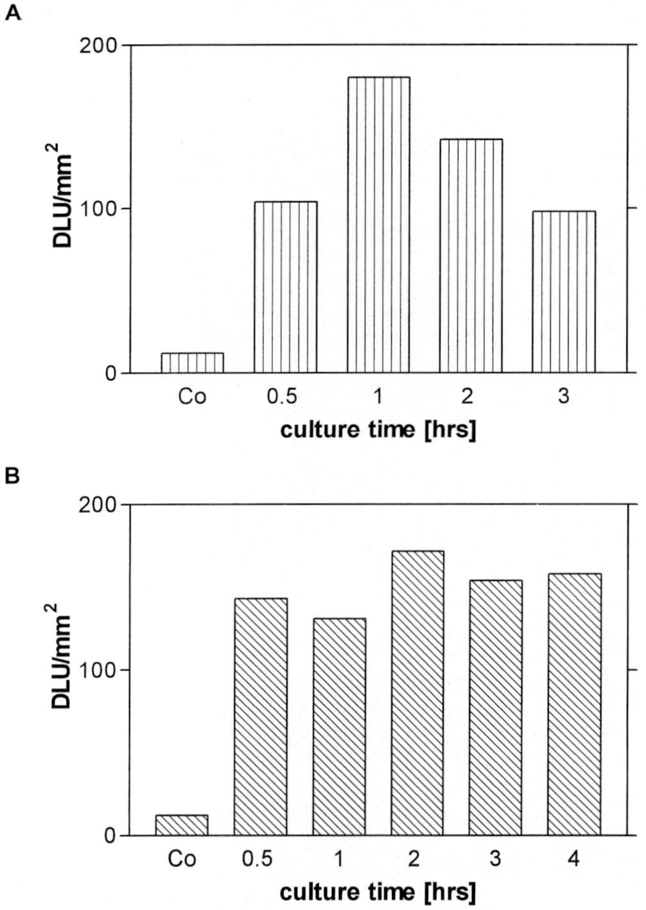

Figure 4. TNFα and IL-1 induction of DNA binding of Ets-1 in synovial fibroblasts analyzed by gel mobility shift assay. Nuclear protein extracts prepared from untreated cells (Co) and from cells treated with TNFα (**A**) or IL-1 (**B**) for various periods of time were incubated with a γ^{32}P end-labeled probe encompassing the ETS-1/PEA-3 motif and separated on a nondenaturing 4% polyacrylamide gel. The shift of radioactivity (i.e., binding of the labeled probe to Ets-1) was measured using a phosphorimager and quantified by computer analyses. Band volumes in digital light units (DLU)/mm^2 are plotted against culture time. See Figure 3 for other definitions.

clear extracts from synovial fibroblasts were prepared from cells incubated for various periods of time (0.5–4 hours) with either TNFα (10 ng/ml) or IL-1 (5 ng/ml). DNA binding activity was undetectable in the absence of either cytokine, while DNA binding was induced by both IL-1 and TNFα in cytokine-treated cells (Figure 4). Remarkably, time courses of activation differed significantly between the two cytokines because IL-1–induced activation was longlasting, being detectable after 4 hours of incubation, when TNFα-induced binding had already declined.

Intracellular localization of Ets-1. To further investigate the regulation of Ets-1 expression, the intracellular localization of Ets-1 in TNFα- and IL-1–treated synovial fibroblasts was analyzed by immunofluorescence (Figure 5). Similar results were obtained with synovial fibroblasts from RA and OA patients. In untreated synovial fibroblasts, Ets-1 was mainly localized in the nucleus (Figure 5A). Treatment with TNFα for 3 hours caused a moderate increase in Ets-1 expression (Figure 5B), while treatment with IL-1 induced a more pronounced up-regulation of Ets-1 (Figure 5C).

DISCUSSION

Several proteolytic enzymes of the MP, cysteine protease, and serine protease classes have been implicated in the destruction of cartilage in the inflamed joint (32) and identified in situ in the lining layer or directly at the cartilage–pannus junction (33–36). MMPs, particularly stromelysin 1 (MMP-3), are believed to be key enzymes involved in cartilage destruction (37,38). The data obtained in the present study revealed that Ets-1, a transcription factor involved in the regulation of MP expression, including stromelysin (39), was overexpressed in situ in a significant proportion of RA synoviocytes, while expression was much less frequently observed in OA synoviocytes.

In line with the important roles of IL-1 and TNFα in the pathogenesis of RA, cultured synovial fibroblasts responded to activation by IL-1 or TNFα by increasing the expression of Ets-1 protein severalfold. Moreover, both cytokines induced specific DNA binding, although with different time courses. Activation by TNFα was rapid and transient, while the effect of IL-1 appeared to be more persistent. These data suggest that among the proinflammatory cytokines, IL-1 may be the more important activator of Ets-1, while the main function of TNFα may be up-regulation and transient activation of this transcription factor. Thus, the interplay of the two cytokines seems to make possible, on the one hand, rapid activation and up-regulation by TNFα, and, on the other hand, maintenance for prolonged periods of high levels of activated Ets-1 (by virtue of the ability of TNFα to induce IL-1 [40]). Since both TNFα and IL-1 are highly expressed in RA, but not OA, synovial membrane (29,41–43), these in vitro data are in line with the ex vivo data obtained by immunohistochemistry and suggest

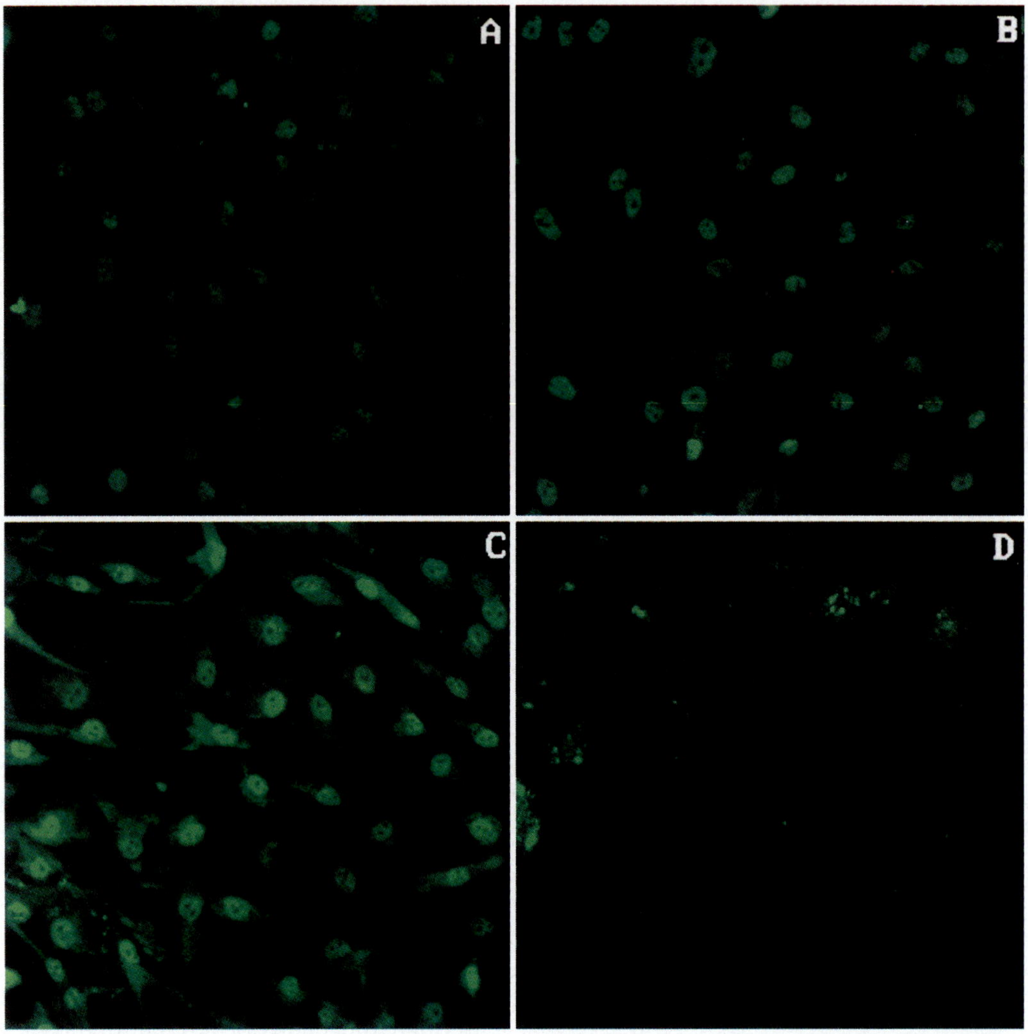

Figure 5. Up-regulation of Ets-1 expression by TNFα and IL-1 in cultured synovial fibroblasts studied by immunofluorescence microscopy. Synovial fibroblasts from a patient with rheumatoid arthritis were cultivated in chamber slides and either left untreated (**A**) or incubated with TNFα (**B**) or IL-1 (**C**) for 3 hours. Permeabilized and fixed cells were then probed with an anti–Ets-1 antibody (**A–C**) or with an anti-CD3 antibody as a control (**D**). (Original magnification × 400.) See Figure 3 for definitions.

that these two cytokines are predominantly responsible for hyperexpression and activation of Ets-1 in RA synovium.

New vessel formation is one of the pathologic features of the RA synovial membrane, and a series of angiogenic growth factors has been found to be overexpressed in RA synovial tissue (44). The pronounced expression of Ets-1 observed in synovial vascular cells indicates activation of the endothelium, and, in fact, Ets-1 has been shown to be abundantly expressed during new blood vessel formation under physiologic conditions and in tumors (45). Moreover, Ets-1 participates in the regulation of tumor invasion, presumably by controlling the transcriptional activation of matrix-degrading protease genes in stromal fibroblasts (46). Interestingly, pronounced expression of Ets-1 was also seen in synovial vascular cells from OA patients, indicating that factors other than IL-1 and TNFα may regulate Ets-1 expression in endothelial cells.

Taken together, our data suggest that Ets-1 may be an important factor in the pathogenesis of RA on several grounds: 1) by virtue of the involvement of Ets-1 in the regulation of MP production, it may be involved in the destructive pathway characteristic of RA; 2) by virtue of its involvement in angiogenesis, it may contribute to pannus expansion; and 3) by virtue of its inducibility by TNFα and IL-1, it appears to be a major mediator molecule downstream of those proinflammatory cytokines, which are known to be of prime pathogenetic importance in RA. Its more pronounced responsiveness to IL-1– versus TNFα-mediated activation signals is in line with observations from some experimental models that IL-1 may be a more important harbinger of cartilage degradation than TNFα (47), although TNFα blockade may indirectly affect IL-1–induced tissue damage (40).

Given that TNFα and IL-1 are crucial mediators of the inflammatory response, Ets-1 might constitute a novel target for therapeutic intervention. Such intervention would affect an important cytokine-mediated pathway centrally involved in the pathogenesis of RA, but leave other pathways (such as defense mechanisms against infectious organisms) unaffected. Further investigations in animal models are required to determine whether specific blockade of Ets-1 expression/activation might represent a novel therapeutic approach in the treatment of RA.

REFERENCES

1. Harris ED Jr. Rheumatoid arthritis: pathophysiology and implications for therapy. N Engl J Med 1990;322:1277–89.
2. Ziff M. Rheumatoid arthritis—its present and future. J Rheumatol 1990;17:127–33.
3. Zvaifler NJ, Tsai V, Alsalameh S, von Kempis J, Firestein GS, Lotz M. Pannocytes: distinctive cells found in rheumatoid arthritis articular cartilage erosions. Am J Pathol 1997;150:1125–38.
4. Gay S, Gay RE, Koopman WJ. Molecular and cellular mechanisms of joint destruction in rheumatoid arthritis: two cellular mechanisms explain joint destruction? Ann Rheum Dis 1993;52 Suppl 1:S39–47.
5. Brennan FM, Maini RN, Feldmann M. Role of pro-inflammatory cytokines in rheumatoid arthritis. Springer Semin Immunopathol 1998;20:133–47.
6. Brennan FM, Maini RN, Feldmann M. TNF alpha—a pivotal role in rheumatoid arthritis? Br J Rheumatol 1992;31:293–8.
7. Arend WP, Dayer J-M. Inhibition of the production and effects of interleukin-1 and tumor necrosis factor α in rheumatoid arthritis. Arthritis Rheum 1995;38:151–60.
8. Maini RN, Elliott M, Brennan FM, Williams RO, Feldmann M. TNF blockade in rheumatoid arthritis: implications for therapy and pathogenesis. APMIS 1997;105:257–63.
9. Elliott MJ, Maini RN, Feldmann M, Kalden JR, Antoni C, Smolen JS, et al. Randomised double-blind comparison of chimeric monoclonal antibody to tumour necrosis factor alpha (cA2) versus placebo in rheumatoid arthritis. Lancet 1994;344:1105–10.
10. Firestein GS, Manning AM. Signal transduction and transcription factors in rheumatic disease. Arthritis Rheum 1999;42:609–21.
11. Westermarck J, Kahari VM. Regulation of matrix metalloproteinase expression in tumor invasion. FASEB J 1999;13:781–92.
12. Schett G, Redlich K, Xu Q, Bizan P, Groger M, Tohidast AM, et al. Enhanced expression of heat shock protein 70 (hsp70) and heat shock factor 1 (HSF1) activation in rheumatoid arthritis synovial tissue: differential regulation of hsp70 expression and hsf1 activation in synovial fibroblasts by proinflammatory cytokines, shear stress, and antiinflammatory drugs. J Clin Invest 1998;102:302–11.
13. Schett G, Steiner CW, Groger M, Winkler S, Graninger W, Smolen J, et al. Activation of Fas inhibits heat-induced activation of HSF1 and up-regulation of hsp70. FASEB J 1999;13:833–42.
14. Lacraz S, Nicod LP, Chicheportiche R, Welgus HG, Dayer JM. IL-10 inhibits metalloproteinase and stimulates TIMP-1 production in human mononuclear phagocytes. J Clin Invest 1995;96: 2304–10.
15. Dayer JM, Burger D. Interleukin-1, tumor necrosis factor and their specific inhibitors. Eur Cytokine Netw 1994;5:563–71.
16. Mort JS, Dodge GR, Roughley PJ, Liu J, Finch SJ, DiPasquale G, et al. Direct evidence for active metalloproteinases mediating matrix degradation in interleukin 1-stimulated human articular cartilage. Matrix 1993;13:95–102.
17. Bondeson J, Foxwell B, Brennan F, Feldmann M. Defining therapeutic targets by using adenovirus: blocking NF-kappaB inhibits both inflammatory and destructive mechanisms in rheumatoid synovium but spares anti-inflammatory mediators. Proc Natl Acad Sci U S A 1999;96:5668–73.
18. Wakisaka S, Suzuki N, Saito N, Ochi T, Sakane T. Possible correction of abnormal rheumatoid arthritis synovial cell function by jun D transfection in vitro. Arthritis Rheum 1998;41:470–81.
19. Gilles F, Raes MB, Stehelin D, Vandenbunder B, Fafeur V. The c-ets-1 proto-oncogene is a new early-response gene differentially regulated by cytokines and growth factors in human fibroblasts. Exp Cell Res 1996;222:370–8.
20. Nunn MF, Seeburg PH, Moscovici C, Duesberg PH. Tripartite structure of the avian erythroblastosis virus E26 transforming gene. Nature 1983;306:391–5.
21. Seth A, Ascione R, Fisher RJ, Mavrothalassitis GJ, Bhat NK, Papas TS. The ets gene family. Cell Growth Differ 1992;3:327–34.
22. Wasylyk B, Hahn SL, Giovane A. The Ets family of transcription factors. Eur J Biochem 1993;211:7–18.
23. Janknecht R, Nordheim A. Gene regulation by Ets proteins. Biochim Biophys Acta 1993;1155:346–56.
24. Crepieux P, Coll J, Stehelin D. The Ets family of proteins: weak modulators of gene expression in quest for transcriptional partners. Crit Rev Oncog 1994;5:615–38.
25. Wasylyk C, Gutman A, Nicholson R, Wasylyk B. The c-Ets oncoprotein activates the stromelysin promoter through the same elements as several non-nuclear oncoproteins. EMBO J 1991;10: 1127–34.
26. Wasylyk C, Wasylyk B. Oncogenic conversion alters the transcriptional properties of ets. Cell Growth Differ 1992;3:617–25.
27. Arnett FC, Edworthy SM, Bloch DA, McShane DJ, Fries JF, Cooper NS, et al. The American Rheumatism Association 1987 revised criteria for the classification of rheumatoid arthritis. Arthritis Rheum 1988;31:315–24.
28. Altman RD, Bloch DA, Bole GG Jr, Brandt KD, Cooke DV, Greenwald RA, et al. Development of clinical criteria for osteoarthritis. J Rheumatol 1987;14:3–6.
29. Steiner G, Tohidast AM, Witzmann G, Vesely M, Studnicka BA, Gal A, et al. Cytokine production by synovial T cells in rheumatoid arthritis. Rheumatology (Oxford) 1999;38:202–13.
30. Kiener HP, Hofbauer R, Tohidast-Akrad M, Walchshofer S, Redlich K, Bitzan P, et al. Tumor necrosis factor α promotes the expression of stem cell factor in synovial fibroblasts and their capacity to induce mast cell chemotaxis. Arthritis Rheum 2000;43: 164–74.
31. Jorcyk CL, Watson DK, Mavrothalassitis GJ, Papas TS. The human ETS1 gene: genomic structure, promoter characterization and alternative splicing. Oncogene 1991;6:523–32.
32. Vincenti MP, Clark IM, Brinckerhoff CE. Using inhibitors of

metalloproteinases to treat arthritis: easier said than done? Arthritis Rheum 1994;37:1115–26.
33. McCachren SS, Haynes BF, Niedel JE. Localization of collagenase mRNA in rheumatoid arthritis synovium by in situ hybridization histochemistry. J Clin Immunol 1990;10:19–27.
34. McCachren SS. Expression of metalloproteinases and metalloproteinase inhibitor in human arthritic synovium. Arthritis Rheum 1991;34:1085–93.
35. Firestein GS, Paine MM, Littman BH. Gene expression (collagenase, tissue inhibitor of metalloproteinases, complement, and HLA–DR) in rheumatoid arthritis and osteoarthritis synovium: quantitative analysis and effect of intraarticular corticosteroids. Arthritis Rheum 1991;34:1094–105.
36. Woolley DE, Crossley MJ, Evanson JM. Collagenase at sites of cartilage erosion in the rheumatoid joint. Arthritis Rheum 1977; 20:1231–9.
37. Krane SM, Conca W, Stephenson ML, Amento EP, Goldring MB. Mechanisms of matrix degradation in rheumatoid arthritis. Ann N Y Acad Sci 1990;580:340–54.
38. Hasty KA, Reife RA, Kang AH, Stuart JM. The role of stromelysin in the cartilage destruction that accompanies inflammatory arthritis. Arthritis Rheum 1990;33:388–97.
39. Wasylyk B, Wasylyk C, Flores P, Begue A, Leprince D, Stehelin D. The c-ets proto-oncogenes encode transcription factors that cooperate with c-Fos and c-Jun for transcriptional activation. Nature 1990;346:191–3.
40. Brennan FM, Chantry D, Jackson A, Maini R, Feldmann M. Inhibitory effect of TNF alpha antibodies on synovial cell interleukin-1 production in rheumatoid arthritis. Lancet 1989;2:244–7.
41. Miyasaka N, Sato K, Goto M, Sasano M, Natsuyama M, Inoue K, et al. Augmented interleukin-1 production and HLA–DR expression in the synovium of rheumatoid arthritis patients: possible involvement in joint destruction. Arthritis Rheum 1988;31:480–6.
42. Saxne T, Palladino MA Jr, Heinegård D, Talal N, Wollheim FA. Detection of tumor necrosis factor α but not tumor necrosis factor β in rheumatoid arthritis synovial fluid and serum. Arthritis Rheum 1988;31:1041–5.
43. Cope AP, Aderka D, Doherty M, Engelmann H, Gibbons D, Jones AC, et al. Increased levels of soluble tumor necrosis factor receptors in the sera and synovial fluid of patients with rheumatic diseases. Arthritis Rheum 1992;35:1160–9.
44. Koch AE. Angiogenesis: implications for rheumatoid arthritis. Arthritis Rheum 1998;41:951–62.
45. Vandenbunder B, Pardanaud L, Jaffredo T, Mirabel MA, Stehelin D. Complementary patterns of expression of c-ets 1, c-myb and c-myc in the blood-forming system of the chick embryo. Development 1989;107:265–74.
46. Wernert N, Gilles F, Fafeur V, Bouali F, Raes MB, Pyke C, et al. Stromal expression of c-Ets1 transcription factor correlates with tumor invasion. Cancer Res 1994;54:5683–8.
47. Bresnihan B, Alvaro-Gracia JM, Cobby M, Doherty M, Domljan Z, Emery P, et al. Treatment of rheumatoid arthritis with recombinant human interleukin-1 receptor antagonist. Arthritis Rheum 1998;41:2196–204.

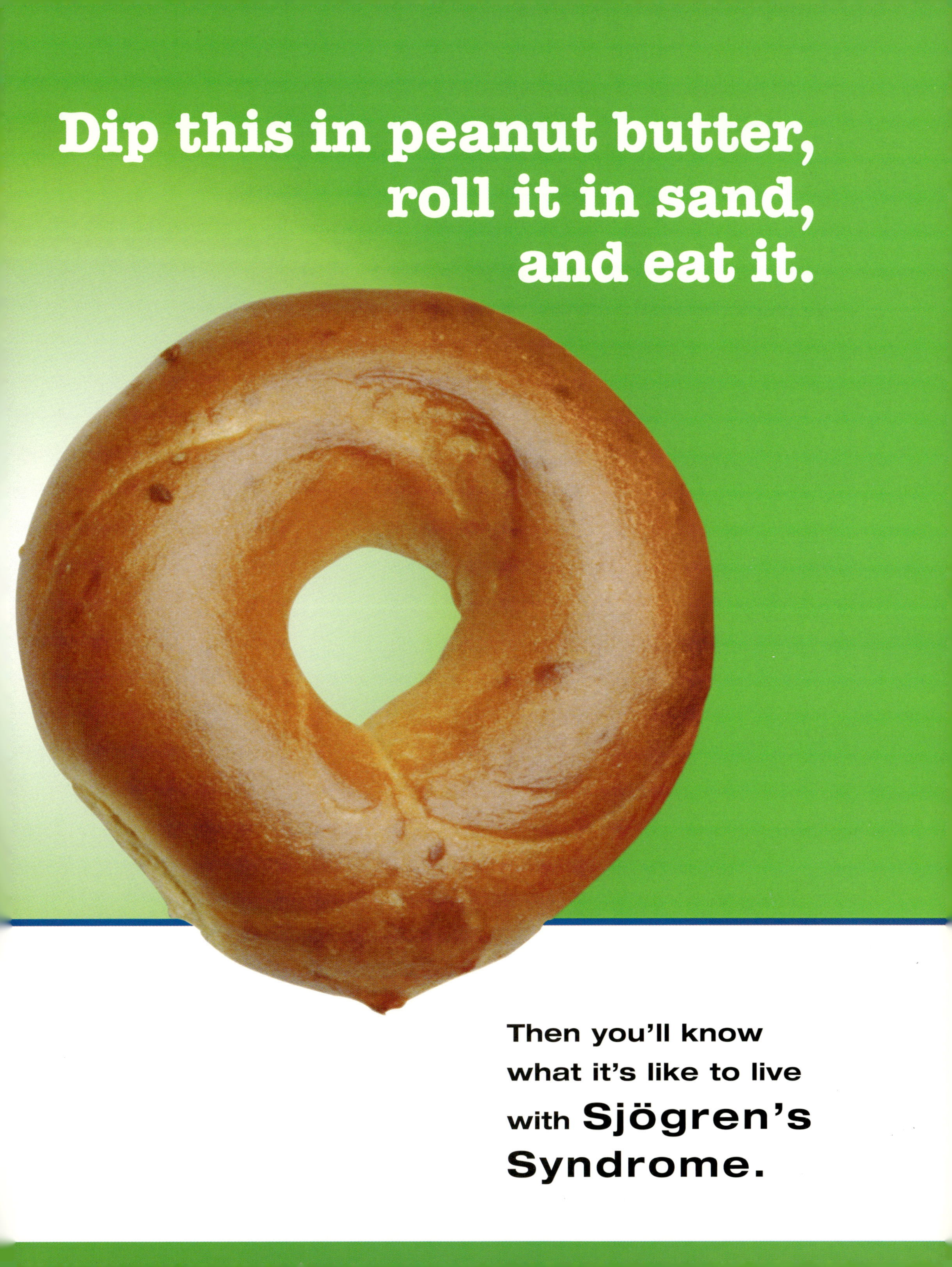
Dip this in peanut butter,
roll it in sand,
and eat it.
Then you'll know
what it's like to live
with Sjögren's
Syndrome.

Evoxac™ (ˈē vō zak)
(cevimeline HCl) 30 mg Capsules

EVOXAC™ Capsules
(cevimeline hydrochloride)

Brief Summary
Consult package insert for full prescribing information.

INDICATIONS AND USAGE: Cevimeline is indicated for the treatment of symptoms of dry mouth in patients with Sjögren's Syndrome.

CONTRAINDICATIONS: Cevimeline is contraindicated in patients with uncontrolled asthma, known hypersensitivity to cevimeline, and when miosis is undesirable, e.g., in acute iritis and in narrow-angle (angle-closure) glaucoma.

WARNINGS:

Cardiovascular Disease: Cevimeline can potentially alter cardiac conduction and/or heart rate. Patients with significant cardiovascular disease may potentially be unable to compensate for transient changes in hemodynamics or rhythm induced by EVOXAC™. EVOXAC™ should be used with caution and under close medical supervision in patients with a history of cardiovascular disease evidenced by angina pectoris or myocardial infarction.

Pulmonary Disease: Cevimeline can potentially increase airway resistance, bronchial smooth muscle tone, and bronchial secretions. Cevimeline should be administered with caution and with close medical supervision to patients with controlled asthma, chronic bronchitis, or chronic obstructive pulmonary disease.

Ocular: Ophthalmic formulations of muscarinic agonists have been reported to cause visual blurring which may result in decreased visual acuity, especially at night and in patients with central lens changes, and to cause impairment of depth perception. Caution should be advised while driving at night or performing hazardous activities in reduced lighting.

PRECAUTIONS:

General: Cevimeline toxicity is characterized by an exaggeration of its parasympathomimetic effects. These may include: headache, visual disturbance, lacrimation, sweating, respiratory distress, gastrointestinal spasm, nausea, vomiting, diarrhea, atrioventricular block, tachycardia, bradycardia, hypotension, hypertension, shock, mental confusion, cardiac arrhythmia, and tremors.

Cevimeline should be administered with caution to patients with a history of nephrolithiasis or cholelithiasis. Contractions of the gallbladder or biliary smooth muscle could precipitate complications such as cholecystitis, cholangitis and biliary obstruction. An increase in the ureteral smooth muscle tone could theoretically precipitate renal colic or ureteral reflux in patients with nephrolithiasis.

Information for Patients: Patients should be informed that cevimeline may cause visual disturbances, especially at night, that could impair their ability to drive safely.

If a patient sweats excessively while taking cevimeline, dehydration may develop. The patient should drink extra water and consult a health care provider.

Drug Interactions: Cevimeline should be administered with caution to patients taking beta adrenergic antagonists, because of the possibility of conduction disturbances. Drugs with parasympathomimetic effects administered concurrently with cevimeline can be expected to have additive effects. Cevimeline might interfere with desirable antimuscarinic effects of drugs used concomitantly.

Drugs which inhibit CYP2D6 and CYP3A3/4 also inhibit the metabolism of cevimeline. Cevimeline should be used with caution in individuals known or suspected to be deficient in CYP2D6 activity, based on previous experience, as they may be at a higher risk of adverse events. In an *in vitro* study, cytochrome P450 isozymes 1A2, 2A6, 2C9, 2C19, 2D6, 2E1, and 3A4 were not inhibited by exposure to cevimeline.

Carcinogenesis, Mutagenesis and Impairment of Fertility: Lifetime carcinogenicity studies were conducted in CD-1 mice and F-344 rats. A statistically significant increase in the incidence of adenocarcinomas of the uterus was observed in female rats that received cevimeline at a dosage of 100 mg/kg/day (approximately 8 times the maximum human exposure based on comparison of AUC data). No other significant differences in tumor incidence were observed in either mice or rats.

Cevimeline exhibited no evidence of mutagenicity or clastogenicity in a battery of assays that included an Ames test, an *in vitro* chromosomal aberration study in mammalian cells, a mouse lymphoma study in L5178Y cells, or a micronucleus assay conducted *in vivo* in ICR mice.

Cevimeline did not adversely affect the reproductive performance or fertility of male Sprague-Dawley rats when administered for 63 days prior to mating and throughout the period of mating at dosages up to 45 mg/kg/day (approximately 5 times the maximum recommended dose for a 60 kg human following normalization of the data on the basis of body surface area estimates). Females that were treated with cevimeline at dosages up to 45 mg/kg/day from 14 days prior to mating through day seven of gestation exhibited a statistically significantly smaller number of implantations than did control animals.

Pregnancy: Pregnancy Category C.

Cevimeline was associated with a reduction in the mean number of implantations when given to pregnant Sprague-Dawley rats from 14 days prior to mating through day seven of gestation at a dosage of 45 mg/kg/day (approximately 5 times the maximum recommended dose for a 60 kg human when compared on the basis of body surface area estimates). This effect may have been secondary to maternal toxicity. There are no adequate and well-controlled studies in pregnant women. Cevimeline should be used during pregnancy only if the potential benefit justifies the potential risk to the fetus.

Nursing Mothers: It is not known whether this drug is secreted in human milk. Because many drugs are excreted in human milk, and because of the potential for serious adverse reactions in nursing infants from EVOXAC™, a decision should be made whether to discontinue nursing or discontinue the drug, taking into account the importance of the drug to the mother.

Pediatric Use: Safety and effectiveness in pediatric patients have not been established.

Geriatric Use: Although clinical studies of cevimeline included subjects over the age of 65, the numbers were not sufficient to determine whether they respond differently from younger subjects. Special care should be exercised when cevimeline treatment is initiated in an elderly patient, considering the greater frequency of decreased hepatic, renal, or cardiac function, and of concomitant disease or other drug therapy in the elderly.

ADVERSE REACTIONS: Cevimeline was administered to 1777 patients during clinical trials worldwide, including Sjögren's patients and patients with other conditions. In placebo-controlled Sjögren's studies in the U.S., 320 patients received cevimeline doses ranging from 15 mg tid to 60 mg tid, of whom 93% were women and 7% were men. Demographic distribution was 90% Caucasian, 5% Hispanic, 3% Black, and 2% of other origin. In these studies, 14.6% of patients discontinued treatment with cevimeline due to adverse events.

The following adverse events associated with muscarinic agonism were observed in the clinical trials of cevimeline in Sjögren's syndrome patients:

Adverse Event	Cevimeline 30 mg (tid) n* = 533	Placebo (tid) n = 164	Adverse Event	Cevimeline 30 mg (tid) n* = 533	Placebo (tid) n = 164
Excessive Sweating	18.7%	2.4%	Urinary Frequency	0.9%	1.8%
Nausea	13.8%	7.9%	Asthenia	0.5%	0.0%
Rhinitis	11.2%	5.4%	Flushing	0.3%	0.6%
Diarrhea	10.3%	10.3%	Polyuria	0.1%	0.6%
Excessive Salivation	2.2%	0.6%			

*n is the total number of patients exposed to the dose at any time during the study

In addition, the following adverse events (≥3% incidence) were reported in the Sjögren's clinical trials:

Adverse Event	Cevimeline 30 mg (tid) n* = 533	Placebo (tid) n = 164	Adverse Event	Cevimeline 30 mg (tid) n* = 533	Placebo (tid) n = 164
Headache	14.4%	20.1%	Conjunctivitis	4.3%	3.6%
Sinusitis	12.3%	10.9%	Dizziness	4.1%	7.3%
Upper Respiratory Tract Infection	11.4%	9.1%	Bronchitis	4.1%	1.2%
Dyspepsia	7.8%	8.5%	Arthralgia	3.7%	1.8%
Abdominal Pain	7.6%	6.7%	Surgical Intervention	3.3%	3.0%
Urinary Tract Infection	6.1%	3.0%	Fatigue	3.3%	1.2%
Coughing	6.1%	3.0%	Pain	3.3%	3.0%
Pharyngitis	5.2%	5.4%	Skeletal Pain	2.8%	1.8%
Vomiting	4.6%	2.4%	Insomnia	2.4%	1.2%
Injury	4.5%	2.4%	Hot Flushes	2.4%	0.0%
Back Pain	4.5%	4.2%	Rigors	1.3%	1.2%
Rash	4.3%	6.0%	Anxiety	1.3%	1.2%

*n is the total number of patients exposed to the dose at any time during the study

The following events were reported in Sjögren's patients at incidences of <3% and ≥1%: constipation, tremor, abnormal vision, hypertonia, peripheral edema, chest pain, myalgia, fever, anorexia, eye pain, earache, dry mouth, vertigo, salivary gland pain, pruritus, influenza-like symptoms, eye infection, post-operative pain, vaginitis, skin disorder, depression, hiccup, hyporeflexia, infection, fungal infection, sialoadenitis, otitis media, erythematous rash, pneumonia, edema, salivary gland enlargement, allergy, gastroesophageal reflux, eye abnormality, migraine, tooth disorder, epistaxis, flatulence, toothache, ulcerative stomatitis, anemia, hypoesthesia, cystitis, leg cramps, abscess, eructation, moniliasis, palpitation, increased amylase, xerophthalmia, allergic reaction.

The following events were reported rarely in treated Sjögren's patients (<1%): Causal relation is unknown:

Body as a Whole Disorders: aggravated allergy, precordial chest pain, abnormal crying, hematoma, leg pain, edema, periorbital edema, activated pain trauma, pallor, changed sensation to temperature, weight decrease, weight increase, choking, mouth edema, syncope, malaise, face edema, substernal chest pain

Cardiovascular Disorders: abnormal ECG, heart disorder, heart murmur, aggravated hypertension, hypotension, arrhythmia, extrasystoles, t wave inversion, tachycardia, supraventricular tachycardia, angina pectoris, myocardial infarction, pericarditis, pulmonary embolism, peripheral ischemia, superficial phlebitis, purpura, deep thrombophlebitis, vascular disorder, vasculitis, hypertension

Digestive Disorders: appendicitis, increased appetite, ulcerative colitis, diverticulitis, duodenitis, dysphagia, enterocolitis, gastric ulcer, gastritis, gastroenteritis, gastrointestinal hemorrhage, gingivitis, glossitis, rectum hemorrhage, hemorrhoids, ileus, irritable bowel syndrome, melena, mucositis, esophageal stricture, esophagitis, oral hemorrhage, peptic ulcer, periodontal destruction, rectal disorder, stomatitis, tenesmus, tongue discoloration, tongue disorder, geographic tongue, tongue ulceration, dental caries

Endocrine Disorders: increased glucocorticoids, goiter, hypothyroidism

Hematologic Disorders: thrombocytopenic purpura, thrombocythemia, thrombocytopenia, hypochromic anemia, eosinophilia, granulocytopenia, leucopenia, leukocytosis, cervical lymphadenopathy, lymphadenopathy

Liver and Biliary System Disorders: cholelithiasis, increased gamma-glutamyl transferase, increased hepatic enzymes, abnormal hepatic function, viral hepatitis, increased serum glutamate oxaloacetic transaminase (SGOT)(also called AST-aspartate aminotransferase), increased serum glutamate pyruvate transaminase (SGPT)(also called ALT-alanine aminotransferase)

Metabolic and Nutritional Disorders: dehydration, diabetes mellitus, hypercalcemia, hypercholesterolemia, hyperglycemia, hyperlipemia, hypertriglyceridemia, hyperuricemia, hypoglycemia, hypokalemia, hyponatremia, thirst

Musculoskeletal Disorders: arthritis, aggravated arthritis, arthropathy, femoral head avascular necrosis, bone disorder, bursitis, costochondritis, plantar fasciitis, muscle weakness, osteomyelitis, osteoporosis, synovitis, tendinitis, tenosynovitis

Neoplasms: basal cell carcinoma, squamous carcinoma

Nervous Disorders: carpal tunnel syndrome, coma, abnormal coordination, dysesthesia, dyskinesia, dysphonia, aggravated multiple sclerosis, involuntary muscle contractions, neuralgia, neuropathy, paresthesia, speech disorder, agitation, confusion, depersonalization, aggravated depression, abnormal dreaming, emotional lability, manic reaction, paroniria, somnolence, abnormal thinking, hyperkinesia, hallucination

Miscellaneous Disorders: fall, food poisoning, heat stroke, joint dislocation, post-operative hemorrhage

Resistance Mechanism Disorders: cellulitis, herpes simplex, herpes zoster, bacterial infection, viral infection, genital moniliasis, sepsis

Respiratory Disorders: asthma, bronchospasm, chronic obstructive airway disease, dyspnea, hemoptysis, laryngitis, nasal ulcer, pleural effusion, pleurisy, pulmonary congestion, pulmonary fibrosis, respiratory disorder

Rheumatologic Disorders: aggravated rheumatoid arthritis, lupus erythematosus rash, lupus erythematosus syndrome

Skin and Appendages Disorders: acne, alopecia, burn, dermatitis, contact dermatitis, lichenoid dermatitis, eczema, furunculosis, hyperkeratosis, lichen planus, nail discoloration, nail disorder, onychia, onychomycosis, paronychia, photosensitivity reaction, rosacea, scleroderma, seborrhea, skin discoloration, dry skin, skin exfoliation, skin hypertrophy, skin ulceration, urticaria, verruca, bullous eruption, cold clammy skin

Special Senses Disorders: deafness, decreased hearing, motion sickness, parosmia, taste perversion, blepharitis, cataract, corneal opacity, corneal ulceration, diplopia, glaucoma, anterior chamber eye hemorrhage, keratitis, keratoconjunctivitis, mydriasis, myopia, photopsia, retinal deposits, retinal disorder, scleritis, vitreous detachment, tinnitus

Urogenital Disorders: epididymitis, prostatic disorder, abnormal sexual function, amenorrhea, female breast neoplasm, malignant female breast neoplasm, female breast pain, positive cervical smear test, dysmenorrhea, endometrial disorder, intermenstrual bleeding, leukorrhea, menorrhagia, menstrual disorder, ovarian cyst, ovarian disorder, genital pruritus, uterine hemorrhage, vaginal hemorrhage, atrophic vaginitis, albuminuria, bladder discomfort, increased blood urea nitrogen, dysuria, hematuria, micturition disorder, nephrosis, nocturia, increased nonprotein nitrogen, pyelonephritis, renal calculus, abnormal renal function, renal pain, strangury, urethral disorder, abnormal urine, urinary incontinence, decreased urine flow, pyuria

In one subject with lupus erythematosus receiving concomitant multiple drug therapy, a highly elevated ALT level was noted after the fourth week of cevimeline therapy. In two other subjects receiving cevimeline in the clinical trials, very high AST levels were noted. The significance of these findings is unknown.

Additional adverse events (relationship unknown) which occurred in other clinical studies (patient population different from Sjögren's patients) are as follows:

cholinergic syndrome, blood pressure fluctuation, cardiomegaly, postural hypotension, aphasia, convulsions, abnormal gait, hyperesthesia, paralysis, abnormal sexual function, enlarged abdomen, change in bowel habits, gum hyperplasia, intestinal obstruction, bundle branch block, increased creatine phosphokinase, electrolyte abnormality, glycosuria, gout, hyperkalemia, hyperproteinemia, increased lactic dehydrogenase (LDH), increased alkaline phosphatase, failure to thrive, abnormal platelets, aggressive reaction, amnesia, apathy, delirium, delusion, dementia, illusion, impotence, neurosis, paranoid reaction, personality disorder, hyperhemoglobinemia, apnea, atelectasis, yawning, oliguria, urinary retention, distended vein, lymphocytosis

MANAGEMENT OF OVERDOSE: Management of the signs and symptoms of acute overdosage should be handled in a manner consistent with that indicated for other muscarinic agonists: general supportive measures should be instituted. If medically indicated, atropine, an anti-cholinergic agent may be of value as an antidote for emergency use in patients who have had an overdose of cevimeline. If medically indicated, epinephrine may also be of value in the presence of severe cardiovascular depression or bronchoconstriction. It is not known if cevimeline is dialyzable.

DOSAGE AND ADMINISTRATION: The recommended dose of cevimeline is 30 mg taken three times a day. There is insufficient safety information to support doses greater than 30 mg tid. There is also insufficient evidence for additional efficacy of cevimeline at doses greater than 30 mg tid.

Rx Only

Manufactured by:
YAMANOUCHI PHARMA TECHNOLOGIES, INC., Palo Alto, CA 94304

for:
SnowBrand Pharmaceuticals, Inc., Rockville, MD 20850

Distributed and Marketed by:
Daiichi Pharmaceutical Corporation, Montvale, NJ 07645

02/2000 Printed in U.S.A.

Reference: 1. Data on file, Daiichi Pharmaceutical Corporation.

ARTHRITIS & RHEUMATISM
Vol. 44, No. 2, February 2001, pp 275–285

Interferon-γ–Inducing Activity of Interleukin-18 in the Joint With Rheumatoid Arthritis

Masahiro Yamamura,[1] Masanori Kawashima,[1] Madoka Taniai,[2] Hiroshi Yamauchi,[2] Tadao Tanimoto,[2] Masashi Kurimoto,[2] Yoshitaka Morita,[1] Yasukazu Ohmoto,[3] and Hirofumi Makino[1]

Objective. **To examine the levels of interleukin-18 (IL-18) bioactivity within the rheumatoid arthritis (RA) joint, and the differential effects of IL-12 and IL-18 on interferon-γ (IFNγ) production by T cell infiltrates.**

Methods. **Expression of IL-18 protein and messenger RNA (mRNA) was determined by enzyme-linked immunosorbent assay and reverse transcriptase–polymerase chain reaction, respectively. The biologic activity of IL-18 was detected on the basis of IFNγ secretion from IL-18–responding human myelomonocytic KG-1 cells. To determine the extent of inhibitory activity on binding of IL-18 to its receptor, a [^{125}I]–IL-18 binding inhibition assay was performed, using a Chinese hamster ovary cell line transfected with a murine IL-18 receptor.**

Results. **The amount of IL-18 protein detected in both the serum and synovial fluid of RA patients was markedly larger than that detected in the serum and synovial fluid of osteoarthritis (OA) patients, and serum IL-18 levels correlated with the levels of serum C-reactive protein. IFNγ production by KG-1 cells was more strongly stimulated in synovial fluid samples from RA patients than in samples from OA patients, and this activity was largely diminished in the presence of anti–IL-18 antibody. In contrast, the activity of IL-18 binding inhibition in the serum and synovial fluid of RA patients was not significantly elevated compared with that in OA patients. RA synovial tissues showed increased expression of IL-18 mRNA and increased IL-18 protein synthesis compared with that in OA tissues. Purified CD14+ macrophages, but not activated fibroblast cell lines, from RA synovium were able to release mature IL-18, although both cell types expressed its transcripts. IL-18 alone showed a negligible effect on IFNγ production by RA synovial tissue cells, in contrast to IL-12, which was directly stimulatory. However, IL-12–induced IFNγ production was synergistically enhanced by IL-18, and yet was >50% reduced by neutralization of endogenous IL-18 with anti–IL-18 antibody.**

Conclusion. **These results indicate that IL-18, produced predominantly by tissue macrophages, primarily potentiates IL-12–induced IFNγ production by T cell infiltrates in RA synovium. Detection of significant IL-18 bioactivity in the joints, despite the presence of IL-18 binding inhibitors, supports an integral role of this cytokine in perpetuating the IFNγ-dominant T cell cytokine response in RA.**

The chronically inflamed synovium of rheumatoid arthritis (RA) is characterized by a massive infiltration of lymphocytes and macrophages, and by an expansion of fibroblast-like synoviocytes. CD4+ T cells are the major cellular component with signs of some activation (1), but their exact role in the pathogenesis of RA has proved controversial. Cytokines produced by activated T cells, such as interleukin-2 (IL-2), IL-4, and interferon-γ (IFNγ), have been detected only at low levels in RA joints (2), in contrast to the abundance of cytokine products from macrophages and fibroblasts, such as IL-1, tumor necrosis factor α (TNFα), and IL-6 (3). However, the involvement of T cell–mediated immune responses in the disease process has been suggested by

Supported in part by grants-in-aid 10670411/12670426 from the Ministry of Education, Science, and Culture of Japan.

[1]Masahiro Yamamura, MD, Masanori Kawashima, MD, Yoshitaka Morita, MD, Hirofumi Makino, MD: Okayama University Medical School, Okayama, Japan; [2]Madoka Taniai, PhD, Hiroshi Yamauchi, PhD, Tadao Tanimoto, PhD, Masashi Kurimoto, PhD: Fujisaki Institute, Hayashibara Company Inc., Okayama, Japan; [3]Yasukazu Ohmoto, PhD: Otsuka Pharmaceutical Company Ltd., Tokushima, Japan.

Address correspondence and reprint requests to Masahiro Yamamura, MD, Department of Medicine III, Okayama University Medical School, 2-5-1 Shikata-cho, Okayama 700-8558, Japan.

Submitted for publication April 27, 2000; accepted in revised form September 27, 2000.

observations of an association between certain HLA–DRB1 genes and disease susceptibility and severity (4), the efficacy of T cell–targeting therapy (5), and evidence of oligoclonal T cell expansion in analyses on the nature of the T cell receptor repertoire (6).

Studies of T cell cytokine patterns in the RA joint at the messenger RNA (mRNA) level and studies using T cell clones indicate the predominance of IFNγ-producing Th1 cells (7–9). By intracellular cytokine staining of peripheral blood and synovial tissue T cells from RA patients, we have confirmed the selective accumulation of Th1 and Th0 cells in the synovium (10). In addition, we have demonstrated that IL-12 is produced mainly by the macrophage-lineage cells localized adjacent to lymphatic aggregates, and can potently and selectively stimulate IFNγ production by RA synovial tissues and IL-2–expanding synovial T cells (11). However, levels of IL-12 expression are very limited. Therefore, the induction of an IFNγ-dominant T cell response within the RA joint may be perpetuated on the basis of the complex interaction between IL-12 and other molecules.

IL-18 was originally identified as an IFNγ-inducing factor derived from Kupffer cells and activated macrophages (12–14), but it is now known to have a wide range of biologic activities, mostly on lymphocytes. IL-18 stimulates the synthesis of IFNγ in T cells and natural killer (NK) cells, the proliferation of activated T cells and their production of IL-2 and granulocyte–macrophage colony-stimulating factor (GM-CSF), the cytotoxic activity of NK cells through up-regulation of the Fas ligand, and the development of Th1-type immune responses (12–18). More recently, IL-18 has been shown to trigger a cascade of inflammatory cytokines, including IL-1β, and chemokines in human blood monocytes through the production of TNFα by T cells and NK cells (19). IL-18 polypeptide is synthesized as the precursor of 193 amino acids, which is cleaved by activated IL-1β–converting enzyme (ICE), the intracellular cysteine proteinase, to generate the mature 18.3-kd protein (20,21).

IL-18 may be involved in various immunologically mediated inflammatory conditions. However, its potentially deleterious properties are thought to be regulated in vivo by inhibitory molecules. IL-18 binding protein (IL-18BP) has recently been identified as a specific inhibitor of IL-18 bioactivity (22,23). Despite its lack of significant homology with IL-18 receptor components, IL-18BP is able to bind to IL-18 protein with high affinity, thereby acting as a soluble decoy receptor. Since it lacks a transmembrane domain, this inhibitor belongs to a novel family of soluble receptor–like proteins. IL-18BP was found to selectively and efficiently abolish IL-18 induction of IFNγ, IL-8, and activation of the transcription factor nuclear factor κB (NF-κB) in vitro (23). This inhibitor is constitutively expressed in healthy human tissue at the mRNA level, but most prominently in the spleen and lungs (22,23). Therefore, the immune response mediated by IL-18 appears to be determined by the net balance of the relative levels of IL-18 and IL-18BP.

Significant levels of expresssion of IL-18 have been previously demonstrated in the synovium of RA patients (24–26). It was suggested that IL-18 could be involved in both Th1 immune responses and macrophage production of inflammatory cytokines such as TNFα, in synergy with IL-12 and IL-15 (25,26). To further elucidate the pathogenic relevance of IL-18 to the disease, the level of IL-18 bioactivity within the joint and the differential effects of IL-12 and IL-18 on IFNγ production by synovial tissue T cells were investigated. We showed in the present study that the biologic activity of mature IL-18, derived mainly from tissue macrophages, was greatly reduced by the presence of IL-18 binding inhibitors in RA joints, but was detectable at significant levels in active disease. In addition, our results suggest that its major effect may be to potentiate the IFNγ-dominant T cell response induced by IL-12.

PATIENTS AND METHODS

Cytokines and cell lines. Recombinant human IL-1β (rHuIL-1β) and rHuTNFα were generously provided by Otsuka Pharmaceutical Company (Tokushima, Japan) and Dainippon Pharmaceutical Company (Osaka, Japan), respectively. Cells from the human myelomonocytic cell line KG-1, which dose-dependently produce IFNγ in response to human IL-18 (27), were maintained at 37°C in RPMI 1640 medium (Life Technologies, Gaithersburg, MD) supplemented with 10% heat-inactivated fetal calf serum (FCS; BioWhittaker, Walkersville, MD). The Chinese hamster ovary–K1 (CHO-K1) cell line was transfected with a murine IL-18 receptor (IL-1 receptor–related protein) expression vector plasmid, hereafter referred to as CHO-K1/mIL-18R, which was maintained at 37°C in Ham's F12 medium (Nissui, Tokyo, Japan) with 5% FCS (22).

Patients and samples. Patients with RA and control patients with osteoarthritis (OA) were diagnosed according to the revised criteria of the American College of Rheumatology (formerly, the American Rheumatism Association) (28,29). Most RA patients were receiving disease-modifying antirheumatic drugs, but none were receiving prednisolone at >5 mg/day. Serum and synovial fluid samples were prepared as described previously (30). Synovial tissue samples were obtained from patients with chronic RA and from patients with

OA (disease duration ≥2 years) at the time of surgical treatment.

Preparation and culture of synovial tissue cells and fibroblast cell lines. Fresh synovial tissues were fragmented and digested for 1 hour with collagenase (Wako Pure Chemical, Osaka, Japan) and DNase (Sigma, St. Louis, MO) in RPMI 1640 medium at 37°C. After removing tissue debris, cells were washed with medium. The resultant single-cell suspensions were adjusted at a density of 2×10^6/ml in 2 ml of Dulbecco's modified Eagle's medium (DMEM; Life Technologies) with 10% FCS, 25 m*M* HEPES (Life Technologies), 100 IU/ml penicillin, and 100 μg/ml streptomycin, and incubated in the wells of 24-well microtiter plates (Costar, Cambridge, MA) at 37°C in a humidified atmosphere containing 5% CO_2. Culture supernatants were harvested 72 hours later and stored at −30°C prior to being used in the IL-18 assay. To isolate mRNA, freshly isolated cells were placed in 4*M* guanidinium isothiocyanate buffer and stored at −30°C.

To determine the differential effects of IL-12 and IL-18 on IFNγ production by T cells in RA synovium, synovial tissue cells were incubated at 2×10^6/ml in DMEM with 10% FCS, with or without 1 ng/ml of IL-12, 1 ng/ml of IL-18, IL-12 plus IL-18, or IL-12 plus 10 μg/ml of anti–IL-18 (125-2H) monoclonal antibody (mAb). Culture supernatants were harvested 72 hours later and stored at −30°C until assayed for IFNγ.

To compare the stimulatory effects of IL-1β and IL-18 on inflammatory cytokine production by RA synovial tissues, cells were incubated at 2×10^6/ml in DMEM with 10% FCS, with or without the indicated concentrations of IL-1β or IL-18. Culture supernatants were harvested 72 hours later and stored at −30°C until assayed for TNFα, IL-1β, IL-6, and IL-8.

Synovial fibroblast cell lines were prepared from RA synovial tissues as described previously (30). Briefly, synovial tissue cells were split weekly after primary cultures had reached confluence, and used after the third passage. The resultant cells were morphologically homogeneous fibroblast-like cells that had typical bipolar configuration under inverse microscopy and lacked CD14+ macrophage-lineage cells as determined by incubation with phycoerythrin-conjugated anti-CD14 mAb (Becton Dickinson, San Jose, CA). Synovial fibroblasts were incubated at a density of 1×10^5/ml in 2 ml DMEM with 10% FCS and allowed to adhere overnight in 24-well microtiter plates. The medium was replaced with DMEM containing 1% FCS with or without 1 ng/ml of IL-1β or 10 ng/ml of TNFα. Culture supernatants were harvested 48 hours later and stored at −30°C until used in the IL-18 assay. For mRNA isolation, cells were lysed in 4*M* guanidinium isothiocyanate buffer after 18 hours of culture. Reagents used for culture were found to contain <200 pg/ml endotoxin as determined by the *Limulus* amebocyte cell lysate assay.

Preparation of purified macrophages and T cells. Macrophages and T cells were purified from RA synovial tissue cells using anti-CD14 mAb (Immunotech, Marseilles, France) and goat anti-mouse antibody–coated flasks or anti-CD3 mAb–coated flasks (AIS MicroCELLector; Applied Immune Sciences, Santa Clara, CA), according to the manufacturer's instructions (30). After removing nonadherent cells, adherent cells were collected by vigorous pipetting. The resulting T cell and macrophage populations were found to be >90% pure, as determined by flow cytometric analysis using fluorescein isothiocyanate–conjugated anti-CD2 mAb (PharMingen, San Diego, CA) and nonspecific esterase staining, respectively. For isolation of mRNA, cells were lysed in 4*M* guanidinium isothiocyanate buffer. Purified macrophages were incubated at a density of 5×10^5/ml in 2 ml of DMEM with 10% FCS. Culture supernatants were harvested 72 hours later and stored at −30°C until used in the IL-18 assay.

Immunoassay for IL-18. Concentrations of mature IL-18 protein were measured by quantitative sandwich enzyme-linked immunosorbent assay (ELISA), as previously described (31). Briefly, ELISA plates (Corning Laboratory Science, Corning, NY) were coated with 20 μg/ml of mouse anti–IL-18 mAb (IgG1κ; 125-2H) in phosphate buffered saline (PBS) for 3 hours at room temperature, followed by blocking with PBS/1% bovine serum albumin (BSA) overnight at 4°C. After washing wells with PBS/0.05% Tween 20, 50 μl of PBS with 1% BSA, 5% FCS, and 1*M* NaCl was dispensed and 50 μl of samples or rHuIL-18 standards was added to each well, followed by incubation for 2 hours at room temperature. After washing, plates were incubated for 2 hours with 0.5 μg/ml peroxidase-conjugated rat anti–IL-18 mAb (IgG2a, κ; 159-12B) in 100 μl of PBS with 1% BSA, 5% FCS, 0.1% CHAPS (Dojin Chemicals, Kumamoto, Japan), and 0.3*M* NaCl, and developed with 0.5 mg/ml of *o*-phenylenediamine (Wako Pure Chemical) in 100 μl of 0.1*M* Na_2HPO_4–citrate buffer, pH 5.0, with 0.003% H_2O_2. The reaction was quenched with 100 μl of 2*N* H_2SO_4, and optical densities at 492 nm were determined. The assay was performed in duplicate and detected concentrations of IL-18 as small as 100 pg/ml.

To eliminate IgG1-directed interferences of human heterophilic anti-mouse antibodies in our assay, MAK33 (Boehringer Mannheim, Mannheim, Germany) was added to serum and synovial fluid samples at a concentration of 200 μg/ml. However, the addition of this interference-eliminating protein is unlikely to be essential, because no significant difference was found between the values of IL-18 determined with and without MAK33 in 20 of our samples that were selected at random.

Bioassay for IL-18. The biologic activity of IL-18 was measured in triplicate by using human myelomonocytic KG-1 cells, as previously described (27). KG-1 cell suspensions were dispensed into the wells of 96-well microtiter plates (Sumitomo Bakelite, Tokyo, Japan) at a density of 3×10^6 cells/ml in 100 μl of RPMI 1640 medium with 10% FCS with or without anti–IL-18 mAb (125-2H), and 100 μl of samples and rHuIL-18 standards were added to each well. The plates were incubated and culture supernatants were harvested 24 hours later. IFNγ concentrations were determined by ELISA using 2 mouse anti-IFNγ mAb (mAb IFNγ-15 and peroxidase-conjugated mAb IFNγ-6). The IL-18 activity in samples was determined by the difference in the levels of IFNγ between cultures without anti–IL-18 mAb and those with anti–IL-18 mAb. The sensitivity of the bioassay was ~100 pg/ml.

IL-18 binding inhibition assay. The capability of samples to inhibit the binding of IL-18 to its receptor was detected in triplicate using CHO-K1/mIL-18R cells, as previously described (22). Briefly, CHO-K1/mIL-18R cells were suspended in RPMI 1640 medium containing 0.1% BSA, 0.1% NaN_3, and 100 m*M* HEPES, pH 7.2 (binding medium). The binding reactions were performed on 5×10^5 CHO-K1/mIL-18R cells for 1 hour at 4°C in 150 μl of binding medium containing serum samples and 1.0 n*M* [^{125}I]–rHuIL-18 with or without 500 n*M* unlabeled rHuIL-18 as a competitor. After incubation, the reaction mixtures were layered over 200 μl of phthalate oil (1:1 dibutyl phthalate:dioctyl phthalate) and centrifuged at 6,000*g* for 5 minutes at 15°C, and the radioactivity counts of the cell pellets, which represent the amounts of cell-bound [^{125}I]–IL-18, were measured in counts per minute using a gamma counter. The binding inhibition rate (%) was calculated by the following equation:

$$\frac{\text{(total binding count [cpm]} - \text{sample binding count [cpm])}}{\text{(total binding count [cpm]} - \text{nonspecific binding count [cpm])}} \times 100.$$

The total binding count and the nonspecific binding count were measured in the absence of samples or when the cold competitor was added to the mixture, respectively.

Immunoassay for TNFα, IL-1β, IL-6, IL-8, and IFNγ. Concentrations of TNFα, IL-1β, IL-6, IL-8, and IFNγ were measured in duplicate by quantitative sandwich ELISA (32). The detection limit for each of these cytokines was ~10 pg/ml.

Isolation of mRNA and reverse transcriptase—polymerase chain reaction (RT-PCR) analysis. The mRNA expression of IL-18 in synovial tissues, macrophages, T cells, and cultured fibroblasts was detected by RT-PCR as described previously (33). Briefly, 0.1 volume of 2*M* sodium acetate, pH 4.0, was added to the lysate of these cells, and vortexed. Total cellular RNA was extracted with phenol–chloroform, ethanol-precipitated with 2*M* sodium acetate, and vacuum-dried. After dissolving RNA in Tris–EDTA buffer, mRNA was isolated by using oligo(dT) latex beads (Oligo-dT30 Super; Takara Shuzo, Otsu, Japan) according to the manufacturer's instructions. Complementary DNA (cDNA) was synthesized from mRNA with Moloney murine leukemia virus reverse transcriptase (US Biochemical, Cleveland, OH) and oligo(dT)$_{15}$ primers (Promega, Madison, WI). Samples of cDNA were PCR amplified for 30 cycles for β-actin and 35 cycles for IL-18, with *rTaq* DNA polymerase (Perkin Elmer, Norwalk, CT) and specific primers in a thermal cycler (TP cycler-100; Toyobo, Osaka, Japan). Each cycle consisted of 1 minute of denaturation at 95°C and 2 minutes of annealing/extension at 65°C for β-actin or at 55°C for IL-18. For comparison of cytokine mRNA expression, cDNA concentrations were normalized to yield approximately equivalent β-actin PCR products. PCR products were electrophoresed on 1.5% agarose gels and visualized by ethidium bromide staining. The sequences of oligonucleotide primers used for PCR were as follows: for IL-18 5′ primer GCTTGAATCTAAATTATCAGTC and 3′ primer GAAGATTCAAATTGCATCTTAT; and for β-actin 5′ primer GTGGGGCGCCCCAGGCACCA and 3′ primer CTCCTTAATGTCACGCACGATTTC.

Statistical analysis. Samples with values below the detection limit for the assay were regarded as negative and assigned a value of 0. The data are expressed as the mean ± SD of the number of patients indicated; bars in the Figures represent the mean and SEM. The statistical significance of differences between 2 groups was determined by Mann-Whitney U test. The correlation coefficient was obtained by Spearman's rank correlation test.

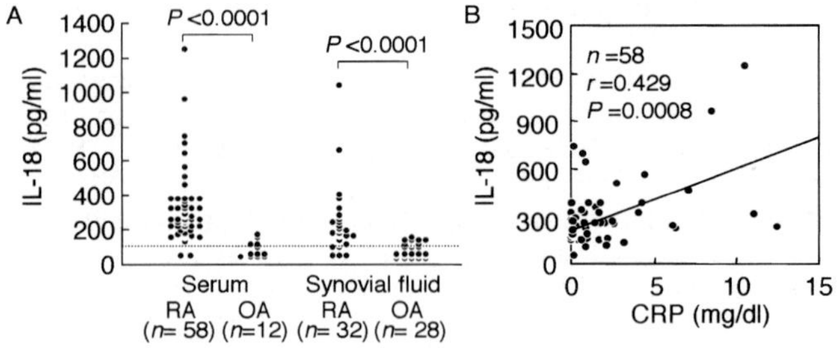

Figure 1. A, Concentrations of interleukin-18 (IL-18) protein in the serum and synovial fluid of rheumatoid arthritis (RA) and osteoarthritis (OA) patients, measured in duplicate by enzyme-linked immunosorbent assay (sensitivity 100 pg/ml [indicated by dotted line]). *n* = number of samples tested. **B,** Correlation between IL-18 and C-reactive protein (CRP) levels in the serum of RA patients. The correlation coefficient was analyzed by Spearman's rank correlation test.

RESULTS

Increased IL-18 levels in the serum and synovial fluid of RA patients. Concentrations of mature IL-18 protein in serum and synovial fluid samples from RA or OA patients were measured by specific ELISA. As shown in Figure 1A, the levels of IL-18 in the serum and synovial fluid of RA patients (mean ± SD 303 ± 210 pg/ml and 225 ± 191 pg/ml, respectively) were markedly higher than the levels in OA patients (83 ± 44 pg/ml and 84 ± 39 pg/ml, respectively). In paired samples from 15 RA patients, IL-18 levels were increased in the synovial fluid compared with the serum (211 ± 151 pg/ml versus 133 ± 84 pg/ml; $P < 0.0001$), indicating local production of this inflammatory cytokine within the joint. In addition, serum IL-18 levels were found to correlate with the levels of serum C-reactive protein (CRP) (Figure 1B), as well as with the erythrocyte sedimentation rate ($r = 0.337$, $P = 0.0098$; $n = 58$). Therefore, IL-18 overproduction in the joint appears to be linked to the disease activity of RA. However, there was no significant correlation between serum IL-18 and rheumatoid factor levels.

IL-18 bioactivity in the synovial fluid of RA patients. The IFNγ-inducing activity of IL-18 in synovial fluid samples from RA patients was determined by using human myelomonocytic KG-1 cells that dose-dependently produce IFNγ in response to human IL-18 (27). Synovial fluid samples from RA patients were able to induce IFNγ production by KG-1 cells more strongly than were those from OA patients (mean ± SEM IFNγ level 68 ± 21 pg/ml versus 34 ± 13 pg/ml), as shown in Figure 2. When the mean level of IL-18 bioactivity in RA synovial fluid was estimated (by taking the difference in IFNγ levels between cultures with and without

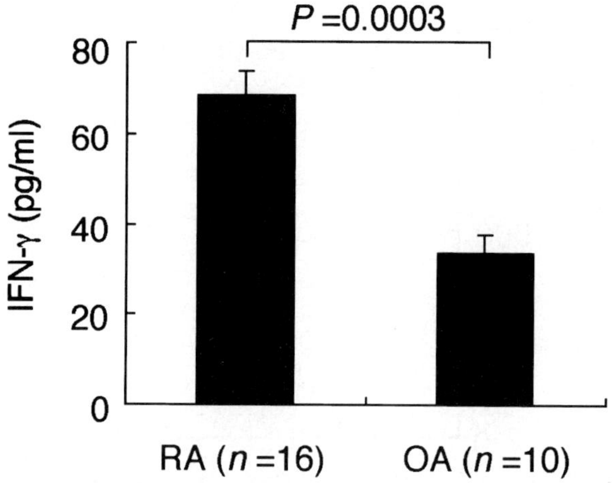

Figure 2. IL-18 bioactivity in the synovial fluid of RA and OA patients, measured in triplicate using human myelomonocytic KG-1 cells that dose-dependently produce interferon-γ (IFN-γ) in response to human IL-18. KG-1 cells (3×10^5/100 μl in RPMI 1640 medium with 10% fetal calf serum) were cultured for 24 hours in the presence of 100 μl of samples with or without anti–IL-18 antibody (125-2H). Concentrations of IFN-γ in culture supernatants were measured by enzyme-linked immunosorbent assay. IL-18 bioactivity in each sample was determined by the difference in IFN-γ levels between cultures with and without anti–IL-18 antibody. Bars show the mean and SEM. n = number of samples tested. See Figure 1 for other definitions.

anti–IL-18 antibodies, using the dose response with rHuIL-18 standards), it was found to be 47 ± 39 pg/ml. Since the IL-18 protein concentration in these samples, as detected by ELISA, was 328 ± 225 pg/ml, there was an ~7-fold difference between the levels of IL-18 protein and the bioactivity of IL-18 in the RA joint. This marked restriction of IL-18 activity indicates the coexistence of effective inhibitors such as IL-18BP.

IL-18 binding inhibitor in the serum and synovial fluid of RA patients. IL-18BP can selectively and efficiently diminish IL-18 activity by acting as a soluble decoy receptor with high affinity (22,23). Levels of such inhibitors present in the serum and synovial fluid from RA or OA patients were measured by IL-18 binding inhibition assay with CHO-K1/mIL-18R cells. Most of the studied samples variously showed inhibitory effects on the binding of [^{125}I]–IL-18 to CHO-K1/mIL-18R cells. As shown in Figure 3, the activity of IL-18 binding inhibition was similar in the serum of both patient groups (RA versus OA 30 ± 7% versus 32 ± 10%), but in the synovial fluid, the inhibitory activity tended to be higher in the RA patients than in the OA patients (39 ± 12% versus 26 ± 14%; P not significant). In patients with RA, the inhibitory activity was significantly elevated in the synovial fluid compared with the serum (P = 0.0488), indicating the accumulation of inhibitors in the joint compartment.

IL-18 production by RA synovial tissue. IL-18 mRNA expression in synovial tissue samples from 8 RA patients and 4 OA patients was examined by RT-PCR. As shown in Figure 4, RA synovial tissues all contained detectable amounts of IL-18 mRNA, whereas only 2 OA tissues displayed noticeable amounts. When cultured for 72 hours without any stimulation, freshly isolated cells from RA synovial tissues released larger amounts of IL-18 protein than did OA tissue cells (409 ± 398 pg/ml versus 160 ± 100 pg/ml) (Figure 5). Therefore, IL-18 may be secreted at substantial levels in the inflamed RA synovium.

To identify the cellular components responsible for this IL-18 overproduction, the macrophage- and T cell–enriched populations from 3 RA synovial tissue samples and the synovial fibroblast cell lines from 5 RA patients were examined for IL-18 mRNA expression by RT-PCR. As shown in Figure 4, fibroblast cell lines as well as tissue macrophages, but not T cells, expressed detectable levels of IL-18 mRNA when stimulated with IL-1β or TNFα. Macrophages cultured at 5×10^5/ml spontaneously secreted 367 ± 186 pg/ml of IL-18 for 72 hours (n = 3). However, neither IL-18 protein nor IL-18 bioactivity was detected, even in cultures of cytokine-

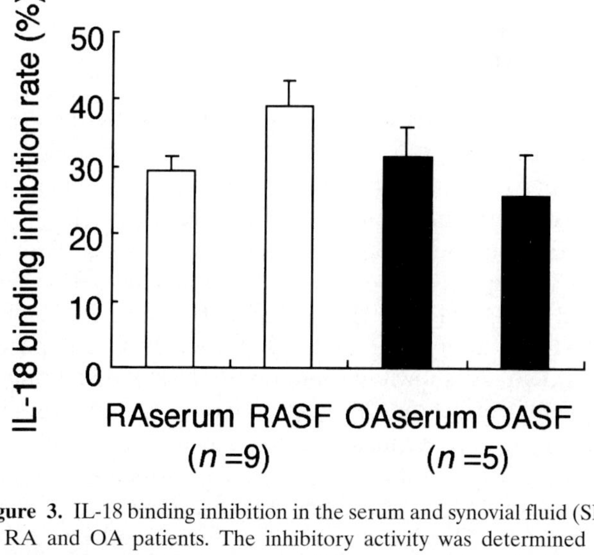

Figure 3. IL-18 binding inhibition in the serum and synovial fluid (SF) of RA and OA patients. The inhibitory activity was determined in triplicate by the ability of serum and SF samples to inhibit the binding of [^{125}I]–IL-18 to the Chinese hamster ovary cell line transfected with a murine IL-18 receptor (IL-1 receptor-related protein) expression vector plasmid. The binding inhibition rate was then calculated as described in Patients and Methods. Bars show the mean and SEM. n = number of samples tested. See Figure 1 for other definitions.

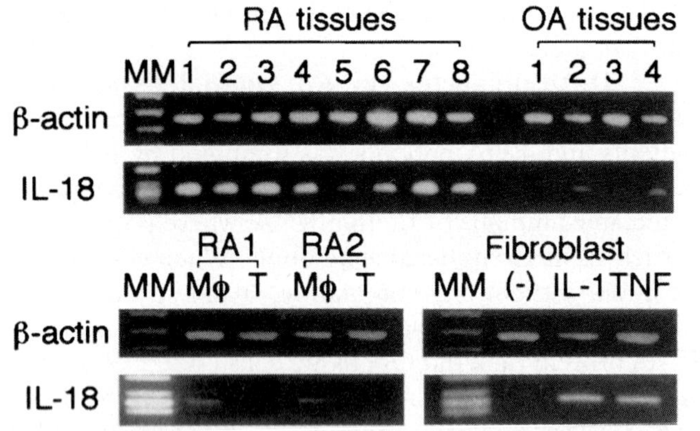

Figure 4. Expression of IL-18 mRNA in synovial tissues from 8 RA and 4 OA patients and in macrophages (Mϕ), T cells (T), and synovial fibroblast cell lines isolated from RA synovial tissues, as detected by reverse transcriptase–polymerase chain reaction (PCR). Macrophages and T cells were purified from RA synovial tissue cells by the panning method, as described in Patients and Methods. Synovial fibroblasts (1×10^5/ml in Dulbecco's modified Eagle's medium with 1% fetal calf serum) were cultured for 18 hours with or without either 1 ng/ml of IL-1β or 10 ng/ml of tumor necrosis factor α (TNF). Complementary DNA was synthesized from poly(A+) RNA isolated from the cells, and was amplified by PCR for 30 cycles for β-actin and for 35 cycles for IL-18. PCR products representing β-actin and IL-18 were stained with ethidium bromide. Shown in the lower panels are the representative results from individual experiments with macrophages and T cells from 3 RA patients and with fibroblasts from 5 RA patients. MM = molecular weight markers (see Figure 1 for other definitions).

activated synovial fibroblasts. Thus, the major source of mature IL-18 in the RA joint is most likely macrophage-lineage tissue cells.

Effect of IL-18 on IFNγ production by RA synovial tissues. IL-12 is a powerful inducer of IFNγ secretion by T cell infiltrates in RA synovium (11). To determine the differential effects of IL-12 and IL-18 on the IFNγ-dominant T cell response in RA, synovial tissue cells were cultured for 72 hours with IL-12 (1 ng/ml), IL-18 (1 ng/ml), IL-12 plus IL-18, or IL-12 plus anti–IL-18 antibodies, and IFNγ levels were compared by ELISA. As shown in Figure 6, IL-18 alone had only a negligible effect on IFNγ production by RA synovial tissues (32 ± 23 pg/ml versus control 30 ± 19 pg/ml, n = 7), in contrast to the effects of IL-12, which was highly stimulatory (1,676 ± 1,064 pg/ml). However, IL-12–stimulated IFNγ production was augmented by exogenous IL-18 in a synergistic manner (levels increased to 2,352 ± 1,032 pg/ml). On the other hand, the level of IL-12–induced IFNγ was >50% reduced by neutralization of endogenous IL-18 with anti–IL-18 antibody treatment (IL-12 2,120 ± 1,154 pg/ml versus IL-12 plus

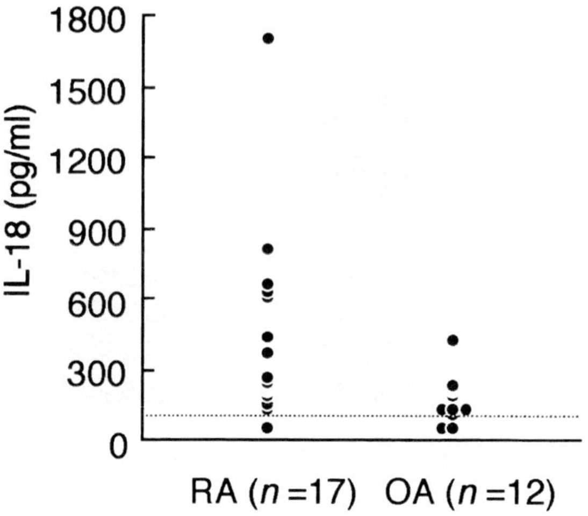

Figure 5. Spontaneous production of IL-18 by RA synovial tissue cells. Freshly isolated synovial tissue cells from RA and OA patients (2×10^6/ml in Dulbecco's modified Eagle's medium with 10% fetal calf serum) were cultured for 72 hours without any stimulation. IL-18 concentrations in culture supernatants were measured in duplicate by enzyme-linked immunosorbent assay (sensitivity 100 pg/ml [indicated by dotted line]). n = number of samples tested (see Figure 1 for other definitions).

anti–IL-18 antibodies 959 ± 522 pg/ml versus control 46 ± 32 pg/ml, n = 7). These findings indicate that the IFNγ-inducing activity of IL-18 itself, at concentrations as much as 1 ng/ml, is very limited on T cells from RA

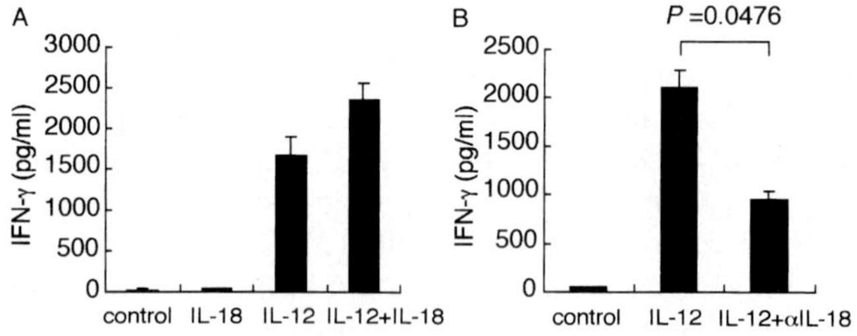

Figure 6. Synergistic effect of IL-12 and IL-18 on IFN-γ production by RA synovial tissue cells. Synovial tissue cells from RA patients (2×10^6/ml in Dulbecco's modified Eagle's medium with 10% fetal calf serum) were cultured for 72 hours with or without 1 ng/ml of IL-12, 1 ng/ml of IL-18, IL-12 plus IL-18, or IL-12 plus 10 μg/ml of anti–IL-18 antibody (αIL-18). IFN-γ concentrations in culture supernatants were measured in duplicate by enzyme-linked immunosorbent assay. **A,** Effect of exogenously added IL-18 on IFN-γ production by RA synovial tissues. **B,** Effect of endogenously produced IL-18 on IL-12–stimulated IFN-γ production by RA synovial tissues. Isotype-matched control monoclonal antibody had no effect. Bars show the mean and SEM of 7 experiments with synovial tissues from different RA patients. See Figures 1 and 2 for other definitions.

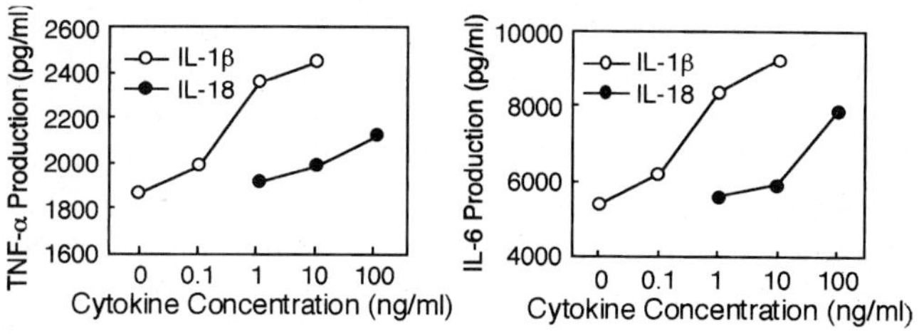

Figure 7. Dose responses of IL-1β and IL-18 on the production of tumor necrosis factor α (TNF-α) and IL-6 by synovial tissue cells from RA patients. Synovial tissue cells from RA patients (2×10^6/ml in Dulbecco's modified Eagle's medium with 10% fetal calf serum) were cultured for 72 hours with or without increasing concentrations of IL-1β or IL-18 as indicated. Concentrations of TNF-α and IL-6 in culture supernatants were measured in duplicate by enzyme-linked immunosorbent assay. Similar results were obtained from 2 additional experiments with synovial tissues from different RA patients. See Figure 1 for other definitions.

synovium, but endogenous IL-18 is a contributory factor in IL-12–induced IFNγ production.

Effect of IL-18 on inflammatory cytokine production by RA synovial tissues. IL-18 shares many biologic functions with IL-12, including the induction of IFNγ synthesis and cytotoxicity, but it also has similarities with IL-1β in terms of its structure, protein-processing mechanism, receptors, and signal transduction pathway (14,34–36). Similar to studies involving IL-1, IL-18 has been shown to induce many cytokines and chemokines from CD14+ monocytes/macrophages, both indirectly and directly (19,26). We therefore compared the activity of IL-18 with that of IL-1β on the expression of inflammatory cytokines in RA synovium. As shown in Figure 7, when RA synovial tissue cells were cultured for 72 hours with or without increasing concentrations of IL-18 or IL-1β, both cytokines were able to dose-dependently stimulate the secretion of TNFα and IL-6. However, IL-18 was found to be much less efficient than IL-1β. Accordingly, at a concentration of 1 ng/ml, IL-1β clearly increased the levels of TNFα, IL-6, and IL-8, whereas IL-18 had, at best, a minute effect on the expression of these cytokines and on the expression of IL-1β (Table 1).

DISCUSSION

IL-18 is an inflammatory cytokine that plays an important role in the Th1-type immune response by promoting IFNγ synthesis in T cells and NK cells, T cell proliferation and cytokine production, NK cell cytotoxic activity, Th1-cell development, and TNFα synthesis in T cells and NK cells, with subsequent induction of proinflammatory cytokines from monocytes (12–19). This cytokine is produced by many different cell types, such as activated macrophages, Kupffer cells, dendritic cells, articular chondrocytes, osteoblasts, and keratinocytes. Evidence for its integral role in the development of immunologically mediated tissue damage has recently accumulated. IL-18 is a critical mediator of the endotoxin-induced liver injury in mice (12,13), and the up-regulated expression of IL-18 mRNA is associated with IFNγ induction and diabetes development in autoimmune nonobese diabetic mice (37). In the intestinal lesion of Crohn's disease, there has been a close correlation between high levels of mature IL-18 protein and Th1-cell–mediated chronic inflammation (38,39). We have demonstrated that the bioactivity of IL-18 is significantly detectable in the inflamed joint of RA, and its major pathogenic role appears to be an enhancement of the IFNγ-dominant T cell cytokine response induced primarily by IL-12.

Levels of mature IL-18 protein, as detected by ELISA, were markedly greater in both the serum and synovial fluid of RA patients than in those of OA patients. In RA, there was a concentration gradient of IL-18 between the joints and the blood circulation, and production of serum IL-18 was related to the level of serum CRP and the erythrocyte sedimentation rate. Therefore, like many other inflammatory cytokines,

Table 1. Effects of interleukin-1β (IL-1β) and IL-18 on the production of tumor necrosis factor α (TNFα), IL-1β, IL-6, and IL-8 by synovial tissue cells from rheumatoid arthritis patients*

Treatment	TNFα, pg/ml	IL-1β, pg/ml	IL-6, pg/ml	IL-8, ng/ml
None	1,605 ± 769	2,233 ± 1,310	6,170 ± 2,887	29.7 ± 14.9
IL-1β (1 ng/ml)	2,128 ± 572	–	8,275 ± 2,374	39.8 ± 14.4
IL-18 (1 ng/ml)	1,650 ± 673	2,330 ± 1,137	6,250 ± 2,933	30.4 ± 14.0

* Freshly isolated synovial tissue cells from rheumatoid arthritis patients (2×10^6/ml in Dulbecco's modified Eagle's medium with 10% fetal calf serum) were cultured for 72 hours with or without 1 ng/ml of either IL-1β or IL-18. Concentrations of TNFα, IL-1β, IL-6, and IL-8 in culture supernatants were measured in duplicate by enzyme-linked immunosorbent assay. Values are the mean ± SD of 4 individual experiments with synovial tissues from different rheumatoid arthritis patients.

local production of IL-18 within the joint can be greatly augmented in proportion to the extent of inflammatory disease activity. Correspondingly, RA synovial tissues expressed IL-18 mRNA more strongly than did OA tissues, and spontaneously released larger amounts of IL-18 protein. These findings are consistent with the results recently reported by Gracie et al (26).

Those authors have also shown, by immunohistochemical staining, that IL-18–producing cells are distributed mostly within and adjacent to lymphatic aggregates, and consist of CD68+ macrophage-lineage cells and activated synovial fibroblasts (26). We also observed that fibroblast cell lines from RA tissues as well as isolated CD14+ tissue macrophages, but not CD3+ T cells, expressed IL-18 transcripts after stimulation with IL-1β or TNFα. However, fibroblasts failed to secrete detectable levels of both IL-18 protein and IL-18 bioactivity, in contrast to macrophages, which effectively produced IL-18. It remains to be determined whether the lack of IL-18 release was due either to the intrinsic defect of ICE activation or to a defect in the IL-18–secreting process in synovial fibroblasts or to a combination of both. In this regard, TNFα-activated fibroblasts were found to produce only small amounts of IL-1β (results not shown). This finding suggests that a defect in ICE activation is more likely, because the synthesis of mature IL-1β also depends on ICE activation (20,21). In any event, the cells most responsible for synovial overproduction of IL-18 are likely to be of the macrophage lineage.

The pathogenic significance of IL-18 in RA was corroborated by the detection of significant IL-18 bioactivity in the joint. Synovial fluid from RA patients was able to induce IFNγ production by IL-18–responsive myelomonocytic KG-1 cells more strongly than that in the synovial fluid from OA patients. However, IL-18 bioactivity was ~7-fold weaker compared with the concentration of IL-18 protein determined by ELISA, suggesting the coexistence of inhibitors of IL-18 activity in the RA joint.

The deleterious potential of IL-18 is thought to be regulated in vivo by a variety of inhibitors. IL-18BP has recently been identified as a soluble decoy receptor with high affinity for IL-18, and has been purified from the sera of endotoxin shock mice or normal human urine (22,23). The functional receptor of IL-18 is composed of 2 subunits, the IL-1 receptor–related protein and the accessory protein-like protein, and the expression of both proteins is required for activation of NF-κB and c-Jun N-terminal kinase, leading to induction of IFNγ and IL-8 (34–36). IL-18BP has the immunoglobulin domain homologous to the third immunoglobulin domain of the decoy type II IL-1 receptor, but lacks a transmembrane domain. This circulating inhibitor is thus categorized as a member of the novel family of soluble receptor-like proteins. Because its transcripts are detected systemically, but most prominently in the spleen and lungs (22,23), IL-18BP may be one of the major in vivo regulators of the inflammatory activities of IL-18.

We showed, by IL-18 binding inhibition assay with CHO-K1/mIL-18R cells, that both serum and synovial fluid samples from RA patients contained inhibitors of IL-18 binding, but we were unable to determine to what extent this activity was attributable to IL-18BP. The activity of IL-18 binding inhibition was higher in the RA synovial fluid than in the RA serum. The accumulation of inhibitors in inflamed joints is considered to be the result of their local production by the synovium or their active effusion from the blood circulation.

The great discrepancy between the bioactivity and the protein levels of IL-18 in RA joints suggests that the majority of IL-18 protein may exist in association with inhibitors such as IL-18BP and soluble IL-18 receptor. However, inhibitor levels appear to be insufficient for complete neutralization of IL-18 functions, since the IFNγ-inducing activity of IL-18 on KG-1 cells could be detected in the synovial fluid. Therefore, there is an excess of local IL-18 production over its inhibitor levels in active RA. Similar imbalances have previously been observed in the RA joint. Typically, 2 essential proinflammatory cytokines, IL-1 and TNFα, and their specific inhibitory molecules, the IL-1 receptor antagonist and soluble TNFα receptors, respectively, are produced in large quantities, but inhibitors are relatively low (40).

We showed that IL-18 markedly potentiated the IL-12–induced production of IFNγ by T cell infiltrates in the RA synovium. Several studies have previously demonstrated that IL-18 can effectively induce the IFNγ-dominant Th1-type immune response in cooperation with IL-12 (16,41–47). However, there has been some controversy about the potency of IL-18 and its interaction with IL-12, presumably relating to the species or differentiating states of T cells or the cytokine dose used in experiments. In our study, IL-18 alone, when added at 1 ng/ml, showed only a negligible effect on IFNγ production by RA synovial tissue, contrasting with the direct stimulatory effects of IL-12, which indicates that the IL-18 responsiveness of tissue-infiltrating T cells is suppressed. The synovium in chronic RA is infiltrated with CD45RO+,CD45RB^{dim},CD27−,CD4+ T cells, i.e., a subset of highly differentiated memory T cells that develops after prolonged antigenic stimulation (48). Restricted T cell cytokine expression, which is characteristic of RA, is thought to be due, in part, to the enrichment of such mature T cells (49). However, IL-18 was able to stimulate synovial IFNγ production in the presence of IL-12, and more importantly, IL-12 induction of IFNγ was >50% reduced by neutralization of endogenous IL-18 with anti–IL-18 antibodies.

These results support the pathogenic role of IL-18 as a potent costimulant for the IFNγ predominance primarily induced by IL-12 within the RA joint. Two major mechanisms underlying this synergism have been elucidated to date. First, IL-12 and IL-18 reciprocally up-regulate the expression of their receptors on T cells (41–43). Second, at the transcriptional level of the IFNγ gene expression, IL-12 mainly activates the transcriptional factor STAT-4 (signal transducer and activator of transcription 4), but IL-18 induces the activation of activator protein 1 and NF-κB (44–47). These combined effects may be required for the efficient induction of the IFNγ response in RA, as has been suggested in studies of IL-18–deficient mice in which the Th1 response is partially defective (50).

It is noteworthy, in this regard, that IL-12–producing cells are exclusively localized to lymphatic infiltrates in RA synovium, and levels of IL-12 p70 in cultured synovial tissues are, accordingly, very low (20.3 $\pm$ 4.3 pg/ml) (11). The restricted distribution of IL-12, in keeping with the low expression of IFNγ in RA joints (2), may be because IL-12 induction depends on T cell help in the form of CD40–CD40 ligand interaction and IFNγ costimulation. In contrast, IL-18–producing macrophages are more diffusely found (24,25), and they released greater amounts in culture (409 $\pm$ 398 pg/ml). These findings, together with the differential effects of IL-12 and IL-18 on synovial IFNγ production, suggest that abundant expression of IL-18 in RA synovium may be important in terms of compensating for a paucity of IL-12 with dominant IFNγ-inducing activity.

IL-18 is structurally related to IL-1 and utilizes an identical signal transduction pathway through its similar receptor system (14,34–36). Like IL-1, IL-18 can initiate a cascade of proinflammatory cytokine production by monocytes/macrophages (19,25). We therefore compared the effects of IL-18 and IL-1β on inflammatory cytokine production from RA synovial tissues. The results showed that IL-18 was capable of stimulating the secretion of cytokines such as TNFα and IL-6, probably from macrophages and fibroblasts, but its activity was much weaker than that of IL-1β. Furthermore, unlike IL-1, IL-18 failed to induce the proliferation of synovial fibroblast cell lines, as determined by the incorporation of 5-bromo-2′-deoxy-uridine (results not shown). Therefore, given the mean estimated IL-18 bioactivity of 47 $\pm$ 39 pg/ml in the joint, the IL-1–like proinflammatory activities of IL-18 could, in a very limited manner, contribute to RA pathology.

In summary, despite the presence of IL-18 binding inhibitors, IL-18 bioactivity is significantly detectable in the joint with active RA, and the major producer of mature IL-18 protein is activated tissue macrophages. The primary role of this pleiotropic inflammatory cytokine in RA synovitis is likely to potentiate the IFNγ-dominant T cell response induced by IL-12. However, recent studies have indicated the contribution of chondrocyte-derived IL-18 to cartilage degradation (51) and the inhibitory effect of osteoblast IL-18 on osteoclast formation via T cell production of GM-CSF (52). Further studies will be necessary for establishing the relevance of IL-18 to the disease process of RA.

ACKNOWLEDGMENTS

The authors thank Dr. H. Okamura (Hyogo College of Medicine, Nishinomiya, Japan) for helpful discussion and Dr. M. Iwahashi (Okayama University Medical School) for technical assistance.

REFERENCES

1. Panayi GS, Lanchbury JS, Kingsley GH. The importance of the T cell in initiating and maintaining the chronic synovitis of rheumatoid arthritis. Arthritis Rheum 1992;35:729–35.
2. Chen E, Keystone EC, Fish EN. Restricted cytokine expression in rheumatoid arthritis. Arthritis Rheum 1993;36:901–10.
3. Firestein GS, Zvaifler NJ. How important are T cells in chronic rheumatoid synovitis? Arthritis Rheum 1990;33:768–73.
4. Gregersen PK. Genetic analysis of rheumatic diseases. In: Kelley WN, Harris ED Jr, Ruddy S, Sledge CB, editors. Textbook of rheumatology. Vol. 1. 5th ed. Philadelphia: WB Saunders; 1997. p. 209–27.
5. Isaacs JD, Watts RA, Hazleman BL, Hale G, Keogan MT, Cobbeld SP, et al. Humanised monoclonal antibody therapy for rheumatoid arthritis. Lancet 1992;340:748–52.
6. Struyk L, Hawes GE, Chatila MK, Breedveld FC, Kurnick JT, van den Elsen PJ. T cell receptors in rheumatoid arthritis. Arthritis Rheum 1995;38:577–89.
7. Miltenburg AM, Vanlaar JM, de Kuiper R, Daha MR, Breedveld FC. T cells cloned from human rheumatoid synovial membrane functionally represent the Th1 subset. Scand J Immunol 1992;35: 603–10.
8. Quayle AJ, Chomarat P, Miossec P, Kjeldsen J, Forre O, Natvig JB. Rheumatoid inflammatory T-cells express mostly Th1 but also Th2 and mixed (Th0-like) cytokine patterns. Scand J Immunol 1993;38:75–82.
9. Simon AK, Seipelt E, Sieper J. Divergent T-cell cytokine patterns in inflammatory arthritis. Proc Natl Acad Sci U S A 1994;91: 8562–6.
10. Morita Y, Yamamura M, Kawashima M, Harada S, Tsuji K, Shibuya K, et al. Flow cytometric single-cell analysis of cytokine

production by CD4+ T cells in synovial tissue and peripheral blood from patients with rheumatoid arthritis. Arthritis Rheum 1998;41:1669–76.
11. Morita Y, Yamamura M, Nishida K, Harada S, Okamoto H, Inoue H, et al. Expression of interleukin-12 in synovial tissue from patients with rheumatoid arthritis. Arthritis Rheum 1998;41: 306–14.
12. Okamura H, Nagata K, Komatsu T, Tanimoto T, Nukata Y, Tanabe F, et al. A novel costimulatory factor for gamma interferon induction found in the livers of mice causes endotoxic shock. Infect Immun 1995;63:3966–72.
13. Okamura H, Tsutsi H, Komatsu T, Yutsudo M, Hakura A, Tanimoto T, et al. Cloning of a new cytokine that induces IFN-γ production by T cells. Nature 1995;378:88–91.
14. Ushio S, Namba M, Okura T, Hattori K, Nukada Y, Akita K, et al. Cloning of the cDNA for human IFN-γ-inducing factor, expression in Escherichia coli, and studies on the biologic activities of the protein. J Immunol 1996;156:4274–9.
15. Kohno K, Kataoka J, Ohtsuki T, Suemoto Y, Okamoto I, Usui M, et al. IFN-γ-inducing factor (IGIF) is a costimulatory factor on the activation of Th1 but not Th2 cells and exerts its effect independently of IL-12. J Immunol 1997;158:1541–50.
16. Micallef MJ, Ohtsuki T, Kohno K, Tanabe F, Ushio S, Namba M, et al. Interferon-γ-inducing factor enhances T helper 1 cytokine production by stimulated human T cells: synergism with interleukin-12 for interferon-gamma production. Eur J Immunol 1996;26: 1647–51.
17. Tsutsui H, Nakanishi K, Matsui K, Higashino K, Okamura H, Miyazawa Y, et al. IFN-γ-inducing factor up-regulates Fas ligand-mediated cytotoxic activity of murine natural killer cell clones. J Immunol 1996;157:3967–73.
18. Tsutsui H, Matsui K, Kawada N, Hyodo Y, Hayashi N, Okamura H, et al. IL-18 accounts for both TNF–α and Fas ligand-mediated hepatotoxic pathways in endotoxin-induced liver injury in mice. J Immunol 1997;159:3961–7.
19. Puren AJ, Fantuzzi G, Gu Y, Su MS, Dinarello CA. Interleukin-18 (IFNγ-inducing factor) induces IL-8 and IL-1β via TNFα production from non-CD14+ human blood mononuclear cells. J Clin Invest 1998;101:711–21.
20. Gu Y, Kuida K, Tsutsui H, Ku G, Hsiao K, Fleming MA, et al. Activation of interferon-γ inducing factor mediated by interleukin-1β converting enzyme. Science 1997;275:206–9.
21. Ghayur T, Banerjee S, Hugunin M, Butler D, Herzog L, Carter A, et al. Caspase-1 processes IFN-γ-inducing factor and regulates LPS-induced IFN-γ production. Nature 1997;386:619–23.
22. Aizawa Y, Akita K, Taniai M, Torigoe K, Mori T, Nishida Y, et al. Cloning and expression of interleukin-18 binding protein. FEBS Lett 1999;445:338–42.
23. Novick D, Kim SH, Fantuzzi G, Reznikov LL, Dinarello CA, Rubinstein M. Interleukin-18 binding protein: a novel modulator of the Th1 cytokine response. Immunity 1999;10:127–36.
24. Kawashima M, Yamamura M, Morita Y, Makino H, Tanimoto T, Kurimoto M. Elevated levels of IFN-γ-inducing factor in synovial fluid of patients with rheumatoid arthritis [abstract]. Arthritis Rheum 1996;39 Suppl 9:S127.
25. Yamamura M, Kawashima M, Morita Y, Makino H, Tanimoto T, Kurimoto M. Increased production of interleukin-18 in synovium from patients with rheumatoid arthritis [abstract]. Arthritis Rheum 1997;40 Suppl 9:S274.
26. Gracie JA, Forsey RJ, Chan WL, Gilmour A, Leung BP, Greer MR, et al. A proinflammatory role for IL-18 in rheumatoid arthritis. J Clin Invest 1999;104:1393–1401.
27. Konishi K, Tanabe F, Taniguchi M, Yamauchi H, Tanimoto T, Ikeda M, et al. A simple and sensitive bioassay for the detection of human interleukin-18/interferon-γ-inducing factor using human myelomonocytic KG-1 cells. J Immunol Methods 1997;209:187–91.
28. Arnett FC, Edworthy SM, Bloch DA, McShane DJ, Fries JF, Cooper NS, et al. The American Rheumatism Association 1987 revised criteria for the classification of rheumatoid arthritis. Arthritis Rheum 1988;31:315–24.
29. Altman R, Asch E, Bloch D, Bole G, Borenstein D, Brandt K, et al. Development of criteria for the classification and reporting of osteoarthritis: classification of osteoarthritis of the knee. Arthritis Rheum 1986;29:1039–49.
30. Okamoto H, Yamamura M, Morita Y, Harada S, Makino H, Ota Z. The synovial expression and serum levels of interleukin-6, interleukin-11, leukemia inhibitory factor, and oncostatin M in rheumatoid arthritis. Arthritis Rheum 1997;40:1096–105.
31. Taniguchi M, Nagaoka K, Kunikata T, Kayano T, Yamauchi H, Nakamura S, et al. Characterization of anti-human interleukin-18 (IL-18)/interferon-gamma-inducing factor (IGIF) monoclonal antibodies and their application in the measurement of human IL-18 by ELISA. J Immunol Methods 1997;206:107–13.
32. Kita M, Ohmoto Y, Hirai N, Yamaguchi N, Imanishi J. Induction of cytokines in human peripheral blood mononuclear cells by mycoplasmas. Microbiol Immunol 1992;36:507–16.
33. Yamamura M, Uyemura K, Deans RJ, Weinberg K, Rea TH, Bloom BR, et al. Defining protective responses to pathogens: cytokine profile in leprosy lesions. Science 1991;254:277–9.
34. Torigoe K, Ushio S, Okura T, Kobayashi S, Taniai M, Kunikata T, et al. Purification and characterization of the human interleukin-18 receptor. J Biol Chem 1997;272:25737–42.
35. Parnet P, Garka KE, Bonnert TP, Dower SK, Sims JE. IL-1Rrp is a novel receptor-like molecule similar to the type I interleukin-1 receptor and its homologues T1/ST2 and IL-1R AcP. J Biol Chem 1996;271:3967–70.
36. Born TL, Thomassen E, Bird TA, Sims JE. Cloning of a novel receptor subset, AcP, required for interleukin-18 signaling. J Biol Chem 1998;273:29445–50.
37. Rothe H, Jenkins NA, Copeland NG, Kolb H. Active stage of autoimmune diabetes is associated with the expression of a novel cytokine, IGIF, which is located near Idd2. J Clin Invest 1997;99: 467–74.
38. Pizarro TT, Michie MH, Bentz M, Woraratanadharm J, Smith MF Jr, Foley E, et al. IL-18, a novel immunoregulatory cytokine, is up-regulated in Crohn's disease: expression and localization in intestinal mucosal cells. J Immunol 1999;162:6829–35.
39. Monteleone G, Trapasso F, Parrello T, Biancone L, Stella A, Iuliano R, et al. Bioactive IL-18 expression is up-regulated in Crohn's disease. J Immunol 1999;163:143–7.
40. Arend WP, Dayer J-M. Cytokines and cytokine inhibitors or antagonists in rheumatoid arthritis. Arthritis Rheum 1990;33: 305–15.
41. Aha H-J, Maruo S, Tomura M, Mu J, Hamaoka T, Nakanishi K, et al. A mechanism underlying synergy between IL-12 and IFN-γ-inducing factor in enhanced production of IFN-γ. J Immunol 1997;159:2125–31.
42. Yoshimoto T, Takeda K, Tanaka T, Ohkusu K, Kashiwamura S, Okamura H, et al. IL-12 up-regulates IL-18 receptor expression on T cells, Th1 cells, and B cells: synergism with IL-18 for IFN-γ production. J Immunol 1998;161:3400–7.
43. Xu D, Chan WL, Leung BP, Hunter D, Schulz K, Carter RW, et al. Selective expression and functions of interleukin-18 receptor on T helper (Th) type 1 but not Th2 cells. J Exp Med 1998;188: 1485–92.
44. Robinson D, Shibuya K, Mui A, Zonin F, Murphy E, Sana T, et al. IGIF does not drive Th1 development but synergizes with IL-12 for interferon-γ production and activates IRAK and NF-γB. Immunity 1997;7:571–81.
45. Barbulescu K, Becker C, Schlaak JF, Schmitt E, Meyer zum Buschenfelde KH, Neurath MF. IL-12 and IL-18 differentially regulate the transcriptional activity of the human IFN-γ promoter in primary CD4+ T lymphocytes. J Immunol 1998;160:3642–7.

46. Carter LL, Murphy KM. Lineage-specific requirement for signal transducer and activator of transcription (Stat) 4 in interferon-γ production from $CD4^+$ versus $CD8^+$ T cells. J Exp Med 1999;189: 1355–60.
47. Kojima H, Aizawa Y, Yanai Y, Nagaoka Y, Takeuchi M, Ohta T, et al. An essential role of NF-κB in IL-18-induced IFN-γ expression in KG-1 cells. J Immunol 1999;162:5063–9.
48. Kohem CL, Brezinschek RI, Wisbey H, Tortorella C, Lipsky PE, Oppenheimer-Marks N. Enrichment of differentiated $CD45RB^{dim}$, CD27− memory T cells in the peripheral blood, synovial fluid, and synovial tissue of patients with rheumatoid arthritis. Arthritis Rheum 1996;39:844–54.
49. Salmon M, Gaston JS. The role of T-lymphocytes in rheumatoid arthritis. Br Med Bull 1995;51:332–45.
50. Takeda K, Tsutsui H, Yoshimoto T, Adachi O, Yoshida N, Kishimoto T, et al. Defective NK cell activity and Th1 response in IL-18-deficient mice. Immunity 1998;8:383–90.
51. Olee T, Hashimoto S, Quach J, Lotz M. IL-18 is produced by articular chondrocytes and induced proinflammatory and catabolic responses. J Immunol 1999;162:1096–100.
52. Udagawa N, Horwood NJ, Elliott J, Mackay A, Owens J, Okamura H, et al. Interleukin-18 (interferon-γ-inducing factor) is produced by osteoblasts and acts via granulocyte/macrophage colony-stimulating factor and not via interferon-γ to inhibit osteoclast formation. J Exp Med 1997;185:1005–12.

ARTHRITIS & RHEUMATISM
Vol. 44, No. 2, February 2001, pp 286–295

Tumor Necrosis Factor Markers Show Sex-Influenced Association With Rheumatoid Arthritis

Joanne M. Meyer,[1] Jinfeng Han,[2] and George Moxley[2]

Objective. **The observation that not all shared-epitope genotypes confer the same risk suggests that a second HLA-region locus may confer risk. Tumor necrosis factor α (TNFα) is a possible candidate. We examined TNFα for sex influences on HLA-associated risk for rheumatoid arthritis (RA).**

Methods. **DRB1 and TNF microsatellite typing of 297 Caucasian RA patients (132 men, 165 women) and 267 Caucasian controls was performed.**

Results. **The TNFab microsatellite haplotype distribution differed among the male RA, female RA, and control groups ($P < 0.01$); the difference was largely an excess of TNFa2b1 haplotypes in the male RA group. However, this did not simply reflect an excess of shared-epitope haplotypes bearing TNFa2b1. In RA, not all shared-epitope–bearing haplotypes had the same TNFab. The *0401-bearing haplotypes commonly had TNFa6b5, TNFa2b1, TNFa10b4, and TNFa11b4, while the *0404-bearing haplotypes had TNFa11b4. In the female RA group, TNFa2b1 was most often on *0401-bearing haplotypes. In the male RA group, there was a surprise: TNFa2b1 was often on HLA haplotypes *without* shared-epitope DRB1 alleles. To estimate the relative strength of associated HLA markers, we performed logistic regression analyses stratified by sex and controlling for a potential confounder, age at disease onset. Among women, TNFa2b3 favored RA (odds ratio 1.932, $P < 0.05$) while TNFa6b5 was protective (odds ratio 0.522, $P < 0.05$). Among males, TNFa2b1 and TNFa11b4 conferred elevated odds ratios (2.58 and 1.681, respectively, $P < 0.05$). However, the odds ratios for TNFa2b1 in men and TNFa2b3 in women were generally well below those for RA-associated DRB1 markers (for example, DRB1*0401 3.553 in male RA patients and 6.991 in female RA patients).**

Conclusion. **Certain TNFab-bearing HLA haplotypes modify RA risk in a manner influenced by sex but independent of DRB1, particularly TNFa2b1 in men.**

Rheumatoid arthritis (RA) has a substantial hereditary component, with familial aggregation (1) and a broad-sense heritability of ~0.6–0.7 (2). Starting with Stastny's observations of Dw4 in United States Caucasians (3), RA has been associated with certain alleles of the DRB1 locus. Since that time, many investigators have distilled the association to a restricted DRB1 allele subset, chiefly of the DR4 group (*0401, *0404, *0405, and *0408) (4), the DR1 group (specifically, *0101) (5), the DR6 group (*1402) (6,7), and the single DR10 allele (*1001) (8,9).

Marker–disease association may occur from either of 2 situations, direct involvement (i.e., the marker is the disease gene) or linkage disequilibrium (i.e., the marker merely indicates the presence of a nearby disease gene). In support of direct involvement, Gregersen and coworkers advanced the shared-epitope hypothesis (10). Simply stated, this hypothesis says that RA risk is explained by similar amino acid sequences encoded by the associated HLA–DR alleles and not by other alleles.

However, 5 observations are not explained by the shared-epitope hypothesis. In populations examined thus far, a substantial proportion of RA patients do not have a shared-epitope DRB1 allele (11–13). Also, some populations have RA associations with DR markers without shared epitopes (such as DR3 and DR9) (14,15). HLA haplotypes bearing shared-epitope alleles do not account for all familial RA: Hasstedt and others noted that in US Caucasian populations showing a shared-epitope DRB1 association, only half of familial

Supported by the Alpha Omicron Pi Foundation, the Arthritis Foundation, and by a Department of Veterans Affairs MERIT award.

[1]Joanne M. Meyer, PhD: Millenium Pharmaceuticals, Cambridge, Massachusetts; [2]Jinfeng Han, BS, George Moxley, MD: McGuire Veterans Administration Medical Center and Medical College of Virginia of Virginia Commonwealth University, Richmond.

Address correspondence and reprint requests to George Moxley, MD, Box 111M, McGuire VAMC, 1201 Broad Rock Boulevard, Richmond, VA 23249.

Submitted for publication June 23, 2000; accepted in revised form September 27, 2000.

RA was HLA-related (as indicated by HLA–B and DR typing) (16). In studies of the influence of sex on RA, several groups have found certain HLA haplotypes (A2;B62;DR4;Dw4) (17,18) and DR genotypes (DRB1*0401,*0404) (19) to be more frequent in male RA patients than in female RA patients. Finally, not all shared-epitope alleles confer the same risk; generally, DR4-group alleles are stronger than DR1 (20), and *0401 is stronger than other DR4-group alleles (21). The shared-epitope hypothesis does not fully explain these observations.

There is also support for the alternative marker–disease association hypothesis, linkage disequilibrium. The HLA region consists of over 4 million basepairs and shows strong allelic association. Several research groups have noted that the DR genotype distribution better fits a recessive mode of inheritance for the HLA-region disease gene than an additive (dominant) mode (22–25). Dizier and coworkers found in a modeling study equating the effects of DR4Dw14 and DR1 that actual DRB1 genotype frequencies fit those predicted with a linkage disequilibrium model but not those predicted with a simple shared epitope model (26). Hasstedt and coworkers concluded that RA may be best explained by a rare HLA-region gene, recessive in men and nearly recessive in women (16).

Which HLA-region gene near DRB1 might be involved? Tumor necrosis factor α (TNFα) is an HLA-region cytokine encoded by a class III locus nestled between those for the second component of complement and HLA–B. Westendorp and coworkers found that the inducible TNFα level has heritable variation, with broad-sense heritability of 0.60 (27). Jacob and coworkers found that TNF variation was related to HLA haplotype (28); persons with DR3 or DR4 tend to have a phenotype of high inducible TNFα, while those with DR2 but not DR3 or DR4 have low inducible TNFα phenotype.

TNFα may be pivotal for RA pathogenesis, directly mediating cartilage and bone damage as well as amplifying the effects of other proinflammatory cytokines, such as interleukin-1 and granulocyte–macrophage colony-stimulating factor (29,30). Experimental therapies directed toward TNFα, such as chimeric monoclonal antibodies or soluble TNF receptors, appear to have remarkable benefit in RA patients (31–33). Recently, Bali et al found that RA multiplex families showed evidence that TNF and the shared epitope contributed independently to RA (34). Finally, 2 studies have noted that RA-affected offspring preferentially inherit some TNFα markers but not others. Such TNFα-associated markers confer risk independent of shared-epitope DRB1 alleles (35,36). Thus, TNFα appears to be involved in both the risk and pathogenesis of RA.

Accordingly, we adopted the hypothesis that TNFα modifies RA risk associated with HLA–DRB1. We examined the frequency distribution of TNFα markers, estimated haplotype frequencies, and did modeling to estimate the strength of associated TNFα markers in predicting RA diagnosis.

PATIENTS AND METHODS

Study subjects. The RA (n = 297), osteoarthritis (n = 145), fibromyalgia (n = 21), bursitis (n = 1), and noninflammatory back pain (n = 1) study subjects were derived from the rheumatology outpatient practice at the Medical College of Virginia of Virginia Commonwealth University and the outpatient rheumatology clinics at the Hunter Holmes McGuire Department of Veterans Affairs Medical Center (VAMC). The normal subjects were derived from the university community (n = 99). This study was approved by the Institutional Review Board of both Virginia Commonwealth University and McGuire VAMC, and all subjects gave their informed consent.

RA diagnosis was classified by the American College of Rheumatology (ACR; formerly, the American Rheumatism Association) 1987 criteria (37). All RA and control subjects were US Caucasians, and by sampling of their grandparents' ancestry, almost all were of northern European origin. However, few grandparents were from Scandinavian countries (12 of the 1,316 grandparents sampled). The demographic and clinical characteristics were described in an earlier publication (38) and are briefly summarized below (see Results).

Typing for HLA–DRB1 and DQB1. DRB1 genotyping methods were outlined in the previous publication (38). The methods included polymerase chain reaction (PCR) amplification followed by dot-blot hybridization with biotinylated sequence-specific oligonucleotides (SSOs) (39) and development with enhanced chemiluminescence (ECL), PCR–restriction fragment length polymorphism (RFLP) (40), and amplification-refractory mutation screening (41). DQB1 was done by similar PCR amplification, dot-blot hybridization with biotinylated SSOs (39) and development with ECL and also by PCR-RFLP (40). DRB1 group and allele assignments are listed in the appendices of our previous publication (see ref. 38).

TNF microsatellite genotypes were assigned by PCR (42) followed by sequencing-type gel electrophoresis and silver-staining; controls included PCR products from templates derived from cell lines of known TNF genotype (43,44). We first typed for TNFa and TNFb microsatellite genotypes. Then, by amplifying the entire TNFab region, we derived the TNFab haplotype from the known TNFa and TNFb genotypes and the TNFab product size (44). For example, in an individual with TNF genotypes a2,a6 and b1,b5 and TNFab product lengths of 202 bp and 214 bp, we reasoned that the TNFab length was consistent with haplotypes TNFa2b1 (202 bp) and TNFa6b5 (214 bp), not a2b5 (206 bp) and a6b1 (210 bp). The TNFab,

TNFc, TNFd, and TNFe frequencies are shown in a table at our Web site at http://views.vcu.edu/~gmoxley/TNFtable.htm. TNF promoter polymorphisms at positions 238 bp and 308 bp upstream of the leader sequence were determined by PCR, dot-blot hybridization with biotinylated probes, incubation with streptavidin–peroxidase, and detection with ECL (ECL Detection Reagents; Amersham Life Science, Rockville, MD) (45).

Statistical analysis. To determine differences in allele frequency among the male RA, female RA, and control groups, a contingency-table χ^2 value was calculated; to ensure that the χ^2 was valid, any alleles with a cell size <5 in any group were pooled with other uncommon alleles. To examine the relative predispositional effect (46), the allele frequencies contributing the most to the χ^2 were deleted, and then the χ^2 was recalculated. Relative risk and confidence intervals were calculated using Haldane's modification of Woolf's relative risk (47).

We did not have family samples from which to deduce haplotypes. Instead, to confirm that alleles of DRB1, DQB1, and TNF loci were in linkage disequilibrium and to estimate haplotype frequencies, we used EH, a linkage utility software program (48). From the numbers with each combination of genotypes, the EH program estimates the allele frequencies for each marker. The haplotype frequencies are estimated assuming either allelic association or none, and the log-likelihood, chi-square, and number of degrees of freedom are also calculated. We adapted and recompiled the EH Pascal source code to allow a larger entry table. When frequency estimates from such maximum-likelihood analyses have been compared with those derived from haplotypes deduced from family data, the estimates were accurate for more frequent haplotypes (49). With 250 individuals, one can reliably estimate haplotype frequencies down to 0.006 (49).

We used statistical modeling to quantify the degree of risk and statistical independence of individual HLA markers. Based on our previous studies and those of others (19,38,50,51), we considered sex and age at onset as potential confounders. We therefore stratified the analyses by sex and included early-onset disease (age younger than 45.4 years) as a potential confounding variable. We first examined multivariate analyses to see whether linkage disequilibrium would substantially interfere with regression analyses. There was no hint of collinearity by PROC REG (SAS System for Windows, Release 6.12; SAS Institute, Cary, NC). We examined interaction among independent variables by PROC CATMOD (SAS System for Windows). Depending on the exact model in women, there was significant interaction between DRB1*0401 and TNFa6b5 ($P < 0.0233$), DRB1*0404 and TNFa11b4 ($P = 0.0003$), DRB1*0101 and TNFa6b5 ($P = 0.0285$), DRB1*0404 and TNFa6b5 ($P = 0.0066$), and DRB1*0401 and TNFa11b4 ($P = 0.0009$); these correspond to common haplotypes. The men showed interaction between DR1 ^{70}QRRAA^{74} and TNFa6b5 ($P = 0.0304$).

We then used PROC LOGISTIC (SAS System for Windows) on sex-stratified multiple logistic regression models to test hypotheses about independence of previously associated alleles of DRB1 and TNF in RA predisposition. Our results were used to predict RA occurrence based on shared-epitope DRB1 alleles (DRB1*0401, *0404, *0408, *0101, and *1001) or shared epitopes, specific TNFab markers (a2b1, a2b3, a6b5, and a11b4), and TNF promoter polymorphisms (−308A). To choose the best-fitting models, we used likelihood comparisons; lower values of this criterion suggest better fitting models. Logistic regression models were developed on a subset of 80% of subjects and confirmed on the remaining 20%. The best models used coding (0, 1, or 2) to represent allele number, but adding interaction terms to represent common HLA shared-epitope haplotypes did not improve fit. We regarded this study as too small to detect significant interactive effects.

RESULTS

Clinical characteristics. The demographic and clinical characteristics of the study subjects have been previously outlined (38). Most RA patients had seropositive disease (86% of men, 78% of women) of long duration (mean 15.7 years in men, 16.2 years in women) and had been treated with slow-acting antirheumatic drugs (mean male number 2.7, female 2.3). The male RA group had a slightly higher frequency of rheumatoid nodules (56.1% versus 34.7%) and met correspondingly more ACR criteria (38); the female RA group had a younger mean age at disease onset (44.9 years versus 49.4 years for men). Early-onset disease, defined as earlier than the median onset in the women (45.4 years), occurred in 49 male RA patients.

TNF microsatellite and promoter alleles. We have previously shown that DRB1 frequencies were not different among normal subjects and patients with osteoarthritis, fibromyalgia, and bursitis (38); similarly, there was no difference in TNFab marker frequencies (after pooling infrequent markers into a single group, $\chi^2 = 8.5$ [10 degrees of freedom (df)], P not significant). Therefore, we pooled normal, osteoarthritis, fibromyalgia, and bursitis subjects into a single control group.

The common TNFab microsatellite marker frequencies among the male RA, female RA, and control groups are shown in Figure 1 (the actual numbers are shown in a table, "Frequency of TNFab haplotypes, TNFc, TNFd, and TNFe alleles, and TNF promoter alleles," at our Web site at http://views.vcu.edu/~gmoxley/HLATNFindex.htm). The distribution of TNFab markers differed among the 3 groups (Figure 1) ($\chi^2 = 32.1$, 16 df, $P < 0.01$); the difference was between the male RA group and the other 2 groups ($\chi^2 = 15.7$ versus the female RA group, $\chi^2 = 26.2$ versus the control group, $P < 0.05$ for both comparisons). The specific TNFab marker responsible for the difference was TNFa2b1, as shown by the relative predispositional effect. The uncorrected relative risk of TNFa2b1 in male RA patients versus controls was 2.0 (Haldane's $\chi^2 = 11.7$, 1 df, $P < 0.001$).

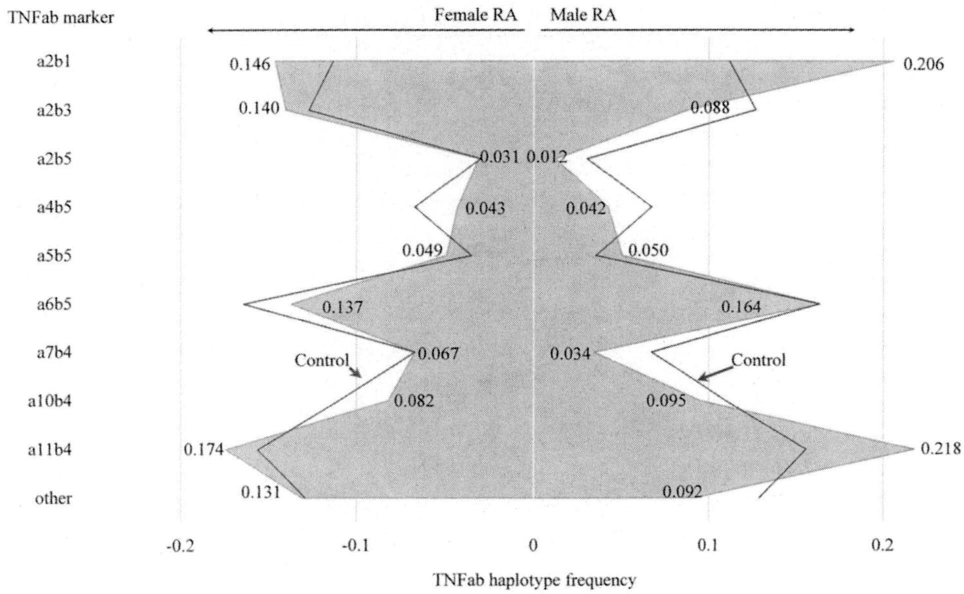

Figure 1. Frequency histogram of tumor necrosis factor ab (TNFab) microsatellite haplotypes. TNF markers are shown on the left. Data for female and male rheumatoid arthritis (RA) patients are plotted as shaded areas, back-to-back, with zero at the center; differences between them are apparent as asymmetries. Control data are plotted as 2 lines on both sides of zero; differences from the RA group are shown by comparing the shaded area to the line.

As others have previously noted (50), this increased relative risk was particularly present in the subset of men with early-onset RA; TNFa2b1 conferred a relative risk of 2.0 versus women with early-onset RA (Haldane's χ^2 = 5.0, $P < 0.05$) and 3.1 versus controls (Haldane's χ^2 = 17.9, $P < 0.05$). Thus, the TNFa2b1 frequency was enriched in the male RA group.

DRB1 allele distribution. From studies of insulin-dependent diabetes mellitus, TNFa2b1 is known to occur on the haplotype bearing HLA–B62 (a split of B15) and DR4 (44). Because others had noted that the HLA haplotype A2;Cw3;Bw62;DR4;Dw4 is enriched among male RA patients (17), we reasoned that TNFa2b1 enrichment might relate to an excess of this haplotype. We therefore predicted that if TNFa2b1 enrichment were due to linkage disequilibrium with a single RA-associated HLA haplotype, there would be a DRB1 frequency difference between the male RA and female RA groups.

The DRB1 allele frequencies in the male RA, female RA, and control groups have been previously reported (see appendix in ref. 38). There was no difference in distribution between the male RA and female RA groups (χ^2 = 15.9, 11 df, P not significant), and the DRB1*0401 frequency was nearly identical in male and female RA patients (men 0.213, women 0.234). Thus, we were unable to explain TNFa2b1 enrichment in male RA patients solely by association with a single RA-associated DRB1 allele.

Linkage disequilibrium among DRB1, DQB1, and TNF markers. We therefore addressed whether TNFa2b1 was found on more than one HLA haplotype bearing an RA-associated DRB1 allele by determining allele association and estimating haplotype frequencies. The data confirmed linkage disequilibrium between DRB1 and TNFab in both the RA patients and the controls. Figure 2 shows estimated frequencies for common haplotypes (see table, "Estimated DRB1-TNFab haplotype frequencies for subjects with rheumatoid arthritis and controls," at our Web site).

Of particular note is that the DRB1*03 group was chiefly associated with the TNFa2b3 marker (7.9% of RA HLA haplotypes bore both markers in RA patients, while 10.5% of control haplotypes had both). The DRB1 allele *0401 was associated with TNFab markers a2b1, a6b5, a10b4, or a11b4. DRB1*0404 was largely associated with the TNFa11b4 marker in both RA patients and controls. DRB1*0101 was found with several TNFab markers that are largely restricted to RA patients (TNFa2b1 and TNFa2b3), while in both RA

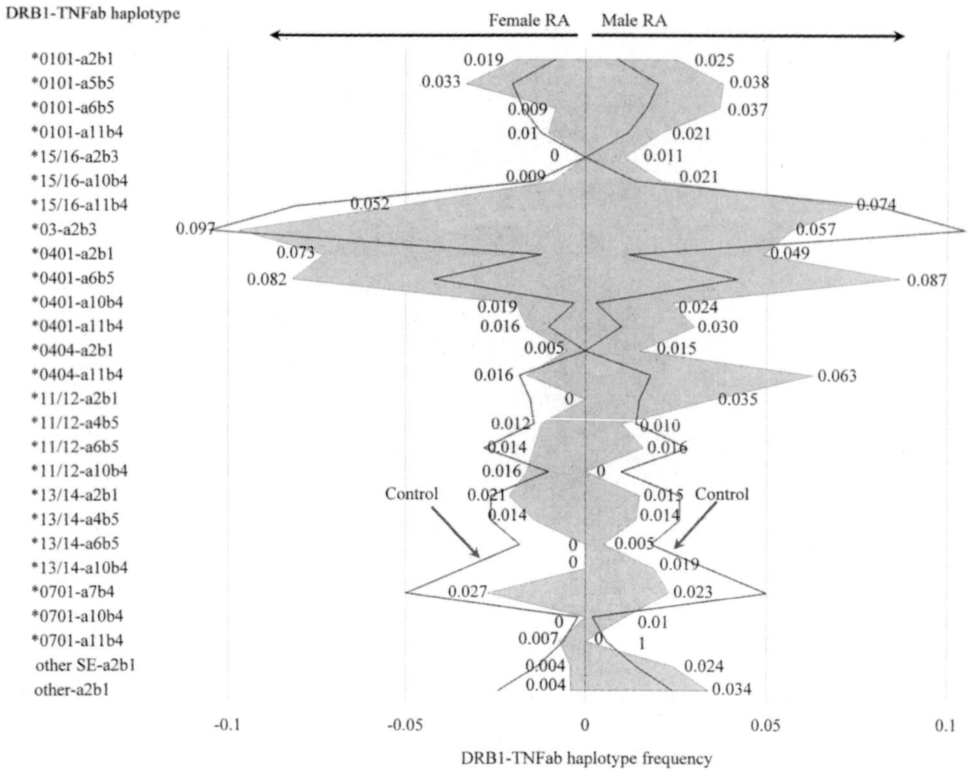

Figure 2. Frequency histogram for HLA–DRB1;TNFab haplotypes (for example, *0101;a2b1 represents the HLA haplotype DRB1*0101;TNFa2b1), plotted as in Figure 1.

patients and controls, *0101 was often found on haplotypes with TNFa5b5, TNFa6b5, TNFa11b4, or other TNFab markers (Table 1). In the group with haplotypes bearing other DRB1 shared-epitope alleles (*0102, *0408, *0405, and *1001), several TNFab markers were found: TNFa2b1, TNFa10b4, TNFa11b4, and others.

Thus, the known linkage disequilibrium reflects a situation of restricted TNFab markers on shared-epitope–bearing HLA haplotypes, not single TNFab markers with each shared-epitope–bearing haplotype. By examining estimated haplotype frequencies in the male RA, female RA, and control groups (Figure 2), the TNFa2b1 in the male RA patients was noted to be on several HLA haplotypes (bearing DRB1*0101, *0401, *0404, *11/12, *13/14, or other shared-epitope DRB1 alleles (*0405, *0408, and *1001).

Analysis of 3-locus linkage disequilibrium among DRB1, DQB1, and TNFab confirmed linkage disequilibrium both in controls and in RA patients (frequencies are shown in a table, "Estimated DRB1-DQB1-TNFab haplotype frequencies for subjects with rheumatoid arthritis and controls," at our Web site). On HLA haplotypes bearing DRB1*0401 and DQB1*0301, the TNFab markers were predominantly TNFa6b5 and, to a lesser degree, TNFa11b4 (Figure 3); on the other hand, HLA haplotypes with DRB1*0401 and DQB1*0302 typically bore TNFa2b1, or less commonly, TNFa10b4. HLA–DRB1*0404;DQB1*0302 haplotypes usually had TNFa11b4, and DRB1*0408;DQB1*0301-bearing haplotypes had TNFa6b5 more frequently than any other TNFab marker. HLA haplotypes with DRB1*0101 and its associated DQB1*0501 allele may have several TNFab markers: a2b1, a6b5, a10b4, a11b4, or others (such as a5b5). In male RA patients, TNFa2b1 was present on haplotypes DRB1*0401;DQB1*0302, DRB1*0404;DQB1*0302, DRB1*0101;DQB1*0501, and others.

As expected (42), there was strong linkage disequilibrium among the TNFab, TNFc, and TNFd markers. The TNF promoter polymorphisms were also in strong linkage disequilibrium with TNFab. The vast majority of HLA haplotypes had the TNF-238G and TNF-308G alleles, but the TNF haplotype −238A; −308G was typically on the HLA haplotypes bearing TNFa2b5 (2.6% of control and 1.7% of RA haplotypes) and the HLA haplotypes bearing DR7 (0.6% of control

Table 1. Multiple logistic regression model with shared-epitope DRB1 alleles and TNF markers (controlling for early disease onset)*

Independent variable	Coefficient (β)	SE	Wald's χ^2	P	Odds ratio	95% CI	No. of positive RA patients (n = 123)	No. of positive controls (n = 120)
Male RA patients								
DRB1*0401	1.268	0.331	14.658	0.0001	3.553	1.855–6.803	53	21
DRB1*0404	0.647	0.368	3.098	0.0784	1.910	0.929–3.922	26	14
DRB1*0408	1.863	0.868	4.608	0.0318	6.441	1.176–35.714	10	2
DRB1*0101	1.395	0.346	16.278	0.0001	4.034	2.049–7.937	40	16
DRB1*1001	1.501	1.207	1.547	0.2136	4.486	0.421–47.619	3	1
TNFa2b1	0.948	0.324	8.554	0.0034	2.580	1.366–4.854	48	24
TNFa2b3	0.120	0.506	0.0564	0.8122	1.128	0.418–3.040	22	30
TNFa6b5	0.094	0.338	0.0766	0.7819	1.098	0.566–2.132	40	34
TNFa11b4	0.519	0.284	3.349	0.0673†	1.681	0.963–2.933	49	35
TNF −308A	0.027	0.438	0.0038	0.9509	1.027	0.435–2.421	31	39
Female RA patients								
DR4 QKRAA‡	1.945	0.326	35.656	0.0001	6.991	3.690–13.16	68	19
DR4 QRRAA‡	1.134	0.357	10.079	0.0015	3.108	1.543–6.250	31	16
DR1 QRRAA‡	0.871	0.295	9.720	0.0018	2.508	1.406–4.464	39	26
DR10 RRRAA‡	2.947	1.126	6.855	0.0088	19.053	2.096–166.7	7	1
TNFa2b1	0.033	0.314	0.011	0.9162	1.034	0.559–1.912	46	35
TNFa2b3	0.669	0.407	2.621	0.1055†	1.932	0.870–4.292	41	31
TNFa6b5	−0.650	0.295	4.868	0.0274	0.522	0.293–0.930	41	47
TNFa11b4	0.115	0.283	0.165	0.6847	1.122	0.645–1.953	53	42
TNF −308A	−0.082	0.376	0.047	0.8282	0.922	0.441–1.927	52	47

* The coefficient (β) is the mathematical weighting of each variable in the model; SE is the standard error of the coefficient (β). Wald's χ^2 is the Wald test statistic calculated from the data, to be compared with the chi-square distribution (1 degree of freedom). P values indicate that the variables are statistically significantly associated with a diagnosis of rheumatoid arthritis (RA). The odds ratio represents the estimated odds ratio of a diagnosis of RA for each allele at the locus; 95% CI is the 95% confidence interval for the estimated odds ratio. TNF = tumor necrosis factor.
† Because TNFa2b3 and TNFa11b4 had been previously shown to be associated (see refs. 35 and 57, respectively), the 1-tailed P value was less than 0.05, showing statistical significance.
‡ DR4 QKRAA = DR4 shared-epitope alleles encoding a shared-epitope DRβ polypeptide chain with ^{70}QKRAA^{74}, representing DRB1*0401; DR4 QRRAA = DR4-group alleles encoding ^{70}QRRAA^{74}, representing alleles *0404, *0405, and *0408; and DR1 QRRAA = DR1-group alleles encoding ^{70}QRRAA^{74}, representing alleles *0101 and *0102; and DR10 RRRAA = *1001 allele encoding ^{70}RRRAA^{74}.

and 1.7% of RA haplotypes). The TNF haplotype −238G;−308A was typically on the HLA haplotypes bearing either TNFa2b3 or TNFa4b5 (controls 11.5% and 2.8%, RA patients 12.8% and 4.7%, respectively). The same −238G;−308A haplotype was found on HLA haplotypes bearing DRB1*03, *11/12, *13/14, or *07

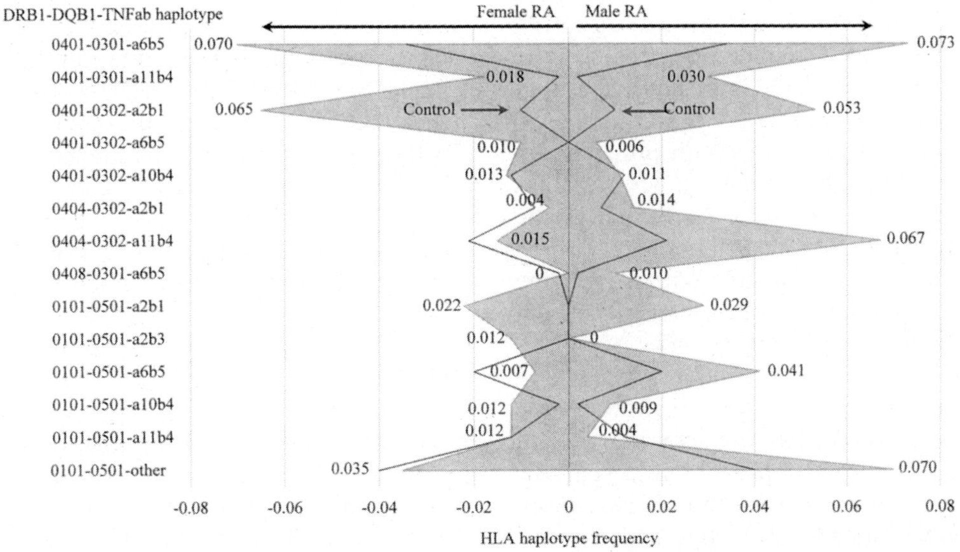

Figure 3. Frequency histogram for HLA–DRB1;DQB1;TNFab haplotypes (for example, 0401;0301;a6b5 represents the HLA haplotype DRB1*0401;DQB1*0301;TNFa6b5), plotted as in Figure 1.

(control frequencies 11.3%, 2.4%, 2.4%, and 1.4%; and RA frequencies 8.4%, 0.7%, 0.9%, and 0.4%, respectively). This confirms that TNF markers are in marked linkage disequilibrium among each other and with DRB1.

Independence of TNF and DRB1 markers in RA susceptibility. Although one cannot statistically separate the biologic effects of one HLA-region allele and another on the same haplotype, one can determine whether a particular TNF marker may confer risk when found on haplotypes without RA-associated DRB1 markers. We therefore examined whether TNFab markers conferred RA risk independently of DRB1. By simply determining the risk in shared-epitope–negative subgroups, we found that TNFa2b1 conferred an elevated relative risk in male RA patients whether compared with female RA patients (relative risk 3.0, Haldane's χ^2 = 5.6, $P < 0.05$) or with control subjects (relative risk 2.7, Haldane's χ^2 = 7.7, $P < 0.05$).

We also examined the degree of association between RA and these HLA markers by developing models based on previously associated markers. The optimal model for predicting RA in men is shown in Table 1. The minimum number of independent variables remaining in the best-fitting model for RA in men included the individual shared-epitope DRB1 alleles (coded 0, 1, or 2 each) plus the TNFa2b1 and TNFa11b4 markers.

For RA in women, the optimal model for predicting the diagnosis of RA is also in Table 1. This included the shared-epitope sequences ^{70}QKRAA^{74} (found on *0401), DR4 ^{70}QRRAA^{74} (found on *0404, *0405, and *0408), DR1 ^{70}QRRAA^{74} (found on *0101 and *0102), and ^{70}RRRAA^{74} (found on *1001), plus the TNFab markers a2b3 and a6b5. Of particular note is that TNFa6b5 was associated with an odds ratio of <1, indicating protection and conflicting with previous observations (35,50). Although the male model findings from the first 80% of patients were confirmed in the remaining 20%, the TNFa6b5 contribution in women was found with only the first panel. When the same logistic regression analyses were done on female subject groups stratified by shared-epitope presence or absence, TNFa6b5 was not a significant independent variable and had protective estimated odds ratios in either group (0.70 and 0.45, respectively) (data not shown).

While TNFa6b5 protection could be a spurious finding, this conflict with previous observations more likely reflects genetic heterogeneity. Interaction terms introduced to represent common haplotypes were not significant, suggesting that DRB1 markers did not influence TNF marker contribution, and vice versa. Of particular note is that, except for DRB1*0404, the odds ratios for TNFab markers were typically lower than those for shared-epitope DRB1 alleles.

DISCUSSION

Taken as a whole, the findings of this study confirm that certain TNFab markers may influence RA risk independently from DRB1 but in a sex-dependent manner. Specifically, the TNF microsatellite marker a2b1 is associated with modest RA risk in male populations (as has been previously reported) (50). The present study extends these observations by finding that such TNFa2b1 alleles in men are found on several HLA haplotypes, including those with and without shared-epitope DRB1 alleles. Our study population does reflect a preponderance of severe disease, particularly in men, so the influences of genetic heterogeneity on severity may confound the disease associations noted.

A central question to explaining how the HLA region contributes to RA pathogenesis is why not all the various associated DRB1 alleles confer the same risk. One potential explanation is that the various shared-epitope DRB1 alleles have similar, but not identical, biologic functions. Another possible explanation is that RA risk may be independently modified by alleles at 2 or more HLA-region loci, sometimes found on the same haplotype, sometimes found alone. There have been hints that certain HLA haplotypes influence RA disease differently from other haplotypes. Some studies have suggested a DRB1 hierarchy in RA, with DRB1*0401 conferring more severe disease (52,53). As noted with our 3-locus linkage disequilibrium studies (Figure 3), the haplotype DRB1*0401;DQB1*0301 typically bears either TNFa6b5 or TNFa11b4. Association of RA severity with a shared epitope is influenced by interaction with TNFa6, predominantly in females (54). Thus, RA severity may be influenced more by certain HLA haplotypes bearing shared-epitope DRB1 alleles than by others. A second HLA-region locus might account for the variation.

One should note that disease associations with HLA markers are largely due to an increased frequency of one or several HLA haplotypes common in the population. Degli-Esposti and coworkers described common HLA haplotypes in the Australian Caucasoid population and designated them according to HLA–B allele and specific class III and DR haplotype (55); for example, the ancestral haplotype 62.1 has B62, Bf*S, C4A*3, C4B*3, and DR4. From extensive studies of TNF microsatellite types in cell lines bearing these ancestral haplotypes (43), one would anticipate that TNFa6b5 association would largely reflect ancestral HLA haplotypes 35.1 and 44.1 (bearing DR5 and DR4, respectively); others have found RA association with an HLA haplotype consistent with B44.1 (A2;Cw5;B44;DRB1*0401; TNFa6b5d4) (56). TNFa11b4 association would arise largely from haplotype 7.1 (bearing DR2), and TNFa2b1 from 35.2, 62.1, and 65.5 (bearing DR1, DR4, and DR1, respectively). Others have noted RA association with the HLA haplotype Cw3;B62;TNFa2b1c2d5 (56), which one would expect to bear DR4 typically.

However, these reported ancestral shared-epitope–bearing haplotypes do not fully explain the male association with TNFa2b1 in the present study; even among shared-epitope–negative haplotypes, there was an enrichment of TNFa2b1 among men. Cell lines without such recognizable ancestral HLA haplotypes also may have TNFa2b1, such as those bearing DR8, DR9, DR16, DR11, DR6, and DR7 (43). Our data showing a female RA association with TNFa2b3 are consistent with other studies showing RA association with the HLA haplotype A1;Cw7;B8;DRB1*0301; TNFa2b3d2 (56). On the other hand, we cannot fully explain why the TNFa6 association with early-onset RA in women, as previously reported (50), was not reproduced in our female RA patients.

This study does not fully explain the observation by Mulcahy et al of an RA association with TNFa2b3 and TNFa6b5, but not with TNFa2b1 (35); among 62 affected individuals, 13 had received a TNFa2b1 allele from a heterozygous parent, while 20 had not. The study involved analyses among multiplex families, so the transmission disequilibrium test was valid for linkage, not association. Relatively few affected offspring were male. In the Mulcahy et al study, the TNFa2b1 transmitted to affected males versus the untransmitted TNFa2b1 was 3 versus 4, TNFa2b3 was 3 versus 2, and TNFa6b5 was 7 versus 1 (O'Gara F: personal communication); this shows that TNFa6b5 was preferentially transmitted to male affected offspring, while TNFa2b1 and TNFa2b3 analyses were not significant. Similarly, Martinez and colleagues reported a TNFa6b5 linkage, but not TNFa2b1 or TNFa3b3, in Spanish families, but nearly all of the probands were female (36). One would predict from our case–control results that TNFa2b1 influence would be restricted to male offspring, and thus, in this context, the previous studies are ambiguous because of low power to detect effects in males.

Therefore, the description of independent risk from TNFab markers in this study seems to largely confirm several previous studies (35,50). Taken as a whole, a hypothesis including both shared-epitope DRB1 alleles and additional sex-influenced HLA susceptibility loci outside DRB1 may better account for various observations among RA populations and families.

ACKNOWLEDGMENTS

The authors are indebted to the members of the Rheumatology Section of the McGuire VAMC and the faculty of the Division of Rheumatology, Allergy, and Immunology for identifying and enlisting subjects, to Nellie Curry and Jean Mallory of the Arthritis Serology Laboratory for valuable laboratory testing, and to Dr. James E. Ames, IV, of the Department of Mathematical Sciences for software assistance.

REFERENCES

1. Wolfe F, Kleinheksel SM, Khan MA. Prevalence of familial occurrence in patients with rheumatoid arthritis. Br J Rheumatol 1988;27 Suppl 2:150–2.
2. Lawrence JS. Rheumatoid arthritis—nature or nurture? Ann Rheum Dis 1970;29:357–79.
3. Stastny P. Mixed lymphocyte cultures in rheumatoid arthritis. J Clin Invest 1976;57:1148–57.
4. Wordsworth BP, Lanchbury JSS, Sakkas LI, Welsh KI, Panayi GS, Bell JI. HLA-DR4 subtype frequencies in rheumatoid arthritis indicate that DRB1 is the major susceptibility locus within the HLA class II region. Proc Natl Acad Sci U S A 1989;86:10049–53.
5. Nichol FE, Woodrow JC. HLA DR antigens in Indian patients with rheumatoid arthritis [letter]. Lancet 1981;1:220–1.
6. Williams RC, Jacobsson LTH, Knowler WC, del Puente A, Kostyu D, McAuley JE, et al. Meta-analysis reveals association between most common class II haplotype in full-heritage Native Americans and rheumatoid arthritis. Hum Immunol 1995;42:90–4.
7. Willkens RF, Nepom GT, Marks CR, Nettles JW, Nepom BS. Association of HLA–Dw16 with rheumatoid arthritis in Yakima Indians: further evidence for the "shared epitope" hypothesis. Arthritis Rheum 1991;34:43–7.
8. Gao X, Gazit E, Livneh A, Stastny P. Rheumatoid arthritis in Israeli Jews: shared sequences in the third hypervariable region of DRB1 alleles are associated with susceptibility. J Rheumatol 1991;18:801–3.
9. Sanchez B, Moreno I, Magarino R, Garzon M, Gonzales MF, Garcia A, et al. HLA-DRw10 confers the highest susceptibility to rheumatoid arthritis in a Spanish population. Tissue Antigens 1990;36:174–6.
10. Gregersen PK, Silver J, Winchester RJ. The shared epitope hypothesis: an approach to understanding the molecular genetics of susceptibility to rheumatoid arthritis. Arthritis Rheum 1987;30: 1205–13.
11. Hillarby MC, Hopkins J, Grennan DM. A re-analysis of the association between rheumatoid arthritis with and without extraarticular features, HLA-DR4, and DR4 subtypes. Tissue Antigens 1991;37:39–41.
12. Boki KA, Panayi GS, Vaughan RW, Drosos AA, Moutsopoulos HM, Lanchbury JS. HLA class II sequence polymorphisms and susceptibility to rheumatoid arthritis in Greeks: the HLA–DRβ shared-epitope hypothesis accounts for the disease in only a minority of Greek patients. Arthritis Rheum 1992;35:749–55.
13. Reveille JD, Alarcón GS, Fowler SE, Pillemer SR, Neuner R, Clegg DO, et al. HLA–DRB1 genes and disease severity in rheumatoid arthritis. Arthritis Rheum 1996;39:1802–7.

14. Sattar MA, Al-Saffar M, Guindi RT, Sugathan TN, White AG, Behbehani K. Histocompatibility antigens (A, B, C, and DR) in Arabs with rheumatoid arthritis. Dis Markers 1990;8:11–5.
15. Massardo L, Jacobelli S, Rodriguez L, Rivero S, Gonzalez A, Marchetti R. Weak association between HLA-DR4 and rheumatoid arthritis in Chilean patients. Ann Rheum Dis 1990;49:290–2.
16. Hasstedt SJ, Clegg DO, Ingles L, Ward RH. HLA-linked rheumatoid arthritis. Am J Hum Genet 1994;55:738–46.
17. Jaraquemada D, Ollier W, Awad J, Young A, Silman A, Roitt IM, et al. HLA and rheumatoid arthritis: a combined analysis of 440 British patients. Ann Rheum Dis 1986;45:627–36.
18. McDermott M, Molloy M, Cashin P, McMahon M, Spencer S, Jennings S, et al. A multicase family study of rheumatoid arthritis in south west Ireland. Dis Markers 1986;4:103–11.
19. MacGregor A, Ollier W, Thomson W, Jawaheer D, Silman A. HLA-DRB1*0401/0404 genotype and rheumatoid arthritis: increased association in men, young age at onset, and disease severity. J Rheumatol 1995;22:1032–6.
20. Lang B, Melchers I, Urlacher A, Tanzi-Fetta RF, Kohlbrenner S, Tongio MM, et al. HLA-DR1 and DRw6 association in DR4-negative rheumatoid arthritis patients. Rheumatol Int 1990;10: 171–5.
21. Gao X, Olsen NJ, Pincus T, Stastny P. HLA–DR alleles with naturally occurring amino acid substitutions and risk for development of rheumatoid arthritis. Arthritis Rheum 1990;33:939–46.
22. Rigby AS, Silman AJ, Voelm L, Gregory JC, Ollier WER, Khan MA, et al. Investigating the HLA component in rheumatoid arthritis: an additive (dominant) mode of inheritance is rejected, a recessive mode is preferred. Genet Epidemiol 1991;8:153–75.
23. Deighton CM, Cavanagh G, Rigby AS, Lloyd HL, Walker DJ. Both inherited HLA-haplotypes are important in the predisposition to rheumatoid arthritis. Brit J Rheumatol 1993;32:893–8.
24. Evans TI, Han J, Singh R, Moxley G. The genotypic distribution of shared-epitope DRB1 alleles suggests a recessive mode of inheritance of the rheumatoid arthritis disease-susceptibility gene. Arthritis Rheum 1995;38:1754–61.
25. Mu H, King MC, Criswell LA. Relative predispositional effects and mode of inheritance of HLA-DRB1 alleles among community-based Caucasian females with rheumatoid arthritis. Genet Epidemiol 1998;15:123–34.
26. Dizier M-H, Eliaou J-F, Babron M-C, Combe B, Sany J, Clot J, et al. Investigation of the HLA component involved in rheumatoid arthritis (RA) by using the marker association-segregation chi-square (MASC) method: rejection of the unifying-shared-epitope hypothesis. Am J Hum Genet 1993;53:715–21.
27. Westendorp RG, Langermans JA, Huizinga TW, Elouali AH, Verweij CL, Boomsma DI, et al. Genetic influence on cytokine production and fatal meningococcal disease. Lancet 1997;349: 170–3.
28. Jacob CO, Fronek Z, Lewis GD, Koo M, Hansen JA, McDevitt HO. Heritable major histocompatibility complex class II-associated differences in production of tumor necrosis factor alpha: relevance to genetic predisposition to systemic lupus erythematosus. Proc Natl Acad Sci U S A 1990;87:1233–7.
29. Brennan FM, Maini RN, Feldmann M. TNF alpha—a pivotal role in rheumatoid arthritis? Br J Rheumatol 1992;31:293–8.
30. Arend WP, Dayer J-M. Inhibition of the production and effects of interleukin-1 and tumor necrosis factor α in rheumatoid arthritis. Arthritis Rheum 1995;38:151–60.
31. Elliott MJ, Maini RN, Feldmann M, Kalden JR, Antoni C, Smolen JS, et al. Randomised double-blind comparison of chimeric monoclonal antibody to tumour necrosis factor alpha (cA2) versus placebo in rheumatoid arthritis. Lancet 1994;344:1105–10.
32. Moreland LW, Baumgartner SW, Schiff MH, Tindall EA, Fleischmann RM, Weaver AL, et al. Treatment of rheumatoid arthritis with a recombinant human tumor necrosis factor receptor (p75)-Fc fusion protein. N Engl J Med 1997;337:141–7.
33. Rankin EC, Choy EH, Kassimos D, Kingsley GH, Sopwith AM, Isenberg DA, et al. The therapeutic effects of an engineered human anti-tumour necrosis factor alpha antibody (CDP571) in rheumatoid arthritis. Br J Rheumatol 1995;34:334–42.
34. Bali D, Gourley S, Kosyu DD, Goel N, Bruce I, Bell A, et al. Genetic analysis of multiplex rheumatoid arthritis families. Genes Immun 1999;1:28–36.
35. Mulcahy B, Waldron-Lynch F, McDermott MF, Adams C, Amos CI, Zhu DK, et al. Genetic variability in the tumor necrosis factor-lymphotoxin region influences susceptibility to rheumatoid arthritis. Am J Hum Genet 1996;59:676–83.
36. Martínez A, Fernández-Arquero M, Pascual-Salcedo D, Conejero L, Alves H, Balsa A, et al. Primary association of tumor necrosis factor–region genetic markers with susceptibility to rheumatoid arthritis. Arthritis Rheum 2000;43:1366–70.
37. Arnett FC, Edworthy SM, Bloch DA, McShane DJ, Fries JF, Cooper NS, et al. The American Rheumatism Association 1987 revised criteria for the classification of rheumatoid arthritis. Arthritis Rheum 1988;31:315–24.
38. Meyer JM, Han J, Singh R, Moxley G. Sex influences on the penetrance of HLA shared-epitope genotypes for rheumatoid arthritis. Am J Hum Genet 1996;58:371–83.
39. Kimura A, Sasazuki T. Eleventh International Histocompatibility Workshop reference protocol for the HLA DNA-typing technique. In: Tsuji K, Aizawa M, Sasazuki T, editors. HLA 1991. Oxford (UK): Oxford University Press; 1992. p. 397–419.
40. Inoko H, Ota M. PCR-RFLP. In: Hui KM, Bidwell JL, editors. Handbook of HLA typing techniques. Boca Raton (FL): CRC Press; 1993. p. 9–70.
41. Jawaheer D, Ollier WER, Thomson W. Multiplex ARMS-RFLP: a simple and rapid method for HLA-DR4 subtyping. Eur J Immunogenet 1993;20:175–87.
42. Jongeneel CV, Briant L, Udalova IA, Sevin A, Nedospasov SA, Cambon-Thomsen A. Extensive genetic polymorphism in the human tumor necrosis factor region and relation to extended HLA haplotypes. Proc Natl Acad Sci U S A 1991;88:9717–21.
43. Udalova IA, Nedospasov SA, Webb GC, Chaplin DD, Turetskaya RL. Highly informative typing of the human TNF locus using six adjacent polymorphic markers. Genomics 1993;16:180–6.
44. Monos DS, Kamoun M, Udalova IA, Csanky E, Cizman B, Turetskaya RL, et al. Genetic polymorphism of the human tumor necrosis factor region in insulin-dependent diabetes mellitus—Linkage disequilibrium of TNFab microsatellite alleles with HLA haplotypes. Hum Immunol 1995;44:70–9.
45. Brinkman BMN, Huizinga TWJ, Kurban SS, van der Velde EA, Schreuder GMT, Hazes JMW, et al. Tumour necrosis factor a gene polymorphisms in rheumatoid arthritis: association with susceptibility to, or severity of, disease? Brit J Rheumatol 1997; 36:516–21.
46. Payami H, Joe S, Farid NR, Stenszky V, Chan SH, Yeo PPB, et al. Relative predispositional effects of marker alleles with disease: HLA-DR alleles and Graves disease. Am J Hum Genet 1989;45: 541–6.
47. Tiwari JL, Terasaki PI. The data and statistical analysis. In: Tiwari JL, Terasaki PI, editors. HLA and disease associations. New York: Springer-Verlag; 1985. p. 18–22.
48. Xie X, Ott J. American Society for Human Genetics annual meeting, 1993 [abstract]. Am J Hum Genet 1993;53:1107.
49. Schipper RF, D'Amaro J, de Lange P, Schreuder GMT, van Rood JJ, Oudshoorn M. Validation of haplotype frequency estimation methods. Hum Immunol 1998;59:518–23.
50. Hajeer A, John S, Ollier WE, Silman AJ, Dawes P, Hassell A, et al. Tumor necrosis factor microsatellite haplotypes are different in male and female patients with RA. J Rheumatol 1997;24:217–9.
51. Bardin T, LeGrand L, Naveau B, Marcelli-Barge A, Debeyre N,

Lathrop GM, et al. HLA antigens and seronegative rheumatoid arthritis. Ann Rheum Dis 1985;44:50–3.
52. Young A, Jaraquemada D, Awad J, Festenstein H, Corbett M, Hay FC, et al. Association of HLA–DR4/Dw4 and DR2/Dw2 with radiologic changes in a prospective study of patients with rheumatoid arthritis: preferential relationship with HLA–Dw rather than HLA–DR specificities. Arthritis Rheum 1984;27:20–5.
53. Weyand CM, McCarthy TG, Goronzy JJ. Correlation between disease phenotype and genetic heterogeneity in rheumatoid arthritis. J Clin Invest 1995;95:2120–6.
54. Mattey DL, Hassell AB, Dawes PT, Ollier WER, Hajeer A. Interaction between tumor necrosis factor microsatellite polymorphisms and the HLA–DRB1 shared epitope in rheumatoid arthritis: influence on disease outcome. Arthritis Rheum 1999;42:2698–704.
55. Degli-Esposti MA, Leaver AL, Christiansen FT, Witt CS, Abraham LJ, Dawkins RL. Ancestral haplotypes: conserved population MHC haplotypes. Hum Immunol 1992;34:242–52.
56. Hajeer AH, Worthington J, Silman AJ, Ollier WER. Association of tumor necrosis factor microsatellite polymorphisms with HLA–DRB1*04–bearing haplotypes in rheumatoid arthritis patients. Arthritis Rheum 1996;39:1109–14.
57. Mu H, Chen JJ, Jiang Y, King M-C, Thomson G, Criswell LA. Tumor necrosis factor α microsatellite polymorphism is associated with rheumatoid severity through an interaction with the HLA–DRB1 shared epitope. Arthritis Rheum 1999;42:438–42.

ARTHRITIS & RHEUMATISM
Vol. 44, No. 2, February 2001, pp 296–306

Recognition of Cell Surface GD3 by Monoclonal Antibody Anti-6C2 in Rheumatoid Arthritis Synovial Fluid

Expression on Human T Cells With Transendothelial Migratory Activity

Toshio Homma,[1] Osamu Hosono,[1] Satoshi Iwata,[1] Susumu Ando,[2] Katsutoshi Sasaki,[3] Tatsunari Nishi,[3] Hiroshi Kawasaki,[1] Hirotoshi Tanaka,[1] and Chikao Morimoto[4]

Objective. **We have previously reported that the anti-6C2 monoclonal antibody (mAb) defines a subset of human CD4+ memory T cells. The present study sought to determine the nature of the 6C2 molecule and the function associated with 6C2+ T cells, and to examine whether this T cell subset is involved in the pathophysiology of rheumatoid arthritis (RA).**

Methods. **Cytofluorographic analysis was performed for identification of T cell surface molecules displaying a distribution similar to that of the 6C2 molecule. T cells in the synovial fluid of RA patients were examined for expression of the 6C2 molecule. Transendothelial migratory activity was assessed by assay using monolayers of human endothelial cells. Specific reactivity of the anti-6C2 mAb was determined by immunoblotting on gangliosides separated by thin-layer chromatography, and flow cytometric analysis of the cells transfected with complementary DNA (cDNA) was performed for determination of the glycosyltransferases involved in biosynthesis of the gangliosides.**

Results. **On human peripheral T cells, the 6C2 molecule was distributed, by and large, in a pattern similar to that of CDw60, or *O*-acetyl-GD3. The majority (>70%) of synovial fluid T cells from patients with RA were found to be 6C2 positive, and those 6C2+ T cells exhibited a transendothelial migratory capacity that was inhibited by pretreatment of T cells with anti-6C2 mAb. Moreover, treatment of T cells with neuraminidase resulted in a loss of 6C2 expression as well as a reduction in the transendothelial migratory activity. Anti-6C2 mAb reacted specifically with GD3, but not with *O*-acetyl-GD3. The reactivity of anti-6C2 mAb was induced on the cell surface only by transfection with cDNA for GD3 synthase.**

Conclusion. **The 6C2 molecule is a disialoganglioside, GD3, and is present on a subset of T cells with transendothelial migratory capacity. The 6C2/GD3 molecules, as well as 6C2/GD3+ T cells, appear to play a role in T cell migration and in the inflammation of RA.**

Functionally heterogeneous human CD4+ lymphocytes have been subdivided into reciprocal subsets based on their expression of unique isoforms of the leukocyte common antigen/T200 family of antigens (CD45/CD45RA and CD45RO) and CD29 (1–6). The subset with the CD4+,CD45RA−,CD29+ ($CD29^{bright}$) phenotype responds maximally to recall antigens, provides a strong helper function for B cell Ig synthesis, and induces CD8+ cells to exert class I major histocompatibility complex–restricted cytotoxicity. In contrast, the CD4+,CD45RA+,CD29− ($CD29^{dim}$) cells perform poorly in these activities. The ability to induce CD8+ cells to suppress Ig synthesis is confined to the latter subset.

We have previously described the development of a monoclonal antibody (mAb), anti-6C2, that defines a

Supported in part by NIH grant AR-33713 and in part by grants from the Ministry of Education, Science, Sport, and Culture and the Ministry of Health and Welfare, Japan.

[1]Toshio Homma, PhD, Osamu Hosono, MD, PhD, Satoshi Iwata, MD, PhD, Hiroshi Kawasaki, MD, PhD, Hirotoshi Tanaka, MD, PhD: University of Tokyo, Tokyo, Japan; [2]Susumu Ando, MD, PhD: Tokyo Metropolitan Institute of Gerontology, Tokyo, Japan; [3]Katsutoshi Sasaki, PhD, Tatsunari Nishi, PhD: Tokyo Research Laboratories, Kyowa Hakko Kogyo Company, Ltd., Tokyo, Japan; [4]Chikao Morimoto, MD, PhD: University of Tokyo, Tokyo, Japan, and Harvard Medical School, Boston, Massachusetts.

Address correspondence and reprint requests to Chikao Morimoto, MD, PhD, Department of Clinical Immunology, Institute of Medical Science, University of Tokyo, 4-6-1, Shirokanedai, Minato-ku, Tokyo 108-8639, Japan.

Submitted for publication May 16, 2000; accepted in revised form September 27, 2000.

subset of CD4+,CD45RO+ memory cells that exhibit maximal responsiveness to soluble recall antigens such as tetanus toxoid and a strong helper function for pokeweed mitogen (PWM)–driven B cell Ig synthesis (7). Biochemical characterization has shown that anti-6C2 precipitated 2 proteins, with relative molecular weights of 180 kd and 95 kd, from ^{125}I-surface–labeled cell lysates, suggesting that the molecule defined by anti-6C2 was the lymphocyte function–associated antigen 1 (LFA-1) complex (CD11a/CD18). In contrast to conventional anti–LFA-1 mAb, however, anti-6C2 did not inhibit cytotoxic killer T cell responses and antigen-induced T cell proliferation, whereas it did inhibit PWM-driven B cell Ig synthesis (7). Moreover, cell distributions defined by this mAb were totally different from those defined by conventional LFA-1 mAb. The above findings suggest that anti-6C2 appears to recognize either a unique epitope of LFA-1 or a molecule other than the LFA-1 complex (7).

In the present study, we further investigated the nature of the 6C2 molecule. Immunofluorescence staining showed that the 6C2 molecule was also present on LFA-1–deficient Epstein-Barr virus (EBV)–transformed B lymphoblastoid cells, suggesting that anti-6C2 recognizes a molecule other than the LFA-1 complex. Immunoreactivity and functional studies suggested that the 6C2 molecule is distinct from CDw60 or is a distinct epitope of CDw60. The majority of 6C2+ T cells were present in the synovial fluid of rheumatoid arthritis (RA) patients. Functional analysis demonstrated that 6C2+ T cells exhibited a transendothelial migratory capacity that was inhibited by anti-6C2, and that treatment of T cells with neuraminidase resulted in loss of anti-6C2 reactivity as well as reduced transendothelial migratory activity. Immunoblot analysis, with separation by thin-layer chromatography (TLC), showed that anti-6C2 reacted with GD3. Moreover, the induction of the 6C2 molecule on the cell surface was observed only by transfection with human GD3 synthase complementary DNA (cDNA), confirming that the 6C2 molecule is cell surface GD3. These results suggest that the 6C2/GD3 molecule, as well as 6C2/GD3+ T cells, play a role in T cell migration and in the inflammation of RA.

PATIENTS AND METHODS

Isolation of lymphoid cell populations. Human peripheral blood mononuclear cells (PBMC) were isolated from healthy volunteer donors and patients with RA by Ficoll-Hypaque density-gradient centrifugation (Pharmacia LKB Biotechnology, Piscataway, NJ). In a similar manner, mononuclear cells were isolated from heparinized synovial fluid drawn under aseptic conditions from 8 patients with RA. All RA patients included in the present study fulfilled the 1987 classification criteria of the American College of Rheumatology (formerly, the American Rheumatism Association) (8). PBMC were depleted of macrophages by adherence to plastic for 1 hour, and T cells were isolated by rosetting with sheep red blood cells as previously described (1,2,7). Further depletion of macrophages was achieved by incubation with 5 m*M* L-leucine methyl ester (9). Of the T cells obtained, >95% were CD3 positive.

Production and characterization of mAb. Production of the IgM mAb anti-6C2 has been previously described (7). Anti-UM4D4, a representative anti-CDw60 IgM mAb reactive with 9-*O*-acetyl-GD3 (10,11) was generously provided in ascites form by Dr. D. A. Fox (University of Michigan, Ann Arbor). Anti–LFA-1 (2F12) has been described elsewhere (12).

Human cell lines. An EBV-transformed B lymphoid cell line established from a patient with hereditary leukocyte adhesion deficiency was generously provided by Dr. M. Minegishi (Tohoku University School of Medicine, Sendai, Japan). In addition, as controls, EBV-transformed B lymphoid cell lines were established from healthy individuals in our laboratory. These cell lines and a human T cell line, H9, were maintained in RPMI 1640 culture medium supplemented with 10% fetal calf serum (FCS) 4 m*M* L-glutamine, 25 m*M* HEPES (Gibco BRL, Grand Island, NY), 0.5% sodium bicarbonate, 100 units/ml penicillin, and 100 μg/ml streptomycin as previously described (7).

Analysis of lymphocyte population with flow cytometry. Cytofluorographic analysis of cell populations was performed by means of both direct and indirect immunofluorescence with fluorescein isothiocyanate (FITC)–conjugated $F(ab')_2$ goat anti-mouse IgG/IgM and phycoerythrin (PE)–conjugated anti-mouse IgM (μ chain; Jackson ImmunoResearch, West Grove, PA), and flow cytometry was performed by using an EPICS XL (Coulter Electronics, Hialeah, FL) (1,2,7). For the analysis, all mAb were utilized in excess dilutions of antibody at 1:200 to 1:1,000. FITC-conjugated CD26 and CD11a and PE-conjugated anti-CD3 were from Coulter Immunotech (Hialeah, FL). FITC-conjugated anti-CDw60 (anti-UM4D4) was from PharMingen (San Diego, CA).

Proliferation assays. PBMC were cultured in triplicate in round-bottomed 96-well culture plates in RPMI 1640 supplemented with 10% FCS, 4 m*M* L-glutamine, 25 m*M* HEPES, 100 μg/ml streptomycin, and 100 units/ml penicillin, in the presence or absence of mAb at various dilutions (indicated in the figure legends) or phytohemagglutinin (1 μg/ml; Gibco BRL) (1,2,7). Following 3 days of culture, cells were incubated with 1 μCi of ^{3}H-thymidine for 18 hours. Cells were harvested and ^{3}H-thymidine incorporation was measured in a beta counter (Matrix 96; Packard, Meriden, CT).

Western blot with gangliosides separated by TLC. Reactivity of anti-6C2 and anti-UM4D4 toward gangliosides was examined by Western blot analysis on gangliosides developed by TLC, as previously described (13). Total gangliosides obtained from monkey brain, containing GM4, GM3, GM2, GM1, GD3, GD1a, GD2, GT1a, GD1b, GT1b, and GQ1b, and a mixture of GD3 and *O*-acetyl-GD3 were applied to a high-performance TLC plate and developed using $CHCl_3$/methanol/0.2% (weight/volume) $CaCl_2$ (volume/volume/volume 50/40/11) as previously described (13). Following development, the plate was coated with 0.4% polyisobutyl methacrylate and incubated with either control mouse IgM, anti-6C2, or anti-UM4D4 for 3 hours at room temperature. Detection was performed with enhanced chemiluminescence (Amersham, Buckinghamshire, UK). Gangliosides were visualized by the resorcinol/HCl reagent (13).

Transfection and expression of sialyl- and fucosyltransferase cDNAs. Namalwa KJM-1, a subline of the human Burkitt lymphoma cell line Namalwa, which expresses abundant GM3 (an acceptor substrate for GD3 synthase) but has no GD3 and GD3 synthase activity, was transfected with the expression vector pAMo alone or with pAMo containing cDNA for human GM3-specific α-2,8-sialyltransferase (GD3 synthase), rat Galβ1,3GlcNAc α-2,3-sialyltransferase (ST3), human Galβ(1-3/1-4)GlcNAc α-2,3-sialyltransferase (ST4), or 1 of 4 human α-1,3-fucosyltransferases (FT3, 4, 6, or 7) (14–16). Transfected cells were examined for expression of the 6C2 molecule on the cell surface by flow cytometric analysis.

Assay for transendothelial migration capacity and adherence to endothelial cells. The transendothelial migration assay used was adapted elsewhere to use 2-chamber culture plates (17,18). Human umbilical vein endothelial cells (HUVEC) were obtained from Clonetics (Walkersville, MD) and maintained on type I collagen–coated dishes in E-STIM endothelial cell culture medium (Becton Dickinson, Bedford, MA). For the transendothelial migration assay, HUVEC were plated on type I collagen–coated BIOCOAT inserts (Becton Dickinson) at a density of 5×10^5 cells/well and cultured for 2 days. Confluent HUVEC monolayers were washed and incubated with T cells (6×10^5 cells/well) in RPMI 1640 containing 0.6% bovine serum albumin for the indicated time period. Following incubation, T cells were recovered from the inserts and bottom wells, and were designated as either nonmigrated or migrated T cells. HUVEC monolayers were washed twice with phosphate buffered saline (PBS) and T cells tightly bound to endothelial cells were removed by incubation with Hanks' balanced salt solution supplemented with 0.5 m*M* EDTA (17).

Migrated and nonmigrated T cells were counted using a hemocytometer. The phenotype of these T cell populations was determined by flow cytometric analysis. Adherence of T cells to endothelial cells was also examined in the absence of transendothelial migration, by incubating T cells (2×10^6 cells/well) on HUVEC monolayers prepared on gelatin-coated 6-well culture plates. Following 6 hours of incubation, nonadherent cells were removed by washing twice with PBS, and adherent T cells were recovered with EDTA, as described above, and counted using a hemocytometer.

Statistical analysis. Comparison of the differences in the migratory capacity of control cells and other groups of cells or between the binding of control T cells and T cells treated with mAb was done by Student's *t*-test. *P* values less than 0.05 were considered significant.

RESULTS

Anti-6C2 reactivity on LFA-1–deficient cells. To further characterize the 6C2 molecule, we first examined the reactivity of anti-6C2 with LFA-1–deficient cells. EBV-transformed B lymphoid cell lines established from normal individuals and from a patient with hereditary leukocyte adhesion deficiency were examined for expression of LFA-1 and the 6C2 molecule by indirect immunofluorescence and flow cytometric analysis. Figure 1A shows representative cytofluorographic profiles of these EBV-transformed B lymphoblastoid cell lines. In cells from 3 normal individuals, 78 ± 15% (mean ± SEM) of cells were reactive with anti–LFA-1 (Figure 1A, upper left), whereas no reactivity was found in cells from an LFA-1–deficient individual (Figure 1A, lower left). In contrast, anti-6C2 reacted with both cell lines. In cells from 3 normal individuals, 44 ± 13% were reactive with anti-6C2 (Figure 1A, upper right), and 54 ± 15% of cells from an LFA-1–deficient individual were reactive with anti-6C2 (Figure 1A, lower right). These findings strongly suggest that anti-6C2 recognizes a molecule other than the LFA-1 complex.

Comparison of the 6C2 molecule with CDw60 (*O*-acetyl-GD3). Since our previous analyses showed that no molecules other than the LFA-1 complex are detected by immunoprecipitation of ^{125}I-surface–labeled cell lysates and sodium dodecyl sulfate–polyacrylamide gel electrophoresis (7), we speculated that the 6C2 molecule may be a nonproteineous molecule preferentially expressed on a subset of T cells. Well-known nonproteineous CD molecules are mostly glycolipids, and of these molecules, only CDw60 (*O*-acetylated ganglioside) has been shown to be present on human T cells (10,11). Therefore, we next examined whether the distribution of the 6C2 molecule within peripheral T cells is similar to that of CDw60.

Figure 1B shows expression of the 6C2 molecule and CDw60 on peripheral T cells. The 6C2 molecule was present on 28 ± 7% of T cells, while CDw60, detected with anti-UM4D4 specific for 9-*O*-acetyl-GD3, was expressed on a somewhat larger population (39 ± 9%) of T cells (Figure 1B). Although the size of the positive T cell population and the intensity of expression were higher in the UM4D4 molecule (CDw60) than in the 6C2 molecule, the reactivity of both antibodies was, by and large, similar. Dual immunostaining for the 6C2 molecule and CDw60 revealed that ~20% of CDw60+ T cells (21 ± 4% of the entire T cell population) were also positive for the 6C2 molecule (Figure 1C). A small population of T cells, representing 7 ± 3%, was 6C2+/CDw60−, and a larger population (16 ± 5%) was 6C2−/CDw60+. Thus, almost two-thirds of the 6C2+ T cells were found within CDw60+ T cells. Therefore, it is possible that anti-UM4D4 mAb may have a higher affinity than that of anti-6C2 mAb.

Several reports showed that one of the character-

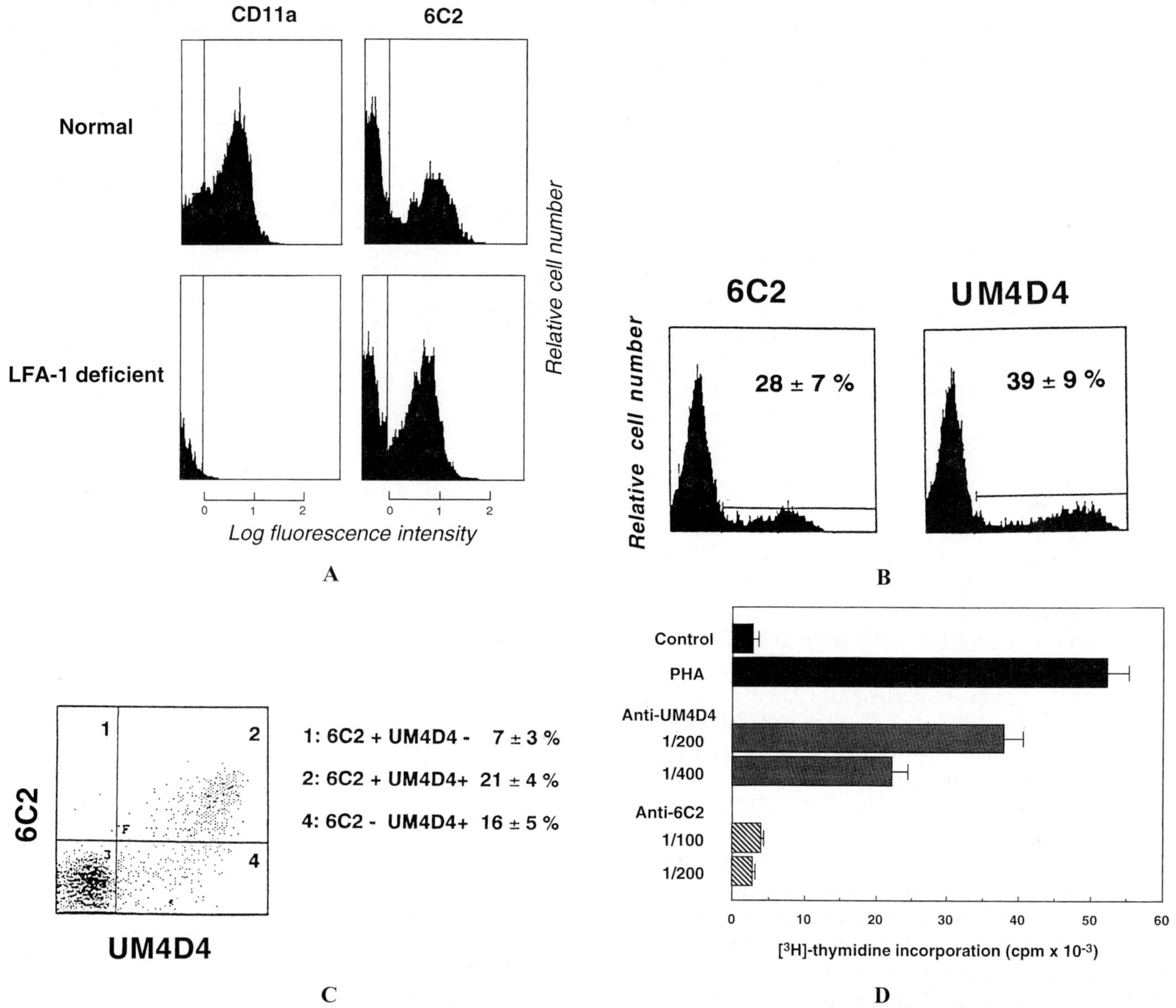

Figure 1. Presence of the 6C2 molecule on lymphocyte function–associated antigen 1 (LFA-1)–deficient, Epstein-Barr virus (EBV)–transformed B lymphoblastoid cells, distribution of the 6C2 molecule and CDw60 in human peripheral T cells, and induction of proliferative response of peripheral blood mononuclear cells (PBMC) by anti-CDw60, but not by anti-6C2 monoclonal antibodies. **A**, EBV-transformed B lymphoblastoid cell lines derived from a normal individual (upper) and from a patient with hereditary LFA-1 deficiency (lower) were examined for reactivity with either anti–LFA-1/CD11a (2F12) or anti-6C2 by indirect immunofluorescence staining. Cytofluorographic profiles are shown with fluorescence intensity in logarithmic scale on the horizontal axis and relative cell number on the vertical axis. Results are representative of 3 separate experiments. Human peripheral T cells were immunostained with either anti-6C2 or anti-UM4D4 (**B**) or both (**C**) and analyzed by flow cytometry for expression of the 6C2 molecule and CDw60 (*O*-acetylated ganglioside). **D**, PBMC were cultured in either the absence or presence of 1 μg/ml of phytohemagglutinin (PHA), anti-UM4D4, or anti-6C2, at the indicated dilutions for 3 days, and ^{3}H-thymidine incorporation was determined. Results are representative of 4 separate experiments. Bars show the mean ± SEM counts per minute of triplicate samples.

istics of anti–*O*-acetylated GD3 mAb is its mitogenic activity for T cells (10,11,19). For example, addition of soluble anti–9-*O*-acetyl-GD3 (anti-UM4D4) (10,11) and anti–7-*O*-acetyl-GD3 (U5) (19) has been shown to induce proliferation of human peripheral T cells. As previously described (10), addition of anti-UM4D4 to

PBMC caused significant proliferation, whereas anti-6C2, added up to a dilution of 1:100, had no proliferative effect (Figure 1D). Taken together, these findings suggest that the 6C2 molecule is distinct from CDw60 or is a distinct epitope of CDw60.

Accumulation of 6C2+ T cells in synovial fluid of patients with RA. Since anti-6C2 preferentially reacted with a subset of CD4+,CD45RO+ memory T cells, and the CDw60 molecule is expressed on the surface of most T cells in synovial fluid from RA patients (10,11), we sought to determine whether 6C2+ T cells are also involved in the chronic inflammation of RA. Mononuclear cells were isolated from the synovial fluid of patients with RA and, along with PBMC from the same patients and from normal individuals, were examined for expression of 6C2 in CD3+ T cells. Figure 2A shows a representative histogram illustrating the marked accumulation of 6C2+ cells in synovial fluid from RA patients. In total, samples from 8 normal individuals and 8 patients with RA were examined for the percentage of 6C2+ cells in CD3+ T cells (Figure 2B). Since the number of CD3+ T cells varied (65–85% in PBMC from normal individuals, and 50–84% and 68–90% in PBMC and synovial mononuclear cells from RA patients, respectively), the values were normalized to the percentage of CD3+ T cells. In peripheral CD3+ T cells from normal individuals, 30.5 ± 7.5% (mean ± SD) of cells were 6C2+ cells. A similar fraction of peripheral CD3+ T cells from 8 RA patients was found to be 6C2+ (31.7 ± 7.4%). In contrast, 78.3 ± 7.0% of CD3+ T cells in the synovial fluid from RA patients were 6C2+. Thus, these observations suggest that 6C2+ T cells accumulate in the synovial fluid of patients with RA.

Transendothelial migratory capacity associated with the 6C2 molecule. Having determined that 6C2-positive T cells accumulate in the synovial fluid of patients with RA, we next examined the functional characteristics of 6C2+ T cells. One of the important properties of memory T cells is transendothelial migratory capacity, which allows T cells to extravasate and accumulate in sites of inflammation (17,20–23). To investigate the transendothelial migratory capacity of 6C2+ T cells, we utilized HUVEC monolayers prepared on the inserts of a 2-chamber culture system (17). Following incubation over HUVEC monolayers, purified T cells migrated through the endothelium, accumulating in the bottom chamber and reaching a plateau at 6 hours of incubation (Figure 3A). Phenotypic analysis of the nonmigrated and migrated T cells demonstrated that almost all of the 6C2+ cells present in the initial T cell population migrated through the endothelium, ac-

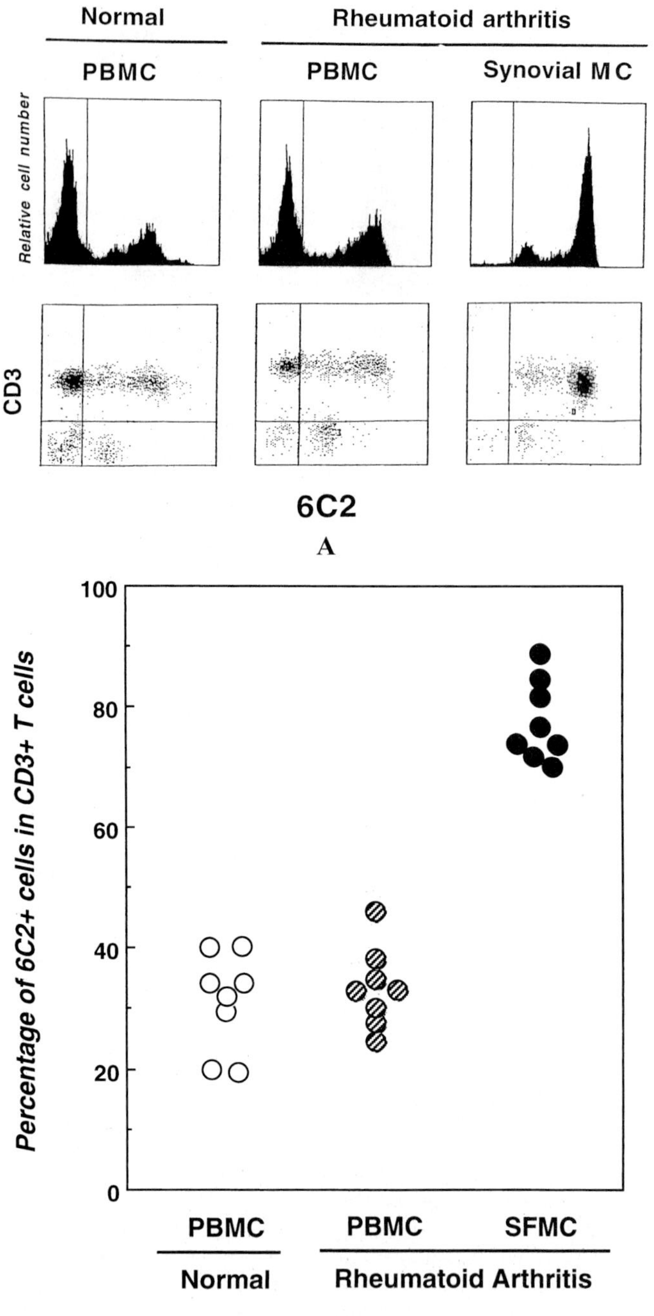

Figure 2. Accumulation of 6C2+ T cells in synovial fluid from patients with rheumatoid arthritis (RA). **A,** expression of 6C2 in peripheral blood mononuclear cells (PBMC) and synovial fluid mononuclear cells (SFMC) from normal individuals and from RA patients. The indicated samples were examined by flow cytometry for 6C2 (upper) or 6C2 and CD3 (lower). Representative cytofluorographic profiles are shown. **B,** Percentage of 6C2+ cells in CD3+ T cells in PBMC and SFMC from normal individuals and from RA patients. Samples from 8 normal individuals and 8 RA patients were examined for 6C2 expression in CD3+ T cells.

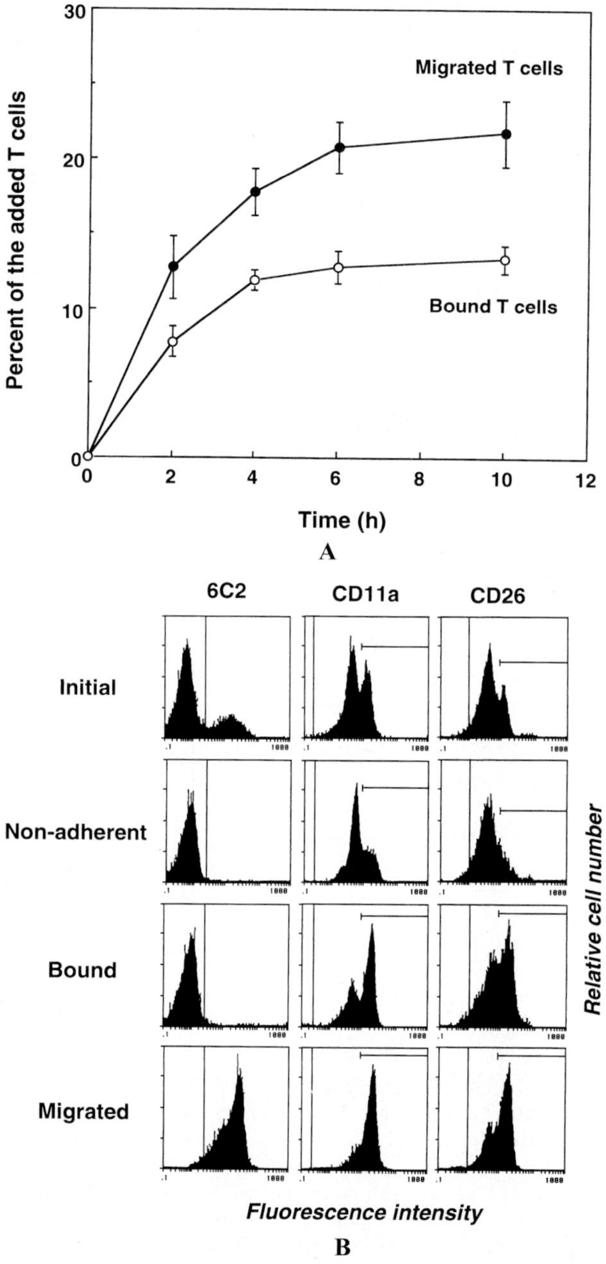

Figure 3. Migration of human peripheral T cells through nonstimulated endothelium. **A,** Time course of transendothelial migration of T cells. Purified T cells were incubated with human umbilical vein endothelial cell (HUVEC) monolayers and, at the indicated times, migrated cells and cells tightly bound to the endothelium were harvested as described in Patients and Methods. Values are the percentage of the added T cells found in each population. Bars show the mean ± SEM of 4 separate experiments. **B,** Expression of 6C2, CD26, and CD11a in the initial, nonadherent, bound, and migrating T cells. Peripheral T cells were incubated with HUVEC monolayers for 5 hours and nonadherent, bound, and migrated T cells were recovered and analyzed for expression of 6C2, CD26, and CD11a by flow cytometry. Representative histograms are shown.

counting for 95% of the migrated cells, suggesting that 6C2+ T cells exhibit greater transendothelial migratory capacity than do 6C2− T cells (Figure 3B). Consistent with the findings of previous studies (17,23), migrated T cells were $CD26^{bright}/CD11a^{bright}$. Of interest is the phenotype of T cells tightly bound to the endothelium, which were recovered by EDTA (Figure 3B). Significant numbers of bound T cells were $CD26^{bright}$ and $CD11a^{bright}$. In marked contrast, no 6C2+ cells were found in bound T cells, suggesting enhanced transendothelial migration of 6C2+ T cells.

To further examine the role of cell surface 6C2 in the transendothelial migratory capacity of T cells, we determined whether the 6C2 epitope was important in the migratory capacity. For this purpose, T cells were incubated with neuraminidase to remove sialic acid, and we then further examined the effects of anti-6C2, anti–LFA-1, and neuraminidase treatment on T cell transmigratory activity. Incubation of T cells with neuraminidase abolished the cell surface anti-6C2 reactivity, whereas expression of CD11a was not affected, demonstrating that the 6C2 epitope was sensitive to the action of neuraminidase (Figures 4A and B). Figure 4B shows that pretreatment with anti-6C2 reduced the number of migrated T cells by ~40%, whereas the number of bound T cells was not affected. This difference was statistically significant in comparison with control migration ($P < 0.05$). It should be noted that pretreatment of T cells with anti-UM4D4 did not affect the transendothelial migration under the same conditions (results not shown).

Pretreatment with anti–LFA-1 caused a greater decrease in the number of both migrated and bound T cells, by ~50% and ~70%, respectively ($P < 0.05$ versus controls), indicating that LFA-1–mediated mechanisms were operative in both the migrated and bound T cells. These findings suggest that LFA-1 is involved in the transendothelial migration of T cells through mediation of binding to the endothelium, whereas T cell surface 6C2 is involved in the steps distant from the initial adhesion to the endothelium. Following neuraminidase treatment, migrated T cells were reduced by 65%, whereas anti-6C2 treatment had no effect on neuraminidase-treated T cells, suggesting that anti-6C2–inhibitable transendothelial migratory capacity requires the presence of the 6C2 epitope on the cell surface (Figure 4B).

Specific reaction of anti-6C2 with GD3, but not with *O*-acetylated GD3. Since our findings indicated that the 6C2 molecule may be closely related to *O*-acetylated gangliosides or may be different from CDw60, we next

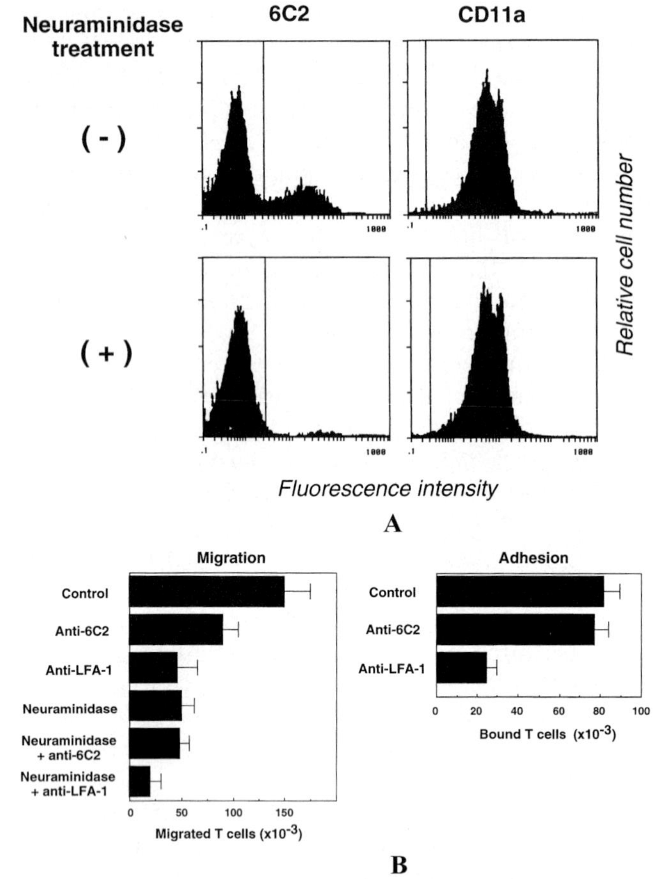

Figure 4. Effects of anti-6C2, anti–LFA-1, and neuraminidase on transendothelial migration and adhesion to the endothelium in T cells. **A,** The effect of neuramanidase treatment of T cells on the expression of 6C2 and the LFA-1 molecule was examined by incubating purified T cells at 2×10^7 cells/ml with 2 m*M* phenylmethylsulfonyl fluoride and *Vibrio cholerae* neuramanidase for 30 minutes at room temperature. Cells were then washed 3 times and stained with anti-6C2 and anti–LFA-1 for flow cytometric analysis (bottom). **B,** The effect of pretreatment of T cells with anti-6C2, anti–LFA-1, and neuraminidase on transendothelial migration and adhesion to the endothelium was examined by incubating purified T cells with saturating concentrations of anti-6C2, anti–LFA-1, or control mouse IgM or neuraminidase for 30 minutes on ice (for antibody) or at room temperature (for neuraminidase). Cells were then washed and utilized in transendothelial migration assay. For the adhesion assay, T cells were incubated with HUVEC cultured on conventional culture plates after antibody treatment. After 5 hours, T cells tightly bound to endothelial cells were recovered and counted. Numbers of migrated and bound T cells are indicated. Bars show the mean and SEM of 3 representative experiments, from a total of 5 separate experiments. The difference was statistically significant in comparison with control migration ($P < 0.05$) and the difference was also significant between control bound T cells and bound T cells treated with anti–LFA-1 monoclonal antibodies ($P < 0.05$). See Figures 1 and 3 for definitions.

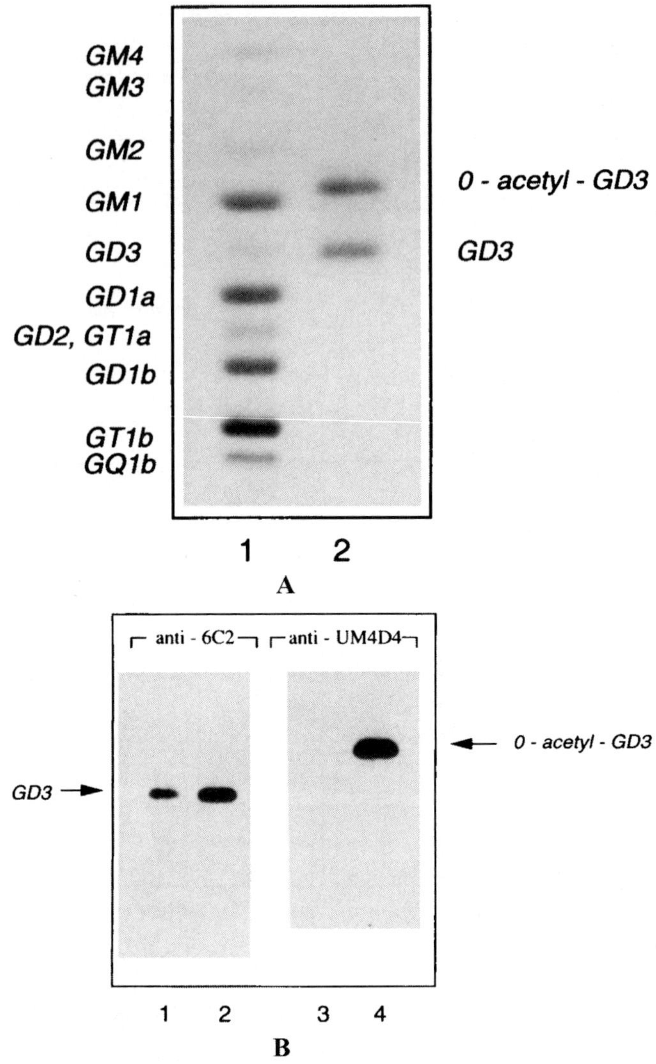

Figure 5. Immunoblotting of anti-6C2 and anti-CDw60 on gangliosides separated by thin-layer chromatography (TLC). **A,** Monkey brain total gangliosides (lane 1) and a mixture of GD3 and *O*-acetyl-GD3 (lane 2) were applied to a high-performance TLC, developed, and visualized by staining with resorcinol as described in Patients and Methods. **B,** Reactivity of anti-6C2 and anti-UM4D4 (anti-CDw60) with gangliosides was examined when monkey brain total gangliosides (lanes 1 and 3) and a mixture of GD3 and *O*-acetyl-GD3 (lanes 2 and 4) were incubated with either anti-6C2 at a dilution of 1:1,600 (lanes 1 and 2) or anti-UM4D4 at a dilution of 1:1,000 (lanes 3 and 4). Bound antibody was detected by enhanced chemiluminescence as described in Patients and Methods.

performed immunoblot analysis on gangliosides developed by TLC (Figure 5). Total gangliosides from monkey brain, containing 11 species of gangliosides, and a mixture of GD3 and *O*-acetyl-GD3 were separated by TLC, and these gangliosides were visualized with the resorcinol/HCl reagent (Figure 5A). Among the gangliosides obtained from monkey brain, anti-6C2 only reacted with GD3 (Figure 5B, lane 1). In the mixture of GD3 and *O*-acetyl-GD3, anti-6C2 was again reactive only with GD3 (Figure 5B, lane 2). In marked contrast, anti-UM4D4 showed no reactivity with the monkey brain total gangliosides (Figure 5B, lane 3), and reacted only with *O*-acetyl-GD3 in the mixture of *O*-acetyl-GD3 and GD3 (Figure 5B, lane 4). Control mouse IgM showed no reactivity with any ganglioside examined (results not shown). These findings strongly suggest that anti-6C2 antibodies specifically recognize GD3.

Anti-6C2 reactivity with GD3 expressed on the cell surface. A final step of the biosynthesis of GD3 is the addition of a sialic acid to a precursor, GM3, catalyzed by a specific sialyltransferase, GD3 synthase (GM3 α-2,8-sialyltransferase). Recently, we have cloned a cDNA for human GD3 synthase by using an expression cloning involving Namalwa KJM-1 cells that express abundant GM3, but no GD3 and GD3 synthase activity (15). Taking advantage of this system, we determined whether anti-6C2 is indeed reactive with the GD3 expressed on the cell surface.

Namalwa KJM-1 cells were transfected with pAMo expression vector containing cDNA for 1 of 3 sialyltransferases (ST3, ST4, and GD3 synthase) or 4 fucosyltransferases (FT3, FT4, FT6, and FT7) (14–16). Transfected cells were examined for anti-6C2 reactivity by immunofluorescence and flow cytometry (Figure 6). Namalwa KJM-1 cells transfected with an empty pAMo vector showed no reactivity with anti-6C2, demonstrating the absence of the 6C2 molecule. Upon transfection with cDNA for various sialyl- or fucosyltransferases, surface expression of the 6C2 molecule was detected only with induction of GD3 synthase activity. These observations, thus, further confirmed that the cell surface structure defined by anti-6C2 is GD3.

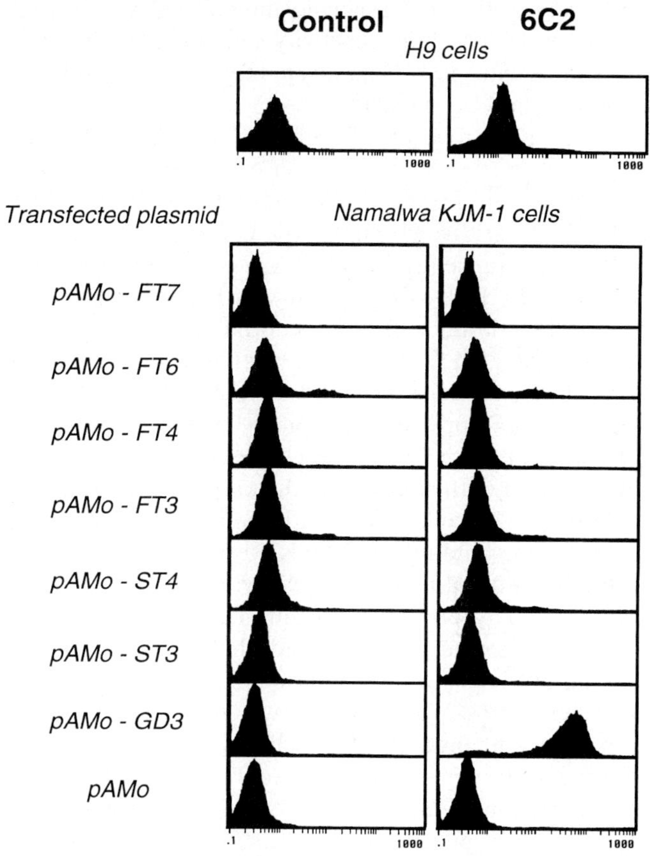

Figure 6. Induction of cell surface anti-6C2 reactivity upon transfection and expression of GD3 synthase cDNA in Namalwa KJM-1 cells. Namalwa KJM-1 cells were transfected with either an empty pAMo vector or pAMo containing cDNA for 1 of 4 fucosyltransferases (FT3, FT4, FT6, and FT7) and 3 sialyltransferases (ST3, ST4, and GD3 synthase) and examined for cell surface expression of the 6C2 molecule by immunostaining and flow cytometry. H9 cells, a human T cell line expressing the 6C2 molecule, is included as a positive control.

DISCUSSION

In the present study, we have shown that the cell surface structure recognized by a mAb, anti-6C2, is GD3, a disialoganglioside preferentially expressed on a subpopulation of T cells, and that 6C2/GD3 molecules may play a role in transendothelial migratory capacity as well as in the inflammation of RA.

In attempting to determine the precise nature of the 6C2 molecule, our present study first examined expression of the 6C2 molecule in LFA-1–deficient cells (Figure 1A). We found the presence of the 6C2 molecule in LFA-1–deficient cells as well as in LFA-1–positive cells. This finding indicates that the cell surface structure recognized by anti-6C2 appears not to be LFA-1 (CD11a/CD18), but rather a distinct molecule other than the LFA-1 complex.

In listing candidate molecules, we drew information as to the nature of the 6C2 molecule from our previous biochemical findings (7). In light of the fact that sodium dodecyl sulfate–polyacrylamide gel electrophoresis of the materials precipitated with anti-6C2 detected no molecules other than ^{125}I-labeled α and β chains of the LFA-1 complex (7), the nonproteineous nature of the 6C2 molecule was suggested. Many of the previously described, nonproteineous cell surface molecules are glycolipids and, of them, *O*-acetylated gangliosides clustered in CDw60 have been reported to be expressed on subpopulations of human T cells (10,11). Flow cytometric analysis revealed that within peripheral T cells, expression of the 6C2 molecule and CDw60 was, by and large, similar in their reactivity (Figures 1B and C), suggesting that the 6C2 molecule may be closely related to *O*-acetylated gangliosides.

A new role for T cell surface 6C2/GD3 was suggested by the results of transendothelial migration assay (Figures 3 and 4). We found that in addition to the $CD26^{bright}/CD11a^{bright}$ phenotype (17,23), peripheral T cells with transendothelial migratory capacity were largely 6C2/GD3+. Of interest was the finding that T cells tightly bound to the endothelium were mostly devoid of 6C2/GD3 expression, whereas significant fractions of these T cells were of the $CD26^{bright}/CD11a^{bright}$ phenotype (Figure 3B), indicating that 6C2/GD3+ T cells are either less adherent to the endothelium or released more efficiently from the endothelium than are 6C2/GD3− T cells. Transendothelial migration and endothelium binding of T cells were differentially affected by pretreatment of T cells with anti-6C2 (Figure 4B). Parallel experiments with anti–LFA-1 caused prominent reduction in both transendothelial migration and binding of T cells to the endothelium, suggesting different roles for 6C2/GD3 and LFA-1 in transendothelial migration and binding of T cells to the endothelium. Moreover, the removal of sialic acid residues from GD3 with neuraminidase resulted in loss of the transendothelial migratory capacity of T cells, supporting the notion that GD3 molecules play a role in transendothelial migratory activity. These observations indicate that within the multistep sequences of transendothelial migration (24), cell surface 6C2/GD3 has an important role at the step following the initial adhesion to the endothelium.

Support for the enhanced transendothelial migratory capacity of 6C2/GD3+ T cells came from the analysis of synovial fluid T cells from RA patients (Figure 2). In all 8 RA patients examined, the percentage of 6C2/GD3+ cells in CD3+ synovial fluid cells was >70%, whereas that in PBMC from both normal individuals and RA patients was <40%. $CD26^{bright}$ T cells were increased in the synovial fluid from RA patients, representing 30% of synovial T cells (25). Thus, in keeping with the present results on transendothelial migratory capacity (Figures 3 and 4), it is likely that 6C2/GD3+ T cells exhibit a greater capacity than do $CD26^{bright}$ T cells to migrate into the sites of inflammation in vivo. Alternatively, it is also likely that T cells that have either migrated in or proliferated within the synovium have been induced to express the 6C2/GD3 molecule as a result of activation within the inflamed environment.

Evidence that the 6C2 molecule is indeed distinct from, but related to, *O*-acetylated gangliosides was provided by immunoblotting on gangliosides separated by TLC (Figure 5). Among 12 species of gangliosides, including *O*-acetylated GD3, anti-6C2 was reactive only with GD3, a disialoganglioside. In parallel analyses, anti-UM4D4, a prototype anti-CDw60 mAb, reacted only with *O*-acetylated GD3, consistent with the findings in a previous report (19). Previously, we demonstrated that Namalwa KJM-1, a subline of the Burkitt's lymphoma cell line Namalwa, expresses abundant GM3, a monosialoganglioside that functions as an acceptor for GD3 synthase–catalized addition of a sialic acid to form GD3, whereas no GD3 and GD3 synthase activity are detectable (15). Upon transfection and expression of cDNAs for 3 sialyltransferases and 4 fucosyltransferases, induction of cell surface anti-6C2 reactivity occurred only with GD3 synthase (Figure 6). Reactivity of anti-6C2 with GD3 is strict, because transfection and expression of these sialyltransferases and fucosyltransferases results in induction of major cell surface structures such as the sialyl-Lewis^x determinant (14–16). Taken together, our present findings established that the cell surface structure recognized by anti-6C2 is GD3.

The presence of gangliosides on human T cells has been documented. Earlier studies have detected the expression of GD3 on 1–2% (26) or up to 15% (27) of resting human T cells and have demonstrated that anti-GD3 mAb, both IgM and $F(ab')_2$ fragments of IgG, induced proliferation of human T cells in a manner independent of accessory cells (27). It has been reported that anti–*O*-acetylated GD3 mAb are also mitogenic for T cells. Upon addition in soluble form, anti-UM4D4, specific for 9-*O*-acetyl-GD3 (10,11), and U5, specific for 7-*O*-acetyl-GD3 (19), induce a proliferative response in PBMC. Moreover, it has been reported that anti-GD3 mAb (R24) stimulation could induce T cell cytotoxicity, cytokine production, and expression of cell surface molecules, such as the interleukin-2 receptor, HLA–DR, CD11a, and CD11c, through multiple signaling pathways, in addition to T cell proliferation (28,29). Moreover, another anti-GD3 mAb (Z21) could deliver a potent costimulatory signal, and the responsiveness of T cells to stimulation via GD3 was dependent on the cell surface expression of this molecule (30).

In the present study, anti-6C2 had no mitogenic activity, in contrast with the previously described mitogenic activity of anti-GD3 mAb, including anti–O-acetyl-GD3 (anti-CDw60) mAb, which indicates that anti-6C2 recognize the different epitope structure on GD3. Recently it was reported that some mAb against

GD3 or *O*-acetyl-GD3 could not induce T cell proliferation at any concentration (31). Therefore, the mitogenic effects of anti-GD3 or anti–*O*-acetyl-GD3 mAb are not general phenomena for these families of antibodies, indicating that a certain epitope of GD3 appears to be important for these mitogenic activity of T cells. The only consequence of transfection and expression of GD3 synthase is the generation of GD3 through the addition of a sialic acid to GM3 (15). Thus, the epitope structure for anti-6C2 is most likely to be carbohydrate moieties.

The exact molecular mechanism through which the 6C2/GD3 molecule participates in transendothelial migration was not determined by the present study. The finding that transendothelial migration was inhibited by anti-6C2 pretreatment of T cells with no effect on T cell binding to the endothelium suggests that cell surface 6C2/GD3 is not involved in the initial stage of T cell adherence to endothelial cells. Thus, a possibility is raised that cell surface 6C2/GD3 may be involved in interactions with the substratum. In this regard, several lines of evidence have indicated that gangliosides play a role in cell adhesion to the substratum (32). Evidence also has been described that the gangliosides GD2 and GD3 are specifically associated with the adhesion plaques of melanoma cells (33), possibly in complex with fibronectin receptor (34).

Gangliosides are sialic acid–containing glycosphingolipids, which are present in the plasma membrane of all eukaryotic cells. They are involved in several important biologic events, such as proliferation, differentiation, signal transduction, and modulation of the immune response (35). In addition, the GD3 disialoganglioside was shown to play an important role in mediating CD95- and ceramide-induced apoptosis (36). Recently, it was reported that some glycosyltransferases are crucial for the biosynthesis of functional P-selectin ligands in Th1 CD4+ T cells which migrate into inflammatory sites through binding to P-selectin (37). In the present study, we demonstrated that the 6C2/GD3 molecule on the surface of T cells is crucial for transendothelial migration. However, the specific ligand for 6C2/GD3 remains unknown. GD3 expression induced by GD3 synthase and slight modifications of GD3, such as *O*-acetylation, could define a subpopulation of T cells with transendothelial migratory activity, which may contribute to the development of inflammatory diseases such as RA. Further studies of the structural and functional relationship of the GD3 molecule may lead to an understanding of the precise mechanism of T cell migration and the pathophysiology of RA, and to the development of rational therapies for RA.

REFERENCES

1. Morimoto C, Letvin NL, Distaso JA, Aldrich WR, Schlossman SF. The isolation and characterization of the human suppressor inducer T cell subset. J Immunol 1985;134:1508–15.
2. Morimoto C, Letvin NL, Boyd AW, Hagen M, Brown HM, Karnacki M, et al. The isolation and characterization of the human helper inducer T cell subset. J Immunol 1985;134:3762–9.
3. Tedder TF, Cooper MD, Clement LT. Human lymphocyte differentiation antigens HB-10 and HB-11. II. Differential production of B cell growth and differentiation factors by distinct helper T cell subpopulations. J Immunol 1985;134:2989–94.
4. Smith SH, Brown MH, Rowe D, Callard RE, Beverly PC. Functional subsets of human helper-inducer cells defined by a new monoclonal antibody, UCHL-1. Immunology 1986;58:63–70.
5. Moore K, Nesbitt AM. Functional heterogeneity of CD4+ T lymphocytes: two subpopulations with counteracting immunoregulatory functions identified with the monoclonal antibodies WR16 and WR19. Immunology 1987;61:159–65.
6. Kalish RS, Morimoto C, Schlossman SF. Generation of CD8 (T8) cytotoxic cells has a preferential requirement of CD4+2H4− inducer cells. Cell Immunol 1988;111:379–89.
7. Torimoto Y, Sugita K, Weinberg DS, Dang NH, Donahue C, Letvin NL, et al. Development of a monoclonal antibody, anti-6C2, which is involved in the interaction of CD4 T helper cells and activated B cells. J Immunol 1991;146:2176–84.
8. Arnett FC, Edworthy SM, Bloch DA, McShane DJ, Fries JF, Cooper NS, et al. The American Rheumatism Association 1987 revised criteria for the classification of rheumatoid arthritis. Arthritis Rheum 1988;31:315–24.
9. Sato T, Tachibana K, Nojima Y, D'Avirro N, Morimoto C. Role of the VLA-4 molecule in T cell costimulation: identification of the tyrosine phosphorylation pattern induced by the ligation of VLA-4. J Immunol 1995;155:2938–47.
10. Higgs JB, Zeldes W, Kozarsky K, Schteingart M, Kan L, Bohlke P, et al. A novel pathway of human T lymphocyte activation: identification by a monoclonal antibody generated against a rheumatoid synovial T cell line. J Immunol 1988;140:3758–65.
11. Fox DA, Millard JA, Kan L, Zeldes WS, Davis W, Higgs J, et al. Activation pathways of synovial T lymphocytes: expression and function of the UM4D4/CDw60 antigen. J Clin Invest 1990;86:1124–36.
12. Tedder TF, Schmidt RE, Rudd CE, Kornacki MM, Ritz J, Schlossman SF. Function of the LFA-1 and T4 molecules in the direct activation of resting human B lymphocytes by T lymphocytes. Eur J Immunol 1986;16:1539–43.
13. Hirabayashi Y, Fujita SC, Kon K, Ando S. Characterization of a novel Le^x-active ganglioside from chick intestinal tissues recognized by murine monoclonal antibody 188Cl. J Biol Chem 1991;266:10268–74.
14. Sasaki K, Watanabe E, Kawashima K, Sekine S, Dohi T, Oshima M, et al. Expression cloning of a novel Galβ(1-3/1-4)GlcNAc α-2,3-sialyltransferase using lectin resistance selection. J Biol Chem 1993;268:22782–7.
15. Sasaki K, Kurata K, Kojima N, Kurosawa N, Ohta S, Hanai N, et al. Expression cloning of a GM3-specific α-2,8-sialytransferase (GD3 synthase). J Biol Chem 1994;269:15950–6.
16. Sasaki K, Kurata K, Funayama K, Nagata M, Watanabe E, Ohta S, et al. Expression cloning of a novel α-1,3-fucosyltransferase that is involved in biosynthesis of the sialyl Lewis x carbohydrate determinants in leukocytes. J Biol Chem 1994;269:14730–7.
17. Masuyama J, Berman JS, Cruikshank WW, Morimoto C, Center DM. Evidence for recent as well as long term activation of T cells

migrating through endothelial cell monolayers in vitro. J Immunol 1992;148:1367–74.
18. Roth SJ, Carr MW, Springer TA. C-C chemokines, but not the C-X-C chemokines interleukin-8 and interferon-γ inducible protein-10, stimulate transendothelial chemotaxis of T lymphocytes. Eur J Immunol 1995;25:3482–8.
19. Kniep B, Claus C, Peter-Katalinic J, Monner DA, Dippold W, Nimtz M. 7-O-acetyl-GD3 in human T-lymphocytes is detected by a specific T-cell-activating monoclonal antibody. J Biol Chem 1995;270:30173–80.
20. Oppenheimer-Marks N, Davis LS, Lipsky PE. Human T lymphocyte adhesion to endothelial cells and transendothelial migration: alteration of receptor use relates to the activation status of both the T cell and the endothelial cell. J Immunol 1990;145:140–8.
21. Oppenheimer-Marks N, Davis LS, Bogue DT, Pamberg J, Lipsky PE. Differential utilization of ICAM-1 and VCAM-1 during the adhesion and transendothelial migration of human T lymphocytes. J Immunol 1991;147:2913–21.
22. Cush JJ, Pietschmann P, Oppenheimer-Marks N, Lipsky PE. The intrinsic migratory capacity of memory T cells contributes to their accumulation in rheumatoid synovium. Arthritis Rheum 1992;35: 1434–44.
23. Brezinscheck RI, Lipsky PE, Galea P, Vita R, Oppenheimer-Marks N. Phenotypic characterization of CD4+ T cells that exhibit a transendothelial migratory capacity. J Immunol 1995;154: 3062–77.
24. Springer TA. Traffic signals for lymphocyte recirculation and leukocyte emigration: the multistep paradigm. Cell 1994;76: 301–14.
25. Mizokami A, Eguchi K, Kawakami A, Ida H, Kawabe Y, Tsukada T, et al. Increased population of high fluorescence 1F7 (CD26) antigen on T cells in synovial fluid of patients with rheumatoid arthritis. J Rheumatol 1996;23:2022–6.
26. Hersey P, Schibeci SD, Townsend P, Burns C, Cheresh DA. Potentiation of lymphocyte responses by monoclonal antibodies to the ganglioside GD3. Cancer Res 1986;46:6083–90.
27. Welte K, Miller G, Chapman PB, Yuasa H, Natoli E, Kunicka JE, et al. Stimulation of T lymphocyte proliferation by monoclonal antibodies against GD3 ganglioside. J Immunol 1987;139:1763–71.
28. Norihisa Y, McVicar DW, Ghosh P, Houghton AN, Longo DL, Creekmore SP, et al. Increased proliferation, cytotoxicity, and gene expression after stimulation of human peripheral blood T lymphocytes through a surface ganglioside (GD3). J Immunol 1994;152:485–95.
29. Ortaldo JR, Mason AT, Longo DL, Beckwith M, Creekmore SP, McVicar DW. T cell activation via the disialoganglioside GD3: analysis of signal transduction. J Leukoc Biol 1996;60:533–9.
30. Schlaak JF, Claus C, Meyer zum Buschenfelde KH, Dippold W. Anti-GD3 antibodies are potent activators of human gamma/delta and alpha/beta positive T cells. Scand J Immunol 1995;41:475–80.
31. Claus C, Schlaak J, Dittmaya M, Meyer zum Buschenfelde K, Dippold W. Inhibition of anti-GD3-ganglioside antibody-induced proliferation of human CD8+ T cells by CD16+ natural killer cells. Eur J Immunol 1994;24:1208–12.
32. Kleinman HK, Martin GR, Fishman PH. Ganglioside inhibition of fibronectin-mediated cell adhesion to collagen. Proc Natl Acad Sci U S A 1979;76:3367–71.
33. Cheresh DA, Harper JR, Schulz G, Reisfeld RA. Localization of the gangliosides GD2 and GD3 in adhesion plaques and on the surface of human melanoma cells. Proc Natl Acad Sci U S A 1984;81:5767–71.
34. Cheresh DA, Pytela R, Pierschbacher MD, Klier FG, Ruoslahti E, Reisfeld RA. An Arg-Gly-Asp-directed receptor on the surface of human melanoma cells exist in a divalent cation-dependent functional complex with the disialoganglioside GD2. J Cell Biol 1987;105:1163–73.
35. Hakomori S, Yamamura S, Handa AK. Signal transduction through glyco(sphingo)lipids: introduction and recent studies on glyco(sphingo)lipid-enriched microdomains. Ann N Y Acad Sci 1998;845:1–10.
36. De Maria R, Lenti L, Malisan F, d'Agostino F, Tomassini B, Zeuner A, et al. Requirement for GD3 ganglioside in CD95- and ceramide-induced apoptosis. Science 1997;277:1652–5.
37. Blander JM, Visintin I, Janeway CA Jr, Medzhitov R. Alpha(1,3)-fucosyltransferase VII and alpha(2,3)-sialytransferase IV are upregulated in activated CD4 T cells and maintained after their differentiation into Th1 and migration into inflammatory sites. J Immunol 1999;163:3746–52.

ARTHRITIS & RHEUMATISM
Vol. 44, No. 2, February 2001, pp 307–314

Rheumatoid Arthritis in Southern Spain

Toward Elucidation of a Unifying Role of the HLA Class II Region in Disease Predisposition

M. Pascual,[1] A. Nieto,[1] M. A. López-Nevot,[2] L. Ramal,[2] L. Matarán,[2] A. Caballero,[3] A. Alonso,[3] J. Martín,[1] and E. Zanelli[4]

Objective. **To evaluate the contributions of HLA–DQ and –DR polymorphisms to susceptibility to rheumatoid arthritis (RA) in a population in southern Spain, and to compare the value of the shared epitope (SE) and RA protection (RAP) models in accounting for the HLA class II region's contribution to RA predisposition.**

Methods. **One hundred sixty RA patients and 153 healthy controls were typed for HLA–DRB1 and –DQB1 using high-resolution DNA techniques. Distributions of predisposing DRB1 alleles in patients and control subjects according to the SE model were compared with distributions of predisposing DQ and protective DERAA-positive DRB1 alleles according to the RAP model.**

Results. **DQ3 (DQB1*03 and *04 combined with DQA1*03) and DQ5 (DQB1*0501/DQA1*0101) alleles predisposed individuals to RA independently of SE-positive DRB1 alleles. DQ3/3-homozygous individuals had the strongest risk of developing RA. DQ3 molecules predisposed to RA more than did DQ5 molecules. The weaker predisposition mediated by DQ5 included the DRB1*1001-carrying haplotype; no DRB1*1001-homozygous patients were observed. DRB1*0401 played a unique role in the contribution of DQ3–DR4 haplotypes to RA, in spite of its low frequency in southern Spain.**

Conclusion. **The low prevalences of RA and of mild disease observed in Spain, and in southern Europe in general, can be explained in great part by the low frequency of DQ3–DR4 haplotypes, especially those carrying DRB1*0401. However, the overall distribution of HLA–DQ and –DR alleles in RA patients compared with control subjects is similar to that in other European and North American populations. A model involving both DQ and DR can best account for the contribution of HLA to RA.**

Supported by grants SAF97-0046 and SAF00-213 from Plan Nacional de I+D (CICYT) and Plan Andaluz de Investigación (grupo CTS-180).

[1]M. Pascual, PhD, A. Nieto, MD, PhD, J. Martín, MD, PhD: Instituto de Parasitología y Biomedicina "López-Neyra," CSIC, Granada, Spain; [2]M. A. López-Nevot, MD, PhD, L. Ramal, PhD, L. Matarán, MD: Hospital Virgen de las Nieves, Granada, Spain; [3]A. Caballero, MD, PhD, A. Alonso, MD, PhD: Hospital Carlos Haya, Málaga, Spain; [4]E. Zanelli, PhD: Leiden University Medical Center, Leiden, The Netherlands.

Address correspondence and reprint requests to J. Martín, MD, PhD, Instituto de Parasitología y Biomedicina "López-Neyra," CSIC, C/ Ventanilla n° 11, 18001 Granada, Spain.

Submitted for publication May 31, 2000; accepted in revised form September 27, 2000.

Rheumatoid arthritis (RA) is a common human autoimmune disease of unknown etiology and poorly understood pathophysiology. Population and family studies have established the important contribution of genetic factors to RA susceptibility and disease progression (1). The most thoroughly examined and well-documented genes associated with predisposition to RA are contained within the HLA class II region (2). Stastny initially reported a significant increase in the DR4–Dw4 specificity among RA patients (3). Later, the DR1 specificity was associated with RA in Mediterranean and Indian populations (4–6), and the DR4–Dw15 specificity was associated with RA in Japanese and Chinese (7,8). After DNA sequencing became available, it was pointed out that DR1 and DR4 alleles associated with RA, i.e., DRB1*0101, *0401, *0404, and *0405, share a common amino acid sequence in their third hypervariable region (HVR3), i.e., $Q^{70}(K/R)RAA^{74}$. This observation led to the "shared epitope" (SE) hypothesis (9). More recently, this motif has been extended to RRRAA to explain the association of DR10 (DRB1*1001) with RA in populations such as the Spanish population (10).

The apparent, but not significant, association of the DRB1*1402 allele, encoding a QRRAA motif, with RA in American Indians has also been regarded as supporting the SE model (11).

Collagen-induced arthritis (CIA) is an accepted experimental model of arthritis that resembles RA. In mice, the H2-Ab and H2-Aa loci (equivalent to DQB1 and DQA1 in humans) control predisposition to CIA, and H2-Eb (equivalent to DR in humans) confers protection (12). A correlation exists between H2-Eb–mediated protection and immunogenicity of peptides derived from the HVR3 region of protective H2-Eβ alleles (13). On the basis of these findings, a novel hypothesis to explain the association of certain HLA haplotypes with RA has been proposed (14). The rheumatoid arthritis protection (RAP) model stresses the importance of both DQ and DR alleles on both chromosomes in disease predisposition. In this model, DQB1 and DQA1 loci confer predisposition, while DRB1 modulates it. Similar to the effect of H2-Eβ peptides on mouse CIA, protection by some DRB1 alleles is mediated through peptides derived from their HVR3 region and binding to predisposing DQ molecules (13).

In the RAP model, the predisposing alleles (DQ^{RA}) are DQB1*0301, *0302, *0303, *0304, *0305, *0401, and *0402 combined with DQA1*0301 (or *0302), but not with *0501; and DQB1*0501 combined with DQA1*0101 (or *0104). The former alleles are linked to DR4 and DR9 and the latter to DR1 and DR10. The most efficient protective DRB1 alleles are referred to as DERAA-positive (DERAA+) because of the amino acid motif found in their HVR3 region; typically, these alleles are DRB1*0103, *0402, *1102, *1103, *1301, and *1302. In support of the model, DQ8 (DQB1*0302/DQA1*0301) transgenic mice are predisposed to severe CIA (15). DRB1 peptides containing the motif DERAA are highly immunogenic in DQ8 mice (16) and interfere with disease incidence and severity in DQ8 transgenic animals (17). Recently, the value of this model was demonstrated in a cross-sectional study involving Dutch and Swiss RA patients and control subjects and in a study involving RA patients from an early arthritis clinic in Leiden, The Netherlands (14,18).

A better understanding of the contribution of HLA to RA requires studies of populations from diverse parts of the world. A few investigators have indicated that RA has less severe characteristics in southern Europe, i.e., Spain (19), Italy (20), Greece (21), and southern France (22), than in northern European countries. The low frequency of DR4, especially DRB1*0401, in these populations has been suggested as an explanation for this mild arthritis (10,20,22,23). Granada is a city in southern Spain that was under Arab rule for more than 7 centuries. As a result of its rich history, the population of Granada is a complex admixture of European, North African, Asian, and Jewish populations. Comparing SE and RAP models in this population represents a unique opportunity to better evaluate the role of the HLA class II region in RA predisposition and to establish common rules applicable to every population.

PATIENTS AND METHODS

Patients and control subjects. The present study included 160 Spanish RA patients and 153 healthy voluntary blood donors from the same geographic origin. Patients were visiting the Rheumatology Department of the Virgen de las Nieves University Hospital in Granada, Spain, and were diagnosed according to the revised criteria of the American College of Rheumatology (formerly, the American Rheumatism Association) (24).

Eighty-three percent of the patients were women. Mean ± SD age at onset and disease duration were 49.7 ± 2.9 and 9.3 ± 5.1 years, respectively. Eighty percent of the patients were positive for rheumatoid factor. The mean ± SD joint erosion score was 4.2 ± 4.0 (joint erosion was measured by the number of eroded joints of hands, up to a total of 11 joints/hand). Disease-related surgery was performed on 10.7% of the patients, and 9.6% of them presented with extraarticular manifestations.

HLA typing. DRB1 and DQB1 typings were done by reverse hybridization with sequence-specific oligonucleotides (Inno-Lipa HLA–DQB and –DRB; Innogenetics, Zwijndrecht, Belgium). DRB1*04, DRB1*11, and DRB1*13 subtypings were performed with sequence-specific primers (Dynal, Oslo, Norway). DQA1 typing was deduced from DQB1 and DRB1 typing on the basis of the strong linkage disequilibrium among HLA class II alleles. Although segregation analysis data were not available, DQB1–DQA1–DRB1 haplotypes were deduced from individual HLA typings on the basis of well-established linkage disequilibrium among alleles within the 3 loci.

Statistical analysis. Statistical analysis was performed by chi-square test or Fisher's exact test, as appropriate. P values less than 0.05 were considered significant. Odds ratios (OR) and 95% confidence intervals were calculated according to Woolf's method or Haldane's modification. Stepwise regression analysis was performed using the software package SPSS 9.0 for Windows (SPSS, Chicago, IL).

RESULTS

Heterogeneity of Granada's population reflected by observed HLA haplotypes. All the HLA class II haplotypes observed in our groups of patients and control subjects and encoding an SE+ DRB1 allele, a DERAA+ DRB1 allele, or an RA-predisposing DQ antigen are listed in Table 1. Their frequencies in patients and control subjects are shown in Table 2.

Although some DQ–DR combinations were rare, all the deduced DQB1–DQA1–DRB1 haplotypes had been previously reported in publications and at HLA International Workshops. Although the overall HLA antigen distribution of Granada's population fell within the Caucasian diversity range, both Table 1 and Table 2 highlight this population's great heterogeneity, which reflects Andalusia's history. The Mediterranean, African, and Asian influences were apparent from HLA haplotypes such as DQB1*0302–DQA1*0301–DRB1*0402, DQB1*0501–DQA1*0101–DRB1*0102, and DQB1*0302–DQA1*0301–DRB1*0405. Another "Asian" haplotype, not listed in the tables but found quite frequently, was DQB1*0601–DQA1*0103–DRB1*1502 (25). Such a large variety of haplotypes has previously been described in other populations, such as the Jewish population (26). A higher frequency of the DQB1*0501–DQA1*0104–DRB1*1001 haplotype was found than had previously been reported in Jews and Algerians (26).

As an indirect consequence of the HLA heterogeneity, no DQB1–DQA1–DRB1 haplotypes were significantly associated with RA (Table 2). The haplotype DQB1*0303–DQA1*0301–DRB1*0901 was in 5 patients but in no control subjects (OR 10.68). Only the increased presence of the haplotype DQB1*0302–DQA1*0301(2)–DRB1*0401 in patients was close to being significant, in spite of this haplotype's very low frequency (OR 3.71). It was therefore of particular interest to investigate which model, SE or RAP, could best account for the contribution of HLA to RA predisposition in this population.

Table 1. Presence of the shared epitope (SE), proposed rheumatoid arthritis (RA)–predisposing DQ antigens, and DERAA motif in DQ–DR haplotypes observed in the present study

DQB1*	DQA1*	DRB1*	SE*	DQ^{RA}†	DERAA‡
0301(2/3/5)	0301(2)	0401(4/5/8/9/10)	+	DQ3	–
0402	0301(2)	0401	+	DQ3	–
0301(2/4)	0301(2)	0402	–	DQ3	+
0301(2)	0301(2)	0403(6/7)	–	DQ3	–
0402	0301(2)	0403	–	DQ3	–
0303	0301	0901	–	DQ3	–
0501	0101	0101(2/4)	+	DQ5	–
0501	0104	1001	+	DQ5	–
0501	0104	1401	–	DQ5	–
0501	0101	1502	–	DQ5	–
0501	0101	0103	–	DQ5	+
0503	0101	0101	+	–	–
0504	0102	0101	+	–	–
0202	0301(2)	0401	+	–	–
0202	0301(2)	0405	+	–	–
0607	0301(2)	0408	+	–	–
0301	0501	1102(3)	–	–	+
0201	0101	1301	–	–	+
0602(3/7)	0103	1301	–	–	+
0501	0102	1302	–	–	+
0603(4/5/6/7/9)	0102	1302	–	–	+
0503	0104	1416	–	–	+
Other			–	–	–

* SE+ alleles are DRB1*0101, *0102, *0104, *0401, *0404, *0405, *0408, *0409, *0410, and *1001.
† RA-predisposing DQ antigen (DQ^{RA}) molecules include DQ3 (encoded by DQB1*0301, *0302, *0303, *0304, *0305, or *0402 combined with DQA1*0301 [or *0302], but not with *0501) and DQ5 (encoded by DQB1*0501 combined with DQA1*0101 or *0104).
‡ Protective DRB1 alleles have a DERAA motif in their third hypervariable region and include DRB1*0103, *0402, *1102, *1103, *1301, *1302, and *1416 in the present study.

Table 2. Frequencies of haplotypes encoding a DQ^{RA} molecule, a shared epitope, or a DERAA motif in rheumatoid arthritis (RA) patients and control subjects*

DQB1*	DQA1*	DRB1*	RA patients (2n = 320), no. (%)	Control subjects (2n = 306), no. (%)	OR (95% CI)
0303	0301	0901	5 (1.6)	0 (0.0)	10.68 (0.58–194.10)
0302	0301(2)	0401	9 (2.8)	2 (0.7)	3.71 (0.91–15.09)
0302	0301(2)	0402	10 (3.1)	5 (1.6)	1.85 (0.65–5.26)
0302	0301(2)	0405	6 (1.9)	3 (1.0)	1.79 (0.48–6.63)
0301	0501	1102	6 (1.9)	3 (1.0)	1.79 (0.48–6.63)
0501	0101	1001	16 (5.0)	9 (2.9)	1.70 (0.75–3.83)
0302	0301(2)	0404	24 (7.5)	14 (4.6)	1.67 (0.85–3.25)
0501	0101	0103	5 (1.6)	3 (1.0)	1.51 (0.39–5.83)
0501	0101	0102	19 (5.9)	13 (4.2)	1.41 (0.69–2.87)
0301	0301(2)	0401	7 (2.2)	5 (1.6)	1.31 (0.43–3.98)
0501	0101	0101	27 (8.4)	25 (8.2)	1.03 (0.59–1.82)
0600	0103	1301	7 (2.2)	8 (2.6)	0.84 (0.31–2.27)
0302	0301(2)	0403	5 (1.6)	6 (2.0)	0.80 (0.26–2.54)
0600	0102	1302	3 (0.9)	10 (3.3)	0.31 (0.09–1.06)
0202	0301(2)	0401	0 (0.0)	1 (0.3)	–
0305	0301(2)	0401	1 (0.3)	0 (0.0)	–
0402	0301(2)	0401	1 (0.3)	0 (0.0)	–
0304	0301(2)	0402	2 (0.6)	0 (0.0)	–
0301	0301(2)	0403	2 (0.6)	0 (0.0)	–
0402	0301(2)	0403	0 (0.0)	1 (0.3)	–
0301	0301(2)	0404	2 (0.6)	0 (0.0)	–
0202	0301(2)	0405	0 (0.0)	1 (0.3)	–
0301	0301(2)	0407	0 (0.0)	2 (0.7)	–
0301	0301(2)	0408	1 (0.3)	0 (0.0)	–
0302	0301(2)	0408	2 (0.6)	0 (0.0)	–
0607	0301(2)	0408	0 (0.0)	1 (0.3)	–
0302	0301(2)	0409	1 (0.3)	0 (0.0)	–
0301	0301(2)	0410	1 (0.3)	0 (0.0)	–
0303	0301(2)	0410	1 (0.3)	0 (0.0)	–
0503	0101	0101	0 (0.0)	1 (0.3)	–
0504	0102	0101	1 (0.3)	0 (0.0)	–
0501	0101	0104	1 (0.3)	0 (0.0)	–
0301	0501	1103	1 (0.3)	2 (0.7)	–
0201	0101	1301	1 (0.3)	0 (0.0)	–
0501	0102	1302	0 (0.0)	1 (0.3)	–
0501	0104	1401	1 (0.3)	0 (0.0)	–
0503	0104	1416	1 (0.3)	0 (0.0)	–
0501	0101	1502	1 (0.3)	0 (0.0)	–
Other	–	–	150 (46.9)	190 (62.1)	–

* DQ^{RA} molecule = RA-predisposing DQ antigen molecule; OR = odds ratio; 95% CI = 95% confidence interval.

Table 3. Contribution of DQ3 and DR4 to RA susceptibility*

	RA patients (n = 160), no. (%)	Control subjects (n = 153), no. (%)	OR (95% CI)	*P*
DQ3+	67 (41.9)	36 (23.5)	2.32 (1.42–3.78)	0.0006
DR4 SE+	47 (29.4)	26 (17.0)	2.01 (1.17–3.45)	0.01
DRB1*0401+	16 (10.0)	8 (5.2)	1.95 (0.82–4.62)	NS
DR4 SE+ (0401−)	31 (19.4)	18 (11.8)	1.78 (0.95–3.33)	NS
DRB1*0403(6/7)+	16 (10.0)	12 (7.8)	1.29 (0.59–2.80)	NS
DRB1*0901+	5 (3.1)	0 (0.0)	10.85 (0.59–198.1)	0.03

* Predisposing DQ3 is DQB1*0301, *0302, *0303, *0304, *0305, and *0402 combined with DQA1*0301 or *0302. DR4 shared epitope (SE)–positive alleles are *0401, *0404, *0405, *0408, and *0409. NS = not significant (see Table 2 for other definitions).

DQ3 versus DR4. In the SE model, certain DRB1*04 alleles predispose to RA. In the RAP model, "DQ3" alleles in linkage disequilibrium with both SE+ and SE− DRB1*04 alleles accounted best for the association of the DQ3–DR4 haplotypes with RA (Table 1). DQ3 was also in linkage disequilibrium with SE− DRB1*0901. Table 3 shows that 41.9% of RA patients carried a DQ3 allele, while only 29.4% of RA patients carried a DR4 SE+ allele. Consequently, the association of DQ3 with RA was stronger than the respective association of DR4 SE ($P = 0.0006$ versus $P = 0.01$). SE− DRB1*0403(6/7) alleles did not predispose to RA less than DR4 SE+ alleles. Five patients versus no control subjects carried an SE− DQ3–DRB1*0901 haplotype (OR 10.85, $P = 0.03$). Two-by-four tables analyses using the method of Svejgaard and Ryder (27) showed that DR4 SE+ alleles were not increased in patients versus control subjects among DQ3-positive individuals (OR 1.18) (Table 4). Conversely, the association of DQ3 with RA in the absence of DR4 SE was almost significant (OR 2.02, $P = 0.06$). Of note, 3 control subjects, but no patients, expressed an SE+ DRB1*04 allele without a DQ3 molecule (2 with a DQB1*0202 allele and 1 with a DQB1*0607 allele) (Table 2). We concluded that DQ3 predisposed to RA more than did DR4 SE in southern Spain.

DQ5 versus DR1 and DR10. Similar analyses were then performed for DQ5, DR1, and DR10, since DQ5 (DQB1*0501/DQA1*0101[4]) is in linkage disequilibrium with DR1 and DR10. Of note, DRB1*0101 and DRB1*1001 differ at 11 amino acid positions in the first domain while in linkage disequilibrium with identical DQ5 alleles (DQA1*0101 and *0104 differ from each other only at position 2, which does not affect the antigen-binding groove). All 4 alleles (DQ5, DRB1*0101, DRB1*0102, and DRB1*1001) tended to be increased in patients versus control subjects, but none of these increases was significant (Table 5). DR10, which has previously been associated with RA in Spain (5,10), was indeed observed in 10.0% of the patients; however, this increase did not reach significance. Not surprisingly, 2 × 4 tables analyses failed to show any preferential association between RA and DQ or DR (Table 6). However, it should be noted that, similar to the case of DQ3 versus DR4 SE, DQ5 tended to predispose to RA in the absence of DR1 and DR10 SE (6 patients versus 3 control subjects),

Table 4. Predisposition to RA by DQ3 independently of DR4 SE*

	RA patients (n = 160), no. (%)	Control subjects (n = 153), no. (%)	OR (95% CI)	*P*
DQ3+, DR4 SE+	47 (29.4)	24 (15.7)	1.18 (0.50–2.79)	NS
DQ3+, DR4 SE−	20 (12.5)	12 (7.8)		
DQ3+, DR4 SE−	20 (12.5)	12 (7.8)	2.02 (0.95–4.31)	0.06
DQ3−, DR4 SE−	93 (58.1)	115 (75.2)		

* DR4 shared epitope (SE)–negative alleles are *0402, *0403, *0406, *0407, and *0901. See Tables 2 and 3 for other definitions and explanations.

Table 5. Contribution of DQ5, DR1, and DR10 to RA susceptibility*

	RA patients (n = 160), no. (%)	Control subjects (n = 153), no. (%)	OR (95% CI)	*P*
DQ5+	63 (39.4)	45 (29.4)	1.55 (0.97–2.49)	NS
DR1 SE+	46 (28.8)	36 (23.5)	1.31 (0.78–2.17)	NS
DR10 SE+	16 (10.0)	9 (5.9)	1.74 (0.75–3.99)	NS

* Predisposing DQ5 is DQB1*0501 combined with DQA1*0101 or *0104. DR1 SE+ alleles are *0101, *0102, and *0104. DR10 SE+ is DRB1*1001. See Tables 2 and 3 for definitions.

Table 6. Tendency of DQ5 to predispose to RA independently of DR1 SE and DR10 SE*

	RA patients (n = 160), no. (%)	Control subjects (n = 153), no. (%)	OR (95% CI)	*P*
DQ5+, DR1(10) SE+	57 (35.6)	42 (27.5)	0.72 (0.18–2.83)	NS
DQ5+, DR1(10) SE−	6 (3.8)	3 (2.0)		
DQ5+, DR1(10) SE−	6 (3.8)	3 (2.0)	2.06 (0.54–7.81)	NS
DQ5−, DR1(10) SE−	96 (60.0)	107 (70.0)		

* DR1(10) shared epitope (SE)–negative alleles are *0103 and *1502. NS = not significant (see Table 2 for other definitions and Table 5 for explanations).

Table 7. Respective contributions of DQ3, DQ5, DR4, and DR1(10) to RA in southern Spain*

	RA patients (n = 160), no. (%)	Control subjects (n = 153), no. (%)	OR (95% CI)†	*P*
DQ3/3	14 (8.8)	3 (2.0)	7.48 (2.20–25.44)	0.0004
DQ3/3 (DRB1*0401−)	5 (3.1)	3 (2.0)	2.84 (0.70–11.39)	NS
DQ3/5	13 (8.1)	6 (3.9)	3.75 (1.37–10.26)	0.008
DQ5/5	9 (5.6)	5 (3.3)	3.11 (1.02–9.50)	0.04
DQ3/x	40 (25.0)	27 (17.6)	2.66 (1.44–4.90)	0.002
DQ5/x	41 (25.6)	34 (22.2)	2.17 (1.21–3.90)	0.009
DQx/x	43 (26.9)	78 (51.0)	1.00	
DR4 SE/DR4 SE	9 (5.6)	1 (0.7)	8.55 (1.48–49.32)	0.006
DR4 SE/DR4 SE (DRB*0401−)	1 (0.6)	1 (0.7)	1.35 (0.13–13.89)	NS
DR1(10) SE/DR4 SE	10 (6.3)	4 (2.6)	3.15 (0.99–9.96)	0.05
DR1(10) SE/DR1(10) SE	8 (5.0)	5 (3.3)	2.09 (0.68–6.40)	NS
DR4 SE/x	28 (17.5)	21 (13.7)	1.79 (0.94–3.42)	NS
DR1(10) SE/x	40 (25.0)	34 (22.2)	1.59 (0.91–2.77)	NS
DRx/x	65 (40.6)	88 (57.5)	1.00	

* See Tables 1–3 and 5 for definitions and explanations.
† OR were calculated by assigning an arbitrary value of 1.00 to the ratios of the numbers of patients and control subjects carrying no predisposing alleles, i.e., DQx/x or DRx/x, where x refers to any DQ or DR alleles other than the ones listed.

while the reciprocal was not true (1 patient and 1 control subject carried DRB1*0101 without DQ5) (Table 2). In concordance with the findings of many studies, we concluded that DQ5, DR1 SE, and DR10 predisposed to RA in southern Spain less than did DQ3 and DR4.

Respective contributions of DQ3, DQ5, DR4, and DR1(10) to RA. Patients and control subjects were then divided according to their number of copies of DQ3 and DQ5 or DR4 and DR1(10) in the RAP or SE model, respectively (Table 7). DQ3/3 homozygotes had the highest risk of developing RA (OR 7.48) and tended to be more predisposed than DQ3-heterozygous (DQ3/x) individuals (OR 2.66). The same was not true for DQ5/5 versus DQ5/x individuals (OR 3.11 versus 2.17). These observations were very consistent with those of previous studies in the Swiss and Dutch populations (14,18). DR4 SE homozygotes were highly predisposed to RA (OR 8.55). However, this association was mostly due to DRB1*0401; 8 of the 9 DR4 SE–homozygous patients were DRB1*0401-positive. Of note, 5 DQ3/3-homozygous patients were DRB1*0401-negative versus only 1 DR4 SE homozygote (OR 2.84 versus 1.35).

Consistent with our analyses shown in Tables 3–6, the *P* values showed that looking at DQ provided a better risk assessment than looking at DR among individuals with different HLA genotypes. To specifically address this issue, a stepwise logistic regression analysis was performed (Table 8). The dependent variable was RA diagnosis, and the tested parameters were DQ3, DQ5, DR4 SE, DR1 SE, and DR10 SE. Clearly, DQ3 predisposed to RA independently of DQ5 in southern Spain, and DQ3 predisposed to RA more than did DQ5 ($P = 0.000023$ for DQ3, $P = 0.002921$ for DQ5) (Table 8). Moreover, there were no significant additive values of DR4 SE, DR1 SE, DR10 SE, or DRB1*0401 to this predisposition.

Mild disease in southern Spain. The increases of DQ3 and DQ5 in the absence of SE+ alleles were due in part to haplotypes that carried DRB1*0103 and *0402 alleles. These alleles are SE−, but also DERAA+. According to the RAP model, they should be protective, especially among DQ5-positive individuals. Indeed, and consistent with our group's previous observations in Swiss and Dutch populations (14,18), 4 of 31 control subjects (13%) and 2 of 33 patients (6%) with 1 copy of predisposing DQ5–DR1 or DQ5–DR10 haplotype carried a protective DRB1*1301 or *1302 allele. Conversely, 5 and 12 patients carried DRB1*0103 or *0402 compared with 3 and 5 control subjects, respectively (Table 2). This apparent failure to observe a protective effect of DRB1*0103 and *0402 could tentatively be explained by

Table 8. Stepwise logistic regression analysis showing the contribution of DQ3 and DQ5 to susceptibility to rheumatoid arthritis*

	Coefficient	Standard error	*P*
Constant	−0.5609	0.1753	
DQ3	0.9534	0.2218	0.000023
DQ5	0.6452	0.2151	0.002921

* DR4 SE, DR1 SE, and DR10 SE were excluded by regression analysis. See Tables 1, 3, and 5 for definitions and explanations.

Table 9. Clinical and demographic parameters by HLA genotype in patients with rheumatoid arthritis*

	Total	DR4/4	DR4/x	DQ3/3	DQ3/x	DQx/x
Age at onset, years	49.7 ± 12.9	47.6 ± 11.3	49.9 ± 13.7	49.0 ± 11.3	50.2 ± 12.1	50.4 ± 15.1
Disease duration, years	9.3 ± 5.1	14.2 ± 8.9	9.7 ± 5.5	13.4 ± 8.6	10.0 ± 5.3	7.4 ± 3.4
RF positivity, %	80.0	87.5	86.8	88.8	83.3	74.5
No. of erosions	4.2 ± 4.0	6.3 ± 5.9	4.4 ± 3.6	6.3 ± 6.0	4.4 ± 3.4	3.4 ± 3.7
Patients undergoing surgery, %	10.7	28.6	12.1	28.6	11.4	4.4

* Except where otherwise indicated, values are the mean ± SD. The letter x refers to any DQ or DR alleles other than the ones listed. RF = rheumatoid factor (see Table 3 for explanations).

the relatively mild disease generally observed among the RA patients from Granada (see Discussion).

Table 9 shows the demographic and clinical characteristics of RA patients according to their HLA genotypes. Overall, the less severe arthritis observed in Granada was evidenced by the low percentage of extraarticular disease manifestations (9.6%), i.e., nodules, vasculitis, pulmonary infarction, Felty's syndrome, and sicca syndrome. This value compares with 80.3% observed in similar, previously published studies (28). Similarly, only 10.7% of the patients had undergone surgery related to their arthritis. Interestingly, DR4/4 or DQ3/3 homozygotes had the highest erosion score (6.3) and the highest percentage of surgery (28.6%), while only 4.4% of the DQx/x patients had undergone disease-related surgery (Table 9).

DISCUSSION

In the present study, we investigated the distributions of HLA–DQ and –DR alleles in RA patients and control subjects from Granada, Spain, a city with a particularly heterogeneous population. We compared the value of the SE and RAP models in accounting for the contribution of the HLA class II region to RA predisposition. Our results indicated that 1) DQ3 and DQ5 are the primary loci associated with RA; 2) DQ3/3 individuals have the highest risk of developing RA (OR 7.48); 3) DQ5 predisposes to RA less than DQ3, even in individuals who carry the DRB1*1001 allele; and 4) DRB1*0401 makes a particular contribution to RA, even in populations in which it is relatively rare. From our analysis, a few rules applicable to every population can be drawn.

HLA–DQ predisposes to RA. HLA–DQ3 and –DQ5 can indeed predispose to RA in the absence of SE+ DRB1 alleles. In the present study, this was mostly due to the increased frequencies of haplotypes DQB1*0303–DQA1*0301–DRB1*0901, DQB1*0302–DQA1*0301–DRB1*0402, and DQB1*0501–DQA1*0101–DRB1*0103 in RA patients compared with control subjects (Tables 2, 4, and 6). The association of DRB1*0901 with RA has already been observed in Singapore (8), Japan (29), and Chile (30). Moreover, 5 patients and no control subjects were homozygous for DQ^{RA} alleles and SE heterozygous (data not shown). Very similar observations have been made in previous studies of Swiss and Dutch RA patients (14,18). The role of HLA–DQ in RA was also stressed by the finding of 3 control subjects and no patients carrying an SE+ DRB1*04 allele without a DQ3 molecule (Table 2). It should be mentioned that, very similarly, the DQB1*0302–DQA1*0301–DRB1*0405 haplotype, but not the DQB1*0202–DQA1*0301–DRB1*0405 haplotype, predisposes to RA in Greece (31).

DQ3 predisposes to RA more than does DQ5. Many studies have pointed out that SE+ DR4 alleles predispose to RA more than do SE+ DR1 alleles (32). This observation is difficult to explain with the SE model, since DRB1*0101, *0102, *0404, *0405, and *0408 share an identical QRRAA motif. On the other hand, our group's present and previous studies (14,18) show that this difference in strength of association can easily be explained by the different DQ alleles in linkage disequilibrium with DR1 and DR4, i.e., DQ5 and DQ3 (Table 8). The stronger predisposing effect of DQ3 compared with that of DQ5 is also seen in its gene dosage effect. DQ3/3 homozygotes have a stronger risk of developing RA than DQ5/5 homozygotes (Table 7). Observations in Dutch and Swiss populations were very similar (14,18). Likewise, DR9/9 homozygotes (i.e., DQ3/3 homozygotes), but not DR9/x individuals, are predisposed to RA in Japan (29). In accordance with the weaker predisposing effect of DQ5, DQ5–DR10/x Spanish individuals only tended to be predisposed to RA in the present study, and not a single RA patient was DR10/10 homozygous. The weaker contribution of DQ5 to RA compared with that of DQ3 is therefore independent of its linkage to DRB1*0101, *0102, *0103, *1001, or *1401, and also independent of the relative frequencies of DQ3 and DQ5 in the populations studied (Tables 2, 5, and 6).

The dichotomy between DQ5 and DQ3 can therefore provide a simple explanation of the weak association of DR1 and DR10 haplotypes with mild RA contrasting with the strong association of DR4-related haplotypes with severe RA. The grouping term "DQ3" is not precisely correct if one is referring to serologic typing, since it includes DQ molecules encoded by both DQB1*03 and DQB1*04 alleles. However, the term does serve to emphasize that all these RA-predisposing molecules have a common DQα1*03 chain. In genetic terms, and in the absence of a molecular basis for explaining the association of HLA class II with RA, one might simply propose that a unique regulation of expression of DQA1*03 is related to the disease process (33). In immunologic terms, one might argue that the different DQ molecules grouped under the term DQ3 might be similar enough, despite being encoded by different DQB1 alleles, to present common autoantigenic determinants recognized by T cells involved in the pathogenesis of RA. In this regard, investigators in our group have isolated highly specific, human T cell clones that are specific for the "protective," DRβ1-derived peptide LEDERAAVD when presented by either DQ8 (DQB1*0302/DQA1*0301) or DQ7 (DQB1*0301/DQA1*0301) (Snijders A: unpublished observations).

DRB1*04 alleles carrying the motif QKRAA have a particular role in RA predisposition. From the original study by Stastny (3), it is clear that the particular allele DRB1*0401 plays a great part in the described influence of SE+ DRB1 alleles in RA. It is by far the most common DRB1*04 allele in North American and northern European populations. Besides the well-established role of the DQB1*0401–DQA1*0302–DRB1*0405 haplotype in RA susceptibility in Asians (7,34), the low frequency of the particular allele DRB1*0401 probably accounts in part for the difficulty of confirming the contribution of SE+ DRB1 alleles to RA in some populations (10,20,22,23). Likewise, in the present study, we have observed this allele only 18 times in patients (5.6% of 320 observed DRB1 alleles) and 8 times in control subjects (Table 2). However, 8 of 9 DR4/4 RA patients were DRB1*0401 positive, and these patients, along with DQ3/3 RA patients, had the highest erosion scores and the highest percentage of disease-related surgery (Table 9).

In accordance with findings of studies by others (35), these observations suggest a particular role for DRB1*04 alleles with the motif QKRAA in RA susceptibility and severity. However, the present study suggests that their role is additive and restricted to DR4/4 (i.e., DQ3/3) homozygotes. One attractive explanation would be the capacity of the QKRAA motif to bind 70-kd heat-shock proteins coupled with its influence on the intracellular trafficking of the DRB1*0401 molecule (36). Of note, the tendency of the DQ5–DRB1*1001 haplotype to predispose to RA more than the DQ5–DRB1*01 haplotypes could also be explained by the same mechanism (Table 5). Indeed, DRB1*0401 and DRB1*1001 are the only alleles reported so far to have this binding property (36).

DERAA+ DRB1 alleles interfere with RA severity. DRB1 alleles carrying the motif DERAA could protect DQ5-positive individuals against RA in Swiss and Dutch populations (14,18). DRB1*1301 and *1302 alleles accounted for most of these observations. Unfortunately, these alleles are rare in Granada; consequently, only 2 patients and 4 control subjects expressed a DQ5 molecule along with DRB1*1301 or *1302 encoded by the second chromosome. The surprise came from the lack of similar protection provided by DRB1*0103 and *0402. This observation is inconsistent with both our model and the SE model. Recently, investigators in our group have found that the effect of DERAA+ DRB1 alleles on the course of early RA is best observed in both DQ3- and DQ5-positive patients (Vos K: unpublished observations). We would like to think that the previously reported protective effect of DERAA+ DRB1 alleles against RA in DQ5-positive individuals was highlighted by the generally more severe disease observed among Dutch patients. In contrast, the mild disease observed among patients in Granada tends to dilute the apparent effect of DERAA+ alleles.

In conclusion, we have evaluated the respective roles of HLA–DQ and –DR in predisposing individuals to RA in a complex, heterogeneous population in which DR4 SE alleles are not as frequent as in other Occidental populations. Our results are consistent with a model in which both DQ and DR influence disease susceptibility. DQ3 (DQB1*03 and *04 combined with DQA1*03) and DQ5 (DQB1*0501 combined with DQA1*0101) are the primary predisposing molecules. However, as shown in our study and those of others, DRB1*0401 has an additional and unique contribution to RA. On the other hand, as shown by our ongoing investigations, the influence of DERAA+ DRB1 alleles is best seen in longitudinal studies involving carefully and regularly monitored patients. Currently, neither the RAP model nor the SE model can totally account for the role of HLA in RA; more investigations involving large data sets from carefully monitored patients are still needed to better understand the contribution of HLA class II genes to the pathogenesis of RA.

REFERENCES

1. Ollier W, Thomson W. Population genetics of rheumatoid arthritis. Rheum Dis Clin North Am 1992;18:741–59.
2. Winchester R. The molecular basis of susceptibility to rheumatoid arthritis. Adv Immunol 1994;56:389–466.
3. Stastny P. Mixed lymphocyte cultures in rheumatoid arthritis. J Clin Invest 1976;57:1148–57.
4. Woodrow JC, Nichol FE, Zaphiropoulos G. DR antigens and rheumatoid arthritis: a study in two populations. Br Med J 1981;283:1287–8.
5. De Juan MD, Belmonte I, Barado J, Martinez-Laso J, Figueroa M, Arnaiz-Villena A, et al. Differential association with rheumatoid arthritis (RA) in Basques: high frequency of DR1 and DR10 and lack of association with HLA-DR4 or any of its subtypes. Tissue Antigens 1994;43:320–3.
6. Taneja V, Mehra NK, Kailash S, Anand C, Malaviya AN. Protective & risk DR phenotypes in Asian Indian patients with rheumatoid arthritis. Indian J Med Res 1992;96:16–23.
7. Maeda H, Juji T, Mitsui H, Sonozaki H, Okitsu K. HLA-DR4 and rheumatoid arthritis in Japanese people. Ann Rheum Dis 1981; 40:299–302.
8. Boey ML, Wee GB, Mohan C, Howe HS, Chan SH, Feng PH. HLA in Singapore Chinese with rheumatoid arthritis. J Rheumatol 1992;19:1517–9.
9. Gregersen PK, Silver J, Winchester RJ. The shared epitope hypothesis: an approach to understanding the molecular genetics of susceptibility to rheumatoid arthritis. Arthritis Rheum 1987;30: 1205–13.
10. Sanchez B, Moreno I, Magarino R, Garzón M, Gonzalez MF, García A, et al. HLA-DRw10 confers the highest susceptibility to rheumatoid arthritis in a Spanish population. Tissue Antigens 1990;36:174–6.
11. Willkens RF, Nepom GT, Marks CR, Nettles JW, Nepom BS. Association of HLA–Dw16 with rheumatoid arthritis in Yakima Indians: further evidence for the "shared epitope" hypothesis. Arthritis Rheum 1991;34:43–7.
12. Gonzalez-Gay MA, Nabozny GH, Bull MJ, Zanelli E, Douhan J III, Griffiths MM, et al. Protective role of major histocompatibility complex class II Eb^d transgene on collagen-induced arthritis. J Exp Med 1994;180:1559–64.
13. Zanelli E, Gonzalez-Gay MA, David CS. Could HLA-DRB1 be the protective locus in rheumatoid arthritis? Immunol Today 1995;16:274–8.
14. Zanelli E, Huizinga TWJ, Guerne P-A, Vischer TL, Tiercy J-M, Verduyn W, et al. An extended HLA-DQ-DR haplotype rather than DRB1 alone contributes to RA predisposition. Immunogenetics 1998;48:394–401.
15. Nabozny GH, Baisch JM, Cheng S, Cosgove D, Griffiths MM, Luthra HS, et al. HLA-DQ8 transgenic mice are highly susceptible to collagen-induced arthritis: a novel model for human polyarthritis. J Exp Med 1996;183:27–37.
16. Zanelli E, Krco CJ, Baisch JM, Cheng S, David CS. Immune response of HLA-DQ8 transgenic mice to peptides from the third hypervariable region of HLA-DRB1 correlates with predisposition to rheumatoid arthritis. Proc Natl Acad Sci U S A 1996;93:1814–9.
17. Das P, Bradley DS, Geluk A, Griffiths MM, Luthra HS, David CS. An HLA-DRB1*0402 derived peptide (HV3 65-79) prevents collagen-induced arthritis in HLA-DQ8 transgenic mice. Hum Immunol 1999;60:575–82.
18. Van der Horst-Bruinsma IE, Visser H, Hazes JMW, Breedveld FC, Verduyn W, Schreuder GM, et al. HLA-DQ-associated predisposition to and dominant HLA-DR-associated protection against rheumatoid arthritis. Hum Immunol 1999;60:152–8.
19. Ronda E, Ruiz MT, Pascual E, Gibson T. Differences between Spanish and British patients in the severity of rheumatoid arthritis: comment on the article by Drosos et al [letter]. Arthritis Rheum 1994;37:147–8.
20. Salvarani C, Macchioni P, Mantovani W, Bragliani M, Collina E, Cremonesi T, et al. HLA-DRB1 alleles associated with rheumatoid arthritis in northern Italy: correlation with disease severity. Br J Rheumatol 1998;37:165–9.
21. Drosos AA, Lanchbury JS, Panayi GS, Moutsopoulos HM. Rheumatoid arthritis in Greek and British patients: a comparative clinical, radiologic, and serologic study. Arthritis Rheum 1992;35:745–8.
22. Benazet JF, Reviron D, Mercier P, Roux H, Roudier J. HLA-DRB1 alleles associated with rheumatoid arthritis in southern France: absence of extraarticular disease despite expression of the shared epitope. J Rheumatol 1995;22:607–10.
23. Balsa A, Minaur NJ, Pascual-Salcedo D, McCabe C, Balas A, Fiddament B, et al. Class II MHC antigens in early rheumatoid arthritis in Bath (UK) and Madrid (Spain). Rheumatology 2000; 39:844–9.
24. Arnett FC, Edworthy SM, Bloch DA, McShane DJ, Fries JF, Cooper NS, et al. The American Rheumatism Association 1987 revised criteria for the classification of rheumatoid arthritis. Arthritis Rheum 1988;31:315–24.
25. Taneja V, Giphart MJ, Verduijn W, Naipal A, Malaviya AN, Mehra NK. Polymorphism of HLA-DRB, -DQA1, and -DQB1 in rheumatoid arthritis in Asian Indians: association with DRB1*0405 and DRB1*1001. Hum Immunol 1996;46:35–41.
26. Martinez-Laso J, Gazit E, Gomez-Casado E, Morales P, Martinez-Quiles N, Alvarez M, et al. HLA-DR and DQ polymorphism in Ashkenazi and non-Ashkenazi Jews: comparison with other Mediterraneans. Tissue Antigens 1996;47:63–71.
27. Svejgaard A, Ryder LP. HLA and disease associations: detecting the strongest association. Tissue Antigens 1994;43:18–27.
28. Seidl C, Käβer UR, Fischer B, Koch U, Meier L, Fischer P, et al. HLA-DR/DQ interaction in patients with erosive rheumatoid arthritis presenting articular and extraarticular disease manifestations. Eur J Immunogenet 1999;26:19–27.
29. Wakitani S, Imoto K, Toda Y, Ogawa R, Ochi T. The homozygote of HLA-DRB1*0901, not its heterozygote, is associated with rheumatoid arthritis in Japanese. Scand J Rheumatol 1998;27:381–2.
30. González A, Nicovani S, Massardo L, Bull P, Rodríguez L, Jacobelli S. Novel genetic markers of rheumatoid arthritis in Chilean patients, by DR serotyping and restriction fragment length polymorphism analysis. Arthritis Rheum 1992;35:282–9.
31. Stavropoulos-Giokas C, Spyropoulou-Vlachou M, Doxiadis IIN, Kaklamanis F, Kaklamani E. The shared epitope versus DR/DQ haplotype hypothesis in rheumatoid arthritis in Greeks [abstract]. Hum Immunol 1999;60 Suppl 1:S48.
32. Nepom GT. Major histocompatibility complex-directed susceptibility to rheumatoid arthritis. Adv Immunol 1998;68:315–32.
33. Maffei A, Harris PE, Reed EF, Del Pozzo G, Ciullo M, Suciu-Foca N, et al. Differential expression of insulin-dependent diabetes mellitus-associated HLA-DQA1 alleles in vivo. Eur J Immunol 1997;27:1549–56.
34. Matsushita S, Nishi T, Oiso M, Yamaoka K, Yone K, Kanai T, et al. HLA-DQ-binding peptide motifs: comparative binding analysis of type II collagen-derived peptides to DR and DQ molecules of rheumatoid arthritis-susceptible and non-susceptible haplotypes. Int Immunol 1996;8:757–64.
35. McDonagh JE, Dunn A, Ollier WER, Walker DJ. Compound heterozygosity for the shared epitope and the risk and severity of rheumatoid arthritis in extended pedigrees. Br J Rheumatol 1997;36:322–7.
36. Auger I, Escola JM, Gorvel JP, Roudier J. HLA-DR4 and HLA-DR10 motifs that carry susceptibility to rheumatoid arthritis bind 70-kD heat shock proteins. Nat Med 1996;2:306–10.

ARTHRITIS & RHEUMATISM
Vol. 44, No. 2, February 2001, pp 315–322

HLA Haplotype Analysis in Finnish Patients With Rheumatoid Arthritis

Juha Tuokko,[1] Sergei Nejentsev,[1] Reijo Luukkainen,[2] Auli Toivanen,[3] and Jorma Ilonen[1]

Objective. **To further characterize the HLA gene products that play an important role in the pathogenesis of rheumatoid arthritis (RA).**

Methods. **One hundred thirty-four haplotypes from 67 Finnish RA patients and 77 control haplotypes were analyzed for HLA–DRB1 loci, associated alleles of the HLA–DQB1 locus, alleles of the type 2 transporter-associated antigen processing (TAP2) genes, and HLA–B27. In addition, a panel of microsatellite markers within the HLA class I and class III regions was studied.**

Results. **The frequency of HLA–DRB1*04 in the haplotypes of RA patients was found to be 34% (45 of 134) compared with 14% (10 of 72) in control haplotypes (P = 0.004). The frequency of HLA–DRB1*13 was decreased in RA haplotypes (4%, or 5 of 134) in contrast to control haplotypes (24%, or 17 of 72) (P = 0.000031). The decrease in DRB1*13 was not secondary to the increase in DRB1*04, since it was also found among DRB1*04-negative haplotypes (P < 0.001). The DRB1*13-associated DQB1*0604 allele was similarly decreased in RA haplotypes (P = 0.025). The TAP2I allele of I/J dimorphism was increased in RA patients (85%, or 114 of 134) as compared with controls (69%, or 49 of 71) (P = 0.011). Of the tumor necrosis factor (TNF) microsatellite alleles, TNFa6 and TNFb5 were found to be increased in RA haplotypes (for a6 27% versus 5% in controls [P = 0.00043], and for b5 43% versus 26% in controls [P = 0.037]).**

Conclusion. **Both protection-associated and susceptibility-associated alleles can be found among HLA class II genes, and the results suggest that loci outside DR/DQ may contribute to the pathogenesis of RA.**

Rheumatoid arthritis (RA) is known to be associated with HLA class II alleles, particularly with HLA–DRB1*04 and its specific subtypes (1,2). These subtypes (0401, 0404, 0405, 0408, 0409, and 0410), as well as DRB1*01 and DRB1*1402, share a similar pattern of amino acids, or the "shared epitope," in their third hypervariable region, from position 67 to position 74, and this has been proposed to provide the molecular basis for genetic susceptibility to RA (3,4). However, a large proportion of patients are DRB1*04 negative, and various alleles with the shared epitope confer different disease risks, suggesting that other genetic elements might also be important in the pathogenesis of RA (5).

The HLA–DQB1 alleles *0301 and *0302 are in strong linkage disequilibrium with HLA–DRB1*04. Zanelli and coworkers have therefore proposed an alternative hypothesis, namely, that instead of DRB1 alleles, DQB1 alleles could be the actual predisposing factors in susceptibility to RA (6). Based on their experimental mouse model of collagen-induced arthritis, the same authors suggested that the HLA–DQ molecules would be the actual arthritogenic peptide–presenting molecules, whereas the HLA–DR molecules would either provide protection or be nonprotective. Contradictory results have been published with regard to which of the 2 DQB1 alleles (*0301 or *0302) is mainly associated with RA. This issue was recently reviewed by Fugger and Svejgaard (7). The conclusion was that DRB1 genes still form the basis of the genetic predisposition to RA, but that the DQB1*0301 allele

Supported by the Academy of Finland, Turku University Central Hospital, the Sigrid Jusélius Foundation, the Turku University Foundation, the Emil and Blida Maunula Foundation, the Finnish Medical Foundation, the Finnish Cultural Foundations, and the Maud Kuistila Foundation.

[1]Juha Tuokko, MD, Sergei Nejentsev, MD, Jorma Ilonen, MD: University of Turku, Turku, Finland; [2]Reijo Luukkainen, MD: Satalinna Hospital, Harjavalta, Finland; [3]Auli Toivanen, MD: Turku University Central Hospital, Turku, Finland.

Address correspondence and reprint requests to Juha Tuokko, MD, Department of Medical Microbiology, University of Turku, Kiinamyllynkatu 13, FIN-20520 Turku, Finland.

Submitted for publication November 23, 1999; accepted in revised form September 27, 2000.

might confer susceptibility to Felty's syndrome, independent of DR4.

In addition to the HLA–DR and –DQ genes, there are several other loci within the HLA gene complex that modify the immune response and thus may be important in defining the risk for RA. Among these are the transporter-associated antigen-processing (TAP) genes, located within the HLA class II gene region between the HLA–DP and –DQ loci. These genes encode proteins that carry antigenic peptides to the endoplasmic reticulum to be loaded into class I molecules (8,9). We have recently found an increased frequency of the TAP2A/A genotype in Finnish patients with RA, which was further associated with HLA–DRB1*04-positive disease (10). With regard to the class I genes, B27 is known to be strongly associated with reactive arthritis and spondylarthropathies, but was also earlier shown to be increased among some subgroups of Finnish RA patients (11,12).

Tumor necrosis factor (TNF) genes are located centromeric to HLA–B within the HLA class III region (13,14). Their polymorphisms have been shown to affect the secretion level of TNFα (15–20), which is an important proinflammatory cytokine in the pathogenesis of RA (21). In addition, a microsatellite marker, D6S273, located within the HLA class III region, was recently reported to be associated with RA, independent of the "shared epitope" (22). The effect of DR4 was not separately reported.

In the present study we used haplotype analyses to clarify further which gene regions and alleles are important in defining susceptibility to RA. We analyzed TAP2 and HLA–DRB1 loci, associated alleles of the HLA–DQB1 locus, and HLA–B27. In addition, a panel of microsatellite markers within the HLA class I and class III regions was assessed.

PATIENTS AND METHODS

Patients and controls. Blood samples were collected from 67 patients with RA from southwest Finland, as well as from either 1 or 2 of their first-degree relatives to enable formation of haplotypes within families. The haplotypes were deduced based on the presence of specific alleles in the patients and their relatives. All diagnoses of RA were based on the criteria of the American College of Rheumatology (formerly, the American Rheumatism Association) (23). Control haplotypes were selected from healthy family members. Haplotypes not inherited by patients were included to represent the background population (24,25). For the HLA–DRB1*04 and TNF haplotype analyses, additional control haplotypes from families with patients with insulin-dependent diabetes mellitus (IDDM) were similarly selected. These included 83 DRB1*04-positive haplotypes analyzed for their TNF microsatellite alleles and 152 DRB1*04 haplotypes that were analyzed for their subtypes and associated DQB1 alleles. In an earlier DNA typing study, DR4 subtyping identified 35 DRB1*04 RA haplotypes (26), which were included in the present analyses of DRB1*04 subtypes (see Table 2); this study of subtypes did not include samples from other family members. DNA isolation was performed from anticoagulated blood samples by a salting out method (27).

HLA typing. HLA–DRB1 alleles were determined by sequence-specific polymerase chain reaction (PCR) amplification (28). The defined HLA–DRB1 alleles positive for the shared epitope were 0401, 0404, 0405, 0408, 0409, 0410, 01, and 1001 (our typing method could not differentiate DRB1*14 subtypes). HLA–DRB1*04 subtyping was performed by using a new modification of the high-resolution, time-resolved fluorometry-based technique (29), utilized also in HLA–DQB1 typing of selected alleles (30). In this method, a region of the DRB1*04 gene is first amplified with DRB1*04-specific primers, of which 1 of each pair is biotinylated. The product is then transferred to 96-well streptavidin-coated microtiter plates, where it is hybridized with a panel of oligonucleotide probes labeled with different lanthanides (europium, samarium, and terbium). Time-resolved fluorescence signals of hybridized probes are finally detected with a fluorometer. A similar kind of procedure was also used for HLA–B27 typing (31).

TAP2 typing. TAP2 analysis was performed as we have described earlier (10). To confirm our method for detection of the TAP2I/J polymorphism, a few homozygous samples for each allele were sequenced. For sequencing, types 1 and 2 primers of the amplification refractory mutation system were used to amplify TAP2 sequences covering TAP2 position 386 (32). Sequencing was made using an Applied Biosystems PRISM dye terminator ready reaction kit and 373 DNA sequencer (Perkin Elmer, Emeryville, CA). Our study included positions 379, 386, 565, 651, 665, and 667 (33). TAP2 alleles were named from A to H on the basis of the nomenclature proposed by Jackson and Capra (34).

Microsatellite typing. Fluorochrome-labeled primers were used to amplify TNFa, TNFb, and TNFc microsatellite sequences (35) as well as the sequences of C12A, C143, and C3211 microsatellites (36). Size determination of PCR products and definition of alleles present in the microsatellite was performed using GeneScan 672 software in an automated DNA sequencer (Applied Biosystems model 373). A panel of samples homozygous for TNF, C12A, C143, and C3211 microsatellite alleles were sequenced to ensure typing results.

Statistical analysis. The number of haplotypes varied between different analyses because the number of haplotypes that could be reliably deduced was different in each case. The frequencies of HLA haplotypes were compared between patients and controls using a chi-square test with continuity correction. Fisher's exact test was used when appropriate. The relative predispositional effect (RPE) method was used to evaluate the relative effects of HLA–DRB1 alleles (37). All other polymorphisms included in the present study were investigated in 3 subgroups of haplotypes (all haplotypes, only DRB1*04 positives, only DRB1*04 negatives) to exclude the possible effect of DRB1*04 as a known marker of RA on our results. Other markers observed to be associated with RA were similarly studied. The chi-square test with continuity correction was also used to study possible linkage disequilibrium between markers associated with RA. In addition, standardized disequilibrium coefficient values were calculated.

RESULTS

A total of 134 haplotypes determined from 67 RA patients (17 male, 50 female) was investigated and compared with 77 control haplotypes not inherited by patients within families. Additional control haplotypes, which were selected from IDDM families, were included when HLA–DRB1*04 haplotypes were analyzed. Fifty-nine percent of RA patients were HLA–DRB1*04 positive and 13% were DRB1*04 homozygous. All patients, except 3 whose positivity or negativity was not known on the basis of clinical data, were positive for rheumatoid factor. Among all RA patients, 93% (62 of 67) had an erosive disease.

HLA–DR and –DQ polymorphisms. The frequency of HLA–DRB1*04 in the haplotypes of RA patients was 34% (45 of 134) compared with 14% (10 of 72) in the control haplotypes (P = 0.004, odds ratio [OR] 3.13, 95% confidence interval [95% CI] 1.39–7.21). HLA–DRB1*13 was found to be decreased in frequency among the RA haplotypes studied; the frequency was 4% (5 of 134) in RA patients in contrast to 24% (17 of 72) in control haplotypes (P = 0.000031, OR 0.13, 95% CI 0.04–0.39).

Table 1 shows the RPEs for DRB1 alleles. Comparison between the number of DR alleles observed in RA haplotypes (shown in the second column of Table 1) and the frequency expected from controls (shown in the third column) revealed that the overall χ^2 value was statistically significant ($P < 10^{-8}$) and the allele with the largest contribution was DRB1*04 (observed number of haplotypes 45 versus expected 18.87; $P < 10^{-7}$). After DRB1*04 was removed from the analysis (round 2 in Table 1), the overall χ^2 was still statistically significant, but the largest deviation was now due to the decreased frequency of DRB1*13 in RA haplotypes (observed number 5 versus expected 24.80; $P < 0.001$). After DRB1*04 and DRB1*13 were removed (round 3 in Table 1), the overall χ^2 value was again statistically significant, with DRB1*03 now showing the largest deviation (observed number 8 versus expected 24.82; $P < 0.001$). Finally, there were no statistically significant differences after DRB1*04, DRB1*13, and DRB1*03 were removed (round 4 in Table 1).

When HLA–DRB1*04 subtypes were analyzed, DRB1*0404 was slightly decreased in frequency among the RA haplotypes (P = 0.041, OR 0.40, 95% CI 0.16–0.97), but when an additional 35 RA DRB1*04

Table 1. Relative predispositional effects of DR alleles in haplotypes of rheumatoid arthritis (RA) patients and controls*

		Round 1: all			Round 2: DR4 removed			Round 3: DR4 and DR13 removed			Round 4: DR3, DR4, and DR13 removed		
DR allele	No. observed	Expected frequency	χ^2	P	Expected frequency	χ^2	P	Expected frequency	χ^2	P	Expected frequency	χ^2	P
1	29	20.76	3.27		16.05	10.45		21.00	3.05		26.97	0.15	
15(2)	14	9.44	2.20		7.30	6.15		9.55	2.07		12.26	0.25	
16(2)	1	3.77	2.04		2.92	1.26		3.82	2.08		4.90	3.10	
3	8	24.54	11.15		18.97	6.03		24.82	11.40	<0.001	–	–	
4	45	18.87	36.18	$<10^{-7}$	–	–		–	–		–	–	
11(5)	4	1.89	2.36		1.46	4.42		1.91	2.29		2.45	0.98	
12(5)	6	3.77	1.32		2.92	3.25		3.82	1.24		4.90	0.25	
13(6)	5	32.08	22.86		24.80	15.81	<0.001	–	–		–	–	
14(6)	1	1.89	0.42		1.46	0.14		1.91	0.43		2.45	0.86	
7	5	5.66	0.08		4.38	0.09		5.73	0.09		7.35	0.75	
8	10	7.55	0.80		5.84	0.12		7.64	0.73		9.81	0.00	
9	5	3.77	0.40		2.92	1.26		3.82	0.36		4.90	0.00	
10	1	0	1.00		0	1.00		0	1.00		0.00	1.00	
Total	134	134	84.08	$<10^{-8}$†	89	49.98	6.311×10^{-7}‡	84	24.74	0.0059§	76	7.34	0.602¶

* Chi-square and P values represent comparisons between the no. of observed RA haplotypes and the frequency of expected haplotypes calculated from the controls.
† Degrees of freedom (df) = 12.
‡ df = 11.
§ df = 10.
¶ df = 9 (P not significant).

Table 2. HLA–DRB1*04 subtypes in haplotypes of patients with rheumatoid arthritis and controls*

	Rheumatoid arthritis		Control	
Haplotype	n	%	n	%
401	46	58	92	57
403	2	3	3	2
404	22	28	57	35
405	0	0	2	1
408	10	13	8	5
Total	80		162	

* Patient haplotypes included an additional 35 haplotypes from our earlier study (26) and controls included an additional 152 DRB1*04 haplotypes selected from families with patients with insulin-dependent diabetes mellitus.

subtypes, as determined in our earlier study (26), were included, the significance of this decrease disappeared (Table 2). The contribution of the DQB1 gene locus in haplotypes was studied by comparing the frequencies of DQB1 alleles that were associated with DRB1 alleles that had been found to be increased or decreased among RA haplotypes. Both of the DRB1*04-associated DQB1 alleles, *0301 (frequency in RA 18% [24 of 134] versus 8% [6 of 77] in controls; P = 0.069, 95% CI 0.94–7.45) and *0302 (in RA 23% [31 of 134] versus 10% [8 of 77] in controls; P = 0.035, 95% CI 1.06–6.55), conferred an almost similar risk, with ORs of 2.58 and 2.60, respectively. The proportion of DRB1*04 subtypes associated with these alleles was also analyzed, and in comparing RA haplotypes with control haplotypes (which totaled 162, including an additional 152 control haplotypes from IDDM families), no significant differences were observed.

Our samples were also typed for DRB1*13-associated DQB1 alleles. DQB1*0604 was found to be decreased in frequency among all RA haplotypes (1 of 134 versus 5 of 77 in controls; P = 0.025, OR 0.11, 95% CI 0.02–0.98). Within DRB1*13 haplotypes, the frequency of DQB1*0604 was 25% (1 of 4) in RA haplotypes in contrast to 50% (5 of 10) in controls (P not significant). All other DR13 haplotypes, except 1 control haplotype that was *0301 positive, were DQB1*0603 positive in both RA and control haplotypes. These results indicate that DRB1*13 together with DQB1*0604 might form an HLA haplotype that is negatively associated with RA.

TAP2 polymorphisms. When the frequencies of TAP2 polymorphisms were compared, the frequency of TAP2I was observed to be increased in RA haplotypes (85% [114 of 134] versus 69% [49 of 71] in controls; P = 0.011, OR 2.56, 95% CI 1.21–5.41) and TAP2J reciprocally decreased in RA haplotypes (15% [20 of 134] versus 31% [22 of 71] in controls; P = 0.011, OR 0.39, 95% CI 0.18–0.82). When other TAP2 dimorphisms were compared, no significant differences between patient and control haplotypes were observed.

TNFa, -b, and -c microsatellite polymorphisms. The TNF alleles a6 and b5 were found to be increased in RA haplotypes (for a6 27% [36 of 134] versus 5% [3 of 65] in controls, P = 0.00043, OR 7.59, 95% CI 2.11–22.22; and for b5 43% [57 of 134] versus 26% [17 of 65] in controls, P = 0.037, OR 2.09, 95% CI 1.04–4.23).

C3211, C12A, and C143 microsatellite polymorphisms. The frequency of the C12A allele 258 was found to be decreased in RA haplotypes (17 of 134 [13%] versus 16 of 60 [27%] in controls; P = 0.029, OR 0.40, 95% CI 0.17–0.92).

HLA–B27. The frequency of HLA–B27 in both control and patient haplotypes was 10% (8 of 77 and 13 of 134, respectively).

Association analyses and linkage disequilibrium between the markers. A significant linkage disequilibrium was detected between DRB1*04 and TNFa6 in the total group of haplotypes and between TNFa6 and b5 in the total group of haplotypes and in each subgroup of haplotypes (Table 3). No linkage disequilibrium between TAP2I and other RA-associated alleles was found, and the separate analyses of TAP2I in DR4-positive and -negative haplotypes also confirmed its independent effect; the frequency of TAP2I was 86% (32 of 37) in DRB1*04-positive RA haplotypes versus 44% (4 of 9) in DRB1*04-positive control haplotypes (P = 0.015), whereas in DRB1*04-negative haplotypes, the respective values were 94% (68 of 72) versus 72% (41 of 57) (P = 0.0011). TAP2A and TAP2I or TAP2J were not in linkage disequilibrium with each other.

Similar analyses of TNF microsatellites revealed no significant differences among DR4-positive haplotypes, whereas in the comparison of DRB1*04-negative haplotypes, the increase in frequency of the a6 allele was still observed (P = 0.0082, OR 7.36, 95% CI 1.49–28.41). The latter result confirms that the association of TNFa6 with RA is not secondary to that of DRB1*04. When TNFa6 was analyzed in terms of DRB1*04 subtypes, it was found to be associated with DRB1*0408. All DRB1*0408 haplotypes (5 of 5) were positive for TNFa6, whereas only 36 of 120 other DRB1*04 subtypes were positive (P = 0.003). No statistically significant differences could be seen in the proportion of TNFa6-positive and -negative haplotypes when various DRB1*04 haplotypes were compared between patients and controls, indicating that no subtype combination of

Table 3. Linkage disequilibrium analyses between markers associated with rheumatoid arthritis (RA) in RA haplotypes, control haplotypes, and total haplotypes

	Haplotype frequency	Δmax	Δstandard	*P*
RA positively associated markers, in their genomic order				
RA haplotypes				
TAP2I;DRB1*04	0.297	0.032	−0.700	0.739
DRB1*04;TNFa6	0.126	0.179	0.189	0.333
TNFa6;TNFb5	0.265	0.149	1.000	3×10^{-5}
Control haplotypes				
TAP2I;DRB1*04	0.061	0.043	−0.747	0.509
DRB1*04;TNFa6	0.016	0.044	0.250	0.791
TNFa6;TNFb5	0.051	0.038	1.000	0.047
Total haplotypes				
TAP2I;DRB1*04	0.209	0.046	−0.217	0.839
DRB1*04;TNFa6	0.085	0.141	0.260	0.048
TNFa6;TNFb5	0.185	0.116	1.000	5.5×10^{-8}
RA negatively associated markers, in their genomic order				
RA haplotypes				
TAP2J;DQB1*0604	0.000	0.015	−0.133	0.543
DQB1*0604;DRB1*13	0.008	0.015	−0.480	0.140
DRB1*13;C12A*258	0.010	0.046	0.086	0.880
Control haplotypes				
TAP2J;DQB1*0604	0.070	0.049	1.000	0.018
DQB1*0604;DRB1*13	0.070	0.064	0.781	0.011
DRB1*13;C12A*258	0.036	0.149	−0.097	0.858
Total haplotypes				
TAP2J;DQB1*0604	0.026	0.030	0.633	0.005
DQB1*0604;DRB1*13	0.031	0.036	0.847	1.3×10^{-6}
DRB1*13;C12A*258	0.020	0.087	0.020	0.886

TNFa6 and DRB1*04 was preferentially increased among RA patients.

Among negatively associated RA markers (TAP2J, DQB1*0604, DRB1*13, and C12A*258), strong linkage disequilibrium was detected between TAP2J and DQB1*0604, as well as between DQB1*0604 and DRB1*13 (Table 3). Although TAP2J was strongly associated with DRB1*13 ($P = 0.0002$ for linkage in total haplotypes), its decrease was detected in both DRB1*13-positive and -negative haplotypes. The only DRB1*13;DQB1*0604 haplotype detected in RA patients was positive for TAP2I, whereas all of these haplotypes in controls were associated with TAP2J (4 of 4). Furthermore, all of these haplotypes in controls were also positive for TAP2F (4 of 4), whereas the only RA haplotype was positive for some other TAP2 allele, which could not be exactly defined. The amino acid combination could have been either val-ala-ala-arg-stop (undescribed combination) or val-ala-ala-arg-gln (TAP2B). Thus, TAP2F together with DRB1*13 and DQB1*0604 appear to form an extended haplotype that is negatively associated with RA.

Among the alleles of C12A, C3211, and C143 microsatellites, allele C12A*258 was decreased in RA haplotypes, and its decrease was independent of other protective markers, whereas C3211*205 and C143*445 alleles were found to be decreased in HLA–DRB1*04 positive RA haplotypes (for *205 6% [2 of 36] versus 33% [3 of 9] in controls [$P = 0.047$], and for *445 19% [6 of 31] versus 67% [4 of 6] in controls [$P = 0.035$]).

Effect of sex on the results. Haplotypes were also compared between male and female patients to see whether markers associated with RA would further be associated with sex. However, no statistically significant deviations could be seen.

DISCUSSION

The present study was designed to further evaluate which polymorphisms within the HLA region are important in RA. Our study also included testing of family members, enabling us to form true HLA haplotypes for investigation into whether the associations revealed by the present study were dependent on the presence of other markers associated with RA.

Our results regarding HLA–DRB1 polymorphisms confirm the known association between DRB1*04 and RA. Both common subtypes of DR4 in Finland, 0401 and 0404, are positive for the "shared epitope" and the ratio between them was not observed to differ significantly between patient and control haplotypes. These results were similar to those obtained in our earlier study (26). In contrast, the DR1 allele, which is a very common allele in the Finnish population (38) and is also positive for the shared epitope, was not found to be associated with RA. The slight observed difference was not significant, even when the effect of other DRB1 alleles associated with RA was excluded from comparison. Interestingly, in the present study, the HLA–DRB1*13 allele was found to be strongly protective against RA. After exclusion of HLA–DRB1*04 from the comparison, the significance still remained, indicating that the decrease in DRB1*13 was not just secondary to the increase in DRB1*04 in RA. DRB1*13 is a subtype of DR6, which has been found to be decreased among RA patients in several earlier studies (39–43). The HLA–DRB1*13 allele carries a DERAA motif in its third hypervariable region, which has been suggested to provide protection against RA, or at least to interfere with disease progression (43).

The DRB1*13 subtypes *1301 and *1302 have been shown to differ in their peptide-binding capacity and also in their DQB1 associations (44,45). Of the DRB1*13 alleles, *1301 is associated with DQB1*0603, and *1302 with *0604 (44). We also studied HLA–DQB1 alleles known to be in linkage disequilibrium with DRB1*13 and found DQB1*0604 to be decreased in DRB1*13 haplotypes of RA patients. Furthermore, the only DRB1*13;DQB1*0604 haplotype in our RA patients carried the TAP2I variant, which was not associated with TAP2F, in contrast to controls, in which all haplotypes were associated with TAP2J and all of these (except 1 that could not be defined due to lack of additional family data) were associated with TAP2F. Although this result was statistically insignificant, it suggests that HLA–DRB1*13, DQB1*0604, TAP2J, and TAP2F together form an extended HLA haplotype that is negatively associated with RA in the Finnish population, but the actual locus responsible for the protective effect remains to be defined.

The TAP2I and TAP2J dichotomy may serve as an additional marker further dissecting TAP2 alleles. Thus, the combination of TAP2J and TAP2F was found to be a part of the protective haplotype. In a dichotomy such as the I/J polymorphism, there is always a reciprocal increase and decrease in the markers. The TAP2J allele decreased among RA haplotypes means that it was part of the protective DRB1*13;DQB1*0604 haplotype, but it was also found to be decreased among DRB1*13-negative haplotypes, which might indicate the primary importance of J-related protection. The lack of association between RA and TAP2I/J markers in our earlier study might be explained by a smaller sample size. Since the TAP2I/J polymorphism in RA has not, to our knowledge, been previously studied, our result might be false positive and therefore it must be confirmed using a larger study sample and in other populations.

Of the HLA class I alleles, B27 has been reported to be associated with RA in the Finnish population and was therefore included in the present study. We could not confirm an increase in HLA–B27 among the RA haplotypes, although it was usually associated with DR1 or DR4 as earlier reported (46). Although B27 was not found to be associated with RA in the present study, it still might affect the outcome of disease, as has been previously described (47).

In the present study, we used microsatellite markers to investigate polymorphisms within TNF sequences in the HLA class III region and their possible associations with susceptibility to RA. The TNF polymorphism has not been studied in Finnish RA patients. Of the TNF microsatellite alleles, TNFa11 was recently reported to be associated with RA severity through an interaction with the HLA–DRB1 shared epitope (48). We did not classify patients according to the severity of the disease, but our study showed a strong association of the TNFa6 allele with RA in DRB1*04-negative haplotypes of patients with RA. Our result is similar to the findings of Martínez et al and Mulcahy et al (49,50), who similarly described an independent association of the TNFa6 allele with RA. The mechanisms behind the TNFa6 association with RA have not been studied, but in IDDM patients, the TNFa6 allele has been reported to be associated with decreased TNFα secretion, whereas the TNFa2 allele was associated with high TNFα-secretion capacity (18). The association of RA-associated TNFa6 with low TNF secretion is not consistent with the known importance of this cytokine in tissue destruction in RA, but we do not know enough about the complex pathogenic mechanisms to draw simple correlations. The genetic polymorphisms actually regulating the level of TNFα secretion should also be analyzed in more detail.

In our study, the TNFb5 allele was also observed to be increased in RA haplotypes, which was expected because of its known linkage with TNFa6. TNFc alleles did not differ in their frequencies between patients and controls, although the c1 allele has been earlier reported to be associated with RA (50). These studies, together with the recently reported association between a microsatellite marker, D6S273, within the class III region and RA (22), suggest that in addition to HLA class II, the class III region polymorphisms also may be relevant to RA pathogenesis. Further studies are needed to resolve the question as to which gene or genes cause the association between these markers within HLA class III and RA.

Additional microsatellites (C12A, C143, and C3211) within the centromeric part of the class I region were included to further investigate whether sequence polymorphisms near the HLA–B locus might play a role in RA. C12A allele 258 was found to be negatively associated with RA, although the association was clearly weaker than that of DRB1*13. Alleles C3211*205 and C143*445 were found to be decreased in RA patients bearing DRB1*04 haplotypes, suggesting that genes within this region might contribute to the susceptibility in DRB1*04-positive RA patients, but this observation also needs confirmation.

It is evident that RA is a polygenic disease, and our results also show that within the HLA region, new susceptibility markers relevant to disease pathogenesis might still be found. In addition, outside the HLA region, new susceptibility genes have already been reported, although they require more exact localization (51–54). Despite the growing interest in regions outside the HLA complex, we have to keep in mind that a lot of data concerning the precise role of the HLA-region genes in the pathogenesis of RA remain to be determined.

ACKNOWLEDGMENTS

We thank Miss Leena Kivistö, Mrs. Terttu Lauren, and Mrs. Ritva Suominen for their excellent technical assistance.

REFERENCES

1. Lanchbury JS. The HLA association with rheumatoid arthritis. Clin Exp Rheumatol 1992;10:301–4.
2. Reveille JD. The genetic contribution to the pathogenesis of rheumatoid arthritis. Curr Opin Rheumatol 1998;10:187–200.
3. Gregersen PK, Silver J, Winchester RJ. The shared epitope hypothesis: an approach to understanding the molecular genetics of susceptibility to rheumatoid arthritis. Arthritis Rheum 1987;30:1205–13.
4. Winchester R, Dwyer E, Rose S. The genetic basis of rheumatoid arthritis: the shared epitope hypothesis. Rheum Dis Clin North Am 1992;18:761–83.
5. Dizier M-H, Eliaou J-F, Babron M-C, Combe B, Sany J, Clot J, et al. Investigation of the HLA component involved in rheumatoid arthritis (RA) by using the marker association-segregation X^2 (MASC) method: rejection of the unifying-shared-epitope hypothesis. Am J Hum Genet 1993;53:715–21.
6. Zanelli E, Gonzalez-Gay MA, David CS. Could HLA-DRB1 be the protective locus in rheumatoid arthritis? Immunol Today 1995;16:274–8.
7. Fugger L, Svejgaard A. The HLA-DQ7 and -DQ8 associations in DR4-positive rheumatoid arthritis patients: a combined analysis of data available in the literature. Tissue Antigens 1997;50:494–500.
8. Spies T, Cerundolo V, Colonna M, Cresswell P, Townsend A, DeMars R. Presentation of viral antigen by MHC class I molecules is dependent on a putative peptide transporter heterodimer. Nature 1992;355:644–6.
9. Kelly A, Powis SH, Kerr L, Mockridge I, Elliot T, Bastin J, et al. Assembly and function of the two ABC transporter proteins encoded in the human major histocompatibility complex. Nature 1992;355:641–4.
10. Tuokko J, Pushnova E, Yli Kerttula U, Toivanen A, Ilonen J. TAP2 alleles in inflammatory arthritis. Scand J Rheumatol 1998;27:225–9.
11. Hakala M, van Assendelft AHW, Ilonen J, Jalava S, Tiilikainen A. Association of different HLA antigens with various toxic effects of gold salts in rheumatoid arthritis. Ann Rheum Dis 1986;45:177–82.
12. Isomäki H, Nissilä M, Koota K, Martio J, Tiilikainen A. HLA-B27 and rheumatoid arthritis [letter]. Lancet 1974;2:1212.
13. Dunham I, Sargent CA, Trowsdale J, Campbell RD. Molecular mapping of the human major histocompatibility complex by pulsed-field gel electrophoresis. Proc Natl Acad Sci U S A 1987;84:7237–41.
14. Carroll MC, Katzman P, Alicot E, Koller BH, Geraghty DE, Orr HT, et al. Linkage map of the human major histocompatibility complex including the tumor necrosis factor genes. Proc Natl Acad Sci U S A 1987;84:8535–9.
15. Bouma G, Crusius JBA, Oudkerk Pool M, Kolkman JJ, von Blomberg BME, Kostense PJ, et al. Secretion of tumour necrosis factor α and lymphotoxin α in relation to polymorphisms in the TNF genes and HLA-DR alleles: relevance for inflammatory bowel disease. Scand J Immunol 1996;43:456–63.
16. Molvig J, Pociot F, Baek L, Worsaae H, Wogensen LD, Christensen P, et al. Monocyte function in IDDM patients and healthy individuals. Scand J Immunol 1990;32:297–311.
17. Pociot F, Molvig J, Wogensen L, Worsaae H, Dalboge H, Baek L, et al. A tumour necrosis factor beta gene polymorphism in relation to monokine secretion and insulin-dependent diabetes mellitus. Scand J Immunol 1991;33:37–49.
18. Pociot F, Briant L, Jongeneel CV, Mölvig J, Worsaae H, Abbal M, et al. Association of tumor necrosis factor (TNF) and class II major histocompatibility complex alleles with the secretion of TNF-α and TNF-β by human mononuclear cells: a possible link to insulin-dependent diabetes mellitus. Eur J Immunol 1993;23:224–31.
19. Whichelow CE, Hitman GA, Raafat I, Bottazzo GF, Sachs JA. The effect of TNF*B gene polymorphism on TNF-α and -β secretion levels in patients with insulin-dependent diabetes mellitus and healthy controls. Eur J Immunogenet 1996;23:425–35.
20. Wilson AG, Symons JA, McDowell TL, McDevitt HO, Duff GW. Effects of a polymorphism in the human tumor necrosis factor α promoter on transcriptional activation. Proc Natl Acad Sci U S A 1997;94:3195–9.
21. Eigler A, Sinha B, Hartmann G, Endres S. Taming TNF: strategies to restrain this proinflammatory cytokine. Immunol Today 1997;18:487–91.
22. Singal DP, Li J, Ye M, Lei K. D6S273 microsatellite polymorphism and susceptibility to rheumatoid arthritis. Tissue Antigens 1998;52:353–8.
23. Arnett FC, Edworthy SM, Bloch DA, McShane DJ, Fries JF, Cooper NS, et al. The American Rheumatism Association 1987

revised criteria for the classification of rheumatoid arthritis. Arthritis Rheum 1988;31:315–24.
24. Falk CT, Rubinstein P. Haplotype relative risks: an easy reliable way to construct a proper control sample for risk calculations. Ann Hum Genet 1987;51:227–33.
25. Thomson G. Mapping disease genes: family-based association studies. Am J Hum Genet 1995;57:487–98.
26. Tuokko J, Reijonen H, Ilonen J, Anttila K, Nikkari S, Möttönen T, et al. Increase of HLA-DRB1*0408 and -DQB1*0301 in HLA-B27 positive reactive arthritis. Ann Rheum Dis 1997;56:37–40.
27. Miller SA, Dykes DD, Polesky HF. A simple salting out procedure for extracting DNA from human nucleated cells. Nucleic Acids Res 1988;16:1215.
28. Olerup O, Zetterquist H. HLA-DR typing by PCR amplification with sequence-specific primers (PCR-SSP) in 2 hours: an alternative to serological DR typing in clinical practice including donor-recipient matching in cadaveric transplantation. Tissue Antigens 1992;39:225–35.
29. Nejentsev S, Sjöroos M, Soukka T, Knip M, Simell O, Lövgren T, et al. Population based genetic screening for estimation of Type 1 diabetes mellitus risk in Finland: selective genotyping of the markers in the HLA-DRB1, HLA-DQA1 and HLA-DRB1 loci. Diabet Med 1999;16:985–92.
30. Sjöroos M, Iitiä A, Ilonen J, Reijonen H, Lövgren T. Triple-label hybridization assay for type-1 diabetes-related HLA alleles. Biotechniques 1995;18:870–7.
31. Välimaa L, Sjöroos M, Luhtala M, Toivanen P, Lövgren T, Ilonen J. Detection of HLA-B27 alleles by group-specific amplification and time-resolved fluorometry. J Immunol Methods 1998;219: 131–7.
32. Powis SH, Tonks S, Mockridge I, Kelly AP, Bodmer JG, Trowsdale J. Alleles and haplotypes of the MHC-encoded ABC transporters TAP1 and TAP2. Immunogenetics 1993;37:373–80.
33. Moins-Teisserenc H, Semana G, Alizadeh M, Loiseau P, Bobrynina V, Deschamps I, et al. TAP2 gene polymorphism contributes to genetic susceptibility to multiple sclerosis. Human Immunol 1995;42:195–202.
34. Jackson DG, Capra JD. TAP2 association with insulin-dependent diabetes mellitus is secondary to HLA-DQB1. Human Immunol 1995;43:57–65.
35. Tuokko J, Koskinen S, Westman P, Yli-Kerttula U, Toivanen A, Ilonen J. Tumour necrosis microsatellites in reactive arthritis. Br J Rheum 1998;37:1203–6.
36. Tamiya G, Ota M, Katsuyama Y, Shiina T, Oka A, Makino S, et al. Twenty-six new polymorphic microsatellite markers around the HLA-B, -C and -E loci in the human MHC class I region. Tissue Antigens 1998;51:337–46.
37. Payami H, Joe S, Farid NR, Stenszky V, Chan SH, Yeo PPB, et al. Relative predispositional effects (RPEs) of marker alleles with disease: HLA-DR alleles and Graves disease. Am J Hum Genet 1989;45:541–6.
38. Sirén MK, Saraneva H, Lokki ML, Koskimies S. Unique HLA antigen frequencies in the Finnish population. Tissue Antigens 1996;48:703–7.
39. Rantapää-Dahlqvist S, Strom H, Bjelle A, Möller E. HLA antigens in rheumatoid arthritis patients with and without a family history of polyarthritis. Scand J Rheumatol 1985;14:375–80.
40. Seidl C, Kässer UR, Fischer P, Koch U, Meier L, Fischer P, et al. HLA-DR/DQ interaction in patients with erosive rheumatoid arthritis presenting articular and extra-articular disease manifestations. Eur J Immunogen 1999;26:19–27.
41. Van Zeben D, Hazes JMW, Zwinderman AH, Cats A, Schreuder GMT, D'Amaro J, et al. Association of HLA–DR4 with a more progressive disease course in patients with rheumatoid arthritis: results of a followup study. Arthritis Rheum 1991;34:822–30.
42. Weyand CM, Hunder NNH, Hicok KC, Hunder GG, Goronzy JJ. HLA–DRB1 alleles in polymyalgia rheumatica, giant cell arteritis, and rheumatoid arthritis. Arthritis Rheum 1994;37:514–20.
43. Zanelli E, Huizinga TW, Guerne PA, Vischer TL, Tiercy JM, Verduyn W, et al. An extended HLA-DQ-DR haplotype rather than DRB1 alone contributes to RA predisposition. Immunogenetics 1998;48:394–401.
44. Brünnler G, Haas JP, Fan LA, Petzl-Erler ML, Volgger A, Yao Z, et al. Promoter polymorphism: 12th International Histocompatibility Workshop study. In: Charron D, editor. HLA. Paris: Medical and Scientific International; 1997. p. 171–5.
45. Davenport MP, Quinn CL, Chicz RM, Green BN, Willis AC, Lane WS, et al. Naturally processed peptides from two disease-resistance-associated HLA-DR13 alleles show related sequence motifs and the effects of the dimorphism at position 86 of the HLA-DRβ chain. Proc Natl Acad Sci U S A 1995;92:6567–71.
46. Ilonen J, Hakala M, Reijonen H, Tiilikainen A. B27-bearing HLA haplotypes in rheumatoid arthritis: characterization in Finnish patients. Hum Immunol 1991;30:7–10.
47. Rantapää-Dahlqvist S, Nordmark LG, Bjelle A. HLA-B27 and involvement of sacroiliac joints in rheumatoid arthritis. J Rheumatol 1984;11:27–32.
48. Mu H, Chen JJ, Jiang Y, King M-C, Thomson G, Criswell LA. Tumor necrosis factor a microsatellite polymorphism is associated with rheumatoid arthritis severity through an interaction with the HLA–DRB1 shared epitope. Arthritis Rheum 1999;42:438–42.
49. Martínez A, Fernández-Arquero M, Pascual-Salcedo D, Conejero L, Alves H, Balsa A, et al. Primary association of tumor necrosis factor–region genetic markers with susceptibility to rheumatoid arthritis. Arthritis Rheum 2000;43:1366–70.
50. Mulcahy B, Waldron Lynch F, McDermott MF, Adams C, Amos CI, Zhu DK, et al. Genetic variability in the tumor necrosis factor-lymphotoxin region influences susceptibility to rheumatoid arthritis. Am J Hum Genet 1996;59:676–83.
51. Baerwald CGO, Panayi GS, Lanchbury JS. Corticotropin releasing hormone promoter region polymorphisms in rheumatoid arthritis. J Rheumatol 1997;24:215–6.
52. Brennan P, Hajeer A, Ong KR, Worthington J, John S, Thomson W, et al. Allelic markers close to prolactin are associated with HLA–DRB1 susceptibility alleles among women with rheumatoid arthritis and systemic lupus erythematosus. Arthritis Rheum 1997; 40:1383–6.
53. Cornélis F, Faure S, Martinez M, Prud'homme JF, Fritz P, Dib C, et al. New susceptibility locus for rheumatoid arthritis suggested by a genome-wide linkage study. Proc Natl Acad Sci U S A 1998;95: 10746–50.
54. Eksdale J, McNicholl J, Wordsworth P, Jonas B, Huizinga T, Field M, et al. Interleukin-10 microsatellite polymorphisms and IL-10 locus alleles in rheumatoid arthritis susceptibility. Lancet 1998; 352:1282–3.

ARTHRITIS & RHEUMATISM
Vol. 44, No. 2, February 2001, pp 323–330

The Association of Cigarette Smoking With Disease Outcome in Patients With Early Inflammatory Polyarthritis

Beverley J. Harrison, Alan J. Silman, Nicola J. Wiles, David G. I. Scott, and Deborah P. M. Symmons

Objective. **Cigarette smoking is known to increase rheumatoid factor (RF) and nodule formation in patients with rheumatoid arthritis (RA). In this study, we examined the influence of smoking on disease outcome at 3 years among patients newly presenting with inflammatory polyarthritis (IP).**

Methods. **We studied 486 patients with IP who were referred to the Norfolk Arthritis Register, of whom 323 (67%) satisfied the American College of Rheumatology 1987 criteria for RA. Smoking status was assessed at baseline. Disease outcome was assessed at 3 years, using measures of joint inflammation, functional disability, and radiologic damage. The influence of smoking on disease outcome was explored using logistic regression techniques, with patients who had never smoked as the referent group. Results are expressed as odds ratios (ORs), with their 95% confidence intervals (95% CIs).**

Results. **Current smokers were significantly more likely to be RF positive at baseline (47%) than were ex-smokers (34%) and never smokers (31%). After 3 years, rheumatoid nodules were significantly more common in smokers (13%) compared with ex-smokers/never smokers (4%), a relationship which persisted after adjusting for age and sex (OR 4.07, 95% CI 1.38–12). In contrast, after adjusting for age and sex, current smokers had significantly *fewer* swollen joints (OR 0.61, 95% CI 0.37–0.98). However, smoking status had no influence on the development of erosions or functional disability.**

Conclusion. **Despite smokers being more likely to develop nodules and to be RF positive, current smokers did *not* have higher levels of radiologic damage, and had *fewer* swollen joints. We hypothesize that this could be due to either the effect of cigarette smoking on the inflammatory response or other factors (e.g., reduced physical activity in smokers) which may limit joint inflammation and damage.**

Of the 10 epidemiologic studies which investigated cigarette smoking as a possible risk factor for the development of rheumatoid arthritis (RA) (1–10), 9 reported that smokers were more likely to develop RA (1,3–10). The strongest association was reported for smoking and seropositive RA. Others have reported that smokers (both with and without RA) are more likely to be rheumatoid factor (RF) positive (11–13). In contrast, there have been few studies on the influence of smoking on disease severity or progression.

The first study to systematically examine the association between smoking and RA severity assessed disease outcome cross-sectionally in 336 patients with established RA who were attending a university outpatient clinic in Iowa (14). After adjustment for potential confounders, smoking (expressed as the number of pack-years) was significantly associated with both being RF positive and having radiologic erosions. The association with erosions was primarily explained by an increased prevalence of RF among smokers. An accompanying editorial suggested that rheumatologists should therefore advise their RA patients to give up smoking (15).

Since then, 3 United Kingdom–based studies of patients with established RA have not shown an association between smoking and an adverse disease outcome (16–18), whereas 1 study showed higher levels of func-

Supported by the Arthritis Research Campaign, UK.

Beverley J. Harrison, MD, MRCP, Alan J. Silman, MD, FRCP, Nicola J. Wiles, BSc, David G. I. Scott, MD, FRCP, Deborah P. M. Symmons, MD, FRCP: University of Manchester, Manchester, UK.

Address correspondence and reprint requests to Beverley J. Harrison, MD, MRCP, ARC Epidemiology Unit, University of Manchester, Stopford Building, Oxford Road, Manchester M13 9PT, UK.

Submitted for publication February 17, 2000; accepted in revised form October 13, 2000.

tional disability among smokers (19). Recently, Wolfe examined the influence of cigarette smoking on disease outcome in a large cross-sectional study of 640 patients from Wichita, Kansas. In that study, patients who had smoked for more than 20 years had higher Larsen scores, although it was found that smoking had no influence on measures of disease activity, disability, or anxiety (20).

However, these reports were based on patients with established disease who were attending hospital clinics and in whom the association of smoking status with disease severity was assessed cross-sectionally. Such studies are subject to misclassification of exposure (smoking) status, which may have changed since disease onset. Further, patients with very mild disease (who may no longer seek medical care) and very severe disease (who may have died or may be unable to participate) are underrepresented. We therefore sought to investigate the influence of cigarette smoking on disease outcome in a large prospective cohort of patients with inflammatory polyarthritis (IP) who were newly presenting to primary care.

In this study, we investigated the influence of smoking status on disease outcome 3 years after the onset of disease in a large cohort of patients newly presenting with IP.

PATIENTS AND METHODS

Setting. Patients were recruited from the Norfolk Arthritis Register (NOAR), a population-based registry of patients newly presenting with IP. The registry covers all adults (ages ≥16 years) who are registered with a general practitioner (GP) in the region of the former Norwich Health Authority. This covers a population of approximately 485,000, predominantly (99%) of European Caucasoid origin. Details of the referral process have been published elsewhere (21).

Briefly, patients who have had swelling of at least 2 joints that has persisted for a minimum of 4 weeks are referred to the registry by their GPs and hospital doctors. Patients are later excluded from the registry if they are found to have an alternative diagnosis (other than RA, psoriatic arthritis, viral arthritis, or undifferentiated IP) that accounts for their symptoms.

Baseline evaluation. All patients were assessed by a research nurse in their own homes within 2 weeks of referral. A detailed history was obtained using a structured questionnaire. The following joints were examined for the presence of soft tissue swelling and/or tenderness: the distal interphalangeal, proximal interphalangeal, metacarpophalangeal, wrists, elbows, shoulders, knees, ankles, and the metatarsophalangeal joints. The presence of rheumatoid nodules was recorded, and patients were asked to complete the Health Assessment Questionnaire (HAQ) which was scored from 0–3 (22). Patients were asked to provide a blood sample, and RF was measured using a tube latex dilution technique. A titer of ≥1:40 was regarded as positive. Patients were then followed up annually for at least 3 years.

Smoking history. At the baseline assessment, patients were asked whether they smoked currently, in the past, or had never smoked. For current and ex-smokers, patients were asked the age at which they started (and stopped) smoking. Using this information, we calculated the number of years the patient had smoked when he or she was first seen. Details of whether patients had started or stopped smoking in the preceding year were recorded at the 1-, 2-, and 3-year followup visits.

Assessment of disease outcome. Disease outcome was assessed in 4 separate ways: persistent joint inflammation, functional disability, rheumatoid nodules, and radiologic damage. Patients were classified as having persistent synovitis if they had soft tissue swelling of at least 1 joint and/or had been treated with disease-modifying antirheumatic drugs (DMARDs) or oral steroids within the previous 3 months. In addition, the total number of swollen joints was counted. Functional disability was determined by the HAQ score at 3 years. The presence or absence of rheumatoid nodules was noted on clinical examination at 3 years.

For assessment of radiologic damage, subjects were asked to have radiographs taken of their hands and feet at the 1-year followup visit. The radiographs were scored by 2 observers (DPMS and BJH) working independently. The following joints were graded from 0–5 using Larsen's system (23): the proximal interphalangeal joints, the metacarpophalangeal joints, the wrists, and the second through fifth metatarsophalangeal joints. A third observer (DGIS) arbitrated in cases of disagreement about whether patients had erosions or not. Those who did not have erosions at that visit had further radiographs taken at the 2-year followup visit. Since this was a community-based cohort that included many patients with mild disease, only those subjects who displayed at least 2 of the 6 American College of Rheumatology (ACR; formerly, the American Rheumatism Association) classification criteria for RA (excluding radiographs) (24) were asked to have radiographs taken. The results of the latest available radiographic assessment were used for analysis.

Transformation of data. For the purposes of analysis, we categorized the data into the following groups: 1) persistent synovitis (present/absent), 2) total number of swollen joints (divided by tertiles), 3) HAQ score (divided by tertiles), 4) nodules (present/absent), 5) radiologic erosions (present/absent), 6) total number of eroded joints (divided by tertiles), and 7) total Larsen score (divided by tertiles).

Statistical analysis. Clinical and demographic variables at baseline and 3 years were compared according to baseline smoking status (never smoked/ex-smoker/current smoker). Differences were compared using the Mann-Whitney U test (2-tailed) for continuous variables, and using the risk difference and 95% confidence intervals (95% CIs) for categorical variables.

Logistic regression techniques were used to evaluate the independent contribution of smoking status to disease outcome, adjusting for age (divided by tertiles) and sex. Smoking status was classified at baseline using 2 methods: 1) never smoked/ex-smoker/current smoker, and 2) never smoked and categories of number of years smoked, divided by tertiles

Table 1. Baseline demographic and clinical characteristics in relation to smoking status in 486 patients newly presenting with inflammatory polyarthritis*

	Never smoked (n = 151)	Ex-smoker (n = 209)	Current smoker (n = 126)	Difference, current vs. ex-/never smokers†
Age, median (range) years	54 (20–86)	57 (19–88)	50 (18–82)	$P = 0.02$
No. (%) females	132 (88)	127 (61)	72 (57)	−15 (−25, −5)
Disease duration, median (range) months	4.6 (1–32)	4.7 (1–36)	5.3 (1–26)	$P = 0.69$
No. (%) with RA	77 (51)	97 (46)	57 (45)	−3 (−13, 7)
No. RF positive/no. tested (%)	32/120 (27)	50/181 (28)	44/104 (42)	15 (4, 26)
HAQ score, median (range)	0.88 (0–3)	0.75 (0–3)	0.81 (0–2.5)	$P = 0.65$
No. of swollen joints, median (range)	8 (0–42)	7 (0–44)	6.5 (0–35)	$P = 0.11$
No. (%) with nodules	13 (9)	14 (7)	10 (8)	0 (−5, 6)

* Rheumatoid arthritis (RA) was defined according to the American College of Rheumatology (formerly, the American Rheumatism Association) 1987 classification criteria (24), applied in list format. RF = rheumatoid factor (positive at a titer ≥1:40); HAQ = Health Assessment Questionnaire.
† Values are either *P* values, which were determined by Mann-Whitney 2-tailed U test, or percentage risk differences (95% confidence interval).

(0–18 years, 19–34 years, and ≥35 years). For dichotomous outcomes, conventional logistic regression was used, and for outcomes with more than 2 categories, ordinal regression techniques were employed. The independent association of each of the explanatory variables with outcome was expressed as the odds ratio (OR) and 95% CI.

RESULTS

Between January 1990 and February 1993, 635 patients were referred to NOAR. Of these, 56 were later excluded because of an alternative diagnosis. Of the remaining 579 patients, 486 (84%) were followed up for 3 years, 24 (4%) died, 41 (7%) declined further participation, and 28 (5%) were lost to followup. The proportion of patients lost to followup did not differ according to smoking status. The 486 patients followed up for 3 years comprise the study population, of whom 432 were assessed at 3 years by a research nurse and the remaining 54 by postal questionnaire.

Of the 486 patients studied, the median disease duration at the initial assessment was 4.8 months, and 406 (84%) had a disease duration of <12 months. The ACR 1987 classification criteria for RA were applied at baseline using both the traditional list format and the classification tree format, which is more sensitive in early disease (24). The proportion of patients who satisfied these criteria was 231 (48%) for the list format (excluding radiographs) and 323 (67%) for the classification tree format.

A total of 368 patients were judged by the research nurse to have satisfied the criteria to be radiographed. Radiographs were available for 335 of these patients (22 patients declined having a radiograph and 11 films were mislaid). The median time from disease onset to the latest available radiograph was 22 months, and was not different among the 3 smoking status groups.

At the initial assessment, 151 patients (31%) had never smoked, 209 (43%) had smoked in the past, and 126 (26%) were current smokers. In the 209 ex-smokers, the median time since the patient stopped smoking was 13 years (interquartile range 4–22). Followup data on smoking status were available for 422 patients. Of the 110 current smokers at baseline, 11 stopped smoking at 1 year, a further 5 stopped at 2 years, and 4 stopped at 3 years. Therefore, 20 of 110 patients (18%) had stopped smoking after disease onset. Only 1 of the never smokers and 4 of the ex-smokers started smoking during the same period of followup.

Table 1 shows the demographic and clinical characteristics of the study patients in relation to smoking status assessed at the same time. Since there were no important differences between ex-smokers and never smokers with respect to any of the characteristics measured at baseline or at 3 years, we combined these 2 groups for the analyses.

As shown in Table 1, current smokers were younger than ex-smokers/never smokers, and were more

Table 2. Clinical outcome at 3 years in relation to smoking status at baseline in 486 patients newly presenting with inflammatory polyarthritis*

	Never smoked (n = 151)	Ex-smoker (n = 209)	Current smoker (n = 126)	Difference, current vs. ex-/never smokers†
No. (%) with persistent disease	106 (70)	147 (70)	79 (63)	−8 (−17, 3)
No. of swollen joints, median (range)	2 (0–36)	1 (0–32)	0 (0–39)	$P = 0.03$
No. (%) with ≥5 swollen joints	46 (31)	59 (28)	26 (21)	−9 (−17, −1)
HAQ score, median (range)	0.63 (0–2.88)	0.5 (0–2.75)	0.63 (0–3)	$P = 0.47$
No. with HAQ score ≥1/no. tested (%)	58/147 (39)	63/206 (31)	52/124 (42)	8 (−2, 18)
No. (%) with nodules	5 (3)	10 (5)	16 (13)	9 (2, 15)
No. (%) treated with DMARDs/steroids	74 (49)	95 (45)	66 (52)	5 (−5, 16)

* Treatment with disease-modifying antirheumatic drugs (DMARDs)/steroids represents current or previous treatment. HAQ = Health Assessment Questionnaire.
† Values are either *P* values, which were determined by Mann-Whitney 2-tailed U test, or percentage risk differences (95% confidence interval).

likely to be male than were patients who had never smoked. Smokers were significantly more likely to be RF positive at baseline (42%) than ex-smokers (28%) and never smokers (27%). However, despite this finding, there were no other clinical differences (number of swollen joints, HAQ score, and presence of nodules) at baseline. Furthermore, there was no association between smoking status and disease characteristics as analyzed separately in males and females (data not shown).

Table 2 shows the clinical aspects of disease outcome at 3 years in relation to smoking status at baseline. The number of swollen joints in current smokers was significantly lower than that in ex-smokers/never smokers, and fewer current smokers had ≥5 swollen joints. There was also a trend toward fewer patients having persistent disease. In contrast, nodules were more frequently observed in smokers (13%) than in ex-smokers (5%) or never smokers (3%). There was no significant difference in HAQ scores according to smoking status. A similar proportion of smokers and nonsmokers had been treated with DMARDs/steroids. Furthermore, the types of DMARDs prescribed did not differ between the smoking status groups.

Radiologic outcome in the 335 patients with available radiographs is shown in Table 3. There was no difference in the frequency of erosions and the number of eroded joints in the smokers. There was a trend toward less radiologic damage (measured by the Larsen score) in current smokers, an effect which was enhanced when the analysis was restricted to patients with radiologic erosions. However, the results did not achieve statistical significance.

Table 3. Radiologic outcome in relation to smoking status at baseline in 335 patients newly presenting with inflammatory polyarthritis*

	Never smoked (n = 117)	Ex-smoker (n = 140)	Current smoker (n = 78)	Difference, current vs. ex-/never smokers†
No. (%) with erosions	49 (42)	53 (38)	35 (45)	5 (−7, 18)
Larsen score, median (range)	5.5 (0–73)	2 (0–56)	2.5 (0–62)	$P = 0.8$
Larsen score, median (range)‡	20 (2–73)	10 (2–56)	15 (2–62)	$P = 0.7$
No. of eroded joints, median (range)‡	3 (1–17)	2 (1–12)	3 (1–18)	$P = 0.4$

* The median time from disease onset to the latest available radiograph was 22 months.
† Values are either *P* values, which were determined by Mann-Whitney 2-tailed U test, or percentage risk differences (95% confidence interval).
‡ Analysis restricted to patients with radiologic erosions (n = 137).

Table 4. Multivariate analysis of the influence of smoking status on clinical outcome at 3 years in patients newly presenting with inflammatory polyarthritis*

Smoking status	No. of swollen joints, OR (95% CI)†	HAQ score, OR (95% CI)‡	Nodules, OR (95% CI)
Never smoked§	1.00	1.00	1.00
Smoked ≥0–18 years	0.66 (0.40, 1.09)	0.62 (0.38, 0.99)	0.78 (0.18, 3.43)
Smoked 19–34 years	0.94 (0.57, 1.53)	0.96 (0.60, 1.53)	1.98 (0.61, 6.39)
Smoked ≥35 years	0.79 (0.46, 1.36)	1.62 (0.96, 2.75)	4.22 (1.31, 13.6)
Never smoked§	1.00	1.00	1.00
Ex-smoker	0.90 (0.59, 1.38)	0.82 (0.54, 1.22)	1.21 (0.39, 3.74)
Current smoker	0.61 (0.37, 0.98)	1.22 (0.76, 1.95)	4.07 (1.38, 12.0)

* Odds ratios (ORs) were adjusted for age and sex. HAQ = Health Assessment Questionnaire; 95% CI = 95% confidence interval.
† Divided by tertiles: 0, 1–4, and ≥5.
‡ Divided by tertiles: 0–0.13, 0.25–1, and ≥1.125.
§ Referent group.

Given the differences in smoking status in relation to age and sex, we examined the influence of smoking status on disease outcome, adjusting for these variables. Table 4 shows the results of multivariate analysis for clinical outcomes at 3 years. After adjusting for age and sex, current smoking was associated with significantly fewer swollen joints at 3 years (OR 0.61, 95% CI 0.37–0.98). However, smokers were more likely to develop rheumatoid nodules, especially those who had smoked for a longer time prior to disease onset (OR 4.22, 95% CI 1.31–13.6 for patients who had smoked ≥35 years). Patients who had smoked for a relatively short period of time (0–18 years) were *less* likely to have high disability scores than patients who had never smoked, whereas those who had smoked for longer (≥35 years) were more likely to be disabled.

Table 5 shows the results of the multivariate analysis for radiologic outcome. After adjusting for age and sex, current smokers had a similar chance of developing erosions and had similar Larsen scores compared with never smokers.

Table 5. Multivariate analysis of the influence of smoking status on radiologic outcome in patients newly presenting with inflammatory polyarthritis*

Smoking status	Erosions, OR (95% CI)	Larsen score, OR (95% CI)†
Never smoked‡	1.00	1.00
Smoked ≥0–18 years	0.57 (0.29, 1.11)	0.61 (0.34, 1.10)
Smoked 19–34 years	1.32 (0.71, 2.44)	0.79 (0.44, 1.41)
Smoked ≥35 years	0.77 (0.40, 1.47)	0.60 (0.33, 1.09)
Never smoked‡	1.00	1.00
Ex-smoker	0.75 (0.44, 1.27)	0.60 (0.37, 0.98)
Current smoker	1.06 (0.58, 1.95)	0.79 (0.45, 1.40)

* Odds ratios (ORs) were adjusted for age and sex. 95% CI = 95% confidence interval.
† Divided by tertiles: 0, 1–8, and ≥9.
‡ Referent group.

DISCUSSION

This is the first study to investigate prospectively the influence of cigarette smoking on disease outcome in patients newly presenting with IP. Smoking status was determined close to the time of disease onset, at a median of 4.8 months from the first reported joint swelling. We have confirmed previous reports of an association between current smoking and being seropositive for RF. Although the frequency of rheumatoid nodules was similar at baseline, smokers were more likely to develop nodules with time. Both RF and nodules are adverse prognostic factors (25). Therefore, we were surprised to find that smokers were less likely to have persistent synovitis at 3 years and had fewer swollen joints. In addition, there was no adverse influence of smoking on radiologic damage (as measured by erosions), the number of eroded joints, and the total Larsen score. This suggests that cigarette smoking combines 2 conflicting influences on disease outcome: a detrimental effect mediated by RF, and an important protective effect, which is, as yet, unexplained.

Saag et al recently investigated the association of the number of pack-years of smoking with disease severity in 336 patients with established RA (14). Their finding of an increase in RF and nodules in smokers is in agreement with the results from our study. However, they found that smokers were more likely to develop erosions, an effect which was explained by an increased prevalence of RF among smokers. Of note, smoking was only associated with the Larsen score at low levels of radiologic damage, and those authors suggested that smoking was therefore associated with the initiation (rather than severity) of erosive damage. In contrast, in a larger study of 640 North American patients, Wolfe reported that higher Larsen scores were found in patients who had smoked for longer periods of time, an effect which was confined to patients who had smoked for more than 20 years (20).

The differences in study design between these studies and the present NOAR study may partly explain the variation in the results. Both the studies by Saag et al and Wolfe were cross-sectional and included patients with established RA (median disease duration 14 years). It is therefore possible that smokers with milder disease were no longer seeking medical care or were less likely to respond to the questionnaire. In the present NOAR study, 18% of smokers stopped smoking after their initial assessment visit. When we analyzed the association of smoking status assessed at 3 years (rather than at baseline), there was no difference in the results (data not shown). However, if we had followed up the patients for a longer period of time, then changes in smoking status may have been found to influence disease outcome with time. We did not collect data on the number of cigarettes smoked, and were therefore unable to examine the influence of smoking defined as the number of pack-years.

Another possible explanation for our findings is that smokers with more severe disease had died prematurely, so that we were unable to detect an association between smoking and more severe disease among those who survived to be followed up at 3 years. Of the 24 patients who died before the 3-year assessment, 4 (17%) were current smokers, 13 (54%) were ex-smokers, and 6 (25%) had never smoked (smoking status was not known in 1 patient). Among these patients, the median HAQ score at baseline was higher in the never smokers (1.75) compared with the ex-smokers (1.5) and current smokers (1.0). Review of the death certificates showed that none of the deaths were related to RA. There is thus no evidence to support the possibility that smokers with more severe disease had died.

There have been 4 other reports, published in letter/abstract form, of the influence of smoking status on disease severity (16–19). All included UK-based patients with established RA. Two of those studies reported a higher prevalence of RF but similar Larsen scores in smokers and nonsmokers (16,17). Three noted similar HAQ scores in smokers (16–18), although Hamilton et al (19) reported that the median HAQ score in current smokers (2.125) was higher than that observed in ex-smokers (2.0) and nonsmokers (1.875). In a larger study of North American patients recently published by Wolfe (20), there was no influence of smoking on the erythrocyte sedimentation rate, tender joint count, or HAQ score. We did not find an association between smoking and functional disability in our study. However, the significance of the HAQ score depends on disease duration, since it predominantly reflects joint inflammation in early disease and joint damage in established disease (26). Further, the HAQ is linked to social deprivation (27), which is also associated with cigarette smoking (28). Therefore, smoking may be associated with HAQ scores in established disease due to a common association with psychosocial variables.

There are 2 explanations for the observation that smokers appear to have a better outcome than nonsmokers. First, the relationship may actually be due to lifestyle factors which are associated with smoking. Alternatively, cigarette smoking may have a direct biologic effect that suppresses the inflammatory process. There are a number of lifestyle characteristics that are associated with smoking, including increased alcohol consumption (29), poor diet (30), and low social class (28). However, these factors would not be expected to *improve* outcome. Smokers tend to be thinner and less physically active, which might exert less stress on the joints and therefore retard damage. We did not measure body mass index or physical activity in the NOAR study. Of interest, smoking has been reported to protect against the development and severity of osteoarthritis (31–33). A proposed explanation for this was that smokers were more likely to have osteopenia such that subchondral bone was more deformable when subjected to impact loads (34). The same factors may underlie the findings of Wolfe and Zwillich (35), who reported that smoking was a significant protective factor for having joint replacement surgery in patients with RA.

Smoking has a number of effects on the immune system. For example, smoking has an antiestrogen action (36), and it has been reported that estrogens can suppress collagen-induced arthritis in mice (an animal model of RA) (37) and may also reduce disease activity in humans with RA (38). We would therefore expect to find that smokers had *more* active disease due to lower estrogen levels, which was not the case in our study. However, smokers also have high levels of androgens (39) and sex hormone binding globulin (40), which may suppress the immune response (41). Immune dysfunction has been reported in smokers with abnormalities in T lymphocytes (42), a reduction in natural killer cells (43), and depression of humoral and cell-mediated immunity (44,45). Spector and Blake proposed that smoking may reduce the number of antigen-presenting cells and therefore ameliorate inflammation (46). A parallel may be drawn between this and the improvement in disease activity which has been reported in patients with inflammatory bowel disease (47,48) and acne (49). Of particular relevance to our study is a recent paper from Manthorpe et al (50) in which they reported that smokers with primary Sjögren's syndrome had lower levels of focal lip sialadenitis/focus scores.

It has previously been reported that smokers with RA are more likely to develop vasculitis (51) and interstitial lung disease (52). In a separate study performed within the NOAR cohort, 77 patients with RA were assessed for the presence of extraarticular disease. In that group of patients, the prevalence of extraarticular disease (including nodules, peripheral neuropathy, vasculitis, and sicca syndrome) was also higher in current smokers (76%) compared with ex-smokers/never smokers (55%): relative risk 1.38, 95% CI 1.00–1.92 (Hailwood S: personal communication). It is possible that the association of smoking with vasculitis and nodules is due to vascular endothelial damage. The mechanisms underlying the association of smoking with joint inflammation may be different, which could explain why we found smoking to be associated with nodules but not with increased joint inflammation. In addition, a dissociation between nodules/vasculitis and synovitis is sometimes recognized clinically.

We have previously reported results from a case–control study performed within the NOAR population to identify risk factors for the development of RA (8). We identified cigarette smoking and a history of blood transfusion as important risk factors. Blood transfusion has also been reported to have a number of effects on the immune system, with an overall tendency toward immunosuppression (53). Recently, Bruinsma et al noted that blood transfusion improved disease activity in patients with RA (54). Therefore, it is possible that the "immunosuppressive" effects of smoking and blood transfusion may both predispose to the development of RA and improve outcome.

In summary, among patients newly presenting with IP, cigarette smoking is associated with an increased prevalence of RF and nodules. Despite this, current smokers did not have a worse prognosis and were less likely to have persistent synovitis. We are keen to determine whether this relationship persists at longer followup times in the NOAR cohort and whether this finding can be confirmed by other investigators in prospective studies of patients with early disease. Further work on the influence of cigarette smoking on the immune system is also warranted.

ACKNOWLEDGMENTS

We are grateful to the Arthritis Research Campaign, UK, for funding this study. We thank the GPs and hospital staff of the Norwich Health Authority for their dedication in referring patients to the Register. We also acknowledge the continued hard work of the NOAR research nurses and staff. We are grateful to Dr. Sarah Hailwood for providing data on extraarticular disease in the NOAR cohort.

REFERENCES

1. Vessey MP, Villard-Mackintosh L, Yeates D. Oral contraceptives, cigarette smoking and other factors in relation to arthritis. Contraception 1987;35:457–64.
2. Hazes JMW, Dijkmans BAC, Vandenbroucke JP, de Vries RRP, Cats A. Lifestyle and the risk of rheumatoid arthritis: cigarette smoking and alcohol consumption. Ann Rheum Dis 1990;49: 980–2.
3. Hernández-Avila M, Liang MH, Willett WC, Stampfer MJ, Colditz GA, Rosner B, et al. Reproductive factors, smoking, and the risk for rheumatoid arthritis. Epidemiology 1990;1:285–91.
4. Heliövaara M, Aho K, Aromaa A, Knekt P, Reunanen A. Smoking and the risk of rheumatoid arthritis. J Rheumatol 1993;20:1830–5.
5. Silman AJ. Smoking and the risk of rheumatoid arthritis. J Rheumatol 1993;20:1815–6.
6. Voigt LF, Koepsell TD, Nelson JL, Dugowson CE, Daling JR. Smoking, obesity, alcohol consumption, and the risk of rheumatoid arthritis. Epidemiology 1994;5:525–32.
7. Masi AT, Fecht T, Aldag JC, Comstock GW, Hoffman S, Malamet RL. History of currently smoking cigarettes, but not years of education, correlated with subsequent development of rheumatoid arthritis: preliminary findings from a community-wide, prospective, nested, case-control study [abstract]. Arthritis Rheum 1996;39 Suppl 9:S301.
8. Symmons DPM, Bankhead CR, Harrison BJ, Brennan P, Barrett EM, Scott DGI, et al. Blood transfusion, smoking, and obesity as risk factors for the development of rheumatoid arthritis: results from a primary care–based incident case–control study in Norfolk, England. Arthritis Rheum 1997;40:1955–61.
9. Karlson EW, Lee I-M, Cook NR, Manson JE, Buring JE, Hennekens CH. A retrospective cohort study of cigarette smoking and risk of rheumatoid arthritis in female health professionals. Arthritis Rheum 1999;42:910–7.
10. Uhlig T, Hagen KB, Kvien TK. Current tobacco smoking, formal education, and the risk of rheumatoid arthritis. J Rheumatol 1999;26:47–54.
11. Mathews JD, Whittingham S, Hooper BM, Mackay JR. Association of autoantibodies with smoking, cardiovascular morbidity, and death in the Busselton population. Lancet 1973;2:754–8.
12. Tuomi T, Heliövaara M, Palosuo T, Aho K. Smoking, lung function, and rheumatoid factors. Ann Rheum Dis 1990;49:753–6.
13. Jónsson T, Thorsteinsson J, Valdimarsson H. Does smoking stimulate rheumatoid factor production in non-rheumatic individuals? APMIS 1998;106:970–4.
14. Saag KG, Cerhan JR, Kolluri S, Ohashi K, Hunninghake GW, Schwartz DA. Cigarette smoking and rheumatoid arthritis severity. Ann Rheum Dis 1997;56:463–9.
15. Deighton C. Smoke gets in your joints? Ann Rheum Dis 1997;56: 453–4.
16. McDonagh JE, Walker DJ. Smoking and rheumatoid arthritis—

observations from a multicase family study: comment on the article by Silman et al [letter]. Arthritis Rheum 1997;40:594.
17. Houssien DA, Scott DL, Jonsson T. Smoking, rheumatoid factors and rheumatoid arthritis [letter]. Ann Rheum Dis 1998;57:175–6.
18. Richards S, Erhardt C, Scott DL. Smoking and disability in rheumatoid arthritis [abstract]. Ann Rheum Dis 1999; EULAR Abstracts 1999:68.
19. Hamilton JD, Thomson E, Porter D, Hunter JA, Madhok R, Capell HA. Lifestyle influences on outcomes in rheumatoid arthritis [abstract]. Ann Rheum Dis 1999;EULAR Abstracts 1999: 89.
20. Wolfe F. The effect of smoking on clinical, laboratory, and radiographic status in rheumatoid arthritis. J Rheumatol 2000;27: 630–7.
21. Symmons DPM, Barrett EM, Bankhead CR, Scott DGI, Silman AJ. The incidence of rheumatoid arthritis in the United Kingdom: results from the Norfolk Arthritis Register. Br J Rheumatol 1994;33:735–9.
22. Fries JF, Spitz P, Kraines RG. Measurement of patient outcome in arthritis. Arthritis Rheum 1980;23:137–45.
23. Larsen A, Dale K, Eek M. Radiographic assessment of rheumatoid arthritis and related conditions by standard reference films. Acta Radiol [Diagn] 1977;18:481–91.
24. Arnett FC, Edworthy SM, Bloch DA, McShane DJ, Fries JF, Cooper NS, et al. The American Rheumatism Association 1987 revised criteria for the classification of rheumatoid arthritis. Arthritis Rheum 1988;31:315–24.
25. Young A, van der Heijde DMFM. Can we predict aggressive disease? Baillieres Clin Rheumatol 1997;11:27–48.
26. Drossaers-Bakker KW, de Buck M, van Zeben D, Zwinderman AH, Breedveld FC, Hazes JMW. Long-term course and outcome of functional capacity in rheumatoid arthritis: the effect of disease activity and radiologic damage over time. Arthritis Rheum 1999; 42:1854–60.
27. McEntegart A, Morrison E, Capell HA, Duncan MR, Porter D, Madhok R, et al. Effect of social deprivation on disease severity and outcome in patients with rheumatoid arthritis. Ann Rheum Dis 1997;56:410–3.
28. Bergen AW, Caporaso N. Cigarette smoking. J Natl Cancer Inst 1999;91:1365–75.
29. Miller NS, Gold MS. Comorbid cigarette and alcohol addiction: epidemiology and treatment. J Addict Dis 1998;17:55–66.
30. Shahar DR, Kristal-Boneh E, Froom P, Harari G, Ribak J. Smoking, diet, and health behaviours among lead-exposed blue-collar workers. Int J Occup Environ Health 1999;5:101–6.
31. Felson DT, Anderson JJ, Naimark A, Hannan MT, Kannel WB, Meenan RF. Does smoking protect against osteoarthritis? Arthritis Rheum 1989;32:166–72.
32. Felson DT, Zhang Y, Hannan MT, Naimark A, Weissman B, Aliabadi P, et al. Risk factors for incident radiographic knee osteoarthritis in the elderly: the Framingham Study. Arthritis Rheum 1997;40:728–33.
33. Samanta A, Jones A, Regan M, Wilson S, Doherty M. Is osteoarthritis in women affected by hormonal changes or smoking? Br J Rheumatol 1993;32:366–70.
34. Radin EL. Mechanical aspects of osteoarthritis. Bull Rheum Dis 1976;26:862–5.
35. Wolfe F, Zwillich SH. The long-term outcomes of rheumatoid arthritis: a 23-year prospective, longitudinal study of total joint replacement and its predictors in 1,600 patients with rheumatoid arthritis. Arthritis Rheum 1998;41:1072–82.
36. Michnovicz JJ, Herschcopf RJ, Naganuma H, Bradlow HL, Fishman J. Increased 2-hydroxylation of estradiol as a possible mechanism for the anti-estrogenic action of cigarettes smoking. N Engl J Med 1986;315:1305–9.
37. Holmdahl R, Jansson L, Andersson M. Female sex hormones suppress development of collagen-induced arthritis in mice. Arthritis Rheum 1986;29:1501–9.
38. Hall GM, Daniels M, Huskisson EC, Spector TD. A randomised controlled trial of the effect of hormone replacement therapy on disease activity in postmenopausal rheumatoid arthritis. Ann Rheum Dis 1994;53:112–6.
39. Khaw KT, Tazuke S, Barrett-Connor E. Cigarette smoking and levels of adrenal androgens in postmenopausal women. N Engl J Med 1988;318:1705–9.
40. Daniel M, Martin AD, Faiman C. Sex hormones and adipose tissue distribution in premenopausal cigarette smokers. Int J Obes Relat Metab Disord 1992;16:245–54.
41. Grossman CJ. Regulation of the immune system by sex steroids. Endocr Rev 1984;5:435–55.
42. Hughes DA, Haslam PL, Townshend PJ, Turner-Warwick M. Numerical and functional alterations in circulatory lymphocytes in cigarette smokers. Clin Exp Immunol 1985;61:459–66.
43. Ginnis LC, Ryu JH, Rogol PR, Sprince NL, Oliver LC, Largon CJ. Natural killer cell activity in cigarette smokers and asbestos workers. Am Rev Respir Dis 1985;131:831–4.
44. Hersey P, Prendergast D, Edwards A. Effects of cigarette smoking on the immune system. Med J Aust 1983;2:425–9.
45. Burton RC. Smoking, immunity and cancer. Med J Aust 1983;2: 411–2.
46. Spector TD, Blake DR. Effect of cigarette smoking on Langerhans' cells [letter]. Lancet 1988;2:1028.
47. De Castella H. Non-smoking: a feature of ulcerative colitis [letter]. Br Med J 1982;284:1706.
48. Roberts CJ, Diggle R. Non-smoking: a feature of ulcerative colitis [letter]. Br Med J 1982;285:440.
49. Mills CM, Peters CJ, Finlay AY. Does smoking influence acne? Clin Exp Dermatol 1993;18:100–1.
50. Manthorpe R, Benoni C, Jacobsson L, Kirtava Z, Larsson A, Liedholm R, et al. Lower frequency of focal lip sialadenitis (focus score) in smoking patients: can tobacco diminish the salivary gland involvement as judged by histological examination and anti-SSA/Ro and anti-SSB/La antibodies in Sjögren's syndrome? Ann Rheum Dis 2000;59:54–60.
51. Struthers GR, Scott DL, Delamere JP, Sheppeard H, Kitt M. Smoking and rheumatoid vasculitis. Rheumatol Int 1981;1:145–6.
52. Saag KG, Kolluri S, Koehnke RK, Georgou TA, Rachow JW, Hunninghake GW, et al. Rheumatoid arthritis lung disease: determinants of radiographic and physiologic abnormalities. Arthritis Rheum 1996;39:1711–9.
53. Bordon JO, Blajchman MA. Immunosuppressive effects of allogenic blood transfusions: implications for patients with cancer. Hematol Oncol Clin North Am 1995;9:205–18.
54. Van der Horst-Bruinsma IE, Huizinga TWJ, Lagaay EM, Hazes JMW, Breedveld FC, Schreuder GMT, et al. The influence of a partially HLA-matched blood transfusion on the disease activity of rheumatoid arthritis. Rheumatol 1999;38:53–8.

ARTHRITIS & RHEUMATISM
Vol. 44, No. 2, February 2001, pp 331–338

Correlation of Power Doppler Sonography With Vascularity of the Synovial Tissue of the Knee Joint in Patients With Osteoarthritis and Rheumatoid Arthritis

Markus Walther, Harry Harms, Veit Krenn, Stephan Radke, Trutz-Peter Faehndrich, and Frank Gohlke

Objective. **To examine the significance of power Doppler sonography (PDS) in the diagnosis of synovial hypertrophy of the knee joint by verifying and comparing the PDS findings with histopathologic findings of synovial membrane vascularity.**

Methods. **The knee joints of 23 patients who were undergoing arthroplasty of the knee joint because of osteoarthritis or rheumatoid arthritis were examined with ultrasound before arthroplasty. The vascularity of the synovial membrane was classified semiquantitatively using PDS. A sample of synovial tissue was obtained during the arthroplasty, and the vascularity of the synovial tissue was evaluated by immunohistochemistry (factor VIII) and was graded qualitatively by a pathologist who was unaware of the PDS findings. The visual qualitative grading by the examiner was controlled by analyzing PDS images and histologic samples using a digital image evaluation system.**

Results. **The correlation between the qualitative PDS results and the qualitative grading of the vascularity by the pathologist was 0.89 by Spearman's ρ ($P < 0.01$). The Pearson correlation coefficient between the digital analysis of the PDS images and the digital analysis of the tissue sections was 0.81 ($P < 0.01$). Digital image analysis and qualitative grading by the examiner had a correlation of 0.89 by Spearman's ρ ($P < 0.01$) for the PDS images. The correlation between the qualitative estimation of vascularity by the pathologist and the digital image analysis was 0.88 by Spearman's ρ ($P < 0.01$).**

Conclusion. **In the present study, PDS proved to be a reliable diagnostic method for qualitative grading of the vascularity of the synovial tissue. In clinical practice, PDS allows further differentiation of the hypertrophic synovium.**

Power Doppler sonography (PDS) was first introduced for cardiologic investigations in the 1980s (1,2). Since it proved useful in cardiology, PDS was soon applied to other medical diagnostic problems (3–11). PDS characteristically encodes the amplitude of the power spectral density of the Doppler signal, rather than the mean Doppler frequency shift as in conventional color Doppler ultrasound methods (12). While conventional color Doppler sonography is well suited for evaluating high-velocity flow in large vessels, it is less effective in detecting low-velocity blood flow at the microvascular level (13–15). The value of PDS in the detection of soft tissue hyperemia was reported by Newman et al in 1994 (16). Recently, its value for estimating the fraction of moving blood in tissue was confirmed (17–19).

There are several studies on the visualization of the synovial membrane with PDS in osteoarthritis (OA) and rheumatoid arthritis (RA) (20–24), but to our knowledge, no study has been published which compares PDS findings and histopathologic findings of vascularity of the synovial membrane. The present study evaluated the correlation between PDS imaging of the vascularity of the knee joint synovial tissue and histopathologic inspection of the same tissue in order to assess the value of PDS in the imaging of synovitis.

Markus Walther, MD, Harry Harms, PhD, Veit Krenn, MD (current address: Charité University Hospital, Berlin, Germany), Stephan Radke, MD, Trutz-Peter Faehndrich, Frank Gohlke, MD, PhD: University of Wuerzburg, Wuerzburg, Germany.

Address correspondence and reprint requests to Frank Gohlke, MD, PhD, Department of Orthopedic Surgery, University of Wuerzburg, Brettreichstrasse 11, 97074 Wuerzburg, Germany.

Submitted for publication June 14, 2000; accepted in revised form September 27, 2000.

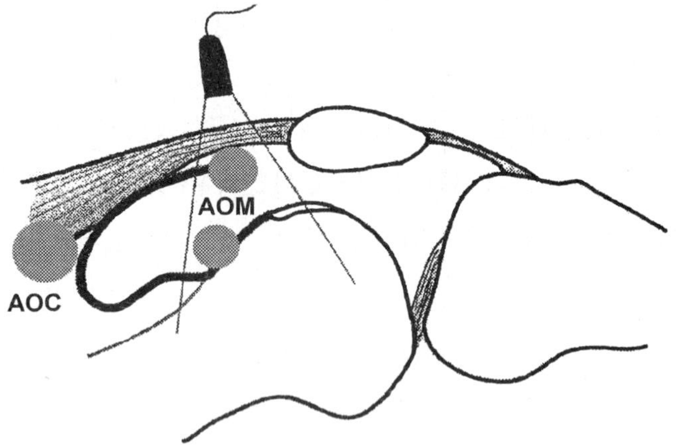

Figure 1. Power Doppler sonography of the synovial membrane of the knee at the upper recesses. AOM = area of measurement and specimen of the synovial tissue; AOC = area of calibration.

PATIENTS AND METHODS

Patients. We evaluated 23 patients (6 men, 17 women), with a mean age of 69 years (range 29–86 years). Ten patients fulfilled at least 4 of the 7 American College of Rheumatology (formerly, the American Rheumatism Association) criteria for RA (25); 13 had OA of the knee joint. All patients had severe knee pain and underwent total knee arthroplasty with synovectomy.

Ultrasound examination. A maximum of 12 hours prior to the operation, the knee joints were examined with an ultrasound real-time scanner (Elegra model; Siemens, Munich, Germany). Ultrasonography was carried out using a 7.5-MHz electronic linear transducer. Standardized anatomical section planes of the scans in the 3 recesses of the knee (suprapatellar and lateral and medial parapatellar) were used as prescribed by Rubaltelli et al (26). The synovial thickness of the suprapatellar recess was documented, as well as the presence of any effusion.

The synovial tissue was visualized using PDS in the suprapatellar recess of the knee joint (27) (Figure 1). Power Doppler settings were standardized with a pulse repetition frequency (PRF) of 1,100 Hz. Although greater low-flow sensitivity can be achieved at lower PRFs (9,16,28), the PRF was adjusted to 1,100 Hz to reduce flash artifact (4,29). This setting worked well in all cases, although in some patients, a lower PRF would have been possible.

For optimum sensitivity, the PDS gain was set as suggested by Rubin and colleagues (17,30). This requires manual elevation of the PDS gain-level until the color box is almost uniformly filled with the first indication of color and with only the minimum amount of the next highest signal just beginning to appear. This procedure can be performed either with the scan wiped clean of gel and contacting only air (6) or after applying the gel-covered transducer to the patient, at the depth of the region of interest (9), which in the present study, was the quadriceps muscle, just superior to the suprapatellar recess (Figure 1). This setting resulted in gains of 63–68 dB (8,23,29,31). Using this method of adjustment (17), depth dependency, effects of blood pressure and medication, as well as heart rate and blood viscosity can be expected to have the same influence on the synovial tissue and the reference tissue of the quadriceps muscle and is therefore of minor importance for the measurement.

Two fully trained and experienced examiners (MW and SR) performed the sonography, which took 10–20 minutes for each patient. Neither examiner was aware of the clinical and laboratory findings in the patients.

Each knee was evaluated and graded on a scale of 1–4 according to the amount of the joint effusion and the thickness of the synovial tissue at the suprapatellar recesses (1 = no effusion/hypertrophic synovial tissue, 2 = mild effusion/hypertrophic synovial tissue, 3 = moderate effusion/hypertrophic synovial tissue, and 4 = marked effusion/hypertrophic synovial tissue).

Both investigators examined blood flow in the synovial tissue using the power Doppler mode. The power Doppler signal of the synovial membrane was graded on a scale of 1–4 as described by Newman et al (23) (1 = normal or minimal tissue perfusion, 2 = mild hyperemia, 3 = moderate hyperemia, and 4 = marked hyperemia), always in relation to the surrounding tissue of the quadriceps muscle (Figure 2). When the scores assigned by the 2 investigators did not match, the investigators examined the patient together and reached a consensus on the findings. The area of PDS was marked preoperatively using a waterproof pencil. The ultrasound examination was transferred to an S-VHS video system.

Histologic examination. Total knee arthroplasty with routine synovectomy was performed with the patient under spinal anesthesia and with a thigh tourniquet. During the procedure, the surgeon took a specimen of the synovial tissue from the suprapatellar recesses (Figure 1), exactly at the site where the PDS had been performed. Synovial tissue sections were stained with hematoxylin and eosin (H&E) and factor VIII (immunohistochemistry). The degree of vascularity was graded on a scale of 1–4 (1 = normal or minimal vascularity, 2 = mild vascularity, 3 = moderate vascularity, and 4 = marked vascularity) by a pathologist (VK) who was unaware of the PDS findings and the patient's clinical diagnosis (see Figure 2).

Digital image analysis of histology samples. Synovial tissue sections stained with H&E and with factor VIII (immunohistochemistry) were evaluated with the use of a microscope–television (TV) system, according to the procedure described by Krenn et al (32). The measurements (10–30/slide) were taken from different regions of interest in which there was good histologic quality of the synovial tissue, and the data were averaged. A Zeiss Axioplan microscope (Zeiss, Wetzlar, Germany) was used, and the stained sections were scanned with a Sony DXC 830b RGB color TV camera (Sony, Tokyo, Japan) and digitized by a Data Translation DT 2871 color frame grabber (Data Translation, Marlboro, MA).

The size of the images was 512 × 512 pixels, with a dynamic range of 8 bits per color channel and a spatial sampling density of 1.3 pixels/μm. The separation algorithms and calculations were performed on a DEC Alpha-433 Workstation (Digital, Santa Barbara, CA).

The brown-colored areas of interest in the tissue (blood vessels) were separated on the images according to the colorimetrics of the TV system (33) by using the differences between the color channels red (R), green (G), and blue (B).

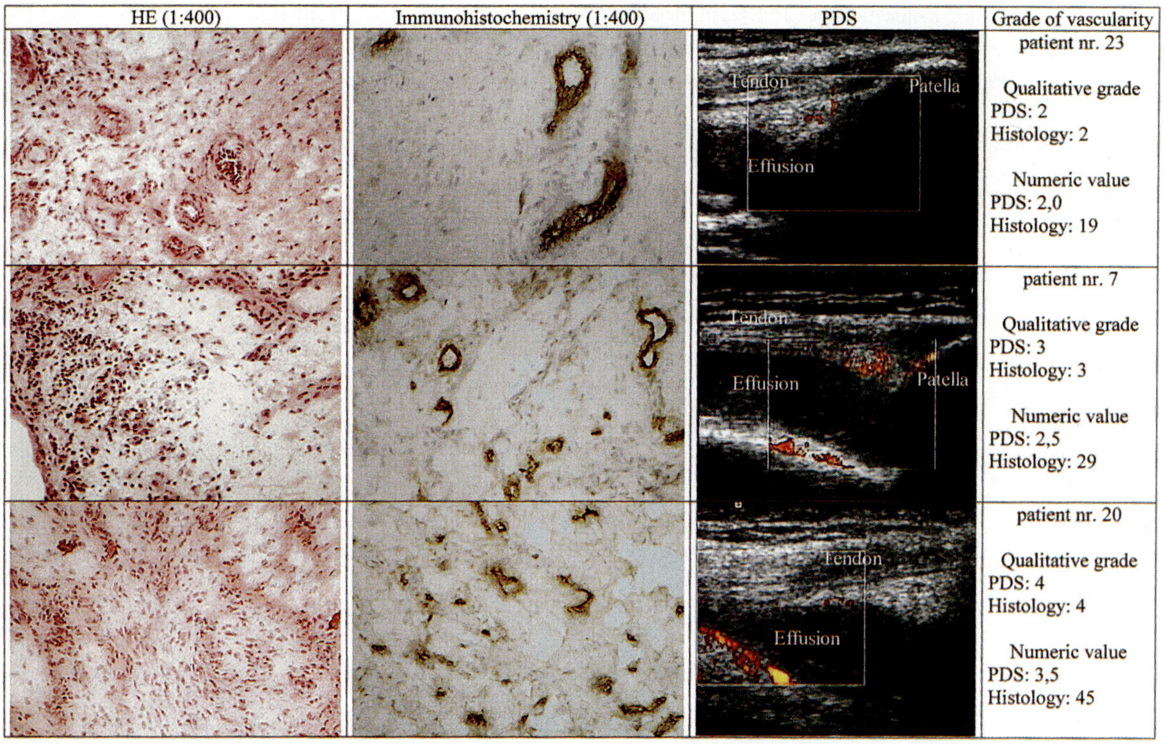

Figure 2. Distinctive features of different grades of vascularity in frozen sections of synovial tissues stained with hematoxylin and eosin (HE) and with factor VIII (immunohistochemistry) and the corresponding power Doppler sonography (PDS) images. Patient numbers (nr.) correspond to those shown in Table 2.

The color brown is represented as a "dirty orange," which means that the red-yellow (orange) color contains a small proportion of blue. Therefore, the relationship $R > G > B$ can be used to distinguish the blood vessels on the images from the surrounding tissue (34).

The average percentage of brown areas in relation to the whole area of the tissue sample is a measure of the vascularity in the section; this percentage was used for further analyses (see Figure 2).

Digital image analysis of PDS images. The S-VHS video tapes were digitized as bitmap-formatted images (24 bit). Representative screen shots of each examination were taken and analyzed for the PDS signal. The areas of calibration on the screen of the Siemens Elegra equipment were analyzed by color measurement (33) on the DEC Alpha-433 Workstation.

PDS does not allow a direct measurement of vascularity. A low level of PDS signal (dark red color) indicates a low number of moving red blood cells; a high number of moving red blood cells is indicated by a more yellow coloration. An increase in the number of detected blood cells leads to a shift from red to yellow in the color marking. The parts of the tissue with no detectable blood cells were gray or white.

The number of red-yellow pixels ($R > G > B$ and B near zero) is a measure of blood flow. Since this number varies from zero to 10,000+, the results were quantified as shown in Table 1, according to the calibration procedure prescribed by Rubin et al (17) and the manufacturer's power Doppler distribution function algorithm.

Statistical analysis. Our main interest was focused on the relationship between the PDS findings and histologic findings of tissue vascularity. In clinical practice, PDS interpretation will, in most cases, lead to qualitative statements.

Table 1. Quantification of red-yellow pixels as a measure of blood flow*

No. of red-yellow pixels	Stage
0–100	0
101–500	0.5
501–1,000	1.0
1,001–1,500	1.5
1,501–2,000	2.0
2,001–2,501	2.5
2,501–3,000	3.0
3,001–5,000	3.5
>5,000	4

* The number of red-yellow pixels is a measure of blood flow; this number varies from 0 to 10,000+. The results were quantified according to the manufacturer's power Doppler distribution function algorithm.

Table 2. Clinical characteristics, medications, and PDS and histologic findings in the knee joint of the study patients*

					Quantitative score		Qualitative score							
Patient/ age/sex	Knee	Clinical diagnosis	Disease duration, years	No. of ACR criteria	Histology, mean ± SD	PDS	Histology	PDS	Effusion	Synovial proliferation	CRP, mg/dl	BP, mm Hg	Heart rate	Cardioactive and antiinflammatory medication
1/59/F	L	RA	12	6	36 ± 12	3.0	2–3	3	2	4	3.5	155/75	66	NSAID, MTX
2/80/M	L	OA	15	–	25 ± 14	2.0	3	2	2	2	0.1	140/85	75	NSAID
3/70/F	R	RA	25	5	29 ± 18	2.5	2–3	2	3	2	2.7	160/80	70	NSAID, MTX, corticosteroids, SSZ
4/29/F	R	RA	5	4	32 ± 11	2.0	3	3	3	3	1.9	140/80	68	NSAID, MTX
5/66/F	R	RA	23	5	41 ± 12	3.0	4	3	3	3	1.0	140/80	82	NSAID
6/76/M	R	OA	8	–	17 ± 7	1.5	1–2	1–2	3	1	0.0	160/100	78	NSAID, ISDN
7/78/F	R	RA	14	5	29 ± 11	2.5	3	3	2	3	0.7	140/60	80	NSAID
8/75/M	R	OA	5	–	14 ± 9	0.5	1–2	1	3	1	0.3	140/90	80	NSAID
9/60/M	R	OA	7	–	10 ± 8	0.5	1	1	2	2	1.1	160/90	85	NSAID
10/78/F	R	OA	27	–	16 ± 10	0.5	2	1	1	1	0.7	170/100	88	NSAID, ACE inhibitor
11/66/F	L	OA	9	–	10 ± 3	1.5	1	1	2	2	0.6	160/90	60	NSAID, ACE inhibitor
12/52/F	R	OA	4	–	23 ± 9	2.5	2–3	2	1	1	1.4	145/90	76	NSAID
13/76/F	R	RA	11	6	41 ± 11	3.0	4	3–4	4	4	5.8	150/80	79	NSAID, MTX, corticosteroids
14/75/F	R	OA	16	–	17 ± 10	0.5	2	2	3	1	0.5	140/70	84	ISDN
15/86/M	R	RA	31	7	33 ± 14	2.5	4	3	3	3	2.4	175/90	78	NSAID, calcium antagonist
16/77/F	L	OA	3	–	18 ± 13	0.5	2–3	1–2	1	2	0.6	125/80	80	Paracetamol, ACE inhibitor
17/65/F	L	OA	15	–	17 ± 6	1.0	1–2	1–2	1	2	1.4	140/60	68	No medication
18/79/F	L	OA	9	–	26 ± 18	3.0	3	3	3	1	0.0	160/90	76	ACE inhibitor
19/76/F	R	OA	8	–	33 ± 21	1.5	2	2	2	1	2.0	160/100	80	NSAID, ACE inhibitor
20/69/F	R	RA	22	5	45 ± 12	3.5	4	4	3	4	1.2	135/80	74	NSAID, ACE inhibitor
21/81/F	L	RA	13	6	42 ± 22	2.0	3–4	2–3	2	2	1.6	140/60	64	NSAID, ACE inhibitor
22/56/F	R	RA	17	5	54 ± 26	3.5	4	4	2	3	1.7	120/70	76	NSAID, MTX, corticosteroids
23/78/M	R	OA	15	–	19 ± 12	2.0	2	2	3	2	0.0	150/80	78	ACE inhibitor

* Rheumatoid arthritis (RA) was assessed according to the number of American College of Rheumatology (ACR) criteria that were met. Osteoarthritis (OA) was determined according to clinical features. C-reactive protein (CRP) levels were determined on the day of power Doppler sonography (PDS). Blood pressure (BP) and heart rate were determined 10 minutes before PDS was performed. NSAID = nonsteroidal antiinflammatory drug; MTX = methotrexate; SSZ = sulfasalazine; ISDN = isosorbide dinitrate; ACE inhibitor = angiotensin-converting enzyme inhibitor.

The assessment by the pathologist judging the vascularity of tissue is also qualitative. The relationship of both variables was analyzed using Spearman's rank correlation test.

In contrast, digital data processing ascribes a numerical value to the power Doppler signal as well as to the vascularity of the tissue. The relationship between these numerical scales was studied using Pearson's correlation test.

The correlation between the qualitative results and the absolute results of the digital image analysis of the PDS and of the tissue section was calculated using Spearman's rank correlation test in order to investigate the reliability of the visual interpretation of the tissue sections and the PDS images by the examiner.

Differences between data for the patients with OA and the patients with RA were investigated with the *t*-test (numerical variables) and the Mann-Whitney U test (qualitative variables).

RESULTS

The characteristics of the study patients, the ultrasound findings including PDS, and the joint effusion, synovial thickness, and histologic findings are shown in Table 2. The correlation between the qualitative results of PDS and the pathologists' estimation of vascularity was 0.89 by Spearman's ρ ($P < 0.01$) (Figure 3).

The visual estimation of vascularity based on PDS images and on tissue sections was compared with the results of digital image processing by Spearman's rank correlation test. The correlation between visual and digital interpretation of PDS was 0.89 by Spearman's ρ

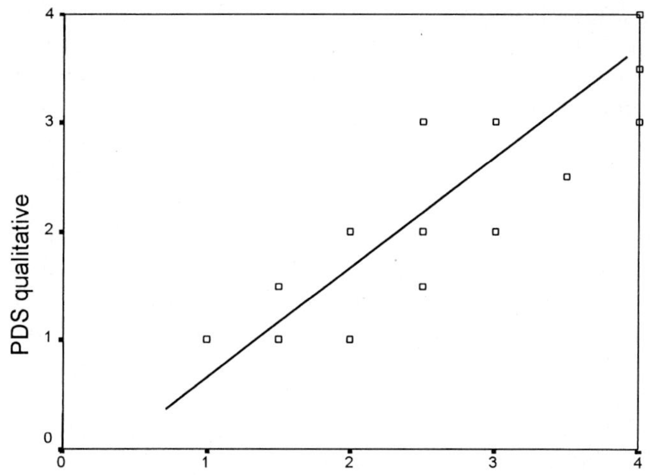

Figure 3. Correlation between the qualitative estimates of blood flow by power Doppler sonography (PDS) and vascularity in the tissue section (Spearman's $\rho = 0.89$, $P < 0.01$).

($P < 0.01$) (Figure 4). The correlation of visual and digital analysis of the factor VIII–stained sections (immunohistochemistry) was 0.88 by Spearman's ρ ($P < 0.01$) (Figure 5). Both values support the reliability of the visual interpretation of the tissue sections and the PDS images by the examiner.

Pearson's correlation between the digital analysis of the PDS images and the digital analysis of the factor VIII–stained tissue sections was 0.81 ($P < 0.01$) (Figure 6).

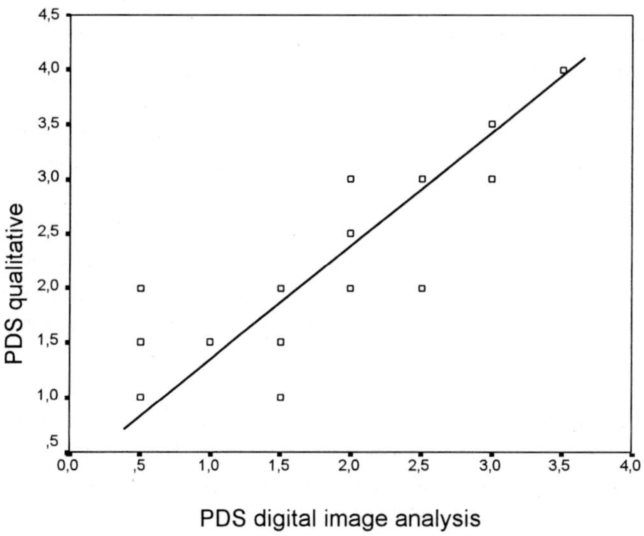

Figure 4. Correlation between the visual (qualitative) interpretation of power Doppler sonography (PDS) images and PDS digital image processing (Spearman's $\rho = 0.89$, $P < 0.01$).

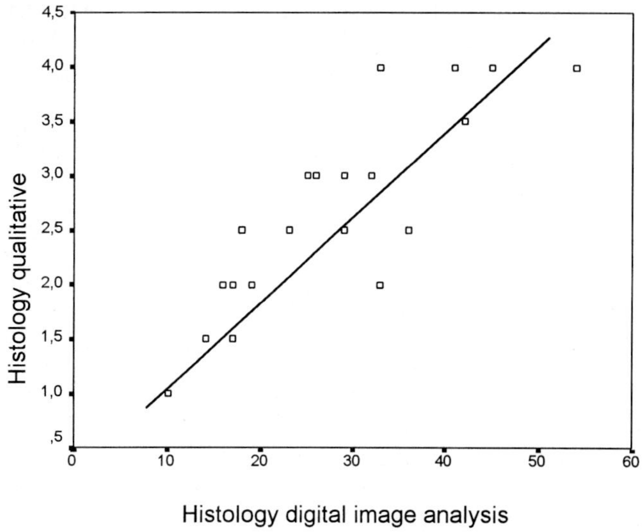

Figure 5. Correlation between the visual and digital image analysis of factor VIII–stained tissue sections (Spearman's $\rho = 0.88$, $P < 0.01$).

We found a correlation between the thickness of the synovial membrane and the PDS signal (Spearman's $\rho = 0.69$, $P < 0.01$). Spearman's ρ for correlation of the thickness of the synovial membrane and vascularity in the tissue section was 0.64 ($P < 0.01$). There was no correlation between synovial proliferation and effusion (Spearman's $\rho = 0.223$, $P = 0.31$).

There was a significant increase in the power Doppler signal for the numerical PDS score ($P < 0.01$)

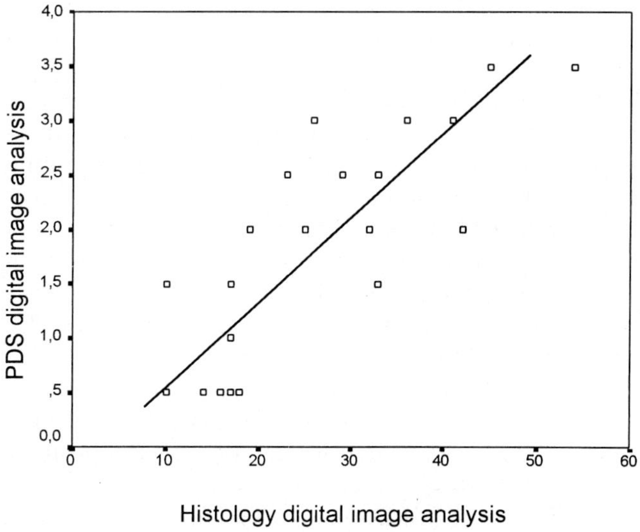

Figure 6. Correlation between the digital analysis of power Doppler sonography (PDS) images and digital analysis of factor VIII–stained tissue sections (Pearson's correlation coefficient r = 0.81, $P < 0.01$).

as well as the qualitative grade ($P < 0.01$) in patients with RA. Digital ($P < 0.01$) and visual ($P < 0.01$) analysis of the immunohistochemistry sections showed a higher degree of vascularity in patients with RA, and hypertrophic synovium was more frequently found in patients with RA ($P < 0.01$). Effusion was found in both groups, but there was no significant between-group difference.

DISCUSSION

Synovial proliferation is the fundamental event in rheumatoid joint lesions (35). Growth of fibroblast-like synoviocytes and metalloproteinase production by fibroblast-like synoviocytes contribute to cartilage and bone destruction associated with hypervascularized tissue containing fibroblastic elements referred to as pannus (36,37). A joint affected by inflammatory tissue as seen in RA requires a specific treatment, such as disease-modifying drugs, local injection of corticosteroids, radionucleotide synoviorthesis, or synovectomy. Visualizing inflammatory tissue is therefore an important element in the diagnosis and monitoring of disease activity in RA.

So far, visualization of synovial tissue and synovial vascularity has been dominated by magnetic resonance imaging (MRI). The ability to differentiate between effusion and synovial proliferation by MRI has been greatly improved by the introduction of the intravenous application of paramagnetic contrast agents (38–44). Van Dijke et al (45) described a technique for measuring abnormal capillary permeability in synovial tissue of arthritic knees of rats, by use of dynamic MRI with an intravenous gadolinium-based blood pool agent. In that study, MRI-derived microvascular characteristics correlated positively with histologic findings. O'Byrne et al (46) compared MRI and histologic findings in a rabbit model of OA and immune arthritis. Those investigators reported that MRI can be used to observe the therapeutic effects of disease-modifying drugs on synovial inflammation and cartilage degradation in rabbit knees. Since enhancement of the synovium is time dependent, the sensitivity of MRI can be reduced by chemical shift artifacts (47). Consequently, for a detailed assessment of disease progression based on serial MRI examinations, precise timing and standardization of the MRI protocol are required (48,49).

The value of PDS in detecting low-velocity blood flow at the microvascular level in several tissues has been demonstrated by Newman et al (16). Strouse et al (50) did not consistently find increased flow in their study of septic arthritis of the hip in children. Their investigations in a rabbit model confirmed their previous findings in children (24). In the latter study, only 23 of 45 examinations of infected knees were unequivocally positive by PDS examinations performed 1–6 days after inoculation. However, several groups of investigators have reported that ultrasound imaging of the synovial tissue is an objective and reliable technique (16,21,23,28,51–53).

Fiocco et al (21) compared conventional ultrasound imaging of synovial proliferation with arthroscopic visualization before and after synovectomy in patients with knee joint synovitis and found a significant correlation between clinical and ultrasound indices. Those authors concluded that sonography can be used as an objective method for monitoring response to therapy in patients with inflammatory knee joint diseases. Silvestri et al (54) used color Doppler to monitor the activity of RA in the knee joint and found a correlation between vascular findings and clinical symptoms.

In the present studies, effusion was found in patients with OA as well as in patients with RA, with no significant between-group differences. The correlation between the thickness of the synovial membrane, the PDS signal, and tissue vascularity is consistent with clinical experience; however, a thick synovial membrane or effusion does not necessarily mean that inflammation is present. There was no correlation between synovial proliferation and the presence of an effusion. Tissue debris, blood clots, and fibrin are known to mimic some ultrasound features of synovial proliferation (21), and these features can be excluded by PDS.

PDS reflects the movement of blood cells within a vessel; however, it does not always indicate increased vascularity or hyperemia of the synovium, which is still a problem in interpreting PDS images (55). PDS findings are influenced by the examiner, the machine, and the acoustical conditions involved in image processing. A sonographic evaluation of the arthritic joint should also be performed. PDS should be used to assist the clinician in determining whether the region of interest shows increased blood flow compared with other tissues (29). This information can be important in distinguishing between hypervascular and fibrous pannus. The value of PDS in the assessment of therapeutic response to the treatment of synovitis of the knee joint was shown by Newman et al (23), who reported a qualitative decrease in synovial perfusion visualized by PDS after intraarticular administration of steroids.

Our study is the first to correlate PDS findings with histologic findings in the synovial tissue, supporting the value of PDS in clinical practice, where the degree of vascularity can be graded according to PDS images. The best correlation was found when a 1–4 grading scale was used by both the sonographer in assessing PDS signals and the pathologist in assessing the degree of vascularity.

Although techniques of digitizing the images and analyzing blood vessels and PDS signals are automatically assumed to be a more accurate approach, this method can be influenced by technical artifacts. Fat cells with intensely colored cell membranes can mimic a high vascularity in the segmentation algorithms of the image analyzing software. Besides technical considerations, the cost of PDS investigations is of increasing concern in our health care systems. The results of the present study, however, indicate that PDS is a powerful tool in the evaluation and objective assessment of synovial tissue perfusion. PDS represents a readily available, easy to handle, and cost effective alternative to dynamic MRI with intravenous gadolinium-based contrast agent. In the future, the use of ultrasound contrast agents and harmonic imaging, both of which greatly enhance color flow sensitivity, may be shown to increase the potential utility of PDS.

In conclusion, PDS provides a reliable and accurate method for visualizing blood flow in the synovial tissue. The highly significant correlation between the PDS findings and the histologic findings supports the value of this technique. Since ultrasound is an easy to handle, safe, inexpensive, and noninvasive procedure that is available in most departments of rheumatology, PDS may continue to play an important role in the diagnosis and monitoring of musculoskeletal disorders.

ACKNOWLEDGMENTS

Thanks to Mrs. J. Pfeuffer for preparing the tissue sections, H. Schmitz, MD, for support in translating the manuscript, Mrs. J. Hinterberger for scanning the tissue sections in the microscope–TV system, and S. Kirschner, MD, for help with compiling the statistics.

REFERENCES

1. Sahn DJ. Instrumentation and physical factors related to visualization of stenotic and regurgitant jets by Doppler color flow mapping. J Am Coll Cardiol 1988;12:1354–65.
2. Tamura T, Sahn DJ, Krabill K. Low flow velocity sensitivity on color flow mapping Doppler: power mode vs. dynamic range reallocation for display [abstract]. J Am Coll Cardiol 1988;11:98A.
3. Breidahl WH, Newman JS, Taljanovic MS, Adler RS. Power Doppler sonography in the assessment of musculoskeletal fluid collections. AJR Am J Roentgenol 1996;166:1443–6.
4. Bude RO, Rubin JM. Power Doppler sonography. Radiology 1996;200:21–3.
5. MacSweeney JE, Cosgrove DO, Arenson J. Colour Doppler energy (power) mode ultrasound. Clin Radiol 1996;51:387–90.
6. Martinoli C, Pretolesi F, Crespi G, Bianchi S, Gandolfo N, Valle M, et al. Power Doppler sonography: clinical applications. Eur J Radiol 1998;27 Suppl 2:S133–40.
7. Murphy KJ, Rubin JM. Power Doppler: it's a good thing. Semin Ultrasound CT MR 1997;18:13–21.
8. Rubin JM, Adler RS. Power Doppler expands standard color capability. Diagn Imaging 1996;12:66–9.
9. Rubin JM, Bude RO, Carson PL, Bree RL, Adler RS. Power Doppler US: a potentially useful alternative to mean frequency-based color Doppler US. Radiology 1994;190:853–6.
10. Rubin JM, Bude RO, Fowlkes JB, Spratt RS, Carson PL, Adler RS. Normalizing fractional moving blood volume estimates with power Doppler US: defining a stable intravascular point with the cumulative power distribution function. Radiology 1997;205: 757–65.
11. Turetschek K, Kollmann C, Dorffner R, Wunderbaldinger P, Mostbeck G. Amplitude-coded color Doppler: clinical applications. Eur Radiol 1999;9:115–21.
12. Kollmann C, Turetschek K, Mostbeck G. Amplitude-coded colour Doppler sonography: physical principles and technique. Eur Radiol 1998;8:649–56.
13. Derchi LE, Martinoli C, Solbiati L, Rizzatto G. Power Doppler: physical and constructive principles and comparison with Doppler color. Radiol Med (Torino) 1997;93:329–35.
14. Eriksson R, Persson HW, Dymling SO, Lindstrom K. Evaluation of Doppler ultrasound for blood perfusion measurements. Ultrasound Med Biol 1991;17:445–52.
15. Teirlinck CJ, Bezemer RA, Kollmann C, Lubbers J, Hoskins PR, Fish P, et al. Development of an example flow test object and comparison of five of these test objects, constructed in various laboratories. Ultrasonics 1998;36:653–60.
16. Newman JS, Adler RS, Bude RO, Rubin JM. Detection of soft-tissue hyperemia: value of power Doppler sonography. AJR Am J Roentgenol 1994;163:385–9.
17. Rubin JM, Adler RS, Fowlkes JB, Spratt S, Pallister JE, Chen JF, et al. Fractional moving blood volume: estimation with power Doppler US. Radiology 1995;197:183–90.
18. Sohn C, Weskott HP. The sensitivity of new color systems in blood-flow diagnosis: the maximum entropy method and angio-color-comparative in vitro flow measurements to determine sensitivity. Surg Endosc 1997;11:1040–4.
19. Weskott HP. Amplitude Doppler US: slow blood flow detection tested with a flow phantom. Radiology 1997;202:125–30.
20. Breidahl WH, Stafford Johnson DB, Newman JS, Adler RS. Power Doppler sonography in tenosynovitis: significance of the peritendinous hypoechoic rim. J Ultrasound Med 1998;17:103–7.
21. Fiocco U, Cozzi L, Rubaltelli L, Rigon C, de Candia A, Tregnaghi A, et al. Long-term sonographic follow-up of rheumatoid and psoriatic proliferative knee joint synovitis. Br J Rheumatol 1996; 35:155–63.
22. Kainberger F, Czerny C, Trattnig S, Lack W, Machold K, Graninger W. MRI und Ultraschall in der Rheumatologie. Radiologe 1996;36:609–16.
23. Newman JS, Laing TJ, McCarthy CJ, Adler RS. Power Doppler sonography of synovitis: assessment of therapeutic response—preliminary observations. Radiology 1996;198:582–4.
24. Strouse PJ, DiPietro MA, Teo EL, Doi K, Chrisp CE. Power Doppler evaluation of joint effusions: investigation in a rabbit model. Pediatr Radiol 1999;29:617–23.
25. Arnett FC, Edworthy SM, Bloch DA, McShane DJ, Fries FJ, Cooper NS, et al. The American Rheumatism Association 1987 revised criteria for the classification of rheumatoid arthritis. Arthritis Rheum 1988;31:315–24.
26. Rubaltelli L, Fiocco U, Cozzi L. Prospective sonographic evalua-

tion of proliferative knee joint synovitis. J Ultrasound Med 1992;13:855–62.
27. Van Holsbeeck M, van Holsbeeck K, Gevers G, Marchal G, van Steen A, Favril A, et al. Staging and follow-up of rheumatoid arthritis of the knee: comparison of sonography, thermography, and clinical assessment. J Ultrasound Med 1988;7:561–6.
28. Newman JS, Adler RS, Rubin JM. Power Doppler sonography: use in measuring alterations in muscle blood volume after exercise. AJR Am J Roentgenol 1997;168:1525–30.
29. Martinoli C, Derchi LE. Gain setting in power Doppler US. Radiology 1997;202:284–5.
30. Adler RS, Rubin JM, Fowlkes JB, Carson PL, Pallister JE. Ultrasonic estimation of tissue perfusion: a stochastic approach. Ultrasound Med Biol 1995;21:493–500.
31. Jain SP, Fan PH, Philpot EF, Nanda NC, Aggarwal KK, Moos S, et al. Influence of various instrument settings on the flow information derived from the power mode. Ultrasound Med Biol 1991;17:49–54.
32. Krenn V, Schedel J, Döring A, Huppertz HI, Gohlke F, Tony HP, et al. Endothelial cells are the major source of sICAM-1 in rheumatoid synovial tissue. Rheumatol Int 1997;17:17–27.
33. Lang H. Farbmetrik und Farbfernsehen. Munich: Oldenbourg; 1978.
34. Harms H, Aus HM. Tissue image segmentation with multicolor, multifocal algorithms. In: Devijver PA, Kittler J, editors. Pattern recognition theory and applications. Nato ASI series Vol. F30. Berlin: Springer; 1987. p. 519–28.
35. Combe B. Inflammation and joint destruction during rheumatoid polyarthritis: what relation? Presse Med 1998;27:481–3.
36. Fassbender HG. What destroys the joint in rheumatoid arthritis? Arch Orthop Trauma Surg 1998;117:2–7.
37. Sarkissian M, Lafyatis R. Integrin engagement regulates proliferation and collagenase expression of rheumatoid synovial fibroblasts. J Immunol 1999;162:1772–9.
38. Adam G, Dammer M, Bohndorf K, Christoph R, Fenke F, Gunther RW. Rheumatoid arthritis of the knee: value of gadopentetate dimeglumine-enhanced MR imaging. AJR Am J Roentgenol 1991;156:125–9.
39. Beckmann N, Bruttel K, Schuurman H, Mir A. Effects of Sandimmune Neoral on collagen-induced arthritis in DA rats: characterization by high resolution three-dimensional magnetic resonance imaging and by histology. J Magn Reson 1998;131:8–16.
40. Carpenter TA, Everett JR, Hall LD, Harper GP, Hodgson RJ, James MF. Visualisation of subchondral erosion in rat monoarticular arthritis by magnetic resonance imaging. Skeletal Radiol 1995;24:341–9.
41. Carpenter TA, Everett JR, Hall LD, Harper GP, Hodgson RJ, James MF, et al. High-resolution magnetic resonance imaging of arthritic pathology in the rat knee. Skeletal Radiol 1994;23: 429–37.
42. Konig H, Sieper J, Wolf KJ. Rheumatoid arthritis: evaluation of hypervascular and fibrous pannus with dynamic MR imaging enhanced with Gd-DTPA. Radiology 1990;176:473–7.
43. Murray JG, Ridley NT, Mitchell N, Rooney M. Juvenile chronic arthritis of the hip: value of contrast-enhanced MR imaging. Clin Radiol 1996;51:99–102.
44. Veale DJ, Reece RJ, Parsons W, Radjenovic A, O'Connor PJ, Orgles CS, et al. Intra-articular primatised anti-CD4: efficacy in resistant rheumatoid knees. A study of combined arthroscopy, magnetic resonance imaging, and histology. Ann Rheum Dis 1999;58:342–9.
45. Van Dijke CF, Peterfy CG, Brasch RC, Lang P, Roberts TP, Shames D, et al. MR imaging of the arthritic rabbit knee joint using albumin-(Gd-DTPA)30 with correlation to histopathology. Magn Reson Imaging 1999;17:237–45.
46. O'Byrne EM, Paul PK, Roberts ED, Blancuzzi V, Wilson D, Goldberg RL, et al. Comparison of magnetic resonance imaging (MRI) and histopathology in rabbit models of osteoarthritis and immune arthritis. Agents Actions 1993;39:C157–9.
47. Konig H, Sieper J, Wolf KJ. Dynamic magnetic resonance imaging in the differentiation of inflammatory joint lesions. Rofo Fortschr Geb Rontgenstr Neuen Bildgeb Verfahr 1990;153:1–5.
48. Kursunoglu Brahme S, Riccio T, Weisman MH, Resnick D, Zvaifler N, Sanders ME, et al. Rheumatoid knee: role of gadopentetate-enhanced MR imaging. Radiology 1990;176:831–5.
49. Yamato M, Tamai K, Yamaguchi T, Ohno W. MRI of the knee in rheumatoid arthritis: Gd-DTPA perfusion dynamics. J Comput Assist Tomogr 1993;17:781–5.
50. Strouse PJ, DiPietro MA, Adler RS. Pediatric hip effusions: evaluation with power Doppler sonography. Radiology 1998;206: 731–5.
51. Chen JF, Fowlkes JB, Carson PL, Rubin JM, Adler RS. Autocorrelation of integrated power Doppler signals and its application. Ultrasound Med Biol 1996;22:1053–7.
52. Martinoli C, Derchi LE, Rizzatto G, Solbiati L. Power Doppler sonography: general principles, clinical applications, and future prospects. Eur Radiol 1998;8:1224–35.
53. Martinoli C, Pretolesi F, Crespi G, Bianchi S, Gandolfo N, Valle M, et al. Power Doppler sonography: clinical applications. Eur J Radiol 1998;27 Suppl 2:S133–40.
54. Silvestri E, Martinoli C, Onetto F, Neumaier CE, Cimmino MA, Derchi LE. Evaluation of rheumatoid arthritis of the knee with Doppler color. Radiol Med (Torino) 1994;88:364–7.
55. Cardinal E, Lafortune M, Burns P. Power Doppler US in synovitis: reality or artifact? Radiology 1996;200:868–9.

VIOXX® (rofecoxib tablets and oral suspension)

Brief Summary of Prescribing Information

INDICATIONS AND USAGE: VIOXX is indicated for: relief of the signs and symptoms of osteoarthritis (OA); management of acute pain in adults; treatment of primary dysmenorrhea.

CONTRAINDICATIONS: VIOXX is contraindicated in patients with known hypersensitivity to rofecoxib or any other component of VIOXX.

VIOXX should not be given to patients who have experienced asthma, urticaria, or allergic-type reactions after taking aspirin or other nonsteroidal anti-inflammatory drugs (NSAIDs). Severe, rarely fatal, anaphylactic-like reactions to NSAIDs have been reported in such patients (see WARNINGS, *Anaphylactoid Reactions* and PRECAUTIONS, *Preexisting Asthma*).

WARNINGS: *Gastrointestinal (GI) Effects—Risk of GI Ulceration, Bleeding, and Perforation:* Serious GI toxicity, such as bleeding, ulceration, and perforation of the stomach, small intestine, or large intestine, can occur at any time, with or without warning symptoms, in patients treated with NSAIDs. Minor upper GI problems, such as dyspepsia, are common and may also occur at any time during NSAID therapy. Therefore, physicians and patients should remain alert for ulceration and bleeding, even in the absence of previous GI tract symptoms. Patients should be informed about the signs and/or symptoms of serious GI toxicity and the steps to take if they occur. The utility of periodic laboratory monitoring has not been demonstrated, nor has it been adequately assessed. Only 1 in 5 patients who develop a serious upper GI adverse event on NSAID therapy is symptomatic. It has been demonstrated that upper GI ulcers, gross bleeding, or perforation caused by NSAIDs, appear to occur in approximately 1% of patients treated for 3–6 months, and in about 2%–4% of patients treated for 1 year. These trends continue thus, increasing the likelihood of developing a serious GI event at some time during the course of therapy. However, even short-term therapy is not without risk.

It is unclear, at the present time, how the above rates apply to VIOXX. Among 3,357 patients who received VIOXX in controlled clinical trials of 6 weeks to 1 year in duration (most were enrolled in 6-month or longer studies) at a daily dose of 12.5 mg to 50 mg, a total of 4 patients experienced a serious upper GI event, using protocol-derived criteria. Two patients experienced an upper GI bleed within 3 months (at Days 62 and 87, respectively) (0.06%). One additional patient experienced an obstruction within 6 months (Day 130) and the remaining patient developed an upper GI bleed within 12 months (Day 322) (0.12%). Approximately 23% of these 3,357 patients were in studies that required them to be ulcer free at study entry. It is unclear if this study population is representative of the general population. Prospective, long-term studies required to compare the incidence of serious, clinically significant upper GI adverse events in patients taking VIOXX vs comparator NSAID products have not been performed.

NSAIDs should be prescribed with extreme caution in patients with a prior history of ulcer disease or GI bleeding. Most spontaneous reports of fatal GI events are in elderly or debilitated patients and therefore special care should be taken in treating this population. **To minimize the potential risk for an adverse GI event, the lowest effective dose should be used for the shortest possible duration.** For high-risk patients, alternate therapies that do not involve NSAIDs should be considered.

Studies have shown that patients with a *prior history of peptic ulcer disease and/or GI bleeding* and who use NSAIDs, have a greater than 10-fold higher risk for developing a GI bleed than patients with neither of these risk factors. In addition to a past history of ulcer disease, pharmacoepidemiologic studies have identified several other cotherapies or comorbid conditions that may increase the risk for GI bleeding, such as: treatment with oral corticosteroids, treatment with anticoagulants, longer duration of NSAID therapy, smoking, alcoholism, older age, and poor general health status.

Anaphylactoid Reactions: As with NSAIDs in general, anaphylactoid reactions have occurred in patients without known prior exposure to VIOXX. In postmarketing experience, rare cases of anaphylactoid reactions and angioedema have been reported in patients receiving VIOXX. VIOXX should not be given to patients with the aspirin triad. This symptom complex typically occurs in asthmatic patients who experience rhinitis with or without nasal polyps, or who exhibit severe, potentially fatal bronchospasm after taking aspirin or other NSAIDs (see CONTRAINDICATIONS and PRECAUTIONS, *Preexisting Asthma*). Emergency help should be sought in cases where an anaphylactoid reaction occurs.

Advanced Renal Disease: No safety information is available regarding the use of VIOXX in patients with advanced kidney disease. Therefore, treatment with VIOXX is not recommended in these patients. If VIOXX therapy must be initiated, close monitoring of the patient's kidney function is advisable (see PRECAUTIONS, *Renal Effects*).

Pregnancy: In late pregnancy, VIOXX should be avoided because it may cause premature closure of the ductus arteriosus.

PRECAUTIONS: *General:* VIOXX cannot be expected to substitute for corticosteroids or to treat corticosteroid insufficiency. Abrupt discontinuation of corticosteroids may lead to exacerbation of corticosteroid-responsive illness. Patients on prolonged corticosteroid therapy should have their therapy tapered slowly if a decision is made to discontinue corticosteroids.

The pharmacologic activity of VIOXX in reducing inflammation, and possibly fever, may diminish the utility of these diagnostic signs in detecting infectious complications of presumed noninfectious, painful conditions.

Hepatic Effects: Borderline elevations of 1 or more liver tests may occur in up to 15% of patients taking NSAIDs, and notable elevations of ALT or AST (~3 or more times the upper limit of normal) have been reported in approximately 1% of patients in clinical trials with NSAIDs. These laboratory abnormalities may progress, may remain unchanged, or may be transient with continuing therapy. Rare cases of severe hepatic reactions, including jaundice and fatal fulminant hepatitis, liver necrosis, and hepatic failure (some with fatal outcome) have been reported with NSAIDs. In controlled clinical trials of VIOXX, the incidence of borderline elevations of liver tests at doses of 12.5 mg and 25 mg daily was comparable to the incidence observed with ibuprofen and lower than that observed with diclofenac. In placebo-controlled trials, approximately 0.5% of patients taking rofecoxib (12.5 mg or 25 mg q.d.) and 0.1% of patients taking placebo had notable elevations of ALT or AST.

A patient with symptoms and/or signs suggesting liver dysfunction, or in whom an abnormal liver test has occurred, should be monitored carefully for evidence of the development of a more severe hepatic reaction while on therapy with VIOXX. Use of VIOXX is not recommended in patients with moderate or severe hepatic insufficiency. If clinical signs and symptoms consistent with liver disease develop, or if systemic manifestations occur (e.g., eosinophilia, rash, etc.), VIOXX should be discontinued.

Renal Effects: Long-term administration of NSAIDs has resulted in renal papillary necrosis and other renal injury. Renal toxicity has also been seen in patients in whom renal prostaglandins have a compensatory role in the maintenance of renal perfusion. In these patients, administration of an NSAID may cause a dose-dependent reduction in prostaglandin formation and, secondarily, in renal blood flow, which may precipitate overt renal decompensation. Patients at greatest risk of this reaction are those with impaired renal function, heart failure, liver dysfunction, those taking diuretics and angiotensin-converting enzyme (ACE) inhibitors, and the elderly. Discontinuation of NSAID therapy is usually followed by recovery to the pretreatment state. Clinical trials with VIOXX at daily doses of 12.5 mg and 25 mg have shown renal effects (e.g., hypertension, edema) similar to those observed with comparator NSAIDs; these occur with an increased frequency with chronic use of VIOXX at doses above the 12.5-mg to 25-mg range (see ADVERSE REACTIONS). Caution should be used when initiating treatment with VIOXX in patients with considerable dehydration. It is advisable to rehydrate patients first and then start therapy with VIOXX. Caution is also recommended in patients with preexisting kidney disease (see WARNINGS, *Advanced Renal Disease*).

Hematologic Effects: Anemia is sometimes seen in patients receiving VIOXX. In placebo-controlled trials, there were no significant differences observed between VIOXX and placebo in clinical reports of anemia. Patients on long-term treatment with VIOXX should have their hemoglobin or hematocrit checked if they exhibit any signs or symptoms of anemia or blood loss. VIOXX does not generally affect platelet counts, prothrombin time, or partial thromboplastin time, and does not inhibit platelet aggregation at indicated dosages.

Fluid Retention and Edema: Fluid retention and edema have been observed in some patients taking VIOXX® (rofecoxib tablets and oral suspension) (see ADVERSE REACTIONS). VIOXX should be used with caution and should be introduced at the lowest recommended dose in patients with fluid retention, hypertension, or heart failure.

Preexisting Asthma: Patients with asthma may have aspirin-sensitive asthma. The use of aspirin in patients with aspirin-sensitive asthma has been associated with severe bronchospasm, which can be fatal. Since cross-reactivity, including bronchospasm, between aspirin and other NSAIDs has been reported in such aspirin-sensitive patients, VIOXX should not be administered to patients with this form of aspirin sensitivity and should be used with caution in patients with preexisting asthma.

Information for Patients: VIOXX can cause discomfort and, rarely, more serious side effects, such as GI bleeding, which may result in hospitalization and even fatal outcomes. Although serious GI tract ulcerations and bleeding can occur without warning symptoms, patients should be alert for the signs and symptoms of ulcerations and bleeding, and should ask for medical advice when observing any indicative signs or symptoms. Patients should be apprised of the importance of this follow-up (see WARNINGS, *Gastrointestinal (GI) Effects—Risk of GI Ulceration, Bleeding, and Perforation)*.

Patients should promptly report signs or symptoms of GI ulceration or bleeding, skin rash, unexplained weight gain, or edema to their physicians.

Patients should be informed of the warning signs and symptoms of hepatotoxicity (e.g., nausea, fatigue, lethargy, pruritus, jaundice, right upper quadrant tenderness, and "flu-like" symptoms). If these occur, patients should be instructed to stop therapy and seek immediate medical therapy.

Patients should also be instructed to seek immediate emergency help in the case of an anaphylactoid reaction (see WARNINGS).

In late pregnancy, VIOXX should be avoided because it may cause premature closure of the ductus arteriosus.

Laboratory Tests: Because serious GI tract ulcerations and bleeding can occur without warning symptoms, physicians should monitor for signs or symptoms of GI bleeding.

Drug Interactions: ACE Inhibitors: Reports suggest that NSAIDs may diminish the antihypertensive effect of ACE inhibitors. In patients with mild to moderate hypertension, administration of 25 mg daily of VIOXX with the ACE inhibitor benazepril, 10 to 40 mg for 4 weeks, was associated with an average increase in mean arterial pressure of about 3 mmHg compared to ACE inhibitor alone. This interaction should be given consideration in patients taking VIOXX concomitantly with ACE inhibitors. *Aspirin:* Concomitant administration of low-dose aspirin with VIOXX may result in an increased rate of GI ulceration or other complications, compared to use of VIOXX alone. At steady state, VIOXX 50 mg once daily had no effect on the antiplatelet activity of low-dose (81 mg once daily) aspirin, as assessed by ex vivo platelet aggregation and serum TXB_2 generation in clotting blood. VIOXX is not a substitute for aspirin for cardiovascular prophylaxis. *Cimetidine:* Coadministration with high doses of cimetidine (800 mg twice daily) increased the C_{max} of rofecoxib by 21%, the $AUC_{0\text{-}120hr}$ by 23%, and the $t_{1/2}$ by 15%. These small changes are not clinically significant and no dose adjustment is necessary. *Digoxin:* Rofecoxib 75 mg once daily for 11 days does not alter the plasma concentration profile or renal elimination of digoxin after a single 0.5-mg oral dose. *Furosemide:* Clinical studies, as well as postmarketing observations, have shown that NSAIDs can reduce the natriuretic effect of furosemide and thiazides in some patients. This response has been attributed to inhibition of renal prostaglandin synthesis. *Ketoconazole:* Ketoconazole 400 mg daily did not have any clinically important effect on the pharmacokinetics of rofecoxib. *Lithium:* NSAIDs have produced an elevation of plasma lithium levels and a reduction in renal lithium clearance. In postmarketing experience, there have been reports of increases in plasma lithium levels. Thus, when VIOXX and lithium are administered concurrently, subjects should be observed carefully for signs of lithium toxicity. *Methotrexate:* VIOXX 75 mg administered once daily for 10 days increased plasma concentrations by 23%, as measured by $AUC_{0\text{-}24hr}$ in patients receiving methotrexate 7.5 mg to 15 mg/week for rheumatoid arthritis. An equivalent magnitude of reduction in methotrexate renal clearance was observed. At 24 hours postdose, a similar proportion of patients treated with methotrexate alone (94%) and subsequently treated with methotrexate coadministered with 75 mg of rofecoxib (88%) had methotrexate plasma concentrations below the measurable limit (5 ng/mL). The effects of the recommended doses for OA (12.5 mg and 25 mg) of VIOXX on plasma methotrexate levels are unknown. Standard monitoring of methotrexate-related toxicity should be continued if VIOXX and methotrexate are administered concomitantly. *Oral Contraceptives:* Rofecoxib did not have any clinically important effect on the pharmacokinetics of ethinyl estradiol and norethindrone. *Prednisone/Prednisolone:* Rofecoxib did not have any clinically important effect on the pharmacokinetics of prednisone or prednisolone. *Rifampin:* Coadministration of VIOXX with rifampin 600 mg daily, a potent inducer of hepatic metabolism, produced an approximate 50% decrease in rofecoxib plasma concentrations. Therefore, a starting daily dose of 25 mg of VIOXX should be considered for the treatment of OA when VIOXX is coadministered with potent inducers of hepatic metabolism. *Warfarin:* Anticoagulant activity should be monitored, particularly in the first few days after initiating or changing VIOXX therapy in patients receiving warfarin or similar agents, since these patients are at an increased risk of bleeding complications. In single- and multiple-dose studies in healthy subjects receiving both warfarin and rofecoxib, prothrombin time (measured as INR) was increased by approximately 8% to 11%. In postmarketing experience, bleeding events have been reported, predominantly in the elderly, in association with increases in prothrombin time in patients receiving VIOXX concurrently with warfarin.

Carcinogenesis, Mutagenesis, Impairment of Fertility: Rofecoxib was not carcinogenic in mice given oral doses up to 30 mg/kg (male) and 60 mg/kg (female) (~5- and 2-fold the human exposure at 25 mg and 50 mg daily based on $AUC_{0\text{-}24}$) and in male and female rats given oral doses up to 8 mg/kg (~6- and 2-fold the human exposure at 25 mg and 50 mg daily based on $AUC_{0\text{-}24}$) for 2 years. Rofecoxib was not mutagenic in an Ames test or in a V-79 mammalian cell mutagenesis assay, nor clastogenic in a chromosome aberration assay in Chinese hamster ovary (CHO) cells, in an in vitro and an in vivo alkaline elution assay, or in an in vivo chromosomal aberration test in mouse bone marrow. Rofecoxib did not impair male fertility in rats at oral doses up to 100 mg/kg (~20- and 7-fold human exposure at 25 mg and 50 mg daily based on $AUC_{0\text{-}24}$) and rofecoxib had no effect on fertility in female rats at doses up to 30 mg/kg (~19- and 7-fold human exposure at 25 mg and 50 mg daily based on $AUC_{0\text{-}24}$).

Pregnancy: Teratogenic Effects: Pregnancy Category C. Rofecoxib was not teratogenic in rats at dosages up to 50 mg/kg/day (~28- and 10-fold human exposure at 25 mg and 50 mg daily based on $AUC_{0\text{-}24}$). There was a slight, nonstatistically significant increase in the overall incidence of vertebral malformations only in the rabbit at doses of 50 mg/kg/day (~1- or <1-fold human exposure at 25 mg and 50 mg daily based on $AUC_{0\text{-}24}$). There are no studies in pregnant women. VIOXX should be used during pregnancy only if the potential benefit justifies the potential risk to the fetus.

Nonteratogenic Effects: Rofecoxib produced periimplantation and postimplantation losses and reduced embryo/fetal survival in rats and rabbits at oral doses ≥10 and ≥75 mg/kg/day, respectively (~9- and 3-fold [rats] and 2- and <1-fold [rabbits] human exposure based on $AUC_{0\text{-}24}$ at 25 mg and 50 mg daily). These changes are expected with inhibition of prostaglandin synthesis and are not the result of permanent alteration of female reproductive function. There was an increase in the incidence of postnatal pup mortality in rats at ≥5 mg/kg/day (~5- and 2-fold human exposure at 25 mg and 50 mg daily based on $AUC_{0\text{-}24}$). In studies in pregnant rats administered single doses of rofecoxib, there was a treatment-related decrease in the diameter of the ductus arteriosus at all doses used (3–300 mg/kg: 3 mg/kg is ~2- and <1-fold human exposure at 25 mg or 50 mg daily based on $AUC_{0\text{-}24}$). As with other drugs known to inhibit prostaglandin synthesis, use of VIOXX during the third trimester of pregnancy should be avoided.

Labor and Delivery: Rofecoxib produced no evidence of significantly delayed labor or parturition in females at doses 15 mg/kg in rats (~10- and 3-fold human exposure as measured by the $AUC_{0\text{-}24}$ at 25 mg and 50 mg). The effects of VIOXX on labor and delivery in pregnant women are unknown. Merck & Co., Inc., maintains a registry to monitor the pregnancy outcomes of women exposed to VIOXX while pregnant. Healthcare providers are encouraged to report any prenatal exposure to VIOXX by calling the Pregnancy Registry at 1-800-986-8999.

Nursing Mothers: Rofecoxib is excreted in the milk of lactating rats at concentrations similar to those in plasma. There was an increase in pup mortality and a decrease in pup body weight following exposure of pups to milk from dams administered VIOXX® (rofecoxib tablets and oral suspension) during lactation. The dose tested represents an approximate 18- and 6-fold human exposure at 25 mg and 50 mg daily based on $AUC_{0\text{-}24}$. It is not known whether this drug is excreted in human milk. Because many drugs are excreted in human milk and because of the potential for serious adverse reactions in nursing infants from VIOXX, a decision should be made whether to discontinue nursing or to discontinue the drug, taking into account the importance of the drug to the mother.

Pediatric Use: Safety and effectiveness in pediatric patients below the age of 18 years have not been evaluated.

Geriatric Use: Of the patients who received VIOXX in OA clinical trials, 1,455 were 65 years of age or older (this included 460 who were 75 years or older). No substantial differences in safety and effectiveness were observed between these subjects and younger subjects. Greater sensitivity of some older individuals cannot be ruled out. Dosage adjustment in the elderly is not necessary; however, therapy with VIOXX should be initiated at the lowest recommended dose. In 1 of these studies (a 6-week, double-blind, randomized clinical trial), VIOXX 12.5 mg or 25 mg once daily was administered to 174 OA patients ≥80 years of age. The safety profile in this elderly population was similar to that of younger patients treated with VIOXX.

ADVERSE REACTIONS: *OA:* Approximately 3,600 patients with OA were treated with VIOXX; approximately 1,400 patients received VIOXX for 6 months or longer, and approximately 800 patients for 1 year or longer. The following paragraph lists all adverse events, regardless of causality, occurring in at least 2% of patients receiving VIOXX in 9 controlled studies of 6 weeks' to 6 months' duration conducted in patients with OA at the therapeutically recommended doses (12.5 mg and 25 mg), which included a placebo and/or positive control group.

Clinical adverse experiences occurring in ≥2.0% of patients treated with VIOXX vs placebo, ibuprofen 2400 mg, or diclofenac 150 mg: *Body as a Whole/Site Unspecified:* abdominal pain, 3.4% (vs 4.1%, placebo; 4.6%, ibuprofen; 5.8%, diclofenac); asthenia/fatigue, 2.2% (vs 1.0%; 2.0%; 2.6%); dizziness, 3.0% (vs 2.2%; 2.7%; 3.4%); influenza-like disease, 2.9% (vs 3.1%; 1.5%; 3.2%); lower extremity edema, 3.7% (vs 1.1%; 3.8%; 3.4%); upper respiratory infection, 8.5% (vs 7.8%; 5.8%; 8.2%). *Cardiovascular System:* hypertension, 3.5% (vs 1.3%; 3.0%; 1.6%). *Digestive System:* diarrhea, 6.5% (vs 6.8%; 7.1%; 10.6%); dyspepsia, 3.5% (vs 2.7%; 4.7%; 4.0%); epigastric discomfort, 3.8% (vs 2.8%; 9.2%; 5.4%); heartburn, 4.2% (vs 3.6%; 5.2%; 4.6%); nausea, 5.2% (vs 2.9%; 7.1%; 7.4%). *Eyes, Ears, Nose, and Throat:* sinusitis, 2.7% (vs 2.0%; 1.8%; 2.4%). *Musculoskeletal System:* back pain, 2.5% (vs 1.9%; 1.4%; 2.8%). *Nervous System:* headache, 4.7% (vs 7.5%; 6.1%; 8.0%). *Respiratory System:* bronchitis, 2.0% (vs 0.8%; 1.4%; 3.2%). *Urogenital System:* urinary tract infection, 2.8% (vs 2.7%; 2.5%; 3.6%).

The general safety profile of VIOXX 50 mg q.d. in OA clinical trials of up to 6 months (476 patients) was similar to that of VIOXX at the recommended OA doses of 12.5 mg and 25 mg q.d., except for a higher incidence of GI symptoms (abdominal pain, epigastric pain, heartburn, nausea, and vomiting), lower extremity edema (6.3%), and hypertension (8.2%).

In the OA studies, the following spontaneous adverse events occurred in >0.1% to 1.9% of patients treated with VIOXX, regardless of causality:

Body as a Whole: abdominal distension, abdominal tenderness, abscess, chest pain, chills, contusion, cyst, diaphragmatic hernia, fever, fluid retention, flushing, fungal infection, infection, laceration, pain, pelvic pain, peripheral edema, postoperative pain, syncope, trauma, upper extremity edema, viral syndrome. *Cardiovascular System:* angina pectoris, atrial fibrillation, bradycardia, hematoma, irregular heartbeat, palpitation, premature ventricular contraction, tachycardia, venous insufficiency. *Digestive System:* acid reflux, aphthous stomatitis, constipation, dental caries, dental pain, digestive gas symptoms, dry mouth, duodenal disorder, dysgeusia, esophagitis, flatulence, gastric disorder, gastritis, gastroenteritis, hematochezia, hemorrhoids, infectious gastroenteritis, oral infection, oral lesion, oral ulcer, vomiting. *Eyes, Ears, Nose, and Throat:* allergic rhinitis, blurred vision, cerumen impaction, conjunctivitis, dry throat, epistaxis, laryngitis, nasal congestion, nasal secretion, ophthalmic injection, otic pain, otitis, otitis media, pharyngitis, tinnitus, tonsillitis. *Immune System:* allergy, hypersensitivity, insect bite reaction. *Metabolism and Nutrition:* appetite change, hypercholesterolemia, weight gain. *Musculoskeletal System:* ankle sprain, arm pain, arthralgia, back strain, bursitis, cartilage trauma, joint swelling, muscular cramp, muscular disorder, muscular weakness, musculoskeletal pain, musculoskeletal stiffness, myalgia, osteoarthritis, tendinitis, traumatic arthropathy, wrist fracture. *Nervous System:* hypesthesia, insomnia, median nerve neuropathy, migraine, muscular spasm, paresthesia, sciatica, somnolence, vertigo. *Psychiatric:* anxiety, depression, mental acuity decreased. *Respiratory System:* asthma, cough, dyspnea, pneumonia, pulmonary congestion, respiratory infection. *Skin and Skin Appendages:* abrasion, alopecia, atopic dermatitis, basal cell carcinoma, blister, cellulitis, contact dermatitis, herpes simplex, herpes zoster, nail unit disorder, perspiration, pruritus, rash, skin erythema, urticaria, xerosis. *Urogenital System:* breast mass, cystitis, dysuria, menopausal symptoms, menstrual disorder, nocturia, urinary retention, vaginitis.

The following serious adverse events have been reported rarely (estimated <0.1%) in patients taking VIOXX, regardless of causality. Cases reported only in the postmarketing experience are indicated in italics.

Cardiovascular: cerebrovascular accident, congestive heart failure, deep venous thrombosis, myocardial infarction, pulmonary embolism, transient ischemic attack, unstable angina. *GI:* cholecystitis, colitis, colonic malignant neoplasm, *duodenal perforation*, duodenal ulcer, *esophageal ulcer, gastric perforation, gastric ulcer*, GI bleeding, *hepatitis,* intestinal obstruction, *jaundice,* pancreatitis. *Hemic and Lymphatic: agranulocytosis, leukopenia,* lymphoma, *thrombocytopenia. Immune System: anaphylactoid reaction, angioedema. Nervous System: aseptic meningitis. Psychiatric: confusion, hallucinations. Skin and Skin Appendages: severe skin reactions, including Stevens-Johnson syndrome. Urogenital System: acute renal failure,* breast malignant neoplasm, *interstitial nepphritis*, prostatic malignant neoplasm, urolithiasis, *worsening chronic renal failure.*

In 1-year controlled clinical trials and in extension studies for up to 86 weeks (~800 patients treated with VIOXX for 1 year or longer), the adverse-experience profile was qualitatively similar to that observed in studies of shorter duration.

Analgesia, Including Primary Dysmenorrhea: Approximately 1,000 patients were treated with VIOXX in analgesia studies. All patients in postdental surgery pain studies received only a single dose of study medication. Patients in primary dysmenorrhea studies may have taken up to 3 daily doses of VIOXX, and those in the postorthopedic surgery pain study were prescribed 5 daily doses of VIOXX.

The adverse-experience profile in the analgesia studies was generally similar to those reported in the OA studies. The following additional adverse experience, which occurred at an incidence of ≥2% of patients treated with VIOXX, was observed in the postdental pain surgery studies: postdental extraction alveolitis (dry socket).

In 110 patients treated with VIOXX (average age ~65 years) in the postorthopedic surgery pain study, the most commonly reported adverse experiences were constipation, fever, and nausea.

DOSAGE AND ADMINISTRATION: VIOXX is administered orally. The lowest dose of VIOXX should be sought for each patient.

OA: The recommended starting dose of VIOXX is 12.5 mg once daily. Some patients may receive additional benefit by increasing the dose to 25 mg once daily. The maximum recommended daily dose is 25 mg.

Management of Acute Pain and Treatment of Primary Dysmenorrhea: The recommended initial dose of VIOXX is 50 mg once daily. Subsequent doses should be 50 mg once daily as needed. Use of VIOXX for more than 5 days in management of pain has not been studied.

VIOXX Tablets may be taken with or without food.

Oral Suspension: VIOXX Oral Suspension 12.5 mg/5 mL or 25 mg/5 mL may be substituted for VIOXX Tablets 12.5 mg or 25 mg, respectively, in any of the above indications. Shake before using.

For more detailed information, consult your Merck representative and read the full Prescribing Information.

MERCK

ARTHRITIS & RHEUMATISM
Vol. 44, No. 2, February 2001, pp 339–342

Development of Fulminant Hepatitis B (Precore Variant Mutant Type) After the Discontinuation of Low-Dose Methotrexate Therapy in a Rheumatoid Arthritis Patient

Satoshi Ito,[1] Kiyoshi Nakazono,[2] Akira Murasawa,[2] Yusaku Mita,[3] Kojiro Hata,[3] Noriko Saito,[1] Masatoshi Kikuchi,[3] Kazukiyo Yoshida,[3] Masaaki Nakano,[1] and Fumitake Gejyo[1]

A 75-year-old female rheumatoid arthritis patient who was positive for hepatitis B surface antigen and for antibodies to hepatitis Be antigen showed liver dysfunction, and therefore methotrexate (MTX) therapy was discontinued. Her drug lymphocyte stimulation test indicated positivity for MTX. Her liver dysfunction improved briefly, but she developed fulminant hepatitis with elevated levels of hepatitis B virus (HBV)/DNA polymerase and subsequently died. HBV/DNA analysis performed with polymerase chain reaction–mutation site–specific assay revealed that the fulminant hepatitis was caused by a precore mutant virus. Sudden reactivation of the immune system by discontinuation of MTX may have led to the attack on infected cells. Even when hepatitis Be antibodies are present, MTX should not be used in patients who have chronic infection with HBV.

Administration or discontinuation of steroid hormone or immunosuppressants sometimes induces recurrence of hepatitis in patients who undergo organ transplantation or chemotherapy for malignant diseases (1,2). Such exacerbation of hepatitis has also been reported in the practice of rheumatology (3–5). In the clinical course of hepatitis B, seroconversion of the hepatitis Be antigen (HBeAg) to anti-HBe antibodies is considered desirable. However, fulminant hepatitis can develop in patients with anti-HBe when a precore mutant virus is present (6–10). Herein we report the case of a female rheumatoid arthritis (RA) patient who developed fulminant hepatitis B after the discontinuation of low-dose methotrexate (MTX) therapy, and whose virus was a precore variant mutant type.

CASE REPORT

The patient developed RA in 1976 when she was 57 years old. D-penicillamine (100 mg/day) was started in 1985, and prednisolone was added at 5 mg/day in 1988. In 1989, D-penicillamine was changed to bucillamine (300 mg/day). When she was admitted to the hospital in 1990, tests for hepatitis B virus (HBV) markers, hepatitis B surface antigen (HBsAg), and anti-HBe yielded positive findings, but the results of her liver function test were within normal limits. Although her creatinine clearance rate was 46.5 ml/minute, MTX (5 mg/week) was added to her treatment regimen and then increased to 7.5 mg/week. Bucillamine was tapered to 100 mg/day. She had also been taking sulindac (200 mg/day). Liver dysfunction was noted in May 1993 and progressed gradually over the next several months. On September 7, 1993, the MTX was discontinued because the patient was found to have elevated transaminase levels (aspartate aminotransferase [AST] 105 IU/liter, alanine aminotransferase [ALT] 112 IU/liter). On September 10, 1993, she was admitted to Senami Hospital because of general malaise.

On physical examination, neither icterus nor ascites was observed. The patient was alert. Her laboratory findings were as follows: white blood cell count 3,800/mm^3, hemoglobin level 11.8 gm/dl, platelet count 12 ×

[1]Satoshi Ito, MD, Noriko Saito, MD, Masaaki Nakano, MD, Fumitake Gejyo, MD: Niigata University School of Medicine, Niigata, Japan; [2]Kiyoshi Nakazono, MD, Akira Murasawa, MD: Rheumatic Center of Niigata Prefectural Senami Hospital, Murakami, Japan; [3]Yusaku Mita, MD, Kojiro Hata, MD, Masatoshi Kikuchi, MD, Kazukiyo Yoshida, MD: Niigata City General Hospital, Niigata, Japan.

Address correspondence and reprint requests to Satoshi Ito, MD, Department of Medicine (II), Niigata University School of Medicine, 1-757 Asahimachi-dori, Niigata 951-8510, Japan.

Submitted for publication April 11, 2000; accepted in revised form October 13, 2000.

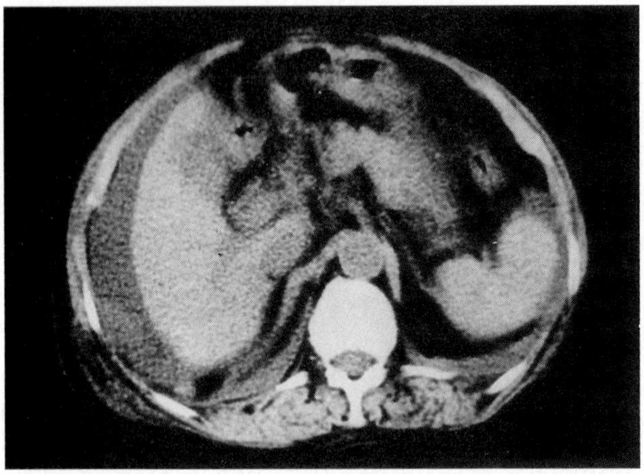

Figure 1. Abdominal computed tomography scan, revealing marked atrophy of the liver with massive ascites.

$10^4/mm^3$, AST 95 IU/liter, ALT 95 IU/liter, lactate dehydrogenase (LDH) 674 IU/liter, alkaline phosphatase (ALP) 362 IU/liter, cholinesterase 2,320 IU/liter (normal 3,600–7,600), total bilirubin 1.49 mg/dl, positive HBsAg, and positive anti-HBe. Antibodies to hepatitis C virus (HCV) were not detected, and she did not have hematuria or proteinuria. Her creatine clearance rate was 38.0 ml/minute, and abdominal ultrasonography revealed no abnormalities.

By September 22, 1993, anorexia had developed,

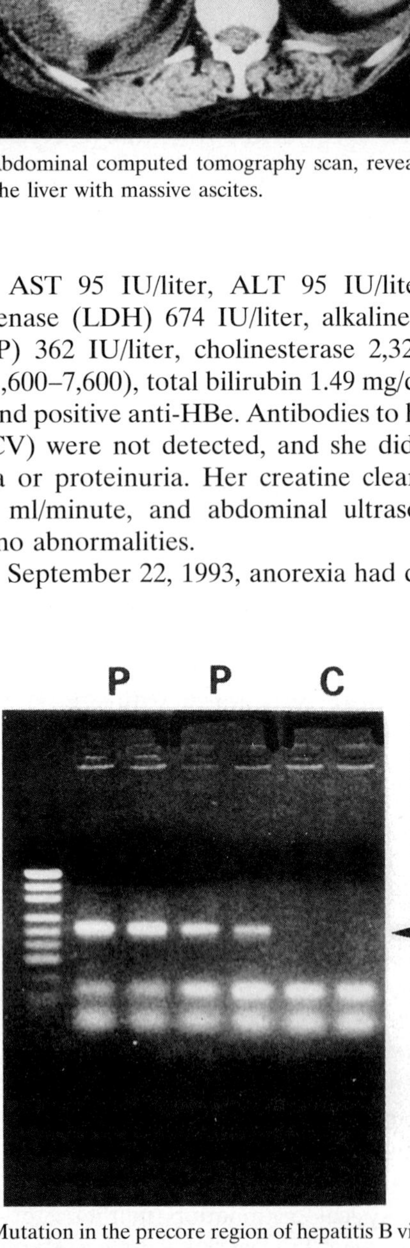

Figure 2. Mutation in the precore region of hepatitis B virus, detected by polymerase chain reaction–mutation site–specific assay. P = patient sample (assay was done in duplicate); C = control sample. The patient's samples showed a band of 203 bp.

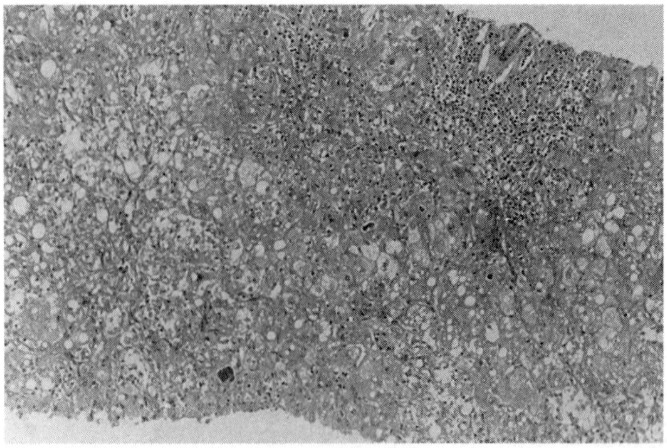

Figure 3. Postmortem needle necropsy, revealing massive necrosis of the liver.

and she showed marked liver dysfunction. Her laboratory findings at this time were as follows: AST 1,501 IU/liter, ALT 1,016 IU/liter, LDH 966 IU/liter, cholinesterase 1,167 IU/liter, total bilirubin 9.7 mg/dl, direct bilirubin 6.6 mg/dl, thrombotest 32%, and hepaplastin test 24%. Fulminant hepatitis was suspected, and she was transferred to Niigata City General Hospital.

Her blood ammonia level was 61 μmoles/liter, arterial ketone body ratio was 0.7 (normal <0.7), hepatocyte growth factor concentration was increased at 1.19 ng/ml (normal <0.39), Fischer's ratio was decreased at 0.84, and α-fetoprotein level was 3 ng/ml (normal <20). She tested positive for HBsAg, negative for anti-HBs antibodies, positive for HBeAg (1.4; normal <1.2), positive for anti-HBe (99.8%; negative <30%, positive >70%), positive for antibodies to hepatitis B core antigen (anti-HBc) (>99%; negative <30%, positive >70%), and negative for IgM–anti-HBc. There was no evidence of hepatitis A virus, HCV, Epstein-Barr virus, cytomegalovirus, or herpes simplex virus infection. Abdominal ultrasonography and a computed tomography (CT) scan revealed ascites.

Findings on her drug lymphocyte stimulation test (DLST) were positive for MTX, but negative for bucillamine and sulindac. We suspected MTX-induced fulminant hepatitis and increased her prednisolone to 80 mg/day, and administered insulin and a branched-chain amino acid solution. Plasma exchange and hemodiafiltration were performed. On September 23, 1993, HBV/DNA polymerase levels tested at Senami Hospital showed 13,628 counts per minute (normal <30), and this abnormally high level was confirmed at Niigata City General Hospital on September 30 (6,862 cpm). Since HBV recurrence was confirmed, treatment with interferon-β (3 million units/day) was started. However, her hepatic condition deteriorated toward failure, and she developed encephalopathy (with symptoms of flapping tremor and triphasic wave on electroencephalography). An additional CT scan on September 28, 1993 showed marked atrophy of the liver with pericardial effusion and massive ascites (Figure 1). She died on October 4, 1993.

Polymerase chain reaction–mutation site–specific assay detected a mutation in the precore region of HBV (Figure 2) (11). Postmortem needle necropsy of the liver revealed massive hepatic necrosis (Figure 3).

DISCUSSION

Steroid withdrawal therapy to achieve seroconversion (HBeAg to anti-HBe) was part of a standard antiviral treatment for hepatitis in Japan (12). In 1989, active type B hepatitis with seroconversion to anti-HBe was reported by Carman and colleagues, who noted that such hepatitis was caused by a precore region variant–type virus (6). The precore region is known to encode proteins of 29 amino acids, but in the variant type, the 28th codon, TGG, changes to a stop codon, TAG (point mutation) (6). Therefore, HBeAg is not secreted in the mutant type (6). Okamoto and colleagues clarified that the mutant precore virus (point mutation) consists of 80% variant mutations and 20% deletion-type and insertion-type mutations (7).

In a subsequent report, Akahane and colleagues proposed that seroconversion of HBeAg to anti-HBe is itself caused by a precore-region point mutation (8). The precore mutant virus was postulated to have a weak proliferative ability, probably due to the lack of HBeAg which can be a target of immune reaction (6–10); that would explain the improvement in the hepatitis after the seroconversion. However, the mutant virus sometimes recovers its ability to proliferate and has strong virulence. With a few exceptions (10), reported cases of fulminant hepatitis have been caused by mutant virus (6–10).

Initially, when we administered MTX in this case, the patient showed seroconversion of HBeAg to anti-HBe and normal liver function. Her liver dysfunction was first thought to be due to the MTX alone, since MTX had not been discontinued at that point and because the DLST yielded positive findings for MTX. Her liver function improved for a while after discontinuation of MTX. However, she later developed fulminant hepatitis with evidence of reactivation of mutant HBV. Fulminant hepatitis caused by the discontinuation of low-dose MTX was previously reported in a patient who was positive for anti-HBe; however, this prior report did not clarify whether the mutant virus was the cause (4).

Abelson and colleagues reported renal dysfunction associated with high-dose MTX (13). Other reports noted that low-dose MTX (1.25–15 mg/week) with nonsteroidal antiinflammatory drugs (NSAIDs) (14), and even MTX without NSAIDs (15), induces renal dysfunction. Our patient showed moderate renal dysfunction, as indicated by a creatinine clearance rate of 46.5 ml/minute, but MTX at a dosage of 7.5 mg/week was continued in conjunction with sulindac. When she was admitted in September 1993, her creatinine clearance rate was decreased to 38.0 ml/minute. The combination of MTX and sulindac apparently accelerated her renal dysfunction and induced the elevated serum concentration of MTX, hepatotoxicity, and marked immunosuppression. Therefore, the mutant virus was activated, and when the sudden discontinuation of MTX activated the immune system, the virus caused fulminant hepatitis.

The target of cytotoxic lymphocytes exists on the core region of HBV, and all precore mutant viruses have a core mutation, which is considered the mechanism for fulminant hepatitis (10). In our patient, it seemed likely that the HBV had already naturally seroconverted when MTX was started. In addition to MTX-associated induction of fulminant hepatitis, induction by mizoribin (an immunosuppressant available only in Japan) was reported in an RA patient with anti-HBe (5). Although the precore region was not analyzed in that case, mutant virus was suspected (5). So far, no reports of fulminant hepatitis have described an association with conventional disease-modifying antirheumatic drugs such as D-penicillamine or sulfasalazine.

We suggest that the use of MTX and other immunosuppressants should be avoided for RA patients with chronic infection with HBV, even when the hepatitis seems to be inactive. If steroids or immunosuppressants must be used for treatment, a gradual dose increase or tapering should be done, and liver function and DNA polymerase levels should be closely monitored. Administration of antiviral drugs should also be considered.

REFERENCES

1. Iwai K, Tashima M, Itoh M, Okazaki T, Yamamoto K, Ohno H, et al. Fulminant hepatitis B following bone marrow transplantation in an HBsAg-negative, HBsAb-positive recipient; reactivation of dormant virus during the immunosuppressive period. Bone Marrow Transplant 2000;25:105–8.
2. Clark FL, Drummond MW, Chambers S, Chapman BA, Patton MW. Successful treatment with lamivudine for fulminant reacti-

vated hepatitis B infection following intensive therapy for high-grade non-Hodgkin's lymphoma. Ann Oncol 1998;9:385–7.
3. Nakanishi K, Ishikawa M, Nakauchi M, Sakurai A, Doi K, Taniguchi Y. Antibody to hepatitis Be positive hepatitis induced by withdrawal of steroid therapy for polymyositis: response to interferon-alpha and cyclosporin A. Intern Med 1998;37:519–22.
4. Flowers MA, Heathcote J, Wanless IR, Sherman M, Reynolds WJ, Cameron RG, et al. Fulminant hepatitis as a consequence of reactivation of hepatitis B virus infection after discontinuation of low-dose methotrexate therapy. Ann Intern Med 1990;112:381–2.
5. Kashiwazaki S, Kondo H, Koike T, Saito T, Kasukawa R, Kashiwagi H, et al. Dose comparison of Bredinine on rheumatoid arthritis: a multicenter post-marketing surveillance study. Jpn J Inflamm 1996;16:269–89.
6. Carman WF, Jacyna MR, Hadziyannis S, Karayiannis P, McGarvey MJ, Makris A, et al. Mutation preventing formation of hepatitis Be antigen in patients with chronic hepatitis B infection. Lancet 1989;2:588–91.
7. Okamoto H, Yotsumoto S, Akahane Y, Yamanaka T, Miyazaki Y, Sugai Y, et al. Hepatitis B viruses with precore region defects prevail in persistently infected hosts along with seroconversion to the antibody against e antigen. J Virol 1990;64:1298–303.
8. Akahane Y, Yamanaka T, Suzuki H, Sugai Y, Tsuda F, Yotsumoto S, et al. Chronic active hepatitis with hepatitis B virus DNA and active e antigen in the serum. Gastroenterology 1990;90:1113–9.
9. Kosaka Y, Takase K, Kojima M, Shimizu M, Inoue K, Yoshiba M, et al. Fulminant hepatitis B: induction by hepatitis B virus mutants defective in the precore region and incapable of encoding e antigen. Gastroenterology 1991;100:1087–94.
10. Ehata T, Omata M, Chaung WL, Yokosuka O, Ito Y, Hosoda K, et al. Mutations in core nucleotide sequence of hepatitis B virus correlate with fulminant and severe hepatitis. J Clin Invest 1993; 91:1206–13.
11. Kinoshita M, Seno T, Fukai T, Shin S, Tsubota A, Kumada H. A detection method for point mutation in the precore region of human hepatitis B virus (HBV)-DNA using mutation-site-specific assay. Clin Chim Acta 1994;228:83–90.
12. Kumada H, Ikeda K, Yoshiba A. Withdrawal therapy of steroid for chronic hepatitis. Kantansui 1983;7:409–16. In Japanese.
13. Abelson HT, Fosburg MT, Beardsley GP, Goorin AM, Gorka C, Link M, et al. Methotrexate-induced renal impairment: clinical studies and rescue from systemic toxicity with high-dose leucovorin and thymidine. J Clin Oncol 1993;1:208–16.
14. Dupuis LL, Koren G, Shore A, Silverman ED, Laxer RM. Methotrexate-nonsteroidal antiinflammatory drug interaction in children with arthritis. J Rheumatol 1990;17:1469–73.
15. Seideman P, Müller-Suur R, Ekman E. Renal effects of low dose methotrexate in rheumatoid arthritis. J Rheumatol 1993;20: 1126–8.

ARTHRITIS & RHEUMATISM
Vol. 44, No. 2, February 2001, pp 343–350

Effects of Intraarticular Glucocorticoids on Macrophage Infiltration and Mediators of Joint Damage in Osteoarthritis Synovial Membranes

Findings in a Double-Blind, Placebo-Controlled Study

Laurel Young,[1] Amel Katrib,[2] Carolyn Cuello,[2] Ute Vollmer-Conna,[2] James V. Bertouch,[1] Peter J. Roberts-Thomson,[3] Michael J. Ahern,[3] Malcolm D. Smith,[3] and Peter P. Youssef[4]

Objective. To investigate the effects of intraarticular glucocorticoid treatment on macrophage infiltration, the expression of the chemokines monocyte chemoattractant protein 1 (MCP-1) and macrophage inflammatory protein 1α (MIP-1α), and the expression of matrix metalloproteinases 1 and 3 (MMPs 1 and 3) and their inhibitors, the tissue inhibitors of metalloproteinases 1 and 2 (TIMPs 1 and 2), in osteoarthritis (OA) synovial membranes.

Methods. Forty patients underwent arthroscopic biopsy before and 1 month after intraarticular injection of glucocorticoids. Twenty-one patients received 120 mg of methylprednisolone acetate (Depo-Medrol; Upjohn, Kalamazoo, MI), and 20 patients received placebo (1 patient received placebo in 1 knee and methylprednisolone acetate in the other). Immunoperoxidase staining for the expression of CD68, MCP-1, MIP-1α, MMP-1, MMP-3, TIMP-1, and TIMP-2 was performed, and the immunostaining was quantified by color video image analysis.

Results. CD68, MCP-1, MIP-1α, MMP-1, MMP-3, TIMP-1, and TIMP-2 immunostaining was observed in all synovial membranes. Intraarticular glucocorticoid treatment was associated with a small (30%) but statistically significant (P = 0.048) reduction in CD68+ macrophage staining in the synovial lining layer, but there was no change in the CD68 expression in the synovial sublining layer. No significant differences were observed for MCP-1, MIP-1α, MMP-1, MMP-3, TIMP-1, and TIMP-2 immunostaining in the synovial lining or sublining layers.

Conclusion. Intraarticular glucocorticoids may reduce CD68+ macrophage infiltration into the synovial lining layer, but not the expression of MCP-1, MIP-1α, MMP-1, MMP-3, TIMP-1, and TIMP-2 in the synovial membrane, in patients with OA.

The incidence of osteoarthritis (OA) of the knee has been reported to be 240 cases per 100,000 person-years (1). OA is a common cause of morbidity and a significant cost to the community (9% of per capita income in the United States) (2). The disease is characterized by cartilage loss and narrowing of the joint space, and it has been generally classified as a degenerative disorder. However, recent studies by our group have demonstrated inflammation in the OA synovial membrane and the expression of proinflammatory cytokines (3) and cell adhesion molecules, even in early disease

Dr. Smith's work was supported by the National Health and Medical Research Council (NHMRC), the Clive and Vera Ramaciotti Trust, and the Rebecca L. Cooper Foundation. Dr. Youssef's work was supported by a postdoctoral research grant from the University of New South Wales, the Arthritis Foundation of Australia, the Royal Australasian College of Physicians, and the NHMRC.

[1]Laurel Young, MB, BS, James V. Bertouch, MD, FRACP: Prince of Wales Hospital, Sydney, New South Wales, Australia; [2]Amel Katrib, MB, BS, FRACP, Carolyn Cuello, BSc (Hons), Ute Vollmer-Conna, PhD: University of New South Wales, Sydney, New South Wales, Australia; [3]Peter J. Roberts-Thomson, DPhil (Oxon), FRACP, Michael J. Ahern, MD, FRACP, Malcolm D. Smith, PhD, FRACP: Repatriation General Hospital, Daw Park, and Flinders Medical Centre, Adelaide, South Australia, Australia; [4]Peter P. Youssef, PhD, FRACP: University of New South Wales, and The Royal Prince Alfred Institute of Rheumatology and Orthopaedics, Camperdown, New South Wales, Australia.

Address correspondence and reprint requests to Peter P. Youssef, PhD, FRACP, The Royal Prince Alfred Institute of Rheumatology and Orthopaedics, QE11 Building, 59 Missenden Road, Camperdown, New South Wales 2050, Australia.

Submitted for publication June 23, 2000; accepted in revised form September 27, 2000.

(4). In studies comparing synovial tissues from OA and rheumatoid arthritis (RA) patients, investigators have observed that OA tissues express and produce chemokines and metalloproteinases, although to a lesser extent than RA tissues (4–6). It is possible that these mediators play a role in the pathogenesis of OA (7).

Chemokines are a group of small molecules produced by synovial macrophages and fibroblast-like synoviocytes that are capable of chemoattracting leukocytes. Monocyte chemoattractant protein 1 (MCP-1) and macrophage inflammatory protein 1α (MIP-1α) are predominantly macrophage chemoattractants that are produced in human OA synovial tissue (4,5) and may play a major role in the entry of macrophages into OA synovial tissue.

The matrix metalloproteinases (MMPs) are a potent family of enzymes produced by macrophages and fibroblasts that can destroy all the components of cartilage. These enzymes are classified according to their substrate specificities for different components of the extracellular matrix. On this basis, MMPs can be divided into 4 groups: the collagenases, which cleave the triple helix of fibrillar collagens; the gelatinases, which can degrade gelatin and type IV collagen in basement membrane; the stromelysins, which are active against a broad spectrum of substrates, such as proteoglycans, laminin, and fibronectin; and the membrane-type (MT) MMPs, which can degrade collagens and are involved in the activation of other MMPs (8).

MMP-1 (collagenase 1) and MMP-3 (stromelysin 1) are among the best studied of the MMPs in OA synovium (9–11) and cartilage (6). The natural inhibitors specific for MMPs, which are produced locally by chondrocytes and fibroblast-like synoviocytes, are called tissue inhibitors of metalloproteinases (TIMPs 1–4). TIMP-1 and TIMP-2 have been studied in OA cartilage, and it has been hypothesized that an imbalance between the MMPs and TIMPs may be important in the development of cartilage loss (6).

Intraarticular glucocorticoids are often used therapeutically in OA, particularly when there is knee involvement (12). In vitro studies demonstrate that glucocorticoids reduce MMP and chemokine production by human fibroblast-like synoviocytes (13). In animal models of OA, glucocorticoids may reduce cartilage damage (14) and stromelysin synthesis by cartilage (15). In a study of intraarticular triamcinolone hexacetonide in 3 patients with RA, investigators observed a reduction in MMP-3 messenger RNA (mRNA) expression in the synovium (16). There are no published data on the in vivo effects of intraarticular glucocorticoids on OA synovium.

Herein we report the findings of a double-blind, placebo-controlled study of intraarticular glucocorticoid treatment on macrophage infiltration, the expression of the chemokines MCP-1 and MIP-1α, and the expression of MMPs 1 and 3 and their inhibitors, TIMPs 1 and 2, in OA synovial tissue.

PATIENTS AND METHODS

Reagents. Methylprednisolone acetate (Depo-Medrol) was purchased from Upjohn (Kalamazoo, MI). Sodium chloride and hydrogen peroxide were purchased from Merck (Melbourne, Victoria, Australia), methanol from Ajax Chemicals (Auburn, New South Wales, Australia), Tris base and diaminobenzidine (DAB) from Sigma (Castle Hill, New South Wales, Australia), bovine serum albumin (BSA) and proteinase K from Boehringer (Mannheim, Germany), normal goat serum, biotinylated goat anti-mouse secondary antibody, and avidin–biotin–horseradish peroxidase complex from Vector Australian Laboratory Services (Rockdale, New South Wales, Australia), methyl green from BDH Chemicals (Sydney, New South Wales, Australia), and Eukitt from Lomb Scientific (Sydney, New South Wales, Australia).

Monoclonal antibodies. All antibodies used were murine monoclonals. Anti–MMP-1 (IgG2a), anti–MMP-3 (IgG1), anti–TIMP-1 (IgG2b), and anti–TIMP-2 (IgG1) antibodies were purchased from ICN Biomedicals (Sydney, New South Wales, Australia). Anti-CD68 (IgG3) antibody and mouse IgG were purchased from Dako (Sydney, New South Wales, Australia). Anti–MIP-1α (IgG2a) and anti–MCP-1 (IgG2a) antibodies were purchased from R&D Systems (Minneapolis, MN). IgG1, IgG2a, IgG2b, and IgG3 antibodies of irrelevant specificities were purchased from Dako and were used as negative controls.

Study protocol. The study protocol is detailed in Figure 1. Patients with symptomatic knee OA were studied. They were randomized into either the active treatment group, which received 120 mg of methylprednisolone acetate intraarticularly, or the placebo group, which received normal saline intraarticularly, at the completion of the first arthroscopy.

Synovial membrane samples were obtained before and 1 month after methylprednisolone acetate or placebo injection. Needle arthroscopic techniques and standard approaches were used to obtain samples, as previously described (17). When possible, repeat biopsy samples were obtained from the area adjacent to the previous biopsy sites.

This project was approved by the ethics committee at the Repatriation General Hospital in Adelaide, and informed consent was obtained from each patient.

Patient assessments. Patients were assessed clinically at the time of the initial arthroscopy and the second arthroscopy 1 month later. These assessments included the Western Ontario and McMaster Universities Osteoarthritis Index (WOMAC) (18) pain score (maximum 20), WOMAC stiffness score (maximum 8), WOMAC total score (maximum 96), and 50-meter walking time (in seconds). The assessments were done by a metrologist who was blinded to the randomization.

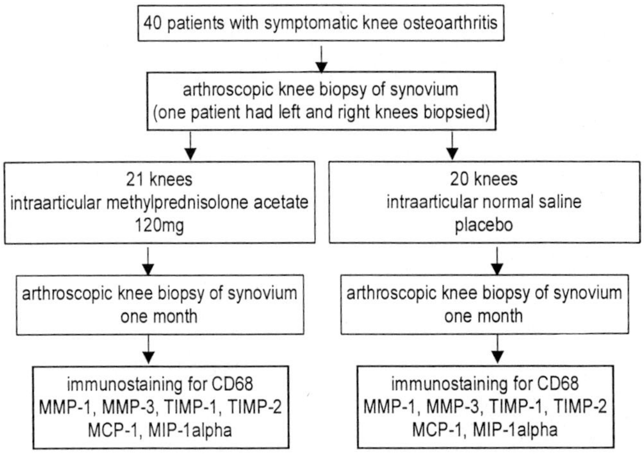

Figure 1. Study protocol. Note, one patient had both knees biopsied and received an injection of methylprednisolone acetate in one knee and placebo in other knee. MMP = matrix metalloproteinase; TIMP = tissue inhibitor of metalloproteinases; MCP-1 = monocyte chemoattractant protein 1; MIP-1α = macrophage inflammatory protein 1α.

Arthroscopies and arthroscopic grading. All arthroscopies were performed by 2 orthopedic surgeons using an inflated tourniquet and continuous irrigation with normal saline; patients were under general anesthesia. All compartments of the knee (medial and lateral tibiofemoral and patellotrochlear) were visualized, and the surgeons were asked to grade the degree of articular cartilage damage at the time of arthroscopy, according to a published method (19). The surgeons were blinded to the randomization. The severity of articular cartilage defects was graded according to depth (0 = no defect, 1 = swelling and softening, 2 = superficial fibrillation, 3 = deep fibrillation, and 4 = exposure to subchondral bone).

All synovial membrane biopsies were performed at the start of the procedure, before intraarticular manipulation was begun, and were taken from the suprapatellar pouch and medial and lateral compartments of the joint using basket forceps.

Tissue processing and immunoperoxidase staining. Synovial membrane tissue was immediately processed for formalin-fixed, paraffin-embedded sections. Adjacent tissue sections (4-μm thickness) were digested and quenched for endogenous peroxidase staining as previously described (20). Slides were incubated in 25 μg/ml of proteinase K for 20 minutes at 37°C. Slides were then incubated with 20% goat serum for 2 hours at room temperature to block nonspecific binding sites, followed by incubation with optimized dilutions of the primary antibody overnight in a humidified chamber at room temperature. All dilutions of the primary antibody were in 2% BSA in Tris buffered saline (TBS).

After further washes with TBS, the sections were incubated with biotinylated goat anti-mouse secondary antibody for 20 minutes at room temperature. The sections were again washed, and an avidin–biotin–horseradish peroxidase complex was added for 60 minutes. After further washes, the sections were incubated with methyl green for 10 minutes, washed with 100% ethanol, placed into xylene, and finally coverslipped with Eukitt.

All sections from the same patient were processed in the same run. Negative controls were performed using irrelevant mouse isotype controls, normal goat serum alone, or by omitting the secondary antibody. Specificity of staining was verified by adsorption of positive staining by preincubation with recombinant protein.

Quantification of immunostaining. The immunostained sections were examined by a computer-assisted color video image analysis system (Video Pro 32; Leading Edge, Sydney, New South Wales, Australia) (21,22). Images were recorded using a solid-state video camera and digitized using a PV100 multimedia 16-bit color video digitizer card in an Intel 80486 DX computer. The resultant image was displayed on an SVGA monitor in a 640 × 480–pixel window with 21-bit resolution. The image windows used by the Video Pro 32 system are composed of up to 640 × 442 pixels that separate into 8-bit brightness and color values for each pixel, so the system can define with great precision the color to be measured.

Thresholds were set for each section to detect and measure the identified reaction product. All sections from a given patient were analyzed in the same sitting, and at least 5 high power fields were measured in a single section from each synovial biopsy sample. The synovial lining and sublining were quantified separately. Measurements of the integrated optical density (proportional to the total amount of protein staining) and the mean optical density (equal to the integrated optical density divided by the area of DAB staining, which is a measure of the average concentration of protein on the positively stained cells) were made by a blinded observer (LY) who was unaware of the order of biopsy sections from any one patient or the patient's randomization. The reproducibility of measurements was within 10% (data not shown). This was mostly due to variability in field selection.

Statistical analysis. Between-group differences and pre- and posttreatment differences were analyzed using the repeated measures analysis of variance option available with

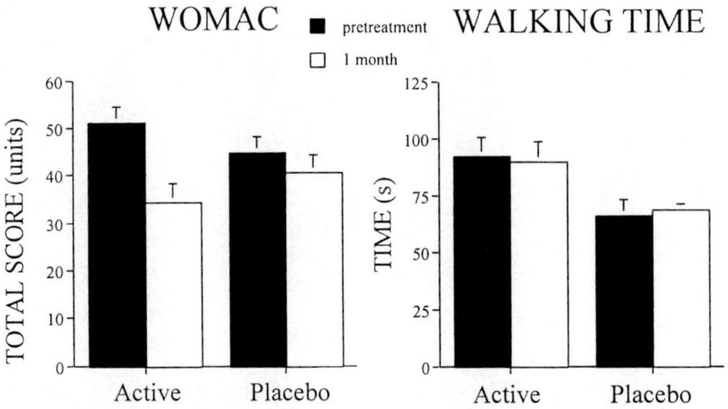

Figure 2. Effects of intraarticular methylprednisolone acetate and placebo administration on clinical scores. Methylprednisolone acetate administration was associated with a significant reduction in the Western Ontario and McMaster Universities Osteoarthritis Index (WOMAC) score (left) but not the 50-meter walking time (right). Placebo treatment did not significantly alter either of these scores.

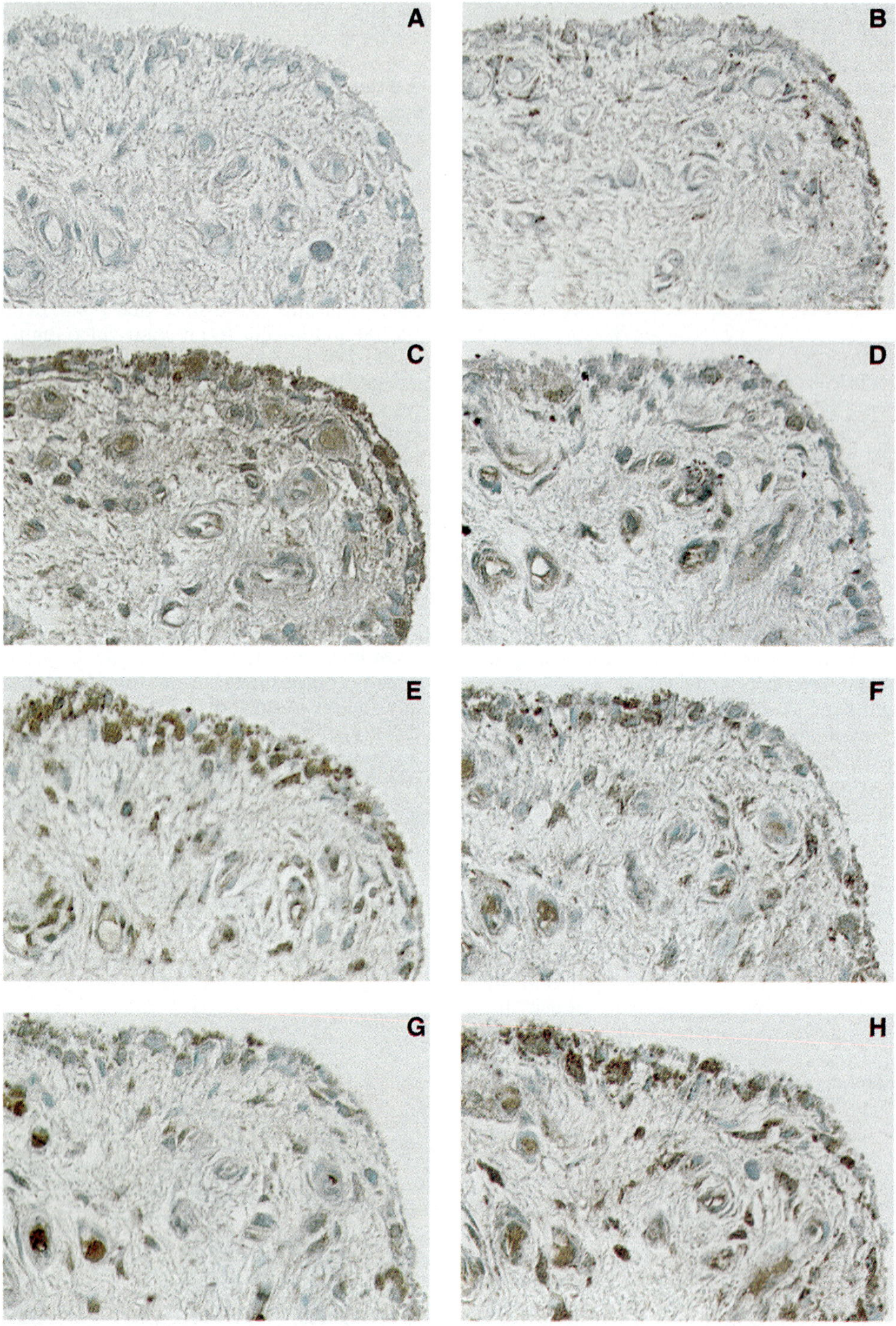

Figure 3. Photomicrographs showing typical immunostaining patterns for chemokines, matrix metalloproteinases, and tissue inhibitors of metalloproteinases in pretreatment osteoarthritic synovium. **A,** Negative control; **B,** CD68; **C,** MCP-1; **D,** MIP-1α; **E,** MMP-1; **F,** MMP-3; **G,** TIMP-1; **H,** TIMP-2 (original magnification $\times$ 120). See Figure 1 for definitions.

the SPSS statistical package (SPSS, Chicago, IL). P values less than 0.05 were considered statistically significant. No adjustments were made for multiple comparisons.

RESULTS

Clinical and laboratory parameters. Forty patients were enrolled in the study. Twenty-one patients (21 knees) received methylprednisolone acetate and 20 patients (20 knees) received placebo. One patient received an injection of methylprednisolone acetate in one knee and placebo in the other. There was no significant difference between the methylprednisolone acetate–treated group and the placebo-treated group with respect to age (mean ± SD 66 ± 11 versus 67 ± 12 years), sex (11 males and 10 females versus 14 males and 6 females), baseline arthroscopy score (13 ± 4.4 versus 11.8 ± 3.8), and baseline WOMAC score (51 ± 15 versus 45 ± 9.9).

The methylprednisolone acetate–treated group had a significantly longer duration of OA (mean ± SD 10 ± 9 years) compared with the placebo-treated group (4.9 ± 5.6 years) ($P < 0.04$). There was a moderate, but statistically significant, reduction in the WOMAC score ($P < 0.05$) in the methylprednisolone acetate–treated group but no significant change in walking time (Figure 2).

Immunohistochemical analysis of synovial membranes. *Pretreatment.* Synovial membrane samples from the knees of all 40 patients were stained with antibodies against MMP-1, MMP-3, TIMP-1, TIMP-2, MCP-1, MIP-1α, and CD68 and analyzed using computer-assisted video image analysis. Immunostaining was observed in all pretreatment biopsy samples, in both the synovial lining and synovial sublining layers (Figure 3).

There were no pretreatment differences between the methylprednisolone acetate group and the placebo group for CD68 (Figure 4), MCP-1 and MIP-1α (Figure 5), MMP-1 and MMP-3 (Figure 6), or TIMP-1 and TIMP-2 (Figure 7) immunostaining.

Posttreatment. After methylprednisolone acetate injection, there was a small reduction (30%) in CD68+ macrophage expression in the synovial lining which was statistically significant ($P = 0.048$). In comparison, there was no significant change in CD68+ immunostaining in the placebo group (Figure 4). MCP-1 and MIP-1α expression did not change significantly between the methylprednisolone acetate–treated and the placebo-treated groups in either the synovial lining layer or synovial sublining layer (Figure 5). Similarly, there were no changes in the expression of MMP-1, MMP-2, TIMP-1, or TIMP-2 (Figures 6 and 7).

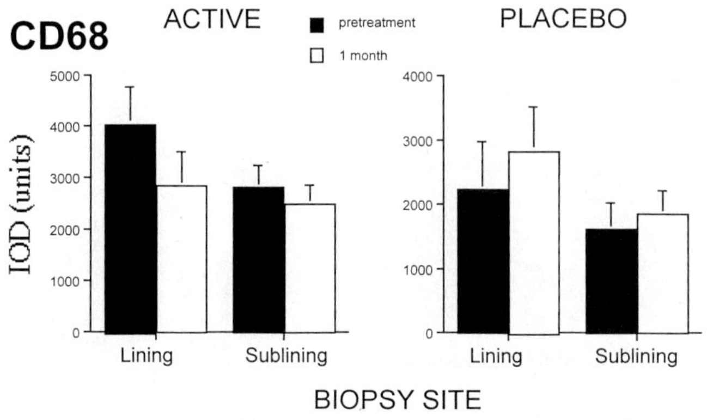

Figure 4. Effects of intraarticular methylprednisolone acetate and placebo administration on the expression of CD68. After injection of methylprednisolone acetate (active), there was a 30% reduction in CD68+ macrophage expression in the synovial lining layer compared with placebo injection; this difference was statistically significant ($P = 0.048$). IOD = integrated optical density.

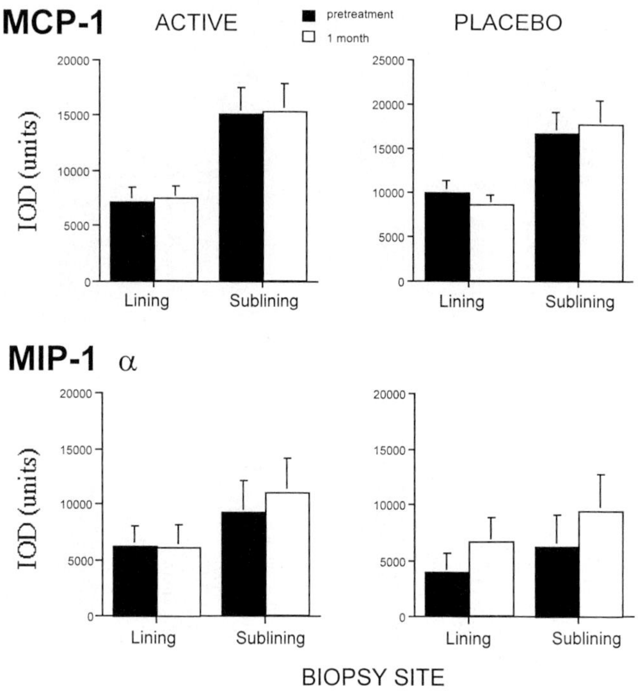

Figure 5. Effects of methylprednisolone acetate and placebo administration on the expression of chemokines. Monocyte chemoattractant protein 1 (MCP-1) and macrophage inflammatory protein 1α (MIP-1α) expression in the synovial lining and sublining layers did not change significantly in either the active-drug group or the placebo group. IOD = integrated optical density.

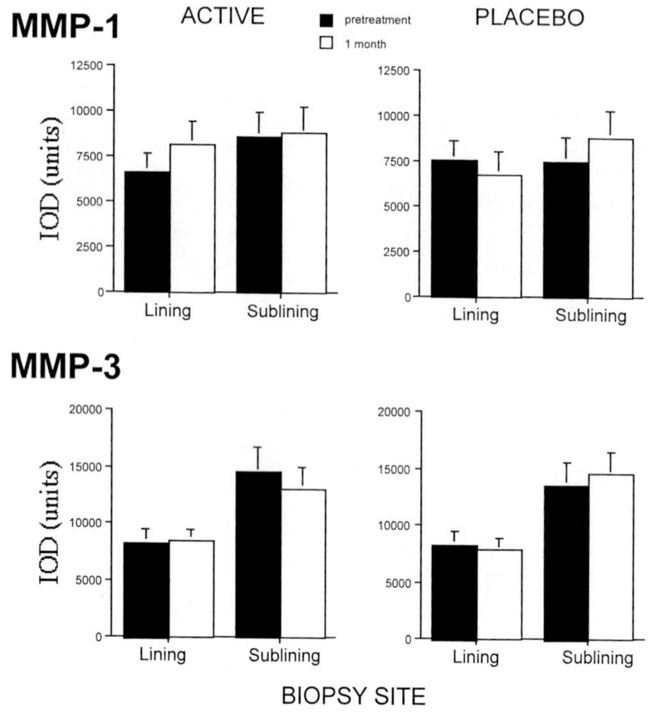

Figure 6. Effects of methylprednisolone acetate and placebo administration on the expression of matrix metalloproteinases (MMPs). MMP-1 and MMP-3 expression in the synovial lining and sublining layers did not change significantly in either the active-drug group or the placebo group. IOD = integrated optical density.

DISCUSSION

Since the first publication of the use of intraarticular glucocorticoid injections by Hollander and colleagues in 1951 (23), there have been a small number of studies of the clinical efficacy of this treatment (24,25). These studies have generally demonstrated a transient analgesic effect, as was observed in the present study. Pathophysiologic studies of the effects of intraarticular glucocorticoids on OA synovial tissue and cartilage in vivo have mostly been performed in animal models. For example, studies in primate and canine models of OA have shown a reduction in cartilage damage and OA progression after intraarticular glucocorticoid administration, associated with a reduction in MMP-3 expression in cartilage and synovium (14,15,26,27) and have also suggested that there is an imbalance between MMP and TIMP expression, which may mediate cartilage destruction (6,28). Those studies did not determine macrophage infiltration.

The present study is the first placebo-controlled in vivo analysis of the effects of intraarticular glucocorticoids on macrophage infiltration and the expression of MMPs and TIMPs in human OA synovial membranes. In contradistinction to the findings of the animal and in vitro studies, we did not observe any alteration in the expression of MMPs or TIMPs after intraarticular glucocorticoid injection.

There are a number of possible explanations for this discordance. It is possible that human OA is different from the OA in the animal models and that intraarticular glucocorticoids do not affect the expression of these factors in human OA synovial membrane and may not alter cartilage degradation mediated by MMP-1 and MMP-3. However, there are some caveats to this statement. First, the patient group entering the methylprednisolone acetate treatment arm had a longer disease duration than the group entering the placebo arm, and this may have biased against finding a difference between the groups. Second, the study was only powered to detect a 30% difference between the 2 groups, which we hypothesized would be biologically significant. However, there did not appear to be a trend toward a reduction in

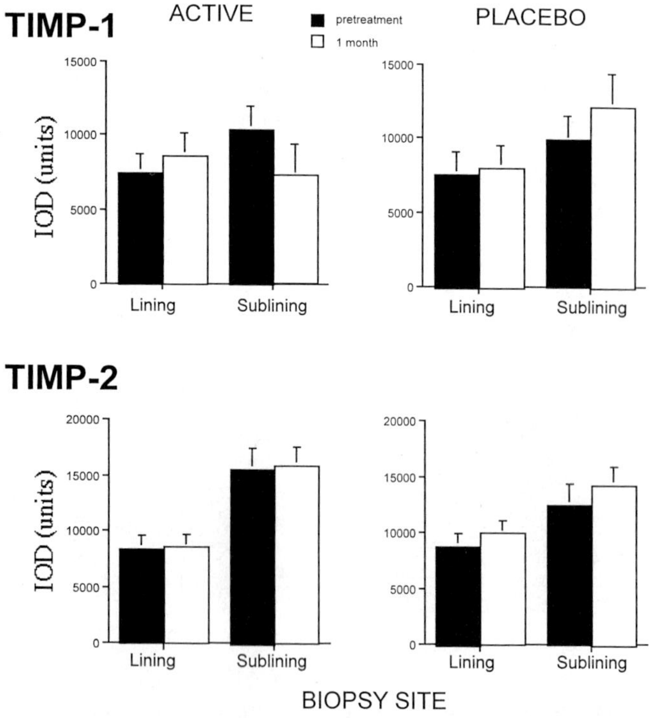

Figure 7. Effects of methylprednisolone acetate and placebo administration on the expression of tissue inhibitors of metalloproteinases (TIMPs). TIMP-1 and TIMP-2 expression in the synovial lining and sublining layers did not change significantly in either the active-drug group or the placebo group. IOD = integrated optical density.

the mediators studied, suggesting that a larger study would be unlikely to demonstrate a difference between the groups.

Interestingly, in a study of 3 RA patients, Firestein et al (16) observed a reduction in MMP-3 and TIMP-1 mRNA in the synovial membrane after intraarticular glucocorticoid injection. The absence of such an effect in the present study suggests that different mechanisms control MMP expression in OA compared with RA. The reason for this discordance remains unclear because the factors that may be controlling MMP-1 and MMP-3 expression (such as the proinflammatory mediators interleukin-1 and tumor necrosis factor) are present in both OA and RA synovial membrane, although to a lesser degree in OA (29). We were also surprised that a reduction in macrophage numbers was not associated with a decrease in the expression of MMPs, TIMPs, and chemokines, since these factors are produced by synovial macrophages. It is probable that a major source of these mediators in OA is the fibroblast-like synoviocyte, which has been shown to be a source of these mediators in RA (4,5,8), and which we postulate may be more resistant to the effects of intraarticular glucocorticoids.

In the present study, we did not determine the effects of intraarticular glucocorticoids on other possible mediators of joint damage, such as the cysteine proteases (cathepsins B, K, and L) (30,31) and the aggrecanases (32). However, in vitro, collagenase is the rate-limiting step in cartilage breakdown, and there appears to be a requirement for the breakdown of the higher structure of collagen before the other enzymes are able to degrade cartilage and proteoglycans (8). Also, because of ethical reasons, we did not study OA cartilage in these patients, and it is possible that intraarticular glucocorticoids may alter MMP expression in OA cartilage, as has been observed in some animal models (14,15).

It is difficult to assess the biologic importance of the reduction in CD68+ macrophages in the synovial lining in the absence of a reduction in CD68+ macrophage numbers in the synovial sublining. It would appear that this reduction is not biologically significant, since it is not associated with a reduction in chemokine and MMP expression, both of which are macrophage products.

In conclusion, the administration of intraarticular glucocorticoids was associated with a small reduction in CD68+ macrophage infiltration in the synovial lining but not the synovial sublining layers in human OA synovial membranes. There was no effect on the expression of MCP-1, MIP-1α, MMP-1, MMP-3, TIMP-1, or TIMP-2. The observations from this study suggest that intraarticular glucocorticoids do not influence the expression of some of the important mediators of cartilage destruction in OA.

REFERENCES

1. Oliveria SA, Felson DT, Reed JI, Cirillo PA, Walker AM. Incidence of symptomatic hand, hip, and knee osteoarthritis among patients in a health maintenance organization. Arthritis Rheum 1995;38:1134–41.
2. Yelin E, Callahan LF, for the National Arthritis Data Work Group. The economic cost and social and psychological impact of musculoskeletal conditions. Arthritis Rheum 1995;38:1351–62.
3. Smith MD, Triantafillou S, Parker A, Youssef PP, Coleman M. Synovial membrane inflammation and cytokine production in patients with early osteoarthritis. J Rheumatol 1997;24:365–71.
4. Koch AE, Kunkel SL, Harlow LA, Mazarakis DD, Haines GK, Burdick MD, et al. Macrophage inflammatory protein-1 alpha: a novel chemotactic cytokine for macrophages in rheumatoid arthritis. J Clin Invest 1994;93:921–8.
5. Koch AE, Kunkel SL, Harlow LA, Johnson B, Evanoff HL, Haines GK, et al. Enhanced production of monocyte chemoattractant protein-1 in rheumatoid arthritis. J Clin Invest 1992;90:772–9.
6. Martel-Pelletier J, McCollum R, Fujimoto N, Obata K, Cloutier J-M, Pelletier J-P. Excess of metalloproteases over tissue inhibitor of metalloprotease may contribute to cartilage degradation in osteoarthritis and rheumatoid arthritis. Lab Invest 1994;70:807–15.
7. Murphy G, Docherty AJP, Hembry RM, Reynolds JJ. Metalloproteinases and tissue damage. Br J Rheumatol 1991;30 Suppl 1:25–31.
8. Vincenti MP, Clark IM, Brinckerhoff CE. Using inhibitors of metalloproteinases to treat arthritis. Arthritis Rheum 1994:37: 1115–26.
9. Zafarullah M, Pelletier J-P, Cloutier J-M, Martel-Pelletier J. Elevated metalloproteinase and tissue inhibitor of metalloproteinase mRNA in human osteoarthritic synovia. J Rheumatol 1993;20: 693–7.
10. Okada Y, Shinmei M, Tanaka O, Naka K, Kimura A, Nakanishi I, et al. Localization of matrix metalloproteinase 3 (stromelysin) in osteoarthritic cartilage and synovium. Lab Invest 1992;66:680–90.
11. McCachren SS. Expression of metalloproteinases and metalloproteinase inhibitor in human arthritic synovium. Arthritis Rheum 1991;34:1085–93.
12. Friedman DM, Morre ME. The efficacy of intraarticular steroids in osteoarthritis: a double blind study. J Rheumatol 1980;7: 1850–6.
13. McGuire MB, Murphy G, Reynolds JJ, Russell RGG. Production of collagenase and inhibitor (TIMP) by normal, rheumatoid and osteoarthritis synovium in vitro: effects of hydrocortisone and indomethacin. Clin Sci (Colch) 1981;61:703–10.
14. Pelletier J-P, Mineau F, Raynauld J-P, Woessner JF Jr, Gunja-Smith Z, Martel-Pelletier J. Intraarticular injections with methylprednisolone acetate reduce osteoarthritic lesions in parallel with chondrocyte stromelysin synthesis in experimental osteoarthritis. Arthritis Rheum 1994;37:414–23.
15. Pelletier J-P, DiBattista JA, Raynauld J-P, Wilhelm S, Martel-Pelletier J. The in vivo effects of intraarticular corticosteroid injections on cartilage lesions, stromelysin, interleukin-1 and oncogene protein synthesis in experimental osteoarthritis. Lab Invest 1995;72:578–88.
16. Firestein GS, Paine MM, Littman BH. Gene expression (collagenase, tissue inhibitor of metalloproteinases, complement, and HLA–DR) in rheumatoid arthritis and osteoarthritis synovium:

quantitative analysis and effect of intraarticular corticosteroids. Arthritis Rheum 1991;34:1094–105.
17. Smith MD, Chandran G, Youssef PP, Darby T, Ahern MJ. Day case knee arthroscopy under regional anaesthesia performed by rheumatologists. Aust N Z J Med 1996;26:108–9.
18. Bellamy N, Buchanan WW, Goldsmith CH, Campbell J, Stitt LW. Validation study of WOMAC: a health status instrument for measuring clinically important patient relevant outcomes to antirheumatic drug therapy in patients with osteoarthritis of the hip or knee. J Rheumatol 1988;15:1833–44.
19. Ayral X, Dougados M, Listrat V, Bonvarlet JP, Simonnet J, Poiraudeau S, et al. Chondroscopy: a new method for scoring chondropathy. Semin Arthritis Rheum 1993;22:289–97.
20. Digirolamo N, McCluskey PJ, Lloyd A, Filipic M, Wakefield D. Increased expression of metalloproteinases in vivo in scleritis tissue and in vitro in cultured scleral fibroblasts. Am J Pathol 1997;150:653–66.
21. Youssef PP, Triantafillou S, Parker A, Coleman M, Roberts-Thomson PJ, Ahern MJ, et al. Effects of pulse methylprednisolone on cell adhesion molecules in the synovial membrane in rheumatoid arthritis: reduced E-selectin and intercellular adhesion molecule 1 expression. Arthritis Rheum 1996;39:1970–9.
22. Youssef PP, Haynes DR, Triantafillou S, Parker A, Gamble JR, Roberts-Thomson PJ, et al. Effects of pulse methylprednisolone on inflammatory mediators in peripheral blood, synovial fluid, and synovial membrane in rheumatoid arthritis. Arthritis Rheum 1997; 40:1400–8.
23. Hollander JL, Brown EM Jr, Jessar RA, Brown CY. Hydrocortisone and cortisone injected into arthritic joints. JAMA 1951;14: 1631–5.
24. Dieppe PA, Sathapatayavongs B, Jones HE, Bacon PA, Ring EF. Intraarticular steroids in osteoarthritis. Rheumatol Rehab 1980; 19:212–7.
25. Friedman DM, Moore ME. The efficacy of intraarticular steroids in osteoarthritis: a double-blind study. J Rheumatol 1980;7:850–6.
26. Gibson T, Burry HC, Poswillo D, Glass J. Effect of intraarticular corticosteroid injections on primate cartilage. Ann Rheum Dis 1976;36:74–9.
27. Pelletier J-P, Martel-Pelletier J. Protective effects of corticosteroids on cartilage lesions and osteophyte formation in the Pond-Nuki dog model of osteoarthritis. Arthritis Rheum 1989;32: 181–93.
28. Dean DD, Martel-Pelletier J, Pelletier J-P, Howell DS, Woessner F. Evidence for metalloproteinases and metalloproteinases inhibitor imbalance in human osteoarthritic cartilage. J Clin Invest 1989;84:678–85.
29. Saha N, Moldovan F, Tardif G, Pelletier J-P, Cloutier J-M, Martel-Pelletier J. Interleukin-1β–converting enzyme/caspase-1 in human osteoarthritic tissues: localization and role in the maturation of interleukin-1β and interleukin-18. Arthritis Rheum 1999; 42:1577–87.
30. Keyszer G, Redlich A, Häupl T, Zacher J, Sparmann M, Ungethüm U, et al. Differential expression of cathepsins B and L compared with matrix metalloproteinases and their respective inhibitors in rheumatoid arthritis and osteoarthritis: a parallel investigation by semiquantitative reverse transcriptase–polymerase chain reaction and immunohistochemistry. Arthritis Rheum 1998;41: 1378–87.
31. Dodds RA, Connor JR, Drake FH, Gowen M. Expression of cathepsin K messenger RNA in giant cells and their precursors in human osteoarthritic synovial tissues. Arthritis Rheum 1999;42: 1588–93.
32. Lark MW, Bayne EK, Flanagan J, Harper CF, Hoerrner LA, Hutchinson NI, et al. Aggrecan degradation in human cartilage. J Clin Invest 1997;100:93–106.

ARTHRITIS & RHEUMATISM
Vol. 44, No. 2, February 2001, pp 351–360

Interleukin-1β Down-Regulates the Expression of Glucuronosyltransferase I, a Key Enzyme Priming Glycosaminoglycan Biosynthesis

Influence of Glucosamine on Interleukin-1β–Mediated Effects in Rat Chondrocytes

Jean-Noel Gouze, Karim Bordji, Sandrine Gulberti, Bernard Terlain, Patrick Netter, Jacques Magdalou, Sylvie Fournel-Gigleux, and Mohamed Ouzzine

Objective. **To assess the variations of galactose-β-1,3-glucuronosyltransferase I (GlcAT-I) expression related to the decrease in proteoglycan synthesis mediated by interleukin-1β (IL-1β) in rat chondrocytes, and to evaluate the influence of glucosamine on the effects elicited by this proinflammatory cytokine.**

Methods. **Rat articular chondrocytes in primary monolayer cultures or encapsulated into alginate beads were treated with recombinant IL-1β in the absence or presence (1.0–4.5 gm/liter) of glucosamine. Variations of GlcAT-I and expression of stromelysin 1 (matrix metalloproteinase 3 [MMP-3]) messenger RNA (mRNA) were evaluated by quantitative multistandard reverse transcriptase–polymerase chain reaction. In vitro enzymatic activity of GlcAT-I was measured by thin-layer chromatography, with radiolabeled UDP-glucuronic acid and a digalactoside derivative as substrates. Proteoglycan synthesis was determined by ex vivo incorporation of Na_2-$^{35}SO_4$. Nitric oxide synthase and cyclooxygenase activities were monitored by the evaluation of nitrite ($NO^-{}_2$) and prostaglandin E_2 (PGE_2) produced in the culture medium, respectively.**

Results. **IL-1β treatment resulted in a marked inhibition of GlcAT-I mRNA expression and in vitro catalytic activity, together with a decrease in proteoglycan synthesis. In addition, glucosamine was able to prevent, in a dose-dependent manner, the inhibitory effects of IL-1β. In the same way, the amino sugar reduced $NO^-{}_2$ and PGE_2 production induced by IL-1β. Finally, the up-regulation of stromelysin 1 (MMP-3) mRNA expression by IL-1β was fully prevented by glucosamine.**

Conclusion. **The results of this study suggest that the deleterious effect of IL-1β on the anabolism of proteoglycan could involve the repression of GlcAT-I, a key enzyme in the biosynthesis of glycosaminoglycan. Glucosamine was highly effective in preventing these IL-1β–mediated suppressive effects. The amino sugar also prevented the production of inflammatory mediators induced by the cytokine. This action could account for a possible beneficial effect of glucosamine on osteoarthritic articular cartilage.**

Glycosaminoglycans (GAG) are ubiquitously distributed among tissues, usually in covalent linkage to proteoglycan core proteins (1). They are linear polymers of repeating disaccharides containing hexosamine and hexuronic acid. In the case of keratan sulfates (KS), hexuronic acid is replaced by galactose. GAG are in-

Presented by Jean-Noel Gouze in partial fulfillment of the requirements for a PhD degree, CNRS-Université Henri Poincaré-Nancy I, Vandœuvre-lès-Nancy, France.

Supported by grants from the Région Lorraine "Jeune Equipe," from the "FR 42 Protéines," and by a Contrat de Programme de Recherche Clinique. Jean-Noel Gouze's work was supported by a grant from the Ministère de la Recherche et de l'Enseignement Supérieur.

Jean-Noel Gouze, BSc, Karim Bordji, PhD, Sandrine Gulberti, BSc, Bernard Terlain, PharmD, Patrick Netter, MD, PhD, Jacques Magdalou, PhD, Sylvie Fournel-Gigleux, PharmD, PhD, Mohamed Ouzzine, PhD: CNRS-Université Henri Poincaré-Nancy I, Vandœuvre-lès-Nancy, France.

Address correspondence and reprint requests to Sylvie Fournel-Gigleux, PhD, Physiopathologie et Pharmacologie Articulaires, UMR CNRS-UHP 7561, Faculté de Médecine, Avenue de la Forêt de Haye, BP 184, F-54505 Vandœuvre-lès-Nancy, France.

Submitted for publication February 4, 2000; accepted in revised form October 23, 2000.

volved in the regulation and maintenance of cell proliferation, cytodifferentiation, and tissue morphogenesis (2,3). They also play a central role in matrix assembly and are especially essential in maintaining the structural and functional integrity of cartilaginous tissue. In particular, sulfated GAG attached to proteoglycans, such as aggrecan, the most abundant proteoglycans in cartilage, contribute to the unique biomechanical properties of this tissue (4). Hexuronic acid–containing GAG are bound to serine residues in the core protein via the common carbohydrate sequence GlcA-β-1,3-Gal-β-1,3-Gal-β-1,4-Xyl-β-1-*O*-Ser, forming the so-called GAG–protein linkage region (1,3). This tetrasaccharide linkage region is shared by chondroitin sulfates, heparan sulfates, and dermatan sulfates.

In contrast, KS are *N*-linked to asparagine in KS-I proteoglycans of cornea, or *O*-linked to serine or threonine via an *N*-acetylgalactosamine residue in skeletal KS-II (5). GAG biosynthesis is initiated by the addition of a xylose moiety to specific serine residues in the core protein. This reaction is followed by the stepwise addition of 2 galactose and 1 glucuronic acid residues, and subsequently by the alternate addition of hexosamine and hexuronic residues. Each step is catalyzed by a specific glycosyltransferase using the corresponding UDP-sugar as donor substrate. The addition of the first glucuronic acid residue on the trisaccharide linkage intermediate is catalyzed by a galactose-β-1,3-glucuronosyltransferase (GlcAT-I), of which the human complementary DNA (cDNA) has recently been cloned by Kitagawa et al (6). GlcAT-I is a member of a family of enzymes catalyzing the transfer of glucuronic acid to a β-linked galactose residue. These glucuronosyltransferases are involved in the biosynthesis of GAG chains as well as in the formation of HNK1, a carbohydrate epitope present on various glycolipids and glycoproteins. They are thought to be different from other glucuronosyltransferases involved in the formation of the repeating disaccharidic unit of GAG (7).

GlcAT-I plays a crucial role in priming hexuronic acid–containing GAG synthesis, and any change in activity could likely affect the rate of synthesis of GAG chains and consequently proteoglycan structure and properties. Joint diseases such as osteoarthritis (OA) or rheumatoid arthritis (RA) are characterized by quantitative and qualitative modifications of proteoglycans and of their GAG chains, leading to alteration of the cartilaginous matrix (8,9). An imbalance between the biosynthesis and degradation of matrix components leads to a progressive destruction of the tissue, finally causing complete damage of the articular surface.

There is convincing evidence that interleukin-1β (IL-1β), a cytokine released by synovial cells and invading macrophages in inflamed joints, plays a decisive role in OA and RA (10). Indeed, the synovial fluid of patients with RA and OA contains elevated levels of IL-1β (11). It is accepted that this cytokine initiates a number of events leading to cartilage damage. This process involves inhibition of biosynthesis of the main matrix components, in particular proteoglycans, together with promotion of their degradation. Cartilage breakdown induced by IL-1β is initiated by the release of matrix metalloproteinases (MMPs), such as stromelysin and collagenase, and by a reduction in the concentration of tissue inhibitors of MMPs (12). Moreover, the proinflammatory effects of IL-1β are attributed to a variety of mediators such as prostaglandin E_2 (PGE_2), produced by the induction of cyclooxygenase 2 (COX-2), or nitric oxide (NO), formed by inducible NO synthase (iNOS) in activated chondrocytes (13,14).

Various studies suggest that an inhibition of proteoglycan synthesis by IL-1β, rather than a stimulation of proteoglycan breakdown, causes the depletion of proteoglycans in cartilage (15,16). However, much research has focused on IL-1β–mediated degradation of proteoglycans, in particular aggrecan, whereas the mechanisms underlying the inhibition of proteoglycan anabolism are much less documented. In this study, we addressed the question of a possible action of this cytokine on the messenger RNA (mRNA) expression and activity of GlcAT-I, a key enzyme involved in the priming of GAG biosynthesis. We show, for the first time, that IL-1β represses both mRNA expression and enzyme activity of GlcAT-I and that these effects are concomitant with a loss of proteoglycan synthesis in rat chondrocytes.

Recent attention to the symptomatic relief afforded by the treatment of OA with glucosamine has spurred new basic scientific research into the effect of this agent on cartilage (17). We found that glucosamine could efficiently prevent the IL-1β–mediated repression of GlcAT-I expression and of proteoglycan anabolism in a dose-dependent manner. In addition, glucosamine was able to antagonize the production of inflammatory mediators induced by IL-1β. These actions could account for the effects of glucosamine derivatives in OA treatment.

MATERIALS AND METHODS

Chemicals. Uridine 5′-diphosphate (UDP)–glucuronic acid (sodium salt) and collagenase B were purchased from

Boehringer-Mannheim (Mannheim, Germany) and UDP U-^{14}C-glucuronic acid (180 mCi/mmole) was from Isotopchim (Ganagobie-Peyruis, France). Na_2-$^{35}SO_4$ was obtained from Amersham (Les Ulis, France). D(+)glucosamine, D(+)glucose, galactosylpyranosyl-β-1,3-D-thio-galactopyranose (Gal-S-Gal), and pronase were supplied by Sigma-Chimie (St Quentin Fallavier, France). Dulbecco's modified Eagle's medium (DMEM), fetal bovine serum (FBS), L-glutamine, gentamicin, reverse transcriptase (RT), and restriction enzymes were obtained from Gibco-BRL (Cergy Pontoise, France). *Taq* polymerase was supplied by Eurobio (Les Ulis, France), and oligonucleotides were synthesized by MWG-Biotech (Ebersberg, Germany). Soluene 350 was obtained from Packard (Rungis, France). Recombinant IL-1β was purchased from Pepro-Tech (Tebu, Le Perray en Yvelines, France).

Chondrocyte cultures and treatments. Male Wistar rats (130–150 gm; Charles River, Saint-Aubin-lès-Elboeuf, France) were housed under controlled temperature and lighting conditions with food and water ad libitum. Articular cartilage isolated from femoral head cap pieces was aseptically dissected, and chondrocytes were obtained after digestion of cartilage fragments in pronase (2% [weight/volume] in 0.15*M* NaCl) followed by an overnight digestion in collagenase B (1.5% [w/v] in DMEM without serum) (18). Experiments were performed with first-passage cultures, 6 days after collagenase treatment. For this purpose, chondrocytes were grown to confluence in 25-cm^2 flasks ($\sim 4 \times 10^6$ chondrocytes per flask) in 5 ml of complete medium (DMEM supplemented with L-glutamine [2 m*M*], gentamicin [50 mg/ml], FBS 10% [volume/volume]). In a first set of experiments, cells were then cultured for 6 hours in FBS-free medium containing glucose (1.0 gm/liter) and glucosamine (1.0, 2.0, or 4.5 gm/liter), and finally stimulated with IL-1β (25 units/ml) for 12 hours. In a second set of experiments, cells were cultured for 6 hours in FBS-free medium containing glucose (4.5 gm/liter) or glucosamine (4.5 gm/liter), and finally stimulated with IL-1β (25 or 250 units/ml) for 12 hours. For RNA isolation and enzymatic assays, cells were harvested, washed once in phosphate buffered saline (Gibco-BRL), pelleted by centrifugation, and kept at −80°C prior to analysis.

For evaluation of proteoglycan synthesis by Na_2-$^{35}SO_4$ incorporation and measurement of NO and PGE_2 production in the culture medium, chondrocytes were suspended in sterile, filtered, low-viscosity alginate solution (1.2% [w/v]) at 6×10^6 cells/ml) and slowly extruded through a 22-gauge needle into a 100-m*M* $CaCl_2$ solution (19). After 2 washes with 0.15*M* NaCl, the encapsulated chondrocytes were maintained in a complete culture medium for 6 days in a humidified atmosphere with 5% CO_2 at 37°C. The IL-1β and glucosamine treatments were performed as described above, and alginate beads were then incubated in medium supplemented with heat-inactivated FBS (2% [v/v]) and 10 μCi/ml of Na_2-$^{35}SO_4$ for 4 hours. Encapsulated chondrocytes were then extensively washed with 0.15*M* NaCl and solubilized in Soluene 350 (0.5*M* quaternary ammonium hydroxide in toluene) overnight. The amount of radiolabeled sulfate that incorporated sulfated GAG was quantitated by liquid scintillation counting (20,21). NO production and PGE_2 assays were performed on samples prepared from chondrocytes cultured under the same conditions but without radiolabeled sulfate (see below).

Enzymatic assays. Membrane-enriched fractions were prepared from chondrocytes by differential ultracentrifugations, according to the procedure of Hogeboom (22), and stored in 100-m*M* HEPES buffer (pH 7.4) containing 0.25*M* sucrose. Protein content was determined by the method of Bradford (23), with bovine serum albumin as standard. Glucuronidation activity for GlcAT-I was measured by the method of Bansal and Gessner (24), using Gal-S-Gal as reporter substrate and radiolabeled UDP–glucuronic acid. Briefly, incubations (40 μl total volume) containing 0.1 m*M* Gal-S-Gal, 0.3 m*M* UDP–glucuronic acid (0.2 μCi), 20 μg microsomal protein, 10 m*M* $MgCl_2$, and 10 m*M* $MnCl_2$ in 100 m*M* sodium acetate buffer (pH 5.0) were carried out at 37°C for 1 hour. Incubations were terminated by addition of 40 μl ethanol, and reaction products were separated by thin-layer chromatography (TLC) on silica plates (Whatman, Clifton, NJ) with *N*-butanol, acetone, acetic acid, aqueous ammonia, and water as the developing solvent system. After scraping the radioactive area visualized by autoradiography, the amount of products formed was quantitated by liquid scintillation counting.

Analysis of GlcAT-I and stromelysin 1 mRNA expression by quantitative RT–polymerase chain reaction (PCR). A partial coding sequence for rat GlcAT-I cDNA was cloned by RT-PCR using chondrocyte poly(A+)RNA as a template. Two degenerate oligonucleotides were designed based on information from amino acid sequence alignment of rat galactose-β-1,3-glucuronosyltransferase (25) with putative proteins in *Caenorhabditis elegans* and *Schistosoma mansoni*, as described by Kitagawa et al (6). These primers were used for PCR amplification of a 210-bp fragment corresponding to nucleotides 560–770 of the human cDNA sequence (GenBank accession number AB009598). This fragment was further extended at the 5′ end by rapid amplification of cDNA ends (5′ RACE system; Gibco-BRL), according to the manufacturer's instructions. The obtained sequence corresponded to nucleotides 268–770 of the human GlcAT-I cDNA and exhibited high homology with an expression sequence tag in the data bank corresponding to the mouse orthologous GlcAT-I.

This sequence information was used to design appropriate oligonucleotide primers for the quantitative multistandard RT-PCR assay developed to evaluate variations of GlcAT-I mRNA levels in rat chondrocytes (26). This method takes advantage of both GlcAT-I and β-actin sequence conservation between mouse and rat species (26). The protocol allowed us to normalize the amounts of GlcAT-I mRNA with respect to those of β-actin mRNA in each sample. Total RNA samples extracted from rat cells were mixed with a constant amount of total RNA prepared from mouse tissue, thus bringing together competitive mouse β-actin with gene sequences of interest and acting as a multistandard source. The mixture was reverse-transcribed using hexamer random primers. Separate PCR amplifications for GlcAT-I, stromelysin 1 (MMP-3), and β-actin were then undertaken with sense and antisense primers corresponding to conserved domains in rat and mouse sequences, allowing the amplification of both sequences with the same efficiency.

For RT-PCR amplification of mouse and rat GlcAT-I, the sense primer extended from nucleotides 268 to 290 and the antisense primer from nucleotides 592 to 620 of the cDNA sequence. These oligonucleotide sequences were identical in

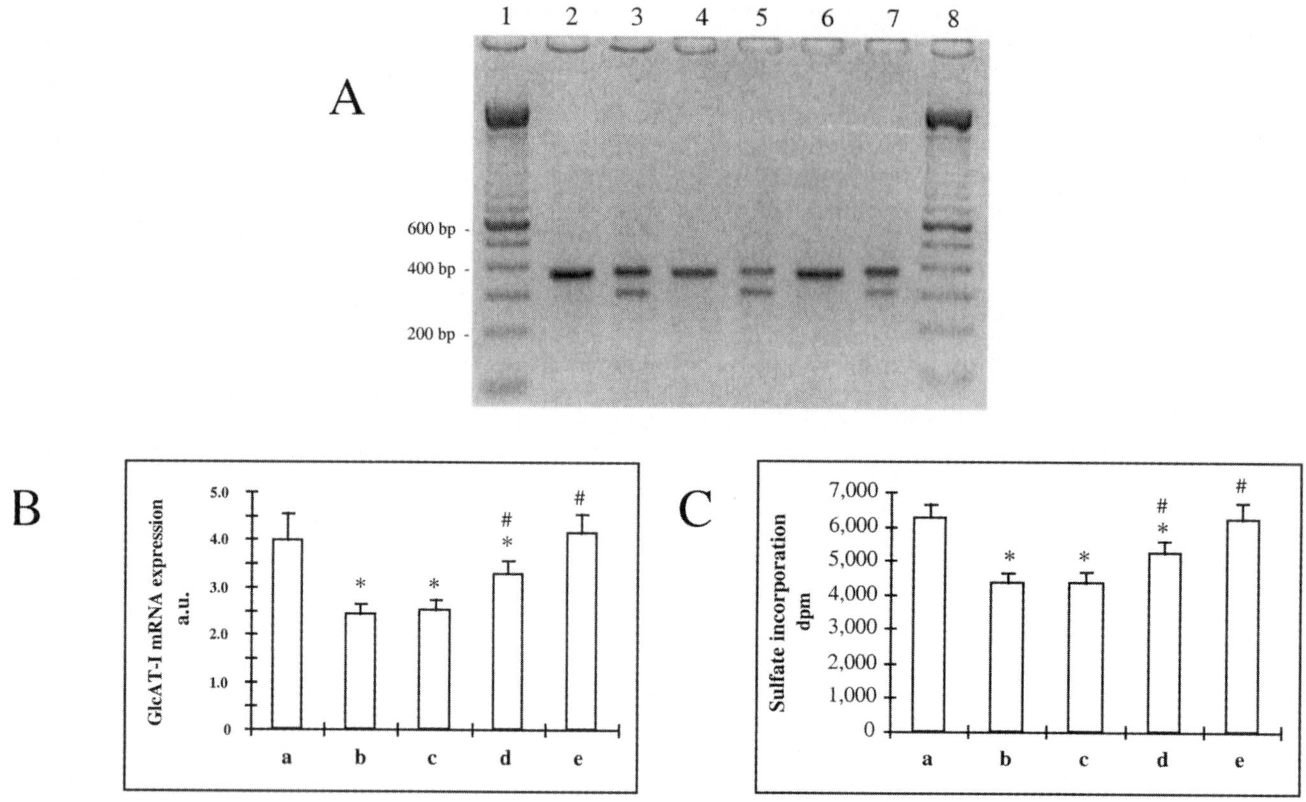

Figure 1. Effect of interleukin-1β (IL-1β) on galactose-β-1,3-glucuronosyltransferase I (GlcAT-I) mRNA expression and proteoglycan synthesis in rat chondrocytes cultured in the presence of increasing doses of glucosamine. **A**, Electrophoretic profile of GlcAT-I reverse transcriptase–polymerase chain reaction (RT-PCR) products amplified from mRNA of rat chondrocytes treated as described below and mixed with mouse mRNA as described in Materials and Methods. Lanes 2, 4, and 6 represent uncut RT-PCR products and lanes 3, 5, and 7 represent *Bam* HI–digested amplicons. Lanes 1 and 8 correspond to molecular weight markers. Lanes 2 and 3, 4 and 5, and 6 and 7 correspond to lanes a, b, and e in Figure 1B after quantitation by scanning densitometry. **B**, Quantitation of the GlcAT-I mRNA expression level. Chondrocytes were maintained in monolayer cultures in Dulbecco's modified Eagle's medium (DMEM) supplemented with glutamine, gentamicin, and fetal bovine serum (FBS) as described in Materials and Methods. Cells were cultured for 6 hours in serum-free medium containing glucose (1.0 gm/liter) and glucosamine (1.0, 2.0, 4.5 gm/liter; c, d, and e, respectively). Treatment with IL-1β (0 units/ml, lane a; 25 units/ml, lanes b–e) for 12 hours was then performed in the same medium. Values correspond to quantitation of the mRNA expression level after scanning densitometry analysis of RT-PCR products as illustrated on **A** and are presented in relative arbitrary units (a.u.). **C**, Variations of proteoglycan synthesis. Chondrocytes were encapsulated in alginate beads and maintained in culture in DMEM supplemented with glutamine, gentamicin, and FBS as described in Materials and Methods. Cells were cultured for 6 hours in medium containing glucose (1.0 gm/liter) and glucosamine (1.0, 2.0, 4.5 gm/liter; lanes c, d, and e, respectively) and 2% (v/v) FBS. Treatment with IL-1β (0 units/ml, lane a; 25 units/ml, lanes b–e) for 12 hours was then carried out in the same medium. Proteoglycan synthesis was evaluated by the measurement of radiolabeled sodium sulfate incorporation in dpm, as described in Materials and Methods. Results are the mean and SD of 3 different assays. $* = P < 0.05$ versus control value (glucose-containing medium, lane a) by Fisher's *t*-test. $\# = P < 0.05$ versus control value (IL-1β treatment, lane b) by Fisher's *t*-test.

rat and mouse, thus allowing the coamplification of both mRNAs. For amplification of rat and mouse β-actin mRNA, the sense primer extended from nucleotides 600 to 623 and the antisense primer from nucleotides 1143 to 1170 of the rat sequence (GenBank accession number X80130). Each amplification product was then distinguished by restriction-site polymorphism: the mouse GlcAT-I RT-PCR product was *Bam* HI digested into 2 fragments (121 and 304 bp), while the rat product remained uncut. A similar approach was used to differentiate mouse and rat β-actin amplification products. Digestion at the single *Xba* I restriction site present in the mouse sequence produced a 144-bp and a 425-bp fragment, whereas the rat β-actin RT-PCR product sequence remained uncut.

For amplification of MMP-3, the mouse and rat sense primers extended from nucleotides 680 to 702 and the antisense primer extended from nucleotides 1366 to 1388 according to the rat sequence (GenBank accession number X02601). The RT-PCR amplification products were distinguished by restriction site polymorphism: the mouse stromelysin 1 product was *Hha* I digested into 2 fragments (318 and 390 bp), while the rat product remained uncut.

Restriction endonuclease–digested RT-PCR products were resolved by agarose gel electrophoresis stained with ethidium bromide. The bands were visualized under ultraviolet light and photographed using a computer-assisted camera. Quantitation of each band was performed by densitometry analysis with National Institutes of Health software. Results are expressed as the ratio (analyzed $gene_{rat}$:β-$actin_{rat}$) $\times$ (β-$actin_{mouse}$:analyzed $gene_{mouse}$), in arbitrary units.

Nitrite assay. NO production was determined spectrophotometrically by measuring the accumulation of nitrite (NO^{-}_{2}), a stable breakdown product of NO, in the culture medium by the Griess reaction using sodium nitrite as standard (27). Briefly, 100 μl of culture supernatant was mixed with 100 μl of Griess reagent (sulfanilamide (1% [w/v]) in 2.5% H_3PO_4 and *N*-naphthylethylenediamine dihydrochloride (0.1% [w/v]) in H_2O) for 5 minutes in 96-well plates. Absorbance at 550 nm was measured on an MR5000 microplate reader (Dynatech, Ann Arbor, MI). Nitrite concentration was calculated from a standard curve of sodium nitrite. Nitrite production was assessed as cumulative nitrite released during incubation with IL-1β and/or glucosamine.

PGE_2 assays. PGE_2, the main metabolite of COX in chondrocytes, was measured in supernatants by an enzyme-linked immunosorbent assay method according to the manufacturer's instructions (Dynatech). This assay showed no cross-reactivity with other prostanoids. Sensitivity was <30 pg/ml. Results were expressed in ng/ml.

Statistical analysis. After comparison of data by analysis of variance, different groups were compared using Fisher's *t*-test. Assays were made in triplicate. *P* values less than 0.05 were considered significant.

RESULTS

Effect of glucosamine on IL-1β–mediated repression of GlcAT-I mRNA expression and proteoglycan anabolism. To investigate the effect of IL-1β and/or glucosamine on GlcAT-I expression, rat articular chondrocytes were isolated, maintained in culture, placed in glucose- and/or glucosamine-containing medium, and challenged with IL-1β. In order to analyze GlcAT-I mRNA expression, we cloned a partial cDNA coding sequence corresponding to 268–770 bp of the human GlcAT-I coding sequence, using mRNA isolated from rat chondrocytes as the template. The rat cDNA sequence obtained showed 88% homology with the human cDNA (6). The newly cloned sequence was used to design appropriate primers for quantitative RT-PCR assay of GlcAT-I mRNA expression in rat chondrocytes, as described in Materials and Methods. A representative RT-PCR experiment is illustrated in Figure 1A.

The effects of increasing doses of glucosamine (1–4.5 gm/liter) on GlcAT-I mRNA expression and on proteoglycan synthesis in chondrocytes cultured in the presence of 1 gm/liter glucose and treated with IL-1β (25 units/ml) were investigated. Treatment of chondrocytes with IL-1β resulted in a significant decrease in GlcAT-I mRNA expression, as illustrated in Figure 1A (compare upper bands in lanes 3 and 5). Quantitation of the variation in mRNA level by scanning densitometry indicated a 38% decrease of GlcAT-I mRNA following IL-1β treatment (Figure 1B, compare lane b with lane a). In addition, as expected, IL-1β produced an inhibition in proteoglycan synthesis (32%; Figure 1C, compare lane b with lane a). Interestingly, the addition of glucosamine prevented IL-1β–mediated inhibitory effects on GlcAT-I mRNA expression (Figure 1B) and on proteoglycan synthesis (Figure 1C) in a dose-dependent manner. A partial restoration of GlcAT-I mRNA expression level and proteoglycan synthesis was observed with the dose of 2.0 gm/liter (Figures 1B and C, compare lane d with lane c), whereas the highest dose of glucosamine (4.5 gm/liter) fully counteracted the inhibitory effects of IL-1β on both variables (Figure 1A, compare lane 7 with lane 5; Figures 1B and C, compare lane e with lane c). The latter dose was therefore selected for the subsequent experiments.

Effect of glucosamine on IL-1β–mediated repression of GlcAT-I expression and activity and proteoglycan anabolism. Figure 2 illustrates the effects of 2 doses of IL-1β (25 units/ml and 250 units/ml) on the GlcAT-I mRNA expression level, GlcAT-I catalytic activity, and on proteoglycan anabolism in chondrocytes cultured in the presence of glucose or glucosamine. Culture of chondrocytes in either glucose- or glucosamine-containing medium did not significantly modify the GlcAT-I mRNA expression level (Figure 2A, compare lane d with lane a). In contrast, IL-1β treatment at a dose of 25 units/ml resulted in a large decrease in GlcAT-I mRNA expression (48%) in rat chondrocytes cultured in glucose-containing medium (Figure 2A, compare lane b with lane a). Increasing the dose of cytokine (to 250 units/ml) did not further enhance this effect (Figure 2A, compare lane c with lane b). Interestingly, the inhibitory effects of Il-1β on GlcAT-I mRNA expression were fully prevented when chondrocytes were cultured in a glucosamine-containing medium (Figure 2A, compare lanes e and f with lane d).

In order to analyze GlcAT-I enzyme activity in membrane-enriched fractions from chondrocytes (Figure 2B), we adapted a TLC method based on the use of radiolabeled UDP–glucuronic acid (24). GlcAT-I activity toward Gal-S-Gal, whose structure mimics that of the natural oligosaccharidic substrate of this enzyme (28), was optimized in terms of pH and concentration of divalent ions. GlcAT-I exhibited a maximum specific activity at pH 5.0 in the presence of 10 m*M* Mn^{2+} and 10

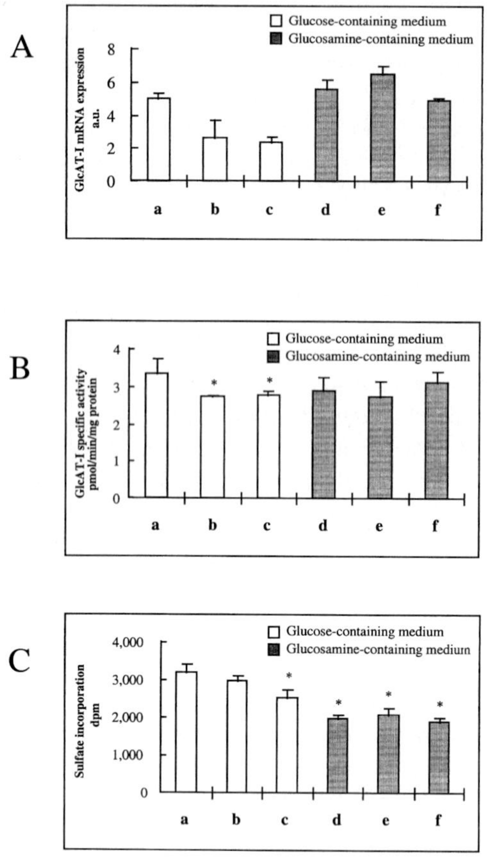

Figure 2. Effect of IL-1β on GlcAT-I mRNA expression and activity and on proteoglycan synthesis in rat chondrocytes cultured in the presence of glucose or glucosamine. Chondrocytes were maintained in monolayer cultures in DMEM supplemented with glutamine, gentamicin, and FBS as described in Materials and Methods. Cells were maintained for 6 hours in serum-free medium containing glucose (4.5 gm/liter; lanes a–c) or glucosamine (4.5 gm/liter; lanes d–f). Treatment with IL-1β (0 units/ml, lanes a and d; 25 units/ml, lanes b and e; 250 units/ml, lanes c and f) for 12 hours was then performed in the same medium. Variations in GlcAT-I mRNA expression (**A**) and enzyme activity toward Gal-S-Gal (**B**) were evaluated by quantitative RT-PCR and thin-layer chromatography, respectively, as described in Materials and Methods. For the determination of the variations of proteoglycan biosynthesis (**C**), chondrocytes were encapsulated in alginate beads and maintained in culture in DMEM supplemented with glutamine, gentamicin, and FBS as described in Materials and Methods. Cells were cultured for 6 hours in medium containing glucose (4.5 gm/liter; lanes a–c) or glucosamine (4.5 gm/liter; lanes d–f) and 2% (v/v) FBS. Treatment with IL-1β (0 units/ml, lanes a and d; 25 units/ml, lanes b and e; and 250 units/ml, lanes c and f) for 12 hours was then performed in the same medium. Proteoglycan synthesis was evaluated by the measurement of radiolabeled sodium sulfate incorporation as described in Materials and Methods. Results are the mean and SD of 3 different assays. * = $P < 0.05$ versus control value (glucose-containing medium, lane a) by Fisher's *t*-test. See Figure 1 for definitions.

m*M* Mg^{2+} (data not shown). The presence of glucosamine instead of glucose in the chondrocyte culture medium did not significantly modify GlcAT-I activity (Figure 2B, compare lane d with lane a). In contrast, as with the mRNA expression level, treatment of chondrocytes cultured in glucose-containing medium with each of the 2 doses of IL-1β led to a decrease in GlcAT-I activity (18%; Figure 2B, compare lanes b and c with lane a), whereas the same treatments had no significant effect when performed in the presence of glucosamine (Figure 2B, compare lanes e and f with lane d).

Furthermore, Figure 2C shows that IL-1β produced a significant concentration-dependent inhibition of proteoglycan synthesis, up to 20% with the highest dose of cytokine (compare lanes b and c with lane a). In contrast, no inhibitory effect of IL-1β on proteoglycan anabolism was observed when the cytokine treatment was performed in the presence of glucosamine (Figure 2C, compare lanes e and f with lane d). On the other hand, glucosamine alone (4.5 gm/liter) produced a significant decrease in proteoglycan synthesis (Figure 2C, compare lane d with lane a).

Taken together, our results provide evidence that IL-1β was able to down-regulate both the mRNA expression and enzyme activity of GlcAT-I in rat chondrocytes and that this effect was concomitant with the inhibition of proteoglycan synthesis. In addition, we found that the cytokine-mediated effects on both GlcAT-I expression and proteoglycan synthesis were prevented when IL-1β was administered in the presence of glucosamine.

Effects of IL-1β on mRNA expression of stromelysin 1 in chondrocytes cultured in the presence or absence of glucosamine. Our results clearly suggested a possible antagonist effect of glucosamine toward the deleterious action of IL-1β on the synthesis of proteoglycan. This prompted us to examine the action of the amino sugar toward the inducing effect of this cytokine on the expression of enzymes involved in the degradation of the cartilaginous matrix. For this purpose, changes in the level of mRNA coding for stromelysin 1 (MMP-3), which is involved in the degradation of the core protein of aggrecan and the collagen network, were evaluated by quantitative RT-PCR, as described for GlcAT-I. Treatment of rat chondrocytes with IL-1β led to a dose-dependent increase in the stromelysin 1 mRNA level, reaching 77% at the highest dose (Figure 3, compare lanes b and c with lane a). In contrast, when the IL-1β challenge was carried out in the presence of glucosamine, no significant variation of stromelysin 1 mRNA expression level was observed (Figure 3, compare lanes e and f with lane d). On the

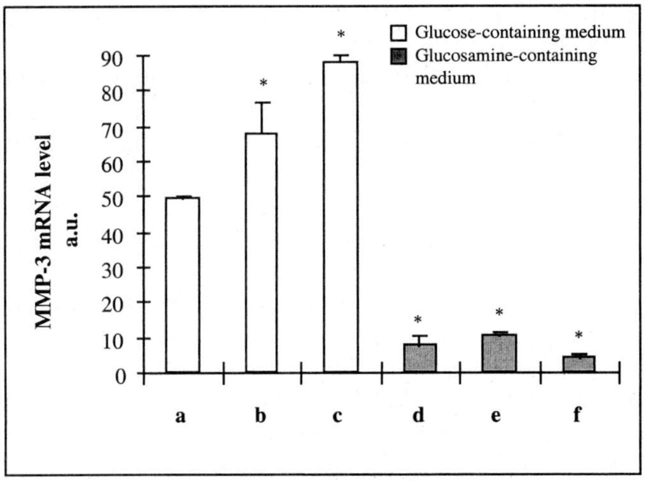

Figure 3. Effect of IL-1β induction on stromelysin 1 mRNA expression in rat chondrocytes. Chondrocytes were maintained in monolayer culture with DMEM supplemented with glutamine, gentamicin, and FBS as described in Materials and Methods. Cells were treated as described in the legend to Figure 2. Quantitation of the stromelysin 1 mRNA level was performed as described in Materials and Methods. Results are the mean and SD of 3 different assays. * = $P < 0.05$ versus control value (glucose-containing medium, lane a) by Fisher's *t*-test. See Figure 1 for definitions.

other hand, in chondrocytes cultured in glucosamine alone, the mRNA expression level of stromelysin decreased significantly (Figure 3, compare lane d with lane a).

Effects of IL-1β on NO synthesis and PGE_2 production in chondrocytes cultured in the presence or absence of glucosamine. In order to investigate the influence of glucosamine on IL-1β–mediated effects, we further examined the variations of known mediators of the inflammatory response, i.e., NO and PGE_2. As expected, treatment of chondrocytes with IL-1β in the presence of glucose induced a strong dose-dependent enhancement of NO production, reaching 200% at a dose of 250 units/ml of cytokine (Figure 4A, compare lanes b and c with lane a). Interestingly, incubation of chondrocytes with IL-1β in a glucosamine-containing medium resulted in an increase in NO production that did not exceed 48% with the highest dose of cytokine (Figure 4A, compare lanes e and f with lane d). It is noteworthy that no significant difference in constitutive NO release was observed when chondrocytes were cultured in the presence of glucosamine, when compared with glucose (Figure 4A, compare lane d with lane a).

On the other hand, as shown in Figure 4B, the production of PGE_2 by chondrocytes cultured in glucosamine-containing medium was significantly lower than that measured when chondrocytes were maintained in glucose-containing medium (mean ± SD 0.62 ± 0.04 μg/ml and 1.63 ± 0.36 μg/ml, respectively; compare lane d with lane a). This observation could result from an inhibitory effect of glucosamine on COX-1, the noninducible isoform. Furthermore, as with NO, IL-1β induced a strong dose-dependent increase in PGE_2 production in the presence of glucose (Figure 4B, compare lanes b and c with lane a). In contrast, this increase was small when the challenge with cytokine was performed in glucosamine-containing medium (142% at 250 units/ml versus 4,600%; compare lane f with lane d and lane c with lane a, respectively).

DISCUSSION

GlcAT-I is a key UDP-glycosyltransferase enzyme involved in the priming of hexuronic acid–GAG chain synthesis. The cDNA coding for the human form

A

B

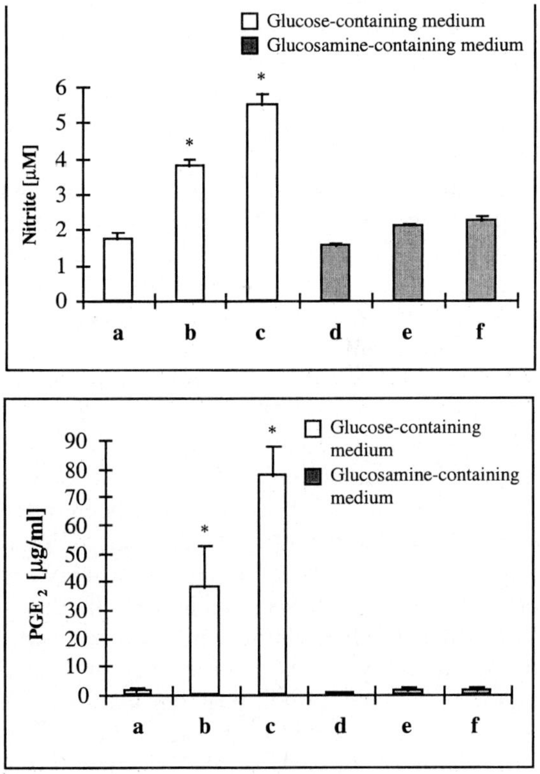

Figure 4. Effect of interleukin-1β (IL-1β) induction on proinflammatory mediators in rat chondrocytes. Chondrocytes encapsulated in alginate beads were cultured and challenged with IL-1β as described in the legend to Figure 2. Production of nitric oxide (**A**) and prostaglandin E_2 (PGE_2) (**B**) in the culture medium was determined as described in Materials and Methods. Results are the mean and SD of 3 different assays. * = $P < 0.05$ versus control value (glucose-containing medium, lane a) by Fisher's *t*-test.

of this enzyme was recently isolated (6), but no information on its regulation is yet available. By cloning the rat orthologous cDNA, we generated appropriate tools for the analysis of GlcAT-I mRNA expression in cultured rat chondrocytes. Furthermore, the development of a specific assay based on the use of a disaccharidic derivative, analogous to the natural digalactosidic substrate of this enzyme (28), allowed us to follow its catalytic activity simultaneously.

A significant finding of this study is that IL-1β markedly down-regulates GlcAT-I expression as well as its enzyme activity in rat chondrocytes. The concomitant inhibition of GlcAT-I expression and proteoglycan synthesis raises the possibility that the reduced expression of this UDP-glucuronosyltransferase responsible for the biosynthesis of the common tetrasaccharidic linkage of GAG could contribute to the deleterious effect of the proinflammatory cytokine on proteoglycan synthesis. Based on the reduced incorporation of radiolabeled precursor sugars, it has been previously suggested that the biosynthesis of GAG chains is affected in IL-1β–challenged chondrocytes (15). However, this is the first demonstration of a direct repressive effect of IL-1β on a glucuronosyltransferase involved in a key step of GAG biosynthesis. It is reasonable to hypothesize that this effect may lead to a reduced content of GAG chains available for further sulfation, thus contributing to the reduced incorporation of radiolabeled sulfate in proteoglycans, traditionally described after IL-1β treatment either in vivo (21) or in cultured cells (29).

Glucosamine is a major component of the repeating disaccharide motif of GAG chains involved in the assembly of the cartilaginous matrix. This amino sugar has recently received attention in the literature (30) and in some clinical studies as a treatment for OA (31,32). The efficacy of glucosamine has been attributed to stimulation of the synthesis of GAG chains and other glycoconjugates (17), although experimental data supporting this hypothesis are limited. In this study, we show that if glucosamine did not by itself increase proteoglycan synthesis, it efficiently prevented the IL-1β–mediated decrease in proteoglycan synthesis in stimulated rat chondrocytes. These results are consistent with those of Bassler et al (17), who reported that glucosamine restored proteoglycan production by human chondrocytes from OA cartilage.

It has been suggested that exogenous addition of glucosamine circumvents glutamine fructose-1-phosphate transaminase, which is responsible for the formation of amino sugars. Since this enzyme is rate-limiting in the hexosamine pathway, a supply of glucosamine provides precursors for glycosyltransferases involved in GAG biosynthesis. In addition, we show here that the mechanisms underlying glucosamine action involve the regulation of GlcAT-I. Our data are strengthened by the fact that the antagonistic effects of glucosamine on IL-1β inductive events were observed at the levels of both GlcAT-I mRNA and enzyme-specific activity. This effect of glucosamine, possibly coordinated with the stimulation of aggrecan core protein synthesis, as suggested by other studies (17), may provide a basis for the restoration of proteoglycan content in IL-1β–stimulated chondrocytes. In accordance with this suggestion, we show that glucosamine is able to antagonize the IL-1β–induced expression of stromelysin 1 as well. Taken together, the data indicate that the corrective effects of glucosamine toward IL-1β–mediated deregulation of enzymes involved either in the catabolism or in the anabolism of proteoglycans may account, at least in part, for the beneficial effect of the drug on pathologic cartilage.

The signaling pathways that mediate the effects of IL-1β and other chondrocyte regulatory factors have only been partially characterized. However, it is accepted that the proinflammatory action of IL-1β involves the mobilization of several transduction pathways, such as the mitogen-activated protein kinase cascade. These various signaling pathways control directly or indirectly the activation of several transcription factors such as activator protein 1 and nuclear factor κB (33). Activation of these factors leads to the up- or down-regulation of the transcriptional activity of a battery of genes associated with inflammation, such as COX-2 and iNOS. In order to provide further insight into the mechanisms underlying glucosamine action, we investigated its influence on the production of mediators of the inflammatory process. Consistent with previous data, our experiments show an enhancement of PGE_2 and NO production in rat chondrocytes treated with IL-1β, likely due to the induction of COX-2 (34) and iNOS (13), respectively.

Interestingly, we found that glucosamine consistently prevents the influence of IL-1β on these variables, further emphasizing a specific effect of the amino sugar in the IL-1β–mediated response. However, the mechanisms that govern the antagonist action remain unclear. Glucosamine could potentially act at many different levels. Complementary to our studies, Sandy et al (30) recently provided evidence for an inhibitory effect of glucosamine on IL-1β–stimulated aggrecanase expression. They suggested that this capacity may involve the inhibition of glycosylphosphatidylinositol (GPI)–linked proteins (35). Such a putative GPI-anchored component may also be part of an upstream receptor/signaling pathway and may regulate the transcription of various genes. In the same way, glucosamine has also been shown to rapidly induce several genes at the transcription level (36). In fact, our study provides evidence that glucosamine modifies the mRNA expression level of GlcAT-I and stromelysin 1. Several studies indicate that the hexosamine pathway may be involved in glucosamine regulation of gene expression (36). Whether this signaling pathway is responsible for glucosamine-mediated effects on GlcAT-I in IL-1β–stimulated chondrocytes requires further investigation.

In conclusion, the results of the present study demonstrate that IL-1β down-regulates the expression of GlcAT-I, a pivotal enzyme of GAG polysaccharide chain biosynthesis, at both the mRNA and enzyme activity levels, possibly contributing to the loss of proteoglycan synthesis elicited by the cytokine. Furthermore, we show that glucosamine not only corrected these effects, but also antagonized the production of various proinflammatory mediators activated by IL-1β, such as NO and PGE_2. Taken together, these results suggest that the pharmacologic effects of glucosamine in the treatment of OA and RA may involve the antagonist action of this amino sugar on the signaling events mediated by IL-1β.

REFERENCES

1. Rodén L. Structure and metabolism of connective tissue proteoglycans. New York: Plenum; 1980.
2. Ruoslahti E. Proteoglycans in cell regulation. J Biol Chem 1989; 264:13369–72.
3. Poole AR. Proteoglycans in health and disease: structures and functions. Biochem J 1986;236:1–14.
4. Vertel BM. The ins and outs of aggrecan. Trends Cell Biol 1995;5:458–64.
5. Tai GH, Nieduszynski IA, Fullwood NJ, Huckerby TN. Human corneal keratan sulfates. J Biol Chem 1997;272:28227–31.
6. Kitagawa H, Tone Y, Tamura J, Neumann KW, Ogawa T, Oka S, et al. Molecular cloning and expression of glucuronosyltransferase I involved in the biosynthesis of the glycosaminoglycan-protein linkage region of proteoglycans. J Biol Chem 1998;273:6615–8.
7. Kitagawa H, Ujikawa M, Sugahara K. Developmental changes in serum UDP-GlcA: chondroitin glucuronosyltransferase activity. J Biol Chem 1996;271:6583–5.
8. Inerot S, Heinegard D, Olsson SE, Telhag H, Audell L. Proteoglycan alterations during developing experimental osteoarthritis in a novel hip joint model. J Orthop Res 1991;9:658–73.
9. Inerot S, Heinegard D, Audell L, Olsson SE. Articular-cartilage proteoglycans in aging and osteoarthritis. Biochem J 1978;169: 143–56.
10. Van de Loo FAJ, Joosten LAB, van Lent PLEM, Arntz OJ, van den Berg WB. Role of interleukin-1, tumor necrosis factor α, and interleukin-6 in cartilage proteoglycan metabolism and destruction: effect of in situ blocking in murine antigen- and zymosan-induced arthritis. Arthritis Rheum 1995;38:164–72.
11. Wood DD, Ihrie EJ, Dinarello CA, Cohen PL. Isolation of an interleukin-1–like factor from human joint effusions. Arthritis Rheum 1983;26:975–83.
12. Goldring MB, Birkhead JR, Suen LF, Yamin R, Mizuno S, Glowacki J, et al. Interleukin-1β–modulated gene expression in immortalized human chondrocytes. J Clin Invest 1994;94:2307–16.
13. Maier R, Bilbe G, Rediske J, Lotz M. Inducible nitric oxide synthase from human articular chondrocytes: cDNA cloning and analysis of mRNA expression. Biochim Biophys Acta 1994;1208: 145–50.
14. Grabowski PS, Wright PK, van 't Hof RJ, Helfrich MH, Ohshima H, Ralston SH. Immunolocalization of inducible nitric oxide synthase in synovium and cartilage in rheumatoid arthritis and osteoarthritis. Br J Rheumatol 1997;36:651–5.
15. Neidel J, Zeidler U. Independent effects of interleukin-1 on proteoglycan synthesis and proteoglycan breakdown of bovine articular cartilage in vitro. Agents Actions 1993;39:82–90.
16. Nietfeld JJ, Wilbrink B, den Otter W, Huber J, Huber-Bruning O. The effect of human interleukin 1 on proteoglycan metabolism in human and porcine cartilage explants. J Rheumatol 1990;17: 818–26.
17. Bassleer C, Rovati L, Franchimont P. Stimulation of proteoglycan production by glucosamine sulfate in chondrocytes isolated from human osteoarthritic articular cartilage in vitro. Osteoarthritis Cartilage 1998;6:427–34.
18. Kuettner KE, Pauli BU, Gall G, Memoli VA, Schenk RK. Synthesis of cartilage matrix by mammalian chondrocytes in vitro. I. Isolation, culture characteristics, and morphology. J Cell Biol 1982;93:743–50.
19. Hauselmann HJ, Aydelotte MB, Schumacher BL, Kuettner KE, Gitelis SH, Thonar EJ. Synthesis and turnover of proteoglycans by human and bovine adult articular chondrocytes cultured in alginate beads. Matrix 1992;12:116–29.
20. De Vries BJ, van den Berg WB, Vitters E, van de Putte LB. Quantitation of glycosaminoglycan metabolism in anatomically intact articular cartilage of the mouse patella: in vitro and in vivo studies with ^{35}S-sulfate, ^{3}H-glucosamine, and ^{3}H-acetate. Rheumatol Int 1986;6:273–81.
21. Decaris E, Guingamp C, Chat M, Philippe L, Grillasca J-P, Abid A, et al. Evidence for neurogenic transmission inducing degenerative cartilage damage distant from local inflammation. Arthritis Rheum 1999;42:1951–60.
22. Hogeboom GH. Fractionation of cell components of animal tissues: general methods for isolation of liver cell components. Methods Enzymol 1955;1:16–9.
23. Bradford MM. A rapid and sensitive method for the quantitation of microgram quantities of protein utilizing the principle of protein-dye binding. Anal Biochem 1976;72:248–54.
24. Bansal SK, Gessner T. A unified method for the assay of uridine diphosphoglucuronyltransferase activity toward various aglycones using uridine diphospho[U-^{14}C]glucuronic acid. Anal Biochem 1980;109:321–9.
25. Terayama K, Oka S, Seiki T, Miki Y, Nakamura A, Kozutsumi Y, et al. Cloning and functional expression of a novel glucuronosyltransferase involved in the biosynthesis of the carbohydrate epitope HNK-1. Proc Natl Acad Sci U S A 1997;94:6093–8.
26. Khiri H, Reynier P, Peyrol N, Lerique B, Torresani J, Planells R. Quantitative multistandard RT-PCR assay using interspecies polymorphism. Mol Cell Probes 1996;10:201–11.
27. Green LC, Wagner DA, Glogowski J, Skipper PL, Wishnok JS, Tannenbaum SR. Analysis of nitrate, nitrite, and [^{15}N]nitrate in biological fluids. Anal Biochem 1982;126:131–8.
28. Wei G, Bai X, Sarkar AK, Esko JD. Formation of HNK-1 determinants and the glycosaminoglycan tetrasaccharide linkage region by UDP-GlcA:galactose-β1,3-glucuronosyltransferases. J Biol Chem 1999;274:7857–64.
29. Cipolletta C, Jouzeau JY, Gegout-Pottie P, Presle N, Bordji K,

Netter P, et al. Modulation of IL-1-induced cartilage injury by NO synthase inhibitors: a comparative study with rat chondrocytes and cartilage entities. Br J Pharmacol 1998;124:1719–27.
30. Sandy JD, Gamett D, Thompson V, Verscharen C. Chondrocyte-mediated catabolism of aggrecan: aggrecanase-dependent cleavage induced by interleukin-1 or retinoic acid can be inhibited by glucosamine. Biochem J 1998;335:59–66.
31. Kelly GS. The role of glucosamine sulfate and chondroitin sulfates in the treatment of degenerative joint disease. Altern Med Rev 1998;3:27–39.
32. Reichelt A, Forster KK, Fischer M, Rovati LC, Setnikar I. Efficacy and safety of intramuscular glucosamine sulfate in osteoarthritis of the knee: a randomised, placebo-controlled, double-blind study. Arzneimittelforschung 1994;44:75–80.
33. Firestein GS, Manning AM. Signal transduction and transcription factors in rheumatic disease. Arthritis Rheum 1999;42:609–21.
34. Lyons-Giordano B, Pratta MA, Galbraith W, Davis GL, Arner EC. Interleukin-1 differentially modulates chondrocyte expression of cyclooxygenase-2 and phospholipase A2. Exp Cell Res 1993;206: 58–62.
35. Sandy JD, Thompson V, Verscharen C, Gamett D. Chondrocyte-mediated catabolism of aggrecan: evidence for a glycosylphosphatidylinositol-linked protein in the aggrecanase response to interleukin-1 or retinoic acid. Arch Biochem Biophys 1999;367: 258–64.
36. Wang J, Liu R, Hawkins M, Barzilai N, Rossetti L. A nutrient-sensing pathway regulates leptin gene expression in muscle and fat. Nature 1998;393:684–8.

ARTHRITIS & RHEUMATISM
Vol. 44, No. 2, February 2001, pp 361–367

Low-Binding Alleles of Fcγ Receptor Types IIA and IIIA Are Inherited Independently and Are Associated With Systemic Lupus Erythematosus in Hispanic Patients

Ricardo Zuñiga,[1] Sonia Ng,[1] Margaret G. E. Peterson,[1] John D. Reveille,[2] Bruce A. Baethge,[3] Graciela S. Alarcón,[4] and Jane E. Salmon[1]

Objective. **To examine the relationship between allelic polymorphisms of IgG receptors (FcγR) and the development of lupus nephritis in a prospective study, and to determine the distribution of FcγR haplotypes (FcγRIIA and FcγRIIIA genotypes) in lupus patients and disease-free control subjects.**

Methods. **We studied 67 Hispanic systemic lupus erythematosus (SLE) patients from a prospective study of outcome and 53 disease-free control subjects. Patients were followed up longitudinally for 3 years. FcγRIIA and FcγRIIIA genotypes were determined using allele-specific polymerase chain reaction.**

Results. **Nephritis was present in 28% of patients at entry into the study and in 69% at the end of 3 years. In the nephritis group (n = 46), as well as the entire SLE cohort, there was a predominance of genotypes with low-binding alleles (FcγRIIa-R131 and FcγRIIIa-F176) at both loci (SLE nephritis patients 89% versus controls 62%; $P < 0.002$; odds ratio 0.20 [95% confidence interval 0.05–0.6] for risk of nephritis in individuals homozygous for either FcγRIIa-H131 or FcγRIIIa-V176). The frequency of individuals homozygous for high-binding alleles at either locus decreased as the burden of disease increased ($P < 0.002$, by Mann-Whitney test). There was no linkage disequilibrium between FcγRIIA and FcγRIIIA in Hispanics, yet in the SLE patients, there was a clear overrepresentation of the FcγRIIa-R131;FcγRIIIa-F176 haplotype (SLE patients 48% versus controls 30%) and a decrease in the frequency of the high-binding haplotype (4% versus 23%) ($P < 0.002$).**

Conclusion. **We observed an increase in the frequency of low-binding FcγR alleles in an SLE population with a high prevalence of renal disease. The apparent selection for the FcγRIIa-R131;FcγRIIIa-F176 haplotype in Hispanic patients suggests that low-binding alleles of both FcγRIIa and FcγRIIIa confer risk for SLE and may act additively in the pathogenesis of disease, whereas the high-binding haplotype FcγRIIa-H131;FcγRIIIa-V176 is protective, particularly in the homozygous state.**

Receptors for the Fc region of IgG (FcγR) provide the link between the humoral and cellular aspects of the immune cascade. Inherited polymorphisms of human FcγR profoundly influence human phagocyte function (1). Single–amino acid substitutions within the extracellular domains of FcγR alter the ability of the receptor to bind IgG and have been associated with risk for, and phenotype of, autoimmune and infectious disease (1).

FcγRIIa, which is expressed on mononuclear phagocytes, neutrophils, and platelets, has 2 codominantly expressed alleles, H131 and R131, which differ at amino acid position 131 in the extracellular domain (histidine or arginine, respectively) and differ substantially in their ability to bind human IgG2 (2,3). H131 is the high-binding allele, R131 the low-binding allele, and heterozygotes have intermediate function (4). Because

Supported in part by grants from the SLE Foundation, Inc., the New York Chapter of the Arthritis Foundation, and the RGK Foundation. Drs. Reveille and Alarcón's work was supported by NIH grant AR-42503. Dr. Salmon's work was supported by NIH grant AR-38889.

[1]Ricardo Zuñiga, MD, Sonia Ng, BS, Margaret G. E. Peterson, PhD, Jane E. Salmon, MD: Hospital for Special Surgery, New York, New York, and Weill College of Medicine of Cornell University, New York, New York; [2]John D. Reveille, MD: University of Texas–Houston Health Sciences Center; [3]Bruce A. Baethge, MD: University of Texas Medical Branch in Galveston; [4]Graciela S. Alarcón, MD, MPH: The University of Alabama at Birmingham.

Address correspondence and reprint requests to Jane E. Salmon, MD, Hospital for Special Surgery, 535 East 70th Street, New York, NY 10021.

Submitted for publication October 4, 1999; accepted in revised form October 13, 2000.

IgG2 is a poor activator of the classical complement pathway, FcγRIIa-H131 is essential for handling IgG2 immune complexes. FcγRIIIa, which is expressed on mononuclear phagocytes and natural killer cells, also has 2 codominantly expressed alleles, F176 and V176, which differ by 1 amino acid at position 176 in the extracellular domain (phenylalanine or valine, respectively) (5). FcγRIIIa alleles differ in IgG1 and IgG3 binding; V/V176 homozygotes bind IgG1 and IgG3 more efficiently than do F/F176 homozygotes.

The interplay between the humoral immune response and FcγR genotypes is a key determinant of the handling of opsonized antigens; such antigen–antibody immune complexes are removed from the circulation by the mononuclear phagocyte system, primarily the liver and spleen. Impaired removal of immune complexes in systemic lupus erythematosus (SLE) leads to tissue deposition of immune complexes, release of inflammatory mediators, influx of inflammatory cells, and target-organ damage, events that are probably crucial to nephritis (6). Indeed, we and others have shown that low-binding alleles of FcγR are enriched in some groups of patients with SLE and nephritis (4–10). There is also evidence from a genome-wide scan for linkage in the region of the FcγR gene cluster on chromosome 1 with SLE (11).

SLE is a heterogeneous disease with a relatively higher prevalence and worse outcome in non-Caucasian populations. These findings have been attributed to both genetic and socioeconomic demographic factors (12–17). Although associations between low-binding alleles of FcγR and lupus nephritis have been described, these have not been demonstrated in all ethnic groups studied (4,5,18–21). Even within ethnic groups where associations have been found, there have been conflicting results, ascribed to population admixture, lack of appropriate internal controls, and the confounding influence of other inherited susceptibility factors. Previously published work has been limited to retrospective and cross-sectional studies that focus mainly on either FcγRIIA or FcγRIIIA. The possibility that associations could be explained by linkage disequilibrium between these 2 genes, with one locus responsible for increased disease severity and the other locus associated because of linkage disequilibrium, has not been examined. The relative importance of interactions between alleles and the potential role of linkage disequilibrium between the 2 genes within the same cluster on chromosome 1q21-23 remains unknown.

In the studies reported here, we examined prospectively the relationship between FcγR genotypes and the development of renal disease, we examined linkage disequilibrium between FcγRIIA and FcγRIIIA, and we assessed the distribution of FcγR haplotypes (FcγRIIA and FcγRIIIA genotypes) in lupus patients and controls. A cohort of Hispanic patients was selected because of the high prevalence and severity of SLE and nephritis in this population (22). We demonstrated that there is no linkage disequilibrium between FcγRIIA and FcγRIIIA in Hispanics, yet there is a clear underrepresentation of the FcγRIIa-H131;FcγRIIIa-V176 haplotype in SLE patients. These observations support our hypothesis that specific FcγR alleles are associated with disease susceptibility.

PATIENTS AND METHODS

Study subjects. The patients were part of a prospective study aimed at determining factors predictive of outcome among SLE patients from different ethnic groups (Hispanic, African American, and Caucasian)—the LUMINA (lupus in minority populations, nature versus nurture) study. Detailed descriptions of the cohort have been reported previously (15,22,23). Hispanic patients and control subjects (Mexican or Central American ancestry) were recruited by the University of Texas–Houston Health Sciences Center and The University of Texas Medical Branch at Galveston. Ethnicity was defined as 4 grandparents of Mexican descent (90% of subjects) or Central American descent (10% of subjects). The Institutional Review Board of each participating center approved the study, and written informed consent was obtained from each subject.

Patients with SLE meeting ≥4 American College of Rheumatology (ACR) criteria for SLE (24), with disease duration of ≤5 years and age ≥14 years, were eligible for the study. Disease-free controls (identified at a blood drive) and patients were living in the geographic catchment area of the participating centers at the time of the study.

Medical records were reviewed prior to enrollment into the study and relevant data abstracted. At enrollment, a complete evaluation was performed; this included a number of questionnaires, a physical examination, and venipuncture. Study visits took place every 6 months for the first 2 years and yearly thereafter. SLE patients were classified as having nephritis if they fulfilled ACR criteria for renal involvement (hematuria [>10 red blood cells/high-power field (hpf)] or proteinuria [>2–3+ or >0.5 gm/24 hours] on >1 occasion) or if they had ≥1 of the following findings: renal biopsy showing World Health Organization class II–V end-stage renal disease due to SLE, granular casts (>3/hpf) or non–red blood cell cellular casts (>3/hpf).

The SLE patients had the following characteristics: 94% female, age 34 ± 13 years (mean ± SD), and disease duration 21 ± 16 months (mean ± SD). SLE patients were assessed for the development of nephritis at each followup study visit for a total of 3 years. Their treating rheumatologist evaluated them every 3 months, more frequently if clinically indicated. Of the 70 Hispanic patients in the LUMINA cohort, 3 died of nephritis and 2 were lost to followup in the last year of data collection for the current study.

FcγR genotyping. Genomic DNA was obtained from anticoagulated peripheral blood. Allele-specific polymerase chain reaction (PCR) assays were used to determine the FcγRIIA and FcγRIIIA genotypes. For FcγRIIA, DNA encoding the extracellular domains of the H131 and R131 forms was amplified with 2 primer pairs. The FcγRIIA-specific reverse (IIaPAN) primer (5′-CCA-TTG-GTG-AAG-AGC-TGC-CCA-TGC-3′) was used in both H131 and R131 allele-specific PCR assays. Two forward primers provided allele specificity, the R-specific forward primer (5′-ATG-GAA-AAT-CCC-AGA-AAT-TCT-CAC-G-3′) differs by 1 nucleotide from the H-specific forward primer (5′-ATG-GAA-AAT-CCC-AGA-AAT-TCT-CAC-A-3′) at the 3′ end.

The PCR reaction was performed in a 96-well thermal cycler (Techne, Princeton, NJ) with 100 ng of genomic DNA in a 50-μl reaction mixture, containing 200 n*M* of each primer, 5.0 nmoles of dNTPs, and 2.5 units of *Taq* DNA polymerase in standard PCR reaction buffer supplemented with 25 μ*M* $MgCl_2$ (Boehringer Mannheim, Indianapolis, IN). After 35 cycles of denaturation (95°C for 1 minute), annealing (61.5°C for 45 seconds), and extension (72°C for 1 minute), 25 μl of each PCR product was assayed on a 1% agarose gel. The appearance of the 800-bp PCR products in the R131 or H131 allele-specific reaction indicated the presence of that allele. For FcγRIIIA genotyping, we utilized the allele-specific PCR assay described elsewhere (6).

Statistical analysis. The distributions of genotypes and haplotypes of patients and controls were compared using a 2 × 2 contingency table. The chi-square test (2-tailed) was used to test for significant associations between FcγR genotypes or haplotypes and the presence of disease. The risk of disease associated with a particular allele or haplotype was expressed as an odds ratio (OR). The Mann-Whitney test was used to test for trends among the groups (SLE nephritis versus SLE non-nephritis versus control). Agreement between the genotypes observed and those predicted by Hardy-Weinberg equilibrium was assessed by a chi-square test. Linkage disequilibrium between FcγRIIA and FcγRIIIA was measured using Levin's delta, which is independent of allele frequency (25,26). Complete disequilibrium, when one allele of a certain polymorphism is linked on the chromosome with a specific allele of the other polymorphism, is indicated by a value of 1. A value of 0 indicates random distribution, that is, the distribution of the allele of one polymorphism is independent of which alleles of the other polymorphism is present on the same chromosome. Logistic regression models were used to predict lupus using the observed allele frequencies. In all analyses, a probability of less than 0.05 was used to reject the null hypothesis. The *P* values presented are uncorrected for multiple comparisons.

RESULTS

Overrepresentation of low-binding FcγRIIa and FcγRIIIa alleles in SLE patients. Of the 70 Hispanic SLE patients from the LUMINA cohort, 67 were studied, along with 53 disease-free control subjects. In the cohort of SLE patients, 28% (19 of 67) had renal disease at enrollment and 27 other patients (40%) developed nephritis within 3 years of enrollment. Only 3 of the 27 patients who developed nephritis (11%) were homozygous for either FcγRIIa-H131 and FcγRIIIa-V176, compared with 19% of patients who had not developed renal disease (n = 21) and 38% of the disease-free population ($P < 0.03$, by chi-square test with 2 × 3 contingency table).

Comparison of the entire group of lupus nephritis patients (those with nephritis at enrollment plus those with nephritis during followup; n = 46) with the controls revealed a similar decrease in those who were homozygous for either high-binding gene (11% versus 38%, respectively; $P < 0.007$). Because optimal FcγR function requires homozygosity for high-binding alleles, we analyzed the trend in distribution of genotypes homozygous for either FcγRIIa-H131 or FcγRIIIa-V176 among the nephritis, non-nephritis, and control groups (11% versus 19% versus 38%). The frequency of individuals homozygous for high-binding alleles at either locus decreased as the burden of disease increased ($P < 0.002$, by Mann-Whitney test). Results of an analysis of the difference between SLE patients with and those without nephritis were not significant, but the number of subjects in each group was small (46 and 21, respectively).

Comparison of the distribution of genotypes at each of the FcγR loci in the entire Hispanic SLE cohort with that in disease-free controls showed that there was an overrepresentation of FcγRIIa-R131 and FcγRIIIa-F176 gene products (Table 1). To examine the combined

Table 1. Distribution of FcγRIIa and FcγRIIIa genotypes*

	No. (%) of disease-free controls (n = 53)	No. (%) of SLE patients (n = 67)
FcγRIIa genotype†		
R131/R131	14 (26)	23 (34)
R131/H131	28 (53)	39 (58)
H131/H131	11 (21)	5 (7)
FcγRIIIa genotype‡		
F176/F176	15 (28)	25 (37)
F176/V176	26 (49)	38 (56)
V176/V176	12 (23)	4 (6)

* The number of homozygous and heterozygous alleles for Fcγ receptor type IIa (FcγRIIa) and FcγRIIIa that were found in the control and systemic lupus erythematosus (SLE) populations was not different from that predicted by the Hardy-Weinberg relationship (for FcγRIIa $P = 0.33$ and $P = 0.98$, respectively; for FcγRIIIa $P = 0.12$ and $P = 0.98$, respectively).

† $P = 0.034$ for SLE patients versus controls, using 2 × 2 contingency tables (FcγRIIa-H131/H131 versus FcγRIIa-R131/R131 and R131/H131).

‡ $P = 0.008$ for SLE patients versus controls, using 2 × 2 contingency tables (FcγRIIIa-V176/V176 versus FcγRIIIa-F176/F176 and F176/V176).

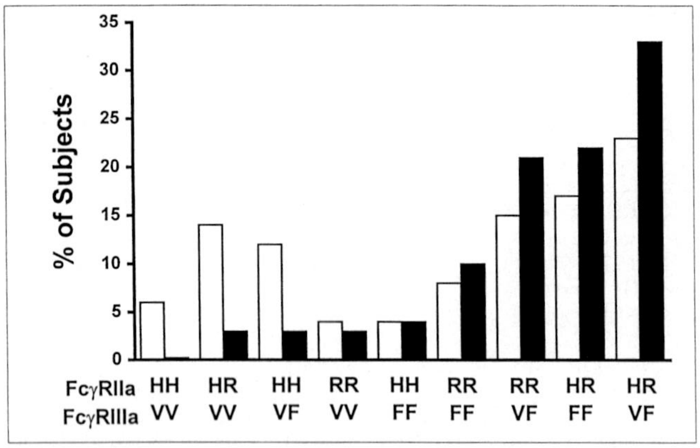

Figure 1. Distribution of Fcγ receptor (FcγR) genotypes in 67 patients with systemic lupus erythematosus (SLE) and in 53 disease-free controls. Solid bars show the percentage of SLE patients with the indicated FcγRIIa;FcγRIIIa genotype, and open bars show the percentage of controls. In the SLE group, there was a predominance of genotypes that included at least 1 low-binding allele at each FcγR locus, FcγRIIa-R131 and FcγRIIIa-F176. The odds ratio for the risk of lupus in individuals homozygous for either high-binding alleles (FcγRIIa-H131 or FcγRIIIa-V176) was 0.26 (95% confidence interval 0.1–0.6) (2 × 2 contingency table $\chi^2 = 9.5$, $P < 0.002$).

effects of the 2 FcγR loci on disease expression, we compared the distribution of the 9 possible genotypes in lupus patients with that in controls. In the patients, there was a predominance of genotypes that included at least 1 low-binding allele at each FcγR locus (87% in all SLE patients versus 62% in controls; $P < 0.002$). The odds ratio for the risk of lupus in individuals homozygous for either FcγRIIa-H131 or FcγRIIIa-V176 was 0.26 (95% confidence interval [95% CI] 0.1–0.6), suggesting a protective role for these alleles (Figure 1). Thus, in an SLE population with a high prevalence of early renal disease, there was an excess of low-binding IgG1, IgG2, and IgG3 genotypes.

Analysis of linkage disequilibrium between FcγRIIA and FcγRIIIA. To assess linkage disequilibrium between the FcγRIIA and FcγRIIIA genes, only individuals homozygous at one or both loci were analyzed so that we could unequivocally assign haplotypes of both variants. We excluded 12 control subjects and 22 SLE patients (11 with nephritis) who were doubly heterozygous. Analysis of the entire Hispanic cohort (patients and controls) indicated that FcγRIIA and FcγRIIIA are not in linkage disequilibrium using Levin's delta ($\delta = 0.078$; 95% CI 0–0.117). Testing for the presence of associations between alleles at the 2 FcγR loci using a chi-square test showed no significant association ($\chi^2 = 0.16$, $P = 0.70$). For this analysis, our power was >0.7 to detect a difference of ≥0.2.

Among disease-free controls, all 4 haplotypes occurred with similar frequency, between 23% and 30% (Table 2). Of 38 FcγRIIa-H131 haplotypes, 19 were associated with FcγRIIIa-V176 and 19 were associated with FcγRIIIa-F176. Of 44 FcγRIIa-R131 haplotypes, 19 were associated with FcγRIIIa-V176 and 25 were associated with FcγRIIIa-F176. The distribution of FcγRIIa alleles was not associated with the distribution of FcγRIIIa alleles; there is no evidence for linkage disequilibrium between loci in the disease-free population ($\chi^2 = 0.38$, $P = 0.54$).

In contrast to our observations in the disease-free population, there was skewing in the distribution of haplotypes detected in the lupus group, with 48% of the haplotypes containing both low IgG binding alleles

Table 2. Distribution of FcγR haplotypes in SLE patients and disease-free controls*

Haplotype	% of SLE patients (n = 45)†	% of SLE patients with nephritis (n = 35)‡	% of control subjects (n = 41)
FcγRIIa-R131;FcγRIIIa-F176	48	42	30
FcγRIIa-H131;FcγRIIIa-F176	26	29	23
FcγRIIa-R131;FcγRIIIa-V176	22	16	23
FcγRIIa-H131;FcγRIIIa-V176	4	3	23

* Only those who were homozygous at one or both Fcγ receptor (FcγR) loci were considered in this analysis in order to assign haplotypes of both variants; 12 control subjects and 22 systemic lupus erythematosus (SLE) patients (11 with nephritis) who were doubly heterozygous were excluded. The number of homozygote and heterozygote alleles for both genes was not different from that predicted by the Hardy-Weinberg relationship in patients and controls ($P > 0.2$ for all groups).
† $P < 0.002$ for SLE patients versus controls, using 4 × 2 contingency tables. Odds ratio for risk of SLE in an individual with an FcγRIIa-H131;FcγRIIIa-V176 haplotype 0.08 (95% confidence interval 0.02–0.3).
‡ $P < 0.002$ for SLE patients with nephritis versus controls, using 4 × 2 contingency tables. Odds ratio for risk of nephritis in an individual with an FcγRIIa-H131;FcγRIIIa-V176 haplotype 0.07 (95% confidence interval 0.09–0.7).

(FcγRIIa-R131;FcγRIIIa-F176) and only 4% containing both high-binding alleles (FcγRIIa-H131;FcγRIIIa-V176) ($P < 0.002$, using 4×2 contingency table) (Table 2). The odds ratio for risk of lupus in an individual with an FcγRIIa-H131;FcγRIIIa-V176 haplotype was 0.08 (95% CI 0.02–0.3), suggesting a protective role for this haplotype. We noted similar findings when the nephritis group was compared with the disease-free controls (Table 2). Our results show a significant association of haplotypes containing low IgG binding alleles of FcγRIIa and FcγRIIIa with lupus in a cohort of Hispanic patients with a high prevalence of nephritis.

That there appeared to be a selection for the FcγRIIa-R131;FcγRIIIa-F176 haplotype in SLE suggested an interaction between FcγRIIa and FcγRIIIa alleles in disease susceptibility. To examine the prediction of disease state by the presence of the FcγR alleles, we ran logistic regression and log-linear analyses. The presence of ≥1 FcγRIIa-R131 allele was associated with lupus when the comparison was lupus versus control ($P = 0.04$). The interaction term between FcγRIIa and FcγRIIIa was not statistically significant ($P = 0.6$). If the association between alleles is ≥0.2, then the power to detect a second factor or interaction term is less than 0.7. When the groups compared were nephritis versus control, FcγRIIIa-F176 was associated with an increasing probability of nephritis ($P < 0.01$). Again, there was no statistically significant second factor or interaction term, but again, there was a low power because the low-binding alleles of FcγRIIa and FcγRIIIa occur together in the lupus group. When the actual number of low-binding alleles at each locus was considered (0, 1, or 2), the interaction term still was not significant ($P = 0.3$). Thus, we have no evidence that the effect of alleles at one locus is influenced by those at another in this group of patients.

DISCUSSION

Genetic factors are considered major determinants of disease outcome and may partly account for the variations in the prevalence, disease manifestations, course, and outcome of SLE among ethnic groups. Our prospective study in a cohort of Hispanic patients is the first to examine the role of both FcγRIIa and FcγRIIIa as predictors of the occurrence of lupus nephritis. In our cohort, 28% had evidence of nephritis at study enrollment, while 69% met the criteria for nephritis after 3 years of followup. There was a striking decrease in the frequency of genotypes homozygous for either FcγR high-binding gene among all patients with SLE. There was a trend toward increased genotypes homozygous for low-binding alleles, comparing nephritis with non-nephritis with controls ($P < 0.002$, by Mann-Whitney test).

Homozygosity for low-binding alleles at either the FcγRIIA or FcγRIIIA locus can lead to impaired binding of immune complexes. The role of specific loci varies with the qualitative nature of the immune response. Differences in the IgG subclass of pathogenic autoantibodies have a profound effect on the relative importance of FcγR alleles on disease severity. For example, anti–double-stranded DNA antibodies, which correlate with renal disease, are predominantly IgG1 and IgG3 subclasses, and therefore support the importance of FcγRIIIA variants as disease-modifying genes. In contrast, in the presence of IgG2-containing immune complexes, FcγRIIA genes play a crucial role in determining disease severity. In either case, optimal handling of pathogenic immune complexes is provided only in the homozygous state for high-binding alleles of FcγRIIa or FcγRIIIa; heterozygotes at either locus have intermediate binding capacity and may therefore be at risk for immune complex deposition (4,5). Thus, we hypothesized that homozygosity at either of these alleles would provide protection against immune complex deposition and resultant tissue injury.

Analysis of the entire lupus cohort indicated that, although FcγRIIA and FcγRIIIA are not in linkage disequilibrium, there was a decreased frequency of both high-binding IgG alleles, FcγRIIa-H131 and FcγRIIIa-V176. In the disease-free population, the 4 possible haplotypes had similar frequencies. In contrast, only 4% of lupus patients had at least 1 copy of the FcγRIIa-H131;FcγRIIIa-V176 haplotype and 48% had an FcγRIIa-R131;FcγRIIIa-F176 haplotype. It is possible that the increased rate of renal disease in this Hispanic population is related to skewing of FcγR haplotypes toward low-binding variants, but our study cannot directly address this point.

Only 21 patients in the cohort did not have renal involvement, and their FcγR genotypes were not significantly shifted toward high-binding alleles. Perhaps other protective genes, as have been described in murine SLE models, may account for the absence of renal disease in this small subset of patients (27). Alternatively, these patients may not be protected from renal disease, but rather, may become symptomatic in the future. Followup of these patients is continuing and may provide this information.

Although the distribution of haplotypes has not been analyzed in other SLE populations, it is notable that in African Americans, another group with a high prevalence of nephritis, FcγRIIa-R131 and FcγRIIIa-F176 variants are increased compared with disease-free African Americans (4). In studies of Caucasian SLE patients, in whom nephritis is less common, alterations in the distribution of FcγR alleles have been a less consistent finding (9,18,28,29). Indeed, genome scans provide evidence for linkage in the region of FcγRIIa with SLE primarily in African Americans (11).

We cannot exclude an alternative explanation for the association of the FcγRIIa-FcγRIIIa haplotype with lupus, which is that these genes may be in linkage disequilibrium with other candidate genes within the FcγR cluster or with neighboring genes on chromosome 1 which encode for other proteins. It is also possible that linkage disequilibrium between FcγRIIa and FcγRIIIa would be detectable with a larger cohort or a different population, given the proximity of the 2 loci (<0.5 kb apart). We recognize that eliminating the double heterozygotes from the analysis may also have altered our results. Nonetheless, the apparent selection for the FcγRIIa-R131; FcγRIIIa-F176 haplotype in this cohort suggests that low-binding alleles of both FcγRIIa and FcγRIIIa confer risk for disease, either lupus or nephritis. Although the phenotypic trait may be determined by alleles at both loci, and the impact of one locus may depend upon the second, we did not find evidence for an interaction between FcγRIIa and FcγRIIIa in predicting risk for SLE.

Our findings support a model in which low affinity for IgG2-containing immune complexes (due to the presence of FcγRIIa-R131 alleles) and low affinity for IgG1 and IgG3 (as a consequence of FcγRIIIa-F176 alleles) result in impaired removal of these circulating immune complexes, their increased tissue deposition, and accelerated organ damage. That the predominant IgG subclasses present in immune deposits of proliferative glomerulonephritis are IgG2 and IgG3 (30,31) is consistent with this model of disease pathogenesis.

We have previously demonstrated that anticardiolipin (aCL) antibodies are predominantly of IgG2 subclass (32). Since aCL opsonize apoptotic cellular debris and, as such, may be poor opsonins in an FcγRIIa-R131 individual, the resultant increased availability of nuclear antigens may promote autoantibody formation in such patients. Recent evidence that FcγRIIa is the main receptor for C-reactive protein (CRP) raises the possibility that handling of nucleosomes that are bound to CRP may also be influenced by allelic polymorphisms (33).

FcγR alleles have been shown to be key determinants of phenotype in SLE (4–10,29,32,34). They mediate responses to autoantigen-containing immune complexes, activation of platelets and monocytes by antiphospholipid antibodies, and phagocytosis of opsonized microbes. The present study, the first to demonstrate that the FcγRIIa;FcγRIIIa haplotype, which contains low-binding variants at both FcγR loci, is overrepresented in an SLE population with a high prevalence of renal disease. Recognition of specific inherited disease-associated haplotypes expands our understanding of disease pathogenesis and provides prognostic markers for disease severity.

REFERENCES

1. Salmon JE, Kimberly RP. Fcγ receptor polymorphisms: clinical aspects. In: Van de Winkel JG, Hogarth PM, editors. The immunoglobulin receptors and their pathological roles in immunity. Dordrecht (The Netherlands): Kluwer Academic; 1998. p. 267–78.
2. Salmon JE, Edberg JC, Brogle NL, Kimberly RP. Allelic polymorphisms of human Fcγ receptor IIA and Fcγ receptor IIIB: independent mechanisms for differences in human phagocyte function. J Clin Invest 1992;89:1274–8.
3. Parren PWHI, Warmerdam PAM, Boeije LCM, Arts J, Westerdaal NAC, Vlug A, et al. On the interaction of IgG subclasses with the low affinity FcγRIIA (CD32) on human monocytes, neutrophils, and platelets: analysis of a functional polymorphism to human IgG2. J Clin Invest 1992;90:1537–46.
4. Salmon JE, Millard S, Schachter LA, Arnett F, Ginzler EM, Gourley MF, et al. FcγRIIA alleles are heritable risk factors for lupus nephritis in African-Americans. J Clin Invest 1996;97: 1348–54.
5. Wu J, Edberg JC, Redecha PB, Bansal V, Guyre PM, Coleman K, et al. A novel polymorphism of FcγRIIIa (CD16) alters receptor function and predisposes to autoimmune disease. J Clin Invest 1997;100:1059–70.
6. Edberg JC, Salmon JE, Kimberly RP. Systemic lupus erythematosus: immunopathology. In: Klippel JH, Dieppe PA, editors. Rheumatology. 2nd ed. Philadelphia: Mosby; 1998. p. 7-2.1–7-2.12.
7. Salmon JE, Ng S, Yoo D-H, Kim T-H, Kim SY, Song GG. Altered distribution of Fcγ receptor IIIA alleles in a cohort of Korean patients with lupus nephritis. Arthritis Rheum 1999;42:818–9.
8. Koene HR, Kleijer M, Swaak AJG, Sullivan KE, Bijl M, Petri MA, et al. The FcγRIIIA-158F allele is a risk factor for systemic lupus erythematosus. Arthritis Rheum 1998;41:1813–8.
9. Manger K, Repp R, Spriewald BM, Rascu A, Geiger A, Wassmuth R, et al. Fcγ receptor IIa polymorphism in Caucasian patients with systemic lupus erythematosus: association with clinical symptoms. Arthritis Rheum 1998;41:1181–9.
10. Song YW, Han C-W, Kang S-W, Baek H-J, Lee E-B, Shin C-H, et al. Abnormal distribution of Fcγ receptor type IIa polymorphisms in Korean patients with systemic lupus erythematosus. Arthritis Rheum 1998;41:421–6.
11. Moser KL, Nease BR, Salmon JE, Yu H, McGuire C, Asundi N, et al. Genome scan of human systemic lupus erythematosus: evidence for linkage on chromosome 1 in African-American pedigrees. Proc Natl Acad Sci U S A 1998;95:14869–74.
12. Ward MM, Pyun E, Studenski S. Long-term survival in systemic lupus erythematosus: patient characteristics associated with poorer outcomes. Arthritis Rheum 1995;38:274–83.
13. Petri M, Perez-Gutthann S, Longenecker JC, Hochberg M. Morbidity of systemic lupus erythematosus: role of race and socioeconomic status. Am J Med 1991;91:345–53.
14. Karlson EW, Daltroy LH, Lew RA, Wright EA, Partridge AJ,

Fossel AH, et al. The relationship of socioeconomic status, race, and modifiable risk factors to outcomes in patients with systemic lupus erythematosus. Arthritis Rheum 1997;40:47–56.
15. Reveille JD, Moulds JM, Ahn C, Friedman AW, Baethge B, Roseman J, et al. Systemic lupus erythematosus in three ethnic groups. I. The effects of HLA class II, C4, and CR1 alleles, socioeconomic factors, and ethnicity at disease onset. Arthritis Rheum 1998;41:1161–72.
16. Zuniga R, Seliger S, Barr G, Appel G, Radhakrishnan J, Salmon J. Prognosis in proliferative lupus nephritis: role of race and socioeconomic status [abstract]. Arthritis Rheum 1998;41:S282.
17. Martin K, Kavanaugh A, Middleton G, Lipsky P. The prevalence of nephritis in Hispanic patients with systemic lupus erythematosus [abstract]. Arthritis Rheum 1994;37:S179.
18. Botto M, Theodoridis E, Thompson EM, Beynon HL, Briggs D, Isenberg DA, et al. Fcγ RIIa polymorphism in systemic lupus erythematosus (SLE): no association with disease. Clin Exp Immunol 1996;104:264–8.
19. Smyth LJ, Snowden N, Carthy D, Papasteriades C, Hajeer A, Ollier WE. Fcγ RIIa polymorphism in systemic lupus erythematosus. Ann Rheum Dis 1997;56:755–6.
20. Oh M, Petri MA, Kim NA, Sullivan KE. Frequency of the Fcγ RIIIA-158F allele in African American patients with systemic lupus erythematosus. J Rheumatol 1999;26:1486–9.
21. Yap SN, Phipps ME, Manivasagar M, Tan SY, Bosco JJ. Human Fcγ receptor IIA (FcγRIIA) genotyping and association with systemic lupus erythematosus (SLE) in Chinese and Malays in Malaysia. Lupus 1999;8:305–10.
22. Alarcón GS, Friedman AW, Straaton KV, Moulds JM, Lisse J, Bastian HM, et al. Systemic lupus erythematosus in three ethnic groups. III. A comparison of characteristics early in the natural history of the LUMINA cohort. Lupus 1999;8:197–209.
23. Alarcón GS, Roseman J, Bartolucci AA, Friedman AW, Moulds JM, Goel N, et al. Systemic lupus erythematosus in three ethnic groups. II. Features predictive of disease activity early in its course. Arthritis Rheum 1998;41:1173–80.
24. Tan EM, Cohen AS, Fries JF, Masi AT, McShane DJ, Rothfield NF, et al. The 1982 revised criteria for the classification of systemic lupus erythematosus. Arthritis Rheum 1982;25:1271–7.
25. Levin ML. The occurrence of lung cancer in man. Acta Unio Int Contra Cancrun 1953;19:531–41.
26. Devlin B, Risch N. A comparison of linkage disequilibrium measures for fine-scale mapping. Genomics 1995;29:311–22.
27. Morel L, Tian XH, Croker BP, Wakeland EK. Epistatic modifiers of autoimmunity in a murine model of lupus nephritis. Immunity 1999;11:131–9.
28. Norsworthy P, Theodoridis E, Botto M, Athanassiou P, Beynon H, Gordon C, et al. Overrepresentation of the Fcγ receptor type IIA R131/R131 genotype in Caucasoid systemic lupus erythematosus patients with autoantibodies to C1q and glomerulonephritis. Arthritis Rheum 1999;42:1828–32.
29. Haseley LA, Wisnieski JJ, Denburg MR, Michael-Grossman AR, Ginzler EM, Gourley MF, et al. Antibodies to C1q in systemic lupus erythematosus: characteristics and relation to FcγRIIA alleles. Kidney Int 1997;52:1375–80.
30. Imai H, Hamai K, Komatsuda A, Ohtani H, Miura AB. IgG subclasses in patients with membranoproliferative glomerulonephritis, membranous nephropathy, and lupus nephritis. Kidney Int 1997;51:270–6.
31. Zuniga R, Markowitz, D'Agati V, Salmon J. IgG subclass glomerular deposition and its relationship to Fcγ receptor IIA alleles in lupus nephritis [abstract]. Arthritis Rheum 1999;42:S174.
32. Sammaritano LR, Ng S, Sobel R, Lo SK, Simantov R, Furie R, et al. Anticardiolipin IgG subclasses: association of IgG2 with arterial and/or venous thrombosis. Arthritis Rheum 1997;40:1998–2006.
33. Bharadwaj D, Stein MP, Volzer M, Mold C, Du Clos TW. The major receptor for C-reactive protein on leukocytes is Fcγ receptor II. J Exp Med 1999;190:585–90.
34. Yee AMF, Phan HM, Zuniga R, Salmon JE, Musher DM. The association between FcγRIIa-R131 allotype and bacteremic pneumococcal pneumonia. Clin Infect Dis 2000;30:25–8.

ARTHRITIS & RHEUMATISM
Vol. 44, No. 2, February 2001, pp 368–375

The Appearance of U1 RNP Antibody Specificities in Sequential Autoimmune Human Antisera Follows a Characteristic Order That Implicates the U1–70 kd and B′/B Proteins as Predominant U1 RNP Immunogens

Eric L. Greidinger and Robert W. Hoffman

Objective. **To observe the order of development of anti–U1 RNP peptide antibodies in humans.**

Methods. **Immunoblots against Jurkat cell lysates were performed on 5,882 serum samples from 3,668 patients referred on clinical grounds for RNP antibody testing to a reference laboratory between 1989 and 1999. In patients from whom multiple samples were drawn, we determined the order in which IgG antibodies to the U1 RNP peptides A, B′/B, C, D, and 70 kd appeared.**

Results. **One hundred sixty-three patients with serial samples were identified in whom antibodies to at least one U1 RNP peptide initially were not present but later appeared. The first RNP antibodies to appear were most often directed against the 70 kd and B′/B peptides ($P < 0.01$). Antibodies to the A and C peptides usually developed after other RNP peptide antibodies, and antibodies to D often emerged only after immunity to multiple other U1 RNP proteins had appeared. B′/B, but not 70 kd, was a frequent early target of spreading after initial immunity to other RNP peptides.**

Conclusion. **Orderly patterns of emergence of U1 RNP peptide antibodies appear to exist in humans. Two peptides, 70 kd and B′/B, show characteristics of early immunogens in the development of human RNP immunity.**

Dr. Greidinger's work was supported by the University of Missouri Research Board and the J. B. Reynolds Foundation. Dr. Hoffman's work was supported by the Department of Veterans Affairs Research Service and by NIH grant AR-43309.

Eric L. Greidinger, MD, Robert W. Hoffman, DO: University of Missouri and Harry S Truman Memorial Veterans Hospital, Columbia, Missouri.

Address correspondence and reprint requests to Eric L. Greidinger, MD, MA427 Health Sciences Center, Columbia, MO 65212.

Submitted for publication June 23, 2000; accepted in revised form October 13, 2000.

The U1 RNP complex was one of the first autoantigens to be defined biochemically (1). This particle, which functions as part of the nuclear messenger RNA splicing machinery, is composed of the U1 RNA and several noncovalently complexed peptides (2). The protein components of the U1 RNP have been classified into subfamilies, including A, B′/B, C, D, and 70 kd, on the basis of size, protein sequence, and immunologic reactivity. The U1 RNP proteins have been further classified into two groups: the Sm proteins, which include B′/B (also known as B1 and B2) and D (also known as D1), and the other, non-Sm proteins. The Sm proteins have been shown to associate with other RNP complexes in addition to U1, unlike the non-Sm proteins (3). Immunity to Sm has been linked with systemic lupus erythematosus (SLE) (4), while anti–U1 RNP immune responses in humans have been linked to SLE, scleroderma, and mixed connective tissue disease (MCTD) (5).

In animal models, immunization with modified forms of individual U1 RNP peptides can lead to the development of antibodies to more than just the immunogen used (6). In such studies, antibodies to the native form of the peptide, and even to other U1 RNP peptides, also develop (7). This migration of immunity from one determinant to other physically associated determinants is known as determinant spreading (8), and can lead to immunity to other parts of the same molecule (intramolecular spreading) or to other associated molecules (intermolecular spreading). Diversification of the anti–U1 RNP immune responses over time in a pattern consistent with spreading has been observed in spontaneous animal models of autoimmunity (9). The presence of intramolecular spreading in animal systems has been viewed as evidence that the immune responses are antigen driven.

To initiate an antigen-driven anti-RNP immune response, two prominent models have received attention: modified self and molecular mimicry. The modified self model proposes that components of the U1 small nuclear RNP develop altered structure in a proimmune context, such that a direct immune response to host antigens is induced (10). The molecular mimicry model proposes that a foreign antigen, such as an infectious agent, provokes an immune response that happens to cross-react with endogenous RNP antigens (11). Apoptosis and oxidative modification have been proposed as mechanisms to generate altered antigen structure in modified self models (12). On the one hand, 70 kd is the only U1 RNP protein antigen that has yet been found to be susceptible to both of these forms of alteration (13,14). On the other hand, immune responses to Epstein-Barr nuclear antigen 1 (EBNA-1) can induce cross-reactivity to a homologous sequence on the B′/B peptide (15).

To assess the relevance of these models to the induction of RNP immunity in humans, the order of emergence of anti-RNP antibodies was examined in a large cohort of patients who had serum samples sent to a clinical immunodiagnostics reference laboratory for RNP peptide antibody measurement. The following criteria were advanced to distinguish immune responses to initial immunogens versus targets of subsequent spreading: 1) initial immunogens should be the first targets of the immune response, 2) immunity to targets of spreading should develop after the response to the initial immunogen has been established, and 3) development of immunity to the initial immunogen should be followed by spreading to its associated targets of spreading.

The results of our investigation suggest that B′/B and 70 kd are predominant early RNP antigens to which immune responses develop. In contrast, the time course of the immune response to the A and C peptides and, particularly, to the D peptide suggests that immunity to these proteins develops most often as a consequence of spreading. Taken together, these observations depict an orderly pattern of evolution of U1 RNP immunity in humans.

PATIENTS AND METHODS

Patients. All human patient data were gathered and used under protocols approved by the University of Missouri Institutional Review Board. Data for all patients who had serum samples analyzed for RNP antibodies between 1989 and 1999 at the University of Missouri Antinuclear Antibody Testing Laboratory were entered into a computerized database (FoxPro; Microsoft, Redmond, WA) on a microcomputer (IBM, Armonk, NY). All patients for whom any positive results for RNP immunoblotting had been entered into the database were identified. All additional serum samples for each such patient were next identified. The dates that each antibody specificity first appeared were determined for each patient. The test dates and results were transferred into an Excel 97 (Microsoft) database. For each patient, the order(s) in which each antibody appeared was recorded. The order for each antibody was calculated as the total of all previously appearing antibodies plus one. Thus, two simultaneously appearing antibodies would be given the same rank. Patients whose first samples had been evaluated before 1989 were excluded. Eight patients who had ambiguous or conflicting records regarding the dates when RNP antibodies first appeared were also excluded.

Serologic testing. Immunoblotting was performed on Jurkat cell lysates as previously described (16). Briefly, 10^8 cells/ml were sonicated in 1 ml gel application buffer and applied to a 13% gel for sodium dodecyl sulfate–polyacrylamide gel electrophoresis separation. Samples were transferred to nitrocellulose, blocked overnight at 4°C with 1% bovine serum albumin in phosphate buffered saline (PBS), and rinsed twice in PBS plus 0.5% Tween 20 prior to incubation with test sera at 1:100 dilutions overnight at 4°C. After 3 washes with PBS–Tween 20, secondary incubations were performed using horseradish peroxidase–conjugated goat anti-human IgG (Cappel, Cochranville, PA) at 1:2,000 for 2 hours at room temperature. After 3 washes with PBS–Tween 20, the nitrocellulose was stained with 0.6 mg/ml 4-chloro-1-naphthol and 0.1 μl/ml H_2O_2 in Tris buffered saline (pH 7.4) for 10 minutes. All chemicals were analytic grade.

Positive control sera for all RNP antigens as well as negative control sera were run with each assay. Antibodies to RNP peptides were judged to be present if distinct bands appeared on immunoblotting, with the test sera corresponding to particular RNP peptide bands identified with the standardized positive control sera in the same experiment. Immunoblots were read without knowledge of the patients' clinical status and prior testing results. The assays reported were performed in batches with sera stored short term at −20°C or long term at −80°C.

Statistical analysis. Independent group proportions were compared using Fisher's exact test. The adherence of group proportions to predicted distributions was assessed with the chi-square test. Comparisons of proportions of matched data were performed with McNemar's test. The 95% confidence intervals for proportions were estimated with the Wald equation. Group means were compared using the Mann-Whitney U test. Statistical significance was set at $P < 0.05$. The Bonferroni correction was used in cases where multiple comparisons were performed. Results were calculated using Prism 3.0 for Windows (GraphPad Software, San Diego, CA) and SPSS 10.0 for Windows (SPSS, Chicago, IL). Binomial probabilities were calculated using the VassarStats Exact Binomial Probability Calculator (http://vassun.vassar.edu/~lowry/binom_stats.html; Web site accessed June 2, 2000).

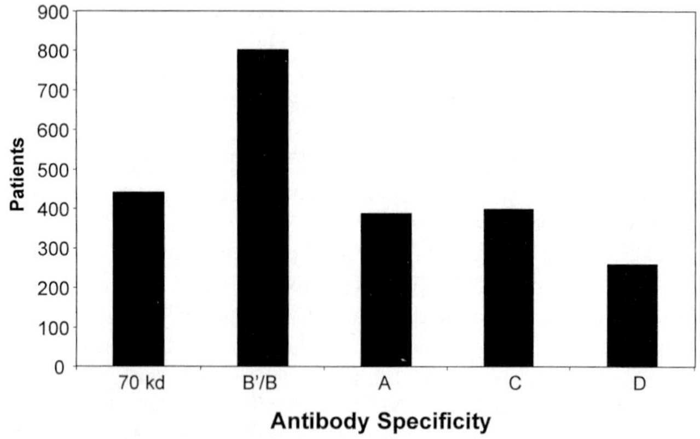

Figure 1. Patients testing positive for U1 RNP peptide IgG antibodies at the University of Missouri Antinuclear Antibody Testing Laboratory between 1989 and 1999. Immunoblotting against Jurkat cell lysates was performed on 5,882 samples from 3,668 patients to detect antibodies to U1 RNP peptides. Antibodies to the indicated peptides were identified in at least one sample for each of the patients tallied. Antibodies to B′/B were detected most frequently in these assays, while antibodies to D were detected least frequently.

RESULTS

Between 1989 and 1999, immunoblot testing for RNP antigens was performed on 5,882 samples (3,668 patients). From this group, antibodies to RNP proteins were detected by immunoblot in 978 patients. This included 441 patients (45.1%) with 70 kd antibodies, 803 (82.1%) with B′/B antibodies, 388 (39.7%) with A antibodies, 399 (40.8%) with C antibodies, and 260 (26.6%) with D antibodies (Figure 1). Sm-specific antibodies (anti–70 kd, A, or C) were present in 814 patients (83.2%), and non–Sm-specific antibodies (anti-B′/B or D) were present in 725 (74.1%). In 699 patients, antibodies to more than one of the tested RNP proteins developed. Immunoblotting was positive for at least one RNP protein on the first serum sample assayed in 869 patients. There were 109 patients who did not have detectable anti-RNP antibodies by immunoblot on the first serum sample evaluated, but who subsequently developed them. An additional 54 patients were initially seronegative for antibodies to at least one U1 RNP peptide and developed antibodies to that peptide in later sera. The date that a patient who previously did not have antibodies to a given specificity was first found to have antibodies to that specificity was termed the date of seroconversion. Of the 163 patients in whom seroconversion was documented, 46 were followed up clinically at the University of Missouri (the remainder were referred from other centers).

For the seroconverters in our cohort, the mean ± SD duration between the most recent prior negative serum sample and the date of initial seroconversion was 460.2 ± 432.5 days. The mean ± SD duration until subsequent seroconversion to additional anti–U1 RNP specificities was 530.9 ± 616.7 days. These prolonged intervals may in part have reflected clinicians' practice of not frequently ordering immunoblots for their patients (an average of <6 assays were ordered per patient during the 10-year span of the study). Eventual loss of immunoblot positivity was observed in 56 seroconverters, including 22 who lost 70 kd antibodies, 22 who lost B′/B antibodies, 28 who lost A antibodies, 27 who lost C antibodies, and 7 who lost D antibodies. Loss of antibody positivity occurred a mean ± SD of 462.2 ± 510.3 days after antibodies to the lost specificity were first noted. Reemergence of intermittently lost antibodies occurred in 16 patients.

Targets of initial seroconversion. The number of patients who seroconverted for each individual U1 RNP peptide specificity tested was 62 for 70 kd, 85 for B′/B, 63 for A, 48 for C, and 19 for D. The order in which peptide seroconversion occurred was determined (Figure 2). The 70 kd and B′/B proteins stood out as frequent initial seroconversion targets, with antibodies to 70 kd appearing at the first time that any RNP antibodies were detected by immunoblot in 43 of 62 cases (mean ± SD 69.4 ± 11.5%), and with antibodies to

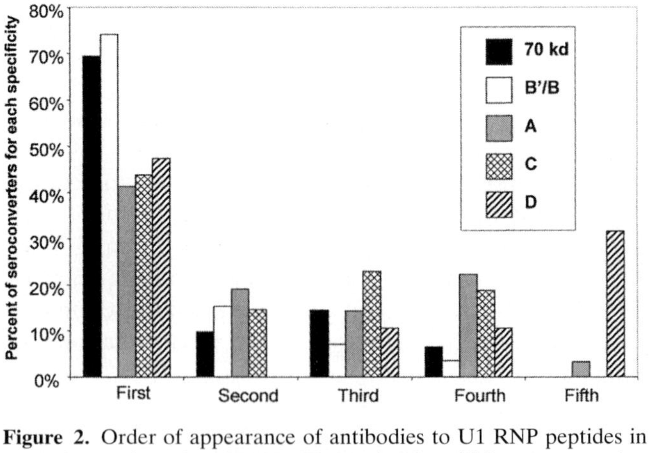

Figure 2. Order of appearance of antibodies to U1 RNP peptides in 163 witnessed seroconverters. The order in which seroconversion occurred was ranked from first through fifth for 70 kd, B′/B, A, C, and D. For each individual peptide, the number of patients in each rank group divided by the total number of seroconverters for that peptide is shown. The majority of 70 kd and B′/B seroconverters developed antibodies to these peptides before any other U1 RNP peptide antibodies emerged. Only antibodies to D frequently appeared fifth.

Table 1. Results of matched group analyses of anti-RNP antibody prevalences among 109 initial seroconverters*

Antibody	First present	First present without concurrent 70 kd	First present without concurrent B′/B	P†	P‡
Anti–70 kd	43	–	14	–	0.006
Anti-B′/B	63	34	–	0.006	–
Anti-A	26	10	8	0.009	<0.0005
Anti-C	21	6	4	<0.0005	<0.0005
Anti-D	9	5	3	<0.0005	<0.0005

* Except where otherwise indicated, values are the number of patients who initially seroconverted. McNemar's test was used to compare the proportion of patients who initially seroconverted to 70 kd or B′/B with the proportion of patients who initially seroconverted for each other individual RNP peptide studied. For each test, the 2 × 2 table depicting the initial seroconverters and noninitial seroconverters for the 2 peptides of the total pool of 109 witnessed initial seroconverters was generated.
† Versus 70 kd, by McNemar's test.
‡ Versus B′/B, by McNemar's test.

B′/B appearing at the first time in 63 of 85 cases (74.1 ± 9.3%). In contrast, antibodies to A, C, and D emerged in the first RNP-positive sera in only 26 of 63 (41.3 ± 12.2%), 21 of 48 (43.8 ± 14.0%), and 9 of 19 (47.4 ± 22.5%) cases, respectively. In many of the cases where A, C, or D antibodies appeared first, they appeared concurrently with 70 kd and/or B′/B. There were only 9 cases in which 70 kd or B′/B antibodies were ultimately detected even though neither had been present at the time of initial seroconversion. In matched group analyses, the prevalences of 70 kd or B′/B antibodies in the first positive sera were significantly greater than those of A, C, or D (Table 1). Initial B′/B antibodies were more prevalent than initial anti–70 kd antibodies.

If antibodies to immunogens develop before determinant spreading occurs, patients observed to seroconvert initially to only a single protein may be especially instructive: frequent targets of initial monospecific seroconversion would be probable immunogens. Of the 47 patients in our cohort for whom monospecific seroconversion was observed, 27 had anti-B′/B antibodies and 11 had anti–70 kd antibodies, but only 5 had anti-A, and 2 each had anti-C and anti-D (Table 2). Thus, the pattern of initial immunity observed was consistent with roles for 70 kd and B′/B as initial immunogens of anti-RNP responses.

Targets of late seroconversion. Late seroconversion was defined as the development of antibodies to individual RNP proteins only after other RNP antibodies had appeared. Frequent late seroconversion to an RNP protein would implicate it as a target of determinant spreading. Late emergence of antibodies to at least one U1 RNP peptide was observed in 88 of the 163 witnessed seroconverters. Of the late seroconverters, 19 were for 70 kd, 22 for B′/B, 37 for A, 27 for C, and 10 for D (Table 2). The proportion of late seroconverters was substantially greater than the proportion of monospecific initial seroconverters for A (mean ± SD 42.0 ± 10.3% versus 10.6 ± 8.8%) and C (30.7 ± 9.6% versus 4.3 ± 5.8%).

While seroconversion to D was uncommon overall, the proportion of D seroconverters who were late seroconverters (52.6 ± 22.5%) was similar to the proportions of A and C seroconverters who were late seroconverters (58.7 ± 12.2% and 56.3 ± 14.0%, respectively). Late seroconversion was less common among 70 kd and B′/B seroconverters (30.6 ± 11.5% and 25.9 ± 9.3%, respectively). Moreover, late seroconversion to the D protein demonstrated features consistent with a target of massive spreading. Immunity to D appeared after immunity to all 4 of the other RNP antigens tested in 6 of 19 cases (31.6%) in which anti-D was ever present. There were only 2 additional patients in whom immunity to all 4 of the other RNP antigens tested developed first—in both of these cases, anti-A was the last antibody specificity to emerge.

The significance of the number of patients in whom anti-D appeared fifth and last was tested against

Table 2. Monospecific and late seroconverters to RNP peptides in the study*

Seroconverters	Peptide: 70 kd	B′/B	A	C	D
Monospecific (n = 47)	11 (23.4)	27 (57.4)	5 (10.6)	2 (4.3)	2 (4.3)
Late (n = 88)†	19 (21.6)	22 (25.0)	37 (42.0)	27 (30.7)	10 (11.4)

* Values are the number (percent) of patients. Shown are patients with a single RNP specificity appearing on the first positive RNP immunoblot after previous negative immunoblots (monospecific seroconverters) and patients with antibodies to an RNP peptide occurring only after other RNP antibodies had previously been detected (late seroconverters).
† Some patients were late seroconverters to multiple specificities.

Table 3. RNP antibodies observed to precede development of anti-D

Antibody	Precedes anti-D*	Prevalence†	P‡
Anti–70 kd	9/10	441/978	0.005
Anti-B′/B	10/10	803/978	0.1
Anti-A	7/10	388/978	0.051
Anti-C	8/10	399/978	0.0122

* Values are the number of times an antibody was observed to develop prior to anti-D/number of instances of late anti-D seroconversion.
† Values are the total number of patients with antibodies to the indicated specificity/total number of RNP-positive patients.
‡ By chi-square test (after Bonferroni correction, P values less than 0.0125 were considered significant).

the null hypothesis that any of the tested antibodies was equally likely to appear last. If any antibody appeared fifth and last in 8 of 163 cases (as observed), and if the actual probability was the same for any of the antibodies to appear last, the binomial probability that at least 6 patients in a cohort of 163 would have anti-D appear last would be <0.4%. Conversely, if each of the individual RNP antibodies had a probability of 6/163 of appearing last (as observed for D), the likelihood that 70 kd (or, equally, B′/B or C) would never appear last in a cohort of 163 patients would be <0.3%. There is no point between these extremes where a probability of ≥5% exists that at least 6 of 163 patients would have anti-D while none of 163 patients would have anti–70 kd, anti-B′/B, and anti-C. We therefore rejected the null hypothesis and concluded that the probability of anti-D emerging last was greater than the probability of other RNP antibodies emerging last.

Spreading to anti-D from non-Sm RNP antibodies. Antibodies to the Sm determinant B′/B developed before anti-D in all 10 cases of late anti-D seroconversion. However, anti-D was also preceded by at least 1 non-Sm RNP antibody in every case. This suggests that spreading of an immune response to the D peptide is promoted by preexisting immunity to the entire U1 RNP, rather than strictly to components of the Sm particle. Specifically, the rate at which anti–70 kd and anti-C antibodies preceded anti-D was significantly greater than the overall prevalence of these antibodies in the total sample (Table 3).

Late emergence of antibodies to the non-Sm proteins was, like anti-D, commonly associated with preexisting immunity to both Sm and non-Sm proteins. Unlike anti-D, however, the rate at which the non-Sm antibodies were preceded by other RNP antibodies merely reflected the overall prevalence of the other antibodies in the population (Table 4).

Determinant spreading by monospecific seroconverters. Finally, we reviewed data for the 11 monospecific seroconverters from whom additional subsequent sera were obtained. Followup sera after the initial appearance of a single RNP antibody were obtained a mean ± SD of 425.0 ± 336.4 days after the anti-RNP peptide response was first seen (502.6 ± 434.3 days in patients with spreading and 372.6 ± 281.8 days in patients without spreading; $P = 0.5$ by Mann-Whitney U test). The most common antigen to be the next target of spreading was B′/B (5 of 5 cases), while initial spreading to any other specificity was observed in only 1 of 5 cases. In cases with initial antibodies to 70 kd, subsequent diversification of the antibody response was common (3 of 4 cases). In 1 case, the initial anti–70 kd responses spread to A and C concurrent with spreading to B′/B. Initial responses to the A protein spread to another specificity (B′/B) in 1 of 4 cases, and initial anti-C responses spread to B′/B in the only monospecific seroconverter for C in our sample from whom additional sera were obtained. Spreading occurred in none of 2 cases with initial monospecific B′/B antibodies. Subsequent sera were not available from the monospecific seroconverters for D. No differences in the intervals between tests were noted between patients positive for the different antibodies.

The frequency with which subsequent sera were assessed in monospecific seroconverters to B′/B or D (2 of 29 cases) was dramatically lower than that for monospecific seroconverters to the non-Sm specificities (9 of 18 cases) ($P = 0.001$ by Fisher's exact test). No difference in utilization of immunoblot testing due to the referral center was found. Fifteen of the 29 Sm peptide seroconverters were followed up at the University of

Table 4. Patterns of emergence of antibodies to individual non-Sm U1 RNP proteins*

Preceded antibody	Total (n = 978)	Non-Sm only (n = 164)	Sm only (n = 253)	Sm and non-Sm (n = 561)	P†
Anti–70 kd	19	0	6	13	0.1
Anti-A	37	8	8	21	0.7
Anti-C	28	4	7	17	0.9
Any anti–non-Sm	69	9	13	47	0.2

* Values are the number of patients in whom the antibodies shown are preceded by Sm and/or non-Sm antibodies.
† Versus total sample, by chi-square test (P values less than 0.05 were considered significant).

Missouri compared with 6 of the 18 other monospecific seroconverters ($P = 0.2$ by Fisher's exact test).

We reviewed clinical data on the 21 monospecific seroconverters followed up at the University of Missouri. Patients were classified as having SLE, MCTD, scleroderma, or "other" based on the assessments documented by their clinicians. (None of the patients in the "other" group had been diagnosed as having any rheumatic diseases.) Followup immunoblotting was frequently performed in patients believed to have MCTD (3 of 3), occasionally performed in patients believed to have SLE or scleroderma (2 of 7 and 1 of 3, respectively), and seldom performed in patients diagnosed as having other diseases (1 of 8). The low frequency with which followup testing was performed in witnessed monospecific Sm seroconverters seemed attributable in part to decreased followup testing of patients diagnosed as having SLE (subsequent testing was performed in none of 5 patients with initial Sm antibodies and in 2 of 2 patients with initial non-Sm antibodies), but also seemed attributable to the substantial absolute number of "other" diagnoses in the initial Sm group (subsequent testing was performed in none of 6 patients with initial Sm antibodies and in 1 of 2 patients with initial non-Sm antibodies).

DISCUSSION

In contrast to prior studies that have examined the longitudinal evolution of RNP immunity in human series (17–21), the cohort in our study was not preselected to already have RNP immunity. Thus, we could observe the order in which initial seroconversion to anti-RNP antibodies developed. Recent reports have suggested that predictable, orderly patterns of emergence of autoantibodies occur in antigen-driven animal models of autoimmune disease (7–9,22), but the order in which RNP immunity develops in humans has not previously been described. Findings of the present study, which we believe contains the largest group for which RNP peptide testing has been reported to date, indicate that orderly patterns of emergence of anti-RNP responses occur in humans as well. We have shown that antibodies to the 70 kd and B′/B polypeptides appear early in the anti-RNP response significantly more frequently than do antibodies to other U1 RNP peptides. We have also shown that antibodies to the D peptide seldom occur in the absence of preexisting or coexisting responses to multiple other U1 RNP antigens. Finally, we see indications that B′/B may be a prominent early target of spreading after initial responses to other U1 RNP peptides.

The early prominence of the 70 kd antigen in anti-RNP responses is consistent with the hypothesis that antigenically modified forms of the 70 kd protein (such as those that occur in apoptosis and under oxidative stress) may be initial immunogens in anti-RNP immunity (12). Studies to further characterize the role of antigenically modified forms of the U1–70 kd peptide as potential initial immunogens, and to define their clinical correlates, are warranted. While the cytomegalovirus gB protein has been reported to share C-terminal epitopes with the 70 kd protein (23), the tendency to develop spreading to other RNP specificities after initial 70 kd immunity is consistent with a role for the RNP particle rather than an indication of the presence of a molecular mimic.

The early prominence of B′/B antibodies in anti-RNP responses suggests that B′/B or B′/B molecular mimics (such as EBNA-1 protein) may also act as initial immunogens in anti-RNP immunity. The anti-B′/B response was found to be different from the anti–70 kd response in two respects. First, anti-B′/B was by far the most common overall target of anti-RNP antibodies. The high prevalence of B′/B antibodies could be due to more potent immunogenicity of the B′/B RNP compared with other RNP proteins, or to a high prevalence of immunity to B′/B molecular mimics. Second, when diversification of an initial anti-RNP response occurred, early spreading to anti-B′/B (in 5 of 5 cases), but not to anti–70 kd (in none of 5 cases), was seen. Initial immunity to 70 kd itself often led to spreading to B′/B, while initial immunity to B′/B was not observed to lead to spreading to any other U1 RNP (although it is true that this was a very small sample). Thus, B′/B, but not 70 kd, showed properties of a prominent target of determinant spreading—that is, after initial responses to other RNP antigens, B′/B appeared to be particularly immunogenic. However, the inability of initial immunity to B′/B to elicit subsequent spreading raises the suspicion that cases of initial immunity to B′/B may be mediated by B′/B molecular mimics rather than by the RNP particle.

The early nature of spreading to anti-B′/B distinguished it from other targets of determinant spreading. When spreading to other RNP specificities occurred, it was almost always preceded by immunity to B′/B (in 60 of 69 cases). This suggests that after the initial development of RNP immunity, spreading of the response to B′/B may be a preferred pathway for inducing more widespread immune reactivity. Although 70 kd appeared to be an efficient initial immunogen, it was no more apt to be a target of subsequent spreading than A or C. Failure to efficiently spread to anti–70 kd responses could reflect a preference for initial immunity to a modified form of the 70 kd antigen that is not typically present during spreading of the subsequent RNP immune response. Since recognition of modified forms of 70 kd has been linked with clinical disease manifestations (12), low production of modified 70 kd antigen could also account for observed cases of loss of anti–70 kd antibodies in patients entering clinical remissions of MCTD (24).

The observation that anti-D responses occur in the context of massive spreading of the U1 RNP response is compatible with prior observations that anti-D antibodies are associated with clinically more severe disease (25). Our findings would suggest that immunoblot detection of anti-D antibody may be a marker for the overall intensity of the autoimmune response. The emergence of anti-D antibodies could indicate that a proimmune context has developed to such an extent that even relatively disfavored potential immunogens have become immunoreactive. One mechanism through which massive RNP spreading might promote D peptide immunogenicity is through the ability of (potentially late-emerging) anti-C antibodies to stabilize the Sm/U1 RNP complex (26). The substantial difference we observed between the prevalences of anti-B′/B and anti-D antibodies in a large population of patients referred for RNP testing has not previously been reported.

Some elements in the design of the current study limit its strength. Sampling errors may skew the conclusions reached. Sera were sent for testing solely at the judgment of the referring clinicians. Thus, the patient sera tested might not reflect the spectrum of RNP responses present in the general population. Also, our findings rely on the results of immunoblot assays that test for antibody recognition of denatured proteins from Jurkat cells instead of native conformations from the physiologically relevant antigen source.

However, the limitations of our study may in part be mitigated by other considerations. While our study group was not obtained by random sampling from a general population, it is a relevant sample, since it consists of all the specimens sent to a referral laboratory for determination of RNP peptide antibodies across a 10-year span. Whether or not this reflects the general population, it is likely to reflect what clinicians treating rheumatic diseases encounter in the course of their practice. While systematic bias may influence which patients were referred for immunoblot testing, we found similar results in patients referred from our own center and in those referred from outside clinicians. Regarding the drawbacks of immunoblot testing, immunoblot results in our laboratory have previously been shown to correlate well with results of enzyme-linked immunosorbent assays for antibodies to 70 kd, A, B′/B, and D (27). In addition, we have confirmed our Jurkat immunoblot results in a subset of sera immunoblotted against HeLa lysates. Finally, while we cannot exclude the possibility that spreading occurs differently to native versus denatured antigens, spreading to diverse epitopes on a single antigen has been observed to occur concurrent with or prior to spreading to other RNP antigens in animal models of autoimmunity (22,28).

The results of this study suggest that at least two distinct antigens may act as initial immunogens of anti-RNP responses: a form of the 70 kd peptide associated with the U1 RNP and a form of the B′/B antigen which may be separate from both the U1 RNP and the D antigens. One would therefore predict that the spectrum of anti-RNP–associated conditions might consist of at least two clinically distinct entities. The fact that a relatively low number of monospecific seroconverters to B′/B at the University of Missouri appeared to develop MCTD (2 of 13), while a relatively high number of these patients (5 of 13) did not appear to develop any known rheumatic disease, is consistent with the possibility that isolated B′/B immunity is related to a distinct disease process. If isolated B′/B immunity is due to molecular mimicry with an infectious agent, the disease process present in some monospecific B′/B-positive patients may be primarily infectious rather than autoimmune in nature. Given the additional role of B′/B immunity as a preferential early target of determinant spreading, it is possible that this same infectious agent could also act as a disease-producing amplifier of endogenous RNP immunity. Further studies may be warranted to identify and characterize the associations of infectious agents with subgroups of patients by their patterns of RNP immunity.

The presence of an orderly pattern of emergence of anti-RNP immunity in humans indicates that the development of an autoimmune disease may occur in a stepwise manner. The recognition of (potentially modified) forms of the 70 kd antigen and the recognition of (potentially infectious mimics of) the B′/B protein may be early points in this progression. By further dissecting the intermediate steps that lead to the expression of anti-RNP–associated clinical syndromes, new approaches to interrupting the expression of clinical disease may be uncovered.

ACKNOWLEDGMENTS

The authors thank Grace Wang, MT, for technical assistance and John E. Hewett, PhD, for statistical expertise.

REFERENCES

1. Holman HR. Partial purification and characterization of an extractable nuclear antigen which reacts with SLE sera. Ann N Y Acad Sci 1965;124:800–6.
2. Kleine Gunnewiek JMT, van de Putte LBA, van Venrooij WJ. The U1 snRNP complex: an autoantigen in connective tissue diseases. An update. Clin Exp Rheumatol 1997;15:549–60.
3. Wooley JC, Zukerberg LR, Chung SY. Polypeptide components of the human small nuclear ribonucleoproteins. Proc Natl Acad Sci U S A 1983;80:5208–12.
4. Tan EM, Kunkel HG. Characteristics of a soluble nuclear antigen precipitating with sera of patients with systemic lupus erythematosus. J Immunol 1966;96:464–71.
5. Sharp GC, Irvin WS, May CM, Holman HR, McDuffie FC, Hess EV, et al. Association of antibodies to ribonucleoprotein and Sm antigens with mixed connective-tissue disease, systemic lupus erythematosus and other rheumatic diseases. N Engl J Med 1976;295:1149–54.
6. Fatenejad S, Mamula MJ, Craft J. Role of intermolecular/intrastructural B- and T-cell determinants in the diversification of autoantibodies to ribonucleoprotein particles. Proc Natl Acad Sci U S A 1993;90:12010–4.
7. James JA, Gross T, Scofield RH, Harley JB. Immunoglobulin epitope spreading and autoimmune disease after peptide immunization: Sm B/B′-derived PPPGMRPP and PPPGIRGP induce spliceosome autoimmunity. J Exp Med 1995;181:453–61.
8. McCluskey J, Farris AD, Keech CL, Purcell AW, Rischmuller M, Kinoshita G, et al. Determinant spreading: lessons from animal models and human disease. Immunol Rev 1998;164:209–29.
9. Fatenejad S, Brooks W, Schwartz A, Craft J. Pattern of anti-small nuclear ribonucleoprotein antibodies in MRL/MP-lpr/lpr mice suggests that the intact U1 snRNP particle is their autoimmunogenic target. J Immunol 1994;152:5523–31.
10. Utz PJ, Anderson P. Posttranslational protein modifications, apoptosis, and the bypass of tolerance to autoantigens. Arthritis Rheum 1998;41:1152–60.
11. Guldner HH, Netter HJ, Szostecki C, Jaeger E, Will H. Human anti-p68 autoantibodies recognize a common epitope of U1 RNA containing small nuclear ribonucleoprotein and influenza B virus. J Exp Med 1990;171:819–29.
12. Greidinger EL, Casciola-Rosen L, Morris SM, Hoffman RW, Rosen A. Autoantibody recognition of distinctly modified forms of the U1–70-kd antigen is associated with different clinical disease manifestations. Arthritis Rheum 2000;43:881–8.
13. Casciola-Rosen L, Andrade F, Ulanet D, Wong WB, Rosen A. Cleavage by granzyme B is strongly predictive of autoantigen status: implications for initiation of autoimmunity. J Exp Med 1999;190:815–26.
14. Casciola-Rosen L, Wigley F, Rosen A. Scleroderma autoantigens are uniquely fragmented by metal-catalyzed oxidation reactions: implications for pathogenesis. J Exp Med 1997;185:71–9.
15. James JA, Kaufman KM, Farris AD, Taylor-Albert E, Lehman TJA, Harley JB. An increased prevalence of Epstein-Barr virus infection in young patients suggests a possible etiology for systemic lupus erythematosus. J Clin Invest 1997;100:3019–26.
16. Pettersson I, Wang G, Smith EI, Wigzell H, Hedfors E, Horn J, et al. The use of immunoblotting and immunoprecipitation of (U) small nuclear ribonucleoproteins in the analysis of sera of patients with mixed connective tissue disease and systemic lupus erythematosus: a cross-sectional, longitudinal study. Arthritis Rheum 1986;29:986–96.
17. Habets WJ, de Rooij DJ, Hoet MH, van de Putte LB, van Venrooij WJ. Quantitation of anti-RNP and anti-Sm antibodies in MCTD and SLE patients by immunoblotting. Clin Exp Immunol 1985;59: 457–66.
18. Combe B, Rucheton M, Graafland H, Lussiez V, Brunel C, Sany J. Clinical significance of anti-RNP and anti-Sm autoantibodies as determined by immunoblotting and immunoprecipitation in sera from patients with connective tissue diseases. Clin Exp Immunol 1989;75:18–24.
19. Ter Borg EJ, Horst G, Limburg PC, Kallenberg CG. Shifts of anti-Sm-specific antibodies in patients with systemic lupus erythematosus: analysis by counter-immunoelectrophoresis, immunoblotting, and RNA-immunoprecipitation. J Autoimmun 1991;4: 155–64.
20. Nyman U, Lundberg I, Hedfors E, Wahren M, Pettersson I. IgG and IgM anti-snRNP reactivity in sequentially obtained serum samples from patients with connective tissue diseases. Ann Rheum Dis 1992;51:1307–12.
21. Ghirardello A, Doria A, Vesco P, Vaccaro E, Bernardi C, Catani C, et al. Blotting patterns of IgG anti-(U1)RNP antibodies in mixed connective tissue disease. Rheumatol Int 1996;16:145–50.
22. Yu M, Johnson JM, Tuohy VK. A predictable sequential determinant spreading cascade invariably accompanies progression of experimental autoimmune encephalomyelitis: a basis for peptide-specific therapy after onset of clinical disease. J Exp Med 1996; 183:1777–88.
23. Curtis HAE, Singh T, Newkirk MM. Recombinant cytomegalovirus glycoprotein gB (UL55) induces an autoantibody response to the U1-70 kDa small nuclear ribonucleoprotein. Eur J Immunol 1999;29:3643–53.
24. Burdt MA, Hoffman RW, Deutscher SL, Wang GS, Johnson JC, Sharp GC. Long-term outcome in mixed connective tissue disease: longitudinal clinical and serologic findings. Arthritis Rheum 1999; 42:899–909.
25. Homma M, Mimori T, Takeda Y, Akama H, Yoshida T, Ogasawara T, et al. Autoantibodies to the Sm antigen: immunological approach to clinical aspects of systemic lupus erythematosus. J Rheumatol 1987;14 Suppl 13:188–93.
26. Satoh M, Richards HB, Hamilton KJ, Reeves WH. Human anti-nuclear ribonucleoprotein antigen autoimmune sera contain a novel subset of autoantibodies that stabilizes the molecular interaction of U1RNP-C protein with the Sm core proteins. J Immunol 1997;158:5017–25.
27. Takeda Y, Wang GS, Wang RJ, Anderson SK, Pettersson I, Amaki S, et al. Enzyme-linked immunosorbent assay using isolated (U) small nuclear ribonucleoprotein polypeptides as antigens to investigate the clinical significance of autoantibodies to these polypeptides. Clin Immunol Immunopathol 1989;50:213–30.
28. Deshmukh US, Lewis JE, Gaskin F, Kannapell CC, Waters ST, Lou Y-H, et al. Immune responses to Ro60 and its peptides in mice. I. The nature of the immunogen and endogenous autoantigen determine the specificities of the induced autoantibodies. J Exp Med 1999;189:531–40.

ARTHRITIS & RHEUMATISM
Vol. 44, No. 2, February 2001, pp 376–383

Anti–Topoisomerase I (Anti–Scl-70) Antibodies in Patients With Systemic Lupus Erythematosus

Hélène A. Elicha Gussin, Georghe P. Ignat, John Varga, and Marius Teodorescu

Objective. **To investigate the presence and clinical significance of anti–Scl-70 antibodies in patients with systemic lupus erythematosus (SLE).**

Methods. **Levels of antibodies against Scl-70 were determined by a commercial clinical enzyme-linked immunosorbent assay (ELISA) during routine evaluation. Results were verified by an additional ELISA with a characterized bovine Scl-70, by ELISA with a recombinant human topoisomerase I, by Western blot, and by double diffusion in agar gel. Disease activity was estimated retrospectively by the Systemic Lupus Activity Measure (SLAM).**

Results. **Of 128 consecutive SLE patients, 25% were positive for anti–Scl-70 antibody; this antibody activity was cognate in nature. No SLE patient could be classified as also having systemic sclerosis. The levels of anti–Scl-70 were significantly correlated with the SLAM score for the entire cohort (r = 0.563, $P < 0.001$) and for 7 individual patients with multiple longitudinal measurements (r = 0.755–0.951, $P < 0.001$; n = 6) (r = 0.378, $P < 0.05$; n = 1). A significant correlation was also found between the levels of anti–Scl-70 and anti–double-stranded DNA antibodies (r = 0.558, $P < 0.001$). Patients with anti–Scl-70 had significantly higher risk of pulmonary hypertension ($P < 0.01$) and renal involvement ($P < 0.001$) than patients without this antibody.**

Conclusion. **Anti–Scl-70 antibody is present in a significant subset of patients with SLE. For this subset, it offers a good correlate of disease activity and suggests increased risk for pulmonary hypertension and nephritis.**

Supported in part by Campus Research Board, University of Illinois at Chicago.

Hélène A. Elicha Gussin, PhD, Georghe P. Ignat, MD, John Varga, MD, Marius Teodorescu, MD, PhD: University of Illinois College of Medicine, Chicago.

Address correspondence and reprint requests to Marius Teodorescu, MD, PhD, Department of Microbiology/Immunology, University of Illinois College of Medicine, 835 South Wolcott Avenue (M/C 790), Chicago, IL 60612.

Submitted for publication June 14, 2000; accepted in revised form October 13, 2000.

Topoisomerase I (topo I; or, Scl-70) is a 67–100-kd nuclear enzyme with nicking-closing activity on DNA (1,2). Anti–Scl-70 autoantibodies are found in 20–35% of patients with systemic sclerosis (SSc), mainly in those with the diffuse form of the disease (3–6). These antibodies have been generally associated with a poor prognosis (7) and have been linked to extensive skin and pulmonary fibrosis (7–9).

The presence of anti–Scl-70 antibodies is generally considered highly specific for SSc (10–12). However, the presence of anti–Scl-70 antibodies detected by enzyme-linked immunosorbent assay (ELISA) has also been reported in 5 of 19 patients (~26%) with systemic lupus erythematosus (SLE) (13–15). In addition, case reports based on double diffusion in agar gel, on immunoprecipitation using ^{35}S-labeled HeLa cell extracts, and on immunoblots have also suggested that anti–Scl-70 may be present in SLE patients with (16) or without (17,18) concomitant features of SSc. Nevertheless, the presence of anti–Scl-70 antibodies in SLE patients has been attributed primarily to an artifact of the ELISA detection method (10). Since >80% of all reported clinical laboratory results are currently based on ELISA, the issue of anti–Scl-70 antibody in SLE needs to be addressed.

In the present study, we evaluated the presence of anti–Scl-70 antibodies in serum specimens from 128 SLE patients tested over the course of 5 years by ELISA. The relationship between the level of anti–Scl-70 antibody and disease activity in SLE patients was investigated retrospectively.

PATIENTS AND METHODS

Patient population. A retrospective review of the charts of 128 consecutive patients seen at the University of Illinois at Chicago Medical Center was performed. The patients met the revised criteria for SLE of the American College of Rheumatology (19). In addition, data regarding the presence and levels of anti–Scl-70 were collected for 89 patients with SSc. Levels of autoantibodies against 8 nuclear antigens (single-stranded DNA [ssDNA; denatured calf thymus DNA], double-stranded DNA [dsDNA; bacteriophage λ DNA], SSA, SSB, Sm, nuclear RNP [nRNP]/Sm, histone, and Scl-70) were routinely determined by ELISA with commercial kits (EL-ANA Profiles, TheraTest/DiaSorin; TheraTest Labs, Chicago, IL). Disease activity and clinical presentation were retrospectively evaluated by the Systemic Lupus Activity Measure (SLAM) (20,21).

Serum specimens. After routine testing, serum specimens were stored in our frozen collection for as long as 5 years. For controls, we used the following: 1) sera without anti–Scl-70, but with very high levels of other antinuclear antibodies (ANA; >100-fold the normal limit of anti-DNA, anti-SSA, anti-SSB, antihistone, anti-nRNP/Sm, and/or anti–ribosomal protein P antibodies); 2) randomly chosen stored sera from 50 blood bank donors (BBD); 3) sera from SSc patients containing relatively high levels of anti–Scl-70 antibodies; and 4) sera from the Centers for Disease Control and Prevention (CDC; Atlanta, GA) specific for a particular nuclear antigen (22): DNA, Sm, nRNP, SSA, SSB, Scl-70, or Jo-1.

Polyacrylamide gels and Western blots. Immunoaffinity-purified bovine Scl-70 (1,000 units/ml) was obtained from Immunovision (Springdale, AR). Lack of contamination was determined by sodium dodecyl sulfate–polyacrylamide gel electrophoresis (SDS-PAGE) and by staining in parallel with Coomassie blue and silver (Silver Stain Plus; Bio-Rad, Hercules, CA). Western blots were performed according to the manufacturer's instructions (Bio-Rad).

ELISA. The disease specificity of ELISA test kits was determined on a minimum of 100 randomly chosen BBD sera. Specificities were 95% for ssDNA; >99% for dsDNA, Sm, SSA, SSB, and Scl-70; and 98% for histone and nRNP. For this study, an ELISA test (Test-Scl-70) was also set up with a characterized Scl-70 antigen as previously described (6). The final values for absorbance at 450 nm were converted into commercial units/ml with the help of an internal standard.

ELISA with recombinant full-length human topo I was performed with the help of a commercial diagnostic kit (Varelisa Scl-70 antibodies; Pharmacia & Upjohn, Kalamazoo, MI) according to the manufacturer's instructions.

Immunoabsorption. Three monospecific patient sera were used to prepare 3 separate specific IgG autoantibody immunoabsorption columns of equal volume (5 ml) for anti–Scl-70, antihistone, and anti-nRNP. The IgG from these sera was purified by protein G affinity chromatography (GammaBind G; Genex, Gaithersburg, MD) according to the manufacturer's instructions. The IgG was coupled to Affi-Prep Hydrazide Support (Bio-Rad) according to the manufacturer's instructions. One hundred–microliter aliquots of Scl-70 antigen solution, followed by 15 ml of phosphate buffered saline (PBS), were passed through the columns at 22°C with the aid of a peristaltic pump. The equally diluted effluents of all 3 columns were collected and coated onto plastic wells (6).

Other methods. Pepsin (23–25) and DNase (26) digestions were performed as described previously. Competitive inhibition assays were performed by mixing 10 μl of serum with 10 μl of antigen solution (700–1,200 μg/ml), or with 10 μl PBS (control). After a 1-hour incubation at room temperature, 980 μl of PBS–Tween 20 was added for a final sample dilution of 1:100.

Double immunodiffusion in agar gel against calf thymus extract containing Scl-70 was performed with the help of a clinical laboratory kit (Inova Gel Scl-70 "S"; Inova Diagnostics, San Diego, CA) according to the manufacturer's instructions.

Statistical analysis. The agreement (kappa statistic) was calculated with the help of the Web site for applied statistics (http://maddog.fammed.wisc.edu/~rbrown/epi.html; website accessed March 2000). Parametric Pearson's correlation coefficients (r) were calculated with the help of CA-Cricket Graph III (Computer Associates International, Islandia, NY), and *P* values were obtained from tables (27). The statistical significance of differences between sets of values was determined by the Kolmogorov-Smirnov test

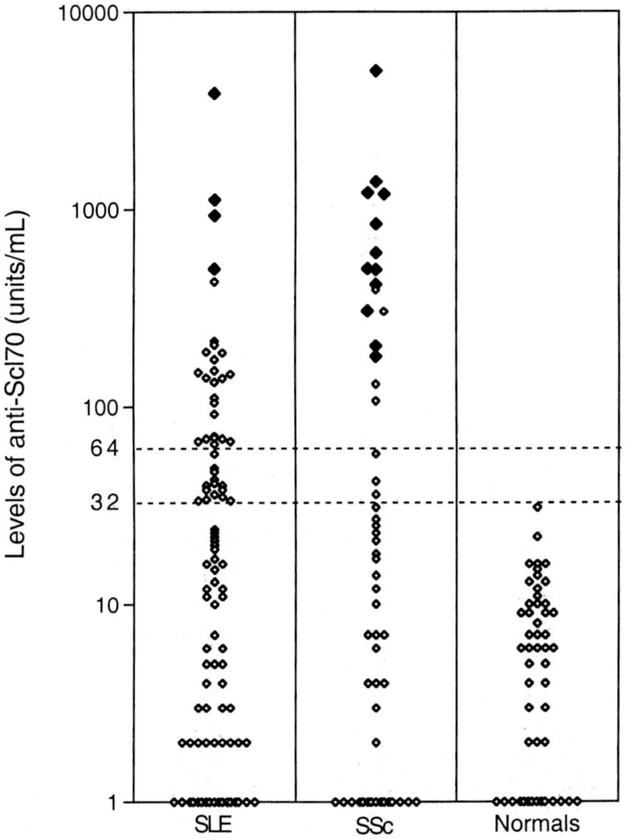

Figure 1. Scattergram of the levels of anti–Scl-70 antibodies in normal subjects and in patients with systemic lupus erythematosus (SLE) and systemic sclerosis (SSc), measured by enzyme-linked immunosorbent assay (ELISA) with a commercial kit. For each SLE patient, the highest recorded value was plotted. For SSc patients, only 1 data point was available. Dark diamonds indicate serum specimens with anti–Scl-70 levels of >64 units/ml by ELISA which were also positive by double diffusion in agar gel. Dashed lines represent 32 units/ml and 64 units/ml, which is the upper limit of normal and twice this limit.

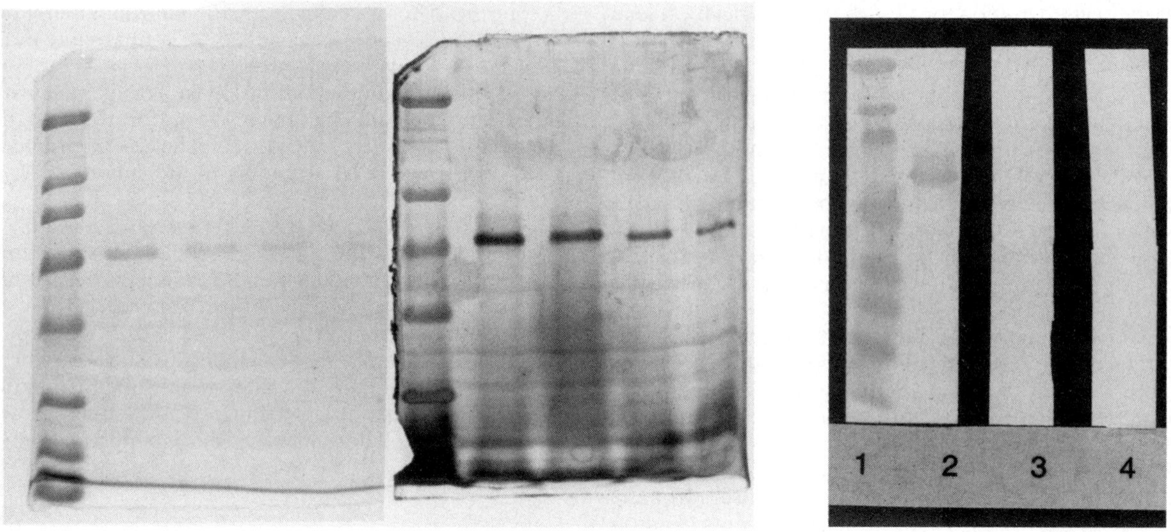

A B

Figure 2. Sodium dodecyl sulfate–polyacrylamide gel electrophoresis of different concentrations of the bovine Scl-70 antigen. Shown are staining by Coomassie blue and silver (**A**) followed by Western blot (**B**) with SSc control serum (lane 2), SLE serum with high levels of anti-nRNP/Sm antibodies (lane 3), and normal human serum (lane 4). Lane 1 contains the MW standard (200, 113, 82, 49, 35, 29.5, 21, and 7.5 kd). See Figure 1 for definitions.

(StatWorks; Cricket Software, Philadelphia, PA) and by chi-square test (27).

RESULTS

Frequency of anti–Scl-70 antibodies in SLE and SSc patients. Twenty-five percent of the SLE patients (32 of 128) had abnormal levels of anti–Scl-70 (up to 3,850 units/ml; normal limit 32 units/ml) at least once during their disease course. None had any clinical findings characteristic of SSc. Among these 32 SLE patients, 25 (19% of all 128 SLE patients) had levels of anti–Scl-70 that were >2-fold the upper limit of normal (Figure 1), and among patients tested before any treatment was implemented, 31% (5 of 16) had levels that exceeded the normal limit by 4–40-fold. Among the patients in the SSc group, 18% (16 of 89) had abnormal levels (≥64 units/ml). However, the levels in SSc patients were significantly higher than those seen in SLE patients ($P = 0.026$, by Kolmogorov-Smirnov test) (Figure 1). Some SLE sera with relatively high levels by ELISA (>64 units/ml) also had anti–Scl-70 by double immunodiffusion (Figure 1, dark diamonds).

We concluded that anti–Scl-70 antibody detected by ELISA was indeed present in a significant proportion of SLE patients; the presence of some of these antibodies was confirmed by double diffusion in agar gel. However, for those serum specimens that were negative for anti–Scl-70 by double immunodiffusion, evidence was needed to determine whether reactivity in ELISA was an artifact of the testing system.

Reproducibility in Test-Scl-70 of results obtained with the commercial ELISA. An ELISA (called Test-Scl-70 to distinguish it from the commercial ELISA) was set up with a purified Scl-70 bovine antigen. In SDS-PAGE, this antigen yielded a unique band with an apparent MW of 70 kd (Figure 2A). A band in the same position was stained by Western blot with an antibody from the serum of an SSc patient, but not by anti-nRNP antibodies (Figure 2B). The upper limit of normal for the Test-Scl-70 ELISA was established with 50 randomly chosen BBD sera by the percentile ranking method (28) at 32 units/ml, for a disease specificity of 100% (28) (the mean + 3SD was 26 units/ml). The test sensitivity was set up to be equal to that of the commercial anti–Scl-70 ELISA used in the routine testing.

The Test-Scl-70 yielded a very strong reaction with the CDC positive control for Scl-70, but reacted within normal limits with the remaining 6 antigen-specific sera from the CDC (Figure 3) (22). Neither the commercial ELISA nor the Test-Scl-70 reacted with sera containing very high levels (>100-fold the normal limit for each) of antibodies against nuclear antigens other

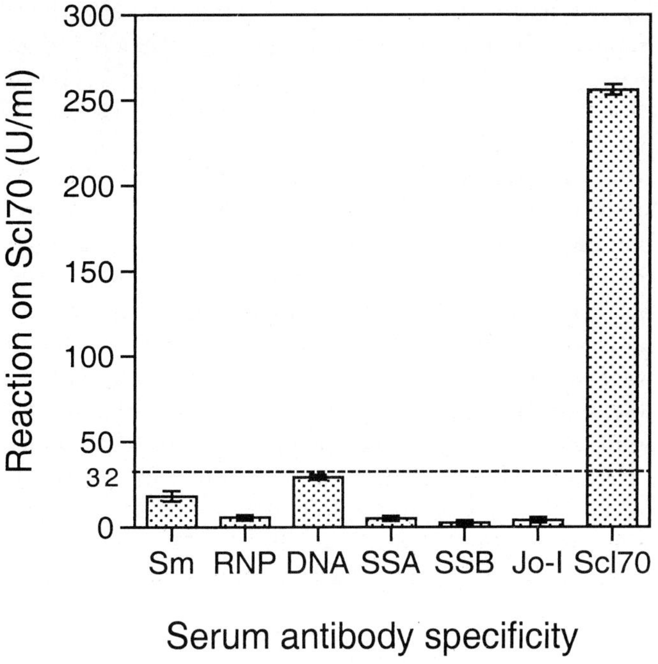

Figure 3. Values (mean ± SD) yielded by standard sera of known specificity from the Centers for Disease Control and Prevention. Sera were tested by an enzyme-linked immunosorbent assay (ELISA) on Test-Scl-70 ELISA wells (the Test-Scl-70 ELISA was set up with a purified Scl-70 bovine antigen). The dashed line indicates the upper limit of normal.

than Scl-70: ssDNA, dsDNA, Sm, nRNP, SSA, SSB, histones, Jo-1, and ribosomal protein P. Also, there was no significant difference in frequency or levels of anti-DNA (ssDNA and dsDNA) between anti–Scl-70–positive and –negative SLE sera (data not shown). Thus, Scl-70 antigen was not contaminated with DNA or other nuclear antigens. There was complete agreement between the recorded positive and negative anti–Scl-70 results obtained with commercial ELISA and Test-Scl-70 ELISA with this antigen (κ = 1.0).

Along with 50 randomly chosen BBD sera, we tested 10 anti–Scl-70–positive SLE sera, 10 anti–Scl-70–negative SLE sera, and 10 anti–Scl-70–positive SSc sera on human recombinant topo I. There was very good agreement between the results with bovine Scl-70 and those with the recombinant antigen (κ = 0.92).

Western blot for anti–Scl-70 in SLE patients. Western blots were performed on 19 SLE sera: 14 from patients with anti–Scl-70 levels of >100 units/ml and 5 from patients with normal levels. The SSc control serum, as well as 12 of the 14 positive SLE specimens, reacted with a unique band at the expected position of 70 kd (Figure 4). None of the SLE sera that were negative by ELISA reacted with the antigen on the blot. There was very good agreement between the results of the commercial ELISA and those of the Western blot (κ = 0.87).

Cognate nature of IgG binding to Scl-70 in ELISA. The possibility was also considered that DNA from SLE patient serum mediated the binding of anti-DNA to Scl-70 and gave the appearance of anti–Scl-70 antibody. First, we determined that pretreatment with DNA of Scl-70–coated wells resulted in the binding of anti-DNA to the wells and that DNase treatment abolished this binding (Table 1). Similarly, the binding to Scl-70 of in vitro–generated DNA–anti-DNA immune complexes (25) (Table 1) was abolished by DNase digestion. However, DNase digestion had no effect on the binding to Scl-70 of IgG from SLE and SSc sera (Table 1). Thus, free DNA or DNA as part of immune complexes did not cause an artifact of binding of anti-DNA antibodies to Scl-70.

In addition to DNA, we considered the possibility that an unknown serum factor might have bound to Scl-70 on the solid phase and attracted an IgG antibody directed against the factor. Therefore, the IgG from 2 SLE sera that were negative for anti–Scl-70 by double diffusion but positive for anti–Scl-70 by ELISA was purified to homogeneity. The concentration was then adjusted to a level similar to that in the serum and tested in triplicate in parallel with the original sera. Essentially all of the anti–Scl-70 antibody activity was accounted for

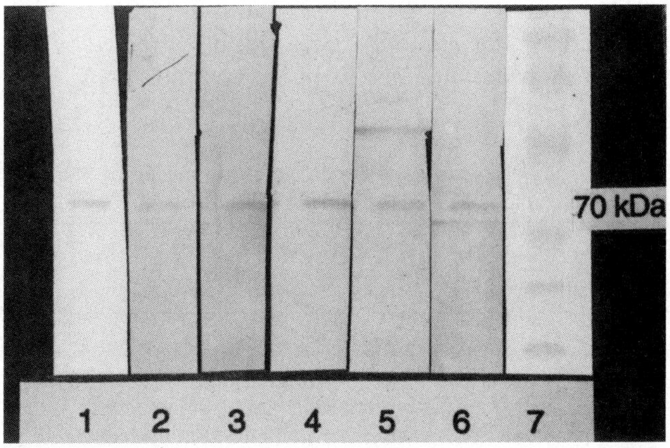

Figure 4. Western blot of the bovine Scl-70 antigen. Shown are SSc control serum (lane 1) and SLE sera with a record of high level of anti–Scl-70 antibodies (lanes 2–6) as primary antibodies. Lane 7 contains the MW standard (200, 113, 82, 49, 35, 29.5, 21, and 7.5 kd). See Figure 1 for definitions.

Table 1. Effect of DNase treatment on the binding to Scl-70 of anti–Scl-70 antibody, DNA and anti-DNA antibodies, and DNA–anti-DNA immune complexes*

Sample	No DNase	DNase treatment
DNA only	0.049	0.041
Blood bank donor serum	0.107	0.094
DNA + anti-DNA antibodies	0.503	0.122
DNA–anti-DNA complex	0.845	0.100
Anti–Scl-70 SLE serum 1	1.657	1.642
Anti–Scl-70 SLE serum 2	0.246	0.245
Anti–Scl-70 SLE serum 3	1.647	1.666
Anti–Scl-70 SSc serum 1	>3.0	>3.0
Anti–Scl-70 SSc serum 2	>3.0	>3.0

* Values are net absorbances at 450 nm. SLE = systemic lupus erythematosus; SSc = systemic sclerosis.

in the IgG fraction (123 units in IgG versus 128 units in serum; 210 units in IgG versus 155 units in serum).

The possibility was also considered that the binding of IgG from SLE patients to Scl-70 could be the result of a nonspecific reaction of the Fcγ to Scl-70 on the solid phase, as we have shown previously for the binding to histone of aggregated IgG and of circulating immune complexes (24,25). Therefore, we determined whether the binding to Scl-70 was associated with the $F(ab')_2$ fragment of the IgG. Pepsin digestion was performed on serum specimens from 6 SLE patients (4 Scl-70 antibody–positive and 2 Scl-70 antibody–negative specimens) and on 2 specimens from SSc patients. In all sera that contained anti–Scl-70 antibody, the activity was present in the $F(ab')_2$ fragments (data not shown).

The antigen specificity of binding was evaluated by free antigen competition (24,25). The binding to Scl-70 of antibodies from 1 SSc and 3 SLE sera was inhibited by >80% by Scl-70, but was not affected by any of the following antigens: RNP/Sm complex, SSA, SSB, histone, and Jo-1. However, these antigens all effectively inhibited the binding of their cognate antibodies (data not shown). Thus, all of the above experiments showed that the binding in ELISA of IgG from SLE sera to Scl-70 was due to anti–Scl-70 antibody function.

Immunoabsorption findings. Effluents of Scl-70 solutions from anti–Scl-70, anti-nRNP, or antihistone immunoaffinity columns were used to coat plastic wells for ELISA. Sera from 2 SSc patients (containing anti–Scl-70), from 3 SLE patients with a record of anti–Scl-70 antibodies, and from 2 SLE patients without anti–Scl-70 were tested on these wells. The antibodies of all SLE or SSc patients did not react with the material in the solution that was passed through the anti–Scl-70 column (Table 2). However, they reacted well with the Scl-70 passed through antihistone and anti-nRNP columns. Thus, absorption of Scl-70 by anti–Scl-70 removed the reactivity from the antigen solution for both SSc and SLE sera.

Correlation of anti–Scl-70 antibody levels with the SLAM score and with levels of other autoantibodies. During the course of the disease, the levels of anti–Scl-70 fluctuated widely in SLE patients. To obviate the potential effect of variations in serum IgG levels, we selected a cohort of 24 patients who had serum levels of anti–Scl-70 antibodies >2-fold the upper limit of normal; 205 open scale measurements were available. A highly significant correlation was found between the level of anti–Scl-70 and the levels of anti-dsDNA ($r = 0.558$, $P < 0.001$) and anti-ssDNA ($r = 0.564$, $P < 0.001$); lower, but still significant, correlations were obtained with histone-binding IgG ($r = 0.472$, $P < 0.001$), anti-Sm ($r = 0.356$, $P < 0.01$), anti-nRNP/Sm ($r = 0.330$, $P < 0.01$), and anti-SSB ($r = 0.280$, $P < 0.05$) antibodies. Levels of anti–Scl-70 antibodies were not

Table 2. Net absorbance at 450 nm ($A_{450\ nm}$) yielded by SSc and SLE sera on wells coated with the Scl-70 antigen passed through immunoabsorption columns*

Disease/patient no.	Antibody specificity	$A_{450\ nm}$ No column	Anti–Scl-70	Antihistones	Anti-nRNP
SSc/1	Scl-70 (5,000 units/ml)	>3.0	0.04	>3.0	>3.0
SSc/2	Scl-70 (129 units/ml)	1.19	0.01	0.75	0.93
SLE/1	Scl-70 (3,000 units/ml), ssDNA, dsDNA, Sm, RNP, SSB, histones	>3.0	0.18	>3.0	>3.0
SLE/2	Scl-70 (1,400 units/ml), histones	>3.0	0.16	>3.0	2.356
SLE/3	Scl-70 (205 units/ml), ssDNA, dsDNA, RNP, SSA, SSB	1.76	0.18	1.02	1.30
SLE/4	ssDNA, Sm, RNP, SSA, histones	0.10	0.04	0.09	0.07
SLE/5	SSA	0.06	0.03	0.04	0.20

* ssDNA = single-stranded DNA; dsDNA = double-stranded DNA (see Table 1 for other definitions).

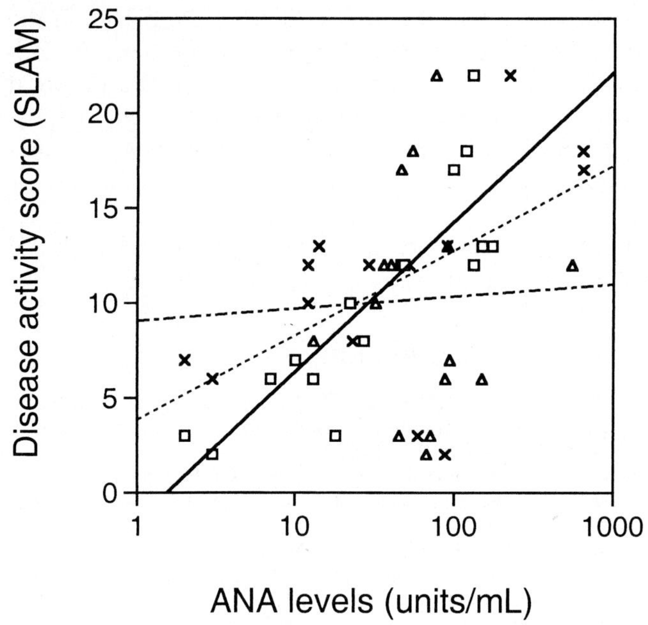

Figure 5. Longitudinal correlations between the Systemic Lupus Activity Measure (SLAM) scores in 1 systemic lupus erythematosus patient with levels of antinuclear antibodies (ANA) against Scl-70 (□), double-stranded DNA (dsDNA) (×), and Sm (△). Correlations were computed according to the logarithmic method for Scl-70 (——) (r = 0.851, $P < 0.001$), dsDNA (– – –) (r = 0.616, $P < 0.001$), and Sm (- - -) (r = 0.041, P not significant).

significantly correlated with levels of anti-SSA antibodies (r = 0.069).

In the 24 patients whose anti–Scl-70 antibody levels exceeded 64 units/ml on at least 1 occasion, the SLAM scores ranged from 2 to 45. The correlation between SLAM score and the levels of anti–Scl-70 antibody was highly significant (r = 0.563, $P < 0.001$). The SLAM score also correlated significantly with levels of anti-dsDNA (r = 0.459, $P < 0.001$), ssDNA (r = 0.327, $P < 0.01$), and histone-binding IgG (r = 0.313, $P < 0.01$), but not with levels of the other antibodies.

Longitudinal correlations between the levels of anti–Scl-70 and the SLAM score were also performed for 7 individual SLE patients whose ANA levels were measured on at least 7 occasions (results for 1 patient are presented in Figure 5). The correlation between anti–Scl-70 levels and the SLAM score was highly significant in 6 of these patients (r = 0.755–0.951, $P < 0.001$ for each); it was lower, but still significant (r = 0.378, $P < 0.05$), for the remaining patient. Moreover, in each of these anti–Scl-70–positive SLE patients, the correlation between disease activity and anti–Scl-70 levels was better than the correlation between disease activity and anti-dsDNA levels (r = 0.340–0.843, $P < 0.05$ to $P < 0.001$).

Clinical features of SLE patients with anti–Scl-70 antibodies. The organ involvement in patients with >2-fold the normal levels of anti–Scl-70 antibody was compared with that in a group of SLE patients matched for age, sex, and race, but with repeatedly normal levels of this antibody. Two significant differences were identified, which could not be attributed to other causes: 1) the presence of pulmonary hypertension in 26% (5 of 19) of the anti–Scl-70–positive patients and in none of the 37 anti–Scl-70–negative patients ($P < 0.01$, by chi-square test), and 2) the higher frequency of renal involvement in anti–Scl-70–positive patients (13 of 19, or 68%) than in anti–Scl-70–negative patients (10 of 37, or 27%) ($P < 0.001$, by chi-square test).

DISCUSSION

We have shown here that a subset of SLE patients (25%) had abnormal levels of anti–Scl-70 antibodies as detected by ELISA. The presence of anti–Scl-70 in the serum of SLE patients was confirmed by ELISA with a characterized Scl-70 antigen, by Western blot, by double diffusion in agar gel, and by immunoabsorption on a specific anti–Scl-70 antibody column. We also showed that this binding was cognate in nature. The levels of anti–Scl-70 antibodies detected by ELISA in this subset of patients correlated significantly with their levels of anti-dsDNA and, when compared with other autoantibodies, offered the best correlation with their disease activity as determined by the SLAM.

The proportion of 26% (5 of 19 patients) in a previous small study of anti–Scl-70 in SLE patients was similar to that obtained in the present study. Our data also confirmed isolated reports of the presence of anti–Scl-70 in SLE patients in studies that used either double immunodiffusion (15,17) or immunoprecipitation (18). The large discrepancy between the proportion of anti–Scl-70–positive SLE patients identified by ELISA and that identified by double diffusion may be the result of the relatively high sensitivity of ELISA (28) compared with that of the topo I inhibition assay (29,30), combined with higher levels of anti–Scl-70 in SSc versus SLE patients (Figure 1). However, other factors may be involved that need further investigation. For example, below the level of 500 units/ml, 4 of 9 SSc specimens were positive by double diffusion (Figure 1), but only 1 of 12 SLE specimens was positive by this method. Differences in epitope recognition and/or antibody avidity and affinity in the solid-phase and liquid-phase assays may explain this discrepancy.

It has been suggested that the relatively high frequency of anti–Scl-70 antibodies detected by ELISA in SLE sera might be due to contaminating antigens (10). All data obtained here, however, showed that the antibodies in SLE sera detected by ELISA were indeed directed against Scl-70, as follows: 1) in ELISA tests and Western blots, the Scl-70 antigen reacted strongly with the anti–Scl-70–specific serum from the CDC and with our internal controls, including anti-nRNP (31–33), but did not react with sera with other ANA specificities (Figure 3); 2) the Test-Scl-70 ELISA, shown to be free of contaminants (Figure 2), confirmed the results of the tests performed with the commercial ELISA; 3) in SLE sera, the presence of anti–Scl-70 was reconfirmed by Western blot (Figure 4) and/or by double diffusion in agar gel; 4) immunoabsorption of the Scl-70 antigen with an anti–Scl-70 antibody from SSc sera also removed the reactivity with SLE sera; and 5) there was good agreement (κ = 0.92) between the results obtained with ELISA tests with native bovine and human recombinant Scl-70 antigens.

The binding of IgG from SLE sera to Scl-70 was cognate in nature and not an artifact of the presence of circulating immune complexes or DNA for the following reasons: 1) it was present in the $F(ab')_2$, unlike the binding of IgG to histone, which usually depends on $Fc\gamma$ (24,25); 2) it was specifically inhibited by free Scl-70; 3) it was not due to the presence of DNA in the reaction (Table 1); 4) most patients with anti-DNA antibodies did not have anti–Scl-70; 5) purified IgG from SLE sera had the same reaction with the Scl-70 antigen and the serum from which it was obtained; and 6) 25% (32 of 128) of the SLE patients in this study (and 31% of the untreated patients) had abnormal levels of anti–Scl-70 antibodies (Figure 1), but only ~2% of SLE patients are known to develop disease overlapping with SSc (15,34).

In our cohort of anti–Scl-70 antibody–positive SLE patients, there was a highly significant correlation between levels of anti–Scl-70 antibodies and disease activity ($r = 0.563$, $P < 0.001$). This correlation was even higher in patients whose sera was measured multiple times (Figure 5), and was seen in spite of the relatively imprecise nature of retrospective clinical data collection for the calculation of the SLAM score. Nevertheless, the validity of our measurement of the disease activity by the SLAM is further supported by the significant correlation between the levels of anti–Scl-70 and anti-dsDNA (a well-established correlate of disease activity in SLE [33,35–37]) ($r = 0.558$, $P < 0.001$).

The presence of anti–Scl-70 in SLE patients, as determined by Western blot and ELISA, suggests that the measurement of anti–Scl-70 has to be placed in the context of clinical manifestations and of other autoantibodies detected simultaneously (35), with two different interpretations. In the context of symptoms characteristic of SSc, this measurement helps in diagnosis and prognosis (5,7); in the context of SLE manifestations and SLE autoantibodies, it provides a very good correlate of disease activity and suggests an increased risk of pulmonary hypertension and renal involvement.

REFERENCES

1. Liu LF, Miller KG. Eukaryotic DNA topoisomerases: two forms of type I DNA topoisomerases from HeLa cell nuclei. Proc Natl Acad Sci U S A 1981;78:3487–91.
2. Stewart L, Redinbo MR, Qiu X, Hol WGH, Champoux JJ. A model for the mechanism of human topoisomerase I. Science 1998;279:1534–41.
3. Douvas AS, Achten M, Tan EM. Identification of a nuclear protein (Scl-70) as a unique target of human antinuclear antibodies in SSc. J Biol Chem 1979;254:1051–4.
4. Shero JH, Bordwell B, Rothfield NF, Earnshaw WC. High titers of autoantibodies to topoisomerase I (Scl-70) in sera from SSc patients. Science 1986;231:737–40.
5. Shoenfeld Y, Grunebaum E, Laufer M, Zurgil N, Bakimer R, Lunderschmidt A, et al. Anti-topoisomerase-I and clinical findings in systemic sclerosis (scleroderma). Isr J Med Sci 1996;32:537–42.
6. Russo K, Hoch S, Dima C, Varga J, Teodorescu M. Circulating anticentromere Cenp-A and Cenp-B antibodies in patients with diffuse and limited systemic sclerosis, systemic lupus erythematosus and rheumatoid arthritis. J Rheumatol 2000;27:142–8.
7. Steen VD, Powell DL, Medsger TA Jr. Clinical correlations and prognosis based on serum autoantibodies in patients with systemic sclerosis. Arthritis Rheum 1988;31:196–203.
8. Weiner ES, Hildebrandt S, Senécal J-L, Daniels L, Noell S, Joyal F, et al. Prognostic significance of anticentromere antibodies and anti–topoisomerase I antibodies in Raynaud's disease: a prospective study. Arthritis Rheum 1991;34:68–77.
9. Weiner ES, Earnshaw WC, Senécal J-L, Bordwell B, Johnson P, Rothfield NF. Clinical associations of anticentromere antibodies and antibodies to topoisomerase I: a study of 355 patients. Arthritis Rheum 1988;31:378–85.
10. Rothfield NF. Autoantibodies in scleroderma. Rheum Dis Clin North Am 1992;18:483–98.
11. Jarzabek-Chorzelska M, Blaszczyk M, Jablonska S, Chorzelski T, Kumar V, Beutner EH. Scl-70 antibody—a specific marker of systemic sclerosis. Brit J Dermatol 1986;115:393–401.
12. Vazquez-Abad D, Tian L, Zanetti M, Rothfield NF. A cross-reactive idiotype in scleroderma. Clin Exp Immunol 1997;108: 420–7.
13. Geisler C, Hoier-Madsen M. An enzyme-linked immunosorbent assay for autoantibodies against the nuclear protein Scl-70. J Immunol Methods 1985;80:211–9.
14. Bronshtein IB, Shuster AM, Golobolov GV, Gromova II, Kvashuk OA, Belostotskaya KM, et al. DNA-specific antiidiotypic antibodies in the sera of patients with autoimmune diseases. FEBS Lett 1992;314:259–63.
15. Watanabe T, Tsuchida T, Kanda N, Tamaki K. Avascular necrosis of bone in systemic lupus erythematosus: the predictive role of precipitating autoantibodies. Scand J Rheumatol 1997;26:184–7.
16. Kameda H, Kuwana M, Hama N, Kaburaki J, Homma M. Coexistence of serum anti-DNA topoisomerase I and anti-Sm antibodies: reports of 3 cases. J Rheumatol 1997;24:400–3.

17. Mukai M, Sagawa A, Atsumi T, Jodo S, Amasaki Y, Nakabayashi T, et al. 3 cases of anti-Scl-70 (topoisomerase I) antibody associated with central nervous system lupus without renal disorder. J Rheumatol 1993;20:1594–7.
18. Stojanov L, Satoh M, Dooley MA, Kuwana M, Jennette JC, Reeves WH. Autoantibodies to topoisomerase I in a patient with systemic lupus erythematosus without features of scleroderma. Lupus 1995;4:314–7.
19. Tan EM, Cohen AS, Fries JF, Masi AT, McShane DJ, Rothfield NF, et al. The 1982 revised criteria for the classification of systemic lupus erythematosus. Arthritis Rheum 1982;25:1271–7.
20. Liang MH, Socher SA, Larson MG, Schur PH. Reliability and validity of six systems for the clinical assessment of disease activity in systemic lupus erythematosus. Arthritis Rheum 1989;32: 1107–18.
21. Cozillius M, Liang MH. Monitoring patients with SLE. In: Lahita RG, editor. Systemic lupus erythematosus. San Diego: Academic Press; 1999. p. 467–76.
22. Smolen JS, Butcher B, Fritzler MJ, Gordon T, Hardin J, Kalden JR, et al. Reference sera for antinuclear antibodies. II. Further definition of antibody specificities in international antinuclear antibody reference sera by immunofluorescence and Western blotting. Arthritis Rheum 1997;40:413–8.
23. Swedler W, Wallman J, Froelich CJ, Teodorescu M. Routine measurement of IgM, IgG, and IgA rheumatoid factors: high sensitivity, specificity and predictive value for rheumatoid arthritis. J Rheumatol 1997;24:1037–44.
24. Elicha Gussin HA, Russo KL, Teodorescu M. The effect of circulating immune complexes on the binding of rheumatoid factor to histones. Ann Rheum Dis 2000;59:351–8.
25. Elicha Gussin HA, Tselentis HN, Teodorescu M. Non cognate binding to histones of IgG from patients with systemic lupus erythematosus. Clin Immunol 2000;96:150–61.
26. Tabor S, Struhl K. Enzymatic manipulations of DNA and RNA: endonucleases. Curr Prot Mol Biol 1994;3:12.5–6.
27. Campbell RC. Statistics for biologists. 2nd ed. Cambridge (UK): Cambridge University Press; 1979.
28. Teodorescu M, Froelich CJ. ELISA and other immunologic techniques in rheumatology. In: Teodorescu M, Froelich CJ, editors. Advanced immunoassays in rheumatology. Boca Raton (FL): CRC Press; 1994. p. 3–26.
29. Vazquez-Abad D, Rothfield NF. Autoantibodies in systemic sclerosis. Int Rev Immunol 1995;12:145–57.
30. Hildebrandt S, Weiner ES, Senecal J-L, Noell GS, Earnshaw WC, Rothfield NF. Autoantibodies to topoisomerase I (Scl-70): analysis by gel diffusion, immunoblot, and enzyme-linked immunosorbent assay. Clin Immunol Immunopathol 1990;57:399–410.
31. White PJ, Gardner WD, Hoch SO. Identification of the immunologically active components of the Sm and RNP antigens. Proc Natl Acad Sci U S A 1981;78:626–30.
32. Conner GE, Nelson D, Wisniewolski R, Lahita RG, Blobel G, Kunkel HG. Protein antigens of the RNA-protein complexes detected by anti-Sm and anti-RNP antibodies found in serum of patients with systemic lupus erythematosus and related disorders. J Exp Med 1982;156:1475–85.
33. Froelich CJ, Wallman J, Skosey JL, Teodorescu M. Clinical value of an integrated ELISA system for the detection of 6 autoantibodies (ssDNA, dsDNA, Sm, RNP/Sm, SSA, and SSB). J Rheumatol 1990;17:192–200.
34. Sharp GC, Hoffman RW. Overlap syndromes: mixed connective tissue disease and Sjogren's syndrome. In: Lahita RG, editor. Systemic lupus erythematosus. New York: Academic Press; 1999. p. 551–73.
35. Teodorescu M, Froelich CJ. Laboratory evaluation of systemic lupus erythematosus. In: Lahita RG, editor. Systemic lupus erythematosus. San Diego: Academic Press; 1999. p. 477–505.
36. Swaak AJG, Aarden LA, Statius van Eps LW, Feltkamp TEW. Anti-dsDNA and complement profiles as prognostic guides in systemic lupus erythematosus. Arthritis Rheum 1979;22:226–35.
37. Ter Borg EJ, Horst G, Hummel EJ, Limburg PC, Kallenberg CGM. Measurement of increases in anti–double-stranded DNA antibody levels as a predictor of disease exacerbation in systemic lupus erythematosus: a long-term, prospective study. Arthritis Rheum 1990;33:634–43.

ARTHRITIS & RHEUMATISM
Vol. 44, No. 2, February 2001, pp 384–388

Detection of Autoantibodies to Killer Immunoglobulin-Like Receptors Using Recombinant Fusion Proteins for Two Killer Immunoglobulin-Like Receptors in Patients With Systemic Autoimmune Diseases

Toshihiro Matsui,[1] Masataka Otsuka,[1] Katsumi Maenaka,[2] Hiroshi Furukawa,[3] Toshio Yabe,[4] Kazuhiko Yamamoto,[5] Kusuki Nishioka,[1] and Tomohiro Kato[1]

Objective. **To investigate the existence of autoantibodies to killer immunoglobulin-like receptors (KIRs), especially p58.1 (KIR2DL1) and p58.2 (KIR2DL3), in patients with systemic autoimmune diseases.**

Methods. **Sera from 30 patients with systemic lupus erythematosus (SLE), 30 patients with rheumatoid arthritis (RA), 22 patients with Behçet's disease, and 20 healthy control subjects were tested for anti-p58.1 and anti-p58.2 antibodies by Western blot analysis using recombinant p58.1 and p58.2 proteins. Furthermore, clinical features and laboratory data were compared between the anti-p58.1/58.2 antibody–positive and –negative patients.**

Results. **Anti-p58.1 antibodies were detected in 7 (23.3%) of the 30 patients with SLE, 9 (30%) of the 30 patients with RA, and 6 (27.3%) of the 22 patients with Behçet's disease. Anti-p58.2 antibodies were detected in the same 22 patients who were positive for the anti-p58.1 antibodies. None of the serum samples from the healthy donors were positive for antibodies to the recombinant p58.1 or p58.2 molecules. Compared with the anti-p58.1/58.2 antibody–negative patients, the anti-p58.1/58.2 antibody–positive patients had significantly elevated levels of serum IgG in all 3 diseases tested, an accelerated erythrocyte sedimentation rate in RA and SLE, and decreased white blood cell counts in RA.**

Conclusion. **This report is the first to describe the presence of autoantibodies to KIR2DL (p58.1 and p58.2) in the sera of patients with systemic autoimmune diseases. Considering the correlation with several clinical features, these autoantibodies may be involved in the pathologic process of the autoimmune diseases.**

The existence of antilymphocyte antibodies (ALA) in patients with systemic autoimmune diseases has been reported (1). The binding of ALA to lymphocytes could affect lymphocyte function by blocking or enhancing the original signaling of their target molecules. However, ALA are poorly understood. In fact, only a few targets of ALA, including CD45, β_2-microglobulin, and HLA class I molecules, have been described thus far (1), even though identification of their targets would be the first step to understanding the function of ALA.

In this context, we recently investigated the antigenicity of T cell costimulatory molecules (B7-1, B7-2, CD28, and CTLA-4), and reported that CTLA-4 (CD152) is one of the targets of ALA in patients with systemic autoimmune diseases (2). Several studies have indicated that the lack of a negative signal through CTLA-4 during T cell activation contributes to the onset or exacerbation of autoimmune diseases. Thus, autoantibodies to CTLA-4 may enhance the autoimmune response. In the present study, we focused on whether

Supported in part by a grant-in-aid from the Ministry of Health and Welfare and the Ministry of Education, Science and Culture, Japan, and by the Japan Rheumatism Foundation.

[1]Toshihiro Matsui, MD, PhD, Masataka Otsuka, BS, Kusuki Nishioka, MD, PhD, Tomohiro Kato, MD, PhD: St. Marianna University School of Medicine, Kawasaki, Japan; [2]Katsumi Maenaka, PhD: The Japanese Red Cross Central Blood Center, Tokyo, Japan, and National Institute of Genetics, Shizuoka, Japan; [3]Hiroshi Furukawa, MD, PhD: The Japanese Red Cross Central Blood Center, Tokyo, Japan, and University of Tokyo Graduate School of Medicine, Tokyo, Japan; [4]Toshio Yabe, PhD: The Japanese Red Cross Central Blood Center, Tokyo, Japan; [5]Kazuhiko Yamamoto, MD, PhD: University of Tokyo Graduate School of Medicine, Tokyo, Japan.

Address correspondence and reprint requests to Toshihiro Matsui, MD, PhD, Rheumatology, Immunology and Genetics Program, Institute of Medical Science, St. Marianna University School of Medicine, 2-16-1, Sugao, Miyamae-ku, Kawasaki, Kanagawa 216-8512, Japan.

Submitted for publication May 2, 2000; accepted in revised form September 27, 2000.

autoantibodies to killer immunoglobulin-like receptors (KIRs) exist in the sera of patients with systemic autoimmune disease.

Natural killer (NK) receptors that recognize HLA class I molecules are classified into 2 groups, immunoglobulin-like receptors and lectin-type receptors. The immunoglobulin-like receptors (KIRs) are further classified into 2 subgroups, the inhibitory form of KIR (KIR2DL) and the activating form of KIR (KIR2DS, or KAR). Both KIR2DL and KIR2DS are expressed on most NK cells and also on a subset of T cells. KIR2DS transduces an activating signal; the cytoplasmic domain of KIR2DS forms a complex with DAP12 and contains an immunoreceptor tyrosine-based activation motif. In contrast, the cytoplasmic domain of KIR2DL contains an immunoreceptor tyrosine-based inhibition motif, and KIR2DL transduces an inhibitory signal. In fact, it is known that the signaling through KIR2DL on NK cells protects HLA class I–expressing cells from the cytotoxic activity of NK cells. Also, the signal through KIR2DL on T cells inhibits T cell receptor–mediated functions (3), and thus may provide a mechanism of peripheral tolerance against self antigens (4,5).

On the basis of these findings, it may be hypothesized that autoantibodies to KIR2DL, if they exist, may affect the progression or maintenance of autoimmunity. Therefore, in this study, we investigated the presence of autoantibodies to KIR2DL in patients with systemic autoimmune diseases. We prepared 2 kinds of recombinant KIR2DL, p58.1 (KIR2DL1) and p58.2 (KIR2DL3), by expressing them in *Escherichia coli*, and tested the reactivity of the serum samples from patients with autoimmune diseases to the recombinant KIR2DL by Western blot analysis. Autoantibodies to KIR2DL were detected in 23.3% of the patients with systemic lupus erythematosus (SLE), 30% of the patients with rheumatoid arthritis (RA), and 27.3% of the patients with Behçet's disease. In addition, compared with the anti-p58.1/58.2 antibody–negative patients, the anti-p58.1/58.2 antibody–positive patients showed significantly elevated levels of serum IgG in all 3 of these diseases, an accelerated erythrocyte sedimentation rate (ESR) in RA and SLE, and decreased white blood cell (WBC) counts in RA.

PATIENTS AND METHODS

Patients and controls. Serum samples were obtained from 30 patients with SLE, 30 patients with RA, and 22 patients with Behçet's disease who were being treated at the hospital of the University of Tokyo or the St. Marianna University School of Medicine. The diseases were diagnosed according to the standard criteria of each respective disease (6–8). Control serum samples were obtained from 20 healthy donors.

Expression and purification of recombinant p58.1 and p58.2 proteins. The complementary DNA (cDNA) fragments that encode the extracellular domain of p58.1 (9) and p58.2 (10) were amplified by polymerase chain reaction (PCR) with a set of primers, 5′-TTTGAATTCCATGAGGGAGTCCACAGAAAAC and 5′-TTTGTCGACCTAGTGCAGGTGTCGGGGGTTAC (underline indicates the restriction enzyme site), by using pKMATHNK1 plasmid and pKMATHNK2 plasmid (11), respectively, as the templates. The PCR products were confirmed, by sequencing, to be those for p58.1 and p58.2.

The cDNA fragments were subcloned into pMAL-c2, together with a nucleotide sequence encoding 6 histidines, $(His)_6$, as a tag. By these constructs, the recombinant p58.1 and p58.2 proteins were produced in *E coli* as fusion proteins with maltose binding protein (MaBP) (MaBP-p58.1 and MaBP-58.2, respectively). The *E coli* (DH5α; ToYoBo, Tokyo, Japan) was transformed with each of these recombinant pMAL plasmids, and then grown in 2XYT medium containing 100 μg/ml ampicillin at 37°C. To induce expression of the fusion proteins, isopropyl 1-β-D-thiogalactoside was added to the medium to a final concentration of 0.3 m*M*, and the *E coli* were incubated at 37°C for 3 hours. The cells were then harvested, lysed in 8*M* urea/phosphate buffered saline (PBS), and sonicated. After centrifugation, the lysate was applied to a column charged with ProBond resin ($NiCl_2$; Invitrogen, San Diego, CA) in a binding buffer (8*M* urea, 20 m*M* sodium phosphate, and 500 m*M* NaCl, pH 7.8). The column was then developed in buffers (8*M* urea, 20 m*M* sodium phosphate, and 500 m*M* NaCl, pH 6.0 and pH 5.3). The $(His)_6$-tagged recombinant proteins were eluted with an elution buffer (8*M* urea, 20 m*M* sodium phosphate, and 500 m*M* NaCl, pH 4.0). The concentration of fusion protein was determined from the absorbance values at 280 nm and 260 nm, which were corrected for background activity at 320 nm using appropriately diluted samples.

The expression of the full length of these recombinant proteins was confirmed by Western blotting (as described below) using antibodies to the N-terminus of MaBP (Santa Cruz Biotechnology, Santa Cruz, CA), and antibodies to horseradish peroxidase–conjugated Ni-NTA (Qiagen, Valencia, CA), which binds to the $(His)_6$ tag located at the C-terminus of the fusion proteins.

Detection of autoantibodies. Serum samples were tested for the presence of autoantibodies to MaBP-p58.1 and MaBP-p58.2 by Western blot analysis, as previously described (2). Briefly, MaBP-p58.1, MaBP-p58.2, and MaBP as a control were separated by 10% sodium dodecyl sulfate–polyacrylamide gel electrophoresis (SDS-PAGE) and transferred onto nitrocellulose membranes. After blocking for 1 hour with PBS containing 3% bovine serum albumin (BSA) and 0.1% Tween 20, and then washing in PBS with 0.1% Tween 20 for 30 minutes, the membranes were incubated with the serum samples for 1 hour. Before being incubated with the membranes, the serum samples had been diluted at 1:200 and preincubated at room temperature for 2 hours with 20 μg/ml of the bacterial lysate, which contained nonrecombinant pMAL-$(His)_6$ product in PBS with 3% BSA and 0.1% Tween 20. After washing the membranes in PBS with 0.1% Tween 20 for 30 minutes, the bound antibodies were reacted with horseradish peroxidase–conjugated goat anti-human IgG (specific for the γ

chain; Zymed, South San Francisco, CA) and visualized with diaminobenzidine.

Serial dilution test. The reactivity of sera to p58.1 and p58.2 was confirmed by a serial dilution test in an enzyme-linked immunosorbent assay (ELISA). Each well of a 96-well microtiter plate (Dynex Technologies, Chantilly, VA) was coated with 10 μg/ml of the individual purified protein or MaBP in a carbonate buffer (50 m*M* sodium carbonate, pH 9.6), followed by blocking with PBS containing 3% BSA and 0.1% Tween 20. To adsorb the reactivity of the serum samples to bacterial proteins and MaBP, the serum samples were diluted and incubated for 2 hours at room temperature with 20 μg/ml of bacterial lysates, which contained nonrecombinant pMAL products in PBS with 3% BSA and 0.1% Tween 20, before being incubated with the coated recombinants. After reacting with the coated recombinants for 8 hours at 4°C, the wells were washed 5 times in PBS with 0.1% Tween 20. Next, the bound antibodies were incubated with horseradish peroxidase–conjugated goat anti-human IgG (Zymed) at a 1:4,000 dilution for 8 hours at 4°C, then reacted with *o*-phenylenediamine as a substrate, and quantitated using a microplate photometer at 492 nm and 630 nm.

Statistical analysis. Laboratory data are expressed as the mean ± SEM. The Mann-Whitney U test was used to examine differences in the clinical parameters of patients with versus those without anti-p58.1/p58.2 antibodies.

RESULTS

Production of recombinant p58.1 and p58.2 proteins. The recombinant p58.1 and p58.2 proteins were produced in *E coli* as fusion proteins with MaBP (MaBP-p58.1 and MaBP-58.2). SDS-PAGE separation and subsequent staining of the 2 purified recombinant proteins

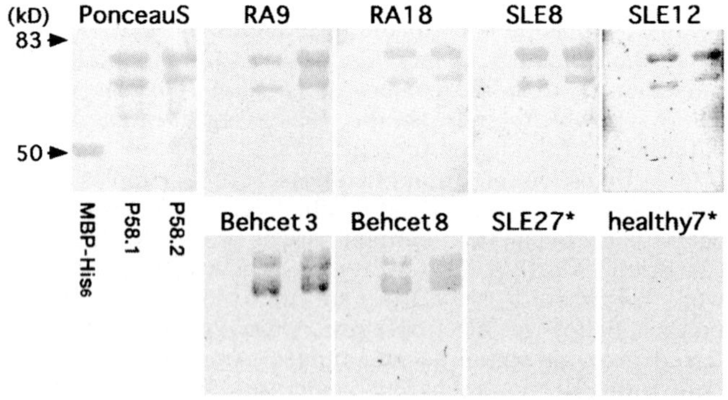

Figure 1. Immunoreactivity of serum samples to recombinant p58.1 (KIR2DL1) and p58.2 (KIR2DL3). Recombinant p58.1 and p58.2 coupled with maltose binding protein (MBP) and control MBP, which contained a LacZα gene product, were separated by sodium dodecyl sulfate–10% polyacrylamide gel electrophoresis and then transferred onto nitrocellulose membranes. Serum samples (diluted at 1:200) were tested by Western blot analysis. The control membrane was stained with Ponceau S. Results from 6 representative positive samples and 2 negative samples (indicated with an asterisk) are shown. RA = rheumatoid arthritis; SLE = systemic lupus erythematosus.

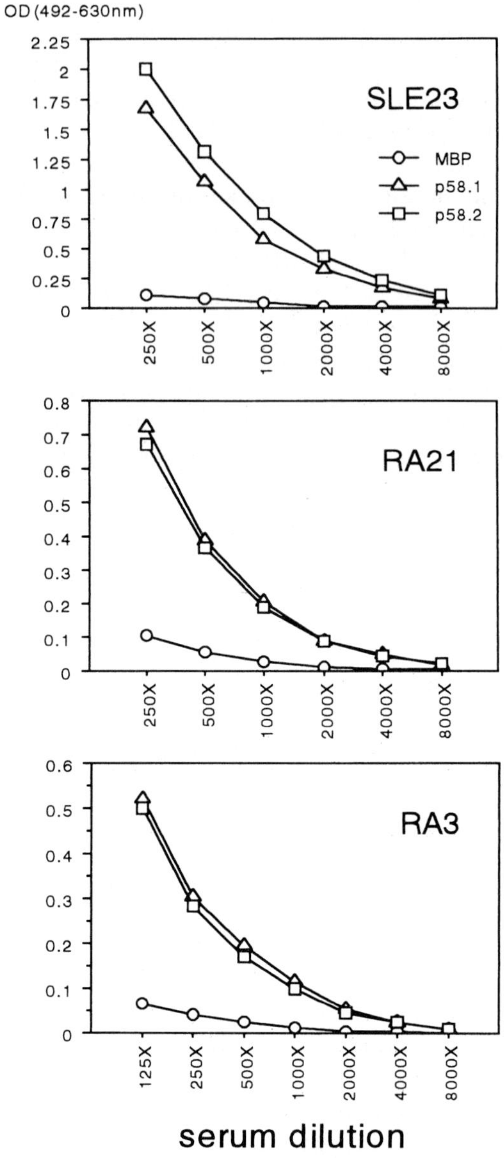

Figure 2. Specific reactivity of serum samples to the p58.1 and p58.2 recombinant proteins. Reactivities to p58.1, p58.2, and MBP as a control were tested by enzyme-linked immunosorbent assay using sequentially diluted sera obtained from the anti-p58.1/p58.2 antibody–positive patients. Three representative cases are shown. OD = optical density (see Figure 1 for other definitions).

with Coomassie brilliant blue showed 2 distinct bands. These 2 bands were reacted with antibodies both to the N-terminus of MaBP and to Ni-NTA, which bound to the $(His)_6$ tag located at the C-terminus of the fusion proteins (results not shown). Since the lower bands had the expected molecular weights, the upper bands were thought to be MaBP-p58.1 and MaBP-p58.2, with an additional modification by *E coli* (Figure 1).

Table 1. Laboratory parameters in the anti-p58.1/p58.2 antibody–positive and –negative patients*

Parameter	RA patients			SLE patients			Behçet's disease patients		
	Antibody negative (n = 21)	Antibody positive (n = 9)	P†	Antibody negative (n = 23)	Antibody positive (n = 7)	P†	Antibody negative (n = 16)	Antibody positive (n = 6)	P†
WBC, mm^3	7,690 ± 394	6,322 ± 692	0.023	7,326 ± 541	7,114 ± 1,444	0.902	7,771 ± 750	5,433 ± 594	0.083
Lymphocytes, mm^3	1,678 ± 128	1,646 ± 265	0.946	1,214 ± 208	1,090 ± 260	0.787	1,940 ± 210	2,043 ± 222	0.461
Hgb, mg/dl	12.8 ± 0.4	12.0 ± 0.4	0.197	13.2 ± 0.3	12.7 ± 0.3	0.326	13.7 ± 0.2	13.5 ± 0.7	0.555
Platelets, $\times 10^4/mm^3$	25.8 ± 1.1	25.8 ± 2.3	0.946	21.1 ± 1.1	20.4 ± 1.9	0.769	24.6 ± 1.1	22.9 ± 2.4	0.338
ESR, mm/hour	30 ± 5	53 ± 10	0.033	23 ± 5	35 ± 5	0.043	15 ± 3	26 ± 9	0.391
IgG, mg/ml	1,193 ± 74	1,740 ± 184	0.014	1,280 ± 108	1,900 ± 185	0.009	1,116 ± 66	1,489 ± 74	0.005
IgA, mg/ml	252 ± 28	284 ± 44	0.689	267 ± 23	282 ± 58	0.825	205 ± 24	276 ± 58	0.364
IgM, mg/ml	128 ± 16	131 ± 18	0.654	93 ± 8	132 ± 44	0.956	128 ± 13	147 ± 22	0.536
RF, units/ml	202 ± 87	169 ± 105	0.910	–	–	–	–	–	–
CH50, units/ml	–	–	–	31.5 ± 1.7	28.3 ± 3.1	0.433	–	–	–
C3, mg/dl	–	–	–	45 ± 2	44 ± 5	0.902	–	–	–
C4, mg/dl	–	–	–	18 ± 2	16 ± 3	0.806	–	–	–
dsDNA, units/ml	–	–	–	18.5 ± 5.4	22.7 ± 9.7	0.602	–	–	–

* Values are the mean ± SEM. RA = rheumatoid arthritis; SLE = systemic lupus erythematosus; WBC = white blood cells; Hgb = hemoglobin; ESR = erythrocyte sedimentation rate; RF = rheumatoid factor; dsDNA = double-stranded DNA.
† By Mann-Whitney U test.

Detection of autoantibodies to the recombinant p58.1 and p58.2 molecules. The purified recombinant proteins were screened by Western blot analysis for anti-p58.1 and anti-p58.2 antibodies. As a result, anti-p58.1 antibodies were detected in the sera of 7 (23.3%) of the 30 patients with SLE, 9 (30%) of the 30 patients with RA, and 6 (27.3%) of the 22 patients with Behçet's disease. Anti-p58.2 antibodies were detected in the same 22 patients who were positive for the anti-p58.1 antibodies (Figure 1). None of the serum samples from the healthy donors was positive for antibodies to the recombinant p58.1 or p58.2 molecules. The serum reactivity to MaBP-p58.1 and MaBP-p58.2 increased in a concentration-dependent manner, but that to MaBP did not, as determined by ELISA (Figure 2). Thus, the specificity of the p58.1 and p58.2 antibody reaction was confirmed (Figure 2).

Comparison of the clinical features and laboratory data between anti-p58.1/58.2 antibody–positive and –negative patients. We compared the clinical features and laboratory data between the anti-p58.1/58.2 antibody–positive and –negative patients with SLE, RA, and Behçet's disease. In each of the 3 diseases, the clinical features did not significantly differ between the anti-p58.1/58.2 antibody–positive and –negative patients. The presence of anti-p58.1/58.2 antibodies did not significantly correlate with either previous pregnancies (antibody-positive patients 64.7% versus antibody-negative patients 74.2%) or a history of blood transfusions (antibody-positive patients 4.5% versus antibody-negative patients 3.5%).

However, with regard to the laboratory data, the anti-p58.1/58.2 antibody–positive patients in each of the 3 disease groups had significantly elevated serum IgG levels (antibody-positive patients versus antibody-negative patients mean ± SEM 1,740 ± 184 mg/ml versus 1,193 ± 74 mg/ml in RA [P = 0.014], 1,900 ± 185 mg/ml versus 1,280 ± 108 mg/ml in SLE [P = 0.009], 1,489 ± 74 mg/ml versus 1,116 ± 66 mg/ml in Behçet's disease [P = 0.005]). Moreover, antibody-positive patients in the RA and SLE groups had an accelerated ESR (RA 53 ± 10 mm/hour versus 30 ± 5 mm/hour [P = 0.033], SLE 35 ± 5 mm/hour versus 23 ± 5 mm/hour [P = 0.043]) and those with decreased WBC counts (6,322 ± $692/mm^3$ versus 7,690 ± $394/mm^3$) compared with antibody-negative patients (P = 0.023) (Table 1).

DISCUSSION

This study is the first to demonstrate the presence of autoantibodies to recombinant KIR2DL, p58.1 and p58.2, in the sera of some patients with systemic autoimmune diseases. Due to the similarity in the amino acid sequence of the extracellular domain of KIR2DL and KIR2DS, the anti-KIR2DL antibodies detected would also bind to KIR2DS and thus would have some effect on their activating signal. However, since the activating signal through KIR2DS is overcome by the inhibitory signal through KIR2DL (12,13), the anti-KIR2DL antibody may mainly affect the activity of KIR2DL, and not KIR2DS. Recently, it has been proposed that KIR2DL plays an inhibitory role in the activation of autoreactive T cells, and thus contributes to the maintenance of peripheral tolerance against self antigens (4,5). Therefore, we speculate that anti-KIR2DL autoantibodies are involved in the breakdown of self tolerance in patients with autoimmune diseases. Our data show that the presence of anti-KIR2DL antibodies is correlated with high levels of serum IgG in RA, SLE, and Behçet's disease, and with an acceleration in the ESR in RA and SLE. This would indicate that these antibodies are associated with increased severity of disease. This may be due to inhibition of KIR2DL signaling in pathogenic T cells by anti-KIR2DL antibodies.

NK cells, as well as some T cells, express KIRs. A reduced number of NK cells and impaired NK cell activity was identified in a subset of SLE and RA patients (14,15). Furthermore, the existence of autoantibodies to NK cells, found in patients with SLE (16), was reported to be associated with impaired NK cell activity (17). From this viewpoint, our findings indicate that KIR2DL would be one of the target molecules for anti–NK cell autoantibodies. In a preliminary experiment, we found that sera from anti-KIR2DL antibody–positive patients slightly enhanced NK cell activity in vitro (results not shown). This may be due to blocking of the KIR2DL signaling by the autoantibody. However, this appears to be discrepant with the findings in the above reports. Since there would be other kinds of autoantibodies to NK cells in addition to those to KIR2DL, more detailed investigation using purified autoantibodies will be needed.

Clinically, it is interesting that a significant elevation in the levels of serum IgG was demonstrated in anti-KIR2DL antibody–positive patients in all 3 of the tested disease groups. Since activated NK cells have been reported to stimulate B cells to secrete immunoglobulin (18), the anti-KIR2DL antibody detected here may block inhibitory signals to NK cells through the KIR2DL molecule. Further studies should help to elucidate this mechanism.

REFERENCES

1. Swaak AJG. Lymphocytotoxic autoantibodies. In: Peter JB, Shoenfeld Y, editors. Autoantibodies. Amsterdam: Elsevier Science; 1996. p. 478–83.
2. Matsui T, Kurokawa M, Kobata T, Oki S, Azuma M, Tohma S, et al. Autoantibodies to T cell costimulatory molecules in systemic autoimmune diseases. J Immunol 1999;162:4328–35.
3. Ferrini S, Cambiaggi A, Meazza R, Sforzini S, Marciano S, Mingari MC, et al. T cell clones expressing the natural killer cell-related p58 receptor molecule display heterogeneity in phenotypic properties and p58 function. Eur J Immunol 1994;24:2294–8.
4. Lanier LL, Phillips JH. Inhibitory MHC class I receptors on NK cells and T cells. Immunol Today 1996;17:86–91.
5. Mingari MC, Moretta A, Moretta L. Regulation of KIR expression in human T cells: a safety mechanism that may impair protective T-cell responses. Immunol Today 1998;19:153–6.
6. Tan EM, Cohen AS, Fries JF, Masi AT, McShane DJ, Rothfield NF, et al. The 1982 revised criteria for the classification of systemic lupus erythematosus. Arthritis Rheum 1982;25:1271–7.
7. Arnett FC, Edworthy SM, Bloch DA, McShane DJ, Fries JF, Cooper NS, et al. The American Rheumatism Association 1987 revised criteria for the classification of rheumatoid arthritis. Arthritis Rheum 1988;31:315–24.
8. International Study Group for Behçet's Disease. Criteria for diagnosis of Behçet's disease. Lancet 1990;335:1078–80.
9. Wagtmann N, Biassoni R, Cantoni C, Verdiani S, Malnati MS, Vitale M, et al. Molecular clones of the p58 NK cell receptor reveal immunoglobulin-related molecules with diversity in both the extra- and intracellular domains. Immunity 1995;2: 439–49.
10. Colonna M, Samaridis J. Cloning of immunoglobulin-superfamily members associated with HLA-C and HLA-B recognition by human natural killer cells. Science 1995;268:405–8.
11. Maenaka K, Juji T, Nakayama T, Wyer JR, Gao GF, Maenaka T, et al. Killer cell immunoglobulin receptors and T cell receptors bind peptide-major histocompatibility complex class I with distinct thermodynamic and kinetic properties. J Biol Chem 1999;274: 28329–34.
12. Bottino C, Sivori S, Vitale M, Cantoni C, Falco M, Pende D, et al. A novel surface molecule homologous to the p58/p50 family of receptors is selectively expressed on a subset of human natural killer cells and induces both triggering of cell functions and proliferation. Eur J Immunol 1996;26:1816–24.
13. Moretta A, Sivori S, Vitale M, Pende D, Morelli L, Augugliaro R, et al. Existence of both inhibitory (p58) and activatory (p50) receptors for HLA-C molecules in human natural killer cells. J Exp Med 1995;182:875–84.
14. Sibbitt WL, Bankhurst AD. Natural killer cells in connective tissue disorders. Clin Rheum Dis 1985;11:507–21.
15. Grunebaum E, Malatzky-Goshen E, Shoenfeld Y. Natural killer cells and autoimmunity. Immunol Res 1989;8:292–304.
16. Rook AH, Tsokos GC, Quinnan GV, Balow JE, Ramsey KM, Stocks N, et al. Cytotoxic autoantibodies to natural killer cells in systemic lupus erythematosus. Clin Immunol Immunopathol 1982; 24:179–85.
17. Sibbitt WL Jr, Froelich CJ, Bankhurst AD. Natural cytotoxicity in systemic lupus erythematosus: mechanisms of suppression by inhibitory serum factors. Clin Exp Immunol 1983;53:363–70.
18. Gray JD, Horwitz DA. Activated human NK cells can stimulate resting B cells to secrete immunoglobulin. J Immunol 1995;154: 5656–64.

ARTHRITIS & RHEUMATISM
Vol. 44, No. 2, February 2001, pp 389–396

The DNA Mismatch Repair Enzyme PMS1 Is a Myositis-Specific Autoantigen

Livia A. Casciola-Rosen,[1] Ann F. Pluta,[2] Paul H. Plotz,[3] Amy E. Cox,[1] Steven Morris,[1] Fredrick M. Wigley,[1] Michelle Petri,[1] Allan C. Gelber,[1] and Antony Rosen[1]

Objective. **The specificity of the autoantibody response in different autoimmune diseases makes autoantibodies useful for diagnostic purposes. It also focuses attention on tissue- and event-specific circumstances that may select unique molecules for an autoimmune response in specific diseases. Defining additional phenotype-specific autoantibodies may identify such circumstances. This study was undertaken to investigate the disease specificity of PMS1, an autoantigen previously identified in some sera from patients with myositis.**

Methods. **We used immunoprecipitation analysis to determine the frequency of autoantibodies to PMS1 in sera from patients with myositis, systemic lupus erythematosus, or scleroderma and from healthy controls. Additional antigens recognized by PMS1-positive sera were further characterized in terms of their susceptibility to cleavage by apoptotic proteases.**

Results. **PMS1, a DNA mismatch repair enzyme, was identified as a myositis-specific autoantigen. Autoantibodies to PMS1 were found in 4 of 53 patients with autoimmune myositis (7.5%), but in no sera from 94 patients with other systemic autoimmune diseases (*P* = 0.016). Additional mismatch repair enzymes (PMS2, MLH1) were targeted, apparently independently. Sera recognizing PMS1 also recognized several other proteins involved in DNA repair and remodeling, including poly(ADP-ribose) polymerase, DNA-dependent protein kinase, and Mi-2. All of these autoantigens were efficiently cleaved by granzyme B, generating unique fragments not observed during other forms of cell death.**

Conclusion. **PMS1 autoantibodies are myositis specific. The striking correlation between an immune response to a group of granzyme B substrates (functioning in DNA repair and remodeling) and the myositis phenotype strongly implies that tissue- and event-specific biochemical events play a role in selecting these molecules for an autoimmune response. Understanding the role of granzyme B cleavage in this response is an important priority.**

Autoantibodies are valuable tools with which to explore the initiating perturbed state in systemic autoimmune diseases (1). Several components of the DNA repair and nucleosome remodeling machinery are targets of the autoimmune response in this spectrum of diseases. Examples include poly(ADP-ribose) polymerase (PARP) (2), several components of DNA-dependent protein kinase (DNA-PK) (including Ku-70, Ku-86, and the catalytic subunit of DNA-PK [DNA-PK_{cs}] [3–5]), and Mi-2 (a component of the nucleosome remodeling and deacetylase machinery) (6–8). Interestingly, in addition to their functioning in a similar process, most of these autoantigens are unified by the fact that they are cleaved by granzyme B and/or caspases during apoptosis (9). In a recent screen of a HeLa cell complementary DNA (cDNA) expression library with a serum from a patient with myositis, autoantibodies that recognize PMS1, a DNA mismatch repair protein which is mutated

Supported by the SLE Foundation and the Scleroderma Research Foundation. Dr. Casciola-Rosen's work was supported by NIH grant AR-44684. Dr. Petri's work was supported by NIH grant AR-43727. Dr. Gelber is the recipient of an Arthritis Foundation Arthritis Investigator Award. Dr. Rosen's work was supported by NIH grant DE-12354 and by a Burroughs Wellcome Fund Translational Research Award. The Johns Hopkins Lupus Cohort received support from the Johns Hopkins University Outpatient Clinical Research Center.

[1]Livia A. Casciola-Rosen, PhD, Amy E. Cox, MS, Steven Morris, MS, Fredrick M. Wigley, MD, Michelle Petri, MD, MPH, Allan C. Gelber, MD, PhD, Antony Rosen, MD: Johns Hopkins University School of Medicine, Baltimore, Maryland; [2]Ann F. Pluta, PhD: University of Maryland, Baltimore, Maryland; [3]Paul H. Plotz, MD: National Institutes of Health, Bethesda, Maryland.

Address correspondence and reprint requests to Livia A. Casciola-Rosen, PhD, and Antony Rosen, MD, Johns Hopkins University School of Medicine, 720 Rutland Avenue, Room 1059, Baltimore, MD 21205.

Submitted for publication July 12, 2000; accepted in revised form September 18, 2000.

Table 1. Demographic characteristics of the patients

Disease (n)	Mean age, years	% female	% African American
Myositis (53)	46.0	58.5	23
Scleroderma (44)	53.8	84	26
SLE (50)*	41.3	90	50

* SLE = systemic lupus erythematosus.

in some patients with hereditary nonpolyposis colorectal cancer, were identified (10). Like many other components of the DNA repair and remodeling machinery, both PMS1 and its close homolog PMS2 are efficiently cleaved by granzyme B during cytotoxic lymphocyte granule–induced apoptosis (9). In the present studies, we investigated the frequency and disease specificity of autoantibodies to the DNA mismatch repair proteins PMS1 and PMS2 in patients with systemic autoimmune diseases.

PATIENTS AND METHODS

Patient cohorts. Sera were obtained from 2 index patients with autoimmune myositis (meeting the Bohan and Peter criteria for dermatomyositis [serum PK] or polymyositis [serum AG]) (11) seen at the Johns Hopkins Medical Institutions, as well as from 51 randomly selected patients with biopsy-proven autoimmune myositis from the National Institutes of Health (NIH) myositis cohort. The NIH patients had dermatomyositis (47%) or polymyositis (45%) which satisfied the Bohan and Peter criteria (11), or eosinophilic myositis (6%) or inclusion body myositis (2%). PMS1-positive sera did not recognize any of the aminoacyl–transfer RNA (aminoacyl-tRNA) synthetases by immunoprecipitation (using reference sera to histidyl-, threonyl-, alanyl-, glycyl-, and isoleucyl-aminoacyl tRNA synthetases as standards). These PMS1-positive patients did not have clinical features of the "synthetase syndrome." Sera from 50 patients with systemic lupus erythematosus (SLE) meeting the American College of Rheumatology (ACR; formerly, the American Rheumatism Association) diagnostic criteria (12) were randomly selected from the Hopkins Lupus Cohort, a prospective study of outcomes in SLE. Sera from 44 patients with scleroderma were randomly selected from stored samples. Thirty-seven of the 44 met ACR criteria for a diagnosis of scleroderma (13), and the remaining 7 had 3 of the 5 features of the CREST syndrome (calcinosis, Raynaud's phenomenon, esophageal dysmotility, sclerodactyly, telangiectasias). Equal numbers of patients with the diffuse and limited forms of scleroderma were included. A summary of demographic characteristics of the patients is presented in Table 1.

Expression cloning of PMS1. Serum PK was used to screen a λGT11 HeLa cell cDNA expression library. Several positive clones were processed to plaque purity, and the inserts were excised by restriction digestion with *Eco*RI. After subcloning into pBluescript II and sequencing, clone 1531 was found to encode the human DNA mismatch repair enzyme PMS1.

Generation of antibody raised against the C-terminus of human PMS1. A peptide corresponding to amino acid residues 903–922 at the C-terminus of human PMS1 (Boston Biomolecules, Woburn, MA) was used to immunize rabbits (Covance Research Products, Denver, PA). Serum from rabbit 3213 contained antibodies that detected PMS1. In some experiments, antibody sc-615 (Santa Cruz Biotechnology, Santa Cruz, CA) was used instead of serum 3213 to detect the C-terminus of PMS1.

Generation of ^{35}S-methionine–labeled autoantigens and cleavage in vitro by granzyme B. ^{35}S-methionine–labeled PMS1, PMS2, and MLH1 were generated by coupled in vitro transcription/translation (IVTT) (14), using the appropriate full-length cDNAs (all generous gifts from Dr. B. Vogelstein, Johns Hopkins University). Radiolabeled PMS1 was diluted in buffer A (consisting of 10 m*M* HEPES [pH 7.4], 2 m*M* EDTA, and 1% Nonidet P40 [NP40]) and incubated in the absence or presence of 70 n*M* granzyme B (15) for 15 minutes at 37°C. Reactions were either terminated, by adding gel buffer and boiling, or were used for immunoprecipitations. In the latter case, the activity of granzyme B was stopped by adding 70 μ*M* chymostatin and placing the reaction mixtures on ice.

Immunoprecipitation of IVTT substrates. Standard immunoprecipitations to test which sera immunoprecipitated radiolabeled substrates were performed as follows. IVTT substrates were diluted with buffer B (consisting of 1% NP40, 20 m*M* Tris [pH 7.4], 150 m*M* NaCl, 1 m*M* EDTA, and 0.2% bovine serum albumin) supplemented with a protease inhibitor cocktail. Serum (2 μl) was added and the mixture was rocked for 1 hour at 4°C, after which immobilized protein A–agarose (Pierce, Rockford, IL) was added. The immunoprecipitates were washed, electrophoresed on 10% sodium dodecyl sulfate (SDS)–polyacrylamide gels, and visualized by fluorography. In experiments in which immunoprecipitations were performed using granzyme B–cleaved PMS1, the reaction mixtures were either incubated on ice or SDS was added (0.7% final concentration) and the samples were boiled for 5 minutes. After boiling, the SDS concentration was decreased to 0.1% by adding buffer B. Immunoprecipitations were then performed as described above.

Immunoblotting to detect cleavage of endogenous HeLa substrates. HeLa cells were cultured and induced to become apoptotic by ultraviolet B irradiation as previously described (16,17). For in vitro incubations in the absence or presence of purified granzyme B, HeLa lysate was prepared (9) and incubated with 42 n*M* granzyme B and 2 m*M* iodoacetamide for 1 hour at 37°C. Reactions were terminated by adding gel buffer and boiling, and samples were electrophoresed on 10% SDS-polyacrylamide gels. Proteins were transferred to nitrocellulose and immunoblotted as previously described (18). Blotted proteins were detected with horseradish peroxidase–labeled secondary antibody and chemiluminescence (Pierce). All experiments were performed on at least 2 separate occasions, using different batches of radiolabeled substrates or HeLa lysates.

Statistical analysis. The significance of the relationship of PMS1 targeting to systemic autoimmune diseases was investigated using Fisher's exact test. Statistical significance was defined as an α level of 0.05.

RESULTS

Detection of PMS1. Serum PK, obtained from a patient with dermatomyositis, was used to screen a λGT11 HeLa cell cDNA expression library. One of the positive clones had an insert of 0.7 kb, which was identical to the human DNA mismatch repair enzyme PMS1. We obtained a full-length cDNA for PMS1 and generated ^{35}S-methionine–labeled PMS1 by coupled IVTT. The labeled 120-kd product was immunoprecipitated by serum PK and rabbit serum 3213 (raised against the C-terminus of PMS1), but not by normal human or preimmune serum from rabbit 3213 (Figure 1). Interestingly, although rabbit anti-PMS1 immunoblotted a molecule of 120 kd in control HeLa cell lysates, serum PK

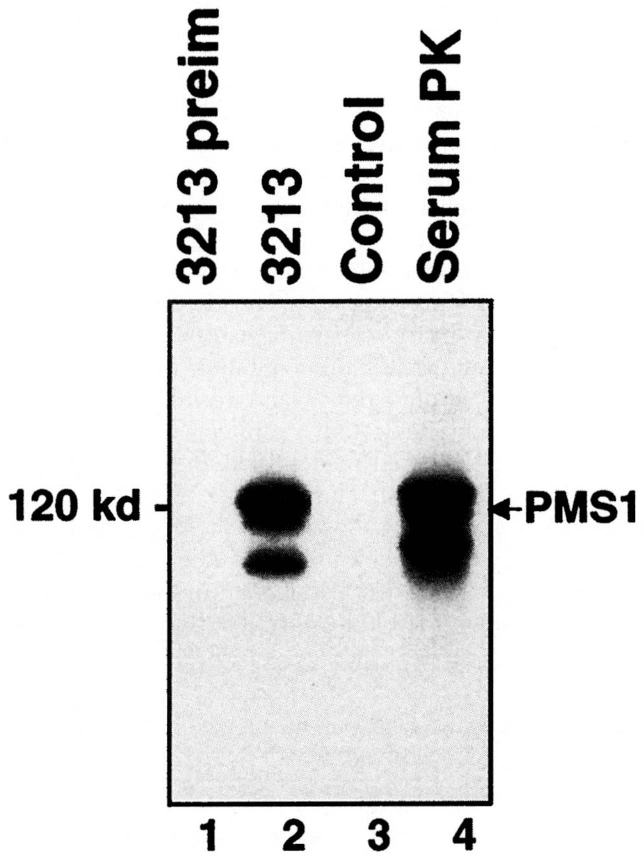

Figure 1. Results of PMS1 immunoprecipitation studies using serum from rabbit 3213 (containing antibodies that detected PMS1), normal human serum, and serum from myositis patient PK. ^{35}S-methionine–labeled PMS1, generated by in vitro transcription/translation, was immunoprecipitated with preimmune (preim) serum from rabbit 3213 (lane 1), rabbit 3213 immune serum (lane 2), normal human serum (lane 3), or serum PK (lane 4). The findings demonstrated that serum PK contains antibodies that immunoprecipitate PMS1.

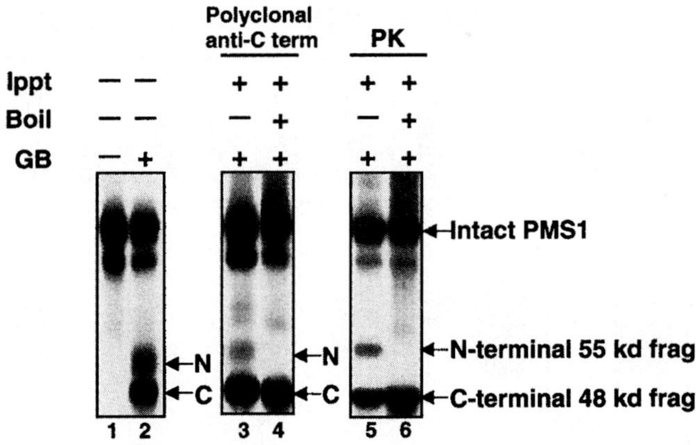

Figure 2. Results of immunoprecipitation studies using rabbit antipeptide antibodies against the N- or C-terminus of PMS1. ^{35}S-methionine–labeled PMS1, generated by in vitro transcription/translation, was incubated in the absence (lane 1) or presence (lane 2) of granzyme B (GB), as described in Patients and Methods. Aliquots of the cleaved PMS1 were used directly for immunoprecipitation (lanes 3 and 5) or were first boiled in the presence of sodium dodecyl sulfate (lanes 4 and 6). Immunoprecipitations were performed using polyclonal rabbit antibody directed against the 48-kd C-terminus of PMS1 (sc-615; Santa Cruz Biotechnology, Santa Cruz, CA) (lanes 3 and 4) or serum PK (lanes 5 and 6). The findings demonstrated that serum PK recognizes the C-terminal fragment (frag) of GB-cleaved PMS1. Ippt = immunoprecipitate.

was not able to immunoblot a similar species, indicating that the epitope recognized by the autoantibody to PMS1 is likely conformational (results not shown).

Recognition of the C-terminus of PMS1 by PMS1 autoantibodies. We have previously observed that PMS1 is efficiently cleaved by granzyme B, generating fragments of 55 kd and 48 kd (9) (Figure 2, lanes 1 and 2). We initially used rabbit antipeptide antibodies raised against the N- or C-terminus of PMS1 to immunoprecipitate these fragments from granzyme B–cleaved ^{35}S-methionine–labeled PMS1 generated by IVTT. The 48-kd fragment was immunoprecipitated by the anti–C-terminal antibody (Figure 2, lane 4), while the 55-kd fragment was recognized by an antibody raised against the N-terminus of PMS1 (results not shown). Interestingly, the anti–C-terminal antibody also immunoprecipitated a small amount of the 55-kd N-terminal fragment (Figure 2, lane 3), suggesting that the N- and C-terminal fragments of PMS1 remain associated even after granzyme B–mediated cleavage. When the cleavage reaction mixture was boiled in SDS (which was subsequently diluted) prior to immunoprecipitation, recognition of the intact protein and the C-terminal 48-kd fragment was improved, but the 55-kd fragment was no longer detected (Figure 2, lane 4). These data demonstrate that

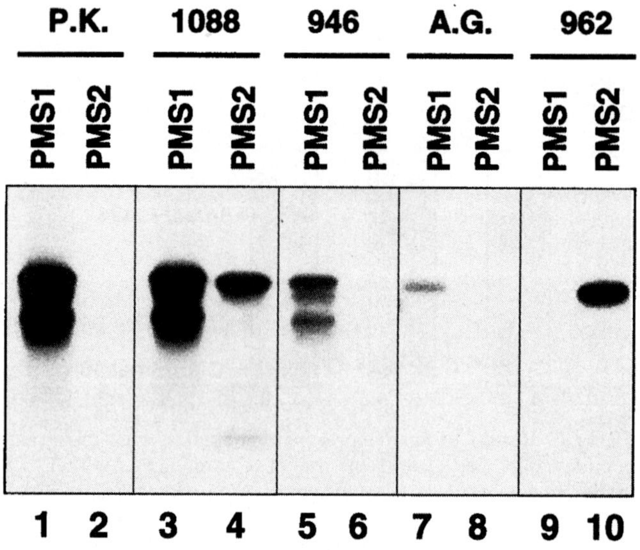

Figure 3. Results of immunoprecipitation studies in 5 myositis patients with a positive reaction to PMS1 and/or PMS2. ^{35}S-methionine–labeled PMS1 and PMS2 were generated by in vitro transcription/translation and immunoprecipitated with the indicated myositis sera.

the N- and C-terminal fragments of PMS1 remain at least partially associated after cleavage by granzyme B, unless separated by denaturation.

Similar immunoprecipitation experiments were performed using human autoantibodies recognizing PMS1 (sera PK [Figure 2] and 1088 [results not shown]). In the absence of boiling, both the 55-kd and the 48-kd fragments were immunoprecipitated by both human sera. In contrast, after boiling of the reaction mixture in SDS to disrupt complexes and diluting prior to immunoprecipitation, the 48-kd C-terminal fragment alone was immunoprecipitated by human sera. These findings confirm that human autoantibodies to PMS1 directly recognize the C-terminal granzyme B fragment, rather than an associated component.

Frequency and specificity of autoantibodies to PMS1. To investigate the frequency of targeting of PMS1 in systemic autoimmune diseases, sera from healthy controls or patients with myositis, SLE, or scleroderma were screened in an immunoprecipitation assay, using ^{35}S-methionine–labeled PMS1 generated by IVTT. Four of 53 sera from patients with autoimmune myositis (7.5%) recognized PMS1 (Figure 3). In contrast, no sera from 94 other patients with systemic autoimmune diseases (50 from patients with SLE and 44 from patients with scleroderma) immunoprecipitated PMS1 ($P = 0.016$ by Fisher's exact test). In addition, none of the 39 healthy control sera immunoprecipitated PMS1. Interestingly, serum from 1 subject who did not have a systemic autoimmune disease, but who had an active zoster eruption, was also positive for antibodies to PMS1 in the immunoprecipitation assay (results not shown). Thus, the occurrence of antibodies to PMS1 was specific for autoimmune myositis as compared with SLE and scleroderma, and the difference was statistically significant. The relatively low frequency of this autoantibody response in myositis patients is in a range similar to that found with several other targeted protein autoantigens in this spectrum of disease (e.g., threonyl-, alanyl-, glycyl-, and isoleucyl-aminoacyl tRNA synthetases [each <2–3%], signal recognition particle [SRP] [~4%], Mi-2 [<8%], and PM-Scl [<8%]) (19).

Recognition of several components of the DNA repair machinery by sera from patients with autoimmune myositis. Sera that recognized PMS1 by immunoprecipitation (sera PK, AG, 1088, and 946) were immunoblotted against lysates of HeLa cells. Although rabbit antibodies against PMS1 recognized their cognate antigen by immunoblotting in HeLa cell lysates, PMS1 was not detected by any of the human sera by immunoblotting. Interestingly, each of these human myositis sera recognized at least 1 other antigen by blotting and/or precipitation (Table 2). Serum PK immunoprecipitated PMS1 and an unidentified 68-kd protein, and immunoblotted Mi-2 (Figure 4, lane 1). The identity of this Mi-2 antibody in serum PK was confirmed by comigration in immunoblots and immunoprecipitation with a standard Mi-2–positive serum (ref. 9 and results not shown). Serum AG immunoblotted several proteins, including DNA-PK_{cs}, PARP, and unidentified antigens of 190 kd and 130 kd (Figure 4, lane 5). The identities of the DNA-PK_{cs} and PARP antibodies in serum AG were confirmed by immunoblotting and documented in an earlier study (16). Serum 946 recognized, in addition to PMS1, an unidentified 125-kd protein (p125) by immuno-

Table 2. Antigens recognized by sera PK, AG, 946, and 1088*

Serum	Antigens recognized
PK	PMS1, Mi-2, 68 kd†
AG	PMS1, DNA-PK_{cs}, PARP, 190 kd,† 130 kd†
946	PMS1, 125 kd†
1088	PMS1, PMS2, MLH1, 85 kd†

* Data were obtained from the immunoblots shown in Figure 4 and from immunoprecipitations using radiolabeled substrates generated by in vitro transcription/translation (Figures 1 and 3 and results not shown). DNA-PK_{cs} = catalytic subunit of DNA-dependent protein kinase; PARP = poly(ADP-ribose) polymerase.
† Unidentified antigens are referred to by molecular weight, as estimated by sodium dodecyl sulfate–polyacrylamide gel electrophoresis.

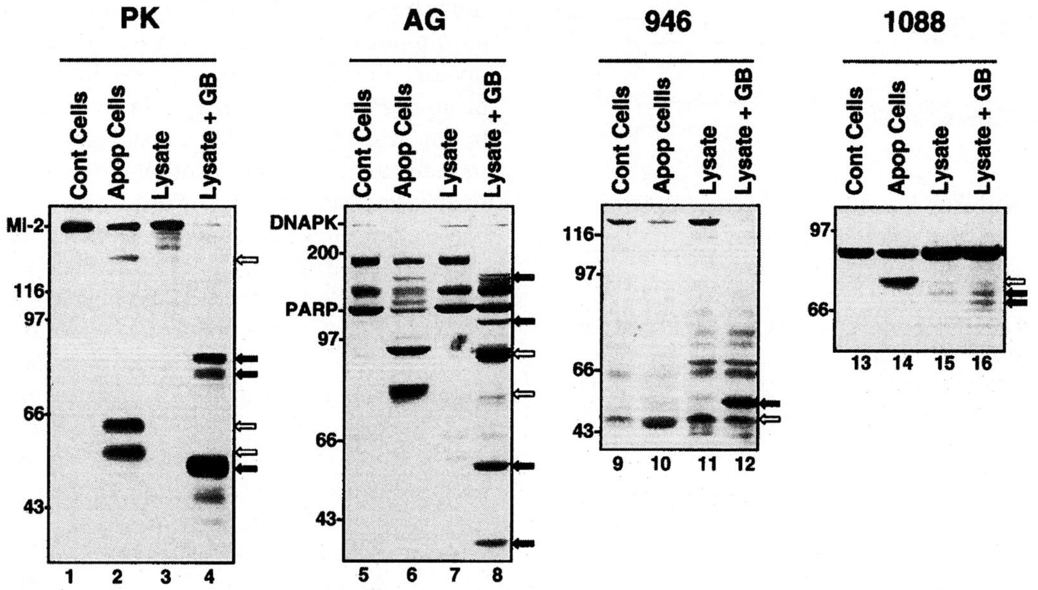

Figure 4. Results of immunoblotting studies of myositis sera that recognized PMS1. Gel samples were prepared from control (Cont) and apoptotic (Apop) (ultraviolet B–irradiated) HeLa cells, and from HeLa lysate incubated in vitro with 42 n*M* granzyme B (GB). Aliquots (75 μg) were electrophoresed in each gel lane, and autoantigens were detected by immunoblotting. **Solid arrows** show the migration positions of GB-specific fragments; **open arrows** denote those fragments detected in cells induced to become apoptotic by ultraviolet B irradiation. The findings demonstrate that sera from myositis patients immunoblot antigens that are uniquely cleaved by GB. DNAPK = catalytic subunit of DNA-dependent protein kinase; PARP = poly(ADP-ribose) polymerase.

blotting (Figure 4, lane 9). Serum 1088 also recognized in vitro–translated PMS2 and MLH1 by immunoprecipitation (see below), and a single 85-kd protein (p85) by immunoblotting (Figure 4, lane 13).

Since many autoantigens are proteolytically cleaved during apoptosis (1,20), we investigated whether the additional antigens recognized by PMS1-positive patient sera were cleaved in apoptotic cells (Figure 4). In every case, the molecules were cleaved in apoptotic cells (Figure 4, lanes 2, 6, 10, and 14), generating stable fragments that were not further processed. Recent studies have demonstrated that ~80% of autoantigens across the spectrum of human autoimmune disease are susceptible to cleavage by granzyme B during cytotoxic lymphocyte granule–induced cell death, generating unique fragments not observed during any other form of apoptotic death (9). We addressed whether the additional antigens recognized by PMS1-positive sera were susceptible to cleavage by granzyme B by adding purified granzyme B to lysates of HeLa cells in which endogenous caspases had been inactivated by alkylating the active site cysteine. In every case, these antigens were efficiently cleaved by granzyme B (Figure 4, solid arrows), and the fragments generated were distinct from those observed in apoptotic cells (Figure 4, open arrows). The immunoblotted cleavage products shown in Figure 4 correspond to those previously reported for Mi-2 (lanes 2 and 4) and DNA-PK and PARP (lanes 6 and 8) (9,15,16).

Autoantibodies to other DNA mismatch repair enzymes. PMS1 belongs to the MutL family of DNA mismatch repair enzymes. All family members have a conserved region of ~300 amino acids at their N-terminus and a very diverse C-terminal region of 300–500 residues that shows no significant homology between family members (Figure 5). We generated radiolabeled PMS2 by IVTT and tested the same series of sera for antibodies to PMS2 by immunoprecipitation (Figure 3 and Table 3). Sera from 2 of 53 patients with myositis (~3.7%) recognized PMS2 by immunoprecipitation. Interestingly, 1 of the positive sera (serum 1088) recognized both PMS1 and PMS2, while the other recognized PMS2 but not PMS1 (Table 3). Although PMS2 antibodies were not found in controls (0 of 29) or scleroderma patients (0 of 44), 1 of 50 SLE patients did have this antibody. This patient did not have clinically apparent myositis either at the time of assay or previously.

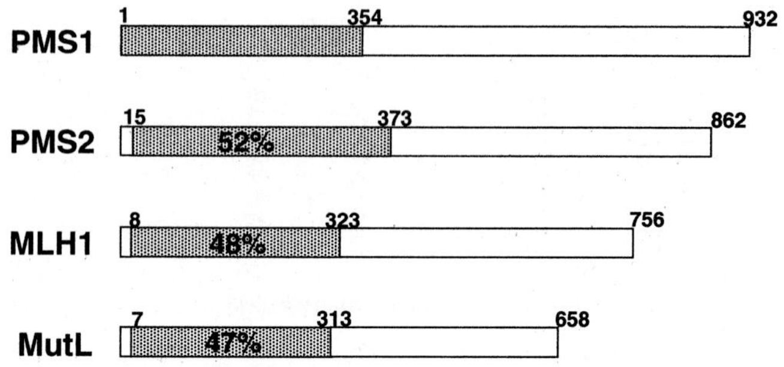

Figure 5. Data showing that PMS1 belongs to a family of DNA mismatch repair enzymes that share a conserved region of ~300 amino acids at the N-terminus (shaded areas) and very diverse C-terminal regions of ~300–500 amino acid residues (open areas).

All myositis sera were also screened in an immunoprecipitation assay against in vitro–translated MLH1. Both of the PMS2-positive myositis sera (sera 962 and 1088) also recognized MLH1. Only 1 of these sera (serum 1088) also immunoprecipitated PMS1. One myositis serum (serum 981) that was negative in the immunoprecipitation assay for PMS1 and PMS2 was positive for antibodies to MLH1. Thus, although there are several examples of myositis sera recognizing multiple MutL-like enzymes, there are also clear examples in which each serum recognizes only 1 of these molecules. These data demonstrate that all of the human MutL homologs may be independently targeted in patients with myositis. The clinical features of those myositis patients with antibodies directed against the DNA mismatch repair enzymes are summarized in Table 3.

DISCUSSION

In these studies, we demonstrated that autoantibodies to PMS1 occur in ~7.5% of patients with autoimmune myositis, but not in patients with other systemic autoimmune diseases. The proportion of sera that are positive for PMS1 is significantly different between the 2 groups ($P = 0.016$). Interestingly, 2 patients with antibodies to PMS1 had dermatomyositis, 1 had polymyositis, and another had eosinophilic myositis with prominent inflammation of the fascia.

Although no unique clinical features are yet apparent in this group of patients, we propose that PMS1 be added to the list of myositis-specific autoantibodies (21). The association of unique autoantibodies with specific clinical states is a common feature in autoimmune myositis (19). For example, antibodies to Mi-2 are associated with typical rash in dermatomyositis, and antibodies to aminoacyl-tRNA synthetases are associated with interstitial lung disease, arthritis, Raynaud's phenomenon, and "mechanic's hands" (referred to as the "synthetase syndrome"). It is possible that unique clinical features associated with antibodies to PMS1 or the other DNA mismatch repair enzymes might yet be found as additional patients with these autoantibodies are identified. Of interest, the 4 patients with antibodies to PMS1 described here did not have antibodies to any of the aminoacyl-tRNA synthetases, although their sera did target several additional autoantigens active in DNA repair and nucleosome remodeling (see below).

In humans, the MutL family of proteins consists of several homologous ATPase proteins, including PMS1, PMS2, and MLH1. These molecules play an essential role in DNA mismatch repair, and mutations in genes encoding these proteins cause cancer susceptibility, as evidenced by the association of these mutations with hereditary nonpolyposis colorectal cancer (10,22,23). Interestingly, antibodies to PMS1, PMS2, and MLH-1 are all found infrequently in myositis pa-

Table 3. Clinical features of the myositis patients with antibodies directed against DNA mismatch repair enzymes*

Patient	Age/sex/race	Symmetric weakness	Biopsy findings	Elevated muscle enzymes	EMG result	Rash	Autoantibodies
PK†	65/F/C	+	DM	+	+	+	PMS1, Mi-2
AG‡	48/M/C	+	NA	+	+	−	PMS1, DNA-PK_{cs}, PARP
981†	45/F/C	+	DM	+	+	+	MLH1
946§	47/F/AA	+	PM	+	+	−	PMS1
962†	55/M/C	+	DM	+	ND	+	PMS2, MLH1
1088	23/F/C	Asymmetric	EM with fasciitis	−	ND	−	PMS1, PMS2, MLH1

* EMG = electromyography; C = Caucasian; NA = not available; AA = African American; ND = not done; EM = eosinophilic myositis (see Table 2 for other definitions).
† Meets Bohan and Peter criteria for definite dermatomyositis (DM).
‡ Meets Bohan and Peter criteria for probable polymyositis (PM); patient also had serologic evidence of systemic lupus erythematosus.
§ Meets Bohan and Peter criteria for definite PM.

tients. Due to the very low frequency of targeting of PMS2 and MLH1, it is not yet clear if these antibodies have specificity for autoimmune myositis. All MutL homologs share a very similar N-terminal domain of ~40 kd, which contains the ATPase function (24) (Figure 5). The function of the C-terminal region of 30–50 kd, which has a very diverse sequence among the various family members, appears to be responsible for dimerization of MutL family members (25), as well as for interactions between MutL and DNA helicase II (26). It is of particular interest that this diverse C-terminal region, rather than the conserved N-terminal region containing the catalytic ATPase, is the target of autoantibodies.

A striking observation made with the myositis sera studied here is that, in addition to recognizing components of the mismatch repair pathway, several sera also recognize other defined autoantigens which function in DNA repair and nucleosome remodeling, including DNA-PK_{cs} (double-strand break repair) (27), PARP (28), and Mi-2 (nucleosome remodeling and deacetylation) (8,29). Interestingly, both the mismatch repair machinery and the Mi-2 deacetylase are methyl directed and include components which recognize and bind specifically to methylated DNA at methyl-CpG (8,30). Thus, MLH1 interacts directly with MBD-4 (a methyl-CpG–binding protein) (31). Similarly, MBD-3 shares this highly conserved methyl-CpG–binding domain and directs the major histone deacetylase complex, containing Mi-2 (a nucleosome-stimulated ATPase belonging to the SWI2/SNF2 family) to effect dynamic changes in chromatin structure associated with transcription, replication, recombination, and repair (8,32). It will be important to define whether the expression and activity of these processes is altered in a muscle-specific manner during initiation and propagation of these diseases.

All of the proteins described above (PMS1, PMS2, MLH1, DNA-PK_{cs}, PARP, and Mi-2), as well as several aminoacyl-tRNA synthetases, SRP-72, U1–70 kd, and PM-Scl, are efficiently cleaved by granzyme B. This feature therefore unifies the majority of proteins recognized by autoantibodies in myositis and demonstrates that they contain a conserved structural motif recognized by the protease. We have previously proposed that the structural motif recognized by granzyme B has an important functional role: granzyme B evolved to cleave this motif, thereby regulating protein function (9). It is of interest that the subset of granzyme B substrates that are targeted in different systemic autoimmune diseases differ, and correlate well with the clinical phenotype. For example, topoisomerase I, centromeric protein B, and fibrillarin are targeted in scleroderma, while La is targeted in SLE and Sjögren's syndrome. This striking correlation between an immune response to specific groups of granzyme B substrates (functioning in unique pathways) and the biologic phenotype strongly implies that tissue- and event-specific biochemical events may play a role in selecting molecules for an autoimmune response. The role of granzyme B sites within these molecules, or their cleavage during cytotoxic lymphocyte–induced death, in this immune response is presently under investigation.

The myositis sera targeting DNA mismatch repair enzymes described here also recognize other substrates that are cleaved during apoptosis and by granzyme B. Many of these additional components are cleaved by caspases during apoptosis, and are cleaved at unique sites by granzyme B, generating novel fragments. Although the identities of these proteins remain unknown, many have molecular sizes of previously defined components of the human DNA repair and remodeling machinery. Since autoantibodies have traditionally been extremely powerful probes of basic biochemical and cell biologic processes (33), it is likely that further study of myositis autoantibodies will provide additional insights into the important processes of DNA repair and chromatin remodeling in humans.

ACKNOWLEDGMENT

The authors thank Nina Lu for help with analysis of data on the myositis cohort.

REFERENCES

1. Rosen A, Casciola-Rosen L. Autoantigens as substrates for apoptotic proteases: implications for the pathogenesis of systemic autoimmune disease. Cell Death Differ 1999;6:6–12.
2. Yamanaka H, Willis EH, Penning CA, Peebles CL, Tan EM, Carson DA. Human autoantibodies to poly (adenosine disphosphate-ribose) polymerase. J Clin Invest 1987;80:900–4.
3. Reeves WH. Antibodies to the p70/p80 (Ku) antigens in systemic lupus erythematosus. Rheum Dis Clin North Am 1992;18: 391–414.
4. Satoh M, Ajmani AK, Stojanov L, Langdon JJ, Ogasawara T, Wang J, et al. Autoantibodies that stabilize the molecular interaction of Ku antigen with DNA-dependent protein kinase catalytic subunit. Clin Exp Immunol 1996;105:460–7.
5. Suwa A, Hirakata M, Takeda Y, Okano Y, Mimori T, Inada S, et al. Autoantibodies to DNA-dependent protein kinase: probes for the catalytic subunit. J Clin Invest 1996;97:1417–21.
6. Ge Q, Nilasena DS, O'Brien CA, Frank MB, Targoff IN. Molecular analysis of a major antigenic region of the 240kDa protein of Mi-2 autoantigen. J Clin Invest 1995;96:1730–7.

7. Seelig HP, Moosbrugger I, Ehrfeld H, Fink T, Renz M, Genth E. The major dermatomyositis-specific Mi-2 autoantigen is a presumed helicase involved in transcriptional activation. Arthritis Rheum 1995;38:1389–99.
8. Wade PA, Gegonne A, Jones PL, Ballestar E, Aubry F, Wolffe AP. Mi-2 complex couples DNA methylation to chromatin remodelling and histone deacetylation. Nat Genet 1999;23:62–6.
9. Casciola-Rosen L, Andrade F, Ulanet D, Wong WB, Rosen A. Cleavage by granzyme B is strongly predictive of autoantigen status: implications for initiation of autoimmunity. J Exp Med 1999;190:815–26.
10. Nicolaides NC, Papadopoulos N, Liu B, Wei YF, Carter KC, Ruben SM, et al. Mutations of two PMS homologues in hereditary nonpolyposis colon cancer. Nature 1994;371:75–80.
11. Bohan A, Peter JB. Polymyositis and dermatomyositis. N Engl J Med 1975;292:403–7.
12. Tan EM, Cohen AS, Fries JF, Masi AT, McShane DJ, Rothfield NF, et al. The 1982 revised criteria for the classification of systemic lupus erythematosus. Arthritis Rheum 1982;25:1271–7.
13. Subcommittee for Scleroderma Criteria of the American Rheumatism Association Diagnostic and Therapeutic Criteria Committee. Preliminary criteria for the classification of systemic sclerosis (scleroderma). Arthritis Rheum 1980;23:581–90.
14. Casciola-Rosen LA, Nicholson DW, Chong T, Rowan KR, Thornberry NA, Miller DK, et al. Apopain/CPP32 cleaves proteins that are essential for cellular repair: a fundamental principle of apoptotic death. J Exp Med 1996;183:1957–64.
15. Andrade F, Roy S, Nicholson DW, Thornberry NA, Rosen A, Casciola-Rosen L. Granzyme B directly and efficiently cleaves several downstream substrates: implications for CTL-induced apoptosis. Immunity 1998;8:451–60.
16. Casciola-Rosen LA, Anhalt GJ, Rosen A. DNA-dependent protein kinase is one of a subset of autoantigens specifically cleaved early during apoptosis. J Exp Med 1995;182:1625–34.
17. Casciola-Rosen LA, Anhalt G, Rosen A. Autoantigens targeted in systemic lupus erythematosus are clustered in two populations of surface structures on apoptotic keratinocytes. J Exp Med 1994;179:1317–30.
18. Casciola-Rosen LA, Miller DK, Anhalt GJ, Rosen A. Specific cleavage of the 70-kDa protein component of the U1 small nuclear ribonucleoprotein is a characteristic biochemical feature of apoptotic cell death. J Biol Chem 1994;269:30757–60.
19. Targoff IN. Immune manifestations of inflammatory muscle disease. Rheum Dis Clin North Am 1994;20:857–80.
20. Utz PJ, Anderson P. Posttranslational protein modifications, apoptosis, and the bypass of tolerance to autoantigens. Arthritis Rheum 1998;41:1152–60.
21. Love LA, Fraser DD, Targoff IN, Dalakas M, Plotz PH, Miller FW. A new approach to the classification of idiopathic inflammatory myopathy: myositis-specific autoantibodies define useful homogenous groups. Medicine (Baltimore) 1991;70:360–74.
22. Bronner CE, Baker SM, Morrison PT, Warren G, Smith LG, Lescoe MK, et al. Mutation in the DNA mismatch repair gene homologue hMLH1 is associated with hereditary non-polyposis colon cancer. Nature 1994;368:258–61.
23. Papadopoulos N, Nicolaides NC, Wei YF, Ruben SM, Carter KC, Rosen CA, et al. Mutation of a mutL homolog in hereditary colon cancer. Science 1994;263:1625–9.
24. Ban C, Yang W. Crystal structure and ATPase activity of MutL: implications for DNA repair and mutagenesis. Cell 1999;95:541–52.
25. Pang Q, Prolla TA, Liskay M. Functional domains of the S. cerevesiae Mlh1p and Pms1p DNA mismatch repair proteins and their relevance to human hereditary nonpolyposis colorectal cancer-associated mutations. Mol Cell Biol 1997;17:4465–73.
26. Hall MC, Jordan JR, Matson SW. Evidence for a physical interaction between the E. coli methyl-directed mismatch repair proteins MutL and UvrD. EMBO J 1998;17:1535–41.
27. Finnie NJ, Gottlieb TM, Blunt T, Jeggo PA, Jackson SP. DNA-dependent protein kinase activity is absent in xrs-6 cells: implications for site-specific recombination and double-strand break repair. Proc Natl Acad Sci U S A 1995;92:320–4.
28. Satoh MS, Lindahl T. Role of poly(ADP-ribose) formation in DNA repair. Nature 1992;356:356–8.
29. Wade PA, Jones PL, Vermaak D, Wolffe AP. A multiple subunit Mi-2 histone deacetylase from Xenopus laevis cofractionates with an associated Snf2 superfamily ATPase. Curr Biol 1998;8:843–6.
30. Kolodner RD. Mismatch repair: mechanisms and relationship to cancer susceptibility. Trends Biochem Sci 1995;20:397–401.
31. Bellacosa A, Cicchillitti L, Schepis F, Riccio A, Yeung AT, Matsumoto Y, et al. MED1, a novel human methyl-CpG–binding endonuclease, interacts with DNA mismatch repair protein MLH1. Proc Natl Acad Sci U S A 1999;96:3969–74.
32. Hendrich B, Abbott C, McQueen H, Chambers D, Cross S, Bird A. Genomic structure and chromosomal mapping of the murine and human Mbd1, Mbd2, Mbd3, and Mbd4 genes. Mamm Genome 1999;10:906–12.
33. Tan EM. Autoantibodies in pathology and cell biology. Cell 1991;67:841–2.

ARTHRITIS & RHEUMATISM
Vol. 44, No. 2, February 2001, pp 397–407

Decreased Ras–Mitogen-Activated Protein Kinase Signaling May Cause DNA Hypomethylation in T Lymphocytes From Lupus Patients

Chun Deng, Mariana J. Kaplan, Jun Yang, Donna Ray, Zhiyong Zhang, W. Joseph McCune, Samir M. Hanash, and Bruce C. Richardson

Objective. **Previous studies have shown that inhibiting T cell DNA methylation causes a lupus-like disease by modifying gene expression. T cells from patients with lupus exhibit diminished levels of DNA methyltransferase (MTase) enzyme activity, hypomethylated DNA, and changes in gene expression similar to those exhibited by T cells treated with methylation inhibitors, suggesting that DNA hypomethylation may contribute to human lupus. Since it is known that DNA MTase levels are regulated by the ras–mitogen-activated protein kinase (MAPK) pathway, this study sought to determine whether decreased ras-MAPK signaling could account for the DNA hypomethylation in lupus T cells.**

Methods. **DNA MTase messenger RNA (mRNA) from lupus patients and from healthy controls was quantitated by Northern analysis, and ras-MAPK signaling was determined by immunoblotting with antibodies to the activated forms of extracellular receptor–associated kinase (ERK). Results were compared with those in T cells in which ras-MAPK signaling was inhibited with a soluble inhibitor of MAPK ERK 1 (MEK1).**

Results. **T cells from patients with active lupus had diminished DNA MTase mRNA levels and decreased signaling through the ras-MAPK pathway. Inhibiting signaling through the ras-MAPK pathway with the MEK1 inhibitor decreased DNA MTase mRNA and enzyme activity to the levels seen in lupus T cells, and resulted in DNA hypomethylation resembling that seen in lupus T cells.**

Conclusion. **These results suggest that a decrease in signaling through the ras-MAPK pathway may be responsible for the decreased MTase activity and DNA hypomethylation in patients with lupus.**

Supported by PHS grants AR-42525, AG-014783, and AI-42753 and by a Veterans Affairs Merit Review grant. Dr. Kaplan's work was supported by an award from Amgen through the Life Sciences Foundation.

Chun Deng, MD, PhD, Mariana J. Kaplan, MD, Jun Yang, MD, PhD, Donna Ray, BS, Zhiyong Zhang, MD, W. Joseph McCune, MD, Samir M. Hanash, MD, PhD, Bruce C. Richardson, MD, PhD: University of Michigan and the Ann Arbor VA Hospital, Ann Arbor, Michigan.

Address correspondence and reprint requests to Bruce Richardson, MD, PhD, 5310 Cancer Center and Geriatrics Center Building, Ann Arbor, MI 48109-0940.

Submitted for publication February 3, 2000; accepted in revised form October 13, 2000.

Although the primary defect in idiopathic human lupus remains unknown, the phenomenon of drug-induced lupus suggests that drug-induced biochemical changes can lead to the development of lupus-like diseases. Thus, elucidation of the mechanisms by which drugs induce lupus may provide clues to the pathogenesis of the idiopathic disease. Our group has demonstrated that some lupus-inducing drugs, including procainamide and hydralazine, inhibit T cell DNA methylation (1). We have also shown that various agents that inhibit DNA methylation in T cells, including procainamide, hydralazine, 5-azacytidine, and ultraviolet light, induce leukocyte function–associated antigen 1 (LFA-1) overexpression (2,3), which makes T cells autoreactive (3,4). Finally, we have demonstrated that adoptive transfer of T cells made autoreactive by treatment with DNA methylation inhibitors (2,4–6) or by transfection with LFA-1 (4) is sufficient to cause a lupus-like disease in unirradiated syngeneic mice. Together, these studies indicate that one mechanism causing a lupus-like disease is the induction of T cell DNA hypomethylation, with subsequent effects on LFA-1 expression and autoreactivity.

To determine the relevance of these studies to human lupus, we investigated T cell DNA methylation in

Table 1. Characteristics of the study patients*

Disease	Number of patients	Sex, no. female/no. male	Age, mean ± SD years (range)	Treatment, no. of patients						
				NSAID	Steroids	Anti-malarial	CYC	AZA	MTX	Gold
RA	10	7/3	50 ± 11 (36–69)	6	4	4	0	0	4	1
Inactive SLE	16	13/3	35 ± 13 (18–65)	2	13	14	2	3	0	0
Active SLE	12	10/2	39 ± 14 (18–61)	2	12	8	2	1	1	0

* NSAID = nonsteroidal antiinflammatory drug; CYC = cyclophosphamide; AZA = azathioprine; MTX = methotrexate; RA = rheumatoid arthritis; SLE = systemic lupus erythematosus.

lupus. We obtained evidence that T cells from patients with active lupus have hypomethylated DNA and an autoreactive T cell subset that overexpresses LFA-1 (7,8). These observations have been confirmed by independent groups (9,10). We have also reported that T cells from lupus patients have a significant decrease in DNA (cytosine-5-)-methyltransferase (MTase) activity, the enzyme mediating maintenance DNA methylation (11). Since treatment with procainamide, a competitive DNA MTase inhibitor, results in a similar decrease in enzyme activity (12), the reduced DNA MTase activity observed in lupus T cells may be an important step in the development of lupus. However, the basis for the reduced MTase activity in lupus is unknown.

We have demonstrated that DNA methyltransferase 1 (Dnmt1) levels increase following T cell stimulation, and our group, as well as others, has reported that Dnmt1 levels are regulated through the ras–mitogen-activated protein kinase (MAPK) signaling pathway and activator protein 1 (AP-1) sites (13–16). The studies presented in this report were undertaken to determine the role of ras-MAPK signaling in the reduced DNA MTase activity and DNA hypomethylation in lupus T cells. We provide evidence that a decrease in signaling through the ras-MAPK pathway may be responsible for the decreased MTase activity and for the hypomethylated DNA in lupus.

PATIENTS AND METHODS

Cells and cell culture. Peripheral blood mononuclear cells (PBMC) were isolated from the venous blood of healthy controls, patients with rheumatoid arthritis (RA), and patients with active and inactive lupus, using density gradient centrifugation as previously described (7). The clinical parameters of these subjects are described in Table 1. Patients with RA met the American College of Rheumatology (ACR; formerly, the American Rheumatism Association) criteria for RA (17), and patients with lupus met the ACR criteria for systemic lupus erythematosus (SLE) (18). Lupus disease activity was assessed as previously described (19) or by the Systemic Lupus Activity Measure (SLAM) (20). Lupus was considered inactive if the activity index was <1 or the SLAM was ≤5. PBMC were stimulated with 1 μg/ml phytohemagglutinin (PHA; Burroughs Wellcome, Greenville, NC) and cultured in interleukin-2 (IL-2) for 7–10 days as previously described (7). Exceptions are noted in the text. In some experiments, the CD8+ population was depleted by lysis with anti-CD8 (PharMingen, San Diego, CA) and complement (Pel-Freeze, Brown Deer, WI) using published protocols (21), and purity was checked by staining with anti–CD4–fluorescein isothiocyanate followed by flow cytometric analysis. Jurkat cells were cultured as previously described (1). Where indicated, the cells were treated with PD 98059 (New England Biolabs, Beverly, MA), a selective inhibitor of MAPK extracellular receptor–associated kinase (ERK) 1 (MEK1) (22). Proliferation was measured using tritiated thymidine (^{3}H-TdR) incorporation as previously described (1).

Flow cytometric cell cycle analysis. For cell cycle analysis, peripheral blood T cells were stimulated with PHA and IL-2 as above, then the cells were stained with propidium iodide (Sigma, St. Louis, MO) as previously described (8). The stained cells were analyzed on a Coulter ELITE flow cytometer (Hialeah, FL), and the percentage of cells in G0/G1,S, and G2/M was determined by DNA content.

RNA isolation and Northern analysis. Total RNA was isolated from T cells using TRIzol reagents from Gibco BRL (Gaithersburg, MD). Twenty micrograms of total RNA was electrophoresed in 1% agarose, 2.2*M* formaldehyde gels and transferred to nylon membranes (Micron Separations, Westboro, MA). Care was taken to include RNA from at least 2 normal controls on each membrane and to calculate the expression of RNA relative to these controls, to avoid variability due to technical differences such as efficiency of random priming and hybridization. The membranes were fixed by baking for 2 hours at 80°C and hybridized with a 2.5-kb human Dnmt1 complementary DNA (cDNA) fragment (encoding the 3′ catalytic domain), kindly donated by Dr. Stephen Baylin (23), or a previously described 2.0-kb β-actin cDNA fragment (8). The cDNA probes were labeled by random priming according to the manufacturer's suggestions (Boehringer Mannheim Biochemicals, Indianapolis, IN) with α-^{32}P-dCTP. After hybridization, the membranes were exposed to Kodak radiographic film or developed on a PhosphorImager (Molecular Dynamics, Sunnyvale, CA). Results are calculated as the ratio of the Dnmt1 band intensity to that of β-actin. Where indicated, the blots were also restripped and hybridized with a cDNA encoding a fragment of histone H4 (24). For comparison between groups, the mean of this ratio was determined for the normal controls, and the results from individual patients are expressed as a percentage of this mean value.

Measurement of MAPK activation. Cultured T cells were treated with 50 ng/ml phorbol myristate acetate (PMA; Sigma) with or without 50 ng/ml ionomycin (Sigma) for 15 minutes, then harvested and disrupted by sonication. Insoluble material was removed by centrifugation at 15,000*g* for 20 minutes, and the supernatant was recovered. Proteins were fractionated through 10–20% polyacrylamide gradient gels (Ready gels; Bio-Rad, Hercules, CA) using 25 μg protein per lane, then electrophoretically transferred to polyvinylidene difluoride membranes (Immobilon-P; Millipore, Bedford, MA). Total MAPK and activated MAPK were quantitated using antibodies to the activated, dually phosphorylated form of human ERKs 1 and 2 (Anti–ACTIVE MAPK; Promega, Madison, WI) and previously described protocols (15). Since the monoclonal antibodies (mAb) to the dually phosphorylated forms of ERKs 1 and 2 react only with the activated form of the proteins, MAPK activation is proportional to the intensity of the band produced by this antibody. Controls included isotype-matched irrelevant antibodies, and similar blots were hybridized with an mAb to ERKs 1 and 2, obtained from Zymed (South San Francisco, CA). Band intensity was measured by densitometry as described (8). The ratio of activated to total MAPK was then determined for each subject, and results are presented as the ratio of PMA-treated to untreated preparations. Care was taken to include at least 1 control for each patient on every blot.

Measurement of DNA MTase activity. DNA MTase enzyme activity was measured as previously described (7), except that 2 μg of a hemimethylated synthetic oligonucleotide was used as substrate (25). All determinations were performed in triplicate.

Measurement of genomic deoxymethylcytosine (d^mC) content. An index of genomic d^mC content was obtained by digesting 4 μg of genomic DNA with the isoschisomers *Hpa* II and *Msp* I (both from Sigma), then fractionating the fragments by electrophoresis. *Hpa* II only cleaves unmethylated CCGG sequences, while *Msp* I cleaves CCGG sequences regardless of their methylation status. The fractionated DNA was stained with propidium iodide, and staining intensity was quantitated by densitometry between 2 kb and 3 kb. The results are expressed as the ratio of the *Hpa* II to *Msp* I digests, which increases as DNA demethylates and is more readily digested by *Hpa* II. *Sss* I assays were similarly used to obtain an index of genomic d^mC content, performed as previously described by our group (16). *Sss* I catalyzes the transfer of methyl groups from S-adenosylmethionine to unmethylated dC residues in CpG pairs. Using S-adenosyl-L-[methyl-^{3}H]methionine as the methyl donor, ^{3}H-TdR incorporation is inversely proportional to the extent of DNA methylation (16).

Statistical analysis. The significance of differences between groups was determined using analysis of variance (ANOVA) or Student's *t*-test. Regression analysis was performed with SySTAT software (Evanston, IL).

RESULTS

Decreased Dnmt1 messenger RNA (mRNA) levels in lupus T cells. To determine if Dnmt1 mRNA levels are decreased in lupus T cells, PBMC were isolated from 7 patients with active lupus, 8 patients with inactive lupus, 5 patients with RA, and normal controls. The control population consisted of 17 healthy individuals (44% women and 56% men), ages 32 ± 7 years (mean ± SD; range 22–47 years). To measure Dnmt1 expression, the PBMC were first stimulated with PHA and IL-2 as described previously (7). Stimulation is essential because little, if any, Dnmt1 mRNA is expressed in unstimulated T cells (15). RNA was isolated, and DNA MTase mRNA was measured by Northern analysis. At least 2 normal control PBMC samples were included on every gel. The filters were then stripped, rehybridized with a β-actin cDNA, and developed as autoradiograms. β-actin was chosen as a control because its expression does not change in lupus T cells (26). To confirm that β-actin levels are not altered in lupus T cells, the β-actin band intensities were compared between the patients with active lupus and the healthy controls, and expressed as the mean ratio of lupus to controls. This ratio was 1.09 ± 0.33 (mean ± SEM). Representative Northern blots are shown in Figure 1A.

All subjects demonstrated Dnmt1 transcripts of the same size. Band intensities were quantitated by densitometry, and relative Dnmt1 levels were calculated as the ratio of the intensity of the Dnmt1 band to that of the β-actin band for each subject. In Figure 1B, the results are expressed relative to the mean band intensity ratio of normal controls, arbitrarily defined as 100%. The results demonstrate that DNA MTase mRNA levels in patients with active lupus were ~50% lower than those in healthy controls and RA patients as well as patients with inactive lupus (P = 0.034 overall by ANOVA; $P < 0.05$ for active lupus versus each of the other 3 groups by pairwise post hoc comparison). This abnormality was detectable for up to 10 days in culture. These mRNA levels are consistent with our prior activity measurements that showed an ~50% decrease in DNA MTase enzyme activity in lupus patients relative to healthy controls and RA patients (7).

The decrease in Dnmt1 mRNA in the T cells from patients with active lupus could not be attributed to corticosteroids, because similar numbers of patients with active and inactive lupus were receiving this drug (Table 1). Furthermore, we have reported that corticosteroids do not affect DNA methylation (7). More subjects with inactive lupus than those with active disease were receiving antimalarial agents, suggesting that these agents were also not contributing to the decrease in Dnmt1 mRNA levels in those with active disease. Similar numbers of patients were also receiving cyclophosphamide. There were

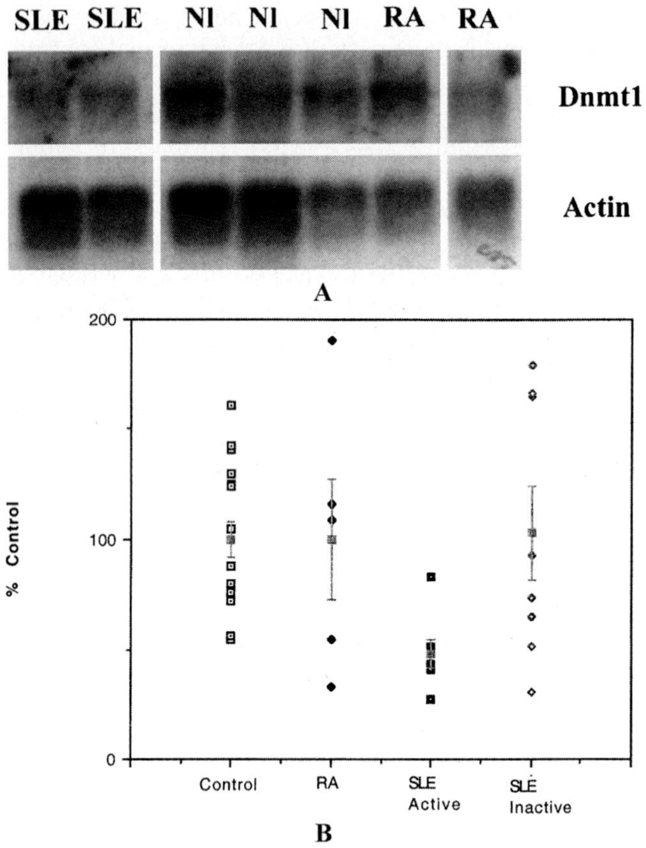

Figure 1. DNA (cytosine-5)-methyltransferase messenger RNA (mRNA) levels in lupus patients and controls. **A,** Peripheral blood mononuclear cells (PBMC) from 2 patients with active systemic lupus erythematosus (SLE), 2 patients with rheumatoid arthritis (RA), and 3 healthy controls (Nl) were stimulated with phytohemagglutin and interleukin-2 as described in Patients and Methods. RNA was then isolated, fractionated by agarose gel electrophoresis, transferred to nylon membranes, hybridized with a ^{32}P-labeled complementary DNA (cDNA) encoding the 3′ half of human DNA methyltransferase 1 (Dnmt1), then developed as an autoradiogram (upper panel). The membranes were then stripped and rehybridized with a ^{32}P-labeled β-actin cDNA (lower panel). **B,** PBMC from 7 patients with active lupus, 8 with inactive lupus, 5 with RA, and 17 normal controls were stimulated and Dnmt1 and β-actin mRNA were detected as in **A.** The ratios of Dnmt1 to actin band densities were normalized to the average of the ratios from at least 2 healthy controls included on each blot. Each point represents a single subject, and some of the points overlap. Bars show the mean ± SEM of the group.

similar numbers of women in the active and inactive lupus groups, thus arguing against a sex-specific effect. In addition, no significant differences in Dnmt1 mRNA levels were observed between healthy men and women (112 ± 17% versus 92 ± 12% [mean ± SEM] for 5 men and 7 women, respectively; compared on the same gels).

Since T cells from patients with active lupus are relatively anergic (for review, see ref. 27), it is possible that the decreased Dnmt1 levels reflected a lower percentage of proliferating cells. To exclude this possibility, cell cycling, as determined by propidium iodide staining, was measured in the stimulated T cells from 5 healthy controls, 5 patients with active lupus, and 4 patients with RA (Figure 2). No differences were seen, indicating that the decrease in DNA MTase was not due to differences in the kinetics of cell cycling.

We then asked if the decrease in Dnmt1 could be due to decreased ras-MAPK signaling. T cells from lupus patients with active and inactive disease and from RA patients were stimulated with PHA and IL-2 as

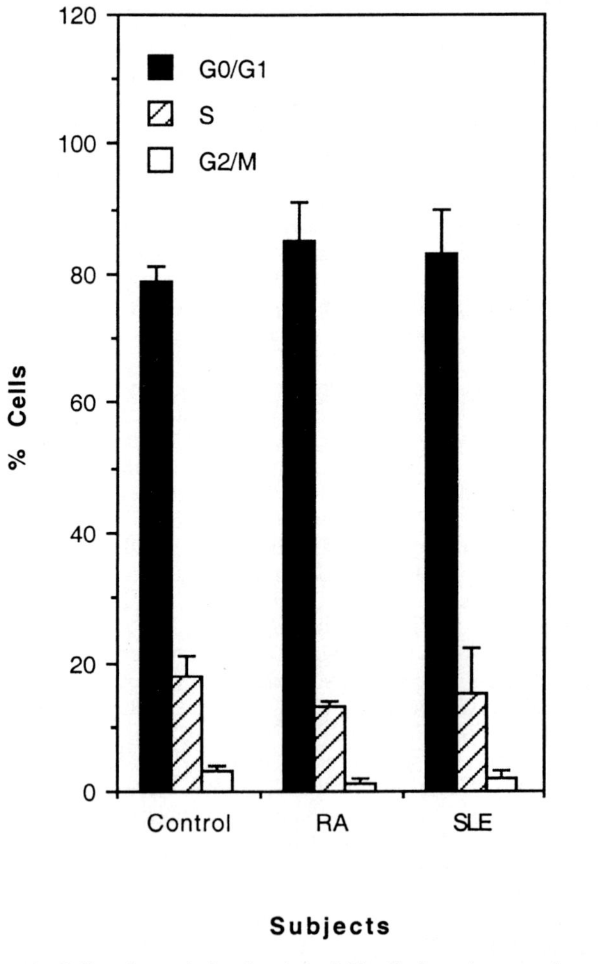

Figure 2. Cell cycle analysis of activated T cells from lupus patients and controls. Phytohemagglutinin- and interleukin-2–stimulated T cells from healthy controls (n = 5), rheumatoid arthritis (RA) patients (n = 4), or patients with active systemic lupus erythematosus (SLE; n = 5) were analyzed by propidium iodide staining and flow cytometric analysis. Results represent the mean and SEM percentage of cells from the subjects in each group.

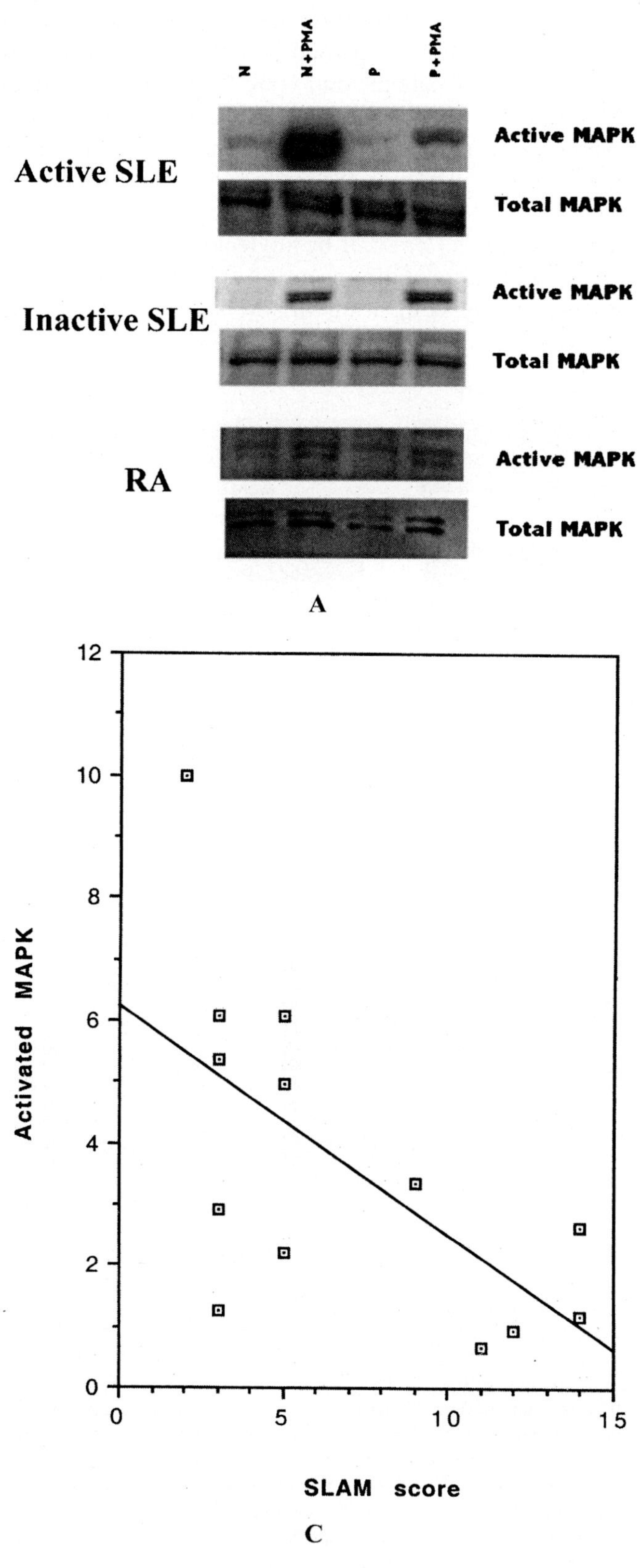

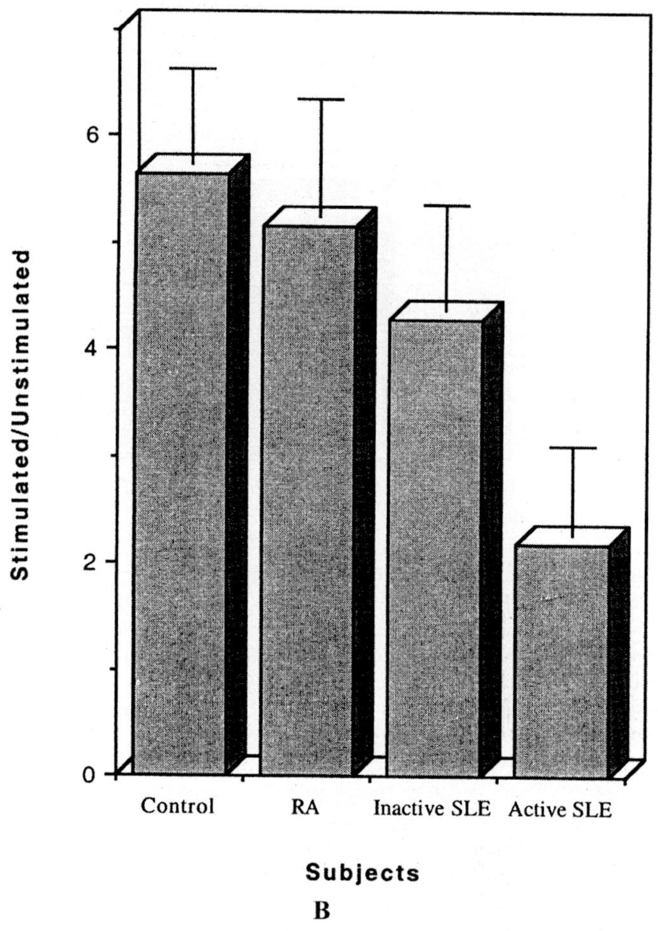

Figure 3. Decreased mitogen-activated protein kinase (MAPK) phosphorylation in lupus T cells. **A,** T cells from a healthy control (N) or from patients (P) with active or inactive systemic lupus erythematosus (SLE) or rheumatoid arthritis (RA) were stimulated with phytohemagglutinin and interleukin-2 as in Figure 1. Aliquots of cells were treated with 50 ng/ml phorbol myristate acetate (PMA) for 15 minutes, then treated (+PMA) and untreated cells were lysed and proteins separated by sodium dodecyl sulfate–polyacrylamide gel electrophoresis using 25 μg protein per lane. The fractionated proteins were transferred to polyvinylidene difluoride membranes and developed as immunoblots using antibodies to the activated, dually phosphorylated form of human extracellular receptor–associated kinases 1 and 2 (Active MAPK) or to framework determinants (Total MAPK). **B,** Quantitative immunoblot analysis of activated and total MAPK was performed as described in Patients and Methods, using T cells from 18 healthy controls, 5 patients with RA, 8 patients with inactive lupus, and 5 patients with active lupus, and the ratio of activated to total MAPK was determined for unstimulated and PMA-stimulated cells from each subject. Results are presented as the ratio of PMA-stimulated to unstimulated preparations, and represent the mean and SEM of the determinations within each group. **C,** Regression analysis comparing the Systemic Lupus Activity Measure (SLAM) score of the patients with lupus with the degree of MAPK phosphorylation.

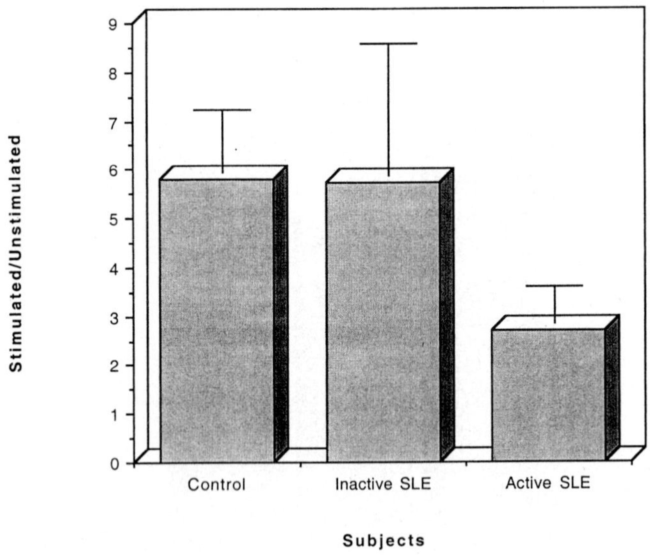

Figure 4. Decreased MAPK phosphorylation in CD4+ lupus T cells. PBMC were isolated from 5 healthy controls, 3 patients with inactive lupus, and 4 patients with active lupus. CD4+ T cells were depleted by treatment with anti-CD8 plus complement, and MAPK activation was studied as in Figure 3B. Cells were ~98% CD4+ at the time of analysis by cytofluorography. Bars show the mean and SEM. See Figures 1 and 3 for definitions.

before. The cells were then treated with PMA, and total MAPK was quantitated by immunoblotting. PMA was used, rather than T cell receptor crosslinking agents, because others have reported abnormalities in early signaling events in lupus T cells (28), which would confound interpretation of the results. No differences in the amount of total MAPK protein was observed between the groups (105%, 99%, and 87%, for active lupus, inactive lupus, and RA T cells, respectively, relative to normal controls). Parallel gels were reacted with an mAb that is reactive with the dually phosphorylated, activated forms of ERKs 1 and 2.

Figure 3A shows that PMA treatment caused significantly less MAPK activation in T cells from a representative lupus patient relative to that in a healthy control. The addition of ionomycin gave identical results (not shown). Kinetic studies demonstrated that both lupus patients and controls had optimal MAPK activation at 15 minutes. For reference, similar studies using T cells from patients with inactive lupus and RA are also shown (Figure 3A), and the results resembled those in the controls. Similar studies were performed on T cells from 18 healthy controls, 5 patients with RA, 8 patients with inactive lupus, and 5 patients with active lupus. The healthy controls consisted of 10 men and 8 women, age 32 ± 7 years (mean ± SD; range 21–49 years). Figure 3B compares the relative amounts of activated MAPK in untreated and PMA-treated T cells from the lupus patients and controls, adjusted for total MAPK protein content from each patient. While PMA caused an increase in MAPK phosphorylation in T cells isolated from all groups, the increase in T cells from lupus patients was the smallest, and significantly less than that in normal controls ($P = 0.01$ by Student's t-test).

The effect of disease activity on MAPK activation was tested by comparing SLAM scores with MAPK

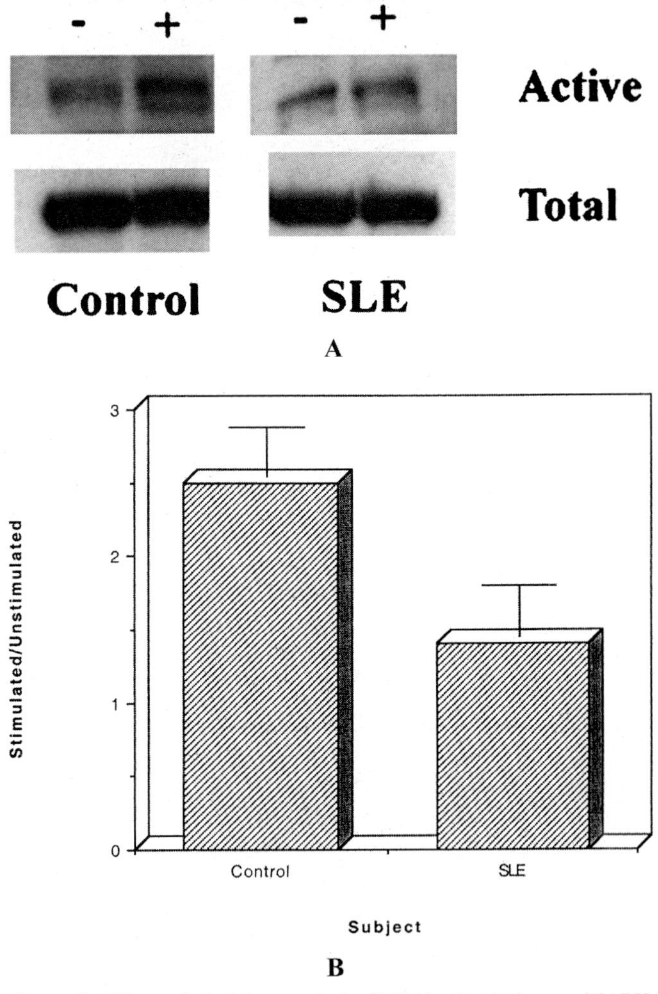

Figure 5. Effect of phytohemagglutin (PHA) stimulation on MAPK signaling in control and lupus T cells. **A,** PBMC from a healthy control and a patient with active lupus were cultured alone (−) or stimulated with interleukin-2 and PHA (+), and 30 minutes later, active MAPK was measured as in Figure 3 (upper panel). Total MAPK was also measured as described in Figure 3, analyzed using a duplicate gel (lower panel). **B,** PBMC from 4 controls and 3 patients with active lupus were stimulated with PHA and analyzed as in **A.** Bars show the mean and SEM of the ratio of activated to total MAPK, as in Figure 3. See Figures 1 and 3 for other definitions.

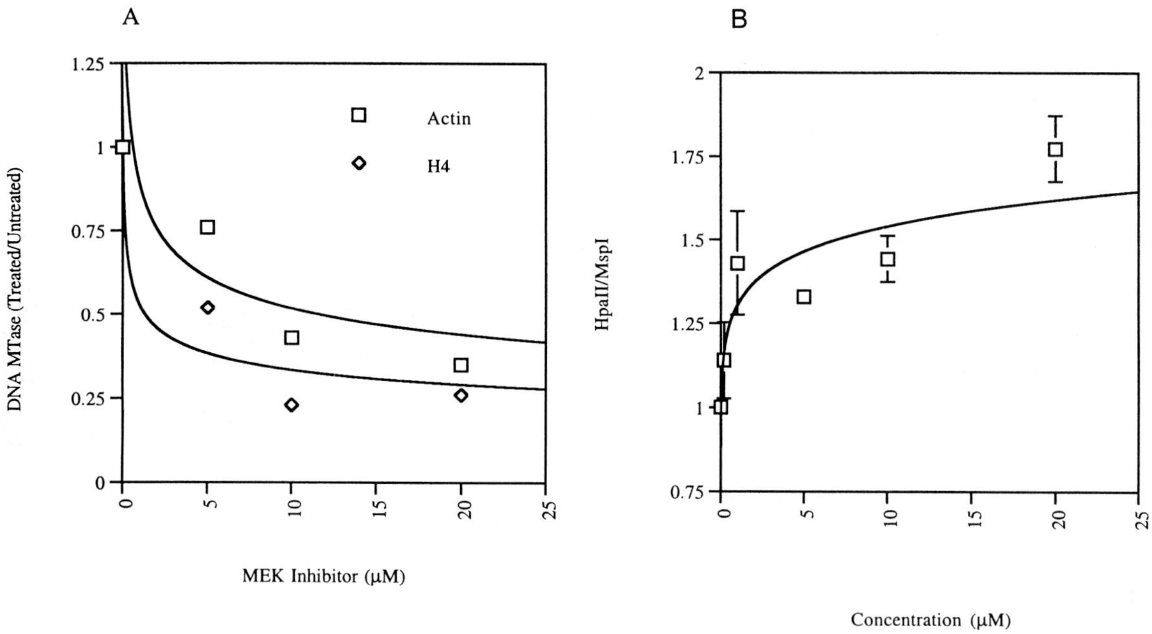

Figure 6. Effect of decreased MAPK signaling on Dnmt1 mRNA and DNA methylation. **A,** Jurkat cells were treated with the indicated concentrations of PD 98059, and 90 minutes later, mRNA was isolated and analyzed for DNA (cytosine-5)-methyltransferase (MTase) and β-actin expression as described in Figure 1, then stripped and restudied for histone H4 expression. Results are expressed as the DNA MTase to β-actin ratio or the DNA MTase to H4 ratio in treated/untreated cells, and are representative of 3 experiments. **B,** Jurkat cells were treated with the indicated concentrations of the MAPK extracellular receptor–associated kinase 1 (MEK1) inhibitor, and 48 hours later, DNA was isolated, digested with *Hpa* II or *Msp* I, then fractionated by electrophoresis and stained with ethidium bromide. Results are presented as the ratio of the *Hpa* II to *Msp* I integrated intensities between 2 kb and 3 kb, and represent the mean ± SEM of 3 independent experiments. See Figures 1 and 3 for other definitions.

activation. Figure 3C shows that as disease activity increased, the degree of MAPK phosphorylation decreased significantly (slope −0.47, $P = 0.004$). This suggests that ras-MAPK signaling is decreased in T cells from patients with active lupus, and may contribute to the decrease in DNA MTase activity. This defect was also stable in culture for up to 10 days.

Since these studies were performed on polyclonal populations containing both CD4+ and CD8+ cells, it was important to determine if the same results could be obtained using purified CD4+ T cells. CD8+ cells were removed by cytolytic depletion, and then the cells were stimulated and cultured as before. These cells were routinely 98% CD4+ by flow cytometric analysis. Figure 4 compares MAPK phosphorylation in PMA-stimulated CD4+ cells from 5 healthy controls, 3 patients with inactive lupus, and 4 patients with active lupus. The CD4+ T cells from patients with active lupus had significantly less MAPK phosphorylation relative to that in healthy controls ($P < 0.05$).

To determine if the defect in MAPK signaling was reflected by differences in the basal phosphorylation of ERKs 1 and 2 in the unstimulated T cells, the ratio of activated to total MAPK was also compared between controls and patients, for unstimulated cells only. There was no difference in this ratio between controls and patients with RA or patients with inactive lupus (mean ± SEM 1.00 ± 0.33 and 1.51 ± 0.33 in RA and inactive lupus patients, respectively, relative to paired controls). In contrast, there was relatively less basal MAPK activation in the T cells from patients with active lupus (0.69 ± 0.12) ($P = 0.049$ versus controls by Student's paired *t*-test).

It was possible that the defect in MAPK signaling was detectable only with PMA stimulation, but not with stimulation using ligands of cell surface receptors. To exclude this possibility, the effect of PHA stimulation on MAPK activation was examined. Preliminary studies demonstrated that MAPK activation was maximal 30 minutes after the addition of PHA. PBMC from 3 patients with active lupus and 4 normal controls (59–83% CD2+) were stimulated with PHA and IL-2 for 30 minutes, and MAPK activation was then measured. Figure 5A shows representative immunoblots from 1 patient and 1 control, and Figure 5B shows the average ratio of activated to total MAPK in the subjects (P = 0.011). The results indicate that a signaling defect resembling that detected using PMA in lupus T cells is detectable with PHA stimulation as well, and is present in freshly isolated PBMC.

Effect of decreased ras-MAPK signaling on T cell DNA methylation. To determine the functional significance of decreased ras-MAPK signaling on T cell DNA methylation, we compared Dnmt1 mRNA expression, enzyme activity, and genomic $d^{m}C$ content in Jurkat T cells treated with PD 98059, a selective MEK1 inhibitor. At the concentrations used in this study, this agent does not affect the activity of at least 18 other known kinases, including those involved in the c-Jun N-terminal kinase (JNK) and p38 cascades, and a >80% inhibition of MEK1 activity is usually achieved at 50 μM (22).

Figure 6A demonstrates that the MEK1 inhibitor decreased the levels of Jurkat mRNA by ~50% relative to those with β-actin and histone H4 (a cell cycle–specific gene), similar to the decrease seen in the lupus patients. Figure 6B compares genomic $d^{m}C$ content in untreated and MEK1 inhibitor–treated Jurkat cells. For this assay, DNA was digested with *Hpa* II and *Msp* I. *Hpa* II recognizes and cuts unmethylated, but not methylated, CCGG sequences, while *Msp* I cuts CCGG sequences regardless of their methylation status. Results are expressed as the ratio of *Hpa* II to *Msp* I digests, and the ratio increases as DNA becomes more hypomethylated and thus more readily digested by *Hpa* II. The results show that treatment with PD 98059 decreased total genomic $d^{m}C$ content (20 μM versus 0 or 0.2 μM; $P < 0.01$).

To confirm that inhibiting ras-MAPK signaling will also decrease DNA MTase enzyme activity, Jurkat cells were treated with 20 μM PD 98059. The level of DNA MTase enzyme activity per μg nuclear protein in the treated cells was 62 ± 2% of controls (mean ± SEM of 3 determinations, each performed in triplicate) ($P <$ 0.01 by univariate t-test of the mean), thus correlating with mRNA levels.

These results were confirmed by treating PHA-stimulated, IL-2–dependent normal T cells with 20 μM PD 98059, then measuring DNA MTase activity (Figure 7). PD 98059 decreased enzyme activity by 58 ± 12% (mean ± SEM of triplicate determinations) ($P < 0.01$). In contrast, no effect was seen on the proliferation of these cells, indicating that the decrease did not represent an effect on cell cycling. *Sss* I assays were used to compare $d^{m}C$ content in the treated and untreated cells. Jurkat cells, as well as normal T cells similarly stimulated

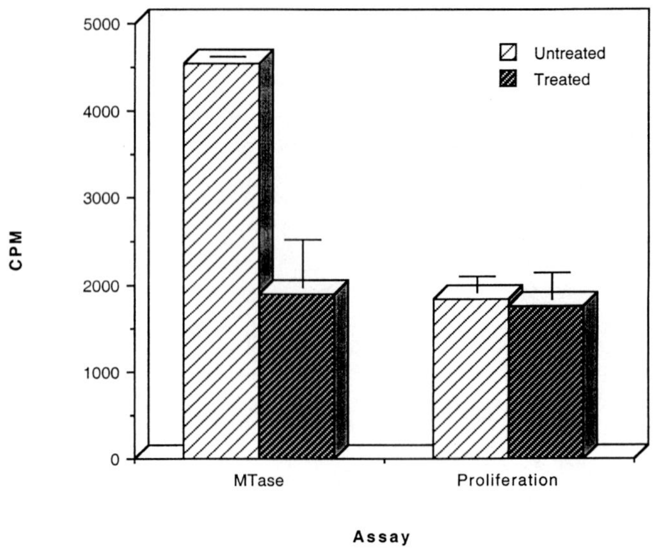

Figure 7. Effect of an MEK1 inhibitor on DNA MTase activity in normal T cells. T cells were stimulated with phytohemagglutinin and interleukin-2 as in Figure 1, then cultured alone (untreated) or with 20 μM PD 98059 (treated) for 24 hours. DNA MTase activity was measured as described in Patients and Methods. Results represent the counts per minute (CPM) of ^{3}H-thymidine incorporated in hemimethylated synthetic oligonucleotides per μg protein, and are presented as the mean and SEM of 3 determinations. Proliferation was measured at the same time by culturing 20,000 untreated or treated cells with ^{3}H-thymidine for 2 hours in microtiter wells, then ^{3}H-thymidine incorporation into DNA was assessed. See Figure 6 for definitions.

with PHA and IL-2, were treated with 20 μM PD 98059 for 24 hours, then DNA was isolated and *Sss* I–catalyzed ^{3}H-TdR incorporation was compared. PD 98059 treatment increased ^{3}H-TdR incorporation by 10.2 ± 1.3% in normal T cells and by 8.8 ± 0.2% in Jurkat T cells (mean ± SEM of duplicate determinations), indicating that inhibiting ras-MAPK signaling inhibits DNA methylation in normal T cells as well as in Jurkat cells.

The observation that inhibiting ras-MAPK signaling causes decreased Dnmt1 mRNA levels and enzyme activity, as well as producing DNA hypomethylation, argues strongly that the decrease in DNA MTase activity and the DNA hypomethylation seen in lupus T cells is due to decreased signaling through the ras-MAPK pathway.

DISCUSSION

The goal of these studies was to determine the mechanism causing a decrease in DNA MTase enzyme activity and DNA hypomethylation in lupus T cells. Since inhibiting DNA MTase was previously shown to be sufficient to cause a lupus-like disease (5,6), early experiments sought evidence for an endogenous inhibitor. However, mixing studies gave no evidence for an inhibitor in lupus T cells (Richardson B et al: unpublished results). More recently, we reported that DNA MTase levels depend on T cell stimulation, and that the levels are regulated, in part, by the ras-MAPK signaling pathway (15,16). In the present studies, we therefore asked if regulation of Dnmt1 by this pathway might be abnormal in lupus T cells.

DNA MTase levels were compared using activated T cells. This was necessary because Dnmt1 is not expressed in unstimulated T cells (15). The results demonstrated a decrease in the amount of Dnmt1 mRNA in lupus T cells, which was almost identical in magnitude to the decrease in enzyme activity previously reported (7). Since we have previously reported a close correlation between the levels of the T cell DNA MTase enzyme and Dnmt1 mRNA levels (15), this suggests that the decrease in enzyme activity is due to a decrease in the level of the mRNA. It should be noted that T cells from patients with active lupus can be refractory to stimulation (27). To avoid this problem, which could result in an artifactual decrease in DNA MTase, the cells were stimulated with PHA and IL-2, then activation was compared by propidium iodide cell cycling studies (also done in a previous study [7]). This strategy confirmed equivalent stimulation between groups. Thus, the DNA MTase decrease is not due to inefficient stimulation of the lupus T cells. Furthermore, the decrease persisted for up to 10 days in culture, suggesting a stable biochemical abnormality.

We next asked if ras-MAPK signaling might be defective in these cells. Decreased MAPK phosphorylation following PMA stimulation was observed in T cells from patients with active lupus, implying that the decrease in DNA MTase could be due to a decrease in ras-MAPK signaling. Inhibiting MEK1 activation caused a similar 50% decrease in Jurkat Dnmt1 mRNA and a corresponding decrease in enzyme activity in Jurkat and normal T cells, and induced DNA hypomethylation resembling that seen in lupus T cells, further suggesting that impaired signaling causes the decrease in Dnmt1 enzyme activity and DNA hypomethylation characteristic of lupus. It should be noted that the MEK1 inhibitor did not completely suppress Dnmt1 expression, implying the existence of other elements providing the remaining promoter activity. Indeed, there is a CpG island, typical of housekeeping genes and containing promoter elements (29), located 5′ to the MTase gene AP-1 sites implicated in ras-MAPK signaling (30), which may also drive this expression.

Other investigators have made observations consistent with the notion of defective ras-MAPK signaling in lupus. For example, IL-2 secretion has been shown to be defective in lupus T cells (31), and IL-2 is regulated, in part, by the ras-MAPK pathway (32,33). Other investigators, using electrophoretic mobility shift assays, have demonstrated that lupus T cells contain less of the AP-1 transcription factor (34), the activation of which is also regulated by this pathway (35). How decreased signaling through the ras-MAPK pathway relates to other signaling abnormalities in lupus T cells (36,37) is unknown at this time.

The mechanism causing the decrease in signaling is unknown. The strategy of stimulating with PMA and measuring MAPK phosphorylation suggests that the defect may lie in protein kinase C, ras, raf, or MEK. Interestingly, preliminary evidence suggests that JNK pathway signaling is normal in patients with active SLE (38), raising the possibility that the defect is unique to the MAPK pathway. The precise mechanisms causing the decrease in signaling, as well as its relationship to lymphocyte subsets and disease activity, will be the subject of future studies.

Recently, additional enzymes modifying DNA methylation have been identified. These include Dnmt3a and Dnmt3b, which mediate de novo methylation (39), as well as a putative demethylase (40). The identification of these enzymes implies that cells have the ability to modify methylation patterns in unstimulated cells, as well as during mitosis through the effects on Dnmt1. Whether these enzymes are expressed in mature T lymphocytes is unknown, and their potential role in the DNA hypomethylation associated with lupus is yet to be determined. However, the observation that inhibiting ras-MAPK signaling decreases Dnmt1 expression to the same extent as that observed in lupus, and that this decrease correlates with DNA hypomethylation in vitro and in vivo, suggests that the defect in Dnmt1 is the primary reason for DNA hypomethylation in SLE.

In summary, these studies suggest a novel mechanism that could contribute to the development of idiopathic lupus, and perhaps to the characteristic disease flares occurring after stresses such as infections (41). In this model, T cells are stimulated to divide by exogenous antigens, but a failure of the cell to adequately up-regulate Dnmt1 results in DNA hypomethylation with subsequent T cell autoreactivity, lasting until the cells more completely remethylate the DNA, or until T cells are suppressed by other immune mechanisms.

Since inhibiting DNA MTase with lupus-inducing drugs has similar effects on T cells, and T cells treated with DNA methylation inhibitors cause a lupus-like disease in vivo, these results suggest a common mechanism for drug-induced and idiopathic lupus.

ACKNOWLEDGMENTS

The authors thank Drs. Gary Kammer, George Tsokos, and C. William Castor for their many helpful discussions and support during the course of these studies. The authors would also like to thank Dr. Steven Baylin for providing the Dnmt1 cDNA, Ms Janet Stevens for her excellent secretarial assistance, and the Department of Pediatrics and the Division of Geriatrics at the University of Michigan Hospital for providing the laboratory space to perform these studies.

REFERENCES

1. Cornacchia E, Golbus J, Maybaum J, Strahler J, Hanash S, Richardson BC. Hydralazine and procainamide inhibit T cell DNA methylation and induce autoreactivity. J Immunol 1988;140:2197–200.
2. Yung R, Chang S, Hemati N, Johnson K, Richardson B. Mechanisms of drug-induced lupus. IV. Comparison of procainamide and hydralazine with analogs in vitro and in vivo. Arthritis Rheum 1997;40:1436–43.
3. Richardson B, Powers D, Hooper F, Yung RL, O'Rourke K. Lymphocyte function–associated antigen 1 overexpression and T cell autoreactivity. Arthritis Rheum 1994;37:1363–72.
4. Yung R, Powers D, Johnson K, Amento E, Carr D, Laing T, et al. Mechanisms of drug-induced lupus. II. T cells overexpressing lymphocyte function-associated antigen 1 become autoreactive and cause a lupus-like disease in syngeneic recipients. J Clin Invest 1996;97:2866–71.
5. Quddus J, Johnson KJ, Gavalchin J, Amento EP, Warren JS, Chrisp C, et al. Treating activated CD4+ T cells with either of two distinct DNA methyltransferase inhibitors, 5-azacytidine or procainamide, is sufficient to induce a lupus-like disease in syngeneic mice. J Clin Invest 1993;92:38–53.
6. Yung RL, Quddus J, Chrisp CE, Johnson KJ, Richardson BC. Mechanisms of drug induced lupus. I. Cloned Th2 cells modified with DNA methylation inhibitors in vitro cause autoimmunity in vivo. J Immunol 1995;154:3025–35.
7. Richardson B, Scheinbart L, Strahler J, Gross L, Hanash S, Johnson M. Evidence for impaired T cell DNA methylation in systemic lupus erythematosus and rheumatoid arthritis. Arthritis Rheum 1990;33:1665–73.
8. Richardson BC, Strahler JR, Pivirotto TS, Quddus J, Bayliss GE, Gross LA, et al. Phenotypic and functional similarities between 5-azacytidine–treated T cells and a T cell subset in patients with active systemic lupus erythematosus. Arthritis Rheum 1992;35:647–62.
9. Corvetta A, Bitta RD, Luchetti MM, Pomponio G. 5-methylcytosine content of DNA in blood, synovial mononuclear cells and synovial tissue from patients affected by autoimmune rheumatic diseases. J Chromatogr 1991;66:481–91.
10. Takeuchi T, Amano K, Sekine H, Koide J, Abe T. Upregulated expression and function of integrin adhesive receptors in systemic lupus erythematosus patients with vasculitis. J Clin Invest 1993;92:3008–16.
11. Bestor T, Laudano A, Mattaliano R, Ingram V. Cloning and sequencing of a cDNA encoding DNA methyltransferase of mouse cells. J Mol Biol 1988;203:971–83.
12. Scheinbart LS, Johnson MA, Gross LA, Edelstein SR, Richardson BC. Procainamide inhibits DNA methyltransferase in a human T cell line. J Rheumatol 1991;18:530–4.
13. Rouleau J, MacLeod AR, Szyf M. Regulation of the DNA methyltransferase by the Ras-AP-1 signaling pathway. J Biol Chem 1995;270:1595–601.
14. MacLeod AR, Rouleau J, Szyf M. Regulation of DNA methylation by the Ras signaling pathway. J Biol Chem 1995;270:11327–37.
15. Yang J, Deng C, Hemati N, Hanash SM, Richardson BC. Effect of mitogenic stimulation and DNA methylation on human T-cell DNA methyltransferase expression and activity. J Immunol 1997;159:1303–9.
16. Deng C, Yang J, Scott J, Hanash S, Richardson BC. Role of the ras-MAPK signaling pathway in the DNA methyltransferase response to DNA hypomethylation. Biol Chem 1998;379:1113–20.
17. Arnett FC, Edworthy SM, Bloch DA, McShane DJ, Fries JF, Cooper NS, et al. The American Rheumatism Association 1987 revised criteria for the classification of rheumatoid arthritis. Arthritis Rheum 1988;31:315–24.
18. Tan EM, Cohen AS, Fries JF, Masi AT, McShane DJ, Rothfield NF, et al. The 1982 revised criteria for the classification of systemic lupus erythematosus. Arthritis Rheum 1982;25:1271–7.
19. Golbus J, Salata M, Greenwood J, Hudson J, Richardson BC. Increased immunoglobulin response to γ-interferon by lymphocytes from patients with systemic lupus erythematosus. Clin Immunol Immunopathol 1988;46:129–40.
20. Liang MH, Socher SA, Larson MG, Schur PH. Reliability and validity of six systems for the clinical assessment of disease activity in systemic lupus erythematosus. Arthritis Rheum 1989;32:1107–18.
21. Richardson BC, Liebling MR, Hudson JL. CD4+ cells treated with DNA methylation inhibitors induce autologous B cell differentiation. Clin Immunol Immunopathol 1990;55:368–81.
22. Alessi DR, Cuenda A, Cohen P, Dudley DT, Saltiel AR. PD098059 is a specific inhibitor of the activation of mitogen-activated protein kinase kinases in vitro and in vivo. J Biol Chem 1995;270:27489–94.
23. Yen RC, Vertino PM, Nelkin BD, Yu JJ, El-Deiry W, Cumaraswamy A, et al. Isolation and characterization of the cDNA encoding human DNA methyltransferase. Nucleic Acids Res 1992;20:2287–91.
24. Lee PJ, Washer LL, Law DJ, Boland CR, Horon IL, Feinberg AP. Limited up-regulation of DNA methyltransferase in human colon cancer reflecting increased cell proliferation. Proc Natl Acad Sci U S A 1996;93:10366–70.
25. Szyf M, Bozovic V, Tanigawa G. Growth regulation of mouse DNA methyltransferase gene expression. J Biol Chem 1991;296:10027–30.
26. Klinman DM, Mushinski JF, Masaaki H, Ishigatsubo Y, Mountz JD, Raveche ES, et al. Oncogene expression in autoimmune and normal peripheral blood mononuclear cells. J Exp Med 1986;163:1292–307.
27. Dayal AK, Kammer GM. The T cell enigma in lupus. Arthritis Rheum 1996;39:23–33.
28. Liossis S-NC, Ding XZ, Dennis GJ, Tsokos GC. Altered pattern of TCR/CD3-mediated protein-tyrosyl phosphorylation in T cells from patients with systemic lupus erythematosus. J Clin Invest 1998;101:1448–57.
29. Antequera F, Bird A. CpG islands. In: Jost JP, Saluz HP, editors. DNA methylation: molecular biology and biological significance. Basel: Birkhäuser Verlag; 1993. p. 169–85.
30. Tucker K, Talbot D, Lee M, Leonhardt H, Jaenisch R. Complementation of methylation deficiency in embryonic stem cells by a

DNA methyltransferase minigene. Biochemistry 1996;93: 12920–25.
31. Kammer GM, Stein RL. T-lymphocyte immune dysfunctions in systemic lupus erythematosus. J Lab Clin Med 1990;273–82.
32. Williams N. T cell inactivation linked to Ras block. Science 1996;271:1234.
33. Umlauf SW, Beverly B, Kang S-M, Brorson K, Tran A-C, Schwartz RH. Molecular regulation of the IL-2 gene: rheostatic control of the immune system. Immunol Rev 1993;133:177–97.
34. Becker H, Stengl G, Stein M, Federlin K. Analysis of proteins that interact with the IL-2 regulatory region in patients with rheumatic diseases. Clin Exp Immunol 1995;99:325–30.
35. Khosravi-Far R, Der CJ. The Ras signal transduction pathway. Cancer Metastasis Rev 1994;13:67–89.
36. Vassilopoulous D, Kovacs B, Tsokos GC. TCR/CD3 complex-mediated signal transduction pathway in T cells and T cell lines from patients with systemic lupus erythematosus. J Immunol 1995;155:2269–81.
37. Kammer GM, Khan IU, Malemud C. Deficient Type I protein kinase A isozyme activity in systemic lupus erythematosus T lymphocytes. J Clin Invest 1994;94:422–30.
38. Rao T, Deng C, Richardson BC. Effects of DNA methylation inhibitors and lupus on T cell signaling pathways [abstract]. Arthritis Rheum 1999;42:S310.
39. Okano M, Xie S, Li E. Cloning and characterization of a family of novel mammalian DNA (cytosine-5) methyltransferases. Nat Genet 1998;19:219–20.
40. Bhattacharya SK, Ramchandani S, Cervoni N, Szyf M. A mammalian protein with specific demethylase activity of mCpG DNA. Nature 1999;397:579–83.
41. Rothfield NF. Systemic lupus erythematosus: clinical and laboratory aspects. In: McCarty DJ, editor. Arthritis and allied conditions. Philadelphia: Lea & Febiger; 1979. p. 691–772.

ARTHRITIS & RHEUMATISM
Vol. 44, No. 2, February 2001, pp 408–418

"Lymphoid" Chemokine Messenger RNA Expression by Epithelial Cells in the Chronic Inflammatory Lesion of the Salivary Glands of Sjögren's Syndrome Patients

Possible Participation in Lymphoid Structure Formation

Georgina Xanthou,[1] Mary Polihronis,[1] Athanasios G. Tzioufas,[1] Spyros Paikos,[1] Paschalis Sideras,[2] and Haralampos M. Moutsopoulos[1]

Objective. **Many studies have shown that the microanatomic organization of infiltrating leukocytes in the salivary gland lesions of patients with Sjögren's syndrome (SS) resembles the structure of lymphoid organs. A newly defined set of chemokines referred to as "lymphoid," which orchestrate leukocyte microenvironmental homing and contribute to the formation of lymphoid structures, provides directional clues. The aim of this study was to investigate the possible existence of "lymphoid" chemokines in the chronic inflammatory lesions of SS patients and thus validate their potential involvement in the disease process.**

Methods. **Twelve patients with primary SS, 3 patients with secondary SS, 4 patients with other autoimmune disorders, and 4 control individuals were the subjects of this study. Reverse transcriptase–polymerase chain reaction analysis was performed in order to examine the messenger RNA (mRNA) expression of "lymphoid" chemokines. Furthermore, in situ hybridization studies revealed chemokine mRNA localization. Immunohistochemistry was also applied in order to identify the cell types that expressed the chemokine mRNA.**

Results. **STCP-1/monocyte-derived chemokine and TARC mRNA were expressed in the majority of patients with primary and secondary SS, in 2 of 4 patients with other autoimmune disorders, and in 2 of 4 controls. BCA-1, ELC, and PARC mRNA were only detected in patients with primary and secondary SS. SLC mRNA was also detected in 1 non-SS patient. The main cellular sources of chemokine mRNA were ductal epithelial cells and infiltrating mononuclear leukocytes.**

Conclusion. **The expression pattern of "lymphoid" chemokine mRNA points further to the role of epithelial cells in the pathogenesis of SS and offers new insight into the potential mechanisms that could be involved in leukocyte attraction and in the in situ formation of secondary lymphoid tissue structures.**

Supported by grant EPET II: 70/3/4440 from the General Secretariat for Research & Technology of the Hellenic Ministry of Development and the Swedish Medical Research Council.

[1]Georgina Xanthou, BSc, Mary Polihronis, PhD, Athanasios G. Tzioufas, MD, Spyros Paikos, DDS, Haralampos M. Moutsopoulos, MD: University of Athens, Athens, Greece; [2]Paschalis Sideras, PhD: Lund University, Lund, Sweden.

Address correspondence and reprint requests to Professor Haralampos M. Moutsopoulos, MD, Department of Pathophysiology, Medical School, University of Athens, M. Asias 75 St., Goudi, Athens 115 27, Greece.

Submitted for publication July 12, 2000; accepted in revised form October 13, 2000.

The major immunopathologic phenomenon observed in Sjögren's syndrome (SS) patients is mononuclear cell infiltration of the salivary and lachrymal glands, resulting in the destruction of epithelial cells, degeneration of the surrounding tissue, and diminished secretion (1,2).

The inflammatory lesions that are formed in minor salivary gland (MSG) biopsy tissue contain focal aggregates with T cells, B lymphocytes, and follicular dendritic cells, which first appear as small clusters around ducts and later enlarge to form structures that resemble organized lymphoid tissues. Recent studies have documented that some of these structures have the appearance and function of germinal centers (3,4). The process of lymphoid tissue formation in nonlymphoid organs has been described in many chronic inflammatory disorders such as insulin-dependent diabetes melli-

Table 1. Primer pairs used in the reverse transcriptase–polymerase chain reaction analysis*

Gene	Chemokine	Forward primer sequence	Reverse primer sequence	Product size, bp
STCP-1 (CCL22)	Stimulated T cell protein 1	CTGCACTCCTGGTTGTCCTC	ACGGTCATCAGAGTAGGCTC	297
BCA-1 (CXCL13)	B cell attracting	GGGCTGCAGCTCCAGACAG-AATGAAGTTC	GGACTCGAGTGGAAATAT-CAGCATCAGGG	356
ELC (CCL19)	EBI1 ligand†	GCTCACACATTCACCGTTG	AGTTGTAAACACCAGGCGG	583
SLC (CCL21)	Secondary lymphoid tissue	GCCGTCGACACAGACATG-GCTCAGTCACTGGCT	GCCTCTAGATGGCCCTTTA-GGGGTCTGTGACCG	407
PARC (CCL18)	Pulmonary/activation regulated	TGACCACTTCTCTGCCTGA-CCAG	GTTGAAGGGAAAGGGGAAA-GGATGA	567
TARC (CCL17)	Thymus/activation regulated	CGCGGATCCGCTCGAGGG-ACCAATGTG	CGCGCGGCCGCTCAAGACC-TCTCAAGGCT	189
LARC (CCL20)	Liver/activation regulated	CGGGATCCACCATGTGCT-GTACCAAGAGTTTG	CGGAATTCCAGTTTTTACA-TGTTCTTGAC	296
GAPDH	Glyceraldehyde phosphate dehydrogenase	ACCACAGTCCATGCCATCAC	TCCACCACCCTGTTGCTGTA	451

* The nomenclature of chemokines is based on their new classification system as presented at the last Keystone Chemokine Symposium (12).
† EBI1 = Epstein-Barr virus–induced gene 1.

tus, Hashimoto's thyroiditis, and rheumatoid arthritis (RA), and is called lymphoid neo-organogenesis (5–8). Many factors have been implicated in the induction of this inflammatory process, such as cytokines, adhesion molecules, and chemokines (9,10). However, a clear understanding of the role of the individual factors and their mechanism of action remains largely unknown.

Chemokines represent an expanding superfamily of structurally related, small (8–10 kd) chemotactic cytokines involved in leukocyte trafficking and activation. Four subtypes have been identified on the basis of the number and spacing of the conserved cysteine residues in the amino-terminal region; these subtypes are CC, CXC, CX3C, and C (X represents nonconserved amino acid residues) (11).

Recently, chemokines have been divided into 2 functionally distinct groups, namely, "inflammatory" chemokines, which attract appropriate effector cells into tissues in response to a particular pathogen or damage, and "lymphoid" chemokines, which are involved in the homeostatic trafficking of leukocytes into different lymphoid compartments. The latter group of "lymphoid" chemokines includes BCA-1, ELC, SLC, STCP-1, PARC, and TARC (see Table 1) (12), which are expressed at high levels in the thymus, lymph nodes, spleen, and other lymphoid organs. T cells, B lymphocytes, and dendritic cells (DCs), depending on their state of differentiation, become receptive to signals delivered by these chemokines and are guided by corresponding receptors to specific microenvironmental niches in lymphoid organs (13).

The homeostatic functions of the aforementioned chemokines were first documented in mice lacking the receptor for BCA-1 (CXCR5), which is expressed by B lymphocytes. Targeted disruption of the CXCR5 gene led to defective formation of primary follicles and germinal centers in the spleen and Peyer's patches as a result of the failure of B lymphocytes to enter the B cell areas (14). In addition, recent studies have described a disrupted distribution of T cells, B lymphocytes, and DCs in secondary lymphoid organs in mice deficient in CCR7, the ligand for ELC and SLC (15).

The identification of this newly defined set of chemokines prompted us to investigate their existence in MSG biopsy samples from patients with SS. In order to test this hypothesis, reverse transcriptase–polymerase chain reaction (RT-PCR) and in situ hybridization analyses were performed. Subsequently, immunohistochemistry was applied on serial sections in order to define the identity of the chemokine messenger RNA (mRNA)–expressing cells. Our results revealed that "lymphoid" chemokine mRNA are expressed in the salivary gland lesions of SS patients. The main sources of chemokine mRNA were ductal epithelial cells and infiltrating mononuclear leukocytes. These observations suggest the possible involvement of "lymphoid" chemokines in the organization of lymphoid structures in SS. Furthermore, a possible inflammatory role, in addition to their homeostatic properties, is discussed.

PATIENTS AND METHODS

Patients. Twelve patients fulfilling the European classification criteria for primary SS (16), 3 patients with secondary SS (2 with systemic lupus erythematosus [SLE] and 1 with

RA), 4 patients with other autoimmune disorders (2 with SLE, 1 with systemic scleroderma, and 1 with RA), and 4 control individuals (patients who were evaluated for dry mouth or dry eyes but did not fulfill the European classification criteria for primary SS) were the subjects of this study. MSG biopsy samples were obtained following the procedure used routinely for diagnosis. The histopathologic grading of each biopsy specimen was performed according to the classification of Chilsolm and Mason (17). None of the patients was undergoing treatment with steroids during the course of this study.

RNA isolation and RT-PCR analysis. Total RNA was isolated from snap-frozen MSG tissue using the SNAP Total RNA isolation kit (Invitrogen, Carlsbad, CA). RNA integrity was checked using RT-PCR with specific primer pairs for the GAPDH housekeeping gene.

RT-PCR was performed using the Access RT-PCR kit (Promega, Madison, WI). Synthesis and amplification of complementary DNA (cDNA) was achieved using ~0.5 μg of RNA. The nucleotide sequences of the primer pairs used in RT-PCR reactions are listed in Table 1. PCR conditions differed for each chemokine tested. PCR products were analyzed on a 1% Tris–borate–EDTA agarose gel. Each RT-PCR reaction was also run using a sample containing water instead of RNA, which served as the negative control.

Southern blot analysis. The RT-PCR results for STCP-1/monocyte-derived chemokine (MDC) gene expression revealed the existence of multiple cDNA bands, which possibly corresponded to nonspecific products, in all MSG samples tested. In order to verify the specificity of the STCP-1/MDC expression, Southern blot hybridization was conducted. The STCP-1/MDC probe was isolated from a plasmid (pBluescript SK[±]; Promega) containing a 300-bp fragment corresponding to the coding region of the gene, and was labeled with ^{32}P-ATP using the Prime-a-Gene labeling system (Promega). Briefly, RT-PCR for the STCP-1/MDC gene was performed in total RNA extracted from MSGs. The cDNA samples were transferred overnight onto a nitrocellulose membrane, which was subsequently prehybridized with appropriate buffer for 2 hours at 65°C (Amersham, Little Chalfont, UK). Hybridization was conducted after adding the labeled STCP-1/MDC probe for 3 hours at 65°C. Posthybridization washes were performed as follows: 2× saline–sodium citrate (SSC)/0.5% sodium dodecyl sulfate (SDS) for 15 minutes at 65°C, 1× SSC/0.5% SDS for 15 minutes at 65°C, and 0.1× SSC/0.5% SDS for 15 minutes at 42°C. Autoradiographs were exposed for 1 hour at room temperature. RNA integrity was confirmed using a labeled probe corresponding to the GAPDH gene.

Cloning of PCR products and in vitro transcription. RT-PCR products of all chemokines tested were ligated into the multiple cloning site of the pGEM-T-Easy vector (Promega), downstream of the T7 and SP6 RNA polymerase promoters, in order to obtain nucleotide riboprobes. The primers used in the RT-PCR experiments to detect "lymphoid" chemokine mRNA expression generated the specific mRNA products for all the chemokines tested, as verified by the GenBank sequence alignment program BLAST. Also, the mRNA products of "lymphoid" chemokines did not show significant homology that could justify crossreactivity between the riboprobes. In this respect, the riboprobes derived from the RT-PCR products corresponded to the specific mRNA for each chemokine and were not subject to nonspecific binding.

Plasmid DNA was used to transform JM-109 competent cells (Promega). After applying Blue-White Colony Screening (Promega), plasmid DNA was isolated from the transformed cells using the Wizard DNA isolation kit (Promega), digested with *Eco* RI, and run on a 1% Tris–acetate–EDTA agarose gel to check the integrity and size of the DNA insert. The DNA plasmids were subsequently linearized using the appropriate restriction enzymes. RNA probes were synthesized with the digoxigenin (DIG) RNA labeling kit

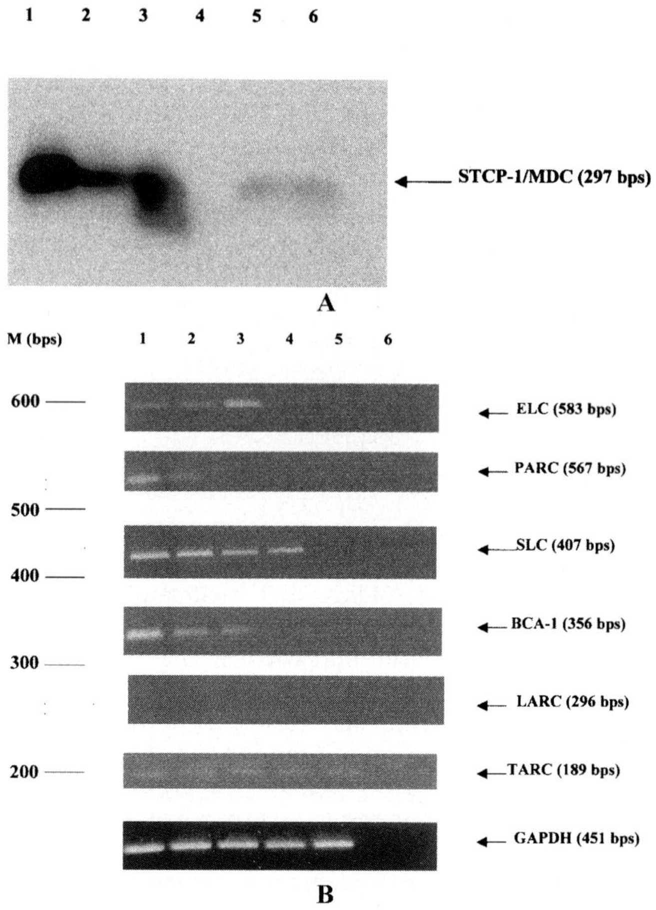

Figure 1. A, Representative results of Southern hybridization analysis of STCP-1/MDC gene expression in minor salivary gland (MSG) biopsy samples. Complementary DNA was transferred onto a nylon membrane and hybridized with a ^{32}P-labeled STCP-1/MDC probe. Lanes 1 and 2, Samples from primary Sjögren's syndrome (SS) patients; lane 3, sample from a secondary SS patient; lane 4, negative control (water instead of RNA); lane 5, sample from a systemic lupus erythematosus patient; lane 6, sample from a control individual (patient with dry eyes and/or dry mouth who did not fulfill the European classification criteria for primary SS). **B,** Detection of chemokine messenger RNA in MSG samples. Each panel shows the results in 2 samples from primary SS patients (lanes 1 and 2), a sample from a secondary SS patient (lane 3), a sample from a patient with another autoimmune disorder (lane 4), a sample from a control individual (lane 5), and a negative control without RNA (lane 6). Values in parentheses are the size of each specific reverse transcriptase–polymerase chain reaction product. M = molecular weight.

(Boehringer-Mannheim, Mannheim, Germany), precipitated with ethanol, dissolved in Tris–EDTA buffer, and stored at −80°C.

In situ hybridization. MSG biopsy samples from the same patients as those used in RT-PCR experiments were fixed with 4% paraformaldehyde phosphate buffered saline (PBS) for 4 hours at 4°C followed by an overnight wash in 30% sucrose/PBS solution. Tissue samples were embedded in paraffin and 6-μm serial sections were prepared, deparaffinized, and rehydrated in distilled H_2O. Sections were then treated with 0.2% Triton X-100/PBS for 5 minutes, 0.2*M* HCl for 20 minutes, and 2× SSC for 10 minutes (at 70°C). A 10-minute wash in diethyl pyrocarbonate/PBS was performed between each step. Subsequently, sections were incubated with 5 μg/ml proteinase K for 30 minutes at 37°C, fixed with 4% paraformaldehyde/PBS for 20 minutes, and acetylated with 0.25% acetic anhydride in 100 m*M* triethanolamine (pH 8) for 15 minutes. Slides were then incubated in hybridization buffer at 37°C for 2 hours, while hybridization was conducted in the same buffer as that containing the DIG-labeled RNA probes, at 42°C overnight. After hybridization, sections were washed with 2× SSC for 15 minutes, 1× SSC for 30 minutes, and 0.1× SSC for 30 minutes, all at 37°C.

Due to the small size of the TARC riboprobe used (198 bp), the sections were incubated with 50 μg/ml RNase in 2× SSC for 30 minutes at 37°C before the posthybridization washes, in order to prevent the formation of nonspecific hybrids between the TARC riboprobe and other small RNA molecules. For detection of the DIG-labeled riboprobes, slides were incubated in a blocking solution for 30 minutes, followed by incubation with anti–DIG–alkaline phosphatase antibody conjugate at room temperature for 60 minutes (Boehringer-Mannheim). The slides were then washed in Tween 20/PBS, and nitroblue tetrazolium/BCIP was used as substrate for color development. Finally, sections were counterstained with nuclear fast red.

Immunohistochemistry. In order to identify the cells that expressed chemokine mRNA, serial sections of paraffin tissue blocks from the same MSG biopsy samples that were used in our in situ hybridization experiments were analyzed by an indirect immunoperoxidase technique. Sections were blocked with 10% nonimmune horse serum for 20 minutes and incubated with the primary antibodies for 90 minutes at room temperature. The following monoclonal primary antibodies were used: anti-CD3 (T cells), anti-CD20 (B cells), anti-CD35 (Clone Ber-MAC-DRC, reactive with DCs and mantle zone lymphoid cells), anti-CD68 (macrophages), anti–MNF-116 (epithelial cells), and anti-CD34 (endothelial cells). All antibodies were purchased from Dako A/S (Glostrup, Denmark) except the anti-CD34 antibody, which was supplied from Immunotech (Marseilles, France). In control sections, irrelevant isotype-matched antibodies were used. Slides were then incubated with biotinylated rabbit anti-mouse antibody (Dako) for 30 minutes at room temperature. Endogenous peroxidase was blocked using 3% H_2O_2 in methanol for 5 minutes. Sections were incubated with avidin–biotin–horseradish peroxidase complex for 30 minutes (Dako). Washes with Tris buffered saline were performed between each step. Subsequently, sections were stained with diaminobenzidine substrate (Dako) and counterstained with Mayer's hematoxylin. Finally, sections were rehydrated through graded series of alcohol and mounted in xylene-diluted mounting medium.

Quantitative analysis. A semiquantitative assessment of the number of cells expressing chemokine mRNA in the MSGs was performed by examining 10 contiguous fields across the whole section at 40× magnification. Positive cells in each section were counted field by field at 16× magnification on a television screen connected to a microscope (Image Pro-Plus 2.1 system; Media Cybernetics, Silver Springs, MD) by 2 independent observers (GX and MP). The percentage of each cell type expressing chemokine mRNA as a portion of the total number of cells of that type in the sections was determined.

Statistical analysis. Results are expressed as the mean ± SD. Student's 2-tailed unpaired *t*-test was used to compare the patient and control groups. *P* values less than or equal to 0.01 were considered statistically significant.

RESULTS

Detection of "lymphoid" chemokine mRNA in MSG samples. TARC mRNA was expressed in 11 of 12 samples from primary SS patients, 2 of 3 secondary SS samples, 2 SLE samples, 1 RA sample, and in 2 of 4 controls. STCP-1/MDC gene expression showed a 297-bp band, among a few nonspecific cDNA products, in 10 of 12 primary SS samples, in 3 of 3 secondary SS samples, in 2 SLE samples, and in 2 of 4 controls. This 297-bp band was confirmed by Southern hybridization analysis to be specific for the STCP-1/MDC gene (Figure 1A). SLC mRNA was detected in all samples from primary SS and secondary SS patients and in 1 SLE sample. Furthermore, RT-PCR products were observed for BCA-1, ELC, and PARC chemokines in primary SS and secondary SS samples only. Finally, LARC mRNA was not expressed in any of the samples tested (Figure 1B). GAPDH gene expression was used to assess the quality of the MSG RNA. RT-PCR results are summarized in Table 2.

Table 2. Chemokine gene expression in minor salivary glands of patients with SS, patients with other autoimmune disorders, and controls*

Chemokine	Primary SS	Secondary SS	Other autoimmune disorders	Control individuals
STCP-1/MDC	10/12	3/3	2/4	2/4
TARC	11/12	2/3	3/4	2/4
SLC	12/12	3/3	1/4	0/4
BCA-1	12/12	3/3	0/4	0/4
ELC	12/12	3/3	0/4	0/4
PARC	10/12	1/3	0/4	0/4
LARC	0/12	0/3	0/4	0/4
GAPDH	12/12	3/3	4/4	4/4

* Values are the number/total number of subjects expressing each chemokine gene among patients with Sjögren's syndrome (SS), patients with other disorders (systemic lupus erythematosus, scleroderma, rheumatoid arthritis), and healthy controls.

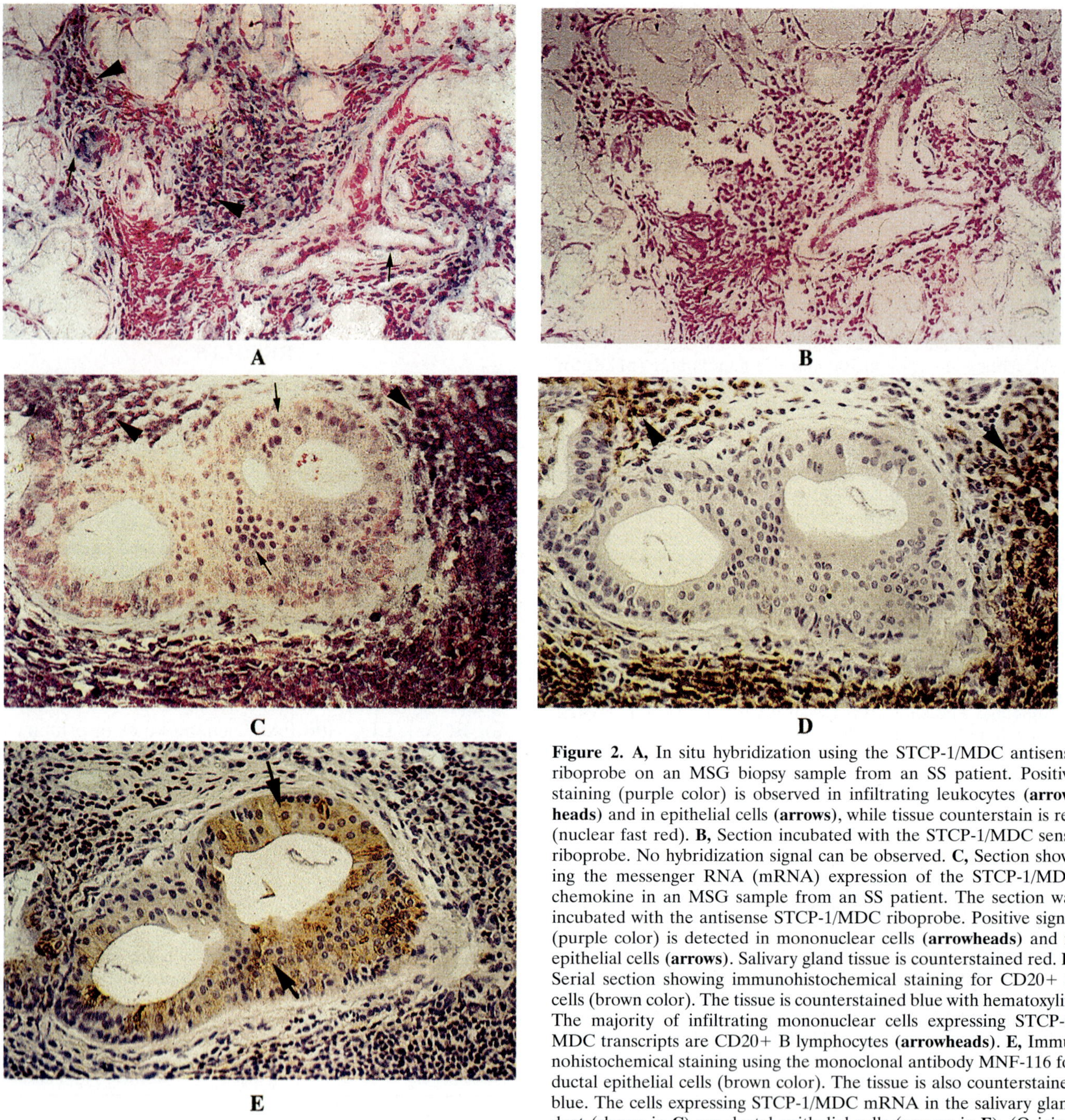

Figure 2. **A,** In situ hybridization using the STCP-1/MDC antisense riboprobe on an MSG biopsy sample from an SS patient. Positive staining (purple color) is observed in infiltrating leukocytes (**arrowheads**) and in epithelial cells (**arrows**), while tissue counterstain is red (nuclear fast red). **B,** Section incubated with the STCP-1/MDC sense riboprobe. No hybridization signal can be observed. **C,** Section showing the messenger RNA (mRNA) expression of the STCP-1/MDC chemokine in an MSG sample from an SS patient. The section was incubated with the antisense STCP-1/MDC riboprobe. Positive signal (purple color) is detected in mononuclear cells (**arrowheads**) and in epithelial cells (**arrows**). Salivary gland tissue is counterstained red. **D,** Serial section showing immunohistochemical staining for CD20+ B cells (brown color). The tissue is counterstained blue with hematoxylin. The majority of infiltrating mononuclear cells expressing STCP-1/MDC transcripts are CD20+ B lymphocytes (**arrowheads**). **E,** Immunohistochemical staining using the monoclonal antibody MNF-116 for ductal epithelial cells (brown color). The tissue is also counterstained blue. The cells expressing STCP-1/MDC mRNA in the salivary gland duct (shown in **C**) are ductal epithelial cells (**arrows** in **E**). (Original magnification × 100 in **A** and **B;** × 200 in **C–E.**) See Figure 1 for other definitions.

Localization of chemokine mRNA in MSG biopsy samples. In situ hybridization studies were conducted in order to investigate the localization of chemokine mRNA in MSG biopsy samples, while immunohistochemistry was subsequently performed to determine their cellular source. STCP-1/MDC mRNA was observed in infiltrating lymphocytes, in cells that resembled DCs, and in epithelial cells in MSGs of SS patients, while no hybridization signal was detected in the sections incubated with the STCP-1/MDC sense riboprobe (Figures 2A and B). The cells that expressed STCP-1/MDC transcripts (Figure 2C) were mainly CD20+ B lympho-

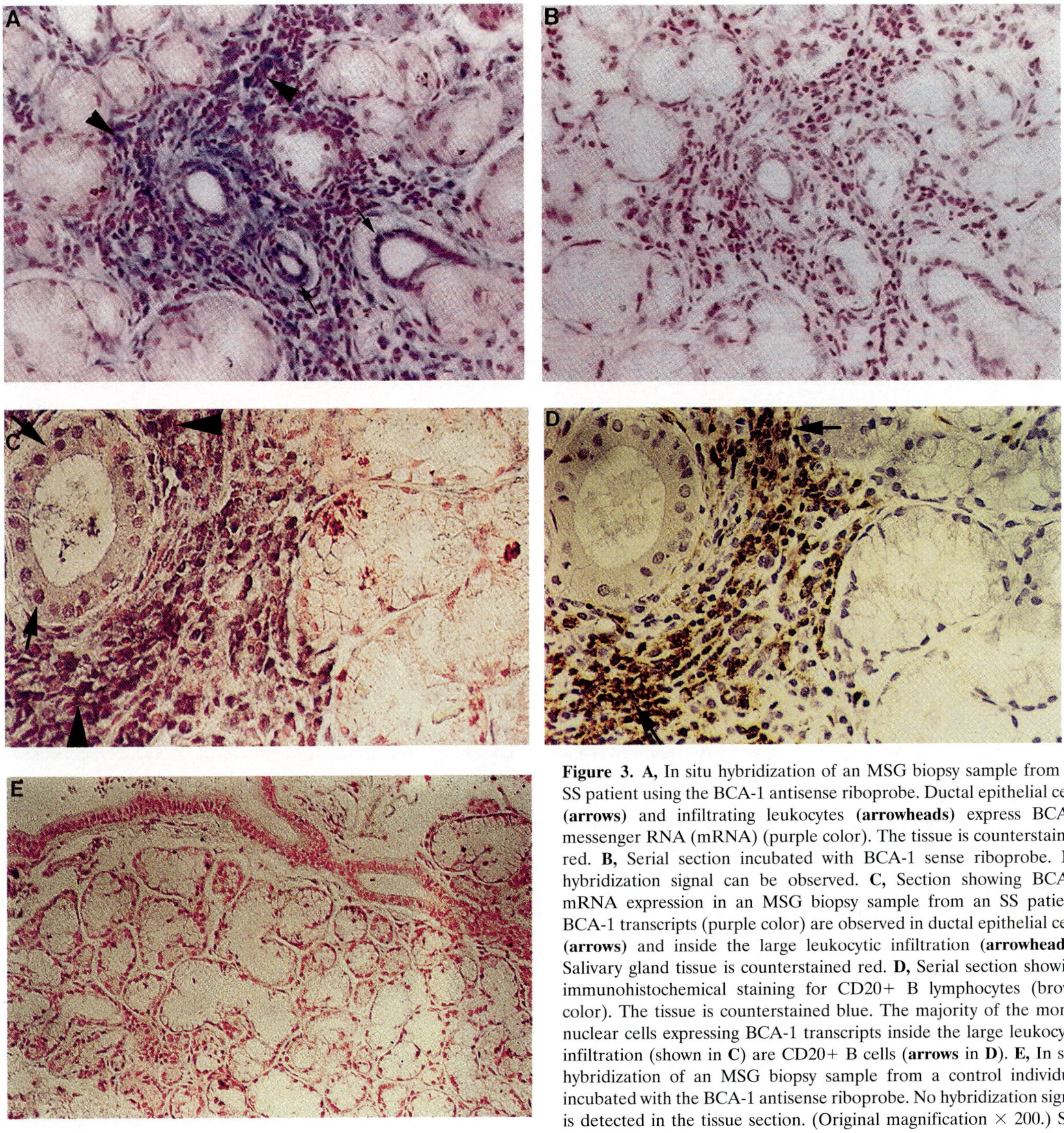

Figure 3. A, In situ hybridization of an MSG biopsy sample from an SS patient using the BCA-1 antisense riboprobe. Ductal epithelial cells **(arrows)** and infiltrating leukocytes **(arrowheads)** express BCA-1 messenger RNA (mRNA) (purple color). The tissue is counterstained red. **B,** Serial section incubated with BCA-1 sense riboprobe. No hybridization signal can be observed. **C,** Section showing BCA-1 mRNA expression in an MSG biopsy sample from an SS patient. BCA-1 transcripts (purple color) are observed in ductal epithelial cells **(arrows)** and inside the large leukocytic infiltration **(arrowheads)**. Salivary gland tissue is counterstained red. **D,** Serial section showing immunohistochemical staining for CD20+ B lymphocytes (brown color). The tissue is counterstained blue. The majority of the mononuclear cells expressing BCA-1 transcripts inside the large leukocytic infiltration (shown in **C**) are CD20+ B cells (**arrows** in **D**). **E,** In situ hybridization of an MSG biopsy sample from a control individual incubated with the BCA-1 antisense riboprobe. No hybridization signal is detected in the tissue section. (Original magnification × 200.) See Figure 1 for other definitions.

cytes (Figure 2D) and ductal epithelial cells (Figure 2E), as observed in adjacent serial sections using immunohistochemistry and cell type–specific markers.

TARC mRNA showed the same pattern of expression as that of STCP-1/MDC (results not shown). TARC and STCP-1/MDC transcripts were also expressed by mononuclear and ductal epithelial cells in 2 samples from SLE patients and in 1 sample from a control individual (results not shown), but the percentage of chemokine mRNA–expressing cells was statisti-

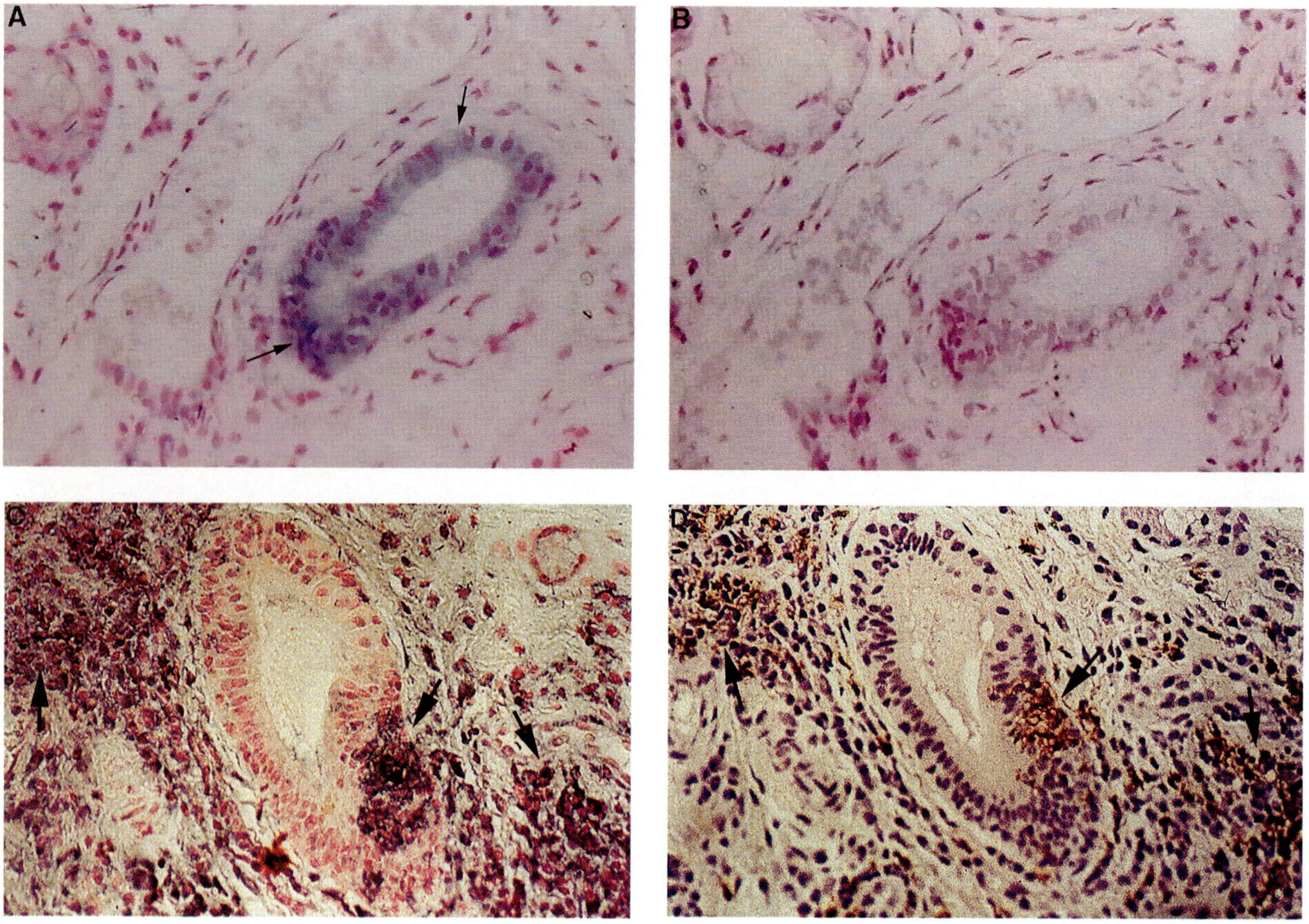

Figure 4. **A,** SLC messenger RNA (mRNA) expression in an MSG biopsy sample from an SS patient, detected using the SLC antisense riboprobe. SLC mRNA (purple color) is observed in ductal epithelial cells **(arrows)**, while no expression can be detected in mononuclear or endothelial cells. **B,** Serial section incubated with the SLC sense riboprobe. No hybridization signal is detected. **C,** In situ expression of PARC mRNA in SS lesions, detected using the PARC antisense riboprobe. Positive signal (purple color) is detected in infiltrating lymphocytes **(arrows)** inside the large lymphocytic infiltration and in mononuclear cells **(arrow)** infiltrating a salivary gland duct. Tissue is counterstained red. **D,** Serial section showing immunohistochemical staining for CD20+ B cells (brown color). Many of the mononuclear cells inside the leukocytic infiltration and in the salivary gland duct expressing PARC mRNA (shown in **C**) are CD20+ B cells (**arrows** in **D**). (Original magnification × 200.) See Figure 1 for other definitions.

cally significantly lower than that of chemokine-expressing cells in samples from SS patients (for quantitative analysis, see Figures 5A and B). The difference between the RT-PCR and in situ hybridization results regarding the mRNA expression of TARC and STCP-1/MDC chemokines in non-SS samples and in control individuals could be due to the following reasons: 1) RT-PCR is a more sensitive technique compared with in situ hybridization, and RT-PCR detected even small amounts of TARC and STCP-1/MDC mRNA which were not detectable with the in situ hybridization technique; and 2) both chemokine mRNA were expressed in MSG biopsy samples from SS and non-SS individuals, but they were up-regulated in SS lesions, and therefore a positive signal is more frequently detected in these samples using in situ hybridization.

BCA-1 mRNA expression was observed in areas with focal mononuclear infiltrates containing B lymphocytes and DC+ cells and in ductal epithelial cells surrounded by infiltrating leukocytes in SS samples (Figure 3A). No hybridization signal was observed for BCA-1 chemokine using the sense riboprobe (Figure 3B). BCA-1 transcripts (Figure 3C) were detected

Table 3. Chemokine messenger RNA–expressing cells in minor salivary glands from Sjögren's syndrome patients*

Chemokine	Mononuclear cells	Ductal cells
BCA-1	20.0	32.0
ELC	14.2	23.5
SLC	–	7.1
STCP-1/MDC	41.0	27.3
PARC	21.24	–
TARC	29.9	22.3

* Values are the percentage of cells expressing messenger RNA for each chemokine.

mainly in ductal epithelial cells and in infiltrating leukocytes, which were identified as CD20+ B lymphocytes using serial sections and cell-type specific antibodies (Figure 3D). BCA-1 mRNA was not detected in any other non-SS sample tested (Figure 3E).

ELC mRNA exhibited the same pattern of expression as that of BCA-1 (results not shown). Low levels of SLC mRNA expression were observed, using the antisense riboprobe, in ductal epithelial cells in MSGs of SS patients, while no signal was detected in mononuclear or endothelial cells (Figure 4A). All sections probed with the SLC sense riboprobe were devoid of a hybridization signal (Figure 4B). Prominent PARC expression was found in lymphocytes and DC+ cells located in lymphocytic infiltrations and in mononuclear cells infiltrating a salivary gland duct in SS lesions (Figure 4C). The majority of the aforementioned mononuclear leukocytes were CD20+ B lymphocytes, as observed in adjacent serial sections (Figure 4D). LARC mRNA was not observed in any of the MSG biopsy samples tested, and this was consistent with the RT-PCR results.

GAPDH gene expression was also investigated in order to assess RNA tissue integrity and assay performance. GAPDH mRNA was abundantly expressed in all MSGs examined using the antisense probe, while no expression was observed in a panel of sections probed with the GAPDH and chemokine sense strands (results not shown). CD3+ T lymphocytes and CD68+ macrophages were also present inside large leukocytic infiltrations, yet their distribution differed from that of the chemokine mRNA–expressing cells. In addition, acinar epithelial cells did not contain detectable mRNA for any of the chemokines analyzed herein.

Quantitative analysis. All of the MSG biopsy samples from the SS patients studied had a focus score between 1.5 and 2.0 according to the classification of Chilsolm and Mason (17). The percentages of chemokine mRNA–expressing cells are presented in Table 3. STCP-1/MDC transcripts were more frequently expressed in ductal epithelial cells (mean ± SD 27.26 ± 3.46%) and in mononuclear leukocytes (41.03 ± 9.87%) in SS samples compared with those expressed by ductal epithelial cells (4.69 ± 1.16%) and mononuclear cells (5.42 ± 1.9%) from non-SS samples (SLE patients and the control individual) ($P < 0.01$). TARC mRNA was also increased in SS ductal epithelial cells (22.3 ± 3.67%) and in mononuclear cells (29.9 ± 3.56%) compared with those detected in non-SS samples (3.78 ±

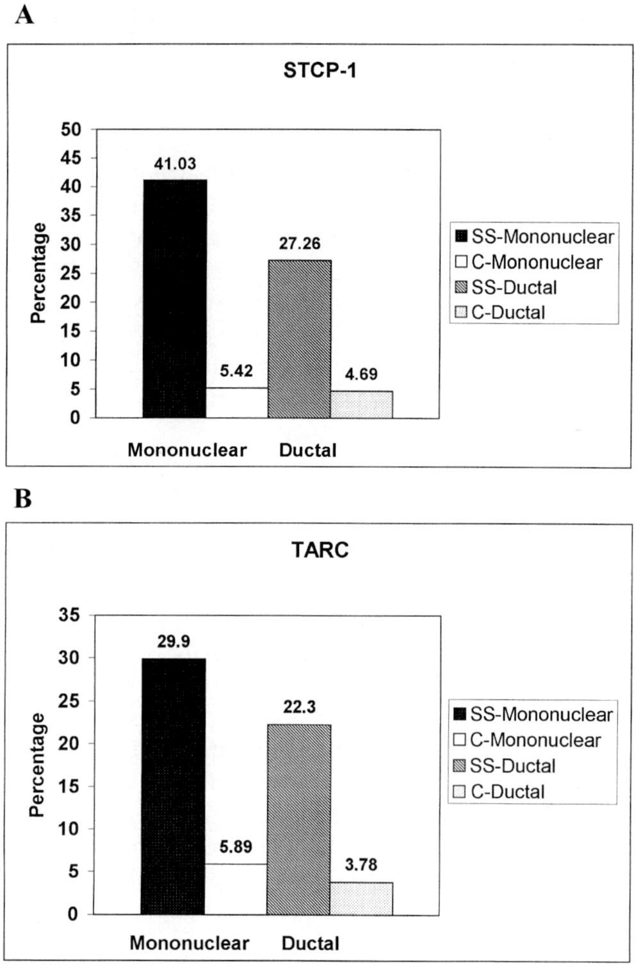

Figure 5. Image analysis of STCP-1/MDC and TARC mRNA expression in MSGs from patients with SS, patients with other autoimmune disorders (systemic lupus erythematosus [SLE]), and controls. **A,** STCP-1/MDC mRNA was more frequently expressed in SS samples compared with samples from SLE patients and the control individual ($P < 0.01$). **B,** TARC mRNA was also significantly increased in SS samples compared with non-SS samples ($P < 0.01$). C = non-SS control samples (see Figure 1 for other definitions).

0.8% and 5.89 ± 1.1%, respectively) ($P < 0.01$) (Figures 5A and B).

DISCUSSION

One of the major questions regarding the immunopathology of SS is the delineation of the mechanisms that govern the accumulation of activated mononuclear leukocytes in the salivary glands, resulting in the ectopic formation of organized lymphoid structures. Since leukocyte migration is largely controlled by chemokines, we investigated the existence of "lymphoid" chemokines that could participate in the recruitment and compartmentalization of infiltrating leukocytes.

In the present study, it was demonstrated that "lymphoid" chemokine–encoding mRNA are expressed in the chronic inflammatory lesions of SS patients. More specifically, STCP-1/MDC and TARC transcripts were detected in B lymphocytes, DC+ cells, and ductal epithelial cells of SS patients, and at lower levels in mononuclear and ductal cells from patients with other autoimmune disorders and from control subjects. In lymphoid organs, both chemokines are expressed by DCs and activated B lymphocytes and attract activated T cells (18,19). The common features of these chemokines could thus explain their similar expression pattern in MSG biopsy tissue. The existence of these chemokine mRNA in SS lesions possibly indicates their participation in the attraction of activated T lymphocytes and the amplification of the immune response. Alternatively, their mRNA expression in samples from patients with other autoimmune diseases and in control individuals could suggest that they may be involved in the attraction of effector cells in response to an inflammatory signal or that they may participate in salivary gland tissue formation and homeostasis.

BCA-1 mRNA was observed in B lymphocytes, DC+ cells, and ductal epithelial cells in primary SS and secondary SS MSG samples. BCA-1 normally participates in the formation of lymphoid follicles (20). In addition, BCA-1 mRNA were recently shown to be expressed by B cells in *Helicobacter pylori*–induced MALT tissue formation and in gastric lymphoma (21). These findings suggest that B lymphocytes and DC+ cells expressing BCA-1 mRNA may be actively involved in the ectopic formation of lymphoid follicles in SS lesions.

SLC is expressed by lymphatic endothelium in many organs and by high endothelial venules (HEVs) and stromal cells in lymphoid organs. SLC induces firm adhesion of T lymphocytes via $\beta 2$ integrin binding to its counter receptor, intercellular adhesion molecule 1 (ICAM-1), on endothelial cells, and thus controls lymphocyte recruitment in secondary lymphoid organs (22). In the present investigation, we found SLC mRNA expression in ductal epithelial cells, and not in endothelial cells, in SS lesions. In a recent study, human SLC transcripts were also not detected in endothelial cells of lymph nodes, but in interdigitating DCs and sinus-lining DCs, using the in situ hybridization technique (23). The absence of SLC transcripts in endothelial cells in our study may be derived from the fact that there were no structures resembling HEVs present in the MSGs tested. Also, the endothelial cells in SS lesions may not have the characteristics and functions of lymphatic endothelium.

In this respect, our findings suggest that epithelial cells may play a role in mediating lymphocyte recruitment in SS lesions. Consistent with this hypothesis, it has recently been demonstrated that SS epithelial cells express ICAM-1, which possibly interacts with its counter receptor expressed on T lymphocytes (24). There are also conflicting data regarding SLC mRNA expression in human mucosal tissues, since some investigators reported its presence in normal salivary glands (22,23), whereas another study demonstrated the presence of SLC transcripts in lymphoid organs only (25). In the present study, SLC transcripts were observed in all SS biopsy samples and in only 1 of the other non-SS samples tested, possibly indicating that SLC is specifically expressed in the chronic inflammatory SS lesions. The lack of SLC mRNA expression in the non-SS samples and in control individuals could be due to the fact that the MSGs studied did not contain lymphoid structures or lymphatic endothelium, which are the usual cell sources of SLC. Future experiments with a larger sample number shall resolve these differences.

PARC and ELC mRNA were also observed in MSGs of SS patients. PARC mRNA was expressed by B lymphocytes and DC+ cells, while ELC mRNA was also detected in ductal epithelial cells. In lymphoid organs, PARC and ELC are produced by DCs and attract naïve and activated T lymphocytes, respectively (26,27). In addition, PARC and ELC mRNA were detected in macrophages and smooth muscle cells in human atherosclerotic plaques, while PARC mRNA was also observed in mononuclear cells in the liver of patients with chronic hepatitis C infection (28,29). Collectively, these findings may indicate that PARC and ELC could have an inflammatory role in SS by mediating the recruitment of naive and activated T cells and promoting their priming and activation.

One of the most interesting findings of this study

is the novel expression of "lymphoid" chemokine mRNA by ductal epithelial cells in MSGs of SS patients. Apart from 2 recent studies that reported the mRNA expression of STCP-1/MDC and SLC by thymic medullary epithelial cells in mice (30,31), epithelial cells have so far not been described to express "lymphoid" chemokines. It is well known that epithelial cells in SS lesions display an activated phenotype, since they express antigen-presenting molecules, apoptotic factors, protooncogenes, and adhesion molecules (24,32–37). Furthermore, glandular epithelial cells express a panel of proinflammatory cytokines and chemokines (38,39). The above data could indicate that epithelial cells in SS lesions are active participants in the induction and perpetuation of the inflammatory process. In this respect, it can be postulated that epithelial cells could be induced by an extrinsic factor, such as locally produced cytokines, to express "lymphoid" chemokine mRNA that mediate, along with other proinflammatory cytokines and chemokines, the attraction of leukocytes, their compartmentalization into lymphoid structures, and the in situ priming of the immune response. Once in the lesion, the recruited leukocytes may also produce "lymphoid" chemokines, resulting in the enhancement of the autoimmune inflammatory response. Consistent with this hypothesis, it has recently been demonstrated that lymphotoxins and tumor necrosis factor α induce the production of "lymphoid" chemokines during the development of lymphoid organs and also mediate their de novo expression in the chronic inflammatory pancreatic lesions of prediabetic nonobese mice (10,40).

The expression of "lymphoid" chemokines by ductal epithelial cells in SS may also be the result of an intrinsic factor such as a viral infection. Viruses have been largely suspected as the etiopathologic factors of SS (41). Many studies have documented the existence of virally encoded chemokines or their analogs, which may enhance viral growth by attracting and infecting effector cells (42). Consistent with this hypothesis, virally infected epithelial cells in SS may express "lymphoid" chemokine mRNA and attract leukocytes which, in turn, destroy infected cells and mediate the degeneration of the glandular tissue. Simultaneously, ductal epithelial cells and DCs residing in lymphoid structures could also promote the infection of mononuclear leukocytes, resulting in viral spreading and perpetuation of the autoimmune disorder.

In conclusion, the results presented in this study describe, for the first time, the expression of "lymphoid" chemokine transcripts in SS lesions and suggest their possible involvement in lymphoid tissue formation. Future studies focusing on the protein levels of these chemokines, as well as their receptors, may provide further insights into their biologic role in both leukocyte homing and inflammation. Finally, the detection of "lymphoid" chemokine mRNA in ductal epithelial cells points further to their pathogenetic role in SS and supports the speculation that they may be not only innocent bystanders, but also active collaborators in their own destruction.

REFERENCES

1. Moutsopoulos HM. Immunopathology of Sjögrens syndrome: more questions than answers. Lupus 1993;2:49–53.
2. Daniels TE, Aufdemorte THB, Greenspan JS. Histopathology of Sjögrens syndrome. In: Talal N, Moutsopoulos HM, Kassan SS, editors. Sjögrens syndrome: clinical and immunological aspects. Berlin: Springer; 1987. p. 258–65.
3. Stott DI, Hiepe F, Hummel M, Steinhauser G, Berek C. Antigen-driven clonal proliferation of B cells within target tissue of an autoimmune disease. J Clin Invest 1998;102:938–46.
4. Xanthou G, Tapinos NI, Polihronis M, Nezis IP, Margaritis LH, Moutsopoulos HM. CD4 cytotoxic and dendritic cells in the immunopathologic lesion of Sjögrens syndrome. Clin Exp Immunol 1999;118:154–63.
5. Ludewig B, Odermatt B, Landmann S, Hengartner H, Zinkernagel RM. Dendritic cells induce autoimmune diabetes and maintain disease via de novo formation of local lymphoid tissue. J Exp Med 1998;188:1493–501.
6. Knecht H, Saremaslani P, Hedinger C. Immunohistological findings in Hashimoto's thyroiditis, focal lymphocytic thyroiditis and thyroiditis de Quervain: comparative study. Virchows Arch A Pathol Anat Histol 1981;393:215–31.
7. Young CL, Adamson TC III, Vaughan JH, Fox RI. Immunohistologic characterization of synovial membrane lymphocytes in rheumatoid arthritis. Arthritis Rheum 1984;27:32–9.
8. Kratz A, Campos-Neto A, Hanson MS, Ruddle N. Chronic inflammation caused by lymphotoxin is lymphoid neogenesis. J Exp Med 1996;183:1461–72.
9. Cuff CA, Sacca R, Ruddle NH. Differential induction of adhesion molecule and chemokine expression by $LT\alpha 3$ and $LT\alpha\beta$ in inflammation elucidates potential mechanisms of mesenteric and peripheral lymph node development. J Immunol 1999;162:5965–72.
10. Ngo NV, Korner H, Gunn MD, Schmidt KN, Riminton DS, Cooper MD, et al. Lymphotoxin α/β and tumor necrosis factor are required for stromal cell expression of homing chemokines in B and T cell areas of the spleen. J Exp Med 1999;189:403–12.
11. Baggiolini M. Chemokines and leukocyte traffic. Nature 1998;392: 565–8.
12. Zlotnik A, Yoshie O. Chemokines: a new classification system and their role in immunity. Immunity 2000;12:121–7.
13. Cyster JG. Chemokines and cell migration in secondary lymphoid organs. Science 1999;286:2098–102.
14. Förster R, Mattis AE, Kremmer E, Wolf E, Brem G, Lipp M. A putative chemokine receptor, BLR1, directs B cell migration to defined lymphoid organs and specific anatomic compartments of the spleen. Cell 1996;87:1037–47.
15. Warnock RA, Cambell JJ, Dorf ME, Matsuzawa A, McEvoy LM, Butcher EC. The role of chemokines in the microenvironmental control of T versus B cell arrest in Peyer's patch high endothelial venules. J Exp Med 2000;191:77–88.
16. Vitali C, Bombardieri S, Moutsopoulos HM, Balestrieri G, Bencivelli W, Bernstein RM, et al. Preliminary criteria for the

classification of Sjögren's syndrome: results of a prospective concerted action supported by the European Community. Arthritis Rheum 1993;36:340–7.
17. Chilsolm DM, Mason DK. Labial salivary gland biopsy in Sjögrens disease. J Clin Pathol 1968;21:656–60.
18. Schaniel C, Pardali E, Sallusto F, Speletas M, Ruedl C, Shimizu T, et al. Activated murine B lymphocytes and dendritic cells produce a novel CC chemokine which acts selectively on activated T cells. J Exp Med 1998;188:451–63.
19. Schaniel C, Sallusto F, Ruedl C, Sideras P, Melchers F, Rolink AG. Three chemokines with potential functions in T lymphocyte-independent and -dependent B lymphocyte stimulation. Eur J Immunol 1999;29:2934–47.
20. Gunn MD, Ngo VN, Ansel KM, Ekland EH, Cyster JG, Williams LT. A B-cell-homing chemokine made in lymphoid follicles activates Burkitt's lymphoma receptor-1. Nature 1998;391:799–803.
21. Mazzucchelli L, Blaser A, Kappeler A, Scärli P, Laissue JA, Baggiolini M, et al. BCA-1 is highly expressed in Helicobacter pylori-induced mucosa-associated lymphoid tissue and gastric lymphoma. J Clin Invest 1999;104:R49–54.
22. Gunn MD, Tangemann K, Tam C, Cyster JG, Rosen SD, Williams LT. A chemokine expressed in lymphoid high endothelial venules promotes the adhesion and chemotaxis of naïve T lymphocytes. Proc Natl Acad Sci U S A 1998;95:258–63.
23. Willimann K, Legler DF, Loetscher M, Roos Stuber R, Delgado Belen M, Clark-Lewis I, et al. The chemokine SLC is expressed in T cell areas of lymph nodes and mucosal lymphoid tissues and attracts activated T cells via CCR7. Eur J Immunol 1998;28: 2025–34.
24. Aziz KE, McCluskey PJ, Wakefield D. Expression of selectins (CD62 E, L, P) and cellular adhesion molecules in primary Sjögren's syndrome: questions to immunoregulation. Clin Immunol Immunopathol 1996;80:55–66.
25. Nagira M, Imai T, Hieshima K, Kusuda J, Ridanpaa M, Takagi S, et al. Molecular cloning of a novel human CC chemokine secondary lymphoid-tissue chemokine that is a potent chemoattractant for lymphocytes and mapped to chromosome 9p13. J Biol Chem 1997;272:19518–24.
26. Yoshida R, Imai T, Hieshima K, Kusuda J, Baba M, Kitaura M, et al. Molecular cloning of a novel human CC chemokine EBI1-ligand chemokine that is a specific functional ligand for EBI1, CCR7. J Biol Chem 1997;272:13803–9.
27. Adema GJ, Hartgers F, Verstraten R, deVries E, Marland G, Menon S, et al. A dendritic-cell-derived C-C chemokine that preferentially attracts naïve T cells. Nature 1997;387:713–7.
28. Reape TJ, Rayner K, Manning CD, Gee AN, Barnette MS, Burnand KG, et al. Expression and cellular localization of CC chemokines PARC and ELC in human atherosclerotic plaques. Am J Pathol 1999;154:365–74.
29. Kusano F, Tanaka Y, Marumo F, Sato C. Expression of C-C chemokines is associated with portal and periportal inflammation in the liver of patients with chronic hepatitis C. Lab Invest 2000;80:415–22.
30. Tanabe S, Lu Z, Luo Y, Quackenbush EJ, Berman MA, Collins-Racie LA, et al. Identification of a new mouse β-chemokine, thymus-derived chemotactic agent 4, with activity on T lymphocytes and mesangial cells. J Immunol 1997;159:5671–79.
31. Chanty D, Romagnani P, Raport CJ, Wood CL, Epp A, Romagnani S, et al. Macrophage-derived chemokine is localized to thymic medullary epithelial cells and is a chemoattractant for CD3 (+), CD8 (low) thymocytes. Blood 1999;94:1890–8.
32. Tzioufas AG, Hantoumi I, Polihronis M, Xanthou G, Moutsopoulos HM. Autoantibodies to La/SSB in patients with primary Sjogrens syndrome (pSS) are associated with upregulation of La/SSB mRNA in minor salivary gland biopsies (MSGs). J Autoimmun 1999;13:429–34.
33. Manoussakis MN, Dimitriou ID, Kapsogeorgou EK, Xanthou G, Paikos S, Polihronis M, et al. Expression of B7 costimulatory molecules by salivary gland epithelial cells in patients with Sjögren's syndrome. Arthritis Rheum 1999;42:229–39.
34. Moutsopoulos HM, Hooks JJ, Chan CC, Dalavanga YA, Skopouli FN, Detrick B. HLA-DR expression in labial minor salivary gland tissues in Sjogren's syndrome. Ann Rheum Dis 1986;45:677–83.
35. Polihronis M, Tapinos NI, Theocharis SE, Economou A, Kittas C, Moutsopoulos HM. Modes of epithelial cell death in Sjogren's syndrome. Clin Exp Immunol 1998;114:485–90.
36. Skopouli FN, Kousvelari EE, Bone R, Schreiber R. C-myc mRNA expression in minor salivary glands of patients with Sjogren's syndrome. J Rheumatol 1992;29:1105–11.
37. Boumba D, Skopouli FN, Moutsopoulos HM. Cytokine mRNA expression in the labial salivary gland tissues from patients with primary Sjögren's Syndrome. Br J Rheumatol 1995;34:326–33.
38. Cuello C, Palladinetti P, Tedla N, di Girolamo N, Lloyd AR, McCluskey PJ, et al. Chemokine expression and leukocyte infiltration in Sjögrens syndrome. Br J Rheumatol 1998;37:779–83.
39. Törnwall J, Lane TE, Fox RI, Fox HS. T cell attractant chemokine expression initiates lacrimal gland destruction in nonobese diabetic mice. Lab Invest 1999;79:1719–26.
40. Hjelmstrom P, Fjell J, Nakagawa T, Sacca R, Cuff CA, Ruddle NH. Lymphoid tissue homing chemokines are expressed in chronic inflammation. Am J Pathol 2000;156:1133–8.
41. Kalden JR, Gay S. Retroviruses and autoimmune rheumatic diseases. Clin Exp Immunol 1994;98:1–5.
42. Pelchen-Matthews A, Signoret N, Klasse PJ, Fraile-Ramos A, Marsh M. Chemokine receptor trafficking and viral replication. Immunol Rev 1999;168:33–49.

ARTHRITIS & RHEUMATISM
Vol. 44, No. 2, February 2001, pp 419–431

Alteration of Peripheral Blood Dendritic Cells in Patients With Primary Sjögren's Syndrome

Yoshio Ozaki, Ryuichi Amakawa, Tomoki Ito, Hiroshi Iwai, Kenichirou Tajima, Kazutaka Uehira, Hideo Kagawa, Yoshiko Uemura, Toshio Yamashita, and Shirou Fukuhara

Objective. **We recently identified 3 fractions of human peripheral blood (PB) dendritic cells (DC), including the monocyte-associated fractions 1 and 2 (CD1a+,CD11c+ and CD1a−,CD11c+, respectively) and the lymphoid-associated fraction 3 (CD1a−,CD11c−). We attempted to determine whether these fractions were altered in Sjögren's syndrome (SS).**

Methods. **We examined 23 patients with primary SS and 22 normal control subjects. DC were purified from PB and analyzed by flow cytometry. Immunohistochemical staining of labial salivary glands of SS patients was performed with monoclonal antibodies against fascin, which is known to be specific for DC.**

Results. **The total numbers of PB DC and fraction 1 DC were decreased in SS. Immunohistochemical staining demonstrated that fascin+,CD11c+,HLA-DR+ mononuclear cells were present and scattered among numerous fascin-hyperfiltrating cells in SS patients. Interferon-γ (IFNγ)–producing Th1 cells were shown to be increased in both PB and salivary glands of patients, indicating the presence of general IFNγ-producing Th1 polarization in SS. Furthermore, numbers of Th1 cells were increased when naive T cells were cocultured with fraction 1 DC in vitro.**

Conclusion. **These findings suggest selective trafficking of fraction 1 DC into focal sites of inflammation and subsequent promotion of Th1 balance, suggesting a novel pathogenesis of SS.**

Supported by a grant-in-aid for scientific research (C) (subject 11670466) from the Japan Society for the Promotion of Science.

Yoshio Ozaki, MD, Ryuichi Amakawa, MD, Tomoki Ito, MD, Hiroshi Iwai, MD, Kenichirou Tajima, MD, Kazutaka Uehira, MD, Hideo Kagawa, MD, Yoshiko Uemura, MD, Toshio Yamashita, MD, Shirou Fukuhara, MD: Kansai Medical University, Moriguchi, Japan.

Address correspondence and reprint requests to Ryuichi Amakawa, MD, First Department of Internal Medicine, Kansai Medical University, 10-15 Fumizono-cho, Moriguchi City, Osaka 570-8506, Japan.

Submitted for publication March 28, 2000; accepted in revised form October 23, 2000.

Sjögren's syndrome (SS) is a chronic autoimmune disease characterized by various immune abnormalities, such as hypergammaglobulinemia, multiple autoantibodies, and focal lymphocytic infiltration of exocrine glands (1–3). SS primarily affects salivary and lacrimal glands, causing xerostomia and sicca syndrome, and thus is categorized as an organ-specific autoimmune disease. The pathogenesis of SS has remained unclear, although many investigators have attempted to demonstrate dysregulation of the cytokine network in patients with SS. Th1 cytokines such as interleukin-2 (IL-2) and interferon-γ (IFNγ) preferentially induce cell-mediated immunity, while Th2 cytokines such as IL-4 and IL-10 primarily support antibody production (4). Although divergence of naive T cells into Th1 and Th2 subsets has been less clearly demonstrated in humans than in mice (5,6), many groups have investigated the presence of a Th1/Th2 imbalance in SS (7–17), and some have suggested that polarized Th1 balance is associated with the immunopathology of SS (7–9,18).

Dendritic cells (DC), which derive from hemopoietic progenitors in the bone marrow, are highly specialized antigen-presenting cells (APC) and constitute a unique cell type with the capacity to prime naive T cells (19–21). Recent progress in the purification and characterization of DC has highlighted the integral roles of this cell type in eliciting primary immune responses in the body. Notably, monocyte-derived DC drive naive T helper cells toward Th1, while lymphoid DC promote differentiation of Th2 cells (22). This suggests that defects in DC-mediated immune responses are involved in the genesis of SS by virtue of causing an imbalance of Th1/Th2.

Recently, we successfully identified 3 fractions of DC in human peripheral blood (PB), based on the differential expression of CD1a and CD11c: the monocyte-associated fraction 1 DC, consisting of CD1a+,CD11c+; the monocyte-associated fraction 2 DC, consisting of CD1a−,CD11c+; and the putative lymphoid-associated fraction 3 DC, consisting of CD1a−,CD11c− (23). These fractions of DC are natural in that they can be directly obtained in pure form without culture or addition of any cytokines in vitro; they thus differ from the relatively artificial DC that have been used in many previous studies (23–25). The 3 fractions of DC are immature and appear to be en route to tissues and lymphoid organs, where they exhibit uptake and presentation of antigens. Therefore, characterization of DC fractions in PB might provide novel findings useful for determining the etiologies of various disease conditions, including SS. In this study, we examined the 3 DC fractions in SS patients and found a decrease in the CD1a+,CD11c+ fraction. We also found this fraction to be capable of inducing IFNγ-producing CD4+ T cells.

PATIENTS AND METHODS

Patients. The individuals enrolled in this study were 23 patients with primary SS (2 men and 21 women, mean age 57.0 years [range 29–74 years]) who had never been treated with steroids or immunosuppressive agents, and 22 age- and sex-matched healthy volunteer donors (controls; 2 men and 20 women, mean age 51.3 years [range 26–72 years]) with no history of autoimmune disease. No patients or volunteers had evidence of infection at the time of study; all underwent routine laboratory examinations and were also examined for a variety of autoantibodies. Informed consent was obtained for this study in accordance with the provisions of the Delcaration of Helsinki.

All SS patients met the criteria of the Research Committee on Sjögren's syndrome of the Ministry of Health and Welfare of Japan (2), as well as the criteria of the European Community (1). Briefly, the diagnosis of SS was based on clinical history and the results of clinical examination, Schirmer I test, rose bengal dye test, biopsies of the sublabial salivary gland, and/or sialography. Patients did not meet the criteria for systemic lupus erythematosus, any other defined connective tissue disease, malignant lymphoma, sarcoidosis, acquired immunodeficiency syndrome, or graft-versus-host disease. Thus, all of the patients were diagnosed as having primary SS. All of the patients presented at our hospital between May 1989 and July 2000.

Media. RPMI 1640 medium supplemented with 2 m*M* L-glutamine, 100 units/ml penicillin, 100 ng/ml streptomycin, and heat-inactivated 10% fetal bovine serum (Irvine Scientific, Santa Ana, CA) was used throughout the experiments.

Enrichment and analyses of the PB DC. PB DC were enriched using a previously described protocol (23). Briefly, the PB mononuclear cells (PBMC) were freshly isolated by Lymphoprep (Nycomed Pharma, Oslo, Norway) gradient centrifugation of heparinized blood. PBMC were incubated with anti-CD3 (HIT3a), anti-CD14 (M5E2), and anti-CD19 (B43) monoclonal antibodies (mAb) from PharMingen (San Diego, CA), and cells binding these mAb were removed using sheep anti-mouse Ig–coated magnetic beads (M-450; Dynal, Oslo, Norway).

The resulting DC-enriched population (CD3−,CD14−,CD19− cells) was stained with phycoerythrin (PE)–labeled anti-CD11c (Leu-M5; Becton Dickinson, San Jose, CA), fluorescein isothiocyanate (FITC)–labeled anti-CD1a (BB-5; BioSource International, Camarillo, CA), peridin chlorophyll protein (PerCP)–labeled anti–HLA–DR (L-243; Becton Dickinson), and a mixture of biotinylated mAb against the following lineage markers (lin): CD3 (M2AB [Exalpha, Boston, MA], which binds to a determinant different from that recognized by previous anti-CD3 mAb), CD14 (UCHM1, which binds to a determinant different from that recognized by previous anti-CD14 mAb; Ancell, Bayport, MN), CD15 (80H5; Immunotech, Marseilles, France), CD16 (3G8; PharMingen), and CD19 (HIB19, which binds to a determinant different from that recognized by previous anti-CD19 mAb; PharMingen), followed by RED613-streptavidin (Life Technologies, Glasgow, UK).

The stained cells were analyzed or sorted by an EPICS ALTRA flow cytometer (Coulter, Hialeah, FL). Consequently, 3 phenotypically distinct fractions of DC were found: fraction 1, CD1a+,CD11c+/lin−,HLA–DR+; fraction 2, CD1a−,CD11c+/lin−,HLA–DR+; and fraction 3, CD1a−,CD11c−/lin−,HLA–DR+ (R2–R4, respectively, in Figure 1).

Absolute numbers (per ml) of DC were calculated by multiplying the percentage contributed by the lin−,HLA–DR+ fraction (designated R1 in Figure 1A) to the total number of flow cytometry events by the count (per ml) of PBMC after negative selection. The absolute number (per ml) of each of the fractions of DC was calculated by multiplying the percentage of each region (R2–R4 in Figure 1B) within the DC by the total number of DC.

Immunohistochemistry. Formalin-fixed, paraffin-embedded sections and frozen sections which had been stored in liquid nitrogen were prepared from biopsied specimens of labial salivary glands of SS patients and normal controls. Hematoxylin and eosin (H&E) staining was performed, and immunohistochemical staining was done with several mAb known to react with DC or lymphocytes, using the avidin–biotin–peroxidase complex method with the LSAB (labeled streptavidin–biotin) kit (Dako, Carpinteria, CA) plus hematoxylin and diaminobenzidine. Monoclonal antibodies against fascin (55K-2; Dako) (26), HLA–DR (LN-3; Nichirei, Tokyo, Japan), CD1a (JPM30; Novocastra, Newcastle upon Tyne, UK), and CD11c (3.9; Ancell) were used for staining of DC. Monoclonal antibodies against latent membrane protein 1 (LMP-1) and Epstein-Barr nuclear antigen 2 (EBNA-2) (CS1-4 and PE2, respectively; both from Dako) were used to detect Epstein-Barr virus (EBV)–infected B cells. Monoclonal antibodies against CD4 and CD8 (MT310 and DK25, respectively; both from Dako) were used for staining of T cells, and monoclonal anti-IFNγ (45.15; Ancell) was used for cytokine staining. Formalin-fixed, paraffin-embedded sections were stained with antifascin, anti–HLA–DR, anti-CD1a, anti–LMP-1, and anti–EBNA-2. Anti-CD11c, anti-CD4, anti-CD8, and anti-IFNγ staining was performed on cryosections.

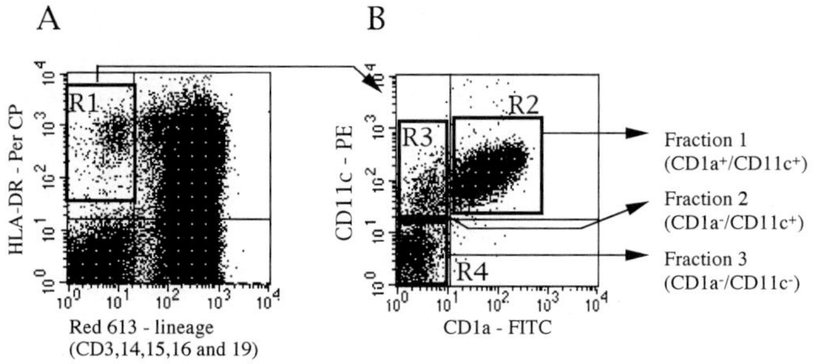

Figure 1. Detection of fractions of peripheral blood dendritic cells (DC). **A,** A DC-enriched population (see Patients and Methods) was stained with fluorescein isiothiocyanate (FITC)–labeled anti-CD1a monoclonal antibody (mAb) (CD1a-FITC), phycoerythrin (PE)–labeled anti-CD11c mAb (CD11c-PE), peridin chlorophyll protein (PerCP)–labeled anti–HLA–DR mAb (HLA-DR-PerCP), and biotinylated mAb against lineage markers (lin) CD3, CD14, CD15, CD16, and CD19, followed by RED613-streptavidin. DC were detected as fractions of the lin−,HLA–DR+ cell population (designated R1). **B,** Three fractions of DC were identified, with phenotypes of CD1a+,CD11c+/lin−,HLA–DR+ (CD1a+/CD11c+), called fraction 1 or R2; CD1a−,CD11c+/lin−,HLA–DR+ (CD1a−/CD11c+), called fraction 2 or R3; and CD1a−,CD11c−/lin−,HLA–DR+ (CD1a−/CD11c−), called fraction 3 or R4).

Determination of IL-4 and IFNγ production by T cells by intracellular cytokine staining. PBMC were stimulated with 10 μg/ml brefeldin A (ICN Biomedicals, Aurora, OH), 25 ng/ml phorbol-12-myristate-13-acetate (PMA), and 1 μg/ml ionomycin for 4 hours. After staining with CD4-PerCP (Leu-3a; Becton Dickinson), these cells were treated with FACS Lysing Solution and FACS Permeabilizing Solution (Becton Dickinson) and simultaneously stained with IL-4–PE and IFNγ-FITC (3010.211 and 25723.11, respectively; both from Becton Dickinson). Cells were washed with phosphate buffered saline (PBS) and resuspended in 500 μl of 1% formaldehyde (in PBS, pH 7.2). Samples were kept at 4°C in the dark and were analyzed within 24 hours of preparation. Mouse isotype controls were included to assess nonspecific interaction. Cells stained by intracellular cytokine staining were counted in a FACScan flow cytometer (Becton Dickinson) by standard methods.

Enzyme-linked immunosorbent assay (ELISA) for cytokines. Serum IL-4 and IFNγ of SS patients and normal controls were measured by ELISA using commercially available kits (Endogen, Woburn, MA).

Allogeneic T cell response induced by fraction 1 or fraction 3 DC. CD4+,CD45RA+ naive T cells were obtained from healthy volunteers by negative selection with anti-CD45RO (UCHL-1; Immunotech), anti-CD8 (T8; Coulter), anti-CD14 (M5E2), anti-CD16 (3G8), anti-CD19 (HIB19), anti–HLA–DR (L-243), and anti-CD11b (ICRF44; PharMingen) mAb followed by sheep anti-mouse Ig–coated magnetic beads. The purity of the cells was demonstrated to be ≥92% by reanalysis using anti-CD4 and anti-CD45RA mAb. Naive T cells (5×10^5) were cultured with or without allogeneic sorted fraction 1 DC or fraction 3 DC (1×10^5 each) in 96-well flat-bottomed culture plates in 200 μl of medium per well. After a 7-day culture, the T cells were washed and subsequently restimulated with PMA (25 ng/ml) and ionomycin (1 μg/ml) for 8 hours. Brefeldin A (2 μg/ml) was added into the cultures for the last 4 hours, and then cells were treated with the intracellular cytokine staining protocol described above.

Autologous T cell response induced by purified protein derivative (PPD)–stimulated fraction 1 DC. Sorted fraction 1 DC (1×10^5) from normal controls were stimulated with or without PPD (10 μg/ml) in 96-well flat-bottomed culture plates in 200 μl of medium per well for 24 hours. Autologous CD4+,CD45RA+ naive T cells (5×10^5) were cultured with these fraction 1 DC in 96-well flat-bottomed culture plates in 200 μl of medium per well. After a 7-day culture, the T cells were washed and subsequently restimulated with PMA (25 ng/ml) and ionomycin (1 μg/ml) for 8 hours. Brefeldin A (2 μg/ml) was added to the cultures for the last 4 hours, and then cells were treated according to the intracellular cytokine staining protocol described above.

Allogeneic coculture of naive T cell and fraction 1 DC from SS patients and normal volunteers. CD4+,CD45RA+ naive T cells (5×10^5) from SS patients or normal controls were cultured with sorted allogeneic fraction 1 DC from SS patients or normal controls in 96-well flat-bottomed culture plates in 200 μl of medium per well. Allogeneic mixed lymphocyte reactions (MLR) were performed on fraction 1 DC from a normal subject with allogeneic naive T cells from a normal subject, on fraction 1 DC from an SS patient with allogeneic naive T cells from a normal subject, on fraction 1 DC from a normal subject with allogeneic naive T cells from an SS patient, and on fraction 1 DC from an SS patient with allogeneic naive T cells from an SS patient. After a 7-day culture, the T cells were washed and subsequently restimulated with PMA (25 ng/ml) and ionomycin (1 μg/ml) for 8 hours. Brefeldin A (2 μg/ml) was added to the cultures for the last 4 hours, and then cells were treated with the intracellular cytokine staining protocol described above.

Statistical analysis. The Mann-Whitney U test was used for statistical analysis with a StatView statistical program (Abacus Concepts, Berkeley, CA). Differences were considered significant when tied P values were less than 0.05.

RESULTS

Clinical characteristics. The clinical characteristics of the patients are shown in Table 1. Most of the patients had high serum IgG and IgA levels and high erythrocyte sedimentation rates (ESRs). Virtually all normal control subjects had normal IgG titers and normal ESRs (data not shown). All 23 patients were positive for antinuclear antibodies (ANA), although the ANA titer varied among patients. All but 1 patient had anti-SSA antibody, and 14 patients had high levels of rheumatoid factors. In the normal control subjects, none of these autoantibodies and rheumatoid factors were detected (data not shown). Five SS patients and a normal subject had mild anemia. Furthermore, there were no significant differences in the total numbers of

Table 1. Clinical and serologic findings for patients with Sjögren's syndrome*

Patient/ age/sex	ANA, log titer	RF, IU/ml	Anti-SSA	Anti-SSB	IgG, mg/dl	IgA, mg/dl	IgM, mg/dl	ESR, mm/hour	CRP, mg/dl
1/68/F	20	45	+	−	2,290	260	336	39	<0.10
2/65/F	640	136	+	+	4,170	619	300	131	<0.10
3/58/F	640	55	+	+	3,560	854	257	118	2.03
4/66/F	320	96	+	+	3,520	468	195	68	0.55
5/45F	80	171	+	+	2,860	384	184	65	<0.10
6/57/F	160	83	+	+	2,010	410	269	54	0.23
7/59/F	320	<20	−	−	2,060	460	313	46	<0.10
8/74/F	20	<20	+	−	1,630	395	146	28	<0.10
9/49/F	20	<20	+	−	1,970	247	205	21	<0.10
10/71/F	320	128	+	−	2,780	528	134	97	<0.10
11/49/F	80	<20	+	−	2,770	195	116	20	0.11
12/49/F	160	<20	+	−	2,003	308	90	50	<0.10
13/47/F	80	<20	+	−	3,207	423	120	102	0.45
14/61/F	20	127	+	−	1,553	187	224	99	<0.10
15/48/M	320	64	+	+	3,591	337	170	64	1.22
16/68/M	20	<20	+	+	2,884	455	401	44	1.00
17/29/F	640	90	+	−	3,520	209	366	29	<0.10
18/72/F	320	<20	+	−	4,390	265	230	87	0.76
19/68/F	80	103	+	+	3,001	170	194	26	<0.10
20/49/F	640	33	+	−	2,674	530	189	33	<0.10
21/50/F	20	29	+	+	2,100	476	260	40	<0.10
22/56/F	40	189	+	−	3,660	319	279	72	0.18
23/53/F	160	<20	+	−	2,902	179	104	44	<0.10

white blood cells or PBMC between SS patients and normal control subjects.

Number of PB DC. The 22 normal control subjects had a mean absolute DC count of 19,173/ml (range 13,566–31,672/ml). SS patients had a significantly lower count (mean 10,810/ml, range 6,784–17,202/ml) (tied $P < 0.01$) (Figure 2). In addition, the percentage of DC within PBMC was lower in patients (mean 0.57%, range 0.41–0.70%) than in control subjects (mean 1.01%, range 0.86–1.32%); this difference was also significant (tied $P < 0.01$).

Frequencies of 3 fractions of DC. Three fractions of DC were identified within the lin−,HLA–DR+ population, based on differential expression of CD1a and CD11c: CD1a+,CD11c+/lin−,HLA–DR+ (fraction 1, designated R2 in Figure 1B), CD1a−,CD11c+/lin−,HLA–DR+ (fraction 2, designated R3), and CD1a−,CD11c−/lin−,HLA–DR+ (fraction 3, designated R4). As shown in Figure 3A, the frequency of fraction 1 DC was significantly lower in SS patients (mean 30.4%, range 10.4–51.1%) than in control subjects (mean 55.9%, range 43.3–74.5%) (tied $P < 0.01$). In contrast, the frequency of fraction 3 DC in patients (mean 59.0%, range 35.6–73.4%) was significantly higher than that in control subjects (mean 36.2%, range 20.1–50.9%) (tied $P < 0.01$). The percentage of fraction 2 DC was similar in patients (mean 10.6%, range 3.9–25.4%) and control subjects (mean 8.0%, range 4.0–13.5%).

The absolute number of fraction 1 DC in patients was significantly lower (mean 3,299/ml, range 1,243–6,365/ml) than that in normal control subjects (mean 10,777/ml, range 6,230–18,059/ml) (tied $P < 0.01$). However, the absolute number of fraction 3 DC in patients (mean 6,398/ml, range 2,416–11,239/ml) was not higher than that in control subjects (mean 6,774/ml, range 3,292–12,270/ml). The counts of fraction 2 DC were similar in the two groups (Figure 3B). Furthermore, the percentage of fraction 1 within PBMC was significantly lower in patients (mean 0.17%, range 0.06–0.30%) than in control subjects (mean 0.63%, range 0.55–0.83%) (tied $P < 0.01$). These findings indicated that the decrease in total blood DC in patients was primarily due to the decrease in fraction 1 DC (Figure 3C).

Infiltration of labial salivary glands of SS patients by fascin-positive mononuclear cells (MNC). H&E staining of labial salivary glands from an SS patient (patient 10 in Table 1) demonstrated infiltration of a number of MNC around the glandular structures (Figure 4A), while such infiltration of MNC was not detected in a normal control subject (Figure 4B). To determine whether infiltrating DC infiltrated were present, immunohistochemical staining of tissue was performed using mAb against fascin, a DC-associated

Table 1. *(Cont'd)*

Hgb, gm/dl	WBCs/μl	PBMC, $\times 10^5$/ml	Total DC/ml†	Fraction 1 DC/ml	Fraction 2 DC/ml	Fraction 3 DC/ml	Intracellular IL-4–producing T cells, %	Intracellular IFNγ-producing T cells, %
13.2	4,500	20.6	11,948	1,243	3,034	7,671	0.78	16.81
9.4	4,000	12.8	6,784	3,466	902	2,416	0.95	20.55
10.7	6,200	26.7	16,554	4,602	713	11,239	1.03	15.57
11.9	6,900	14.6	7,154	1,424	916	4,814	1.04	20.56
12.0	3,700	22.2	9,102	1,337	1,539	6,226	1.59	19.05
13.0	3,800	12.9	7,152	1,279	679	5,194	1.07	12.19
12.6	6,000	28.2	17,202	5,813	2,085	9,304	0.91	17.3
12.0	4,300	16.7	10,688	3,644	1,689	5,355	3.66	19.51
12.8	9,100	25.3	12,903	4,812	875	7,216	0.71	10.07
10.3	3,300	12.9	8,901	1,609	887	6,405	1.22	16.25
11.4	3,800	18.6	7,812	3,381	994	3,437	0.88	20.02
13.8	3,300	14.3	9,844	3,856	628	5,361	0.47	16.12
11.3	7,800	20.3	12,874	4,634	653	7,587	1.13	9.25
13.4	4,000	16.2	8,710	3,391	723	4,596	0.70	12.88
15.3	7,900	21.5	13,520	6,365	912	6,242	1.11	10.43
14.3	6,700	22.0	10,957	1,594	1,320	8,041	1.32	18.44
12.7	3,600	13.9	8,382	2,582	960	4,839	0.07	11.42
10.1	4,700	24.2	11,039	3,974	751	6,314	0.41	14.16
16.2	7,200	22.0	14,890	4,765	1,343	8,782	1.45	17.09
14.7	6,200	21.4	12,705	3,002	1,731	7,972	0.89	11.54
10.9	5,200	16.0	11,180	3,173	436	7,571	0.53	16.22
11.4	4,900	17.3	9,270	3,404	1,077	4,969	2.56	15.55
12.2	4,100	18.9	9,053	2,535	922	5,596	2.53	15.36

* Normal values are as follows: antinuclear antibodies (ANA) <20, rheumatoid factor (RF) <20, anti-SSA and anti-SSB negative, IgG 1,237–1,711 in men and 1,285–1,855 in women, IgA 153–341 in men and 162–346 in women, IgM 58–152 in men and 89–241 in women, erythrocyte sedimentation rate (ESR) ≤15 in men and ≤20 in women, C-reactive protein (CRP) <0.10, hemoglobin (Hgb) 12.9–17.2 in men and 11.3–15.4 in women, and white blood cells (WBCs) 3,000–8,500. PBMC = peripheral blood mononuclear cells; DC = dendritic cells; IL-4 = interleukin-4; IFNγ = interferon-γ (see Patients and Methods for an explanation of fractions 1–3).

† Absolute numbers (per ml) of PB DC were calculated by multiplying the percentage contributed by the lineage marker–negative (lin−), HLA–DR+ fraction (designated R1 in Figure 1A) to the total number of flow cytometry events by the count (per ml) of PBMC after negative selection.

marker. Fascin-positive MNC were present and scattered among numerous fascin-negative MNC (Figure 4D), while such cells were not detected in salivary glands of a normal control subject (Figure 4C). The fascin-positive cells were mostly observed in areas surrounding the tubular ducts. The epithelial cells of the tubular ducts were also positive for fascin in both the patient and the normal control subject. Immunohistochemical staining of the specimens prepared by serial cutting indicated that the infiltrated fascin-positive cells were HLA–DR+ but CD1a− (Figures 4E and F). Furthermore, CD11c+ cells were also detected at a frequency similar to that of fascin-positive cells in the patient (Figure 4G). Both fascin-positive cells and CD11c+ cells showed dendritic projections on the cell surface, suggesting that these cells were DC. Similar results were obtained for another 6 patients and 2 normal subjects (data not shown).

Increased number of IFNγ-producing CD4+ T cells in PB of SS patients. IFNγ and IL-4 production by CD4+ T cells was examined by intracellular staining. Figure 5A shows representative results for a patient and

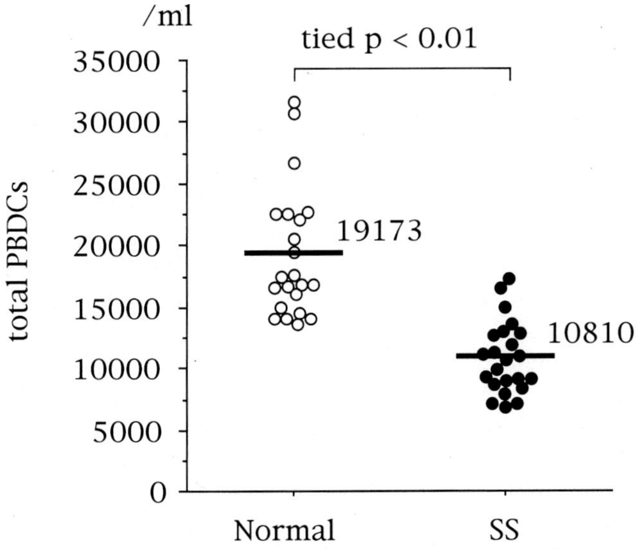

Figure 2. Reduction of the total number of peripheral blood dendritic cells (total PBDCs) in Sjögren's syndrome (SS). The mean number in patients with SS was significantly lower (10,810/ml) than that in 22 normal control subjects (19,173/ml) (tied $P < 0.01$).

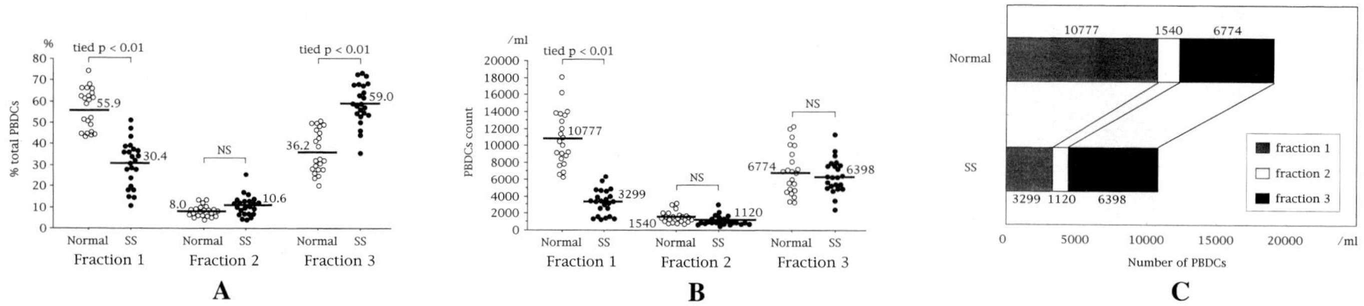

Figure 3. Frequencies and absolute numbers of the 3 fractions of dendritic cells (DC). **A,** Frequencies of fraction 1 and fraction 3 DC among total peripheral blood DC (total PBDCs) in patients with Sjögren's syndrome (SS) differed from those in normal control subjects. The mean frequency of fraction 1 DC in patients with SS was significantly lower than that in normal control subjects (30.4% versus 55.9%; tied $P < 0.01$), while the mean frequency of fraction 3 DC was significantly higher in patients with SS (59.0% versus 36.2%; tied $P < 0.01$). The mean percentages of fraction 2 DC were similar for patients and normal control subjects (10.6% versus 8.0%, respectively; *P* not significant [NS]). The Mann-Whitney U test was used for statistical analysis. **B,** The mean number of fraction 1 DC in patients was significantly lower than that in normal control subjects (3,299/ml versus 10,777/ml; tied $P < 0.01$). However, the mean number of fraction 3 DC in patients was not larger than that in normal control subjects (6,398/ml versus 6,774/ml; *P* NS), and the mean number of fraction 2 DC in patients was similar to that in normal control subjects (1,120/ml versus 1,540/ml; *P* NS). **C,** Histograms indicate absolute numbers of the 3 DC fractions. The decrease in total PBDCs was shown to be due to a selective decrease in the number of fraction 1 DC in patients with SS.

a normal control subject. The percentage of IFNγ-producing CD4+ T cells among total CD4+ T cells in the PB was significantly higher in patients (mean 15.49%, range 9.25–20.56%) than in normal subjects (mean 7.62%, range 4.83–12.25%) (tied $P < 0.01$). However, the percentage of IL-4–producing CD4+ T cells was similar and low in both patients (mean 1.17%, range 0.7–3.7%) and control subjects (mean 1.15%, range 0.2–3.0%), although 3 patients and 1 normal control subject exhibited significant increases. The titers of IFNγ and IL-4 in serum were measured by means of ELISA. In contrast to the results of intracellular staining, the titer of both cytokines was very low in patients as well as in control subjects (data not shown). Figure 5B indicates the percentages of the respective cytokine-producing T cells in each dot blot profile.

Infiltration of labial salivary glands of SS patients by IFNγ-producing T cells. To examine whether IFNγ-producing CD4+ T cells infiltrated labial salivary glands of SS patients, immunohistochemical staining was performed using mAb against CD4, CD8, and IFNγ. As shown in Figure 6A, numerous CD4+ T cells were found within the interstitial area of salivary glands from an SS patient. In contrast, CD8+ T cells were found to be scattered within the same area, but the frequency was much lower than that of CD4+ T cells (Figure 6B). In addition, a number of IFNγ-producing MNC were detected within the interstitial regions (Figure 6C). Based on the relative frequency of CD4+ T cells, CD8+ T cells, and IFNγ-producing cells, most of the infiltrated IFNγ-producing cells were considered to be CD4+ T cells.

Differentiation of naive T cells into Th1 driven by fraction 1 DC. It has recently been demonstrated that monocyte-derived DC drive naive T helper cells to differentiate into Th1 cells (22). To show that fraction 1 DC, which are monocyte-associated DC, have the capacity to instruct naive CD4+ T cells to differentiate into Th1 cells, freshly prepared naive T helper cells (5×10^5) from normal subjects were cultured with allogeneic fraction 1 DC or fraction 3 DC (1×10^5 each) from normal subjects.

The percentages of IFNγ- or IL-4–producing CD4+ T cells were determined by intracellular staining after a 7-day culture (Figure 7A). Numbers of IFNγ-producing T cells were significantly increased when T cells were cocultured with allogeneic fraction 1 DC versus coculture with allogeneic fraction 3 DC (tied $P = 0.049$) (Figure 7B). However, when naive T helper cells were cocultured with allogeneic fraction 3 DC (which were CD1a−,CD11c− [and which have recently been demonstrated to be IFNα-producing cells]), numbers of single producers of IL-4 and double producers of IFNγ and IL-4 were significantly increased, but numbers of single producers of IFNγ were only slightly increased (Figures 7A and B and data not shown). These findings indicated that fraction 1 DC had specific Th1-inducing capacity, while fraction 3 DC were potent inducers of Th2 cells, at least in terms of allogeneic responses. In addition, when naive T helper cells were cocultured with autologous fraction 1 DC pretreated with PPD, a dramatic increase in the number of IFNγ-producing T cells was observed, demonstrating that Th1-inducing capacity

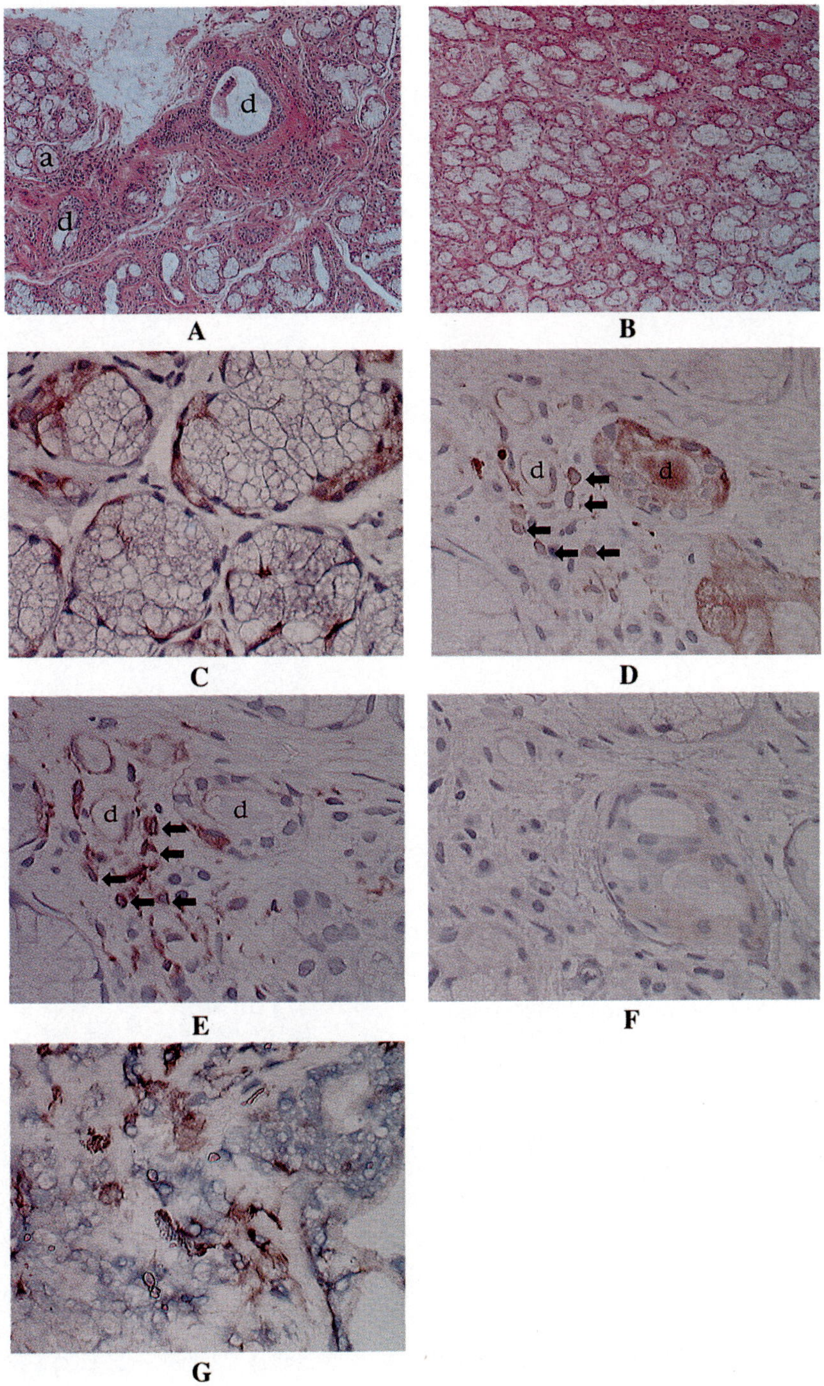

Figure 4. Histologic findings for dendritic cells (DC) of labial salivary glands from a patient with Sjögren's syndrome (SS) and a normal subject. Immunohistochemical staining of the same biopsied specimen (from patient 10, see Table 1) with antifascin monoclonal antibody (mAb), anti–HLA–DR mAb, and anti-CD1a mAb demonstrated infiltration of fascin+,HLA–DR+,CD1a− mononuclear cells (MNC) (**arrows**) within the aggregates of lymphoid cells around the tubular ducts (**d**) of the secretory glands. CD11c+ MNC also infiltrated the inflammatory cells at a frequency similar to that of fascin+,HLA–DR+,CD1a− MNC. Antifascin, anti–HLA–DR, and anti-CD1a stainings were performed on formalin-fixed paraffin-embedded sections. Anti-CD11c staining was carried out on cryosections. **A,** Hematoxylin and eosin (H&E) staining (patient 10). **a** indicates acini. **B,** H&E staining (normal subject). **C,** Staining with antifascin mAb (normal subject). **D,** Staining with antifascin mAb (patient 10). **E,** Staining with anti–HLA–DR mAb (patient 10). **F,** Staining with anti-CD1a mAb (patient 10). **G,** Staining with anti-CD11c mAb (patient 10). (Original magnification × 10 in **A** and **B**; × 50 in **C–G**.)

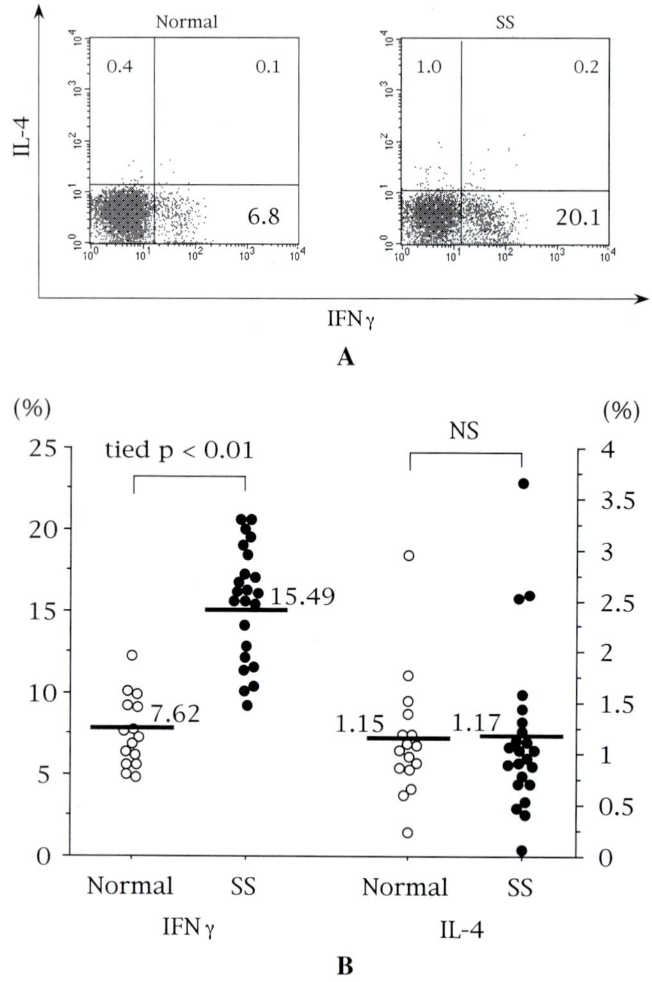

Figure 5. Intracellular double staining of interferon-γ (IFNγ) and interleukin-4 (IL-4) in peripheral blood CD4+ T cells. **A,** Representative results of intracellular staining. The percentage of IFNγ-producing CD4+ T cells in patients with Sjögren's syndrome (SS) was significantly higher than that in normal control subjects (mean 15.49% versus 7.62% of CD4+ T cells; tied $P < 0.01$, by Mann-Whitney U test). **B,** Percentages of the respective cytokine-producing T cells are indicated in each dot-blot profile. NS = not significant.

of fraction 1 DC could be exhibited in an antigen-specific manner (Figures 7C and D).

No functional impairment of fraction 1 DC from SS patients. To investigate whether fraction 1 DC from SS patients were functionally altered, allogeneic MLR was performed using fraction 1 DC and naive CD4+ T cells from patients and normal subjects. When naive CD4+ T cells from a normal subject were cocultured with allogeneic fraction 1 DC from a normal subject, 26% of IFNγ-producing T cells were induced (Figure 8A), while coculture of naive CD4+ T cells from a normal subject with fraction 1 DC from an SS patient resulted in induction of 22% of IFNγ-producing T cells (Figure 8B). These findings indicated that fraction 1 DC

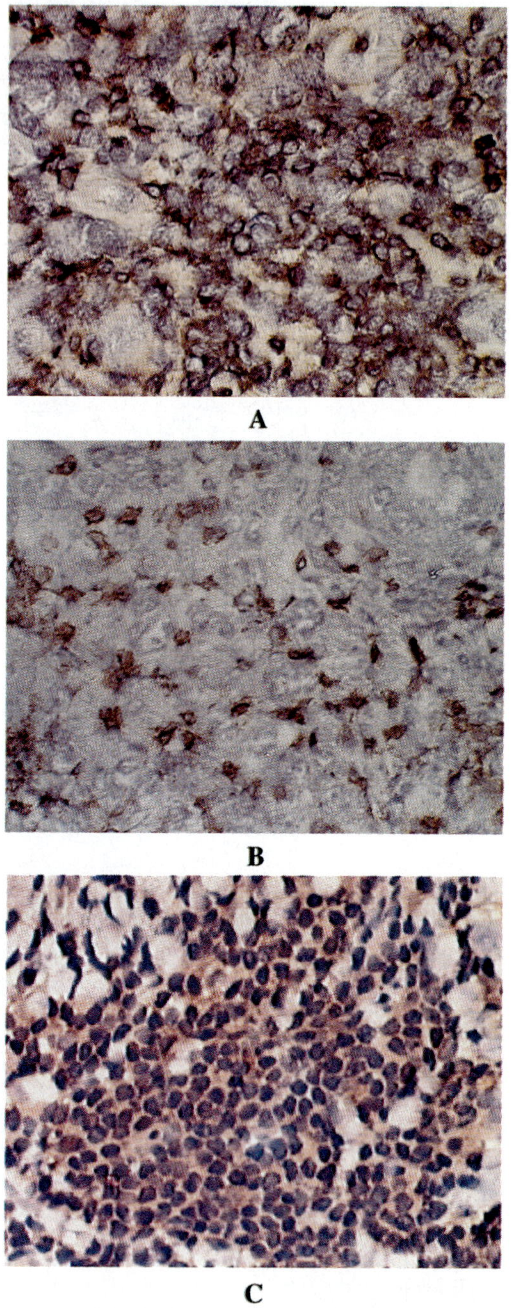

Figure 6. Histologic findings for T cells of labial salivary glands from a patient with Sjögren's syndrome. Immunohistochemical staining of the biopsied specimen with **A,** anti-CD4 monoclonal antibodies (mAb), **B,** anti-CD8 mAb, and **C,** anti–interferon-γ (anti-IFNγ) mAb demonstrated that the majority of infiltrated cells around the tubular ducts of the secretory glands were IFNγ-producing CD4+ T cells. (Original magnification × 50.)

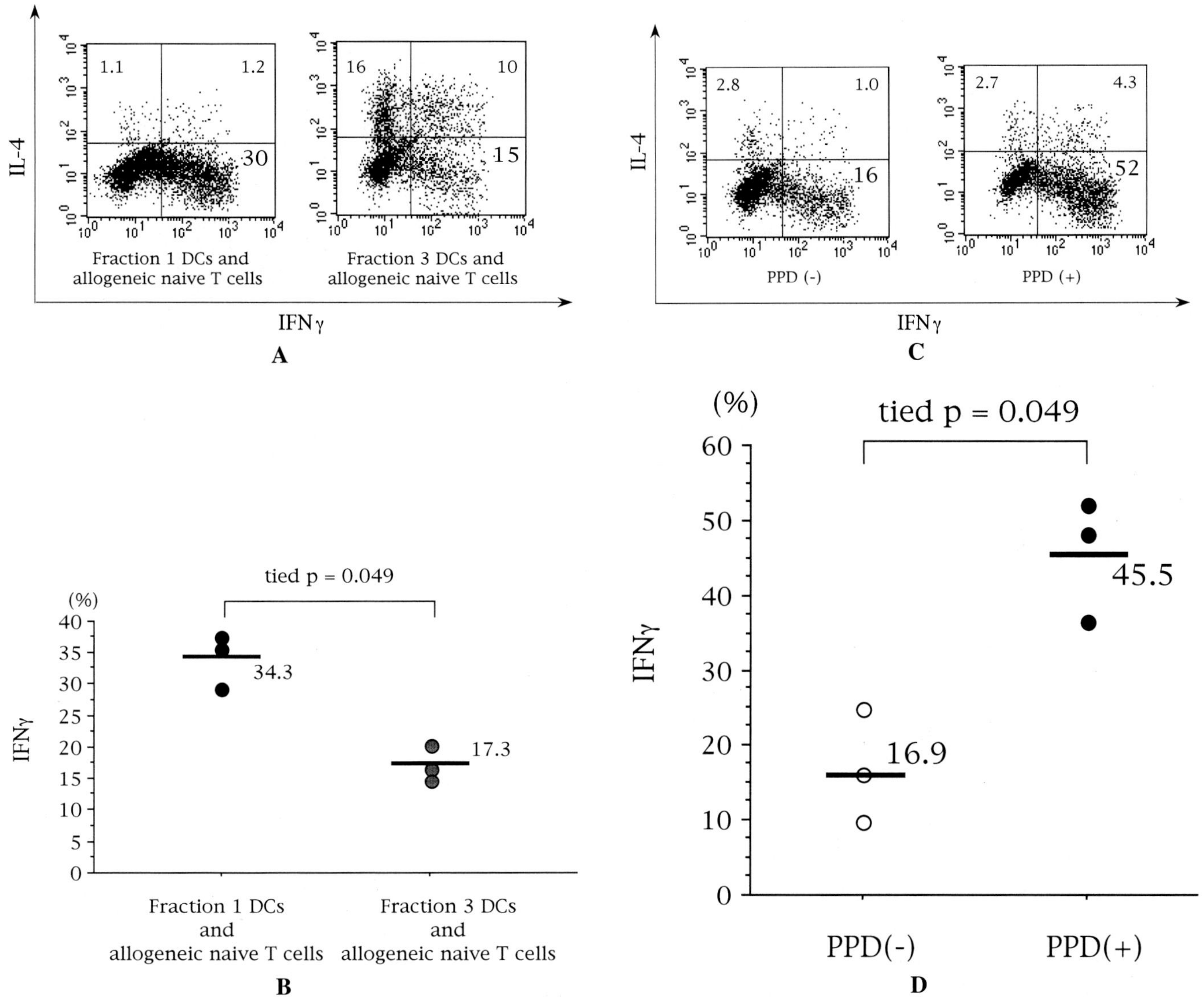

Figure 7. In vitro differentiation of allogeneic and autologous naive T cells into Th1 cells driven by fraction 1 dendritic cells (DC). **A** and **B,** Allogeneic mixed lymphocyte reactions (MLR) using fraction 1 or fraction 3 DC. Freshly prepared naive T cells (5×10^5) from normal volunteers were cultured with allogeneic fraction 1 DC or fraction 3 DC (1×10^5 each) from normal subjects. Interferon-γ (IFNγ) and interleukin-4 (IL-4) production was measured by intracellular staining after a 7-day culture. Three independent experiments were performed. **A,** Representative results of intracellular staining. **B,** Numbers of IFNγ-producing T cells were significantly increased when naive T cells were cocultured with fraction 1 DC versus coculture with fraction 3 DC (tied $P = 0.049$, by Mann-Whitney U test). **C** and **D,** Autologous MLR of fraction 1 DC pretreated with purified protein derivative (PPD). Fraction 1 DC (1×10^5) from normal subjects were stimulated with PPD for 24 hours. Freshly prepared autologous naive T cells (5×10^5) from normal subjects were cultured with PPD-pretreated fraction 1 DC. IFNγ and IL-4 production was measured by intracellular staining after a 7-day culture. Three independent experiments were performed. **C,** Representative results of intracellular staining. **D,** Numbers of IFNγ-producing T cells were significantly increased when naive T cells were cocultured with stimulated autologous fraction 1 DC versus coculture with nonstimulated fraction 1 DC (tied $P = 0.049$, by Mann-Whitney U test). **A** and **C**, Percentages of the respective cytokine-producing T cells are indicated in each dot-blot profile.

from the patient were functionally normal, especially in terms of Th1 polarization. In contrast, when naive CD4+ T cells from the same patient were cocultured with fraction 1 DC from either a normal subject or another SS patient, 39% (Figure 8C) or 40% (Figure 8D), respectively, of IFNγ-producing T cells were produced. These findings indicated that naive CD4+ T cells from the patient were more prone to be skewed toward

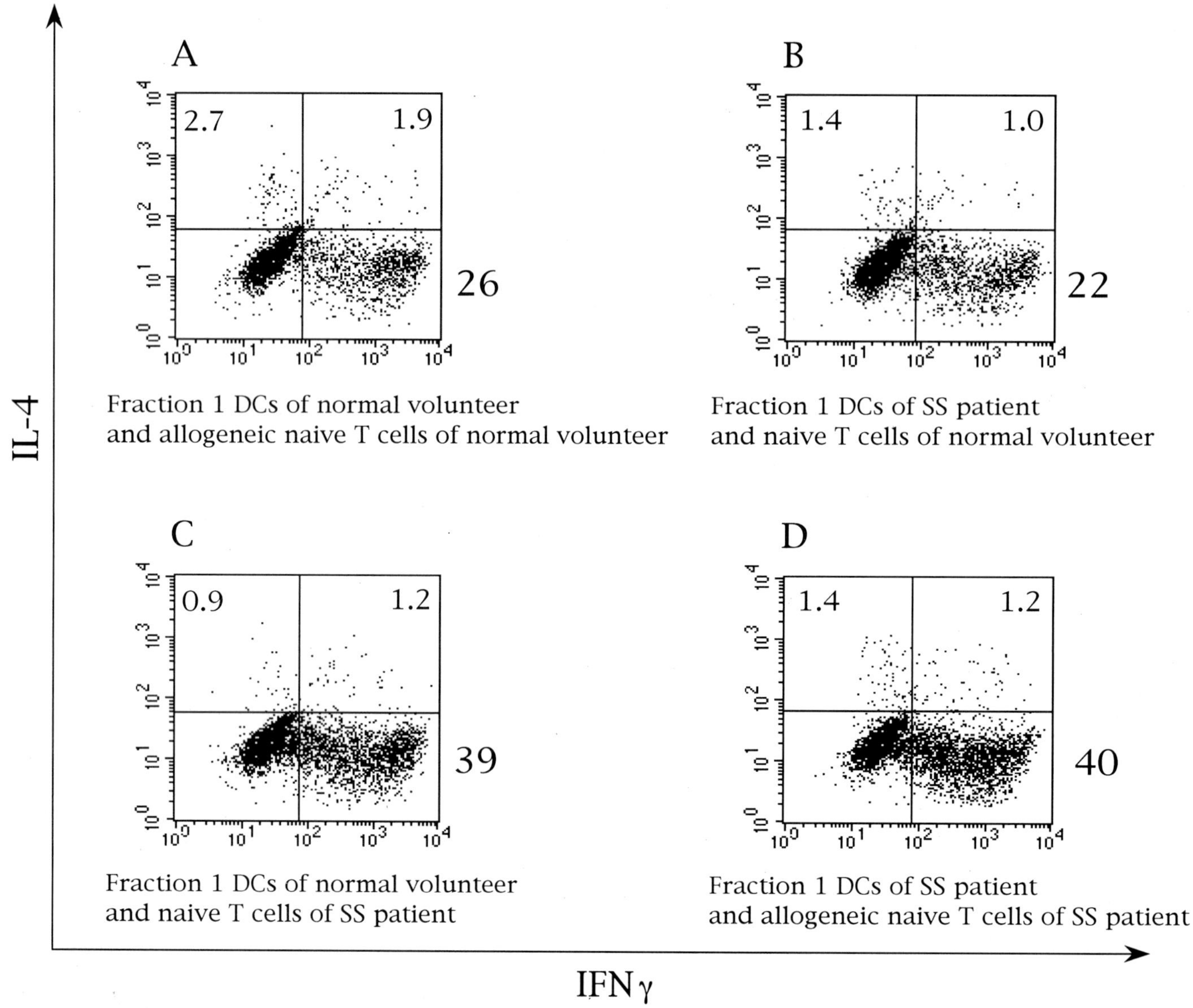

Figure 8. Differential induction of cytokine-producing T cells resulting from coculture of fraction 1 dendritic cells (DC) and naive T cells from patients with Sjögren's syndrome (SS) and normal subjects. Shown are results of mixed lymphocyte reactions of **A,** fraction 1 DC from a normal subject with allogeneic naive T cells from a normal subject, **B,** fraction 1 DC from an SS patient with allogeneic naive T cells from a normal subject, **C,** fraction 1 DC from a normal subject with allogeneic naive T cells from an SS patient, and **D,** fraction 1 DC from an SS patient with allogeneic naive T cells from an SS patient. Percentages of the respective cytokine-producing T cells are indicated in each dot-blot profile. Values are the results from 1 of the 3 experiments. IL-4 = interleukin-4; IFNγ = interferon-γ.

Th1 than normal counterparts, implicating the presence of some intrinsic defects in naive CD4+ T cells from the patient. Similar results were obtained using cells from two other patients (data not shown).

DISCUSSION

Despite extensive studies, the etiology of SS has long remained unclear. This seems to be related to the lack of information concerning the mechanism for breakdown of self tolerance in SS patients. DC are specialized APC and play central roles in eliciting primary immune responses (19–21). Thus, it is possible that DC are involved in breakdown of self tolerance, resulting in the genesis of SS.

In this study, we demonstrated that there were fewer circulating DC in the PB of SS patients than in that of healthy subjects. This decrease was shown to be due to selective reduction of the number of fraction 1 DC. Immunohistochemical analysis of labial salivary glands from SS patients demonstrated infiltration of fascin+,HLA–DR+,CD11c+,CD1a− MNC around the tubular ducts of the secretory glands. Fascin is known to be specific to mature DC among hemopoietic cells, although it is induced in B cells after EBV infection (26–28). The infiltrating fascin-positive cells were negative for EBNA-2 and LMP-1 (data not shown), excluding the possibility that they were EBV-infected B cells. However, the epithelial cells of the tubular ducts were also found to express fascin protein in both patients and normal control subjects, in accordance with a previous report (26).

These findings strongly suggest that the infiltrating fascin-positive cells were DC. This raises the possibility that the decrease in fraction 1 DC in PB may have been caused by selective trafficking of this cell type to affected tissues such as salivary glands. Notably, however, the infiltrating cells were CD11c+,CD1a−, a finding inconsistent with the phenotype of freshly isolated fraction 1 DC, which was CD11c+,CD1a+. This discrepancy might reflect a down-regulation of CD1a in fraction 1 DC during the process of recruitment, since it has been shown that expression of CD1a in DC is normally reduced upon maturation (29–31). Although it is also possible that the CD11c+,CD1a− cells were fraction 2 DC that were recruited from PB, the finding of a dramatic decrease in fraction 1 DC in PB from SS patients may favor the former possibility. We speculate that the selective trafficking of fraction 1 DC from PB to salivary gland might be continuous, resulting in the decrease in the number of fraction 1 DC in PB.

Many previous studies have investigated the production of various cytokines in focal lesions or in PB of patients with SS with the purpose of determining the factors involved in the pathophysiology of SS. Although a series of studies suggested that polarized Th1 responses are generally associated with the pathogenesis of SS (7–10), the results of such studies were not conclusive, since Th2 cytokines such as IL-4 and IL-10 were also detected in some studies (10–17). Furthermore, the mechanisms responsible for Th1 balance have remained unclear. In this study, we found an increased frequency of IFNγ-producing CD4+ T cells in the PB of all 23 SS patients by intracellular staining, although we detected neither IFNγ nor IL-4 in serum by ELISA. This indicated that predominant Th1 balance was consistently present in PB in SS patients, although 3 patients were found to produce IL-4 as well as IFNγ.

In view of the intrinsic properties of DC, we speculate that the IFNγ-producing CD4+ T cells found in the PB of SS patients had been generated in regional lymph nodes, presumably by interacting with fraction 1 DC that might have been recruited from salivary glands. It is technically difficult, however, to demonstrate in the clinical setting that fraction 1 DC are actively transported to regional lymph nodes via afferent lymphatic vessels from secretory glands. The IFNγ-producing CD4+ T cells found in PB were probably en route to salivary glands, because numerous IFNγ+ cells as well as CD4+ T cells were detected in the salivary glands of the patients, but not in those of the normal control subjects. The transported IFNγ+ cells would presumably meet antigens in the salivary glands and thereby actively secrete IFNγ, causing inflammatory reactions there.

We next examined whether the observed Th1 polarization might actually be related to the fraction 1 DC. Indeed, in vitro coculture of fraction 1 DC and allogeneic naive CD4+ T cells induced IFNγ-producing Th1 cells, while fraction 3 DC facilitated the induction of IL-4–producing Th2 cells rather than IFNγ-producing Th1 cells. Furthermore, it was demonstrated that fraction 1 DC preincubated with PPD instructed autologous naive CD4+ T cells to produce IFNγ, indicating that the Th1 polarizing effect of fraction 1 DC could be exerted in an antigen-specific manner. These findings are consistent with the finding that monocyte-associated DC, which fraction 1 DC appear to be, have the capacity to drive naive T cells to differentiate into Th1 cells (22).

Based on these findings, we hypothesize that fraction 1 DC play essential roles in initiating Th1 immune responses in SS patients, and that preferential trafficking of fraction 1 DC into salivary or lacrimal glands is an early event in the pathogenesis of SS. However, the factors triggering recruitment of fraction 1 DC remain unknown. A clue to the answer may reside in the chemokine receptor—or homing receptor—system, since it has been shown that selective recruitment of immature and mature DC might depend on differential expression of distinct chemokine receptors (32). Relevant to this, one of the most critical issues to be addressed is the nature of target autoantigens associated with disruption of self tolerance.

Remarkably, we obtained intriguing results from MLR assays using fraction 1 DC and naive CD4+ T cells from patients and normal individuals. The results indicated that fraction 1 DC from patients were not functionally altered, while PB naive CD4+ T cells from patients were abnormal because they were more susceptible to Th1-inducible stimuli of fraction 1 DC than were those from normal individuals. These findings suggest that functional defects of naive CD4+ T cells might also contribute to the pathophysiology of SS. The essential basis of the defects, however, remains to be clarified.

Clinical characteristics of SS include the presence of ANA, anti-SSA or anti-SSB antibodies, polyclonal hypergammaglobulinemia, and high ESRs (1–3). Of these, anti-SSA and anti-SSB antibodies are considered relatively specific to SS (1). All patients in this study were positive for ANA, and 21 of 23 patients had anti-SSA antibody. Furthermore, other parameters such as the serum IgG or IgA level and the ESR were elevated in most cases. Further detailed studies will be required to determine whether these clinical parameters were directly associated with the decrease in circulating fraction 1 DC or the increase in the number of Th1 cells in PB. Notably, in myasthenia gravis, which is also categorized as an organ-specific autoimmune disease, IFNγ is thought to play a role in modulating the anti–acetylcholine receptor antibody response via B7–CD28 and CD27–CD27L costimulation pathways (33).

In conclusion, we have demonstrated that in SS, fraction 1 DC were selectively decreased in PB, and that this was associated with infiltration of fascin+,CD11c+ DC in salivary glands. We also found that the numbers of IFNγ-producing Th1 cells were increased in the PB as well as in the salivary glands of patients, and that this appeared to be generated by interaction with fraction 1 DC. Furthermore, the current study findings suggested the presence of intrinsic defects of naive T cells in patients with SS. These findings suggest a novel mechanism of SS in which DC may play central roles. DC may therefore be a target of new basic or clinical approaches to SS.

ACKNOWLEDGMENTS

We are grateful to Ms Sachiko Miura and Ms Takako Akamatsu for their technical assistance, and to Ms Rie Okuda for secretarial assistance.

REFERENCES

1. Vitali C, Bombardieri S, Moutsopoulos HM, Balestrieri G, Bencivelli W, Bernstein RM, et al. Preliminary criteria for the classification of Sjögren's syndrome: results of a prospective concerted action supported by the European Community. Arthritis Rheum 1993;36:340–7.
2. Homma M, Tojo T, Akizuki M, Yamagata H. Criteria for Sjögren's syndrome in Japan. Scand J Rheumatol Suppl 1986;61:26–7.
3. Fox RI. Clinical features, pathogenesis, and treatment of Sjögren's syndrome. Curr Opin Rheumatol 1996;8:438–45.
4. Mosmann TR, Coffman RL. TH1 and TH2 cells: different patterns of lymphokine secretion lead to different functional properties. Annu Rev Immunol 1989;7:145–73.
5. Yamamura M, Uyemura K, Deans RJ, Weinberg K, Rea TH, Bloom BR, et al. Defining protective responses to pathogens: cytokine profiles in leprosy lesions. Science 1991;254:277–9.
6. Salgame P, Abrams JS, Clayberger C, Goldstein H, Convit J, Modlin RL, et al. Differing lymphokine profiles of functional subsets of human CD4 and CD8 T cell clones. Science 1991;254: 279–82.
7. Fox RI, Kang HI, Ando D, Abrams J, Pisa E. Cytokine mRNA expression in salivary gland biopsies of Sjögren's syndrome. J Immunol 1994;152:5532–9.
8. Ohyama Y, Nakamura S, Matsuzaki G, Shinohara M, Hiroki A, Fujimura T, et al. Cytokine messenger RNA expression in the labial salivary glands of patients with Sjögren's syndrome. Arthritis Rheum 1996;39:1376–84.
9. Konttinen YT, Kemppinen P, Koski H, Li TF, Jumppanen M, Hietanen J, et al. Th1 cytokines are produced in labial salivary glands in Sjögren's syndrome, but also in healthy individuals. Scand J Rheumatol 1999;28:106–12.
10. Al-Janadi M, al-Balla S, al-Dalaan A, Raziuddin S. Cytokine profile in systemic lupus erythematosus, rheumatoid arthritis, and other rheumatic diseases. J Clin Immunol 1993;13:58–67.
11. Villarreal GM, Alcocer-Varela J, Llorente L. Cytokine gene and CD25 antigen expression by peripheral blood T cells from patients with primary Sjögren's syndrome. Autoimmunity 1995;20:223–9.
12. Boumba D, Skopouli FN, Moutsopoulos HM. Cytokine mRNA expression in the labial salivary gland tissues from patients with primary Sjögren's syndrome. Br J Rheumatol 1995;34:326–33.
13. Ogawa N, Dang H, Lazaridis K, McGuff HS, Aufdemorte TB, Talal N. Analysis of transforming growth factor beta and other cytokines in autoimmune exocrinopathy (Sjögren's syndrome). J Interferon Cytokine Res 1995;15:759–67.
14. Brookes SM, Cohen SBA, Price EJ, Webb LM, Feldmann M, Maini RN, et al. T cell clones from a Sjögren's syndrome salivary gland biopsy produce high levels of IL-10. Clin Exp Immunol 1996;103:268–72.
15. Sun DI, Emmert-Buck MR, Fox PC. Differential cytokine mRNA expression in human labial minor salivary glands in primary Sjögren's syndrome. Autoimmunity 1998;28:125–37.
16. Hagiwara E, Pando J, Ishigatsubo Y, Klinman DM. Altered frequency of type 1 cytokine secreting cells in the peripheral blood of patients with primary Sjögren's syndrome. J Rheumatol 1998; 25:89–93.
17. Halse A, Tengner P, Wahren-Herlenius M, Haga H, Jonsson R. Increased frequency of cells secreting interleukin-6 and interleukin-10 in peripheral blood of patients with primary Sjögren's syndrome. Scand J Immunol 1999;49:533–8.
18. Price EJ, Venables PJ. The etiopathogenesis of Sjögren's syndrome. Semin Arthritis Rheum 1995;25:117–33.
19. Steinman RM. The dendritic cell system and its role in immunogenicity. Annu Rev Immunol 1991;9:271–96.
20. Banchereau J, Steinman RM. Dendritic cells and the control of immunity. Nature 1998;392:245–52.
21. Inaba K, Metlay JP, Crowley MT, Steinman RM. Dendritic cells pulsed with protein antigens in vitro can prime antigen-specific, MHC-restricted T cells in situ. J Exp Med 1990;172:631–40.
22. Rissoan MC, Soumelis V, Kadowaki N, Grouard G, Briere F, de Waal Malefyt R, et al. Reciprocal control of T helper cell and dendritic cell differentiation. Science 1999;283:1183–6.
23. Ito T, Inaba M, Inaba K, Toki J, Sogo S, Iguchi T, et al. A CD1a+/CD11c+ subset of human blood dendritic cells is a direct precursor of Langerhans cells. J Immunol 1999;163:1409–19.
24. Freudenthal PS, Steinman RM. The distinct surface of human blood dendritic cells, as observed after an improved isolation method. Proc Natl Acad Sci U S A 1990;87:7698–702.
25. Zhou LJ, Tedder TF. Human blood dendritic cells selectively

express CD83, a member of the immunoglobulin superfamily. J Immunol 1995;154:3821–35.
26. Ross R, Ross XL, Schwing J, Langin T, Reske-Kunz AB. The actin-bundling protein fascin is involved in the formation of dendritic processes in maturing epidermal Langerhans cells. J Immunol 1998;160:3776–82.
27. Mosialos G, Yamashiro S, Baughman RW, Matsudaira P, Vara L, Matsumura F, et al. Epstein-Barr virus infection induces expression in B lymphocytes of a novel gene encoding an evolutionarily conserved 55-kilodalton actin-bundling protein. J Virol 1994;68: 7320–8.
28. Mosialos G, Birkenbach M, Ayehunie S, Matsumura F, Pinkus GS, Kieff E, et al. Circulating human dendritic cells differentially express high levels of a 55-kd actin-bundling protein. Am J Pathol 1996;148:593–600.
29. Romani N, Lenz A, Glassel H, Stossel H, Stanzl U, Majdic O, et al. Cultured human Langerhans cells resemble lymphoid dendritic cells in phenotype and function. J Invest Dermatol 1989;93:600–9.
30. Mackensen A, Herbst B, Kohler G, Wolff-Vorbeck G, Rosenthal FM, Veelken H, et al. Delineation of the dendritic cell lineage by generating large numbers of Birbeck granule-positive Langerhans cells from human peripheral blood progenitor cells in vitro. Blood 1995;86:2699–707.
31. Bjorck P, Flores-Romo L, Liu YJ. Human interdigitating dendritic cells directly stimulate CD40-activated naive B cells. Eur J Immunol 1997;27:1266–74.
32. Dieu MC, Vanbervliet B, Vicari A, Bridon JM, Oldham E, Ait-Yahia S, et al. Selective recruitment of immature and mature dendritic cells by distinct chemokines expressed in different anatomic sites. J Exp Med 1998;188:373–86.
33. Balasa B, Sarvetnick N. Is pathogenic humoral autoimmunity a Th1 response? Lessons from (for) myasthenia gravis. Immunol Today 2000;21:19–23.

ARTHRITIS & RHEUMATISM
Vol. 44, No. 2, February 2001, pp 432–441

Treatment With a Consensus Peptide Based on Amino Acid Sequences in Autoantibodies Prevents T Cell Activation by Autoantigens and Delays Disease Onset in Murine Lupus

Bevra H. Hahn,[1] Ram R. Singh,[2] Weng Kee Wong,[1] Betty P. Tsao,[1] Ken Bulpitt,[1] and Fanny M. Ebling[1]

Objective. **To test the hypothesis that an artificial peptide, based on an algorithm describing T cell stimulatory sequences from the V_H regions of murine IgG antibodies to DNA, is an effective tolerogen in vivo in the (NZB/NZW)F_1 (BWF1) mouse model of systemic lupus erythematosus.**

Methods. **Using proliferative T cell responses to 439 Ig peptides, an algorithm was constructed that describes the amino acid sequences likely to stimulate BWF1 T cells. Stimulatory (pConsensus [pCONS]) or nonstimulatory (pNegative [pNEG]) peptides were synthesized. Groups of 10-week-old (healthy) or 20-week-old (diseased) BWF1 mice received monthly intravenous injections of 1,000 μg of peptide or saline. Ex vivo splenic T cell responses and in vivo clinical effects were measured.**

Results. **Tolerance was induced by pCONS, but not by pNEG, with respect to ex vivo T cell proliferation and T cell help for antibodies to DNA. T cell help for IgG anti-DNA was impaired not only after T cell stimulation by pCONS but also after stimulation by some peptides from nucleosomal and Ro antigens. Treatment with pCONS significantly delayed the onset of nephritis and inhibited increases in the plasma levels of total IgG, IgG antibodies to DNA, nucleosome, cardiolipin, interferon-γ, and interleukin-4. In contrast, antibody responses to an exogenous antigen were not impaired. Survival was significantly prolonged in both healthy and diseased mice treated with pCONS.**

Conclusion. **Induction of immune tolerance in response to treatment with pCONS in autoreactive T cell helper populations is highly effective in delaying the appearance of multiple autoantibodies, cytokine increases, and nephritis in BWF1 mice, and dramatically prolongs survival. A striking effect is the ability of the peptide to tolerize T cell help for anti-DNA that is induced by multiple, structurally unrelated self antigens.**

Induction of immune tolerance in response to self antigens in patients with autoimmune disorders might suppress disease, thus avoiding the toxic effects of current nonspecific immunosuppressive treatments. Induction of tolerance in response to selected peptides from autoantigens prevents or reverses disease in rodents with experimental allergic encephalomyelitis, diabetes, and systemic lupus erythematosus (SLE) (1–4). SLE is probably initiated by the pathogenic functions of autoantibodies and immune complexes (5); antigens and antibodies provide the amino acid sequences for peptides that activate T cell help for antibody-forming B cells. Activation of T cell help by Ig-derived peptides occurs spontaneously in (NZB/NZW)F_1 (BWF1) female mice with SLE (6,7). Induction of peptide-specific immune tolerance in T cell proliferation to individual T cell stimulatory peptides derived from pathogenic anti-DNA antibodies did not prolong the survival of BWF1 mice in a recent study (8); however, administration of a combination of these wild autoantibody IgG peptides in a tolerogenic regimen delayed the appearance of antibodies to DNA and the development of nephritis in BWF1 mice. Indeed, life was prolonged 6–10 weeks, but only

Supported by PHS grants P-60-AR-36834, R0-1-AR-33962, and R0-1-AI/AR-46776, awards from the Arthritis Foundation, and a gift from the Paxson Foundation.

[1]Bevra H. Hahn, MD, FACR, Weng Kee Wong, MD, Betty P. Tsao, PhD, Ken Bulpitt, MD, Fanny M. Ebling, PhD: University of California Los Angeles; [2]Ram R. Singh, MD: University of Cincinnati College of Medicine, Cincinnati, Ohio.

Address correspondence and reprint requests to Bevra H. Hahn, MD, FACR, UCLA Rheumatology, 1000 Veteran Avenue, Los Angeles, CA 90095.

Submitted for publication April 19, 2000; accepted in revised form October 13, 2000.

when treatment was initiated prior to the manifestations of clinical disease (8).

In the work reported here, we constructed an artificial peptide ("consensus" peptide [pCONS]) based on an algorithm that defines the T cell stimulatory amino acid sequences from the V_H regions of multiple BWF1 IgG antibodies to DNA. Treatment of young BWF1 female mice with a tolerogenic regimen using pCONS prevented activation of T cell help for anti-DNA by peptides from multiple self antigens, delayed the appearance of multiple autoantibodies, and prolonged survival by 25–30 weeks. Treatment with pCONS was effective when initiated either at 10 weeks (before disease) or at 20 weeks (disease present). Since SLE patients have circulating T cells that are activated by similar peptides from human anti-DNA (9), a similar strategy might suppress pathogenic anti-self responses in this disease in humans.

MATERIALS AND METHODS

Mice. BWF1 and BALB/c mice were bred in colonies in the Division of Rheumatology at the University of California, Los Angeles (UCLA) or purchased from Jackson Laboratories (Bar Harbor, ME) and were maintained in accordance with the guidelines of the UCLA Animal Research Committee. All studies were performed in female mice.

Peptides. Four hundred thirty-nine 12-mer and 15-mer peptides representing the V_H regions of 4 different IgG2a or IgG2b anti-DNA monoclonal antibodies from nephritic BWF1 mice (3 encoded by V_H J558, 1 encoded by V_H 7183) (10,11) were synthesized for the purpose of screening spleen cells from nonimmunized BWF1 female mice to determine the ability of each peptide to stimulate spontaneous T cell proliferation in vitro. Peptides for screening were synthesized as described previously (7). Peptides used to confirm screening assays and those used as therapy were synthesized by a macrocrown method (Chiron Biochemicals, San Diego, CA), purified to a single peak on high-performance liquid chromatography, and analyzed by mass spectroscopy for expected amino acid content.

Assays to test the ability of individual peptides to stimulate proliferation in naïve splenic T cells of BWF1 mice. Proliferation assays were performed using standard methods (8). Briefly, spleen cells were pooled from 6–12-week-old nonimmunized BWF1 female mice (n = 4–6 per group for each experiment) and enriched for T cells over nylon wool columns. T cells (5×10^6) were cultured with $5–10 \times 10^5$ syngeneic antigen-presenting cells (APC) in 200-μl volumes with or without 10 μM of each test peptide or 10 μM of nonstimulatory or stimulatory control peptides or 1 μg of concanavalin A. (If T cell responses were increased <10-fold by concanavalin A, the experiment was discarded.) Assays were set up in triplicate. BWF1 mononuclear spleen cells purified on Ficoll-Hypaque and irradiated were used as APC. After 3 days of incubation, cells were harvested and the proliferation was measured 16 hours following labeling with tritiated thymidine. Results were reported as the mean stimulation index, in disintegrations per minute (dpm in cultures with peptides, divided by the dpm in cultures without peptides) for each set of triplicate assays.

Calculation of algorithm for consensus peptide. Each of the 439 peptides screened was defined as stimulatory or nonstimulatory based on the ability to increase proliferation of naïve BWF1 splenic T cells at least 3-fold in at least 2 experiments. Among the peptides, 21% were stimulatory. All peptides were statistically analyzed for the presence of amino acids at each position that correlated with stimulatory responses. For each amino acid, or each combination of amino acids, we formed a 2×2 contingency table containing the number of peptides with positive stimulatory indices and the number of peptides with nonstimulatory indices; statistical differences were analyzed using a chi-square test (*P* values less than 0.05 were taken as significant). The analysis was also performed taking into account the position of each amino acid or combination. The software used in the analysis is STATA 5.0 (Stata Corporation, College Station, TX). An algorithm was constructed to indicate the stimulatory or nonstimulatory amino acids at each position in a 12-mer peptide (see Results for algorithm).

Assays to test the ability of individual peptides to stimulate production of IgG anti-DNA. The ability of each peptide to activate T cell help for IgG anti-DNA production was tested by coculturing splenic T and B cells with or without peptides. In general, splenic T cells from BWF1 female mice aged 6–12 weeks have the most vigorous proliferative responses, and B cells from 24–30-week old female mice produce the highest number of antibody-forming cells (AFC) that make IgG anti–double-stranded DNA (anti-dsDNA). Single cell suspensions of spleen cells were passed over Ficoll-Hypaque, then enriched for T or B cells with the Vario MACS magnetic purification system using microbead-coated antibodies (Miltenyi, Auburn, CA). Purity of the isolated T and B cell populations was determined by fluorescence-activated cell sorter analysis and was found to vary from 92% to 99%. T cells from nonimmunized 6–12-week-old BWF1 mice were cocultured with B cells from nonimmunized 24–30-week-old BWF1 mice, at a ratio of 10 T cells to 1 B cell, in 96-well microtiter plates; assays were performed in quadruplicate.

After 5 days of incubation at 37°C, cells were transferred to microtiter plates coated with calf thymus dsDNA, and spots of IgG anti-DNA were identified after incubation with alkaline phosphatase–conjugated anti-mouse IgG, followed by incubation with BCIP and 0.6% agarose. Blue spots were enumerated and reported as the number of AFC per 10^5 BWF1 B cells. Development of IgG anti-dsDNA spots was blocked most efficiently by dsDNA; single-stranded DNA (ssDNA) only partially blocked the spots, but cardiolipin or hen egg lysozyme (HEL) did not block the spots, even in BWF1 mice immunized with HEL (7,12,13). (In mice immunized with HEL, IgG anti-HEL spots were blocked by HEL, but not by dsDNA or ssDNA). Data for each experiment were recorded as the mean of each set of quadruplicate assays.

Antibody responses to an exogenous antigen. Twelve-week-old BWF1 mice received 1,000 μg of pCONS or saline intravenously once monthly for 3 doses. Two weeks later, each mouse was immunized intraperitoneally with 20 μg of HEL in Freund's complete adjuvant, which was boosted twice with

Table 1. Algorithm describing T cell stimulatory sequences of the artificial peptide*

Amino acid position														
1	2	3	4	5	6	7	8	9	10	11	12	13	14	15
F	–	Q	–	Q	–	(L)	H	H (F)	H (L)	–	–	–	–	–
W		N		N		(I)	K	K (W)	K (I)					
Y		E		E		(V)	R	R (Y)	R (V)					
		D		D		(M)			(M)					

* Amino acids are indicated as stimulatory (no parentheses), inhibitory (in parentheses), or unrestricted (–) at each position in the 15-mer peptide.

intraperitoneal injections of 20 μg HEL in Freund's incomplete adjuvant. T and B cells were purified and pooled from spleens harvested 2 weeks after the final immunization and cocultured at a ratio of 10:1 (T to B cells), with or without the immunodominant HEL peptide p106. Five days later, the numbers of cells secreting IgG anti-HEL were measured in ELISPOT; these techniques have been reported previously (7).

Clinical studies. BWF1 female mice received 1,000 μg of pCONS or pNEG dissolved in phosphate buffered saline once a month intravenously (IV) throughout their lifetimes, or the same volume of IV saline, beginning at either 10 or 20 weeks of age. Measurements of outcome included survival (checked daily), proteinuria (measured once every 2 weeks), azotemia (measured once a month), and plasma levels of total IgG and of IgG antibodies to dsDNA, cardiolipin, and nucleosomes, measured in enzyme-linked immunosorbent assay (ELISA) every 8–10 weeks. Proteinuria was estimated on a fresh, early-morning urine sample using Albustix and recorded on a scale of negative to 3+. Azotemia was estimated using a drop of whole blood applied to Azostix. Clinical glomerulonephritis was defined as ≥2+ proteinuria on 2 consecutive samples and a blood urea nitrogen level >15 mg/dl. All these measurements of clinical disease are standard in our laboratory (6,8,10,11). Kaplan-Meier survival curves were generated for each treatment group and compared with that for the saline-treated controls using a log-rank test (Stata Corporation).

Assays for T cell tolerance. Six-to-10-week-old BWF1 female mice received 1,000 μg of test peptides or saline IV. Two weeks later, spleen cells were harvested and enriched for T cells as described above. T cells were incubated with APC from spleens of untreated mice and proliferation was measured as described above. To measure tolerance in a spontaneous T cell help assay, groups of 4–6 mice received p33B or pCONS IV. Two weeks later, spleens were harvested. T-enriched cells were cocultured with B-enriched cells from untreated 24-week-old BWF1 mice for 5 days, with and without different concentrations of various peptides, after which IgG anti-DNA spots were developed and enumerated, as described above.

Assays for cytokine levels in plasma. Plasma was obtained at 8–10-week intervals from BWF1 female mice injected monthly with pCONS, pNEG, or saline and from healthy, unmanipulated BALB/c female mice and stored at −20°C. The following cytokine levels were measured in triplicate in individual plasma samples, using commercial ELISA kits and following manufacturer's instructions: interleukin-2 (IL-2) interferon-γ (IFNγ) and IL-4 (all from PharMingen, San Diego, CA). Each plasma sample was assayed in 2 or 3 separate experiments; a standard curve was constructed for each experiment using recombinant cytokines.

Statistical analysis. For comparisons of data on more than 2 groups, analysis of variance (ANOVA) was used, and Tukey's pairwise comparison was performed to identify those groups responsible for the mean difference. *P* values less than 0.05 were considered significant.

RESULTS

Derivation of an algorithm describing stimulatory peptides. The ability of 439 12-mer or 15-mer peptides to induce T cell proliferation ≥3-fold above the background levels in spleen cells from nonimmunized, young BWF1 mice was measured. A 2 × 2 contingency table was made, containing the number of peptides that were stimulatory and the number that were nonstimulatory, and chi-square analysis was used to determine statistically significant differences ($P < 0.05$). The analysis took into account the position of each amino acid or combination of amino acids. For example, 33% of peptides containing F (phenylalanine), W (tryptophane), or Y (tyrosine) at position 1 (p1) were stimulatory, compared with 20% of peptides without those amino acids at p1 ($P < 0.01$). In contrast, only 12% of peptides with F, W, or Y at p9 were stimulatory, compared with 23% of peptides without those amino acids at p9 ($P < 0.02$). Thus, the presence of F, W, or Y at p1 favors the ability of a peptide to stimulate BWF1 T cells, whereas the same amino acids at p9 are relatively inhibitory. The algorithm constructed to describe stimulatory, inhibitory, or unrestricted amino acids at each position in a 15-mer peptide is shown in Table 1. Synthetic peptides were constructed to fit or violate the algorithm and then tested for their ability to induce T cell proliferation and T cell help for IgG anti-DNA production in lymphocytes from BWF1 female mice.

The peptide fitting the algorithm was FIEWNKLRFRQGLEW (amino acids fitting the algorithm are underlined); this was designated pCONS.

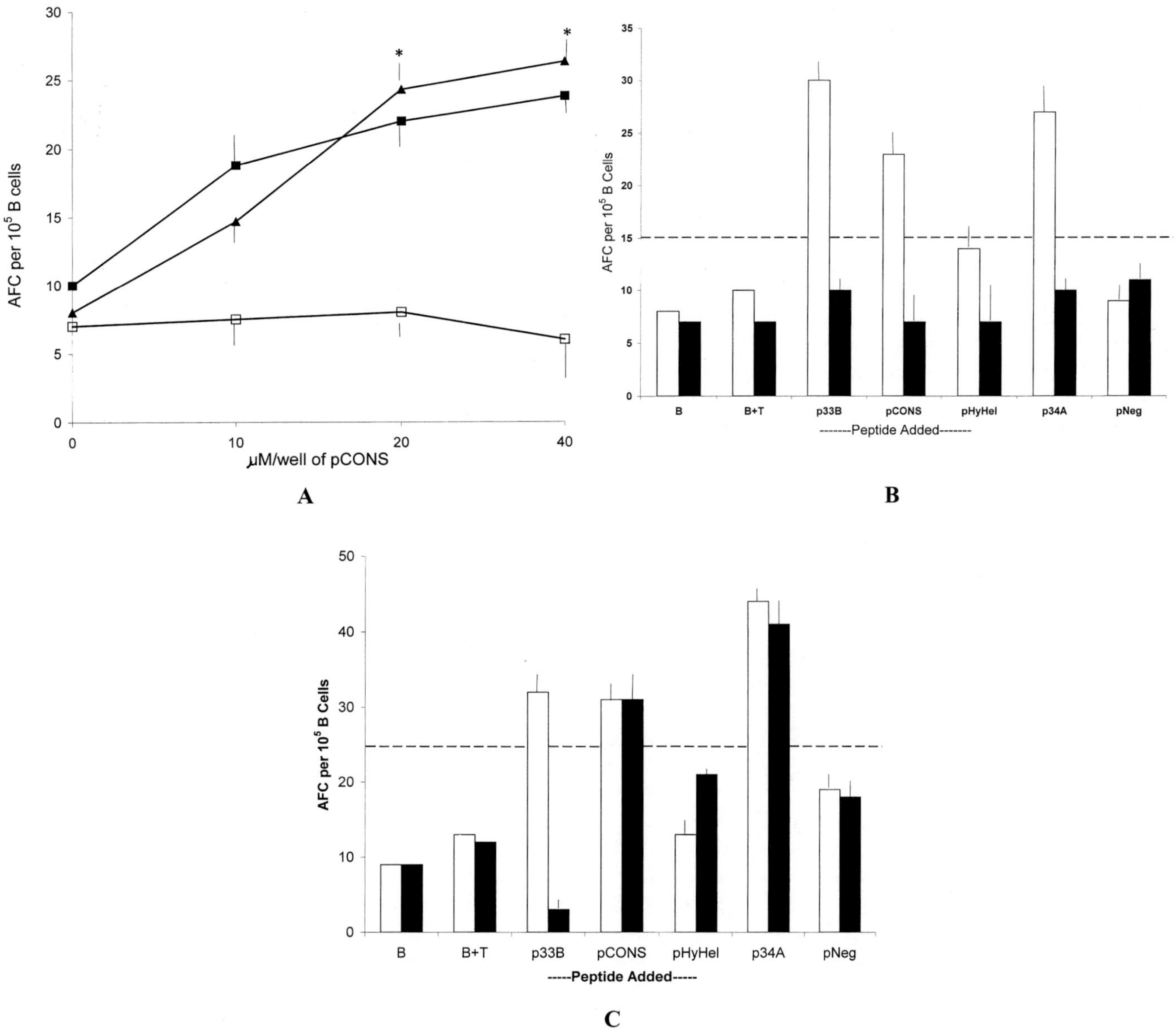

Figure 1. A, Treatment with pConsensus (pCONS) prevents activation of T cell help for production of IgG anti–double-stranded DNA (anti-dsDNA). Mice treated with 1 intravenous (IV) injection of 1,000 μg of pCONS or pNegative (pNEG) or saline-treated female littermates were killed 2 weeks after injections. T cells were purified from spleens and cocultured with B cells from 28–32-week-old untreated (NZB/NZW)F_1 (BWF1) female mice. In saline-treated mice (▲) and mice treated with pNEG (■), addition of pCONS to cultures resulted in increased antibody-forming cells (AFC) making IgG anti-dsDNA, from means of 7–10 to means of 25–27 AFC per 10^5 B cells, as shown on the Y axis. In contrast, T cells from mice treated with pCONS (□) could not be activated to give help by incubation with pCONS in vitro. $* = P < 0.05$ by analysis of variance. **B,** Suppression of T cell help by pCONS was not peptide specific. Spleen cells from mice treated with pCONS 2 weeks earlier (or spleen cells from saline-treated littermates) were cultured with B cells from untreated mice with and without 20 μM/well of Ig peptides. IgG anti-DNA AFC were increased more than 2-fold above background levels in saline-treated mice (open bars) but were not increased in pCONS-treated mice (black bars). Bars represent the mean and SEM of 3 experiments. None of the stimulatory Ig peptides could activate T cell help after treatment with pCONS. There was no response to pNEG; pHyHEL was nonstimulatory, I-E^d–restricted control peptide from a BALB/c Ig V_H. **C,** Suppression of T cell help by p33B was peptide specific. Splenic T cells from mice treated with 1,000 μg IV of p33B 2 weeks earlier (or saline-treated littermates) were cultured with BWF1 B cells from untreated mice, with and without 20 μM/well of various peptides. Data are presented as in **B**. In saline-treated mice (open bars), T cell help was activated by addition of p33B, pCONS, or p34A. In mice treated with p33B (black bars), T cell help could not be activated by p33B but could be activated by other peptides; p33B tolerance was specific for that peptide. The dashed line in **B** and **C** indicates a 2-fold increase above background levels with B plus T cells without peptide stimulation. Bars indicate the mean and SEM of 3 experiments. Each group in each experiment contained spleen cells pooled from 4–6 mice.

Preliminary data suggested that pCONS was restricted by the major histocompatibility complex class II molecules I-A^d and I-E^d. Immunization with pCONS induced proliferative responses in spleen cells from 4 of 5 BALB/c mice, but 0 of 9 NZW mice, indicating that pCONS is restricted by I-E^d and/or I-A^d and not by I-E^z or I-A^z. In BALB/c cells, proliferation in response to pCONS was abrogated 50–100% by incubation with monoclonal antibodies to either I-A^d or I-E^d, suggesting that both molecules can present this peptide.

The peptide poorly fitting the algorithm was AIAWAKARARQGLEW, designated pNEG. BWF1 spleen cells did not proliferate spontaneously when incubated with pNEG. Immunization of BALB/c mice, but not NZW mice, with pNEG in Freund's complete adjuvant resulted in weak proliferation (2–4-fold), suggesting that I-A^d or I-E^d can present pNEG.

In September 2000, the sequences of pCONS and pNEG were compared with those in the nonredundant GenBank database, which contains 690,000 nucleotide sequences dynamically translated in all reading frames. Based on this BLAST search, there were no matches.

The effects of pCONS and pNEG were compared with those of 2 wild peptides, similar to pCONS in sequence, which stimulate T cell proliferation in naïve BWF1 mice: p33B (FITWVKQRTGQGLEW), located at amino acid positions 33–47 in the first complementary-determining region (CDR1) framework 2 (Fr2) region of V_H of monoclonal IgG BWF1 anti-DNA BWds3 (10), and p34A (FMNWVKQSGHGKS), located at amino acid positions 34–46 in the V_H of anti-DNA monoclonal antibody A6.1, and restricted by I-E^d (11). In addition, they were compared with the effects of a nonstimulatory, I-E^d–restricted peptide, pHyHEL (VKQRPGHGLEWIGEI) from the CDR1/Fr2 V_H region of a murine monoclonal antibody against HEL (6,14).

Effects of peptides on naïve BWF1 splenic T cells in vitro. In vitro, the numbers of AFC making IgG anti-dsDNA in spleen cells from unmanipulated BWF1 female mice increased 2–4-fold above baseline values when pCONS, p33B, or p34A were added at the institution of cultures, but not after addition of pNEG or pHyHEL (Figures 1A and B). Production of IgG AFC depends on T cell help. Addition of stimulatory peptides to B cells plus APC depleted of T cells did not increase the levels of AFC above background levels. Addition of pCONS, p33B, or p34A, but not pNEG or pHyHEL, induced proliferation 3–8-fold above baseline levels in splenic T cells from young nonimmunized BWF1 female mice (data not shown). There were no obvious differences in the immunostimulatory capacities of pCONS and stimulatory wild Ig peptides; all of these peptides induced similar quantities of T cell proliferation.

Table 2. Antibody production in response to hen egg lysozyme (HEL) in mice tolerized with or without pConsensus (pCONS)*

Immunization, treatment	HEL p106 in culture	Anti-HEL response, mean ± SEM AFC per 10^6 B cells
No immunization		
Saline	−	0
	+	0
pCONS	−	0
	+	0
HEL immunization		
Saline	−	57 ± 2
	+	213 ± 4
pCONS	−	97 ± 2†
	+	197 ± 8

* Values are the mean ± SEM antibody-forming cells (AFC) per 10^6 B cells in triplicate cultures (1 of 2 similar experiments are shown). Twelve-week-old mice were treated monthly with pCONS or saline for 3 doses, then immunized with HEL in Freund's complete adjuvant, boosted twice at 2-week intervals with HEL in Freund's incomplete adjuvant. Spleens were harvested 1 week later. Cells from 4–5 mice in each group were pooled, purified into T and B cell populations, and cocultured at 10:1 ratios of T:B cells with or without the immunodominant HEL peptide, p106. AFC secreting IgG anti-HEL were enumerated 5 days later in ELISPOT. Background of nonimmune B plus T cells without peptides is zero in the anti-HEL system. (Details of the methods used are discussed in ref. 7.)

† $P < 0.001$ versus nontolerized immunized mice, by Student's t test.

Induction of immune tolerance in T cell help for anti-DNA. Treatment with high doses (300–1,000 μg) of Ig peptides induces T cell tolerance to Ig peptides, as demonstrated by decreased T cell proliferation (8). Using a similar regimen with pCONS, we showed induction of tolerance in T cell help for IgG anti-DNA production. BWF1 female mice were treated at 10 weeks of age with a single injection of 1,000 μg of pCONS or pNEG; saline-treated littermates served as controls. Splenic T cells were harvested 2 weeks later (mice were not immunized with peptides). The effects on T cell help are shown in Figure 1. As shown in Figure 1A, IgG anti-DNA AFC from T and B cells stimulated in vitro with pCONS increased ~3-fold when T cells were from saline- or pNEG-treated mice, compared with no increase in mice treated with pCONS. Treatment with pCONS also eliminated peptide-specific T cell proliferation (data not shown), as we have shown previously using wild Ig peptides as tolerogens (8). Therefore, pCONS (but not pNEG) induced unresponsiveness in T cell help for anti-DNA as well as in T cell proliferation to Ig peptides.

As shown in Figure 1B, a single treatment with

pCONS abrogated the T cell help induced by pCONS, p33B, or p34A. In contrast, as shown in Figure 1C, treatment with p33B induced peptide-specific unresponsiveness in production of anti-DNA. Therefore, treatment with the artificial peptide pCONS resulted in failure of T cell help for anti-DNA induced by multiple Ig peptides; treatment with the wild peptide p33B resulted in tolerance to p33B only.

In contrast to the effect on the anti-DNA response, repeated tolerogenic doses of pCONS did not impair the ability of mice to respond to an exogenous antigen, HEL, as shown in Table 2. The number of IgG anti-HEL AFC was higher in pCONS-treated than in saline-treated mice in the absence of in vitro stimulation with HEL p106, and the numbers of AFC were nearly identical in cells from tolerized and nontolerized mice stimulated with HEL p106. Therefore, tolerization with pCONS can prevent responses to self Ig peptides without abrogating responses to an exogenous antigen.

In vivo effects of treatment pCONS and pNEG. Effect of treatment with pCONS on survival in BWF1 female mice is shown in Figure 2. Mice were given monthly IV doses of 1,000 μg of pCONS, pNEG, or saline, beginning either at 10 weeks of age (no IgG anti-DNA detectable, no proteinuria) or at 20 weeks of age (IgG anti-DNA and nephritis present). In mice treated from 10 weeks of age (Figure 2A), pNEG did not change survival; pNEG was not studied in the 20-week-old group. In both age groups, pCONS improved survival. In mice treated from 10 weeks of age, all untreated and pNEG-treated mice died by 50 weeks of age, compared with 35% of the pCONS-treated mice. All mice that died in all groups, including the pCONS-treated mice, had clinical nephritis. Log-rank tests of Kaplan-Meier survival curves showed that survival was significantly longer in the group treated with pCONS compared with mice treated with saline ($P < 0.002$). In mice treated beginning at 20 weeks of age (Figure 2B), differences in survival were significant by log-rank analysis of the Kaplan-Meier curves ($P < 0.0005$). In both 10- and 20-week-old groups, prolonged survival correlated with delayed clinical nephritis (data not shown). For example, at 40 weeks in the group treated from 10 weeks of age, 100% of untreated mice had clinical nephritis compared with 25% treated with pCONS ($P <$ 0.001 by chi-square test). Data were similar in the group treated from 20 weeks of age.

Plasma from the 10-week-old group was tested at 10, 20, and 30 weeks of age for levels of several cytokines (Figure 3). Levels of IFNγ and IL-4, which increased with the development of disease in saline-treated mice, rose significantly less in pCONS-treated mice ($P < 0.05$ at 30 weeks by ANOVA). IL-2 levels decreased similarly in treated and untreated mice (data not shown).

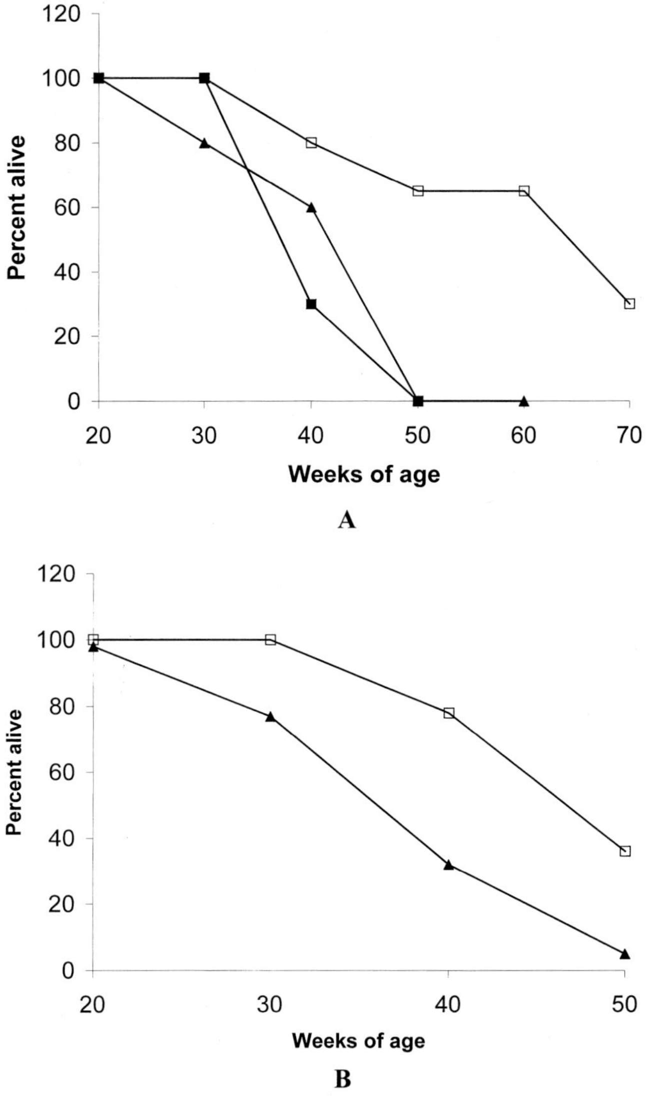

Figure 2. Treatment with pCONS increased survival in mice treated from 10 weeks or 20 weeks of age. **A,** Survival in BWF1 female mice treated from 10 weeks of age with monthly injections of saline (▲), 1,000 μg of pNEG (■), or 1,000 μg of pCONS (□) is indicated as the percentage of mice in each group alive at each time point. The pNEG group contained 5 mice, the saline-treated group 15 mice, and the pCONS group 15 mice. Treatment with pCONS resulted in prolonged survival. Log-rank analysis of Kaplan-Meier survival curves showed that survival was significantly higher in the pCONS group compared with the saline group ($P < 0.002$). **B,** Survival in BWF1 female mice treated from 20 weeks of age with saline (▲) or pCONS (□) was compared. Each group contained 20 mice. Log-rank analysis of Kaplan-Meier survival curves showed significantly higher survival in the pCONS group ($P < 0.0005$). See Figure 1 for definitions.

Plasma levels of total IgG (Figure 4A) and of IgG antibodies to nucleosomes, DNA, and cardiolipin (Figure 4B) rose at a significantly lower rate in pCONS-tolerized mice than in controls. Differences at 40 weeks between pCONS-treated mice and either saline- or pNEG-treated mice were significant ($P < 0.05$ by ANOVA).

Effect of peptide treatments on T cell responses to peptides from self antigens other than Ig. Since treatment with pCONS delayed the appearance of multiple autoan-

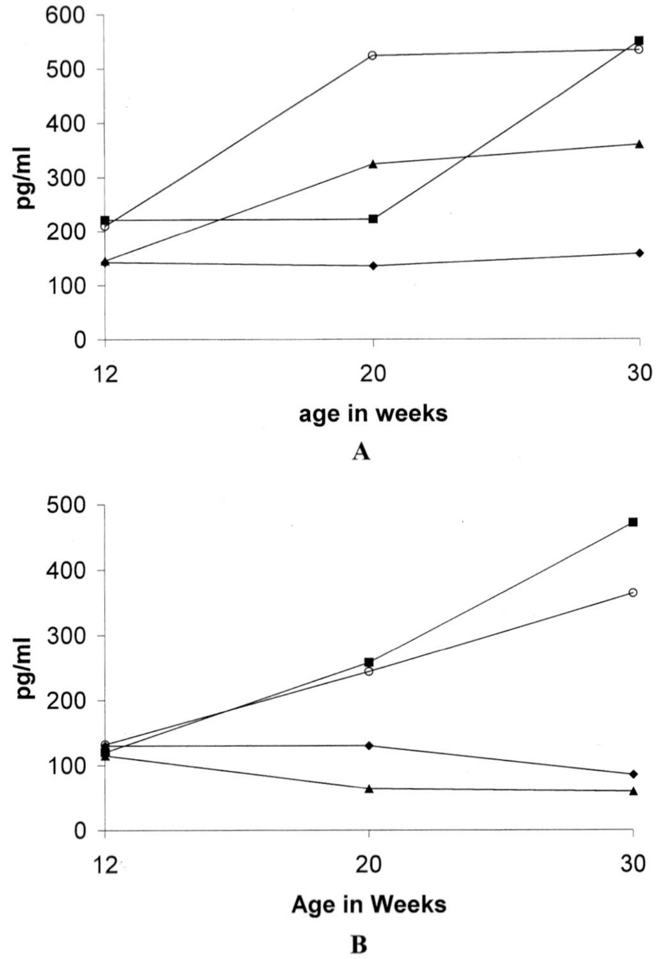

Figure 3. Effect of peptide treatment on plasma cytokine levels. **A,** Mean levels of interferonγ (IFNγ) in plasma of normal BALB/c mice (◆), saline-treated BWF1 mice (■), and BWF1 mice treated monthly with intravenous pCONS (▲) or pNEG (○). Each group at each time point contains 5–13 mice; means of 3 experiments are shown. The SEM ranged from 3% to 12%. **B,** Mean levels of interleukin-4 (IL-4) are shown. Each group contains 6–22 mice. At 30 weeks of age, the levels of IFNγ and IL-4 in BALB/c and pCONS-treated BWF1 mice are significantly lower than the levels in saline- or pNEG-treated BWF1 mice ($P < 0.05$ by analysis of variance). See Figure 1 for other definitions.

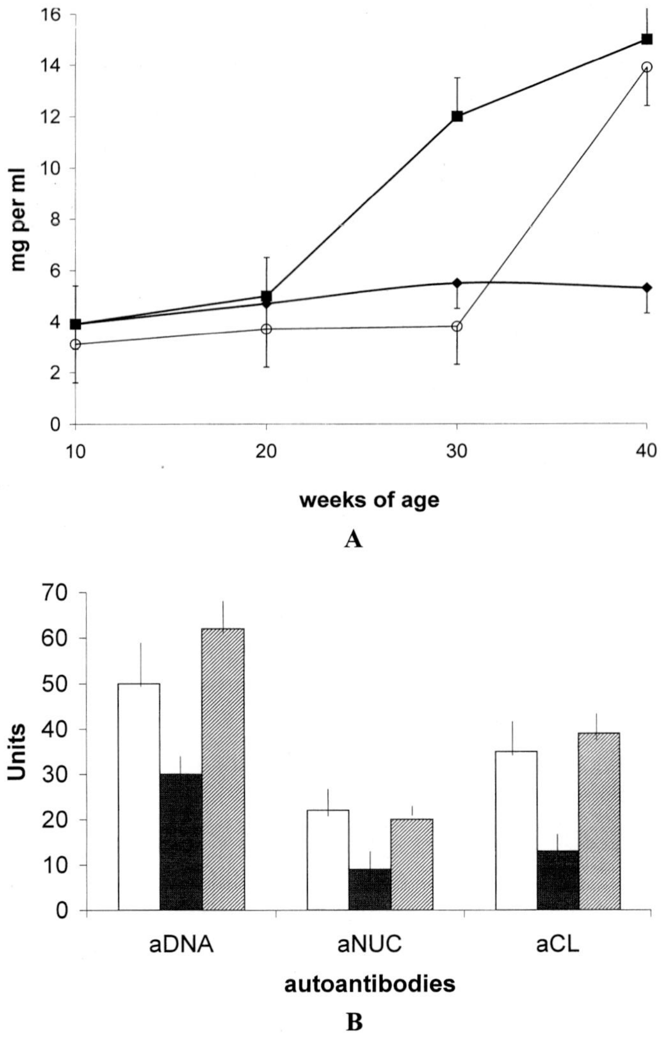

Figure 4. **A,** Treatment with pCONS prevented the increase in plasma levels of IgG that characterize spontaneous disease in BWF1 female mice. Mean and SEM levels of IgG are shown for 4–9 mice in each group—saline-treated mice (■) or mice treated monthly with intravenous doses of 1,000 μg of pCONS (◆) or pNEG (○). The SEM varied from 1% to 10%. Differences are statistically significant at 40 weeks by analysis of variance ($P < 0.05$), comparing pCONS-treated with either pNEG-treated or untreated BWF1 mice. **B,** Treatment with pCONS resulted in lower levels of all autoantibodies tested. Data were pooled from mice beginning treatment at either 10 or 20 weeks of age. The mean plasma levels of various IgG autoantibodies at 40 weeks of age are indicated on the y axis (5–20 mice in each group). The mean levels in saline-treated mice are shown by open bars, in pCONS-treated mice by black bars, and in pNEG-treated BWF1 mice by hatched bars. Bars show the mean and SEM. Levels were significantly lower in pCONS-treated mice compared with untreated mice ($P < 0.05$ or better by Student's t test). Quantities of specific IgG autoantibodies are expressed in units, with each test standardized to pooled plasma of positive and negative controls in each enzyme-linked immunosorbent assay. aDNA = anti–double-stranded DNA; aNUC = antinucleosome; aCL = anticardiolipin (see Figure 1 for other definitions).

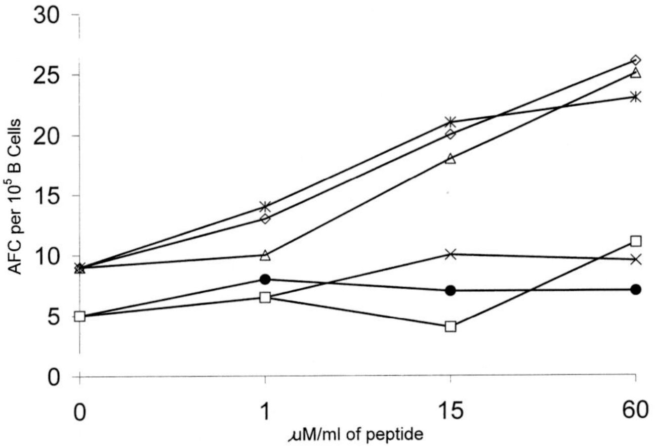

Figure 5. Tolerance induced by pCONS was broad, preventing T cell activation by multiple peptides from self antigens other than IgG. After treatment with pCONS, T cells from spleens of saline-treated, but not pCONS-treated, mice could activate B cell production of IgG anti-DNA when incubated with various concentrations of pCONS (saline-treated [◇], pCONS-treated [□]), histone 3 peptide 91-105 (saline [△], pCONS [×]), or Ro-480 peptide (saline [✳], pCONS [●]). Bars show the mean and SEM of 2 experiments, with each group containing splenic T cells from 4–6 mice in each experiment. See Figure 1 for definitions.

tibodies, induced tolerance in T cell help activated by different Ig peptides, and prolonged survival more effectively than did treatment with single or combination wild Ig peptides studied previously (8), it seems likely that pCONS affects a broad autoreactive T cell repertoire. We next tested whether treatment with pCONS influenced T cell responses to self peptides from antigens other than IgG, using peptides from histone and Ro that are reported to stimulate murine T cells (15,16). As shown in Figure 5, in vivo treatment with pCONS abolished T cell help for IgG anti-DNA to BWF1 B cells when T cells were activated by the peptides histone 3 (91–105; QSSAVMALQEASEAY) or Ro-480 (CAIALREYRKKMDI). Several other tested peptides from the anti-DNA IgG, from histone 3, and from the Ro antigen (kindly supplied by Dr. Judith James, Oklahoma Research Foundation, Oklahoma City) could not stimulate BWF1 T cells from nonimmunized mice.

DISCUSSION

This is the first report of the sequence and clinical utility of the unique synthetic peptide, pCONS. In the present study, pCONS administered repeatedly as a tolerogen was highly effective in delaying the appearance of multiple autoantibodies characteristic of spontaneous SLE-like disease in BWF1 female mice, even when IgG anti-DNA and proteinuria were present before therapy was instituted. This benefit probably results from the ability of pCONS to impair autoreactive T cell help—not only help stimulated by pCONS but also help stimulated by other self peptides, including some from nucleosomes and the Ro antigen. This contrasts with the peptide-specific inhibition of T cell help induced by tolerance to a wild peptide and might explain the relatively weak clinical effects of such peptides when used as tolerogens (8). These effects on T cell help in vitro were measured in spleen cells from mice treated only once with high-dose IV pCONS; whether these effects change in mice treated repeatedly requires further study. Antibody responses of BWF1 T and B cells to HEL were not abrogated in mice treated with pCONS, suggesting that the response to an external antigen was not tolerized.

Why would the tolerogen affect the anti-self response but not the anti–external antigen response? We have previously reported that the sequences of some V_H peptides frequently found in murine antibodies to DNA derived from the gene family V_H J558 (which includes peptides located in amino acid positions 33–47, to which the sequence of pCONS is similar) are found primarily in murine autoantibodies, particularly anti-DNA (7). Therefore, a tolerogen such as pCONS may primarily influence autoantibody production, because exogenous antigens activate T cell help for B cells that make Ig containing other sequences.

The most important finding was that repeatedly tolerizing lupus mice with pCONS greatly improved their survival. Other investigators have manipulated lupus-like disease in mice by administration of wild-type self peptides. Induction of neonatal tolerance in normal BALB/c mice with a peptide from an anti-DNA V_H CDR1 region (TGYYMQWVKQSPEKLEWIG) was associated with lower quantities of anti-DNA when autoantibodies were induced by immunization with peptide or idiotype (17). Our experiments differed from others because tolerance was induced in a mouse strain with genetically determined spontaneous murine lupus, an artificial rather than a wild peptide was used, and disease was delayed in mice tolerized at either 10 or 20 weeks of age; at 20 weeks, disease was clinically evident. Injection of a peptide from the V_H CDR3 of another anti-DNA improved survival in BWF1 mice, probably by inducing a regulatory idiotype circuit (18). Administration of a soluble peptide identified from a peptide display library as a strong binder of a murine anti-DNA monoclonal antibody protected mice from deposition of the pathogenic anti-DNA, probably by binding the monoclonal antibody before it could attach to glomeruli (19). In contrast to the studies reported previously (18,19), our experiments appear to have influenced disease by induction of immune tolerance in T cell help for autoantibodies.

Induction of tolerance to each of several peptides from H3 and H4 histones (components of nucleosome) in (Swiss-Webster × NZW)F_1 lupus mice (a strain with spontaneous lupus similar to that in BWF1 mice) reduced the levels of antinucleosome and anti-DNA; tolerance to some peptides reduced histologic renal damage and tolerance to one peptide prolonged life in older mice with established nephritis (4). These experiments are similar to ours, except that the peptides were different (I-A and I-E restrictions probably differ in the 2 strains), our studies measured effects on survival when animals were treated before or after the onset of disease, and the effect of pCONS on survival in younger mice was particularly dramatic.

Taken together, it is clear that administration of selected self peptides that alter autoantibody production or deposition is effective clinically in mitigating the outcomes of murine lupus, whether the peptides are derived from antigen or from antibody.

The effects of tolerizing with pCONS on the plasma levels of IFNγ and IL-4 were striking. It is somewhat hazardous to interpret the changes in plasma levels of these cytokines, which are subject to considerable variation related to factors such as the time of release, capture by both cell-bound and soluble receptors, and failure to mirror immune responses occurring in target organs. However, our observations, that tolerance with pCONS significantly delayed the rise in levels of these cytokines that occur in spontaneous BWF1 disease, suggest that cells of both the Th1 and Th2 type participate in disease development. This is consistent with other reports that have shown that inhibition of the Th1 cytokine IFNγ or of the Th2 cytokines IL-4, IL-6, or IL-10 delays the onset of SLE in mouse models (20–25). Apparently, the induction of tolerance delays the cytokine bursts that characterize spontaneous disease.

Patients with SLE have circulating T cells that can be activated by various peptides from Ig of human anti-DNA (9). This response is detected in higher proportions of SLE patients than in their first-degree relatives or in normal controls. Therefore, a strategy similar to the Ig peptide therapy that was demonstrated herein to be effective in BWF1 mice might be useful in the treatment of patients with autoantibody-mediated diseases such as SLE.

REFERENCES

1. Karin N, Binah O, Grabie N, Mitchell DJ, Felzen B, Solomon MD, et al. Short peptide-based tolerogens without self-antigenic or pathogenic activity reverse autoimmune diseases. J Immunol 1998;160:5188–94.
2. Nicholson LB, Greer JM, Sobel RA, Lees MB, Kuchroo VK. An altered peptide ligand mediates immune deviation and prevents autoimmune encephalomyelitis. Immunity 1995;3:397–405.
3. Tisch R, Wang B, Serreze DV. Induction of glutamic acid decarboxylase 65-specific Th2 cells and suppression of autoimmune diabetes at late stages of disease is epitope dependent. J Immunol 1999;163:1178–87.
4. Kalyaperumal A, Michaels MA, Datta SK. Antigen-specific therapy of murine lupus nephritis using nucleosomal peptides: tolerance spreading impairs pathogenic function of autoimmune T and B cells. J Immunol 1999;162:5775–83.
5. Tsao B, Kronenberg M, Cheroutre H, Hahn BH. Failed self-tolerance and autoimmunity in mice transgenic for an IgG anti-DNA. J Immunol 1992;149:350–8.
6. Singh RR, Kumar V, Ebling FM, Southwood S, Sette A, Sercarz EE, et al. T cell determinants from autoantibodies to DNA can upregulate autoimmunity in murine lupus. J Exp Med 1995;181:2017–27.
7. Singh RR, Hahn BH, Tsao BP, Ebling FM. Evidence for multiple mechanisms of polyclonal T cell activation in murine lupus. J Clin Invest 1998;102:1841–9.
8. Singh RR, Ebling FM, Sercarz EE, Hahn BH. Immune tolerance to autoantibody-derived peptides delays development of murine lupus. J Clin Invest 1995;96:2990–6.
9. Williams WM, Staines NA, Muller S, Isenberg DA. Human T cell responses to autoantibody variable region peptides. Lupus 1995; 4:464–71.
10. Ohnishi K, Ebling FM, Mitchell B, Singh RR, Hahn BH, Tsao BP. Comparison of pathogenic and nonpathogenic murine antibodies to DNA: antigen binding and structural characteristics. Int Immunol 1994;6:817–30.
11. Tsao BP, Ebling FM, Roman C, Panosian-Sahakian N, Calame K, Hahn BH. Structural characteristics of the variable regions of immunoglobulin genes encoding a pathogenic autoantibody in murine lupus. J Clin Invest 1990;85:530–40.
12. Ando DG, Ebling FM, Hahn BH. Detection of native and denatured DNA antibody forming cells by the enzyme-linked immunospot assay: a clinical study of (New Zealand black × New Zealand white) F_1 mice. Arthritis Rheum 1986;29:1139–46.
13. Ando DG, Sercarz EE, Hahn BH. Mechanisms of T and B cell collaboration in the in-vitro production of anti-DNA antibodies in the N2B/N2WF murine SLE model. J Immunol 1987;138:3185–90.
14. Hartman AB, Mallett CP, Sheriff S, Smith-Gill SJ. Unusual joining sites in the H and L chains of an anti-lysozyme antibody. J Immunol 1998;141:932–6.
15. Scofield RH, Kaufman KM, Baber U, James JA, Harley JB, Kurien BT. Immunization of mice with human 60-kd Ro peptides results in epitope spreading if the peptides are highly homologous between human and mouse. Arthritis Rheum 1999;42:1017–24.
16. Kaliyaperumal A, Mohan C, Wu W, Datta SK. Nucleosomal peptide epitopes for nephritis-inducing T helper cells of murine lupus. J Exp Med 1996;183:2459–63.
17. Waisman A, Ruiz PJ, Israeli E, Eilat E, Konen-Waisman S, Zinger H, et al. Modulation of murine systemic lupus erythematosus with peptides based on complementary determining regions of a pathogenic anti-DNA monoclonal antibody. Proc Natl Acad Sci U S A 1997;94:4620–5.
18. Jouanne C, Avrameas S, Payell-Brogard M. A peptide derived from a polyreactive monoclonal anti-DNA natural antibody can modulate lupus development in (NZB × NZW)F1 mice. Immunol 1999;96:333–9.
19. Gaynor B, Putterman C, Valadon P, Spatz L, Scharff MD,

Diamond B. Peptide inhibition of glomerular deposition of an anti-DNA antibody. Proc Natl Acad Sci U S A 1997;94:1955–60.
20. Jacob CO, van der Meide PH, McDevitt HO. In vivo treatment of (NZB × NZW)F1 lupus-like nephritis with monoclonal antibody to gamma interferon. J Exp Med 1987;166:798–803.
21. Ozmen L, Roman D, Rountoulakis M, Schmid G, Ryffel B, Garotta G. Experimental therapy of systemic lupus erythematosus: the treatment of NZB/W mice with mouse soluble interferon-gamma receptor inhibits the onset of glomerulonephritis. Eur J Immunol 1995;25:6–12.
22. Haas C, Tyffel B, Le Hir M. IFN-gamma receptor deletion prevents autoantibody production and glomerulonephritis in lupus-prone (NZB×NZW)F1 mice. J Immunol 1998;160:3713–8.
23. Finck BK, Chan B, Wofsy D. Interleukin 6 promotes murine lupus in NZB/NZW mice. J Clin Invest 1994;94:585–91.
24. Ishida H, Muchamuel T, Sakaguchi S, Andrade S, Menon S, Howard M. Continuous administration of anti-interleukin 10 antibodies delays onset of autoimmunity in NZB/W F1 mice. J Exp Med 1994;179:305–10.
25. Nakajima A, Hirose S, Yagita H, Okumura K. Roles of IL-4 and IL-12 in the development of lupus in NZB/W F1 mice. J Immunol 1997;158:1466–72.

ARTHRITIS & RHEUMATISM
Vol. 44, No. 2, February 2001, pp 442–450

Molecular and Cellular Mediators of Interleukin-1–Dependent Acute Inflammatory Arthritis

Kate E. Lawlor, Ian K. Campbell, Kristy O'Donnell, Li Wu, and Ian P. Wicks

Objective. To examine the molecular and cellular mechanisms in a model of acute inflammatory monarticular arthritis induced by methylated bovine serum albumin (mBSA) and interleukin-1 (IL-1).

Methods. Mice were injected intraarticularly with mBSA on day 0 and subcutaneously with recombinant human IL-1β on days 0–2. At day 7, knee joints were removed and assessed histologically. Flow cytometry and RNase protection were used to analyze IL-1–dependent events.

Results. C57BL/6 (B6), 129/Sv, and (B6 × 129/Sv)F_1 hybrid mice, all H-2^b strains, were susceptible to mBSA/IL-1–induced arthritis, whereas C3H/HeJ (H-2^k) mice were not. B6 mice lacking T and B cells (RAG-$1^{-/-}$) or major histocompatibility complex (MHC) class II antigens (MHCII$^{-/-}$), and B6 mice treated with a CD4+ T cell–depleting monoclonal antibody, were resistant to disease. In contrast, B cell–deficient (*μMT*/*μMT*) mice developed arthritis at an incidence and severity similar to that of controls. RelB-deficient (RelB$^{-/-}$) bone marrow chimeric mice had arthritis that was significantly reduced in incidence and severity. In B6 mice, flow cytometry demonstrated an IL-1–dependent leukocyte infiltration into the synovial compartment and RNase protection assays revealed induction of messenger RNA (mRNA) for the chemokines monocyte chemoattractant protein 1, macrophage inhibitory protein 2 (MIP-2), RANTES, MIP-1α, and MIP-1β, in vivo and in vitro.

Conclusion. Arthritis induced by mBSA/IL-1 is strain specific and dependent on CD4+ T lymphocytes and at least partially on RelB, but not on B lymphocytes or antibody. IL-1 contributes to leukocyte recruitment to the synovium and directly induces chemokine mRNA production by synovial cells. This model of acute monarticular arthritis is particularly suitable for further investigations into cell-mediated immunity in arthritis and the role of IL-1.

Animal models of arthritis, such as collagen-induced arthritis (CIA) in mice, have proven invaluable for use in examining immune mechanisms in chronic inflammatory joint diseases, such as rheumatoid arthritis (RA). However, models of acute arthritis provide a more rapid and potentially simplified approach to investigating pathogenesis. Methylated bovine serum albumin/interleukin-1 (mBSA/IL-1)–induced arthritis was first described by Staite et al in 1990 (1). A mild inflammatory reaction resulting from intraarticular (IA) injection of mBSA was exacerbated by subcutaneous (SC) injection of recombinant human IL-1 and led to the development of synovitis and pannus tissue, which rapidly peaked in severity on day 7 and was almost completely resolved by day 28. It was speculated that mBSA either caused a nonspecific local inflammatory reaction in synovium, which was exacerbated by IL-1, or was an antigen recognized by the adaptive immune system (1). The acute onset of mBSA/IL-1–induced arthritis, the restriction of disease to a defined joint, and the presence of pathology in all mBSA-injected joints are major experimental advantages and led us to examine this model further.

IL-1 is a pleiotropic cytokine that is thought to mediate inflammation and cartilage destruction in RA. IL-1 has multiple biologic actions on leukocytes and connective tissue, including synovial cell proliferation

Supported by the Reid Charitable Trusts, the Arthritis Foundation of Australia, and the National Health and Medical Research Council of Australia.

Kate E. Lawlor, BSc(Hons), Ian K. Campbell, BSc(Hons), PhD, Kristy O'Donnell, BAppSc, BSc(Hons), Li Wu, MB, MMedSc, PhD, Ian P. Wicks, MBBS, PhD, FRACP: The Walter and Eliza Hall Institute of Medical Research, Parkville, Victoria, Australia.

Address correspondence and reprint requests to Ian P. Wicks, MBBS, PhD, FRACP, Reid Rheumatology Laboratory, Division of Autoimmunity and Transplantation, The Walter and Eliza Hall Institute, Post Office, The Royal Melbourne Hospital, Victoria 3050, Australia.

Submitted for publication May 11, 2000; accepted in revised form October 13, 2000.

and production of cytokines and matrix metalloproteinases (2,3). Systemic administration of IL-1 accelerated and exacerbated the development of murine CIA (4). In rabbits and mice, IA injection of IL-1 alone led to cellular infiltration of the joint and transient loss of cartilage proteoglycan (5,6). Gene transfer of human IL-1β into the rabbit synovium resulted in severe arthritis (7), while IL-1 receptor antagonist–deficient mice of the BALB/c background developed a spontaneous chronic inflammatory polyarthropathy, resembling RA (8). IL-1 therefore may influence the course of arthritis through both local and systemic effects and has become a major therapeutic target in RA (9).

This study aimed to characterize molecular and cellular mechanisms in mBSA/IL-1–induced arthritis. We report that the model is dependent on CD4+ T lymphocytes and partly on RelB-expressing cells, but not on B lymphocytes or antibody. The model was strain dependent and, in an important finding, B6, 129/Sv, and B6 × 129/Sv (H-2^b) mice developed disease at a similar incidence and severity, making it suitable for studies involving gene knockout mice derived from B6 or 129/Sv embryonic stem cells. Further investigations of the mechanisms whereby systemic IL-1 exacerbates a weak local inflammatory reaction revealed that IL-1β stimulates chemokine messenger RNA (mRNA) induction in synovial cells and results in inflammatory cell infiltration into the synovium.

MATERIALS AND METHODS

Mice. Congenic inbred C57BL/6 (B6; H-2^b), 129/Sv (H-2^b), (B6 × 129/Sv)F$_1$ hybrid (H-2^b), nonobese diabetic (NOD; H-2^{g7}), and C3H/HeJ (H-2^k) mice were obtained from the Walter and Eliza Hall Institute (WEHI) Animal Supplies. Recombinase activating gene 1–deficient mice (RAG-1$^{-/-}$) (10) were provided by L. Corcoran (WEHI). Major histocompatibility complex class II–deficient mice (MHCII$^{-/-}$) generated from B6 embryonic stem cells (11) were provided by W. Heath (WEHI), and B cell–deficient $\mu MT/\mu MT$ mice (12) were provided by D. Tarlinton (WEHI). All gene knockout mice were backcrossed onto B6 mice for ≥8 generations. All mice were ≥8 weeks of age at the time of experimentation, were fed standard rodent chow and water ad libitum, and were housed (≤6 mice/cage) in sawdust-lined cages. All animal procedures were approved by the institutional ethics committee.

Arthritis induction with mBSA/IL-1. The procedure used for induction of arthritis was based on that previously described (1). Mice were anesthetized, and 10 μl of 20 mg/ml mBSA (Sigma, St Louis, MO) was injected IA into the knee joint. Control joints received the same volume of vehicle (normal saline). Mice were next injected SC into the rear footpad with 20 μl of 12.5 μg/ml recombinant human IL-1β (specific activity 5 × 10^8 units/mg; Amgen, Thousand Oaks, CA) in normal saline/normal mouse serum (0.5% volume/volume), and the injection was repeated on the next 2 days.

Histologic assessment of arthritis. The mice were killed on day 7 and the knee joints were excised and fixed in 10% (volume/volume) neutral buffered formalin for at least 2 days, decalcified, and processed to paraffin. Frontal tissue sections (4 μm) were cut at 4 depths ~100 μm apart and stained with hematoxylin and eosin to assess joint pathology.

Arthritis was assessed by an investigator who was blinded to the experimental groups, and 5 components of arthritis were graded for severity from 0 (normal) to 5 (severe), based on the scoring system of Staite et al (1). Joint space exudate was graded according to the presence and relative numbers of inflammatory cells in the joint space, particularly neutrophils and monocytes/macrophages, interspersed with fibrin-like material. Synovitis was defined as thickening of the synovial lining layer and soft tissue inflammation in the infrapatellar fatpad, joint capsule, and the area adjacent to the periosteal sheath. Pannus was defined as the encroachment of hyperplastic synovium over the articular surface or bone at the cartilage–bone junction. Cartilage degradation was evaluated on patellofemoral and tibiofemoral articular surfaces. Bone degradation was evaluated as the extent and depth of subchondral and periosteal bone erosion.

Based on the above histologic scores, joints were classified as demonstrating inflammatory arthritis if there was a joint space exudate score ≥1 and a synovitis score ≥2. Destructive arthritis was defined for joints that scored ≥2 for pannus or ≥1 for either cartilage degradation or bone degradation. The overall mean histologic severity score (of a maximum possible score of 25) for an experimental group was calculated by averaging the sum of the 5 histopathologic features, with each individual feature scored at 4 section depths per joint.

Depletion of CD4+ T lymphocytes in mBSA/IL-1–induced arthritis. To investigate the role of CD4+ T lymphocytes in mBSA/IL-1–induced arthritis, groups of mice were injected intraperitoneally 2 days prior to mBSA administration with either 300 μg of the CD4-depleting monoclonal antibody (mAb) GK1.5, provided by T. Mandel (WEHI), or an equal amount of isotype control mAb (GL121; a gift from DNAX, Palo Alto, CA). Injections of mAb were repeated on the day of disease induction (day 0). Depletion of peripheral CD4+ T lymphocytes was ~98% in GK1.5-treated mice (confirmed by flow cytometric analysis of blood obtained on day 7; data not shown).

Generation of RelB knockout bone marrow chimeras. Briefly, unseparated bone marrow cells (5 × 10^6) from B6 Ly5.2 RelB$^{-/-}$ (13) or wild-type B6 Ly5.2 mice were injected intravenously into lethally γ-irradiated (2 × 5.5 Gy) B6 Ly5.1 recipient mice (14). Effective reconstitution was determined by flow cytometric analysis, with 89 ± 2% (mean ± SEM) of peripheral blood leukocytes in RelB$^{-/-}$ bone marrow chimeras (n = 6) expressing H-2K (the gene used to disrupt RelB expression) (13) at >4 weeks posttransfer.

T cell proliferation assay. Popliteal lymph node (LN) cells (4 × 10^5/well) in 200-μl RPMI 1640 supplemented with 5% (v/v) fetal bovine serum (FBS; Trace Biosciences, Sydney, Australia) and 50 μM 2-mercaptoethanol were incubated in a 96-well plate at 37°C (5% CO_2) for 72 hours with 0–30 μg/ml of mBSA that had been boiled for 10 minutes. Cultures were pulsed with 1 μCi of ^{3}H-thymidine/well (Amersham, Little Chalfont, UK) during the last 8 hours of incubation and cells were harvested with an Inotech (Rockville, MD) cell harvester. ^{3}H-thymidine incorporation was determined on a microplate scintillation counter (Canberra Packard, Melbourne, Australia) as a measure of T cell proliferation.

Immunohistochemical staining of CD4 in synovial tissue. Joints were removed from mBSA/IL-1–treated mice at day 7, fixed in 4% (weight/volume) paraformaldehyde in phosphate buffered saline (PBS), and demineralized as described (15). Joints were immersed in Tissue-Tek embedding medium (Miles Scientific, Elkhart, IN), snap-frozen in liquid nitrogen, and stored at −70°C. Frontal sections (6 μm) were cut at −30°C, fixed in cold acetone, rehydrated in PBS, and quenched for endogenous peroxidase activity using 0.3% (v/v) H_2O_2 in methanol for 30 minutes. Tissue sections were blocked for 30 minutes (10% [v/v] Fcγ receptor III/II block [rat anti-mouse CD16/CD32] in 10% [v/v] normal rat serum [NRS]/PBS + avidin D blocking reagent [Avidin/Biotin Blocking Kit; Vector, Burlingame, CA]). Biotinylated anti-mouse CD4 mAb (clone GK1.5) diluted in 10% (v/v) NRS with biotin blocking reagent (Vector) was applied and incubated for 2 hours. ABC peroxidase working solution (Vectrastain Elite ABC Kit Universal; Vector) was applied for 30 minutes and peroxidase activity was detected with NovaRed (NovaRed Substrate Kit; Vector). Sections were counterstained in Mayer's hematoxylin. Negative controls included NRS without primary antibody. All incubations were performed in a humidified atmosphere at room temperature.

Flow cytometric analysis of infiltrating cells. Patellae from mBSA-injected knee joints of B6 mice that received either SC IL-1β or vehicle were dissected on day 7. Fat and muscle fragments were discarded and the synovium was minced into 2-mm pieces and digested into 1 cell suspension using 2.4 mg/ml dispase (Boehringer, Mannheim, Germany), 1 mg/ml collagenase type II (Sigma), and 100 μg/ml DNase I (Boehringer Mannheim, Indianapolis, IN) in RPMI 1640. The suspension was agitated gently at 37°C for 30 minutes and then washed through a 70-μM nylon cell strainer with RPMI 1640 containing 10% (v/v) FBS. Nonadherent cells were collected after overnight culture at 37°C, 5% CO_2, washed in PBS/2% (v/v) FBS, and stained with phycoerythrin–conjugated anti-mouse CD3 (clone 29B; Sigma) mAb and either fluorescein isothiocyanate–conjugated anti-mouse CD4 (clone H129.19; Sigma) or CD8 (clone CTCD8a; Caltag, Burlingame, CA) mAb. Cells were analyzed using a Becton Dickinson FACScan and CellQuest software (Becton Dickinson, San Jose, CA).

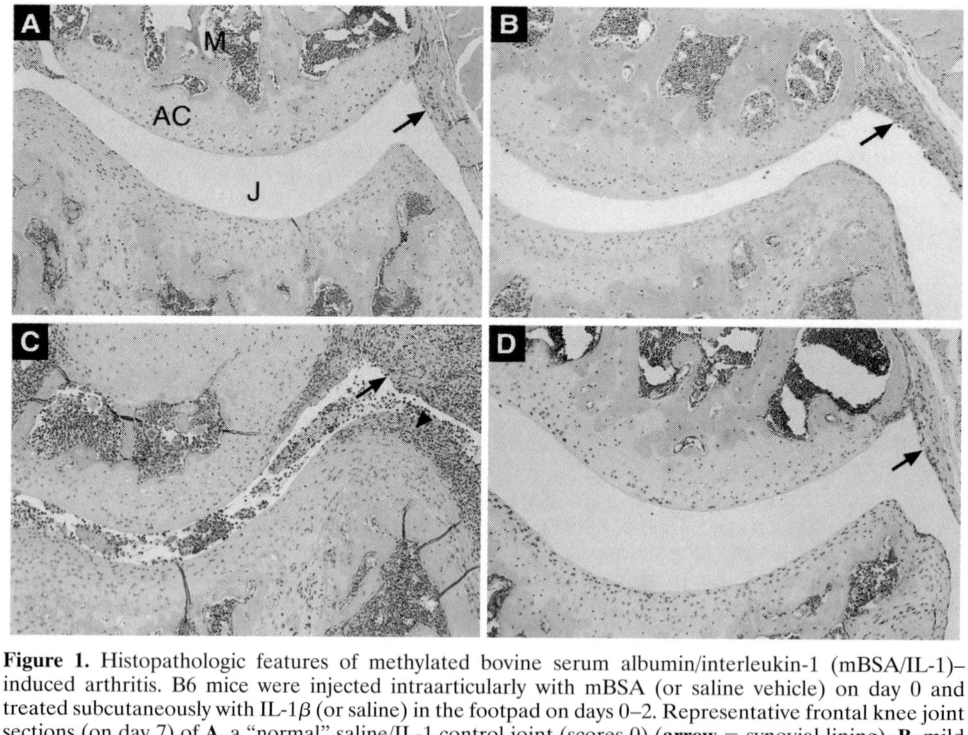

Figure 1. Histopathologic features of methylated bovine serum albumin/interleukin-1 (mBSA/IL-1)–induced arthritis. B6 mice were injected intraarticularly with mBSA (or saline vehicle) on day 0 and treated subcutaneously with IL-1β (or saline) in the footpad on days 0–2. Representative frontal knee joint sections (on day 7) of **A,** a "normal" saline/IL-1 control joint (scores 0) (**arrow** = synovial lining), **B,** mild inflammatory synovial reaction in a mBSA/saline–treated joint (**arrow**), and **C,** the typical mBSA/IL-1–induced arthritic response, with a moderate exudate in the joint space and marked synovitis visible in the joint capsule (**arrow**). Hypertrophic synovium, pannus tissue (**arrowhead**), and underlying articular cartilage and bone loss are also evident. **D,** Section illustrating the normal appearance of the MHCII$^{-/-}$ mouse joint (mBSA/IL-1–treated), which is also representative of responses in RAG-1$^{-/-}$ and CD4+ T cell–depleted mice (**arrow** = synovial lining). **AC** = articular cartilage; **J** = joint space; **M** = bone marrow. (Hematoxylin and eosin stained; original magnification ×100.)

Table 1. Strain specificity in methylated bovine serum albumin/interleukin-1 (mBSA/IL-1)–induced arthritis*

Strain	MHC haplotype (H-2)†	Arthritis incidence‡		Histologic score§
		Inflammatory	Destructive	
B6	b	18/20	18/20	14.3 ± 1.3
129/Sv	b	5/7	6/7	11.1 ± 2.5
B6 × 129/Sv	b	9/10	9/10	11.7 ± 1.6
NOD	g7	6/10	7/10	7.6 ± 1.6
C3H/HeJ	k	0/10	0/10	0.9 ± 0.1

* Mice were injected intraarticularly with mBSA on day 0 and subcutaneously with IL-1β into the rear footpad on days 0–2, and knees were histologically assessed at day 7.
† MHC = major histocompatibility complex.
‡ Incidence = number of responsive joints/total number of joints examined. Inflammatory arthritis was defined as an exudate scored ≥1 and synovitis scored ≥2; destructive arthritis was defined as pannus scored ≥2, or cartilage or bone degradation scored ≥1.
§ Values are the mean ± SEM of the sum of the 5 histopathologic features scored (maximum total score 25; see Materials and Methods).

RNase protection analysis of chemokine expression. B6 mice were injected IA with mBSA and SC with either IL-1β or saline. On day 7, synovial tissue was dissected from the knee joints, snap-frozen, and ground into a powder using a mortar and pestle. Total RNA was extracted using RNAzol B reagent (Tel-Test, Friendswood, TX). For in vitro IL-1 stimulation studies, patellae from mBSA/IL-1 arthritic joints were placed into 24-well tissue culture plates in RPMI 1640 + 10% (v/v) FBS and synovial explant fibroblasts were allowed to expand. At confluence, synovial cells were replated in 6-well plates and recombinant human IL-1β was added at 35 ng/ml. Total RNA was isolated at 0, 1, 2, and 4 hours (in duplicate) using RNAzol B added directly to the monolayer.

RNA was analyzed for chemokine expression using the RiboQuant RNAse Protection System (PharMingen, San Diego, CA) according to the manufacturer's instructions. The murine chemokine template set mCK5 (PharMingen) was used to obtain radiolabeled antisense RNA probes for lymphotactin, RANTES, eotaxin, macrophage inhibitory protein 1α (MIP-1α), MIP-1β, MIP-2, monocyte chemoattractant protein 1 (MCP-1), and L32 and GAPDH control RNA. Dried polyacrylamide gels were visualized after an overnight exposure by phosphorimager (Molecular Dynamics, Sunnyvale, CA) using Image Quant software.

Statistical analysis. Where appropriate, data are expressed as the mean ± SEM. The Mann-Whitney 2-sample rank test was used to compare mean histologic severity scores of test and control groups. Student's *t*-test (1-tailed) was used to analyze T cell proliferation assays. *P* values less than 0.05 were considered significant.

RESULTS

Histologic characteristics of mBSA/IL-1–induced arthritis. Acute monarticular arthritis was inducible in B6 mice by IA injection of mBSA (0.2 mg) into the knee joint on day 0, along with daily SC injection of IL-1β (250 ng) into the rear footpad on days 0–2 (hereinafter referred to as the mBSA/IL-1 group). At 7 days after the mBSA injection, the overall disease severity, determined by the sum of individual histologic scores (see Materials and Methods), was 14.3 ± 1.3 (mean ± SEM) of a possible score of 25. Ipsilateral and contralateral injections of IL-1β yielded similar levels of arthritis in the mBSA-injected joints (13.2 ± 1.6 and 15.9 ± 1.0, respectively; n = 8 per group) as previously reported (1), suggesting that IL-1β acts systemically.

Joints of mice injected IA with saline (vehicle) and treated SC with IL-1β (saline/IL-1 group) on days 0–2 appeared normal, with a thin synovial membrane and acellular joint space (Figure 1A). Joints treated IA with mBSA and SC with saline (mBSA/saline) developed a weak inflammatory reaction, with mild synovitis (Figure 1B, arrow). In contrast, mBSA/IL-1 treatment induced a marked arthritis that typically scored 3–4 for each of the 5 pathologic features graded (Figure 1C). A simplified classification system was also devised to indicate inflammatory versus destructive arthritis (see Materials and Methods). Based on these criteria, 90% of B6 mouse joints had inflammatory and/or destructive arthritis (Table 1).

Strain specificity of mBSA/IL-1–induced arthritis. The mBSA/IL-1–induced arthritis model was originally described for B6 mice (1) as a modification of mBSA antigen-induced arthritis (AIA) (16). Because AIA is strain specific, we examined strain dependence in

Table 2. Involvement of lymphocytes and RelB in mBSA/IL-1–induced arthritis*

Experiment, group	Arthritis incidence		Histologic score
	Inflammatory	Destructive	
1			
B6 control	9/10	10/10	14.7 ± 1.2
RAG-1$^{-/-}$	0/8	0/8	1.5 ± 0.3†
2			
B6 control	9/10	10/10	13.8 ± 1.4
MHCII$^{-/-}$	0/10	0/10	0.6 ± 0.2†
3			
B6 + GL121‡	15/16	15/16	12.3 ± 1.2
B6 + GK1.5	0/16	0/16	1.1 ± 0.2†
4			
B6 control	6/6	6/6	16.1 ± 1.8
$\mu MT/\mu MT$	6/6	6/6	15.7 ± 0.9
5§			
B6 reconstituted	13/14	13/14	12.5 ± 1.1
RelB$^{-/-}$ BM chimera	5/10	4/10	7.0 ± 1.3†

* See Table 1 for definitions and explanations.
† $P < 0.005$ versus control.
‡ Isotype control for GK1.5.
§ Representative of 2 experiments.
¶ BM = bone marrow.

the mBSA/IL-1 model. B6 (H-2^b) and 129/Sv (H-2^b) strains and B6 × 129/Sv crosses were most susceptible to mBSA/IL-1–induced arthritis, with 70–90% of joints developing inflammatory and/or destructive arthritis of comparable severity (Table 1). In contrast, NOD (H-2^{g7}) mice showed less severe disease (mean ± SEM score 7.6 ± 1.6), while C3H/HeJ (H-2^k) mice were resistant (Table 1). Susceptibility to mBSA/IL-1–induced arthritis is therefore genetically regulated and is not simply the result of a nonspecific innate immune response.

Dependence of arthritis on CD4+ T lymphocytes but not on B lymphocytes. To further investigate adaptive immune mechanisms, we examined the importance of lymphocytes in mBSA/IL-1–induced arthritis using RAG-$1^{-/-}$ mice, which lack mature T and B lymphocytes (10). None of the joints from these mice developed either inflammatory or destructive arthritis (Table 2, experiment 1). The importance of CD4+ T lymphocytes in mBSA/IL-1–induced arthritis was investigated next. MHCII$^{-/-}$ mice, which lack MHC class II antigen and are severely depleted of CD4+ T lymphocytes (11), were assessed (Table 2, experiment 2). Neither inflammatory nor destructive arthritis developed in the MHCII$^{-/-}$ mice, and the mean histologic score (0.6 ± 0.2) was significantly lower ($P < 0.005$) than that in control mice (13.8 ± 1.4). The requirement for CD4+ T lymphocytes was confirmed by treatment of B6 mice with CD4+ cell–depleting mAb (GK1.5) immediately prior to and

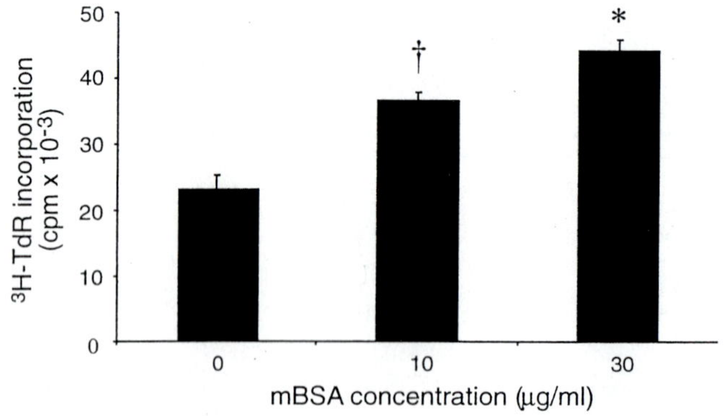

Figure 2. Proliferation of draining lymph node (LN) cells from mBSA/IL-1–treated mice in response to mBSA. B6 mice were injected intraarticularly with mBSA on day 0 and subcutaneously with IL-1β (days 0–2) as described in Materials and Methods. On day 7, the popliteal LN were removed and the cells (4 × 10^5/well) incubated for 72 hours in vitro with increasing concentrations of mBSA (0–30 μg/ml). During the last 8 hours of incubation, cells were pulsed with ^{3}H-thymidine (^{3}H-TdR). Bars show the mean and SEM cpm (n = 5 wells). † = $P < 0.001$; * = $P < 0.01$, versus control. Results are representative of 3 experiments. See Figure 1 for other definitions.

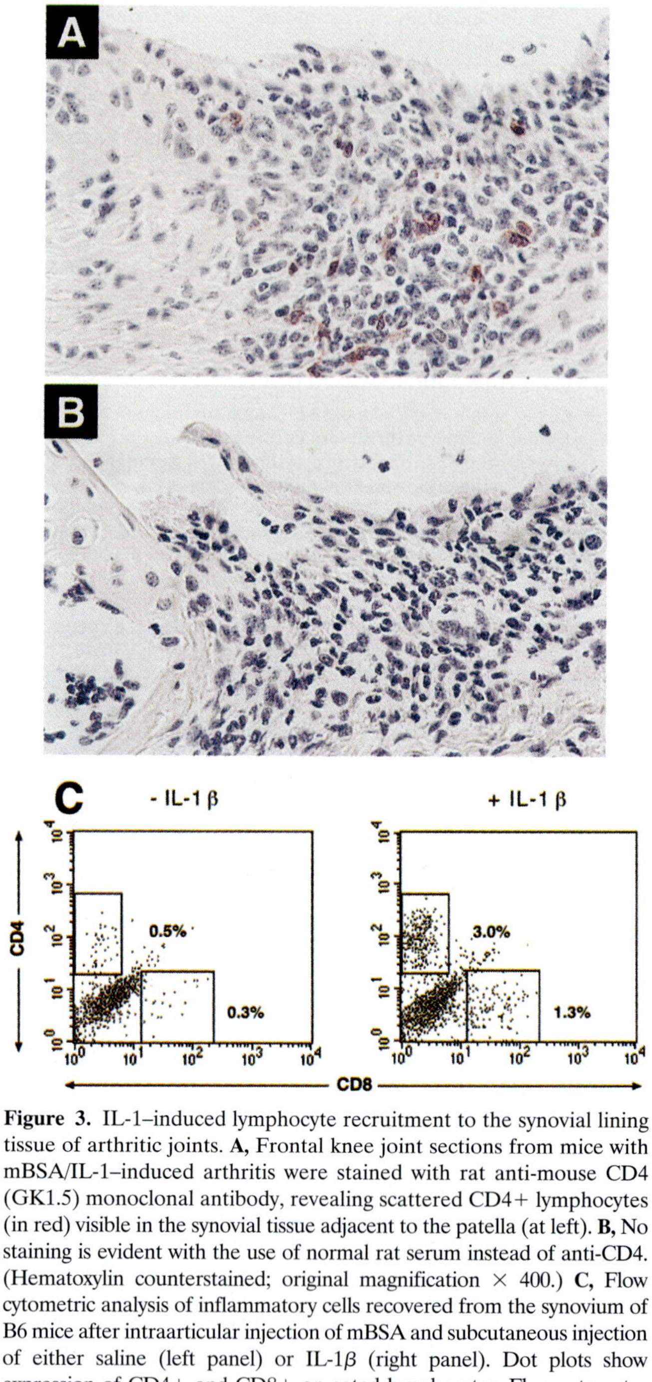

Figure 3. IL-1–induced lymphocyte recruitment to the synovial lining tissue of arthritic joints. **A,** Frontal knee joint sections from mice with mBSA/IL-1–induced arthritis were stained with rat anti-mouse CD4 (GK1.5) monoclonal antibody, revealing scattered CD4+ lymphocytes (in red) visible in the synovial tissue adjacent to the patella (at left). **B,** No staining is evident with the use of normal rat serum instead of anti-CD4. (Hematoxylin counterstained; original magnification × 400.) **C,** Flow cytometric analysis of inflammatory cells recovered from the synovium of B6 mice after intraarticular injection of mBSA and subcutaneous injection of either saline (left panel) or IL-1β (right panel). Dot plots show expression of CD4+ and CD8+ on gated lymphocytes. Flow cytometry results are representative of 2 experiments. See Figure 1 for definitions.

during disease induction (Table 2, experiment 3). Histologically, the joints from the mBSA/IL-1–treated RAG-$1^{-/-}$, MHCII$^{-/-}$, and CD4+ T cell–depleted B6 mice appeared normal, apart from limited synovial

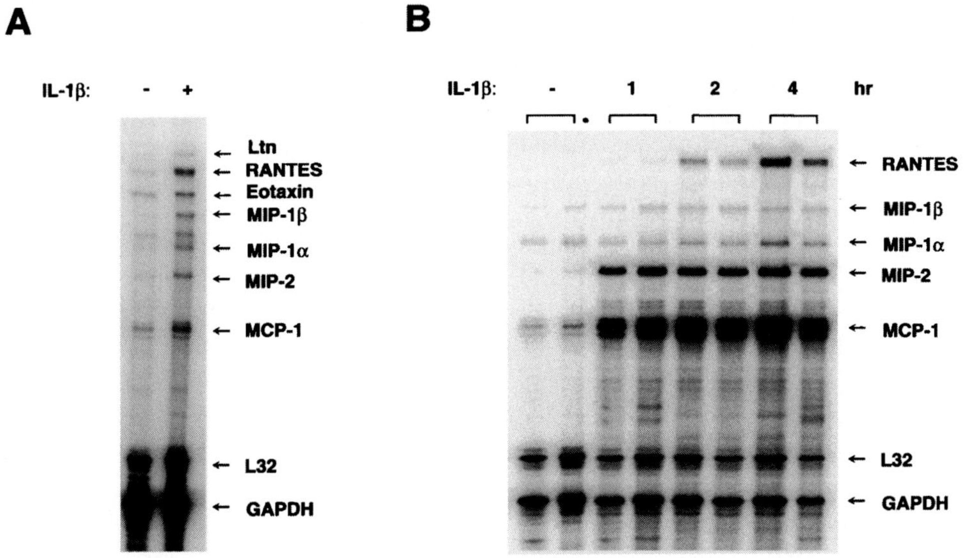

Figure 4. Chemokine mRNA expression in mBSA/IL-1–induced arthritis, and the effect of IL-1. **A**, Synovium was dissected on day 7 from the knee joints of mice treated with mBSA either with or without IL-1β. Total RNA was extracted and production of chemokine mRNA assessed. Each lane represents synovial tissue pooled from 5 mice. **B**, Synovial fibroblasts derived from explant patella cultures were stimulated, in duplicate, with IL-1β (35 ng/ml) for the times indicated. Similar results were obtained in 3 separate experiments. L32 and GAPDH represent RNA loading controls in each case. Ltn = lymphotactin; MIP-1β = macrophage inhibitory protein 1β; MCP-1 = monocyte chemoattractant protein 1 (see Figure 1 for other definitions).

hyperplasia (see Figure 1D, for example). To evaluate the role of B lymphocytes in mBSA/IL-1–induced arthritis, *μMT/μMT* mice, which lack mature B lymphocytes and do not produce IgM or IgG antibodies (12), were examined. The monarthritis induced in these mice was similar to that observed in control animals (Table 2, experiment 4). Arthritis induced by mBSA/IL-1 is therefore dependent on CD4+ T lymphocytes, but not on B lymphocytes or antibody.

Dose-dependent stimulation of a T cell proliferative response to mBSA. In view of the in vivo dependence of the model on T cells, we sought evidence for mBSA-specific T cells in the draining popliteal LN of mBSA/IL-1–treated B6 mice. Figure 2 shows that T cells proliferated in a dose-dependent manner in response to mBSA.

Increased synovial CD4+ and CD8+ T cells in response to IL-1. To investigate the recruitment of lymphocytes into the synovial compartment, immunoperoxidase staining was first performed on frozen knee joint sections. Figure 3A depicts CD4 staining (red cells) within the subsynovial tissue of an arthritic joint. Staining was also observed within the periosteal lining tissue and infrapatellar fatpad (not shown). No staining was observed when NRS was used in lieu of anti-CD4 mAb (Figure 3B). The effect of IL-1 on the number of CD4+ and CD8+ lymphocytes infiltrating the synovium of mBSA/IL-1 arthritic joints was next evaluated by flow cytometric analysis of dissociated synovial tissue. The majority of nonadherent cells were polymorphonuclear neutrophils, monocytes, and macrophages (not shown). Cells within the lymphocyte gate were analyzed for CD4 and CD8 expression. IL-1β increased the number of CD4+ lymphocytes by ~6-fold and CD8+ cells by ~4-fold in the synovial tissue of mBSA/IL-1–treated mice, compared with that of control (mBSA/saline–treated) mice (Figure 3C).

IL-1 stimulation of chemokine expression by synovial cells. Chemokines play an important role in recruitment of immune cells to sites of inflammation (17). To examine the effect of IL-1β on chemokine expression in the synovium during acute arthritis, synovial tissue (comprising a heterogeneous population of resident and infiltrating cells) was extracted from either mBSA/IL-1– or mBSA/saline–treated mice for RNase protection analysis (RPA). The chemokines lymphotactin, RANTES, MIP-1α, MIP-1β, MIP-2, and MCP-1 were all up-regulated by IL-1β in the synovial compartment (Figure 4A). To more specifically examine the effect of IL-1 on synovial fibroblast chemokine production, synovial explant cells were stimulated in vitro with IL-1β. Figure 4B shows RPA of chemokine mRNA during the course of IL-1β stimulation. Synovial fibroblasts constitutively expressed MCP-1, MIP-1α, MIP-1β, and MIP-2 mRNA. IL-1β markedly up-regulated MCP-1 and MIP-2 mRNA levels by 1 hour, and RANTES by 2 hours. MIP-1α and MIP-1β also appeared to be weakly up-regulated by IL-1β. Interestingly, the chemokines lymphotactin and eotaxin were detected only in the synovium removed directly from mBSA/IL-1–treated joints and not in cultured synovial fibroblasts treated with IL-1.

Importance of RelB in mBSA/IL-1–induced arthritis. RelB, a member of the nuclear factor κB (NF-κB)/Rel family of transcription factors, is expressed at high levels in myeloid-related interdigitating dendritic cells (DC) and at lower levels in macrophages and T and B cells (18–20). To examine the importance of RelB, we tested RelB$^{-/-}$ bone marrow chimeric mice in the mBSA/IL-1–induced arthritis model. Bone marrow chimeric mice were constructed by transfer of Ly5.2 RelB$^{-/-}$ bone marrow cells into lethally irradiated wild-type B6 Ly5.1 mice, creating mice with a normal nonhemopoietic compartment but with RelB$^{-/-}$ bone marrow–derived cells. The histologic joint score for each pathologic feature was reduced in the RelB$^{-/-}$ bone marrow chimeras compared with wild-type reconstituted mice (Figure 5). Both inflammatory and destructive arthritis features were reduced in the RelB$^{-/-}$ bone marrow chimeric mouse joints (50% and 40%, respectively; n = 10) compared with wild-type reconstituted mice (>90% incidence of inflammatory/destructive arthritis; n = 14) (Table 2, experiment 5). In summary, RelB$^{-/-}$ bone marrow chimeric mice still developed arthritis, but with a significantly reduced incidence and severity.

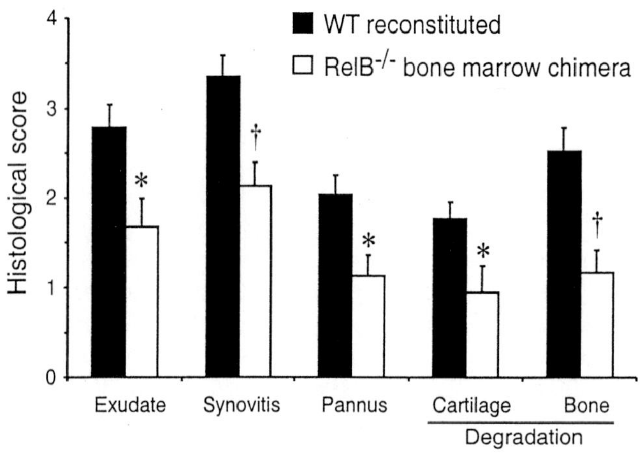

Figure 5. Involvement of RelB expression in mBSA/IL-1–induced arthritis. Pathologic features of knee joints of B6 (wild-type; WT) reconstituted and RelB$^{-/-}$ bone marrow B6 chimeric mice injected intraarticularly with mBSA (day 0) and treated subcutaneously with IL-1β (days 0–2) were evaluated on day 7. The severity of each feature of arthritis—joint space exudate, synovitis, pannus formation, and cartilage and bone degradation—was graded from 0 (normal) to 5 (severe) (see Materials and Methods). Values are the mean and SEM scores for wild-type reconstituted (n =14) and RelB$^{-/-}$ bone marrow chimeric (n = 10) mouse joints. * = $P < 0.05$; † = $P < 0.005$. Results are representative of 2 experiments. See Figure 1 for other definitions.

DISCUSSION

Arthritis induced by mBSA/IL-1 was first described in 1990 (1). However, despite the potential usefulness of this novel model for the rapid assessment of mediators of inflammation in acute arthritis, the underlying immune mechanisms have not been reported. In view of the rapid onset of inflammatory arthritis and the predominance of polymorphonuclear neutrophils and mononuclear cells in arthritic joints, it is possible that arthritis was due to activation of innate immunity. We therefore examined the role of molecular and cellular mediators and found that mBSA/IL-1–induced arthritis is restricted to specific mouse strains and is dependent on CD4+ T lymphocytes, but not on B lymphocytes. Responsive mouse strains included B6, 129/Sv, and B6 × 129/Sv crosses, each of H-2^b haplotype at the MHC class II locus. Susceptibility of B6, 129/Sv, and B6 × 129/Sv mice to mBSA/IL-1–induced arthritis is a major advantage of the model for gene knockout and chimeric mouse studies, since gene knockout mice are frequently derived on these backgrounds.

CD4+ T lymphocytes are important cellular mediators in RA (21) and in murine CIA (22) and AIA (23). The absence of disease in RAG-1$^{-/-}$ and MHCII$^{-/-}$ mice highlights the role of lymphocytes (and possibly MHC class II) in mBSA/IL-1–induced arthritis. The absolute dependence of the model on CD4+ T lymphocytes was demonstrated by the protection achieved via depletion of CD4+ T lymphocytes. Dose-dependent T cell proliferation in draining LN cells in response to mBSA was confirmed. The finding that B lymphocytes or antibodies were not required for mBSA/IL-1–induced arthritis contrasts with models of chronic arthritis, which are dependent on both cellular and humoral immunity (24–27). Together, these findings suggest that mBSA/IL-1–induced arthritis is a model of a T cell–dependent adaptive immune response confined to the local joint/LN environment, which is enhanced by systemic IL-1.

The influence of IL-1 on the induction and progression of acute inflammatory arthritis is intriguing. Systemic (ipsilateral or contralateral) SC footpad injections of IL-1β induced local joint pathology, as previously reported (1). IL-1β stimulation in vitro increased T cell proliferation in LN cells from mBSA/IL-1–treated mice (data not shown), confirming previous observations (28). We found that systemic IL-1β induced CD4+/CD8+ lymphocyte infiltration of the synovium in mBSA-treated joints, suggesting that IL-1β influences leukocyte trafficking. Constitutive or induced tissue-specific expression of chemokines mediates, in part, the recruitment of leukocytes to sites of inflammation (29). The chemokines RANTES, MIP-1α, MIP-1β, and MCP-1 are members of the CC or β chemokine group and act mainly on monocytes, macrophages, and lymphocytes, whereas MIP-2 is a CXC or α chemokine and acts primarily on neutrophils (30). These chemokines were all up-regulated in response to IL-1β, both in vivo and in vitro. The expression of eotaxin and lymphotactin was confined to the synovial tissue taken directly from arthritic joints and not in cultured synovial fibroblasts. Eotaxin, a member of the CC family, is a powerful eosinophil attractant; however, basophils and some T lymphocytes also express receptors for eotaxin (31). The C chemokine, lymphotactin, recruits lymphocytes and natural killer cells (32). Presumably, the expression of these 2 chemokines in synovial tissue is due to the presence of tissue macrophages or infiltrating immune cells. Systemic IL-1 may therefore regulate leukocyte trafficking via induction of chemokines in target tissues, as recently proposed for tumor necrosis factor α (33).

RelB, a member of the NF-κB/Rel family of transcription factors, is of particular interest in RA, as RelB expression correlates with maturation and activation of myeloid-related DC populations (34) and RelB^{+} differentiated DC are expressed in rheumatoid synovial tissue (35). Expression of RelB is restricted to lymphoid tissues, with high expression in interdigitating DC and lower expression in macrophages and T and B cells (18–20). RelB$^{-/-}$ mice lack a subset of interdigitating DC and have impaired antigen-presenting cell function, as well as a defect in cellular immunity (36). RelB$^{-/-}$ mice develop an inflammatory syndrome with severe myeloid hyperplasia and splenomegaly shortly after birth and die prematurely (37). Bone marrow chimeric RelB$^{-/-}$ mice are viable, and studies using these mice allow distinction between hemopoietic and nonhemopoietic cellular contributions to disease. Our study allowed assessment of the contribution of RelB to acute arthritis. The reduction in acute arthritis in RelB$^{-/-}$ bone marrow chimeras indicates a substantial, but not essential, role for RelB-expressing cells. Residual disease in RelB$^{-/-}$ bone marrow chimeras may be caused by the presence of other NF-κB/Rel family members (38). Further studies are needed to specifically address which RelB-bearing cell(s) mediate these effects.

In conclusion, mBSA/IL-1–induced arthritis is an acute CD4+ T cell–dependent model of inflammatory monarthritis that is useful for investigating cell-mediated immune mechanisms and the actions of IL-1. IL-1 influences both adaptive immune responses and local chemokine production in this model. The model of mBSA/IL-1–induced arthritis can be directly applied to mouse strains (B6 and 129/Sv) that are commonly used to generate gene knockout and bone marrow chimeric mice. Examination of RelB mutant bone marrow chimeric mice illustrated the involvement of RelB in acute arthritis. The model may also be useful for understanding progression from acute to chronic arthritis and mechanisms of disease resolution.

ACKNOWLEDGMENTS

We thank L. Corcoran, W. Heath, D. Tarlinton, and A. D'Amico for the provision of mice, A. Milligan for animal care, S. Mihajlovic for histologic analysis, and D. Advani for assistance with figures.

REFERENCES

1. Staite ND, Richard KA, Aspar DG, Franz KA, Galinet LA, Dunn CJ. Induction of an acute erosive monarticular arthritis in mice by interleukin-1 and methylated bovine serum albumin. Arthritis Rheum 1990;33:253–60.
2. Miller LC, Dinarello CA. Biologic activities of interleukin-1 relevant to rheumatic diseases. Pathol Immunopathol Res 1987;6: 22–36.
3. Arend WP, Dayer J-M. Cytokines and cytokine inhibitors or antagonists in rheumatoid arthritis. Arthritis Rheum 1990;33: 305–15.
4. Hom JT, Bendele AM, Carlson DG. In vivo administration with IL-1 accelerates the development of collagen-induced arthritis in mice. J Immunol 1988;141:834–41.
5. Pettipher ER, Higgs GA, Henderson B. Interleukin 1 induces leukocyte infiltration and cartilage proteoglycan degradation in the synovial joint. Proc Natl Acad Sci U S A 1986;83:8749–53.
6. Van de Loo AA, van den Berg WB. Effects of murine recombinant interleukin 1 on synovial joints in mice: measurement of patellar cartilage metabolism and joint inflammation. Ann Rheum Dis 1990;49:238–45.
7. Ghivizzani SC, Kang R, Georgescu HI, Lechman ER, Jaffurs D, Engle JM, et al. Constitutive intra-articular expression of human

IL-1 beta following gene transfer to rabbit synovium produces all major pathologies of human rheumatoid arthritis. J Immunol 1997;159:3604–12.
8. Horai R, Saijo S, Tanioka H, Nakae S, Sudo K, Okahara A, et al. Development of chronic inflammatory arthropathy resembling rheumatoid arthritis in interleukin 1 receptor antagonist-deficient mice. J Exp Med 2000;191:313–20.
9. Gabay C, Arend WP. Treatment of rheumatoid arthritis with IL-1 inhibitors. Springer Semin Immunopathol 1998;20:229–46.
10. Mombaerts P, Iacomini J, Johnson RS, Herrup K, Tonegawa S, Papaioannou VE. RAG-1-deficient mice have no mature B and T lymphocytes. Cell 1992;68:869–77.
11. Köntgen F, Suss G, Stewart C, Steinmetz M, Bluethmann H. Targeted disruption of the MHC class II Aa gene in C57BL/6 mice. Int Immunol 1993;5:957–64.
12. Kitamura D, Roes J, Kuhn R, Rajewsky K. A B cell-deficient mouse by targeted disruption of the membrane exon of the immunoglobulin mu chain gene. Nature 1991;350:423–6.
13. Burkly L, Hession C, Ogata L, Reilly C, Marconi LA, Olson D, et al. Expression of relB is required for the development of thymic medulla and dendritic cells. Nature 1995;373:531–6.
14. Wu L, D'Amico A, Winkel KD, Suter M, Lo D, Shortman K. RelB is essential for the development of myeloid-related $CD8\alpha^-$ dendritic cells but not of lymphoid-related $CD8\alpha^+$ dendritic cells. Immunity 1998;9:839–47.
15. Jonsson R, Tarkowski A, Klareskog L. A demineralization procedure for immunohistopathological use: EDTA treatment preserves lymphoid cell surface antigens. J Immunol Methods 1986; 88:109–14.
16. Brackertz D, Mitchell GF, Mackay IR. Antigen-induced arthritis in mice. I. Induction of arthritis in various strains of mice. Arthritis Rheum 1977;20:841–50.
17. Taub DD, Oppenheim JJ. Chemokines, inflammation and the immune system. Ther Immunol 1994;1:229–46.
18. Carrasco D, Ryseck RP, Bravo R. Expression of relB transcripts during lymphoid organ development: specific expression in dendritic antigen-presenting cells. Development 1993;118:1221–31.
19. Lernbecher T, Kistler B, Wirth T. Two distinct mechanisms contribute to the constitutive activation of RelB in lymphoid cells. EMBO J 1994;13:4060–9.
20. Weih F, Carrasco D, Bravo R. Constitutive and inducible Rel/NF-κB activities in mouse thymus and spleen. Oncogene 1994;9: 3289–97.
21. Panayi GS, Lanchbury JS, Kingsley GH. The importance of the T cell in initiating and maintaining the chronic synovitis of rheumatoid arthritis. Arthritis Rheum 1992;35:729–35.
22. Ranges GE, Sriram S, Cooper SM. Prevention of type II collagen-induced arthritis by in vivo treatment with anti-L3T4. J Exp Med 1985;162:1105–10.
23. Petrow PK, Thoss K, Katenkamp D, Brauer R. Adoptive transfer of susceptibility to antigen-induced arthritis into severe combined immunodeficient (SCID) mice: a role of CD4+ and CD8+ T cells. Immunol Invest 1996;25:341–53.
24. Cooke TD, Jasin HE. The pathogenesis of chronic inflammation in experimental antigen-induced arthritis. I. The role of antigen on the local immune response. Arthritis Rheum 1972;15:327–37.
25. Seki N, Sudo Y, Yoshioka T, Sugihara S, Fujitsu T, Sakuma S, et al. Type II collagen-induced murine arthritis. I. Induction and perpetuation of arthritis require synergy between humoral and cell-mediated immunity. J Immunol 1988;140:1477–84.
26. Kouskoff V, Korganow AS, Duchatelle V, Degott C, Benoist C, Mathis D. Organ-specific disease provoked by systemic autoimmunity. Cell 1996;87:811–22.
27. Campbell IK, Hamilton JA, Wicks IP. Collagen-induced arthritis in C57BL/6 (H-2^b) mice: new insights into an important disease model of rheumatoid arthritis. Eur J Immunol 2000;30: 1568–75.
28. Lichtman AH, Chin J, Schmidt JA, Abbas AK. Role of interleukin 1 in the activation of T lymphocytes. Proc Natl Acad Sci U S A 1988;85:9699–703.
29. Kim CH, Broxmeyer HE. Chemokines: signal lamps for trafficking of T and B cells for development and effector function. J Leukoc Biol 1999;65:6–15.
30. Rossi D, Zlotnik A. The biology of chemokines and their receptors. Annu Rev Immunol 2000;18:217–42.
31. Baggiolini M. Chemokines and leukocyte traffic. Nature 1998;392: 565–8.
32. Hedrick JA, Saylor V, Figueroa D, Mizoue L, Xu Y, Menon S, et al. Lymphotactin is produced by NK cells and attracts both NK and T cells in vivo. J Immunol 1997;158:1533–40.
33. Sedgwick JD, Riminton DS, Cyster JG, Körner H. Tumor necrosis factor: a master-regulator of leukocyte movement. Immunol Today 2000;21:110–3.
34. Pettit AR, Quinn C, MacDonald KP, Cavanagh LL, Thomas G, Townsend W, et al. Nuclear localization of RelB is associated with effective antigen-presenting cell function. J Immunol 1997;159: 3681–91.
35. Pettit AR, MacDonald KPA, O'Sullivan B, Thomas R. Differentiated dendritic cells expressing nuclear RelB are predominantly located in rheumatoid synovial tissue perivascular mononuclear cell aggregates. Arthritis Rheum 2000;43:791–800.
36. Weih F, Warr G, Yang H, Bravo R. Multifocal defects in immune responses in RelB-deficient mice. J Immunol 1997;158:5211–8.
37. Weih F, Carrasco D, Durham SK, Barton DS, Rizzo CA, Ryseck RP, et al. Multiorgan inflammation and hematopoietic abnormalities in mice with a targeted disruption of RelB, a member of the NF-κB/Rel family. Cell 1995;80:331–40.
38. Campbell IK, Gerondakis S, O'Donnell K, Wicks IP. Distinct roles for the NF-κB1 (p50) and c-Rel transcription factors in inflammatory arthritis. J Clin Invest 2000;105:1799–806.

ARTHRITIS & RHEUMATISM
Vol. 44, No. 2, February 2001, pp 451–462

Increased Production of Intracellular Interleukin-1 Receptor Antagonist Type I in the Synovium of Mice With Collagen-Induced Arthritis

A Possible Role in the Resolution of Arthritis

Cem Gabay,[1] Liliana Marinova-Mutafchieva,[2] Richard O. Williams,[2] Jason P. Gigley,[3] Debra M. Butler,[2] Marc Feldmann,[2] and William P. Arend[3]

Objective. **To examine the patterns of production of interleukin-1 receptor antagonist (IL-1Ra) isoforms and of IL-1β during arthritis in vivo.**

Methods. **Arthritis was induced in DBA/1 mice by immunization with type II collagen, and the production of IL-1Ra isoforms was examined in whole joints and in dissected synovial tissues by reverse transcription–polymerase chain reaction (RT-PCR), RNase protection assay, Western blotting, immunostaining, and in situ hybridization. Production of IL-1β also was examined using similar approaches.**

Results. **Production of IL-1Ra increased in the joints during collagen-induced arthritis (CIA). By RT-PCR, secreted IL-1Ra messenger RNA (mRNA) was detected in normal joints, whereas intracellular IL-1Ra type I (icIL-1Ra1) mRNA was only produced in inflamed joints. Western blot studies showed that icIL-1Ra1 protein levels increased in the joints during the course of CIA and that icIL-1Ra3 protein was also present in low amounts. RNase protection assays showed that the IL-1β:IL-1Ra mRNA ratio was increased in inflamed joints through day 14 of arthritis, whereas a reverse pattern was present at later time points (from day 20 to day 60). Consistent with this finding, immunohistochemistry and in situ hybridization studies confirmed that icIL-1Ra1 was only present in inflamed joints. The histologic evaluation of CIA during the course of the disease indicated a resolution of acute inflammation, since icIL-1Ra1 production increased and the ratio of IL-1β to total IL-1Ra decreased.**

Conclusion. **Production of IL-1Ra isoforms, particularly icIL-1Ra1, is stimulated in inflamed joints during CIA in mice. The combination of decreased production of IL-1β and elevated levels of icIL-1Ra1 during the course of CIA was associated with a reduction in inflammatory activity. These results suggest that icIL-1Ra1 may play a role in the resolution of murine CIA.**

Interleukin-1 (IL-1) is a proinflammatory cytokine that plays a major role in acute and chronic inflammation (for review, see ref. 1). In particular, IL-1 has been proposed to participate in the early events of rheumatoid arthritis (RA), including in the migration of inflammatory cells and in the release of enzymes leading to progressive joint destruction (for review, see ref. 2). IL-1 receptor antagonist (IL-1Ra) is a member of the IL-1 family and binds to cell surface IL-1 receptors without inducing any intracellular responses. IL-1Ra prevents the binding of IL-1 to its membrane-bound receptors and acts as a natural cytokine inhibitor. IL-1Ra has been shown to possess antiinflammatory prop-

Dr. Gabay's work was supported by Swiss National Science Foundation grants 3231-054954.98 and 3200-054955.98. Drs. Marinova-Mutafchieva, Williams, Butler, and Feldmann's work was supported by the Arthritis Research Campaign, UK. Dr. Arend's work was supported by NIH grant AR-40135 and by the Rocky Mountain Chapter of the Arthritis Foundation.

[1]Cem Gabay, MD: University Hospital of Geneva, Geneva, Switzerland; [2]Liliana Marinova-Mutafchieva, MD, PhD, Richard O. Williams, PhD, Debra M. Butler, PhD, Marc Feldmann, MD, PhD: Kennedy Institute of Rheumatology, London, UK; [3]Jason P. Gigley, BA, William P. Arend, MD: University of Colorado Health Sciences Center, Denver, Colorado.

Address correspondence and reprint requests to Cem Gabay, MD, Division of Rheumatology, University Hospital of Geneva, 26 Avenue Beau-Sejour, 1211 Geneva 14, Switzerland.

Submitted for publication May 29, 2000; accepted in revised form September 18, 2000.

erties in several animal models of inflammatory diseases, including arthritis (for review, see ref. 3). In addition, the therapeutic administration of IL-1Ra was recently shown to have a beneficial effect on clinical and radiologic parameters in patients with RA (4).

The role of endogenous IL-1Ra in suppressing arthritis has recently been demonstrated in experimental animal models. The administration of neutralizing $F(ab')_2$ anti–IL-1Ra antibodies led to enhanced leukocyte infiltration and protein leakage in lipopolysaccharide (LPS)–induced arthritis in rabbits (5). IL-1Ra knockout mice exhibited an earlier onset of collagen-induced arthritis (CIA) and more severe arthritis, often accompanied by bony erosions (6). Finally, the absence of IL-1Ra by gene deletion in BALB/cA mice was associated with the spontaneous development of chronic polyarthritis, reproducing some of the clinical and biologic features of RA (7).

Consistent with these findings in experimental models of arthritis, several studies have suggested that local and systemic production of IL-1Ra is inadequate in patients with RA. Production of IL-1Ra by isolated synovial cells was relatively low in comparison with IL-1 (8). Isolated CD14+ synovial macrophages produced less IL-1Ra per cell than did alveolar macrophages or in vitro–derived macrophages (8). In addition, up to 90% of the cells at the cartilage–pannus junction in RA patients stained positive for IL-1α, whereas only 10% of these cells expressed IL-1Ra (9). Patients with RA exhibited a lower ratio of IL-1Ra to IL-1β in plasma at both baseline and after surgery in comparison with controls (10). Taken together, these results suggest that a relatively deficient local and systemic production of IL-1Ra in comparison with IL-1 may predispose to the perpetuation of inflammation in rheumatoid joints.

IL-1Ra encompasses 4 different isoforms derived from the same gene (for review, see ref. 3). One isoform, the 17-kd secreted IL-1Ra (sIL-1Ra), is glycosylated and secreted with a molecular weight that varies between 22 kd and 25 kd (11). The 3 other IL-1Ra isoforms do not possess a leader sequence and therefore remain intracellular (icIL-1Ra types 1, 2, and 3). The icIL-1Ra1 isoform is generated by an alternate splice into the leader sequence area of sIL-1Ra and has a molecular weight of 18 kd (12). The sequence of icIL-1Ra2 messenger RNA (mRNA) contains an additional exon encoding for 21 amino acids, thus producing a predicted 26-kd protein (13). The 16-kd icIL-1Ra3 is produced by alternative translation initiation primarily from sIL-1Ra mRNA (14). Macrophages cultured from rheumatoid synovial tissue were shown to produce primarily sIL-1Ra, whereas cultured synovial fibroblasts contained only icIL-1Ra1 mRNA (8). The presence of both icIL-1Ra1 and icIL-1Ra3 has been described in mouse tissues (15,16), whereas the production of icIL-1Ra2 mRNA and protein has not yet been demonstrated in murine cells. However, the production of IL-1Ra isoforms in the joints and their relationship to disease activity in vivo has not previously been examined.

CIA is a well-established animal model of RA that has been used extensively to assess the biologic significance of both pro- and antiinflammatory mediators. The objective of the studies described herein was to examine the production of IL-1Ra isoforms and IL-1β during the course of CIA, that is, during both induction and remission phases.

MATERIALS AND METHODS

Animals. Male DBA/1 mice (ages 8–10 weeks at the time of immunization) were used in the present experiments. Mice were housed at low numbers per cage. Studies were conducted in parallel at the University of Colorado Health Sciences Center (Denver, CO) and at the Kennedy Institute of Rheumatology (London, UK). The experiments were approved by the ethics committees for animal use at both institutions. Mice were fed water and high-lipid chow ad libitum.

Induction of CIA. Bovine type II collagen was prepared at the Kennedy Institute of Rheumatology or was purchased from Dr. Marie Griffiths (University of Utah, Salt Lake City, UT). Bovine type II collagen was dissolved in 0.1*M* acetic acid overnight at 4°C. For the studies conducted at the University of Colorado Health Sciences Center, wild-type DBA/1 mice were immunized intradermally at the base of the tail with 100 μg of collagen in an equal volume with Freund's complete adjuvant (CFA) containing H37Ra *Mycobacterium tuberculosis* (Difco, Detroit, MI). On day 21, a booster injection with 100 μg of collagen emulsified in Freund's incomplete adjuvant (Difco) was given at the base of the tail.

For the experiments performed at the Kennedy Institute of Rheumatology, DBA/1 mice were immunized intradermally at the base of the tail with a single injection of 200 μg of bovine type II collagen emulsified in an equal volume of CFA (Difco). The incidence of arthritis in mice at both institutions varied between 80% and 100%.

Clinical assessment of disease. The severity of arthritis was scored on a 3-point scale, where 0 = normal appearance, 1 = mild swelling and/or erythema, and 2 = pronounced swelling and erythema. For some experiments, mice were killed at different times during the course of arthritis, after the appearance of the first signs of joint inflammation. As controls, naive mice and immunized mice without clinical signs of arthritis were also studied.

Preparation of total RNA from whole joints and from synovial tissues. Arthritic and control mice were killed according to the experimental protocol. The inflamed joints and the clinically unaffected contralateral joints were dissected and used for preparation of total RNA. For some experiments, the knee joints were also dissected, and the synovial membranes were prepared and snap-frozen. Total RNA was extracted with TRIzol (Life Technologies, Gaithersburg, MD).

Reverse transcription–polymerase chain reaction (RT-PCR). One microgram of total RNA was treated with Ampgrade DNase I (Life Technologies). RT-PCR was performed using the primers for murine icIL-1Ra1, murine sIL-1Ra, and murine GAPDH, as recently described (16).

RNase protection assays. Using an approach recently described for human IL-1Ra mRNA (17), a riboprobe was created that would distinguish between the 2 major IL-1Ra mRNA isoforms (sIL-1Ra and icIL-1Ra1) as 2 different protected-size products following RNase treatment. RT-PCR was performed on total RNA from LPS-stimulated murine peritoneal macrophages, using a forward primer specific for the icIL-1Ra1 sequence 5′ IL-1Ra (GCA-TGA-ATT-CAG-GGG-CAG-TTC-CAC-CCT-GGG-AAG-GT) and a reverse primer complementary to the common sequence 3′ IL-1Ra (GCA-TAA-GCT-TCT-GGA-GCT-TGA-TAT-CAT-CTC-CAG). Riboprobes for IL-1β and GAPDH mRNA were created using the following primers: for 5′ IL-1β GCA-TGA-ATT-CAA-CTT-CAG-GCA-GGC-AGT-ATC-AC; for 3′ IL-1β GCA-TAA-GCT-TCA-GCA-GGT-TAT-CAT-CAT-CAT-CC; for 5′ GAPDH GCA-TGA-ATT-CAG-CCC-ATC-ACC-ATC-TTC-CAG-GAG-CG; and for 3′ GAPDH GCA-TAA-GCT-TGT-GAA-GAC-ACC-AGT-AGA-CTC-CAC-G.

The PCR products were cleaved with *Eco* RI and *Hind* III, gel purified, and cloned into pBluescript SK+ (Stratagene, San Diego, CA). Plasmids containing the probes were linearized with *Eco* RI and transcribed with T7 RNA polymerase and ^{32}P-labeled CTP. RNase protection assays were performed as recently described (15), and quantification of cytokine and GAPDH mRNA fragments was performed with a PhosphorImager using ImageQuant software (Molecular Dynamics, Sunnyvale, CA).

Western blot analysis. Total proteins from whole joints and dissected synovial tissues were prepared using TRIzol (15). The concentration of proteins was determined using a protein assay kit (Bio-Rad, Richmond, CA). Western blot analyses were performed using a horseradish peroxidase–labeled goat anti-murine IL-1Ra antibody that recognizes all murine IL-1Ra isoforms (15). Recombinant murine icIL-1Ra1 and sIL-1Ra were included as controls.

Histology studies. Mice were killed according to the experimental protocol, and hind paws with clinical evidence of arthritis were removed above the ankle joint. The paws were immediately frozen in OCT embedding matrix on dry ice and isopentane and were stored at −70°C. In some cases, normal paws were included as a control.

For immunohistochemistry studies, sections were performed using an adhesive tape as previously described (18). Briefly, frozen paws were mounted laterally on the chuck of a motor-driven cryostat. After trimming the tissue, transparent adhesive tape was applied to the tissue surface by pressure, and sagittal sections of whole hind paws (8 μm thickness) were obtained. The adhesive tape containing the tissue section was then attached to a microscopic slide and processed for immunohistochemistry.

For in situ hybridization studies, adhesive tape was also applied to the tissue surface prior to sectioning. The tissue sections were then ultraviolet light–crosslinked to a slide (Instrumedics, Hackensack, NJ) and processed as described below.

Immunohistochemistry studies. Immunolocalization of IL-1Ra in the joints was carried out as previously described (18). For detection of IL-1Ra, tissue sections were incubated overnight at 4°C with 5 μg/ml of goat anti-mouse IL-1Ra antibodies. Control staining was performed in parallel with normal goat serum. The expression of IL-1β was detected using a hamster anti-mouse IL-1β monoclonal antibody (Genzyme, Cambridge, MA) that recognizes both mature IL-1β and pro–IL-1β (18).

Microscopic analysis. Specimens were examined using an Olympus BH2 microscope and analyzed by computer image analysis (AnalySIS; Soft Imaging System, Munster, Germany) in a blinded manner. To localize and identify areas with positively stained cells within the isolated and fixed whole paw, entire tissue sections were examined. Five digital images (400× magnification) per specimen of synovial tissue from a metatarsophalangeal joint were recorded, and quantitative analysis was performed according to the color cell separation. The results are expressed as the mean region of interest, representing the percentage of area covered with positively stained cells per image at a magnification of 400×. For each cytokine, 3 semiserial sections, spaced 10 sections apart, were examined.

In addition to immunohistochemical staining, sections from all hind limbs were also stained with hematoxylin and eosin and Safranin O in order to assess the histopathologic severity of arthritis.

In situ hybridization studies. A plasmid containing the probe for icIL-1Ra1 mRNA was used to generate a digoxigenin-labeled complementary riboprobe for in situ hybridization (16). A digoxigenin-labeled sense probe was used as a negative control. In situ hybridization studies were performed as recently described (16). Briefly, tissue sections were fixed for 40 minutes in 2% paraformaldehyde in phosphate buffered saline. The slides were treated for 15 minutes at room temperature with 5 μg/ml of proteinase K, rinsed, and then treated for 10 minutes at room temperature with 0.2*N* HCl. Sections were hybridized overnight at 42°C with 100 ng of the riboprobes, followed by increasing stringency washes at 42°C. Slides were then incubated with alkaline phosphatase–conjugated antidigoxigenin antibodies (Boehringer, Indianapolis, IN), followed by the addition of NBT/BCIP substrate (Dako, Carpinteria, CA) supplemented with 10 μg/ml of levamisole. Nuclear fast red (Dako) was used as the counterstain.

Statistical analysis. Comparison of cytokine mRNA levels between the different groups was performed using Student's *t*-test. Tukey's multiple comparison test was used to compare differences in the levels of IL-1β and IL-1Ra expression, as assessed by immunostaining, between days 5 and 60 of clinical arthritis.

RESULTS

IL-1Ra isoform and IL-1β mRNA levels in normal and inflamed joints. To examine the production of IL-1Ra isoforms in normal and inflamed joints ~1 week after the onset of CIA, total RNA was prepared from

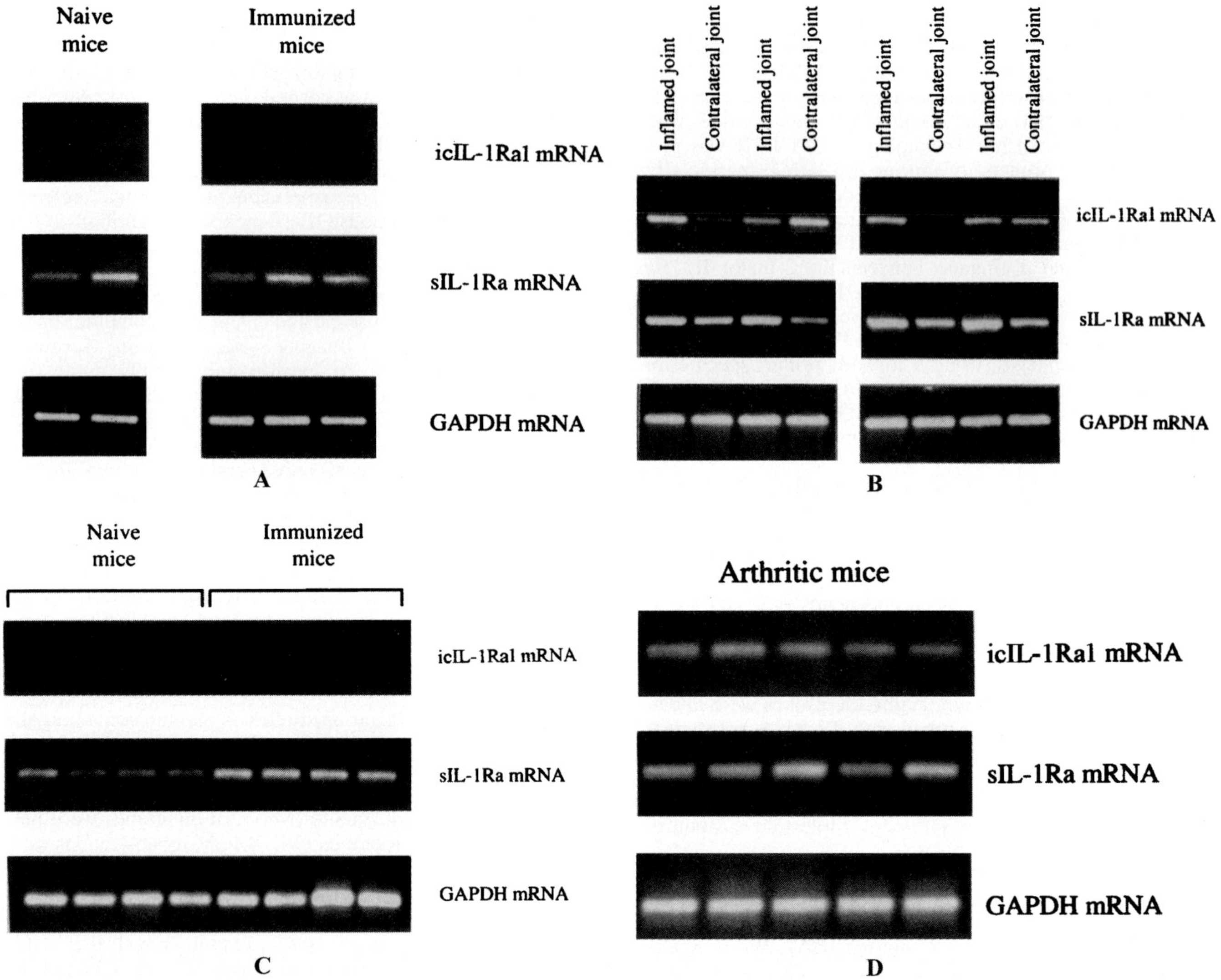

Figure 1. The presence of interleukin-1 receptor antagonist (IL-1Ra) mRNA isoforms in whole joints and in dissected synovium of mice with collagen-induced arthritis (CIA). Whole joints were dissected from 2 naive DBA/1 mice and from mice immunized with 2 intradermal injections of collagen (see Materials and Methods), including 3 immunized mice examined prior to the onset of clinical signs of arthritis **(A)** and 4 mice examined after 1 week of CIA **(B).** Both inflamed and clinically uninvolved contralateral joints were collected from mice with CIA. Dissected synovial membranes were obtained from 4 naive DBA/1 mice and from mice immunized with a single intradermal injection of collagen, including 4 mice without clinical signs of arthritis (14 days after immunization) **(C)** and 5 mice with CIA for 4 days **(D).** Total RNA was prepared and examined by reverse transcription–polymerase chain reaction (PCR) using primers for the IL-1Ra isoforms intracellular IL-1Ra1 (icIL-1Ra1) and secreted IL-1Ra (sIL-1Ra) and for GAPDH. PCR products were analyzed by ethidium bromide/agarose gel electrophoresis. The results are representative of 3 different experiments.

dissected joints, and RT-PCR was performed using primers specific for murine sIL-1Ra and icIL-1Ra1 mRNA. Isoform sIL-1Ra mRNA was present at low levels in the joints of both naive mice and immunized mice prior to the development of CIA (Figure 1A). The levels of sIL-1Ra mRNA were increased in inflamed joints (Figure 1B). In contrast, we found that icIL-1Ra1 mRNA was detected only in the joints of mice with overt CIA, in both clinically inflamed joints and unaffected contralateral joints (Figure 1B).

To determine which IL-1Ra isoforms were produced in the synovium, the knees of mice with and without arthritis were dissected, and the synovial membranes were collected to prepare total RNA. Inflamed

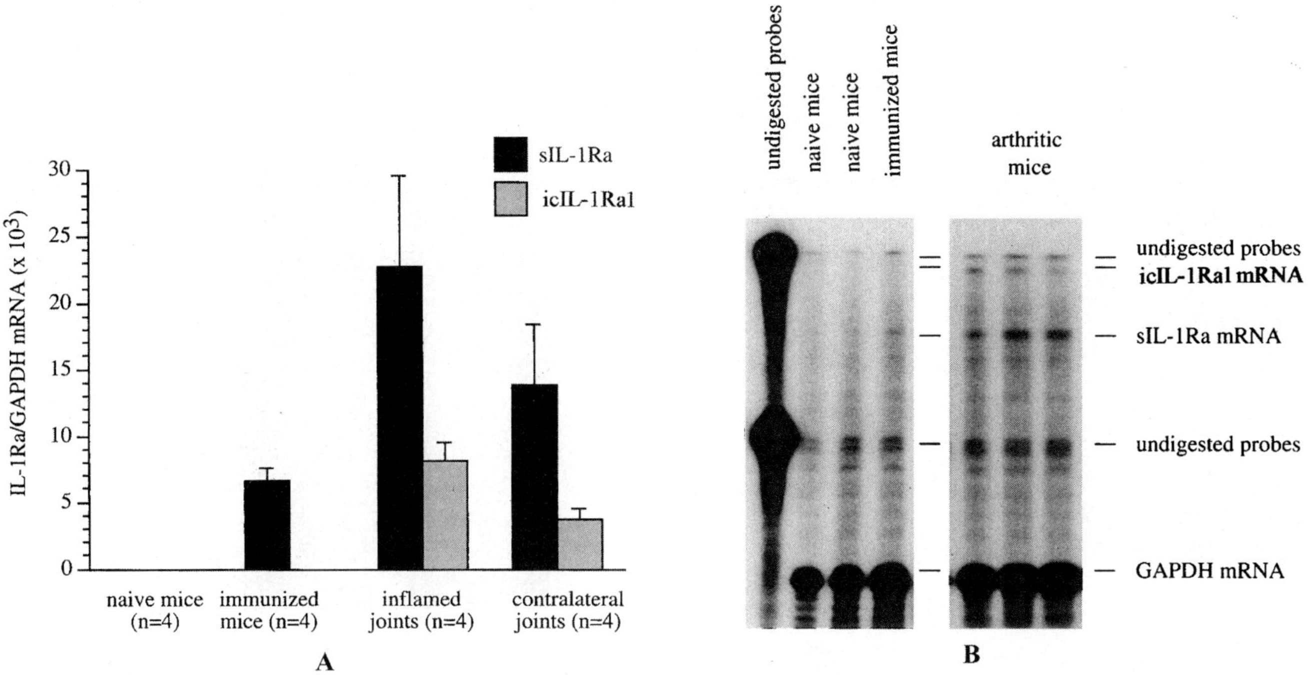

Figure 2. Quantification of IL-1Ra mRNA isoform levels in whole joints and in synovial membranes. Whole joints were dissected from naive DBA/1 mice and from mice immunized with 2 injections (see Materials and Methods), including mice without clinical signs of arthritis and mice with CIA for 1 week (both inflamed and contralateral, clinically uninvolved joints). Total RNA was prepared and levels of IL-1Ra isoform and GAPDH mRNA were examined by RNase protection assay (see Materials and Methods). Quantitative analysis for mRNA extracted from whole joints was performed by PhosphorImager (**A**). Values are the mean and SEM mRNA ratios of sIL-1Ra and icIL-1Ra1 to GAPDH (n = number of mice per group). RNase protection assays were also performed on total RNA from dissected synovium obtained from either naive mice or from mice immunized with a single intradermal injection of collagen (see Materials and Methods). Material from naive mice and immunized mice without arthritis was pooled to obtain 10 μg of total RNA for each assay. The gels were dried and autoradiography was immediately performed (**B**). Results represent pooled material from 4 mice/lane for the naive mice and for the immunized mice before the onset of arthritis and from 1 mouse/lane for the arthritic mice. See Figure 1 for definitions.

synovium was prepared from mice at 4 days after the onset of clinical arthritis. The results of RT-PCR studies showed that, as in whole joints, sIL-1Ra mRNA was present in the synovium of both naive mice and immunized mice before the occurrence of CIA, as well as in mice with clinical arthritis. In contrast, icIL-1Ra1 mRNA was detected only in arthritic mice (Figures 1C and D). Similar results were obtained when synovium from inflamed joints was examined 14 or 20 days after the onset of arthritis (results not shown).

The mRNA levels of the 2 major IL-1Ra isoforms were quantitated by RNase protection assay. Neither IL-1Ra mRNA isoform was detected in the joints of naive mice, and sIL-1Ra mRNA, but not icIL-1Ra1

Table 1. Levels of IL-1β and IL-1Ra isoform mRNA in the joints of immunized DBA/1 mice*

Group	IL-1β: GAPDH ($\times 10^3$)	sIL-1Ra: GAPDH ($\times 10^3$)	icIL-1Ra1: GAPDH ($\times 10^3$)	IL-1β: IL-1Ra (s + ic)
Nonarthritic mice (n = 4)	6.6 ± 1	10.3 ± 4.4	ND	0.63
Inflamed joints (n = 4)	98.8 ± 17.7	22.7 ± 6.9	8.1 ± 1.5	3.25
Contralateral uninflamed joints (n = 4)	4.4 ± 0.9	13.9 ± 4.5	3.7 ± 0.8	0.25

* All tissues were obtained 1 week after the onset of arthritis for the groups of inflamed or contralateral clinically uninflamed joints. The results were obtained by RNase protection assay, with quantification by PhosphorImager. Values are the mean ± SEM. IL-1β = interleukin-1β; IL-1Ra = interleukin-1 receptor antagonist; sIL-1Ra = secreted IL-1Ra; icIL-1Ra1 = intracellular IL-1Ra1; ND = not detected.

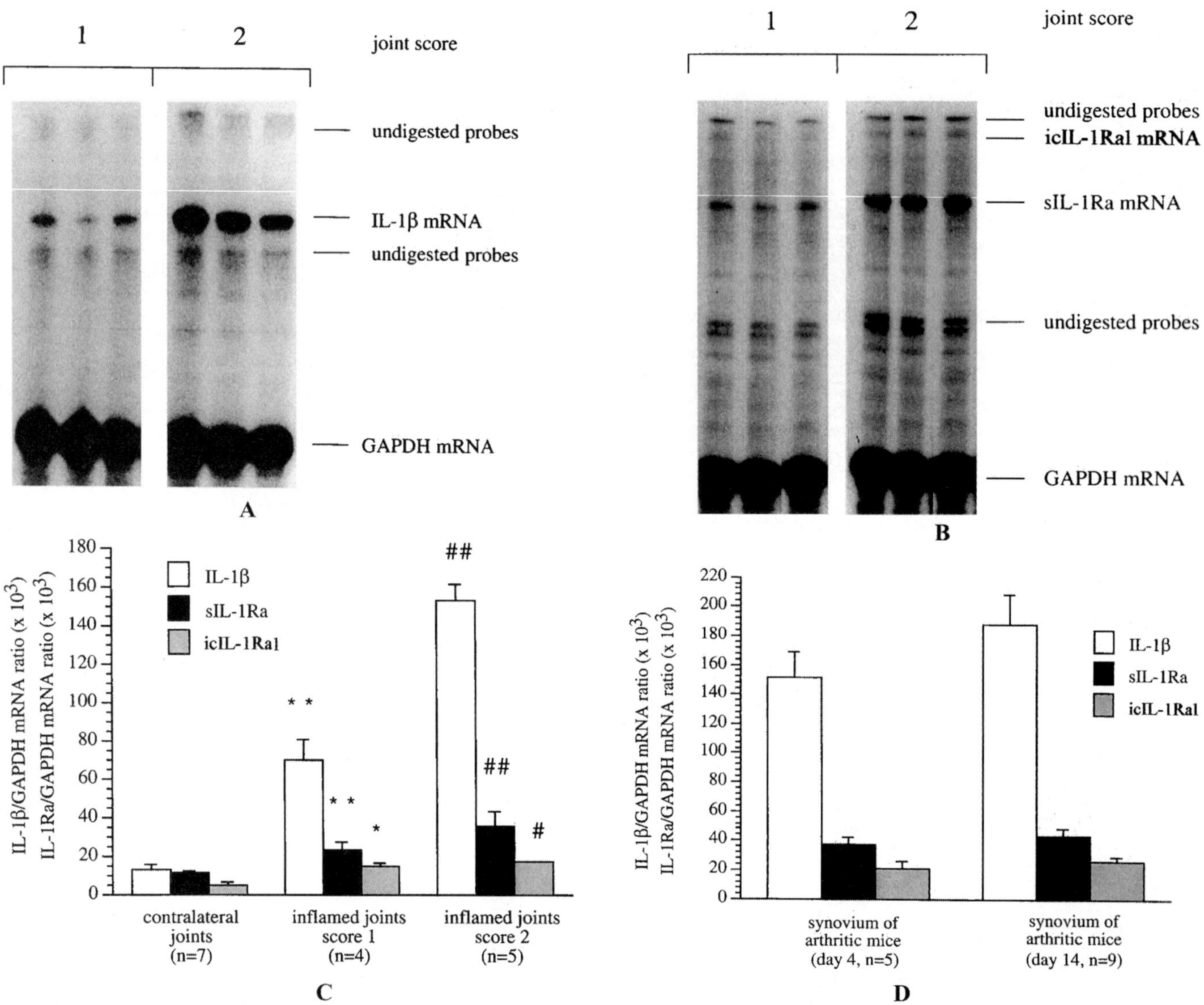

Figure 3. Ratios of IL-1β to IL-1Ra isoform mRNA in the joints of mice with CIA. Total RNA was prepared from inflamed and contralateral, clinically uninvolved joints of mice with CIA for 1 week (immunized with 2 injections of collagen). A clinical arthritis score was determined for the inflamed joints (see Materials and Methods). Levels of IL-1β and of IL-1Ra isoform mRNA were examined by RNase protection assay. **A** and **B,** The mRNA ratios for IL-1β to GAPDH and IL-1Ra isoform to GAPDH in 3 mice with a joint score of 1 or 2, respectively. Quantitative analysis was performed by PhosphorImager. **C,** The mRNA ratios for IL-1β to GAPDH, sIL-1Ra to GAPDH, and icIL-1Ra1 to GAPDH. Values are the mean $\pm$ SEM (n = number of mice per group). $* = P < 0.05$ and $** = P < 0.01$ versus contralateral joints and $\# = P < 0.05$ and $\#\# = P < 0.01$ versus arthritic joints with a clinical score of 1, by Student's *t*-test. **D,** The mRNA ratios of IL-1β to IL-1Ra isoforms were also examined in dissected synovium from mice with CIA for 4 and 14 days. These mice were immunized with a single injection of collagen. Values are the mean and SEM (n = number of mice per group). See Figure 1 for definitions.

mRNA, was detected in the joints of immunized mice before the occurrence of clinical signs of arthritis. In mice with clinical signs of arthritis (1 week after onset), the levels of sIL-1Ra mRNA further increased, whereas the presence of icIL-1Ra1 mRNA was detected at lower levels in arthritic mice in both the inflamed and in the clinically uninvolved contralateral joints (Figure 2A). Similar results were observed when the RNase protection assay was performed on dissected synovium (Figure 2B).

To compare the balance of agonist and antagonist in the joints during CIA, the levels of IL-1β mRNA were also measured by RNase protection assay, and the IL-1β:IL-1Ra isoform mRNA ratio was determined over time. IL-1β mRNA levels were measured because this cytokine has been shown to play a major role in CIA using neutralizing antibodies to IL-1β, IL-1β gene knockout, and IL-1β–converting enzyme knockout mice (for review, see ref. 1).

By RT-PCR, IL-1β mRNA was present both in the joints and in the dissected synovial membranes of naive mice (results not shown). In contrast, by RNase protection assay, IL-1β mRNA was not detected in normal joints, but was present in the joints of immunized mice before the appearance of arthritis, as well as in the clinically uninvolved contralateral joints of arthritic mice (results not shown). In mice with CIA (1 week after onset), the levels of IL-1β mRNA were strongly increased in inflamed joints.

Analysis of the IL-1β:IL-1Ra isoform mRNA ratio showed that the balance was in favor of IL-1β mRNA in inflamed joints, as compared with clinically unaffected contralateral joints as well as with the joints of nonarthritic mice (Table 1). In a subsequent experiment including mice with arthritis of ~1 week's duration, we observed that the IL-1β:IL-1Ra mRNA ratio increased according to the degree of clinical signs of inflammation (Figures 3A–C). The ratio between pro- and antiinflammatory mediators was also examined in the dissected synovial membranes of mice on days 4 and 14 of arthritis. Consistent with the results obtained in whole joints, the IL-1β:IL-1Ra ratio was increased in the synovium of arthritic mice (Figure 3D).

IL-1Ra protein isoforms in normal and inflamed joints. Total proteins were isolated from the dissected synovium, and Western blot analysis was performed using goat polyclonal anti-murine IL-1Ra antibodies that recognize all known IL-1Ra species (15). The different isoforms were identified on the basis of apparent molecular weight. The results showed that icIL-1Ra1 protein was detected only in inflamed joints. Examination of levels of icIL-1Ra1 in synovial membranes collected at different time points revealed that the intensity of the icIL-1Ra1 bands increased during the course of the disease up to 20 days after the onset of CIA, suggesting that this protein accumulated in the inflamed synovium (Figure 4A). Another intracellular isoform (16-kd icIL-1Ra3) was also detected in inflamed synovium. However, the intensities of the bands of icIL-1Ra3 were much lower that those of icIL-1Ra1. The icIL-1Ra1 protein was also present at later time points (days 30 and 60), although in lower amounts than at day 15 (Figure 4B). In contrast, sIL-1Ra protein was not detected in any of the tested samples.

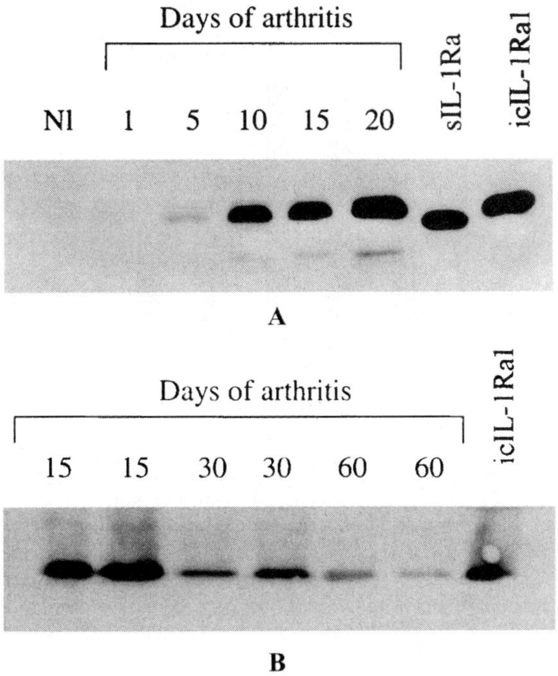

Figure 4. Western blot analysis of IL-1Ra isoforms in the synovium of mice with CIA. Total proteins were extracted from the dissected synovium obtained from the knees of mice with CIA at different time points during the course of the disease (1 mouse per time point; mice immunized with a single injection of collagen) **(A)** and from whole joints on days 15, 30, and 60 of arthritis (2 mice per time point; mice immunized with 2 injections of collagen) **(B)**. Twenty micrograms of protein was heated in reducing buffer and electrophoresed in a 17% polyacrylamide gel, followed by electrophoretic transfer to a polyvinylidene difluoride membrane. Western blot analysis was performed using horseradish peroxidase–conjugated polyclonal goat anti-mouse IL-1Ra. Joint extract from a naive mouse (Nl), as well as recombinant murine icIL-1Ra1 and sIL-1Ra, were included as controls. See Figure 1 for definitions.

Immunolocalization and kinetics of IL-1Ra and IL-1β protein expression during the course of CIA. The kinetics of IL-1Ra and IL-1β immunolocalization in the synovium during the course of arthritis is presented in Figure 5A. IL-1Ra and IL-1β proteins were not detected in joints from naive mice or in clinically uninflamed joints from immunized mice before the onset of arthritis (14–23 days after immunization). In early arthritis (day 1), there was limited expression of IL-1β and IL-1Ra in the synovial tissue; IL-1Ra was usually observed in the same joints in which IL-1β–positive cells were detected (data not shown). On day 5 of arthritis, the numbers of IL-1β–expressing cells and IL-1Ra–expressing cells were

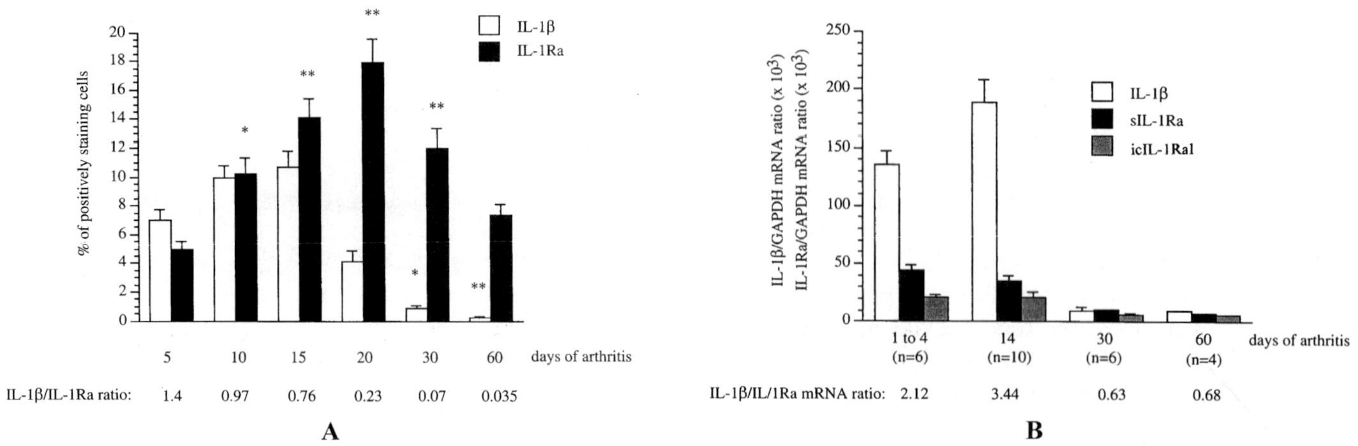

Figure 5. Kinetics of IL-1Ra and IL-1β proteins and mRNA in the joints of mice with CIA. DBA/1 mice were immunized with a single injection of bovine type II collagen emulsified in Freund's complete adjuvant. At different time points during the course of CIA, limbs were removed postmortem and frozen sections were obtained. Immunohistochemistry studies were performed using goat anti-murine IL-1Ra antibodies that recognize all of the IL-1Ra isoforms, as well as a hamster anti-murine IL-1β antibody **(A)**. Values are the mean and SEM of 10 sections. $* = P < 0.05$ and $** = P < 0.001$ versus values on day 5 of arthritis, by Student's *t*-test. Kinetics of IL-1Ra and IL-1β mRNA levels in extracts of whole joints of DBA/1 mice immunized with 2 injections of collagen were determined by RNase protection assay **(B)**. Quantitative analysis was performed by PhosphorImager. Values are the mean and SEM mRNA ratios of IL-1β to GAPDH, sIL-1Ra to GAPDH, and icIL-1Ra1 to GAPDH (n = number of mice per group). See Figure 1 for definitions.

comparable. Peak IL-1β expression occurred on days 10 and 15, while on day 20, a significant reduction in synovial cells staining positively for IL-1β was observed. In contrast, the levels of IL-1Ra expression progressively increased until day 20 of arthritis. On days 30 and 60, synovial cells staining positively for IL-1β were barely detectable. In contrast, at the same late time points, IL-1Ra–positive cells were still readily observed.

Kinetics of IL-1β and IL-1Ra mRNA levels in whole joints were also examined by RNase protection assay. Consistent with the results of immunohistochemistry studies for proteins, there was a disproportionate decrease in IL-1β mRNA levels, with a reversal in the ratio of IL-1β to IL-1Ra mRNA on days 30 and 60 (Figure 5B).

Cells expressing IL-1Ra were localized predominantly to the synovial lining layer and the zone of pannus formation, although scattered cells were also present in the subintima. Positively stained cells had either a macrophage or fibroblast-like morphology (Figure 6), whereas neutrophils, chondrocytes, and endothelial cells remained negative. Although the antibodies used to detect IL-1Ra cannot distinguish between the different IL-1Ra protein isoforms, the presence of a cytoplasmic staining pattern suggested that positive cells were producing icIL-1Ra. A similar pattern was previously observed for IL-1β, a cytokine produced in the cytoplasm, whereas secreted cytokines typically exhibited a perinuclear staining pattern (18). A similar pattern of localization of IL-1Ra–expressing cells and cells positive for F4/80 was observed, but not of cells expressing the CD4 marker, in sequential sections (data not shown). This finding suggested that among infiltrating leukocytes, macrophages rather than T lymphocytes were the main sources of IL-1Ra. IL-1Ra and IL-1β proteins exhibited similar patterns of localization in the inflamed synovium (intima and subintima), although there was a tendency for IL-1β to be expressed by small aggregates of cells in the subintima.

Histopathologic evolution of CIA. The evolution of histologic lesions in the joints of mice with CIA was consistent with the results of previous studies (19,20). Analysis of joints removed on days 14 and 23 after immunization, before any clinical evidence of arthritis, revealed one-third to be normal, with two-thirds exhibiting fibrin deposition and synovial hyperplasia localized in the marginal zone (results not shown). Five days after arthritis onset, the joint pathology was characterized by acute synovitis, with intense infiltration of polymorphonuclear cells. In the advanced stage of arthritis (day 15 or 20 after disease onset), the pathologic process was characterized by chronic synovitis with the predominant infiltrating cells being mononuclear. The cartilage itself showed severe degenerative changes, with fragmentation of the surface and many necrotic chondrocytes. In

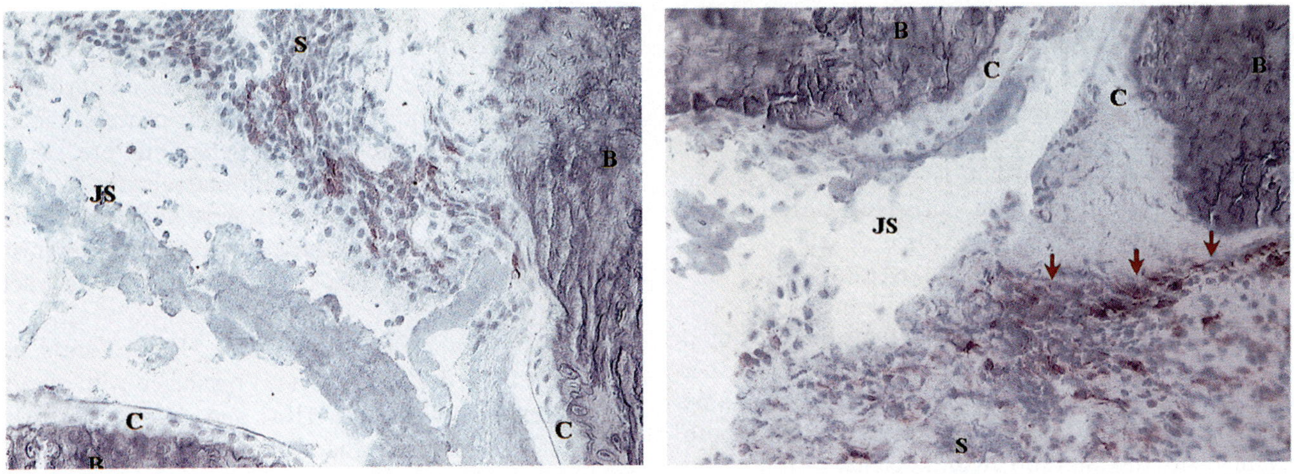

Figure 6. Immunolocalization of IL-1Ra within inflamed joints. DBA/1 mice were immunized with a single injection of bovine type II collagen emulsified in Freund's complete adjuvant. Sagittal sections of undecalcified mouse paws with clinical arthritis for 10 days were used for immunoperoxidase staining of IL-1Ra (reddish-brown cells). IL-1Ra–positive cells were localized in the lining layer **(A),** at the bone–cartilage–pannus junction **(arrows) (B),** and in some scattered cells in the subintima. **S** = synovium; **B** = bone; **JS** = joint space; **C** = cartilage. (Original magnification × 150.) See Figure 1 for definitions.

the late stages of arthritis (30 and 60 days after disease onset), the synovium became fibrotic, with synovial cells oriented in a columnar or palisading manner and infiltrates of mononuclear cell predominating. Destruction of cartilage was evident, together with focal fibrous ankylosis.

Localization of icIL-1Ra1 mRNA in the synovium of mice with CIA. To confirm the presence of icIL-1Ra1 within arthritic joints, in situ hybridization was employed with an antisense riboprobe that specifically recognized icIL-1Ra1 mRNA (16). Sagittal tissue sections of the knee joints of mice with CIA (day 10 of arthritis) and of naive mice were examined. Consistent with our previous results, icIL-1Ra1 mRNA was not detected in normal joints (Figure 7A), but was found in the inflamed synovium (Figures 7B and C). A sense probe showed no positive-staining cells (data not shown). This analysis further established that icIL-1Ra1 mRNA was present within the inflamed synovial membrane.

DISCUSSION

The results of our studies show that 3 different IL-1Ra isoforms were present in the joints of mice with

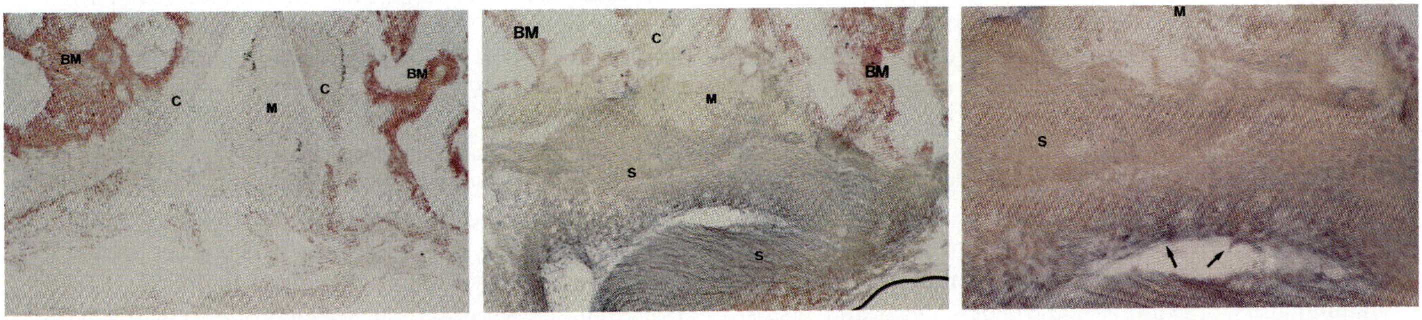

Figure 7. Expression of icIL-1Ra1 mRNA within the inflamed joints of mice with CIA. DBA/1 mice were immunized with 2 injections of collagen. Frozen sections of knee joints from naive mice **(A)** and mice with CIA for 10 days **(B and C)** were used to determine the presence of icIL-1Ra1 mRNA by in situ hybridization. Slides were counterstained with nuclear fast red. The presence of icIL-1Ra1 mRNA is shown by the purple staining **(arrows). BM** = bone marrow; **C** = cartilage; **M** = meniscus; **S** = synovium. (Original magnification × 100 in **A** and **B**; × 400 in **C.**) See Figure 1 for definitions.

CIA: sIL-1Ra, icIL-1Ra1, and icIL-1Ra3; isoform icIL-1Ra2 was not detected. By RT-PCR, we found that sIL-1Ra mRNA was constitutively produced at low levels in normal joints of DBA/1 mice, a strain that is susceptible to CIA. By RNase protection assay, we observed that sIL-1Ra mRNA levels increased during CIA. In contrast to sIL-1Ra, icIL-1Ra1 mRNA and protein were only detected in the joints of arthritic mice. The production of either IL-1Ra isoform in the dissected synovial membranes confirmed the results obtained in whole joints, indicating that the inflamed synovial membrane is a major source of IL-1Ra in CIA. The production of IL-1Ra isoforms followed the same pattern in experiments performed independently at both the University of Colorado Health Sciences Center and the Kennedy Institute of Rheumatology and employing different immunization protocols.

Immunohistochemistry and Western blot studies showed that levels of icIL-1Ra1 increased within the inflamed synovium, particularly at later time points. In addition, macrophages and fibroblasts were the predominant types of cells at later time points, suggesting that these cells may contribute significantly to the production of icIL-1Ra1. Previous studies have shown that stimulated murine macrophages and human synovial fibroblasts produce icIL-1Ra1 mRNA and protein in culture (8,16,21). In addition, we observed that cultured murine synovial fibroblasts also produce icIL-1Ra1 mRNA and protein (Gabay C, Arend WP: unpublished observations).

The levels of IL-1β and IL-1Ra in the joints and synovium varied during the course of CIA. The results of RNase protection assays showed that IL-1β mRNA levels were significantly increased early in the inflamed joints of mice with CIA and that the ratio of IL-1β to IL-1Ra was higher in inflamed than in clinically quiescent joints. In addition, the IL-1β mRNA levels correlated with the severity of arthritis as assessed by the joint score. These findings suggest that early in CIA, an imbalance in the IL-1 system may contribute to the inflammatory process. However, IL-1Ra levels, particularly icIL-1Ra1 protein, increased during the later course of CIA, whereas levels of IL-1β mRNA and protein decreased at later time points (from day 20). These changes in the IL-1β:IL-1Ra balance were associated with a progressive reduction in the level of inflammatory activity, as judged by clinical and histologic criteria.

In addition, circulating levels of the acute-phase protein, serum amyloid A, which were elevated through day 14 of arthritis, decreased at later time points, correlating with the clinical resolution of CIA (Gabay et al: unpublished observations). Histopathologic studies showed a decrease in synovial inflammation beyond day 14 of CIA with the presence of repair processes including fibrous synovitis. These observations are strongly indicative of a protective role for endogenous IL-1Ra in CIA and suggest that icIL-1Ra1, most likely produced by synovial macrophages and fibroblasts, may be important in the process that leads to resolution of the acute synovitis.

Two other intracellular IL-1Ra isoforms have recently been described. One is produced with an additional exon between icIL-1Ra1 and sIL-1Ra first exons (icIL-1Ra2) (13), and the other is derived by alternative translation initiation from the sIL-1Ra mRNA (icIL-1Ra3) (14). The mRNA of icIL-1Ra2 has been described in human cells, such as stimulated neutrophils, monocytes, and fibroblasts, as well as in resting keratinocytes (22). However, we did not detect icIL-1Ra2 mRNA in either normal or inflamed joints, or in isolated murine fibroblasts and macrophages by RT-PCR. In addition, Western blot analysis revealed no protein that migrated at 26 kd, the expected size of icIL-1Ra2 (13). In contrast, icIL-1Ra3 was detected in inflamed joints, although at lower levels than icIL-1Ra1.

A possible discrepancy was noted between levels of icIL-1Ra1 mRNA and protein. Levels of icIL-1Ra1 protein increased significantly in the inflamed synovium after 15 days of arthritis, whereas levels of icIL-1Ra1 mRNA did not vary. Similarly, 18-kd icIL-1Ra1 protein was still present after 60 days of arthritis, although levels of icIL-1Ra1 mRNA were markedly decreased. These findings suggest that icIL-1Ra1 protein accumulates inside cells in the probable presence of low rates of synthesis. This conclusion is supported by the observation that the levels of icIL-1Ra1 mRNA were rather low in normal mouse skin and intestine, whereas high amounts of icIL-1Ra1 protein were readily detected in these organs by Western blot analysis (16).

Low levels of sIL-1Ra mRNA were detected in the joints of naive mice by RT-PCR. In contrast, the presence of sIL-1Ra mRNA was not detected in the joints of naive mice by RNase protection assay. Differences in sensitivity between these two methods are likely to account for this finding. The failure to detect sIL-1Ra protein in the synovial tissue extracts of mice with CIA is in apparent contradiction to elevated levels of sIL-1Ra mRNA. It is possible that sIL-1Ra protein diffuses into adjacent tissues and eventually reaches the circulation. Also, sIL-1Ra protein could have been washed away during preparation of the synovial tissue extracts. However, this possibility is less likely, since mature sIL-1Ra protein was also virtually absent in whole joint extracts. Alternatively, posttranscription mechanisms may have contributed to the apparent discrepancy between detected levels of sIL-1Ra mRNA and protein.

The biologic function of intracellular variants of IL-1Ra remains unclear. The icIL-1Ra1 isoform binds IL-1 receptors with the same affinity as sIL-1Ra and is able to inhibit the biologic effects of IL-1 in vitro (15). However, because of its intracellular localization, icIL-1Ra1 cannot interact with cell surface IL-1 receptors unless secreted by living cells, which has been described to occur (23,24). The icIL-1Ra1 isoform may also be released by dying cells within the synovial membrane, since apoptotic cells have been described in the synovium in both RA and CIA (25,26). Alternatively, icIL-1Ra1 may play a unique role inside cells, without interacting with membrane-bound IL-1 receptors (27).

In conclusion, our results show that different IL-1Ra isoforms are produced in the joints during CIA and that high levels of icIL-1Ra1 are present in the inflamed synovium during the resolution of CIA, strongly suggesting a regulatory role for this isoform. Furthermore, this study is the first to show that the level of disease activity correlates with the ratio of IL-1β to IL-1Ra, strongly suggesting that the balance between agonist and antagonist may play an important role in the degree and severity of inflammation. The CIA model may provide an extremely valuable experimental system in which to better understand the biologic function of IL-1Ra isoforms in vivo.

ACKNOWLEDGMENTS

We would like to thank Dr. W. A. Franklin, Dr. W. Huffer, and K. E. Fox (Department of Pathology, University of Colorado Health Sciences Center, Denver) for assisting with the in situ hybridization studies.

REFERENCES

1. Dinarello CA. Biologic basis for interleukin-1 in disease. Blood 1996;87:2095–147.
2. Arend WP, Dayer J-M. Inhibition of the production and effects of interleukin-1 and tumor necrosis factor α in rheumatoid arthritis. Arthritis Rheum 1995;38:151–60.
3. Arend WP, Malyak M, Guthridge CJ, Gabay C. Interleukin-1 receptor antagonist: role in biology. Annu Rev Immunol 1998;16: 27–55.
4. Bresnihan B, Alvaro-Gracia JM, Cobby M, Doherty M, Domljan Z, Emery P, et al. Treatment of rheumatoid arthritis with recombinant human interleukin-1 receptor antagonist. Arthritis Rheum 1998;41:2196–204.
5. Fukumoto T, Matsukawa A, Ohkawara S, Takagi K, Yoshinaga M. Administration of neutralizing antibody against rabbit IL-1 receptor antagonist exacerbates lipopolysaccharide-induced arthritis in rabbits. Inflamm Res 1996;45:479–85.
6. Ma Y, Thornton S, Boivin GP, Hirsh D, Hirsch R, Hirsch E. Altered susceptibility to collagen-induced arthritis in transgenic mice with aberrant expression of interleukin-1 receptor antagonist. Arthritis Rheum 1998;41:1798–805.
7. Horai R, Saito S, Tanioka H, Nakae S, Sudo K, Okahara A, et al. Development of chronic inflammatory polyarthropathy resembling rheumatoid arthritis in interleukin-1 receptor antagonist–deficient mice. J Exp Med 2000;191:313–20.
8. Firestein GS, Boyle DL, Yu C, Paine MM, Whisenand TD, Zvaifler NJ, et al. Synovial interleukin-1 receptor antagonist and interleukin-1 balance in rheumatoid arthritis. Arthritis Rheum 1994;37:644–52.
9. Deleuran BW, Chu CQ, Field M, Brennan FM, Katsikis P, Feldmann M, et al. Localization of interleukin-1 alpha, type 1 interleukin-1 receptor and interleukin-1 receptor antagonist in the synovial membrane and cartilage/pannus junction in rheumatoid arthritis. Br J Rheumatol 1992;31:801–9.
10. Chikanza IC, Roux-Lombard P, Dayer J-M, Panayi G. Dysregulation of the in vivo production of interleukin-1 receptor antagonist in patients with rheumatoid arthritis. Arthritis Rheum 1995; 38:642–8.
11. Hannum CH, Wilcox CJ, Arend WP, Joslin FG, Dripps DJ, Heimdal PL, et al. Interleukin-1 receptor antagonist activity of a human interleukin-1 inhibitor. Nature 1990;343:336–40.
12. Haskill S, Martin G, van Le L, Morris J, Peace A, Bigler CF, et al. cDNA cloning of an intracellular form of the human interleukin 1 receptor antagonist associated with epithelium. Proc Natl Acad Sci U S A 1991;88:3681–5.
13. Muzio M, Polentarutti N, Sironi M, Poli G, De Gioia L, Introna M, et al. Cloning and characterization of a new isoform of the interleukin 1 receptor antagonist. J Exp Med 1995;182:623–8.
14. Malyak M, Guthridge JM, Hance KR, Dower SK, Freed JH, Arend WP. Characterization of a low molecular weight isoform of IL-1 receptor antagonist. J Immunol 1998;161:1997–2003.
15. Gabay C, Porter B, Fantuzzi G, Arend WP. Mouse IL-1 receptor antagonist isoforms: complementary DNA cloning and protein expression of intracellular isoform and tissue distribution of secreted and intracellular IL-1 receptor antagonist in vivo. J Immunol 1997;159:5905–13.
16. Gabay C, Smith MF Jr, Arend WP. The human intracellular interleukin-1 receptor antagonist promoter regulates gene expression in keratinocytes and gastrointestinal epithelial cells in vivo. Cytokine 1999;11:361–70.
17. Gabay C, Porter B, Guenette D, Bilir B, Arend WP. IL-4 and IL-13 enhance the effect of interleukin-1 on IL-1 receptor antagonist production by human primary hepatocytes and HepG2 cells: differential regulation for C-reactive protein. Blood 1999;93: 1299–1307.
18. Marinova-Mutafchieva L, Williams RO, Mason LJ, Mauri C, Feldmann M, Maini RN. Dynamics of proinflammatory cytokine expression in the joints of mice with collagen-induced arthritis (CIA). Clin Exp Immunol 1997;107:507–12.
19. Stuart JM, Townes AS, Kang AH. Collagen autoimmune arthritis. Annu Rev Immunol 1984;2:199–218.
20. Thornton S, Duwel LE, Boivin GP, Ma Y, Hirsch R. Association of the course of collagen-induced arthritis with distinct patterns of cytokine and chemokine messenger RNA expression. Arthritis Rheum 1999;42:1109–18.
21. Krzesicki RF, Hatfield CA, Bienkowski MJ, McGuire J, Winterrowd GE, Chapman DL, et al. Regulation of expression of IL-1

receptor antagonist protein in human synovial and dermal fibroblasts. J Immunol 1993;150:4008–18.
22. Muzio M, Polentarutti N, Facchetti F, Peri G, Doni A, Sironi M, et al. Characterization of type II intracellular IL-1 receptor antagonist (IL-1ra3): a depot IL-1ra. Eur J Immunol 1999;29:781–8.
23. Levine SJ, Wu T, Shelhamer JH. Extracellular release of the type I intracellular IL-1 receptor antagonist from human airway epithelial cells: differential effects of IL-4, IL-13, IFNγ, and corticosteroids. J Immunol 1997;158:5949–57.
24. Lee RT, Briggs WH, Cheng GC, Rossiter HB, Libby P, Kupper T. Mechanical deformation promotes secretion of IL-1α and IL-1 receptor antagonist. J Immunol 1997;159:5084–8.
25. Firestein GS, Yeo M, Zvaifler NJ. Apoptosis in rheumatoid arthritis synovium. J Clin Invest 1995;96:1631–8.
26. Matsuno T. Time course apoptosis in collagen-induced arthritis. Int J Tissue React 1998;20:37–43.
27. Watson JM, Lofquist AK, Rinehart CA, Olsen JC, Makarov SS, Kaufman DG, et al. The intracellular IL-1 receptor antagonist alters IL-1-inducible gene expression without blocking exogenous signaling by IL-1β. J Immunol 1995;155:4467–75.

ARTHRITIS & RHEUMATISM
Vol. 44, No. 2, February 2001, pp 463–468

Antineutrophil Cytoplasmic Antibodies Reacting With the Pro Form of Proteinase 3 and Disease Activity in Patients With Wegener's Granulomatosis and Microscopic Polyangiitis

Kimberly A. Russell, David N. Fass, and Ulrich Specks

Objective. **Antineutrophil cytoplasmic antibodies (ANCA) directed against proteinase 3 (PR3) are diagnostic markers for the small vessel vasculitides Wegener's granulomatosis (WG) and microscopic polyangiitis (MPA). Correlation of disease activity with PR3 ANCA levels, as determined by standard methods, is not apparent in every patient. PR3 ANCA react with yet to be identified conformational epitopes. We have identified PR3 ANCA subsets that react differentially with mature recombinant PR3 (rPR3; lacking the N-terminal activation dipeptide) and the pro form of this enzyme (pro-rPR3). The present study was performed to determine the association of these PR3 ANCA subsets with disease activity.**

Methods. **Sera from 61 PR3 ANCA–positive patients with WG or MPA were assayed by capture enzyme-linked immunosorbent assay using pro-rPR3 and rPR3 as target antigens, and were correlated with disease activity as determined by the Birmingham Vasculitis Activity Score (BVAS).**

Results. **Median levels of PR3 ANCA reacting with pro-rPR3 were higher during active (n = 32) than during inactive (n = 29) disease ($P = 0.016$). Reactivity with mature rPR3 was not significantly different ($P = 0.71$). Serial followup in individual patients also indicated better correlation of PR3 ANCA reactivity with pro-rPR3 than with mature rPR3.**

Conclusion. **PR3 ANCA subsets reactive with epitopes accessible on pro-PR3 correlate better with disease activity than do subsets reactive with epitopes accessible only on mature PR3. This observation may explain why ANCA levels determined with current standard methods are suboptimal for monitoring disease activity. It raises new questions about the primary target of the PR3 ANCA immune response in patients with small vessel vasculitis.**

Supported in part by the Mayo Foundation. Dr. Russell's work was supported by NIH training grant HL-07897-02-B. Dr. Specks' work was supported by Clinician-Scientist award AHA-94004360 from the American Heart Association and by grant-in-aid AHA-9708006-A from the Minnesota Affiliate of the American Heart Association.

Kimberly A. Russell, MD, David N. Fass, PhD, Ulrich Specks, MD: Mayo Clinic and Foundation, Rochester, Minnesota.

Address correspondence and reprint requests to Ulrich Specks, MD, Thoracic Diseases Research Unit, Guggenheim Building 642 A, Mayo Clinic and Foundation, 200 First Street SW, Rochester, MN 55905.

Submitted for publication August 1, 2000; accepted in revised form September 27, 2000.

Antineutrophil cytoplasmic antibodies (ANCA) generating a characteristic granular cytoplasmic immunofluorescence pattern (cANCA) on ethanol-fixed neutrophil cytospin preparations have emerged as a major diagnostic adjunct in the evaluation of patients with suspected small vessel vasculitis, particularly Wegener's granulomatosis (WG). The neutrophil granule serine protease, proteinase 3 (PR3), has been identified as the primary target antigen for cANCA (for review, see ref. 1).

Clinical observations and extensive in vitro experiments suggest that cANCA may play a significant role in the pathogenesis of the vasculitis of WG (for review, see refs. 1 and 2). When large cohorts of patients are evaluated, the median cANCA levels, as determined by standard indirect immunofluorescence techniques, appear to correlate with categories of disease activity and disease extent (3,4). However, cANCA titers by themselves do not reflect the organ involvement in individual patients, i.e., patients with high titers may have limited disease, whereas patients with low titers may have fulminant generalized disease (4). In the majority of patients, cANCA levels correlate with disease activity, decreasing as the disease improves and increasing as relapses occur (5). The persistence or recurrence of cANCA represents an independent risk factor for clinical relapse (6). However, not all increases in cANCA are inevitably followed by a relapse of disease (7). Consequently, the utility of cANCA determination as a direct marker of disease activity remains controversial, and treatment decisions cannot be made solely on the basis of cANCA titer changes.

Different solid-phase assay systems for PR3 ANCA detection have become available and are used in clinical practice (8,9). The extent to which the PR3 ANCA levels as measured by the various solid-phase assay techniques correlate with disease activity remains unclear. Limited studies examining the relationship between cANCA titers and enzyme-linked immunosorbent assay (ELISA) absorbance values have found a rather poor correlation between the two (8).

Most cANCA recognize conformational epitopes on the PR3 molecule (10). To determine whether the intact conformation of N-terminal–processed mature PR3 is required for recognition by all PR3 ANCA (highest sensitivity), we designed recombinant PR3 (rPR3) variants expressed in 293 cells that have the conformation of N-terminal–unprocessed proenzyme (pro-PR3) and of N-terminal–processed mature PR3 (11). Using these 2 variants as target antigens in the capture ELISA, we discovered that, indeed, only the mature PR3 was recognized by all PR3 ANCA tested (11). Eighty-five percent of PR3 ANCA recognized both pro-PR3 and mature PR3, but 15% of PR3 ANCA exclusively recognized the mature form. This indicates that some patients have PR3 ANCA that recognize epitopes that are accessible only on the mature form of PR3. No serum sample was found to react exclusively with pro-PR3 (11). Some serum samples contained equivalent PR3 ANCA reactivity with mature PR3 and pro-PR3, whereas others had largely divergent reactivity with the 2 substrates. Reactivity with pro-PR3 was generally lower than reactivity with mature PR3 (11).

To better understand the clinical significance of this phenomenon, we undertook the present study, comparing the PR3 ANCA reactivity with mature PR3 and pro-PR3 with the clinical disease activity of the patient at the time of sampling, as well as with cANCA titers as determined by standard immunofluorescence techniques.

Table 1. Characteristics of the patient population*

	Total (n = 61)	Active disease (n = 32)	Inactive disease (n = 29)
No. of males	39	19	20
No. of females	22	13	9
Age, years			
Range	17–87	17–82	22–87
Mean	49	53	49
Diagnosis			
No. with WG	57	30	27
No. with MPA	4	2	2
No. with active organ involvement at time of serum sampling			
Ear, nose, throat		20	
Lung		18	
Kidney		8	
Eye		2	
Joints		1	
Skin		0	
CNS		1	

* WG = Wegener's granulomatosis; MPA = microscopic polyangiitis; CNS = central nervous system.

PATIENTS AND METHODS

Patients. Serum samples from 61 PR3 ANCA–positive patients evaluated at Mayo Clinic Rochester were used in this study. The mean (±SD) age of the patients was 49 ± 16.5 years (range 17–87 years) with a male-to-female ratio of 1.65. Fifty-seven patients had WG and 4 had microscopic polyangiitis (MPA), according to the definitions of the Chapel Hill Consensus Conference (12). All patients fulfilled the American College of Rheumatology 1990 criteria for WG (13). The clinical characteristics of the patients and the presence of active organ involvement at the time of serum sampling are summarized in Table 1.

Patients with active disease were either newly diagnosed or were experiencing a generalized or localized flare. Disease activity at the time of serum sampling was determined according to the Birmingham Vasculitis Activity Score (BVAS) (14).

ANCA detection methods. Titers of cANCA were determined using standard indirect immunofluorescence with ethanol-fixed neutrophil cytospin preparations (15). All patients had been confirmed to have PR3 ANCA by indirect immunofluorescence using HMC-1/PR3 cells and HMC-1/VEC control cells, as well as by capture ELISA with purified neutrophil PR3 (Athens Research, Athens, GA) as target antigen (16,17).

For the determination of PR3 ANCA reactivity with mature and pro-PR3, we used the capture ELISA with the rPR3 variants, rPR3-S176A (pro-rPR3) or Δ-rPR3-S176A (mature rPR3), secreted into the media supernatants of stably transfected 293 cells as target antigens (11). A net absorbance of ≤0.100 is considered positive in this assay (11). All readings fell within the linear range of the assay.

Statistical analysis. The Mann-Whitney U test was used to evaluate the differences in median net absorbance values among groups of patients in the various disease activity categories. For all statistical tests, a P value of less than 0.05 was considered significant.

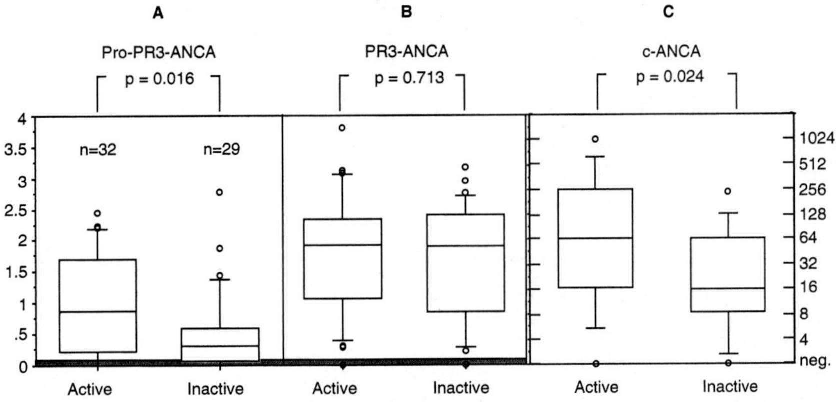

Figure 1. Antineutrophil cytoplasmic antibody (ANCA) reactivity and clinical disease activity. Median optical densities for proteinase 3 (PR3) ANCA binding with both the pro form of recombinant PR3 (pro-rPR3) and the mature form of rPR3 are shown for patients with active clinical disease (n = 32) and for those with complete remission (n = 29). Data are shown as box plots. Horizontal bars represent the median of the data in each category; lower and upper ends of the boxes represent the 25th and 75th percentiles, respectively; lower and upper bars represent the 10th and 90th percentiles, respectively. Outliers are represented by open circles. The shaded area in **A** and **B** represents the normal (negative) optical density range for the capture enzyme-linked immunosorbent assay (<0.100). PR3 ANCA binding to pro-rPR3 was significantly greater in patients with active clinical disease (P = 0.016) **(A)**. PR3 ANCA binding to mature rPR3 was equivalent for both groups (P = 0.71) **(B)**. For comparison, cytoplasmic ANCA (cANCA) titers are also shown **(C)**. The median cANCA titer was significantly higher for patients with active disease than for patients with inactive disease (P = 0.024).

RESULTS

To determine whether PR3 ANCA reactivity with mature rPR3 or with pro-PR3 is related to clinical disease activity, we evaluated serum samples from 61 patients with WG or PR3 ANCA–associated MPA by capture ELISA. The assays were performed in parallel, using either pro-rPR3 or mature rPR3 variants from culture supernatants of stably transfected 293 cells as target antigen (11). Only the first serum sample obtained from each patient was used for this analysis.

Patients were categorized into 2 groups according to disease activity at the time of sampling. Thirty-two patients with various degrees of disease activity were classified as having active disease. Their median BVAS was 8.5 (range 2–27). Twenty-nine patients had no sign of disease activity at the time their serum samples were obtained. Their BVAS was 0.

The median net capture ELISA absorbance of PR3 ANCA reacting with pro-PR3 (Figure 1A) in patients with active disease was significantly higher than that in patients with inactive disease (0.879 versus 0.312; P = 0.016). In contrast, the median net absorbance values of PR3 ANCA reacting with the mature rPR3 variant (Figure 1B) were not different for patients with active disease versus those with inactive disease (1.926 versus 1.912; P = 0.713). As a comparison, the median cANCA titer (Figure 1C) was 1:64 for patients with active disease and 1:16 for patients without active disease (P = 0.024).

No significant relationship between specific organ involvement or extent of disease and any of the PR3 ANCA reactivities was detected, largely because of the small numbers of patients in each group. However, for patients with active lung involvement, PR3 ANCA reactivity with pro-PR3 was lower in those with active necrotizing granulomatous lesions (median 0.34, n = 9) compared with those with active capillaritis and alveolar hemorrhage (median 1.79, n = 5). The median BVAS was 7 for patients with necrotizing granulomatous lung lesions compared with 10 for the patients with active capillaritis. PR3 ANCA reactivity with mature PR3 (2.01 versus 1.96) or cANCA titers (1:64 versus 1:32) did not appear to discriminate between these two groups.

In patients from whom serial serum samples were available, the disease activity appeared to correlate better with PR3 ANCA reactivity with pro-PR3 than

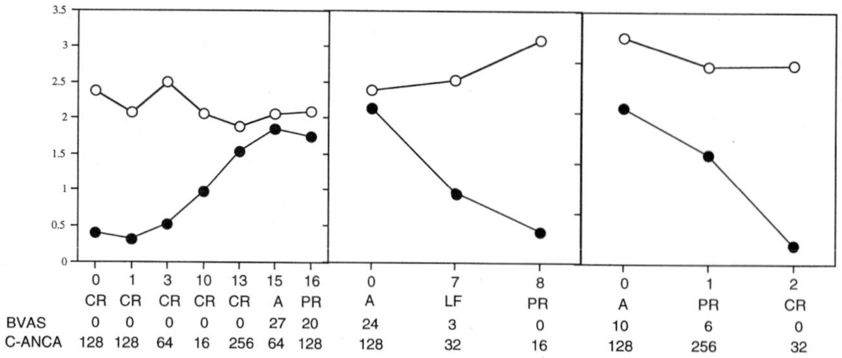

Figure 2. Proteinase 3 (PR3) antineutrophil cytoplasmic antibody (ANCA) binding to the pro form of recombinant PR3 (pro-rPR3) (●), but not to the mature form of rPR3 (○), appears to correlate with disease activity in individual patients. Shown are sequential data for 3 patients. The time of serum sampling (months) is shown at the bottom. Disease activity status is indicated as follows: CR = complete remission; A = active disease; PR = partial remission; LF = localized flare. Disease activity status according to the Birmingham Vasculitis Activity Score (BVAS) is also shown.

with mature PR3 or with the cANCA titers. Figure 2 shows examples of findings in patients who experienced changes in their disease activity during the followup period.

To determine whether PR3 ANCA reactivity with mature PR3 or pro-PR3 was related to the overall duration of disease, we compared the serum samples from patients with disease of <1 year's duration with those with >1 year's duration. We also compared sera from patients in whom the active disease episode was the first disease manifestation with sera from those in whom the active disease episode represented a relapse. No significant differences were detected for any of the comparisons.

DISCUSSION

Our findings indicate that PR3 ANCA reactivity with pro-PR3 is more closely related to clinical disease activity in patients with PR3 ANCA-associated small vessel vasculitis than is the reactivity with mature PR3. This unexpected observation raises compelling questions about what is measured in cANCA determinations. Furthermore, it needs to be reconciled with current hypotheses of the potential pathogenic role of the PR3 ANCA autoimmune response.

It has been suggested that cANCA titers correlate reasonably well with clinical disease activity. Yet, there are sufficient exceptions to warrant caution against relying on cANCA titers as the sole surrogate marker of activity (5). The cANCA data obtained from the present series are consistent with those of previous reports. The correlation of cANCA titers with PR3 ANCA levels determined by direct ELISA techniques using purified mature PR3 as target antigen is weak (8), and information about the correlation of PR3 ANCA ELISA readings with clinical disease activity is scarce.

PR3 ANCA recognize conformational epitopes that are yet to be identified (10). Like neutrophil elastase, cathepsin G, or lymphocyte granzymes, PR3 undergoes several posttranslational intracellular processing steps (for review, see refs. 18 and 19). In granules, it is stored, presumably, in its fully enzymatically active form. The activation of granule serine proteases of hematopoietic cells depends on the removal of an N-terminal activation dipeptide. This prompts a conformational change that renders the active site pocket of the enzyme accessible for substrates.

The primary purpose of compartmentalization of enzymes such as PR3 within the cell is to protect the cell from autodigestion and to allow the release of the enzymes on demand. Within the granules, these enzymes are stored in a manner that keeps the active site pocket inaccessible to potential substrates. For related enzymes, such as murine mast cell proteases, this is achieved by binding of the protease to granule matrix proteoglycans, from which these proteases dissociate in response to the pH change associated with degranulation (20). This implies that these proteases are maintained in their inactive conformation within the granules even after their N-terminal propeptide has been removed.

This concept is supported by the following observation: histochemistry staining with the substrate naphthol AS-D chloroacetate indicates that a portion of the PR3 stored in granules has enzymatic activity (21). However, this activity can be removed by washing the cells in aqueous solutions prior to fixation. If immunofluorescence using anti-PR3 antibodies is performed before and after washing cells in aqueous solution, the immunologically detectable signal of PR3 remains essentially unchanged (Russell et al: unpublished data). It is therefore likely that most of the PR3 stored in granules is maintained in its inactive conformation. Consequently, cANCA determination by immunofluorescence largely measures the binding of ANCA to PR3 in azurophil granules that may mimic its pro form conformation. This could explain the poor correlation between cANCA titers and ELISA readings (8).

PR3 ANCA are thought to be pathogenic for small vessel vasculitis (1). However, this role remains a subject of controversy. It is not obvious when, where, or under which conditions PR3 ANCA can interact with PR3 in vivo, since the enzyme is mostly compartmentalized intracellularly. Several possible mechanisms have been proposed. The most widely accepted hypothesis is based on the interaction of PR3 ANCA with PR3 expressed on the surface of activated neutrophils (1). Variable amounts of PR3 are expressed on the surface of resting neutrophils, and PR3 surface expression is increased after cytokine stimulation of neutrophils, a situation that occurs in vivo at times of infection or tissue repair (22,23). In analogy to neutrophil elastase and cathepsin G (24), surface-expressed PR3 can be expected to be enzymatically active and, consequently, in its mature enzyme conformation. Our data suggest that PR3 ANCA reacting with pro-PR3 are more closely related to disease activity than are those reacting with mature PR3. Consequently, the question needs to be extended to include how PR3 ANCA can have access to pro-PR3 in vivo.

Apoptosis of unprimed neutrophils is associated with translocation of azurophil granules to the cell surface (25). Furthermore, once translocation of granules occurs, ANCA can bind to apoptotic unprimed neutrophils (25). Consequently, it is possible that PR3 ANCA gain access to PR3 packaged in azurophil granules in the pro form conformation during apoptosis of neutrophils. Furthermore, release of pro-PR3 from hematopoietic cell lines in culture as well as from bone marrow cells has been reported (26,27). The secreted pro-PR3 was found to have an inhibitory effect on the proliferation of granulopoietic progenitor cells, and therefore, the release of pro-PR3 has been proposed as a biologically relevant feedback mechanism involved in the suppression of granulopoiesis (27). Hence, it is possible that PR3 ANCA bind to conformational epitopes expressed on pro-PR3 in vivo, both at times of accelerated neutrophil production and at times of neutrophil apoptosis, i.e., during active inflammation.

The autoimmune response leading to the primary formation and persistent production of PR3 ANCA remains poorly understood. It is possible that exposure to foreign antigens, such as microbial antigens, that display conformational epitopes similar to those of pro-PR3 may elicit an antibody response that cross-reacts with epitopes of pro-PR3. The observed PR3 ANCA reactivity with mature PR3 may be a result of subsequent epitope spreading (28). Our initial analysis of PR3 ANCA reactivity with pro-PR3 and mature PR3 and disease duration did not uncover statistically significant relationships. This may be explained by the fact that PR3 ANCA levels from one patient cannot be compared with those from other patients (4). Long-term followup of individual patients may be required to uncover such relationships.

A prospective study that monitors a large cohort of patients from initial diagnosis through various remissions and flares is currently under way. More detailed in vitro studies to corroborate the speculative possible explanations of our intriguing observation are also in progress in our laboratory.

ACKNOWLEDGMENTS

We thank Ms Amber M. Hummel for maintaining the rPR3-expressing cell lines and Ms Margaret A. Viss for preparing the cDNA constructs.

REFERENCES

1. Hewins P, Cohen Tervaert JW, Savage CO, Kallenberg CG. Is Wegener's granulomatosis an autoimmune disease? Curr Opin Rheumatol 2000;12:3–10.
2. Nowack R, Flores-Suarez LF, van der Woude FJ. New developments in pathogenesis of systemic vasculitis. Curr Opin Rheumatol 1998;10:3–11.
3. Cohen Tervaert JW, van der Woude FJ, Fauci AS, Ambrus JL, Velosa J, Keane WF, et al. Association between active Wegener's granulomatosis and anticytoplasmic antibodies. Arch Intern Med 1989;149:2461–5.
4. Nölle B, Specks U, Lüdemann J, Rohrbach MS, DeRemee RA, Gross WL. Anticytoplasmic autoantibodies: their immunodiagnostic value. Ann Intern Med 1989;111:28–40.
5. Cohen Tervaert JW, Stegeman CA, Kallenberg CGM. Serial

ANCA testing is useful in monitoring disease activity of patients with ANCA-associated vasculitides. Sarcoidosis Vasc Diffuse Lung Dis 1996;13:241–5.
6. Stegeman CA, Cohen Tervaert JW, de Jong PE, Kallenberg CG, the Dutch Co-Trimoxazole Wegener Study Group. Trimethoprim-sulfamethoxazole (co-trimoxazole) for the prevention of relapses of Wegener's granulomatosis. N Engl J Med 1996;335:16–20.
7. Kerr GS, Fleisher TA, Hallahan CW, Leavitt RY, Fauci AS, Hoffman GS. Limited prognostic value of changes in antineutrophil cytoplasmic antibody titer in patients with Wegener's granulomatosis. Arthritis Rheum 1993;36:365–71.
8. Wang G, Csernok E, de Groot K, Gross WL. Comparison of eight commercial kits for quantitation of antineutrophil cytoplasmic antibodies (ANCA). J Immunol Meth 1997;208:203–11.
9. Lim LC, Taylor JG 3rd, Schmitz JL, Folds JD, Wilkman AS, Falk RJ, et al. Diagnostic usefulness of antineutrophil cytoplasmic autoantibody serology: comparative evaluation of commercial indirect fluorescent antibody kits and enzyme immunoassay kits. Am J Clin Pathol 1999;111:363–9.
10. Bini P, Gabay JE, Teitel A, Melchior M, Zhou J-L, Elkon KB. Antineutrophil cytoplasmic autoantibodies in Wegener's granulomatosis recognize conformational epitopes on proteinase 3. J Immunol 1992;149:1409–15.
11. Sun J, Fass DN, Viss MA, Hummel AM, Tang H, Homburger HA, et al. A proportion of proteinase 3-specific anti-neutrophil cytoplasmic antibodies only react with proteinase 3 after cleavage of its N-terminal activation dipeptide. Clin Exp Immunol 1998;114: 320–6.
12. Jennette JC, Falk RJ, Andrassy K, Bacon PA, Churg J, Gross WL, et al. Nomenclature of systemic vasculitides: proposal of an international consensus conference. Arthritis Rheum 1994;37: 187–92.
13. Leavitt RY, Fauci AS, Bloch DA, Michel BA, Hunder GG, Arend WP, et al. The American College of Rheumatology 1990 criteria for the classification of Wegener's granulomatosis. Arthritis Rheum 1990;33:1101–7.
14. Luqmani RA, Bacon PA, Moots RJ, Janssen BA, Pall A, Emery P, et al. Birmingham Vasculitis Activity Score (BVAS) in systemic necrotizing vasculitis. QJM 1994;87:671–8.
15. Specks U, Wheatley CL, McDonald TJ, Rohrbach MS, DeRemee RA. Anticytoplasmic autoantibodies in the diagnosis and follow-up of Wegener's granulomatosis. Mayo Clin Proc 1989;64: 28–36.
16. Specks U, Wiegert EM, Homburger HA. Human mast cells expressing recombinant proteinase 3 (PR3) as substrate for clinical testing for anti-neutrophil cytoplasmic antibodies (ANCA). Clin Exp Immunol 1997;109:286–95.
17. Sun J, Fass DN, Hudson JA, Viss MA, Homburger HA, Specks U. Capture-ELISA based on recombinant proteinase 3 (PR3) is sensitive for PR3-ANCA testing and allows detection of PR3 and PR3-ANCA/PR3 immune complexes. J Immunol Methods 1998; 211:111–23.
18. Jenne DE. Structure of the azurocidin, proteinase 3, and neutrophil elastase genes: implications for inflammation and vasculitis. Am J Respir Crit Care Med 1994;150:S147–54.
19. Gullberg U, Andersson E, Garwicz D, Lindmark A, Olsson I. Biosynthesis, processing and sorting of neutrophil proteins: insight into neutrophil granule development. Eur J Haematol 1997;58: 137–53.
20. Matsumoto R, Sali A, Guildyal N, Karplus M, Stevens RL. Packaging of proteases and proteoglycans in the granules of mast cells and other hematopoietic cells. J Biol Chem 1995;270: 19524–31.
21. Braun MG, Csernok E, Rögener-Schwarz W, Ludwig WD, Müller-Hermelink HK, Gross WL, et al. Monoclonal antibody WGM1 directed against proteinase 3: an immunohistochemical marker for naphthol ASD chloroacetate. Hematol Oncol 1996;14:83–90.
22. Csernok E, Ernst M, Schmitt W, Bainton DF, Gross WL. Activated neutrophils express proteinase 3 on their plasma membrane in vitro and in vivo. Clin Exp Immunol 1994;95:244–50.
23. Halbwachs-Mecarelli L, Bessou G, Lesavre P, Lopez S, Witko-Sarsat V. Bimodal distribution of proteinase 3 (PR3) surface expression reflects a constitutive heterogeneity in the polymorphonuclear neutrophil pool. FEBS Lett 1995;374:29–33.
24. Owen CA, Campbell MA, Sannes PL, Boukedes SS, Campbell EJ. Cell surface-bound elastase and cathepsin G on human neutrophils: a novel, non-oxidative mechanism by which neutrophils focus and preserve catalytic activity of serine proteinases. J Cell Biol 1995;131:775–89.
25. Gilligan HM, Bredy B, Brady HR, Hebert MJ, Slayter HS, Xu Y, et al. Antineutrophil cytoplasmic autoantibodies interact with primary granule constituents on the surface of apoptotic neutrophils in the absence of neutrophil priming. J Exp Med 1996;184: 2231–41.
26. Rao NV, Rao GV, Marshall BC, Hoidal JR. Biosynthesis and processing of proteinase 3 in U937 cells. J Biol Chem 1996;271: 2972–8.
27. Sköld S, Rosberg B, Gullberg U, Olofsson T. A secreted proform of neutrophil proteinase 3 regulates the proliferation of granulopoietic progenitor cells. Blood 1999;93:849–56.
28. Vanderlugt CJ, Miller SD. Epitope spreading. Curr Opin Immunol 1996;8:831–6.

ARTHRITIS & RHEUMATISM
Vol. 44, No. 2, February 2001, pp 469–473

Elevated Interleukin-4 and Interleukin-13 Production by T Cell Lines From Patients With Churg-Strauss Syndrome

M. Kiene, E. Csernok, A. Müller, C. Metzler, A. Trabandt, and W. L. Gross

Objective. **To investigate cytokine production patterns of T cell lines (TCL) from patients with Churg-Strauss syndrome (CSS).**

Methods. **Short-term polyclonal TCL were generated from peripheral blood of patients with CSS or Wegener's granulomatosis (WG) and healthy controls (HC). TCL were established in the presence of interleukin-2 (IL-2) and phytohemagglutinin and were phenotypically characterized by flow cytometry. Th1/Th2 cytokine production by stimulated TCL (72 hours) was analyzed by enzyme-linked immunosorbent assay.**

Results. **TCL that represented the progeny of in vivo–activated T cells from CSS patients displayed a heterogeneous immunophenotype, with a predominance of CD4+ T cells when compared with WG TCL, which were predominantly CD8+. All CSS TCL shared the ability to produce large amounts of interferon-γ (IFNγ), IL-4, and IL-13 compared with HC ($P = 0.014$ for all 3). Production of IL-4 and IL-13 was higher in CSS TCL than in WG TCL ($P = 0.014$ for both). IL-5 production was up-regulated in WG TCL compared with CSS TCL ($P = 0.014$). Compared with HC, WG TCL showed increased production of IFNγ ($P = 0.021$), IL-5 ($P = 0.043$), and IL-13 ($P = 0.021$).**

Conclusion. **Our results indicate that, while there is evidence for both a type 1 and a type 2 response in CSS, type 2 cytokine production pattern appears to predominate in this disease when compared with WG and HC.**

Supported by a grant from Sonderforschungsbereich 367 (Project A8) and by grant FKZ-01-VM-9306 from the Bundesministerium für Forschung und Technologie.

M. Kiene, MD, E. Csernok, PhD, A. Müller, PhD, C. Metzler, MD, A. Trabandt, MD, W. L. Gross, MD, PhD: University of Lübeck, Lübeck, Germany, and Rheumaklinik Bad Bramstedt, Bad Bramstedt, Germany.

Address correspondence and reprint requests to A. Müller, PhD, Department of Rheumatology, University of Lübeck, Ratzeburger Allee 160, D-23538 Lübeck, Germany.

Submitted for publication February 25, 2000; accepted in revised form September 18, 2000.

Churg-Strauss syndrome (CSS), also known as allergic granulomatosis and angiitis, is characterized by eosinophilia and extravascular granulomas, as well as pulmonary and systemic small vessel vasculitis (1). Mainly because of the significant atopic component (2), CSS can be clearly distinguished from Wegener's granulomatosis (WG). However, there is very little available information regarding the immunopathogenesis of CSS. We have demonstrated that, similar to findings in WG (3), soluble interleukin-2 receptor (sIL-2R) is a serum marker for CSS, and eosinophilic cationic protein levels have been found to be up-regulated and correlated with the eosinophil blood count in this disease (4). Furthermore, an elevated level of IL-5 in serum and bronchoalveolar fluid of CSS patients has been reported (5). Impaired eosinophilic apoptosis has been suggested as a possible disease mechanism in CSS (6). Interferon-α (IFNα) may be an effective treatment in CSS (7), potentially acting by decreasing the number of blood eosinophils and lymphocytes. In patients with idiopathic hypereosinophilic syndrome, which is clinically related to CSS, elevated sIL-2R levels have been observed as well (8).

Based on these findings and the clinical characteristics, we thus hypothesized that not only might activated T cells play a pivotal role in the pathogenesis of CSS, but the T cell cytokine pattern might also be skewed toward a disease-potentiating Th2 immune response. Our data from the present study indicate that peripheral blood–derived, short-term polyclonal T cell lines (TCL) from CSS patients differ substantially from WG TCL and healthy control (HC) TCL in their phenotype and, more importantly, their cytokine profile. Moreover, our results show that, while there is evidence for both a type 1 (characterized by IFNγ) and a type 2 response in CSS, in quantitative terms a type 2 cytokine pattern (characterized by IL-4, IL-5, and IL-13) appears to predominate.

Table 1. Clinical features of the 5 Churg-Strauss syndrome patients from whom T cell lines were derived*

Patient/ age/ sex†	Active disease manifestation‡	DEI	Disease duration, months	ANCA titer	Positive histologic findings	ESR, mm/hour	CRP, mg/dl	Eosinophil count, /μl§	IgE, IU/ml¶	Therapy
1/28/F	G, L	4	36	1:512	Yes	52	5.8	1400	206	CS
2/68/M	H, P	4	40	1:256	No	12	0.5	350	11	CS
3/59/M	E, L, A, P, G, B	11	4	1:256	No	22	1.3	230	151	MTX + CS
4/40/M	L, C	4	14	1:64	No	16	2.5	100	<10	CYC + CS
5/55/F	P, B, L	5	4	1:64	Yes	19	0.9	1200	58	CYC + CS

* DEI = Disease Extent Index (20); ANCA = antineutrophil cytoplasmic antibodies (classic or perinuclear); ESR = erythrocyte sedimentation rate; CRP = C-reactive protein; CS = corticosteroids; MTX = methotrexate; CYC = cyclophosphamide.
† Patient 1 had a relapse, patient 2 was in stable remission, and patients 3, 4, and 5 were in partial remission.
‡ Based on the extended ELK classification: G = gut; L = lungs; H = heart; P = polyneuropathy; E = ear, nose, throat; A = arthritis/arthralgia; B = constitutional symptoms; C = central nervous system. Manifestations are those that were present at the time of blood sampling, despite therapy.
§ Normal 5–360.
¶ Normal <100.

PATIENTS AND METHODS

Patients. The study subjects were 5 patients with CSS, 4 patients with WG (disease controls), and 4 healthy subjects. The clinical characteristics of the patients are shown in Tables 1 and 2. All CSS and WG patients had disease that was consistent with the definitions proposed by the Chapel Hill Consensus Conference (9) and that fulfilled the criteria of the American College of Rheumatology (10,11). With the exception of 1 patient with WG, all patients were receiving steroid treatment, which might have biased cytokine production in a systematic manner.

Cell preparation and generation of TCL. Peripheral blood mononuclear cells (PBMC) were obtained from EDTA-anticoagulated blood by Ficoll-Paque (Pharmacia, Freiburg, Germany) density-gradient centrifugation (400*g* for 35 minutes at room temperature) and extensive washing. Purified PBMC (1×10^6/ml) were then cultured with 20 units/ml of recombinant human IL-2 (rHuIL-2; Genzyme, Cambridge, MA) in complete medium (RPMI 1640 supplemented with 5% fetal calf serum, 5% human serum, 1% L-glutamate, and 1% penicillin/streptomycin; Gibco, Karlsruhe, Germany and Sigma, Deisenhofen, Germany) for 5 days, in order to select for activated T cells. The blast cells were isolated by centrifugation on discontinuous Percoll gradients and cultured at a concentration of 10^5 cells/ml in RPMI 1640 supplemented with phytohemagglutinin (2 μg/ml; Sigma) for 15–20 days. Afterwards, TCL were phenotyped using a standard flow cytometry technique.

Flow cytometry. Fluorescein isothiocyanate (FITC)–conjugated anti-CD3, phycoerythrin (PE)–conjugated anti-CD4, and peridin chlorophyll protein–conjugated anti-CD8 were obtained from Becton Dickinson (Heidelberg, Germany). FITC-conjugated IgG1 and PE-conjugated IgG2a were used as irregular isotype controls. Each TCL was incubated with 10 μl of the appropriate monoclonal antibody for 30 minutes at room temperature, after which phosphate buffered saline (PBS; Gibco) with 0.5% bovine serum albumin (Sigma) and 0.5% NaN_3 (Merck, Darmstadt, Germany) was added. The cells were centrifuged (1,000 revolutions per minute, 10 minutes at 4°C) and resuspended in PBS containing 1% paraformaldehyde (Sigma). Analyses were performed within 24 hours, with an EPICS Profile II flow cytometer (Coulter, Krefeld, Germany).

Stimulation of TCL. After 3 washes, the cells were resuspended in RPMI 1640 at a final concentration of 1×10^6/ml. TCL from each patient and HC were stimulated with phorbol myristate acetate (PMA, 10 ng/ml; Sigma) and anti-CD3 antibody (100 ng/ml; Ortho Diagnostics, Raritan, NJ). The supernatants were harvested 72 hours later and stored at −70°C.

Enzyme-linked immunosorbent assay (ELISA) for IFNγ, IL-4, IL-5, IL-10, and IL-13. Culture supernatants of the TCL of each patient or HC were assayed for IFNγ, IL-4, IL-5, IL-10, and IL-13 content with commercial ELISAs obtained from the following sources: Genzyme (IFNγ), R&D Systems, Wiesbaden, Germany (IL-4), Becton Dickinson (IL-5 and

Table 2. Clinical features of the 4 Wegener's granulomatosis patients from whom T cell lines were derived*

Patient/ age/sex†	Active disease manifestation	DEI	Disease duration, months	ANCA titer	Positive histologic findings	ESR, mm/hour	CRP, mg/dl	Therapy
1/71/M	E, K, H, P, C, B	11	1	1:2,048	Yes	118	1.2	CYC + CS
2/57/F	E, L, K, A, P, B	11	1	1:512	Yes	105	1	None
3/43/M	E, Ey, K, A, B	9	71	1:64	Yes	22	0.6	CYC + CS
4/33/M	K, A, L	6	32	1:8	Yes	39	0.8	CYC + CS

* K = kidney; Ey = eye (see Table 1 for explanations and other definitions).
† Patients 1 and 2 had progressive active disease; patients 3 and 4 had a relapse.

Table 3. Predominant Th phenotype and Th1 (IFNγ) and Th2 (IL-4) cytokine production patterns of polyclonal TCL following stimulation with PMA and anti-CD3 for 72 hours*

TCL source	Predominant Th phenotype (CD4:CD8 ratio)†	IFNγ, pg/ml	IL-4, pg/ml	IFNγ:IL-4
CSS	CD4 (1.7)	275 ± 59	38 ± 17	7.2 (Th0-like)
WG	CD8 (0.3)	256 ± 32	1.0 ± 0.5	256 (Th1-like)
HC	CD4 (1.1)	26 ± 18	0.5 ± 0.3	52 (Th1-like)

* Values are the mean of the means (±SEM) of 5 T cell lines (TCL) from each subject. The interferon-γ:interleukin-4 (IFNγ:IL-4) ratio was calculated and then, using a previously reported scheme (13), the cytokine pattern was classified (i.e., IFNγ:IL-4 >10 = Th1-like, IFNγ:IL-4 1–10 = Th0-like, and IFNγ:IL-4 <1 = Th2-like). PMA = phorbol myristate acetate; CSS = Churg-Strauss syndrome; WG = Wegener's granulomatosis; HC = healthy controls.

† The expression of T cell receptor α/β (TCRα/β) and TCR γ/δ was also determined, by flow cytometry. All TCL, from both patient groups as well as from controls, showed an average of ≥93% TCRα/β expression. Contamination with monocytes (CD14) was always <1%. There were no statistically significant differences between groups.

IL-13), and Diaclone Research, Besançon, France (IL-10). According to the manufacturers, the assays used do not exhibit cross-reactivity with any of the other cytokines investigated. The minimum detectable amounts (pg/ml) were as follows: IFNγ 15.6, IL-4 0.09, IL-5 15.6, IL-10 12.5, IL-13 7.8.

Statistical analysis. Unless otherwise noted, all data are expressed as the mean ± SEM. Population means were compared using the Mann-Whitney U test. *P* values less than 0.05 were considered significant. Relationships between phenotype, cytokine levels, and clinical variables were examined by determining the Spearman rank order correlation coefficient.

RESULTS

Establishment and characterization of TCL from IL-2–expanded PBMC. All TCL were of the CD3 phenotype and consisted of different proportions of CD4+ and CD8+ T cell subpopulations. Among CSS TCL, an average of 63% of the T cells exhibited CD4 surface molecules, whereas the remaining population of T cells (37%) was CD8+. CSS TCL displayed a nonsignificant trend toward a higher number of CD4+ T cells and a lower number of CD8+ T cells when compared with HC (53% CD4+ cells and 47% CD8+ cells in HC; $P > 0.05$ versus patients with CSS). The phenotype of WG TCL was characterized by a predominance of CD8+ T cells (75%) and a lower number of CD4+ T cells (25%). The differences in the proportions of CD4+ and CD8+ T cells in CSS versus WG TCL were statistically significant ($P = 0.028$ for CD4+ cells, $P = 0.021$ for CD8+ cells). In addition, WG TCL displayed an increased percentage of CD8+ T cells when compared with HC ($P = 0.043$ for both).

Cytokine production by TCL from PB. We assessed the ability of short-term polyclonal TCL obtained from PB of CSS patients, WG patients, and HC to produce IFNγ, IL-4, IL-5, IL-10, and IL-13 in response to stimulation with PMA and anti-CD3 antibody. For comparison between TCL from CSS patients and TCL from WG patients, we first determined the mean cytokine production values in at least 5 TCL from each subject. Statistical differences were then calculated based upon the mean of the mean values in each of the 5 CSS patients, 4 WG patients, and 4 HC.

IFNγ production. TCL from CSS patients produced more IFNγ than did those from HC (mean ± SEM 274.8 ± 59.0 pg/ml versus 26.4 ± 18.1 pg/ml; $P = 0.014$) (Table 3). Similarly, TCL from WG patients showed increased IFNγ production (256.5 ± 31.9 pg/ml) when compared with those from HC ($P = 0.021$) (Table 3).

IL-4 production. TCL from patients with CSS showed elevated IL-4 production (37.5 ± 16.7 pg/ml) when compared with production of IL-4 in TCL from HC (0.54 ± 0.28 pg/ml) and from patients with WG (1.02 ± 0.48 pg/ml) (Table 3 and Figure 1). Both of these differences were statistically significant ($P = 0.014$).

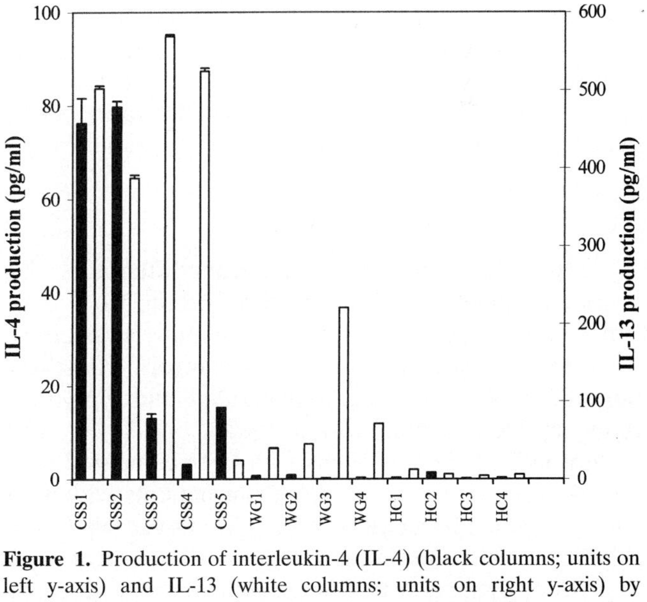

Figure 1. Production of interleukin-4 (IL-4) (black columns; units on left y-axis) and IL-13 (white columns; units on right y-axis) by peripheral blood–derived short-term polyclonal T cell lines (TCL) from patients with Churg-Strauss syndrome (CSS; n = 5), patients with Wegener's granulomatosis (WG; n = 4), and healthy controls (HC; n = 4). Values are the mean and SEM of at least 5 TCL from each subject.

IL-5 production. IL-5 production by CSS TCL (6.9 ± 2.2 pg/ml) was not significantly different from that observed with HC TCL (6.9 ± 4.7 pg/ml). WG TCL showed significantly increased IL-5 production (31.4 ± 8.3 pg/ml) compared with that observed in TCL from CSS patients and from HC (P = 0.014 and P = 0.043, respectively).

IL-10 production. IL-10 production by TCL from patients as well as HC was negligible, i.e., below the 12.5-pg/ml cutoff value for the ELISA. Because of these low values, the relevance of a statistically significant difference in IL-10 production between CSS and WG TCL (3.18 ± 0.9 pg/ml and 0.53 ± 0.21 pg/ml, respectively; P = 0.014) remains questionable. In addition, levels in neither CSS TCL nor WG TCL differed significantly from those in HC TCL (1.08 ± 0.66 pg/ml).

IL-13 production. IL-13 was the cytokine produced in the highest amounts in CSS TCL (443.9 ± 59.6 pg/ml) when compared with WG TCL (94.1 ± 42.8 pg/ml; P = 0.014) and with HC TCL (7.1 ± 1.7 pg/ml; P = 0.014) (Figure 1). Furthermore, the difference between IL-13 production in WG TCL and that in HC TCL was also statistically significant (P = 0.021).

Correlation between clinical and immunologic parameters. Among CSS patients, the only significant positive correlation between TCL cytokine production and clinical or laboratory features was between IL-4 levels and the absolute number of eosinophils (r = 0.7, $P < 0.05$). There were no correlations between cytokine levels and clinical or laboratory findings in the patients with WG. We did not observe any significant correlation between clinical features and the CD4:CD8 ratio among the CSS TCL or the WG TCL.

DISCUSSION

Our data demonstrate significant differences with respect to phenotype and cytokine profile of T cells between CSS patients and WG patients, as well as between CSS patients and healthy controls. Classification of the TCL according to phenotype and IFNγ:IL-4 ratio revealed a polarization toward a CD4+, Th0 pattern in TCL from patients with CSS, compared with a CD8+, Th1 pattern in TCL from patients with WG and a CD4+, Th1 pattern in HC. Moreover, we found significant increases in IL-4 and IL-13 production in TCL from patients with CSS in comparison with those derived from patients with another granulomatous disease (WG) or from healthy controls. In addition, a positive correlation between IL-4 production and the eosinophil count in CSS supports our assumption that CSS is a Th2-associated disease, in contrast to the more Th1-associated cytokine pattern found in WG.

We observed a weak polarization toward the CD4+ phenotype in CSS TCL and a strong polarization toward the CD8+ phenotype in WG TCL, whereas the HC TCL showed no substantial preference for CD4 or CD8. However, because of the in vitro generation of the TCL and the possibility that the phenotypes may not be representative of the in vivo situation, care must be taken with respect to the interpretation of these findings.

We took two different approaches to examine potential differences between CSS, WG, and HC in terms of the immunoregulatory cytokine profile of TCL. First, we used a method similar to that used in previous studies utilizing either the IFNγ:IL-4 ratio (12) or the IL-4:IFNγ ratio (13) to investigate whether there is a preference for Th1 or Th2. We classified the TCL according to their IFNγ:IL-4 ratio, whereby those with ratios of >10 were considered to have a Th1 pattern, those with ratios of 1–10 were considered to have a Th0 pattern, and those with ratios of <1 were considered to have a Th2 pattern (13). With this strategy, we observed a predominant Th1 profile for all WG TCL examined as well as for most of the HC TCL (60%), whereas the majority of CSS TCL (60%) belonged to the Th0 type. Interestingly, WG and CSS TCL produced about the same amount of IFNγ, i.e., in the range of 260–280 pg/ml. The increased IL-4 production by CSS TCL compared with WG TCL could provide a likely explanation for the differences in predominant Th type. With regard to IL-4, we additionally observed that within the CSS group the patients with longer disease duration displayed substantially higher production. However, although the division of TCL according to the IFNγ:IL-4 ratio revealed substantial differences, it is difficult to make assumptions about the importance of these findings, because there is no standardization of Th grading with respect to the IFNγ:IL-4 ratio, and the sensitivity of the grading limits is not known.

Second, as a direct approach, we investigated production of other cytokines (IL-5, IL-10, and IL-13) and compared the data for each. This revealed that CSS TCL displayed not only elevated IL-4 but even higher IL-13 production, when compared with WG or HC TCL (Figure 1). The notion of a more Th2-polarized immune response in CSS, based on this exaggerated IL-4 and IL-13 production, is also supported by the findings of studies on potential pathogenic roles of both IL-4 and IL-13 in Th2-associated allergic diseases. IL-13 is believed to play a role as a central mediator of allergic asthma (14). Since IL-13 and IL-4 have been reported to display common receptor units and signal transduction pathways (15), a similar function of these molecules may be imputed on that ground. Interestingly, CSS patients produced no or very little IL-5, compared with significantly higher IL-5 production in WG. With respect to this cytokine, our findings differ somewhat from those presented in a case report of a patient with CSS (5) as well as from data reported for idiopathic eosinophilia (16), stating that IL-5, based on its eosinophil differentiating properties, is one of the main, if not the only, molecule aggravating eosinophilia and/or the course of a type 2 immune response, respectively.

For WG, the data from this study support previous findings (17,18) by demonstrating significantly elevated IFNγ production by polyclonal PB TCL compared with TCL from HC. Further, our results showed that WG TCL produced not only more IFNγ but also more IL-5 and IL-13, when compared with HC. *Staphylococcus*-specific HLA–DR–restricted CD4+ PB lymphocyte–derived TCL from WG patients exhibited a predominant Th2 pattern (high IL-4 and IL-10, low IFNγ production) (19). Therefore, one could speculate that not only is the cytokine profile of T cells in vasculitic WG dominated by a Th1-like reaction, but there are hints of the presence of Th2-like reactions as well.

Because of the small number of patients studied, the findings presented herein need to be confirmed in a larger cohort. Further investigations are under way to more extensively and more precisely characterize differences in immunopathogenesis between CSS and WG.

ACKNOWLEDGMENTS

We thank Monika Backes and Inga Goldt for their skillful technical assistance, and we are grateful to the patients and healthy blood donors for their cooperation.

REFERENCES

1. Churg J, Strauss L. Allergic granulomatosis, allergic angiitis and polyarteritis nodosa. Am J Pathol 1951;27:277–301.
2. Guillevin L, Cohen P, Gayraud M, Lhote F, Jarrousse B, Casassus P. Churg-Strauss syndrome: clinical study and long-term follow-up of 96 patients. Medicine (Baltimore) 1999;78:26–37.
3. Schmitt WH, Heesen C, Csernok E, Rautmann A, Gross WL. Elevated serum levels of soluble interleukin-2 receptor in patients with Wegener's granulomatosis: association with disease activity. Arthritis Rheum 1992;35:1088–96.
4. Schmitt WH, Csernok E, Kobayashi S, Klinkenborg A, Reinhold-Keller E, Gross WL. Churg-Strauss syndrome: serum markers of lymphocyte activation and endothelial damage. Arthritis Rheum 1998;41:445–52.
5. Tsukadaira A, Okubo Y, Kitano K, Horie S, Momose T, Takashi S, et al. Eosinophil active cytokines and surface analysis of eosinophils in Churg-Strauss syndrome. Allergy Asthma Proc 1999;20:39–44.
6. Müschen M, Warskulat U, Perniok A, Even J, Moers C, Kismet B, et al. Involvement of soluble CD95 in Churg-Strauss syndrome. Am J Pathol 1999;155:915–25.
7. Tatsis E, Schnabel A, Gross WL. Interferon-α treatment of four patients with the Churg-Strauss syndrome. Ann Intern Med 1998; 129:370–4.
8. Prin L, Ameisen JC, Plumas J, Gruart V, Loiseau S, Bletry O, et al. High levels of soluble interleukin-2 receptor in the serum of 30 patients with idiopathic hypereosinophilic syndrome. Br J Haematol 1990;74:223–9.
9. Jennette JC, Falk RJ, Andrassy K, Bacon PA, Churg J, Gross WL, et al. Nomenclature of systemic vasculitides: proposal of an international consensus conference. Arthritis Rheum 1994;37: 187–92.
10. Masi AT, Hunder GG, Lie JT, Michel BA, Bloch DA, Arend WP, et al. The American College of Rheumatology 1990 criteria for the classification of the Churg-Strauss syndrome (allergic granulomatosis and angiitis). Arthritis Rheum 1990;33:1094–100.
11. Leavitt RY, Fauci AS, Bloch DA, Michel BA, Hunder GG, Arend WP, et al. The American College of Rheumatology 1990 criteria for the classification of Wegener's granulomatosis. Arthritis Rheum 1990;33:1101–7.
12. Voll RE, Roth EA, Girkontaite I, Fehr H, Herrmann M, Lorenz HM, et al. Histone-specific Th0 and Th1 clones derived from systemic lupus erythematosus patients induce double-stranded DNA antibody production. Arthritis Rheum 1997;40:2162–71.
13. Lagier B, Lebel B, Bousquet J, Pene J. Different modulation by histamine of IL-4 and IFN-γ release according to the phenotype of human Th0, Th1 and Th2 clones. Clin Exp Immunol 1997;108: 545–51.
14. Wills-Karp M, Luyimbazi J, Xu X, Schofield B, Neben TY, Karp CL, et al. Interleukin-13: central mediator of allergic asthma. Science 1998;282:2258–61.
15. Murata T, Obiri NI, Puri NK. Structure of and signal transduction through IL-4 and IL-13 receptors. Int J Mol Med 1998;1:551–7.
16. Simon HU, Plötz SG, Dummer R, Blaser K. Abnormal clones of T cells producing interleukin-5 in idiopathic eosinophilia. N Engl J Med 1999;341:1112–20.
17. Csernok E, Trabandt A, Müller A, Wang GC, Moosig F, Paulsen J, et al. Cytokine profiles in Wegener's granulomatosis: predominance of type 1 (Th1) in the granulomatous inflammation. Arthritis Rheum 1999;42:742–50.
18. Lúdvíksson BR, Sneller MC, Chua KS, Talar-Williams C, Langford CA, Ehrhardt RO, et al. Active Wegener's granulomatosis is associated with HLA-DR$^+$ CD4$^+$ T cells exhibiting an unbalanced Th1-type T cell cytokine pattern: reversal with IL-10. J Immunol 1998;160:3602–9.
19. Mayet WJ, Märker-Hermann E, Schlaak J, Meyer zum Büschenfelde KH. Irregular cytokine pattern of CD4+ lymphocytes in response to S. aureus in patients with Wegener's granulomatosis. Scand J Immunol 1999;49:585–94.
20. Reinhold-Keller E, Kekow J, Schnabel A, Schmitt WH, Heller M, Beigel A, et al. Influence of disease manifestation and antineutrophil cytoplasmic antibody titer on the response to pulse cyclophosphamide therapy in patients with Wegener's granulomatosis. Arthritis Rheum 1994;37:919–24.

ARTHRITIS & RHEUMATISM
Vol. 44, No. 2, February 2001, pp 474–480

Blockade of Endogenous Transforming Growth Factor β Signaling Prevents Up-Regulated Collagen Synthesis in Scleroderma Fibroblasts

Association With Increased Expression of Transforming Growth Factor β Receptors

Hironobu Ihn, Kenichi Yamane, Masahide Kubo, and Kunihiko Tamaki

Objective. **To elucidate the role of transforming growth factor β (TGFβ) in the increased expression of the collagen gene in scleroderma fibroblasts.**

Methods. **Dermal fibroblasts from 10 patients with diffuse systemic sclerosis (SSc) of recent onset and from 10 healthy individuals were studied. The production of active and total (active + latent) TGFβ1 levels from cultured dermal fibroblasts was measured using a TGFβ1 enzyme-linked immunosorbent assay system. Expression of the TGFβ type I and type II receptor proteins in dermal fibroblasts was determined by immunoblotting, and the level of expression of human α2(I) collagen messenger RNA (mRNA) was evaluated by Northern blot analysis. The transcriptional activity of the human α2(I) collagen gene was examined with chloramphenicol acetyltransferase (CAT) assays using the −772 COL1A2/CAT construct.**

Results. **SSc fibroblasts expressed increased levels of TGFβ type I and type II receptors but secreted amounts of TGFβ similar to those secreted by normal fibroblasts. The blockade of TGFβ signaling with anti-TGFβ antibodies or a TGFβ1 antisense oligonucleotide abolished the increased mRNA expression, as well as the up-regulated transcriptional activity of the human α2(I) collagen gene in SSc fibroblasts.**

Conclusion. **These results suggest that TGFβ plays a crucial role in the pathogenesis of SSc and raise the possibility of a therapeutic approach with anti-TGFβ antibodies or a TGFβ1 antisense oligonucleotide.**

Excessive extracellular matrix (ECM) deposition in the skin, lung, or other organs is a hallmark of systemic sclerosis (SSc) (1). The pathogenesis of SSc is still poorly understood, but increasing evidence suggests that activation of lesional fibroblasts contributes to the fibrotic process (2,3). Numerous differences between cultured SSc and healthy skin fibroblasts that can contribute to excessive ECM deposition in vivo have been demonstrated, such as elevated expression of collagens type I, III, VI, and VII, fibronectin, and glycosaminoglycans (3–9), of tissue inhibitor of metalloproteinase (10,11), and of intercellular adhesion molecules (12,13). SSc and healthy skin fibroblasts also differ in their response to transforming growth factor β (TGFβ). TGFβ stimulates platelet-derived growth factor α receptor expression in SSc fibroblasts, but not in healthy skin fibroblasts (14). In addition, SSc fibroblasts are less sensitive to the stimulatory effects of cytokines that regulate collagen production, such as TGFβ, oncostatin M, and interleukin-4 (15–17).

The mechanism of dermal fibroblast activation in SSc is presently unknown. However, many of the characteristics of SSc fibroblasts resemble those of healthy fibroblasts stimulated by TGFβ (18,19), suggesting that the dermal fibroblast activation in SSc may be a result of

Supported by grant 10770391 for scientific research from the Ministry of Education, Japan, by the Research for Progressive Systemic Sclerosis project of the Ministry of Health and Welfare, by a grant for basic dermatologic research from Shiseido Co., Ltd, Japan, and by the Lydia O'Learly Memorial Foundation, Japan.

Hironobu Ihn, MD, PhD, Kenichi Yamane, MD, Masahide Kubo, MD, PhD, Kunihiko Tamaki, MD, PhD: University of Tokyo, Tokyo, Japan.

Address correspondence and reprint requests to Hironobu Ihn, MD, PhD, Department of Dermatology, Faculty of Medicine, University of Tokyo, 7-3-1 Hongo, Bunkyo-ku, Tokyo 113, Japan.

Submitted for publication July 19, 2000; accepted in revised form October 13, 2000.

stimulation by autocrine TGFβ. This notion is supported by our recent finding that SSc fibroblasts express elevated levels of TGFβ receptor type I and type II messenger RNA (mRNA) and that this correlates with elevated levels of α2(I) collagen mRNA (20).

The present study was undertaken to further confirm this hypothesis. First, we investigated the levels of TGFβ production, and also of TGFβ receptors, in SSc and control fibroblasts. We then investigated the type I collagen mRNA expression and transcriptional activity of the gene in the absence or presence of TGFβ signaling blockade, using TGFβ neutralizing antibodies or a TGFβ1 antisense oligonucleotide. The results support the notion that the blockade of TGFβ signaling inhibits the up-regulation of collagen synthesis in SSc fibroblasts and that this increased collagen synthesis may be regulated by elevated expression of TGFβ receptors in these fibroblasts.

MATERIALS AND METHODS

Cell cultures. After institutional approval of the study design, human dermal fibroblasts were obtained by skin biopsy from the affected areas (dorsal forearm) of 10 randomly selected patients with diffuse cutaneous SSc of <2 years' duration. Control fibroblasts were obtained from skin biopsy specimens from 10 healthy donors. Informed consent was obtained from all subjects. The controls were matched with each SSc patient for age, sex, and biopsy site, and their specimens were processed in parallel. Primary explant cultures were established in 25-cm^2 culture flasks in modified Eagle's medium (MEM) supplemented with 10% fetal calf serum (FCS), 2 m*M* L-glutamine, and 50 μg/ml amphotericin (21). Fibroblast cultures independently isolated from different individuals were maintained as monolayers at 37°C in 90% air, 10% CO_2 and studied between the third and sixth subpassages.

Measurement of TGFβ1 levels. The fibroblasts were grown to confluence in 6-well plates. The culture medium was removed, washed with MEM to remove excess TGFβ1, and replaced with serum-free MEM. After incubation for 24 hours, the fibroblast supernatants were collected and centrifuged for 5 minutes. The production of active and total (active + latent) TGFβ1 levels from cultured dermal fibroblasts was measured using a TGFβ1 enzyme-linked immunosorbent assay system (Amersham, Tokyo, Japan) (22). This system is designed to measure biologically active TGFβ1. Total TGFβ1 was assayed after acid activation by addition of 1*N* HCl to samples.

Western blot analysis. For the preparation of cell lysates from dermal fibroblasts, cells were placed in MEM and 0.1% bovine serum albumin (BSA) for 24 hours. Then the medium was removed, and the cells were washed with phosphate buffered saline. The cells were lysed by scraping into solubilization buffer (50 m*M* Tris Cl [pH 8], 150 m*M* NaCl, 2 m*M* EDTA, 50 m*M* NaF, 1% Nonidet P40, 1 mM sodium orthovanadate, 0.2 m*M* phenylmethylsulfonyl fluoride, 10 μg/ml aprotinin, 10 μg/ml leupeptin, and 10 μg/ml pepstatin). The lysates were incubated for 30 minutes at 4°C and then centrifuged for 5 minutes at 4°C. Protein concentrations of lysates were determined using a Bio-Rad (Hercules, CA) protein assay reagent.

Immunoblotting was performed as described previously (23). Briefly, cell lysates (20 μg) were electrophoresed on a 4/20% gradient sodium dodecyl sulfate–polyacrylamide gel, transferred onto nitrocellulose filters, and probed with the indicated primary antibodies. Then the filters were incubated overnight with horseradish peroxidase–conjugated goat anti-rabbit IgG, and immunoreactive bands were visualized using an enhanced chemilunescence system (Amersham) according to the manufacturer's recommendations. The densities of bands were measured with a densitometer.

RNA preparation and Northern blot analysis. Fibroblasts were grown to confluence in MEM supplemented with 10% FCS and incubated for 24 hours in serum-free medium (MEM plus 0.1% BSA) before addition of the indicated reagent. Total RNA was extracted and analyzed by Northern blotting as described previously (24). Filters were sequentially hybridized with radioactive probes for α2(I) procollagen and G3PDH. The filters were scanned with a Phosphoimager (Molecular Dynamics, Sunnyvale, CA).

Plasmid construction. Generation of a −772 COL1A2/CAT construct consisting of the human collagen α2(I) gene fragment (+58 to −772 bp relative to the transcription start site) linked to the chloramphenicol acetyltransferase (CAT) reporter gene was done as previously described (21). Plasmids used in transient transfection assays were purified twice on CsCl gradients. At least 2 different plasmid preparations were used for each experiment.

Transient transfection and CAT assay. Human fibroblasts were grown to 90% confluence in 100-mm dishes in Dulbecco's MEM with 10% FCS. Monolayers were washed, and cells were transfected using the calcium phosphate technique (21) with 10 μg of −772 COL1A2/CAT constructs. Control vector (pSV-β-galactosidase; Promega, Madison, WI) was cotransfected to normalize for transfection efficiency. After incubation overnight, the medium was replaced with MEM containing 0.1% BSA or with MEM containing 10% FCS, and incubation was continued for 48 hours. Cells were harvested in 0.25*M* Tris HCl (pH 8) and fractured by freeze–thawing. Extracts, normalized for protein content as measured by the Bio-Rad reagent, were incubated with butyryl-CoA and ^{14}C-chloramphenicol for 90 minutes at 37°C. Butyrated chloramphenicol was extracted using an organic solvent (2:1 mixture of tetramethylpentadecane and xylene) and quantitated by scintillation counting. Each experiment was performed in duplicate.

Treatment of dermal fibroblasts with anti-TGFβ antibodies or the antisense TGFβ1 oligonucleotide. We used a pan-specific neutralizing TGFβ antibody (R&D Systems, Min-

Table 1. Levels of active and total (active + latent) transforming growth factor β1 (TGFβ1) secreted by fibroblasts into culture supernatants*

	Active TGFβ1, ng/ml	Total TGFβ1, ng/ml
Systemic sclerosis fibroblasts	0.073 ± 0.021	0.381 ± 0.031
Normal fibroblasts	0.062 ± 0.031	0.435 ± 0.082

* Values are mean ± SEM.

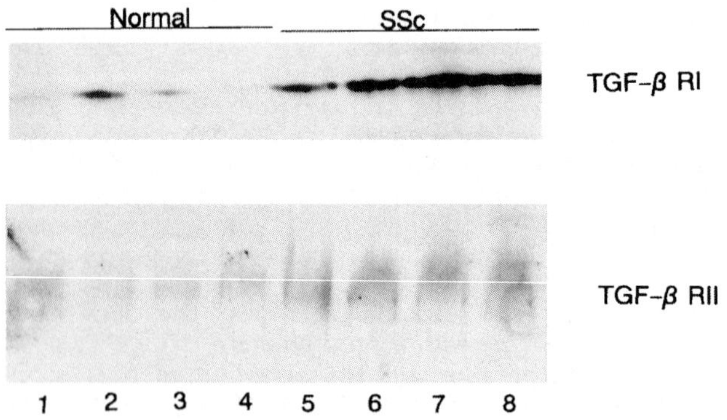

Figure 1. Increased expression of transforming growth factor β type I and type II receptors (TGF-β RI and TGF-β RII) by systemic sclerosis (SSc) fibroblasts. Representative results of immunoblot detection of TGF-β RI and RII in human dermal fibroblasts are shown. Cell lysates were electrophoresed through a 4/20% sodium dodecyl sulfate–polyacrylamide gel, transferred to a nitrocellulose membrane, and probed with anti–TGF-β RI or anti–TGF-β RII antibodies. Lanes 1–4, Cell lysates from normal dermal fibroblasts. Lanes 5–8, Cell lysates from SSc fibroblasts. Reactivities were determined and compared using a densitometer.

neapolis, MN), which has been shown to inhibit TGFβ activity specifically (20). We also used a TGFβ1 19-mer antisense oligonucleotide (GAGGGCGGCATGGGGAGG), which overlaps the promoter and transcriptional start site of the TGFβ1 gene. This same sequence, which is specific for the TGFβ1 isoform, has been found to be sufficient to block TGFβ1 transcription in vitro (25) and in vivo (26). A sense oligonucleotide served as control. Fibroblasts were grown to confluence and the culture medium was removed, washed with MEM to remove excess TGFβ1, and replaced with serum-free MEM. Various amounts of TGFβ antibodies or antisense or sense TGFβ1 oligonucleotide were added, and RNA isolation or cell extraction was performed 48 hours later.

Statistical analysis. Statistical analysis was performed using the Mann-Whitney *U* test for comparisons of means. *P* values less than 0.05 were considered significant.

RESULTS

Production of TGFβ1 by SSc and control fibroblasts. In order to investigate the role of autocrine TGFβ signaling in activated SSc fibroblasts, we exam-

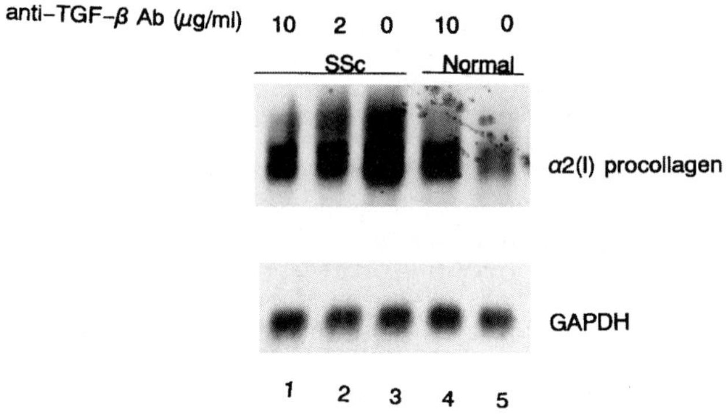

A

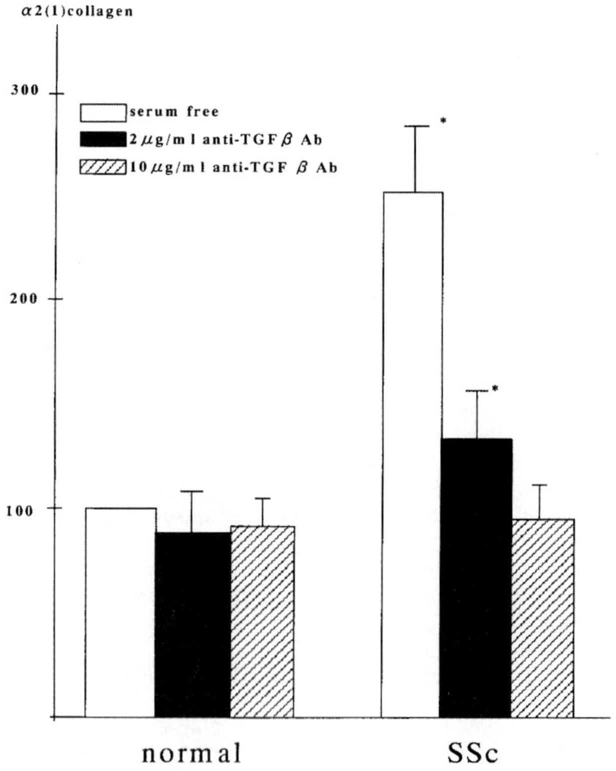

B

Figure 2. Effects of anti–TGF-β antibodies (Ab) on expression of the α2(I) collagen gene. Levels of mRNA for the α2(I) collagen gene in the presence or absence of anti–TGF-β antibodies were investigated by Northern blot analysis. **A,** Representative Northern blots. Lane 1, SSc fibroblasts treated with 10 μg/ml anti–TGF-β antibody. Lane 2, SSc fibroblasts treated with 2 μg/ml anti–TGF-β antibody. Lane 3, Untreated SSc fibroblasts. Lane 4, Normal fibroblasts treated with 10 μg/ml anti–TGF-β antibody. Lane 5, Untreated normal fibroblasts. **B,** Quantitative analysis of α2(I) collagen mRNA levels. Values represent the band density relative to that of untreated normal dermal fibroblasts, which was set at 100. The mean and SEM results from studies of 7 pairs of normal and SSc fibroblasts are shown. * = $P < 0.01$ versus normal fibroblasts under the same conditions. See Figure 1 for other definitions.

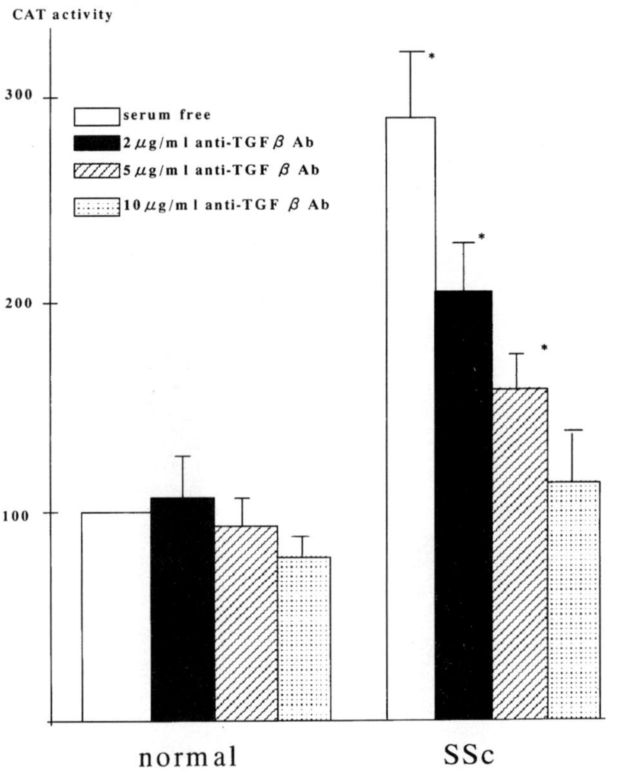

Figure 3. Effects of anti-TGF-β antibodies (Ab) on the transcriptional activity of the human $\alpha 2$(I) collagen gene. The plasmid carrying a −772 deletion of the human $\alpha 2$(I) collagen promoter was used in transient transfections of cells in the absence or presence of anti–TGF-β antibodies. Values represent the $\alpha 2$(I) promoter activities relative to that of untreated normal dermal fibroblasts, which was set at 100. The mean and SEM results from 5 separate experiments are shown. $* P < 0.01$ versus normal fibroblasts under the same conditions. CAT = chloramphenicol acetyltransferase (see Figure 1 for other definitions).

ined the production of TGFβ by SSc and control fibroblasts. A previous study showed that SSc fibroblasts produced an amount of TGFβ equivalent to that produced by control fibroblasts (27). In that study, TGFβ levels were determined by a growth inhibition assay using mink lung epithelial cells, which suggested that the investigators were measuring levels of the active form of TGFβ (27). In the present study, the production of total TGFβ1 (active + latent forms), as well as the active form of TGFβ1, was examined. The production of TGFβ1 was determined in conditioned medium from fibroblast lines derived from the involved skin of SSc patients or the normal skin of control donors.

As shown in Table 1, both groups' fibroblasts produced detectable levels of active TGFβ1 as well as total TGFβ1. The serum-free tissue culture medium alone contained no measurable TGFβ1. There was no significant difference between the amount of total TGFβ1 or the amount of active TGFβ1 produced by SSc fibroblasts and by control fibroblasts.

Increased expression of TGFβ type I and type II receptors by SSc fibroblasts. In the previous study (20), we examined the expression of TGFβ receptor mRNA in SSc and control dermal fibroblasts. We demonstrated that SSc fibroblasts expressed increased levels of TGFβ type I and type II receptor mRNA. In the present study, we wished to examine expression of TGFβ receptor proteins in SSc fibroblasts. The expression of the TGFβ type I and type II receptor proteins in 8 pairs of SSc and normal fibroblasts was measured (Figure 1). SSc fibroblasts expressed increased levels of the TGFβ type I receptor protein (2.3-fold increase; $P < 0.01$) and of the TGFβ type II receptor protein (2.6-fold increase; $P < 0.01$).

Effects of anti-TGFβ antibodies on expression of the collagen gene. To further examine the possibility that the dermal fibroblast activation in SSc may be a result of stimulation by autocrine TGFβ, we investigated the effects of anti-TGFβ antibodies on the expression of the human $\alpha 2$(I) collagen gene. As seen in Figure 2, SSc fibroblasts showed increased expression of the human $\alpha 2$(I) collagen gene. Upon treatment with anti-TGFβ antibodies, normal fibroblasts showed little reduction in human $\alpha 2$(I) collagen mRNA expression (~10% decrease; Figure 2B). In contrast, SSc fibroblasts treated with anti-TGFβ antibodies showed a marked, dose-dependent reduction in expression of human $\alpha 2$(I) collagen mRNA. Treatment with preimmune rabbit IgG had no effect on the expression of human $\alpha 2$(I) collagen mRNA (data not shown). In previous studies, SSc fibroblasts exhibited elevated activity of human $\alpha 1$(I) and $\alpha 2$(I) promoters (15,28). Therefore, we examined the effects of anti-TGFβ antibodies on the promoter activity of the human $\alpha 2$(I) collagen gene. As seen in Figure 3, normal fibroblasts treated with anti-TGFβ antibodies showed little reduction in the promoter activity of the human $\alpha 2$(I) collagen gene (~15% decrease). However, SSc fibroblasts treated with anti-TGFβ antibodies showed a marked, dose-dependent reduction in this activity.

Effects of the TGFβ1 antisense oligonucleotide on the expression of the collagen gene. Our results suggested that the blockade of TGFβ signaling inhibits up-regulation of collagen synthesis in SSc fibroblasts. We further explored this hypothesis by using a TGFβ1 antisense oligonucleotide, which is specific for the TGFβ1 isoform, to block TGFβ1 transcription in human dermal fibroblasts. The 19-mer TGFβ1 antisense oligonucleotide used in these experiments was previously

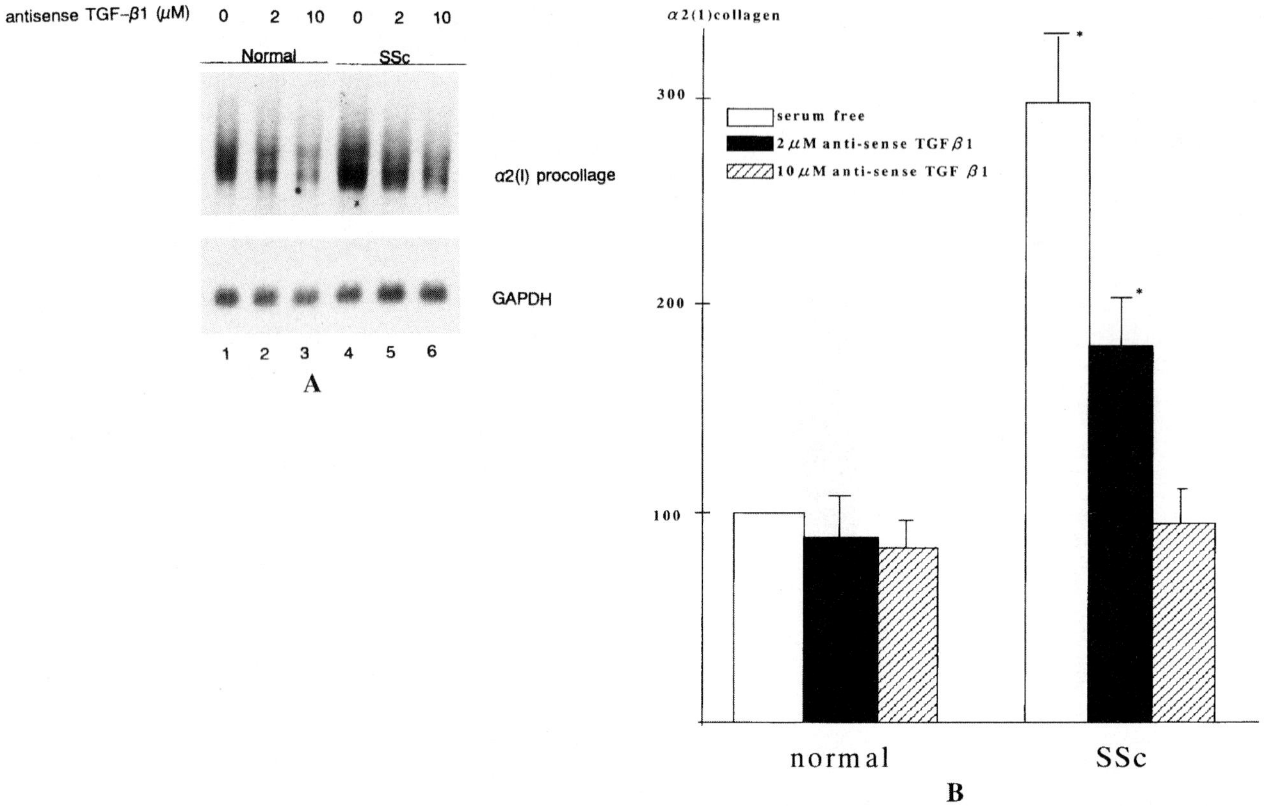

Figure 4. Effects of a TGF-β antisense oligonucleotide on expression of the α2(I) collagen gene. Levels of mRNA for the α2(I) collagen gene in the presence or absence of a TGF-β antisense oligonucleotide were investigated by Northern blot analysis. **A,** Representative Northern blots. Lane 1, Untreated normal fibroblasts. Lane 2, Normal fibroblasts treated with 2 *μM* antisense TGF-β1. Lane 3, Normal fibroblasts treated with 10 *μM* antisense TGF-β1. Lane 4, Untreated SSc fibroblasts. Lane 5, SSc fibroblasts treated with 2 *μM* antisense TGF-β1. Lane 6, SSc fibroblasts treated with 10 *μM* antisense TGF-β1. **B,** Quantitative analysis of α2(I) collagen mRNA levels. Values represent the band density relative to that of untreated normal dermal fibroblasts, which was set at 100. The mean and SEM results from studies of 7 pairs of normal and SSc fibroblasts are shown. * $P < 0.01$ versus normal fibroblasts under the same conditions. See Figure 1 for definitions.

shown to block the action of TGFβ in vitro (25) and in vivo (26). As shown in Figure 4, this antisense oligonucleotide caused little decrease in the expression of human α2(I) collagen mRNA by normal fibroblasts. However, increasing concentrations of the TGFβ1 antisense oligonucleotide caused a progressive decrease in the expression of human α2(I) collagen mRNA by SSc fibroblasts. The sense oligonucleotide had no such inhibitory effect (data not shown).

Furthermore, we determined the effect of the TGFβ1 antisense oligonucleotide on the promoter activity of the human α2(I) collagen gene. As shown in Figure 5, normal fibroblasts treated with the TGFβ1 antisense oligonucleotide showed little reduction in the promoter activity of the human α2(I) collagen gene. However, SSc fibroblasts treated with this antisense oligonucleotide showed a marked, dose-dependent reduction in the promoter activity of the human α2(I) collagen gene.

DISCUSSION

TGFβ is a multifunctional peptide that regulates cell growth and differentiation (29). It is important in the developmental process, regulating the immune response and playing a fundamental role in ECM formation (29). TGFβ has been shown to induce many tissue repair factors, and its pathogenetic role in the development of fibrosis is becoming increasingly clear (30). The principal effect of TGFβ on mesenchymal cells is its stimulation of ECM deposition. TGFβ has been shown to increase expression of collagen types I, III, VI, VII, and X, fibronectin, and proteoglycans (18). Stimulation of ECM production by TGFβ is further enhanced by its

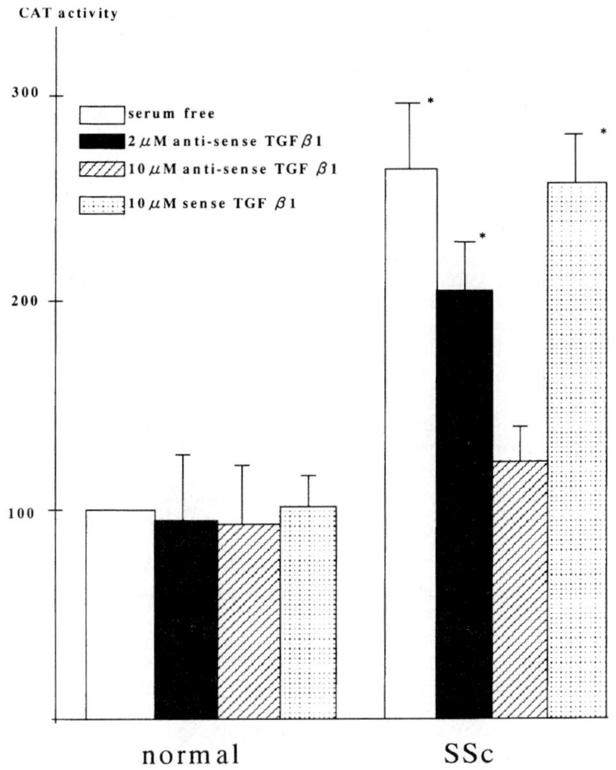

Figure 5. Effects of a TGF-β antisense oligonucleotide on the transcriptional activity of the human α2(I) collagen gene. The plasmid carrying a −772 deletion of the human α2(I) collagen promoter was used in transient transfections of cells in the absence or presence of anti–TGF-β antibodies. Values represent the α2(I) promoter activities relative to that of untreated normal dermal fibroblasts, which was set at 100. The mean and SEM results from 5 separate experiments are shown. * $P < 0.01$ versus normal fibroblasts under the same conditions. CAT = chloramphenicol acetyltransferase (see Figure 1 for other definitions).

inhibitory effect on matrix degradation, decreasing synthesis of proteases and increasing levels of protease inhibitors (18).

Various types of cells, including immune, endothelial, and mesenchymal cells, may serve as sources of TGFβ in fibrotic lesions. Moreover, sustained production of TGFβ in fibrotic lesions is thought to be maintained by autoinduction (31). It has been recognized that activated cells in fibrotic lesions may contribute to disease progression, but the mechanism of this activation is still unknown. One possible mechanism may involve the establishment of an autocrine TGFβ loop (20). This loop may be initiated in vivo by exposure to certain cytokines or environmental stimuli and may continue to operate under cell culture conditions.

A previous study showed that the amount of the active form of TGFβ produced by SSc fibroblasts was equivalent to that produced by control fibroblasts (27). In the present study, we first measured the production of not only the active form of TGFβ1 but also total TGFβ1 (active + latent forms) by SSc and control fibroblasts. There was no difference between the amount of active TGFβ1 produced by SSc fibroblasts and that produced by control fibroblasts, which is consistent with a previous report (27). Furthermore, there was no difference in the amount of total TGFβ1 produced by SSc fibroblasts and control fibroblasts.

In our previous study, both type I and II TGFβ receptor mRNA expression levels were higher in SSc fibroblasts than in healthy fibroblasts (20). In the present investigation, we examined the expression of the TGFβ receptor proteins in SSc fibroblasts, and SSc fibroblasts were shown to express increased levels of TGFβ type I and type II receptor proteins (Figure 1). These results, along with our previous findings (20), suggest that, although SSc fibroblasts express TGFβ in quantities similar to those produced by healthy fibroblasts, the levels of TGFβ type I and type II receptors produced by SSc fibroblasts are greater than those produced by normal fibroblasts.

The blockade of TGFβ signaling with anti-TGFβ antibodies abolished the increased expression of human α2(I) collagen mRNA in SSc fibroblasts (Figure 2). This result was also confirmed by an experiment using a TGFβ1 antisense oligonucleotide (Figure 4). SSc fibroblasts have been reported to exhibit elevated activity of the human α2(I) promoter (15,28). Therefore, we also investigated the effect of anti-TGFβ antibodies or the TGFβ1 antisense oligonucleotide on the transcriptional activity of the human α2(I) collagen gene. Treatment of SSc fibroblasts with anti-TGFβ antibodies abolished the increased promoter activity of the human α2(I) collagen gene in SSc fibroblasts, in a dose-dependent manner (Figure 3). This finding was also supported by the results of another experiment using a TGFβ1 antisense oligonucleotide (Figure 5).

A recent study demonstrated the antisclerotic effect of TGFβ antibodies in a mouse model of scleroderma (32). The present study showed blockade of TGFβ signaling by anti-TGFβ antibodies or a TGFβ1 antisense oligonucleotide in vitro. These results confirm the crucial role of TGFβ in the pathogenesis of SSc and raise the possibility of the development of a therapy for this disease using an approach that involves anti-TGFβ antibodies or a TGFβ1 antisense oligonucleotide.

REFERENCES

1. LeRoy EC. Systemic sclerosis (scleroderma). In: Wyngaarden JB, Smith LH, Bennett JC, editors. Cecil text book of medicine. 19th ed. Philadelphia: WB Saunders; 1992. p. 1530–5.
2. Kulozik M, Hogg A, Lankat-Buttgereit B, Kreig T. Co-localization of transforming growth factor $\beta 2$ with $\alpha 1(I)$ procollagen mRNA in tissue sections of patients with systemic sclerosis. J Clin Invest 1990;86:917–22.
3. Jelaska A, Arakawa M, Broketa G, Korn JH. Heterogeneity of collagen synthesis in normal and systemic sclerosis skin fibroblasts: increased proportion of high collagen–producing cells in systemic sclerosis fibroblasts. Arthritis Rheum 1996;39:1338–46.
4. LeRoy EC. Increased collagen synthesis by scleroderma skin fibroblasts in vitro: a possible defect in the regulation or activation of the scleroderma fibroblast. J Clin Invest 1974;54:880–9.
5. Buckingham RB, Prince RK, Rodnan GP, Taylor F. Increased collagen accumulation in dermal fibroblast cultures from patients with systemic sclerosis (scleroderma). J Lab Clin Med 1978;92: 5–21.
6. Peltonen J, Kähäri L, Uitto J, Jimenez SA. Increased expression of type VI collagen genes in systemic sclerosis. Arthritis Rheum 1990;33:1829–35.
7. Xu W, LeRoy EC, Smith EA. Fibronectin release by systemic sclerosis and normal dermal fibroblasts in response to TGF-β. J Rheumatol 1991;18:241–6.
8. Ludnicka L, Varga J, Christiano AM, Iozzo RV, Jimenez SA, Uitto J. Elevated expression of type VII collagen in the skin of patients with systemic sclerosis: regulation by transforming growth factor-beta. J Clin Invest 1994;93:1709–15.
9. Falanga V, Tiegs SL, Alstadt SP, Roberts AB, Sporn MB. Transforming growth factor beta: selective increase in glycosaminoglycan synthesis by cultures of fibroblasts from patients with progressive systemic sclerosis. J Invest Dermatol 1987;89:100–4.
10. Kirk TZ, Mark ME, Chua CC, Chua BH, Mayes MD. Myofibroblasts from scleroderma skin synthesize elevated levels of collagen and tissue inhibitor of metalloproteinase (TIMP-1) with two forms of TIMP-1. J Biol Chem 1995;270:3423–8.
11. Mattila L, Airola K, Ahonen M, Hietarinta M, Black M, Saarialho-Kere U, et al. Activation of tissue inhibitor of metalloproteinase-3 (TIMP-3) mRNA expression in scleroderma skin fibroblasts. J Invest Dermatol 1998;110:416–21.
12. Abraham D, Lupoli S, McWhirter A, Plater-Zyberk C, Piela TH, Korn JH, et al. Expression and function of surface antigens on scleroderma fibroblasts. Arthritis Rheum 1991;34:1164–72.
13. Ihn H, Sato S, Fujimoto M, Kikuchi K, Kadono T, Tamaki K, et al. Circulating intercellular adhesion molecule-1 in the sera of patients with systemic sclerosis: enhancement by inflammatory cytokines. Br J Rheumatol 1997;36:1270–5.
14. Yamakage A, Kikuchi K, Smith EA, LeRoy EC, Trojanowska M. Selective upregulation of platelet-derived growth factor α receptors by transforming growth factor β in scleroderma fibroblasts. J Exp Med 1992;175:1227–34.
15. Kikuchi K, Hartl EA, Smith EA, LeRoy EC, Trojanowska M. Direct demonstration of transcriptional activation of collagen gene expression in systemic sclerosis fibroblasts: insensitivity to TGF-β stimulation. Biochem Biophys Res Commun 1992;187:45–50.
16. Duncan MA, Hasan A, Berman B. Oncostatin M stimulates collagen and glycosaminoglycan production by cultured normal dermal fibroblasts: insensitivity of sclerodermal and keloidal fibroblasts. J Invest Dermatol 1995;104:128–33.
17. Lee KS, Ro YJ, Ryoo YW, Kwon HJ, Song JY. Regulation of interleukin-4 on collagen gene expression by systemic sclerosis fibroblasts in culture. J Dermatol Sci 1996;12:110–7.
18. Massagué J. The transforming growth factor-β family. Annu Rev Cell Biol 1990;6:597–641.
19. LeRoy EC, Smith EA, Kahaleh MB, Trojanowska M, Silver RM. A strategy for determining the pathogenesis of systemic sclerosis: is transforming growth factor β the answer? Arthritis Rheum 1989;32:817–25.
20. Kawakami T, Ihn H, Xu W, Smith E, LeRoy EC, Trojanowska M. Increased expression of TGF-β receptors by scleroderma fibroblasts: evidence for contribution of autocrine TGF-β signaling to scleroderma phenotype. J Invest Dermatol 1998;110:47–51.
21. Ihn H, Ohnishi K, Tamaki T, LeRoy EC, Trojanowska M. Transcriptional regulation of the human $\alpha 2(I)$ collagen gene: combined action of upstream stimulatory and inhibitory cis-acting elements. J Biol Chem 1996;271:26717–23.
22. Shirai Y, Kawata S, Tamura S, Ito N, Tsushima H, Takaishi K, et al. Plasma transforming growth factor-$\alpha 1$ in patients with hepatocellular carcinoma. Cancer 1994;73:2275–9.
23. Ihn H, Trojanowska M. Sp3 is a transcriptional activator of the human $\alpha 2(I)$ collagen gene. Nucleic Acids Res 1997;25:3712–7.
24. Ihn H, LeRoy EC, Trojanowska M. Oncostatin M stimulates transcription of the human $\alpha 2(I)$ collagen gene via the Sp1/Sp3-binding site. J Biol Chem 1997;272:24666–72.
25. Falanga V, Greenberg AS, Ochoa SM, Roberts AB, Falabella A, Yamaguchi Y. Stimulation of collagen synthesis by anabolic steroid stanozol. J Invest Dermatol 1998;111:1193–7.
26. Brunet CL, Sharpe PM, Ferguson MWJ. Inhibition of TGF-$\beta 3$ (but not TGF-$\beta 1$ or TGF-$\beta 2$) activity prevents normal and mouse embryonic palate fusion. Int J Dev Biol 1995;39:345–55.
27. Needleman BW, Choi J, Burrows-Mezu A, Fontana JA. Secretion and binding of transforming growth factor β by scleroderma and normal dermal fibroblasts. Arthritis Rheum 1990;33:650–6.
28. Hitraya EG, Jiménez SA. Transcriptional activation of the $\alpha 1(I)$ procollagen gene in systemic sclerosis dermal fibroblasts: role of intronic sequences. Arthritis Rheum 1996;39:1347–54.
29. Roberts AB, Sporn MB. Physiological actions and clinical applications of transforming growth factor-β (TGF-β). Growth Factors 1993;8:1–9.
30. Border WA, Noble NA. Transforming growth factor β in tissue fibrosis. N Engl J Med 1994;331:1286–92.
31. Obberghen-Schilling EV, Roche NS, Flanders KC, Sporn MB, Roberts AB. Transforming growth factor $\beta 1$ positively regulates its own expression in normal and transformed cells. J Biol Chem 1988;263:7741–6.
32. Yamamoto T, Takagawa S, Katayama I, Nishioka K. Anti-sclerotic effect of transforming growth factor-β antibody in a mouse model of bleomycin-induced scleroderma. Clin Immunol 1999;92:6–13.

ARTHRITIS & RHEUMATISM
Vol. 44, No. 2, February 2001, pp 481–485

Widespread Pain Among 11-Year-Old Finnish Twin Pairs

Marja Mikkelsson,[1] Jaakko Kaprio,[2] Jouko J. Salminen,[3] Lea Pulkkinen,[4] and Richard J. Rose[5]

Objective. To examine the prevalence of widespread musculoskeletal pain (WSP) symptoms in 11-year-old Finnish twins and to determine the relative role of genetic and environmental factors in the etiology of WSP.

Methods. Data on current pain items were collected from 1995 to 1998 from a national sample of Finnish families with 11-year-old twins born between 1984 and 1987. The presence of WSP was determined using a validated questionnaire method. Pairwise similarity was computed for 583 monozygotic (MZ) pairs, 588 same-sex dizygotic (DZ) pairs, and 618 opposite-sex DZ twin pairs. Variance components for genetic and environmental factors were estimated using biometric structural equation modeling techniques.

Results. The prevalence of WSP was 9.9%, with no sex difference. The majority of twin pairs with WSP were discordant. The tetrachoric correlations for male MZ (r = 0.38), male DZ (r = 0.37), female MZ (r = 0.59), female DZ (r = 0.54), and opposite-sex pairs (r = 0.43) showed little difference by zygosity. Female pairs were more concordant than male pairs among both MZ and DZ twins. Biometric model-fitting indicated that genetic factors did not account for the pattern of twin similarity. Among boys 35%, and among girls 56%, of the variation in liability to WSP could be attributed to shared familial environmental effects. The remainder was attributed to unshared environmental effects.

Conclusion. Genetic factors seem to play at most a minor role in WSP in 11-year-old twins, and environmental factors shared by family members account for a substantial proportion of the variability in WSP.

Supported by grants AA-09203 and AA-00145 from the National Institute on Alcohol Abuse and Alcoholism and by the Academy of Finland Centre of Excellence Programme and the Wilhelm & Else Stockmann Foundation.

[1]Marja Mikkelsson, MD, PhD: The Rheumatism Foundation Hospital, Heinola, Finland; [2]Jaakko Kaprio, MD, PhD: University of Helsinki, Helsinki, Finland, and the University of Oulu, Oulu, Finland; [3]Jouko J. Salminen, MD, PhD: University Hospital of Turku, Turku, Finland; [4]Lea Pulkkinen, PhD: University of Jyväskylä, Jyväskylä, Finland; [5]Richard J. Rose, PhD: Indiana University, Bloomington.

Address correspondence and reprint requests to Professor Jaakko Kaprio, MD, PhD, The Finnish Twin Cohort Study, Department of Public Health, P.O. Box 41, University of Helsinki, FIN-00014 Helsinki, Finland.

Submitted for publication April 19, 2000; accepted in revised form October 13, 2000.

Widespread musculoskeletal pain (WSP), as determined in the American College of Rheumatology (ACR) criteria for fibromyalgia (FM), includes persistent pain symptoms for at least 3 months in both sides of the body, above and below the waist, and in the axial skeleton (1). The prevalence of WSP has been estimated to be ~11% among adult populations in England and Wales (2) and the US (3). The persistence of WSP after a median of 27 months of followup has been reported to be 35% (4). In Finland, the prevalence of WSP, occurring at least once a week, among 9–12-year-old schoolchildren was 7.5% (5), with a 1-year persistence of 29.7%. Whether WSP is more dependent on environmental factors than genetic factors has not been studied. One subset of persons with WSP has FM, and familial aggregation of FM has been found (6–9). In addition, a case report on adult monozygotic (MZ) twins having FM has been published (10). In terms of FM, an autosomal-dominant inheritance pattern has been suggested (6), whereas in 1999 Yunus et al found evidence of a possible gene for FM that is linked with the HLA region (9). For a complex trait without a clear mode of inheritance, it is necessary to first establish whether the trait aggregates in families, and to what degree it is inherited. Twins can be used to estimate the genetic contribution to a trait through the comparison of MZ pairs (those who share all their genes) with dizygotic (DZ) pairs, who have an average of 50% of their genes in common.

SUBJECTS AND METHODS

Subjects. This study is part of a longitudinal study of behavioral development and health habits in 5 consecutive birth cohorts of Finnish twin children, called FinnTwin12. Data on pain items were collected from 4 of the 5 nationwide birth cohorts because the relevant items were not included in the first year of data collection. Baseline data collection is now complete, but followup of the families continues. From 1995 to 1998, Finnish families (n = 2,487) with twins born between 1984 and 1987 were identified from the nation's Central Population Registry as part of the younger Finnish Twin Cohort (11). Approximately 85% of the identified families in these 4 cohorts returned an initial questionnaire on the twins' childhood development and medical history. Both Finnish- and Swedish-speaking families were included in the study, and all received their questionnaires in their native language. After families had returned the initial questionnaire, the twins were mailed their own personal questionnaire during the late autumn of each year. Each twin received a separate questionnaire with a return envelope with prepaid postage. Items covered included their leisure time activities, health habits, pubertal development, pains, and symptoms. The response rate among twins was 95.9% (4,034 individual responses). Eighty-eight individuals had to be dropped from analyses because their cotwins had not replied or the questionnaire response of at least one cotwin was not usable, thus leaving 3,946 responses from 1,973 pairs.

Comparisons of twin similarity were limited to pairs with confirmed zygosity, with complete data from both cotwins in each pair (n = 1,789 pairs). Sample sizes for these comparisons were 583 MZ pairs, 588 same-sex DZ pairs, and 618 opposite-sex DZ twin pairs. Zygosity was determined from validated (12) items on twins' perceived similarity and confusability of appearance, as reported by the twins and their parents in the mailed questionnaires; additional items useful for diagnosis of zygosity were added from a study of zygosity in young twins (13). In some pairs, photographs and evaluations from face-to-face interviews have provided additional zygosity information. Zygosity could not be assigned at the time of analysis on 184 same-sex pairs.

Measures and variables. The questions on pain were taken from a questionnaire developed by us (5). The brief test–retest reliability of the questions in detecting those who have pain at least once a week has been found to be satisfactory (κ = 0.9). The concurrent validity of the questionnaire compared with interviews has also been studied; the observed agreement of results with the pain questionnaire with the interview technique was 86% and κ was 0.67 (5).

The goal of the pain questions was to classify the frequency of pain symptoms during the previous months according to the body area. The following body areas were distinguished: neck and shoulder region, upper extremities, upper back and chest, low back, buttocks, and lower extremities. The body area concerned was marked in a drawing beside the question to help the child recognize the named area. A 5-level frequency classification (pain seldom or never, once a month, once a week, more than once a week, almost daily) was used, and the questions on the questionnaire asked about the frequency of pain in the given areas since the previous summer (approximately a 3-month period for all subjects). WSP was classified according to the ACR 1990 criteria for FM (1) and by noting that the frequency of pain was at least once a week. WSP classification also required that pain occurred above and below the waist, on both sides of the body, and in the axial skeleton.

Pain due to injury was excluded. However, in the first age group (born in 1984), a question on pain due to injury was included, but children did not indicate the area concerned. Thus, we could not differentiate whether WSP classification was biased by pain due to injury. Of those who were born between 1985 and 1987, WSP due to injury was excluded and the percentages of children with WSP due to injury were calculated. The annual percentages were 24%, 18%, and 28%. There were 37 children with WSP born in 1984 who reported pain due to injury but were included in the study. This means that the results may include ~7–10 children with WSP due to injury whom we could not recognize and exclude.

Statistical methods. To estimate genetic and environmental contributions to WSP, biometric modeling was used. The basic model is one in which the individual's deviation from the population mean is assumed to result from both genetic and environmental effects. Genetic effects may be due to additive genetic effects (i.e., the allele-specific average effects at a locus, summed over all relevant loci) or nonadditive effects (due to interactions within a locus-dominance or between loci, known as epistasis). Environmental effects can be further divided into shared and nonshared effects. Shared environmental effects refer to those that are common to both twins, or more generally those shared by family members living in the same household, while nonshared effects are unique to each twin (i.e., not shared by family members). In terms of variability, the corresponding phenotypic variance is assumed to result from genetic and environmental variances. Data from twins can be used to model and estimate these variance components.

Under the current study design of twins reared together, it is possible to model 4 separate parameters: an additive genetic (A) component, nonadditive effects (D), and shared (C) and nonshared (E) environmental components. The influence of these components on the phenotype is given by parameters (h, d, c, and e) that are equivalent to the standardized regression coefficients of the phenotype on the corresponding variance component (A, D, C, and E, respectively) (14). The square of these parameters is an estimate of the proportion of variance due to each component. One can fit models based on the different combinations of these parameters: AE, ACE, ADE, and CE, but effects due to dominance and shared environmental effects cannot be simultaneously modeled with data limited to that from twins reared together (14). Because we had data on twins of both sexes and opposite-sex twin pairs, additional hypotheses regarding gender-specific effects could be tested (14).

For dichotomous variables (presence/absence of WSP), tetrachoric correlations among twin pairs were computed and models were fitted to these tetrachoric correlations using weighted least squares, which is an asymptotically distribution-free procedure. In computing tetrachoric correlations, it is assumed that the distribution underlying the dichotomous trait is continuous and normal, with a threshold that distinguishes symptomatic subjects from healthy ones (15). Model fitting was carried out using the Mx program (16) to build structural equation models for multiple groups. Chi-square goodness-of-fit statistics were used to assess how well a model fit the data. The superiority of alternative, hierarchically nested models was assessed by the difference in chi-square values of the models, which is itself distributed as chi-square with degrees of freedom equal to the difference in degrees of freedom of the models to be compared. This was done to

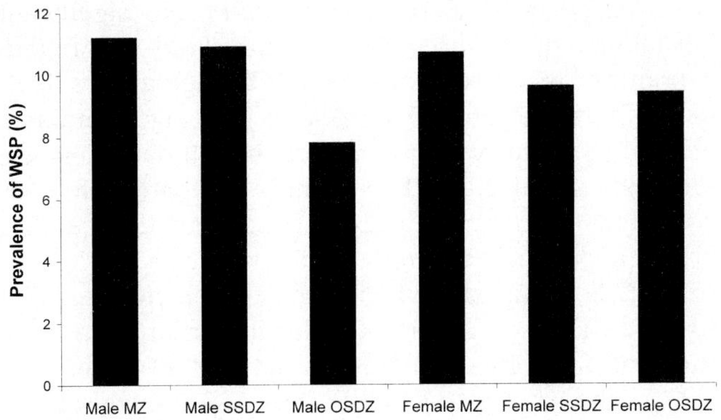

Figure 1. Prevalence of widespread pain (WSP) in the twins in the FinnTwin12 study by sex and twin pair type (monozygotic [MZ], same-sex dizygotic [SSDZ], or opposite-sex dizygotic [OSDZ]).

compare models where different components of variance have been specified. Based on the best model, variance components were computed and 95% confidence intervals estimated.

RESULTS

A total of 355 subjects of the total 3,578 individual twins fulfilled the criteria for WSP, thus yielding a prevalence among 11-year-old twins of 9.9%. The prevalence among girls was 9.9% and that among boys was 10.0%. Figure 1 shows the prevalence of WSP by zygosity of the pairs and sex of the subject. The prevalence of WSP did not vary by zygosity or sex.

Table 1 shows the concordance and discordance for WSP. Both the probandwise concordances, i.e., the proportion of cases that occur in concordant pairs, and the tetrachoric correlations of liability in MZ and DZ twins indicated little difference between MZ and DZ pairs, but among girls the probandwise concordances and correlations were greater than among boys. The correlations were significantly different from 0. This pattern of correlations suggests that WSP is correlated within twin pairs, but there is little genetic influence. This was assessed in more detail through modeling.

Table 1. Concordance and discordance for WSP in twin pairs from the FinnTwin12 study*

	Boys		Girls		
	MZ	DZ	MZ	DZ	OSDZ
No. of concordant pairs	9	9	12	9	13
No. of discordant pairs	48	51	38	34	80†
Total no. of pairs	294	317	289	271	618
Total no. of twins with WSP	66	69	62	52	106
Probandwise concordance	0.27	0.26	0.39	0.35	0.25
Tetrachoric correlation	0.38	0.37	0.59	0.54	0.43

* MZ = monozygotic; DZ = dizygotic; OSDZ = opposite-sex dizygotic.
† 35 boys and 45 girls with widespread pain (WSP) in these 80 discordant pairs.

Model fitting started with estimating parameters that indicate the relative strengths of genetic and environmental influences. First, we fit a full-sex differences model (ACE) in which estimates for h, c, and e are allowed to differ in magnitude between boys and girls. This fit the data well ($\chi^2 = 7.49$, degrees of freedom [df] 10, $P = 0.68$), but, because the estimates for the genetic component, h ($h^2 < 7\%$), in boys and girls were nonsignificant, we dropped these from the model. The CE model with sex-specific effects fit the data just as well with fewer parameters ($\chi^2 = 7.60$, df 12, $P = 0.82$). This was the model against which we tested other submodels.

A model in which estimates of c and e parameters were constrained to be equal in magnitude across sexes did not fit as well ($\chi^2 = 10.25$, df 13, $P = 0.67$), with a χ^2 difference of 2.65 (difference in df 1, $P = 0.10$). We also fit a sex differences CE model in which an additional parameter is estimated that represents the extent to which the same shared environmental influences are expressed in boys and girls. This did not result in an improvement in fit, with the model χ^2 value being 7.48 (df 11, $P = 0.76$).

Table 2 shows the parameter estimates and 95% confidence intervals for the final model of shared and nonshared environmental effects differing in magnitude between boys and girls. Of the variation in liability to WSP, 35% among boys and 56% among girls could be attributed to shared familial effects, and the remainder was attributed to unshared environmental effects.

Table 2. Parameter estimates for best-fitting biometric model to data on widespread pain (WSP) in Finnish twin children age 11*

Sex	Proportion of variance in liability to WSP attributed to shared environmental effects	Proportion of variance in liability to WSP attributed to unshared environmental effects
Boys	35.4 (19.8–50.6)	64.6 (49.4–80.2)
Girls	55.6 (39.1–69.6)	44.4 (30.4–60.9)

* Values are the percentage (95% confidence intervals).

DISCUSSION

This study investigated the pattern of familial aggregation of WSP in a large set of twins assessed within a narrow age range. The analysis indicates that there is substantial familial aggregation of WSP, but genetic factors are not of major importance. Rather, there are nongenetic familial influences that result in the same degree of similarity in both MZ and DZ twin pairs. Genetic modeling suggested that for boys about one-third, and for girls about one-half, of the interindividual variation in liability to WSP was accounted for by familial factors. The genetic modeling was based on the threshold model, which assumes that there is variation in the susceptibility or liability to the trait on a single dimension. Multiple environmental factors and multiple genes, each with a small effect, are assumed to contribute to the liability. Given that single genes for widespread pain or related disorders have not been identified, and that the environmental risk factors are largely unknown, the threshold model can be considered reasonable for providing estimates of the relative role of genetic and environmental effects.

A role for genetic factors could not be totally excluded, but a model including additive genetic factors suggests that genetic factors account for at most 10% of total variance. Because the relative influence of genetic factors on a trait may vary depending on age, the later influence of genetic factors on WSP and FM cannot be excluded by the results of this study. Environmental factors unique to each twin pair, unrelated to sex, were associated with WSP, but the relative influence of shared environmental factors was greater among girls.

This study showed similar prevalences of WSP in MZ and DZ twins and in both sexes. A sex difference in subjects of this age has not been found in previous studies (17), although, in adults, women have more WSP than men (2). The comparison of MZ and DZ similarity by the classic twin model presumes that the prevalence of the trait being studied does not vary by twin type. More specifically, it assumes that the shared environmental variance does not differ by zygosity (14). In our study, nearly all pairs were living together in the same household, and most attended the same school, sharing the same physical and social environments. There were insufficient numbers of pairs living in separate homes or attending different schools to permit further analysis.

There are no previous studies about the genetics of WSP. However, determinants of the pressure pain threshold, which has been found to be low both in adults (18) and in children with WSP (19,20), have been studied among adult twins (21). In the latter study, dolorimeter measurements of the pressure pain threshold among 269 female MZ pairs and 340 female DZ pairs showed equally strong correlations for both MZ ($r = 0.57$) and DZ pairs ($r = 0.51$). No significant heritability of the pressure pain threshold was found. The intraclass correlations did not change after adjustment for numerous covariates such as age, smoking, alcohol use, analgesic use, general health questionnaire score, or social class. The authors of that study concluded that "learned patterns of behavior within families are an important determinant of perceived sensitivity to pain" (21). Thus, shared environmental factors seemed to have the most important influence on pressure pain threshold, as well as on WSP in the present study.

The concept of WSP is based on consensual criteria (1). Subjects fulfilling the criteria for WSP may have different pathophysiology for WSP. Thus, heterogeneity of the phenotype might exist, which should be taken into account when interpreting the results. In addition, the ACR criteria were originally developed for adults. However, the criteria have been used in studies on children (22), and population-based studies have shown surprisingly similar symptoms of WSP and FM in children (17,20,23) as in adults in the general population (3) and in clinics (24).

In this study, determination of WSP was based on a questionnaire, which had good test–retest reliability. However, unlike previous adult studies, we used an additional criterion for pain frequency (pain at least once a week) during the prior months. Although the recall error with regard to timing is possible, it was minimized with a clear definition ("since the summer"). The 3-month period was used because the questionnaire was originally developed for evaluating WSP and FM, and the definition of FM includes the requirement of WSP for at least 3 months. The exclusion of pain due to injury was decided because children at the age of 11 often have several small injuries. We were interested in nonspecific pain. However, this might have caused bias due to variation of the individuals' own opinion of the cause of pain.

Although the prevalence of WSP was as high in boys as in girls, and the modeling indicated that variability specific to one sex could not be detected, the point estimates of components of variance (shared versus unshared family effects) differed by sex. Thus, there may be factors external to the family that contribute relatively more to boys' WSP than to girls' WSP.

The results highlight the need for evaluation of family and other environmental factors when dealing with children with multiple pain symptoms. Such factors as psychosocial problems, including stressful roles or recently experienced major life events, enmeshment between child and mother, and other evidence of family dysfunction have been associated with recurrent musculoskeletal pain in children (25). Lower family education and chronic family difficulties (26) and psychosocial factors (27) have been associated with persistent musculoskeletal pain. Learned pain behavior may also play a role (28). In the present study, essentially all the children were cohabiting with 1 or both parents and shared all familial influences as well as most nonfamilial influences, including neighborhood and school influences. So, to the degree that such contextual variables contribute to the reports of symptomatic pain at this age, these twins may well be exhibiting maximum concordance. As the twins age, the relative contribution of genetic and shared environmental factors may change.

ACKNOWLEDGMENTS

We are grateful to Kauko Heikkilä and Olli Lounela for database management.

REFERENCES

1. Wolfe F, Smythe HA, Yunus MB, Bennett RM, Bombardier C, Goldenberg DL, et al. The American College of Rheumatology 1990 criteria for the classification of fibromyalgia: report of the Multicenter Criteria Committee. Arthritis Rheum 1990;33:160–72.
2. Croft P, Rigby AS, Boswell R, Schollum J, Silman A. The prevalence of chronic widespread pain in the general population. J Rheumatol 1993;20:710–3.
3. Wolfe F, Ross K, Anderson J, Russell IJ, Hebert L. The prevalence and characteristics of fibromyalgia in the general population. Arthritis Rheum 1995;38:19–28.
4. Macfarlane GJ, Thomas E, Papageorgiou AC, Schollum J, Croft PR, Silman AJ. The natural history of chronic pain in the community: a better prognosis than in the clinic? J Rheumatol 1996;23:1617–20.
5. Mikkelsson M, Salminen JJ, Kautiainen H. Non-specific musculoskeletal pain in preadolescents: prevalence and 1-year persistence. Pain 1997;73:29–35.
6. Pellegrino MJ, Waylonis GW, Sommer A. Familial occurrence of primary fibromyalgia. Arch Phys Med Rehabil 1989;70:61–3.
7. Buskila D, Neumann L, Hazanov I, Carmi R. Familial aggregation in the fibromyalgia syndrome. Semin Arthritis Rheum 1996;26: 605–11.
8. Roizenblatt S, Tufik S, Goldenberg J, Pinto LR, Hilário MO, Feldman D. Juvenile fibromyalgia: clinical and polysomnographic aspects. J Rheumatol 1997;24:579–85.
9. Yunus MB, Khan MA, Rawlings KK, Green JR, Olson JM, Shah S. Genetic linkage analysis of multicase families with fibromyalgia syndrome. J Rheumatol 1999;26:408–12.
10. Järvinen P, Aho K. Fibromyalgia in a pair of identical twins. Clin Exp Rheumatol 1990;8:615–6.
11. Kaprio J, Koskenvuo M, Rose RJ. Population-based twin registries: illustrative applications in genetic epidemiology and behavioral genetics from the Finnish Twin Cohort Study. Acta Genet Med Gemellol (Roma) 1990;39:427–39.
12. Sarna S, Kaprio J, Sistonen P, Koskenvuo M. Diagnosis of twin zygosity by mailed questionnaire. Hum Hered 1978;28:241–54.
13. Goldsmith HH. A zygosity questionnaire for young twins: a research note. Behav Genet 1991;21:257–69.
14. Neale MC, Cardon LR. Methodology for genetic studies of twins and families. Dordrecht (The Netherlands): Kluwer Academic; 1992.
15. Falconer DS. Introduction to quantitative genetics. 2nd ed. Harlow (UK): Longman; 1981.
16. Neale MC. Mx: statistical modelling [computer program and manual]. Richmond (VA): Medical College of Virginia, Department of Psychiatry; 1994.
17. Mikkelsson M, Sourander A, Piha J, Salminen JJ. Psychiatric symptoms in preadolescents with musculoskeletal pain and fibromyalgia. Pediatrics 1997;100:220–7.
18. Granges G, Littlejohn G. Pressure pain threshold in pain-free subjects, in patients with chronic regional pain syndromes, and in patients with fibromyalgia syndrome. Arthritis Rheum 1993;36: 642–6.
19. Buskila D, Press J, Gedalia A, Klein M, Neumann L, Boehm R, et al. Assessment of nonarticular tenderness and prevalence of fibromyalgia in children. J Rheumatol 1993;20:368–70.
20. Mikkelsson M. Musculoskeletal pain and fibromyalgia in preadolescents: prospective 1-year follow-up study [dissertation]. Turku (Finland): Annales Universitatis Turkuensis, Ser D, Medica-Odontologica; 1998.
21. MacGregor AJ, Griffiths GO, Baker J, Spector TD. Determinants of pressure pain threshold in adult twins: evidence that shared environmental influences predominate. Pain 1997;73:253–7.
22. Buskila D. Fibromyalgia in children: lessons from assessing nonarticular tenderness. J Rheumatol 1996;23:2017–9.
23. Mikkelsson M. One year outcome of preadolescents with fibromyalgia. J Rheumatol 1999;26:674–82.
24. Wolfe F. The relation between tender points and fibromyalgia symptom variables: evidence that fibromyalgia is not a discrete disorder in the clinic. Ann Rheum Dis 1997;56:268–71.
25. Sherry DD, McGuire T, Mellins E, Salmonson K, Wallace CA, Nepom B. Psychosomatic musculoskeletal pain in childhood: clinical and psychological analyses of 100 children. Pediatrics 1991;88:1093–9.
26. Flatø B, Aasland A, Vandvik IH, Førre Ø. Outcome and predictive factors in children with chronic idiopathic musculoskeletal pain. Clin Exp Rheumatol 1997;15:569–77.
27. Aasland A, Flatø B, Vandvik IH. Psychosocial factors in children with idiopathic musculoskeletal pain: a prospective, longitudinal study. Acta Paediatr 1997;86:740–6.
28. McGrath PA. The multidimensional assessment and management of recurrent pain syndromes in children. Behav Res Ther 1987;25: 251–62.

ARTHRITIS & RHEUMATISM
Vol. 44, No. 2, February 2001, pp 486–489

CONCISE COMMUNICATIONS

Synovial stimulatory protein fragments copurify with woodchuck hepatitis virus: implications for the etiology of arthritis in chronic hepatitis B virus infection

Arthritis pain is a common complaint among those chronically infected with hepatitis B virus (HBV). Biopsy-proven polyarteritis nodosa was reported to occur in as many as one-third to one-half of those who were persistently infected with HBV (1,2). Even acute arthritis has been observed following acute HBV infection (2). These syndromes have been associated with hepatitis B surface antigen (HBsAg)–anti-HBsAg immune complexes in serum, synovial fluid and membranes, and diseased vessels (3).

Previously, it has been shown that the secretion of enveloped HBV and woodchuck hepatitis virus (WHV) is dependent upon the cellular endoplasmic reticulum enzyme α-glucosidase I (4). In the course of studying WHV derived from chronically infected woodchucks that had been treated with the glucosidase inhibitor *N*-nonyl DNJ, a protein determined to be an N-terminal fragment of "synovial stimulatory protein" (referred to as p205) was found to be associated with WHV subviral and/or viral particles.

WHV was purified from serum samples derived from the study described by Block et al (4). Briefly, WHV and polypeptides associated with woodchuck M286 were resolved through 12.5% sodium dodecyl sulfate–polyacrylamide gel electrophoresis (SDS-PAGE), as shown in Figure 1, after partial purification by sedimentation through 20% sucrose, resuspension in 1× phosphate buffered saline (150 m*M* NaCl, 10 m*M* Na_2HPO_4, 1.5 m*M* K_2HPO_4 [pH 7.12]), and resolution through a Zorbax GF-450 high-performance liquid chromatography (HPLC) sizing column (DuPont Laboratories, Wilmington, DE). The HPLC elution fraction containing species with MW >450 kd (void peak) was stained with silver following resolution through SDS-PAGE, and the results are shown in Figure 1.

Lanes 1 and 2 show the proteins associated with mock-infected, untreated animals after pelleting through either 20% sucrose and HPLC or 20% sucrose alone, respectively. As shown in lane 1, sera from mock-infected, untreated animals contained very little protein that stained with silver. In contrast, lanes 3–6 show the polypeptides found in the HPLC void peak from woodchuck M286 either before treatment (lane 3) or after 1, 2, or 3 weeks of treatment (lanes 4–6, respectively). Several polypeptides specific to the infected woodchuck serum samples are indicated by arrows. Surprisingly, the polypeptide originally thought to be the WHV-M, based on its MW of 36 kd, was determined to have 92% homology with a proteolytic fragment of synovial stimulatory protein (p205) (Table 1). The WHV-M protein was later identified as having an MW of 42 kd (data not shown).

The p205 fragment was found only in samples from which WHV was purified, and not in control samples from uninfected woodchucks. Interestingly, this peptide fragment appeared 1 week after drug treatment and disappeared during the study period. Although the peptide fragment may have been induced by treatment, it was also seen in untreated animals (data not shown). Moreover, the amount of p205 fragment copurifying with WHV particles decreased as a function of glucosidase inhibitor treatment. For example, lanes 3–6 in Figure 1 show polypeptides associated with WHV particles purified from serum from the same chronically infected animal prior to glucosidase inhibition and at 1, 2, and 3 weeks of inhibition, respectively. Other experiments confirmed that glucosidase was inhibited in the treated animals in a dose-dependent manner, and there was no detectable toxicity associated with the treatment (4). Clearly, however, the p205 polypeptide fragment was no longer recovered from the WHV particles purified from animal sera after 3 weeks of glucosidase inhibition.

Although these results are preliminary and are derived from a small number of animals (n = 4), they are thought

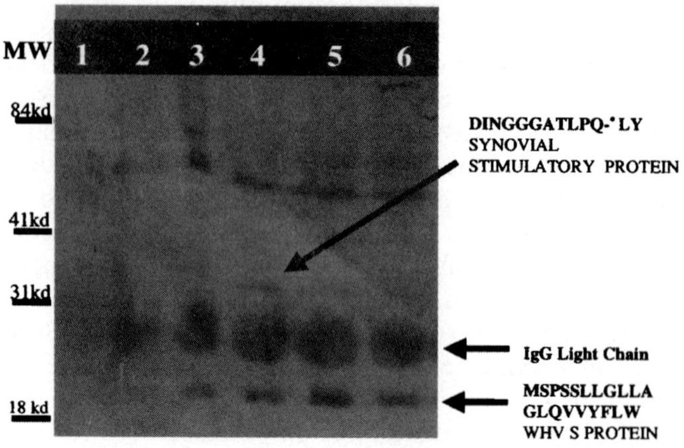

Figure 1. Polypeptides associated with woodchuck hepatitis virus (WHV). WHV particles were purified from the serum of woodchuck M286 as described in the text and resolved through 12.5% sodium dodecyl sulfate–polyacrylamide gel electrophoresis. Polypeptides were detected by silver staining. Serum from an uninfected woodchuck after 20% sucrose and high-performance liquid chromatography gel filtration (lane 1) and serum from an uninfected woodchuck after 20% sucrose alone (lane 2) are shown as controls. The polypeptides associated with woodchuck M286 before glucosidase inhibition and after 1, 2, and 3 weeks of 25 mg/kg/day of the glucosidase inhibitor N-nonyl DNJ are shown in lanes 3–6, respectively. **Arrows** indicate the IgG light chain as well as polypeptides of interest that were excised and subjected to N-terminal amino acid sequencing. These polypeptides were determined to have the indicated sequences (see Table 1). In our sequence analysis, the position indicated by the asterisk was determined to be either a K or a P. Because of this uncertainty, it was not used in the sequence search.

Table 1. Amino acid sequence of selected woodchuck hepatitis virus (WHV)–associated polypeptides*

Polypeptide MW (in kd) and closest match	Amino acid sequence
22	MSPSSLLGLLAGLQVVYFLW
sAg	MSPSSLLGLLAGLQVVYFLW
36	DINGGGATLPQ-*LY
Synovial stimulatory protein	DINGGGATLPQP LY

* Polypeptides were resolved through sodium dodecyl sulfate–polyacrylamide gels, as shown in Figure 1. Selected polypeptides were excised from the gel and subjected to amino terminal sequence analysis (see ref. 10). The amino acids determined for 2 of the polypeptides are shown with their closest matches from the Swiss-Prot Annotated Protein Sequence database (accession no. P80697, 5, and 11). In our sequence analysis, the position indicated by an asterisk was determined to be either a K or a P. Because of this uncertainty, it was not used in the sequence search. sAg = WHV surface antigen.

provoking. P205 is a newly characterized and microsequenced polypeptide (with a native MW of 205 kd) that has been isolated from the synovial fluid of patients with rheumatoid arthritis (RA) (5–6). P205 was reported to have homology with the IgG heavy chain and rheumatoid factor binding region, and was also reported to have bioactivity characterized by induction of T lymphocyte proliferation. It was suggested that p205 is secreted by synovial cells and that it might play a role in the etiology of human RA (5,6). We found that a 36-kd peptide fragment of p205 copurified with the woodchuck subviral particles. The origin of the peptide fragment remains unknown. Although proteolysis of the 205-kd protein may be the result of drug treatment, the finding of the peptide in untreated (but infected) animals suggests another mechanism.

The copurification of p205 with WHV raises the possibility that viral and cytokine polypeptides may interact in a way that is related to the etiology of arthritis syndromes in HBV-infected individuals. Glucosidase inhibition has been shown to reduce the amount of enveloped WHV in the serum of chronically infected woodchucks (4). Moreover, although surface antigen (the major viral envelope glycoprotein) secretion from hepatocytes is not immediately influenced by glucosidase inhibition (Figure 1), the secretion of HBV M and L antigens is extremely sensitive (7,8). Thus, it is possible that p205 association with WHV is mediated by the HBV M or L polypeptides. Alternatively, the synthesis or secretion of p205 itself could be reduced by glucosidase inhibition.

More work is needed to determine whether the copurification of a p205 fragment with WHV is biologically relevant or merely adventitious. However, given that the finding of arthritis pain in association with hepatitis infection coincides with a recent report of another glucosidase inhibitor depressing the severity of arthritis-like symptoms in an experimental model of the disease (9), it is tempting to propose a role for the binding of p205 and HBV in the etiology of arthritis-like syndromes. In this case, the possibility should also be considered that glucosidase inhibitors might have therapeutic value in the treatment of such syndromes.

Anand Mehta, DPhil
Xuanyong Lu, PhD
Timothy Block, PhD
Jefferson Medical College
Philadelphia, PA
Anthony Willis, DPhil, FRS
Raymond Dwek, DPhil, FRS
Oxford University
Oxford, UK
Bud Tennant, DVM
Cornell University
Ithaca, NY
Baruch Blumberg, MD, PhD
Fox Chase Cancer Center
Philadelphia, PA

1. Heathcote EJ, Dudley FJ, Sherlock S. Association of polyarteritis and Australia antigen. Gut 1972;13:319–20.
2. Schumacher HR, Gall EP. Arthritis in acute hepatitis and chronic active hepatitis: pathology of the synovial membrane with evidence for the presence of Australia antigen in synovial membranes. Am J Med 1974;57:655–64.
3. Wands JR, Mann EA, Isselbacher KJ. The pathogenesis of arthritis associated with acute hepatitis B surface antigen positive hepatitis: complement activation and characterization of circulating immune complexes. J Clin Invest 1975;55:930–6.
4. Block TM, Lu X, Mehta S, Blumberg BS, Tennant B, Ebling M, et al. Treatment of woodchucks chronically infected with woodchuck hepatitis virus with protein folding inhibitors. Nat Med 1998;4: 610–4.
5. Hain NAK, Stuhlmuller B, Hahn GR, Kalden JR, Deutzmann R, Burmester ER. Biochemical characterization and microsequencing of a 205 kDa synovial protein stimulatory for T cells and reactive with rheumatoid containing sera. J Immunol 1996;157: 1773–80.
6. Bläss S, Schumann F, Hain NAK, Engel JM, Stuhlmüller B, Burmester GR. p205 is a major target of autoreactive T cells in rheumatoid arthritis. Arthritis Rheum 1999;42:971–80.
7. Mehta A, Lu X, Block TM, Blumberg BS, Dwek RA. Similar glycoproteins with drastically different sensitivities to glycosylation processing. Proc Natl Acad Sci U S A 1997;94:1822–7.
8. Lu X, Mehta A, Dadmarz M, Blumberg B, Dwek RA, Block TM. Aberrant trafficking of hepatitis B virus glycoproteins in cells in which N-glycan processing is inhibited. Proc Natl Acad Sci U S A 1997;94:2380–5.
9. Van den Broek LA, Kat-Van Den Nieuwenhof MW, Butters TD, van Boeckel CA. Synthesis of alpha-glucosidase I inhibitors showing antiviral (HIV-1) and immunosuppressive activity. J Pharm Pharmacol 1996;48:172–8.
10. Mattu TS, Pleass RJ, Willis AC, Kilian M, Wormald MR, Lellouch AC, et al. The glycosylation and structure of human serum IgA1, Fab, and Fc regions and the role of N-glycosylation on Fcalpha receptor interactions. J Biol Chem 1998;273:2260–72.

The rate of recurrence of isolated congenital heart block: a population-based study

Isolated congenital heart block (CHB) is a potentially life-threatening disease caused by maternal antibodies to SSA and/or SSB. The rate of recurrence of CHB is not well known. Herein, we report the familial occurrence of CHB in Finland and discuss the rationale for the prophylaxis of CHB.

We reviewed the hospital registries and the pacemaker insertion registries of the 5 university hospitals in Finland for patients born between 1950 and 1999 and diagnosed with heart block before the age of 15 years. The obstetric case records of the mothers and the hospital records of the neonates, children, and adults were reviewed to verify the time of detection of heart block and to demonstrate any associated cardiac malformations. Patients were included in the study only if the heart block was second (1 case) or third degree, diagnosed by ultrasound during pregnancy or by electrocardiogram during the first day of life, and there were no intracardiac malformations considered to be causally related to CHB (1).

The mothers of these children (and adults) were contacted personally, by mail, and/or by telephone, and familial data were collected. If the mothers were not contacted or had died, the data were collected from close relatives and/or from the population registry of Finland. A subset of cases reported previously by us (2) was included in the present study.

We identified 101 offspring with isolated CHB. There were 2 twins concordant and 2 twins discordant for CHB. Of the 91 mothers who had given birth to at least 1 child with CHB, 2 could not be identified, and from 5 mothers familial data were not available. The final analysis consisted of data from 84 (92%) of all 91 affected mothers.

Before the birth of the first child with CHB (index delivery), these mothers had borne 57 children and after the index delivery, 47 children had been born. Of these 47 children, 8 had CHB. Thus, the risk of recurrence of CHB was 17% (8 of 47), and the familial occurrence was 9% (10 of

108, i.e., 8 recurrences + 2 concordant twins/57 children born before and 47 after the index delivery + 4 twins). Of the 33 pregnancies immediately subsequent to the index delivery, 6 (18%) were complicated by CHB.

Although isolated CHB defined using stringent inclusion criteria is practically always immune mediated (3), our results may not be generalizable to all studies in which maternal antibodies to SSA and/or SSB are an inclusion criterion. However, our findings are quite similar to previously reported results. In a review including 5 studies published between 1981 and 1987 and reporting sibling data from 64 index cases, the risk of recurrence was 1 in 3 (4). In a multicenter study by Scott et al, this risk was 20% (4 of 20) (5). Waltuck and Buyon recruited 57 mothers of children with CHB from many different sources, and reported that 4 (15%) of 26 subsequent pregnancies in 23 women were complicated by CHB (6). A recent study reported data from the Research Registry for Neonatal Lupus including 105 affected mothers whose sera contained anti-SSA and/or SSB; 8 (16%) of the 49 pregnancies immediately subsequent to the birth of a child with CHB resulted in a second child with CHB (7).

In this nationwide study, we identified the majority of children with isolated CHB born in Finland between 1950 and 1999 and collected familial data from practically all mothers of these children. We consider that our study had no selection bias, and the number of pregnancies studied was sufficiently large. The 17% rate of recurrence of CHB found in this study may be considered high by affected mothers.

Many of the mothers in this study have been worried that they might give birth to another child with CHB and have reduced their planned family size. CHB is a serious disease associated with high mortality (16%) and considerable morbidity in later life (1). Although the management of CHB in children is usually successful, the disease is often a great burden for the whole family. CHB is also an expensive disease for the community, requiring frequent followup visits, hospitalizations, pacemaker insertions, and sometimes even cardiac transplantation.

The ultimate goal of the management of CHB is prevention. There are, however, several problems in preventing CHB, including the identification of mothers at risk of having a child with CHB (3,8). In general, a woman with antibodies to SSA and/or SSB has a low chance (1–2%) of having a child with CHB (9). The group of women who probably have the highest risk of having an infant with CHB are those with a previously affected child. Should these women receive prophylaxis for CHB during pregnancy, and are there any effective treatments?

There are occasional case reports on possible prevention of CHB recurrence by administering corticosteroids, plasmapheresis, or intravenous gamma globulin to the mother before and during the second trimester of pregnancy (4,10,11). Successful early treatment to prevent the development of possible CHB has been reported by Rosenthal et al (12) and Manthorpe et al (13). In these 2 case reports, serial fetal echocardiograms were performed in high-risk pregnancies, and when pericardial effusion and premature atrial contractions (12) or first- and second-degree heart block (13) were noted, the mothers were given 4 mg dexamethasone orally daily. Both of these children had first-degree heart block after birth, but were otherwise healthy.

Due to lack of controlled studies, treatments to prevent CHB are considered purely experimental. However, given the high mortality and morbidity and the considerable risk of recurrence associated with CHB, they could be an option for pregnant women with a previously affected child. Frequent fetal echocardiograms starting at the 16th gestational week and the institution of dexamethasone only when an abnormality is found would be, at present, the most rational approach.

Supported by the Helsinki University Hospital Research Foundation.

Heiki Julkunen, MD
Peijas Hospital
Vantaa, Finland
Marianne Eronen, MD
Helsinki University Hospital
Helsinki, Finland

1. Eronen M, Siren MK, Ekblad H, Tikanoja T, Julkunen H, Paavilainen T. Short and long-term outcome of children with congenital complete heart block diagnosed in utero or as a newborn. Pediatrics 2000;106:86–91.
2. Julkunen H, Kaaja R, Wallgren E, Teramo K. Isolated congenital heart block: fetal and infant outcome and familial incidence of heart block. Obstet Gynecol 1993;82:11–6.
3. Julkunen H, Kaaja R, Siren MK, Mack C, McCready S, Holthöfer H, et al. Immune-mediated congenital heart block (CHB): identifying and counseling patients at risk for having children with CHB. Semin Arthritis Rheum 1998;28:97–106.
4. Buyon J, Roubey R, Swersky S, Pompeo L, Parke A, Baxi L, et al. Complete congenital heart block: risk of occurrence and therapeutic approach to prevention. J Rheumatol 1988;15:1104–8.
5. Scott JS, Maddison PJ, Taylor PV, Esscher E, Scott O, Skimmer RP. Connective-tissue disease, antibodies to ribonucleoprotein, and congenital heart block. N Engl J Med 1983;309:209–12.
6. Waltuck J, Buyon P. Autoantibody-associated congenital heart block: outcome in mothers and children. Ann Intern Med 1994; 120:544–51.
7. Buyon JP, Hiebert R, Copel J, Craft J, Friedman D, Katholi M, et al. Autoimmune-associated congenital heart block: demographics, mortality, morbidity and recurrence rates obtained from a national neonatal lupus registry. J Am Coll Cardiol 1998;31:1658–66.
8. Press J, Uziel Y, Laxer RM, Luy L, Hamilton RM, Silverman ED. Long-term outcome of mothers of children with complete congenital heart block. Am J Med 1996;100:328–32.
9. Lee LA. Neonatal lupus erythematosus. J Invest Dermatol 1993; 100:9S–13S.
10. Barclay CS, French MA, Ross LD, Sokol RJ. Successful pregnancy following steroid therapy and plasma exchange in a woman with anti-Ro (SS-A) antibodies: case report. Br J Obstet Gynaecol 1987;94:369–71.
11. Kaaja R, Julkunen H, Ämmälä P, Teppo AM, Kurki P. Congenital heart block: successful prophylactic treatment with intravenous gamma globulin and corticosteroid therapy. Am J Obstet Gynecol 1991;165:1333–4.
12. Rosenthal D, Druzin M, Chin C, Dubin A. A new therapeutic approach to the fetus with congenital complete heart block: preemptive, targeted therapy with dexamethasone. Obstet Gynecol 1998;92:689–91.
13. Manthorpe R, Gudmundsson S, Salomonsson S, Wahren-Herlenius M, Brucato A, Theander E. Sjögren's syndrome—successful treatment of fetal AV-block: a case report [abstract]. Scand J Rheumatol 2000;29 Suppl 114:P97.

Lupus band test yields negative results in primary antiphospholipid syndrome

The appropriate classification of patients with antiphospholipid syndrome (APS) as having either primary APS or systemic lupus erythematosus (SLE)–associated APS sometimes raises puzzling questions (1,2), but may have practical implications, especially for management of pregnancies. The nonlesional lupus band test (LBT) is considered to yield "a very useful piece of diagnostic information in difficult cases of SLE" (3). Although the LBT's specificity for SLE has been discussed (3), the test's relevance has been recently reaffirmed (4). We prospectively performed the LBT on patients with primary APS and on others with SLE.

Twenty-six consecutive patients with primary APS were studied. All fulfilled the preliminary classification criteria for definite APS (5), and we applied strict criteria to exclude possible SLE (2). Our study included 21 women and 5 men with a mean ± SD age of 36.5 ± 8.6 years (range 24–54 years). The LBT was performed a mean ± SD of 62 ± 71 months (range 3–275 months) after the first documented thrombotic or obstetric event. Except for 2 women presenting with miscarriages only, all patients had histories of (usually recurrent) thrombotic events. Arteries were affected in 18 of these 24 patients and veins in 11 (both were affected in 5). Among the 18 patients with arterial involvement, 7 fulfilled the criteria for Sneddon's syndrome (6). Six of the 19 women with arterial or venous involvement had a history of either fetal death or ≥3 unexplained consecutive spontaneous abortions.

The 26 patients with primary APS were definitely positive for antiphospholipid antibodies, i.e., anticardiolipin antibodies (high titers in 13 patients, medium titers in 12), mainly of the IgG isotype, and/or lupus anticoagulant (in 13 patients). Titers of antinuclear antibodies (ANA) determined on HEp-2 cells were as follows: negative (≤1:50) in 16 patients, low positive (1:80–1:160) in 3, and medium positive (1:200–1:320) in 7. By definition, all patients with primary APS were seronegative for antibodies to double-stranded DNA (dsDNA) by *Crithidia* fluorescence or Farr assays (2), while 3 patients with medium positive ANA titers had low or borderline titers of antibodies to dsDNA by enzyme-linked immunosorbent assay (ELISA), as reported by others (7).

The results were compared with those of 13 consecutive patients with SLE (11 women and 2 men) fulfilling the 1997 update of the revised criteria of the American College of Rheumatology (8). Their mean ± SD age at the time of the study was 32.5 ± 14 years (range 17–65 years). The LBT was performed a mean ± SD of 71 ± 57 months (range 1–180 months) after disease onset. In 10 patients, SLE was clearly active at the time of the study. For the 13 patients with SLE, ANA titers were as follows: low positive (1:100) in 1, medium positive (1:200) in 1, and highly positive (≥1:1,000) in 11. All but 2 SLE patients had antibodies to dsDNA, as shown by *Crithidia* fluorescence and/or Farr assays. At the time of the study, 2 SLE patients had associated APS according to the Sapporo criteria (5).

After we obtained informed consent, the LBT was performed on nonlesional, sun-exposed skin of the patients' forearms. Fisher's exact test was used for statistics. Direct immunofluorescence findings are summarized in Table 1.

Results of the LBT were negative in all patients with primary APS, except in 1 patient who had weak granular IgM deposits at the dermo–epidermal junction. At the time of the study, this woman had low positive (1:80) ANA titers, negative titers of antibodies to dsDNA by ELISA, medium positive IgG titers, and negative titers of IgM anticardiolipin antibodies. A further LBT performed 3 years later had a negative result, and her clinical and serologic status remained unchanged after a total followup period of 8 years. However, the LBT yielded a positive result in 62% of SLE patients. This finding is in accord with the 70% positive result (105 of 149 patients) for the LBT

Table 1. Results of lupus band test performed on nonlesional, sun-exposed skin*

Antibody positivity	Patients with primary APS (n = 26)	Patients with SLE (n = 13)	*P*
Anti-IgG	0 (0)	7 (54)	<0.001
Anti-IgM	1 (4)	8 (62)	<0.001
Anti-IgA	0 (0)	3 (23)	NS
Anti-C1q	0 (0)	6 (46)	0.001
Anti-C3	0 (0)	1 (8)	NS
Any antibody above	1 (4)	8 (62)	<0.001

* Except where otherwise indicated, values are the number (percent) of patients. Primary APS = primary antiphospholipid syndrome; SLE = systemic lupus erythematosus; NS = not significant.

in our retrospective SLE data bank, as well as with reports in the literature (3).

We conclude that the LBT gives a negative result in nearly all patients with primary APS defined by strict criteria. In addition to other tests, such as the determination of IgG antibodies directed to nucleosomes (9), the LBT may be useful for classifying patients with APS into the categories of primary versus SLE-related APS.

Jean-Charles Piette, MD
Eduardo Marinho, MD
Du Le Thi Huong, MD
Zahir Amoura, MD
Camille Francès, MD
Hôpital Pitié-Salpêtrière
Paris, France

1. Hughes GRV. The antiphospholipid syndrome: ten years on. Lancet 1993;342:341–4.
2. Piette JC. 1996 Diagnostic and classification criteria for the antiphospholipid/cofactors syndrome: a "mission impossible"? Lupus 1996;5:354–63.
3. Sontheimer RD, Provost TT. Cutaneous manifestations of lupus erythematosus. In: Wallace DJ, Hahn BH, editors. Dubois' lupus erythematosus. 5th ed. Baltimore (MD): Williams & Wilkins, 1997. p. 569–623.
4. Cardinali C, Caproni M, Fabbri P. The utility of the lupus band test on sun-protected non-lesional skin for the diagnosis of systemic lupus erythematosus. Clin Exp Rheumatol 1999;17:427–32.
5. Wilson WA, Gharavi AE, Koike T, Lockshin MD, Branch DW, Piette JC, et al. International consensus statement on preliminary classification criteria for definite antiphospholipid syndrome: report of an international workshop. Arthritis Rheum 1999;42:1309–11.
6. Francès C, Papo T, Wechsler B, Laporte JL, Biousse V, Piette JC. Sneddon syndrome with or without antiphospholipid antibodies: a comparative study in 46 patients. Medicine (Baltimore) 1999;78:209–19.
7. Krause I, Cohen J, Blank M, Bakimer R, Cartman A, Hohmann A, et al. Distribution of two common idiotypes of anticardiolipin antibodies in sera of patients with primary antiphospholipid syndrome, systemic lupus erythematosus and monoclonal gammopathies. Lupus 1992;1:91–6.
8. Hochberg MC. Updating the American College of Rheumatology revised criteria for the classification of systemic lupus erythematosus [letter]. Arthritis Rheum 1997;40:1725.
9. Amoura Z, Koutouzov S, Chabre H, Cacoub P, Amoura I, Musset L, et al. Presence of antinucleosome autoantibodies in a restricted set of connective tissue diseases: antinucleosome antibodies of the IgG3 subclass are markers of renal pathogenicity in systemic lupus erythematosus. Arthritis Rheum 2000;43:76–84.

ARTHRITIS & RHEUMATISM
Vol. 44, No. 2, February 2001, pp 490–492

LETTERS

Monoclonal expansion of B cells in Sjögren's syndrome: comment on the article by Martin et al

To the Editor:

We read with interest the report by Martin et al, in which it is reported that lymphomatous B cells from the affected salivary glands of patients with Sjögren's syndrome (SS) produce monoclonal IgMκ rheumatoid factors (RF) (1). This supports the notion that surface immunoglobulin is an important tool for the initial evaluation of nonmalignant B cell clones, which in the future will probably undergo lymphomagenesis. The authors underplay the significance of previous work, since the oligo-monoclonal B lymphocyte process in SS has been studied extensively. Apart from the first description of IgMκ-containing B cells in SS patients with lymphoma (2,3), a large body of knowledge has been mounted with regard to B cell monoclonal expansion in SS. Previous studies from our institution have clearly indicated that patients with SS often have circulating mixed monoclonal IgMκ cryoglobulins with RF reactivity (4). Furthermore, it has been shown that most of the B cells infiltrating the minor salivary glands of SS patients with monoclonal cryoglobulins belong to a single clone (5). Finally, patients with mixed monoclonal cryoglobulinemia are at increased risk of developing lymphoma, as was shown in a 5-year followup study (6). These studies provide indirect evidence that B lymphocytes producing monoclonal RF are found in patients with SS several years before the development of lymphoma. This is reinforced by the presence of cross-reactive idiotypes in the kappa light chain of monoclonal RF of patients with SS and those with Waldenström's macroglobulinemia (7).

The etiology of the longstanding monoclonal expansion of B cells in salivary glands of SS patients is largely unknown. Antigenic selection via the surface immunoglobulin bearing appropriate V_H structures, coupled with additional oncogenic events, such as p53 mutation (8), is an attractive model for further investigation. In this regard, the hypothesis of a putative antigen internalization, either directly or captured by specific antibodies, should be explored. Molecular analysis of B cell infiltration of the salivary glands of SS patients presenting with mixed monoclonal cryoglobulins in their serum may prove to be very useful in elucidating the mechanisms that govern the transition from the polyclonal reactivity to monoclonal expansion.

M. Voulgarelis, MD
A. G. Tzioufas, MD
H. M. Moutsopoulos, MD
National University of Athens
Athens, Greece

1. Martin T, Weber J-C, Levallois H, Labouret N, Soley A, Koenig S, et al. Salivary gland lymphoma in patients with Sjögren's syndrome may frequently develop from rheumatoid factor B cells. Arthritis Rheum 2000;43:908–16.
2. Zulman J, Jaffe R, Talal N. Evidence that the malignant lymphoma of Sjogren's syndrome is a monoclonal B-cell neoplasm. N Engl J Med 1978;299:1215–20.
3. Schmid U, Helbron D, Lennert K. Development of malignant lymphoma in myoepithelial sialadenitis (Sjogren's syndrome). Virchows Arch 1982;385:11–43.
4. Tzioufas AG, Manoussakis MN, Costello R, Silis M, Papadopoulos NM, Moutsopoulos HM. Cryoglobulinemia in autoimmune rheumatic diseases: evidence of circulating monoclonal cryoglobulins in patients with primary Sjögren's syndrome. Arthritis Rheum 1986;29:1098–104.
5. Moutsopoulos HM, Tzioufas AG, Bai MK, Papadopoulos NM, Papadimitriou CS. Association of serum IgM kappa monoclonicity in patients with Sjogren's syndrome with an increased proportion of kappa positive plasma cells infiltrating the labial minor salivary glands. Ann Rheum Dis 1990;49:929–31.
6. Tzioufas AG, Boumba DS, Skopouli FN, Moutsopoulos HM. Mixed monoclonal cryoglobulinemia and monoclonal rheumatoid factor cross-reactive idiotypes as predictive factors for the development of lymphoma in primary Sjögren's syndrome. Arthritis Rheum 1996;39:767–72.
7. Katsikis PD, Youinou PY, Galanopoulou V, Papadopoulos NM, Tzioufas AG, Moutsopoulos HM. Monoclonal process in primary Sjogren's syndrome and cross-reactive idiotype associated with rheumatoid factor. Clin Exp Immunol 1990;82:509–14.
8. Tapinos NI, Polihronis M, Moutsopoulos HM. Lymphoma development in Sjögren's syndrome: novel p53 mutations. Arthritis Rheum 1999;42:1466–72.

Reply

To the Editor:

We thank Dr. Voulgarelis and colleagues for their interest in our report. We of course acknowledge the important contributions of Dr. Moutsopoulos and his group in the field of monoclonal B cell proliferation in salivary glands of patients with SS, and we have referred to their work several times (refs. 3, 5, and 7 in our report). In the introduction and discussion sections of our report, we summarize the previous indirect evidence suggesting that these B cells could express RF. However, because of their special relevance with regard to this issue, we emphasized the recent molecular studies (1–3) showing that the Ig V-region gene repertoire used by myoepithelial sialadenitis– and salivary gland lymphoma–associated clones is biased toward V genes known to be involved in RF production. Still, prior to our study, there was no reported evidence directly linking the V-region sequences expressed by SS lymphomas to the binding specificity of the antibodies they encoded.

Thierry Martin, MD, PhD
Jean-Louis Pasquali, MD, PhD
University Hospital Strasbourg
Strasbourg, France

1. Bahler DW, Swerdlow SH. Clonal salivary gland infiltrates associated with myoepithelial sialadenitis (Sjögren's syndrome) begin as nonmalignant antigen-selected expansions. Blood 1998;91:1864–72.
2. Stott DI, Hiepe F, Hummel M, Steinhauser G, Berek C. Antigen-driven clonal proliferation of B cells within the target tissue of an autoimmune disease. J Clin Invest 1998;102:938–46.
3. Bahler DW, Miklos JA, Swerdlow SH. Ongoing Ig gene hypermutation in salivary gland mucosa-associated lymphoid tissue-type lymphomas. Blood 1997;89:3335–44.

Is the anti–topoisomerase I autoantibody response associated with a distinct amino acid sequence in the HLA–DQβ1 domain?

To the Editor:

In 1996, Horiki et al reported on the distribution of HLA–DQB1 alleles among anti–topoisomerase I (anti–topo I)–positive patients with an overlap syndrome of systemic sclerosis (SSc) and rheumatoid arthritis (RA) (1). The production of anti–topo I autoantibodies is strongly associated with HLA class II. Since the correlation between anti–topo I production and HLA–DRw11 in patients with SSc was first confirmed by Genth and colleagues in 1990, in a study of German patients (2), various studies supporting their findings (i.e., correlation with DRB1*1101–*1104) have been published in the UK and the US (3,4). In contrast, no correlation with a specific HLA–DQB1 allele has yet been identified, although some reports have described a significant correlation between anti–topo I and DQB1 alleles in general (5–7).

After obtaining informed consent, we studied anti–topo I by enzyme-linked immunosorbent assay in 72 Japanese patients with silicosis. Four patients were found to be anti–topo I positive patients (8). The following HLA–DQB1 alleles were identified in these 4 patients: *0402 and *0302, *0402 and *0401, *0402 and *0402, and *0601 and *0302, respectively. These findings are similar to the results obtained in the study by Horiki et al (1), in which all 4 Japanese patients with anti–topo I–positive SSc/RA overlap syndrome had the DQB1*04 allele. However, studies on DQB1 alleles among anti–topo I–positive Caucasian Americans, African Americans, and Choctaw Indians with SSc have not confirmed the involvement of DQB1*04 (5–7).

Previous studies have shown a correlation between anti–topo I antibodies and DQB1*0301 or *0601, and in some cases *0302 has been mentioned (5–7). Therefore, we sought common features among various DQB1 alleles, including DQB1*04, which was detected among Japanese patients in our study and by Horiki and colleagues. Arnett et al (5) suggested the importance of tyrosine at position 30 of the DQβ1 domain. Position 30 of DQB1*04, *0301, and *0601 is also tyrosine. Although the ^{71}TRAELDT^{77} motif is thought to be associated with the production of anti–topo I antibodies, DQB1*04 lacks this motif.

Consequently, we investigated the amino acid sequence of alleles that are thought to be involved in anti–topo I autoantibody production. The results revealed some common positioning of distinct amino acids among the *0301, *0303, *0306, *0401, *0402, *0601, and *0602 alleles; i.e., positions 14, 30, 57, and 77 of the DQβ1 domain of these alleles are methionine, tyrosine, aspartic acid, and threonine, respectively (Figure 1). However, *0302 has been detected only rarely in anti–topo I–positive patients and possesses alanine at position 57, instead of aspartic acid. The β1 domain of HLA class II takes on a spiral or folded shape, and the above-mentioned amino acids that come into contact with an antigen are located at certain distances within the domain. Therefore, we suggest that alleles having the 4 above-mentioned amino acids (or at least 3 of these amino acids) within the DQβ1 domain can efficiently present topo I antigens, and thus facilitate autoantibody production.

These findings suggest that HLA–DQB1 is clearly involved in the production of anti–topo I autoantibodies. Furthermore, as is the case with DQB1*04 alleles, there is linkage disequilibrium between racial groups, as postulated by Reveille et al (7).

Supported by Kawasaki Medical School grant 10-603 and by a grant-in/aid for scientific research from the Japanese Ministry of Education, Science, Sports and Culture (1999).

Ayako Ueki, MD, PhD
Yumika Isozaki, PhD
Akiko Tomokuni, PhD
Takemi Otsuki, MD, PhD
Fuminori Hydoh, MD, PhD
Haruko Sakaguchi, PhD
Kawaski Medical School
Kurashiki, Japan
Shinichiro Tanaka, MD, PhD
Okayama National Hospital
Okayama, Japan
Masayasu Kusaka, MD, PhD
Kusaka Hospital
Bizen-cho, Okayama, Japan

```
                   10                20           30         40          50             60          70            80          90
DQB1*0501  RDSPEDFVYQ  FKG L CYFTING  TERVRGVTR H  IYNREEYVRF  DSDVGVYRAV  TPQGRP V AEY  WNSQKEVLEG  ARASVD R VCR  HNYEVAYRGI  L

DQB1*0301  ----------  --A M -------  -----Y--- Y  -------A--  ----E-----  --L-P- D ---  ---------R  T--EL- T ---  ---QLEL-TT  -
DQB1*0302  ----------  --- M -------  -----L--- Y  -------A--  ----------  --L-P- A ---  ---------R  T--EL- T ---  ---QLEL-TT  -
DQB1*0303  ----------  --- M -------  -----L--- Y  -------A--  ----------  --L-P- D ---  ---------R  T--EL- T ---  ---QLEL-TT  -
DQB1*0306  ----------  --- M -------  -----L--- Y  -------A--  ----------  --L-P- D ---  ----------  ------ T ---  ---QLEL-TT  -
DQB1*0401  --------F-  --- M -------  --------- Y  -------A--  ----------  --L--L D ---  -----DI---  ------ T ---  ---QLEL-TT  -
DQB1*0402  --------F-  --- M -------  -----G--- Y  -------A--  ----------  --L--L D ---  -----DI--E  D----- T ---  ---QLEL-TT  -
DQB1*0601  --P-----L-  --A M -------  -----Y--- Y  ------D---  ----------  ------ D ---  -----DI--R  T--EL- T ---  ------F---  -
DQB1*0602  --------F-  --- M -------  -----L--- Y  -------A--  ----------  ------ D ---  ----------  T--EL- T ---  ------F---  -
DQB1*0603                              ---L--- Y  -------A--  ----------  ------ D ---  ----------  T--EL- T -
DQB1*0604  ----------  --- M -------  -----L--- Y  -------A--  ----------  ------ - ---  ---------R  T--EL- T ---  -----G----  -
```

Figure 1. HLA–DQB1 alleles with the distinct amino acid sequence in the HLA–DQβ1 domain, i.e., methionine at position 14, tyrosine at position 30, aspartic acid at position 57, and threonine at position 77.

1. Horiki T, Moriuchi J, Takaya M, Uchiyama M, Hoshina Y, Inada K, et al. The coexistence of systemic sclerosis and rheumatoid arthritis in five patients: clinical and immunogenetic features suggest a distinct entity. Arthritis Rheum 1996;39:152–6.
2. Genth E, Mierau R, Genetzky P, von Mühlen CA, Kaufmann S, von Wilmowsky H, et al. Immunogenetic associations of scleroderma-related antinuclear antibodies. Arthritis Rheum 1990;33:657–65.
3. Fanning GC, Welsh KI, Bunn C, du Bois R, Black CM. HLA association in three mutually exclusive autoantibody subgroups in UK systemic sclerosis patients. Br J Rheumatol 1998;37:201–7.
4. Falkner D, Wilson J, Medsger TA, Morel PA. HLA and clinical associations in systemic sclerosis patients with anti-Th/To antibodies. Arthritis Rheum 1998;41:74–80.
5. Arnett FC. HLA and autoimmunity in scleroderma (systemic sclerosis). Int Rev Immunol 1995;12:107–28.
6. Harvey GR, McHugh NJ. Serologic abnormalities in systemic sclerosis. Curr Opin Rheumatol 1999;11:495–502.
7. Reveille JD. Molecular genetics of systemic sclerosis. Curr Opin Rheumatol 1995;7:522–8.
8. Tomokuni A, Ueki A. Detection of anti-topoisomerase I autoantibody in patients with silicosis. Submitted for publication.

Clinical Images: Arthritis induced by South American blastomycosis

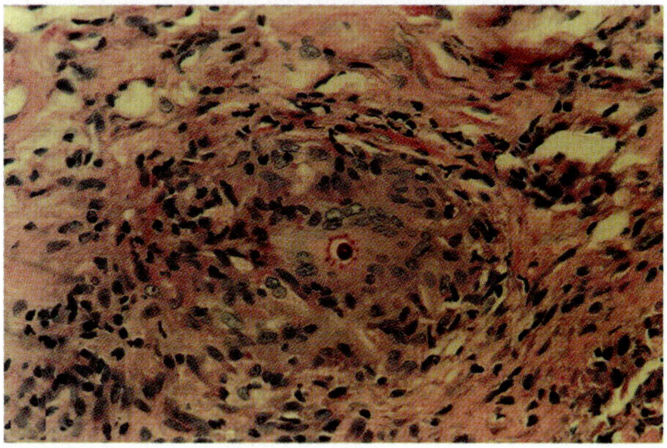

A

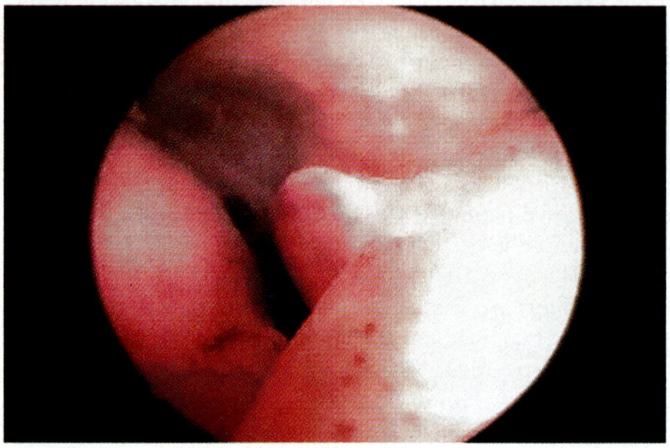

B

The patient, a 52-year-old man who lived on a farm, developed arthritis in his knees, which was treated with nonsteroidal antiinflammatory drugs for 6 months. The arthritis did not remit, and he was subsequently seen in our unit. A synovial biopsy with arthroscopy was performed (**A**). Note the presence of a marked synovial cellular inflammatory reaction with *Paracoccidioides brasiliensis* organisms at the center, exhibiting the typical double-wall membrane with peripheral buds. The corresponding arthroscopic image (**B**) shows vascular congestion and synovial hypertrophy. The patient was treated with sulfadiazine 3 gm/day for 6 months, with complete resolution of the clinical symptoms.

Morton A. Scheinberg, MD, PhD, FACP
Moises Cohen, MD
Federal University of São Paulo
Center for Clinical Immunology–LID Laboratory
Cohen Institute
Sao Paulo, Brazil

Brief Summary of
Prescribing Information as of February 2000

ARAVA™ Tablets
(leflunomide)
10 mg, 20 mg, 100 mg

CONTRAINDICATIONS AND WARNINGS

PREGNANCY MUST BE EXCLUDED BEFORE THE START OF TREATMENT WITH ARAVA. ARAVA IS CONTRAINDICATED IN PREGNANT WOMEN, OR WOMEN OF CHILDBEARING POTENTIAL WHO ARE NOT USING RELIABLE CONTRACEPTION. (SEE CONTRAINDICATIONS AND WARNINGS.) PREGNANCY MUST BE AVOIDED DURING ARAVA TREATMENT OR PRIOR TO THE COMPLETION OF THE DRUG ELIMINATION PROCEDURE AFTER ARAVA TREATMENT.

INDICATIONS AND USAGE

ARAVA is indicated in adults for the treatment of active rheumatoid arthritis (RA) to reduce signs and symptoms and to retard structural damage as evidenced by X-ray erosions and joint space narrowing (see CLINICAL STUDIES).

Aspirin, nonsteroidal anti-inflammatory agents and/or low dose corticosteroids may be continued during treatment with ARAVA (see PRECAUTIONS – Drug Interactions – NSAIDs). The combined use of ARAVA with antimalarials, intramuscular or oral gold, D penicillamine, azathioprine, or methotrexate has not been adequately studied (see WARNINGS – Immunosuppression Potential).

CONTRAINDICATIONS

ARAVA is contraindicated in patients with known hypersensitivity to leflunomide or any of the other components of ARAVA.

ARAVA can cause fetal harm when administered to a pregnant woman. Leflunomide, when administered orally to rats during organogenesis at a dose of 15 mg/kg, was teratogenic (most notably anophthalmia or microophthalmia and internal hydrocephalus). The systemic exposure of rats at this dose was approximately 1/10 the human exposure level based on AUC. Under these exposure conditions, leflunomide also caused a decrease in the maternal body weight and an increase in embryolethality with a decrease in fetal body weight for surviving fetuses. In rabbits, oral treatment with 10 mg/kg of leflunomide during organogenesis resulted in fused, dysplastic sternebrae. The exposure level at this dose was essentially equivalent to the maximum human exposure level based on AUC. At a 1 mg/kg dose, leflunomide was not teratogenic in rats and rabbits. When female rats were treated with 1.25 mg/kg of leflunomide beginning 14 days before mating and continuing until the end of lactation, the offspring exhibited marked (greater than 90%) decreases in postnatal survival. The systemic exposure level at 1.25 mg/kg was approximately 1/100 the human exposure level based on AUC.

ARAVA is contraindicated in women who are or may become pregnant. If this drug is used during pregnancy, or if the patient becomes pregnant while taking this drug, the patient should be apprised of the potential hazard to the fetus.

WARNINGS

Immunosuppression Potential

ARAVA is not recommended for patients with severe immunodeficiency, bone marrow dysplasia, or severe, uncontrolled infections.

There have been rare reports of pancytopenia in patients receiving ARAVA. In most of these cases, patients received concomitant treatment with methotrexate or other immunosuppressive agents, or they had recently discontinued these therapies; in some cases, patients had a prior history of a significant hematologic abnormality. If ARAVA is used in such patients, it should be administered with caution and with frequent clinical and hematologic monitoring. The use of ARAVA in combination therapy with methotrexate has not been adequately studied in a controlled setting.

If evidence of bone marrow suppression occurs in a patient taking ARAVA, treatment with ARAVA should be stopped, and cholestyramine or charcoal should be used to reduce the plasma concentration of leflunomide active metabolite (see PRECAUTIONS – General – Need for Drug Elimination).

In any situation in which the decision is made to switch from ARAVA to another anti-rheumatic agent with a known potential for hematologic suppression, it would be prudent to monitor for hematologic toxicity, because there will be overlap of systemic exposure to both compounds. ARAVA washout with cholestyramine or charcoal may decrease this risk, but also may induce disease worsening if the patient had been responding to ARAVA treatment.

Skin Reactions

Rare cases of Stevens-Johnson syndrome and toxic epidermal necrolysis have been reported in patients receiving ARAVA. If a patient taking ARAVA develops any of these conditions, ARAVA therapy should be stopped, and a drug elimination procedure is recommended (see PRECAUTIONS - General - Need for Drug Elimination).

Hepatotoxicity

In clinical trials, ARAVA treatment was associated with elevations of liver enzymes, primarily ALT and AST, in a significant number of patients; these effects were generally reversible. Most transaminase elevations were mild (≤2-fold ULN) and usually resolved while continuing treatment. Marked elevations (>3-fold ULN) occurred infrequently and reversed with dose reduction or discontinuation of treatment. The following table shows liver enzyme elevations seen with monthly monitoring in clinical trials US301 and MN301. It was notable that the absence of folate use in MN302 was associated with a considerably greater incidence of liver enzyme elevation on methotrexate.

Table 4. Liver Enzyme Elevations >3-fold Upper Limits of Normal (ULN)

	US301			MN301			MN302*	
	LEF	PL	MTX	LEF	PL	SSZ	LEF	MTX
ALT (SGPT) >3-fold ULN	8	3	5	2	1	2	13	83
(n %)	(4.4)	(2.5)	(2.7)	(1.5)	(1.1)	(1.5)	(2.6)	(16.7)
Reversed to ≤2-fold ULN:	8	3	5	2	1	2	12	82
Timing of Elevation								
0-3 Months	6	1	1	2	1	2	7	27
4-6 Months	1	1	3	-	-	-	1	34
7-9 Months	1	1	1	-	-	-	-	16
10-12 Months	-	-	-	-	-	-	5	6
AST (SGOT) >3-fold ULN	4	2	1	2	0	5	7	29
(n %)	(2.2)	(1.7)	(0.6)	(1.5)	-	(3.8)	(1.4)	(5.8)
Reversed to ≤2-fold ULN:	4	2	1	2	-	4	5	29
Timing of Elevation								
0-3 Months	2	1	-	2	-	4	3	10
4-6 Months	1	1	1	-	-	1	1	11
7-9 Months	1	-	-	-	-	-	-	8
10-12 Months	-	-	-	-	-	-	3	-

*Only 10% of patients in MN302 received folate. All patients in US301 received folate.

At minimum, ALT (SGPT) should be performed at baseline and monitored initially at monthly intervals then, if stable, at intervals determined by the individual clinical situation.

Guidelines for dose adjustment or discontinuation based on the severity and persistence of ALT elevation are recommended as follows: For confirmed ALT elevations >2-fold ULN, dose reduction to 10 mg/day may allow continued administration of ARAVA. If elevations >2 but ≤3-fold ULN persist despite dose reduction, liver biopsy is recommended if continued treatment is desired. If elevations >3-fold ULN persist despite dose reduction, ARAVA should be discontinued and cholestyramine should be administered (see PRECAUTIONS - General - Need for Drug Elimination) with close monitoring, including retreatment with cholestyramine as indicated.

Rare elevations of alkaline phosphatase and bilirubin have been observed. Trial US301 used ACR Methotrexate Liver Biopsy Guidelines for monitoring therapy. One of 182 patients receiving leflunomide and 1 of 182 patients receiving methotrexate underwent liver biopsy at 106 and 50 weeks respectively. The biopsy for the leflunomide subject was Roegnik Grade IIIA and for the methotrexate subject, Roegnik Grade I.

Pre-existing Hepatic Disease

Given the possible risk of increased hepatotoxicity, and the role of the liver in drug activation, elimination and recycling, the use of ARAVA is not recommended in patients with significant hepatic impairment or evidence of infection with hepatitis B or C viruses.

Malignancy

The risk of malignancy, particularly lymphoproliferative disorders, is increased with the use of some immunosuppression medications. There is a potential for immunosuppression with ARAVA. No apparent increase in the incidence of malignancies and lymphoproliferative disorders was reported in the clinical trials of ARAVA, but larger and longer-term studies would be needed to determine whether there is an increased risk of malignancy or lymphoproliferative disorders with ARAVA.

Use in Women of Childbearing Potential

There are no adequate and well-controlled studies evaluating ARAVA in pregnant women. However, based on animal studies, leflunomide may increase the risk of fetal death or teratogenic effects when administered to a pregnant woman (see CONTRAINDICATIONS). Women of childbearing potential must not be started on ARAVA until pregnancy is excluded and it has been confirmed that they are using reliable contraception. Before starting treatment with ARAVA, patients must be fully counseled on the potential for serious risk to the fetus.

The patient must be advised that if there is any delay in onset of menses or any other reason to suspect pregnancy, they must notify the physician immediately for pregnancy testing and, if positive, the physician and patient must discuss the risk to the pregnancy. It is possible that rapidly lowering the blood level of the active metabolite by instituting the drug elimination procedure described below at the first delay of menses may decrease the risk to the fetus from ARAVA.

Upon discontinuing ARAVA, it is recommended that all women of childbearing potential undergo the drug elimination procedure described below. Women receiving ARAVA treatment who wish to become pregnant must discontinue ARAVA and undergo the drug elimination procedure described below which includes verification of M1 metabolite plasma levels less than 0.02 mg/L (0.02 µg/mL). Human plasma levels of the active metabolite (M1) less than 0.02 mg/L (0.02 µg/mL) are expected to have minimal risk based on available animal data.

Drug Elimination Procedure

The following drug elimination procedure is recommended to achieve non-detectable plasma levels (less than 0.02 mg/L or 0.02 µg/mL) after stopping treatment with ARAVA:

1) Administer cholestyramine 8 grams 3 times daily for 11 days. (The 11 days do not need to be consecutive unless there is a need to lower the plasma level rapidly.)
2) Verify plasma levels less than 0.02 mg/L (0.02 µg/mL) by two separate tests at least 14 days apart. If plasma levels are higher than 0.02 mg/L, additional cholestyramine treatment should be considered.

Without the drug elimination procedure, it may take up to 2 years to reach plasma M1 metabolite levels less than 0.02 mg/L due to individual variation in drug clearance.

PRECAUTIONS

General

Need for Drug Elimination

The active metabolite of leflunomide is eliminated slowly from the plasma. In instances of any serious toxicity from ARAVA, including hypersensitivity, use of a drug elimination procedure as described in this section is highly recommended to reduce the drug concentration more rapidly after stopping ARAVA therapy. If hypersensitivity is the suspected clinical mechanism, more prolonged cholestyramine or charcoal administration may be necessary to achieve rapid and sufficient clearance. The duration may be modified based on the clinical status of the patient.

Cholestyramine given orally at a dose of 8 g three times a day for 24 hours to three healthy volunteers decreased plasma levels of M1 by approximately 40% in 24 hours and by 49 to 65% in 48 hours.

Administration of activated charcoal (powder made into a suspension) orally or via nasogastric tube (50 g every 6 hours for 24 hours) has been shown to reduce plasma concentrations of the active metabolite, M1, by 37% in 24 hours and by 48% in 48 hours.

These drug elimination procedures may be repeated if clinically necessary.

Renal Insufficiency

Single dose studies in dialysis patients show a doubling of the free fraction of M1 in plasma. There is no clinical experience in the use of ARAVA in patients with renal impairment. Caution should be used when administering this drug in this population.

Vaccinations

No clinical data are available on the efficacy and safety of vaccinations during ARAVA treatment. Vaccination with live vaccines is, however, not recommended. The long half-life of ARAVA should be considered when contemplating administration of a live vaccine after stopping ARAVA.

Information for Patients

The potential for increased risk of birth defects should be discussed with female patients of childbearing potential. It is recommended that physicians advise women that they may be at increased risk of having a child with birth defects if they are pregnant when taking ARAVA, become pregnant while taking ARAVA, or do not wait to become pregnant until they have stopped taking ARAVA and followed the drug elimination procedure (as described in WARNINGS – Use In Women of Childbearing Potential – Drug Elimination Procedure).

Patients should be advised of the possibility of rare, serious skin reactions. Patients should be instructed to inform their physicians promptly if they develop a skin rash or mucous membrane lesions.

Patients should be advised of the potential hepatotoxic effects of ARAVA and of the need for monitoring liver enzymes.

Patients who are receiving other immunosuppressive therapy concurrently with ARAVA, who have recently discontinued such therapy before starting treatment with ARAVA, or who have had a history of a significant hematologic abnormality, should be advised of the potential for pancytopenia and of the need for frequent hematologic monitoring. They should be instructed to notify their physicians promptly if they notice symptoms of pancytopenia (such as easy bruising, proneness to infections, paleness or unusual tiredness).

Laboratory Tests

At minimum, ALT (SGPT) should be performed at baseline and monitored initially at monthly intervals then, if stable, at intervals determined by the individual clinical situation. In patients who are at an increased risk of hematologic toxicity (see WARNINGS - Immunosuppression Potential), more vigilant monitoring, including hematologic monitoring, is warranted.

Due to a specific effect on the brush border of the renal proximal tubule, ARAVA has a uricosuric effect. A separate effect of hypophosphaturia is seen in some patients. These effects have not been seen together, nor have there been alterations in renal function.

Carcinogenesis, Mutagenesis, and Impairment of Fertility

No evidence of carcinogenicity was observed in a 2-year bioassay in rats at oral doses of leflunomide up to the maximally tolerated dose of 6 mg/kg (approximately 1/40 the maximum human M1 systemic exposure based on AUC). However, male mice in a 2-year bioassay exhibited an increased incidence in lymphoma at an oral dose of 15 mg/kg, the highest dose studied (1.7 times the human M1 exposure based on AUC). Female mice, in the same study, exhibited a dose-related increased incidence of bronchoalveolar adenomas and carcinomas combined beginning at 1.5 mg/kg (approximately 1/10 the human M1 exposure based on AUC). The significance of the findings in mice relative to the clinical use of ARAVA is not known.

Leflunomide was not mutagenic in the Ames Assay, the Unscheduled DNA Synthesis Assay, or in the HGPRT Gene Mutation Assay. In addition, leflunomide was not clastogenic in the *in vivo* Mouse Micronucleus Assay nor in the *in vivo* Cytogenetic Test in Chinese Hamster Bone Marrow Cells. However, 4-trifluoromethylaniline (TFMA), a minor metabolite of leflunomide, was mutagenic in the Ames Assay and in the HGPRT Gene Mutation Assay, and was clastogenic in the *in vitro* Assay for Chromosome Aberrations in the Chinese Hamster Cells. TFMA was not clastogenic in the *in vivo* Mouse Micronucleus Assay nor in the *in vivo* Cytogenetic Test in Chinese Hamster Bone Marrow Cells.

Leflunomide had no effect on fertility in either male or female rats at oral doses up to 4.0 mg/kg (approximately 1/30 the human M1 exposure based on AUC).

Pregnancy

Pregnancy Category X. See CONTRAINDICATIONS section. Pregnancy Registry: To monitor fetal outcomes of pregnant women exposed to leflunomide, health care providers are encouraged to register such patients by calling 1-877-311-8972.

Nursing Mothers

ARAVA should not be used by nursing mothers. It is not known whether ARAVA is excreted in human milk. Many drugs are excreted in human milk, and there is a potential for serious adverse reactions in nursing infants from ARAVA. Therefore, a decision should be made whether to proceed with nursing or to initiate treatment with ARAVA, taking into account the importance of the drug to the mother.

Use in Males

Available information does not suggest that ARAVA would be associated with an increased risk of male-mediated fetal toxicity. However, animal studies to evaluate this specific risk have not been conducted. To minimize any possible risk, men wishing to father a child should consider discontinuing use of ARAVA and taking cholestyramine 8 grams 3 times daily for 11 days.

Drug Interactions

Cholestyramine and Charcoal

Administration of cholestyramine or activated charcoal in patients (n=13) and volunteers (n=96) resulted in a rapid and significant decrease in plasma M1 (the active metabolite of leflunomide) concentration (see PRECAUTIONS – General – Need for Drug Elimination).

Hepatotoxic Drugs

Increased side effects may occur when leflunomide is given concomitantly with hepatotoxic substances. This is also to be considered when leflunomide treatment is followed by such drugs without a drug elimination procedure. In a small (n=30) combination study of ARAVA with methotrexate, a 2- to 3-fold elevation in liver enzymes was seen in 5 of 30 patients. All elevations resolved, 2 with continuation of both drugs and 3 after discontinuation of leflunomide. A >3-fold increase was seen in another 5 patients. All of these also resolved, 2 with continuation of both drugs and 3 after discontinuation of leflunomide. Three patients met "ACR criteria" for liver biopsy (1: Roegnik Grade I, 2: Roegnik Grade IIIa). No pharmacokinetic interaction was identified (see CLINICAL PHARMACOLOGY).

NSAIDs

In *in vitro* studies, M1 was shown to cause increases ranging from 13 - 50% in the free fraction of diclofenac and ibuprofen at concentrations in the clinical range. The clinical significance of this finding is unknown, however, there was extensive concomitant use of NSAIDs in clinical studies and no differential effect was observed.

Tolbutamide

In *in vitro* studies, M1 was shown to cause increases ranging from 13 - 50% in the free fraction of tolbutamide at concentrations in the clinical range. The clinical significance of this finding is unknown.

Rifampin

Following concomitant administration of a single dose of ARAVA to subjects receiving multiple doses of rifampin, M1 peak levels were increased (~40%) over those seen when ARAVA was given alone. Because of the potential for ARAVA levels to continue to increase with multiple dosing, caution should be used if patients are to be receiving both ARAVA and rifampin.

Pediatric Use

The safety and efficacy of ARAVA in the pediatric population have not been studied. Use of ARAVA in patients less than 18 years of age is not recommended.

Geriatric Use

No dosage adjustment is needed in patients over 65.

ADVERSE REACTIONS

Adverse reactions associated with the use of leflunomide in RA include diarrhea, elevated liver enzymes (ALT and AST), alopecia and rash. In the controlled studies, the following adverse events were reported, regardless of causality. (See Table 5.)

2000 Annual Meeting Presentations Now Online!

For the first time ever, ACR members will be able to access six of the most popular sessions at this year's Annual Scientific Meeting on the ACR Web site, www.rheumatology.org, for free.

This is a tremendous benefit for members who were unable to attend the annual meeting, who missed a session due to a scheduling conflict, or who would like to hear the session again.

The following sessions have been selected to highlight the most recent advances in the specialty, as well as basic science research discoveries that impact the care and treatment of patients:

Paul Klemperer, MD, Memorial Lectureship
Innate Immunity: New Roles in Host Defense and Rheumatic Disease
Sunday, October 28, 2000, 5:30 – 7:00 PM
Speaker: John P. Atkinson, MD

State-of-the-Art Lecture
Steroid-Induced Osteoporosis
Monday, October 30, 2000, 2:15 – 3:15 PM
Speaker: Kenneth G. Saag, MD

State-of-the-Art Lecture
Fibromyalgia: Advances in Understanding and Improvements in Management
Tuesday, October 31, 2000, 4:00 – 5:00 PM
Speaker: Daniel J. Clauw, MD

ACR Special Lecture
Rheumatoid Arthritis and Atherosclerotic Cardiovascular Disease: Shared Disease Mechanism
Tuesday, October 31, 2000, 5:45 – 6:45 PM
Speaker: Cornelia M. Weyand, MD, PhD

ARHP Concurrent Session
Innovative Approaches to Acute Low Back Pain Management
Wednesday, November 1, 2000, 11:00 AM – 12:00 NN

Role of Case Management in Managed Care	Donna A. Levitt, MSN, MA, CRNP
Developing an Integrative Low Back Pain Program	Terence Starz, MD
Analysis and Interpretation of Outcome Measures	Molly T. Vogt, PhD

State-of-the-Art Lecture
Early Rheumatoid Arthritis
Thursday, November 2, 2000, 7:30 – 8:30 AM
Speaker: Josef S. Smolen, MD

The six webcast presentations are posted free of charge on the ACR Web site at www.rheumatology.org.

Supported by an educational grant from Merck & Co., Inc.

SALAGEN® Tablets
(pilocarpine hydrochloride)

Brief Summary

Consult package insert for full prescribing information

INDICATIONS AND USAGE: SALAGEN® Tablets are indicated for 1) the treatment of symptoms of dry mouth from salivary gland hypofunction caused by radiotherapy for cancer of the head and neck; and 2) the treatment of symptoms of dry mouth in patients with Sjogren's syndrome.

CONTRAINDICATIONS: SALAGEN® Tablets are contraindicated in patients with uncontrolled asthma, known hypersensitivity to pilocarpine, and when miosis is undesirable, e.g., in acute iritis and in narrow-angle (angle closure) glaucoma.

WARNINGS:

Cardiovascular Disease: Patients with significant cardiovascular disease may be unable to compensate for transient changes in hemodynamics or rhythm induced by pilocarpine. Pulmonary edema has been reported as a complication of pilocarpine toxicity from high ocular doses given for acute angle-closure glaucoma. Pilocarpine should be administered with caution in and under close medical supervision of patients with significant cardiovascular disease.

Ocular: Ocular formulations of pilocarpine have been reported to cause visual blurring which may result in decreased visual acuity, especially at night and in patients with central lens changes, and to cause impairment of depth perception. Caution should be advised while driving at night or performing hazardous activities in reduced lighting.

Pulmonary Disease: Pilocarpine has been reported to increase airway resistance, bronchial smooth muscle tone, and bronchial secretions. Pilocarpine hydrochloride should be administered with caution to and under close medical supervision in patients with controlled asthma, chronic bronchitis, or chronic obstructive pulmonary disease requiring pharmacotherapy.

PRECAUTIONS:

General: Pilocarpine toxicity is characterized by an exaggeration of its parasympathomimetic effects. These may include: headache, visual disturbance, lacrimation, sweating, respiratory distress, gastrointestinal spasm, nausea, vomiting, diarrhea, atrioventricular block, tachycardia, bradycardia, hypotension, hypertension, shock, mental confusion, cardiac arrhythmia, and tremors.

The dose-related cardiovascular pharmacologic effects of pilocarpine include hypotension, hypertension, bradycardia, and tachycardia.

Pilocarpine should be administered with caution to patients with known or suspected cholelithiasis or biliary tract disease. Contractions of the gallbladder or biliary smooth muscle could precipitate complications including cholecystitis, cholangitis, and biliary obstruction.

Pilocarpine may increase ureteral smooth muscle tone and could theoretically precipitate renal colic (or "ureteral reflux"), particularly in patients with nephrolithiasis.

Cholinergic agonists may have dose-related central nervous system effects. This should be considered when treating patients with underlying cognitive or psychiatric disturbances.

Renal Insufficiency: The pharmacokinetics of orally administered pilocarpine in patients with renal and hepatic disease is not known.

Information for Patients: Patients should be informed that pilocarpine may cause visual disturbances, especially at night, that could impair their ability to drive safely.

If a patient sweats excessively while taking pilocarpine hydrochloride and cannot drink enough liquid, the patient should consult a physician. Dehydration may develop.

Drug Interactions: Pilocarpine should be administered with caution to patients taking beta adrenergic antagonists because of the possibility of conduction disturbances. Drugs with parasympathomimetic effects administered concurrently with pilocarpine would be expected to result in additive pharmacologic effects. Pilocarpine might antagonize the anticholinergic effects of drugs used concomitantly. These effects should be considered when anticholinergic properties may be contributing to the therapeutic effect of concomitant medication (e.g., atropine, inhaled ipratropium).

While no formal drug interaction studies have been performed, the following concomitant drugs were used in at least 10% of patients in either or both Sjogren's efficacy studies: acetylsalicylic acid, artificial tears, calcium, conjugated estrogens, hydroxychloroquine sulfate, ibuprofen, levothyroxine sodium, medroxyprogesterone acetate, methotrexate, multivitamins, naproxen, omeprazole, paracetamol, and prednisone.

Carcinogenesis, Mutagenesis, Impairment of Fertility: No definitive long term animal studies have evaluated the carcinogenic potential of pilocarpine. No evidence that pilocarpine has the potential to cause genetic toxicity was obtained in a series of studies that included: 1) bacterial assays (Salmonella and E. coli) for reverse gene mutations; 2) an *in vitro* chromosome aberration assay in a Chinese hamster ovary cell line; 3) an *in vivo* chromosome aberration assay (micronucleus test) in mice; and 4) a primary DNA damage assay (unscheduled DNA synthesis) in rat hepatocyte primary cultures.

Oral administration of pilocarpine to male and female rats at a dosage of 18 mg/kg/day (approximately 5 times the maximum recommended dose for a 50 kg human when compared on the basis of body surface area (mg/m^2) estimates) resulted in impaired reproductive function, including reduced fertility, decreased sperm motility, and morphologic evidence of abnormal sperm. It is unclear whether the reduction in fertility was due to effects on male animals, female animals, or both males and females. In dogs, exposure to pilocarpine at a dosage of 3 mg/kg/day (approximately 3 times the maximum recommended dose for a 50 kg human when compared on the basis of body surface area (mg/m^2) estimates) for six months resulted in evidence of impaired spermatogenesis. The data obtained in these studies suggest that pilocarpine may impair the fertility of male and female humans.

SALAGEN® Tablets should be administered to individuals who are attempting to conceive a child only if the potential benefit justifies potential impairment of fertility.

Pregnancy: Teratogenic effects.

Pregnancy Category C: Pilocarpine was associated with a reduction in the mean fetal body weight and an increase in the incidence of skeletal variations when given to pregnant rats at a dosage of 90 mg/kg/day (approximately 26 times the maximum recommended dose for a 50 kg human when compared on the basis of body surface area (mg/m^2) estimates). These effects may have been secondary to maternal toxicity. In another study, oral administration of pilocarpine to female rats during gestation and lactation at a dosage of 36 mg/kg/day (approximately 10 times the maximum recommended dose for a 50 kg human when compared on the basis of body surface area (mg/m^2) estimates) resulted in an increased incidence of stillbirths; decreased neonatal survival and reduced mean body weight of pups were observed at dosages of 18 mg/kg/day (approximately 5 times the maximum recommended dose for a 50 kg human when compared on the basis of body surface area (mg/m^2) estimates) and above. There are no adequate and well-controlled studies in pregnant women. SALAGEN® Tablets should be used during pregnancy only if the potential benefit justifies the potential risk to the fetus.

Nursing Mothers: It is not known whether this drug is excreted in human milk. Because many drugs are excreted in human milk and because of the potential for serious adverse reactions in nursing infants from SALAGEN® Tablets, a decision should be made whether to discontinue nursing or to discontinue the drug, taking into account the importance of the drug to the mother.

Pediatric Use: Safety and effectiveness in pediatric patients have not been established.

Geriatric Use: Head and Neck Cancer Patients: In the placebo-controlled clinical trials (see Clinical Studies section in full prescribing information) the mean age of patients was approximately 58 years (range 19 to 80). Of these patients, 97/369 (61/217 receiving pilocarpine) were over the age of 65 years. In the healthy volunteer studies, 15/150 subjects were over the age of 65 years. In both study populations, the adverse events reported by those over 65 years and those 65 years and younger were comparable. Of the 15 elderly volunteers (5 women, 10 men), the 5 women had higher C_{max}'s and AUC's than the men.

Sjogren's Syndrome Patients: In the placebo-controlled clinical trials, the mean age of patients was approximately 55 years (range 21 to 85). The adverse events reported by those over 65 years and those 65 years and younger were comparable except for notable trends for urinary frequency, diarrhea, and dizziness (see **ADVERSE REACTIONS** section).

ADVERSE REACTIONS: Head & Neck Cancer Patients: In controlled studies, 217 patients received pilocarpine, of whom 68% were men and 32% were women. Race distribution was 91% Caucasian, 8% Black, and 1% of other origin. Mean age was approximately 58 years. The majority of patients were between 50 and 64 years (51%), 33% were 65 years and older and 16% were younger than 50 years of age.

The most frequent adverse experiences associated with SALAGEN® Tablets were a consequence of the expected pharmacologic effects of pilocarpine.

Adverse Event	10 mg t.i.d. (30mg/day) n=121	5 mg t.i.d. (15mg/day) n=141	placebo (t.i.d.) n=152
Sweating	68%	29%	9%
Nausea	15	6	4
Rhinitis	14	5	7
Diarrhea	7	4	5
Chills	15	3	<1
Flushing	13	8	3
Urinary Frequency	12	9	7
Dizziness	12	5	4
Asthenia	12	6	3

In addition, the following adverse events (≥3% incidence) were reported at dosages of 15-30 mg/day in the controlled clinical trials: Headache (11%), dyspepsia (7%), lacrimation (6%), edema (5%), abdominal pain (4%), amblyopia (4%), vomiting (4%), pharyngitis (3%), hypertension (3%).

The following events were reported with treated head and neck cancer patients at incidences of 1% to 2% at dosages of 7.5 to 30 mg/day: abnormal vision, conjunctivitis, dysphagia, epistaxis, myalgias, pruritus, rash, sinusitis, tachycardia, taste perversion, tremor, voice alteration.

The following events were reported rarely in treated head and neck cancer patients (<1%): Causal relation is unknown.

Body odor, hypothermia, mucous membrane abnormality, bradycardia, ECG abnormality, palpitations, syncope, anorexia, increased appetite, esophagitis, gastrointestinal disorder, tongue disorder, leukopenia, lymphadenopathy, anxiety, confusion, depression, abnormal dreams, hyperkinesia, hypoesthesia, nervousness, paresthesias, speech disorder, twitching, increased sputum, stridor, yawning, seborrhea, deafness, eye pain, glaucoma, dysuria, metrorrhagia, urinary impairment.

In long-term treatment were two patients with underlying cardiovascular disease of whom one experienced a myocardial infarct and another an episode of syncope. The association with drug is uncertain.

Sjogren's Syndrome Patients: In controlled studies, 376 patients received pilocarpine, of whom 5% were men and 95% were women. Race distribution was 84% Caucasian, 9% Oriental, 3% Black, and 4% of other origin. Mean age was 55 years. The majority of patients were between 40 and 69 years (70%), 16% were 70 years and older and 14% were younger than 40 years of age. Of these patients, 161/629 (89/376 receiving pilocarpine) were over the age of 65 years. The adverse events reported by those over 65 years and those 65 years and younger were comparable except for notable trends for urinary frequency, diarrhea, and dizziness. The incidences of urinary frequency and diarrhea in the elderly were about double those in the non-elderly. The incidence of dizziness was about three times as high in the elderly as in the non-elderly. These adverse experiences were not considered to be serious. In the 2 placebo-controlled studies, the most common adverse events related to drug use were sweating, urinary frequency, chills, and vasodilatation (flushing). The most commonly reported reason for patient discontinuation of treatment was sweating. Expected pharmacologic effects of pilocarpine include the following adverse experiences associated with SALAGEN® Tablets:

Adverse Event	5 mg q.i.d. (20 mg/day) n=255	Placebo (q.i.d.) n=253
Sweating	40%	7%
Urinary Frequency	10	4
Nausea	9	9
Flushing	9	2
Rhinitis	7	8
Diarrhea	6	7
Chills	4	2
Increased Salivation	3	0
Asthenia	2	2

In addition, the following adverse events (≥3% incidence) were reported at dosing of 20 mg/day in the controlled clinical trials: Headache (13%), flu syndrome (9%), dyspepsia (7%), dizziness (6%), pain (4%), sinusitis (4%), abdominal pain (3%), pharyngitis (2%), rash (2%), infection (2%).

The following events were reported in Sjögren's patients at incidences of 1% to 2% at dosing of 20 mg/day: accidental injury, allergic reaction, back pain, blurred vision, constipation, increased cough, edema, epistaxis, face edema, fever, flatulence, glossitis, lab test abnormalities including chemistry, hematology, and urinalysis, myalgia, palpitation, pruritus, somnolence, stomatitis, tachycardia, tinnitus, urinary incontinence, urinary tract infection, vaginitis, vomiting.

The following events were reported rarely in treated Sjogren's patients (<1%): Causal relation is unknown.

Chest pain, cyst, death, moniliasis, neck pain, neck rigidity, photosensitivity reaction, angina pectoris, arrhythmia, ECG abnormality, hypotension, hypertension, intracranial hemorrhage, migraine, myocardial infarction, anorexia, bilirubinemia, cholelithiasis, colitis, dry mouth, eructation, gastritis, gastroenteritis, gastrointestinal disorder, gingivitis, hepatitis, abnormal liver function tests, melena, nausea & vomiting, pancreatitis, parotid gland enlargement, salivary gland enlargement, sputum increased, taste loss, tongue disorder, tooth disorder, hematuria, lymphadenopathy, abnormal platelets, thrombocythemia, thrombocytopenia, thrombosis, abnormal WBC, peripheral edema, hypoglycemia, arthralgia, arthritis, bone disorder, spontaneous bone fracture, pathological fracture, myasthenia, tendon disorder, tenosynovitis, aphasia, confusion, depression, abnormal dreams, emotional lability, hyperkinesia, hypesthesia, insomnia, leg cramps, nervousness, paresthesias, abnormal thinking, tremor, bronchitis, dyspnea, hiccup, laryngismus, laryngitis, pneumonia, viral infection, voice alteration, alopecia, contact dermatitis, dry skin, eczema, erythema nodosum, exfoliative dermatitis, herpes simplex, skin ulcer, vesiculobullous rash, cataract, conjunctivitis, dry eyes, ear disorder, ear pain, eye disorder, eye hemorrhage, glaucoma, lacrimation disorder, retinal disorder, taste perversion, abnormal vision, breast pain, dysuria, mastitis, menorrhagia, metrorrhagia, ovarian disorder, pyuria, salpingitis, urethral pain, urinary urgency, vaginal hemorrhage, vaginal moniliasis.

The following adverse experiences have been reported rarely with ocular pilocarpine: A-V block, agitation, ciliary congestion, confusion, delusion, depression, dermatitis, middle ear disturbance, eyelid twitching, malignant glaucoma, iris cysts, macular hole, shock, and visual hallucination.

MANAGEMENT OF OVERDOSE: Fatal overdosage with pilocarpine has been reported in the scientific literature at doses presumed to be greater than 100 mg in two hospitalized patients. 100 mg of pilocarpine is considered potentially fatal. Overdosage should be treated with atropine titration (0.5 mg to 1.0 mg given subcutaneously or intravenously) and supportive measures to maintain respiration and circulation. Epinephrine (0.3 mg to 1.0 mg, subcutaneously or intramuscularly) may also be of value in the presence of severe cardiovascular depression or bronchoconstriction. It is not known if pilocarpine is dialyzable.

DOSAGE AND ADMINISTRATION:

Head & Neck Cancer Patients:

The recommended initial dose of SALAGEN® Tablets is one tablet (5 mg) taken three times a day. Dosage should be titrated according to therapeutic response and tolerance. The usual dosage range is up to 3-6 tablets or 15-30 mg per day. (Not to exceed 2 tablets per dose.) Although early improvement may be realized, at least 12 weeks of uninterrupted therapy with SALAGEN® Tablets may be necessary to assess whether a beneficial response will be achieved. The incidence of the most common adverse events increases with dose. The lowest dose that is tolerated and effective should be used for maintenance.

Sjögren's Syndrome Patients:

The recommended dose of SALAGEN® Tablets is one tablet (5 mg) taken four times a day. Efficacy was established by 6 weeks of use.

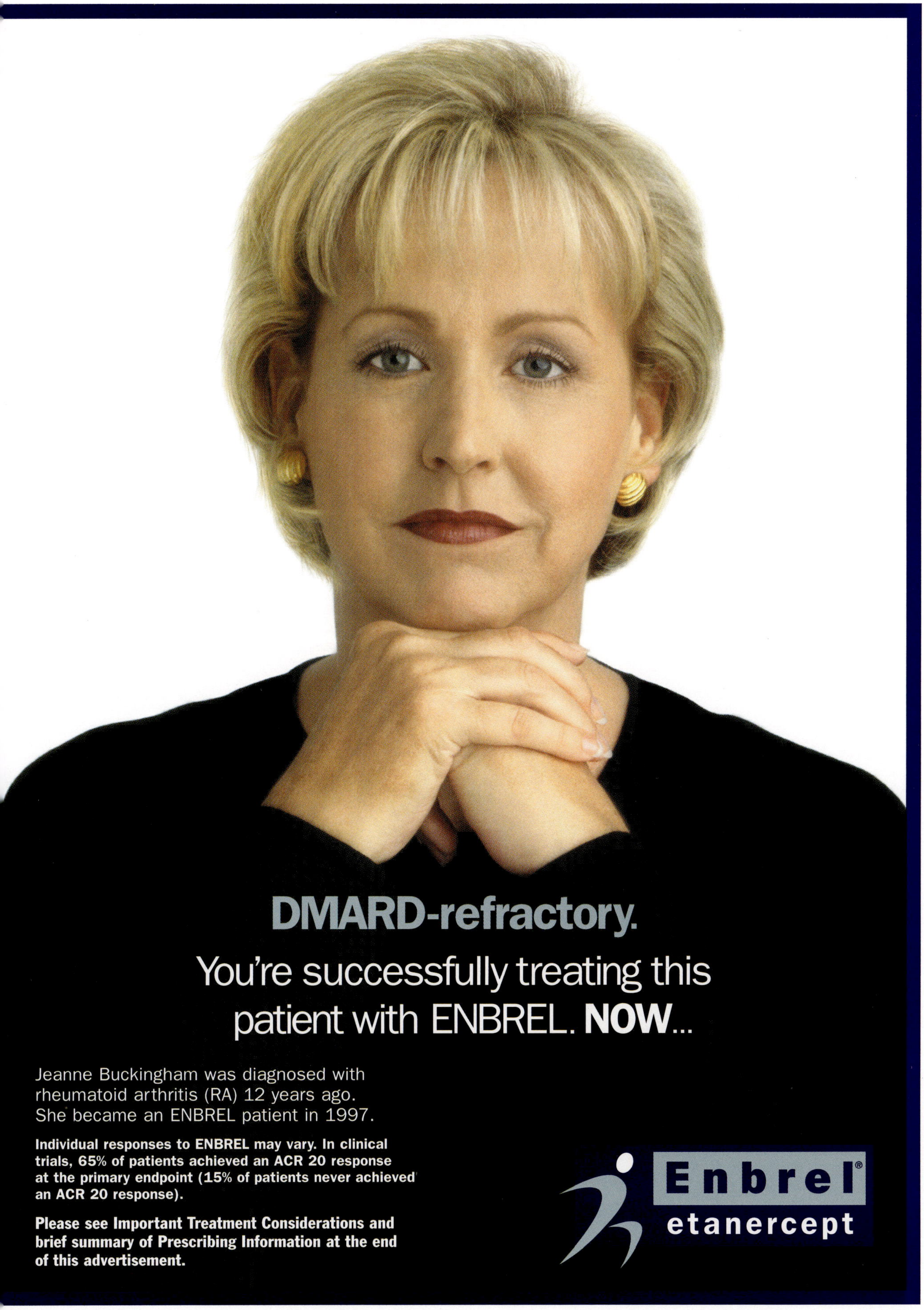
DMARD-refractory.
You're successfully treating this patient with ENBREL. NOW...
Jeanne Buckingham was diagnosed with rheumatoid arthritis (RA) 12 years ago. She became an ENBREL patient in 1997.
Individual responses to ENBREL may vary. In clinical trials, 65% of patients achieved an ACR 20 response at the primary endpoint (15% of patients never achieved an ACR 20 response).
Please see Important Treatment Considerations and brief summary of Prescribing Information at the end of this advertisement.
Enbrel®
etanercept

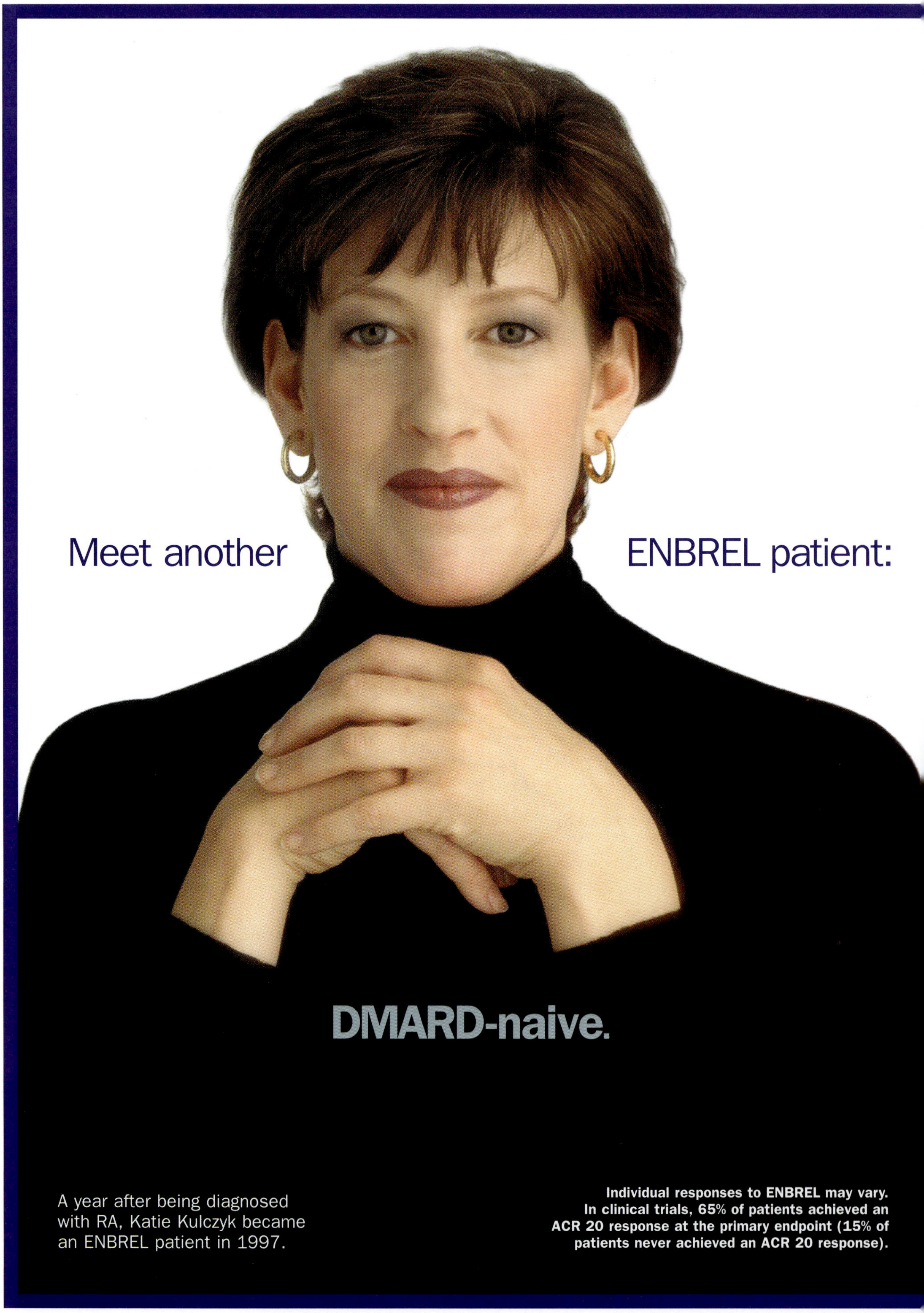
Meet another ENBREL patient:
DMARD-naive.
A year after being diagnosed with RA, Katie Kulczyk became an ENBREL patient in 1997.
Individual responses to ENBREL may vary. In clinical trials, 65% of patients achieved an ACR 20 response at the primary endpoint (15% of patients never achieved an ACR 20 response).

Enbrel®
etanercept

BRIEF SUMMARY
See package insert for full Prescribing Information.

INDICATIONS AND USAGE

ENBREL is indicated for reducing signs and symptoms and delaying structural damage in patients with moderately to severely active rheumatoid arthritis. ENBREL can be used in combination with methotrexate in patients who do not respond adequately to methotrexate alone.

ENBREL is indicated for reducing signs and symptoms of moderately to severely active polyarticular-course juvenile rheumatoid arthritis in patients who have had an inadequate response to one or more DMARDs.

CONTRAINDICATIONS

ENBREL should not be administered to patients with sepsis or with known hypersensitivity to ENBREL or any of its components.

WARNINGS

IN POSTMARKETING REPORTS, SERIOUS INFECTIONS AND SEPSIS, INCLUDING FATALITIES, HAVE BEEN REPORTED WITH THE USE OF ENBREL. MANY OF THESE SERIOUS EVENTS HAVE OCCURRED IN PATIENTS WITH UNDERLYING DISEASES THAT IN ADDITION TO THEIR RHEUMATOID ARTHRITIS COULD PREDISPOSE THEM TO INFECTIONS. PATIENTS WHO DEVELOP A NEW INFECTION WHILE UNDERGOING TREATMENT WITH ENBREL SHOULD BE MONITORED CLOSELY. ADMINISTRATION OF ENBREL SHOULD BE DISCONTINUED IF A PATIENT DEVELOPS A SERIOUS INFECTION OR SEPSIS. TREATMENT WITH ENBREL SHOULD NOT BE INITIATED IN PATIENTS WITH ACTIVE INFECTIONS INCLUDING CHRONIC OR LOCALIZED INFECTIONS. PHYSICIANS SHOULD EXERCISE CAUTION WHEN CONSIDERING THE USE OF ENBREL IN PATIENTS WITH A HISTORY OF RECURRING INFECTIONS OR WITH UNDERLYING CONDITIONS WHICH MAY PREDISPOSE PATIENTS TO INFECTIONS, SUCH AS ADVANCED OR POORLY CONTROLLED DIABETES (see **PRECAUTIONS, ADVERSE REACTIONS, Infections**).

Neurologic Events- Rare cases of central nervous system demyelinating disorders have been described in spontaneous adverse event reports (see **ADVERSE REACTIONS**). The causal relationship to ENBREL therapy remains unclear. However, while no clinical trials have been performed evaluating ENBREL therapy in multiple sclerosis, other TNF antagonists administered to patients with multiple sclerosis have been associated with increases in disease activity. Prescribers should exercise caution in considering the use of ENBREL in patients with preexisting or recent onset of central nervous system demyelinating disorders. **Hematologic Events-** Rare reports of pancytopenia, including aplastic anemia, some with a fatal outcome, have been reported in patients with rheumatoid arthritis treated with ENBREL (see **ADVERSE REACTIONS**). The causal relationship to ENBREL therapy remains unclear. Although no high risk group has been identified, caution should be exercised in patients being treated with ENBREL who have a previous history of significant hematologic abnormalities. All patients should be advised that if they develop signs and symptoms suggestive of blood dyscrasias or infection (e.g., persistent fever, bruising, bleeding, pallor) while on ENBREL, they should seek immediate medical attention. If significant hematologic abnormalities are confirmed, consideration should be given to discontinuation of ENBREL therapy.

PRECAUTIONS: General-Allergic reactions associated with administration of ENBREL during clinical trials have been reported in <2% of patients. If an anaphylactic reaction or other serious allergic reaction occurs, administration of ENBREL should be discontinued immediately and appropriate therapy initiated. **Information to Patients-**If a patient or caregiver is to self-administer ENBREL, he/she should be instructed in injection techniques and how to measure the correct dose to help ensure the proper administration of ENBREL (see **How to Use ENBREL, Instructions for Preparing and Giving an Injection**). The first injection should be performed under the supervision of a qualified health care professional. The patient's or caregiver's ability to self-inject subcutaneously should be assessed. A puncture-resistant container for disposal of needles and syringes should be used. Patients and caregivers should be instructed in the technique as well as proper syringe and needle disposal, and be cautioned against reuse of these items. **Immunosuppression-**The possibility exists for anti-TNF therapies, including ENBREL, to affect host defenses against infections and malignancies since TNF mediates inflammation and modulates cellular immune responses. In a study of 49 patients with RA treated with ENBREL, there was no evidence of depression of delayed-type hypersensitivity, depression of immunoglobulin levels, or change in enumeration of effector cell populations. The impact of treatment with ENBREL on the development and course of malignancies, as well as active and/or chronic infections is not fully understood (see **WARNINGS, ADVERSE REACTIONS, Infections** and **Malignancies**). The safety and efficacy of ENBREL in patients with immunosuppression have not been evaluated. **Immunizations-**No data are available on the effects of vaccination in patients receiving ENBREL. Live vaccines should not be given concurrently with ENBREL. No data are available on the secondary transmission of infection by live vaccines in patients receiving ENBREL (see **PRECAUTIONS, Immunosuppression**). It is recommended that JRA patients, if possible, be brought up to date with all immunizations in agreement with current immunization guidelines prior to initiating ENBREL therapy. Two JRA patients developed varicella infection and signs and symptoms of aseptic meningitis, which resolved without sequelae. Patients with a significant exposure to varicella virus should temporarily discontinue ENBREL therapy and be considered for prophylactic treatment with Varicella Zoster Immune Globulin. **Autoantibody Formation-**Treatment with ENBREL may result in the formation of autoimmune antibodies (see **ADVERSE REACTIONS, Autoantibodies**). **Drug Interactions-**Specific drug interaction studies have not been conducted with ENBREL. **Carcinogenesis, Mutagenesis, and Impairment of Fertility-**Long-term animal studies have not been conducted to evaluate the carcinogenic potential of ENBREL or its effect on fertility. Mutagenesis studies were conducted in vitro and in vivo, and no evidence of mutagenic activity was observed. **Pregnancy (Category B)-**Developmental toxicity studies have been performed in rats and rabbits at doses ranging from 60- to 100-fold higher than the human dose and have revealed no evidence of harm to the fetus due to ENBREL. There are, however, no studies in pregnant women. Because animal reproduction studies are not always predictive of human response, this drug should be used during pregnancy only if clearly needed. **Nursing Mothers-**It is not known whether ENBREL is excreted in human milk or absorbed systemically after ingestion. Because many drugs and immunoglobulins are excreted in human milk, and because of the potential for serious adverse reactions in nursing infants from ENBREL, a decision should be made whether to discontinue nursing or to discontinue the drug. **Geriatric Use-**A total of 197 RA patients ages 65 years or older have been studied in clinical trials. No overall differences in safety or effectiveness were observed between these patients and younger patients. Because there is a higher incidence of infections in the elderly population in general, caution should be used in treating the elderly. **Pediatric Use**-ENBREL is indicated for treatment of polyarticular-course juvenile rheumatoid arthritis in patients who have had an inadequate response to one or more DMARDs. For issues relevant to pediatric patients, in addition to other sections of the label, see also **PRECAUTIONS, Immunizations,** and **ADVERSE REACTIONS, Adverse Reactions in Pediatric Patients.** ENBREL has not been studied in children <4 years of age.

ADVERSE REACTIONS: ENBREL has been studied in 1197 patients with RA, followed for up to 36 months. The proportion of patients who discontinued treatment due to adverse events was approximately 4% in both ENBREL and placebo-treated patients. **Injection Site Reactions-**In controlled trials, 37% of patients treated with ENBREL developed injection site reactions. All injection site reactions were described as mild to moderate (erythema and/or itching, pain, or swelling) and generally did not necessitate drug discontinuation. Injection site reactions generally occurred in the first month and subsequently decreased in frequency. The mean duration of injection site reactions was 3 to 5 days. Seven percent of patients experienced redness at a previous injection site when subsequent injections were given. In post-marketing experience, injection site bleeding and bruising have also been observed in conjunction with ENBREL therapy. **Infections-**In controlled trials, there were no differences in rates of infection among patients treated with ENBREL and those treated with placebo or MTX. The most common type of infection was upper respiratory infection, which occurred in 16% of placebo-treated patients and 29% of patients treated with ENBREL. When the longer observation of patients on ENBREL was accounted for, the event rate was similar in both groups. In placebo-controlled trials in DMARD-refractory RA, no increase in the incidence of serious infections was observed (approximately 1% in both placebo and ENBREL-treated groups). The rates of infections for the ENBREL arm in Study III were similar. In all clinical trials in RA, 50 of 1197 subjects exposed to ENBREL for up to 36 months experienced serious infections, including pyelonephritis, bronchitis, septic arthritis, abdominal abscess, cellulitis, osteomyelitis, wound infection, pneumonia, foot abscess, leg ulcer, diarrhea, sinusitis, and sepsis. Serious infections, including sepsis and death, have also been reported during post-marketing use of ENBREL. Some have occurred within a few weeks after initiating treatment with ENBREL. Many of the patients had underlying conditions (e.g., diabetes, congestive heart failure, history of active or chronic infections) in addition to their rheumatoid arthritis (see **WARNINGS**). Data from a sepsis clinical trial not specifically in patients with RA suggest that ENBREL treatment may increase mortality in patients with established sepsis. **Malignancies-**Seventeen malignancies of various types were observed in 1197 RA patients treated in clinical trials with ENBREL for up to 36 months. The observed rates and incidences were similar to those expected for the population studied. **Autoantibodies-**Patients had serum samples tested for autoantibodies at multiple timepoints. In Studies I and II, the percentage of patients evaluated for antinuclear antibodies (ANA), the percentage of patients who developed new positive ANA (≥1:40) was higher in patients treated with ENBREL (11%) than in placebo-treated patients (5%). The percentage of patients who developed new positive anti-double-stranded DNA antibodies was also higher by radioimmunoassay (15% of patients treated with ENBREL compared to 4% of placebo-treated patients) and by crithidia lucilae assay (3% of patients treated with ENBREL compared to none of placebo-treated patients). The proportion of patients treated with ENBREL who developed anticardiolipin antibodies was similarly increased compared to placebo-treated patients. In Study III, no pattern of increased autoantibody development was seen in ENBREL patients compared to MTX patients. No patients in placebo- and active-controlled trials developed clinical signs suggestive of a lupus-like syndrome. The impact of long-term treatment with ENBREL on the development of autoimmune diseases is unknown. **Other Adverse Reactions-**The following table summarizes events reported in at least 3% of all patients with higher incidence in patients treated with ENBREL compared to controls in placebo-controlled RA trials (including the combination methotrexate trial), and relevant events from Study III.

Percent of RA Patients Reporting Adverse Events in Controlled Clinical Trials*

	Placebo Controlled		Active Controlled (Study III)	
	Percent of patients		Percent of patients	
Event	Placebo† (n=152)	ENBREL (n=349)	MTX (n=217)	ENBREL (n=415)
Injection site reaction	10	37	7	34
Infection	32	35	72	64
Non-upper respiratory infection**	32	38	60	51
Upper respiratory infection**	16	29	39	31
Headache	13	17	27	24
Nausea	10	9	29	15
Rhinitis	8	12	14	16
Dizziness	5	7	11	8
Pharyngitis	5	7	9	6
Cough	3	6	6	5
Asthenia	3	5	12	11
Abdominal pain	3	5	10	10
Rash	3	5	23	14
Peripheral edema	3	2	4	8
Respiratory disorder	1	5	NA	NA
Dyspepsia	1	4	10	11
Sinusitis	2	3	3	5
Vomiting	–	3	8	5
Mouth ulcer	1	2	14	6
Alopecia	1	1	12	6
Pneumonitis ("MTX lung")	–	–	2	0

* *Includes data from the 6-month study in which patients received concurrent MTX therapy.*

† *The duration of exposure for patients receiving placebo was less than the ENBREL-treated patients.*

** *Includes data from two of the three placebo-controlled trials.*

Among patients with rheumatoid arthritis treated in placebo-controlled trials, serious adverse events occurred at a frequency of 4% in 349 patients treated with ENBREL compared to 5% of 152 placebo-treated patients. In Study III, serious adverse events occurred at a frequency of 6% in 415 patients treated with ENBREL compared to 8% of 217 MTX-treated patients. Among patients with RA in placebo-controlled, active-controlled, and open-label trials of ENBREL, malignancies (see **ADVERSE REACTIONS, Malignancies**) and infections (see **ADVERSE REACTIONS, Infections**) were the most common serious adverse events observed. Other infrequent serious adverse events observed included heart failure, myocardial infarction, myocardial ischemia, cerebral ischemia, hypertension, hypotension, cholecystitis, pancreatitis, gastrointestinal hemorrhage, bursitis, depression, dyspnea, deep vein thrombosis, pulmonary embolism, membranous glomerulonephropathy, polymyositis, and thrombophlebitis.

Adverse Reaction Information from Spontaneous Reports-Adverse events have been reported during post-approval use of ENBREL. Because these events are reported voluntarily from a population of uncertain size, it is not always possible to reliably estimate their frequency or establish a causal relationship to ENBREL exposure.

In post-marketing experience, patients being treated for RA have reported developing additional manifestations of RA while receiving ENBREL therapy. There are uncommon reports of joint pain, generalized pain, fatigue, and dry mouth. There have also been rare reports of patients developing pulmonary disease, ocular inflammation, anorexia, cutaneous vasculitis, subcutaneous nodules, and dry eyes.

Additional adverse events are listed by body system below:

Body as a whole:	fever, flu syndrome, angioedema, weight gain
Cardiovascular:	chest pain, vasodilation (flushing)
Digestive:	diarrhea, altered sense of taste
Hematologic/Lymphatic:	adenopathy, anemia, leukopenia, thrombocytopenia, pancytopenia, aplastic anemia (see **WARNINGS**)
Nervous:	stroke, paresthesias, seizures and central nervous system events suggestive of multiple sclerosis or isolated demyelinating condition such as transverse myelitis or optic neuritis (see **PRECAUTIONS**)
Respiratory:	dyspnea, worsening of prior lung disorder
Skin:	urticaria, pruritis

Adverse Reactions in Pediatric Patients-In general, the adverse events in pediatric patients were similar in frequency and type as those seen in adult patients. Differences from adults and other special considerations are discussed in the following paragraphs.

Severe adverse reactions reported in 69 JRA patients ages 4 to 17 years included varicella (see also **PRECAUTIONS, Immunizations**), gastroenteritis, depression/personality disorder, cutaneous ulcer, esophagitis/gastritis, group A streptococcal septic shock, type I diabetes mellitus, and soft tissue and post-operative wound infection.

Forty-three of 69 (62%) children with JRA experienced an infection while receiving ENBREL during 3 months of study (part 1 open-label), and the frequency and severity of infections was similar in 58 patients completing 12 months of open-label extension therapy. The types of infections reported in JRA patients were generally mild and consistent with those commonly seen in outpatient pediatric populations.

The following adverse events were reported more commonly in 69 JRA patients receiving 3 months of ENBREL compared to the 349 adult RA patients in placebo-controlled trials. These included headache (19% of patients, 1.7 events per patient year), nausea (9%, 1.0 events per patient year), abdominal pain (19%, 0.74 events per patient year), and vomiting (13%, 0.74 events per patient year).

In post-marketing experience, very rare cases of cutaneous vasculitis in children with JRA have been reported. A causal relationship to ENBREL therapy for this condition has not been established.

OVERDOSAGE: The maximum tolerated dose of ENBREL has not been established in humans. Toxicology studies have been performed in monkeys at doses up to 30 times the human dose with no evidence of dose-limiting toxicities. No dose-limiting toxicities have been observed during clinical trials of ENBREL. Single IV doses up to 60 mg/m² have been administered to healthy volunteers in an endotoxemia study without evidence of dose-limiting toxicities. The highest dose level evaluated in RA patients has been a single IV loading dose of 32 mg/m² followed by SC doses of 16 mg/m² (~25 mg) administered twice weekly. In one RA trial, one patient mistakenly self-administered 62 mg ENBREL SC twice weekly for 3 weeks without experiencing adverse effects.

RX only

This Brief Summary is based on document 0311-06, issued 10/00.

Manufactured by:
Immunex Corporation
Seattle, Washington 98101
U.S. License Number 1132

Marketed by Immunex Corporation and Wyeth-Ayerst Pharmaceuticals

IMMUNEX® WYETH-AYERST LABORATORIES

For more information, please call 1-888-436-2735.

61746-00

RHEUMATOLOGY **South-Central Michigan**

Seeking associate for an excellent hospital-employed opportunity. Current Rheumatologist is extremely busy serving a patient population of 300,000. Good mix of rheumatology cases. All support services readily available. Flexible hours. Affiliated with 448-bed not-for-profit community hospital. Located in Jackson, just 30 miles West of Ann Arbor and 30 miles South of Lansing. Jackson offers excellent schools, very affordable housing and all cultural and recreational amenities. Competitive salary plus bonus and full benefits package.

Contact: Michelle Neuman 800/572-3732 Fax: 314/821-2722
Email: Mprosp1234@aol.com No J-1 visa applicants.

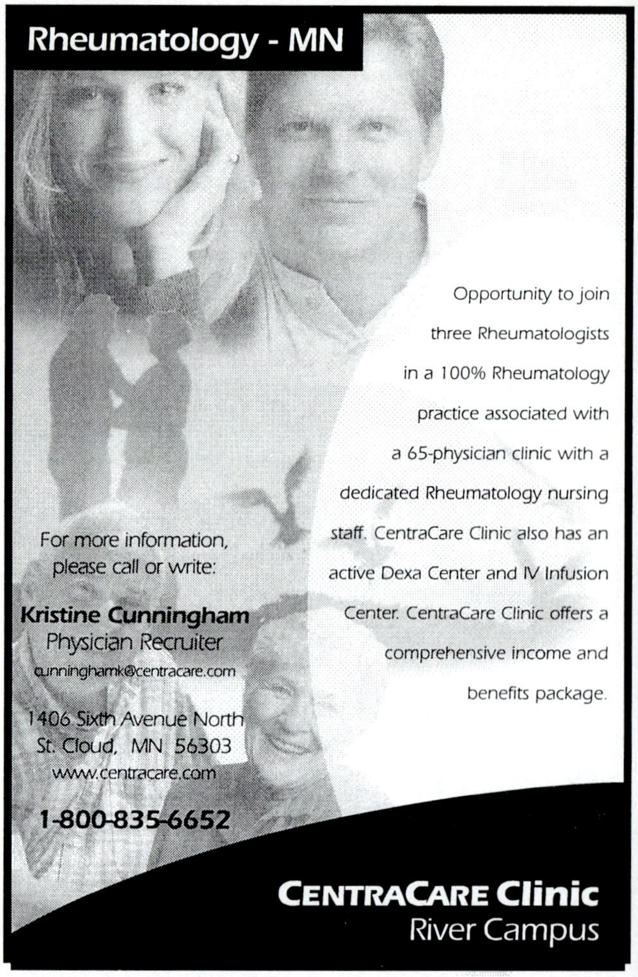

PHYSICIAN RESEARCHER: We seek a rheumatologist/researcher to join our research program in hormonally mediated induction of autoimmunity. Candidates should have a proven research record in the molecular biology of the immune system to join a multidisciplinary research effort designed to characterize the impact of female hormones on autoreactive B-cells. Documented experience with animal immunization and surgery, lymphocyte isolation and purification, flow cytometry, immunoblotting, RT-PCR, and sequencing required. Candidates should be BC in Rheumatology with a strong commitment to research. The candidate will be expected to establish independent, funded research program, but must also have the ability to interact collaboratively. Salary range will be commensurate with experience. Send CV and three letters of recommendation to: Betty Diamond, MD, Director, Rheumatology Division, Albert Einstein College of Medicine, 1300 Morris Park Avenue, Bronx, NY 10461.

GEISINGER HEALTH SYSTEM

......Has 2 Diverse Practice Opportunities in its Division of Rheumatology

Danville, PA

GEISINGER CLINIC is inviting applications for a Board Certified Rheumatologist to join our very busy 5-person Rheumatology Department at the Geisinger Medical Center in Danville, PA. The Geisinger Medical Center is a multispecialty tertiary care center with a Trauma Center, Children's Hospital, Women's Pavilion, Rehabilitation Center, and Basic/Clinical Research Center. This unique 100% rheumatology position involves a combination of clinical practice, clinical research, and teaching rheumatology fellows and residents. We have an accredited Rheumatology Fellowship Program as part of our 23 residency and fellowship programs. A previous track record in Industry-sponsored Clinical Research would be a plus. To get a better flavor of our Department, visit its web site at: http://www.geisinger.org/medicine/rheum.htm ~ Discover the joys of beautiful Central Pennsylvania. Refer to Position No. 001002run1.ar

Wilkes-Barre, PA

The Geisinger Health System is seeking a BC/BE rheumatologist to take over a busy, well established 100% rheumatology practice at its GEISINGER WYOMING VALLEY MEDICAL CENTER location. This is a clinic practice, and referrals are supported through a very active rehabilitation program along with a very busy orthopaedic surgery group. There is a Rehabilitation Center in the community that also receives the support of our program. Work in a busy clinic, attached to a full-service Medical Center licensed at 177 beds. The Geisinger Health System's GWV Medical Center is a multi-specialty group situated in one of the most scenic and conveniently located regions of Northeastern Pennsylvania. Philadelphia Phillies baseball and Pittsburgh Penguins hockey semi-pro teams, and a new 8,500-seat ice hockey arena, along with proximity to the Pocono Mountains, will complement your recreational lifestyle. We are located approximately two hours from New York and Philadelphia. Refer to Position No. 990701rhe.ar

Geisinger Health System comprises 75 practice sites, covering 40 of Pennsylvania's 67 counties. Practice medicine in a physician-led, not-for-profit health system with 600 physicians, and over 200 mid-level providers. We offer competitive salary and comprehensive benefits. A/A/E/O/E - Women and members of minorities are encouraged to apply.

For information on any of the above positions, please contact:

Nancy Shipman, Professional Staffing Dept. ~ Geisinger Health System, Danville, PA 17822-2428

Phone: 800 - 845-7112 ~ Fax: 800 - 622-2515 ~ E-Mail: nshipman@geisinger.edu

Paediatric Rheumatology

UNIVERSITY OF CALGARY

Creating the future of health.

The Department of Paediatrics and the Calgary Regional Health Authority invite applications for a full-time academic physician in Paediatric Rheumatology to be responsible for teaching, research and patient care. The CRHA comprises four teaching hospitals situated in the city of Calgary, and serves residents of southern Alberta, British Columbia and Saskatchewan. The Department of Paediatrics is part of the rapidly growing Faculty of Medicine which is in the process of building a major new research facility. A new Alberta Children's Hospital and an adjacent research and education building is expected to open in 2004. Calgary is a vibrant, multicultural city (population ~850,000) near the Rocky Mountains, Banff National Park and Lake Louise.

Qualifications include a MD, certification in Paediatrics, eligibility for or certification in Rheumatology, a demonstrated record of research and teaching and eligibility for licensure in the Province of Alberta.

Please forward a curriculum vitae and the names of three referees by **March 2, 2001** to:

Dr. R. Brent Scott
Professor and Head, Department of Paediatrics
University of Calgary
1820 Richmond Road S.W.
Calgary, Alberta, Canada T2T 5C7

In accordance with Canadian immigration requirements, priority will be given to Canadian citizens and permanent residents of Canada. The University of Calgary respects, appreciates and encourages diversity.

www.ucalgary.ca

Temple University School of Medicine

ASSISTANT/ASSOCIATE PROFESSOR

Department of Medicine – Rheumatology: Full-time faculty position available at Assistant/Associate Professor level. Applicants should be board eligible/certified in Rheumatology. Candidates will be expected to participate in patient care, teaching and research. Send CV and letter of interest to:

Steven Berney, MD
Temple University School of Medicine
Chief, Section of Rheumatology
8th floor, Jones Hall
1316 West Ontario St.
Philadelphia, PA 19140.

Temple University is an affirmative action/equal opportunity employer and strongly encourages applications from women and minorities.

BOISE, IDAHO:

Exceptionally busy arthritis and osteoporosis center needs a second BC/BE Rheumatologist in a 100% rheumatology practice in one of the fastest growing communities in the country. Low managed care penetration with a service area of approximately 350,000. State-of-the-art equipment including x-ray and a Delphi Hologic bone densitometer on-site. Boise offers metropolitan amenities including the ballet, philharmonic and opera. Experience the best of outdoor Idaho: snow skiing, golfing, boating, camping, whitewater rafting, fishing, hunting and much more! Combine a lucrative practice with an unparalleled quality of life for the entire family. Contact: Daryl MacCarter, MD, FACP at (208) 887-9500 or send CV to Idaho Arthritis & Osteoporosis Center, 520 S. Eagle Road, Suite 3211, Meridian, ID 83642.

KAISER PERMANENTE

A Great History.
A Greater Future.

What has 50 years of medical excellence brought our professionals at The Permanente Medical Group Inc.? A longstanding reputation for progress that not only offers them the stability they need for a fulfilling career, but also the freedom to explore innovative ideas on the horizon. We currently have an exceptional opportunity in Northern California.

RHEUMATOLOGY
San Francisco Bay Area

For more information, please contact Mazie Blanks, Physician Recruiter, Physician Recruitment Services, Dept A159, 1814 Franklin Street, 4th Floor, Oakland, CA 94612; Phone: (800) 777-4912; Fax: (510) 873-5006. Email: Mazie.Blanks@kp.org.

KAISER PERMANENTE®

www.kp.org/ca • EEO/AA Employer

RHEUMATOLOGIST - NORTHERN UTAH

Ogden, Utah - One BC/BE Rheumatologist is needed to join two others in a group practice. Strong community need for this position. Large referral base of primary care physicians. Office space is located in the medical office building next to McKay-Dee Hospital. Employment position with IHC's Physician Division. Guaranteed salary and full benefits. Moving expenses are negotiable. Ogden, home of Weber State University, is a strong family oriented, growing community situated at the base of the Wasatch Mountains. It is a 35 minute drive from Salt Lake City and a few minutes drive from Snowbasin Ski Resort, site of the 2002 Olympic downhill and giant slalom ski events. Send/fax CV to IHC Physician Services, Attn: Wilf Rudert, 36 S. State Street, 20th Floor, Salt Lake City, UT 84111. 800-888-3134 #1. Fax: 801-442-2999. E-mail: comdixon@ihc.com. Internet: http://www.ihc.com/phys_recruit.

IHC

WASHINGTON - ***Group Health Permanente*** **is currently seeking a board eligible/certified rheumatologist with superb clinical skills to join a five-person department with office based in downtown Seattle. The rheumatology service is largely consultative and is part of a multispecialty group practice that includes over 800 physicians. Opportunities exist for university affiliation and collaboration in clinical trials. Please email your CV with cover letter to:**

Pamela Cereghino at cereghino.p@ghc.org or fax to 206-448-6191. Visit our website at www.ghc.org. For more information, give us a call at 1-800-543-9323.

An equal opportunity employer.

Rheumatologist Faculty Position

The Division of Rheumatology at Stony BrookUniversity is seeking a physician-scientist for a full-time academic position at the Instructor/Assistant or Associate Professor level. Excellent opportunity for the right candidate. Must be board-certified in Internal Medicine and board-eligible/certified in Rheumatology. Specific interest in bone diseases or angiogenesis are preferred.

Please send letter of interest and curriculum vitae to Dr. Barry L. Gruber, Chief of Rheumatology, Room 040, T16 Health Sciences Center, Stony Brook University, Stony Brook, NY 11794-8161.
AA/EOE

STONY BROOK
STATE UNIVERSITY OF NEW YORK

RHEUMATOLOGY

S.F. BAY AREA	WISCONSIN
Hospital sponsored solo rheumatology position associated with 300+ bed hospital. Neotiable income guarantee including start-up expenses and overhead.	Lake Michigan resort community to join another rheumatologist with 100 physician health system. No call. Salary, bonus and benefits. Employee position.

Donohue and Associates
Phone: 1-800-831-5475
Fax: 314-984-8246
E-mail: donohueandassoc@aol.com

RHEUMATOLOGIST

Join two Rheumatologists in a growing 100% rheumatology practice which is part of a well-established 175-physician multi-specialty group. Partnership offered after two years.

A full range of support services is available including physicians in 36 specialties, inhouse laboratory and radiology services, including MRI and CT, centralized billing and computerized medical record system. Ideal location between Tampa and Orlando with unlimited recreational activities including golf, tennis, boating and fishing. Great community and no State income tax!

Professional Services / WATSON CLINIC LLP
1600 Lakeland Hills Boulevard / Lakeland, Fl 33805
Fax: (863) 680-7951 / Phone: (800) 854-7786

Classified Advertising

Place your ad in

Arthritis & Rheumatism Professional Opportunities

The official publication of the American College of Rheumatology

Reach your targeted audience by advertising in the

PROFESSIONAL OPPORTUNITIES

section of Arthritis & Rheumatism

For closing dates and further information call:
212-685-5010
or fax
212-685-6126
or e-mail
arivera@pminy.com
and get your best recruitment ad buy today!

Sales Office:

Pharmaceutical Media, Inc.
Arthritis & Rheumatism
Classified Advertising
Attn: Aileen Rivera
30 E. 33rd Street, 4th Fl.
New York, New York 10016

Display space such as 1/8, 1/4, 1/2 and full page sizes available, CALL TODAY to reserve your space.

AN OFFICIAL JOURNAL OF THE AMERICAN COLLEGE OF RHEUMATOLOGY

Arthritis & Rheumatism

VOLUME 44, NUMBER 3

MARCH 2001

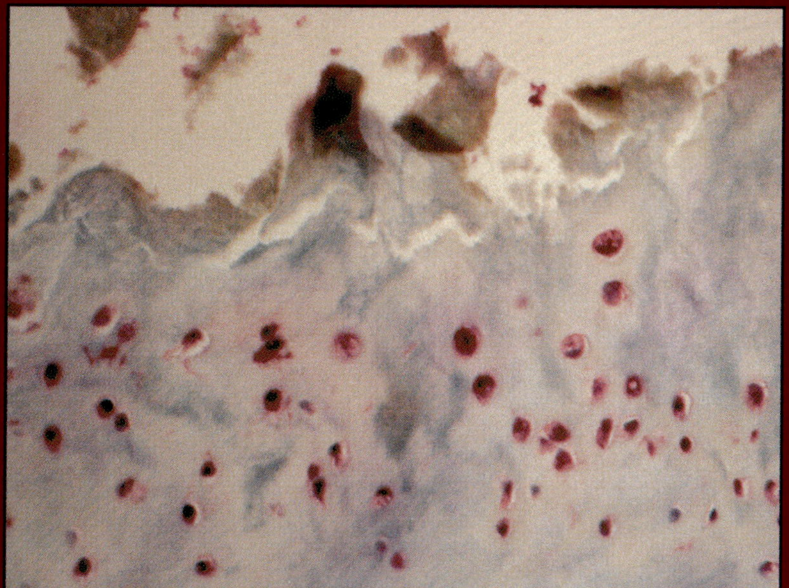

WILEY
InterScience®
www.interscience.wiley.com

EDUCATION TREATMENT RESEARCH
AMERICAN COLLEGE OF RHEUMATOLOGY
www.arthritisrheum.org

She's got RA.

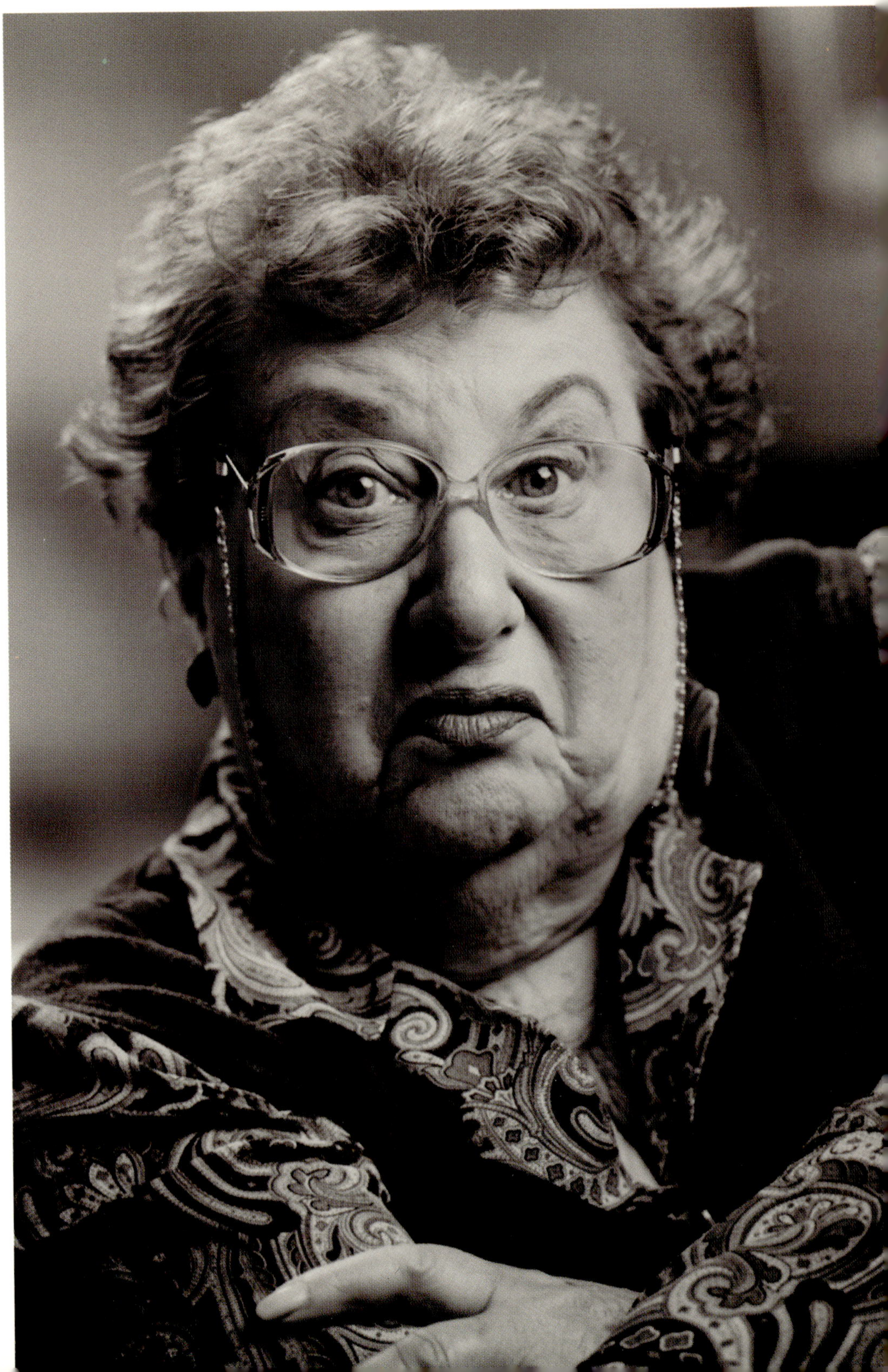

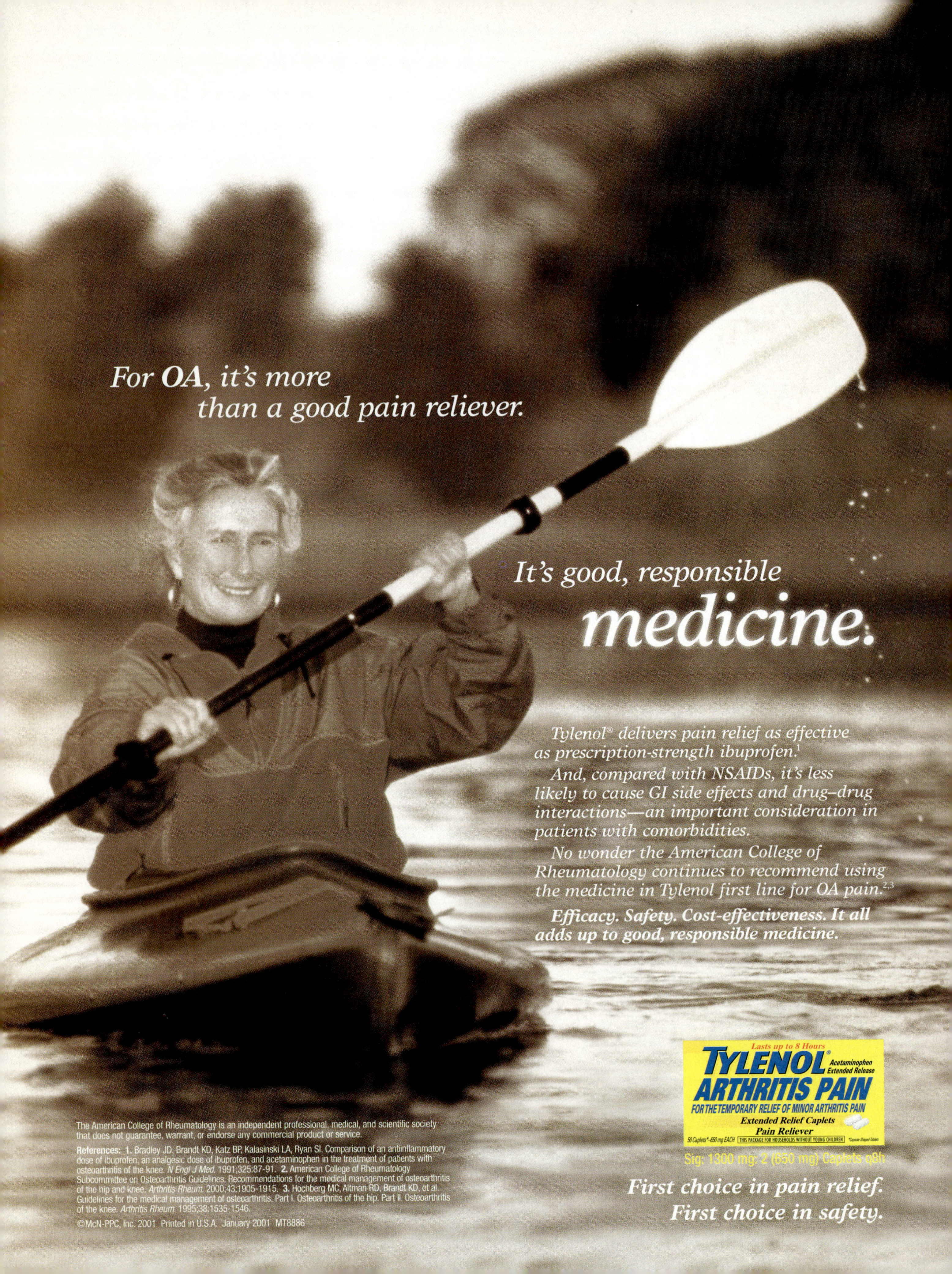

For OA, it's more
than a good pain reliever.
It's good, responsible
medicine.
Tylenol® delivers pain relief as effective as prescription-strength ibuprofen.[1]
And, compared with NSAIDs, it's less likely to cause GI side effects and drug–drug interactions—an important consideration in patients with comorbidities.
No wonder the American College of Rheumatology continues to recommend using the medicine in Tylenol first line for OA pain.[2,3]
Efficacy. Safety. Cost-effectiveness. It all adds up to good, responsible medicine.
Lasts up to 8 Hours
TYLENOL®
Acetaminophen Extended Release
ARTHRITIS PAIN
FOR THE TEMPORARY RELIEF OF MINOR ARTHRITIS PAIN
Extended Relief Caplets
Pain Reliever
50 Caplets*–650 mg EACH
THIS PACKAGE FOR HOUSEHOLDS WITHOUT YOUNG CHILDREN
*Capsule-Shaped Tablets
Sig: 1300 mg: 2 (650 mg) Caplets q8h
First choice in pain relief.
First choice in safety.
The American College of Rheumatology is an independent professional, medical, and scientific society that does not guarantee, warrant, or endorse any commercial product or service.
References: 1. Bradley JD, Brandt KD, Katz BP, Kalasinski LA, Ryan SI. Comparison of an antiinflammatory dose of ibuprofen, an analgesic dose of ibuprofen, and acetaminophen in the treatment of patients with osteoarthritis of the knee. N Engl J Med. 1991;325:87-91. 2. American College of Rheumatology Subcommittee on Osteoarthritis Guidelines. Recommendations for the medical management of osteoarthritis of the hip and knee. Arthritis Rheum. 2000;43:1905-1915. 3. Hochberg MC, Altman RD, Brandt KD, et al. Guidelines for the medical management of osteoarthritis. Part I. Osteoarthritis of the hip. Part II. Osteoarthritis of the knee. Arthritis Rheum. 1995;38:1535-1546.
©McN-PPC, Inc. 2001 Printed in U.S.A. January 2001 MT8886

Arthritis & Rheumatism

An Official Journal of the American College of Rheumatology
www.arthritisrheum.org and www.interscience.wiley.com

ARTHRITIS & RHEUMATISM (Print ISSN 0004-3591; Online ISSN 1529-0131 at Wiley InterScience, www.interscience.wiley.com) is published monthly, except semi-monthly in February, April, June, August, October, and December by Wiley-Liss, Inc., a division of John Wiley & Sons, Inc., 605 Third Avenue, New York, NY 10158-0012. **Send subscription inquiries to:** John Wiley & Sons, Inc., Subscription Department, 9th Floor, 605 Third Avenue, New York, NY 10158-0012, (212) 850-6645. **Advertising sales contact:** Susan Tagliaferro, Accounts Representative, Pharmaceutical Media, Inc., 30 East 33rd Street, New York, NY 10016, phone (212) 685-5010. **Offprint sales and inquiries** should be directed to the Customer Service Department, John Wiley and Sons, 605 Third Avenue, New York, NY 10158-0012, (212) 850-8776. For 2001, Volumes 44 and 45; institutional rate in U.S., $560; outside U.S., $720; personal subscription rate in U.S., $207; outside U.S., $249. (Subscriptions outside North America are sent by air.) Payment must be made in U.S. dollars drawn on a U.S. bank. **Change of Address:** Please forward to the subscriptions address listed above 6 weeks prior to move; enclose present mailing label with change of address. **Claims** for undelivered copies will be accepted only after the following issue has been received. Please enclose a copy of the mailing label or cite your subscriber reference number in order to expedite handling. Missing copies will be supplied when losses have been sustained in transit and where reserve stock permits. Send claims to John Wiley & Sons, Inc., Customer Service, 605 Third Avenue, New York, NY 10158-0012. If claims are not resolved satisfactorily, please write to Caroline Rothaug, Subscription Fulfillment and Sales, John Wiley & Sons, Inc., 605 Third Avenue, New York, NY 10158-0012. **Cancellations:** Subscription cancellations will not be accepted after the first issue has been mailed. Periodicals postage paid at New York, N.Y., and at additional mailing offices. Printed in U.S.A. Copyright © 2001 American College of Rheumatology. POSTMASTER: Send address changes to Arthritis & Rheumatism, Subscription Systems and Distribution, John Wiley & Sons, Inc., 605 Third Avenue, New York, NY 10158-0012.

Introducing Genzyme Biosurgery

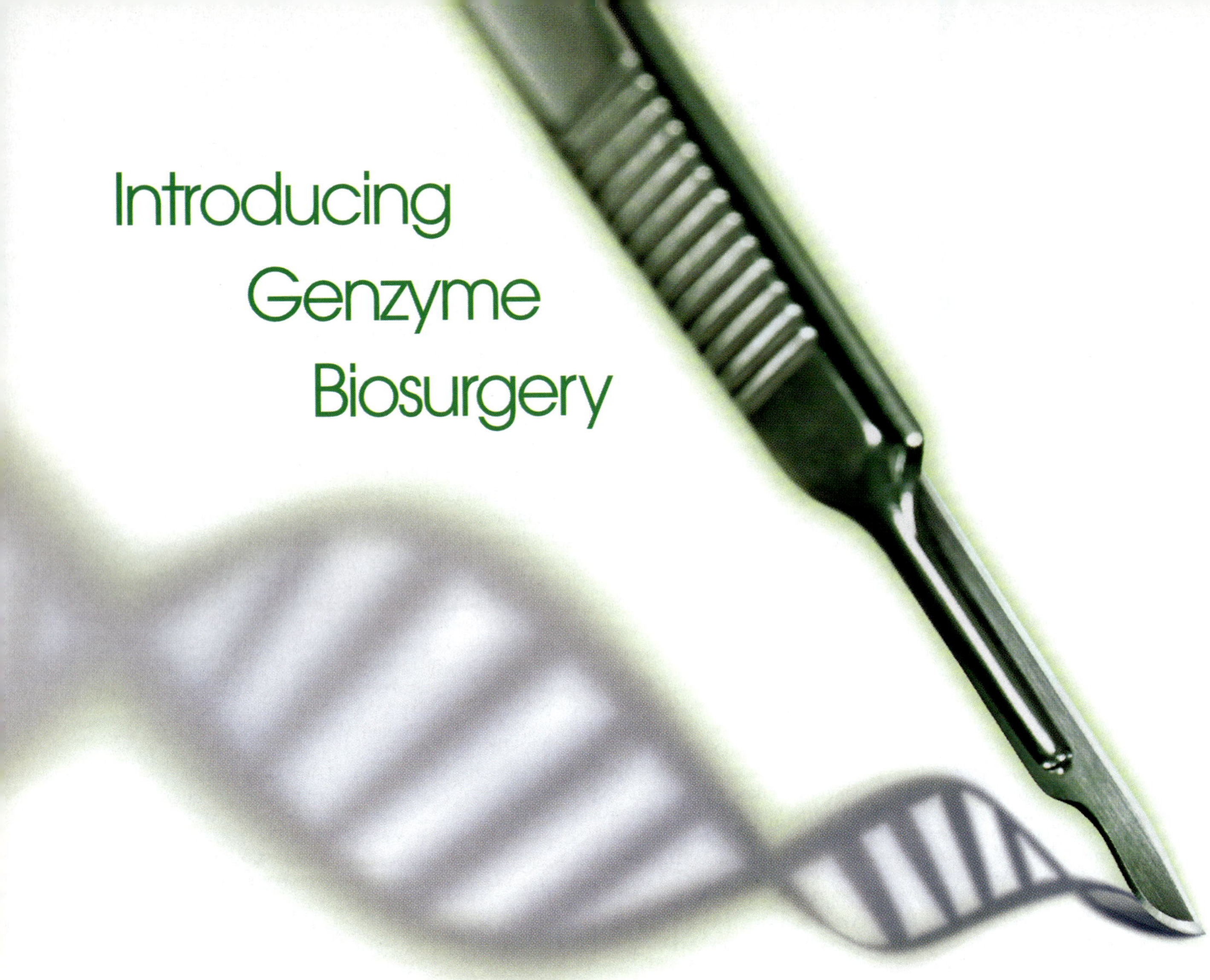

Where cutting-edge research becomes cutting-edge reality

When it comes to biotechnology in the operating room, a lot of companies have been talking but not delivering.

Except one.

One new organization has been busy fulfilling the promise of biotechnology in orthopaedic surgery. Making the cutting edge practical today with FDA-approved products utilizing advanced biomaterials and cell therapy—exciting products that change the standard of care and shape the future of orthopaedics.

Introducing Genzyme Biosurgery.
Not just talking about the future.
Delivering it.

genzyme
BIOSURGERY
Bringing biotechnology to surgery
www.genzymebiosurgery.com

A division of
Genzyme Corporation
One Kendall Square
Cambridge, MA 02139-1562 USA
Tel 800-367-7874

 Code No. 25-1358 2000-11

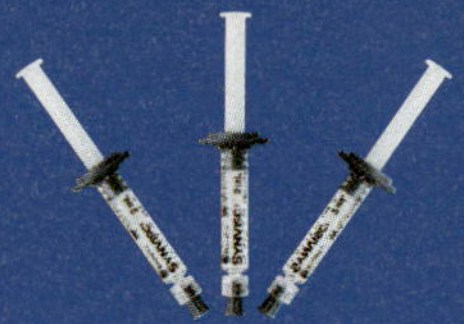

Arthritis & Rheumatism

An Official Journal of the American College of Rheumatology
www.arthritisrheum.org and www.interscience.wiley.com

VOLUME 44 **MARCH 2001** **NO. 3**

Special Articles

Review: Involvement of the Hypothalamic–Pituitary–Adrenal/Gonadal Axis and the Peripheral Nervous System in Rheumatoid Arthritis: Viewpoint Based on a Systemic Pathogenetic Role
Rainer H. Straub and Maurizio Cutolo 493

Editorial: Treatment of Polyarteritis Nodosa, Microscopic Polyangiitis, and Churg-Strauss Syndrome: Where Do We Stand?
Carol A. Langford 508

Winners of the 2000 American College of Rheumatology Slide Competition
Catherine M. Meyer and the ACR Audiovisual Aids Subcommittee 513

Rheumatoid Arthritis

A Randomized Two-Year Study of the Effects of Dynamic Strength Training on Muscle Strength, Disease Activity, Functional Capacity, and Bone Mineral Density in Early Rheumatoid Arthritis
Arja Häkkinen, Tuulikki Sokka, Antero Kotaniemi, and Pekka Hannonen 515

Increased Mortality in Adults With a History of Juvenile Rheumatoid Arthritis: A Population-Based Study
Anthony R. French, Tom Mason, Audrey M. Nelson, W. Michael O'Fallon, and Sherine E. Gabriel 523

Indirect Medical Costs in Early Rheumatoid Arthritis: Composition of and Changes in Indirect Costs Within the First Three Years of Disease
S. Merkesdal, J. Ruof, O. Schöffski, K. Bernitt, H. Zeidler, and W. Mau 528

Influence of Shared Epitope–Negative HLA–DRB1 Alleles on Genetic Susceptibility to Rheumatoid Arthritis
Denis Reviron, Aleth Perdriger, Eric Toussirot, Daniel Wendling, Nathalie Balandraud, Sandrine Guis, Gilbert Semana, Pierre Tiberghien, Pierre Mercier, and Jean Roudier 535

Lymph Draining From Foot Joints in Rheumatoid Arthritis Provides Insight Into Local Cytokine and Chemokine Production and Transport to Lymph Nodes
Waldemar L. Olszewski, J. Pazdur, E. Kubasiewicz, M. Zaleska, Conrad J. Cooke, and Norman E. Miller .. 541

Levels of Interleukin-18 and Its Binding Inhibitors in the Blood Circulation of Patients With Adult-Onset Still's Disease
Masanori Kawashima, Masahiro Yamamura, Madoka Taniai, Hiroshi Yamauchi, Tadao Tanimoto, Masashi Kurimoto, Shoji Miyawaki, Tetsuki Amano, Tsutomu Takeuchi, and Hirofumi Makino 550

Shift Toward T Helper 1 Cytokines by Type II Collagen–Reactive T Cells in Patients With Rheumatoid Arthritis
Sung-Hwan Park, Do-June Min, Mi-La Cho, Wan-Uk Kim, Jeehee Youn, Won Park, Chul-Soo Cho, and Ho-Youn Kim 561

Infection Efficiency of Type 5 Adenoviral Vectors in Synovial Tissue Can Be Enhanced With a Type 16 Fiber
Paulien H. Goossens, Menzo J. E. Havenga, Elsbet Pieterman, Angelique A. Lemckert, Ferdinand C. Breedveld, Abraham Bout, and Tom W. J. Huizinga 570

Osteoarthritis and Cartilage

Osteopontin: An Intrinsic Inhibitor of Inflammation in Cartilage
Mukundan G. Attur, Mandar N. Dave, Steven Stuchin, Aaron J. Kowalski, German Steiner, Steven B. Abramson, David T. Denhardt, and Ashok R. Amin 578

Matrix Metalloproteinase and Proinflammatory Cytokine Production by Chondrocytes of Human Osteoarthritic Cartilage: Associations With Degenerative Changes
Lynne C. Tetlow, Daman J. Adlam, and David E. Woolley 585

Peroxisome Proliferator–Activated Receptor γ Activators Inhibit Interleukin-1β–Induced Nitric Oxide and Matrix Metalloproteinase 13 Production in Human Chondrocytes
Hassan Fahmi, John A. Di Battista, Jean-Pierre Pelletier, François Mineau, Pierre Ranger, and Johanne Martel-Pelletier 595

Cyclic Tensile Strain Suppresses Catabolic Effects of Interleukin-1β in Fibrochondrocytes From the Temporomandibular Joint
Sudha Agarwal, Ping Long, Robert Gassner, Nicholas P. Piesco, and Michael J. Buckley 608

Systemic Lupus Erythematosus

The Fcγ Receptor IIIA–158F Allele Is a Major Risk Factor for the Development of Lupus Nephritis Among Caucasians but Not Non-Caucasians
Victoria A. Seligman, Charlyn Suarez, Raymond Lum, Sven E. Inda, Doris Lin, Hongzhe Li, Jean L. Olson, Michael F. Seldin, and Lindsey A. Criswell 618

Immunoglobulin V_κ Light Chain Gene Analysis in Patients With Sjögren's Syndrome
Claudia Heimbächer, Arne Hansen, Axel Pruss, Annett Jacobi, Karin Reiter, Peter E. Lipsky, and Thomas Dörner 626

Polymorphisms of the *Ro52* Gene Associated With Anti–Ro 52-kd Autoantibodies in Patients With Primary Sjögren's Syndrome
Britt Nakken, Roland Jonsson, and Anne Isine Bolstad 638

Long-Term Outcome of Mothers of Children With Isolated Heart Block in Finland
Heikki Julkunen and Marianne Eronen 647

Scleroderma

The Disability Index of the Health Assessment Questionnaire Is a Predictor and Correlate of Outcome in the High-Dose Versus Low-Dose Penicillamine in Systemic Sclerosis Trial
Philip J. Clements, Weng Kee Wong, Eric L. Hurwitz, Daniel E. Furst, Maureen Mayes, Barbara White, Fredrick Wigley, Michael Weisman, Walter Barr, Larry Moreland, Thomas A. Medsger, Jr., Virginia Steen, Richard W. Martin, David Collier, Arthur Weinstein, Edward Lally, John Varga, Steven R. Weiner, Brian Andrews, Micha Abeles, and James R. Seibold 653

Cytochrome P2 Polymorphisms and Susceptibility to Scleroderma Following Exposure to Organic Solvents
A. Povey, M. J. Guppy, M. Wood, C. Knight, C. M. Black, and A. J. Silman 662

Vasculitis

Long-Term Followup of Polyarteritis Nodosa, Microscopic Polyangiitis, and Churg-Strauss Syndrome: Analysis of Four Prospective Trials Including 278 Patients
Martine Gayraud, Loïc Guillevin, Philippe le Toumelin, Pascal Cohen, François Lhote, Philippe Casassus, Bernard Jarrousse, and the French Vasculitis Study Group 666

Mechanisms of Disease: Models and Genetics

Invasiveness of Synovial Fibroblasts Is Regulated by p53 in the SCID Mouse In Vivo Model of Cartilage Invasion
Thomas Pap, Karlfried R. Aupperle, Steffen Gay, Gary S. Firestein, and Renate E. Gay 676

Variations in Susceptibility to Proteoglycan-Induced Arthritis and Spondylitis Among C3H Substrains of Mice: Evidence of Genetically Acquired Resistance to Autoimmune Disease
Tibor T. Glant, Tamás Bárdos, Csaba Vermes, Raman Chandrasekaran, Juan C. Valdéz, Jeffrey M. Otto, David Gerard, Sonja Velins, György Lovász, Jian Zhang, Katalin Mikecz, and Alison Finnegan 682

Elevated Proapoptotic Bax and Caspase 3 Activation in the NOD.*scid* Model of Sjögren's Syndrome
Reiji Masago, Sonomi Aiba-Masago, Norman Talal, Fabio Jimenez Zuluaga, Ibtisam Al-Hashimi, Michael Moody, C. Allen Lau, Ammon B. Peck, Jason Brayer, Michael G. Humphreys-Beher, and Howard Dang 693

Cysteine Protease Activity Is Up-Regulated in Inflamed Ankle Joints of Rats With Adjuvant-Induced Arthritis and Decreases With In Vivo Administration of a Vinyl Sulfone Cysteine Protease Inhibitor
Sandra L. Biroc, Steffen Gay, Klaus Hummel, Catherine Magill, James T. Palmer, Donna R. Spencer, Susan Sa, Jeffrey L. Klaus, Beat A. Michel, David Rasnick, and Renate E. Gay 703

Activation of a Fibroblast-Specific Enhancer of the Proα2(I) Collagen Gene in Tight-Skin Mice
Christopher P. Denton, Bing Zheng, Xu Shiwen, Zhaoping Zhang, George Bou-Gharios, Heidi Eberspaecher, Carol M. Black, and Benoit de Crombrugghe 712

Development of the Tight-Skin Phenotype in Immune-Deficient Mice
Tatjana D. Dodig, Kristine T. Mack, Deborah F. Cassarino, and Stephen H. Clark 723

Concise Communications

Prolonged Remission Without Treatment After Autologous Stem Cell Transplantation for Refractory Childhood Systemic Lupus Erythematosus
N. M. Wulffraat, E. A. M. Sanders, S. S. M. Kamphuis, G. T. Rijkers, W. Kuis, M. Lilien, and I. C. M. Slaper-Cortenbach 728

Up-Regulated Expression of Transforming Growth Factor β Receptors in Dermal Fibroblasts in Skin Sections From Patients With Localized Scleroderma
Masahide Kubo, Hironobu Ihn, Kenichi Yamane, and Kunihiko Tamaki 731

Letters
Updating the American College of Rheumatology Preliminary Classification Criteria for Systemic Sclerosis: Addition of Severe Nailfold Capillaroscopy Abnormalities Markedly Increases the Sensitivity for Limited Scleroderma
Lilian Scussel Lonzetti, France Joyal, Jean-Pierre Raynauld, André Roussin, Jean-Richard Goulet, Éric Rich, Denis Choquette, Yves Raymond, and Jean-Luc Senécal 735
Possible Role of Antiidiotypes in the Loss of Anti–Topoisomerase I Antibodies: Comment on the Article by Kuwana et al
Haraldine A. Stafford, Zi-Jian Pan, and Camille J. Anderson 737
Reply
Masataka Kuwana and Junichi Kaburaki 737
ACR Announcements 22A

Cover image: The figure on the cover (from Tetlow et al, page 588) depicts staining for matrix metalloproteinase 8 (MMP-8) in osteoarthritic cartilage. In this specimen, MMP-8 is localized to chondrocytes in the superficial zone near the articular surface. In concert with data on staining for other MMPs and interleukin-1 and tumor necrosis factor α, these findings help elucidate the phenotype of chondrocytes in osteoarthritis and the process of cartilage destruction.

Erosion in rheumatoid arthritis

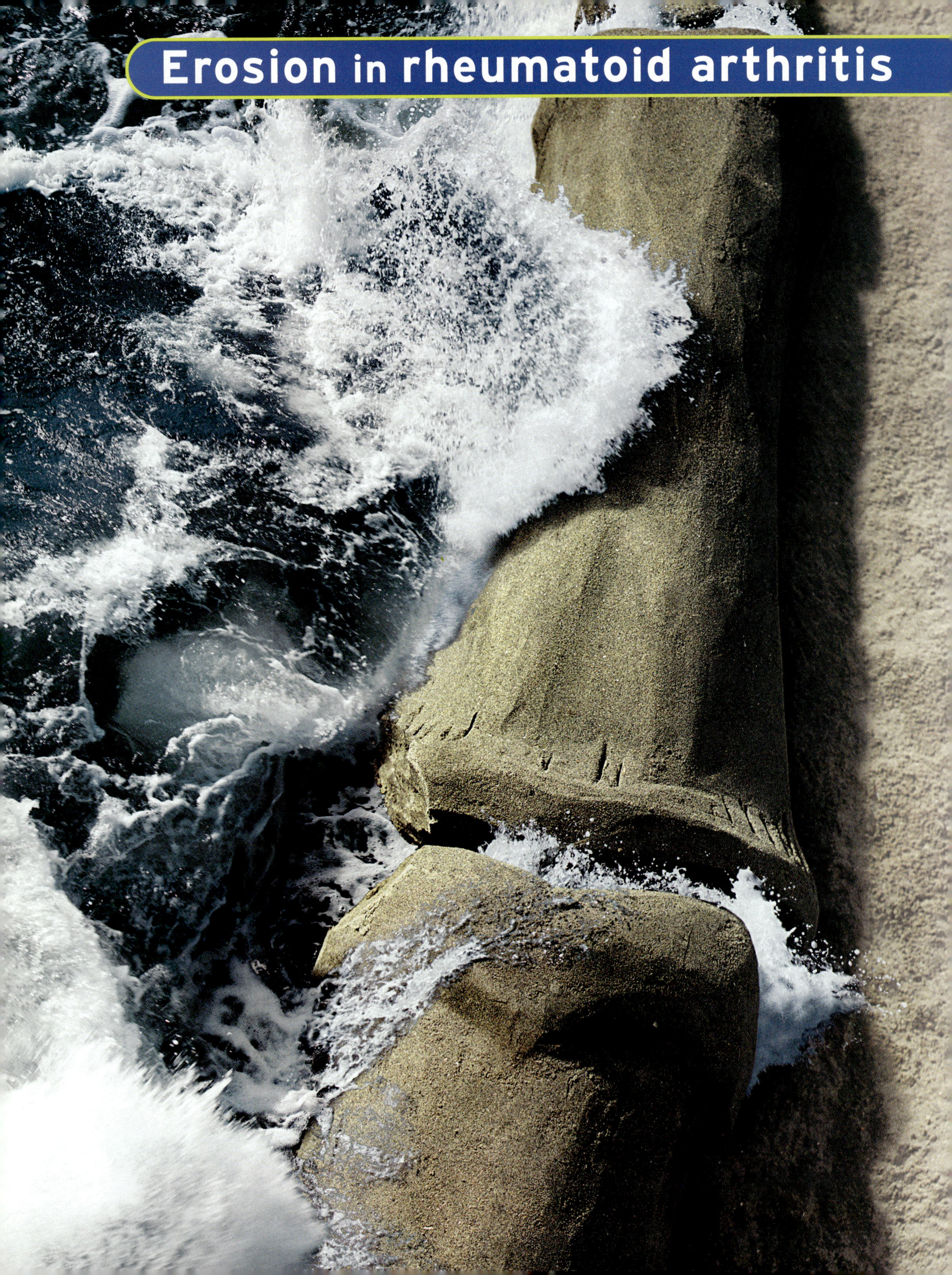

The critical role of IL-1

The pathogenesis of RA is a complex process that leads to joint inflammation and bone erosion. It's known to include several interdependent and variable interactions between proinflammatory and anti-inflammatory mechanisms.[1,2] Cytokines have been found to play a key role in promoting this disease process. The two pivotal cytokines in the pathogenesis of RA are interleukin-1 (IL-1) and tumor necrosis factor-alpha (TNF-α).[3,4]

IL-1 has been implicated in a destructive tide of events

In the RA disease process, IL-1 and TNF-α act synergistically to induce other cytokines and COX-2. Moreover, TNF-α induces IL-1,[5] IL-1 induces TNF-α,[6] and IL-1 induces IL-1.[7] This activity increases the production of PGE_2[8] and other arachidonic acid metabolites from synoviocytes[9,10] and accounts for much of the pain and swelling associated with RA.[11]

IL-1 is involved in many facets of the RA disease process. Proinflammatory cytokines cause neutrophils, monocytes, and lymphocytes to migrate to the synovium. In immunohistologic studies of macrophages accumulating in the synovial tissue, IL-1 production has been demonstrated in the cartilage-pannus junction as well as in the lining and sublining layers.[12,13]

Once in the synovium, neutrophils are activated and release mediators that stimulate mononuclear leukocytes, synoviocytes, and chondrocytes. These cells release IL-1 (more specifically, IL-1β) and other pro- and anti-inflammatory cytokines.[3,9,11]

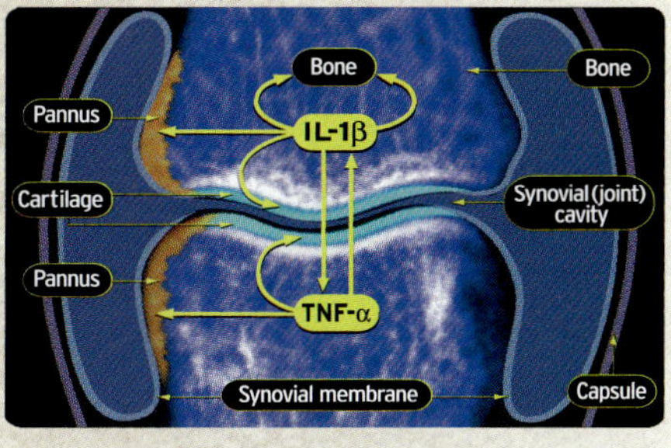

Then, once IL-1 and TNF-α are present, other interleukins (IL-6, IL-8, and IL-10) stimulate local fibroblast proliferation and recruit leukocytes. Although inflamed synovial cells express TNF-α, it is secreted to a far lesser extent than IL-1.[4,14] Early in the RA disease process, IL-1 causes cartilage degradation by inducing rapid loss of proteoglycans and stimulating the production of neutral proteinases in chondrocytes.[1,15] Since IL-1 also stimulates osteoclasts, bone resorption occurs.[16]

Higher levels of IL-1 seen with bone erosion

Animal studies, preclinical research, and early clinical studies all support the dominant role that IL-1 plays in cartilage damage and bone resorption, and suggest that TNF-α is more responsible for the inflammation in RA.[4,15,16]

In animal studies, joint swelling and cartilage damage are still present in TNF-α knockout mice (which cannot produce TNF-α), while there is an impressive reduction of cartilage damage, bone erosion, and chronic synovial infiltration in IL-1–deficient mice.[4]

These findings are supported by clinical evidence that patients with RA who have bone erosions also have higher IL-1 levels in their synovial fluid than RA patients who do not have bone erosions. Together, these findings point to the primary role of IL-1 in the bone and cartilage erosion seen in RA.[17]

The IL-1 gene family consists of IL-1α, IL-1β, and IL-1 receptor antagonist (IL-1Ra), which is the naturally occurring cytokine antagonist that normally balances the destructive effects of IL-1α and IL-1β in rheumatoid arthritis.[18,19] However, in RA, production of IL-1 cannot be sufficiently countered by endogenous IL-1Ra alone; this leads to the damaging bone and cartilage effects seen in rheumatoid joints.[20]

Amgen is conducting research in the area of rheumatology to develop new and important therapies.

www.Interleukin-1.com

AMGEN®

Advancing the science of rheumatology

References

1. Cush JJ, Lipsky PE. Cellular basis for rheumatoid inflammation. *Clin Orthop.* 1991;265:9-22.
2. Arend WP. Interleukin-1 receptor antagonist. *Adv Immunol.* 1993;54:167-227.
3. Buchan G, Barrett K, Turner M, Chantry D, Maini RN, Feldmann M. Interleukin-1 and tumour necrosis factor mRNA expression in rheumatoid arthritis: prolonged production of IL-1α. *Clin Exp Immunol.* 1998; 73:449-455.
4. van den Berg WB. Joint inflammation and cartilage destruction may occur uncoupled. *Springer Semin Immunopathol.* 1998;20:149-164.
5. Dinarello CA, Cannon JG, Wolff SM, et al. Tumor necrosis factor (cachectin) is an endogenous pyrogen and induces production of interleukin 1. *J Exp Med.* 1986;163(6): 1433-1450.
6. Philip R, Epstein LB. Tumour necrosis factor as immunomodulator and mediator of monocyte cytotoxicity induced by itself, γ-interferon and interleukin-1. *Nature.* 1986;323(6083):86-89.
7. Dinarello CA, Ikejima T, Warner SJC, et al. Interleukin 1 induces interleukin 1, I: induction of circulating interleukin 1 in rabbits in vivo and in human mononuclear cells in vitro. *J Immunol.* 1987;139(6):1902-1910.
8. Dayer J-M, de Rochemonteix B, Burrus B, Demczuk S, Dinarello CA. Human recombinant interleukin 1 stimulates collagenase and prostaglandin E_2 production by human synovial cells. *J Clin Invest.* 1986;77:645-648.
9. Koch AE, Kunkel SL, Strieter RM. Cytokines in rheumatoid arthritis. *J Invest Med.* 1995;43:28-38.
10. Crofford LJ, Wilder RL, Ristimake AP. Cyclooxygenase-1 and -2 expression in rheumatoid synovial tissues: effects of interleukin-1β, phorbol ester, and corticosteroids. *J Clin Invest.* 1994;93(3):1095-1101.
11. Harris ED Jr. Rheumatoid arthritis: pathophysiology and implications for therapy. *New Engl J Med.* 1990;322:1277-1289.
12. Chu CQ, Field M, Allard S, Abney E, Feldmann M, Maini RN. Detection of cytokines at the cartilage/pannus junction in patients with rheumatoid arthritis: implications for the role of cytokines in cartilage destruction and repair. *Br J Rheumatol.* 1992;31(10):653-661.
13. Wood NC, Dickens E, Symons JA, Duff GW. In situ hybridization of interleukin-1 in CD14-positive cells in rheumatoid arthritis. *Clin Immunol Immunopathol.* 1992;62(3):295-300.
14. van den Berg WB, Joosten LAB, van de Loo FAJ. TNFα and IL-1β are separate targets in chronic arthritis. *Clin Exp Rheumatol.* 1999;17(suppl 18):S105-S114.
15. van Lent PLEM, van de Loo FAJ, Astrid EM, et al. Major role for interleukin 1 but not for tumor necrosis factor in early cartilage damage in immune complex arthritis in mice. *J Rheumatol.* 1995;22:2250-2258.
16. Dinarello CA, Moldawer LL. *Proinflammatory and Anti-inflammatory Cytokines in Rheumatoid Arthritis: A Primer for Clinicians.* Thousand Oaks, Calif: Amgen Inc.; 1999:34.
17. Eastgate JA, Symons JA, Wood NC, Grinlinton FM, di Giovine FS, Duff GW. Correlation of plasma interleukin 1 levels with disease activity in rheumatoid arthritis. *Lancet.* 1988;2:706-709.
18. Arend WP, Joslin FG, Massoni RJ. Effects of immune complexes on production by human monocytes of interleukin 1 or an interleukin 1 inhibitor. *J Immunol.* 1985;134:3868-3875.
19. Seckinger P, Lowenthal JW, Williamson K, Dayer J-M, MacDonald HR. A urine inhibitor of interleukin 1 activity that blocks ligand binding. *J Immunol.* 1987;139:1546-1549.
20. Arend WP, Malyak M, Guthridge CJ, Gabay C. Interleukin-1 receptor antagonist: role in biology. *Annu Rev Immunol.* 1998;16:27-55.

For patients with moderate to severe pain requiring opioid therapy for more than a few days

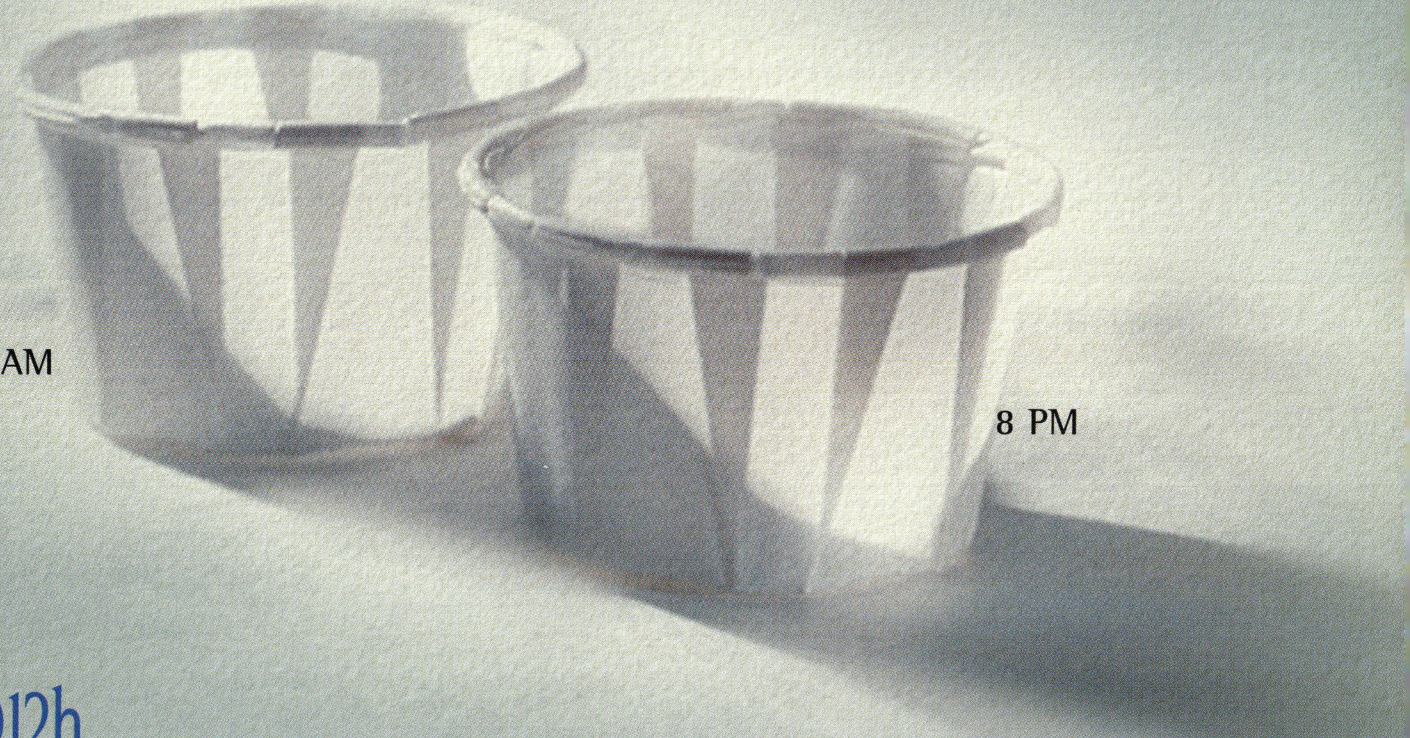

Q12h

OxyContin® CII

(OXYCODONE HCl CONTROLLED-RELEASE) TABLETS

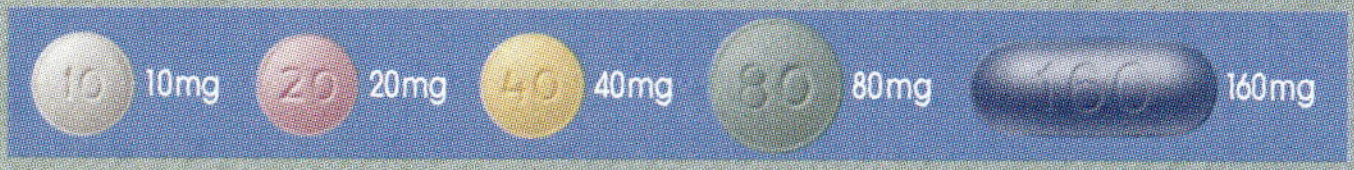

Small, color-coded tablets (actual size)

OxyContin 80 and 160 mg Tablets for use only in opioid-tolerant patients requiring daily oxycodone equivalent dosages of 160 mg and 320 mg respectively.

OxyContin® Tablets are to be swallowed whole, and are not to be broken, chewed or crushed. Taking broken, chewed or crushed OxyContin Tablets could lead to the rapid release and absorption of a potentially toxic dose of oxycodone.

One OxyContin 160 mg Tablet is comparable to two 80 mg tablets when taken on an empty stomach. With a high fat meal, however, there is a 25% greater peak plasma concentration following one 160 mg tablet. Dietary caution should be taken when patients are initially titrated to 160 mg tablets.

The most serious risk associated with opioids, including OxyContin, is respiratory depression.

Common opioid side effects are constipation, nausea, sedation, dizziness, vomiting, pruritus, headache, dry mouth, sweating and weakness.

OxyContin Tablets are contraindicated in patients with known hypersensitivity to oxycodone, or in any situation where opioids are contraindicated. **(Please see Contraindications section in package insert.)**

For more information about pain management and prevention, visit our Web site: **www.partnersagainstpain.com**

Please read attached professional prescribing information.

Co-promoted by Purdue Pharma L.P. and Abbott Laboratories

PURDUE

B6571

PUR-4000733

OxyContin® CII

(OXYCODONE HCl CONTROLLED-RELEASE) TABLETS

10 mg 20 mg 40 mg 80 mg* 160 mg*

*80 mg and 160 mg For use in opioid tolerant patients only.

Brief Summary on OxyContin® (oxycodone hydrochloride controlled-release) Tablets.

Before prescribing, see complete prescribing information, including DOSAGE AND ADMINISTRATION

INDICATIONS AND USAGE:

For the management of moderate to severe pain where use of an opioid analgesic is appropriate for more than a few days.

CONTRAINDICATIONS:

OxyContin® is contraindicated in patients with known hypersensitivity to oxycodone, or in any situation where opioids are contraindicated. This includes patients with significant respiratory depression (in unmonitored settings or the absence of resuscitative equipment), and patients with acute or severe bronchial asthma or hypercarbia. OxyContin is contraindicated in any patient who has or is suspected of having paralytic ileus.

WARNINGS:

OxyContin® TABLETS ARE TO BE SWALLOWED WHOLE, AND ARE NOT TO BE BROKEN, CHEWED OR CRUSHED. TAKING BROKEN, CHEWED OR CRUSHED OxyContin TABLETS COULD LEAD TO THE RAPID RELEASE AND ABSORPTION OF A POTENTIALLY TOXIC DOSE OF OXYCODONE.

Respiratory Depression

Respiratory depression, the chief hazard from all opioid agonist preparations, occurs most frequently in elderly or debilitated patients, usually following large initial doses in non-tolerant patients, or when opioids are given in conjunction with other agents that depress respiration.

Oxycodone should be used with extreme caution in patients with significant chronic obstructive pulmonary disease or cor pulmonale, and in patients having a substantially decreased respiratory reserve, hypoxia, hypercapnia, or preexisting respiratory depression. In such patients, even usual therapeutic doses of oxycodone may decrease respiratory drive to the point of apnea. In these patients alternative non-opioid analgesics should be considered, and opioids should be employed only under careful medical supervision at the lowest effective dose.

Head Injury

The respiratory depressant effects of opioids include carbon dioxide retention and secondary elevation of cerebrospinal fluid pressure, and may be markedly exaggerated in the presence of head injury, intracranial lesions, or other sources of preexisting increased intracranial pressure. Oxycodone produces effects which may obscure neurologic signs of further increases in intracranial pressure in patients with head injuries.

Hypotensive Effect

OxyContin®, like all opioid analgesics, may cause severe hypotension in an individual whose ability to maintain blood pressure has been compromised by a depleted blood volume, or after concurrent administration with drugs such as phenothiazines or other agents which compromise vasomotor tone. OxyContin may produce orthostatic hypotension in ambulatory patients. OxyContin, like all opioid analgesics, should be administered with caution to patients in circulatory shock, since vasodilation produced by the drug may further reduce cardiac output and blood pressure.

PRECAUTIONS:

Special precautions regarding OxyContin® 80 mg and 160 mg Tablets

OxyContin® 80 mg and 160 mg Tablets are for use only in opioid tolerant patients requiring daily oxycodone equivalent dosages of 160 mg or more for the 80 mg tablet and 320 mg or more for the 160 mg tablet. Care should be taken in the prescription of this tablet strength. Patients should be instructed against use by individuals other than the patient for whom it was prescribed, as such inappropriate use may have severe medical consequences.

One OxyContin® 160 mg tablet is comparable to two 80 mg tablets when taken on an empty stomach. With a high fat meal, however, there is a 25% greater peak plasma concentration following one 160 mg tablet. Dietary caution should be taken when patients are initially titrated to 160 mg tablets.

General — OxyContin® tablets are intended for use in patients who require oral pain therapy with an opioid agonist of more than a few days duration. As with any opioid analgesic, it is critical to adjust the dosing regimen individually for each patient.

Selection of patients for treatment with OxyContin should be governed by the same principles that apply to the use of similar controlled-release opioid analgesics. Opioid analgesics given on a fixed-dosage schedule have a narrow therapeutic index in certain patient populations, especially when combined with other drugs, and should be reserved for cases where the benefits of opioid analgesia outweigh the known risks of respiratory depression, altered mental state, and postural hypotension. Physicians should individualize treatment in every case, using non-opioid analgesics, prn opioids and/or combination products, and chronic opioid therapy with drugs such as OxyContin in a progressive plan of pain management such as outlined by the World Health Organization, the Agency for Health Care Policy and Research, and the American Pain Society.

Use of OxyContin is associated with increased potential risks and should be used only with caution in the following conditions: acute alcoholism; adrenocortical insufficiency (e.g., Addison's disease); CNS depression or coma; delirium tremens; debilitated patients; kyphoscoliosis associated with respiratory depression; myxedema or hypothyroidism; prostatic hypertrophy or urethral stricture; severe impairment of hepatic, pulmonary or renal function; and toxic psychosis.

The administration of oxycodone, like all opioid analgesics, may obscure the diagnosis or clinical course in patients with acute abdominal conditions. Oxycodone may aggravate convulsions in patients with convulsive disorders, and all opioids may induce or aggravate seizures in some clinical settings.

Interactions with other CNS Depressants

OxyContin, like all opioid analgesics, should be used with caution and started in a reduced dosage (1/3 to 1/2 of the usual dosage) in patients who are concurrently receiving other central nervous system depressants including sedatives or hypnotics, general anesthetics, phenothiazines, other tranquilizers, and alcohol. Interactive effects resulting in respiratory depression, hypotension, profound sedation, or coma may result if these drugs are taken in combination with the usual doses of OxyContin.

Interactions with Mixed Agonist/Antagonist Opioid Analgesics

Agonist/antagonist analgesics (i.e., pentazocine, nalbuphine, butorphanol, and buprenorphine) should be administered with caution to a patient who has received or is receiving a course of therapy with a pure opioid agonist analgesic such as oxycodone. In this situation, mixed agonist/antagonist analgesics may reduce the analgesic effect of oxycodone and/or may precipitate withdrawal symptoms in these patients.

Ambulatory Surgery

OxyContin is not recommended pre-operatively (preemptive analgesia) or for the management of pain in the immediate post-operative period (the first 12 to 24 hours following surgery) for patients not previously taking the drug, because its safety in this setting has not been established.

Patients who are already receiving OxyContin tablets as part of ongoing analgesic therapy may be safely continued on the drug if appropriate dosage adjustments are made considering the procedure, other drugs given and the temporary changes in physiology caused by the surgical intervention (see **PRECAUTIONS**; *Drug-Drug Interactions*).

Post-Operative Use

Morphine and other opioids have been shown to decrease bowel motility. Ileus is a common post-operative complication, especially after intra-abdominal surgery with opioid analgesia. Caution should be taken to monitor for decreased bowel motility in post-operative patients receiving opioids. Standard supportive therapy should be implemented.

Use in Pancreatic/Biliary Tract Disease

Oxycodone may cause spasm of the sphincter of Oddi and should be used with caution in patients with biliary tract disease, including acute pancreatitis. Opioids like oxycodone may cause increases in the serum amylase level.

Tolerance and Physical Dependence

Tolerance is the need for increasing doses of opioids to maintain a defined effect such as analgesia (in the absence of disease progression or other external factors). Physical dependence is the occurrence of withdrawal symptoms after abrupt discontinuation of a drug or upon administration of an antagonist. Physical dependence and tolerance are not unusual during chronic opioid therapy.

Significant tolerance should not occur in most of the patients treated with the lowest doses of oxycodone. It should be expected, however, that a fraction of cancer patients will develop some degree of tolerance and require progressively higher dosages of OxyContin to maintain pain control during chronic treatment. Regardless of whether this occurs as a result of increased pain secondary to disease progression or pharmacological tolerance, dosages can usually be increased safely by adjusting the patient's dose to maintain an acceptable balance between pain relief and side effects. The dosage should be selected according to the patient's individual analgesic response and ability to tolerate side effects. Tolerance to the analgesic effect of opioids is usually paralleled by tolerance to side effects, except for constipation.

Physical dependence results in withdrawal symptoms in patients who abruptly discontinue the drug or may be precipitated through the administration of drugs with opioid antagonist activity (see **OVERDOSAGE**). If OxyContin is abruptly discontinued in a physically dependent patient, an abstinence syndrome may occur. This is characterized by some or all of the following: restlessness, lacrimation, rhinorrhea, yawning, perspiration, chills, myalgia, and mydriasis. Other symptoms also may develop, including: irritability, anxiety, backache, joint pain, weakness, abdominal cramps, insomnia, nausea, anorexia, vomiting, diarrhea, or increased blood pressure, respiratory rate, or heart rate.

If signs and symptoms of withdrawal occur, patients should be treated by reinstitution of opioid therapy followed by a gradual, tapered dose reduction of OxyContin combined with symptomatic support.

Information for Patients/Caregivers

If clinically advisable, patients receiving OxyContin should be given the following information by the physician:

1. OxyContin tablets were designed to work properly only if swallowed whole. They may release all their contents at once if broken, chewed or crushed, resulting in a risk of overdose.
2. Report episodes of breakthrough pain and adverse experiences occurring during therapy. Individualization of dosage is essential to make optimal use of this medication.
3. Do not adjust the dose of OxyContin without consulting the prescribing professional.
4. OxyContin may impair mental and/or physical ability required for the performance of potentially hazardous tasks (e.g., driving, operating heavy machinery).
5. Do not combine OxyContin with alcohol or other central nervous system depressants (sleep aids, tranquilizers) except by the orders of the prescribing physician, because additive effects may occur.
6. Women of childbearing potential who become, or are planning to become, pregnant should consult their physician regarding the effects of analgesics and other drug use during pregnancy on themselves and their unborn child.
7. OxyContin is a potential drug of abuse. Patients should protect it from theft, and it should never be given to anyone other than the individual for whom it was prescribed.
8. Patients may pass empty matrix "ghosts" (tablets) via colostomy or in the stool; this is of no concern since the active medication has already been absorbed.
9. If patients have been receiving treatment with OxyContin for more than a few weeks and cessation of therapy is indicated, it may be appropriate to taper the OxyContin dose, rather than abruptly discontinue it, due to the risk of precipitating withdrawal symptoms. Their physician can provide a dose schedule to accomplish a gradual discontinuation of the medication.

Laboratory Monitoring

Due to the broad range of plasma concentrations seen in clinical populations, the varying degrees of pain, and the development of tolerance, plasma oxycodone measurements are usually not helpful in clinical management. Plasma concentrations of the active drug substance may be of value in selected, unusual or complex cases.

Interactions with Alcohol and Drugs of Abuse

Oxycodone may be expected to have additive effects when used in conjunction with alcohol, other opioids or illicit drugs which cause central nervous system depression.

Use in Drug and Alcohol Addiction

OxyContin is an opioid with no approved use in the management of addictive disorders. Its proper usage in individuals with drug or alcohol dependence, either active or in remission, is for the management of pain requiring opioid analgesia.

Drug-Drug Interactions

Opioid analgesics, including OxyContin, may enhance the neuromuscular blocking action of skeletal muscle relaxants and produce an increased degree of respiratory depression.

Oxycodone is metabolized in part to oxymorphone via CYP2D6. While this pathway may be blocked by a variety of drugs (e.g., certain cardiovascular drugs and antidepressants), such blockade has not yet been shown to be of clinical significance with this agent. Clinicians should be aware of this possible interaction, however.

Use with CNS Depressants

OxyContin, like all opioid analgesics, should be started at 1/3 to 1/2 of the usual dosage in patients who are concurrently receiving other central nervous system depressants including sedatives or hypnotics, general anesthetics, phenothiazines, centrally acting anti-emetics, tranquilizers, and alcohol because respiratory depression, hypotension, and profound sedation or coma may result. No specific interaction between oxycodone and monoamine oxidase inhibitors has been observed, but caution in the use of any opioid in patients taking this class of drugs is appropriate.

Mutagenicity/Carcinogenicity

Oxycodone was not mutagenic in the following assays: Ames Salmonella and E. Coli test with and without metabolic activation at doses of up to 5000 μg, chromosomal aberration test in human lymphocytes in the absence of metabolic activation at doses of up to 1500 μg/ml and with activation 48 hours after exposure at doses of up to 5000 μg/ml, and in the in vivo bone marrow micronucleus test in mice (at plasma levels of up to 48 μg/ml). Mutagenic results occurred in the presence of metabolic activation in the human chromosomal aberration test (at greater than or equal to 1250 μg/ml) at 24 but not 48 hours of exposure and in the mouse lymphoma assay at doses of 50 μg/ml or greater with metabolic activation and at 400 μg/ml or greater without metabolic activation. The data from these tests indicate that the genotoxic risk to humans may be considered low.

Studies of oxycodone in animals to evaluate its carcinogenic potential have not been conducted owing to the length of clinical experience with the drug substance.

Pregnancy

Teratogenic Effects—Category B: Reproduction studies have been performed in rats and rabbits by oral administration at doses up to 8 mg/kg (48 mg/m^2) and 125 mg/kg (1375 mg/m^2), respectively. These doses are 3 and 47 times a human dose of 160 mg/day (90 mg/m^2), based on mg/kg of a 60 kg adult (0.5 and 15 times this human dose based upon mg/m^2). The results did not reveal evidence of harm to the fetus due to oxycodone. There are, however, no adequate and well-controlled studies in pregnant women. Because animal reproduction studies are not always predictive of human response, this drug should be used during pregnancy only if clearly needed.

Nonteratogenic Effects—Neonates whose mothers have been taking oxycodone chronically may exhibit respiratory depression and/or withdrawal symptoms, either at birth and/or in the nursery.

Labor and Delivery

OxyContin is not recommended for use in women during and immediately prior to labor and delivery because oral opioids may cause respiratory depression in the newborn.

Nursing Mothers

Low concentrations of oxycodone have been detected in breast milk. Withdrawal symptoms can occur in breast-feeding infants when maternal administration of an opioid analgesic is stopped. Ordinarily, nursing should not be undertaken while a patient is receiving OxyContin since oxycodone may be excreted in the milk.

Pediatric Use

Safety and effectiveness in pediatric patients below the age of 18 have not been established with this dosage form of oxycodone. However, oxycodone has been used extensively in the pediatric population in other dosage forms, as have the excipients used in this formulation. No specific increased risk is expected from the use of this form of oxycodone in pediatric patients old enough to safely take tablets if dosing is adjusted for the patient's weight. **It must be remembered that OxyContin tablets cannot be crushed or divided for administration.**

Geriatric Use

In controlled pharmacokinetic studies in elderly subjects (greater than 65 years) the clearance of oxycodone appeared to be slightly reduced. Compared to young adults, the plasma concentrations of oxycodone were increased approximately 15%. In clinical trials with appropriate initiation of therapy and dose titration, no untoward or unexpected side effects were seen based on age, and the usual doses and dosing intervals are appropriate for the geriatric patient. As with all opioids, the starting dose should be reduced to 1/3 to 1/2 of the usual dosage in debilitated, non-tolerant patients.

Hepatic Impairment

A study of OxyContin in patients with hepatic impairment indicates greater plasma concentrations than those with normal function. The initiation of therapy at 1/3 to 1/2 the usual doses and careful dose titration is warranted.

Renal Impairment

In patients with renal impairment, as evidenced by decreased creatinine clearance (<60 mL/min.), the concentrations of oxycodone in the plasma are approximately 50% higher than in subjects with normal renal function. Dose initiation should follow a conservative approach. Dosages should be adjusted according to the clinical situation.

Gender Differences

In pharmacokinetic studies, opioid-naive females demonstrate up to 25% higher average plasma concentrations and greater frequency of typical opioid adverse events than males, even after adjustment for body weight. The clinical relevance of a difference of this magnitude is low for a drug intended for chronic usage at individualized dosages, and there was no male/female difference detected for efficacy or adverse events in clinical trials.

Rectal Administration

OxyContin Tablets are not recommended for administration per rectum. A study in normal volunteers showed a significantly greater AUC and higher C_{max} during this route of administration.

ADVERSE REACTIONS:

Serious adverse reactions which may be associated with OxyContin® tablet therapy in clinical use are those observed with other opioid analgesics, including: respiratory depression, apnea, respiratory arrest, and (to an even lesser degree) circulatory depression, hypotension, or shock (see **OVERDOSAGE**).

The non-serious adverse events seen on initiation of therapy with OxyContin are typical opioid side effects. These events are dose-dependent, and their frequency depends upon the dose, the clinical setting, the patient's level of opioid tolerance, and host factors specific to the individual. They should be expected and managed as a part of opioid analgesia. The most frequent (>5%) include constipation, nausea, somnolence, dizziness, vomiting, pruritus, headache, dry mouth, sweating, and asthenia.

In many cases the frequency of these events during initiation of therapy may be minimized by careful individualization of starting dosage, slow titration, and the avoidance of large swings in the plasma concentrations of the opioid. Many of these adverse events will cease or decrease in intensity as OxyContin therapy is continued and some degree of tolerance is developed.

In clinical trials comparing OxyContin with immediate-release oxycodone and placebo, the most common adverse events (>5%) reported by patients (pts) at least once during therapy were:

	OxyContin (n=227)		Immediate-Release (n=225)		Placebo (n=45)	
	# Pts	(%)	# Pts	(%)	# Pts	(%)
Constipation	52	(23)	58	(26)	3	(7)
Nausea	52	(23)	60	(27)	5	(11)
Somnolence	52	(23)	55	(24)	2	(4)
Dizziness	29	(13)	35	(16)	4	(9)
Pruritus	29	(13)	28	(12)	1	(2)
Vomiting	27	(12)	31	(14)	3	(7)
Headache	17	(7)	19	(8)	3	(7)
Dry Mouth	13	(6)	15	(7)	1	(2)
Asthenia	13	(6)	16	(7)	—	—
Sweating	12	(5)	13	(6)	1	(2)

The following adverse experiences were reported in OxyContin treated patients with an incidence between 1% and 5%. In descending order of frequency they were anorexia, nervousness, insomnia, fever, confusion, diarrhea, abdominal pain, dyspepsia, rash, anxiety, euphoria, dyspnea, postural hypotension, chills, twitching, gastritis, abnormal dreams, thought abnormalities, and hiccups.

The following adverse reactions occurred in less than 1% of patients involved in clinical trials:

General: accidental injury, chest pain, facial edema, malaise, neck pain, pain

Cardiovascular: migraine, syncope, vasodilation, ST depression

Digestive: dysphagia, eructation, flatulence, gastrointestinal disorder, increased appetite, nausea and vomiting, stomatitis, ileus

Hemic and Lymphatic: lymphadenopathy

Metabolic and Nutritional: dehydration, edema, hyponatremia, peripheral edema, syndrome of inappropriate antidiuretic hormone secretion, thirst

Nervous: abnormal gait, agitation, amnesia, depersonalization, depression, emotional lability, hallucination, hyperkinesia, hypesthesia, hypotonia, malaise, paresthesia, seizures, speech disorder, stupor, tinnitus, tremor, vertigo, withdrawal syndrome with or without seizures

Respiratory: cough increased, pharyngitis, voice alteration

Skin: dry skin, exfoliative dermatitis, urticaria

Special Senses: abnormal vision, taste perversion

Urogenital: dysuria, hematuria, impotence, polyuria, urinary retention, urination impaired

DRUG ABUSE AND DEPENDENCE (Addiction):

OxyContin® is a mu-agonist opioid with an abuse liability similar to morphine and is a Schedule **II** controlled substance. Oxycodone products are common targets for both drug abusers and drug addicts. Delayed absorption, as provided by OxyContin tablets, is believed to reduce the abuse liability of a drug.

Drug addiction (drug dependence, psychological dependence) is characterized by a preoccupation with the procurement, hoarding, and abuse of drugs for non-medicinal purposes. Drug dependence is treatable, utilizing a multi-disciplinary approach, but relapse is common. Iatrogenic "addiction" to opioids legitimately used in the management of pain is very rare.

OxyContin consists of a dual-polymer matrix, intended for oral use only. Parenteral venous injection of the tablet constituents, especially talc, can be expected to result in local tissue necrosis and pulmonary granulomas.

OVERDOSAGE:

Acute overdosage with oxycodone can be manifested by respiratory depression, somnolence progressing to stupor or coma, skeletal muscle flaccidity, cold and clammy skin, constricted pupils, bradycardia, hypotension, and death.

In the treatment of oxycodone overdosage, primary attention should be given to the re-establishment of a patent airway and institution of assisted or controlled ventilation. Supportive measures (including oxygen and vasopressors) should be employed in the management of circulatory shock and pulmonary edema accompanying overdose as indicated. Cardiac arrest or arrhythmias may require cardiac massage or defibrillation.

The pure opioid antagonists such as naloxone or nalmefene are specific antidotes against respiratory depression from opioid overdose. Opioid antagonists should not be administered in the absence of clinically significant respiratory or circulatory depression secondary to oxycodone overdose. They should be administered cautiously to persons who are known, or suspected to be, physically dependent on any opioid agonist including OxyContin®. In such cases, an abrupt or complete reversal of opioid effects may precipitate an acute abstinence syndrome. The severity of the withdrawal syndrome produced will depend on the degree of physical dependence and the dose of the antagonist administered. Please see the prescribing information for the specific opioid antagonist for details of their proper use.

SAFETY AND HANDLING:

OxyContin® tablets are solid dosage forms that pose no known health risk to health-care providers beyond that of any controlled substance. As with all such drugs, care should be taken to prevent diversion or abuse by proper handling.

STORAGE: Store at 25°C (77°F); excursions permitted between 15°-30°C (59°-86°F).

CAUTION: DEA Order Form Required.

Manufactured by The PF Laboratories, Inc., Totowa, N.J. 07512

Distributed by Purdue Pharma L.P., Stamford, CT 06901-3431

U.S. Patent Numbers 4,861,598; 4,970,075; 5,266,331; 5,508,042; 5,549,912; and 5,656,295

March 17, 2000 L4909-BS

Notes to Contributors

(Note: the information that follows is also available online at www.arthritisrheum.org and www.interscience.wiley.com)

Manuscripts for publication, letters, news, and notes should be sent to:
David S. Pisetsky, MD, PhD, Editor, *Arthritis & Rheumatism*
2400 Pratt Street, Room 0311 Terrace Level
Duke University Medical Center Box 3806
Durham, NC 27710
phone (919) 668-0488, fax (919) 668-0744, e-mail jennifer.deyton@duke.edu

Articles are accepted for publication on the condition that they are submitted to this journal only. Articles should definitely pertain to the field of rheumatic disease.

Manuscripts not in compliance with the following instructions may be subject to a delay in the review process.

Format and organization

______ Submit 5 copies of the manuscript, including tables and figures. For figures that are charts, graphs, or other line art that retains its readability when photocopied, the figures should be sent in the form of 1 photocopy attached to each copy of the manuscript, plus 1 high-quality original that will be used for printing if the manuscript is accepted. For radiographs, micrographs, and other halftone photographs, 5 high-quality glossy prints (not photocopies) should be sent (see Illustrations section below).

______ A cover letter with the corresponding author's signature should accompany the manuscript. Note in cover letter what type of manuscript is enclosed (Full-Length Article, Brief Report, Case Report, Concise Communication, or Letter to the Editor). Confirm that the manuscript has not been submitted or is not simultaneously being submitted elsewhere for either print or electronic publication, and that no portion of the data has been or will be published, in print or electronic form, in proceedings or transactions of meetings or symposium volumes. The publication of data in abstracts, and presentation in oral or poster sessions at meetings, do not constitute previous publication. Indicate any financial support or other benefits from commercial sources for the work reported on in the manuscript, or any other financial interests that any of the authors may have, which could create a potential conflict of interest or the appearance of a conflict of interest with regard to the work. Corresponding author should include address, telephone number, fax number, and E-mail address if applicable.

______ Type the manuscript in standard 12-point type on 8½ × 11″ paper with 1″ margins, double spaced throughout, including references, tables, and figure legends.

______ Number all sheets in succession, including references, tables, and figure legends. Title page is page 1.

______ On the first page, type the title, name(s) of the author(s) and their major degrees, grant supporter(s), address for reprint requests, and corresponding author's telephone and fax numbers and E-mail address.

Full-Length Articles and Brief Reports

Definition: Full-Length Articles are descriptions of original research that add to the body of knowledge in arthritis and the rheumatic diseases. Brief Reports are short papers of investigations into disease mechanisms, reports of clinical experience, therapeutic trials, or research and/or clinical contributions to diagnosis, treatment, etiopathology, and epidemiology of rheumatic diseases.

______ On the second page of Full-Length Articles and Brief Reports, include an abstract of less than 250 words. The abstract should be divided into the following sections: Objective, Methods, Results, and Conclusion.

______ On the third page, begin the introduction (no heading is necessary).

______ Follow this plan of organization: Materials and Methods (or Patients and Methods), Results, Discussion, References, Tables, and Figure Legends.

______ Full-Length Articles should not exceed 15 typed manuscript pages from introduction through discussion (not including references, tables, and figure legends).

______ Brief Reports should not exceed 9 manuscript pages from introduction through references, and should contain no more than 3 tables and/or figures and no more than 15 references.

Case Reports

Definition: Case Reports are reports of single cases that contribute to the body of knowledge of rheumatic diseases by reporting in-depth observations and/or laboratory investigations that may reveal etiopathogenetic mechanisms of a broader significance, or by presenting a concise discussion of an infrequently encountered problem that emphasizes a particular clinical point not generally available in the literature. Emphasis will be placed on the scholarship of discussion.

______ On the second page of Case Reports, include an abstract of less than 150 words. The abstract should not be divided into sections as required for Full-Length Articles and Brief Reports.

______ On the third page, begin the introduction (no heading is necessary).

______ After the introduction, include a description of the case, followed by a general discussion.

______ Case Reports should not exceed 9 manuscript pages from introduction through references, and should contain no more than 3 tables and/or figures and no more than 15 references.

Radiologic/Dermatologic Vignettes and Clinical Images

______ Radiologic Vignettes are short articles describing cases with interesting and significant radiologic features. The Vignette should present a case description with clinical findings, radiologic findings, differential diagnosis, final diagnosis, and discussion. No abstract is necessary. Page length should be less than that for a Brief Report or Case Report; up to 3 figures may be included. Dermatologic Vignettes describe cases with interesting and significant dermatologic features and should have a format similar to that of Radiologic Vignettes.

______ Clinical Images are photographic depictions (clinical, radiologic, or pathologic) of interesting rheumatologic phenomena. The image and accompanying caption should be short enough to fit on half a page of the journal (i.e., no more than one half page of double-spaced typewritten text, with the image preferably oriented horizontally). All images must be in black and white. There is no page charge for Clinical Images.

Letters to the Editor/Concise Communications

Definitions: Letters to the Editor should be limited to commentaries on previous articles published in *Arthritis & Rheumatism* and issues affecting rheumatology and the American College of Rheumatology. Concise Communications should be very short reports of cases or research findings, with no abstract, subheads, or acknowledgments section.

______ Letters to the Editor and Concise Communications should be double spaced throughout.

______ Length of Letters to the Editor and Concise Communications should be no more than 4 pages, including references.

______ Only 1 table or figure may accompany a Letter to the Editor or Concise Communication.

Content

______ Do not use new technical words, laboratory slang, words not defined in dictionaries, or abbreviations or terminology not consistent with internationally accepted guidelines.

______ Define any abbreviations the first time they are used. A list of standard abbreviations appears on pages 1903–1905 of the November 1998 issue.

______ In order to make the description of patients as clear as possible and to facilitate comparisons with other studies, the Methods section should include, whenever possible, a short paragraph detailing the proportion of patients who satisfy the ACR classification criteria for the particular disease described.

Compliance with research ethics standards

______ For articles reporting prospective research involving human or animal subjects, note in the Methods section that the study has been approved by the appropriate institutional review board or, if there is not an institutional review board or comparable formal ethics review committee, that the Declaration of Helsinki principles have been followed.

Illustrations

______ For illustrations that are photographs (as opposed to line art), send 5 packaged sets in labeled envelopes. For line art that reproduces well on a photocopier, include 1 copy with each copy of the manuscript, and also send 1 high-quality original to be used for printing.

______ Do not write on the back of any figure, but attach a label to each with the figure number and first author's name. Include on the label an arrow indicating which end is the top of the figure.

______ Lettering and symbols on figures should be large enough, and shading distinct enough, to remain readable after figure size is reduced to one column width.

______ Do not attach illustrations to the manuscript with a paperclip.

______ Obtain releases from any patients whose pictures will be printed in the journal. Blinders on the eyes are not a substitute for patient's permission.

______ Radiographs, micrographs, other halftones, and linecuts should be no more than 3¼″ square.

______ **Color figures:** Authors are entitled to one free page of color. Additional are billed to the author at the special reduced rate of $500 per page. All color figures will be reproduced in full color in the online edition of the journal at no cost to authors. Authors are encouraged to submit color illustrations that highlight the text and convey essential scientific information. For best reproduction, bright, clear colors should be used. Dark colors against a dark background do not reproduce well; please place your color images against a white background whenever possible. Please contact Jennifer Nowak at [jnowak@wiley.com] for further information.

Tables

______ Refer to current issues of the Journal for table style.

______ Provide each table with an explanatory title so that it is intelligible without specific reference to the text.

______ Provide each table column with an appropriate heading.

______ Indicate clearly any units of measure on a table.

References

______ Limit the length of the reference list by using only key references.

______ Double space references.

______ Compile references numerically according to the order of the citation.

______ Use abbreviations for titles of medical periodicals that conform to those in *Index Medicus*.

______ In 1997, the Journal changed its reference style to conform to the style suggested in the Uniform Requirements for Manuscripts Submitted to Biomedical Journals. All new submissions should use the new reference style, which can be found in the article "Uniform Requirements for Manuscripts Submitted to Biomedical Journals" (N Engl J Med, January 23, 1997, pp 309–15).

Assignment of reviewers

______ Authors are asked to suggest potential reviewers of their manuscript. If there are individuals they would prefer not to review their manuscript, they may also so indicate.

Related manuscripts/Duplicate publication

______ If the authors are aware of any related manuscript that has been or will be published by or submitted to another journal or to *Arthritis & Rheumatism* (e.g., another manuscript resulting from the same study), a copy of the other manuscript should be sent along with the one that is being submitted for publication in *Arthritis & Rheumatism*.

______ Articles are received only for exclusive publication in *Arthritis & Rheumatism* with the understanding that they have not been published elsewhere (in part or in full, in other words or in the same words, in letter or article form, in print or electronic form, or otherwise), are not at the time of submission under consideration by another journal or other publication, and will not be submitted elsewhere unless rejected by *Arthritis & Rheumatism.* If an author violates this requirement or engages in other similar misconduct, the Editor may, in addition to rejecting the manuscript, impose a moratorium on the acceptance of new manuscripts from the author and, if the misconduct is deemed sufficiently serious, may refer the matter to the author's academic institution or hospital and/or the appropriate state or local disciplinary body.

Disclosure of interest

______ The American College of Rheumatology's Board of Directors officially adopted Conflict of Interest Guidelines for *Arthritis & Rheumatism* on July 7, 1995. These guidelines, as they relate to authors, are as follows.

______ A cover letter to the Editor accompanying a submitted manuscript must disclose information about financial support and consulting activities, for *all* authors, that might be interpreted as constituting a possible conflict of interest for the described studies.

______ *All* authors of manuscripts (basic or clinical research, case reports, letters, reviews, editorials or commentary) accepted for publication will be asked to sign a full disclosure form regarding possible conflicts of interest for that individual, any member of his/her immediate family, or any other individual or entity with whom the author has a significant relationship, including: (a) ownership or control of stock in a company developing or distributing a product studied or discussed in the manuscript, or a competing product; (b) service as a consultant or advisor to a company developing or distributing a product studied or discussed in the manuscript, or a competing product; (c) the existence of any patent/license/royalty arrangements for any material studied or discussed in the manuscript; (d) any other possible financial benefit, such as derived income from a diagnostic test or product described or discussed in the manuscript, or frequent legal work as an expert witness or consultant in cases related to the content of the manuscript.

______ The Editor and Associate Editors will decide whether any of this information constitutes a possible conflict of interest, or the appearance thereof, and should be divulged in a footnote.

Publication procedures

______ In accordance with the 1978 Copyright Law, authors are requested to sign a provisional copyright transfer statement at the time manuscript revisions are requested.

______ Contributors are provided with page proofs and asked to check for errors and for editorial queries. Although the correction of editorial and typographical errors will be made without charge, the cost of excessive additional alterations may be charged to the author.

______ Authors are requested to return one set of proofs, the original manuscript and illustrations, and the reprint order within 48 hours. Publication of the article may be delayed if the proofs are not sent back on time.

Page charge

______ A $70 per page charge will be assessed for publication in *Arthritis & Rheumatism*. Instructions for payment will be sent to authors along with the proofs. In extreme cases of inability to pay, the page charge may be reduced or waived. There is no page charge for solicited articles, letters to the editor, or book reviews. Questions regarding the page charge should be directed to the Managing Editor, *Arthritis & Rheumatism*, 1800 Century Place, Suite 250, Atlanta, GA 30345-4300.

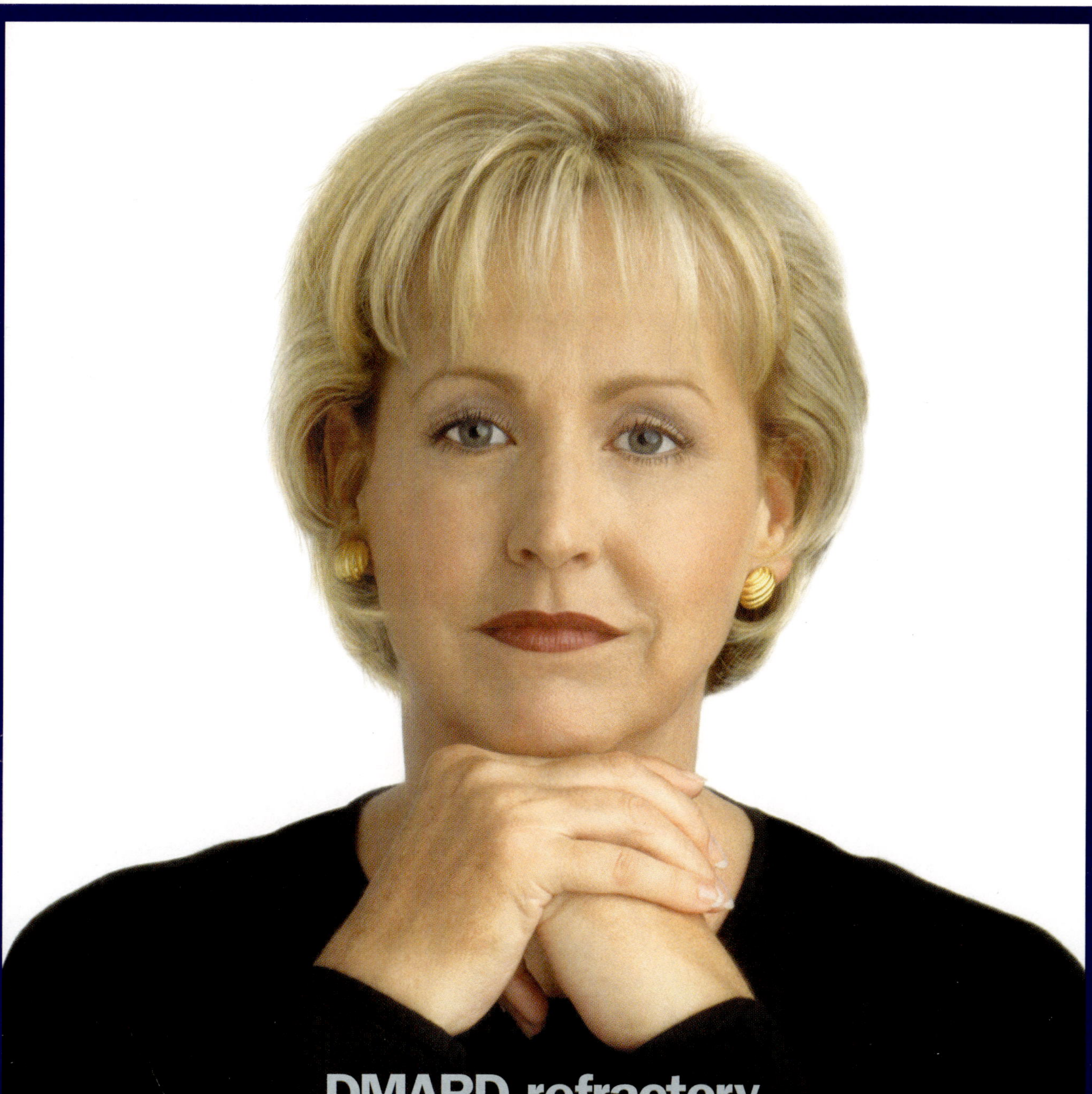

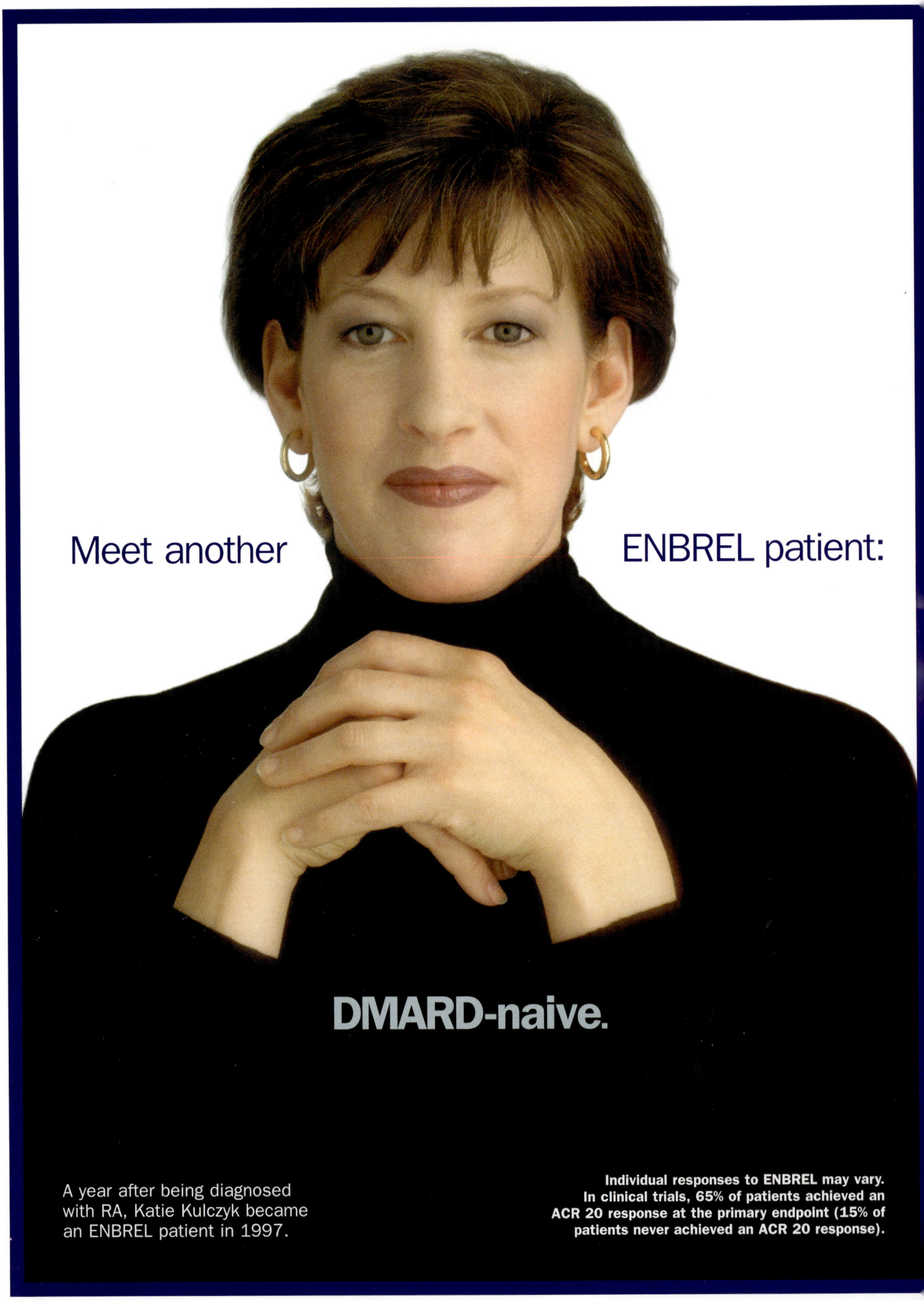
Meet another ENBREL patient:
DMARD-naive.
A year after being diagnosed with RA, Katie Kulczyk became an ENBREL patient in 1997.
Individual responses to ENBREL may vary. In clinical trials, 65% of patients achieved an ACR 20 response at the primary endpoint (15% of patients never achieved an ACR 20 response).

Important Treatment Considerations

IN POSTMARKETING USE, SERIOUS INFECTIONS AND SEPSIS, INCLUDING FATALITIES, HAVE BEEN REPORTED. MANY OF THESE EVENTS OCCURRED IN PATIENTS PREDISPOSED TO INFECTIONS, SUCH AS THOSE WITH ADVANCED OR POORLY CONTROLLED DIABETES. DISCONTINUE ENBREL IN PATIENTS WITH SERIOUS INFECTIONS OR SEPSIS. DO NOT START ENBREL IN THE PRESENCE OF SEPSIS, INFECTION (INCLUDING CHRONIC OR LOCALIZED), OR ALLERGY TO ENBREL OR ITS COMPONENTS. USE CAUTION IN PATIENTS PREDISPOSED TO INFECTION.

Rare cases of CNS demyelinating disorders have been reported, although the causal relationship to ENBREL remains unclear. Exercise caution when considering ENBREL for patients with these disorders. Rare cases of pancytopenia, including aplastic anemia, some fatal, have been reported in RA patients. Exercise caution in patients who have a previous history of significant hematologic abnormalities. Although the causal relationship to ENBREL remains unclear, advise patients to seek immediate medical attention if they develop signs or symptoms of blood dyscrasias or infection. If significant hematologic abnormalities are confirmed, consider discontinuing ENBREL.

The most frequent adverse events in placebo-controlled clinical trials (n=349) were injection site reactions (ISR) (37%), infections (35%), and headache (17%). Only the rate of ISR was higher than that of placebo. The most frequent adverse events in the methotrexate-controlled trial (n=415) were infections (64%), ISR (34%), and headache (24%). Only the rate of ISR was higher than that of MTX. In all RA patients treated in clinical trials (n=1,197), malignancies were rare (1%).

References: 1. ENBREL Prescribing Information, Immunex Corporation, Seattle, Wash. **2.** Data on file, Immunex Corporation, Seattle, Wash.

Enbrel®
etanercept

FREEDOM TO MOVE ON™

Please see brief summary of Prescribing Information at the end of this advertisement.

ACR ANNOUNCEMENTS

AMERICAN COLLEGE OF RHEUMATOLOGY
1800 Century Place, Suite 250, Atlanta, Georgia 30345-4300

ACR Meetings

Annual Meetings
November 10–15, 2001, San Francisco
October 24–29, 2002, New Orleans
October 23–28, 2003, Orlando
October 7–12, 2004, San Antonio
November 12–17, 2005, San Diego

State-of-the-Art Clinical Symposium
April 20–22, 2001, Chicago

Summer Clinical Meeting
June 21–24, 2001, Santa Barbara

For additional information, contact the ACR office.

Nominations for ACR Awards of Distinction and Masters Due May 15

Nominations for the 2001 ACR Awards of Distinction and ACR Masters are due May 15. To nominate someone for one of the Awards of Distinction (Paulding Phelps Award, Distinguished Service Award, Distinguished Rheumatologist Award, Distinguished Investigator Award, Henry Kunkel Young Investigator Award, Clinical Young Investigator Award, and Presidential Gold Medal), the sponsor must submit a nomination form, a letter of nomination, two additional letters of recommendation, and a copy of the nominee's curriculum vitae. To nominate someone for Master status, the sponsor must submit a nomination form and two letters of nomination from voting members of the ACR. The letters should explain how the nominee has set the highest professional standards in advancing the art and science of rheumatology. Nominees must have reached the age of 65 before November 1, 2001. Nomination forms for Awards of Distinction and Masters are available from the Member Services Department at the ACR office and in the Membership section of the ACR Web site. Completed nomination packets should be sent to Joseph D. Croft, Jr., MD, Chair, Committee on Nominations and Appointments, c/o the ACR office.

ACR Rheumatology Fellow Award Nominations Due May 31

Ten clinical or research fellows who are in a rheumatology fellowship training program will receive the ACR Rheumatology Fellow Awards (formerly known as the Senior Rheumatology Scholar Awards) at the 2001 Annual Scientific Meeting in San Francisco. To nominate a fellow for this $1,500 award, the program director or supervisor should submit a nomination form, the nominee's curriculum vitae, and copies of any abstracts the nominee submits to the Annual Scientific Meeting. A nomination form is enclosed with the Call for Abstracts and is available from the Member Services Department at the ACR office and in the Membership section of the ACR Web site. These awards are supported by an unrestricted educational grant from Merck & Co., Inc.

ACR Invites Nominations for Leadership Positions

The ACR encourages all members to participate in forming policy and conducting activities of the College by assuming positions of leadership in the organization. Appointments will become effective at the 2001 Annual Scientific Meeting in November. Positions are available on the following committees: Communications and Marketing, Continuing Medical Education, Educational Products, Finance, Government Affairs, Journal Publications, Nominations and Appointments, Research, Rheumatologic Care, and Rheumatology Training and Workforce Issues. Positions are also available on the Research and Education Foundation Board of Directors and on the ACR Board of Directors. Two officer positions—Vice President and Secretary/Treasurer— are available as well. Members are invited to submit names of candidates to serve as officers, on committees, or on the Board of Directors. For more information, contact the Director of Membership by phone at (404) 633-3777 or by e-mail at membership@rheumatology.org. Nomination forms are available from the Member Services Department at the ACR office and in the Membership section of the ACR Web site. Nominations should be submitted by June 1 to Joseph D. Croft, Jr., MD, Chair, Committee on Nominations and Appointments, c/o the ACR office.

American Board of Internal Medicine Certification and Recertification Examinations

The ABIM 2001 Certification Examination in Rheumatology will be held November 7, 2001. The registration period is January 1–April 1, 2001; the late registration period is April 2–June 1, 2001. The ABIM's Recertification Program, which has been renamed the Program for Continuous Professional Development (CPD), consists of an at-home, open-book self-evaluation process and a proctored final examination which will be administered twice each year in May and November. To register for the examination, Diplomates must be enrolled in the CPD Program and be in at least year 6 of their certification cycle. For the 2001 Recertification Examinations in Internal Medicine, its Subspecialties, and Added Qualifications, the final examination will be administered May 1 (registration deadline March 1) and November 7 (registration deadline September 1). For additional information and registration forms, contact Registration Section, American Board of Internal Medicine, 510 Walnut Street, Suite 1700, Philadelphia, PA 19106-3699, phone 800-441-2246 or 215-446-

3500, fax 215-446-3590, e-mail request@abim.org, or visit the ABIM's Web site at www.abim.org.

Education Programs

First Annual Jerry Jacobs Lectureship: New Trends in the Treatment of Inflammatory Disorders. March 31, 2001, New York, NY. Sponsored by Columbia University College of Physicians & Surgeons and Babies & Children's Hospital, New York Presbyterian Hospital, The University Hospital of Columbia and Cornell. For additional information, contact Center for Continuing Education, Columbia University College of Physicians & Surgeons, 630 West 168th Street, Unit 39, New York, NY 10032, phone 212-305-3334, fax 212-781-6047, e-mail, cme@columbia.edu, or visit the Web site http://cpmcnet.columbia.edu/dept/cme.

First Joint Meeting of the International Bone and Mineral Society and the European Calcified Tissue Society. June 5–10, 2001, Madrid, Spain. For additional information, contact Lucia Calvo, IBMS/ECTS 2001, c/o Tilcsa OPC, SL, Londres 17, 28028 Madrid, Spain, phone 34-91-361-2600, fax 34-91-355-9208, e-mail ibms-ects2001@tilesa.es, or visit the Web site http://www.intercongres-2001.com.

20th International League of Associations for Rheumatology (ILAR) World Congress. August 26–31, 2001, Edmonton, Alberta. Canada. The theme of the congress will be Therapy for the 21st Century. For additional information, contact ILAR Secretariat, Health Care Communications, Suite 906, 50 Burnhamthorpe Road West, Mississauga, Ontario, L5B 3C2, Canada. phone 800-535-3330 (from within Canada) or 905-273-3080, fax 905-273-3611, e-mail healthcarecomm@sympatico.ca.

II International Scientific Conference for Students and Young Scientists, October 11–13, 2001, Lviv, Ukraine. Sponsored by Lviv State Medical University. Official language will be English. Abstract deadline is August 1, 2001. For additional information, contact Organizing Committee, II International Scientific Conference for Students and Young Scientists, Lviv State Medical University, Albanska St. 6/2, 79017 Lviv, Ukraine, phone 380-322-753634, fax 380-322-757531, e-mail snt@meduniv.lviv.ua, or visit the Web site http://www.meduniv.lviv.ua/sss.

Controversies in Diagnosis, Management, and Costs of Osteoarticular Implications of Obesity. October 12–13, 2001, Brussels, Belgium. For additional information, contact Prof. Dr. M. Szpalski, Centre Hospitalier Molière Longchamps, Rue Marconi 142, 1180 Brussels, Belgium, fax 32-2-348-5694.

ARTHRITIS & RHEUMATISM
Vol. 44, No. 3, March 2001, pp 493–507

Arthritis & Rheumatism

Official Journal of the American College of Rheumatology
www.arthritisrheum.org and www.interscience.wiley.com

REVIEW

Involvement of the Hypothalamic–Pituitary–Adrenal/Gonadal Axis and the Peripheral Nervous System in Rheumatoid Arthritis

Viewpoint Based on a Systemic Pathogenetic Role

Rainer H. Straub[1] and Maurizio Cutolo[2]

Introduction

Rheumatoid arthritis (RA) is a multifactorial disease that results in severe destruction in the microenvironment of the synovial tissue, cartilage, and juxtaarticular bone. A hallmark of local inflammation is the secretion of huge amounts of proinflammatory immune mediators such as cytokines, e.g., tumor necrosis factor (TNF) and interleukin 1 (IL-1). Local secretion of cytokines and activation of immunocompetent cells in the microenvironment are followed by a systemic reaction. As a result of involvement of nonarticular structures, the endocrine system and the nervous system participate directly in the pathophysiology of RA (1,2). Since mediators of the endocrine system (e.g., steroid hormones) and the peripheral nervous system (e.g., norepinephrine or substance P) reach synovial target cells, which are provided with specific receptors, these systemic feedback systems have the potential to modulate the local inflammatory process in RA (3,4). During the last 15 years, there has been a dramatic increase in our understanding about systemic feedback responses of the neuroendocrine and peripheral nervous system on target immune cells during inflammatory diseases such as RA (1,5,6). Furthermore, it has been shown that psychological stress modulates disease activity in RA and juvenile chronic arthritis (7,8).

In this review, we will discuss 1) the physiologic response of the endocrine system and the nervous system during inflammation and the effects of their specific mediators on immune mechanisms (the physiologic situation in RA), 2) the occurrence of alterations of the systemic responses of the endocrine system and the nervous system in RA (the pathologic situation), 3) a scenario in which events including both local immune mechanisms and systemic neuroendocrine immune mechanisms simultaneously contribute to the pathogenesis of RA (systemic pathogenetic viewpoint), and 4) alternative, neuroendocrine immune–based approaches to the therapy of RA (examples of possible clinical pharmacologic trials).

Presently known aspects of the pathogenesis of RA

At present, there is no consensus concerning the triggering factor in RA and whether it is an autoantigen or a non-self stimulus. No single agent has consistently been found as *the* sole pathogenic stimulus in the disease. As a result, one possibly has to accept the concept that many different stimuli can initiate RA; among them are a large list of autoantigens (for review, see ref. 9) and various infectious agents such as bacteria (10) or viruses (11). Since post hoc relics of the trigger of the local articular inflammation are seldom found in synovial fluid or tissue, a significant diagnostic problem arises. Furthermore, the same triggers may be present in various rheumatic diseases, which leads to a general lack

Supported in part by the Deutsche Forschungsgemeinschaft (Str 511/5-2) and the Italian Ministry of the University and Research.
[1]Rainer H. Straub, MD: University Hospital, Regensburg, Germany; [2]Maurizio Cutolo, MD: Division of Rheumatology, Department of Internal Medicine, University of Genoa, Genoa, Italy.
Address correspondence and reprint requests to Rainer H. Straub, MD, Laboratory of Neuroendocrinoimmunology, Division of Rheumatology, Department of Internal Medicine I, University Hospital, 93042 Regensburg, Germany.
Submitted for publication August 3, 2000; accepted in revised form October 13, 2000.

of specificity. From this point of view, the triggering stimulus might "target" different organs depending on the individual genetic background, and may be less important as compared with the relatively uniform proinflammatory reaction that follows the initiation phase.

With respect to the above-mentioned possible causative agents, the adaptive immune system plays a significant role in the phase of initiation (or activation) of the disease: T cells (12), B cells (13), and antigen-presenting cells (i.e., macrophages) (12) interact with one another, attempting to eliminate causative agents. The importance of adaptive immune processes is exemplified by the known association between HLA class II alloantigens and RA (14), including the concept of shared epitopes (15). However, besides these adaptive immune responses, the pathogenesis of RA is characterized by a relatively uniform reaction with sustained macrophage activation in the absence of infection (16), abnormalities in apoptosis (17), and growth of immature synovial fibroblasts with invasive properties (18). In this phase of the disease, uniform invasion of neutrophils (19) and mast cells (20) and activation of endothelial cells with neovascularization (21) are other important features of the destructive process.

There currently is not a suitable theory that explains the maintenance of this uniform chronic proinflammatory state in RA. Thus, a fundamental question arises as to whether the chronic proinflammatory state depends on sustained stimulation of synovial target cells by a persistent trigger or whether normally present physiologic inhibitory systems become deficient. In this review, it is demonstrated that the two main systemic inhibitory systems, the hypothalamic–pituitary–adrenal (HPA) axis and the hypothalamic–autonomic nervous system (HANS) axis, become clearly deficient in patients with RA. The alteration of these axes, together with changes of gonadal hormones, may contribute significantly to the perpetuation of RA, leading to smoldering inflammation in the chronic phase of the disease.

Induction of a systemic neuroendocrine and neuronal response by local inflammation

Upon local inflammation during RA, huge amounts of paracrine factors, for example, cytokines such as TNF, IL-2, IL-6, IL-8, IL-12, and many others, are released into the systemic circulation (measurable in the serum). Besides these immune mediators, activated cells circulate throughout the whole body. Furthermore, at the local site of inflammation, primary sensory afferent nerve fibers are activated by chemical, mechanical,

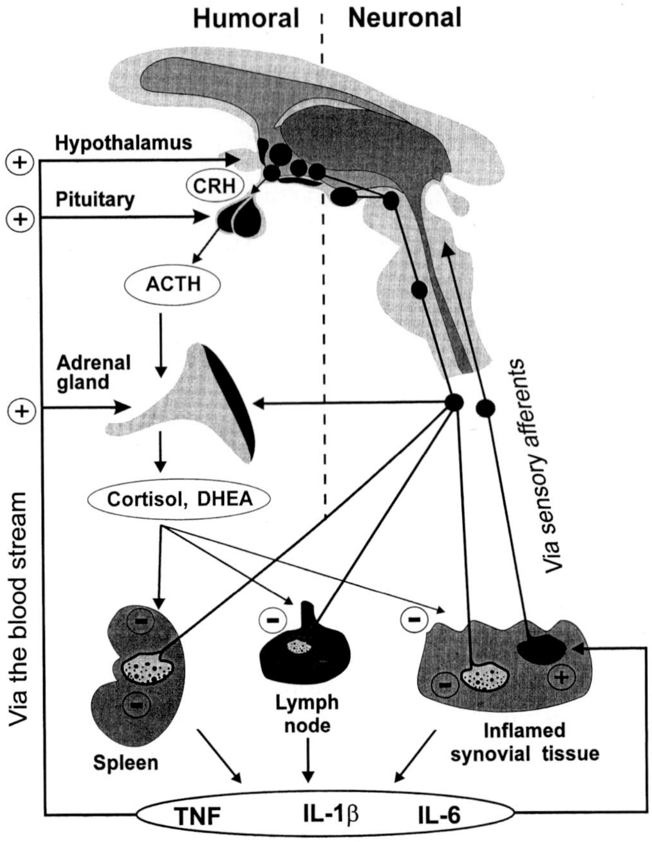

Figure 1. Antiinflammatory feedback pathways during systemic inflammation. The humoral hypothalamic–pituitary–adrenal axis, which regulates adrenal hormones, is shown on the left side, and the efferent neuronal hypothalamic–autonomic nervous system axis, which influences local neurotransmitter release, on the right. Cytokines released in the periphery stimulate the central nervous system directly via the blood stream or via receptors on sensory nerves. This leads to activation of the humoral and neuronal antiinflammatory feedback pathways in order to dampen inflammation in the periphery. Minus signs indicate inhibition; plus signs indicate stimulation. CRH = corticotropin-releasing hormone; ACTH = adrenocorticotropic hormone; DHEA = dehydroepiandrosterone; TNF = tumor necrosis factor; IL-1β = interleukin-1β.

thermal, and immune stimuli and release neurotransmitters in the vicinity of nerve terminals (2). All three mechanisms (immune mediators, activated cells, afferent sensory nerves) *announce* a proinflammatory situation to the central nervous system (CNS) and other organs (liver, adrenal glands, gonadal glands, etc.).

The "side effect" of this local inflammation is a systemic feedback response of the CNS, the sacred central organ, which must be sheltered from peripheral inflammation. Upon strong proinflammatory stimulation, the CNS reacts with activation of the HPA axis and the HANS axis (for review, see refs. 5, 22, and 23) (Figure 1). With respect to the HPA axis, this has been demonstrated by a cytokine-induced increase of adrenocorticotropic hormone (ACTH) and adrenal steroids (5,24) (Figure 1). With respect to the HANS axis, a cytokine-induced increase of the firing rate at the sympathetic splenic nerves has been demonstrated (25) (Figure 1). Such an increase of the firing rate at the sympathetic nerves will lead to increased secretion of neurotransmitters into the vicinity of the nerve terminals. However, with respect to the hypothalamic–pituitary–gonadal (HPG) axis, the same proinflammatory cytokines, e.g., IL-1, TNF, or endotoxin, inhibit secretion of gonadotropin-releasing hormone from the hypothalamus, luteinizing hormone from the pituitary gland (26), and thus, consequently, testosterone production in men and estrogen production in women. Physiologically, during systemic inflammation, the reproductive system is inhibited and the HPA axis and HANS axis are activated.

In general, the CNS responses via the HPA axis and via the HANS axis are thought to dampen inflammation in the periphery (5,6,22,23). As discussed in detail below, the CNS tries to inhibit peripheral inflammation using two parallel pathways: 1) the HPA axis with the main antiinflammatory hormone cortisol, and 2) the sympathetic nervous system with the main antiinflammatory neurotransmitters norepinephrine (via β-adrenoceptors), adenosine (via adenosine 2 [A2] receptors), and endogenous opioids. It will be shown that both axes have a stronger antiinflammatory impact when they act in parallel. However, in RA, these axes are obviously altered, which leads to a loss of the CNS-mediated antiinflammatory influence on local articular inflammation. The alterations of the HPA and HANS axes contribute to the pathogenesis of RA.

Table 1. Immunomodulation by adrenal/gonadal hormones and sympathetic and sensory neurotransmitters*

Hormone or neurotransmitter	Modulation of innate and adaptive immune functions
Cortisol	Inhibition of oxidative burst, phagocytosis, collagenase production, antigen presentation, COX-2, IL-1, IL-2, IL-6, IL-12, IFNγ, TNF, NF-κB, etc.
DHEA	Inhibition of oxygen radical production, IL-1, IL-6, TNF
Testosterone	Inhibition of IL-6, NK cell activity
Estrogen	Stimulation of immunoglobulin production (physiologic concentration), inhibition of IL-1, IL-6, TNF (pharmacologic concentration)
cAMP	Inhibition of oxygen radicals, phagocytosis, HLA class I and II expression, IL-2, IL-12, IFNγ, TNF (but increases Th2 pathways)
Norepinephrine (α_2)	Inhibition of intracellular cAMP (increase of TNF)
Norepinephrine (β)	Inhibition of oxygen radicals, phagocytosis, NK cell activity, HLA class II expression, IL-2, IFNγ, IL-12, TNF (but increases Th2 pathways)
Adenosine (A1)	Inhibition of intracellular cAMP
Adenosine (A2)	Inhibition of oxygen radicals, phagocytosis, NK cell activity, IL-8, IL-12, IFNγ, TNF (but increases Th2 pathways)
Substance P	Stimulation of oxygen radicals, phagocytosis, chemotaxis of monocytes, NK cell activity, IL-1, IL-2, IL-4, IL-8, IL-10, IL-12, TNF, immunoglobulin production, prostaglandin E_2

* See ref. 116. COX-2 = cyclooxygenase 2; IL-1 = interleukin-1; IFNγ = interferon-γ; TNF = tumor necrosis factor; NF-κB = nuclear factor κB; DHEA = dehydroepiandrosterone; NK cell = natural killer cell.

Role of adrenal/gonadal hormones and neurotransmitters for immunomodulation: a short overview (Table 1)

Cortisol (adrenal hormone). The multiple antiinflammatory effects of cortisol and its synthetic derivatives have been studied extensively over the last 50 years. It is obvious that this hormone has multiple antiinflammatory activities, including, among others, inhibition of cytokines, of phagocytosis, of the oxidative burst, and of inducible cyclooxygenase 2 (6) (Table 1). In addition, cortisol induces a more Th2-directed immune response in vivo, with an increase of the antiinflammatory cytokine IL-10 (27). This has been exemplified in studies of glucocorticoid therapy in animals with arthritis and in patients with RA. In conclusion, high physiologic concentrations of cortisol (10^{-6}–$10^{-5}M$) are antiinflammatory.

Dehydroepiandrosterone (adrenal hormone). Two other adrenal hormones, which are secreted upon ACTH stimulation, are dehydroepiandrosterone (DHEA) and its sulfated derivative DHEAS. DHEA is the active hormone, which can be converted to downstream androgens in peripheral cells such as macrophages (28). Since androgens such as testosterone have antiinflammatory properties, DHEA and DHEAS, the androgen precursors, contribute to the hormone pool in order to maintain antiinflammatory conditions in the periphery, when the gonadal glands undergo gradual involution during aging. Furthermore, DHEA may have its own intracellular receptor to exert direct antiinflammatory effects in animals and humans (29,30) (Table 1).

Androgens (gonadal hormone). Generally, androgens, in physiologic concentrations, tend to suppress the immune response (for review, see ref. 31) (Figure 2). Studies have shown that both physiologic ($10^{-8}M$) and pharmacologic (or high physiologic) ($10^{-6}M$) concentrations of testosterone inhibit IL-1β secretion by peri-

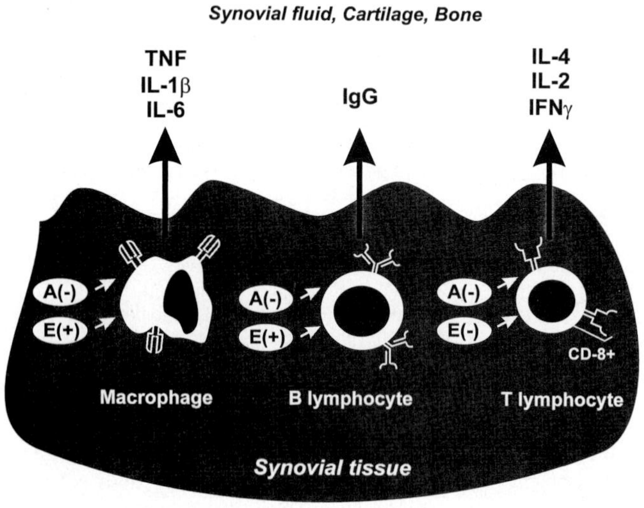

Figure 2. Major stimulatory (plus signs) or inhibitory (minus signs) effects (direct and indirect) of androgens (A) and estrogens (E) on cytokine/immunoglobulin production by synovial/immune cells in synovial tissue of patients with rheumatoid arthritis. IFNγ = interferon-γ (see Figure 1 for other definitions).

pheral blood mononuclear cells (PBMC) obtained from patients with RA (32). In addition, physiologic concentrations of testosterone inhibit IL-1 synthesis in primary cultured human synovial macrophages (33). In other studies, dihydrotestosterone has been found to repress the expression and activity of the human IL-6 gene promoter in human fibroblasts, thus supporting the concept of antiinflammatory/immunosuppressive effects of androgens (34). Testosterone treatment does not appear to directly affect isolated B or T cells. However, in a followup study of patients with systemic lupus erythematosus (SLE), testosterone suppressed both anti–double-stranded DNA IgG and total IgG production by PBMC (35). Low serum and synovial fluid androgen levels have been observed in RA patients (36,37).

Estrogens (gonadal hormone). Generally, estrogens, in physiologic concentrations, serve to enhance immune responses and, particularly, may act as an important stimulator of human humoral immunity (for review, see ref. 38) (Figure 2). It has been reported that 17β-estradiol enhances IgG and IgM production by PBMC, both in men and in women, without altering cell viability or proliferation (39). A more recent study confirmed that 17β-estradiol has the capacity to increase the production of polyclonal IgG, including anti–double-stranded DNA IgG, in PBMC of SLE patients by enhancing B cell activity via IL-10 (40). The effects of estrogens on cytokine production (IL-1, IL-6, TNF) seem to be bimodal, with decreased synthesis when high-dose pharmacologic concentrations ($10^{-6}M$) are used and increased cytokine production when physiologic concentrations ($\leq 10^{-8}M$) are used (41,42). Recently, it has been demonstrated that estrogens are able to enhance secretion of matrix metalloproteinases from human fibroblast-like synoviocytes (43). Serum levels of estrogens in RA patients are not changed, which is in sharp contrast to androgen levels (44).

Conversion of steroid hormones in peripheral target cells. Since steroid hormones can be converted along defined pathways to downstream hormones in the periphery, multiple secondary effects may arise depending on local regulation of steroid conversion. We have recently demonstrated that conversion of DHEA occurs in macrophages and depends on the state of differentiation and presence of endotoxin (28). In postmenopausal women and aged men, the availability of adrenal DHEA is important to maintain a significant level of sex hormones in the periphery. It is not known whether, under certain circumstances, macrophages or other peripheral immune cells are able to synthesize steroid hormones in adequate amounts using cholesterol, as has been demonstrated in thymocytes (45). Furthermore, we do not exactly know the importance of degradation of, for example, cortisol by 11β-hydroxysteroid dehydrogenase in the synovial tissue, which changes the activity of the steroid hormones in the local microenvironment (46).

Effectors of the sympathetic nervous system. The adrenal hormone epinephrine, the sympathetic neurotransmitter norepinephrine, and the sympathetic neurotransmitter adenosine (after conversion from ATP) play dual immunomodulatory roles due to their binding to different G protein–coupled receptor subtypes (Figure 3). Epinephrine preferentially binds β-adrenoceptors (receptor 1 in Figure 3; at high physiologic concentrations also α-adrenoceptors shown as receptor 2 in Figure 3), and norepinephrine binds preferentially α-adrenoceptors (receptor 2 in Figure 3; at high physiologic concentrations also β-adrenoceptors shown as receptor 1 in Figure 3). Adenosine preferentially binds A1 receptors (receptor 2 in Figure 3). At high physiologic concentrations it also binds A2 receptors (receptor 1 in Figure 3). Ligation of β-adrenoceptors or A2 receptors increases intracellular cAMP levels, and ligation of α_2-adrenoceptors or A1 receptors decreases intracellular cAMP levels (Figure 3).

Generally, an elevated sympathetic tone due to increased firing rates at sympathetic nerves results in increased levels of epinephrine, norepinephrine, and adenosine (after conversion from ATP) in the systemic

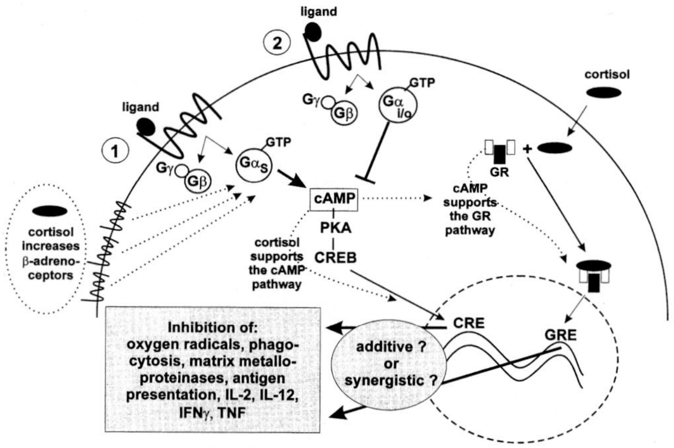

Figure 3. Synergistic antiinflammatory pathways of cortisol and sympathetic neurotransmitters. These mediators support one another in order to exert antiinflammatory effects (demonstrated by dotted lines). Upon ligation of cortisol to the glucocorticoid receptor (GR), this complex translocates into the nucleus and binds to DNA (at the GR-responsive element [GRE]). This leads to inhibition of downstream proinflammatory mechanisms. The GR pathway is supported by cAMP (dotted line). On the other hand, it is known that upon ligation of a ligand to receptor 1 ①, $G\alpha_S$ is activated, which increases intracellular cAMP levels (the ligand may be norepinephrine or adenosine). This pathway is supported by cortisol, which increases, for example, β-adrenoceptors and stabilizes the downstream pathway via protein kinase A (PKA) and the cAMP-responsive element binding protein (CREB). Stabilizing this pathway yields higher concentrations of CREB, which can bind to CRE. Binding of a ligand to receptor 2 ② stimulates $G\alpha_{i/O}$, which leads to decreased intracellular cAMP levels (solid line with bar). Since the affinities of norepinephrine and adenosine to the two receptors are markedly different, low concentrations of norepinephrine or adenosine preferentially stimulate receptor 2, whereas high concentrations of these neurotransmitters stimulate both receptors. Thus, adequately high levels of these neurotransmitters are needed for the antiinflammatory effect. IFNγ = interferon-γ (see Figure 1 for other definitions).

circulation and in the vicinity of the nerve terminal. This leads to an increase of intracellular cAMP in multiple peripheral target cells (Figure 3). Elevation of cAMP by these mechanisms has been repeatedly demonstrated to induce many antiinflammatory effects on target immune mechanisms (Table 1). Thus, it is important to estimate the local concentration of these sympathetic effector molecules, because one would expect a prominent antiinflammatory activity only at high physiologic concentrations 10^{-6}–$10^{-5}M$. With respect to sympathetic nerve fibers, this means the presence of nerves at a high fiber density would yield a high enough antiinflammatory concentration of norepinephrine. The importance of a β-adrenergic agonist (cAMP increase) has been recently demonstrated in an animal model of arthritis (47). Furthermore, sympathetic nerve terminals bear vesicles with endogenous opioids, which are able to inhibit release of the proinflammatory substance P from afferent sensory nerve fibers (2).

Substance P (neurotransmitter of sensory afferents). It is currently widely accepted that substance P is a proinflammatory neurotransmitter (Table 1). For example, substance P stimulates IL-1 (48), IL-2 (49), TNF (48), and nuclear factor κB (50) from various cell types. This indicates that it is a potent proinflammatory agent. Its proinflammatory role in acute arthritis has been demonstrated (51).

Simultaneous activation of the HPA axis and the HANS axis. It is a known feature of asthma therapy that parallel topical (or systemic) treatment with a β-adrenergic agonist and a glucocorticoid has an additive or even synergistic effect in elimination of bronchial obstruction (52). Simultaneous activation of the HPA axis with an increase of cortisol and of the HANS axis with an increase of norepinephrine would have an additive effect with respect to the increase of intracellular cAMP (Figure 3), as has been demonstrated in various cells (53–55). Furthermore, cortisol supports production of norepinephrine and epinephrine from sympathetic nerve terminals and the adrenal medulla, respectively, by stimulating the synthesizing enzymes (56,57). Thus, a parallel increase of cortisol and norepinephrine with local concentrations of 10^{-6}–$10^{-5}M$ would have a more antiinflammatory effect than either substance alone. This indicates that possibly both antiinflammatory systems, the HPA axis and the HANS axis, must be simultaneously activated to exert the full antiinflammatory effect. Presumably, an uncoupling of the two axes may be deleterious in chronic inflammatory diseases.

Observed alterations in functions of the HPA axis, the HPG axis, and the peripheral nervous system in RA

Above, we have reviewed the normally occurring physiologic reactions of the CNS and the released hormones and neurotransmitters following a systemic proinflammatory stimulus. We indicated that high physiologic concentrations of cortisol, DHEA, androgens, and sympathetic neurotransmitters are antiinflammatory, particularly when they act in parallel (Table 1). The following section will discuss the alterations of these different axes in patients with RA.

Changes at the central level of the hypothalamus and pituitary gland. *Corticotropin-releasing hormone (CRH) and ACTH secretion.* In the acute situation (day 1 of IL-6 therapy), IL-6 stimulates the hypothalamus, which leads to a strong ACTH response in humans (24) and rats (58). This has been also demonstrated with other cytokines, such as IL-1 in rats (59), IL-2 in humans (60), and TNF in humans (61) and rats (62). However, long-term administration of cytokines such as IL-6 results in a blunted ACTH response in humans (24). Furthermore, acute adjuvant-induced arthritis leads to strong activation of CRH, whereas chronic arthritis is accompanied by low hypothalamic CRH but elevated arginine vasopressin levels (63). This indicates that adaptive changes occur at the level of the hypothalamus and pituitary gland when cytokines are chronically elevated (i.e., during chronic inflammation). Such a situation may lead to relatively low secretion of CRH and ACTH despite elevated levels of cytokines.

Although adaptation of the hypothalamus seems to be a known physiologic principle, we do not know the cytokine concentration and the amount of time necessary to induce an adaptive process at the level of the hypothalamus or pituitary gland in RA. Since these patients do not have constantly elevated levels of stimulating cytokines, adaptive changes at this level may be absent. Only 1 study has demonstrated a defective ACTH response (48 hours after the stress of major surgery) in RA (64), but in a similar study by others, this was not confirmed (65). The topic has been reviewed extensively (63), and we agree that the CRH/ACTH response in RA is probably not markedly altered. Any inherent abnormality lies in the inability to increase cortisol production in response to chronic inflammation, which is more a peripheral problem of the adrenal glands.

Follicle-stimulating hormone and luteinizing hormone secretion. Secretion of the gonadotropins follicle-stimulating hormone and luteinizing hormone seems to be significantly elevated in patients with RA, due to low levels of peripheral sex hormones (37). This indicates that possible defects are not at the level of the hypothalamus or the pituitary gland, but, similar to the CRH/ACTH response, in the periphery.

Changes at the peripheral level of the adrenal and gonadal glands: inappropriately low peripheral hormones in relation to inflammation. *The adrenal gland*. In patients with RA, a number of studies have shown that cortisol secretion is inappropriately low in relation to serum concentrations of proinflammatory cytokines and general inflammation (66–72). In other chronic inflammatory diseases, there is a similar reduction of cortisol relative to the inflammatory potency of the specific disease, as exemplified in Crohn's disease (73), Sjögren's syndrome (74), SLE (75), and others. Thus, we believe that there is inappropriately low secretion of adrenal cortisol in relation to continuous inflammation in chronic inflammatory diseases such as RA. It must be remembered that the number of glucocorticoid receptors seems to be normal or even elevated in PBMC of patients with RA without prior glucocorticoid therapy (76). This may further support the concept of inadequately low secretion of cortisol in this disease.

Furthermore, there is a significant decrease of serum levels of adrenal androgens in patients with RA (37,77,78). A very similar decrease of adrenal androgens, particularly DHEAS, has been observed in other chronic inflammatory diseases, such as Crohn's disease and ulcerative colitis (73), SLE (79), systemic sclerosis (80), and polymyalgia rheumatica (81,82). Again, chronic inflammatory diseases are characterized by inappropriately low secretion of adrenal androgens. From the present point of view, the reduced production of adrenal hormones is not disease specific and seems to depend particularly on the extent and duration of systemic inflammation.

The gonadal glands. Generally, proinflammatory cytokines (IL-1, TNF) inhibit important early and intermediate steps of sex hormone production, such as P450ssc and the P450c17 enzyme activity in Leydig cells (83). This would probably lead to reduction of sex hormones in gonadal glands. In contrast, the same proinflammatory cytokines (IL-1, TNF) and IL-6 have been found to stimulate the activity of the aromatase enzyme complex in nongonadal tissue, which leads to conversion of androgens to downstream estrogens in the periphery (84) (Figure 4). Accordingly, in macrophage-rich tissue, a significant correlation between aromatase activity and IL-6 production was found, resulting in lower androgen and higher estrogen levels (85). This would result in a high estrogen:androgen ratio, as has been observed in the synovial fluid of male and female RA patients (86). During inflammatory conditions, the reduced sex hormone production at the level of the gonadal glands is followed by low serum and body fluid levels of androgens. However, estrogen levels remain relatively normal because the proinflammatory cytokines stimulate production of estrogens from precursors in peripheral cells (breast cells, osteoblasts, fat cells, macrophages) (Figure 4).

Changes at the peripheral level of the sympathetic and sensory nervous systems. It was indicated above that the simultaneous presence of cortisol and norepinephrine in an inflammatory lesion may lead to stronger antiinflammatory activity as compared with that resulting from the presence of either substance

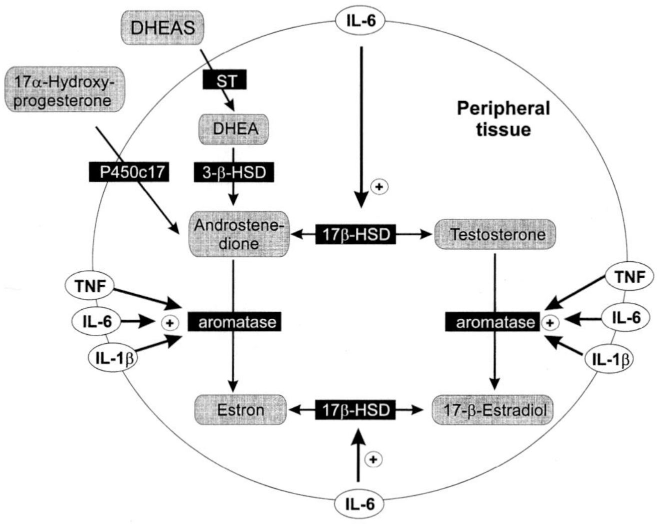

Figure 4. Activation of the aromatase complex by cytokines in the periphery. Locally produced inflammatory cytokines (i.e., IL-1β, IL-6, TNF) are able to stimulate aromatase activity in peripheral tissues (i.e., breast cells), leading to increased conversion of androgens (testosterone and androstenedione) to estrogens (estrone and 17β-estradiol, respectively). In addition, IL-6 has been found to mediate an increase in reductive 17β-hydroxysteroid dehydrogenase (17β-HSD) activity that converts estrone to the biologically more active 17β-estradiol. In general, the above-mentioned cytokines favor the production of 17β-estradiol, which is proinflammatory at the local site, in relation to androgens. DHEAS = sulfated derivative of DHEA; ST = sulfatase; P450c17 = 17-α-hydroxylase/17,20-lyase; + = stimulatory (see Figure 1 for other definitions).

alone (coupling of the HPA axis and the HANS axis). Thus, we believe that it is important to elucidate the local changes in the sympathetic nervous system during RA. In contrast to lipophilic steroids, which reach nearly every site in the body, hydrophilic neurotransmitters are secreted at defined locations. With respect to norepinephrine, this can lead to very high concentrations ($\sim 10^{-5}M$) in the vicinity of nerve terminals (87).

The sympathetic nervous system. Many studies have been carried out to delineate the impact of the sympathetic nervous system in animal models of arthritis. In these studies, α_2-adrenergic and A1 receptor mechanisms are involved in sensitization of primary afferent sensory nerve fibers, leading to release of proinflammatory substance P into the lumen of the joint (for review, see ref. 88). In contrast, other studies have indicated that experimental arthritis is attenuated by administration of β-adrenergic agonists (47,89). In this respect, the sympathetic nervous system plays a *dual role*, which presumably depends on the ligation of sympathetic neurotransmitters at either α_2- or β-adrenoceptors and A1 or A2 adenosine receptors, respectively (Figure 5). The differential effects of sympathetic neurotransmitters (norepinephrine, epinephrine, adenosine; see above) are consistent with the concept that stimulation of β-adrenoceptors or A2 receptors increases intracellular cAMP, which inhibits production of proinflammatory cytokines such as TNF, interferon-γ, IL-2, and IL-12 (Table 1). This effect is completely opposite when α_2-adrenoceptors or A1 receptors are stimulated (Table 1). We believe that the local concentration of these immunomodulating sympathetic neurotransmitters is of primary importance. Therefore, a complete loss of sympathetic nerve fibers due to experimental sympathectomy may even reduce inflammation, because α_2-adrenergic pathways are then eliminated (90).

The question remains as to whether the above-mentioned sympathetic mechanisms play a significant role in the human disease. Experimental plasma extravasation, swelling, redness, and hyperalgesia in rats occur within minutes, and these symptoms are probably not comparable with long-term chronic inflammation in RA. Studies in this respect have never focused on important immune mechanisms such as TNF-induced secretion of matrix metalloproteinases and degradation of cartilage during chronic disease. Furthermore, the investigated models of adjuvant- or type II collagen–induced arthritis are characterized by a self-limiting disease, which normally heals within 40–80 days. These animal models probably represent models of the RA initiation (or activation) phase, but not of the chronic phase of the disease.

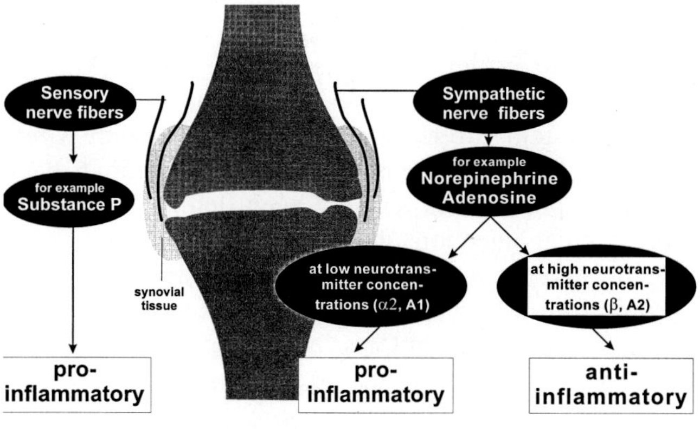

Figure 5. Influence of sympathetic and sensory nerve fibers on inflammation in the synovial tissue. Proinflammatory and antiinflammatory mechanisms are depicted. Substance P of sensory nerve fibers and norepinephrine/adenosine at low concentrations are proinflammatory, whereas norepinephrine/adenosine at high concentrations are antiinflammatory. $\alpha 2$ = α_2-adrenergic, β = β-adrenergic, A1 = adenosine receptor 1.

In this regard, it is important to study human subjects with RA. One such study demonstrated low levels of β-adrenoceptors on synovial lymphocytes of patients with RA, which may lead to decreased intracellular cAMP levels (low numbers of receptor 1 in Figure 3) and thus, to a proinflammatory state of these cells (91). Others did not confirm the low numbers of β-adrenoceptors, but found decreased expression and activity of the G-protein receptor–coupled kinases in PBMC of patients with RA (92). Such a reduction of the kinase activity would result in a stabilization of not only the β-adrenoceptor signaling pathway (Figure 3), but also chemokine and substance P pathways (92). This has been demonstrated by increased cAMP production and inhibition of TNF secretion by β_2-adrenergic stimulation in PBMC of RA patients (92).

The beneficial therapeutic effect of cAMP-inducing agents in RA has been demonstrated in one study by injecting a β-adrenergic agonist or a synthetic analog of cAMP into the joint (93). Furthermore, it is important to mention that low-dose methotrexate (MTX) exerts its antiinflammatory effects by inducing accumulation of extracellular adenosine, which binds A2 receptors and increases intracellular cAMP (94). In the report of these studies, it was mentioned that inhibition of purine and pyrimidine synthesis by MTX does not explain the therapeutic effect of the substance when it is used at low doses. Recent studies by the same group demonstrated that other antirheumatic drugs, such as sulfasalazine or salicylates, also exert their antiinflammatory effects by increasing extracellular adenosine concentrations (95). The possible immunosuppressive effect of adenosine in RA is further substantiated by therapeutic inhibition of the degrading enzyme of adenosine, the adenosine deaminase (96).

Another possible effect of the local sympathetic nervous system is release of endogenous opioids which are colocalized in the sympathetic nerve terminals (23). In this respect, it has recently been demonstrated that intraarticular injection of the predominantly μ-opioid–specific agonist morphine attenuates inflammation in chronic RA (97). One should remember that the sympathetic neurotransmitters norepinephrine (via β), adenosine (via A2), or endogenous opioids (via μ) can exert antiinflammatory effects only when sympathetic nerve fibers are present in the synovial tissue. A recent extensive study of patients with long-term RA (mean duration 10 years) demonstrated a highly significant reduction of sympathetic nerve fibers in RA as compared with osteoarthritis (OA), which was dependent on the degree of inflammation in the RA patients (98). This study confirmed the findings of an earlier small study in RA (99). It may be that reduction of sympathetic nerve fibers in the chronic disease leads to uncoupling of the local inflammation from the antiinflammatory input by the CNS (98). Furthermore, retraction of sympathetic nerve fibers may lead to low concentrations of sympathetic neurotransmitters in the area of the synovial lining layer, which would promote a proinflammatory response due to binding of sympathetic neurotransmitters at α_2-adrenoceptors and A1 receptors (Table 1). This may be a situation in which sympathectomy could provide benefit.

The sensory nervous system. With respect to the sensory nervous system, the situation is more clear because there is general consensus about the proinflammatory role of its major neurotransmitter, substance P (Table 1) (51). Local administration of substance P antagonists (51) markedly reduces the severity of inflammation in animal models. Furthermore, substance P sensitizes articular afferent nerve fibers in normal and inflamed rat knee joints (for review, see ref. 100), which leads to increased sensitivity to mechanical pressure, pain, and continuous increased substance P release into the lumen of the joint. Silent nociceptors become sensitive to mechanical pressure following experimental inflammation, which leads to an extension of the receptive field. In addition, large joints project to several spinal levels, and the processing of the nociceptive input from the inflamed joint shows a large amplification in the spinal cord. Thus, it seems that effects via substance P serve to continuously sense painful stimuli in the periphery (for review, see ref. 100). The analgesic drug capsaicin, which destroys the nerve terminals of primary sensory afferents, is now approved by the US Food and Drug Administration for the topical relief of pain due to RA.

The question remains as to whether primary sensory afferent fibers are still present in the inflamed synovial tissue. Similar to findings with sympathetic nerve fibers, levels of substance P fibers have been found to be reduced in RA synovial tissue (101). In a recent comparative study, somewhat higher levels of substance P fibers were found in RA patients versus OA patients (98). The direct comparison of substance P–positive fibers and sympathetic fibers revealed a preponderance of ~10:1 for primary sensory afferents as compared with sympathetic efferents; this preponderance of sensory afferents depends on local inflammation (98). In conclusion, such a preponderance may lead to an unfavorable proinflammatory situation, supporting the disease process of RA.

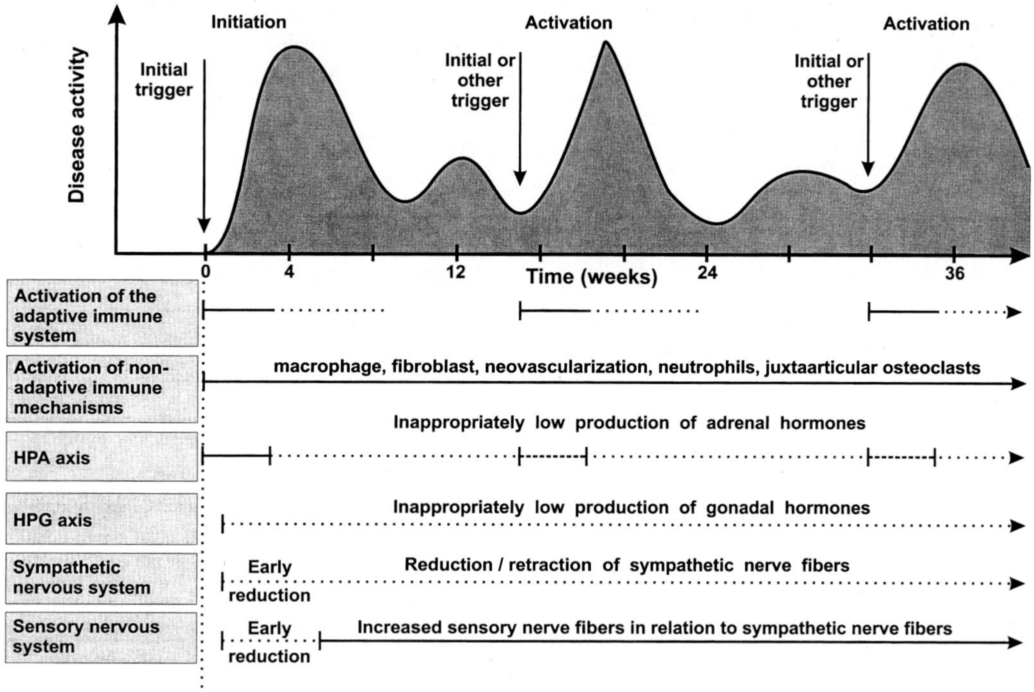

Figure 6. Synthesized scenario of the pathogenesis of chronic disease in rheumatoid arthritis. An initial trigger starts the disease, which leads to activation of the adaptive immune system. After elimination of the initial trigger, the adaptive immune system moves into a state of immunologic memory, which can be activated after reexposure to the initial trigger or another arthrophilic trigger (activation is indicated by a solid line and memory state by a dotted line). During the initial activation and thereafter, the nonadaptive immune system and many local nonimmune cells are continuously stimulated in a sort of wound healing (continuous solid line). This involves macrophages, fibroblasts (scar formation = pannus formation), neovascularization, invasion by neutrophils, and activation of juxtaarticular osteoclasts. During the initial phase, the hypothalamic–pituitary–adrenal (HPA) axis is probably able to produce huge amounts of adrenal steroids (solid line with bars at the ends). This HPA axis stimulation will be terminated by adaptation of the HPA axis within 3–6 weeks (dotted line). Thereafter, the disease is characterized by inadequately low production of adrenal/gonadal steroids in relation to systemic inflammation throughout the chronic phase (dotted line). During short episodes of activation of the disease, the HPA axis is able to mount a stronger response, which is, however, inadequate in relation to inflammation (dashed lines with bars at the ends). Relatively early after the initiation of the disease, the activity of the hypothalamic–pituitary–gonadal (HPG) axis is reduced (dotted line). Furthermore, during the early phase of the disease, sensory and sympathetic nerve fibers retract from synovial tissue (Early reduction). Sensory nerve fibers seem to reinvade the synovial tissue (sprouting: continuous solid line), which is in contrast to sympathetic nerve fibers (dotted line). At the local site, all of the above-mentioned mechanisms contribute to a more proinflammatory situation, which resembles a sort of chronic wound healing. However, in this process, final termination of wound healing does not occur.

Consequences of altered functions of the HPA axis, the HPG axis, and the peripheral nervous system in RA: a scenario for the pathogenesis and development of RA

In the initiation (or activation) phase of the disease, innate and adaptive immune pathways are activated to eliminate a possible trigger of RA in the synovial microenvironment. It is of course important to note that the trigger must be arthrophilic, as has been demonstrated for some bacteria and viruses. In this phase of the disease, a strong proinflammatory immune response against the local trigger leads to activation of distant organs, e.g., the CNS, the pituitary gland, the adrenal glands, and the liver (Figure 6). In the early phase of such a proinflammatory response, the antiinflammatory feedback is strong in order to control inflammation in the distant joints. However, after several weeks, inflammation cannot be adequately controlled because the HPA and HPG axes will produce inappropriately low amounts of antiinflammatory steroid hor-

Table 2. Treatment options from the perspective of neuroendocrine immune pathogenetic mechanisms

Target	Therapy
Substitution of the adrenal glands	Cortisol and analogs; dehydroepiandrosterone
Substitution of the gonadal glands	Testosterone (male patients); progesterone (estrogens)
Substitution of the local sympathetic nervous system (the antiinflammatory pathway)	Local adenosine (increase with methotrexate, sulfasalazine, salicylates); local opioids (μ-opioidergic such as morphine); local β-adrenergic agonists; local cAMP-elevating mechanisms
Blockade of substance P	Neurokinin receptor antagonists; capsaicin locally

mones in relation to inflammation (Figure 6). In particular, serum cortisol and adrenal/gonadal androgen levels are low in RA, but serum estrogen levels remain normal (102). Simultaneously, during the acute phase of the disease, the number of sympathetic nerve fibers and sensory nerve fibers decreases over a period of ~14 days (103) (Figure 6). Regeneration of nerve fibers (sprouting) after the acute inflammation will be incomplete and may be restricted to sensory nerve fibers (103,104). As a result, there are nearly normal levels of substance P–positive nerve fibers during long-term disease, but extremely low levels of sympathetic nerve fibers (98).

Thus, both steroid hormones and antiinflammatory neurotransmitters of the sympathetic nervous system (antiinflammatory only at high concentrations!) are secreted in inappropriately low amounts (Figure 6). This may lead to a continuous imbalance in the synovial microenvironment and perpetuation of the disease, even in a situation without the persistence of the initial trigger. In this scenario of RA pathogenesis, the known pathogenic mechanisms in the local synovial microenvironment (local immune mechanisms) are considered together with the concept of severe alteration of the two main systemic antiinflammatory feedback pathways, the HPA axis and the HANS axis (Figure 6).

Treatment options from a neuroendocrine immune perspective

New therapeutic approaches must take into consideration the known alterations of the systemic antiinflammatory feedback pathways in RA (Table 2). Concerning endocrine–immune interactions, substitution of cortisol in patients with RA is the most important principle due to the inadequately low secretion of this hormone in relation to inflammation. At present, low-dose cortisol replacement (≤7.5 mg prednisolone/day) is a mainstay in the treatment of RA. Furthermore, substitution of adrenal androgens such as DHEA seems to exert beneficial effects in chronic inflammatory diseases (105,106). In a large double-blind placebo-controlled study of patients with moderately active SLE, it was demonstrated that DHEA exerted glucocorticoid-sparing effects (107). In a small short-term (4-month) open-label study of patients with RA, no effect of DHEA on disease activity was found, but the study did not focus on bone mineral density and other long-term parameters of outcome (108). Positive clinical effects, for example, the maintenance of bone mineral density and protection from atherosclerosis, should be expected after at least 1 year, but not within 4 months.

Since DHEA is peripherally converted to appropriate amounts of testosterone and estrogens in target cells (i.e., macrophages) (28), administration of DHEA may be a substitute for either estrogen or testosterone replacement therapy in male and elderly female patients with RA (109). We believe that hormone replacement therapy with DHEA (or testosterone in male patients) should be considered more often in the therapy of patients with RA when respective hormone levels are significantly decreased (110). This is particularly true for patients who are simultaneously receiving corticosteroid therapy and are at higher risk for osteoporosis. Long-term studies are needed to evaluate the possible effects of hormone replacement therapy even in patients without overt osteoporosis, but with low serum levels of DHEA.

Normal serum levels of estrogens in RA patients, and the described immune-enhancing properties of estrogens, have represented a poor stimulus to test estrogen replacement therapy in RA. Considerable interest has been devoted to the use of oral contraceptives, which may have a protective effect against the development of RA. The results of many controlled studies with oral contraceptives have been contradictory. A recent study showed that only current use of oral contraceptives at the time of RA initiation might protect against progression to inflammatory polyarthritis (111). At the present time, no consensus has been achieved regarding oral contraceptive administration and its relationship to the prevention or development of RA (112,113). However, if there is any effect, it certainly would be a small one because oral contraceptives are only weak modulators of RA. Probably, the use of selective estrogen receptor modulators (SERM) should be taken into account. A candidate SERM should induce bone formation without inducing proinflammatory effects on immune cells.

Considering the well-demonstrated immunosuppressive activities exerted by androgens, male hormones and their derivatives seem to be the most promising therapeutic approach. Recent studies have supported the positive effects of adjuvant androgen replacement therapy at least in male RA patients (110), which further indicates the involvement of low androgen levels in the pathogenesis of the disease (72). Interestingly, the antirheumatic drug cyclosporin A may exert some of its antiinflammatory effects by enhancing local levels of testosterone and its metabolites in synovial target cells, which may be the reason for drug-induced hypertrichosis (114).

Substitution of the local sympathetic nervous system should be directed to mechanisms that enhance intracellular cAMP levels in target immune cells (Table 1). In this respect, a local increase of adenosine or norepinephrine could be a goal of treatment. Indeed, increased extracellular adenosine exerts a marked antiinflammatory effect via A2 receptors as a consequence of therapy with low-dose MTX (94) and with sulfasalazine or salicylates (95). Thus, low-dose MTX is another important mainstay in the therapy of RA, which might support the suggestion that loss of sympathetic nerve fibers, leading to low levels of adenosine, should represent an important pathogenetic factor in the disease. Local substitution of μ-opioidergic agonists and β-adrenergic agonists may be further important principles (47,93,97). Finally, since substance P is the most important proinflammatory neurotransmitter, its inhibition by neurokinin 1 antagonists or local capsaicin should be considered in local RA therapy.

Based on these treatment options, we wish to propose some clinical pharmacologic trials to be carried out in patients with RA. These possible future trials, which should include multicenter studies conducted in a placebo-controlled and double-blind manner, are as follows: 1) systemic combination therapy for at least 1 year with low-dose MTX, low-dose corticosteroids plus DHEA in comparison with MTX, and corticosteroids alone (outcome measures: joint score, parameters of systemic inflammation, radiologic joint damage, bone mineral density); 2) systemic combination therapy in male patients for at least 1 year with low-dose MTX, low-dose corticosteroids plus testosterone in comparison with MTX, and corticosteroids alone (outcome measures: joint score, parameters of systemic inflammation, radiologic joint damage, bone mineral density); 3) systemic combination therapy for at least 1 year with low-dose MTX, low-dose corticosteroids plus an antidepressant drug (e.g., low-dose amitriptyline or the new substance P antagonist MK-869 [115]) in comparison with MTX, and corticosteroids alone (outcome measures: joint score, parameters of systemic inflammation, radiologic joint damage, bone mineral density); 4) local therapy with a combination of a corticosteroid plus low-dose morphine in comparison with a corticosteroid alone (outcome measures: joint swelling, pain score, duration of effect).

These are 4 examples of possible clinical trials which reflect the view of the authors. The list is certainly far from complete due to space constraints. However, these proposals demonstrate that there are treatment options that offer additional strategies based on an approach that focuses on neuroendocrine immune factors.

Summary

From the compendium presented above, the following statements become evident: 1) Inappropriately low secretion of cortisol in relation to inflammation is a typical feature of the inflammatory disease in patients with RA. 2) The secretion of adrenal androgens is significantly reduced, which is a problem in postmenopausal women and elderly men due to a lack of downstream sex hormones. 3) Serum levels of testosterone are markedly reduced in RA. 4) Sympathetic nerve fibers are markedly reduced in the synovial tissue of patients with RA, whereas proinflammatory sensory fibers (substance P) are present. 5) Substance P serves to continuously sense painful stimuli in the periphery, and the nociceptive input from the inflamed joint shows a large amplification in the spinal cord. This leads to continuous pain with stabilization of the afferent sensory input and continuous release of proinflammatory substance P into the lumen of the joint.

From these facts it is obvious that alterations of the systemic antiinflammatory feedback systems contribute significantly to the pathogenesis of RA. Disease therapy directed at these alterations must provide a mechanism to replace the adrenal glands (glucocorticoids), the gonadal glands (androgens), and the sympathetic nervous system (adenosine increase by low-dose MTX, sulfasalazine, and salicylates) in order to integrate their immunosuppressive effects at the local site of synovial inflammation. Although local processes of the adaptive immune system are important in pathogenesis in the acute phase of RA, these mechanisms may be less important during the chronic phase of the disease in the absence of a specific trigger. We believe that a defect of systemic antiinflammatory feedback systems is an important factor in the perpetuation of RA. This review reinforces the belief that combined therapeutic approaches on a neuroendocrine immune basis are of crucial importance in a pathogenetically oriented therapy of RA.

ACKNOWLEDGMENT

We acknowledge the authors of the many interesting articles that regrettably could not be cited due to space constraints.

REFERENCES

1. Masi AT, Bijlsma JW, Chikanza IC, Pitzalis C, Cutolo M. Neuroendocrine, immunologic, and microvascular systems interactions in rheumatoid arthritis: physiopathogenetic and therapeutic perspectives. Semin Arthritis Rheum 1999;29:65–81.
2. Konttinen YT, Kemppinen P, Segerberg M, Hukkanen M, Rees R, Santavirta S, et al. Peripheral and spinal neural mechanisms in arthritis, with particular reference to treatment of inflammation and pain. Arthritis Rheum 1994;37:965–82.
3. Cutolo M, Accardo S, Villaggio B, Clerico P, Indiveri F, Carruba G, et al. Evidence for the presence of androgen receptors in the synovial tissue of rheumatoid arthritis patients and healthy controls. Arthritis Rheum 1992;35:1007–15.
4. Matucci-Cerinic MM, Konttinen Y, Generini S, Cutolo M. Neuropeptides and steroid hormones in arthritis. Curr Opin Rheumatol 1998;10:220–35.
5. Besedovsky HO, Del Rey A. Immune-neuro-endocrine interactions. Endocr Rev 1996;17:64–102.
6. Munck A, Guyre PM. Glucocorticoid physiology, pharmacology and stress. Adv Exp Med Biol 1986;196:81–96.
7. Walker JG, Littlejohn GO, McMurray NE, Cutolo M. Stress system response and rheumatoid arthritis: a multilevel approach. Rheumatology (Oxford) 1999;38:1050–7.
8. Herrmann M, Schölmerich J, Straub RH. Stress and rheumatic diseases. Rheum Dis Clin North Am 2000;26:818–27.
9. Bläß S, Engel J-M, Burmester G-R. The immunologic homunculus in rheumatoid arthritis. Arthritis Rheum 1999;42:2499–506.
10. Ebringer A, Wilson C, Tiwana H. Is rheumatoid arthritis a form of reactive arthritis? J Rheumatol 2000;27:559–63.
11. Takeda T, Mizugaki Y, Matsubara L, Imai S, Koike T, Takada K. Lytic Epstein-Barr virus infection in the synovial tissue of patients with rheumatoid arthritis. Arthritis Rheum 2000;43:1218–25.
12. Janossy G, Panayi G, Duke O, Bofill M, Poulter LW, Goldstein G. Rheumatoid arthritis: a disease of T-lymphocyte/macrophage immunoregulation. Lancet 1981;2:839–42.
13. Van de Putte LB, Meijer CJ, Lafeber GJ, Kleinjan R, Cats A. Lymphocytes in rheumatoid and nonrheumatoid synovial fluids: nonspecificity of high T-cell and low B-cell percentages. Ann Rheum Dis 1975;35:451–5.
14. McMichael AJ, Sasazuki T, McDevitt HO, Payne RO. Increased frequency of HLA-Cw3 and HLA-Dw4 in rheumatoid arthritis. Arthritis Rheum 1977;20:1037–42.
15. Roudier J, Petersen J, Rhodes GH, Luka J, Carson DA. Susceptibility to rheumatoid arthritis maps to a T-cell epitope shared by the HLA-Dw4 DR beta-1 chain and the Epstein-Barr virus glycoprotein gp110. Proc Natl Acad Sci U S A 1989;86:5104–8.
16. Carson DA. Rheumatoid arthritis: pathogenesis and future therapies. Annual Scientific Meeting of the American College of Rheumatology; 1999 Nov 13–17; Boston.
17. Firestein GS, Nguyen K, Aupperle KR, Yeo M, Boyle DL, Zvaifler NJ. Apoptosis in rheumatoid arthritis: p53 overexpression in rheumatoid arthritis synovium. Am J Pathol 1996;149: 2143–51.
18. Müller-Ladner U, Kriegsmann J, Franklin BN, Matsumoto S, Geiler T, Gay RE, et al. Synovial fibroblasts of patients with rheumatoid arthritis attach to and invade normal human cartilage when engrafted into SCID mice. Am J Pathol 1996;149:1607–15.
19. Weissmann G, Korchak H. Rheumatoid arthritis: the role of neutrophil activation. Inflammation 1984;8 Suppl:S3–14.
20. Crisp AJ, Chapman CM, Kirkham SE, Schiller AL, Krane SM. Articular mastocytosis in rheumatoid arthritis. Arthritis Rheum 1984;27:845–51.
21. Koch AE, Polverini PJ, Leibovich SJ. Stimulation of neovascularization by human rheumatoid synovial tissue macrophages. Arthritis Rheum 1986;29:471–9.
22. Chrousos GP. The hypothalamic-pituitary-adrenal axis and immune-mediated inflammation. N Engl J Med 1995;332:1351–62.
23. Straub RH, Westermann J, Schölmerich J, Falk W. Dialogue between CNS and immune system in lymphoid organs. Immunol Today 1998;19:409–13.
24. Mastorakos G, Chrousos GP, Weber JS. Recombinant interleukin-6 activates the hypothalamic-pituitary-adrenal axis in humans. J Clin Endocrinol Metab 1993;77:1690–4.
25. Niijima A, Hori T, Aou S, Oomura Y. The effects of interleukin-1 beta on the activity of adrenal, splenic and renal sympathetic nerves in the rat. J Auton Nerv Syst 1991;36:183–92.
26. Battaglia DF, Bowen JM, Krasa HB, Thrun LA, Viguie C, Karsch FJ. Endotoxin inhibits the reproductive neuroendocrine axis while stimulating adrenal steroids: a simultaneous view from hypophyseal portal and peripheral blood. Endocrinology 1997; 138:4273–81.
27. Van der Poll T, Barber AE, Coyle SM, Lowry SF. Hypercortisolemia increases plasma interleukin-10 concentrations during human endotoxemia—a clinical research center study. J Clin Endocrinol Metab 1996;81:3604–6.
28. Schmidt M, Kreutz M, Löffler G, Schölmerich J, Straub RH. Conversion of dehydroepiandrosterone to downstream steroid hormones in macrophages. J Endocrinol 2000;164:161–9.
29. Daynes RA, Araneo BA, Ershler WB, Maloney C, Li GZ, Ryu SY. Altered regulation of IL-6 production with normal aging: possible linkage to the age-associated decline in dehydroepiandrosterone and its sulfated derivative. J Immunol 1993;150: 5219–30.
30. Straub RH, Konecna L, Hrach S, Rothe G, Kreutz M, Schölmerich J, et al. Serum dehydroepiandrosterone (DHEA) and DHEA sulfate are negatively correlated with serum interleukin-6 (IL-6), and DHEA inhibits IL-6 secretion from mononuclear cells in man in vitro: possible link between endocrinosenescence and immunosenescence. J Clin Endocrinol Metab 1998;83:2012–7.
31. Cutolo M, Sulli A, Villaggio B, Seriolo B, Accardo S. Relations between steroid hormones and cytokines in rheumatoid arthritis and systemic lupus erythematosus. Ann Rheum Dis 1998;57: 573–7.
32. Li ZG, Danis VA, Brooks PM. Effect of gonadal steroids on the production of IL-1 and IL-6 by blood mononuclear cells in vitro. Clin Exp Rheumatol 1993;11:157–62.
33. Cutolo M, Accardo S, Villaggio B, Barone A, Sulli A, Balleari E, et al. Androgen metabolism and inhibition of interleukin-1 synthesis in primary cultured human synovial macrophages. Mediators Inflamm 1995;4:138.
34. Keller ET, Chang C, Ershler WB. Inhibition of NFkappaB activity through maintenance of IkappaBalpha levels contributes to dihydrotestosterone-mediated repression of the interleukin-6 promoter. J Biol Chem 1996;271:26267–75.
35. Kanda N, Tsuchida T, Tamaki K. Testosterone suppresses anti-DNA antibody production in peripheral blood mononuclear cells

from patients with systemic lupus erythematosus. Arthritis Rheum 1997;40:1703–11.
36. Spector TD, Perry LA, Tubb G, Silman AJ, Huskisson EC. Low free testosterone levels in rheumatoid arthritis. Ann Rheum Dis 1988;47:65–8.
37. Cutolo M, Balleari E, Giusti M, Monachesi M, Accardo S. Sex hormone status of male patients with rheumatoid arthritis: evidence of low serum concentrations of testosterone at baseline and after human chorionic gonadotropin stimulation. Arthritis Rheum 1988;31:1314–7.
38. Cutolo M, Wilder R. Different roles for androgens and estrogens in the susceptibility to autoimmune rheumatic diseases. Rheum Dis Clin North Am 2000;26:825–39.
39. Kanda N, Tamaki K. Estrogen enhances immunoglobulin production by human PBMCs. J Allergy Clin Immunol 1999;103: 282–8.
40. Kanda N, Tsuchida T, Tamaki K. Estrogen enhancement of anti–double-stranded DNA antibody and immunoglobulin G production in peripheral blood mononuclear cells from patients with systemic lupus erythematosus. Arthritis Rheum 1999;42: 328–37.
41. Hu SK, Mitcho YL, Rath NC. Effect of estradiol on interleukin 1 synthesis by macrophages. Int J Immunopharmacol 1988;10: 247–52.
42. Polan ML, Kuo A, Loukides J, Bottomly K. Cultured human luteal peripheral monocytes secrete increased levels of interleukin-1. J Clin Endocrinol Metab 1990;70:480–4.
43. Khalkhali-Ellis Z, Seftor EA, Nieva DRC, Handa RJ, Price RH Jr, Kirschmann DA, et al. Estrogen and progesterone regulation of human fibroblast-like synoviocyte function in vitro: implications in rheumatoid arthritis. J Rheumatol 2000;27:1622–31.
44. Seriolo B, Cutolo M, Garnero A, Accardo S. Relationships between serum 17 beta-oestradiol and anticardiolipin antibody concentrations in female patients with rheumatoid arthritis. Rheumatology (Oxford) 1999;38:1159–61.
45. Lechner O, Wiegers GJ, Oliveira-Dos-Santos AJ, Dietrich H, Recheis H, Waterman M, et al. Glucocorticoid production in the murine thymus. Eur J Immunol 2000;30:337–46.
46. Hennebold JD, Daynes RA. Inhibition of skin 11beta-hydroxysteroid dehydrogenase activity in vivo potentiates the anti-inflammatory actions of glucocorticoids. Arch Dermatol Res 1998;290:413–9.
47. Malfait AM, Malik AS, Marinova-Mutafchieva L, Butler DM, Maini RN, Feldmann M. The beta2-adrenergic agonist salbutamol is a potent suppressor of established collagen-induced arthritis: mechanisms of action. J Immunol 1999;162:6278–83.
48. Lotz M, Vaughan JH, Carson DA. Effect of neuropeptides on production of inflammatory cytokines by human monocytes. Science 1988;241:1218–21.
49. Rameshwar P, Gascon P, Ganea D. Stimulation of IL-2 production in murine lymphocytes by substance P and related tachykinins. J Immunol 1993;151:2484–96.
50. Lieb K, Fiebich BL, Berger M, Bauer J, Schulze-Osthoff K. The neuropeptide substance P activates transcription factor NF-kappa B and kappa B-dependent gene expression in human astrocytoma cells. J Immunol 1997;159:4952–8.
51. Levine JD, Clark R, Devor M, Helms C, Moskowitz MA, Basbaum AI. Intraneuronal substance P contributes to the severity of experimental arthritis. Science 1984;226:547–9.
52. Motulsky HJ, Insel PA. Adrenergic receptors in man: direct identification, physiologic regulation, and clinical alterations. N Engl J Med 1982;307:18–29.
53. Oikarinen J, Hamalainen L, Oikarinen A. Modulation of glucocorticoid receptor activity by cyclic nucleotides and its implications on the regulation of human skin fibroblast growth and protein synthesis. Biochim Biophys Acta 1984;799:158–65.
54. Gruol DJ, Campbell NF, Bourgeois S. Cyclic AMP-dependent protein kinase promotes glucocorticoid receptor function. J Biol Chem 1986;261:4909–14.
55. DiBattista JA, Martel-Pelletier J, Cloutier JM, Pelletier JP. Modulation of glucocorticoid receptor expression in human articular chondrocytes by cAMP and prostaglandins. J Rheumatol Suppl 1991;27:102–5.
56. Schubert D, LaCorbiere M, Klier FG, Steinbach JH. The modulation of neurotransmitter synthesis by steroid hormones and insulin. Brain Res 1980;190:67–79.
57. Ehrhart-Bornstein M, Hinson JP, Bornstein SR, Scherbaum WA, Vinson GP. Intraadrenal interactions in the regulation of adrenocortical steroidogenesis. Endocr Rev 1998;19:101–43.
58. Naitoh Y, Fukata J, Tominaga T, Nakai Y, Tamai S, Mori K, et al. Interleukin-6 stimulates the secretion of adrenocorticotropic hormone in conscious, freely-moving rats. Biochem Biophys Res Commun 1988;155:1459–63.
59. Besedovsky HO, del Rey A, Sorkin E, Dinarello C. Immunoregulatory feedback between interleukin-1 and glucocorticoid hormones. Science 1986;233:652–4.
60. Lotze MT, Frana LW, Sharrow SO, Robb RJ, Rosenberg SA. In vivo administration of purified human interleukin 2. I. Half-life and immunologic effects of the Jurkat cell line-derived interleukin 2. J Immunol 1985;134:157–66.
61. Michie HR, Spriggs DR, Manogue KR, Sherman ML, Revhaug A, O'Dwyer ST, et al. Tumor necrosis factor and endotoxin induce similar metabolic responses in human beings. Surgery 1988;104:280–6.
62. Nakamura H, Motoyoshi S, Kadokawa T. Anti-inflammatory action of interleukin 1 through the pituitary-adrenal axis in rats. Eur J Pharmacol 1988;151:67–73.
63. Harbuz MS, Jessop DS. Is there a defect in cortisol production in rheumatoid arthritis? Rheumatology (Oxford) 1999;38:298–302.
64. Chikanza IC, Petrou P, Kingsley G, Chrousos G, Panayi GS. Defective hypothalamic response to immune and inflammatory stimuli in patients with rheumatoid arthritis. Arthritis Rheum 1992;35:1281–8.
65. Eijsbouts A, van den HF, Laan R, de Waal MM, Hermus A, Sweep C, et al. Similar response of adrenocorticotrophic hormone, cortisol and prolactin to surgery in rheumatoid arthritis and osteoarthritis [letter]. Br J Rheumatol 1998;37:1138–9.
66. Cash JM, Crofford LJ, Gallucci WT, Sternberg EM, Gold PW, Chrousos GP, et al. Pituitary-adrenal axis responsiveness to ovine corticotropin releasing hormone in patients with rheumatoid arthritis treated with low dose prednisone. J Rheumatol 1992;19: 1692–6.
67. Van den Brink HR, Blankenstein MA, Koppeschaar HP, Bijlsma JW. Influence of disease activity on steroid hormone levels in peripheral blood of patients with rheumatoid arthritis. Clin Exp Rheumatol 1993;11:649–52.
68. Gudbjornsson B, Skogseid B, Oberg K, Wide L, Hallgren R. Intact adrenocorticotropic hormone secretion but impaired cortisol response in patients with active rheumatoid arthritis: effect of glucocorticoids. J Rheumatol 1996;23:596–602.
69. Templ E, Koeller M, Riedl M, Wagner O, Graninger W, Luger A. Anterior pituitary function in patients with newly diagnosed rheumatoid arthritis. Br J Rheumatol 1996;35:350–6.
70. Cutolo M, Foppiani L, Prete C, Ballarino P, Sulli A, Villaggio B, et al. Hypothalamic-pituitary-adrenocortical axis function in premenopausal women with rheumatoid arthritis not treated with glucocorticoids. J Rheumatol 1999;26:282–8.
71. Gutierrez MA, Garcia ME, Rodriguez JA, Mardonez G, Jacobelli S, Rivero S. Hypothalamic-pituitary-adrenal axis function in patients with active rheumatoid arthritis: a controlled study using insulin hypoglycemia stress test and prolactin stimulation. J Rheumatol 1999;26:277–81.
72. Kanik KS, Chrousos GP, Schumacher HR, Crane ML, Yarboro CH, Wilder RL. Adrenocorticotropin, glucocorticoid, and andro-

gen secretion in patients with new onset synovitis/rheumatoid arthritis: relations with indices of inflammation. J Clin Endocrinol Metab 2000;85:1461–6.
73. Straub RH, Vogl D, Gross V, Lang B, Schölmerich J, Andus T. Association of humoral markers of inflammation and dehydroepiandrosterone sulfate or cortisol serum levels in patients with chronic inflammatory bowel disease. Am J Gastroenterol 1998; 93:2197–202.
74. Johnson EO, Vlachoyiannopoulos PG, Skopouli FN, Tzioufas AG, Moutsopoulos HM. Hypofunction of the stress axis in Sjogren's syndrome. J Rheumatol 1998;25:1508–14.
75. Zietz B, Reber T, Oertel M, Glück T, Schölmerich J, Straub RH. Altered function of the hypothalamic stress axes in patients with moderately active systemic lupus erythematosus. II. Dissociation between androstenedione, cortisol, or dehydroepiandrosterone and interleukin 6 or tumor necrosis factor. J Rheumatol 2000;27: 911–8.
76. Sanden S, Tripmacher R, Weltrich R, Rohde W, Hiepe F, Burmester GR, et al. Glucocorticoid dose dependent downregulation of glucocorticoid receptors in patients with rheumatic diseases. J Rheumatol 2000;27:1265–70.
77. Masi AT, Josipovic DB, Jefferson WE. Low adrenal androgenic-anabolic steroids in women with rheumatoid arthritis (RA): gas-liquid chromatographic studies of RA patients and matched normal control women indicating decreased 11-deoxy-17-ketosteroid excretion. Semin Arthritis Rheum 1984; 14:1–23.
78. Sambrook PN, Eisman JA, Champion GD, Pocock NA. Sex hormone status and osteoporosis in postmenopausal women with rheumatoid arthritis. Arthritis Rheum 1988;31:973–8.
79. Lahita RG, Bradlow HL, Ginzler E, Pang S, New M. Low plasma androgens in women with systemic lupus erythematosus. Arthritis Rheum 1987;30:241–8.
80. Straub RH, Zeuner M, Lock G, Schölmerich J, Lang B. High prolactin and low dehydroepiandrosterone sulphate serum levels in patients with severe systemic sclerosis. Br J Rheumatol 1997; 36:426–32.
81. Nilsson E, de la Torre B, Hedman M, Goobar J, Thorner A. Blood dehydroepiandrosterone sulphate (DHEAS) levels in polymyalgia rheumatica/giant cell arteritis and primary fibromyalgia. Clin Exp Rheumatol 1994;12:415–7.
82. Straub RH, Glück T, Cutolo M, Georgi J, Helmke K, Schölmerich J, et al. The adrenal steroid status in relation to inflammatory cytokines (interleukin-6 and tumour necrosis factor) in polymyalgia rheumatica. Rheumatology (Oxford) 2000;39:624–31.
83. Hales DB. Interleukin-1 inhibits Leydig cell steroidogenesis primarily by decreasing 17 alpha-hydroxylase/C17-20 lyase cytochrome P450 expression. Endocrinology 1992;131:2165–72.
84. MacDiarmid F, Wang D, Duncan LJ, Purohit A, Ghilchick MW, Reed MJ. Stimulation of aromatase activity in breast fibroblasts by tumor necrosis factor alpha. Mol Cell Endocrinol 1994;106: 17–21.
85. Purohit A, Ghilchik MW, Duncan L, Wang DY, Singh A, Walker MM, et al. Aromatase activity and interleukin-6 production by normal and malignant breast tissues. J Clin Endocrinol Metab 1995;80:3052–8.
86. Castagnetta L, Cutolo M, Granata OM, Di Falco M, Bellavia V, Carruba G. Endocrine end-points in rheumatoid arthritis. Ann N Y Acad Sci 1999;876:180–91; discussion 191–2.
87. Bevan JA. Some functional consequences of variation in adrenergic synaptic cleft width and in nerve density and distribution. Fed Proc 1977;36:2439–43.
88. Janig W, Levine JD, Michaelis M. Interactions of sympathetic and primary afferent neurons following nerve injury and tissue trauma. Prog Brain Res 1996;113:161–84.
89. Laemont KD, Schaefer CJ, Juneau PL, Schrier DJ. Effects of the phosphodiesterase inhibitor rolipram on streptococcal cell wall-induced arthritis in rats. Int J Immunopharmacol 1999; 21:711–25.
90. Lee A, Coderre TJ, Basbaum AI, Levine JD. Sympathetic neuron factors involved in bradykinin-induced plasma extravasation in the rat. Brain Res 1991;557:146–8.
91. Baerwald CG, Laufenberg M, Specht T, von Wichert P, Burmester GR, Krause A. Impaired sympathetic influence on the immune response in patients with rheumatoid arthritis due to lymphocyte subset-specific modulation of beta 2-adrenergic receptors. Br J Rheumatol 1997;36:1262–9.
92. Lombardi MS, Kavelaars A, Schedlowski M, Bijlsma JW, Okihara KL, van de Pol M, et al. Decreased expression and activity of G-protein-coupled receptor kinases in peripheral blood mononuclear cells of patients with rheumatoid arthritis. FASEB J 1999;13:715–25.
93. Trang LE, Lovgren O, Roch-Norlund AE, Horn RS, Walaas O. Cyclic nucleotides in joint fluid in rheumatoid arthritis and in Reiter's syndrome. Scand J Rheumatol 1979;8:91–6.
94. Cronstein BN. The mechanism of action of methotrexate. Rheum Dis Clin North Am 1997;23:739–55.
95. Cronstein BN, Montesinos MC, Weissmann G. Salicylates and sulfasalazine, but not glucocorticoids, inhibit leukocyte accumulation by an adenosine-dependent mechanism that is independent of inhibition of prostaglandin synthesis and p105 of NFkappaB. Proc Natl Acad Sci U S A 1999;96:6377–81.
96. Carrera CJ, Terai C, Lotz M, Curd JG, Piro LD, Beutler E, et al. Potent toxicity of 2-chlorodeoxyadenosine toward human monocytes in vitro and in vivo: a novel approach to immunosuppressive therapy. J Clin Invest 1990;86:1480–8.
97. Stein A, Yassouridis A, Szopko C, Helmke K, Stein C. Intraarticular morphine versus dexamethasone in chronic arthritis. Pain 1999;83:525–32.
98. Miller LE, Jüsten H-P, Schölmerich J, Straub RH. The loss of sympathetic nerve fibers in the synovial membrane of patients with rheumatoid arthritis is accompanied by increased norepinephrine release from synovial cells. FASEB J 2000;14: 2097–2107.
99. Pereira da Silva JA, Carmo-Fonseca M. Peptide containing nerves in human synovium: immunohistochemical evidence for decreased innervation in rheumatoid arthritis. J Rheumatol 1990;17:1592–9.
100. Schaible HG, Grubb BD. Afferent and spinal mechanisms of joint pain. Pain 1993;55:5–54.
101. Mapp PI, Kidd BL, Gibson SJ, Terry JM, Revell PA, Ibrahim NB, et al. Substance P-, calcitonin gene-related peptide- and C-flanking peptide of neuropeptide Y-immunoreactive fibres are present in normal synovium but depleted in patients with rheumatoid arthritis. Neuroscience 1990;37:143–53.
102. Cutolo M, Sulli A, Seriolo B, Accardo S, Masi AT. Estrogens, the immune response and autoimmunity. Clin Exp Rheumatol 1995; 13:217–26.
103. Imai S, Tokunaga Y, Konttinen YT, Maeda T, Hukuda S, Santavirta S. Ultrastructure of the synovial sensory peptidergic fibers is distinctively altered in different phases of adjuvant induced arthritis in rats: ultramorphological characterization combined with morphometric and immunohistochemical study for substance P, calcitonin gene related peptide, and protein gene product 9.5. J Rheumatol 1997;24:2177–87.
104. Ahmed M, Bjurholm A, Schultzberg M, Theodorsson E, Kreicbergs A. Increased levels of substance P and calcitonin gene–related peptide in rat adjuvant arthritis: a combined immunohistochemical and radioimmunoassay analysis. Arthritis Rheum 1995;38:699–709.
105. Van Vollenhoven RF, Engleman EG, McGuire JL. Dehydroepiandrosterone in systemic lupus erythematosus: results of a double-blind, placebo-controlled, randomized clinical trial. Arthritis Rheum 1995;38:1826–31.

106. Andus T, Klebl F, Rogler G, Schölmerich J, Straub RH. Successful treatment of refractory ulcerative colitis with dehydroepiandrosterone (DHEA)—an open controlled pilot trial [abstract]. Gastroenterology 2000;188:A116.
107. Petri M, Lahita R, McGuire J, van Vollenhoven R, Strand V, Kunz A, et al. Results of the GL701 (DHEA) multicenter steroid-sparing SLE study [abstract]. Arthritis Rheum 1997;40: S327.
108. Giltay EJ, van Schaardenburg D, Gooren LJ, von Blomberg BM, Fonk JC, Touw DJ, et al. Effects of dehydroepiandrosterone administration on disease activity in patients with rheumatoid arthritis [letter]. Br J Rheumatol 1998;37:705–6.
109. Robinzon B, Cutolo M. Should dehydroepiandrosterone replacement therapy be provided with glucocorticoids? Rheumatology (Oxford) 1999;38:488–95.
110. Cutolo M, Balleari E, Giusti M, Intra E, Accardo S. Androgen replacement therapy in male patients with rheumatoid arthritis. Arthritis Rheum 1991;34:1–5.
111. Brennan P, Bankhead C, Silman A, Symmons D. Oral contraceptives and rheumatoid arthritis: results from a primary care-based incident case-control study. Semin Arthritis Rheum 1997;26: 817–23.
112. Masi AT, Feigenbaum SL, Chatterton RT. Hormonal and pregnancy relationships to rheumatoid arthritis: convergent effects with immunologic and microvascular systems. Semin Arthritis Rheum 1995;25:1–27.
113. Bijlsma JW, van den Brink HR. Estrogens and rheumatoid arthritis. Am J Reprod Immunol 1992;28:231–4.
114. Cutolo M, Giusti M, Villaggio B, Barone A, Accardo S, Sulli A, et al. Testosterone metabolism and cyclosporin A treatment in rheumatoid arthritis. Br J Rheumatol 1997;36:433–9.
115. Kramer MS, Cutler N, Feighner J, Shrivastava R, Carman J, Sramek JJ, et al. Distinct mechanism for antidepressant activity by blockade of central substance P receptors. Science 1998;281: 1640–5.
116. Straub RH. Tables of molecular and functional neuroendocrine immune interactions. Eching (Germany): Biozol; 2000.

ARTHRITIS & RHEUMATISM
Vol. 44, No. 3, March 2001, pp 508–512

EDITORIAL

Treatment of Polyarteritis Nodosa, Microscopic Polyangiitis, and Churg-Strauss Syndrome: Where Do We Stand?

Carol A. Langford

In 1866, Kussmaul and Maier described a unique illness they named "periarteritis nodosa" in recognition of the nodularity and inflammation that involved the small muscular arteries (1). Ferrari introduced the term "polyarteritis nodosa (PAN)" in 1903 to illustrate the transmural arterial inflammation that occurs in this disease (2). Despite the subsequent work of many investigators, including an important paper in this issue of *Arthritis & Rheumatism* (3), many questions regarding the treatment of PAN remain unanswered.

Developments in nomenclature have complicated the conduct and interpretation of therapeutic trials in PAN. Wohlwill in 1923 (4) and Davson et al in 1948 (5) described glomerular and small vessel disease in patients with PAN that they termed "microscopic polyarteritis." Although some authors adopted this terminology, most continued to include glomerulonephritis as a manifestation of PAN. In 1993, a committee of clinicians and pathologists convened in Chapel Hill, North Carolina, with the goal of reaching a consensus on the names and definitions for the common forms of noninfectious systemic vasculitis (6). Under this nomenclature, "polyarteritis nodosa" is restricted to disease with necrotizing inflammation of the medium-sized and small arteries but without involvement of smaller vessels (Table 1). Patients with glomerulonephritis or necrotizing vasculitis with few or no immune complexes affecting the small vessels (i.e., arterioles, venules, or capillaries) are considered to have "microscopic polyangiitis" (MPA).

The designation of MPA as a discrete entity has been a subject of controversy, especially concerning the separation from Wegener's granulomatosis (WG). Clinically, these two diseases have many similarities, including small vessel vasculitis of the lung, glomerulonephritis, and the presence of antineutrophil cytoplasmic antibodies (ANCA) (Table 2). Furthermore, the glomerular lesion of MPA, a focal crescentic glomerulonephritis with few or no immune complexes, is histologically identical to WG (7). In the definitions set forth at the Chapel Hill Consensus Conference, the diagnosis of WG is restricted to patients with necrotizing granulomatous inflammation (Table 1). Granulomatous inflammation does not have to be histologically proven in this nomenclature system and can be inferred by noninvasive evaluations. Clinical manifestations, however, do not always predict the presence of granulomatous inflammation. In one series, only 42% of 126 upper airways biopsy tissues from patients with known WG revealed granulomas (8). Granulomatous inflammation is also often not observed in lung biopsy tissues from patients with WG and pulmonary hemorrhage (9).

The distinction between WG and MPA may be particularly difficult in certain clinical settings, such as patients with sinus mucosal thickening, pulmonary hemorrhage, and glomerulonephritis. In one series, 13% of patients with MPA were found to have upper respiratory tract disease (10), while, in another series, such involvement was said to exclude this diagnosis (11). In addition, there are reports of patients who meet the definition for MPA but later develop characteristic clinical and histologic features of WG (12). These issues highlight the lack of a universally accepted definition for MPA.

In series of patients with PAN described prior to the separate designation of MPA, those with untreated disease had a poor prognosis, with a 5-year survival rate of <15% (13,14). Corticosteroids (CS) were the first applied treatment and were found to improve 5-year survival rates to 48–57% (13–16). Beneficial effects were also observed with the introduction of combined therapy with cyclophosphamide (CYC) and CS (14,17), particularly in patients with severe disease (18). However, some investigators found that the use of CYC did not improve outcome beyond that of treatment with CS alone (15).

Carol A. Langford, MD, MHS: National Institute of Allergy and Infectious Diseases, NIH, Bethesda, Maryland.

Address correspondence and reprint requests to Carol A. Langford, MD, MHS, Laboratory of Immunoregulation, National Institute of Allergy and Infectious Diseases, National Institutes of Health, Bethesda, MD 20892.

Submitted for publication October 18, 2000; accepted in revised form October 23, 2000.

Table 1. Chapel Hill Consensus Conference definitions of polyarteritis nodosa, microscopic polyangiitis, Wegener's granulomatosis, and Churg-Strauss syndrome (6)

Polyarteritis nodosa (classic polyarteritis nodosa)	Necrotizing inflammation of medium-sized or small arteries without glomerulonephritis or vasculitis in arterioles, capillaries, or venules
Microscopic polyangiitis (microscopic polyarteritis)	Necrotizing vasculitis, with few or no immune deposits, affecting small vessels (i.e., capillaries, venules, or arterioles). *Necrotizing arteritis involving small and medium-sized arteries may be present. Necrotizing glomerulonephritis is very common. Pulmonary capillaritis often occurs.*
Wegener's granulomatosis	Granulomatous inflammation involving the respiratory tract, and necrotizing vasculitis affecting small to medium-sized vessels (e.g., capillaries, venules, arterioles, and arteries). *Necrotizing glomerulonephritis is common.*
Churg-Strauss syndrome	Eosinophil-rich and granulomatous inflammation involving the respiratory tract, and necrotizing vasculitis affecting small to medium-sized vessels, and associated with asthma and eosinophilia.

Such findings raise questions about the optimal therapeutic strategy for PAN and the necessity for CYC use in all patients.

The most recent literature on the treatment of PAN has come from trials performed by the French Vasculitis Study Group (FVSG). These studies, which began in 1980, represent the largest experience on the therapy of PAN and have presented a valuable body of information. In the first trial performed by the FVSG, patients with PAN and Churg-Strauss syndrome (CSS) were randomized to receive prednisone plus plasma exchanges either alone or in combination with daily CYC (19). Study recruitment was halted after 71 patients had entered the study because the interim analysis at 3 years demonstrated a greater efficacy of the CYC arm on disease control; fewer relapses also occurred in the group who had received CYC. No difference, however, was observed in the cumulative 10-year survival rate regardless of whether the patient had initially received CYC. Examination of the survival curves from later studies similarly failed to demonstrate a difference in survival based on the initial use of CYC therapy (20). While these studies supported the effectiveness of CYC in PAN and CSS, they did not determine whether CYC is necessary in all instances.

To explore whether disease severity could guide treatment, the FVSG sought to identify the factors associated with a poor prognosis in PAN and CSS (20). From a univariate and multivariate analysis, the Five-Factors Score (FFS) was derived. This score integrated items that had been found to be associated with an increased mortality and included a serum creatinine level of >1.58 mg/dl, proteinuria of >1 gm/day, gastrointestinal (GI) tract involvement (defined as bleeding,

Table 2. Comparison of the clinical and histologic features of 4 different forms of systemic vasculitis*

Characteristic	Wegener's granulomatosis	Microscopic polyangiitis	Polyarteritis nodosa	Churg-Strauss syndrome
Size of affected vessels	Small vessels; small and medium-sized arteries	Small vessels; small and medium-sized arteries	Medium-sized and small arteries	Small vessels; small and medium-sized arteries
Granulomatous inflammation	Yes	No	No	Yes
Organ system involved, % of patients				
Upper airways disease	95	No	No	50–60
Pulmonary disease	85	50–70	No	40–70
Pulmonary hemorrhage	5–15	10–50	No	<3
Glomerulonephritis	80	90	No	10–25
Gastrointestinal tract	<5	30	25–40	30–50
Nervous system	20–50	60–70	50–70	70–80
Cardiac	10	10–15	5–30	10–15
Relapsing course, % of patients	50	35	20	30–50
Hepatitis associated	No	No	Yes	No
Eosinophilia	Rare	Rare	Rare	Yes
Arteriographic microaneurysms	No	Uncertain	Yes	No
ANCA, % of patients	>85%	50–80	<20	50–70

* Frequencies reflect data combined from the following sources: for Wegener's granulomatosis, ref. 39; for microscopic polyangiitis, refs. 10, 11, 33, 35, and 42–44; for polyarteritis nodosa, refs. 13–15, 25, and 44; for Churg-Strauss syndrome, refs. 22, 23, 43, and 44. ANCA = antineutrophil cytoplasmic antibodies.

perforation, infarction, or pancreatitis), central nervous system (CNS) involvement, and cardiomyopathy. A score of 0 was given when none of the 5 factors was present, a score of 1 when 1 factor was present, and a score of 2 when ≥2 factors were present. Among 336 patients enrolled in 5 prospective trials, a 46% 5-year mortality rate was observed in patients with an FFS score of >2, compared with a rate of 12% in patients with a score of 0 (20).

Important information has been gained from the PAN studies performed by the FVSG; several issues, however, have complicated their interpretation. While these trials have been prospective, randomized, and standardized, they have generally been of insufficient size to draw definitive conclusions with regard to differences between treatment arms. For some series, cohorts from different treatment trials have been combined to examine outcome. Although this increases the sample size, the use of diverse therapeutic regimens from patient to patient may confound the analysis.

The lack of a homogenous disease population has been another area of potential concern. From work pioneered by the FVSG, it has been recognized that antiviral agents together with minimization of immunosuppression are important in the treatment of hepatitis B virus (HBV)–associated PAN (21). Despite this very different therapeutic approach, patients with HBV-associated PAN have continued to be combined with those who have noninfectious PAN in longitudinal analyses. In studies by the FVSG, patients with CSS have also been included. While the investigators have discussed the clinical and histopathologic differences between PAN and CSS (22,23), they have suggested that the similarity in prognosis supports this trial design (20). The separation of PAN and MPA may further affect the homogeneity of the study population because a substantial number of enrolled patients have glomerulonephritis. These methodologic issues highlight the challenges that are faced in conducting clinical trials in rare diseases. PAN and CSS are among the least common forms of systemic vasculitis. With the Chapel Hill Consensus Conference reclassification, PAN in particular appears to be exceedingly rare (24). Even with such formidable obstacles, the work of these investigators has continued, and their efforts to better understand these rare diseases are to be commended.

In the current issue of *Arthritis & Rheumatism*, Gayraud and colleagues from the FVSG present data on the long-term followup of 278 patients with PAN and CSS enrolled in 4 prospective trials between 1980 and 1993. With a mean patient followup time of 7.3 years (range 3 months to 16 years), this paper contains the most comprehensive longitudinal data for patients with PAN and provides an extension of their previous analyses in 1992 and 1996 (20,25). Outcome was examined as it relates to the type of vasculitis, the treatments administered, and the presence of prognostic factors as assessed by the FFS and the Birmingham Vasculitis Activity Score (BVAS) at the time of diagnosis. In addition, the investigators went back to their cohort and reclassified them as having PAN, HBV-related PAN, MPA, or CSS according to the criteria of the American College of Rheumatology, the Chapel Hill Consensus Conference, and their own recommendations for the diagnosis of MPA.

The findings from this study indicate that the initial treatment for patients with severe vasculitis should consist of CS together with CYC. In combined data from 215 patients treated across 4 different protocols, survival was found to be comparable for those who received CS or CS plus CYC. However, when these same patients were stratified according to FFS, those with a score of ≥2 had prolonged survival when treated with CYC. A tendency toward prolonged survival with CYC treatment was also observed for patients with a BVAS score of >30. Overall, the death rate reflected disease severity as assessed by both the FFS and the BVAS. No relationship was observed between disease severity and relapse. Treatment with CYC also did not appear to prevent relapses.

The use of daily versus intermittent CYC therapy in systemic vasculitis continues to be a topic of some controversy. For WG, findings of 3 prospective trials suggest an increased rate of disease relapse with intermittent administration of CYC (26–28). However, PAN may be pathophysiologically distinct from WG and thus could respond differently to intermittent CYC. In a randomized trial by the FVSG comparing intermittent with daily CYC in 25 patients with good-prognosis PAN or CSS (FFS = 0), no superiority of efficacy could be established between the 2 regimens (29). Haubitz et al also conducted a prospective trial in which 47 patients with either WG or MPA and renal involvement were randomized to receive either intermittent or daily CYC (30). No difference in patient survival, remission rate, time of remission, relapse rate, or outcome of renal function was observed between the 2 groups. While these results appear encouraging, both studies are of insufficient size to demonstrate equivalence.

Reduction of bladder cancer risk has been frequently cited as a rationale for favoring intermittent CYC, but to date there remains limited long-term experience with this administration schedule. Talar-Williams et al found that the mean time from the first daily CYC dose to the development of transitional cell carcinoma of the bladder was 9 years (31); the study population described by Gayraud and colleagues has not yet reached this point. While intermittent administration may lower the cumulative CYC dose, the benefit of a lowered cumulative dose is not clear. In the only trial in which a risk analysis has been performed, the total dose of CYC was not found to be an independent risk factor for the development of bladder cancer (31).

In the abstract of their paper, Gayraud et al conclude that the initial treatment intensity should reflect disease severity. While mortality was associated with disease severity, 15 patients taking CS alone died of uncontrolled disease, and only patients treated with CS had uncontrolled disease. These data suggest that caution should be used when deciding to treat a patient with CS alone and that this should be considered only in the absence of manifestations that could result in mortality or severe morbidity.

As discussed by the investigators in this and previous publications, clinical judgment is needed when assessing the presence of severe disease (11,32). Few people would dispute that the renal, GI, cardiac, and neurologic parameters contained within the FFS reflect severe disease in major organ sites. However, the FFS is not all-inclusive, and the presence of severe disease must be assessed in the context of the individual patient, particularly with regard to MPA. In the study on which the FFS was based, no patients had pulmonary hemorrhage; thus, the impact of this manifestation could not be tested (20). Pulmonary hemorrhage is potentially life-threatening, and current clinical experience supports the use of CS plus CYC in patients with this manifestation of small vessel vasculitis.

The FFS also does not address the possibility that certain manifestations, in particular glomerulonephritis, may require a cytotoxic agent to control disease. In 3 British studies of microscopic polyarteritis performed prior to the Chapel Hill Consensus Conference, combined therapy with CS and a cytotoxic agent appeared to improve outcome (33–35). Hogan et al found that the risk of death in patients with ANCA-associated MPA and necrotizing crescentic glomerulonephritis was 5.56 times lower in the CYC-treated patients than in those treated with CS alone (10). In WG, there is strong evidence that CS alone is insufficient to treat patients with glomerulonephritis (36,37). The only 2 regimens used to date that have effectively induced remission of active WG-related glomerulonephritis are prednisone in combination with either CYC or methotrexate (38–40). These data would suggest that a patient with an ANCA-associated necrotizing glomerulonephritis and few or no immune complexes should initially be treated with CS and a cytotoxic agent, even if the creatinine level is <1.58 mg/dl and proteinuria is <1 gm/day.

CSS presents unique problems in management, ones that are often related to the severity of reactive airways disease (23). In examining long-term outcome, Gayraud et al found that the survival curve for patients with CSS paralleled that of PAN and MPA. While there appear to be many instances in which the use of CS alone may effectively treat CSS, life-threatening manifestations can occur. The data reported by these investigators suggest that patients with manifestations of severe disease, particularly involving the heart, GI tract, CNS, or kidneys, should initially be treated with CYC combined with CS.

An important contribution of the article by Gayraud and colleagues lies in its outlook toward future studies. Despite advances in therapy, the overall mortality of people with certain vasculitic diseases is significantly higher than that of the general population, as demonstrated in this study. A plan to explore treatment strategies adapted to the type of vasculitis, its severity, and predicted outcome has much merit. In WG, there have been successful therapeutic approaches based on minimizing exposure to CYC through staged regimens (41) or, alternatively, the use of methotrexate and CS to induce remission in patients with less severe disease (40). To date, CYC remains the only cytotoxic agent for which there has been a published prospective experience in the treatment of PAN, MPA, or CSS. This collaborative group's planned investigation of other immunosuppressive agents as well as the specific indications for CYC remains of great importance. In the years to come, we will continue to follow their progress and await their findings with interest.

REFERENCES

1. Kussmaul A, Maier K. Ueber eine bisher nicht beschriebene eigenthumliche Arterienerkrankung (Periarteritis nodosa), die mit Morbus Brightii und rapid fortschreitender allgemeiner Muskellahmung einhergeht. Dtsch Arch Klin 1866;1:484–518.
2. Ferrari E. Ueber Polyarteritis acuta nodosa (sogenannte Periarteritis nodosa), und ihre Beziehungen zur Polymyositis und Polyneuritis acuta. Beitr Pathol Anat 1903;34:350–86.
3. Gayraud M, Guillevin L, Toumelin PL, Cohen P, Lhote F, Casassus P, et al. Long-term followup of polyarteritis nodosa, microscopic polyangiitis, and Churg-Strauss syndrome: analysis of four prospective trials including 278 patients. Arthritis Rheum 2001;44:668–77.

4. Wohlwill F. Über die nur mikroskopisch erkennbare Form der Periarteritis nodosa. Virchows Arch 1923;246:377–411.
5. Davson J, Ball J, Platt R. The kidney in periarteritis nodosa. QJM 1948;17:175–202.
6. Jennette JC, Falk RJ, Andrassy K, Bacon PA, Churg J, Gross WL, et al. Nomenclature of systemic vasculitides: proposal of an international consensus conference. Arthritis Rheum 1994;37:187–92.
7. Jennette JC, Falk RJ. The pathology of vasculitis involving the kidney. Am J Kidney Dis 1994;24:130–41.
8. Devaney KO, Travis WD, Hoffman GS, Leavitt RY, Lebovics R, Fauci AS. Interpretation of head and neck biopsies in Wegener's granulomatosis: a pathologic study of 126 biopsies in 70 patients. Am J Surg Pathol 1990;14:555–64.
9. Travis WD, Colby TV, Lombard C, Carpenter HA. A clinicopathologic study of 34 cases of diffuse pulmonary hemorrhage with lung biopsy confirmation. Am J Surg Pathol 1990;15:315–33.
10. Hogan SL, Nachman PH, Wilkman AS, Jennette JC, Falk RJ. Prognostic markers in patients with antineutrophil cytoplasmic autoantibody-associated microscopic polyangiitis and glomerulonephritis. J Am Soc Nephrol 1996;7:23–32.
11. Guillevin L, Durand-Gasselin B, Cevallos R, Gayraud M, Lhote F, Callard P, et al. Microscopic polyangiitis: clinical and laboratory findings in eighty-five patients. Arthritis Rheum 1999;42:421–30.
12. Bosch X. Microscopic polyangiitis (microscopic polyarteritis) with late emergence of generalised Wegener's granulomatosis. Ann Rheum Dis 1999;58:644–7.
13. Frohnert PP, Sheps SG. Long-term follow-up study of periarteritis nodosa. Am J Med 1967;43:8–14.
14. Leib ES, Restino C, Paulus HE. Immunosuppressive and corticosteroid therapy of polyarteritis nodosa. Am J Med 1979;67:941–7.
15. Cohen RD, Conn DL, Illstrup DM. Clinical features, prognosis and response to treatment in polyarteritis. Mayo Clin Proc 1980; 55:146–55.
16. Sack M, Cassidy JT, Bole GG. Prognostic factors in polyarteritis. J Rheumatol 1975;2:411–20.
17. Fauci AS, Katz P, Haynes BF, Wolff SM. Cyclophosphamide therapy of severe systemic necrotizing vasculitis. N Engl J Med 1979;301:235–8.
18. Fauci AS, Doppman JL, Wolff SM. Cyclophosphamide-induced remissions in advanced polyarteritis nodosa. Am J Med 1978;64: 890–4.
19. Guillevin L, Jarrousse B, Lok C, Lhote F, Jais JP, Le Thi Huong Du D, et al, and the Cooperative Study Group for Polyarteritis Nodosa. Longterm followup after treatment of polyarteritis nodosa and Churg-Strauss angiitis with comparison of steroids, plasma exchange and cyclophosphamide to steroids and plasma exchange: a prospective randomized trial of 71 patients. J Rheumatol 1991;18:567–74.
20. Guillevin L, Lhote F, Gayraud M, Cohen P, Jarrousse B, Lortholary O, et al. Prognostic factors in polyarteritis nodosa and Churg-Strauss syndrome: a prospective study in 342 patients. Medicine (Baltimore) 1996;75:17–28.
21. Guillevin L, Lhote F, Cohen P, Sauvaget F, Jarrousse B, Lortholary O, et al. Polyarteritis nodosa related to hepatitis B virus: a prospective study with long-term observation of 41 patients. Medicine (Baltimore) 1995;74:238–53.
22. Lanham JG, Elkon KB, Pusey CD, Hughes GR. Systemic vasculitis with asthma and eosinophilia: a clinical approach to Churg-Strauss syndrome. Medicine (Baltimore) 1984;63:65–81.
23. Guillevin L, Cohen P, Gayraud M, Lhote F, Jarrousse B, Casassus P. Churg-Strauss syndrome: clinical study and long-term follow-up of 96 patients. Medicine (Baltimore) 1999;78:26–37.
24. Watts RA, Jolliffe VA, Carruthers DM, Lockwood M, Scott DGI. Effect of classification on the incidence of polyarteritis nodosa and microscopic polyangiitis. Arthritis Rheum 1996;39:1208–12.
25. Guillevin L, Lhote F, Jarrousse B, Fain O. Treatment of polyarteritis nodosa and Churg-Strauss syndrome: a meta-analysis of 3 prospective controlled trials including 182 patients over 12 years. Ann Med Interne (Paris) 1992;143:405–16.
26. Hoffman GS, Leavitt RY, Fleisher TA, Minor JR, Fauci AS. Treatment of Wegener's granulomatosis with intermittent high-dose intravenous cyclophosphamide. Am J Med 1990;89:403–10.
27. Reinhold-Keller E, Kekow J, Schnabel A, Schmitt WH, Heller M, Beigel A, et al. Influence of disease manifestation and antineutrophil cytoplasmic antibody titer on the response to pulse cyclophosphamide therapy in patients with Wegener's granulomatosis. Arthritis Rheum 1994;37:919–24.
28. Guillevin L, Cordier J-F, Lhote F, Cohen P, Jarrousse B, Royer I, et al. A prospective, multicenter, randomized trial comparing steroids and pulse cyclophosphamide versus steroids and oral cyclophosphamide in the treatment of generalized Wegener's granulomatosis. Arthritis Rheum 1997;40:2187–98.
29. Gayraud M, Guillevin L, Cohen P, Lhote F, Cacoub P, Deblois P, et al. Treatment of good-prognosis polyarteritis nodosa and Churg-Strauss syndrome: comparison of steroids and oral or pulse cyclophosphamide in 25 patients. Br J Rheumatol 1997;36:1290–7.
30. Haubitz M, Schellong S, Göbel U, Schurek HJ, Schaumann D, Koch KM, et al. Intravenous pulse administration of cyclophosphamide versus daily oral treatment in patients with antineutrophil cytoplasmic antibody–associated vasculitis and renal involvement: a prospective, randomized study. Arthritis Rheum 1998;41:1835–44.
31. Talar-Williams C, Hijazi YM, Walther MM, Linehan WM, Hallahan CW, Lubensky I, et al. Cyclophosphamide-induced cystitis and bladder cancer in patients with Wegener granulomatosis. Ann Intern Med 1996;124:477–84.
32. Guillevin L, Lhote F. Treatment of polyarteritis nodosa and microscopic polyangiitis. Arthritis Rheum 1998;41:2100–5.
33. Adu D, Howie AJ, Scott DG, Bacon PA, McGonigle RJ, Michael J. Polyarteritis and the kidney. QJM 1987;62:221–37.
34. Rodgers H, Guthrie JA, Brownjohn AM, Turney JH. Microscopic polyarteritis: clinical features and treatment. Postgrad Med J 1989;65:515–8.
35. Savage CO, Winearls CG, Evans DJ, Rees AJ, Lockwood CM. Microscopic polyarteritis: presentation, pathology and prognosis. QJM 1985;56:467–83.
36. Hollander D, Manning RT. The use of alkylating agents in the treatment of Wegener's granulomatosis. Ann Intern Med 1967;67: 393–8.
37. Hoffman GS. Wegener's granulomatosis. Curr Opin Rheumatol 1993;5:11–7.
38. Fauci A, Haynes B, Katz P, Wolff S. Wegener's granulomatosis: prospective clinical and therapeutic experience with 85 patients for 21 years. Ann Intern Med 1983;98:76–85.
39. Hoffman GS, Kerr GS, Leavitt RY, Hallahan CW, Lebovics RS, Travis WD, et al. Wegener granulomatosis: an analysis of 158 patients. Ann Intern Med 1992;116:488–94.
40. Sneller MC, Hoffman GS, Talar-Williams C, Kerr GS, Hallahan CW, Fauci AS. An analysis of forty-two Wegener's granulomatosis patients treated with methotrexate and prednisone. Arthritis Rheum 1995;38:608–13.
41. Langford CA, Talar-Williams C, Barron KS, Sneller MC. A staged approach to the treatment of Wegener's granulomatosis: induction of remission with glucocorticoids and daily cyclophosphamide switching to methotrexate for remission maintenance. Arthritis Rheum 1999;42:2666–73.
42. Specks U. Pulmonary vasculitis. In: Schwarz MI, King TE, editors. Interstitial lung disease. 3rd ed. Hamilton (Ontario): BC Decker; 1998. p. 507–34.
43. Jennette JC, Falk RJ. Small-vessel vasculitis. N Engl J Med 1997;337:1512–23.
44. Lhote F, Guillevin L. Polyarteritis nodosa, microscopic polyangiitis, and Churg-Strauss syndrome: clinical aspects and treatment. Rheum Dis Clin North Am 1995;21:911–47.

Evoxac™ (ˈē vō zak)
(cevimeline HCl) 30 mg Capsules

EVOXAC™ Capsules
(cevimeline hydrochloride)

Brief Summary
Consult package insert for full prescribing information.

INDICATIONS AND USAGE: Cevimeline is indicated for the treatment of symptoms of dry mouth in patients with Sjögren's Syndrome.

CONTRAINDICATIONS: Cevimeline is contraindicated in patients with uncontrolled asthma, known hypersensitivity to cevimeline, and when miosis is undesirable, e.g., in acute iritis and in narrow-angle (angle-closure) glaucoma.

WARNINGS:
Cardiovascular Disease: Cevimeline can potentially alter cardiac conduction and/or heart rate. Patients with significant cardiovascular disease may potentially be unable to compensate for transient changes in hemodynamics or rhythm induced by EVOXAC™. EVOXAC™ should be used with caution and under close medical supervision in patients with a history of cardiovascular disease evidenced by angina pectoris or myocardial infarction.

Pulmonary Disease: Cevimeline can potentially increase airway resistance, bronchial smooth muscle tone, and bronchial secretions. Cevimeline should be administered with caution and with close medical supervision to patients with controlled asthma, chronic bronchitis, or chronic obstructive pulmonary disease.

Ocular: Ophthalmic formulations of muscarinic agonists have been reported to cause visual blurring which may result in decreased visual acuity, especially at night and in patients with central lens changes, and to cause impairment of depth perception. Caution should be advised while driving at night or performing hazardous activities in reduced lighting.

PRECAUTIONS:
General: Cevimeline toxicity is characterized by an exaggeration of its parasympathomimetic effects. These may include: headache, visual disturbance, lacrimation, sweating, respiratory distress, gastrointestinal spasm, nausea, vomiting, diarrhea, atrioventricular block, tachycardia, bradycardia, hypotension, hypertension, shock, mental confusion, cardiac arrhythmia, and tremors.

Cevimeline should be administered with caution to patients with a history of nephrolithiasis or cholelithiasis. Contractions of the gallbladder or biliary smooth muscle could precipitate complications such as cholecystitis, cholangitis and biliary obstruction. An increase in the ureteral smooth muscle tone could theoretically precipitate renal colic or ureteral reflux in patients with nephrolithiasis.

Information for Patients: Patients should be informed that cevimeline may cause visual disturbances, especially at night, that could impair their ability to drive safely.

If a patient sweats excessively while taking cevimeline, dehydration may develop. The patient should drink extra water and consult a health care provider.

Drug Interactions: Cevimeline should be administered with caution to patients taking beta adrenergic antagonists, because of the possibility of conduction disturbances. Drugs with parasympathomimetic effects administered concurrently with cevimeline can be expected to have additive effects. Cevimeline might interfere with desirable antimuscarinic effects of drugs used concomitantly.

Drugs which inhibit CYP2D6 and CYP3A3/4 also inhibit the metabolism of cevimeline. Cevimeline should be used with caution in individuals known or suspected to be deficient in CYP2D6 activity, based on previous experience, as they may be at a higher risk of adverse events. In an *in vitro* study, cytochrome P450 isozymes 1A2, 2A6, 2C9, 2C19, 2D6, 2E1, and 3A4 were not inhibited by exposure to cevimeline.

Carcinogenesis, Mutagenesis and Impairment of Fertility: Lifetime carcinogenicity studies were conducted in CD-1 mice and F-344 rats. A statistically significant increase in the incidence of adenocarcinomas of the uterus was observed in female rats that received cevimeline at a dosage of 100 mg/kg/day (approximately 8 times the maximum human exposure based on comparison of AUC data). No other significant differences in tumor incidence were observed in either mice or rats.

Cevimeline exhibited no evidence of mutagenicity or clastogenicity in a battery of assays that included an Ames test, an *in vitro* chromosomal aberration study in mammalian cells, a mouse lymphoma study in L5178Y cells, or a micronucleus assay conducted *in vivo* in ICR mice.

Cevimeline did not adversely affect the reproductive performance or fertility of male Sprague-Dawley rats when administered for 63 days prior to mating and throughout the period of mating at dosages up to 45 mg/kg/day (approximately 5 times the maximum recommended dose for a 60 kg human following normalization of the data on the basis of body surface area estimates). Females that were treated with cevimeline at dosages up to 45 mg/kg/day from 14 days prior to mating through day seven of gestation exhibited a statistically significantly smaller number of implantations than did control animals.

Pregnancy: Pregnancy Category C.

Cevimeline was associated with a reduction in the mean number of implantations when given to pregnant Sprague-Dawley rats from 14 days prior to mating through day seven of gestation at a dosage of 45 mg/kg/day (approximately 5 times the maximum recommended dose for a 60 kg human when compared on the basis of body surface area estimates). This effect may have been secondary to maternal toxicity. There are no adequate and well-controlled studies in pregnant women. Cevimeline should be used during pregnancy only if the potential benefit justifies the potential risk to the fetus.

Nursing Mothers: It is not known whether this drug is secreted in human milk. Because many drugs are excreted in human milk, and because of the potential for serious adverse reactions in nursing infants from EVOXAC™, a decision should be made whether to discontinue nursing or discontinue the drug, taking into account the importance of the drug to the mother.

Pediatric Use: Safety and effectiveness in pediatric patients have not been established.

Geriatric Use: Although clinical studies of cevimeline included subjects over the age of 65, the numbers were not sufficient to determine whether they respond differently from younger subjects. Special care should be exercised when cevimeline treatment is initiated in an elderly patient, considering the greater frequency of decreased hepatic, renal, or cardiac function, and of concomitant disease or other drug therapy in the elderly.

ADVERSE REACTIONS: Cevimeline was administered to 1777 patients during clinical trials worldwide, including Sjögren's patients and patients with other conditions. In placebo-controlled Sjögren's studies in the U.S., 320 patients received cevimeline doses ranging from 15 mg tid to 60 mg tid, of whom 93% were women and 7% were men. Demographic distribution was 90% Caucasian, 5% Hispanic, 3% Black, and 2% of other origin. In these studies, 14.6% of patients discontinued treatment with cevimeline due to adverse events.

The following adverse events associated with muscarinic agonism were observed in the clinical trials of cevimeline in Sjögren's syndrome patients:

Adverse Event	Cevimeline 30 mg (tid) n* = 533	Placebo (tid) n = 164	Adverse Event	Cevimeline 30 mg (tid) n* = 533	Placebo (tid) n = 164
Excessive Sweating	18.7%	2.4%	Urinary Frequency	0.9%	1.8%
Nausea	13.8%	7.9%	Asthenia	0.5%	0.0%
Rhinitis	11.2%	5.4%	Flushing	0.3%	0.6%
Diarrhea	10.3%	10.3%	Polyuria	0.1%	0.6%
Excessive Salivation	2.2%	0.6%			

*n is the total number of patients exposed to the dose at any time during the study

EVOXAC™ Capsules
(cevimeline hydrochloride)

In addition, the following adverse events (≥3% incidence) were reported in the Sjögren's clinical trials:

Adverse Event	Cevimeline 30 mg (tid) n* = 533	Placebo (tid) n = 164	Adverse Event	Cevimeline 30 mg (tid) n* = 533	Placebo (tid) n = 164
Headache	14.4%	20.1%	Conjunctivitis	4.3%	3.6%
Sinusitis	12.3%	10.9%	Dizziness	4.1%	7.3%
Upper Respiratory Tract Infection	11.4%	9.1%	Bronchitis	4.1%	1.2%
Dyspepsia	7.8%	8.5%	Arthralgia	3.7%	1.8%
Abdominal Pain	7.6%	6.7%	Surgical Intervention	3.3%	3.0%
Urinary Tract Infection	6.1%	3.0%	Fatigue	3.3%	1.2%
Coughing	6.1%	3.0%	Pain	3.3%	3.0%
Pharyngitis	5.2%	5.4%	Skeletal Pain	2.8%	1.8%
Vomiting	4.6%	2.4%	Insomnia	2.4%	1.2%
Injury	4.5%	2.4%	Hot Flushes	2.4%	0.0%
Back Pain	4.5%	4.2%	Rigors	1.3%	1.2%
Rash	4.3%	6.0%	Anxiety	1.3%	1.2%

*n is the total number of patients exposed to the dose at any time during the study

The following events were reported in Sjögren's patients at incidences of <3% and ≥1%: constipation, tremor, abnormal vision, hypertonia, peripheral edema, chest pain, myalgia, fever, anorexia, eye pain, earache, dry mouth, vertigo, salivary gland pain, pruritus, influenza-like symptoms, eye infection, post-operative pain, vaginitis, skin disorder, depression, hiccup, hyporeflexia, infection, fungal infection, sialoadenitis, otitis media, erythematous rash, pneumonia, edema, salivary gland enlargement, allergy, gastroesophageal reflux, eye abnormality, migraine, tooth disorder, epistaxis, flatulence, toothache, ulcerative stomatitis, anemia, hypoesthesia, cystitis, leg cramps, abscess, eructation, moniliasis, palpitation, increased amylase, xerophthalmia, allergic reaction.

The following events were reported rarely in treated Sjögren's patients (<1%): Causal relation is unknown:

Body as a Whole Disorders: aggravated allergy, precordial chest pain, abnormal crying, hematoma, leg pain, edema, periorbital edema, activated pain trauma, pallor, changed sensation to temperature, weight decrease, weight increase, choking, mouth edema, syncope, malaise, face edema, substernal chest pain

Cardiovascular Disorders: abnormal ECG, heart disorder, heart murmur, aggravated hypertension, hypotension, arrhythmia, extrasystoles, t wave inversion, tachycardia, supraventricular tachycardia, angina pectoris, myocardial infarction, pericarditis, pulmonary embolism, peripheral ischemia, superficial phlebitis, purpura, deep thrombophlebitis, vascular disorder, vasculitis, hypertension

Digestive Disorders: appendicitis, increased appetite, ulcerative colitis, diverticulitis, duodenitis, dysphagia, enterocolitis, gastric ulcer, gastritis, gastroenteritis, gastrointestinal hemorrhage, gingivitis, glossitis, rectum hemorrhage, hemorrhoids, ileus, irritable bowel syndrome, melena, mucositis, esophageal stricture, esophagitis, oral hemorrhage, peptic ulcer, periodontal destruction, rectal disorder, stomatitis, tenesmus, tongue discoloration, tongue disorder, geographic tongue, tongue ulceration, dental caries

Endocrine Disorders: increased glucocorticoids, goiter, hypothyroidism

Hematologic Disorders: thrombocytopenic purpura, thrombocythemia, thrombocytopenia, hypochromic anemia, eosinophilia, granulocytopenia, leucopenia, leukocytosis, cervical lymphadenopathy, lymphadenopathy

Liver and Biliary System Disorders: cholelithiasis, increased gamma-glutamyl transferase, increased hepatic enzymes, abnormal hepatic function, viral hepatitis, increased serum glutamate oxaloacetic transaminase (SGOT)(also called AST-aspartate aminotransferase), increased serum glutamate pyruvate transaminase (SGPT)(also called ALT-alanine aminotransferase)

Metabolic and Nutritional Disorders: dehydration, diabetes mellitus, hypercalcemia, hypercholesterolemia, hyperglycemia, hyperlipemia, hypertriglyceridemia, hyperuricemia, hypoglycemia, hypokalemia, hyponatremia, thirst

Musculoskeletal Disorders: arthritis, aggravated arthritis, arthropathy, femoral head avascular necrosis, bone disorder, bursitis, costochondritis, plantar fasciitis, muscle weakness, osteomyelitis, osteoporosis, synovitis, tendinitis, tenosynovitis

Neoplasms: basal cell carcinoma, squamous carcinoma

Nervous Disorders: carpal tunnel syndrome, coma, abnormal coordination, dysesthesia, dyskinesia, dysphonia, aggravated multiple sclerosis, involuntary muscle contractions, neuralgia, neuropathy, paresthesia, speech disorder, agitation, confusion, depersonalization, aggravated depression, abnormal dreaming, emotional lability, manic reaction, paroniria, somnolence, abnormal thinking, hyperkinesia, hallucination

Miscellaneous Disorders: fall, food poisoning, heat stroke, joint dislocation, post-operative hemorrhage

Resistance Mechanism Disorders: cellulitis, herpes simplex, herpes zoster, bacterial infection, viral infection, genital moniliasis, sepsis

Respiratory Disorders: asthma, bronchospasm, chronic obstructive airway disease, dyspnea, hemoptysis, laryngitis, nasal ulcer, pleural effusion, pleurisy, pulmonary congestion, pulmonary fibrosis, respiratory disorder

Rheumatologic Disorders: aggravated rheumatoid arthritis, lupus erythematosus rash, lupus erythematosus syndrome

Skin and Appendages Disorders: acne, alopecia, burn, dermatitis, contact dermatitis, lichenoid dermatitis, eczema, furunculosis, hyperkeratosis, lichen planus, nail discoloration, nail disorder, onychia, onychomycosis, paronychia, photosensitivity reaction, rosacea, scleroderma, seborrhea, skin discoloration, dry skin, skin exfoliation, skin hypertrophy, skin ulceration, urticaria, verruca, bullous eruption, cold clammy skin

Special Senses Disorders: deafness, decreased hearing, motion sickness, parosmia, taste perversion, blepharitis, cataract, corneal opacity, corneal ulceration, diplopia, glaucoma, anterior chamber eye hemorrhage, keratitis, keratoconjunctivitis, mydriasis, myopia, photopsia, retinal deposits, retinal disorder, scleritis, vitreous detachment, tinnitus

Urogenital Disorders: epididymitis, prostatic disorder, abnormal sexual function, amenorrhea, female breast neoplasm, malignant female breast neoplasm, female breast pain, positive cervical smear test, dysmenorrhea, endometrial disorder, intermenstrual bleeding, leukorrhea, menorrhagia, menstrual disorder, ovarian cyst, ovarian disorder, genital pruritus, uterine hemorrhage, vaginal hemorrhage, atrophic vaginitis, albuminuria, bladder discomfort, increased blood urea nitrogen, dysuria, hematuria, micturition disorder, nephrosis, nocturia, increased nonprotein nitrogen, pyelonephritis, renal calculus, abnormal renal function, renal pain, strangury, urethral disorder, abnormal urine, urinary incontinence, decreased urine flow, pyuria

In one subject with lupus erythematosus receiving concomitant multiple drug therapy, a highly elevated ALT level was noted after the fourth week of cevimeline therapy. In two other subjects receiving cevimeline in the clinical trials, very high AST levels were noted. The significance of these findings is unknown.

Additional adverse events (relationship unknown) which occurred in other clinical studies (patient population different from Sjögren's patients) are as follows:

cholinergic syndrome, blood pressure fluctuation, cardiomegaly, postural hypotension, aphasia, convulsions, abnormal gait, hyperesthesia, paralysis, abnormal sexual function, enlarged abdomen, change in bowel habits, gum hyperplasia, intestinal obstruction, bundle branch block, increased creatine phosphokinase, electrolyte abnormality, glycosuria, gout, hyperkalemia, hyperproteinemia, increased lactic dehydrogenase (LDH), increased alkaline phosphatase, failure to thrive, abnormal platelets, aggressive reaction, amnesia, apathy, delirium, delusion, dementia, illusion, impotence, neurosis, paranoid reaction, personality disorder, hyperhemoglobinemia, apnea, atelectasis, yawning, oliguria, urinary retention, distended vein, lymphocytosis

MANAGEMENT OF OVERDOSE: Management of the signs and symptoms of acute overdosage should be handled in a manner consistent with that indicated for other muscarinic agonists: general supportive measures should be instituted. If medically indicated, atropine, an anti-cholinergic agent may be of value as an antidote for emergency use in patients who have had an overdose of cevimeline. If medically indicated, epinephrine may also be of value in the presence of severe cardiovascular depression or bronchoconstriction. It is not known if cevimeline is dialyzable.

DOSAGE AND ADMINISTRATION: The recommended dose of cevimeline is 30 mg taken three times a day. There is insufficient safety information to support doses greater than 30 mg tid. There is also insufficient evidence for additional efficacy of cevimeline at doses greater than 30 mg tid.

Rx Only

Manufactured by:
YAMANOUCHI PHARMA TECHNOLOGIES, INC., Palo Alto, CA 94304

for:
SnowBrand Pharmaceuticals, Inc., Rockville, MD 20850

Distributed and Marketed by:
Daiichi Pharmaceutical Corporation, Montvale, NJ 07645

02/2000 Printed in U.S.A.

Reference: 1. Data on file, Daiichi Pharmaceutical Corporation.

ARTHRITIS & RHEUMATISM
Vol. 44, No. 3, March 2001, pp 513–514

Winners of the 2000 American College of Rheumatology Slide Competition

Catherine M. Meyer and the ACR Audiovisual Aids Subcommittee

The members of the Audiovisual Aids Subcommittee of the American College of Rheumatology (ACR) have selected 7 slides as winners of the 2000 Slide Competition (Figures 1–7). The slides were chosen from a large number of submissions from our members worldwide. They include a computed tomography scan illustrating sacroiliitis; a magnetic resonance image of the chest in a patient with Takayasu's arteritis; photomicrographs illustrating renal pathology in Goodpasture's syndrome; abnormalities in the gallbladder of a patient with Churg-Strauss syndrome; and a slide showing profound clubbing of the fingers in hypertrophic osteoarthropathy. There are also two pediatric slides: one showing linear scleroderma in the arm of a child, and the other, which is a composite photograph, showing anterior and posterior views of a child with osteogenesis imperfecta.

These slides, along with several other of this year's submissions, will be added to the Clinical Slide Collection on the Rheumatic Diseases itself, or to the Slide Archive. The Archive was created 1 year ago as a repository for high-quality images of conditions already covered in the Clinical Slide Collection or illustrating unusual rheumatologic manifestations. We are currently digitizing our collections. We will continue to produce the hard-copy collection but will also eventually publish a larger collection of slides in CD-ROM and electronic formats. Also in the future, we plan to produce an imaging/radiology supplement and to make physical examination and arthrocentesis resources available on the ACR Web site.

We congratulate this year's winners and thank them and all others who submitted slides this year. We encourage you to continue to send high-quality slides that might enhance our teaching collections. If you have slides to submit for consideration, please send them to Catherine Meyer, MD, Chair, ACR Audiovisual Aids Subcommittee, Mercy Hospital and Medical Center, 2525 S. Michigan Avenue, Chicago, IL 60616.

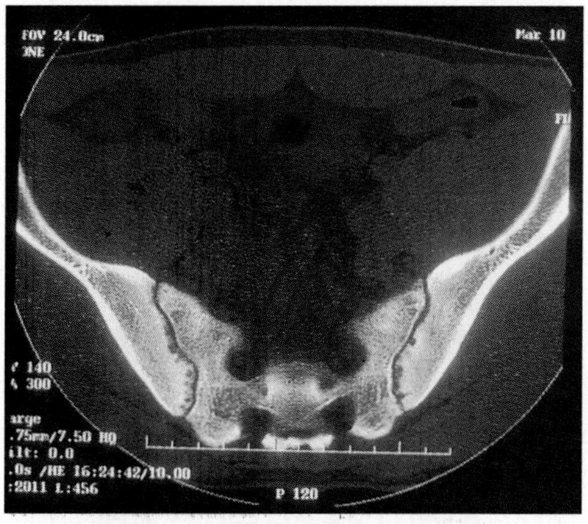

Figure 1. Sacroiliitis (CT scan). This computed tomography scan shows bilateral sacroiliitis with multiple erosions and a "string of pearls" appearance. Submitted by S. Louis Bridges, MD, PhD, Birmingham, AL.

Members of the Audiovisual Aids Subcommittee of the American College of Rheumatology Committee on Educational Products: Catherine M. Meyer, MD (Chair), Chicago, Illinois; Dennis W. Boulware, MD, Birmingham, Alabama; Eric L. Matteson, MD, Rochester, Minnesota; Marc L. Miller, MD, Portland, Maine; Thomas A. Pressly, MD, Shreveport, Louisiana.

Submitted for publication November 15, 2000; accepted December 7, 2000.

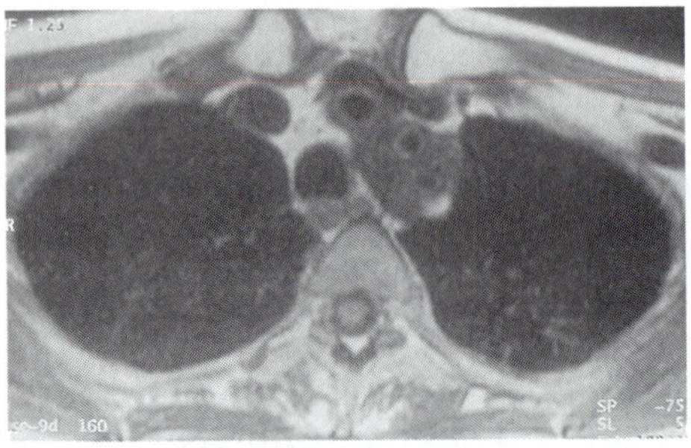

Figure 2. Takayasu's arteritis: chest (MRI). This MRI of the chest of a patient with Takayasu's arteritis shows a soft tissue infiltrate encasing the origins of the left subclavian and left common carotid arteries. This soft tissue infiltrate represents an inflammatory perivascular reaction. Serial scans can demonstrate regression of the infiltrate with successful treatment. Submitted by Lachy McLean, MD, PhD, MRCP, FRACP, Auckland, New Zealand.

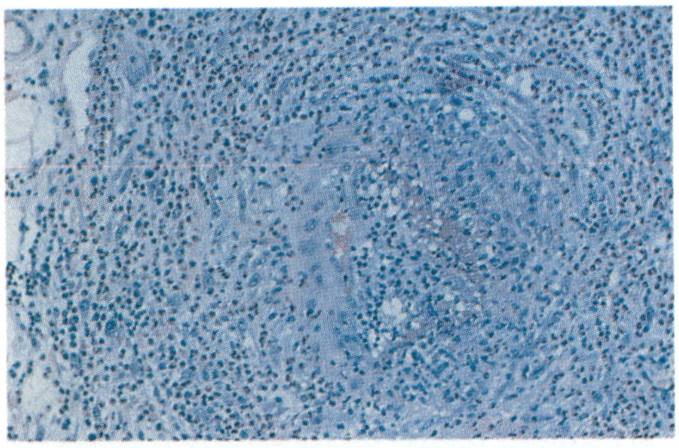

Figure 4. Churg-Strauss syndrome: gallbladder (photomicrograph). Inflammation is present in an artery in the gallbladder serosa. Also seen are subendothelial fibrin accumulation and transmural non-necrotizing and granulomatous inflammation with perivascular eosinophils (hematoxylin and eosin, medium power). Submitted by Johannes Björnsson, MD, Rochester, MN.

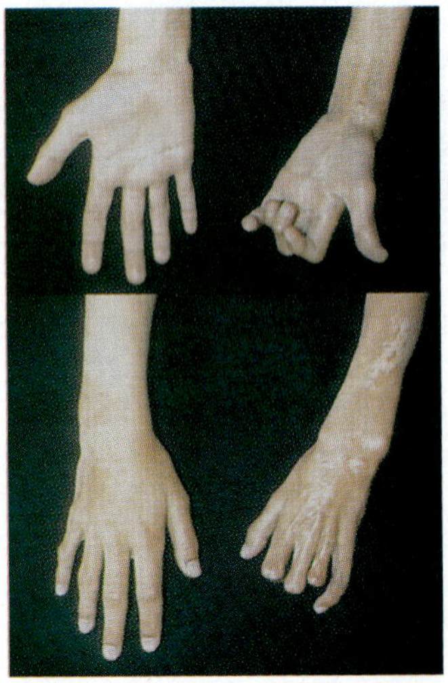

Figure 6. Linear scleroderma: arm. Linear scleroderma of the left hand and forearm is seen in this 11-year-old girl. Hypopigmentation and tightening of the skin, diffuse atrophy, and soft tissue contractures are evident. Submitted by José A. Melo Gomes, MD, Lisbon, Portugal.

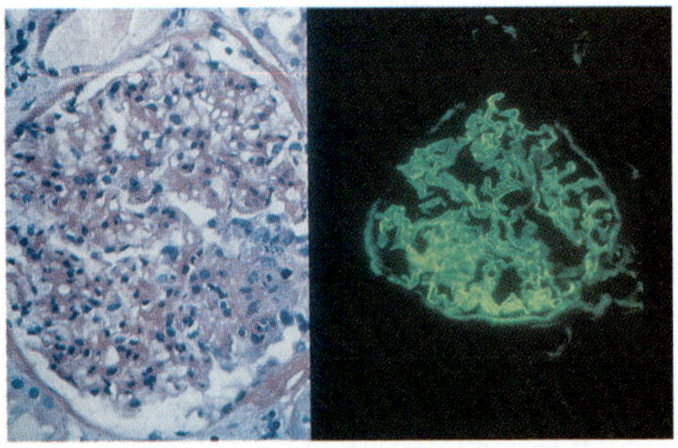

Figure 3. Goodpasture's syndrome: kidney (photomicrographs). Left, Glomerulus with diffuse mesangial inflammation and segmental necrosis. No crescents are seen (hematoxylin and eosin, medium power). Right, Immunofluorescence demonstrates linear staining of the glomerular basement membrane, typical of Goodpasture's syndrome. Submitted by Dana Kageyama, MD, and Michael Maricic, MD, Tucson, AZ.

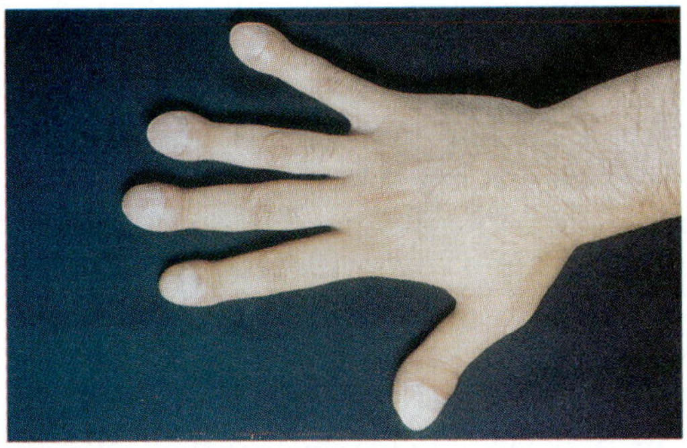

Figure 5. Hypertrophic osteoarthropathy: clubbing. Severe clubbing of the fingers and marked periostitis with overlying soft tissue swelling at the wrist are seen in this 27-year-old man. The condition had progressed over a 15-year period. There was no evidence of an underlying malignancy or cardiac or pulmonary disease. Submitted by Eric Matteson, MD, Rochester, MN.

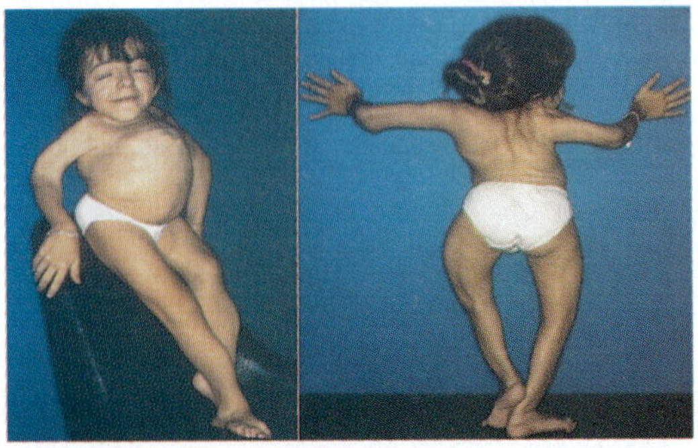

Figure 7. Osteogenesis imperfecta. This 13-year-old girl with type III osteogenesis imperfecta has severe chest and limb deformities due to multiple fractures. Submitted by José A. Melo Gomes, MD, Lisbon, Portugal.

ARTHRITIS & RHEUMATISM
Vol. 44, No. 3, March 2001, pp 515–522

A Randomized Two-Year Study of the Effects of Dynamic Strength Training on Muscle Strength, Disease Activity, Functional Capacity, and Bone Mineral Density in Early Rheumatoid Arthritis

Arja Häkkinen,[1] Tuulikki Sokka,[1] Antero Kotaniemi,[2] and Pekka Hannonen[1]

Objective. **To evaluate the impact of a 2-year program of strength training on muscle strength, bone mineral density (BMD), physical function, joint damage, and disease activity in patients with recent-onset (<2 years) rheumatoid arthritis (RA).**

Methods. **In this prospective trial, 70 RA patients were randomly assigned to perform either strength training (all major muscle groups of the lower and upper extremities and trunk, with loads of 50–70% of repetition maximum) or range of motion exercises (without resistance) twice a week; all were encouraged to engage in recreational activities 2–3 times a week. All patients completed training diaries (evaluated bimonthly) and were examined at 6-month intervals. All were treated with medications to achieve disease remission. Maximum strength of the knee extensors, trunk flexors and extensors, and grip strength was measured with dynamometers. BMD was measured at the femoral neck and lumbar spine by dual x-ray densitometry. Disease activity was determined by the Disease Activity Score, the extent of joint damage by the Larsen score, and functional capacity by the Health Assessment Questionnaire (HAQ); walking speed was also measured.**

Results. **Sixty-two patients (31 per group) completed the study. Strength training compliance averaged 1.4–1.5 times/week. The maximum strength of all muscle groups examined increased significantly (19–59%) in the strength-training group, with statistically significant improvements in clinical disease activity parameters, HAQ scores, and walking speed. While muscle strength, disease activity parameters, and physical function also improved significantly in the control group, the changes were not as great as those in the strength-training group. BMD in the femoral neck and spine increased by a mean ± SD of 0.51 ± 1.64% and by 1.17 ± 5.34%, respectively, in the strength-training group, but decreased by 0.70 ± 2.25% and 0.91 ± 4.07% in the controls. Femoral neck BMD in the 17 patients with high initial disease activity (and subsequent use of oral glucocorticoids) remained constantly at a statistically significantly lower level than that in the other 45 patients.**

Conclusion. **Regular dynamic strength training combined with endurance-type physical activities improves muscle strength and physical function, but not BMD, in patients with early RA, without detrimental effects on disease activity.**

Supported by grants from Central Finland Health Care District and from the Yrjö Jahnsson Foundation, Finland.

[1]Arja Häkkinen, PhD, Tuulikki Sokka, MD, PhD, Pekka Hannonen, MD, PhD: Central Finland Health Care District, Jyväskylä, Finland; [2]Antero Kotaniemi, MD, PhD: Rheumatism Foundation Hospital, Heinola, Finland.

Address correspondence and reprint requests to Arja Häkkinen, PhD, Department of Physical Medicine and Rehabilitation, Central Hospital, Keskussairaalantie 19, FIN-40620 Jyväskylä, Finland.

Submitted for publication June 21, 2000; accepted in revised form November 9, 2000.

Persistent synovitis with joint swelling and limited joint mobility in rheumatoid arthritis (RA) patients may result in the stretching of tendons, ligaments, and joint capsules, with subsequent joint instability and decreases in muscle mass and strength. Furthermore, joint effusions directly inhibit contraction of the surrounding muscle groups, and if a muscle contracts while the joint is malaligned, it will not be able to generate its peak contractile force. Moreover, the compromises in biomechanical integrity of the joint and its surrounding tissues result in pain, altered loading response, and patterns of motion that are often energy insufficient and further limit the patient's physical activities (1).

With regard to osseous tissues, the disease duration (2–5), physical inactivity, impaired function (5–7), and the inflammatory process itself contribute to bone loss in diseases such as RA. The concomitant use of corticosteroids further enhances the development of both muscle atrophy and decrease in bone mineral density (BMD) (1,8,9). The vicious circle that results in losses of muscle strength, BMD, and functional capacity in RA is finally catalyzed by the generalized fatigue that is associated with inflammation, resulting in further limitations in physical activity.

Thus, the loss of muscle strength and functional capacity (6,10–12) as well as the accelerated bone loss (13) may develop early in the course of RA. Various clinical trials examining the effects of exercise training programs on BMD in healthy subjects have been described (14). Some studies show that exercise does not lead to maintenance or improvement in BMD (15,16), while others report positive results (17–19). The earlier studies indicate that the important osteogenic exercise stimulus is high strain rates and high peak forces in versatile movements. Moreover, the number of loading cycles probably increases in significance if the repetitive loading magnitude is low on the loaded side (20). Exercise is reportedly an important tool for reducing pain, stiffness, and joint tenderness in RA patients (21–23). Nevertheless, although physical activity is also of central importance in maintaining or increasing muscle strength in patients with RA, long-term studies regarding the effects of strength training on muscle performance (24,25) and BMD (23,24) are few. There is a definite need for additional longitudinal studies to determine the adaptation of the muscles and bones to various types of exercise training in patients with RA.

Therefore, the purpose of the present study was to investigate whether the 24-month strength training program used to increase muscle strength and physical function in patients with early RA also produces positive effects on BMD in these patients.

PATIENTS AND METHODS

Subjects. Seventy patients with recent-onset RA according to the 1987 criteria of the American College of Rheumatology (formerly, the American Rheumatism Association) (26) volunteered to participate in the 24-month study. Patients had been referred to the rheumatology unit at Jyväskylä Central Hospital for diagnosis and therapy. None of the patients had taken glucocorticoids or disease-modifying antirheumatic drugs (DMARDs) previously. The patients were randomly assigned to either the dynamic strength–training group or the control group. The randomization was carried out using clusters of 4 patients who had been stratified according to age (<50 years and ≥50 years) and sex to ensure that the demographic data of the study groups remained comparable.

This study was approved by the local ethics committee, and the participants gave their written informed consent.

Training programs. The patients in the dynamic strength–training group were personally instructed to perform a strength-training program for 24 months. The training program included exercises for the upper and lower extremities, using elastic bands for resistance, as well as abdominal and back muscle exercises, using dumbbells. The exercises for extremities were performed in a sitting or a standing position and the trunk exercises in a supine position. Subjects were instructed to exercise twice a week, with moderate loads (50–70% of the repetition maximum), 2 sets per exercise, and 8–12 repetitions per set. The exercise duration was ~45 minutes. The intensity of the strength training was reevaluated every 6 months. In addition, the patients were encouraged to engage in recreational physical activities, such as walking, cycling, skiing, and swimming for an average of 2–3 times a week for 30–45 minutes each time.

The patients in the control group were instructed to perform range of motion and stretching exercises twice a week, without using additional resistance, to maintain their joint mobility. They were free to continue their recreational physical activities with the exception of strength training of any kind.

All subjects completed training diaries during the entire 2 years of followup. Diaries were mailed to the investigators every second month for evaluation.

Measurements. *Muscle strength.* The maximum unilateral concentric strength of the knee extensors was measured using the David 200 dynamometer (Outokumpu, Finland) (27). The subject was seated with the hips in a fixed position and the knee in 110° of flexion. The ankle was supported just above the malleoli. The load in the weight stack of the machine was gradually increased until the subject was unable to perform a full knee extension (starting from knee flexion of 110° to full extension) in order to record the subject's 1 repetition maximum (in kg). Maximum isometric forces of the trunk flexors and extensors were measured by an isometric strain-gauge dynamometer (28). With the subject in a standing position and the hips fixed at the level of the anterior superior iliac spine, a 5-cm–wide strap was tightened around the shoulders at the level of the clavicle during trunk flexion and at the level of the spina scapulae during trunk extension.

Isometric grip strength was measured by a Digitest dynamometer (Oulu, Finland) (29). The results of dynamic knee extension and isometric grip strength tests are expressed as the sum of the right and left side. Before the leg and trunk strength tests, the subjects warmed up with a bicycle ergometer and, thereafter, performed a few submaximal contractions on the strength dynamometer to become familiar with the testing procedure. In all strength measurements, the subjects received verbal encouragement to exert maximum force. The highest value obtained for 3–4 trials was used for the final analysis.

Bone mineral density. BMD was measured at the Rheumatism Foundation Hospital (Heinola, Finland) using dual x-ray absorptiometry bone densitometry (Lunar DPX; Lunar Corporation, Madison, WI) in duplicate measurements at months 0, 12, and 24. The measurement sites were lumbar vertebrae L2–L4 and the left proximal femur. Quality assurance tests for densitometry were run daily. The precision of the method was previously tested on adults, and the coefficient of variation was calculated to be 1.0% for the spine and 1.8% for the femoral neck.

Functional capacity. Functional capacity was assessed by patient self-report, using the Health Assessment Questionnaire (HAQ) (30). Maximum walking speed (in meters/second) over a distance of 30 meters was measured. The time used for initial acceleration was included in the calculation.

Clinical health status. The modified Disease Activity Score (DAS), including 28 tender and 28 swollen joints (DAS28), the patient's assessment of general health (on a 0–100-mm visual analog scale [VAS]) and the erythrocyte sedimentation rate were used to evaluate clinical disease activity (31). Pain, as assessed with a 1–100-mm VAS, and morning stiffness (minutes) were also evaluated.

Joint radiology. Radiographic damage in the peripheral small joints was scored according to the method described by Larsen et al (32,33). The score ranged from 0 to 100, and included the 10 metacarpophalangeal joints, 8 metatarsophalangeal joints (second to fifth), and both wrists (all scored 0–5).

Statistical analysis. Means and standard deviations are given as descriptive statistics. Changes in muscle strength, BMD, and disease activity at the end of the training are expressed as percentages of the baseline values. Statistical comparisons between the study groups were performed with the unpaired *t*-test. The effects of strength training were analyzed by multivariate analysis of variance with repeated measures. Multiple linear regression analyses were used to explore the relationship between BMD and the demographic and disease-related risk factors.

RESULTS

Two patients from the strength-training group and 3 from the control group dropped out of the study after the baseline measurements (2 discontinued the exercises, 1 fell ill with cancer, 1 drowned, and 1 was involved in an accident and had neurologic symptoms). One patient from the strength-training group (whose data are included for the first year) dropped out of the study after the first year because of a lack of motivation for the training. The diagnosis changed for 3 patients (spondylarthrosis, psoriatic arthritis, and longstanding RA), and their data were excluded from the analysis. At baseline, there were no significant differences in demographic, strength, or clinical variables between the patients who completed the trial and those who dropped out.

At baseline, the study groups were comparable with regard to demographic variables (Table 1). After the initial measurements, therapy with DMARDs was instituted. All patients were initially treated with sulfasalazine, except for 1 patient in each group, who received gold sodium thiomalate because of allergies to sulfonamides. During the 24-month trial, the initial DMARD was changed in 15 and 19 patients in the strength-training group and the control group, respectively, because of inefficacy and/or adverse events.

Table 1. Baseline characteristics of the rheumatoid arthritis patients, by exercise group*

Variable	Strength-training group (n = 31)	Control group (n = 31)
No. of males:no. of females	13:18	11:20
Age, mean ± SD years	49 ± 10	49 ± 11
Weight, mean ± SD kg	74 ± 14	72 ± 11
Height, mean ± SD cm	169 ± 8	167 ± 9
Duration of symptoms, mean ± SD months	10 ± 10	8 ± 12
No. of current smokers	8	2
No. consuming 1–5 alcoholic drinks/week	8	10
No. of postmenopausal women	8	13
Time since menopause, mean ± SD years	8.4 ± 3.6	7.6 ± 5.6

* See Patients and Methods for a description of the exercise groups.

During the last 12 months of the study, 2 patients in the strength-training group and 10 in the control group were also treated for short periods with low-dose prednisolone (2.5–7.5 mg/day).

If the BMD measurements revealed osteopenia, treatment with alendronate (10 mg/day) was instituted. Thus, 3 patients in the strength-training group and 9 in the control group received bisphosphonate therapy for a mean ± SD of 6.2 ± 4.8 months and 8.3 ± 3.9 months, respectively.

The reported compliance with the exercise program averaged 1.5 times/week during the first 12 months and 1.4 times/week during months 13–24 in the strength-training group instead of the planned 2 times/week. The mean ± SD time used for various types of physical exercises during the first year were 240 ± 124 minutes/week for the strength-training group (including the strength-training exercise program) and 205 ± 103 minutes/week for the control group. During the second year, the corresponding values were 249 ± 121 and 187 ± 107 minutes/week. Three male patients in the strength-training group started to exercise in the gym instead of at home with the elastic bands.

Both groups had moderate disease activity at baseline, before initiation of DMARDs (Table 2). During the followup period, the parameters of disease activity improved statistically significantly in both groups. However, a significant between-group difference in favor of the strength-training group was observed.

Table 2. Parameters of disease activity and joint destruction in rheumatoid arthritis patients at baseline and after 6, 12, 18, and 24 months, by exercise group*

Parameter	Strength-training group (n = 31)	Control group (n = 31)	Difference between groups (95% CI)
ESR (mm/hour)			
Baseline	24.4 ± 17.8	24.8 ± 15.7	−0.4 (−8.8 to 8.2)
6 months	9.7 ± 9.5	16.7 ± 12.7	−7.0 (−12.7 to −1.3)†
12 months	9.5 ± 7.5	17.3 ± 16.1	−7.8 (−14.1 to −1.4)†
18 months	8.4 ± 7.2	15.5 ± 10.9	−7.1 (−11.9 to −2.3)‡
24 months	10.9 ± 9.8	15.4 ± 11.5	−4.5 (−10.0 to 0.9)
Pain (0–100-mm VAS)			
Baseline	41.7 ± 19.5	41.3 ± 27.1	0.4 (−11.6 to 12.4)
6 months	20.0 ± 16.4	28.6 ± 23.1	−8.6 (−18.9 to 1.5)
12 months	21.1 ± 20.6	24.2 ± 22.7	−3.1 (−14.3 to 8.1)
18 months	14.6 ± 13.5	24.5 ± 21.3	−9.9 (−19.2 to −0.6)†
24 months	13.7 ± 16.2	24.9 ± 22.8	−11.2 (−21.4 to −0.96)†
Morning stiffness (minutes)			
Baseline	72.4 ± 54.5	81.5 ± 90.4	−9.1 (46.9 to 28.9)
6 months	31.8 ± 41.1	62.9 ± 75.5	−31.1 (−62.0 to −25.7)†
12 months	22.3 ± 31.8	42.5 ± 65.8	−20.2 (−46.9 to 6.4)
18 months	18.3 ± 25.6	36.4 ± 51.3	−18.1 (−39.4 to 3.1)
24 months	16.3 ± 21.3	37.7 ± 43.8	−21.4 (−39.2 to −3.5)†
DAS28 index (0–10 scale)			
Baseline	4.4 ± 1.1	4.9 ± 1.1	−0.5 (−1.1 to 0.003)
6 months	2.4 ± 1.0	3.4 ± 1.2	−1.0 (−1.7 to −0.5)§
12 months	2.3 ± 1.0	3.0 ± 1.2	−0.7 (−1.3 to −0.2)†
18 months	2.0 ± 1.0	3.0 ± 1.9	−1.0 (−1.5 to −0.4)§
24 months	2.2 ± 1.2	2.7 ± 1.2	−0.5 (−1.2 to −0.004)
Larsen score (0–100 scale)			
Baseline	0.9 ± 1.8	1.2 ± 2.0	−0.3 (−1.4 to 0.6)
6 months	1.3 ± 2.3	1.3 ± 2.2	−0.0 (−1.6 to 0.7)
12 months	1.4 ± 2.9	2.3 ± 2.7	−0.9 (−2.2 to 0.7)
18 months	–	–	–
24 months	1.5 ± 3.4	3.1 ± 3.5	−1.6 (−3.1 to 0.4)

* One patient from the strength-training group dropped out of the study after the first year because of a lack of motivation for the training. See Patients and Methods for a description of the exercise groups. Values are the mean ± SD. 95% CI = 95% confidence interval; ESR = erythrocyte sedimentation rate; VAS = visual analog scale; DAS28 = Disease Activity Score in 28 swollen and 28 tender joints.
† $P < 0.05$.
‡ $P < 0.01$.
§ $P < 0.001$.

The maximum muscle strength values did not differ statistically between the groups at baseline (Figure 1). During the 24-month strength training, the mean ± SD knee extension strength per body mass increased by 59 ± 44% ($P < 0.001$) and 31 ± 27% ($P < 0.001$) in the strength-training group and the control group, respectively. The corresponding increases in trunk extension strength per body mass were 19 ± 28% ($P < 0.001$) versus 1 ± 19% (P not significant), trunk flexion strength 24 ± 19% ($P < 0.001$) versus 20 ± 43% ($P = 0.007$), and grip strength 50 ± 57% ($P < 0.001$) versus 24 ± 49% ($P < 0.001$) in the strength-training group and the control group, respectively. With the exception of trunk flexion strength, the muscle strength increases were significantly in favor of the strength-training group ($P = 0.002–0.025$).

The study groups did not differ with regard to the extent of joint damage at baseline (Table 2). During the 24-month followup, the joint damage index increased only slightly in both study groups. Thus, the difference between the groups at the end of the study was also not significant.

As shown in Table 3, there were no significant intergroup differences in BMD at either of the measured sites at baseline. During the 24-month strength-training intervention, the femoral neck BMD was increased by 0.51 ± 1.64% (mean ± SD) in the strength-training group and decreased by 0.70 ± 2.25% in the controls. For BMD of the spine, these changes were an increase of 1.17 ± 5.34% and a decrease of 0.91 ± 4.07%, respectively. At the femoral neck, the intergroup difference was significant ($P = 0.024$).

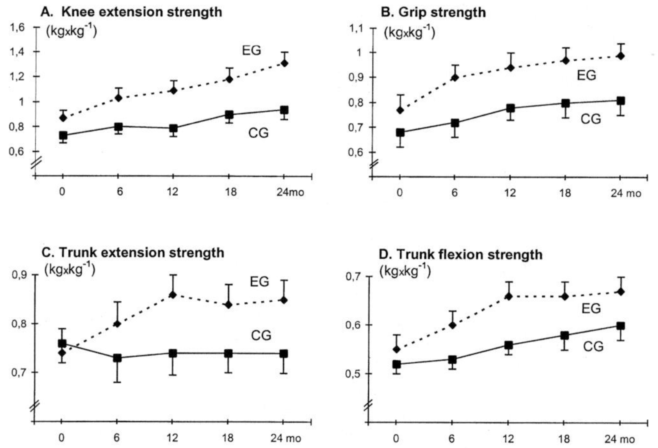

Figure 1. Changes in mean levels of maximum knee extension (**A**), grip (**B**), trunk extension (**C**), and trunk flexion (**D**) strength at 0, 6, 12, 18, and 24 months in patients with early rheumatoid arthritis randomly assigned to strength-training exercise (EG) or range of motion exercise (controls; CG).

Seventeen of the 62 patients were treated for various periods with prednisolone and/or alendronate during the followup because of active disease and osteopenia, respectively. When these 17 subjects were removed from the analysis, the comparison of BMD values in the remaining patients (28 strength-training and 18 control subjects) showed no statistically significant between-group differences at either of the evaluated sites (Table 3).

However, when the group that took prednisolone and/or alendronate (n = 17) was compared with the group that did not (n = 45), there was a significant intergroup difference for BMD at the femoral neck for all 3 time points (P = 0.002–0.006). For BMD of the spine, there was a minor, but not statistically significant, difference between the groups. Both the femoral neck and spine BMD values remained unchanged in both users and nonusers during the followup. At baseline, the mean ± SD duration of RA symptoms in the users was 6.3 ± 4.2 months and the age 53 ± 7 years, compared with 12.0 ± 12.7 months (P not significant) and 48 ± 11 years (P = 0.045) in the nonusers. The users had statistically significantly lower HAQ scores ($P < 0.021$–0.047) during the followup compared with the nonusers. Further, their DAS28 index correlated negatively with the femoral neck BMD at month 24 (r = −0.38, $P <$ 0.003).

The initial functional capacity, as measured by the HAQ and walking speed, was comparable between the groups at baseline (Table 4). The HAQ scores improved statistically significantly in both groups during the followup period. However, there were statistically significant between-group differences in the HAQ scores in favor of the strength-training group at months 18 and 24. The mean ± SD walking speed increased by 16 ± 17% ($P < 0.001$) in the strength-training group and by 9 ± 12% (P = 0.025) in the control group (Table 4).

DISCUSSION

The results of the present study show that even minimally supervised at-home strength training for 24 months led to significant increases in maximum strength

Table 3. BMD in the femoral neck and lumbar spine at baseline and after 12 and 24 months in the entire rheumatoid arthritis study cohort and in patients of both groups who did and did not take prednisolone and/or alendronate*

	All study patients		All study patients not taking prednisolone and/or alendronate		All study patients	
	Strength-training group (n = 31)	Control group (n = 31)	Strength-training group (n = 28)	Control group (n = 18)	Taking prednisolone and/or alendronate (n = 17)	Not taking prednisolone and/or alendronate (n = 45)
Femoral neck BMD						
Baseline	0.95 ± 0.12	0.95 ± 0.12	0.98 ± 0.01	0.99 ± 0.13	0.88 ± 0.12	0.98 ± 0.11†
12 months	0.96 ± 0.12	0.95 ± 0.13	0.99 ± 0.10	0.99 ± 0.14	0.88 ± 0.11	0.99 ± 0.12‡
24 months	0.96 ± 0.12	0.93 ± 0.13	0.98 ± 0.11	0.98 ± 0.15	0.87 ± 0.10	0.98 ± 0.12‡
Lumbar spine BMD						
Baseline	1.23 ± 0.20	1.20 ± 0.20	1.25 ± 0.19	1.21 ± 0.15	1.16 ± 0.20	1.24 ± 0.17
12 months	1.24 ± 0.20	1.18 ± 0.16	1.24 ± 0.18	1.22 ± 0.14	1.16 ± 0.21	1.23 ± 0.17
24 months	1.24 ± 0.19	1.18 ± 0.15	1.24 ± 0.18	1.21 ± 0.15	1.16 ± 0.21	1.22 ± 0.16

* One patient from the strength-training group dropped out of the study after the first year because of a lack of motivation for the training. See Patients and Methods for a description of the exercise groups and the parameters for prednisolone and alendronate therapy. Values are the mean ± SD. BMD = bone mineral density.
† P = 0.006.
‡ P = 0.002.

Table 4. Parameters of functional capacity in patients with rheumatoid arthritis at baseline and after 6, 12, 18, and 24 months, by exercise group*

Parameter	Strength-training group (n = 31)	Control group (n = 31)	Difference between groups (95% CI)
HAQ index (0–3 scale)			
Baseline	0.60 ± 0.53	0.77 ± 0.55	−0.17 (−0.4 to 0.1)
6 months	0.25 ± 0.36	0.47 ± 0.51	−0.22 (0.4 to 0.003)
12 months	0.20 ± 0.31	0.41 ± 0.48	−0.21 (−0.4 to 0.003)
18 months	0.15 ± 0.26	0.39 ± 0.45	−0.24 (−0.4 to −0.006)†
24 months	0.13 ± 0.21	0.35 ± 0.45	−0.22 (−0.4 to −0.004)‡
Walking speed (meters/second)			
Baseline	1.9 ± 0.5	1.9 ± 0.4	0.00 (−0.18 to 0.32)
6 months	2.2 ± 0.6	2.0 ± 0.6	0.20 (−0.006 to 0.51)
12 months	2.2 ± 0.5	2.0 ± 0.6	0.20 (−0.008 to 0.47)
18 months	2.3 ± 0.5	2.1 ± 0.5	0.20 (−0.009 to 0.45)
24 months	2.4 ± 0.5	2.1 ± 0.6	0.30 (−0.10 to 0.47)

* One patient from the strength-training group dropped out of the study after the first year because of a lack of motivation for the training. See Patients and Methods for a description of the exercise groups. Values are the mean ± SD. 95% CI = 95% confidence interval; HAQ = Health Assessment Questionnaire.
† $P < 0.01$.
‡ $P < 0.05$.

and general physical function in patients with early RA, without exacerbating the disease. Despite the substantial training effects on muscle strength, the BMD values remained, as expected, relatively unchanged over the 2-year study period.

In the strength-training group, maximum strength of the muscle groups evaluated increased by 19–59%. The corresponding change in the controls was 1–31%. In fact, the increases in muscle strength in favor of the strength-training group continued throughout the 24-month followup period. However, 1.4–1.5 weekly strength training sessions carried out in this study exceeded the normal daily tension levels of the muscles sufficiently to facilitate muscle performance (the overload principle). Although the exercise adherence in the experimental group was 70–75% of the planned rate, it was at the level achieved in other prospective interventions (24,34). The present frequency of strength training did not inhibit the motivation of the patients for continuous training and left time and energy for other physical activities as well.

The control subjects were also able to increase their muscle strength. The improvement in muscle strength values in the controls was most probably due to an increase in the intensity of their physical activities, which was facilitated by a decrease in disease activity over time. The production of maximal voluntary muscle force is an unusual event, especially in RA patients, and for this reason, motor learning and improved coordination in strength measurements must be taken into account (35,36). However, the increases in muscle strength in the control group were significantly inferior to those in the strength-training group, thus demonstrating the advantage of the applied dynamic strength–training regimen.

Osteoporosis is a well known extraarticular complication of RA (37). Although bone remodeling aberrations in RA have not been thoroughly defined, decreased physical activity and high levels of clinical disease activity as well as glucocorticoid treatment have been recognized as the most important contributory factors for the development of osteopenia (38–40). Most of the patients in the present study of early RA had normal BMD values at baseline. Thus, a realistic target for physical training was the maintenance of BMD and the prevention of disease-related bone loss. In addition to aerobic recreational physical activities, strength training consisted of exercises performed mostly in the supine, sitting, or standing positions using an elastic band for resistance. It seems that the "smooth" movements generally recommended for RA patients by, for example, the Arthritis Foundation (41,42) and applied in the present study were sufficient to maintain, but insufficient to increase, BMD values. Previous studies on biking, swimming, or rowing (43–45) suggest that these typical non–weight-bearing exercises do not generate the necessary ground-reaction forces on the skeleton to increase BMD. Although our exercise modality has not been proven to be beneficial for bone density, it has many other benefits, such as increased muscle strength and walking speed, which in turn, may result in a lower risk of falling and an increase in daily activity levels.

Statistically significantly lower femoral neck BMD was found in the 17 patients who had more active disease compared with the value in the other 45 patients with less active RA. The difference between the groups was present at baseline—before the institution of glucocorticoid treatment—and persisted at months 12 and 24. A minor, not statistically significant, difference in spine BMD was also detected between these groups. On the other hand, during the 24-month followup, the contribution of glucocorticoids to inflammation and of alendronate to bone resorption apparently had a positive influence on these subjects to maintain their BMD at the baseline level by improving their capacity for physical activity. Some studies suggest that patients with clinically active disease receiving steroid therapy lose BMD significantly more rapidly than patients with inactive disease (3,6). In the present study, the bone loss due to active disease was noted even before the initiation of glucocorticoids, which indicates that RA patients need early and effective treatment with DMARDs.

The progressive loss of function starts to develop early in RA. Inflammation disturbs bodily functions, which leads to restrictions in daily activities, tasks, and behaviors (46–48). In fact, one of the core aims of therapy for RA is the prevention or delay of disability. Dynamic strength training seems to be effective in improving muscle strength and, concomitantly, physical function, as demonstrated in this study by improvements in walking speed and self-reported physical function (HAQ). On the other hand, individually tailored dynamic muscle strength training had no negative effects on disease activity or structural joint damage.

In conclusion, the present study showed that a 24-month dynamic strength–training period results in increases in muscle strength and physical function, but it imposes only minor effects on BMD in the spine and femoral neck. High levels of disease activity, on the other hand, appear to play a central role in the loss of BMD in early RA. To improve long-term outcomes, patients with RA need to be assessed early in the disease course, and individualized therapies that include physical exercise as an integral element should be initiated in most cases.

REFERENCES

1. Hicks EJ. Exercise in patients with inflammatory arthritis and connective tissue disease. Rheum Dis Clin North Am 1990;16: 845–70.
2. Laan R, Buijs W, Verbeek A, Draad M, Corstens L, van de Putte L, et al. Bone mineral density in patients with recent onset rheumatoid arthritis: influence of disease activity and functional capacity. Ann Rheum Dis 1993;52:21–6.
3. Kröger H, Honkanen R, Saarikoski S, Alhava E. Decreased axial bone mineral density in perimenopausal women with rheumatoid arthritis: a population based study. Ann Rheum Dis 1994;53: 18–23.
4. Celiker R, Gökce-Kutsal Y, Cindas A, Ariyurek M, Renda N, Koray Z, et al. Osteoporosis in rheumatoid arthritis: effect of disease. Clin Rheumatol 1995;14:429–33.
5. Hansen M, Florescu A, Stoltenberg M, Podenphant J, Pedersen-Zbinden B, Horslev-Petersen K, et al. Bone loss in rheumatoid arthritis: influence of disease activity, duration of the disease, functional capacity, and corticosteroid treatment. Scand J Rheumatol 1996;25:367–76.
6. Gough A, Lilley J, Ayre S, Holder R, Emery P. Generalized bone loss in patients with early rheumatoid arthritis. Lancet 1994;344: 23–7.
7. Eggelmeijer F, Camps J, Valkema R, Papapoulos S, Pauwels B, Dijkmans B, et al. Bone mineral density in ambulant, non-steroid treated female patients with rheumatoid arthritis. Clin Exp Rheumatol 1993;11:381–5.
8. Sambrook P, Cohen M, Eisman J, Pocock N, Champion G, Yeates M. Effects of low-dose corticosteroids on bone mass in rheumatoid arthritis: a longitudinal study. Ann Rheum Dis 1989;48:535–8.
9. Rothstein J, Delitto A, Sinacore D, Rose S. Muscle function in rheumatic disease patients treated with corticosteroids. Muscle Nerve 1983;6:128–35.
10. Pincus T, Callahan LF, Sale WG, Brooks AL, Payne LE, Vaughn WK. Severe functional declines, work disability, and increased mortality in seventy-five rheumatoid arthritis patients studied over nine years. Arthritis Rheum 1984;27:864–72.
11. Ekblom B, Lövgren O, Alderin M, Fridström M, Satterström G. Physical performance in patients with rheumatoid arthritis. Scand J Rheumatol 1974;3:121–5.
12. Wolfe F, Hawley D, Cathey M. Clinical and health status measures over time: prognosis and outcome assessment in rheumatoid arthritis. J Rheumatol 1991;18:1290–7.
13. Häkkinen A, Sokka T, Kotaniemi A, Paananen M-L, Mälkiä E, Kautiainen H, et al. Muscle strength characteristics and central bone mineral density in women with rheumatoid arthritis compared with healthy women. Scand J Rheumatol 1999;28:145–51.
14. Wolff I, van Croonenborg J, Kemper H, Kostence P, Twisk J. The effect of exercise training programs on bone mass: a meta-analysis of published controlled trials in pre- and postmenopausal women. Osteoporosis Int 1999;9:1–12.
15. Cavanaugh D, Cann E. Brisk walking does not stop bone loss in postmenopausal women. Bone 1988;9:201–4.
16. Heinonen A, Sievänen H, Kannus P, Oja P, Vuori I. Effects of unilateral strength training and detraining on bone mineral mass and estimated mechanical characteristics of the upper limb bones in young women. J Bone Miner Res 1996;11:490–501.
17. Hatori M, Hasegawa A, Adachi H, Shinozaki A, Hayashi R, Okano H, et al. The effects of walking at aerobic threshold level on vertebral bone loss in postmenopausal women. Calcif Tissue Int 1993;52:411–4.
18. Lohman T, Going S, Pamenter R, Hall M, Bouden T, Houtcooper L, et al. Effects of resistance training on regional and total bone mineral density in premenopausal women: a randomized prospective study. J Bone Miner Res 1995;10:1015–24.
19. Snow-Harter C, Bouxsein M, Carter D, Marcus R. Effects of resistance and endurance exercise on bone mineral status of young women: a randomized exercise intervention trial. J Bone Miner Res 1992;7:647–57.
20. Heinonen A. Exercise as an osteogenic stimulus. Stud Sport Phys Educ Health 1997;49:1–69.

21. Komatireddy G, Leitch R, Cella K, Browning G, Minor M. Efficacy of low load resistive muscle training in patients with rheumatoid arthritis functional class II and III. J Rheumatol 1997;24:1531–9.
22. Stenström C. Home exercise in rheumatoid arthritis functional class II: goal setting versus pain attention. J Rheumatol 1994;21: 527–34.
23. Häkkinen A, Sokka T, Kotaniemi A, Kautiainen H, Jäppinen I, Laitinen L, et al. Dynamic strength training in patients with recent onset rheumatoid arthritis increases muscle strength but not bone mineral density. J Rheumatol 1999;26:1257–63.
24. Westby M, Wade J, Rangno K, Berkowitz J. A randomized controlled trial to evaluate the effectiveness of an exercise program in women with rheumatoid arthritis taking low dose prednisolone. J Rheumatol 2000;27;1674–80.
25. Häkkinen A, Häkkinen K, Hannonen P. Effects of strength training on neuromuscular function and disease activity in patients with recent-onset inflammatory arthritis. Scand J Rheumatol 1994;23:237–42.
26. Arnett FC, Edworthy SM, Bloch DA, McShane DJ, Fries JF, Cooper NS, et al. The American Rheumatism Association 1987 revised criteria for the classification of rheumatoid arthritis. Arthritis Rheum 1988;31:315–24.
27. Häkkinen K, Komi P, Kauhanen H. Scientific evaluation of specific loading of the knee extensors with variable resistance, isokinetic and barbell exercises. In: Marconnet P, Komi P, editors. Medicine and sport science. Basel: Karger; 1987. p. 224–37.
28. Rantanen P, Airaksinen O, Penttinen E. Paradoxical variation of strength determinants with different rotation axes of trunk flexion and extension strength tests. Eur J Appl Physiol 1994;68:322–6.
29. Mathiowetz V, Candidate P. Reliability and validity of grip and pinch strength measurements. Phys Rehabil Med 1991;4:201–12.
30. Fries JF, Spitz P, Kraines RG, Holman HR. Measurement of patient outcome in arthritis. Arthritis Rheum 1980;23:137–45.
31. Prevoo MLL, van 't Hof MA, Kuper HH, van Leeuwen MA, van de Putte LBA, van Riel PLCM. Modified disease activity scores that include twenty-eight–joint counts: development and validation in a prospective longitudinal study of patients with rheumatoid arthritis. Arthritis Rheum 1995;38:44–8.
32. Larsen A, Dale K, Eek M. Radiographic evaluation of rheumatoid arthritis and related conditions by standard reference films. Acta Radiol 1977;18:481–91.
33. Larsen A. How to apply Larsen score in evaluating radiographs of rheumatoid arthritis in long-term studies. J Rheumatol 1995;22: 1974–5.
34. Heinonen A, Oja P, Sievänen H, Pasanen M, Vuori I. Effect of two training regimens on bone mineral density in healthy perimenopausal women: a randomized controlled trial. J Bone Miner Res 1998;13:483–90.
35. Moritani T, deVries H. Neural factors versus hypertrophy in the time course of muscle strength gain. Am J Phys Med 1979;58: 115–30.
36. Rutherford O, Jones D. The role of learning and coordination in strength training. Eur J Appl Physiol 1986;55:100–5.
37. Deodhar A, Woolf A. Bone mass measurement and bone metabolism in rheumatoid arthritis: a review. Br J Rheumatol 1995;35: 309–22.
38. Als O, Godfredsen A, Riis B, Christiansen C. Are disease duration and degree of functional impairment determinants of bone mass in rheumatoid arthritis? Ann Rheum Dis 1985;44:406–11.
39. Haugeberg G, Uhlig T, Falch JA, Halse JI, Kvien TK. Bone mineral density and frequency of osteoporosis in female patients with rheumatoid arthritis: results from 394 patients in the Oslo County rheumatoid arthritis register. Arthritis Rheum 2000;43: 522–30.
40. Laan R, van Riel P, van de Putte L, van Erning L, van 't Hof M, Lemmens A. Low-dose prednisone induces rapid reversible axial bone loss in patients with rheumatoid arthritis. Ann Intern Med 1993;119:963–8.
41. Boulware D, Byrd S. Optimizing exercise programs for arthritis patients. Physician Sportsmed 1993;21:104–20.
42. Shephard R, Shek P. Autoimmune disorders, physical activity, and training, with particular reference to rheumatoid arthritis. Exerc Immunol Rev 1997;3:53–67.
43. Heinonen A, Sievänen H, Kannus P, Oja P, Vuori I. Effects of unilateral strength training and detraining on bone mineral mass and estimated mechanical characteristics of the upper limb bones in young women. J Bone Miner Res 1996;11:490–501.
44. Orwoll E, Ferar J, Oviatt S, McClung R, Huntington K. The relationship of swimming exercise to bone mass in men and women. Arch Intern Med 1989;149:2197–200.
45. Taaffe D, Snow-Harter C, Connolly D, Robinson T, Brown M, Marcus R. Differential effects of swimming versus weight-bearing activity on bone mineral status of eumenorrheic athletes. J Bone Miner Res 1995;10:586–93.
46. Hansen T, Hansen G, Langgaard A, Rasmussen J. Longterm physical training in rheumatoid arthritis: a randomized trial with different training programs and blinded observers. Scand J Rheumatol 1996;22:107–12.
47. Wolfe F, Cathey M. The assessment and prediction of functional disability in rheumatoid arthritis. J Rheumatol 1991;18:1298–306.
48. Fitzpatrick F, Badley E. An overview of disability. Br J Rheum 1996;35:184–7.

ARTHRITIS & RHEUMATISM
Vol. 44, No. 3, March 2001, pp 523–527

Increased Mortality in Adults With a History of Juvenile Rheumatoid Arthritis

A Population-Based Study

Anthony R. French, Tom Mason, Audrey M. Nelson, W. Michael O'Fallon, and Sherine E. Gabriel

Objective. **To assess mortality in a population-based cohort of adults with a history of juvenile rheumatoid arthritis (JRA).**

Methods. **The Rochester Epidemiology Project database was used to identify all cases of JRA diagnosed among Rochester, Minnesota residents under the age of 16 between January 1, 1960 and December 31, 1993. Fifty-seven patients in this cohort are now adults (ages 18–53 years, mean age 34.3 years), and this subgroup was contacted for a long-term followup study. The average length of followup from the time of diagnosis was 25.6 years.**

Results. **Four deaths occurred in this cohort of 57 adults with a history of JRA. All 4 deceased patients had other autoimmune illnesses and died of complications of these diseases. The observed frequency of 4 deaths was significantly greater ($P < 0.0026$ by one-sample log-rank test) than the 1 death that would be expected among Minnesota whites of similar age and sex, and corresponds to a mortality rate of 0.27 deaths per 100 years of patient followup compared with an expected mortality rate of 0.068 deaths per 100 years of followup in the general population.**

Conclusion. **The results indicate a significant, unexpected increase in mortality in this population-based cohort of adults with a history of JRA in comparison with the rate in the general population. The deaths in this group were all associated with other autoimmune disorders, suggesting that special emphasis should be given to the diagnosis and treatment of other autoimmune diseases, including immunodeficiencies, in JRA patients. The frequency of deaths in this cohort suggests that JRA patients are at substantial risk for mortality, and highlights the need for longitudinal followup and care into adulthood.**

Juvenile rheumatoid arthritis (JRA) is a childhood rheumatic disease with the potential for long-term morbidity. JRA has often been considered a fairly benign disease that generally resolves by adulthood. It is now clear that this prognosis is too optimistic (1–4). Wallace and Levinson (3), in a summary of several longitudinal studies, demonstrated that 31–55% of JRA patients continued to have active disease after 10 years of followup. In addition, adults with a history of JRA may experience long-term physical and psychosocial impairments, including poorer health perception and decreased physical functioning (1).

We have previously reported on the psychosocial outcomes and health status of a population-based cohort of 50 adults with a history of JRA (5). In that study, adults who had had JRA were found to have greater physical disability, increased bodily pain and fatigue, poorer health perception, and increased levels of unemployment compared with healthy control subjects. We now report an unexpected, increased mortality within a population-based cohort of adults with a history of JRA. After an average of 25.6 years of followup, 4 of the patients within this cohort were deceased. All 4 had other autoimmune illnesses and died of complications from these diseases. This suggests that adults with a

Supported in part by a research grant from the Mayo Foundation.

Anthony R. French, MD, PhD, Tom Mason, MD, Audrey M. Nelson, MD, W. Michael O'Fallon, PhD, Sherine E. Gabriel, MD, MSc: Mayo Clinic, Rochester, Minnesota.

Address correspondence and reprint requests to Sherine E. Gabriel, MD, MSc, Department of Health Sciences Research, Mayo Clinic, 200 First Street SW, Rochester, MN 55905.

Submitted for publication June 16, 2000; accepted in revised form November 9, 2000.

Table 1. Demographic characteristics of the population-based cohort of adults with a history of juvenile rheumatoid arthritis (JRA) and the deceased patients within this group

	Cohort (n = 57)	Deceased (n = 4)
Mean ± SD age at diagnosis, years	8.7 ± 4.8	7.2 ± 5.5
Number (%) female	41 (72)	2 (50)
Number (%) with pauciarticular JRA	39 (68)	1 (25)
Number (%) with polyarticular JRA	11 (19)	1 (25)
Number (%) with systemic JRA	7 (12)	2 (50)
Mean age at followup or death, years (minimum, maximum)	34.3 (18, 53)	26.8 (18, 40)
Mean ± SD followup, years	25.6 ± 9.0	19.6 ± 10.7

history of JRA experience an increase not only in morbidity, but also in mortality, compared with the general population.

PATIENTS AND METHODS

Study cohort. The Rochester Epidemiology Project database was used to identify all cases of JRA (based on the American College of Rheumatology criteria [6]) that were diagnosed among Rochester, Minnesota residents under the age of 16 between January 1, 1960 and December 31, 1993 (7). The Rochester Epidemiology Project provides the unique capability to perform population-based epidemiologic research in Olmsted County, Minnesota, due to several factors, including 1) the relative isolation of the county from other urban areas, 2) the long-standing centralization of health care to a handful of providers including a major tertiary care center, and 3) centralized records accumulated in a single dossier with a master-list of diagnoses. Patients who were diagnosed with JRA during this 33-year period and whose birth date was prior to December 31, 1980, thus now classifying them as adults, were eligible for inclusion in this long-term followup study. All eligible participants were sent a letter describing the rationale, methods, and goals of the study, a consent form, and a survey. A second mailing was sent to those individuals who did not reply within 1 month. If there still was no response, telephone contact was attempted.

Statistical analysis. The number of deaths within the cohort was compared with the expected number of deaths in age- and sex-matched Minnesota whites, using a one-sample log-rank test.

RESULTS

Patient characteristics. Sixty-five patients were identified as having been diagnosed with JRA while living in Rochester, Minnesota during this 33-year period (7). Fifty-nine of these 65 patients were now adults, with birth dates prior to December 31, 1980, and were eligible for inclusion in this long-term followup study. Two of the 59 patients (1 male and 1 female, both with pauciarticular JRA) could not be approached regarding participation in this study because they refused research authorization to their medical records and were therefore not included in the followup analysis. Forty-eight of the potential 57 participants were contacted between August 1999 and January 2000. Five patients (3 male and 2 female, of whom 2 had pauciarticular JRA, 2 had polyarticular JRA, and 1 had systemic JRA) either did not respond or could not be located during this period. The most recent previous followup on these 5 patients occurred between March 1995 and November 1999 and that information was utilized in the analysis. Four patients were deceased at the time of the study.

The patients ranged in age (in 1999 or at the time of death) from 18 years to 53 years (average age 34.3 years) and were followed up from the time of diagnosis for an average of 25.6 years (median 26.3 years, range 7.7–39.1 years). The demographic characteristics of this cohort are described in Table 1. As would be expected, the group was predominantly female. It is noteworthy that nearly 70% of the patients in this population-based cohort had pauciarticular JRA. Table 1 also lists the characteristics of the 4 deceased patients and demonstrates that they were disproportionately affected by polyarticular (25%) and systemic (50%) JRA. Although men comprised only 28% of the cohort, they made up 50% of the deaths. All 4 deceased patients had other

Table 2. Associated autoimmune diseases in deceased adults with a history of JRA*

Patient/sex/JRA subtype	Age at diagnosis, years	Age at death, years	Other autoimmune diseases
Patient 1/F/polyarticular	4.7	40.2	Chronic autoimmune hepatitis; insulin-dependent diabetes mellitus (steroid-induced)
Patient 2/M/systemic	14.5	29.1	CVID
Patient 3/M/pauciarticular	7.8	19.9	Insulin-dependent diabetes mellitus; Graves' disease; lymphocytic myocarditis
Patient 4/F/systemic	1.8	18.0	Antipolysaccharide antibody deficiency (variant of CVID)

* JRA = juvenile rheumatoid arthritis; CVID = common variable immunodeficiency.

associated autoimmune problems, as delineated in Table 2 and discussed below.

Deceased patients. *Patient 1.* Patient 1 was a woman whose polyarticular JRA was diagnosed at 4 years of age and who had persistent arthritis throughout adulthood that required several orthopedic operations. She developed chronic autoimmune hepatitis at age 16 and underwent extensive immunosuppressive therapy, including azathioprine for 6 years and corticosteroids for 22 years. She developed steroid-induced insulin-dependent diabetes mellitus (IDDM) at age 36. Her autoimmune hepatitis progressed to liver failure with worsening encephalopathy requiring a liver transplant at age 39. She developed complications from her liver transplant (including celiac and hepatic artery thromboses) and died 17 months posttransplant at age 40 after experiencing ventricular fibrillation and cardiac arrest during endoscopic retrograde cholangiopancreatography.

Patient 2. Patient 2 was a man whose systemic JRA was diagnosed at 14 years of age. Corticosteroids were not used in treating his JRA. He was diagnosed with asthma at age 2. He experienced multiple sinopulmonary infections and was subsequently diagnosed with common variable immunodeficiency (CVID) at age 11 and received immunoglobulin therapy for several years. This patient transferred his care to another medical institution as an adult (age 24), where he underwent a bone marrow transplant for his immunodeficiency at age 28. He developed multiorgan failure secondary to his bone marrow transplant and died at age 29.

Patient 3. Patient 3 was a man whose pauciarticular JRA was diagnosed at 7 years of age. His JRA was not treated with corticosteroids. He had previously developed Graves' disease at age 4 and underwent a thyroidectomy at that time. In addition, he also had developed IDDM at age 4, which was poorly controlled, with glycosylated hemoglobin values ranging from 12.2% to 16.3% during the 4 years preceding his death. He died at age 19 from an apparent severe hypoglycemic reaction, but on autopsy he was also found to have lymphocytic myocarditis.

Patient 4. Patient 4 was a woman whose systemic JRA was diagnosed at 21 months of age. Her JRA was not treated with corticosteroids. She experienced multiple sinopulmonary infections throughout her 18 years of life (23 episodes of otitis media with the last episode occurring at age 16, 4 episodes of sinusitis, more than 10 pneumonias documented by chest radiograph, recurrent herpes simplex, and 9 episodes of pharyngitis). She was investigated several times for an immunodeficiency disorder and found to have normal immunoglobulin levels on 4 separate occasions (mean IgG level 950 mg/dl) with normal T and B cell populations as well as normal complement levels. She had negative results on a sweat chloride test. She died at age 18 from overwhelming streptococcal pneumoniae septicemia. Although not diagnosed prior to her death, this patient appeared to have had antipolysaccharide antibody deficiency, a variant of CVID with normal immunoglobulin levels. Both her mother and her sister were subsequently diagnosed with antipolysaccharide antibody deficiency with no response to any of 12 serotypes in the pneumococcal vaccine.

Mortality analysis. The observed incidence of 4 deaths in this population-based cohort of adults with a history of JRA was significantly higher than the 1 death that would be expected among age- and sex-matched Minnesota whites, as determined by a one-sample log-rank test ($P < 0.0026$). The 7% mortality observed over a mean followup period of 25.6 years corresponds to a mortality rate of 0.27 deaths per 100 years of patient followup (95% confidence interval 0.07–0.7 deaths per 100 years of patient followup).

DISCUSSION

Our long-term followup of a population-based cohort of adults with a history of JRA suggests that these patients experienced an increased mortality compared with that in the general population. This unexpected finding is even more surprising given the predominance of pauciarticular JRA in this population-based group. The observed mortality in this cohort was substantial, with a 4-fold increase over the expected mortality for similar age- and sex-matched Minnesota whites ($P < 0.0026$). The major strength of this observation is that it is drawn from a very long followup of a population-based group, which should more accurately reflect the natural history of JRA than would a referral-based cohort. The most obvious limitation of our study is the small size of our cohort.

Previous estimates of mortality associated with JRA have been primarily based on deaths in children with the disease. Baum and Gutowska (8) reported a mortality of 1.1% in children with JRA in the United States (n = 23 deaths in 2,055 children with JRA) and a higher rate of 4.2% at 8 European centers (n = 158 deaths in 3,776 children with JRA). A large cohort assembled from 23 pediatric rheumatology centers (22 US and 1 Canadian) reported 33 deaths among 11,287 JRA patients, corresponding to 0.29 deaths per 100 patients (3). Five deaths occurred in 472 children with JRA over a 23-year period in Cincinnati (3). A similar

Table 3. Mortality rate (number of deaths/100 years of patient followup) in longitudinal studies of children with juvenile rheumatoid arthritis

Study, first author (year)	No. of patients	Average followup, years	Number of deaths	Mean age at death, years	% systemic subtype among deceased patients	Mortality, no. dead/years of followup
Goel (1974)	100	9.1*	9	8.5	89	0.99
Ansell (1976)	243	15	17	NA†	59	0.47
Stoeber (1981)	433	15	31	NA†	94	0.48

* Average length of followup not explicitly stated, but derived from information within the report.
† NA = not available.

rate of mortality (0.9%) was reported in England, with 18 deaths in 2,100 children with juvenile chronic arthritis (JCA) (3).

Three longitudinal reports that focused primarily on childhood deaths among children with JCA included enough information to derive comparable mortality rates with respect to numbers of deaths per 100 years of patient followup (9–11) (see Table 3). All 3 of these referral-based European studies listed infection or amyloidosis as the primary cause of death. In the study with the highest reported mortality rate, nearly 80% of children who died were being treated with steroids (10).

In contrast to these earlier reports of deaths in children with JRA, none of the deaths in our population-based cohort of JRA patients occurred in childhood; all occurred after the patients had reached adulthood. A recent Scandinavian study also reported no childhood deaths in a population-based cohort of 124 children with JCA who were followed up for an average of 7.1 years until an average age of 17.7 years (4).

We were able to find only 2 previous reports of mortality in adults with a history of JRA. Calabro and colleagues (12) reported a 3% mortality in a referral-based cohort of 100 JRA patients followed up over a 25-year period. The 3 deaths included an 8-year-old girl with systemic JRA who died of renal failure, a 19-year-old boy with polyarticular JRA who died from postsurgical sepsis, and a 25-year-old man with polyarticular JRA who committed suicide. Zak and coworkers (13) reported 2 deaths in a referral-based cohort of 93 JCA patients followed up for an average of 26 years. One death was the result of sepsis and the other related to human immunodeficiency virus. Both of these studies reported lower mortality rates in adults with a history of JRA than that observed in our cohort. The differences may be partially attributable to losses in followup, but these discrepancies highlight the need for larger, longitudinal studies to clarify the long-term outcomes, including mortality, associated with JRA.

All 4 deceased patients in our cohort died from complications of associated autoimmune diseases, suggesting that their JRA was a manifestation of more widespread immune system dysregulation. The deaths disproportionately occurred in patients with polyarticular or systemic JRA, implying that more severely affected JRA patients may be at greater risk for other autoimmune illnesses. Previously reported JRA-associated deaths in children also occurred disproportionately in systemic JRA patients, but, in contrast to our findings in adults, those deaths were not primarily related to complications of associated autoimmune diseases (3).

Two of the JRA patients in our cohort who died had CVID or antipolysaccharide antibody deficiency, a variant of CVID with normal immunoglobulin levels. An association between CVID and JRA has been previously described. In a series of 103 patients with CVID, of which one-third were children or adolescents, 22% of the patients had associated autoimmune diseases, including 3 patients with JRA (14). Hausser and coworkers (15) found that 9 of 30 children with CVID had associated autoimmune disorders, including 2 with polyarticular JRA.

Two of the deceased JRA patients in our cohort had IDDM, although 1 case appears to have been steroid-induced. An association between these 2 diseases has been previously noted (16–18). Rudolf and coworkers (18) reported that 7 of 200 diabetic children at a large referral center had JRA, which is much higher than the expected prevalence of JRA of ~1 per 1,000 children in the general population (7). Interestingly, 6 of the 7 children with JRA in this series had polyarticular disease.

Two other autoimmune phenomena found in our deceased patients included Graves' disease and autoimmune hepatitis. Fewer reports in the literature link these autoimmune manifestations with JRA, but several case reports have noted an association between autoimmune thyroid disease and JRA, including a 15-year-old girl with Hashimoto's thyroiditis, diabetes mellitus, and JRA (16). These 2 autoimmune disorders have also been associated with other rheumatologic diseases such as mixed connective tissue disease (19).

Lymphocytic myocarditis can occur as a manifestation of autoimmune disease or as an isolated entity often following a viral illness. It is not possible to determine whether the lymphocytic myocarditis, observed during the autopsy of patient 3, was the result of an autoimmune or postviral process. In light of the patient's extensive history of multiple autoimmune illnesses, including Graves' disease, IDDM, and JRA, his lymphocytic myocarditis may have been another manifestation of diffuse autoimmune dysregulation.

The frequency of deaths in this population-based cohort of adults with a history of JRA demonstrates that these patients may be at risk for substantial mortality and may benefit from longitudinal followup and care into adulthood. Interestingly, in this cohort, the deaths were all associated with other autoimmune diseases. This evidence of more generalized immune system dysregulation suggests that special attention should be focused on the diagnosis and treatment of other autoimmune disorders, including immunodeficiencies, in JRA patients. These unexpected observations in our small population-based study suggest that larger, longitudinal studies are needed to more definitively define the long-term outcomes, including associated mortality, in JRA.

ACKNOWLEDGMENT

We are grateful for the statistical assistance provided by Mr. James Kuiper.

REFERENCES

1. David J, Cooper C, Hickey L, Lloyd J, Dore C, McCullough C, et al. The functional and psychological outcomes of JCA in young adulthood. Br J Rheumatol 1994;33:876–81.
2. Graham TB, Lovell DJ. Outcome in pediatric rheumatic disease. Curr Opin Rheumatol 1997;9:434–9.
3. Wallace CA, Levinson JE. Juvenile rheumatoid arthritis: outcome and treatment for the 1990s. Rheum Dis Clin North Am 1991;17: 891–905.
4. Gare BA, Fasth A. The natural history of JCA: a population based cohort study. J Rheumatol 1995;22:295–307.
5. Peterson LS, Mason T, Nelson AM, O'Fallon WM, Gabriel SE. Psychosocial outcomes and health status of adults who have had juvenile rheumatoid arthritis: a controlled, population-based study. Arthritis Rheum 1997;40:2235–40.
6. Cassidy JT, Levinson JE, Bass JC, Baum J, Brewer EJ Jr, Fink CW, et al. A study of classification criteria for a diagnosis of juvenile rheumatoid arthritis. Arthritis Rheum 1986;29:274–81.
7. Peterson LS, Mason T, Nelson AM, O'Fallon WM, Gabriel SE. Juvenile rheumatoid arthritis in Rochester, Minnesota 1960–1993: is the epidemiology changing? Arthritis Rheum 1996; 39:1385–90.
8. Baum J, Gutowska G. Death in juvenile rheumatoid arthritis. Arthritis Rheum 1977;20:253–5.
9. Ansell BM, Wood PHN. Prognosis in juvenile chronic polyarthritis. Clin Rheum Dis 1976;2:397–412.
10. Goel KM, Shanks RA. Follow-up study of 100 cases of juvenile rheumatoid arthritis. Ann Rheum Dis 1974;33:25–31.
11. Stoeber E. Prognosis in juvenile chronic arthritis: follow-up of 433 children. Eur J Pediatr 1981;135:225–8.
12. Calabro JJ, Marchesano JM, Parrino GR. Juvenile rheumatoid arthritis: long-term management and prognosis. J Musculoskeletal Med 1989;6:17–32.
13. Zak M, Hassager C, Lovell DJ, Nielsen S, Henderson CJ, Pedersen FK. Assessment of bone mineral density in adults with a history of juvenile chronic arthritis: a cross-sectional long-term followup study. Arthritis Rheum 1999;42:790–8.
14. Cunningham-Rundles C. Clinical immunologic analyses of 103 patients with common variable immunodeficiency. J Clin Immunol 1989;9:22–33.
15. Hausser C, Virelizier JL, Buriot D, Griscelli C. Common variable hypogammaglobulinemia in children. Am J Dis Child 1983;137: 833–7.
16. Fisher M, Nussbaum M, Abrams CAL, Shenker IR. Diabetes mellitus, Hashimoto's thyroiditis and juvenile rheumatoid arthritis. Am J Dis Child 1980;134:93–4.
17. Jenkins EA, Hull RG, Gray RES, Hall MA, Ansell BM. Diabetes mellitus and myasthenia gravis in a patient with systemic-onset juvenile chronic arthritis. J R Soc Med 1989;82:368–9.
18. Rudolf MC, Genel M, Tamborlane WV, Dwyer JM. Juvenile rheumatoid arthritis in children with diabetes mellitus. J Pediatr 1981;99:519–24.
19. Inoue K, Okajima T, Tanaka E, Ando B, Takeshita M, Masuda A, et al. A case of Graves' disease associated with autoimmune hepatitis and mixed connective tissue disease. Endocr J 1999;46: 173–7.

ARTHRITIS & RHEUMATISM
Vol. 44, No. 3, March 2001, pp 528–534

Indirect Medical Costs in Early Rheumatoid Arthritis

Composition of and Changes in Indirect Costs Within the First Three Years of Disease

S. Merkesdal,[1] J. Ruof,[1] O. Schöffski,[2] K. Bernitt,[1] H. Zeidler,[1] and W. Mau[1]

Objective. **To investigate 1) the magnitude of indirect costs, 2) changes in cost components, and 3) correlations between changes in cost and social, clinical, and occupational variables within the first 3 years of rheumatoid arthritis (RA).**

Methods. **We evaluated the indirect costs per person-year in 133 consecutive gainfully employed outpatients with early RA, in a prospective multicenter followup study. Costs due to RA-related sick leave, work disability, and other work loss were assessed using the human capital approach. Variables associated with reduction in lost productivity were tested by multivariate logistic regression analysis.**

Results. **Mean ± SEM annual indirect costs were $11,750 ± 1,120 per person. During the 3-year period of observation, a marked reduction in the costs associated with sick leave was seen, which exceeded the increase in costs due to work disability and other work loss. This phenomenon resulted in an overall reduction in indirect costs of 21%. The final logistic regression model of reduced loss of productivity included 3 variables: no problems with standing (odds ratio [OR] 7.1), no problems with working speed (OR 4.1), and no problems with outdoor work (OR 3.1).**

Conclusion. **High indirect costs in early RA were demonstrated. An overall decrease of costs can be seen in the first 3 years, due to the reduction in sick leave. Since the absence of problems due to strenuous working conditions was found to be associated with a reduction in indirect costs, it is assumed that early intensified vocational rehabilitation, apart from controlling disease activity by adequate treatment, might help to reduce indirect costs.**

Supported by grant 07068223 from the German Ministry of Research and Technology.

[1]S. Merkesdal, MD, J. Ruof, MD, MPH, K. Bernitt, H. Zeidler, MD, PhD, W. Mau, MD, PhD: Hannover Medical School, Hannover, Germany; [2]O. Schöffski, PhD, MPH: University of Hannover, Hannover, Germany.

Address correspondence and reprint requests to S. Merkesdal, MD, Hannover Medical School, Division of Rheumatology, 30623 Hannover, Germany.

Submitted for publication February 14, 2000; accepted in revised form November 9, 2000.

Given the necessity to optimize the distribution of scarce financial resources for health care, a number of cost-of-illness studies investigating the economic impact of chronic diseases have been conducted in recent years. As a chronic progressive disease, rheumatoid arthritis (RA) presents a tremendous burden both for patients and for society as a whole. Remarkably high costs of disease have been reported for RA (1–7).

Indirect costs are of major importance in RA. Analyses of RA-related costs have shown that indirect costs (due to loss of productivity) account for 50–85% of the overall costs of the disease (1–3). The main components of these high indirect costs in RA are work disability, with rates between 37% and 60% (8,9), and sick leave, with 36% of RA patients being on sick leave at the time of assessment (according to cross-sectional data from an epidemiologic survey of RA in France [10]). There are data indicating that both sickness-related absence and loss of employment might constitute important components of indirect costs even in the early phase of RA. Within the first 4 years, up to 42% of patients have to stop working (11–13), and cross-sectional data from a Dutch study show a markedly lower employment rate among RA patients with disease duration of <6 years compared with the Dutch general population (14). Sick leave from work due to RA, occurring in the first year of disease, was reported by 3 of 4 patients, with an average of 11 days absent per month among men and 8 days among women (15).

To date, there has been no systematic analysis of the different components of indirect costs in the early phase of RA. Furthermore, the correlation between changes in these costs and clinical, occupational, social, and psychological outcome variables has yet to be investigated. The present prospective study provides information about the magnitude of RA-associated indirect costs within the first 3 years of disease, about changes in cost components, and about the correlation of changes in these costs with different outcome variables.

PATIENTS AND METHODS

Study design. The data for the present cost analysis were derived from a multicenter prospective study assessing disease course and work disability in early RA (15). Figure 1 presents the design of the study. Assessment times were designated time 0 (enrollment), time 1 (first examination), time 2 (reexamination at 12 months), and time 3 (reexamination at 12 months). The mean ± SEM observation time was 2.5 ± 0.2 years. The centers in Germany in which the study was conducted, and the participating investigators, were as follows: Medical School of Hannover (H. Zeidler, W. Mau), Ev. Fachkrankenhaus Ratingen (R. Rau, G. Herborn), Klinik Niedersachsen Bad Nenndorf (H. G. Pott), Schloßpark-Klinik Berlin (R. Alten), and Klinikum Südstadt Rostock (M. Keysser).

Patients. The original cohort comprised 317 consecutive outpatients with early RA (<12 months since first symptom of joint swelling) who fulfilled the traditional or tree format of the American College of Rheumatology (formerly, the American Rheumatism Association) 1987 criteria for RA (16). One hundred fifty-four of the 317 patients were either older than 65 years at time 0 (84 patients), already receiving disability payments for reasons other than RA (4 patients), not employed due to job loss (6 patients), or not employed for other reasons (e.g., homemakers) (60 patients). Information on work history prior to onset of symptoms was recorded for 140 of these 154 patients, only 64 of whom were younger than 65 years. Of the 163 patients who were gainfully employed at time 0, 30 (18%) were lost to followup during the 2 years of the study: 10 moved to distant areas and 20 refused reexaminations. Thus, 133 patients who were employed outside the home at time 0 and who participated in the followup were included in the cost analysis. Baseline characteristics did not differ significantly between these 133 patients and the 184 who were not included (data not shown). Demographic, clinical, and occupational variables of the 133 patients at time 1 are shown in Table 1.

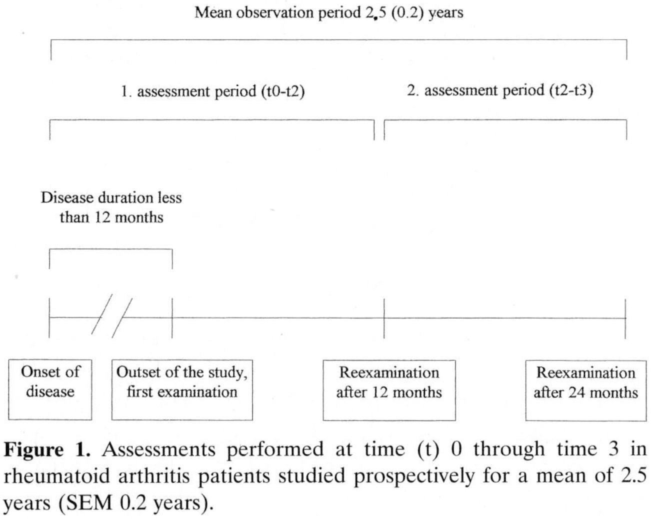

Figure 1. Assessments performed at time (t) 0 through time 3 in rheumatoid arthritis patients studied prospectively for a mean of 2.5 years (SEM 0.2 years).

Table 1. Demographic, clinical, and occupational variables in the 133 patients at the first examination*

Demographic variables	
Female	84 (63)
Age, mean ± SEM years	47 ± 0.8
>9 years of education	61 (46)
Clinical variables	
Disease duration, mean ± SEM months	7 ± 0.3
No. of swollen joints, mean ± SEM	11 ± 0.6
ESR, mean ± SEM mm/hour	30 ± 2.2
Rheumatoid factor positive	75 (56)
Erosive changes	50 (38)
Occupational variables	
Blue-collar worker	44 (34)
White-collar worker	86 (66)
Working hours/week, mean ± SEM	34 ± 0.9
Gross income, mean ± SEM $/month	2,090 ± 1,170

* Except where otherwise indicated, values are the number (%).

Data collection. Demographic, occupational, and social variables, including reasons for changes in employment status, number of sickness-related work days lost, and patient and household income for the periods time 0–time 1, time 1–time 2, and time 2–time 3 were assessed by means of standardized interviews. Clinical data on all patients were obtained at time 1, time 2, and time 3.

The German social security system. The German social security system is based on funding by companies providing compulsory health insurance, social security pension insurance funds, and state welfare. During at least the first 6 weeks of sick leave, an unchanged basic salary is paid by the employer. After week 6 and for a maximum of 78 weeks' cumulative duration of sick leave due to the same disease within 3 years, the companies providing compulsory health insurance provide ~70–90% of the lost income. Before this 78-week limit is reached, the patient should be referred to a comprehensive multidisciplinary rehabilitation program if restoration of work ability is feasible. After a maximum of 78 weeks of sick leave, the income depends on the determination of work disability and on formal criteria of the social security pension insurance fund or the labor office. Patients who meet criteria for work disability receive a disability pension provided by the social security pension insurance fund, and those who meet criteria for unemployment compensation receive payments by the state welfare department. Patients not meeting any formal criteria (e.g., minimum duration of work and payment to the compulsory insurance system) receive state welfare at the basic subsistence level.

Cost estimation. The indirect costs of illness were evaluated by means of the human capital approach. According to guidelines for socioeconomic evaluation (17), a top-down procedure was used in order to estimate costs from a societal perspective. The human capital approach takes into account all costs to society that arise from lost productivity (relating to paid work) in subjects of working age. All types of work loss due to RA were taken into account.

The mean cumulative number of work days lost during the periods time 0–time 2 and time 2–time 3 was calculated separately for each RA-related cause: 1) sick leave as certified by a physician, 2) work disability (i.e., total cessation of employment with social security pension), and 3) other work loss without social security payment. Lost productivity due to work disability and other work loss was counted from the day the individual patient left the labor force until the day the patient resumed working or reached retirement age (65 years).

Valuation of loss of productivity was performed according to guidelines for socioeconomic evaluation using population data (17): An estimate of the loss of productivity was then obtained by multiplying the ratio of the number of work days lost/year by the gross income of all gainfully employed workers/year. The result was then divided by the total number of labor force participants, multiplied by 365 days. These figures are based on gainful (paid) employment only. On the basis of 1994, 1995, and 1996 population data (time 2) (18), the costs of lost productivity were calculated at approximately \$93 (US) per person per day (range \$91–94), e.g., gross income of all gainfully employed workers in 1995 = \$1.060 billion and number of labor force participants in 1995 = 31.209 million, yielding the equation $\$1{,}060{,}460{,}000{,}000/31{,}209{,}000 \times 365 = \$93$. Costs were converted to US dollars for reasons of better comparability with other studies, by applying an average of 1.51 German marks to 1 US dollar for the period 1994–1996 (according to the statistics of the German National Bank).

The cumulative number of days of lost productivity was calculated separately for each patient and each cause of RA-related work loss and was subsequently valuated. Since the defined followup periods (time 0–time 2 and time 2–time 3) were of different lengths, the pertinent costs that were incurred in these periods were compared in terms of annual costs. The results are presented as mean ± SEM annual costs per patient at risk for loss of productivity. The analysis takes into account only lost productivity arising while a patient represents "human capital" to society (up to the retirement age of 65 years).

Sensitivity analyses. Variation of the valuation of lost productivity has an impact on overall indirect costs. The following issues may have influenced the amount of indirect costs calculated: 1) valuation of lost productivity of RA patients based on the average income in Germany, 2) 18% dropout rate among the patients, and 3) exclusion of patients not in the labor force at the time of symptom onset. In order to address these issues, sensitivity analyses were applied. First, costs were recalculated valuating lost productivity according to individual income. Subsequently, the costs were estimated assuming that inclusion of the patients who dropped out of the study might have resulted in a 20% higher or lower average income than that of the 133 patients included. Finally, indirect costs were recalculated for all consecutive patients with RA who had a history of employment prior to the onset of RA symptoms.

Outcomes definition. In order to identify indicators for a favorable change in RA-related costs, a multivariate regression analysis was performed for assessment of the correlation between changes in the cost factor "lost productivity" and a series of clinical, occupational, social, and psychological variables. The dichotomous outcome changes in lost productivity from the period time 0–time 2 to the period time 2–time 3 was defined as follows: a favorable outcome was assumed when 1) a ≥20% reduction in sickness-related absence was found in patients who had had >21 days of sick leave or 2) no change in sickness-related absence was found in patients who had had <21 days of sick leave. In contrast, an unfavorable outcome was assumed when 1) a ≥20% increase in sickness-related absence was found in patients who had had <21 days of sick leave, 2) no changes in sickness-related absence were found in patients who had had >21 days of sick leave, or 3) patients had stopped working because of the disease (work disability or other work loss).

Generally, the independent variables were dichotomized in order to yield 2 groups: the 25% of patients with the best outcome (highest functional scores) and the other 3 quartiles combined. A favorable change in these variables was assumed if a patient stayed in the quartile with the best outcome or if 20% improvement in the symptoms occurred. Stability of poor symptoms or worsening of symptoms was assumed in all other cases. Independent occupational variables were dichotomized according to the categories "difficulties" and "no difficulties" with required job tasks during followup. In order to control for a possible positive influence of treatment, medication variables were analyzed. Usage of disease-modifying antirheumatic drugs (DMARDs) was assessed on the basis of the drug with the longest duration of application in the period time 0–time 3. In addition, the variables "DMARD-therapy at time 3" and "corticosteroids at time 3" were recorded. The average daily dosage of corticosteroids and the duration of any DMARD therapy between time 0 and time 3 were documented. Psychological assessment was based on a depression scale, with possible scores ranging from 0 (no depression) to 48 (highest level of depression) (19).

Statistical analysis. Statistical analyses were performed using an SPSS 7.0 database. In univariate pretesting, a P value of <0.1 was required for inclusion into stepwise backward multivariate analyses. Multivariate testing was performed in 3 subgroups: clinical and psychological variables, medication, and occupational variables ($P < 0.1$). For the final model, the level of significance was set at $P < 0.05$. All parameters identified at a significance level of $P < 0.1$ in the multivariate subgroup models were included in the final analyses ($P < 0.05$). Odds ratios (OR) with 95% confidence intervals are presented for the variables in the final model.

RESULTS

Of the 133 patients who were participating in the labor force at the time of onset of RA symptoms, 78 (59%) continued working until time 3, 23 (17%) stopped working and received disability payments, 12 (9%) lost work because of RA but did not receive a disability pension, and 20 (15%) left the labor force for reasons

Table 2. Mean ± SEM number of days of lost productivity per year in the periods time 0–time 2, time 2–time 3, and time 0–time 3

		Sick leave			Work disability			Other work loss			
Period	No. of patients at risk for lost productivity	No. of patients experiencing sick leave	Lost-productivity days per patient experiencing sick leave	Lost-productivity days per gainfully employed patient	No. of patients experiencing work disability	Lost-productivity days per patient experiencing work disability	Lost-productivity days per gainfully employed patient	No. of patients experiencing other work loss	Lost-productivity days per patient experiencing other work loss	Lost-productivity days per gainfully employed patient	Total
Time 0–time 2	133	109	139 ± 12	113 ± 11	14	119 ± 12	13 ± 4	6	199 ± 17	9 ± 4	135 ± 11
Time 2–time 3	113	40	90 ± 8	27 ± 6	9	171 ± 14	49 ± 10	6	298 ± 22	30 ± 8	106 ± 13
Time 0–time 3	133	112	103 ± 10	82 ± 8	23	155 ± 14	27 ± 6	12	189 ± 18	17 ± 6	126 ± 11

unrelated to RA (data not shown). Over the entire observation period (time 0–time 3), an average of 82 days of sick leave per person-year was reported, accounting for mean annual costs of $7,640 (Tables 2 and 3). Twenty-seven days of lost productivity per person-year due to work disability and 17 days due to other RA-related loss of work accounted for indirect costs of $2,520 and $1,590, respectively. These cost components totaled an average indirect cost of $11,750 per person-year (due to 126 days of lost productivity) for the whole period.

At the beginning of the first period studied, all 133 gainfully employed patients were at risk for days of lost productivity, compared with 113 patients who were still at risk at the beginning of the second period (133 patients − 14 patients with work disability − 6 patients with other work loss between time 0 and time 2).

When the periods time 0–time 2 and time 2–time 3 were compared, a change in the relation of cost components per person-year was seen. Lost productivity due to sick leave accounted for 84% of overall lost productivity within the first assessment period, compared with only 25% in the second assessment period. In contrast, lost productivity related to work disability or other work loss increased from the first to the second period. The marked, 4.2-fold reduction in lost productivity due to sick leave (from 113 days in the first period to 27 days in the second period) exceeded the 3.6-fold increase found for lost productivity due to work disability and other work loss (for lost productivity days due to work disability and other work loss, respectively, 13 days and 9 days in the first period, versus 49 days and 30 days in the second period). This resulted in an overall decrease in lost productivity of 21% (from 135 lost productivity days to 106 lost productivity days).

Sensitivity analyses revealed that indirect overall costs might range from $7,180 to $11,750. Valuation of lost productivity using individuals' earnings resulted in 24% lower costs per patient (mean ± SEM $8,980 ± 770) compared with the costs obtained according to standardized evaluation ($11,750 ± 1,120). Calculating indirect costs according to the assumption that the individual average income might be 20% higher or lower than the average of $2,090 due to the patients who were lost to followup yielded a range of $7,180–10,780. Inclusion of the 64 patients who were not employed at the time of symptom onset but had a history of employment prior to onset and were younger than 65 years yielded lower costs per patient with RA ($7,930), since only 6 patients started working after the onset of RA symptoms; thus, overall costs remained basically unchanged, and relative costs per patient decreased.

Correlations between reduced loss of productivity and clinical, occupational, and treatment variables are shown in Table 4. While reduced numbers of affected joints and improvement in physical function, pain, and depression scores were related to a favorable outcome in terms of lost productivity in univariate analyses, pain reduction was the only clinical parameter that remained (highly) significant in multivariate analyses. With regard to

Table 3. Mean ± SEM costs (US dollars) per person-year, for gainfully employed patients

Period	Sick leave	Work disability	Other work loss	Total
Time 0–time 2	10,530 ± 990	1,210 ± 360	840 ± 370	12,580 ± 1,030
Time 2–time 3	2,520 ± 580	4,570 ± 960	2,800 ± 780	9,890 ± 1,210
Time 0–time 3	7,640 ± 740	2,520 ± 550	1,590 ± 480	11,750 ± 1,120

Table 4. Univariate and multivariate logistic regression of potential variables associated with reduction of lost productivity*

	Reduction of lost productivity†		Univariate analysis		Multivariate analysis of subgroups‡	
Subgroup, independent variable	Yes	No	*P*	OR	*P*	OR
Clinical parameters						
Female sex	27 (39)	16 (36)	NS			
Age (years) at time 1	45 ± 1.1	48 ± 1.5	NS			
Improvement of tender joints	49 (72)	23 (51)	0.05	2.2	NS	
Improvement of swollen joints	50 (74)	22 (49)	0.006	3.1	NS	
Improvement of pain score (VAS)	58 (85)	25 (56)	0.0005	4.9	0.0008	5.2
Improvement of physical functioning	42 (63)	17 (38)	0.02	2.6	NS	
Improvement of ESR	56 (82)	36 (80)	NS			
Improvement of depression	29 (63)	25 (46)	0.02	2.6	NS	
Medical treatment						
Steroids at time 3	18 (25)	22 (51)	0.01	0.4	0.03	0.4
Average daily steroid dosage (mg prednisolone)	4.8 ± 2.0	9.3 ± 3.7	NS			
Treatment with DMARDs (% of disease duration)	66 ± 3.0	67 ± 2.8	NS			
Longest DMARD: methotrexate	19 (27)	24 (56)	0.005	0.3	0.01	0.4
Longest DMARD: sulfasalazine	18 (27)	10 (22)	NS			
Longest DMARD: gold salts (IM)	16 (24)	6 (13)	NS			
DMARD treatment at time 3	49 (72)	40 (89)	0.05	0.3	NS	
No problems due to specified labor condition						
Working hours	40 (76)	20 (35)	0.0000	7.5	NS	
Shift work	49 (94)	54 (93)	NS			
Contract work	49 (94)	54 (93)	NS			
Time pressure	14 (88)	15 (94)	NS			
Rigid schedule	47 (89)	41 (72)	0.008	3.8	NS	
Working speed	38 (72)	23 (40)	0.0000	6.7	0.004	4.1
Colleagues without consideration of illness	22 (49)	23 (47)	NS			
Outdoor work	47 (89)	36 (64)	0.001	4.6	0.04	3.1
Cold/heat exposure	39 (74)	26 (46)	0.0009	4.0	NS	
Sitting	42 (79)	40 (71)	NS			
Walking	35 (66)	19 (34)	0.0001	5.7	NS	
Standing	37 (70)	12 (21)	0.0000	10.0	0.0004	7.1
Overhead work	43 (81)	30 (54)	0.0006	4.5	NS	
Kneeling	45 (85)	34 (61)	0.001	4.5	NS	
Bending	38 (72)	25 (45)	0.0000	6.0	NS	
Climbing stairs	42 (79)	21 (38)	0.0000	7.3	NS	
Using grip force	28 (53)	8 (14)	0.0003	8.2	NS	
Manual precision work/writing	36 (68)	22 (39)	0.002	3.5	NS	
Carrying heavy loads	35 (66)	23 (41)	0.008	3.0	NS	
Other strenuous work	43 (81)	36 (64)	0.004	3.7	NS	

* OR = odds ratio; NS = not significant ($P > 0.1$), VAS = visual analog scale, ESR = erythrocyte sedimentation rate; DMARDs = disease-modifying antirheumatic drugs; IM = intramuscular.
† Age at time 1, daily steroid dosage, and % of disease duration treated with DMARDs are the mean ± SEM; other values are the number (%).
‡ Only parameters that were significant in the univariate analysis were tested in the multivariate analysis of the subgroups.

the analysis of medication variables, less frequent use of steroids, less frequent use of methotrexate (as the longest DMARD taken in the period time 1–time 3), and less frequent use of DMARDs at time 3 were seen in patients who had a favorable work loss outcome. In the occupational analysis, patients with a favorable outcome less frequently reported problems with regard to most of the working conditions assessed.

All variables identified in the subgroup analyses were tested in the final logistic regression model. The variables in the clinical and psychological characteristics subgroup and the medication subgroup did not contribute significantly to the explanation of the variance in indirect costs. Strong associations between the occupational characteristics "no problems with standing," "no problems with speed of performance," and "no problems with outdoor work" and the reduction of lost productivity were found (OR 7.1, 4.1, and 3.1, respectively) (Table 5).

DISCUSSION

In the present study high indirect annual costs of $11,750 were identified even in the early phase of RA. The

Table 5. Final model of the mulitvariate logistic regression analysis for reduction of lost productivity*

Independent variable	OR (95% CI)
No problems with standing	7.1 (2.4–21.1)
No problems with working speed	4.1 (1.6–10.9)
No problems with outdoor work	3.1 (1.1–9.1)

* R^2 = 0.43. OR = odds ratio; 95% CI = 95% confidence interval.

comparability of the results of the present study with those of other studies is limited (20), mainly due to differences in methods of cost estimation, valuation of lost productivity, and basic characteristics of the study populations.

To date, there has only been 1 published study on indirect costs in early RA (21). This study, conducted in Sweden, showed costs that were clearly lower ($5,610 per patient per year) than those found in the present investigation. An explanation might be that costs related to short-term sick leave were not taken into account, and the authors discuss an underestimation of indirect costs due to the valuation method applied. Furthermore, the present study focused on gainfully employed patients who were at risk of loss of productivity at the onset of symptoms, possibly leading to higher indirect costs.

Results of studies focusing on annual indirect costs in advanced RA differ widely (between $1,200 and $21,000 per patient) (1–4,22,23). Liang and coworkers (23) demonstrated approximate indirect costs of $10,000 expressed in 1995 terms, similar to the results of the present study. Studies from Great Britain and Canada (1,4) showed lower costs than those found in the present study. Annual indirect costs of $4,100 US (1) and $2,165 Cdn (corresponding to $1,670 US) in the late 1980s (4) and $1,597 Cdn (corresponding to $1,200 US) in the early 1990s (4) were found. A conservative approach to estimating the incidence of lost productivity was applied in the British study (1); only work disability was considered, probably leading to a finding of lower overall indirect costs. The lower indirect costs reported by the Canadian group (4) can be explained mainly by the markedly higher average age in the Canadian sample compared with the present cohort (61 years versus 47 years), with indirect costs decreasing substantially in patients over 65 years old.

Two cost-of-illness studies showed higher average indirect costs (3,22). The results of the American study (3) are based on the estimation of lost wages; this method yields results that are not directly comparable with those derived using the human capital approach. Still, expressing indirect costs in 1995 terms would result in even higher costs than were found in the present study (approximately $16,000). In the Swedish intervention study (22), the reported indirect annual costs of RA were clearly higher than in our study, amounting to $21,000 per patient. This might be due to a markedly higher valuation of a day of lost productivity compared with the present study ($150 versus $93). A decrease in indirect costs after initiation of DMARD therapy was shown.

A comparison with the results of other investigations shows that overall indirect costs incurred within the first 3 years of RA equal those arising in advanced stages of the disease. While one might expect that indirect costs would increase as the disease progresses, this assumption is not supported by the findings of the present study. In fact, an overall reduction in indirect costs of 21% within the first 3 years was found in the present study. This is due to the fact that the decrease in costs caused by sick leave exceeds the increase in costs due to work disability and other RA-related work loss.

The number of RA-related hospital days was not assessed separately from other RA-related work-absence days. Since lost-productivity days are not valuated differently, the results of the present cost estimation are not influenced by the number of work-absence days in which the patient was hospitalized.

There are no comparable data available in the literature for the outcome lost productivity. However, in studies focusing on work disability in patients with early RA, physically demanding work and nonadministrative jobs were found to be important predictive factors for RA-related work disability (11,12,24). These observations support the assumption that patient coping with strenuous working conditions might be related to the occurrence of lost productivity, and thus to indirect costs as well.

The present study focused on the estimation of indirect costs from the societal perspective, using the human capital approach. Traditionally, the human capital approach has been used in cost-of-illness studies for the assessment of indirect costs from society's perspective (25,26), but the following limitation has to be considered: This approach has the disadvantage that homemakers, children, students, unemployed persons, and retirees are not taken into account since they do not receive salaries. An additional valuation of unpaid work (i.e., via opportunity costs) (25,26) was not applied in the present study because the study focused on details of paid work in the course of the disease, and hence only patients who were in the labor force at the outset of the study were considered.

In conclusion, high indirect costs in early RA, reaching the extent of those associated with advanced RA, were demonstrated in this study. Examination of the change in indirect costs in the first 3 years of the disease revealed a decrease due to a reduced frequency of sick leave. Given the positive correlation between favorable cost changes and absence of problems due to strenuous working conditions, we would assume that apart from controlling disease activity by adequate treatment, improvement of working conditions, e.g., by early intensified vocational rehabilitation, could be an approach to reducing indirect costs in the future. Further studies are necessary to evaluate the cost-effectiveness of such interventions.

ACKNOWLEDGMENTS

The authors thank all of the investigators involved in the multicenter data collection (see Patients and Methods). In particular, we would like to express our gratitude to Ms Helga Weber and Ms Martina Bornmann for their support in establishing the cohort.

REFERENCES

1. McIntosh E. The cost of rheumatoid arthritis. Br J Rheumatol 1996;35:781–90.
2. Yelin EH. The cost of rheumatoid arthritis: absolute, incremental, and marginal estimates. J Rheumatol Suppl 1996;44:47–51.
3. Meenan RF, Yelin EH, Henke CJ, Curtis DL, Epstein WV. The costs of rheumatoid arthritis: a patient-oriented study of chronic disease costs. Arthritis Rheum 1978;21:827–33.
4. Clarke AE, Zowall H, Levinton C, Assimakopoulos H, Sibley JT, Haga M, et al. Direct and indirect medical costs incurred by Canadian patients with rheumatoid arthritis: a 12 year study. J Rheumatol 1997;24:1051–60.
5. Gabriel SE, Crowson CS, Campion ME, O'Fallon WM. Indirect and nonmedical costs among people with rheumatoid arthritis and osteoarthritis compared with nonarthritic controls. J Rheumatol 1997;24:43–8.
6. Gabriel SE, Crowson CS, Luthra HS, Wagner JL, O'Fallon WM. Modeling the lifetime costs of rheumatoid arthritis. J Rheumatol 1999;26:1269–74.
7. Rothfuss J, Mau W, Zeidler H, Brenner MH. Socioeconomic evaluation of rheumatoid arthritis and osteoarthritis: a literature review. Semin Arthritis Rheum 1997;26:771–9.
8. Yelin EH. Musculoskeletal conditions and employment. Arthritis Care Res 1995;8:311–7.
9. Fex E, Larsson BM, Nived K, Eberhardt K. Effect of rheumatoid arthritis on work status and social and leisure time activities in patients followed 8 years from onset. J Rheumatol 1998;25:44–50.
10. Sany J, Dropsy R, Daures JP. Cross-sectional epidemiological survey of rheumatoid arthritis patients seen in private practice in France: descriptive results (1629 cases). Rev Rhum Engl Ed 1998;65:462–70.
11. Doeglas D, Suurmeijer T, Krol B, Sanderman R, van Leeuwen M, van Rijswijk M. Work disability in early rheumatoid arthritis. Ann Rheum Dis 1995;54:455–60.
12. Eberhardt K, Larsson BM, Nived K. Early rheumatoid arthritis: some social, economical, and psychological aspects. Scand J Rheumatol 1993;22:119–23.
13. Mau W, Bornmann M, Weber H, Weidemann HF, Hecker H, Raspe HH. Prediction of permanent work disability in a follow-up study of early rheumatoid arthritis: results of a tree structured analysis using RECPAM. Br J Rheumatol 1996;35:652–9.
14. Van Jaarsveld CHM, Jacobs JWG, Schrijvers AJP, van Albada-Kuipers GA, Hofman DM, Bijlsma JWJ. Effects of rheumatoid arthritis on employment and social participation during the first years of disease in the Netherlands. Br J Rheumatol 1998;37:848–53.
15. Mau W, Bornmann M, Weber H. The occurrence of sick leave in the first year of rheumatoid arthritis: a comparison with the members of the compulsory health insurance. Z Rheumatol 1997;56:1–7.
16. Arnett FC, Edworthy SM, Bloch DA, McShane DJ, Fries JF, Cooper NS, et al. The American Rheumatism Association 1987 revised criteria for the classification of rheumatoid arthritis. Arthritis Rheum 1988;31:315–24.
17. Graf von der Schulenburg JM, Greiner W, Schöffski O, Schumacher MAI, Bestehorn K, Brecht JG, et al. Consensusgroup "Health Economics." PharmacoEconomics Outcomes News 1996;56:4-6.
18. Statistisches Bundesamt. Statistical yearbook 1996 for the Federal Republic of Germany. Wiesbaden: Metzler Poeschel; 1996.
19. Von Zerssen D, Koeller DM. Paranoid-Depressivitäts-Skala: Klinische Selbstbeurteilungs-Skalen (Ksb-S) aus dem Münchener Psychiatrischen Information System (PSYCHIS München). Weinheim (Germany): Beltz; 1976.
20. Ruof J, Hülsemann JL, Stucki G. Evaluation of costs in rheumatic diseases: a literature review. Curr Opin Rheumatol 1999;11:104–9.
21. Kobelt G, Eberhardt K, Jönsson L, Jönsson B. Economic consequences of the progression of rheumatoid arthritis in Sweden. Arthritis Rheum 1999;42:347–56.
22. Magnusson S. Treatment of rheumatoid arthritis: does it affect society's cost for the disease? Br J Rheumatol 1996;35:791–5.
23. Liang MH, Larson M, Thompson M, Eaton H, McNamara E, Katz R, et al. Costs and outcomes in rheumatoid arthritis and osteoarthritis. Arthritis Rheum 1984;27:522–9.
24. Allaire SH, Anderson JJ, Meenan RF. Reducing work disability associated with rheumatoid arthritis: identification of additional risk factors and persons likely to benefit from intervention. Arthritis Care Res 1996;9:349–57.
25. Schöffski O, Glaser P, Graf von der Schulenburg JM. Gesundheitsökonomische Evaluationen: Grundlagen und Standortbestimmung. Berlin, Heidelberg: Springer-Verlag; 1998.
26. Koopmanschap MA. Complementary analyses in economic evaluation of health care [dissertation]. Rotterdam: Erasmus University; 1994.

ARTHRITIS & RHEUMATISM
Vol. 44, No. 3, March 2001, pp 535–540

Influence of Shared Epitope–Negative HLA–DRB1 Alleles on Genetic Susceptibility to Rheumatoid Arthritis

Denis Reviron,[1] Aleth Perdriger,[2] Eric Toussirot,[3] Daniel Wendling,[3] Nathalie Balandraud,[4] Sandrine Guis,[5] Gilbert Semana,[6] Pierre Tiberghien,[7] Pierre Mercier,[8] and Jean Roudier[9]

Objective. **Most patients with rheumatoid arthritis (RA) express the shared epitope (SE). It is not known whether SE-negative HLA–DRB1 alleles influence the development of RA. This study examined the influence of SE-negative HLA–DR alleles (DRB1*X) on the development of RA in 3 different French populations.**

Methods. **HLA–DRB1 alleles were defined by polymerase chain reaction with sequence-specific oligonucleotide hybridization or sequence-specific primers. SE-negative alleles were classified according to the electric charge of their P4 pocket. HLA–DRB1 alleles *0103, *0402, *07, *08, *11 (except *1107), *12, and *13 have a neutral or negative P4 charge and are called DRB1*XP4n. HLA–DRB1*03, *0403, *0406, *0407, *0901, *1107, *14, *15, and *16 have a positive P4 charge and are called DRB1*XP4p.**

Results. **Among the SE-negative subjects, DRB1 genotypes with 1 or 2 DRB1*XP4n alleles were significantly overrepresented in the control subjects compared with the RA patients, whereas DRB1*XP4p/XP4p genotypes were equally represented in the patients and controls. In single-dose SE–positive subjects, SE/XP4n genotypes were equally represented in the patients and controls. However, SE/XP4p genotypes were significantly overrepresented in the RA patients.**

Conclusion. **The DRB1*X allele polymorphism influences susceptibility to RA. Alleles that have a neutral or negative electric charge in their P4 pocket (DRB1*XP4n), such as DRB1*0103, *0402, *07, *08, *11 (except *1107), *12, and *13, protect against RA. Alleles that have a positive electric charge in their P4 pocket (DRB1*XP4p), such as DRB1*03, *0403, *0406, *0407, *0901, *1107, *14, *15, and *16, have no influence on the predisposition to RA.**

Rheumatoid arthritis (RA), a chronic inflammatory joint disease, is strongly associated with HLA–DRB1 alleles whose third hypervariable region contains the shared epitope (SE), a conserved 5–amino acid motif (1). The most common SE-positive alleles in Western Europe are DRB1*0401, *0404, *0405, *0408, *0101, *0102, and *1001. A dose effect has been observed in SE-positive HLA–DRB1 genotypes. Indeed, SE/SE (double-dose) genotypes confer a higher risk than do SE/X (single-dose) genotypes (2,3). SE/X (single-dose) genotypes confer a higher risk than do X/X (SE-negative) genotypes. This dose effect is still unexplained.

In this study, we tested the hypothesis that, in addition to the predisposing effect of SE-positive alleles, SE-negative alleles might also influence the predisposition to RA. We focused on polymorphic residues of the P4 pocket. Indeed, the β1 chains of HLA–DR molecules contain polymorphic residues contributing to 5 binding pockets: P1, P4, P6, P7, and P9. These pockets influence the peptide-binding specificity of different class II molecules (4). The SE contributes to the P4 pocket. Of the 4 polymorphic residues of the P4 pocket, only 3 (residues 70, 71, and 74) are contained in the SE. Residue 13 is encoded by the first hypervariable region of DRB1.

Supported by grants from INSERM, PHRC 1997, Societé Française de Rhumatologie, Association de Recherche sur la Polyarthrite.

[1]Denis Reviron, MD, PhD: EFS Alpes Méditerranée, Marseilles, France, and INSERM E9940, Faculté de Médecine, Marseilles, France; [2]Aleth Perdriger, MD, PhD: University Hospital, Rennes, France; [3]Eric Toussirot, MD, PhD, Daniel Wendling, MD: Hôpital Minjoz, Besançon, France; [4]Nathalie Balandraud, MD: INSERM E9940, Faculté de Médecine, Marseilles, France; [5]Sandrine Guis, MD: Hôpital La Conception, Marseilles, France; [6]Gilbert Semana, MD, PhD: EFS Bretagne, Rennes, France; [7]Pierre Tiberghien, MD, PhD: EFS Bourgogne Franche Comté, Besançon, France; [8]Pierre Mercier, MD: EFS Alpes Méditerranée, Marseilles, France; [9]Jean Roudier, MD, PhD: INSERM E9940, Faculté de Médecine, Marseilles, France, and Hôpital La Conception, Marseilles, France.

Address correspondence and reprint requests to Jean Roudier, MD, PhD, INSERM EPI9940, Faculté de Médecine, 13005 Marseilles, France.

Submitted for publication February 11, 2000; accepted in revised form October 23, 2000.

Table 1. Polymorphic residues of HLA–DR pocket 4 (DRβ1 chain)*

	DRB1*																			
													0801							1301
													0802	1101						1302
		0404				0301	0403			1501			0803	1104						1304
		0405		0101		0302	0406			1502			0804	1106						1102
	0401	0408	1001	0102	1402	1109	0407	0901	1401	1503	1601	0701	0805	1305	1201	1303	1309	0402	0103	1103
β-chain position																				
13	H	H	F	F	S	S	H	F	S	R	R	Y	G	S	G	S	S	H	F	S
70	Q	Q	R	Q	Q	Q	Q	R	R	Q	D	D	D	D	D	D	Q	D	D	D
71	K	R	R	R	R	K	R	R	R	A	R	R	R	R	R	K	A	E	E	E
74	A	A	A	A	A	R	E	E	E	A	A	Q	L	A	A	A	A	A	A	A
78	Y	Y	Y	Y	Y	Y	Y	V	Y	Y	Y	V	Y	Y	Y	Y	Y	Y	Y	Y
Electric charge	++	++	++	+	+	++	+	+	+	+	+	N	N	N	N	N	N	−	−−	−−
Type	SE	SE	SE	SE	SE	XP4p	XP4p	XP4p	XP4p	XP4p	XP4p	XP4n	XP4n	XP4n	XP4n	XP4n	XP4n	XP4n	XP4n	XP4n

* Two kinds of DRB1*X alleles are distinguished according to the electric charge in their P4 pocket: DRB1*X P4 positive (XP4p) and DRB1*X P4 neutral or negative (XP4n). N = neutral; SE = shared epitope.

PATIENTS AND METHODS

Patients and controls. Two hundred RA patients and 200 controls from Marseilles (Southern France), 120 RA patients and 101 controls from Besançon (Eastern France), and 197 RA patients and 200 controls from Rennes (Western France) were studied. In these 3 populations, RA is associated with SE-positive HLA–DR alleles (5–7). Every RA patient fulfilled at least 4 of the 1987 American College of Rheumatology (formerly, the American Rheumatism Association) criteria for RA (8).

The 3 control groups comprised voluntary bone marrow/blood donors from the same geographic area. All patients and controls were European Caucasians.

HLA genotyping. HLA–DRB1 typing was done using polymerase chain reaction (PCR) and sequence-specific oligonucleotide hybridization with ddUTP-labeled probes (SSOP) according to the Twelfth International Histocompatibility Workshop reference protocol (9), and/or PCR and sequence-specific primers (10). All subjects were first typed for generic DRB1 loci to define a generic DRB1 type. Then, a 2-step specific amplification using primers for group-specific amplification and hybridization with particular sets of SSOP was achieved to define the DRB1-specific typing for each group of alleles.

P4 pocket polymorphism. Amino acids 13, 70, 71, 74, and 78 in the β chain determine the specificity of the P4 pocket. We defined 2 types of DRB1*X alleles according to the total electric charge in their P4 pocket: DRB1*X P4 positive (XP4p) and DRB1*X P4 neutral or negative (XP4n) (Table 1). This allowed us to distinguish 6 genotypes of DRB1: SE/SE, SE/XP4p, SE/XP4n, XP4p/XP4p, XP4p/XP4n, and XP4n/XP4n. It must be noted that SE-positive alleles have a positively charged P4 pocket.

Statistical analysis. Statistical significance of the differences in genotype frequency between patients and controls was evaluated by chi-square test with 1 degree of freedom or by Fisher's test if any value in the 2 × 2 contingency table was <5. The P values were corrected (P_{corr}) by the number of comparisons made (Bonferroni correction). Odds ratios (OR) and 95% confidence intervals were calculated according to Woolf's method; Haldane's correction was used when any value was null (11).

Table 2. DRB1 genotype frequencies according to the electric charge in their P4 pocket in 200 RA patients versus 200 controls in the Marseilles population*

	RA patients		Controls					
DRB1/DRB1	No.	%	No.	%	OR	95% CI	P	P_{corr}
SE/SE	39	19.5	7	3.5	6.7	2.9–15.3	<0.0001	<0.0001
SE/X	114		56					
SE/XP4p	55	27.5	16	8.0	4.4	2.4–7.9	<0.0001	<0.001
SE/XP4n	59	29.5	40	20.0	1.7	1.1–2.7	<0.02	NS
X/X	47		137					
XP4p/XP4p	16	8.0	20	10.0	0.8	0.4–1.6	NS	NS
XP4p/XP4n	16	8.0	73	36.5	0.2	0.1–0.3	<0.0001	<0.0001
XP4n/XP4n	15	7.5	44	22.0	0.3	0.2–0.5	<0.0001	<0.0001

* RA = rheumatoid arthritis; OR = odds ratio; 95% CI = 95% confidence interval; P_{corr} = corrected P value (n = 6 comparisons); SE = shared epitope; XP4p = positive P4 charge; XP4n = negative P4 charge; NS = not significant.

Table 3. DRB1 genotype frequencies according to the electric charge in their P4 pocket in 120 RA patients versus 101 controls in the Besançon population*

	RA patients		Controls					
DRB1/DRB1	No.	%	No.	%	OR	95% CI	*P*	P_{corr}
SE/SE	31	25.8	6	5.9	5.5	2.1–16.8	<0.0001	<0.001
SE/X	57		28					
SE/XP4p	29	24.2	7	6.9	4.3	1.7–12.1	<0.0001	<0.001
SE/XP4n	28	23.3	21	20.8	1.2	0.6–2.3	NS	NS
X/X	32		67					
XP4p/XP4p	10	8.3	8	7.9	1.1	0.4–3.1	NS	NS
XP4p/XP4n	17	14.2	33	32.7	0.3	0.2–0.7	<0.005	<0.03
XP4n/XP4n	5	4.2	26	25.7	0.2	0.1–0.4	<0.001	<0.002

* See Table 2 for definitions.

RESULTS

DRB1 genotype frequencies in RA patients and controls from Marseilles (Table 2). *DRB1*SE/X individuals.* DRB1*SE/XP4p genotypes were significantly associated with RA (OR 4.4, $P_{corr} < 0.001$). Conversely, DRB1*SE/XP4n genotypes were not differently distributed between the RA patients and controls (OR 1.7, P_{corr} not significant [NS]). The distributions of SE/XP4p and SE/XP4n genotypes in patients and controls were different ($P < 0.02$). Thus, it seems that in individuals with DRB1*SE/XP4n, the presence of DRB1*XP4n contradicts the susceptibility effect of the SE.

*DRB1*X/X individuals.* Two genotype groups were significantly underrepresented in RA patients: DRB1*XP4p/XP4n (OR 0.2, $P_{corr} < 0.0001$) and DRB1*XP4n/XP4n (OR 0.3, $P_{corr} < 0.0001$). The distribution of DRB1*X/X genotypes with an XP4n allele between patients and controls was significantly different from that of DRB1*XP4p/XP4p genotypes ($P < 0.01$). Therefore, genotypes containing DRB1*XP4n seem to protect against RA.

DRB1*XP4p/XP4p genotypes were not differently distributed between RA patients and controls (OR 0.8, P_{corr} NS). Therefore, DRB1*XP4p does not predispose to RA. The Marseilles data suggest that DRB1*XP4n alleles exert a protective effect against RA, independent of the presence of an SE-positive allele. Conversely, DRB1*XP4p alleles do not predispose to RA.

DRB1 genotype frequencies in RA patients and controls from Besançon (Table 3) and Rennes (Table 4). The Besançon and Rennes data, highly similar to the Marseilles data, also suggest that DRB1*XP4n alleles exert a protective effect against RA, independent of the presence of an SE-positive allele. Conversely, the data from these 2 groups indicate that DRB1*XP4p alleles do not predispose individuals to RA.

Influence of different DRB1*XP4p alleles in individuals with SE/XP4p (Table 5). In the 3 populations that we studied, DRB1*03 and DRB1*15 were the most common XP4p alleles. No XP4p allele was overrepresented in RA patients versus controls in any of the 3 populations.

Table 4. DRB1 genotype frequencies according to the electric charge in their P4 pocket in 197 RA patients versus 200 controls in the Rennes population*

	RA patients		Controls					
DRB1/DRB1	No.	%	No.	%	OR	95% CI	*P*	P_{corr}
SE/SE	59	29.9	11	5.5	7.3	3.6–15.4	<0.0001	<0.0001
SE/X	106		77					
SE/XP4p	58	29.4	36	18.0	1.9	1.2–3.1	<0.01	<0.05
SE/XP4n	48	24.4	41	20.5	1.2	0.8–2.0	NS	NS
X/X	32		112					
XP4p/XP4p	13	6.6	25	12.5	0.5	0.2–1.0	<0.05	NS
XP4p/XP4n	15	7.6	58	29.0	0.2	0.1–0.4	<0.0001	<0.0001
XP4n/XP4n	4	2.0	29	14.5	0.1	0.1–0.4	<0.0001	<0.0001

* See Table 2 for definitions.

Table 5. DRB1 XP4p allele frequency in individuals with SE/XP4p*

	Marseilles group				Besançon group				Rennes group			
	RA patients		Controls		RA patients		Controls		RA patients		Controls	
	No.	%	No.	%	No.	%	No.	%	No.	%	No.	%
DRB1*SE/XP4p	55	100	16	100	29	100	7	100	58	100	36	100
DRB1*SE/03	19	34.5	8	50.0	6	20.7	3	42.9	28	48.3	12	33.3
DRB1*SE/15	20	36.4	6	37.5	12	41.4	3	42.9	22	37.9	17	47.2
DRB1*SE/16	5	9.1	1	6.3	3	10.3	0	0.0	2	3.4	1	2.8
DRB1*SE/14	2	3.6	0	0.0	5	17.2	1	14.3	3	5.2	3	8.3
DRB1*SE/0901	4	7.3	0	0.0	0	0.0	0	0.0	0	0.0	1	2.8
DRB1*SE/0403	5	9.1	1	6.3	2	6.9	0	0.0	1	1.7	0	0.0
DRB1*SE/0407	0	0.0	0	0.0	1	3.4	0	0.0	2	3.4	2	5.6

* See Table 2 for definitions.

Influence of DRX alleles on SE/DRX genotypes containing DRB1*0401 or DRB1*0101 (Table 6). DRB1*0401 and DRB1*0101 were the most common SE-positive alleles in the 3 populations tested. Therefore, the influence of SE-negative alleles on individual SE-positive alleles was tested on DRB1*0401 and DRB1*0101 (Table 6).

DRB1*0401/XP4p genotypes were significantly associated with RA in the 3 populations, whereas DRB1*0401/XP4n genotypes were not. Because of the small number of individuals in this analysis, the difference between the distribution of DRB1*0401/XP4p and DRB1*0401/XP4n genotypes in patients and controls was significant in the Rennes group only ($P < 0.01$). Similarly, DRB1*0101/XP4p genotypes were significantly associated with RA in the first 2 populations, whereas DRB1*0101/XP4n genotypes were not. Because of the small number of individuals in this analysis, the difference between the distribution of DRB1*0101/XP4p and DRB1*0101/XP4n genotypes in patients and controls was significant in the Besançon group only ($P < 0.05$).

XP4n alleles and protection against extraarticular disease. Early RA studies have suggested that the SE increases the severity of RA (12). In this study, we compared the frequency of extraarticular disease (nodules and/or vasculitis) between patients with SE/XP4p and those with SE/XP4n. This analysis performed on the

Table 6. Influence of the DRX allele on SE/DRX genotypes containing DRB1*0401 or DRB1*0101*

Group, DRB1/DRB1†	RA patients		Controls		OR	95% CI	P	P_{corr}‡
	No.	%	No.	%				
Marseilles group								
DRB1*0401/XP4p	14	7.0	2	1.0	7.5	1.7–33.2	<0.003	<0.02
DRB1*0401/XP4n	11	5.5	6	3.0	1.9	0.7–5.2	NS	NS
DRB1*0101/XP4p	25	12.5	8	4.0	3.4	1.5–7.8	<0.003	<0.02
DRB1*0101/XP4n	22	11.0	17	8.5	1.3	0.7–2.6	NS	NS
Besançon group								
DRB1*0401/XP4p	10	8.3	1	1.0	9.1	1.1–72.3	<0.02	<0.05
DRB1*0401/XP4n	6	5.0	5	5.0	1.0	0.3–3.4	NS	NS
DRB1*0101/XP4p	13	10.8	2	2.0	6.0	1.3–27.3	<0.01	<0.04
DRB1*0101/XP4n	14	11.7	13	12.9	0.9	0.4–2.1	NS	NS
Rennes group								
DRB1*0401/XP4p	37	18.8	12	6.0	3.6	1.8–7.2	<0.0002	<0.001
DRB1*0401/XP4n	17	8.6	20	10.0	0.9	0.4–1.7	NS	NS
DRB1*0101/XP4p	11	5.6	14	7.0	0.8	0.3–1.8	NS	NS
DRB1*0101/XP4n	16	8.1	12	6.0	1.4	0.6–3.0	NS	NS

* See Table 2 for definitions.

† For the Marseilles group, the differences between the distributions, in patients and controls, of DRB1*0401/XP4p and DRB1*0401/XP4n and of DRB1*0101/XP4p and DRB1*0101/XP4n were NS. For the Besançon group, only the difference between the distributions of DRB1*0101/XP4p and DRB1*0101/XP4n was significant ($P < 0.05$). For the Rennes group, only the difference between the distributions of DRB1*0401/XP4p and DRB1*0401/XP4n was significant ($P < 0.01$).

‡ n = 4 comparisons.

pooled population of patients from the 3 geographic areas (517 patients) suggests that extraarticular disease was less common in the patients with SE/XP4n (17%) than in the patients with SE/XP4p (29%) ($P < 0.02$).

DISCUSSION

In this study, we tested whether SE-negative HLA–DRB1 alleles (DRB1*X alleles) may influence susceptibility to RA. DRB1*X alleles were classified in 2 groups according to the charge of their P4 pocket: DRB1*XP4 positive (DRB1*XP4p) and DRB1*XP4 neutral or negative (DRB1*XP4n). DRB1 genotypes were studied in 3 different French populations: Marseilles, a port on the Mediterranean whose population is of Greek descent; Besançon, in northeastern France, whose population is more Central European; and Rennes, in Bretagne, whose population is of Celtic origin.

In these 3 different areas of France, the association of RA with HLA–DR is not exactly the same. In Rennes, Besançon, and Marseilles, 80% of the patients with RA express SE-positive HLA–DR alleles. However, these alleles are not the same: in Rennes (Western France, Celtic population), DRB1*0401 is the most common SE-positive allele, expressed by 54% of the patients, and far exceeding the distribution of DRB1*01 (28%) and DRB1*0404 (12%) (6). Conversely, in Marseilles (Southeastern France, Latin/Greek population), DRB1*01 is the most common SE-positive allele in the patients (41%), in comparison with DRB1*0401 (25%) and DRB1*0404 (13%) (5). In Besançon (Northeastern France), the most common SE-positive allele in the patients is DRB1*01 (35%), slightly more than the frequencies of DRB1*0401 (28%) and DRB1*0404 (14%) (7). These differences parallel the differences in HLA–DR gene frequencies in each control population: DRB1*01 is a Mediterranean allele, whereas DRB1*0401 is Northern European.

Our main finding, validated in these 3 populations, is that alleles whose P4 pocket is negative or neutral (DRB1*XP4n alleles), which include HLA–DRB1*0103, *0402, *07, *08, *11 (except *1107), *12, and *13, protect against RA. This is true whether or not the other HLA–DR allele in the genotype contains the SE. Conversely, DRB1*XP4p alleles, which include DRB1*03, *0403, *0406, *0407, *0901, *1107, *14, *15, and *16, have no influence on the predisposition to RA.

Our data suggest that prediction of RA susceptibility through HLA–DR genotyping could be improved by distinguishing the 3 groups of alleles: SE-positive alleles (susceptible), XP4p alleles (neutral), and XP4n alleles (dominantly protective). According to this classification, HLA–DR genotypes predictive of RA are SE/SE and SE/XP4p, with relative risks of ~4, neutral genotypes are SE/XP4n and XP4p/XP4p, with relative risks of ~1, and protective genotypes are XP4n/XP4n and XP4p/XP4n, with relative risks of ~0.25.

Our data also raise the issue of the protective effect of XP4n alleles. How can an HLA–DRB1 allele with a neutral or negatively charged P4 pocket dominantly protect against RA? The simplest model for such protection is that XP4n alleles are able to bind peptides that XP4p or SE-positive alleles cannot bind, because a positively charged side chain on the peptide can only bind a neutral or negative P4 pocket. This could occur in the periphery and allow CD4 T cell recognition of particular antigens presented by HLA–DR, and/or could occur in the thymus, which could lead to selection of a particular repertoire by a positively charged peptide presented by HLA–DR.

Thus, our data obtained from 3 different populations in France suggest that HLA–DR–associated susceptibility to RA can be evaluated by analysis of the electric charge of the P4 pocket of both HLA–DR molecules expressed by a given individual. This can be seen as an extension of the shared epitope hypothesis; indeed, the shared epitope hypothesis suggests that SE-positive alleles (which have positively charged P4 pockets) are associated with an increased risk of developing RA, but does not consider the influence of SE-negative alleles on susceptibility. We show that among the SE-negative alleles, those with a negatively charged P4 pocket protect against the development of RA. This distinction allows more accurate evaluation, by HLA–DRB1 genotyping, of the risk of developing RA.

REFERENCES

1. Gregersen PK, Silver J, Winchester RJ. The shared epitope hypothesis: an approach to understanding the molecular genetics of susceptibility to rheumatoid arthritis. Arthritis Rheum 1987;30: 1205–13.
2. Wordsworth P, Pile K, Buckely J, Lanchbury J, Ollier B, Lathrop M, et al. HLA heterozygosity contributes to susceptibility to rheumatoid arthritis. Am J Hum Genet 1992;51:585–91.
3. Jawaheer D, Thomson W, MacGregor AJ, Carthy D, Davidson J, Dyer PA, et al. "Homozygosity" for the HLA–DR shared epitope contributes the highest risk for rheumatoid arthritis concordance in identical twins. Arthritis Rheum 1994;37:681–6.
4. Stern LJ, Brown JH, Jardetzky TS, Gorga JC, Urban RJ, Strominger JL, et al. Crystal structure of the human class II MHC protein HLA-DR1 complexed with an influenza virus peptide. Nature 1994;368:215–21.
5. Reviron D, Tezenas du Montcel S, Foutrier C, Guis S, Benazet JF,

Auquier P, et al. HLA-DRB1, DMA and DMB gene polymorphisms in rheumatoid arthritis. Human Immunol 1999;60:245–9.
6. Perdriger A, Guggenbuhl P, Chales G, Le Dantec P, Yaouanq J, Genetet B, et al. The role of HLA-DR-DR and HLA-DP-DP interactions in genetic susceptibility to rheumatoid arthritis. Human Immunol 1996;46:42–8.
7. Toussirot E, Auge B, Tiberghien P, Chabod J, Cedoz JP, Wendling D. HLA-DRB1 alleles and shared amino acid sequences in disease susceptibility and severity in patients from eastern France with rheumatoid arthritis. J Rheumatol 1999;26:1446–51.
8. Arnett FC, Edworthy SM, Bloch DA, McShane DJ, Fries JF, Cooper NS, et al. The American Rheumatism Association 1987 revised criteria for the classification of rheumatoid arthritis. Arthritis Rheum 1988;31:315–24.
9. Charron D, Fauchet R. Twelfth International Histocompatibility Workshop reference protocol Addendum 12-1994. Charron D, Fauchet R, editors. Paris (France): HLA et Médecine; 1994. p. 1–18.
10. Ollerup O, Zetterquist H. HLA-DR typing PCR amplification with sequence specific primers (PCR-SSP) in two hours: an alternative to DR serological typing in clinical practice including donor-recipient matching in cadaveric transplantation. Tissue Antigens 1992;39:225–35.
11. Haldane JBS. The estimation and significance of the logarithm of a ratio of frequencies. Ann Hum Genet 1955;20:309–15.
12. Harrison B, Thomson W, Symmons D, Ollier B, Wiles N, Payton T, et al. The influence of HLA–DRB1 alleles and rheumatoid factor on disease outcome in an inception cohort of patients with early inflammatory arthritis. Arthritis Rheum 1999;42:2174–83.

ARTHRITIS & RHEUMATISM
Vol. 44, No. 3, March 2001, pp 541–549

Lymph Draining From Foot Joints in Rheumatoid Arthritis Provides Insight Into Local Cytokine and Chemokine Production and Transport to Lymph Nodes

Waldemar L. Olszewski,[1] J. Pazdur,[2] E. Kubasiewicz,[2] M. Zaleska,[3] Conrad J. Cooke,[4] and Norman E. Miller[4]

Objective. **Rheumatoid arthritis (RA) is characterized by inflammatory reactions in joints and adjacent tissues unaccompanied by clinically evident changes in lymphatics and lymph nodes draining the inflamed areas. The explanation for this phenomenon, which contrasts with infectious processes in joints and soft tissues that evoke major changes in the lymphatic system, is unclear. To determine which inflammatory factors produced in the joints of RA patients are transported in lymph to lymph nodes, we measured levels of immunoglobulins, cytokines, and chemokines in prenodal lymph from the foot joints of RA patients and quantified their rate of transport to regional lymph nodes.**

Methods. **Lymph was collected from the cannulated lymphatics draining the foot joints, tendons, fascia, and skin of 20 RA patients. Lymph flow rate and concentrations of proteins and immunoglobulins were measured. Cytokine and chemokine levels were quantified by enzyme-linked immunosorbent assays. Results were compared with those obtained in 20 control subjects.**

Results. **In the cannulated vessel, the mean ± SEM lymph flow rate in RA patients was almost 2-fold that in control subjects (22.6 ± 3.2 ml/24 hours versus 13.2 ± 1.1 ml/24 hours; $P < 0.01$). Lymph concentrations of total protein, IgG, and IgM were 1.80 ± 0.14 gm/dl, 384 ± 45 mg/dl, and 32.0 ± 1.5 mg/dl, respectively, in RA patients and 1.66 ± 0.14 gm/dl, 238 ± 32 mg/dl, and 15.0 ± 1.3 mg/dl, respectively, in control subjects. The corresponding lymph:serum (L:S) ratios were 0.21 ± 0.02, 0.22 ± 0.02, and 0.15 ± 0.02, respectively, in RA patients and 0.22 ± 0.02, 0.19 ± 0.02, and 0.11 ± 0.02, respectively, in control subjects. The L:S ratios of <1 and the absence of significant differences between groups suggested a lack of local production of immunoglobulins. In RA patients, lymph concentrations (in pg/ml) were as follows: interleukin-1β (IL-1β) 14.8 ± 3.9, IL-6 511 ± 143, tumor necrosis factor α (TNFα) 9.9 ± 1.1, IL-1 receptor antagonist (IL-1Ra) 4,274 ± 737, IL-10 13.3 ± 4.4, IL-8 846 ± 174, IL-15 6.2 ± 0.9, granulocyte–macrophage colony-stimulating factor (GM-CSF) 2.30 ± 0.15, vascular endothelial growth factor (VEGF) 80.4 ± 8.6, and macrophage inflammatory protein 1α (MIP-1α) 171 ± 34. In control subjects, these values were as follows: IL-1β 1.50 ± 0.25, IL-6 79.0 ± 14.6, TNFα 4.4 ± 1.1, IL-1Ra 208 ± 52, IL-10 0.0, IL-8 216 ± 83, IL-15 5.00 ± 0.45, GM-CSF 0.40 ± 0.05, VEGF 42.0 ± 2.4, and MIP-1α 3.4 ± 1.7 ($P < 0.05$ versus RA patients for all except IL-15). The L:S ratio was >1 in all RA patient samples for IL-1β, IL-6, IL-1Ra, IL-8, GM-CSF, IL-10, IL-15, TNFα, and MIP-1α, indicating local production of cytokines. Great variability in lymph cytokine concentrations, presumably reflecting differences in the intensity of local inflammation, was not reflected in serum cytokine concentrations. Intravenously infused methylprednisolone decreased lymph cytokine levels to normal within 12 hours. In contrast, their concentrations in serum showed little or no change.**

Conclusion. **High lymph concentrations of cyto-**

Supported by grant 4PO5B 028 14 from the Committee for Scientific Research, Poland.

[1]Waldemar L. Olszewski, MD: Polish Academy of Sciences, Warsaw, Poland, and St. Bartholomew's & Royal London School of Medicine and Dentistry, London, UK; [2]J. Pazdur, MD, E. Kubasiewicz, MD: Institute of Rheumatology, Warsaw, Poland; [3]M. Zaleska, MD: Polish Academy of Sciences, Warsaw, Poland; [4]Conrad J. Cooke, MD, Norman E. Miller, MD: St. Bartholomew's & Royal London School of Medicine and Dentistry, London, UK.

Address correspondence and reprint requests to Waldemar L. Olszewski, MD, Department of Surgical Research, Medical Research Center, Polish Academy of Sciences, 5 Pawinski Street, 02 106 Warsaw, Poland.

Submitted for publication November 30, 1999; accepted in revised form November 9, 2000.

kines and chemokines, exceeding those in serum, were found in RA patients. The L:S concentration ratios of >1 indicate the local production of these cytokines and chemokines in the inflamed tissues. High flow rates of lymph containing high cytokine concentrations through the regional lymph nodes are likely to affect node lymphocytes and dendritic cells. Analysis of cytokines in lymph should provide insight into events in inflamed tissues in RA and in regional lymph nodes.

Rheumatoid arthritis (RA) is characterized by inflammatory reactions in joints without clinically detectable changes in the regional lymphatics and nodes, as opposed to infectious processes in joints that evoke major reactions in the lymphatic system. The question arises as to which products of immune cells are absorbed from inflamed joints and adjacent tissues into the lymphatics and flow in lymph to lymph nodes.

In RA, the synovial tissue lining the joints contains infiltrating immune cells and activated resident fibroblasts. These cells produce an array of pro- and antiinflammatory cytokines, which are important regulators of cell activation and differentiation. There are several lines of evidence indicating that cytokines and chemokines accumulating in synovial fluid and synovial tissue contribute to the pathogenesis of synovitis. The synovial fluid contains high concentrations of cytokines (1). The presence of the same cytokines has been demonstrated by immunohistochemical methods and in situ hybridization in cultures of explanted synovial cells and in synovial tissue (2).

The joints and connective tissues of the extremity are drained by a network of lymphatics that removes mobile tissue fluid from the intercellular space (3). Collection of tissue fluid (which is called lymph after entering the lymphatics) and examination of its composition provide insight into the humoral and cellular events occurring in the inflammatory focus. We have developed a method for the continuous collection of lymph from the lower extremity that enables lymph sampling for periods of days or weeks (4). Quantification of cytokines and other analytes in both lymph and serum collected simultaneously provides information about the blood–tissue cytokine gradient, and thus about local production. Lymph is a protein-poor fluid that, relative to serum, has low concentrations of immunoglobulins, antibodies, and blocking proteins, obviating some of the problems of measuring biologically active substances. Synovial fluid contains high levels of molecular rheumatoid factor (RF), anticytokine antibodies, soluble cytokine receptors, and cellular debris, which can block various epitopes of cytokines in enzyme-linked immunosorbent assays (ELISAs). These factors render largely unreliable the cytokine bioassays in synovial fluid obtained by joint puncture.

These problems might be largely avoided if pure synovial tissue fluid could be investigated. Lymph-draining joints and adjacent tissues contain synovial fluid produced in the inflamed synovial membrane, but are deprived of the joint cavity fluid. Furthermore, lymph flow rate and lymph cytokine concentrations provide information about the delivery to lymph nodes of peripherally produced cytokines likely to influence node cellular reactions.

In the present study, we collected afferent lymph draining the foot joints of RA patients for 72 hours and measured the concentrations of several cytokines and chemokines. The transport rates of cytokines from the inflamed tissues to the regional lymph nodes were calculated. In addition, we studied the effects of administered glucocorticoids on cytokine levels in lymph and serum.

PATIENTS AND METHODS

Patients. We studied 20 patients (16 women and 4 men, ages 37–67 years [median 42 years]) diagnosed as having RA according to the 1987 revised criteria of the American College of Rheumatology (formerly, the American Rheumatism Association) (5). These patients were randomly selected from a group of RA patients (in remission of disease symptoms and not receiving any treatment) in our registry. Patients had varying Steinbrocker stages of disease (1 with stage 0, 3 with stage I, 5 with stage II, 4 with stage II/III, 2 with stage III, 3 with stage III/IV, and 2 with stage IV) (6). All had swollen feet and painful foot and ankle joints. The duration of RA ranged from 6 months to 32 years (median 6 years). Patients had not been treated with antirheumatic drugs for at least 3 months prior to the study, with the exception of occasional administration of nonsteroidal antiinflammatory drugs to relieve symptoms, and had not received glucocorticoids or immunosuppressive agents for the previous 6 months. Patients with evident cardiovascular, pulmonary, gastrointestinal, renal, or hematologic changes were excluded. All patients provided informed consent.

Control subjects. Control subjects were 20 randomly selected healthy individuals (ages 24–28 years, median 25 years) without any history of RA who were undergoing studies of lymph lipids. They did not receive any drugs either prior to or at the time of lymph and serum sampling for our investigations, and all provided informed consent. The study was approved by the local ethics committee.

Collection of lymph and blood. Prenodal lymph was collected by cannulating a lymphatic vessel on the anteromedial aspect of the lower leg, 5 cm above the medial malleolus, as previously described (4). Briefly, we made a 1-cm skin incision under strictly sterile conditions with 1% xylocaine for

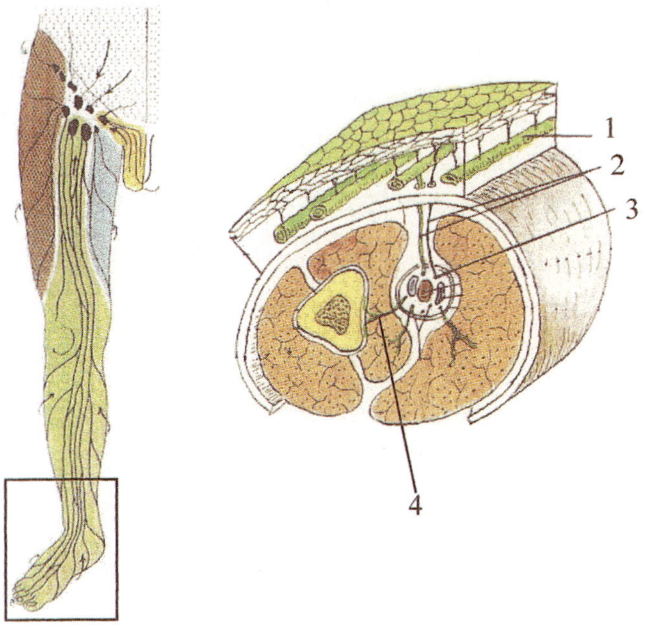

Figure 1. The network of lymphatic vessels draining foot joints, subcutaneous tissues, and skin. Since superficial and deep vessels are interconnected, cannulated collecting trunks in the calf contain lymph from all foot tissues. Normal lymph pressure during lymphangion contractions reaches 10–40 mm Hg. Cannulation of lymphatics and external drainage of lymph to atmospheric pressure directs the lymph stream from most areas to the cannula. The 24-hour lymph output from a cannulated lymphatic ranges from 5 ml to 60 ml. Any event developing in the tissues drained by the cannulated lymphatics that changes local tissue fluid chemistry and cellularity is reflected in lymph composition (see refs. 4 and 17). The box encloses the region of the extremity drained by the cannulated lymphatic vessel. 1 indicates lymphatic plexus of skin, 2 indicates lymphatics connecting the deep and superficial lymphatic systems, 3 indicates perivascular space where tissue fluid accumulates, and 4 indicates lymphatics draining bone and joints. Reproduced, with permission, from Kubik S. Atlas of the lymphatics of the lower limbs. Paris: Servier; 1999. p. 15.

local anesthesia. A lymphatic lying on the fascia was exposed under the operating microscope and was cannulated in a retrograde manner. This vessel drained lymph from the joint capsules, tendons, ligaments, subcutaneous tissue, and skin of the foot (Figure 1) (4). The external tip of the cannula was placed in a calibrated test tube, and lymph was collected continuously for 72 hours. Patients were kept ambulatory. Lymph samples were taken at 12-hour intervals. In 2 patients, samples were collected at 2-hour intervals for studying the effect of methylprednisolone on lymph composition. At the end of the study, the cannula was withdrawn and the lymphatic vessel sealed by external pressure. There was no edema, lymph leakage, or other subsequent side effect. Lymph was centrifuged, and aliquots of the supernatant were frozen and stored at −70°C until used. Blood samples were drawn from an antecubital vein at the times of lymph sampling, allowed to clot, and centrifuged. Serum aliquots were frozen and stored at −70°C until used.

Total protein, immunoglobulins, and acute-phase proteins. Total protein concentration was measured according to the Lowry method (7). Routine quantitative protein electrophoresis was performed. IgG, IgM, C3c, and transferrin concentrations were measured by radial immunodiffusion (Boehringer, Mannheim, Germany).

ELISA for interleukin-1β (IL-1β), IL-1 receptor antagonist (IL-1Ra), IL-6, IL-8, IL-10, IL-15, tumor necrosis factor α (TNFα), vascular endothelial growth factor (VEGF), macrophage inflammatory protein 1α (MIP-1α), and granulocyte–macrophage colony-stimulating factor (GM-CSF). Lymph and serum concentrations of IL-1β, IL-1Ra, IL-6, IL-8, IL-10, IL-15, TNFα, VEGF, MIP-1α, and GM-CSF were measured by enzyme immunometric assays (Quantikine; R&D Systems Europe, Abingdon, UK). Each serum sample and lymph sample was examined in duplicate.

Effects of glucocorticoids on lymph and serum cytokine levels. In 2 patients, a 1-gm bolus of methylprednisolone (Upjohn, Brussels, Belgium) was infused intravenously (IV) in 500 ml of 0.9% NaCl for 2 hours. Lymph and blood samples were obtained every 2 hours, and cytokine levels were measured.

Statistical analysis. Results were expressed as the mean ± SEM. The lymph:serum (L:S) ratio was calculated for each pair of lymph and serum samples. The differences in lymph and serum values for RA patients and control subjects were evaluated using Student's *t*-test or Wilcoxon's rank sum test. The choice of test was based on the normality of the distribution of the considered parameters. Modifications of tests for paired data were used when comparisons were made within the same group. Because of the large number of comparisons, the Bonferroni correction was used to obtain an overall significance level of less than 0.05.

RESULTS

Lymph flow. The mean ± SEM lymph flow in the cannulated vessel was 22.6 ± 3.2 ml/24 hours in the RA patients, which was significantly higher than that in the control subjects (13.2 ± 1.1 ml/24 hours) ($P < 0.01$).

Lymph proteins. In RA patients, the total protein concentration of lymph was 1.80 ± 0.14 gm/dl, while that of serum was 7.40 ± 0.20 gm/dl (mean ± SEM L:S ratio 0.21 ± 0.1). These values did not differ significantly from those in control subjects, which were 1.66 ± 0.14 gm/dl and 7.30 ± 0.1 gm/dl, respectively (L:S ratio 0.22 ± 0.1). By electrophoresis, α_1, α_2, and gamma globulins in lymph and serum were found at higher concentrations in RA patients than in control subjects ($P < 0.05$) (Table 1). Beta globulin concentrations were higher only in lymph ($P < 0.05$). The percentages of various globulins in lymph were higher in RA patients than in control subjects; however, there was a concurrent increase in serum globulins in RA patients. Thus, the L:S ratios for RA patients remained unchanged compared with those for control subjects (Table 2).

The lymph IgM and IgG concentrations were

Table 1. Protein concentrations in lymph and serum of patients with rheumatoid arthritis (RA) and control subjects*

	RA patients (n = 20)		Control subjects (n = 20)	
Protein	Lymph	Serum	Lymph	Serum
Total, gm/dl	1.80 ± 0.14	7.40 ± 0.20	1.66 ± 0.14	7.30 ± 0.10
Globulins, %				
α_1	5.30 ± 0.26†	4.50 ± 0.26‡	2.45 ± 0.10	2.50 ± 0.05
α_2	7.80 ± 0.26†	12.40 ± 0.64‡	4.50 ± 0.20	7.40 ± 0.21
β	14.10 ± 1.24†	12.40 ± 0.40	6.90 ± 0.28	14.0 ± 0.57
γ	16.00 ± 1.02†	22.10 ± 1.00‡	9.10 ± 0.15	8.9 ± 0.21
IgM, mg/dl	32.0 ± 1.5§	236 ± 25¶	15.0 ± 1.3	124 ± 13
IgG, mg/dl	384 ± 45#	1,708 ± 104**	238 ± 32	890 ± 53
CRP, mg/dl	0.92 ± 0.19††	4.84 ± 0.76‡‡	0.50 ± 0.02	0.09 ± 0.02

* Values are the mean ± SEM. CRP = C-reactive protein.
† $P < 0.05$ versus control lymph.
‡ $P < 0.05$ versus control serum.
§ $P = 0.0088$ versus control lymph.
¶ $P = 0.05$ versus control serum.
# $P = 0.05$ versus control lymph.
** $P = 0.0021$ versus control serum.
†† P not significant versus control lymph.
‡‡ $P = 0.0001$ versus control serum.

significantly higher in RA patients than in control subjects ($P = 0.0088$ and $P = 0.05$, respectively) (Table 1). There were also significant increases in serum IgM and IgG concentrations in RA patients compared with control subjects ($P = 0.05$ and $P = 0.0021$, respectively). The lymph C-reactive protein (CRP) concentrations in RA patients were only slightly elevated (P not significant), while the serum CRP concentrations in RA patients significantly exceeded those in control subjects ($P = 0.0001$). The lymph and serum concentrations for C3c and transferrin were also higher in RA patients than in control subjects (data not shown). However, when the L:S ratios were compared, no statistically significant differences were observed between the RA patients and the control subjects (data not shown).

Proinflammatory cytokines in lymph and serum. *IL-1β*. Lymph IL-1β concentrations in RA patients greatly exceeded those in control subjects ($P = 0.0097$), while serum concentrations did not differ significantly (Table 3). There were wide interindividual variations in lymph concentrations that were not observed in serum concentrations. The IL-1β L:S ratio in RA patients was >30-fold that in control subjects ($P = 0.0013$) (Table 2).

TNFα. The lymph concentrations of TNFα were higher in RA patients than in control subjects ($P = 0.037$) (Table 3). TNFα concentrations were also higher in RA patients' lymph than in their serum ($P = 0.049$). The serum TNFα concentration in RA patients was significantly increased compared with that in control subjects ($P = 0.0048$). The mean ± SEM TNFα L:S ratio in RA patients was 3.8 ± 1.2 compared with 1.9 ± 0.02 in control subjects ($P = 0.05$) (Table 2).

Table 2. Lymph:serum ratios of proteins and cytokines in RA patients and control subjects*

Protein or cytokine	RA patients (n = 20)	Control subjects (n = 20)
Total protein	0.21 ± 0.02	0.22 ± 0.02
Globulins		
α_1	0.98 ± 0.04	1.15 ± 0.02
α_2	0.69 ± 0.02	0.59 ± 0.02
β	0.97 ± 0.08	0.50 ± 0.05
γ	0.75 ± 0.03	1.03 ± 0.06
IgM	0.15 ± 0.02	0.11 ± 0.02
IgG	0.22 ± 0.02	0.19 ± 0.02
CRP	0.23 ± 0.03	0.28 ± 0.01
IL-1β	13.9 ± 0.4†	0.4 ± 0.02
TNFα	3.8 ± 1.2‡	1.9 ± 0.02
IL-6	38.0 ± 14.8§	9.2 ± 0.015
IL-15	2.7 ± 0.5	5.0 ± 0.4
GM-CSF	4.2 ± 0.35¶	1.0 ± 0.06
VEGF	0.29 ± 0.02	2.4 ± 0.1
IL-1Ra	4.8 ± 0.8#	1.1 ± 0.04
IL-10	1.1 ± 0.1	0.0
IL-8	390 ± 153#	10.0 ± 0.62
MIP-1α	168 ± 39#	3.4 ± 1.66

* Values are the mean ± SEM. RA = rheumatoid arthritis; CRP = C-reactive protein; IL-1β = interleukin-1β; TNFα = tumor necrosis factor α; GM-CSF = granulocyte–macrophage colony-stimulating factor; VEGF = vascular endothelial growth factor; IL-1Ra = IL-1 receptor antagonist; MIP-1α = macrophage inhibitory protein 1α.
† $P = 0.0013$ versus control subjects.
‡ $P = 0.05$ versus control subjects.
§ $P = 0.0036$ versus control subjects.
¶ $P = 0.0078$ versus control subjects.
# $P < 0.05$ versus control subjects.

Table 3. Proinflammatory cytokine concentrations in lymph and serum of RA patients and control subjects*

	RA patients (n = 20)		Control subjects (n = 20)	
Cytokine, pg/ml	Lymph	Serum	Lymph	Serum
IL-1β	14.8 ± 3.9†	0.8 ± 0.3	1.50 ± 0.25	3.4 ± 1.0
TNFα	9.9 ± 1.1‡	4.7 ± 0.64	4.4 ± 1.1	2.0 ± 0.1
IL-6	511 ± 143§	37.00 ± 7.33	79.0 ± 14.6	3.5 ± 1.4
IL-15	6.2 ± 0.9	5.20 ± 1.86	5.00 ± 0.45	0.30 ± 0.01
GM-CSF	2.30 ± 0.15¶	0.70 ± 0.09	0.40 ± 0.05	0.20 ± 0.06
VEGF	80.4 ± 8.6	298 ± 11	42.0 ± 2.4	36.0 ± 9.5

* Values are the mean ± SEM. See Table 2 for definitions.
† $P = 0.0044$ and $P = 0.0097$ versus RA serum and versus control lymph, respectively.
‡ $P = 0.049$ and $P = 0.037$ versus RA serum and versus control lymph, respectively.
§ $P = 0.0006$ (Bonferroni correction) and $P = 0.026$ versus RA serum and versus control lymph, respectively.
¶ $P = 0.0018$ and $P = 0.0022$ versus RA serum and versus control lymph, respectively.

Table 4. Antiinflammatory cytokine and chemokine concentrations in lymph and serum of RA patients and control subjects*

Cytokine, pg/ml	RA patients (n = 20) Lymph	RA patients (n = 20) Serum	Control subjects (n = 20) Lymph	Control subjects (n = 20) Serum
IL-1Ra	4,274 ± 737†	1,688 ± 537	208 ± 52	258 ± 66
IL-10	13.3 ± 4.4‡	8.3 ± 1.1	0.0	0.0
IL-8	846 ± 174§	192 ± 91	216 ± 83	13 ± 4
MIP-1α	171 ± 34¶	1.6 ± 0.8	3.4 ± 1.7	0.0

* Values are the mean ± SEM. See Table 2 for definitions.
† P = 0.001 and P = 0.0357 versus RA serum and versus control lymph, respectively.
‡ P not significant and $P < 0.0001$ versus RA serum and versus control lymph, respectively.
§ P = 0.0078 and P = 0.0286 versus RA serum and versus control lymph, respectively.
¶ P = 0.032 and P = 0.0006 (Bonferroni correction) versus RA serum and versus control lymph, respectively.

IL-6. In RA patients, IL-6 concentrations were higher in lymph than in serum (P = 0.0006), and these lymph IL-6 concentrations were also higher than lymph and serum IL-6 concentrations in control subjects (P = 0.026 [Table 3] and P = 0.0011, respectively). There were wide interindividual variations in lymph, but not in serum, IL-6 levels. The L:S ratio in RA patients was 38 ± 14.8, which was significantly greater than that in control subjects (P = 0.0036) (Table 2).

IL-15. Lymph and serum IL-15 concentrations were higher in RA patients than in control subjects (Table 3). However, these differences were not statistically significant. The L:S ratio in RA patients was 2.7 ± 0.5 and did not differ significantly from that in control subjects (5.0 ± 0.4) (Table 2).

GM-CSF. In RA patients, lymph GM-CSF concentrations were higher than those in serum (P = 0.0018) (Table 3). In addition, RA patients' lymph and serum concentrations were higher than those in control subjects (P = 0.0022 [Table 3] and P = 0.039, respectively). The L:S ratio in RA patients was 4.2 ± 0.35, which was significantly higher than that in control subjects (1.0 ± 0.06) (P = 0.0078) (Table 2).

VEGF. The VEGF concentration in RA patients was lower in lymph than in serum, although it exceeded the normal value (Table 3). A high concentration of VEGF was observed in RA patients' sera, significantly higher than that in control sera ($P < 0.05$). The L:S ratio in RA patients was 0.29 ± 0.02, significantly lower than that in control subjects (2.4 ± 0.1) (Table 2).

Antiinflammatory cytokines. *IL-1Ra.* The concentration of IL-1Ra in lymph was significantly higher than that in serum in RA patients (P = 0.001) (Table 4), and both were higher than the corresponding concentrations in control subjects (P = 0.0357 and P = 0.0008, respectively). The L:S ratio in RA patients was 4.8 ± 0.8, which was higher than that in control subjects (1.1 ± 0.04) ($P < 0.05$) (Table 2).

IL-10. The concentration of IL-10 in lymph was higher than that in serum in RA patients, but the difference was not statistically significant (Table 4). No IL-10 was detectable in lymph or serum from control subjects.

Chemokines. *IL-8.* The concentration of IL-8 in lymph was significantly higher than that in serum in RA patients (P = 0.0078) (Table 4). Lymph concentrations in RA patients significantly exceeded those in control subjects' lymph and serum (P = 0.0286 and P = 0.0001, respectively). The L:S ratio was high in all RA patients (390 ± 153) (Table 2). This extremely high ratio was due to individual lymph concentrations of >1,500 pg/ml and serum concentrations as low as 5–10 pg/ml.

MIP-1α. Lymph MIP-1α concentrations were significantly higher than those in serum in RA patients (P = 0.032) (Table 4). Both concentrations were significantly higher than those in control subjects (P = 0.0006 and P = 0.01, respectively). The L:S ratio was 168 ± 39, higher than the corresponding value in control subjects (3.4 ± 1.66) ($P < 0.05$) (Table 2).

Effects of methylprednisolone on lymph cytokine levels. Lymph levels of IL-1β, TNFα, IL-1Ra, IL-6, and IL-10, but not those of IL-15, decreased rapidly after administration of methylprednisolone, reaching their lowest values at 12 hours after IV infusion (Figure 2). In contrast, no reductions of IL-10, IL-1Ra, or IL-15 were recorded in serum, while serum levels of IL-1β, TNFα, and IL-6 decreased slightly at 12 hours after IV infusion in one patient, although not in the other.

Total mass of cytokines transported in lymph to lymph nodes. The output of a substance is its concentration multiplied by the flow rate. The lymph flow rate increased in RA patients by a factor of 2 compared with that in control subjects, and the mean ± SEM concentrations of IL-1, TNFα, IL-6, GM-CSF, IL-10, IL-8, and MIP-1α increased by 10 ± 2, 2.25 ± 0.5, 13 ± 4, 5.3 ± 1.2, 13.3 ± 2.0, 3.9 ± 0.4, and 50 ± 8, respectively. Consequently, cytokine outputs reaching lymph nodes from the inflamed tissues were increased in these patients by mean factors of approximately 20, 5, 26, 10, 26, 8, and 100, respectively.

DISCUSSION

Our results show for the first time that lymph draining from the inflamed joints and foot connective

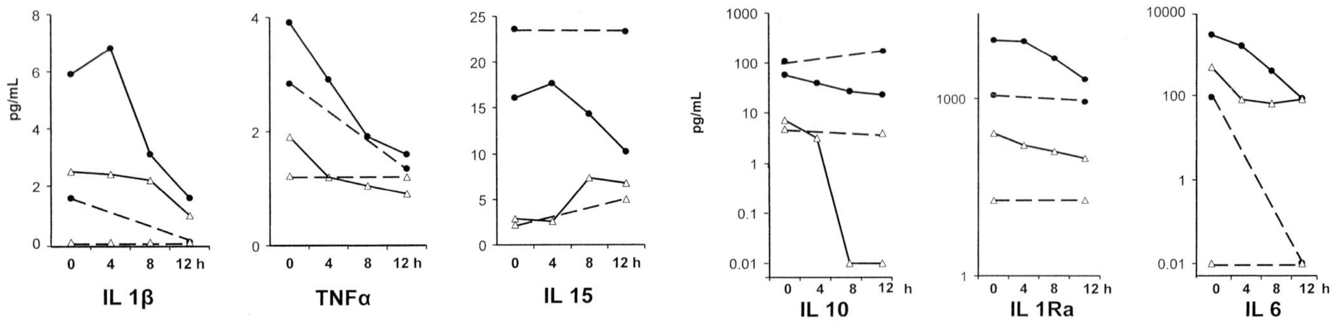

Figure 2. Lymph (solid lines) and serum (broken lines) cytokine levels of patient 1 (●) and patient 2 (△) before (time 0) and after intravenous infusion of 1.0 gm of methylprednisolone. **A,** Arithmetic scale. **B,** Logarithmic scale. A substantial decrease occurred in lymph concentrations, but not in serum concentrations, of interleukin-1β (IL 1β), tumor necrosis factor α (TNFα), IL-10, IL-1 receptor antagonist (IL 1Ra), and IL-6. Only a small effect of methylprednisolone on IL-15 concentration was recorded. Lymph cytokine levels provide greater insight into tissue events than do serum cytokine levels.

tissue of RA patients contains very high levels of cytokines and chemokines, exceeding the serum levels by severalfold. This cannot be explained by filtration from blood and must be attributed to local production by the synovial cells and fibroblasts. These regulatory polypeptides are delivered directly to lymph nodes via the afferent lymphatics. Serum concentrations of cytokines were only slightly elevated; thus, blood remained only a poor supplier of cytokines to the lymph nodes. Glucocorticoids rapidly decreased lymph, but not serum, cytokine levels, supporting the notion that most of the cytokines are produced locally. Our lymph drainage method provides new insights into the events in the inflamed tissues and may be useful for establishing improved treatment protocols for various antiinflammatory drugs, especially in drug-resistant cases.

The immune events develop in nonlymphoid tissues between parenchymal cells in the intercellular space in the vicinity of blood capillaries in the mobile tissue fluid and ground matrix. This area is drained by initial lymphatics, which form a dense network that leads into collecting lymphatic trunks (3,8). These trunks can be cannulated, and the lymph so obtained contains all the humoral and cellular elements of the intercellular space (9). The joints and neighboring tissues are drained by a dense network of lymphatics (10) (Figure 1). Therefore, lymph originating in that area should contain all the factors absorbed from the inflamed joint tissues. Continuous collection of lymph enables tissue changes, as well as the local effects of drugs, to be monitored over time.

During the inflammatory process in a given tissue, the capillary transport of immune cells and humoral components from plasma to the intercellular space increases. Moreover, the infiltrating cells actively produce and release cytokines and chemokines. Subsequently, the concentrations of proteins, immune polypeptides, and immune cells rise in the intercellular space (11–16). The inflammatory products are washed out from the intercellular space into the lymphatics and are delivered to the regional lymph nodes, where the immune reaction is triggered.

As in any local inflammatory reaction, capillary permeability and filtration are increased in RA, and consequently, lymph production and protein concentration are high. In our patients, the lymph concentrations of IgG, IgM, CRP, C3c, and transferrin were found to be high; as expected, however, the L:S ratios remained within normal limits owing to the concomitant increases in serum concentrations. Interestingly, the L:S ratios remained <1, suggesting that there was little or no local production of these proteins (the bulk of lymph immunoglobulins originating from the filtered plasma). This finding is in apparent contrast to reports of local production of immunoglobulins by infiltrating B cells and plasmacytes present in the synovial fluid. In our in vitro studies on protein synthesis by cells from inflammatory foci, we found these cells' contribution to the lymph immunoglobulin concentration to be very low compared with the high transcapillary flux of these proteins produced elsewhere (Olszewski WL, et al: unpublished observations). Moreover, only a few migrating cells in lymph (T lymphocytes, Langerhans' cells, and B cells) synthesize proteins and could contribute their level of these proteins to lymph. The normal concentration of cells is 5–120/μl (14) and is only about twice that number in RA patients (Olszewski WL, et al: unpublished observations).

Although the bulk of lymph immune proteins originated from the capillary filtrate, cytokines seemed to be produced locally. Many cytokines have been measured in synovial fluid, and high levels of some of them, including IL-1 and IL-6, have been consistently detected (17,18). In another approach, explanted synovial membranes or partially purified fibroblasts or monocytes from joints were placed directly into culture medium, and cytokine production was measured (2). Spontaneous production of cytokines under such circumstances might indicate production in vivo. However, cells that have been removed from their normal environment might begin to express cytokines that are suppressed in vivo (2). Draining lymph from the joints and their neighboring tissues overcomes these problems, since the concentrations and activities of lymph components should be similar to those of synovial fluid. This should be particularly true of low molecular weight products such as cytokines, which can readily diffuse in the tissue. Some cytokines will interact with their receptors and become internalized, and as a consequence, be undetectable in fluids. However, this applies more to the measurement of cytokines in cell-rich synovial fluid than in lymph, which contains rather few cells.

Studying lymph also obviates problems that can result from the viscosity of synovial fluid, which can interfere with antibody–cytokine interactions in ELISAs. Since the RF titer in lymph is low (Olszewski WL, et al: unpublished observations), one can avoid the overestimation of cytokine levels in ELISAs that results from nonspecific binding of the Fc region with anticytokine antibodies (19). Compared with serum, lymph contains low levels of inhibitory proteins and antibodies. Their concentrations in synovial fluid are the product of cellular synthesis and release and cellular disintegration, while the lymph cytokine mass represents their net efflux from the joint. In addition, knowledge of the masses of cytokines and chemokines delivered in lymph to the local lymph nodes should throw light on the possible mechanism of activation of lymph node cells in RA and other conditions.

In contrast to our findings for immunoglobulins, we found that the concentrations of IL-1β, TNFα, IL-6, GM-CSF, IL-1Ra, IL-8, and MIP-1α in lymph were several times higher than in the serum of RA patients. They were also higher than the corresponding lymph concentrations in control subjects. These findings indicate that the measured cytokines and chemokines were synthesized and released locally in the inflamed tissues. In contrast, serum cytokine levels in RA patients were only slightly elevated compared with those in control subjects, and only for TNFα, IL-15, IL-10, IL-1Ra, IL-6, GM-CSF, and IL-8, but not for IL-1β or MIP-1α.

Interestingly, under normal conditions, levels of IL-1Ra, IL-6, TNFα, IL-8, IL-15, VEGF, monocyte chemotactic protein 1 (MCP-1), MIP-1α, and RANTES are higher in lymph than in serum (14,15). The sources of cytokines in limbs are most likely keratinocytes, fibroblasts, and endothelial, Langerhans', and synovial cells. However, their levels are only 2–3-fold those in serum, while even hundredfold concentrations were reached in RA patients.

The preferential source of the cytokines in RA patients was the infiltrating synovial monocytes, which have been shown to produce IL-1, IL-6, IL-8, IL-10, TNFα, GM-CSF, transforming growth factor β (TGFβ), platelet-derived growth factor, basic fibroblast growth factor, IL-1Ra, VEGF, MCP-1, and MIP-1α (1,20–30). Activated fibroblasts can also produce high levels of cytokines and chemokines during synovitis (1). Synovial T cells produce rather little IL-4, IL-5, or IL-6 (31). This expression is transient in the absence of continuing stimulation. However, a low level of expression does not rule out a potentially important regulatory role. Neutrophils present in synovium at high density produce IL-1Ra (19) and VEGF (32,33). Activated granulocytes adhere to synovial endothelial cells and release VEGF into the circulation. This may have contributed to the high serum VEGF concentration that was not reflected in lymph. Although the VEGF concentration was raised in our RA patients' lymph, it remained below that in serum. The contributions of B cells, plasma cells, and dendritic cells to synovial cytokine production have not been established.

An important observation corroborating our conclusions that the concentration and output of cytokines and chemokines in lymph draining from inflamed joints and connective tissue reflect the local production of these inflammatory mediators was the effect of an IV bolus of the glucocorticoid methylprednisolone. The lymph cytokine concentrations decreased within 12 hours to almost normal values. In contrast, the serum concentrations were only slightly affected. An inhibitory influence of glucocorticoids on activator protein 1 (AP-1) and nuclear factor κB (NF-κB) proteins has been documented (34,35).

The inflammatory process in joints and connective tissue in RA clearly involves sending stimulatory signals to the local lymph nodes via the lymph. Enlargement of inguinal and iliac lymph nodes has been observed only occasionally (36,37). Under normal conditions, cytokines constitutively produced in skin, joints, and connective tissue of the foot reach the regional lymph nodes and regulate the level of cellular "alert" (16,17). Interruption of afferent lymphatics, and thereby, interruption of the flow of cytokines, specifically TNFα, to lymph nodes, leads to node atrophy (38,39).

In RA patients, the delivery of cytokines to lymph nodes was increased by severalfold to hundredfold. The question arises of how the inflowing cytokines and chemokines affect the lymph node cells. Cytokines exert their effects by activating cellular signal transduction pathways, with the production of second messengers and the triggering of cascades of activation agents (40). The transcription factors AP-1, NF-κB, and signal transducer and activator of transcription (STAT) play an important role in mediating gene activation by cytokines and are also important in regulating the expression of the cytokines themselves. Increased expression of AP-1 protein Fos has been detected in arthritis. Synovial fluid activates NF-κB in resting monocytes (1). Most cytokines and inflammatory mediators activate janus kinase/STAT pathways. Activation of STAT results in changes in cell phenotype and has been implicated in the activation of genes that are important in inflammatory responses (41).

It is poorly understood why there is only a minor clinically evident reaction of lymph nodes in RA in the presence of acute changes in the joints. One possibility is that the cytokine inhibitors IL-1Ra, TGFβ, and IL-10 in lymph block the proinflammatory cytokines. This is the subject of our present investigations.

Our results indicate that our model should be useful not only for studies of the pathogenesis and natural history of RA, but also for assessing the efficacy of drugs and for titrating drug dosages in resistant cases. In responsive cases, our model could enable drug dosages to be attenuated, thereby minimizing side effects. Further studies are in progress concerning the effects of steroid hormone administration on cytokines and chemokines in RA lymph.

ACKNOWLEDGMENT

The cooperation of St. Bartholomew's Medical School is greatly appreciated.

REFERENCES

1. Ivashkin LB. Cytokine expression and cell activation in inflammatory arthritis. Adv Immunol 1996;63:337–76.
2. Feldmann M, Brennan FM, Chantry D, Haworth C, Turner M, Katsikis P, et al. Cytokine assays: role in evaluation of the pathogenesis of autoimmunity. Immunol Rev 1991;119:105–23.
3. Kubik S. The anatomy of the lymphatic system. Recent Results Cancer Res 1974;46:5–17.
4. Olszewski WL. Collection and physiological measurements of lymph and interstitial fluid in man. Lymphology 1977;10:137–41.
5. Arnett FC, Edworthy SM, Bloch DA, McShane DJ, Fries JF, Cooper NS, et al. The American Rheumatism Association 1987 revised criteria for the classification of rheumatoid arthritis. Arthritis Rheum 1988;31:315–24.
6. Steinbrocker O, Traeger CH, Batterman RC. Therapeutic criteria in rheumatoid arthritis. JAMA 1949;140:659–62.
7. Lowry OH, Rosebrough NJ, Farr AL, Randall RJ. Protein measurement with the Folin phenol reagent. J Biol Chem 1951;193: 265–75.
8. Ittaviani G, Azzali G. Ultrastructure des capillaires lymphatique. In: Comel M, Szszt L, editors. Morphologie und Histochemie der Gefasswand. Pt 2. Basel: Karger; 1966.
9. Taylor AE, Gibson WH, Granger HJ, Guyton AC. The interaction between intracapillary and tissue forces in the overall regulation of interstitial fluid volume. Lymphology 1973;6:192–5.
10. Shdanov DA. Die Lymphgefasse des Tarsalgelenkes, Kniegelenkes und Huftgelenkes des Menschen. Anat Anz 1930;69:194–210.
11. Olszewski WL, Engeset A. Hemolytic complement in peripheral lymph of normal man. Clin Exp Immunol 1978;32:392–6.
12. Olszewski WL, Engeset A. Immune proteins, enzymes and electrolytes in human peripheral lymph. Lymphology 1978;11:56–60.
13. Olszewski WL, Engeset A. Immune proteins and other biochemical constituents of peripheral lymph in patients with malignancy and postirradiation lymphedema. Lymphology 1978;11:174–8.
14. Plachta J, Olszewski WL, Grzelak I, Engeset A, Cholewka W. Identification of interleukin 1 in normal human lymph derived from skin. Lymphokine Res 1988;7:93–6.
15. Olszewski WL, Jamal S, Manokaran G, Galkowska H, Grzelak I, Zaleska M. Lymph cytokines in obstructive lymphedema—a sign of chronic inflammatory reaction. Lymphology 1998;31:126–9.
16. Olszewski WL, Grzelak I, Ziolkowska A, Engeset A. Immune cell traffic from blood through the normal skin to lymphatics. Clin Dermatol 1995;13:473–83.
17. Miyasaka N, Sato K, Goto M, Sasano M, Natsuyama M, Inoue K, et al. Augmented interleukin-1 production and HLA–DR expression in the synovium of rheumatoid arthritis patients: possible involvement in joint destruction. Arthritis Rheum 1988;31:480–6.
18. Field M, Chu C, Feldmann M, Maini RN. Interleukin-6 localisation in the synovial membrane in rheumatoid arthritis. Rheumatol Int 1991;11:45–50.
19. Malyak M, Swaney RE, Arend WP. Levels of synovial fluid interleukin-1 receptor antagonist in rheumatoid arthritis and other arthropathies: potential contribution from synovial fluid neutrophils. Arthritis Rheum 1993;36:781–9.
20. Wood NC, Dickens E, Symons JA, Duff GW. In situ hybridization of interleukin-1 in CD14-positive cells in rheumatoid arthritis. Clin Immunol Immunopathol 1992;62:295–300.
21. Katsikis PD, Chu CQ, Brennan FN, Maini RN, Feldmann M. Immunoregulatory role of interleukin 10 in rheumatoid arthritis. J Exp Med 1994;179:1517–27.
22. De Benedetti F, Massa M, Pignatti P, Albani S, Novick D, Martini A. Serum soluble interleukin 6 (IL-6) receptor and IL-6/soluble IL-6 receptor complex in systemic juvenile rheumatoid arthritis. J Clin Invest 1994;93:2114–9.
23. Campbell IK, Novak U, Cebon J, Layton JE, Hamilton JA. Human articular cartilage and chondrocytes produce hemopoietic colony-stimulating factors in culture in response to IL-1. J Immunol 1991;147:1238–46.
24. Bucala R, Ritchlin C, Winchester R, Cerami A. Constitutive production of inflammatory and mitogenic cytokines by rheumatoid synovial fibroblasts. J Exp Med 1991;173:569–74.

25. Chomarat P, Vannier E, Dechanet J, Rissoan MC, Banchereau J, Dinarello CA, et al. Balance of IL-1 receptor antagonist/IL-1β in rheumatoid synovium and its regulation by IL-4 and IL-10. J Immunol 1995;154:1432–9.
26. Wahl SM, Allen JB, Welch GR, Wong HL. Transforming growth factor β in synovial fluids modulates FcγRIII (CD16) expression on mononuclear phagocytes. J Immunol 1992;148:485–90.
27. Llorente L, Richaud-Patin Y, Fior R, Alcocer-Varela J, Wijdenes J, Fourrier BM, et al. In vivo production of interleukin-10 by non–T cells in rheumatoid arthritis, Sjögren's syndrome, and systemic lupus erythematosus: a potential mechanism of B lymphocyte hyperactivity and autoimmunity. Arthritis Rheum 1994; 37:1647–55.
28. Koch AE, Kunkel SL, Harlow LA, Mazarakis DD, Haines GK, Burdick MD, et al. Macrophage inflammatory protein-1α: a novel chemotactic cytokine for macrophages in rheumatoid arthritis. J Clin Invest 1994;93:921–6.
29. Lotz M, Kekow J, Carson DA. Transforming factor β and cellular immune responses in synovial fluids. J Immunol 1990;144:4189–94.
30. Fava RA, Olsen NJ, Spencer-Green G, Yeo KT, Berse B, Jackman RW, et al. Vascular permeability factor/endothelial growth factor (VPF/VEGF): accumulation and expression in human synovial fluids and rheumatoid synovial tissue. J Exp Med 1994;180:341–6.
31. Simon AK, Siepelt E, Sieper J. Divergent T-cell cytokine patterns in inflammatory arthritis. Proc Natl Acad Sci U S A 1994;91: 8562–6.
32. Webb NJ, Myers CR, Watson CJ, Bottomley MJ, Brenchley PE. Activated human neutrophils express vascular endothelial growth factor (VEGF). Cytokine 1998;10:254–7.
33. Taichman NS, Young S, Cruchley AT, Taylor P, Paleolog E. Human neutrophils secrete vascular endothelial growth factor. J Leukoc Biol 1997;62:397–400.
34. Scheinman RI, Cogswell PG, Lofquist AK, Baldwin AS. Role of transcriptional activation of I kappa B alpha in mediation of immunosuppression by glucocorticoids. Science 1995;270:283–6.
35. Auphan N, DiDonato JA, Rosette C, Helmberg A, Karin A. Immunosuppression by glucocorticoids: inhibition of NFκB activity through induction of IκB synthesis. Science 1995;270:286–90.
36. Kyle VM, de Silva M, Hurst G. Rheumatoid lymphedema. Clin Rheumatol 1982;1:126–7.
37. Lacroix HR, Gruwez JA, Casteels-van Daele M, Dequeker J. Lymphedema of the leg associated with rheumatoid arthritis. Lymphology 1991;24:68–70.
38. Wolfe JHN, Rutt D, Kinmonth JB. Lymphatic obstruction and lymph node changes—a study of the rabbit popliteal node. Lymphology 1983;16;19–22.
39. Cumberbatch M, Kimber I. Tumor necrosis factor alpha is required for accumulation of dendritic cells in draining lymph nodes and for optimal contact sensitization. Immunology 1995;84:31–5.
40. Taniguchi T. Cytokine signaling through nonreceptor protein tyrosine kinases. Science 1995;268:251--6.
41. Firestein GS, Manning AM. Signal transduction and transcription factors in rheumatic disease. Arthritis Rheum 1999;42:609–21.

ARTHRITIS & RHEUMATISM
Vol. 44, No. 3, March 2001, pp 550–560

Levels of Interleukin-18 and Its Binding Inhibitors in the Blood Circulation of Patients With Adult-Onset Still's Disease

Masanori Kawashima,[1] Masahiro Yamamura,[1] Madoka Taniai,[2] Hiroshi Yamauchi,[2] Tadao Tanimoto,[2] Masashi Kurimoto,[2] Shoji Miyawaki,[3] Tetsuki Amano,[4] Tsutomu Takeuchi,[5] and Hirofumi Makino[1]

Objective. **Interleukin-18 (IL-18) is a proinflammatory cytokine that is involved in immunologically mediated tissue damage, but its bioactivity is regulated in vivo by its soluble decoy receptor, IL-18 binding protein (IL-18BP). This study was undertaken to determine levels of IL-18 and IL-18 binding inhibition in the blood of patients with adult-onset Still's disease (ASD).**

Methods. **Serum concentrations of IL-18 in ASD patients were compared by enzyme-linked immunosorbent assay (ELISA) with those in patients with other systemic rheumatic diseases and healthy controls. The biologically active mature protein of IL-18 was detected by Western blot analysis with anti–IL-18 antibody and its induction of interferon-γ (IFNγ) secretion from IL-18–responding human myelomonocytic KG-1 cells. The inhibitory activity on IL-18 binding to its receptor was determined by ^{125}I–IL-18 binding inhibition assay using the Chinese hamster ovary cell line transfected with a murine IL-18 receptor (CHO-K1/mIL-18R).**

Results. **Concentrations of serum IL-18 were extremely elevated in patients with active ASD compared with those in patients with rheumatoid arthritis, systemic lupus erythematosus, systemic sclerosis, polymyositis/dermatomyositis, Sjögren's syndrome, or healthy individuals. Levels of IL-18 were found to correlate with serum ferritin values and disease severity in ASD. Western blot analysis revealed that serum samples from patients with active ASD contained an 18-kd polypeptide of IL-18, corresponding in size to the mature form. Accordingly, the samples were able to induce IFNγ secretion from KG-1 cells, which was largely abolished by neutralizing anti–IL-18 antibody. However, the level of IL-18 bioactivity was more than 10-fold weaker than the concentration of IL-18 protein measured by ELISA. Serum samples from patients with active ASD showed an inhibitory effect on the binding of ^{125}I–IL-18 to CHO-K1/mIL-18R cells, and this activity was associated with elevation of IL-18.**

Conclusion. **These data indicate that systemic overproduction of IL-18 may be closely related to the pathogenesis of ASD, despite the restriction on its inflammatory activity by IL-18 binding inhibitors such as IL-18BP. The disease activity appears to be determined on the basis of the relative levels of IL-18 and its specific inhibitors.**

Interleukin-18 (IL-18) was originally described as an interferon-γ (IFNγ)–inducing factor that was expressed in the liver of mice treated with *Propionibacterium acnes* and subsequently challenged with lipopolysaccharide (1,2). IL-18 is produced mainly by activated macrophage-lineage cells such as Kupffer cells (2,3). The secretion of biologically active IL-18 protein depends on activation of IL-1β–converting enzyme (ICE); IL-18 polypeptide is synthesized as the precursor of 193 amino acids, which is cleaved by ICE to generate the mature 18.3-kd protein (4). IL-18 has a wide range of biologic activities: it potentiates the development of Th1-type immune responses (2,5), stimulates the synthesis of IFNγ in T cells and natural killer (NK) cells (2,3,5–7), promotes the proliferation of activated T cells and their production of IL-2 and granulocyte–

Supported in part by grants-in-aid 10670411 and 12670426 from the Ministry of Education, Science, and Culture of Japan.

[1]Masanori Kawashima, MD, Masahiro Yamamura, MD, Hirofumi Makino, MD: Okayama University Medical School, Okayama, Japan; [2]Madoka Taniai, PhD, Hiroshi Yamauchi, PhD, Tadao Tanimoto, PhD, Masashi Kurimoto, PhD: Hayashibara Company, Okayama, Japan; [3]Shoji Miyawaki, MD: Kurashiki Medical Center, Kurashiki, Japan; [4]Tetsuki Amano, MD: Aioi City Hospital, Aioi, Japan; [5]Tsutomu Takeuchi, MD: Saitama Medical School, Kawagoe, Japan.

Address correspondence and reprint requests to Masahiro Yamamura, MD, Department of Medicine III, Okayama University Medical School, 2-5-1 Shikata-cho, Okayama 700-8558, Japan.

Submitted for publication May 2, 2000; accepted in revised form November 8, 2000.

macrophage colony-stimulating factor (GM-CSF) (1–3,5,6), and augments the cytotoxic activity of NK cells through up-regulation of Fas ligand (1–3,8). Such inflammatory properties are considered to be involved in immunologically mediated tissue damage. IL-18 has a pivotal role in bringing about endotoxin-induced liver injury in mice (1,2,9), and the detection of IL-18 messenger RNA (mRNA) has been associated with IFNγ induction and diabetes development in NOD mice (10). In the intestinal lesions of Crohn's disease, the synthesis of mature IL-18 protein appears to be responsible for Th1 cell–mediated chronic inflammation by inducing local production of IFNγ (11,12). In the joints of patients with rheumatoid arthritis (RA), increased expression of IL-18 may contribute to maintaining both Th1 responses and macrophage production of inflammatory cytokines such as tumor necrosis factor α (TNFα) and GM-CSF (13,14).

More recently, IL-18 binding protein (IL-18BP) has been identified as a specific inhibitor for IL-18 (15,16). The functional receptor of IL-18 (IL-18R) consists of 2 components, similar to IL-1R: the IL-1 receptor–related protein (IL-1Rrp) and the accessory protein-like (IL-1AcPL); coexpression of both molecules is important in inducing the activation of the transcriptional factor nuclear factor κB (NF-κB) and c-Jun N-terminal kinase (17–19). There is no significant similarity between IL-18BP and IL-18R components, but IL-18BP has the immunoglobulin domain homologous to the third Ig domain of the decoy receptor of IL-1, type II IL-1R. Since it lacks a transmembrane domain, IL-18BP appears to exist only as a soluble circulating protein and thus belongs to a novel family of soluble receptor–like proteins including osteoprotegerin and cytokine-like factor 1 (16). The major function of IL-18BP is to regulate the inflammatory activity of IL-18 by acting as its soluble decoy receptor (15,16). IL-18BP can effectively diminish IL-18–induced NF-κB activation, with subsequent synthesis of IFNγ and IL-8 in vitro. This inhibitor is constitutively expressed in various normal human tissues at the mRNA level, most prominently in the spleen and lungs (15,16).

Adult-onset Still's disease (ASD) is a form of polyarthritis associated with systemic manifestations such as a high spiking fever, an evanescent salmon-colored rash, and sore throat. It is considered identical to the systemic form of juvenile RA (20). ASD often involves organ failure, including lymphadenopathy, liver injury, pleuritis, pericarditis, pneumonitis, and disseminated intravascular coagulation, which occasionally have an effect on patient outcome (21–24). Laboratory studies reveal evidence of nonspecific inflammation, such as an elevated erythrocyte sedimentation rate (ESR), leukocytosis, anemia, increased levels of serum acute-phase reactants with hypoalbuminemia, and an elevation of hepatic enzyme levels. A markedly raised level of serum ferritin is highly supportive of the diagnosis of ASD and correlates well with its disease activity (21,25,26). Although the pathogenesis has not yet been made clear, immunologically mediated inflammation occurs in active ASD. Several inflammatory cytokines such as IL-6 have been detected at high levels in the blood of juvenile or adult patients with Still's disease (27–32). Therefore, we measured concentrations of serum IL-18 protein in patients with active ASD by immunoassay and found that IL-18 was extremely elevated compared with other systemic rheumatic diseases such as RA. We further examined the presence of biologically active mature IL-18 protein and the regulation of its activity by IL-18 binding inhibitors in this systemic inflammatory disease.

PATIENTS AND METHODS

Patients and samples. Serum samples were obtained from 16 patients with ASD; 135 patients with other systemic rheumatic diseases, including RA (n = 34), systemic lupus erythematosus (SLE; n = 33), systemic sclerosis (SSc; n = 19), polymyositis/dermatomyositis (PM/DM; n = 21), and Sjögren's syndrome (SS; n = 28), as disease controls; and 53 healthy controls. Study patients with ASD (13 women and 3 men) satisfied both the criteria of Cush et al (33) and those of Yamaguchi et al (24); the patients all presented with a spiking fever (≥39°C), arthralgia or arthritis, and the typical rash, and were negative for rheumatoid factor or antinuclear antibody. Their mean ± SD age was 40 ± 18 years (range 16–73 years), and the mean duration of disease was 2.7 ± 1.7 years (range 1 month–7 years). Fourteen of the ASD patients showed evidence of liver injury as suggested by elevated hepatic enzyme levels and/or hepatomegaly, 11 had splenomegaly, and 10 had lymphadenopathy. Most patients had received nonsteroidal antiinflammatory drugs (NSAIDs) as first-line agents, but in 13 patients, corticosteroids (5–60 mg/day of prednisolone) were used to control systemic manifestations. Methotrexate was given to 2 patients due to an insufficient response to corticosteroid therapy. Patients with other rheumatic diseases were diagnosed according to the American College of Rheumatology (formerly, the American Rheumatism Association) criteria for the classification of RA (34), SLE (35), and SSc (36); the criteria for the diagnosis of PM and DM by Bohan and Peter (37); and the criteria for the classification of SS by Vitali et al (38). RA patients were receiving NSAIDs, disease-modifying antirheumatic drugs, and/or prednisolone (≤5 mg/day), but they had active disease as indicated by elevated levels of serum C-reactive protein (CRP; mean ± SD 35 ± 34 mg/liter). Patients with SLE, although receiving various doses of daily prednisolone (5–40 mg/day), had active disease at the time of blood collection, as indicated by Systemic Lupus Disease

Activity Index (SLEDAI) scores of >8 (39). Patients with SSc or SS did not receive prednisolone.

Cell lines. Cells of the human myelomonocytic cell line KG-1, which dose dependently produce IFNγ in response to human IL-18 (40), were maintained at 37°C in RPMI 1640 medium supplemented with 10% heat-inactivated fetal calf serum (FCS; BioWhittaker, Walkersville, MD). The Chinese hamster ovary–K1 (CHO-K1) cell line was transfected with a murine IL-18R (IL-1Rrp) expression vector plasmid, named CHO-K1/mIL-18R, and was maintained at 37°C in Ham's F12 medium (Nissui Pharmaceutical, Tokyo, Japan) with 5% FCS (15).

Immunoassay for IL-18. Concentrations of antigenic IL-18 were measured in duplicate by specific enzyme-linked immunosorbent assay (ELISA) as previously described (41). Briefly, ELISA plates (Corning, Corning, NY) were coated with 20 μg/ml of mouse monoclonal anti–IL-18 antibody (anti–IL-18 mAb;125-2H) in phosphate buffered saline (PBS) for 3 hours at room temperature, followed by blocking overnight with PBS–1% bovine serum albumin (BSA) at 4°C. After washing with PBS–0.05% Tween 20, 50 μl of PBS with 1% BSA, 5% FCS, and 1*M* NaCl was dispensed and 50 μl of samples or recombinant human IL-18 (rHuIL-18) standards was added to each well, followed by incubation for 2 hours at room temperature. After washing, plates were incubated for 2 hours with 0.5 μg/ml of peroxidase-conjugated rat anti–IL-18 mAb (159-12B) in 100 μl of PBS with 1% BSA, 5% FCS, 0.1% CHAPS (Dojin Chemicals, Kumamoto, Japan), and 0.3*M* NaCl, and developed with 0.5 mg/ml of *o*-phenylenediamine (Wako, Osaka, Japan) in 100 μl of 0.1*M* Na_2HPO_4-citrate buffer (pH 5.0) with 0.003% H_2O_2. The reaction was quenched with 100 μl of 2*N* H_2SO_4, and optical densities at 492 nm were determined. The assay could detect as little as 100 pg/ml of IL-18.

Immunoassay for TNFα, IL-1β, IL-6, and IFNγ. Cytokine concentrations were measured in duplicate by the quantitative sandwich ELISA, using ELISA kits provided by Dr. Y. Ohmoto (Otsuka Pharmaceutical, Tokushima, Japan). The detection limit for each of these cytokines was ~10 pg/ml.

Western blotting for IL-18. Serum samples were 10-fold diluted with distilled water, separated on a 12.5% sodium dodecyl sulfate–polyacrylamide gel, and electrophoretically transferred onto a nitrocellulose membrane (Hybond-C pure; Amersham, Buckinghamshire, UK) for 1 hour. The membrane was blocked with blocking solution (Blockace; Yukijirushi Nyugyo, Sapporo, Japan). After washing with TBS buffer (50 m*M* Tris [pH 7.5], 200 m*M* NaCl, and 0.05% Tween 20), the membrane was incubated overnight at 4°C with 0.4 μg/ml of goat polyclonal anti–IL-18 antibody (*sc-6177*; Santa Cruz Biotechnology, Santa Cruz, CA) in TBS buffer with 10% Blockace with or without IL-18–specific competitors (Blocking Peptide, *sc-6177p*). After washing with TBS buffer, the membrane was incubated for 1 hour at room temperature with 0.2 μg/ml of alkaline phosphatase–conjugated donkey polyclonal anti-goat IgG antibody (*sc-2059*) in TBS buffer with 10% Blockace. Finally, the enzyme activity was detected by using an alkaline phosphatase substrate staining kit (AP substrate kit II; Vector Laboratories, Burlingame, CA) according to the manufacturer's instructions.

Bioassay for IL-18. The biologic activity of IL-18 was measured in triplicate by using human myelomonocytic KG-1 cells (40). Then, 100 μl of KG-1 cell suspensions, adjusted at a density of 3×10^6 cells/ml in RPMI 1640 medium with 10% FCS with or without anti–IL-18 mAb (125-2H), were dispensed into the wells of 96-well microtiter plates (Sumitomo Bakelite, Tokyo, Japan), and 100 μl of samples and rHuIL-18 standards was added to each well. The plates were incubated at 37°C in a humidified atmosphere containing 5% CO_2, and culture supernatants were harvested 24 hours later. Concentrations of IFNγ were determined by a sandwich ELISA using 2 mouse anti-IFNγ mAb (mAb-IFNγ-15 and peroxidase-conjugated mAb-IFNγ-6). The activity of IL-18 was determined by the difference in IFNγ levels between those cultures with and without anti–IL-18 mAb. The sensitivity of the bioassay was ~100 pg/ml.

IL-18 binding inhibition assay. The activity of samples to inhibit the binding of IL-18 to its receptor was detected as previously described (15). Briefly, CHO-K1/mIL-18R cells were suspended in RPMI 1640 medium containing 0.1% BSA, 0.1% NaN_3, and 100 m*M* HEPES (pH 7.2) (binding medium). The binding reactions were performed on 5×10^5 CHO-K1/mIL-18R cells for 1 hour at 4°C in 150 μl of binding medium containing serum samples and 1.0 n*M* ^{125}I–rHuIL-18 with or without 500 n*M* unlabeled rHuIL-18 as a competitor. After incubation, the reaction mixtures were layered over 200 μl of phthalate oil (dibutylphthalate:dioctylphthalate = 1:1), centrifuged at 6,000*g* for 5 minutes at 15°C, and the radioactivity counts of the cell pellets, which represent the amounts of cell-bound ^{125}I–IL-18, were measured as cpm using a gamma counter. The binding inhibition rate was calculated using the following equation: binding inhibition rate (%) =

$$\frac{\text{Total binding count (cpm)} - \text{sample binding count (cpm)}}{\text{Total binding count (cpm)} - \text{nonspecific binding count (cpm)}} \times 100$$

The total binding count and the nonspecific binding count were measured in the absence of samples or when the cold competitor was added to the mixture, respectively.

Detection of IL-18 mRNA expression in blood monocytes and T cells by reverse transcriptase–polymerase chain reaction (RT-PCR). Mononuclear cells were freshly isolated from heparinized venous blood from 5 patients with active ASD and 5 healthy individuals by Ficoll density-gradient centrifugation. Peripheral blood monocytes and T cells were purified by positive selection using anti-CD14 or anti-CD3 antibody–coated magnetic beads (Dynabeads M-450 CD3 and CD14; Dynal, Oslo, Norway), respectively. The purity of monocyte and T cell populations was found to be >95% by flow cytometric analysis using fluorescein isothiocyanate–conjugated anti-CD2 mAb (PharMingen, San Diego, CA) and nonspecific esterase staining, respectively. Cells were immediately lysed in guanidinium thiocyanate buffer. The mRNA expression of IL-18 was detected by RT-PCR, as described previously (42). Briefly, 0.1 volume of 2*M* Na-acetate (pH 4.0) was added to the cell lysate and vortexed. Total cellular RNA was extracted with phenol/chloroform, ethanol-precipitated with 2*M* Na-acetate, and vacuum dried. The complementary DNA (cDNA) was synthesized from RNA with Molony murine leukemia virus reverse transcriptase (US Biochemical, Cleveland, OH) and oligo-$(dT)_{15}$ primers (Promega, Madison, WI).

Samples of cDNA were PCR amplified for 30 cycles for β-actin and for 35 cycles for IL-18 with *rTaq* DNA

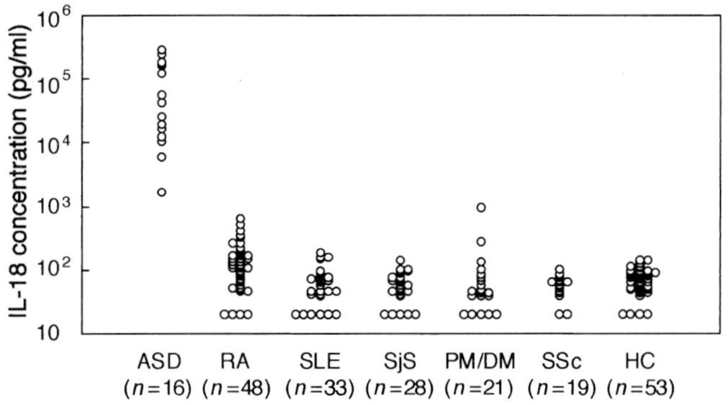

Figure 1. Concentrations of serum interleukin-18 (IL-18) in adult-onset Still's disease (ASD) and other systemic rheumatic diseases, measured in duplicate by enzyme-linked immunosorbent assay. Serum samples were obtained from patients with ASD, rheumatoid arthritis (RA), systemic lupus erythematosus (SLE), systemic sclerosis (SSc), polymyositis/dermatomyositis (PM/DM), Sjögren's syndrome (SjS), or healthy controls (HC).

polymerase (Promega, Madison, WI) and specific primers in a thermal cycler (TP cycler-100; Toyobo, Osaka, Japan). Each cycle consisted of 1 minute of denaturation at 95°C and 2 minutes of annealing/extension at 65°C for β-actin or at 55°C for IL-18. For comparison of cytokine mRNA expression, cDNA concentrations were normalized to yield approximately equivalent β-actin PCR products. PCR products were electrophoresed on 1.5% agarose gel and visualized by ethidium bromide staining. The sequences of oligonucleotide primers used for PCR were as follows: for IL-18, 5′ primer GCTTGAATCTAAATTATCAGTC and 3′ primer GAAGATTCAAATTGCATCTTAT; for β-actin, 5′ primer GTGGGGCGCCCCAGGCACCA and 3′ primer CTCCTTAATGTCACGCACGATTTC.

Statistical analysis. Samples with values below the detection limit for the assay were regarded as negative and assigned a value of 0. The data are expressed as the mean ± SD of the number of patients indicated. The statistical significance of differences between 2 groups was determined by Mann-Whitney U-test. The correlation coefficient was obtained by Spearman's rank correlation test.

RESULTS

Markedly elevated concentrations of serum IL-18 in patients with active ASD. Concentrations of serum IL-18 in patients with active ASD were compared by specific ELISA with those in patients with other systemic rheumatic diseases including RA, SLE, SSc, PM/DM, and SS, and in healthy individuals. As shown in Figure 1, serum IL-18 levels in ASD patients (mean ± SD 99,000 ± 99,800 pg/ml) were much higher than the levels in patients with RA (146 ± 124 pg/ml), SLE (68 ± 40 pg/ml), SSc (59 ± 18 pg/ml), PM/DM (104 ± 195 pg/ml), or SS (63 ± 27 pg/ml), or in healthy controls (74 ± 26 pg/ml); these differences were all statistically significant ($P < 0.005$).

To confirm the disease specificity of IL-18 elevation in ASD, serum IL-18 levels in febrile patients with

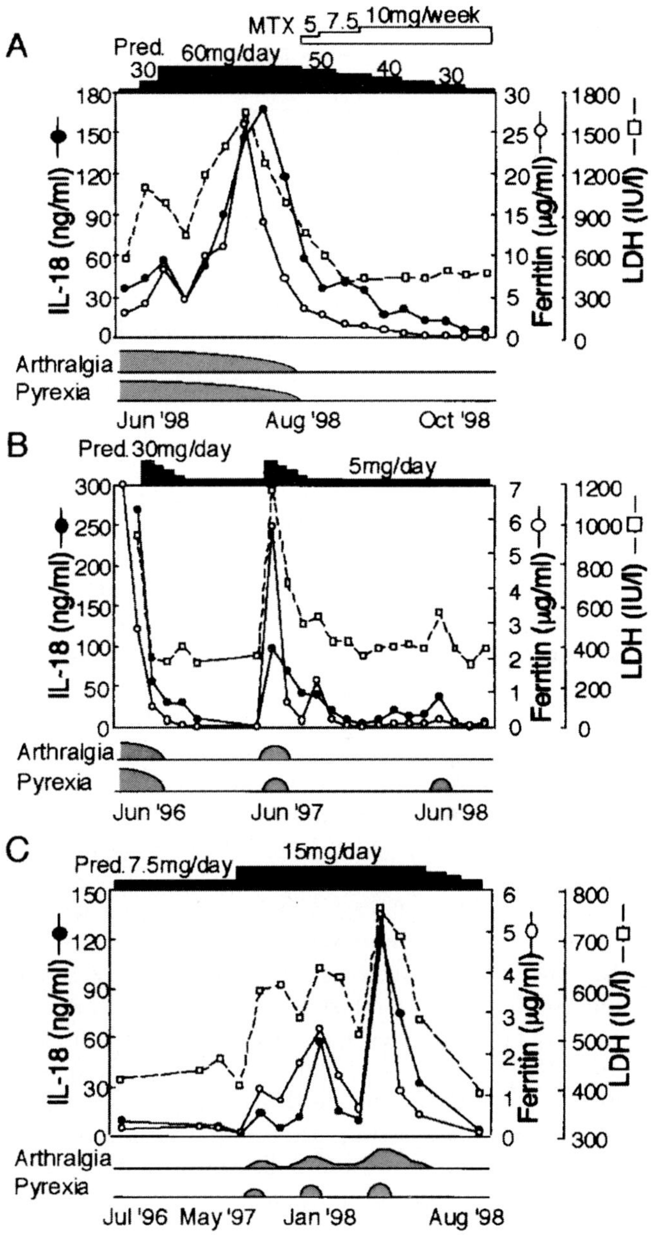

Figure 2. Changes in serum IL-18 levels in patients during the clinical course of ASD. Shown are the IL-18 levels of 3 patients with ASD (**A**, **B**, and **C**) whose levels were serially monitored, together with clinical manifestations such as fever and arthralgia and serum levels of ferritin and lactate dehydrogenase (LDH). Concentrations of IL-18 were determined by enzyme-linked immunosorbent assay. Pred. = prednisolone; MTX = methotrexate (see Figure 1 for other definitions).

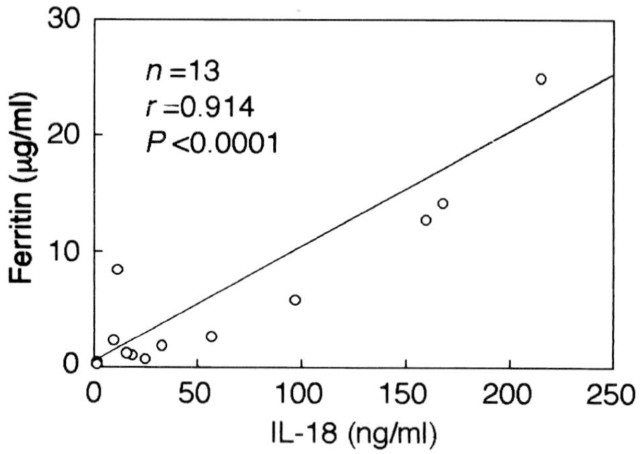

Figure 3. Correlation between IL-18 and ferritin levels in the serum of patients with active ASD. Serum samples were obtained from 13 patients with active ASD. Concentrations of IL-18 were determined by enzyme-linked immunosorbent assay. The correlation coefficient was analyzed by Spearman's rank correlation test. See Figure 1 for definitions.

bacterial infection or malignancy such as solid tumors and multiple myeloma were measured by ELISA. The mean ± SD values of IL-18 in 14 patients with bacterial infection and 22 patients with malignancy were 299 ± 137 pg/ml and 261 ± 135 pg/ml, respectively. Their levels were significantly greater than those of healthy controls, but were much lower than those of patients with ASD.

To investigate the relevance of IL-18 to the disease process of ASD, serum levels of IL-18 were serially monitored in 3 ASD patients (Figure 2). Their disease activity was assessed by the major clinical symptoms such as pyrexia and arthralgia as well as laboratory findings including serum levels of ferritin, lactate dehydrogenase (LDH), CRP, and the ESR. The level of serum IL-18 became both rapidly and markedly elevated when pyrexia and arthralgia developed, but gradually reduced after such manifestations disappeared with corticosteroid or additional methotrexate therapy. Furthermore, IL-18 levels were closely related to values of ferritin, LDH, CRP, and the ESR throughout observation of the disease course. However, even a few weeks after normalization of these indicators of inflammatory reaction, IL-18 was still detectable beyond the value in healthy controls.

Since serum ferritin levels are clinically used as a sensitive indicator for the disease activity of ASD, concentrations of ferritin were compared with those of IL-18 in 13 patients with active disease. The results clearly showed a positive correlation between these 2 values (Figure 3). However, IL-18 levels did not significantly correlate with CRP or ESR values. Taken together, these findings indicate that IL-18 overproduction appears to be intimately associated with the disease process of ASD.

Serum concentrations of other proinflammatory cytokines in ASD patients. Because increased production of several proinflammatory cytokines has been reported in juvenile or adult patients with Still's disease (27–32), serum levels of cytokines such as IL-1β, TNFα, IL-6, and IFNγ in ASD patients were determined by specific ELISA and compared with those in patients with active RA. As shown in Table 1, mean values of IL-6 and IFNγ were higher in the ASD patient group than in the RA group, whereas levels of TNFα and IL-1β were lower; however, these differences were not statistically significant ($P > 0.05$). It is noteworthy to indicate that the magnitude of the difference in IL-18 levels between these 2 patient groups was overwhelming in comparison with that of IL-6 or IFNγ levels; the difference was more than 600-fold for IL-18 (Figure 1), although it was less than 50-fold for IL-6 and IFNγ. Therefore, abnormal production of IL-18 appears to be highly specific for ASD. Of interest, IFNγ was detected at significant levels only in the active phase of disease in ASD patients but was undetectable during remission (data not shown), implicating IL-18 as an important inducer of IFNγ production in this inflammatory condition.

Detection of the mature 18-kd peptide of IL-18 in the serum of patients with active ASD. To confirm the synthesis of mature IL-18 protein in active ASD, total serum proteins from the patients were examined by Western blot analysis with anti–IL-18 antibody. The mature form of IL-18 has been shown to have a molecular weight of 18.3 kd (1–3). As shown in Figure 4, an 18-kd protein was determined by polyclonal anti–IL-18 antibody in patients with active ASD, and the staining of this band was eliminated in the presence of an excess amount of IL-18–specific blocking peptides, indicating the production of mature IL-18. In addition, serial

Table 1. Concentrations of IL-1β, TNFα, IL-6, and IFNγ in the serum from patients with active ASD and RA*

	IL-1β, pg/ml	TNFα, pg/ml	IL-6, pg/ml	IFNγ, pg/ml
ASD (n = 16)	0.7 ± 2.9	11.2 ± 14.5	19.4 ± 43.2	153.7 ± 563.5
RA (n = 34)	2.1 ± 7.5	13.5 ± 42.2	2.0 ± 3.5	3.7 ± 15.6

* Serum samples were obtained from patients with active adult-onset Still's disease (ASD) and rheumatoid arthritis (RA). Concentrations of interleukin-1β (IL-1β), tumor necrosis factor α (TNFα), IL-6, and interferon-γ (IFNγ) were measured in duplicate by enzyme-linked immunosorbent assay. Values are the mean ± SD.

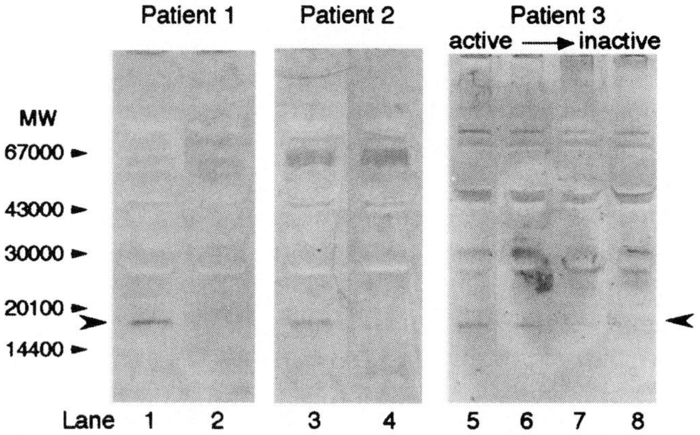

Figure 4. Detection of the mature form of IL-18 protein in the serum of ASD patients by Western blot analysis. Serum proteins from patients with active ASD were separated on a sodium docecyl sulfate–12.5% polyacrylamide gel and electrophoretically transferred onto a nitrocellulose membrane. The membrane was incubated with 0.4 μg/ml of goat polyclonal anti–IL-18 antibody with or without blocking peptide, followed by incubation with 0.2 μg/ml of alkaline phosphatase–conjugated donkey polyclonal anti-goat IgG antibody. Finally, the enzyme activity was detected using an alkaline phosphatase substrate staining kit. The mature form of IL-18 with a molecular weight of 18 kd is indicated by the **arrowhead** (lanes 1, 3, and 5–8). Bands of IL-18 weighing 18 kd were abolished in the presence of blocking peptide (lanes 2 and 4), confirming the specific detection of IL-18 with anti–IL-18 antibody. Shown are the results with samples from 2 patients with active ASD and with samples serially obtained from an ASD patient. See Figure 1 for definitions.

determination of the mature IL-18 protein in an ASD patient showed that the amount of serum 18-kd peptide gradually diminished in parallel with improvement in the disease severity.

Detection of IL-18 bioactivity in the serum of patients with active ASD. Having demonstrated the presence of the mature form of IL-18 protein, we examined serum samples from 6 patients with active ASD for IL-18 bioactivity by using KG-1 cells that dose dependently produce IFNγ in response to human IL-18 (40). All samples were able to stimulate IFNγ production by KG-1 cells, and this activity was largely neutralized by anti–IL-18 antibody (125-2H) (data not shown). In contrast, serum samples from healthy controls were not stimulatory for KG-1 cells (data not shown). Thus, significant IL-18 bioactivity was found in the blood of patients with active ASD. However, levels of IL-18 bioactivity were 7.3–42.7–fold (mean ± SD 18.2 ± 13.7–fold) lower than those of IL-18 protein measured by specific ELISA, although there was a direct correlation between these 2 values ($r = 0.919$, $P = 0.0096$) (Figure 5). This finding strongly suggests the coexistence of effective inhibitory molecules for IL-18 bioactivity in the serum of patients with active ASD.

Activity of IL-18 binding inhibition in the serum of ASD patients. IL-18BP is a recently identified molecule that efficiently regulates the inflammatory activity of IL-18 as a soluble decoy receptor (15,16). The inhibitory activity on IL-18 binding to its receptor was determined by IL-18 binding inhibition assay with CHO-K1/mIL-18R cells. Serum samples from 14 ASD patients were able to variously inhibit the binding of ^{125}I–IL-18 to CHO-K1/mIL-18R cells, whereas such inhibitory effects were mostly undetectable in those from healthy individuals (Figure 6A). A strong correlation was found between levels of IL-18 and its binding inhibition in ASD patients (Figure 7). In addition, serum inhibitory activity was found to change in parallel with IL-18 protein level during the disease course in 3 ASD patients (Figure 6B). These data indicate that IL-18 binding inhibitors such as IL-18BP may be induced in vivo in an attempt to confine the inflammatory effect of IL-18.

IL-18 mRNA expression in blood monocytes from patients with active ASD. Because the synthesis of IL-18 appears to be systemically aggravated during the active phase of ASD, IL-18 mRNA expression in freshly isolated peripheral blood monocytes and T cells from 5 patients

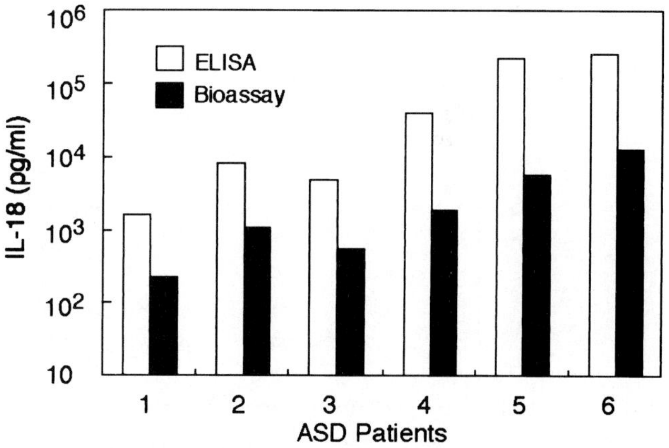

Figure 5. Bioactivity of IL-18 in the serum of 6 patients with active ASD, measured in triplicate using human myelomonocytic KG-1 cells, which produce interferon-γ (IFNγ) in response to IL-18, in a dose-dependent manner. The KG-1 cells were incubated for 24 hours with 100 μl of samples and recombinant human IL-18 standards with or without anti–IL-18 antibody. IFNγ concentrations in culture supernatants were measured by enzyme-linked immunosorbent assay (ELISA). IL-18 bioactivity was determined by the difference in IFNγ levels between those cultures with and without anti–IL-18 antibody, and was quantified by using IL-18 standards. Bioactivity of IL-18 in each sample is compared with the concentration of IL-18 protein determined by ELISA. See Figure 1 for other definitions.

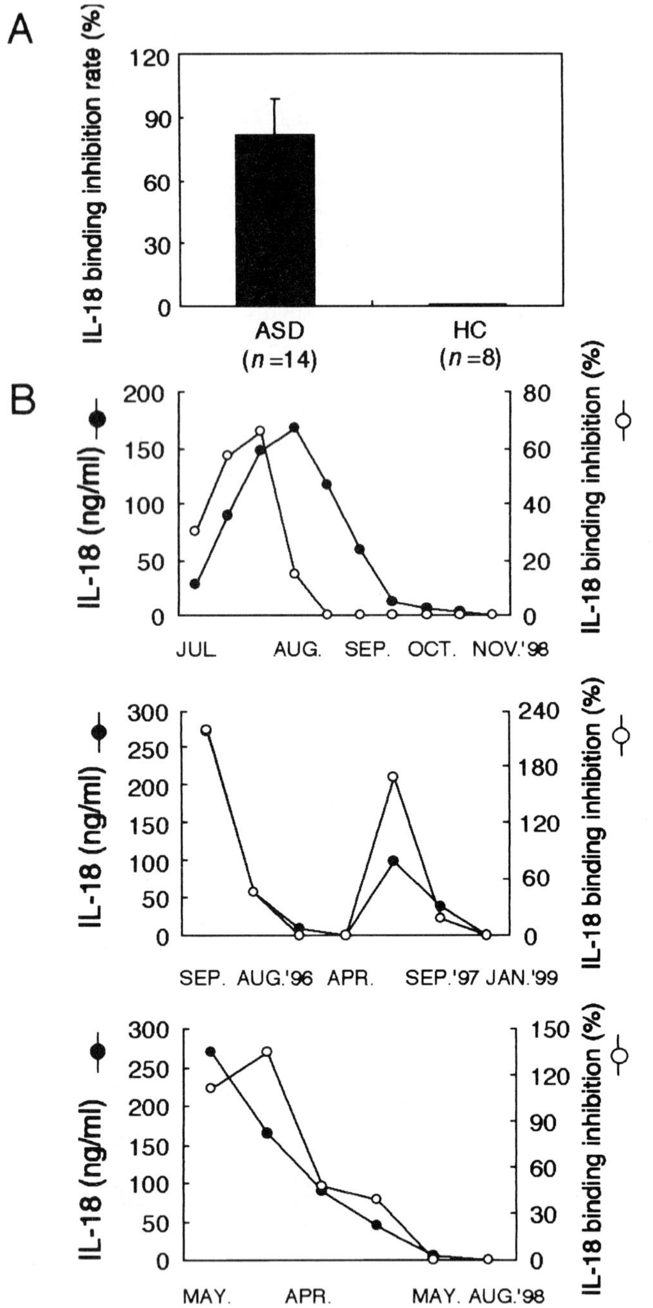

Figure 6. Activity of IL-18 binding inhibition, determined by IL-18 binding inhibition assay with a Chinese hamster ovary cell line transfected with a murine IL-18 receptor. **A,** Activity of IL-18 binding inhibition in the serum of patients with active ASD and healthy controls. Values are the mean and SD. **B,** Changes in levels of IL-18 protein and IL-18 binding inhibition during the clinical course of 3 ASD patients. See Figure 1 for definitions.

with active ASD was compared, by RT-PCR, with that in the corresponding cells of healthy individuals. Blood monocytes, but not T cells, from ASD patients contained

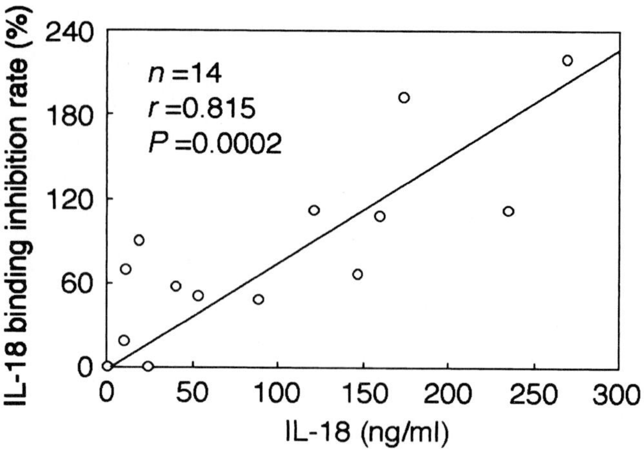

Figure 7. Correlation between IL-18 and IL-18 binding inhibitors in the serum of patients with active ASD. IL-18 and IL-18 binding inhibitors were measured by enzyme-linked immunosorbent assay and by IL-18 binding inhibition assay with a Chinese hamster ovary cell line transfected with a murine IL-18 receptor, respectively. The correlation coefficient was analyzed by Spearman's rank correlation test. See Figure 1 for definitions.

significant amounts of IL-18 mRNA, whereas IL-18 mRNA was undetectable in both cell types from any healthy controls (Figure 8). However, IL-18 protein was not detected in culture supernatants of monocytes from these patients by ELISA (results not shown).

DISCUSSION

In this study, we have demonstrated that the proinflammatory cytokine IL-18 is markedly elevated in the blood of ASD patients during the acute phase of the disease, and their peripheral blood monocytes may be primed to produce IL-18. Although its biologic activity appears to be considerably restricted by induction of IL-18 binding inhibitors, this cytokine is believed to contribute to

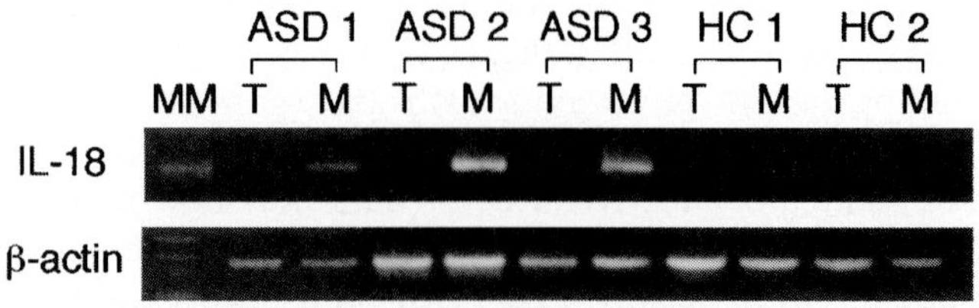

Figure 8. Expression of IL-18 mRNA in peripheral blood monocytes (M) and T cells (T) from ASD patients. Mononuclear cells were isolated from peripheral blood from 5 patients with active ASD and 5 healthy controls, and monocytes and T cells were purified by positive selection using anti-CD14– or anti-CD3–coated magnetic beads, respectively. Shown are representative results with the cells from 3 ASD patients and 2 healthy controls. See Figure 1 for other definitions.

the disease process of ASD by generating an inflammatory cytokine cascade including TNFα, IL-6, and IFNγ.

In ASD patients, serum IL-18 was drastically elevated in conjunction with the development of clinical manifestations, such as a high spiking fever, arthralgia or arthritis, and often a rash. Laboratory studies also revealed the presence of a systemic inflammatory reaction, indicated by increased levels of serum CRP and the ESR. However, shortly after the disease was successfully controlled by corticosteroid therapy or the addition of methotrexate, IL-18 levels diminished and then gradually normalized. Of interest, IL-18 levels were closely correlated with serum ferritin levels within the studied group of patients with active ASD and through the clinical course of each patient. A marked hyperferritinemia has been recognized as being most pathognomonic for ASD, and ferritin levels are used to monitor the disease activity (24–26). Therefore, IL-18 induction appears to be related to the process of this systemic inflammatory disease.

Previously, several inflammatory cytokines have been described as being involved in juvenile or adult Still's disease. Studies of the juvenile onset disease have demonstrated enhanced production of IL-1 by blood mononuclear cells (27), correlation of increased serum IL-6 levels with joint inflammation and thrombocytosis (28), large amounts of IL-6 and soluble IL-6R complex circulating in the peripheral blood (29), and an elevation of serum IL-1β, TNFα, IL-6, and IL-7 (30,31). In ASD patients, IL-6, TNFα, and IFNγ have been detected at high levels in the blood, with IL-6 being most associated with both systemic and articular manifestations (32). In our study, serum IL-6 and IFNγ were mostly detected at higher levels in ASD patients than in RA patients, although the difference between the groups was not statistically significant, and IL-1β and TNFα were measurable in some of the patients. These inflammatory cytokines are believed to be involved in the pathophysiology of ASD; for example, IL-1, TNFα, and IL-6 are well known as inducers of serum acute-phase reactants. Nonetheless, IL-18 elevation in active ASD was much greater than that found in other systemic rheumatic diseases, including RA, and in febrile patients with bacterial infection and malignancy. Thus, overproduction of IL-18 may be the event specific for the disease of ASD.

The pathogenic significance of IL-18 in ASD is further supported by the detection of its biologically active mature protein in active disease. Serum IL-18 protein determined by Western blot analysis had a molecular weight of 18 kd, corresponding to that of the mature form (2,3). Accordingly, serum samples from patients with active ASD were able to induce IFNγ production by IL-18–responding KG-1 cells, which was largely blocked by anti-IL-18 antibody. In addition, a significant amount of circulating IFNγ was detected in the active phase of the disease, but it became undetectable soon after satisfactory treatment. These findings indicate that IFNγ elevation in active ASD may be caused by the circulation of bioactive IL-18.

The inflammatory cytokine IFNγ, known as a potent macrophage-activating factor, is produced mainly by T cells and NK cells. High levels of serum IFNγ are thus thought to represent the in vivo activation of inflammatory Th1-type CD4+ T cells, cytotoxic CD8+ T cells, and/or NK cells. In addition to stimulating their IFNγ production (6,7), IL-18 can promote diverse functions of these cell types, such as T cell differentiation toward Th1 type (5), T cell proliferation and cytokine production (3), and NK cell cytotoxicity through Fas ligand induction (6,8). More recently, IL-18 has been shown to initiate the proinflammatory cascade independently of IFNγ. It stimulates CD14+ monocytes to secrete inflammatory cytokines, such as IL-1β, IL-8, macrophage inflammatory protein 1α, and monocyte chemotactic protein 1, indirectly through its induction of TNFα from CD4+ T cells and NK cells (43). Therefore, IL-18 overproduction can elicit T cell– and NK cell–mediated inflammatory reactions via both IFNγ-dependent and -independent pathways.

The contribution of IL-18 to Th1 cell–mediated inflammation has recently been demonstrated in human diseases such as RA and Crohn's disease (10–14). Our determination of serum IL-18 concentrations showed its increased level in patients with RA, particularly in patients with early and active disease, in comparison with healthy controls and those with other rheumatic diseases such as SLE, SS, and SSc. This finding likely reflects the local production of IL-18 and its contribution to Th1 cell activation in the joints of patients with RA. It is thus possible that IL-18 overproduction may induce the systemic Th1-type immune response in ASD. However, a recent report showed a mixed Th1/Th2 cytokine response by blood mononuclear cells from patients with juvenile-onset Still's disease (44), suggesting the absence of the predominant activation of Th1 cells over Th2 cells in ASD. This may be due to the concomitant production of cytokines antagonizing the Th1 response, such as IL-4 and IL-10, or the deficiency of costimulants to effective Th1 cell activation, such as IL-12 and CD40. Recently, IL-18 has been shown to stimulate T cell production of Th2 cytokines as well as IFNγ (45), supporting the former possibility. In NOD mice, administration of IL-18 suppressed Th1-type destructive insulitis by counterregulating Th1 cell activation (46). Therefore, it is most likely that IL-18 may generate the systemic inflammation in ASD by activating the innate immune response involving NK cells and macrophages, rather than the Th1 response.

We found that the activity of IL-18 binding inhibition was increased in the serum of patients with active ASD. IL-18BP, a soluble decoy receptor for IL-18 with high affinity, has been identified as a major inhibitor of IL-18 activity in vivo, and was shown to effectively inhibit IL-18 induction of activation of the transcriptional factor NF-κB and production of cytokines such as IFNγ and IL-8 in KG-1 cells and blood mononuclear cells by preventing IL-18 binding to its receptor (15,16). It remains unclear at present whether IL-18BP is most responsible for the activity of IL-18 binding inhibition found in ASD, but the coexistence of such specific inhibitors could explain the restriction of IL-18 bioactivity, as shown by the relatively low IFNγ secretion from KG-1 cells stimulated with serum IL-18 of patients with ASD. Because levels of IL-18 binding inhibition correlated well with those of IL-18 protein, the in vivo production of inhibitors may be induced by IL-18 itself as its own major negative feedback mechanism. However, this regulation appears to be only partial in active ASD, since IFNγ-inducing activity on KG-1 cells was still detectable in the serum.

The balance between inflammatory molecules and their inhibitors is disturbed in many pathologic conditions. For example, in the joints of patients with active RA, the 2 essential proinflammatory cytokines, IL-1 and TNFα, and their specific inhibitors, such as the IL-1 receptor antagonist and soluble TNFα receptors, are produced at high levels, but levels of inhibitors are relatively low (47). Therefore, the disease activity of ASD may be associated with the relative levels of IL-18 and IL-18 binding inhibitors. IL-18 production predominates in active disease, but IL-18 activity can be neutralized by its inhibitors during remission.

Blood monocytes from patients with active ASD expressed IL-18 mRNA more strongly than the cells from healthy controls, but failed to secrete detectable amounts of IL-18 protein. Because activated macrophages are known to be the major producer of human IL-18 (2,3), it is speculated that systemic activation of these lineage cells may be responsible for IL-18 overproduction in active ASD; circulating monocytes are already committed, readily differentiated into tissue macrophages, and then substantially release IL-18. However, organ sources of IL-18 are so far undetermined in this inflammatory disease.

In the murine model of endotoxin shock, IL-18 elevation is associated with extensive liver damage and is derived mainly from Kuppfer cells and activated macrophages (1,2). More recently, it has been demonstrated in hemophagocytic lymphohistocytosis that serum IL-18 levels are extremely high and the spleen strongly expresses transcripts of IL-18 (48). In this regard, ASD is often complicated by hepatomegaly with liver damage, splenomegaly, and lymphadenopathy. In a review of 228 cases of ASD, hepatomegaly was found in 40.6% of the patients, elevated hepatic enzyme levels in 71.6%, splenomegaly in 51.7%, and lymphadenopathy in 60.3% (21). The majority of our ASD patients showed evidence of liver and spleen involvement. It is thus conceivable that in ASD, blood monocytes may be distributed to the reticuloendothelial system, including the liver, spleen, and lymph nodes, in which they functionally develop into potent IL-18–producing tissue macrophages.

There was a significant correlation between serum ferritin and IL-18 levels in ASD patients. Hyperferritinemia is mainly attributable to increased ferritin release from the liver and spleen in ASD (26). The reticuloendothelial cells, such as Kuppfer cells and splenic macrophages, release the iron acquired by erythrophagocytosis in the form of ferritin, and the ferritin synthesis, without increased body iron storage, is stimulated in inflammatory states (49–51). Therefore, there is a possibility that IL-18 could be a powerful autocrine or paracrine stimulator of ferritin synthesis. On the other hand, the clearance of ferritin has been suggested to be impaired in ASD, due to decreased expression of the hepatic ferritin receptor and increased synthesis of the desialylated isoform (26). IL-18 may be an inhibitor of ferritin clearance. It is also conceivable that both IL-18 and ferritin could be released by leakage through the damaged membrane of reticuloendothelial cells because liver injury, splenomegaly, and lymphadenopathy are often observed in ASD.

In conclusion, overproduction of IL-18 protein appears to be intimately associated with the pathophysiology of ASD. Despite the significant induction of IL-18 binding inhibitors, the biologic activity of IL-18 can be detected in the serum of patients with active ASD. Since IL-18 has the potential to induce the systemic inflammatory reactions and tissue damage found in ASD, neutralization of its inflammatory activities, e.g., by using IL-18BP, may have implications for reducing the severity of the disease.

ACKNOWLEDGMENTS

The authors thank Dr. H. Okamura (Hyogo College of Medicine, Nishinomiya, Japan) for helpful discussion; Dr. Y. Ohmoto (Otsuka Pharmaceutical, Tokushima, Japan) for the gift of the ELISAs for IL-1β, TNFα, IL-6, and IFNγ; and Dr. Y. Yamanishi (Hiroshima University School of Medicine, Hiroshima, Japan) for providing clinical samples.

REFERENCES

1. Okamura H, Nagata K, Komatsu T, Tanimoto T, Nukata Y, Tanabe F, et al. A novel costimulatory factor for gamma interferon induction found in the livers of mice causes endotoxic shock. Infect Immun 1995;63:3966–72.
2. Okamura H, Tsutsi H, Komatsu T, Yutsudo M, Hakura A, Tanimoto T, et al. Cloning of a new cytokine that induces IFN-γ production by T cells. Nature 1995;378:88–91.
3. Ushio S, Namba M, Okura T, Hattori K, Nukada Y, Akita K, et al. Cloning of the cDNA for human IFN-γ-inducing factor, expression in Escherichia coli, and studies on the biologic activities of the protein. J Immunol 1996;156:4274–9.
4. Gu Y, Kuida K, Tsutsui H, Ku G, Hsiao K, Fleming MA, et al. Activation of interferon-γ inducing factor mediated by interleukin-1β converting enzyme. Science 1997;275:206–9.
5. Robinson D, Shibuya K, Mui A, Zonin F, Murphy E, Sana T, et al. IGIF does not drive Th1 development but synergizes with IL-12 for interferon-gamma production and activates IRAK and NF-κB. Immunity 1997;7:571–81.
6. Micallef MJ, Ohtsuki T, Kohno K, Tanabe F, Ushio S, Namba M, et al. Interferon-γ-inducing factor enhances T helper 1 cytokine production by stimulated human T cells: synergism with interleukin-12 for interferon-gamma production. Eur J Immunol 1996;26: 1647–51.
7. Zhang T, Kawakami K, Qureshi MH, Okamura H, Kurimoto M, Saito A. Interleukin-12 (IL-12) and IL-18 synergistically induce the fungicidal activity of murine peritoneal exudate cells against Cryptococcus neoformans through production of gamma interferon by natural killer cells. Infect Immun 1997;65:3594–9.
8. Tsutsui H, Nakanishi K, Matsui K, Higashino K, Okamura H, Miyazawa Y, et al. IFN-γ-inducing factor up-regulates Fas ligand-mediated cytotoxic activity of murine natural killer cell clones. J Immunol 1996;157:3967–73.
9. Tsutsui H, Matsui K, Kawada N, Hyodo Y, Hayashi N, Okamura H, et al. IL-18 accounts for both TNF-α- and Fas ligand-mediated hepatotoxic pathways in endotoxin-induced liver injury in mice. J Immunol 1997;159:3961–7.
10. Rothe H, Jenkins NA, Copeland NG, Kolb H. Active stage of autoimmune diabetes is associated with the expression of a novel cytokine, IGIF, which is located near *Idd2*. J Clin Invest 1997;99: 469–74.
11. Pizarro TT, Michie MH, Bentz M, Woraratanadharm J, Smith MF Jr, Foley E, et al. IL-18, a novel immunoregulatory cytokine, is up-regulated in Crohn's disease: expression and localization in intestinal mucosal cells. J Immunol 1999;162:6829–35.
12. Monteleone G, Trapasso F, Parrello T, Biancone L, Stella A, Iuliano R, et al. Bioactive IL-18 expression is up-regulated in Crohn's disease. J Immunol 1999;163:143–7.
13. Yamamura M, Kawashima M, Morita Y, Makino H, Tanimoto T, Kurimoto M. Increased production of interleukin-18 in synovium from patients with rheumatoid arthritis [abstract]. Arthritis Rheum 1997;40 Suppl 9:S274.
14. Gracie JA, Forsey RJ, Chan WL, Gilmour A, Leung BP, Greer MR, et al. A proinflammatory role for IL-18 in rheumatoid arthritis. J Clin Invest 1999;104:1393–401.
15. Aizawa Y, Akita K, Taniai M, Torigoe K, Mori T, Nishida Y, et al. Cloning and expression of interleukin-18 binding protein. FEBS Lett 1999;445:338–42.
16. Novick D, Kim SH, Fantuzzi G, Reznikov LL, Dinarello CA, Rubinstein M. Interleukin-18 binding protein: a novel modulator of the Th1 cytokine response. Immunity 1999;10:127–36.
17. Torigoe K, Ushio S, Okura T, Kobayashi S, Taniai M, Kunikata T, et al. Purification and characterization of the human interleukin-18 receptor. J Biol Chem 1997;272:25737–42.
18. Parnet P, Garka KE, Bonnert TP, Dower SK, Sims JE. IL-1Rrp is a novel receptor-like molecule similar to the type I interleukin-1 receptor and its homologues T1/ST2 and IL-1R AcP. J Biol Chem 1996;271:3967–70.
19. Born TL, Thomassen E, Bird TA, Sims JE. Cloning of a novel receptor subunit, AcPL, required for interleukin-18 signaling. J Biol Chem 1998;273:29445–50.
20. Bywaters EGL. Still's disease in the adult. Ann Rheum Dis 1971;30:121–33.
21. Ohta A, Yamaguchi M, Kaneoka H, Nagayoshi T, Hiida M. Adult Still's disease: review of 228 cases from the literature. J Rheumatol 1987;14:1139–46.
22. Reginato AJ, Schumacher HR Jr, Baker DG, O'Connor CR, Ferreiros J. Adult onset Still's disease: experience in 23 patients and literature review with emphasis on organ failure. Semin Arthritis Rheum 1987;17:39–57.
23. Pouchot J, Sampalis JS, Beaudet F, Carette S, Decary F, Salusinsky-Sternbach M, et al. Adult Still's disease: manifestations, disease course, and outcome in 62 patients. Medicine (Baltimore) 1991;70:118–36.
24. Yamaguchi M, Ohta A, Tsunematsu T, Kasukawa R, Mizushima Y, Kashiwagi H, et al. Preliminary criteria for classification of adult Still's disease. J Rheumatol 1992;19:424–30.
25. Ota T, Higashi S, Suzuki H, Eto S. Increased serum ferritin levels in adult Still's disease. Lancet 1987;1:562–3.
26. Van Reeth C, le Moel G, Lasne Y, Revenant MC, Agneray J, Kahn MF, et al. Serum ferritin and isoferritins are tools for diagnosis of active adult Still's disease. J Rheumatol 1994;21: 890–5.
27. Martini A, Ravelli A, Notarangelo LD, Maccario R, Lanfranchi A, Rondena D, et al. Enhanced interleukin 1 and depressed interleukin 2 production in juvenile arthritis. J Rheumatol 1986;13: 598–603.
28. De Benedetti F, Massa M, Robbioni P, Ravelli A, Burgio GR, Martini A. Correlation of serum interleukin-6 levels with joint involvement and thrombocytosis in systemic juvenile rheumatoid arthritis. Arthritis Rheum 1991;34:1158–63.
29. De Benedetti F, Massa M, Pignatti P, Albani S, Novick D, Martini A. Serum soluble interleukin 6 (IL-6) receptor and IL-6/soluble IL-6 receptor complex in systemic juvenile rheumatoid arthritis. J Clin Invest 1994;93:2114–9.
30. Mangge H, Kenzian H, Gallistl S, Neuwirth G, Liebmann P, Kaulfersch W, et al. Serum cytokines in juvenile rheumatoid arthritis: correlation with conventional inflammation parameters and clinical subtypes. Arthritis Rheum 1995;38:211–20.
31. De Benedetti F, Massa M, Pignatti P, Kelley M, Faltynek CR, Martini A. Elevated circulating interleukin-7 levels in patients with systemic juvenile rheumatoid arthritis. J Rheumatol 1995;22: 1581–5.
32. Hoshino T, Ohta A, Yang D, Kawamoto M, Kikuchi M, Inoue Y, et al. Elevated serum interleukin 6, interferon-γ, and tumor necrosis factor α levels in patients with adult Still's disease. J Rheumatol 1998;25:396–8.
33. Cush JJ, Medsger TA Jr, Christy WC, Herbert DC, Cooperstein LA. Adult-onset Still's disease: clinical course and outcome. Arthritis Rheum 1987;30:186–94.
34. Arnett FC, Edworthy SM, Bloch DA, McShane DJ, Fries JF, Cooper NS, et al. The American Rheumatism Association 1987

revised criteria for the classification of rheumatoid arthritis. Arthritis Rheum 1988;31:315–24.
35. Tan EM, Cohen AS, Fries JF, Masi AT, McShane DJ, Rothfield NF, et al. The 1982 revised criteria for the classification of systemic lupus erythematosus. Arthritis Rheum 1982;25:1271–7.
36. Subcommittee for Scleroderma Criteria of the American Rheumatism Association Diagnostic and Therapeutic Criteria Committee. Preliminary criteria for the classification of systemic sclerosis (scleroderma). Arthritis Rheum 1980;23:581–90.
37. Bohan A, Peter JB. Polymyositis and dermatomyositis. N Engl J Med 1975;292:344–7.
38. Vitali C, Bombardieri S, Moutsopoulos HM, Balestrieri G, Bencivelli W, Bernstein RM, et al. Preliminary criteria for the classification of Sjögren's syndrome: results of a prospective concerted action supported by the European Community. Arthritis Rheum 1993;36:340–7.
39. Bombardier C, Gladman DD, Urowitz MB, Caron D, Chang CH, and the Committee on Prognosis Studies in SLE. Derivation of the SLEDAI: a disease activity index for lupus patients. Arthritis Rheum 1992;35:630–40.
40. Konishi K, Tanabe F, Taniguchi M, Yamauchi H, Tanimoto T, Ikeda M, et al. A simple and sensitive bioassay for the detection of human interleukin-18/interferon-γ-inducing factor using human myelomonocytic KG-1 cells. J Immunol Methods 1997;209:187–91.
41. Taniguchi M, Nagaoka K, Kunikata T, Kayano T, Yamauchi H, Nakamura S, et al. Characterization of anti-human interleukin-18 (IL-18)/interferon-γ-inducing factor (IGIF) monoclonal antibodies and their application in the measurement of human IL-18 by ELISA. J Immunol Methods 1997;206:107–13.
42. Yamamura M, Uyemura K, Deans RJ, Weinberg K, Rea TH, Bloom BR, et al. Defining protective responses to pathogens: cytokine profiles in leprosy lesions. Science 1991;254:277–9.
43. Puren AJ, Fantuzzi G, Gu Y, Su MS, Dinarello CA. Interleukin-18 (IFNγ-inducing factor) induces IL-8 and IL-1β via TNFα production from non-CD14+ human blood mononuclear cells. J Clin Invest 1998;101:711–21.
44. Raziuddin S, Bahabri S, Al-Dalaan A, Siraj AK, Al-Sedairy S. A mixed Th1/Th2 cell cytokine response predominates in systemic onset juvenile rheumatoid arthritis: immunoregulatory IL-10 function. Clin Immunol Immunopathol 1998;86:192–8.
45. Hoshino T, Yagita H, Ortaldo JR, Wiltrout RH, Young HA. In vivo administration of IL-18 can induce IgE production through Th2 cytokine induction and up-regulation of CD40 ligand (CD154) expression on CD4+ T cells. Eur J Immunol 2000;30:1998–2006.
46. Rothe H, Housmann A, Casteels K, Okamura H, Kurimoto M, Burkart V, et al. IL-18 inhibits diabetes development in nonobese diabetic mice by counterregulation of Th1-dependent destructive insulitis. J Immunol 1999;163:1230–6.
47. Arend WP, Dayer J-M. Cytokines and cytokine inhibitors or antagonists in rheumatoid arthritis. Arthritis Rheum 1990;33:305–15.
48. Takada H, Ohga S, Mizuno Y, Suminoe A, Matsuzaki A, Ihara K, et al. Oversecretion of IL-18 in haemophagocytic lymphohistiocytosis: a novel marker of disease activity. Br J Haematol 1999;106:182–9.
49. Kondo H, Saito K, Grasso JP, Aisen P. Iron metabolism in the erythrophagocytosing Kupffer cell. Hepatology 1988;8:32–8.
50. Sibille JC, Kondo H, Aisen P. Interactions between isolated hepatocytes and Kupffer cells in iron metabolism: a possible role for ferritin as an iron carrier protein. Hepatology 1988;8:296–301.
51. Campbell CH, Solgonick RM, Linder MC. Translational regulation of ferritin synthesis in rat spleen: effects of iron and inflammation. Biochem Biophys Res Commun 1989;160:453–9.

SALAGEN® Tablets
(pilocarpine hydrochloride)

Brief Summary

Consult package insert for full prescribing information

INDICATIONS AND USAGE: SALAGEN® Tablets are indicated for 1) the treatment of symptoms of dry mouth from salivary gland hypofunction caused by radiotherapy for cancer of the head and neck; and 2) the treatment of symptoms of dry mouth in patients with Sjogren's syndrome.

CONTRAINDICATIONS: SALAGEN® Tablets are contraindicated in patients with uncontrolled asthma, known hypersensitivity to pilocarpine, and when miosis is undesirable, e.g., in acute iritis and in narrow-angle (angle closure) glaucoma.

WARNINGS:

Cardiovascular Disease: Patients with significant cardiovascular disease may be unable to compensate for transient changes in hemodynamics or rhythm induced by pilocarpine. Pulmonary edema has been reported as a complication of pilocarpine toxicity from high ocular doses given for acute angle-closure glaucoma. Pilocarpine should be administered with caution in and under close medical supervision of patients with significant cardiovascular disease.

Ocular: Ocular formulations of pilocarpine have been reported to cause visual blurring which may result in decreased visual acuity, especially at night and in patients with central lens changes, and to cause impairment of depth perception. Caution should be advised while driving at night or performing hazardous activities in reduced lighting.

Pulmonary Disease: Pilocarpine has been reported to increase airway resistance, bronchial smooth muscle tone, and bronchial secretions. Pilocarpine hydrochloride should be administered with caution to and under close medical supervision in patients with controlled asthma, chronic bronchitis, or chronic obstructive pulmonary disease requiring pharmacotherapy.

PRECAUTIONS:

General: Pilocarpine toxicity is characterized by an exaggeration of its parasympathomimetic effects. These may include: headache, visual disturbance, lacrimation, sweating, respiratory distress, gastrointestinal spasm, nausea, vomiting, diarrhea, atrioventricular block, tachycardia, bradycardia, hypotension, hypertension, shock, mental confusion, cardiac arrhythmia, and tremors.

The dose-related cardiovascular pharmacologic effects of pilocarpine include hypotension, hypertension, bradycardia, and tachycardia.

Pilocarpine should be administered with caution to patients with known or suspected cholelithiasis or biliary tract disease. Contractions of the gallbladder or biliary smooth muscle could precipitate complications including cholecystitis, cholangitis, and biliary obstruction.

Pilocarpine may increase ureteral smooth muscle tone and could theoretically precipitate renal colic (or "ureteral reflux"), particularly in patients with nephrolithiasis.

Cholinergic agonists may have dose-related central nervous system effects. This should be considered when treating patients with underlying cognitive or psychiatric disturbances.

Renal Insufficiency: The pharmacokinetics of orally administered pilocarpine in patients with renal and hepatic disease is not known.

Information for Patients: Patients should be informed that pilocarpine may cause visual disturbances, especially at night, that could impair their ability to drive safely.

If a patient sweats excessively while taking pilocarpine hydrochloride and cannot drink enough liquid, the patient should consult a physician. Dehydration may develop.

Drug Interactions: Pilocarpine should be administered with caution to patients taking beta adrenergic antagonists because of the possibility of conduction disturbances. Drugs with parasympathomimetic effects administered concurrently with pilocarpine would be expected to result in additive pharmacologic effects. Pilocarpine might antagonize the anticholinergic effects of drugs used concomitantly. These effects should be considered when anticholinergic properties may be contributing to the therapeutic effect of concomitant medication (e.g., atropine, inhaled ipratropium).

While no formal drug interaction studies have been performed, the following concomitant drugs were used in at least 10% of patients in either or both Sjogren's efficacy studies: acetylsalicylic acid, artificial tears, calcium, conjugated estrogens, hydroxychloroquine sulfate, ibuprofen, levothyroxine sodium, medroxyprogesterone acetate, methotrexate, multivitamins, naproxen, omeprazole, paracetamol, and prednisone.

Carcinogenesis, Mutagenesis, Impairment of Fertility: No definitive long term animal studies have evaluated the carcinogenic potential of pilocarpine. No evidence that pilocarpine has the potential to cause genetic toxicity was obtained in a series of studies that included: 1) bacterial assays (Salmonella and E. coli) for reverse gene mutations; 2) an *in vitro* chromosome aberration assay in a Chinese hamster ovary cell line; 3) an *in vivo* chromosome aberration assay (micronucleus test) in mice; and 4) a primary DNA damage assay (unscheduled DNA synthesis) in rat hepatocyte primary cultures.

Oral administration of pilocarpine to male and female rats at a dosage of 18 mg/kg/day (approximately 5 times the maximum recommended dose for a 50 kg human when compared on the basis of body surface area (mg/m^2) estimates) resulted in impaired reproductive function, including reduced fertility, decreased sperm motility, and morphologic evidence of abnormal sperm. It is unclear whether the reduction in fertility was due to effects on male animals, female animals, or both males and females. In dogs, exposure to pilocarpine at a dosage of 3 mg/kg/day (approximately 3 times the maximum recommended dose for a 50 kg human when compared on the basis of body surface area (mg/m^2) estimates) for six months resulted in evidence of impaired spermatogenesis. The data obtained in these studies suggest that pilocarpine may impair the fertility of male and female humans.

SALAGEN® Tablets should be administered to individuals who are attempting to conceive a child only if the potential benefit justifies potential impairment of fertility.

Pregnancy: Teratogenic effects.

Pregnancy Category C: Pilocarpine was associated with a reduction in the mean fetal body weight and an increase in the incidence of skeletal variations when given to pregnant rats at a dosage of 90 mg/kg/day (approximately 26 times the maximum recommended dose for a 50 kg human when compared on the basis of body surface area (mg/m^2) estimates). These effects may have been secondary to maternal toxicity. In another study, oral administration of pilocarpine to female rats during gestation and lactation at a dosage of 36 mg/kg/day (approximately 10 times the maximum recommended dose for a 50 kg human when compared on the basis of body surface area (mg/m^2) estimates) resulted in an increased incidence of stillbirths; decreased neonatal survival and reduced mean body weight of pups were observed at dosages of 18 mg/kg/day (approximately 5 times the maximum recommended dose for a 50 kg human when compared on the basis of body surface area (mg/m^2) estimates) and above. There are no adequate and well-controlled studies in pregnant women. SALAGEN® Tablets should be used during pregnancy only if the potential benefit justifies the potential risk to the fetus.

Nursing Mothers: It is not known whether this drug is excreted in human milk. Because many drugs are excreted in human milk and because of the potential for serious adverse reactions in nursing infants from SALAGEN® Tablets, a decision should be made whether to discontinue nursing or to discontinue the drug, taking into account the importance of the drug to the mother.

Pediatric Use: Safety and effectiveness in pediatric patients have not been established.

Geriatric Use: Head and Neck Cancer Patients: In the placebo-controlled clinical trials (see Clinical Studies section in full prescribing information) the mean age of patients was approximately 58 years (range 19 to 80). Of these patients, 97/369 (61/217 receiving pilocarpine) were over the age of 65 years. In the healthy volunteer studies, 15/150 subjects were over the age of 65 years. In both study populations, the adverse events reported by those over 65 years and those 65 years and younger were comparable. Of the 15 elderly volunteers (5 women, 10 men), the 5 women had higher C_{max}'s and AUC's than the men.

Sjogren's Syndrome Patients: In the placebo-controlled clinical trials, the mean age of patients was approximately 55 years (range 21 to 85). The adverse events reported by those over 65 years and those 65 years and younger were comparable except for notable trends for urinary frequency, diarrhea, and dizziness (see **ADVERSE REACTIONS** section).

ADVERSE REACTIONS: Head & Neck Cancer Patients: In controlled studies, 217 patients received pilocarpine, of whom 68% were men and 32% were women. Race distribution was 91% Caucasian, 8% Black, and 1% of other origin. Mean age was approximately 58 years. The majority of patients were between 50 and 64 years (51%), 33% were 65 years and older and 16% were younger than 50 years of age.

The most frequent adverse experiences associated with SALAGEN® Tablets were a consequence of the expected pharmacologic effects of pilocarpine.

Adverse Event	10 mg t.i.d. (30mg/day) n=121	5 mg t.i.d. (15mg/day) n=141	placebo (t.i.d.) n=152
Sweating	68%	29%	9%
Nausea	15	6	4
Rhinitis	14	5	7
Diarrhea	7	4	5
Chills	15	3	<1
Flushing	13	8	3
Urinary Frequency	12	9	7
Dizziness	12	5	4
Asthenia	12	6	3

In addition, the following adverse events (≥3% incidence) were reported at dosages of 15-30 mg/day in the controlled clinical trials: Headache (11%), dyspepsia (7%), lacrimation (6%), edema (5%), abdominal pain (4%), amblyopia (4%), vomiting (4%), pharyngitis (3%), hypertension (3%).

The following events were reported with treated head and neck cancer patients at incidences of 1% to 2% at dosages of 7.5 to 30 mg/day: abnormal vision, conjunctivitis, dysphagia, epistaxis, myalgias, pruritus, rash, sinusitis, tachycardia, taste perversion, tremor, voice alteration.

The following events were reported rarely in treated head and neck cancer patients (<1%): Causal relation is unknown.

Body odor, hypothermia, mucous membrane abnormality, bradycardia, ECG abnormality, palpitations, syncope, anorexia, increased appetite, esophagitis, gastrointestinal disorder, tongue disorder, leukopenia, lymphadenopathy, anxiety, confusion, depression, abnormal dreams, hyperkinesia, hypoesthesia, nervousness, paresthesias, speech disorder, twitching, increased sputum, stridor, yawning, seborrhea, deafness, eye pain, glaucoma, dysuria, metrorrhagia, urinary impairment.

In long-term treatment were two patients with underlying cardiovascular disease of whom one experienced a myocardial infarct and another an episode of syncope. The association with drug is uncertain.

Sjogren's Syndrome Patients: In controlled studies, 376 patients received pilocarpine, of whom 5% were men and 95% were women. Race distribution was 84% Caucasian, 9% Oriental, 3% Black, and 4% of other origin. Mean age was 55 years. The majority of patients were between 40 and 69 years (70%), 16% were 70 years and older and 14% were younger than 40 years of age. Of these patients, 161/629 (89/376 receiving pilocarpine) were over the age of 65 years. The adverse events reported by those over 65 years and those 65 years and younger were comparable except for notable trends for urinary frequency, diarrhea, and dizziness. The incidences of urinary frequency and diarrhea in the elderly were about double those in the non-elderly. The incidence of dizziness was about three times as high in the elderly as in the non-elderly. These adverse experiences were not considered to be serious. In the 2 placebo-controlled studies, the most common adverse events related to drug use were sweating, urinary frequency, chills, and vasodilatation (flushing). The most commonly reported reason for patient discontinuation of treatment was sweating. Expected pharmacologic effects of pilocarpine include the following adverse experiences associated with SALAGEN® Tablets:

Adverse Event	5 mg q.i.d. (20 mg/day) n=255	Placebo (q.i.d.) n=253
Sweating	40%	7%
Urinary Frequency	10	4
Nausea	9	9
Flushing	9	2
Rhinitis	7	8
Diarrhea	6	7
Chills	4	2
Increased Salivation	3	0
Asthenia	2	2

In addition, the following adverse events (≥3% incidence) were reported at dosing of 20 mg/day in the controlled clinical trials: Headache (13%), flu syndrome (9%), dyspepsia (7%), dizziness (6%), pain (4%), sinusitis (4%), abdominal pain (3%), pharyngitis (2%), rash (2%), infection (2%).

The following events were reported in Sjögren's patients at incidences of 1% to 2% at dosing of 20 mg/day: accidental injury, allergic reaction, back pain, blurred vision, constipation, increased cough, edema, epistaxis, face edema, fever, flatulence, glossitis, lab test abnormalities including chemistry, hematology, and urinalysis, myalgia, palpitation, pruritus, somnolence, stomatitis, tachycardia, tinnitus, urinary incontinence, urinary tract infection, vaginitis, vomiting.

The following events were reported rarely in treated Sjogren's patients (<1%): Causal relation is unknown.

Chest pain, cyst, death, moniliasis, neck pain, neck rigidity, photosensitivity reaction, angina pectoris, arrhythmia, ECG abnormality, hypotension, hypertension, intracranial hemorrhage, migraine, myocardial infarction, anorexia, bilirubinemia, cholelithiasis, colitis, dry mouth, eructation, gastritis, gastroenteritis, gastrointestinal disorder, gingivitis, hepatitis, abnormal liver function tests, melena, nausea & vomiting, pancreatitis, parotid gland enlargement, salivary gland enlargement, sputum increased, taste loss, tongue disorder, tooth disorder, hematuria, lymphadenopathy, abnormal platelets, thrombocythemia, thrombocytopenia, thrombosis, abnormal WBC, peripheral edema, hypoglycemia, arthralgia, arthritis, bone disorder, spontaneous bone fracture, pathological fracture, myasthenia, tendon disorder, tenosynovitis, aphasia, confusion, depression, abnormal dreams, emotional lability, hyperkinesia, hypesthesia, insomnia, leg cramps, nervousness, paresthesias, abnormal thinking, tremor, bronchitis, dyspnea, hiccup, laryngismus, laryngitis, pneumonia, viral infection, voice alteration, alopecia, contact dermatitis, dry skin, eczema, erythema nodosum, exfoliative dermatitis, herpes simplex, skin ulcer, vesiculobullous rash, cataract, conjunctivitis, dry eyes, ear disorder, ear pain, eye disorder, eye hemorrhage, glaucoma, lacrimation disorder, retinal disorder, taste perversion, abnormal vision, breast pain, dysuria, mastitis, menorrhagia, metrorrhagia, ovarian disorder, pyuria, salpingitis, urethral pain, urinary urgency, vaginal hemorrhage, vaginal moniliasis.

The following adverse experiences have been reported rarely with ocular pilocarpine: A-V block, agitation, ciliary congestion, confusion, delusion, depression, dermatitis, middle ear disturbance, eyelid twitching, malignant glaucoma, iris cysts, macular hole, shock, and visual hallucination.

MANAGEMENT OF OVERDOSE: Fatal overdosage with pilocarpine has been reported in the scientific literature at doses presumed to be greater than 100 mg in two hospitalized patients. 100 mg of pilocarpine is considered potentially fatal. Overdosage should be treated with atropine titration (0.5 mg to 1.0 mg given subcutaneously or intravenously) and supportive measures to maintain respiration and circulation. Epinephrine (0.3 mg to 1.0 mg, subcutaneously or intramuscularly) may also be of value in the presence of severe cardiovascular depression or bronchoconstriction. It is not known if pilocarpine is dialyzable.

DOSAGE AND ADMINISTRATION:

Head & Neck Cancer Patients:

The recommended initial dose of SALAGEN® Tablets is one tablet (5 mg) taken three times a day. Dosage should be titrated according to therapeutic response and tolerance. The usual dosage range is up to 3-6 tablets or 15-30 mg per day. (Not to exceed 2 tablets per dose.) Although early improvement may be realized, at least 12 weeks of uninterrupted therapy with SALAGEN® Tablets may be necessary to assess whether a beneficial response will be achieved. The incidence of the most common adverse events increases with dose. The lowest dose that is tolerated and effective should be used for maintenance.

Sjögren's Syndrome Patients:

The recommended dose of SALAGEN® Tablets is one tablet (5 mg) taken four times a day. Efficacy was established by 6 weeks of use.

Manufactured by Boehringer Ingelheim Pharmaceuticals, Inc., Ridgefield, CT 06877

For MGI PHARMA, INC., Bloomington, MN 55438-2318

ARTHRITIS & RHEUMATISM
Vol. 44, No. 3, March 2001, pp 561–569

Shift Toward T Helper 1 Cytokines by Type II Collagen–Reactive T Cells in Patients With Rheumatoid Arthritis

Sung-Hwan Park,[1] Do-June Min,[1] Mi-La Cho,[1] Wan-Uk Kim,[1] Jeehee Youn,[2] Won Park,[3] Chul-Soo Cho,[1] and Ho-Youn Kim[1]

Objective. **To investigate the impact of type II collagen (CII)–reactive T cells on the Th1/Th2 cytokine balance in patients with rheumatoid arthritis (RA).**

Methods. **T cell proliferative responses to bovine CII were examined in synovial fluid mononuclear cells (SFMC) and peripheral blood mononuclear cells (PBMC) by mixed lymphocyte culture. CII-reactive T cell lines were generated from the SFMC and PBMC. Interferon-γ (IFNγ), interleukin-12 (IL-12), and IL-4 were measured by enzyme-linked immunosorbent assay in the SF, sera, and culture supernatants of PBMC and SFMC that had been stimulated with CII.**

Results. **The frequency of CII-reactive T cells was higher in the PBMC from RA patients than in that from osteoarthritis patients and healthy control subjects. In RA patients, CII-reactive T cells were more prevalent in SFMC than in PBMC. The mean level of IFNγ and the ratio of IFNγ to IL-4 were significantly higher in the culture supernatants of T cells stimulated with CII; these differences were more prominent in SFMC. Levels of IL-12 in the culture supernatants of SFMC and PBMC stimulated with CII were significantly higher than those in unstimulated supernatants. T cell responsiveness correlated well with the level of type 1 cytokines in culture supernatants from RA T cells stimulated with CII. In the CII-reactive cell lines, the increased production of IFNγ was consistent with clonal expansion.**

Conclusion. **CII-reactive T cells are more abundant in SFMC than in PBMC and are strongly associated with a shift toward Th1 cytokine in the inflamed joints of RA patients. Our results suggest that a skewing toward type 1 cytokines by CII-reactive T cells may play an important role in the chronic inflammatory process of RA.**

Rheumatoid arthritis (RA) is characterized by joint destruction as a result of chronic synovial inflammation. Many investigators have described the importance of a T cell–mediated autoimmune response in the initiation and maintenance of this inflammation (1–3). Although the aberrations of T cell homeostasis, such as contraction in diversity and clonal outgrowths of CD4 T cells, have the potential to create the conditions for chronic inflammation, the role of T cells in the maintenance of synovial inflammation, which eventually leads to cartilage degradation, remains a subject of controversy (1).

Studies of T cells in patients with RA have focused on the potential role of the initiation of the immune response to an immunodominant arthritogenic antigen. Type II collagen (CII) is a major component of hyaline cartilage, and autoimmunity to CII in RA has been well established. In animal models, synergy between antibodies to CII and collagen-reactive T cells is required to induce a chronic arthritis (4). Antibody to CII and CII-reactive T cells has been detected in the synovial fluid (SF) of patients with joint disease (5–8). Oligoclonal T cell expansion in the inflamed joints of RA patients is probably antigen driven, at least in part, by intraarticular components such as CII (6).

The balance between T cells that are able to

Supported by grant G-035649 from the Ministry of Health and Welfare of the Republic of Korea and by a grant from the Catholic Research Institutes of Medical Science.

[1]Sung-Hwan Park, MD, Do-June Min, MD, Mi-La Cho, MS, Wan-Uk Kim, MD, Chul-Soo Cho, MD, Ho-Youn Kim, MD: Catholic University of Korea, Seoul, Korea; [2]Jeehee Youn, PhD: Hanyang University, Seoul, Korea; [3]Won Park, MD: Inha University, Inchon, Korea.

Address correspondence and reprint requests to Ho-Youn Kim, MD, Center for Rheumatic Diseases, Catholic Research Institute of Medical Science, Kang-Nam St. Mary's Hospital, Department of Internal Medicine, Catholic University of Korea, Seoul, Korea.

Submitted for publication March 7, 2000; accepted in revised form October 13, 2000.

produce interferon-γ (IFNγ) and interleukin-4 (IL-4) is considered to be important in the induction or prevention of autoimmunity (9). It has been believed that CII may play an important role in the induction of IL-1, IL-6, and tumor necrosis factor α production by synovial fluid mononuclear cells (SFMC) or peripheral blood mononuclear cells (PBMC) in RA (10,11). The detection of Th1 and Th2 cytokines in RA and a shift toward lymphocytes with Th1 cytokine profiles in activated SFMC have provided evidence that supports the role of Th1 cytokine–producing T cells in the chronic inflammatory process of RA (12–16).

In our previous studies, we demonstrated that T cell responses to bovine CII, synthetic immunodominant peptide (peptide 255–274), and human CII were enhanced in RA, particularly in the joint (5). Those results suggested that CII-reactive T cells might play an important role in the pathogenesis of RA. One recent study has shown that CII, a major autoantigen candidate in RA, can elicit an IFNγ response in vitro (17). However, it is not as well known that CII can act as an inducer of type 1 cytokine production in the chronic inflammatory process in RA.

In the present study, we sought to elucidate the pathologic effect of CII-reactive T cells on the cytokine balance in patients with RA. We examined the proliferative response of T cells and Th1/Th2 cytokine production by SFMC and PBMC in the presence of CII.

PATIENTS AND METHODS

Patients. Informed consent was obtained from 40 patients (8 men and 32 women) with RA who fulfilled the 1987 revised criteria of the American College of Rheumatology (formerly, the American Rheumatism Association) (18), and paired samples of serum and SF were obtained after a 48-hour medication washout period. In the case of methotrexate, patients skipped 1 dose if the weekly schedule for taking the drug fell within the 48-hour period before sampling.

The mean age of the RA patients was 42.9 years. The mean disease duration was 78.4 months (range 3.5–396 months); 30 of the 40 patients (75%) were positive for rheumatoid factor. In 34 of the 40 patients (85%), erosive changes were noted on radiographs of the hands. All patients had clinically active synovitis at the time of arthrocentesis. The majority of patients were being treated with nonsteroidal antiinflammatory drugs, prednisolone (≤7.5 mg/day), and slow-acting antirheumatic drugs (methotrexate, sulfasalazine, hydroxychloroquine, and gold salts).

Controls. Twenty-six patients with osteoarthritis (OA; 5 men and 21 women) and 39 healthy subjects (8 men and 31 women) served as controls. The mean age of the OA patients was 56.3 years; the mean age of the healthy subjects was 45.3 years. There was no difference in age or sex distribution among the RA, OA, and healthy control groups.

Antigens. We used native CII, which was obtained by limited pepsin digestion of bovine cartilage (19). Lyophilized bovine CII (generous gift from Dr. Andrew H. Kang, University of Tennessee, Memphis) was dissolved in 0.1*N* acetic acid at 1 mg/ml, dialyzed against 50 m*M* Tris, 0.2*M* NaCl, and then sterilized by filtering through a 0.2-μm micropore filter. Ovalbumin (40 μg/well) and phytohemagglutinin (PHA; 1 μg/well) (Gibco BRL, Grand Island, NY) were used as the negative and positive controls, respectively.

T cell proliferation assays. SF was aspirated from knee joint effusions, and blood samples were obtained by venipuncture at the same visit. Mononuclear cells in PB and SF were isolated by density-gradient centrifugation on Ficoll-Hypaque (SG 1077). Cell viability was >95% by trypan blue exclusion. Cells were resuspended in RPMI 1640 supplemented with 10% fetal calf serum, 100 units/ml of penicillin, 100 mg/ml of streptomycin, and 2 m*M* L-glutamine.

Cells were then separated immunomagnetically into T cells and non–T cells using anti-CD3 microbeads (Miltenyi Biotec, Auburn, CA). Non–T cells were irradiated (3,000 rads) and used as antigen-presenting cells. T cells (1×10^6/ml) were cocultured with irradiated non–T cells (1×10^6/ml) in the presence or absence of 40 μg/well of bovine CII in 96-well round-bottomed microtiter wells (Nunc, Roskilde, Denmark) in triplicate. In this study, we used a single antigen, bovine CII, because the T cell response to bovine CII correlates strongly with that of human CII and its immunodominant peptide CII (peptide 255–274) ($r = 0.72$, $P < 0.001$ and $r = 0.72$, $P < 0.001$, respectively) (5). The optimal culture time and concentration of CII were 5 days and 40 μg/well, as previously described (5).

The plates were incubated at 37°C in 5% CO_2 for 5 days. Before the last 12 hours of culture, 0.5 μCi of ^{3}H-thymidine (NEN, Boston, MA) was added to each well. After the cells were harvested, the incorporated radioactivity was counted in a beta-scintillation counter. Data are presented as stimulation indices (SIs), which were calculated as the ratio of the counts per minute in the presence of CII to the cpm in the absence of CII. T cell proliferative responses were considered positive if the SI was ≥2.

Generation of CII-reactive T cell lines. SFMC and PBMC from a patient with RA and PBMC from a healthy subject who had a positive proliferative response to CII were plated in 96-well U-bottomed plates (Nunc) at a density of 1×10^5 cells/well in the presence of 40 μg/well of CII. After 3 days of culture, recombinant IL-2 (10 units/ml) was added. On day 10, cultures were restimulated with irradiated autologous PBMC (1×10^5 cells/well; used as antigen-presenting cells) in the presence of CII, followed by the addition of 10 units/ml of recombinant IL-2 after 72 hours. The culture supernatants from CII-reactive T cell lines were collected every 10 days, and T cells were restimulated every 10 days for a total of 15 stimulations, using autologous PBMC and CII. In each culture for the generation of T cell lines, T cell proliferative responses to CII were performed as described above.

Detection of cytokines. An enzyme-linked immunosorbent assay (ELISA) was used to detect the amount of cytokines in the SF, sera, and culture supernatants of SFMC and PBMC. Culture supernatants were collected after 24 hours for IFNγ and IL-4 determinations and after 72 hours for IFNγ, IL-4, and IL-12 determinations. ELISA kits for IFNγ, IL-4, and IL-12 were obtained from Diaclone Research (Besançon, France).

No interference of rheumatoid factor was found by absorption of rheumatoid factor on IgG agarose (Sigma, St. Louis, MO). The detection limits were 1 pg/ml for IL-4, 6.25 pg/ml for IL-12, and 12.5 pg/ml for IFNγ.

Statistical analysis. Wilcoxon's signed rank test was used to analyze matched pairs. Absolute levels of response were compared using Student's *t*-test, or the Mann-Whitney U test if the results were not normally distributed. Correlation coefficients were determined by Spearman's rank correlation test.

RESULTS

Increased frequency of CII-reactive T cells in SFMC from RA patients. The number of positive T cell responses (SI ≥2) to CII in PBMC was higher in RA patients (13 of 40, or 32.5%) than in OA patients (1 of 26, or 3.8%) and healthy control subjects (1 of 39, or 2.6%) (P = 0.011 versus OA and P = 0.002 versus healthy controls). In addition, RA patients had significantly higher mean SI values for the T cell response to CII in PBMC than did OA patients and healthy controls (RA 1.80 versus OA 1.35 [$P < 0.001$] and versus healthy controls 1.41 [P = 0.001]).

In SFMC from RA patients, the frequency of positive T cell proliferative responses to CII was significantly greater (61.5% versus 32.5%; P = 0.006) and the mean SI was higher (2.73 versus 1.80; P = 0.001) than in the corresponding PBMC (Figure 1).

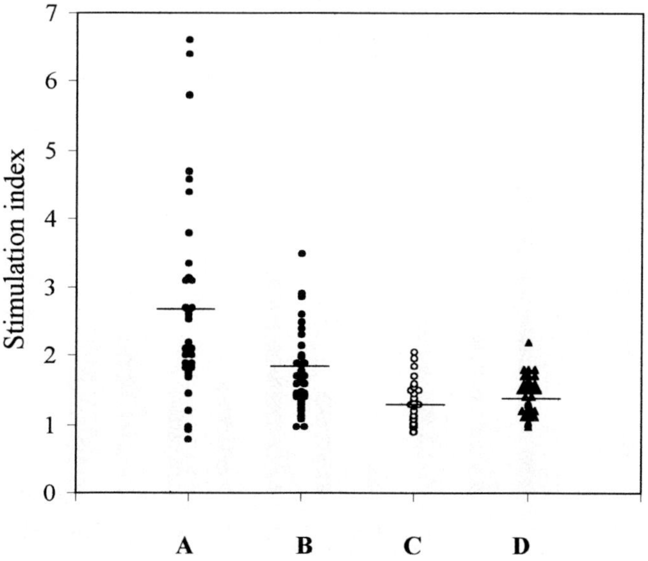

Figure 1. T cell proliferative responses to bovine type II collagen (CII). **A,** Synovial fluid mononuclear cells (SFMC) from rheumatoid arthritis (RA) patients; **B,** peripheral blood mononuclear cells (PBMC) from RA patients; **C,** PBMC from osteoarthritis (OA) patients; **D,** PBMC from healthy control subjects. The frequency of positive T cell responses to CII and the mean stimulation index were significantly increased in RA patients compared with OA patients and with healthy controls. The presence of CII-reactive T cells was more conspicuous in SFMC from the RA patients.

Table 1. Levels of Th1/Th2 cytokines in synovial fluid and serum from patients with rheumatoid arthritis*

	Synovial fluid (n = 37)	Serum (n = 37)	P
IFNγ (pg/ml)	86.25 ± 67.44	20.7 ± 16.36	<0.001
IL-4 (pg/ml)	13.80 ± 7.22	13.04 ± 9.07	0.351
IFNγ:IL-4 ratio	7.38 ± 9.49	2.03 ± 2.80	<0.001
IL-12 (pg/ml)	26.7 ± 41.7	9.9 ± 27.4	0.004

* In synovial fluid, the levels of Th1 cytokines and the ratio of interferon-γ (IFNγ) to interleukin-4 (IL-4) were significantly higher than in paired sera. Values are the mean ± SD.

Association of CII-reactive T cells with the levels of type 1 cytokines in RA. The levels of IFNγ and IL-12 in SF were significantly higher than those in paired sera, while the levels of IL-4 in SF and sera were comparable (Table 1). The ratio of the concentration of IFNγ to that of IL-4 was significantly higher in SF than in paired sera (7.38 versus 2.03; $P < 0.001$). The concentration of type 1 cytokines and the mean SI to CII tended to be higher in the SF from RA patients than in their sera.

Type 1 cytokine production of CII-reactive T cells in RA. Supernatants of SFMC from 11 RA patients were further evaluated after 24 hours of culture with and without CII stimulation. The levels of IFNγ were significantly higher in the culture supernatants from SFMC stimulated with CII for 24 hours than in those without CII stimulation (180.2 pg/ml versus 36.0 pg/ml; P = 0.003). No differences were found between the concentrations of IFNγ in culture supernatants of ovalbumin-stimulated and unstimulated T cells from the PBMC and SFMC obtained from RA patients (PBMC 38.3 pg/ml versus 29.1 pg/ml and SFMC 42.3 pg/ml versus 36.0 pg/ml, respectively).

CII-stimulated PBMC from the 11 RA patients produced significantly more IFNγ than did PBMC from 9 OA patients and 12 healthy controls, as determined at 24 hours (mean level in RA patients 120.1 pg/ml versus 77.0 pg/ml in OA patients [P = 0.031] and 72.4 pg/ml in healthy controls [P = 0.004]). The concentrations of IFNγ were also higher in the culture supernatants of CII-stimulated SFMC than in the culture supernatants of the CII-stimulated paired PBMC from RA patients (180.2 pg/ml versus 120.1 pg/ml; P = 0.045) (Figure 2A). Similarly, RA patient (n = 11) SFMC and PBMC that had been stimulated with CII for 72 hours also showed

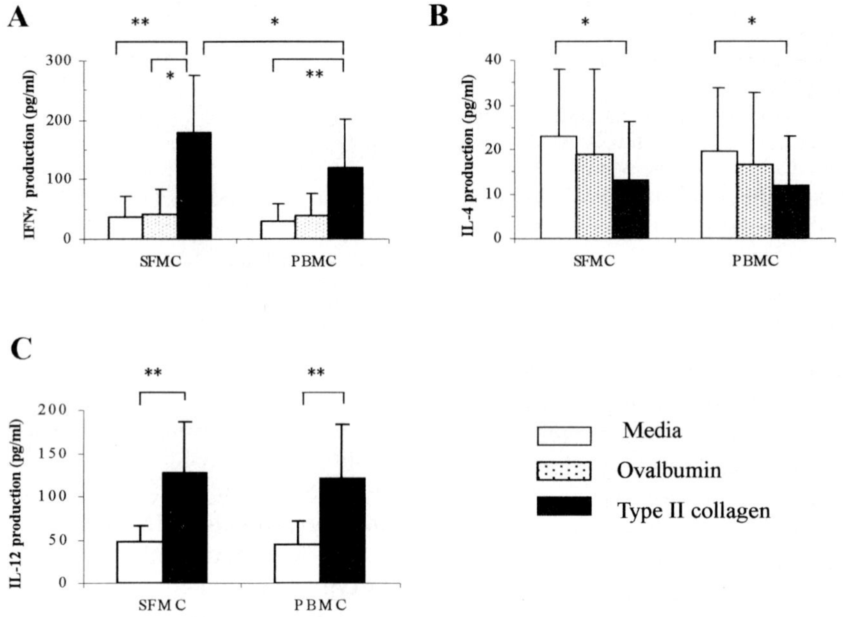

Figure 2. Increased production of Th1 cytokines by CII-stimulated SFMC and PBMC obtained from RA patients. T cells from SFMC and PBMC from 11 patients with RA were stimulated for 24 hours with bovine CII. Values shown are the mean and SD. **A,** Interferon-γ (IFNγ) production was higher in CII-stimulated SFMC and PBMC than in unstimulated SFMC and PBMC. The level of IFNγ was higher in the culture supernatants of CII-stimulated SFMC than in CII-stimulated PBMC. **B,** Interleukin-4 (IL-4) production was lower in CII-stimulated PBMC and SFMC than in unstimulated PBMC and SFMC. **C,** IL-12 production in CII-stimulated PBMC and SFMC from 8 RA patients was higher than that in unstimulated PBMC and SFMC. * = $P < 0.05$; ** = $P < 0.01$. See Figure 1 for other definitions.

significant production of IFNγ in the culture supernatants (data not shown).

IL-4 production in CII-stimulated PBMC from the 11 RA patients was lower than that in unstimulated PBMC (11.8 pg/ml versus 19.7 pg/ml; $P = 0.046$). In contrast with RA, IL-4 production in CII-stimulated PBMC from the OA patients and healthy controls was similar to that in unstimulated PBMC (data not shown). No differences were found between the concentrations of IL-4 in culture supernatants of ovalbumin-stimulated and unstimulated T cells in PBMC and SFMC from RA patients (for PBMC 16.7 pg/ml versus 19.7 pg/ml and for SFMC 19.0 pg/ml versus 23.0 pg/ml in stimulated and unstimulated culture supernatants, respectively).

IL-4 production in CII-stimulated SFMC from the 11 RA patients was also lower than that in unstimulated SFMC (12.5 pg/ml versus 23.0 pg/ml; $P = 0.004$). No differences in the concentration of IL-4 in supernatants of CII-stimulated SFMC and paired PBMC from RA patients were observed (Figure 2B). However, the

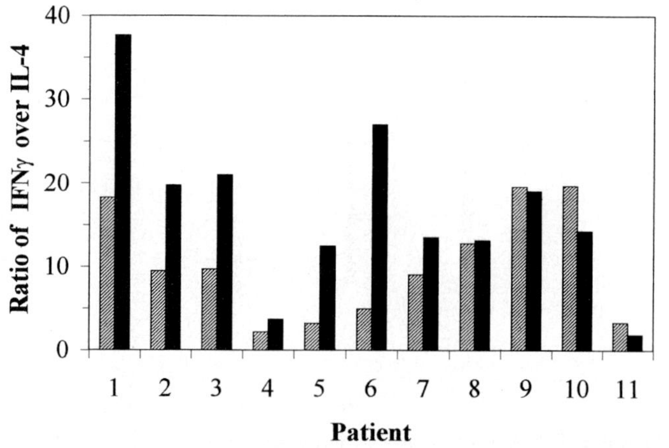

Figure 3. Ratio of the production of interferon-γ (IFNγ) to interleukin-4 (IL-4) in SFMC (solid bars) compared with PBMC (gray bars). In 8 of 11 RA patients, this ratio was higher in the SFMC culture supernatants than in supernatants from paired PBMC. The IFNγ:IL-4 ratio was calculated by dividing the concentration of IFNγ by that of IL-4 in the culture supernatants of bovine CII–stimulated SFMC and PBMC (mean ± SD 14.9 ± 10.09 versus 10.27 ± 7.16, respectively; $P = 0.035$). See Figure 1 for other definitions.

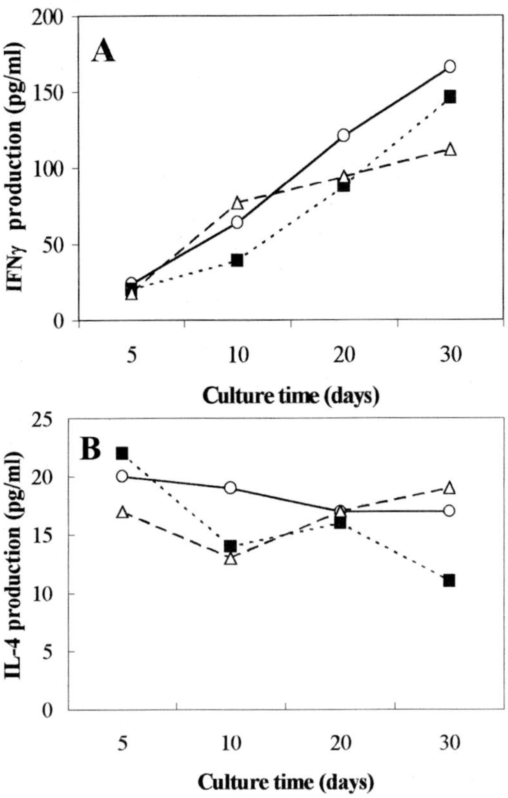

Figure 4. The concentration of interferon-γ (IFNγ) and interleukin-4 (IL-4) according to the clonal expansion of CII-reactive T cell lines in SFMC (○) and PBMC (■) from an RA patient and PBMC from a healthy control subject (△). CII-reactive T cells were restimulated with autologous irradiated PBMC in the presence of CII every 10 days. The increase in IFNγ production was consistent with the clonal expansion of CII-reactive T cells. See Figure 1 for other definitions.

levels of IFNγ:IL-4 were significantly higher in the culture supernatants of 24-hour CII-stimulated SFMC from RA patients than in those without CII stimulation (14.9 versus 1.9; $P = 0.008$). In addition, the IFNγ:IL-4 production ratio was also higher in the culture supernatants of SFMC than of paired PBMC (14.9 versus 10.2; $P = 0.035$) (Figure 3).

The levels of IL-12 in the culture supernatants of SFMC and paired PBMC (n = 8 RA patients) stimulated with CII for 72 hours were significantly higher than those without CII stimulation (for SFMC 127.1 pg/ml versus 46.8 pg/ml [$P = 0.007$] and for PBMC 119.6 pg/ml versus 43.5 pg/ml [$P = 0.009$]) (Figure 2C). Although the supernatants of CII-stimulated SFMC contained more IL-12 than the paired PBMC, this difference did not reach statistical significance ($P > 0.05$).

In CII-reactive T cell lines generated from the SFMC and PBMC from a patient with RA and from the PBMC from a healthy subject, the levels of IFNγ and the ratio of IFNγ:IL-4 production were considerably increased, which is consistent with clonal expansion of CII-reactive cell lines (Figure 4). In contrast to the concentration of IFNγ, the concentrations of IL-4 did not change. The proliferative response to CII showed an SI of 3.5 on day 5, increasing to 14.7 on day 30. Peripheral T cell responses to CII in the RA patient and the healthy control showed similar patterns, increasing from 2.6 to 11.4 and from 2.3 to 10.9, respectively. On day 3, the concentrations of IFNγ and IL-4 in the culture supernatants of CII-stimulated SFMC were 24 pg/ml and 20 pg/ml, respectively. On day 30, the IFNγ:IL-4 production ratio was increased to 9.76 (IFNγ 166 pg/ml and IL-4 17 pg/ml). Similar changes in the concentrations of IFNγ and IL-4 were also noted in the culture supernatants of CII-reactive T cell lines from the PBMC from the RA patient and the healthy control. The IFNγ:IL-4 production ratio in the culture supernatants of CII-reactive T cell lines from the healthy control on day 30 was lower than from the PBMC from the RA patient (13.27 versus 5.89). On day 150, the concentrations of IFNγ and IL-4 in the CII-stimulated supernatant of SFMC from the RA patient were 387 pg/ml and 4 pg/ml, respectively, and the SI was further increased to 46.9.

Positive correlations between type 1 cytokines in the CII-stimulated culture supernatants and T cell responses to CII. To investigate the correlations between a particular cytokine and the proliferative response of T cells to CII, we analyzed the cytokine concentrations in the culture supernatants that had a proliferative response to CII. The SI with PBMC from 11 RA patients correlated with the level of IFNγ (r = 0.829, $P = 0.042$) and IL-12 (r = 0.886, $P = 0.019$), and the SI in the SFMC from the RA patients correlated with the level of IFNγ (r = 0.893, $P = 0.007$) and the ratio of IFNγ:IL-4 (r = 0.886, $P < 0.001$) (Figure 5). However, there was no correlation between the IL-4 levels and the SI values.

DISCUSSION

In the case of chronic inflammatory autoimmune diseases such as RA, diabetes mellitus, and multiple sclerosis, pathogenic and protective roles have been ascribed to Th1 cells and Th2 cells, respectively (1–3,20). A shift toward T cells with a Th1 cytokine profile has been reported in the early stage of RA. Since Th1 and Th2 cytokines are believed to have mutual regulatory interactions, the balance between T cells with the Th1 or

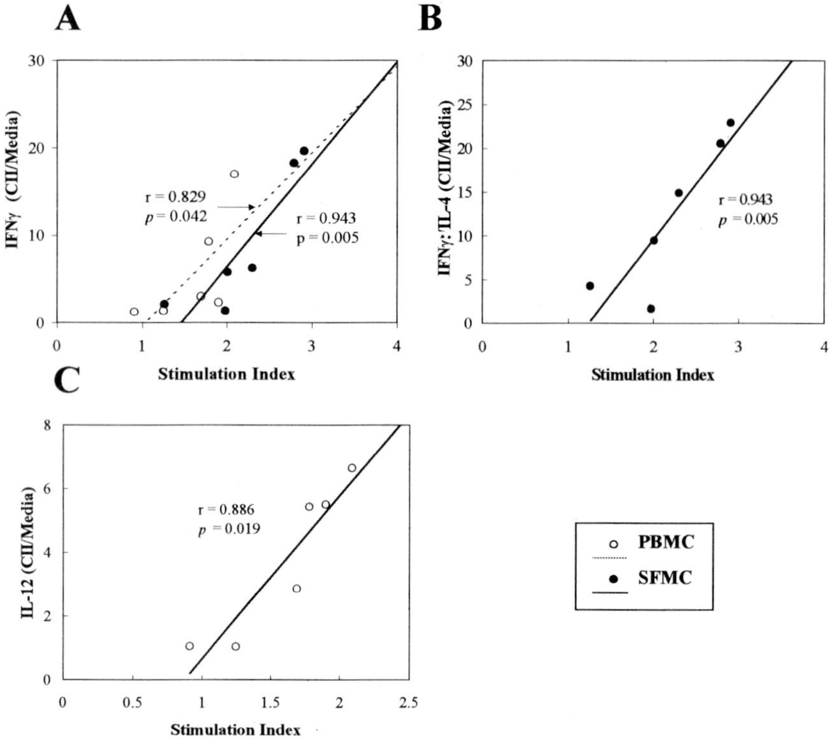

Figure 5. Correlations between the increases in cytokine production by CII stimulation and the stimulation index. The increases in **A**, interferon-γ (IFNγ) and **C**, interleukin-12 (IL-12) production as well as the **B**, IFNγ:IL-4 ratio were positively correlated with the T cell proliferative response to CII in PBMC and SFMC from patients with RA.

Th2 phenotype is considered to be an important regulatory mechanism of T cell function (20,21). Several cytokines produced during the initial presentation of antigen to naive T cells regulates the development of Th1 and Th2 cells. IL-12 and IFNγ cause a shift toward Th1 responses, whereas IL-4 directs the development toward Th2 cells. The chronic immune response in RA might be driven by activated Th1 cells without sufficient Th2 cell differentiation to down-regulate the inflammation (9,15), and the imbalance between Th1 and Th2 cells is thought to be of pathogenic significance. However, the major factors contributing to the skewing of Th1 cytokines remain unclear.

In the present study, CII-reactive T cells were more prevalent in SFMC than in PBMC from RA patients. A shift toward a type 1 cytokine profile was more prominent in SF, as compared with paired PB samples. This shift was also found in the culture supernatants of PBMC and SFMC in the presence of CII and more evident in the SFMC from RA patients. In particular, the production of type 1 cytokines (IFNγ and IL-12) by CII-stimulated PBMC and SFMC from RA patients was higher than the production without stimulation, and the levels of IFNγ were higher in the culture supernatants of CII-stimulated SFMC than in those of CII-stimulated PBMC. The increased production of IFNγ was consistent with the progression of CII-reactive T cell lines. Moreover, T cell responsiveness to CII in PBMC and SFMC correlated with the levels of IFNγ and IL-12 and the ratio of IFNγ:IL-4.

Taken together, our observations suggest that CII-reactive T cells, especially in the joints, are strongly associated with a skewing toward type 1 cytokine profiles. We found no difference in IL-4 levels in the sera and SF from RA patients. CII-induced IL-4 production by PBMC and SFMC from RA patients was also similar and was lower than the production by unstimulated PBMC and SFMC. Our findings further support the notion that CD4+ T cells derived from rheumatoid synovium express higher levels of IFNγ than do PB-derived CD4+ T cells, whereas the expression of IL-4 in these cell populations was comparable (22), and there was no significant difference in the frequency of IL-4–producing cells between SF and PB CD4+ or CD8+ T cells (9). Although previous reports have shown low levels of IL-4 in the serum and SF of RA patients (23,24), recent reports have demonstrated elevated levels of IL-4 (25,26). Therefore, the difference in IL-4 levels between this study and previously published studies may be the result of differences in the detection limits of the ELISAs used as well as differences in the characteristics of the RA patients studied.

It has been observed that the T cell response to recall antigen (27) and the autologous mixed lymphocyte reaction (28) are decreased in patients with RA. Considering the general hyporesponsiveness of RA T cells, a new methodologic approach has been suggested in order to demonstrate cellular response to specific antigen and cytokine production (5,17). In the present study, we prepared T cells using 2 methods: a sheep erythrocyte rosetting technique and magnetic bead (anti-CD3) separation. The findings of T cell proliferation to CII and the secretion of cytokines were not different with the 2 methods we used. We concluded that the magnetic bead system has less influence on cell function, which has been documented in several previous reports (29,30), and we therefore used the magnetic bead system for the preparation of T cells, which is a relatively simple procedure.

Although the proliferative responses to phytohemagglutinin (5) and tetanus toxoid (obtained from the Swiss Serum and Vaccine Institute, Berne, Switzerland) were lower in RA patients than in OA patients and healthy controls in our culture system, the difference was not statistically significant (data not shown). This result supports the recent report that the response of PBMC to purified protein derivative (PPD) and tetanus toxoid did not differ significantly between healthy controls and patients with early RA or late RA (31). Our culture conditions were different from those in previous studies in terms of the dose of antigen and the number of antigen-presenting cells (17,32).

It has been reported that the kinetics of cytokine secretion by PBMC from the blood of RA patients are different from those of healthy subjects (33). In our studies, the IL-4 concentration rose quickly during the first 8 hours of incubation and reached a maximum after 24 hours; the IFNγ concentration, however, increased constantly during the 72-hour incubation period. A 24-hour period of stimulation was found to be optimal for the induction of IL-4 production and a 72-hour period of stimulation for the induction of IFNγ production in the initial experiments (data not shown). It has been recommended that the production of IFNγ in response to standard recall antigens requires longer culture times for cells from patients with RA (17). To investigate the Th1/Th2 cytokine balance, we decided to measure the culture supernatants after 24 hours, 72 hours, 10 days, 20 days, and 30 days of culture. As expected, the CII-induced production of IFNγ increased persistently with increasing culture times, but the CII-induced production of IL-4 did not significantly change.

The finding that CII-reactive T cells are associated with a shift toward type 1 cytokines illustrates a novel pathway in the maintenance of the chronic inflammatory process of RA. Dolhain et al (12) reported that highly significant correlation coefficients were found between the percentage of cytokine-producing cells and the amount of that specific cytokine in the cell culture supernatant from SFMC obtained from RA patients. Although CII-reactive T cell lines have not yet been characterized, clonal expansion of CII-reactive cells might contribute to the production of IFNγ and the subsequent up-regulation of HLA–DR expression. An enhanced HLA–DR–mediated CII-reactive T cell response may elicit a cascade of inflammatory cytokines through the interaction between T cells and antigen-presenting cells. As a result, an increase in the production of IFNγ over that of IL-4 by the CII-reactive T cell lines may further recruit and activate synovial T cells, which then amplify and perpetuate the inflammation.

The cytokine milieu of RA is influenced by the duration and activity of the disease (16,17,25,31,34). It has been reported that the T cell response to CII is more prevalent and stronger in early RA than in late RA (5). Just as the PPD-induced IFNγ production decreases with increasing disease duration, general T cell reactivity decreases gradually during the course of RA (17). In the present study, samples from patients with new-onset synovitis were very few, and we could not conclude whether there was an association between cytokine balance and disease duration. In comparisons of RA disease activity with T cell responsiveness to CII, levels of C-reactive protein correlated well with SI values for CII in SFMC (data not shown). The study, however, was not designed to address this question. Because the clinical status, including the disease activity, erosive state, and presence of HLA–DR susceptibility alleles, may be involved in CII-induced production of type 1 cytokines, further detailed study is required.

Genetic predisposition to RA is linked to the class II major histocompatibility complex alleles, such as HLA–DRB1*0401, 0404, 0405, and 0101, which possess a shared epitope (35–37). Furthermore, the CII peptide (peptide 256–271) has been shown to bind to a restricted population that includes the HLA–DR molecules associated with susceptibility to RA (38,39). In addition, the T cell response to CII is HLA–DR restricted (17,32), suggesting that the HLA–DR status is important for the development of autoimmunity to CII, especially in the recognition of human CII peptide (peptide 256–271). Furthermore, a recent study identified an association between the magnitude of the IFNγ response to CII and the presence of HLA–DRB1*0401 and HLA–DQ8 (17). However, in agreement with the results reported by Kammer and Trentham (40), no preferential response was apparent in subgroups of RA patients categorized according to the presence or absence of the HLA–DR shared epitope (5). This finding suggests that the skewing of Th1 cytokine levels might be more important than the HLA–DR status in the activation of CII-reactive T cells. Interactions of T cells with bystander cytokines, adhesion molecules, and perhaps, antigens have been proposed as pathways whereby the T cell memory component is maintained in the absence of the initiating antigen (3). The question concerning the cause of the activation of CII-reactive T cells that participate in disease induction and/or perpetuation in vivo remains unanswered.

Taken together, our findings show that CII-reactive T cells were more prevalent in SFMC than in PBMC from patients with RA. A shift toward a type 1 cytokine profile was observed in cells from the joints of patients with RA and correlated positively with the T cell response to CII, demonstrating that oligoclonal expansion of CII-reactive T cells in RA joints contributes to the skewing toward type 1 cytokines. CII-reactive T cell responses, followed by skewing toward type 1 cytokines, may play an important role in the perpetuation of the inflammatory process in RA. Interventions aimed at CII-reactive T cells might be helpful in the treatment of RA, especially early in the course of the disease.

REFERENCES

1. Weyand CM, Goronzy JJ. T-cell responses in rheumatoid arthritis: systemic abnormalities-local disease. Curr Opin Rheumatol 1999; 11:210–7.
2. Weyand CM, Klimiuk PA, Goronzy JJ. Heterogeneity of rheumatoid arthritis: from phenotypes to genotypes. Springer Semin Immunopathol 1998;20:5–22.
3. McInnes IB, Liew FY. Interleukin 15: a proinflammatory role in rheumatoid arthritis synovitis. Immunol Today 1998;19:75–9.
4. Vermeire K, Heremans H, Vandeputte M, Huang S, Billiau A, Matthys P. Accelerated collagen-induced arthritis in IFN-γ receptor-deficient mice. J Immunol 1997;158:5507–13.
5. Kim H-Y, Kim W-U, Cho M-L, Lee SK, Youn J, Kim S-I, et al. Enhanced T cell proliferative response to type II collagen and synthetic peptide CII (255–274) in patients with rheumatoid arthritis. Arthritis Rheum 1999;42:2085–93.
6. Sekine T, Kato T, Masuko-Hongo K, Nakamura H, Yoshino S, Nishioka K, et al. Type II collagen is a target antigen of clonally expanded T cells in the synovium of patients with rheumatoid arthritis. Ann Rheum Dis 1999;58:446–50.
7. He X, Kang AH, Stuart JM. Accumulation of T cells reactive to type II collagen in synovial fluid of patients with rheumatoid arthritis. J Rheumatol 2000;27:589–93.
8. Kim WU, Yoo WH, Park W, Kang YM, Kim SI, Park JH, et al. IgG antibodies to type II collagen reflect inflammatory activity in patients with rheumatoid arthritis. J Rheumatol 2000;27:575–81.
9. Isomaki P, Luukkainen R, Lassila O, Toivanen P, Punnonen J. Synovial fluid T cells from patients with rheumatoid arthritis are refractory to the T helper type 2 differentiation-inducing effects of interleukin-4. Immunol 1999;96:358–64.
10. Goto M, Yoshinoya S, Miyamoto T, Sasano M, Okamoto M, Nishioka K, et al. Stimulation of interleukin-1α and interleukin-1β release from human monocytes by cyanogen bromide peptides of type II collagen. Arthritis Rheum 1988;31:1508–14.
11. Jeng KCG, Liu MT, Lan JL, Wu CH, Wong DW, Cheung BMH. Collagen induces cytokine production by synovial fluid mononuclear cells in rheumatoid arthritis. Immunol Lett 1995;45:13–7.
12. Dolhain RJEM, van der Heiden AN, ter Haar NT, Breedveld FC, Miltenburg AMM. Shift toward T lymphocytes with a T helper 1 cytokine–secretion profile in the joints of patients with rheumatoid arthritis. Arthritis Rheum 1996;39:1961–9.
13. Kusaba M, Honda J, Fukuda T, Oizumi K. Analysis of type 1 and type 2 T cells in synovial fluid and peripheral blood of patients with rheumatoid arthritis. J Rheumatol 1998;25:1466–71.
14. Ronnelid J, Berg L, Rogberg S, Nilsson A, Albertsson K, Klareskog L. Production of T-cell cytokines at the single-cell level in patients with inflammatory arthritides: enhanced activity in synovial fluid compared to blood. Br J Rheumatol 1998;37:7–14.
15. Van der Graaff WL, Prins AP, Niers TM, Dijkmans BA, van Lier RA. Quantitation of interferon-γ and interleukin-4 producing T cells in synovial fluid and peripheral blood of arthritis patients. Rheumatol 1999;38:214–20.
16. Roon JA, Verhoef CM, van Roy JL, Gmelig-Meyling FH, Huber-Bruning O, Lafeber FP, et al. Decrease in peripheral type 1 over type 2 T cell cytokine production in patients with rheumatoid arthritis correlates with an increase in severity of disease. Ann Rheum Dis 1997;56:656–60.
17. Berg L, Ronnelid J, Sanjeevi CB, Lampa J, Klareskog L. Interferon-γ production in response to in vitro stimulation with collagen type II in rheumatoid arthritis is associated with HLA-DRB1*0401 and HLA-DQ8. Arthritis Res 2000;2:75–84.
18. Arnett FC, Edworthy SM, Bloch DA, McShane DJ, Fries JF, Cooper NS, et al. The American Rheumatism Association 1987 revised criteria for the classification of rheumatoid arthritis. Arthritis Rheum 1988;31:315–24.
19. Stuart JM, Cremer MA, Kang AH, Townes AS. Collagen-induced arthritis in rats: evaluation of early immunologic events. Arthritis Rheum 1979;22:1344–51.
20. Verhoef CM, van Roon JA, Vianen ME, Bruijnzeel-Koomen CA, Lafeber FP, Bijlsma JW. Mutual antagonism of rheumatoid arthritis and hay fever: a role for type 1/type 2 T cell balance. Ann Rheum Dis 1998;57:275–80.
21. Steiner G, Tohidast-Akrad M, Witzmann G, Vesely M, Studnika-Benke A, Gal A, et al. Cytokine production by synovial T cells in rheumatoid arthritis. Rheumatol 1999;38:202–13.
22. Morita Y, Yamamura M, Kawashima M, Harada S, Tsuji K, Shibuya K, et al. Flow cytometric single-cell analysis of cytokine production by CD4+ T cells in synovial tissue and peripheral blood from patients with rheumatoid arthritis. Arthritis Rheum 1998;41:1669–76.
23. Miossec P, Naviliat M, Dupuy d'Angeac A, Sany J, Banchereau J.

Low levels of interleukin-4 and high levels of transforming growth factor β in rheumatoid synovitis. Arthritis Rheum 1990;33:1180–7.
24. Cicuttini FM, Byron KA, Maher D, Wootton AM, Muirden KD, Hamilton JA. Serum IL-4, IL-10 and IL-6 levels in inflammatory arthritis. Rheumatol Int 1995;14:201–6.
25. Ribbens C, Bonnet V, Kaiser MJ, Andre B, Kaye O, Franchimont N, et al. Increased synovial fluid levels of soluble CD23 are associated with an erosive status in rheumatoid arthritis. Clin Exp Immunol 2000;120:194–9.
26. Mantas C, Direskeneli H, Eksioglu-Demiralp E, Akoglu T. Serum levels of Th2 cytokines IL-4 and IL-10 in Behçet's disease [letter]. J Rheumatol 1999;26:510–2.
27. Verwilghen J, Vertessen S, Stevens EA, Dequeker J, Ceuppens JL. Depressed T-cell reactivity to recall antigens in rheumatoid arthritis. J Clin Immunol 1990;10:90–8.
28. Pope RM, McChesney L, Talal N, Fischbach M. Characterization of the defective autologous mixed lymphocyte response in rheumatoid arthritis. Arthritis Rheum 1984;27:1234–44.
29. Stanciu LA, Shute J, Holgate ST, Djukanovic R. Production of IL-8 and IL-4 by positively and negatively selected CD4+ and CD8+ human T cells following a four-step cell separation method including magnetic cell sorting (MACS). J Immunol Methods 1996;189:107–15.
30. Semple JW, Allen D, Chang W, Castaldi P, Freedman J. Rapid separation of CD4+ and CD19+ lymphocyte populations from human peripheral blood by a magnetic activated cell sorter (MACS). Cytometry 1993;14:955–60.
31. Macht LM, Elson CJ, Kirwan JR, Gaston JS, Lamont AG, Thompson JM, Thompson SJ. Relationship between disease severity and responses by blood mononuclear cells from patients with rheumatoid arthritis to human heat-shock protein 60. Immunology 2000;99:208–14.
32. Snowden N, Reynolds I, Morgan K, Holt L. T cell responses to human type II collagen in patients with rheumatoid arthritis and healthy controls. Arthritis Rheum 1997;40:1210–8.
33. Ruschen S, Stellberg W, Warnatz H. Kinetics of cytokine secretion by mononuclear cells of the blood from rheumatoid arthritis patients are different from those of healthy controls. Clin Exp Immunol 1992;89:32–7.
34. Kanik KS, Hagiwara E, Yarboro CH, Schumacher HR, Wilder RL, Klinman DM. Distinct patterns of cytokine secretion characterize new onset synovitis versus chronic rheumatoid arthritis. J Rheumatol 1998;25:16–22.
35. Kim HY, Kim TG, Park SH, Lee SH, Cho CS, Han H. Predominance of HLA-DRB1*0405 in Korean patients with rheumatoid arthritis. Ann Rheum Dis 1995;54:988–90.
36. Kim HY, Min JK, Yang HI, Park SH, Hong YS, Jee WH, et al. The impact of HLA-DRB1*0405 on disease severity in Korean patients with seropositive rheumatoid arthritis. Br J Rheumatol 1996;36:440–3.
37. Dessen A, Lawrence CM, Cupo S, Zaller DM, Wiley DC. X-ray crystal structure of HLA-DR4 (DRA*0101, DRB1*0401) complexed with a peptide from human collagen II. Immunity 1997;7: 473–81.
38. Fugger L, Rothbard JB, Sonderstrup-McDevitt G. Specificity of an HLA-DRB1*0401-restricted T cell response to type II collagen. Eur J Immunol 1996;26:928–33.
39. Diab BY, Lambert NC, L'Faqihi FE, Loubet-Lescoulie P, de Preval C, Coppin HU. Human collagen II peptide 256-271 preferentially binds to HLA-DR molecules associated with susceptibility to rheumatoid arthritis. Immunogenetics 1999;49:36–44.
40. Kammer GM, Trentham DE. HLA–DR4 is not a requisite for autoimmunity to collagen in rheumatoid arthritis. Arthritis Rheum 1984;27:489–94.

ARTHRITIS & RHEUMATISM
Vol. 44, No. 3, March 2001, pp 570–577

Infection Efficiency of Type 5 Adenoviral Vectors in Synovial Tissue Can Be Enhanced With a Type 16 Fiber

Paulien H. Goossens,[1] Menzo J. E. Havenga,[2] Elsbet Pieterman,[1] Angelique A. Lemckert,[2] Ferdinand C. Breedveld,[1] Abraham Bout,[2] and Tom W. J. Huizinga[1]

Objective. **To obtain an adenoviral vector with increased infection efficiency in the synovial tissue compared with conventional vectors based on adenovirus serotype 5 (Ad5), without compromising the specificity of infection.**

Methods. **Coxsackie adenovirus receptor (CAR) expression was assessed in cultured synoviocytes. Chimeric adenoviruses based on Ad5 but carrying the DNA encoding the fiber of adenovirus from subgroup B (Ad11, 16, 35) or D (Ad24, 28, 33, 45, or 47) were constructed and produced on PER.C6 cells. The gene transfer efficiency of these chimera was tested on cultured synoviocytes and peripheral blood mononuclear cells (PBMC).**

Results. **No surface expression of CAR protein was observed on synoviocytes. CAR messenger RNA expression of synoviocytes was found to be low. Of all fiber chimeric vectors tested, vectors carrying the fiber of Ad16 (Ad5.fib16) were most potent, yielding ~150 times increased transgene expression in cultured synoviocytes compared with those of Ad5. Flow cytometry showed that the increase in transgene expression was caused by the transduction of higher percentages of synoviocytes and higher gene expression per synoviocyte. Experiments with 500 virus particles/cell of Ad5.GFP or Ad5.fib16.GFP resulted in an infection efficiency of 0.6% and 1% in PBMC and 43% and 76% in synoviocytes, respectively.**

Conclusion. **Synoviocytes hardly express CAR, which hampers Ad5-mediated gene transfer. Ad5.fib16 is superior to Ad5 vectors for transducing synoviocytes, without compromising the specificity of infection. Our data suggest that Ad5.fib16-mediated gene transfer to synovial tissue improves the therapeutic window.**

Rheumatoid arthritis (RA) is a systemic, chronic, progressive inflammatory disease that specifically affects the synovial tissue of diarthrodal joints (1). The disease is characterized by joint pain, swelling, and destruction of bone and cartilage, leading to functional failure of the joint. Especially when a limited number of joints is involved, local treatment of a joint can be considered. A promising new local treatment in RA is the transfer of therapeutic genes to the synovial tissue by adenovirus (Ad) vectors. The feasibility of gene transfer to the synovial tissue after intraarticular administration of Ad5-based vectors has been demonstrated in several animal models (2–6).

In most of these animal models, Ad-induced inflammation was observed in the synovial tissue after intraarticular injection of vectors. This implies that gene therapy for local treatment of the rheumatic joint may induce a flare of the preexisting arthritis. In rabbits, it was shown that the induction of inflammation in the synovial tissue depends on the dose of Ad administered (7). The aim of this study was to develop an adenoviral vector that can infect synoviocytes more efficiently compared with Ad5, so that the same percentage of cells can be infected with a lower dose of the virus.

The cellular tropism of Ad5 depends on the binding of the knob of the Ad5 fiber to a cellular Ad receptor (8). In general, the fiber is a trimeric protein with a shaft of varying lengths and a globular fiber knob that protrudes from the 12 pentons of the viral capsid. Different Ad serotypes have been found to bind to different receptors, such as the Coxsackie adenovirus receptor (CAR) (9,10), sialic acid (11), and possibly other as-yet-unknown receptors. Since the primary re-

[1]Paulien H. Goossens, MD, Elsbet Pieterman, Ferdinand C. Breedveld, MD, Tom W. J. Huizinga, MD, PhD: Leiden University Medical Center, Leiden, The Netherlands; [2]Menzo J. E. Havenga, PhD, Angelique A. Lemckert, Abraham Bout, PhD: Crucell B. V., Leiden, The Netherlands.

Address correspondence and reprint requests to Tom W. J. Huizinga, Leiden University Medical Center, Department of Rheumatology, C4-R, PO Box 9600, 2300 RC Leiden, The Netherlands.

Submitted for publication August 31, 2000; accepted in revised form November 9, 2000.

ceptor for Ad5 is CAR, it can be envisioned that cells deficient for CAR are difficult targets for Ad5-mediated gene transfer (12). In human airway epithelium with a low expression of CAR, it has been demonstrated that a low infection efficiency can be circumvented by modifying the Ad fiber to bind to cell surface receptors other than CAR (13). To our knowledge, strategies to improve gene transfer to synoviocytes have not been explored.

This study shows that CAR expression on the surface of synoviocytes is undetectable. To find a vector with increased capacity of gene transfer to synoviocytes, Ad5-based vectors that carry the DNA coding for the fiber shaft and fiber knob of other Ad serotypes were constructed. We found that the efficiency of gene transfer to synoviocytes increases when Ad5 vectors carrying the fiber of Ad16 (Ad5.fib16) are used. Ad16 belongs to the group B adenoviruses, which do not use CAR for infection of the cell (14).

Due to the small pore size of the cartilage matrix and since the adenovirus is ~100 nm in size, the joint can be depicted as a closed compartment leaving predominantly cells in the synovial membrane and cells in the synovial fluid as targets for Ad infection. This study shows that whereas Ad5.fib16-mediated gene transfer to synoviocytes is highly efficient, mononuclear cells in the synovial fluid are hardly transduced. Thus, the current data indicate that efficient and specific gene transfer can be achieved when Ad5.fib16 vectors are used for gene transfer to the synovial tissue.

MATERIALS AND METHODS

Synoviocytes. Synovial tissue was collected from patients with RA according to the criteria of the American College of Rheumatology (formerly, the American Rheumatism Association) (15), at the time of joint replacement surgery or synovectomy. The synovial tissues were digested and the obtained synoviocytes were cultured in Iscove's modified Dulbecco's medium (IMDM) supplemented with L-glutamine (Life Technologies, Paisley, UK) and 10% fetal calf serum (FCS) according to standard methods (6). Synoviocytes were used between passages 1 and 5.

Coxsackie adenovirus receptor. As a positive control, A549 cells were used. Protein expression of CAR was determined by flow cytometry (16). Reverse transcriptase–polymerase chain reaction (RT-PCR) was used to quantify RNA levels of CAR. One microgram of total RNA pretreated with RT was synthesized using RNAsin (Promega, Madison, WI) in a 25-μl reaction. After this reaction, PCRs for CAR and β-actin were performed in 1 reaction in a final volume of 40 μl using 1.125 μl complementary DNA (cDNA), 10 μM dNTP, and 0.2 μl *Taq* DNA polymerase (Promega). For the amplification of CAR from the cDNA, oligonucleotides CAR-sense (5′-AGCCTTCAGGTGCGAGATGTTACG-3′) and CAR-antisense (5′-TACGACAGCAAAAGATGATAA-GAC-3′) were used. For amplification of β-actin, the primers β-actin–sense and antisense (5′-GGGTCAGAAGGATTCC-TATG-3′ and 5′-GGTCTCAAACATGATCTGGG-3′) were used (all primers from Gibco, Paisley, UK). Samples were harvested after 10, 15, 20, 25, and 30 cycles.

Construction of pBr/Ad.BamRΔFIB. Plasmid pBr/Ad.Bam-rITR contains the Ad serotype 5 sequence from the *Bam* HI site (nt 21562) until the 3′-end. This plasmid was used as a template for PCR to delete fiber sequences (nt 31042–32787). For this purpose, a PCR was performed using oligonucleotides "NY-up" (5′-CGA**CATATG**TAG**ATGCAT**TA-GTTTGTGTTATGTTTCAACGTG-3′), which contains both an *Nde* I site and an *Nsi* I site) (boldface), and "NY-down" (5′-GGAGACCACTGCCATGTTG-3′). The expected 2,200-bp DNA fragment was digested with *Sbf* I (present just upstream of "NY-down"), and *Nde* I and was subsequently cloned into an SbfI- and *Nde* I–digested pBr/Ad.Bam-rITR. The resulting plasmid, pBr/Ad.BamRΔFIB, thus lacks part of the fiber starting from the *Nde* I site until the stop codon, but instead contains a unique *Nsi* I site directly after the fiber stop codon. The restriction sites *Nde* I and *Nsi* I were introduced into the tail of degenerate oligonucleotides used to amplify fiber sequences from alternative Ad serotypes and for subsequent cloning into pBr/Ad.BamRΔFIB. The human wild-type Ad5, 11, 16, 24, 28, 33, 35, 45, and 47 were propagated on PER.C6 cells (17), after which virus DNA was isolated from crude lysate as described previously (18). The plasmid library generated was coded pBr/Ad.BamRΔFIBXX (where XX represents the serotype number from which the fiber was amplified). The amplified sequences inserted in the pBr/Ad.BamRΔFIBXX constructs were sequenced to confirm the existence of an open reading frame. Protein sequences were aligned and putative fiber domains, such as the trimerization domain, were localized.

To maximize the change of generating fiber chimeric recombinant Ad, an additional cloning step was performed. All pBr/Ad.BamRΔFIBXX constructs as well as plasmid pBr/Ad.AflII–*Bam* HI were digested with *Bam* HI and *Pac* I, separated on gels, and isolated using agarase enzyme (Roche, Almere, The Netherlands) according to the instructions supplied by the manufacturer. The fragments obtained were subsequently cloned (3-point ligation) into a *Pac* I–digested pWE.pac cosmid using a packaging kit and the instructions provided by the manufacturer (Stratagene, Amsterdam, The Netherlands). Cosmid pWE.Pac was generated from pWE15 (Westburg, Leusden, The Netherlands) by inserting a synthetic DNA fragment containing a *Pac* I restriction site into the *Eco* RI sites. Cosmids obtained were verified with restriction enzyme analysis. The cosmid library generated was coded pWe/Ad.AflII-rITR.pac/FibXX. To generate recombinant Ad, 2 DNA molecules were cotransfected: (a) pWe/Ad.AflII-rITR.pac/FibXX linearized with *Pac* I, and (b) a plasmid-encoding Ad5 sequence in which the E1 region was replaced by a marker gene. This plasmid, coded either pClip or pAdapt, contained Ad serotype 5 sequence from nt 1 to 454 (left intron and packaging signal), a cassette for transgene expression containing the cytomegalovirus promoter (nt −601 to −14: pClip or nt −735 to +95: pAdapt), a polylinker, SV40 intron/polyA from pcDNA1 (*Hha* I–*Avr* II fragment; Invitrogen, San Diego, CA), and a second Ad5 sequence ranging from nt 3511

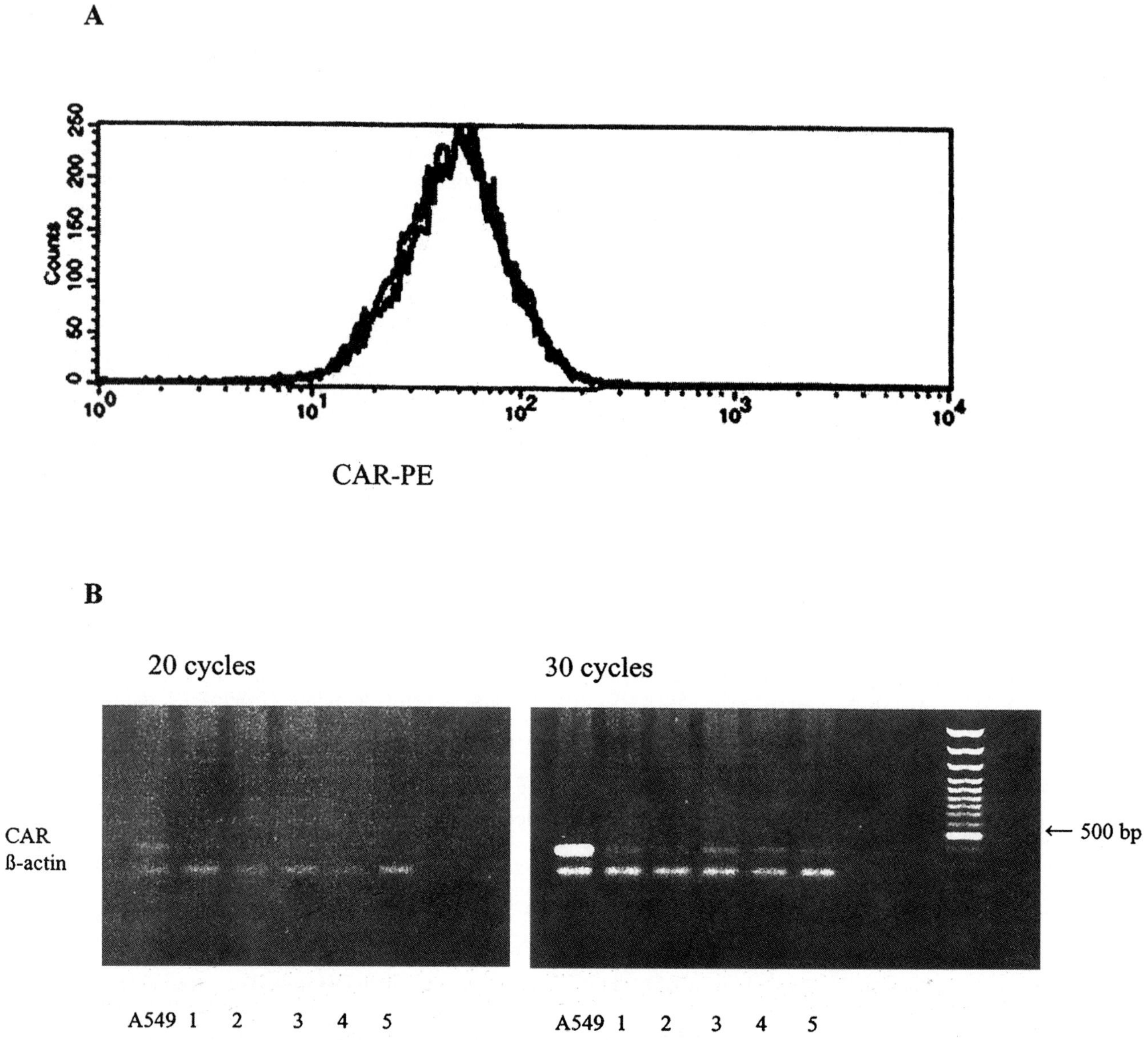

Figure 1. Coxsackie adenovirus receptor (CAR) expression on synoviocytes. CAR expression on synoviocytes was measured on the level of protein expression by flow cytometry (**A**) and in the synoviocytes of 5 rheumatoid arthritis patients on the level of mRNA expression by reverse transcriptase–polymerase chain reaction (**B**). A549 cells served as positive controls. PE = phycoerythrin

to 6095. pAdapt lacks the SV40 intron sequences. The Ad5 sequence (nt 3511–6095) enables the generation of recombinant Ad through homologous recombination with pWe/Ad.AflII-rITR.pac/FibXX.

To determine the presence of the correct fiber, viral DNA isolated from purified batches was subjected to DNA amplification using subgroup-specific oligonucleotides and enzyme restriction analysis (data not shown). Moreover, hemagglutination assays were performed on purified virus using erythrocytes derived from rats and rhesus monkeys. The hemagglutination assay has been described previously (19).

Generation and production of recombinant fiber chimeric Ad. To generate recombinant virus, both plasmids described above were transfected in PER.C6 cells using lipofectamine according to the instructions provided by the manufacturer (Life Technologies, Gibco BRL, Grand Island, NY). For production, 9 × T175 flasks containing a 70% confluent PER.C6 cell layer were each inoculated with 2–5 ml of virus. Upon reaching full cytopathic effect (usually within 2 days), virus was pooled and purified using the 2-step cesium chloride purification process. The production yields in virus particles (VP)/ml of fiber chimeric viruses were determined by high-

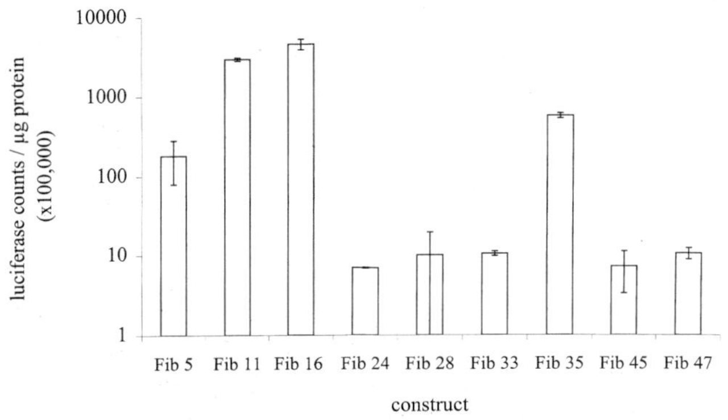

Figure 2. Luciferase gene expression after infection with chimeric adenovirus (Ad). Synoviocytes were incubated with 500 virus particles/cell of Ad5 vectors (group C) or with chimeric Ad vectors with group B fibers (Fib) (Ad serotypes 11, 16, and 35) or group D fibers (Ad serotypes 24, 28, 33, 45, and 47). Luciferase expression was measured 3 days postinfection. Values are the mean ± SEM, corrected for background.

performance liquid chromatography (20) and ranged between 2.2×10^{11} VP/ml and 5.1×10^{12} VP/ml.

Cell transduction. Synoviocytes were seeded at 1.5×10^4 per well in 1 ml for LacZ and luciferase experiments (12-well plate; Cellstar Greiner, Alphen a/d Rijn, The Netherlands) or 5.0×10^4 per well in 2 ml for green fluorescent protein (GFP) experiments (6-well plate). Twenty-four hours after seeding, cells were incubated with an increasing dose of VP/ml in fresh IMDM–10% FCS for variable time periods. Subsequently, synoviocytes were washed twice with phosphate buffered saline and incubated with IMDM–10% FCS and 10% normal human serum at 37°C, 10% CO_2. Cells were analyzed for transgene expression 2 or 3 days postinfection. Details on detection of LacZ, luciferase, and GFP have been reported previously (21–25).

Specificity of infection. Peripheral blood mononuclear cells (PBMC) from healthy blood donors were isolated by Ficoll-Hypaque density gradient centrifugation. Then, 30,000 PBMC were incubated overnight with 500 VP/cell of Ad5.GFP or Ad5.fib16.GFP. Cells were stained 48 hours postinfection with the cell surface markers for T cells (CD3-phycoerythrin [CD3-PE]), B cells (CD19-PE), plasma cells (CD38-PE), natural killer (NK) cells (CD16/56-PE), or monocytes (CD14-PE). The percentage of cells that express GFP, the mean amount of GFP expression, and the cell surface markers (all antibodies from Becton Dickinson, Mountain View, CA) were determined by flow cytometry.

RESULTS

Coxsackie Ad receptor. The CAR is known to be involved in the binding of Ad5 to a cell. Surface expression of the CAR was assessed by flow cytometry on the cultured synoviocytes of 3 RA patients. Also, Northern blotting on messenger RNA (mRNA) extracted from synoviocytes was performed to analyze for transcription of CAR. Neither flow cytometry (Figure 1A) nor mRNA analysis (data not shown) demonstrated expression of CAR in primary human synoviocytes. Since both assays may be too insensitive to detect a low level of CAR expression or transcription and minute amounts of CAR may be sufficient for adequate Ad5 gene transfer, PCR analysis was performed. Complementary DNA was generated from mRNA extracted from RA synoviocytes. This cDNA was analyzed for the presence of CAR and, as a control for the quality of the mRNA, for β-actin. In synoviocytes, a clear β-actin signal was found after 15 cycles and for CAR after 30 cycles. In contrast, A549 cells, which were highly positive in both flow cytometric and Northern analyses, were found to express CAR after 20 cycles of PCR (Figure 1B). This indicates that synoviocytes from RA patients express extremely low levels of CAR, especially when compared with a cell line that is very transducible with Ad5 vectors, i.e., A549 cells. Synoviocytes from 3 osteoarthritis patients gave results similar to synoviocytes from RA patients (data not shown).

In vitro infection efficiency of synoviocytes. Cultured synoviocytes were incubated overnight with different chimeric Ad vectors harboring the luciferase gene at 500 VP/cell. Luciferase activity was measured 3 days postinfection. Figure 2 shows that the Ad5-based vectors carrying a fiber derived from B-group Ad (Ad serotypes 11, 16, and 35) yielded a higher activity of luciferase compared with Ad5. In contrast, Ad5-based vectors carrying a fiber derived from D-subgroup Ad (Ad serotypes 24, 28, 33, 45, and 47) induced lower transgene expression in synoviocytes than Ad5.

Experiments with the group B fiber chimeric vectors were repeated using synoviocytes from different RA patients. Student's paired, 2-tailed *t*-test showed that Ad5.fib11, Ad5.fib16, and Ad5.fib35 gave significantly higher levels of transgene expression than Ad5 ($P < 0.005$). On average, Ad5.fib11.luc, Ad5.fib16.luc, and Ad5.fib35.luc produced 28 (SD 18; n = 3), 161 (SD 192; n = 9), and 4 (SD 2; n = 3) times more gene expression than Ad5.luc, respectively.

To determine the effect of incubation time with the vectors on infection of synoviocytes, time series experiments were performed in which Ad5.fib16.luc was compared with Ad5.luc. Figure 3 shows that Ad5.fib16.luc produced higher gene expression than Ad5.luc at all time points, indicating an increased virus attachment to synoviocytes.

Luciferase activity experiments do not provide data on the percentage of cells that are infected. Therefore, experiments were repeated with other reporter

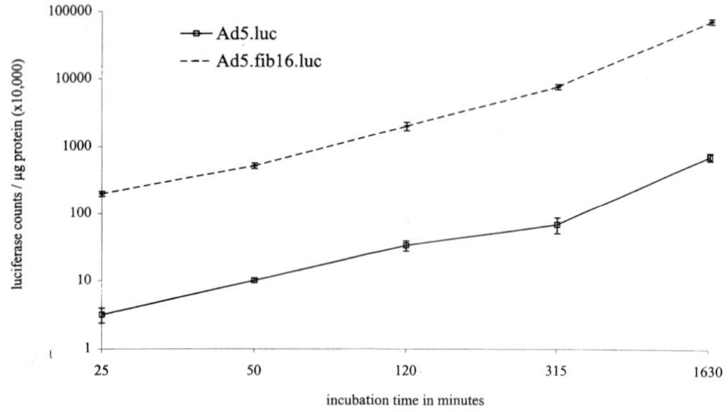

Figure 3. Time series experiment. Synoviocytes were incubated for indicated time periods with 500 virus particles/cell of adenovirus (Ad) (Ad5.luc or Ad5.fib16.luc). Synoviocytes were harvested 3 days postinfection and luciferase activity was measured. Values are corrected for background.

genes, i.e., LacZ and GFP. Experiments in which LacZ was used as a marker gene were performed in triplicate, with 2 or 48 hours virus exposure time points in synoviocytes derived from 6 RA patients. Forty-eight hours postinfection, the synoviocytes were stained for β-galactosidase expression and the percentage of blue cells per well was estimated. Synoviocytes incubated for 2 hours with 500 VP/cell of Ad5.lacZ or Ad5.fib16.lacZ yielded on average 1.3% (SD 0.3) and 19.4% (SD 2.0) of LacZ-positive cells, respectively. After 48 hours, the percentages of blue cells increased to 8.0% (SD 1.3) and 76.2% (SD 5.5), respectively. Experiments in which GFP was used as a marker were performed on synoviocytes from 3 different RA patients. Synoviocytes were incubated overnight with 50, 500, or 5,000 VP of Ad5.GFP or Ad5.fib16.GFP per cell. Flow cytometric analyses showed that Ad5.fib16.GFP consistently infected a higher percentage of synoviocytes than Ad5.GFP, with a higher mean GFP production (Figure 4).

Fiber-16 chimera. For clinical applications, it is important that a production process can be controlled and is reproducible. To test for the reproducibility of Ad5.fib16 production, different batches were generated independently. For this fiber chimeric vector, the virus yield obtained from 9 × T175 flasks ranged from 4.8×10^{11} to 4.6×10^{12} VP/ml (n = 17) as determined by high-performance liquid chromatography. To test for the efficiency of the production, end point titration of the vectors was performed on 911 cells (26). On these cells, Ad5.fib16 vectors demonstrated a mean ± SEM VP:infective units ratio of 114.3 ± 64.8 (n = 17). These results show that fiber chimeric viruses can be propagated reproducibly on PER.C6 helper cells to titers comparable with those found with recombinant Ad5. End point titration of Ad5 vectors yielded a VP:IU ratio of 7.1 ± 6.7 (n = 11). The VP:IU ratios indicate that Ad5.fib16 infects 911 cells less efficiently than does Ad5.

Specificity of the vectors. As discussed above, the joint can be observed as a closed compartment. Therefore, only synoviocytes and cells in the synovial fluid are targets for the Ad vector after intraarticular administration. Cells in the synovial fluid consist mainly of polymorphonuclear cells (PMN) and mononuclear cells. The time needed to allow reporter gene expression is longer than the time in which we are able to culture PMN. Consequently, we were not able to test infection of PMN with Ad vectors. In our test system, PBMC were used as a model for synovial fluid mononuclear cells.

The PBMC of 2 healthy controls were incubated overnight with 500 VP per cell of either Ad5.GFP or

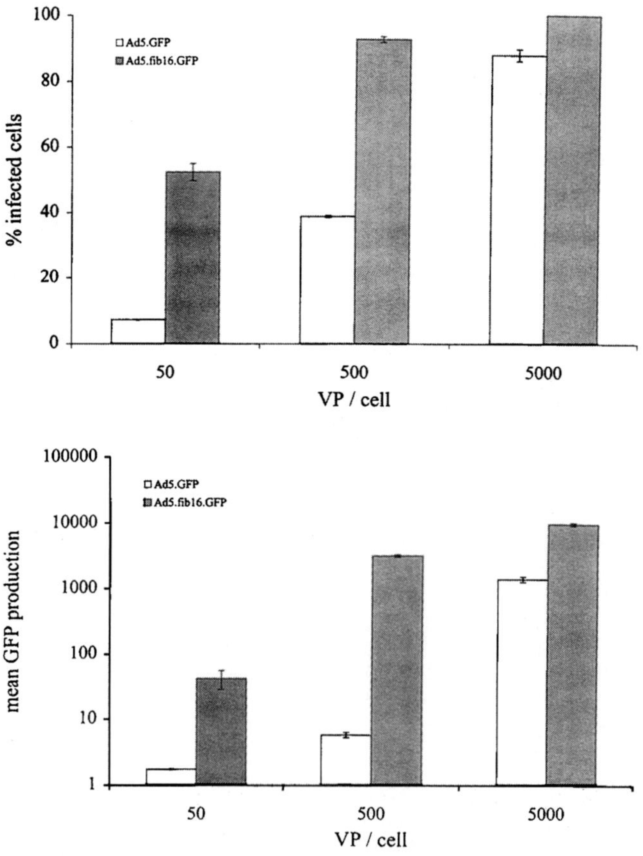

Figure 4. Percentage of adenovirus [Ad]–infected synoviocytes, and green fluorescent protein (GFP) production. Synoviocytes were incubated overnight with the indicated concentrations of Ad5.GFP or Ad5.fib16.GFP. GFP expression was measured 3 days postinfection. Values are the mean ± SEM. Ad5.fib16 = Ad5 vector carrying fibor of Ad16; VP = virus particles.

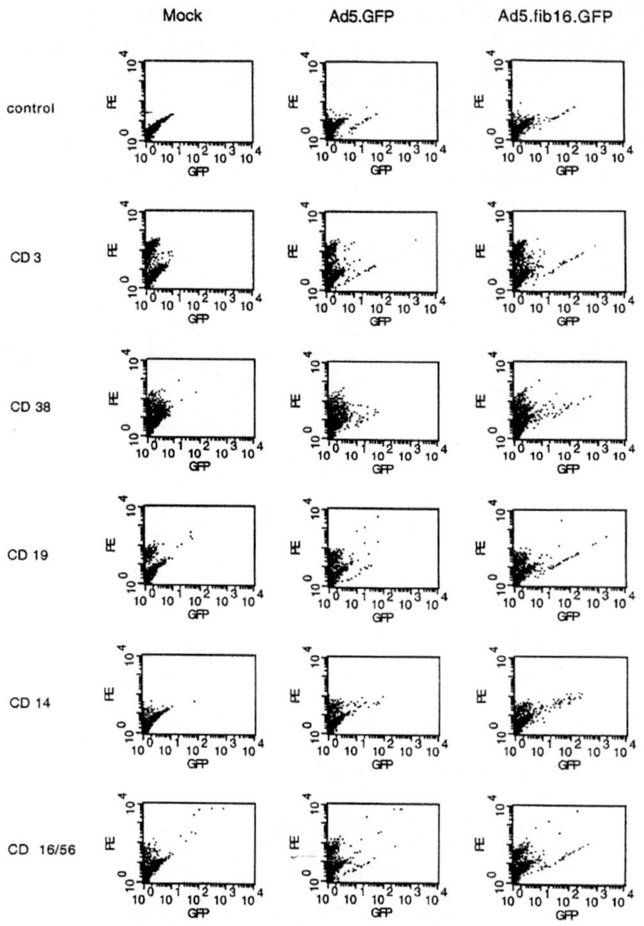

Figure 5. Specificity of peripheral blood mononuclear cell (PBMC) infection. To assess the cell specificity of the infection, PBMC were incubated overnight with 500 VP Ad5.GFP or Ad5.fib16.GFP per cell. Three days postinfection, cells were stained for cell surface markers. GFP expression and cell surface markers were assessed by flow cytometry. PE = phycoerythrin (see Figure 4 for other definitions).

Ad5.fib16.GFP. Forty-eight hours postinfection, cells were harvested and analyzed simultaneously for GFP and the expression of the cell surface markers CD3 (T cells), CD14 (monocytes and macrophages), CD19 (B cells), CD38 (plasma cells, activated T cells), or CD16/56 (NK cells). Upon transduction with Ad5.GFP, a mean of 0.6% (SD 0.04%) of all PBMC were positive for GFP, with a mean GFP expression of 19 units. GFP expression was restricted to CD14-positive cells, indicating that only monocytes were transduced. Upon transduction with Ad5.fib16.GFP, 1.0% (SD 0.2%) of all PBMC were positive for GFP, with a mean GFP expression of 77 units. GFP expression was restricted to cells positive for CD14 or CD38, indicating transduction of monocytes and plasma cells (Figure 5). In parallel, synoviocytes were transduced with the same virus that was used to transduce the PBMC. These synoviocytes showed 43% GFP-positive cells, with a mean GFP expression of 1.3×10^2 units for Ad5.GFP, and 76% GFP-positive cells, with a mean GFP expression of 1.9×10^3 units for Ad5.fib16.GFP.

DISCUSSION

Ad5 infects cells by attachment of the knob of the Ad fiber to cellular receptors such as CAR (9). Lack of expression of CAR appears to be a rate-limiting step in the infection efficiency of Ad5 (27) since CAR represents a high-affinity receptor for this virus. In this study, synoviocytes from different patients were found to be negative for expression of CAR protein on their surface. Moreover, RT-PCR showed that extremely low levels of CAR mRNA are present in human primary synoviocytes. These results are consistent with the relatively low transduction efficiency we usually find on synoviocytes using Ad5 vectors. Although CAR is absent or very low, transgene expression can be obtained with Ad5, probably due either to receptor-independent uptake of the virus because of the high multiplicities of infection used, or through the binding of Ad to alternative receptors, i.e., major histocompatibility complex class I a2 domain (28).

Although many different strategies to improve Ad vectors for certain cell types are under investigation, we exploited the natural diversity of Ad serotypes. An important reason to use building blocks, i.e., fibers, already present in nature is the hypothesis that such vectors can be generated in high titers. The data presented indicate that we have identified a vector (Ad5.fib16) that is superior to Ad5 for transfection of synoviocytes, both in the amount of cells transduced as well as in the amount of transgene expressed per transduced cell. The increase in transgene expression per cell can probably be explained by multiple infections of the same cell. Although Ad5.fib16 consistently proved to be the best vector based on transgene expression, other Ad5-based vectors carrying fibers derived from other B-group Ad were also better than Ad5. The observation that none of the D-group chimeric Ad5-based vectors did better compared with Ad5 might indicate that these vectors have an even stricter requirement for CAR. Alternatively, D-group viruses might display a lower affinity compared with Ad5 for another receptor collectively shared between Ad5 (subgroup C) and subgroup D Ad.

Titration assays on 911 cells indicate that the

infection efficiency of these cells with Ad5.fib16 vectors is worse compared with Ad5. Although some Ad receptors have been identified, reports in the literature demonstrate that receptor usage might be complex between subgroups of Ad as well as within a subgroup (11,19). For many of the 51 human Ad identified (29), including members of subgroup B, the attachment molecules are unknown. Because the receptors are unknown, the fiber chimeric vectors generated need to be compared based on equal amounts of virus particles. Another concern when equal amounts of virus particles are used is the chance that small differences in the quality of virus production contribute to the differences observed in transgene expression. To exclude this possibility, different batches of Ad5.fib16 carrying different marker genes were used.

As discussed earlier (30), Ad itself can cause inflammation. The increased infection efficiency obtained with Ad5.fib16 might prove sufficient to lower the viral load and thus limit the chance of inducing a flare of arthritis. Although little is known about the persistence of infective Ad particles after administration in the joint, it can be hypothesized that Ad that are able to infect cells within a short period are more favorable than vectors that infect slowly. The results of the time series experiments performed showed that the increased infection efficiency of Ad5.fib16 was consistent for all virus exposure times compared with Ad5. More important, the results demonstrated that a 25-minute virus exposure is already sufficient to achieve a relatively high transduction efficiency.

To investigate whether the specificity of Ad5.fib16 is similar to that of Ad5, experiments on human PBMC were performed. The results obtained are consistent with the literature, showing that ~10% of all monocytes were infected with Ad5.GFP (31,32). Lymphocytes, plasma cells, and NK cells did not show expression of the reporter gene after incubation with Ad5.GFP. PBMC incubated overnight with 500 VP/cell of Ad5.fib16.GFP showed ~1% GFP-positive mononuclear cells. These GFP-positive PBMC were monocytes and plasma cells but not T or B lymphocytes or NK cells. The percentage of Ad5.fib16.GFP-infected PBMC is low compared with the 76% GFP-positive cells in experiments performed simultaneously in synoviocytes. Besides, gene expression in GFP-positive PBMC was 96% lower than that in GFP-positive synoviocytes. This indicates that a high degree of efficiency can be obtained with Ad5.fib16.

In conclusion, the increased transduction efficiency, together with the maintenance of specificity and the short time frame required for transduction, makes Ad5.fib16 a powerful new tool for transducing synoviocytes. Since these parameters are also important for in vivo use, it can be envisioned that Ad5.fib16 improves the therapeutic window of gene-based strategies for the treatment of RA.

ACKNOWLEDGMENTS

The authors wish to thank all orthopedic surgeons of the Leiden University Medical Center, but especially Rob Nelissen and Prof. Dr. P. M. Rozing, for collecting synovial tissue during joint replacement surgery.

REFERENCES

1. McCarty DJ, Koopman WJ. Arthritis and allied conditions: a textbook of rheumatology. 12th ed. Philadelphia: Lea & Febiger; 1993.
2. Chernajovsky Y, Annenkov A, Herman C, Triantaphyllopoulos K, Gould D, Dreja H, et al. Gene therapy for rheumatoid arthritis: theoretical considerations. Drugs Aging 1998;12:29–41.
3. Roessler BJ, Allen ED, Wilson JM, Hartman JW, Davidson BL. Adenoviral-mediated gene transfer to rabbit synovium in vivo. J Clin Invest 1993;92:1085–92.
4. Ikeda T, Kubo T, Arai Y, Nakanishi T, Kobayashi K, Takahashi K, et al. Adenovirus mediated gene delivery to the joints of guinea pigs. J Rheumatol 1998;25:1666–73.
5. Whalen JD, Lechman EL, Carlos CA, Weiss K, Kovesdi I, Glorioso JC, et al. Adenoviral transfer of the viral IL-10 gene periarticularly to mouse paws suppresses development of collagen-induced arthritis in both injected and uninjected paws. J Immunol 1999;162:3625–32.
6. Goossens PH, Schouten GJ, 't Hart BA, Bout A, Brok HPM, Kluin PM, et al. Feasibility of adenovirus-mediated nonsurgical synovectomy in collagen-induced arthritis-affected rhesus monkeys. Hum Gene Ther 1999;10:1139–49.
7. Ghivizanni SC, Kang R, Hatton C, Tio C, Lechman ER, Emmert A, et al. In vivo delivery of genes encoding soluble receptors for IL-1 and TNFα results in a synergistic therapeutic effect in antigen-induced arthritis in the rabbit knee [abstract]. Arthritis Rheum 1996;39:S308.
8. Fields BN, Knipe DM, Howley PM. Fields virology. 3rd ed. Philadelphia: Lippincott-Raven; 1996.
9. Bergelson JM, Cunningham JA, Droguett G, Kurt-Jones EA, Krithivas A, Hong JS, et al. Isolation of a common receptor for Coxsackie B viruses and adenoviruses 2 and 5. Science 1997;275: 1320–3.
10. McDonald D, Stockwin L, Matzow T, Zajdel MB, Blair G. Coxsackie and adenovirus receptor (CAR)-dependent and major histocompatibility complex (MHC) class I-independent uptake of recombinant adenoviruses into human tumour cells. Gene Ther 1999;6:1512–9.
11. Arnberg N, Edlund K, Kidd AH, Wadell G. Adenovirus type 37 uses sialic acid as a cellular receptor. J Virol 2000;74:42–8.
12. Wirtz S, Galle PR, Neurath MF. Efficient gene delivery to the inflamed colon by local administration of recombinant adenoviruses with normal or modified fibre structure. Gut 1999;44:800–7.
13. Zabner J, Chillon M, Grunst T, Moninger TO, Davidson BL, Gregory R, et al. A chimeric type 2 adenovirus vector with a type 17 fiber enhances gene transfer to human airway epithelia. J Virol 1999;73:8689–95.
14. Roelvink PW, Lizonova A, Lee JGM, Li Y, Bergelson JM, Finberg

RW, et al. The coxsackie virus-adenovirus receptor protein can function as a cellular attachment protein for adenovirus serotypes from subgroups A, C, D, E, and F. J Virol 1998;72:7909–15.
15. Arnett FC, Edworthy SM, Bloch DA, McShane DJ, Fries JF, Cooper NS, et al. The American Rheumatism Association 1987 revised criteria for the classification of rheumatoid arthritis. Arthritis Rheum 1988;31:315–24.
16. Rea D, Schagen FHE, Hoeben RC, Mehtali M, Havenga MJE, Toes REM, et al. Adenoviruses activate human dendritic cells without polarization toward a T-helper type 1-inducing subset. J Virol 1999;73:10245–53.
17. Fallaux FJ, Bout A, van der Velde I, van den Wollenberg DJ, Hehir KM, Keegan J, et al. New helper cells and matched early region 1-deleted adenovirus vectors prevent generation of replication-competent adenoviruses. Hum Gene Ther 1998;9:1909–17.
18. Zhang WW, Koch PE, Roth JA. Detection of wild-type contamination in a recombinant adenoviral preparation by PCR. Biotechniques 1995;18:444–7.
19. Shayakhmetov DM, Papayannopoulou T, Stamatoyannopoulos G, Lieber A. Efficient gene transfer into human CD34(+) cells by a retargeted adenovirus vector. J Virol 2000;74:2567–83.
20. Shabram PW, Giroux DD, Goudreau AM, Gregory RJ, Horn MT, Huyghe BG, et al. Analytical anion-exchange HPLC of recombinant type-5 adenoviral particles. Hum Gene Ther 1997;8:453–65.
21. Bonnerot C, Rocancourt D, Briand P, Grimber G, Nicolas JF. A beta-galactosidase hybrid protein targeted to nuclei as a marker for developmental studies. Proc Natl Acad Sci U S A 1987;84: 6795–9.
22. De Wet JR, Wood KV, DeLuca M, Helinski DR, Subramani S. Firefly luciferase gene: structure and expression in mammalian cells. Mol Cell Biol 1987;7:725–37.
23. De Wet JR, Wood KV, Helinski DR, DeLuca M. Cloning of firefly luciferase cDNA and the expression of active luciferase in Escherichia coli. Proc Natl Acad Sci U S A 1985;82:7870–3.
24. Chalfie M, Tu Y, Euskirchen G, Ward WW, Prasher DC. Green fluorescent protein as a marker for gene expression. Science 1994;263:802–5.
25. Prendergast FG, Mann KG. Chemical and physical properties of aequorin and the green fluorescent protein isolated from Aequorea forskalea. Biochemistry 1978;17:3448–53.
26. Fallaux FJ, Kranenburg O, Cramer SJ, Houweling A, van Ormondt H, Hoeben RC, et al. Characterization of 911: a new helper cell line for the titration and propagation of early region 1-deleted adenoviral vectors. Hum Gene Ther 1996;7:215–22.
27. Kaner RJ, Worgall S, Leopold PL, Stolze E, Milano E, Hidaka C, et al. Modification of the genetic program of human alveolar macrophages by adenovirus vectors in vitro is feasible but inefficient, limited in part by the low level of expression of the coxsackie/adenovirus receptor. Am J Respir Cell Mol Biol 1999; 20:361–70.
28. Hong SS, Galaup A, Peytavi R, Chazal N, Boulanger P. Enhancement of adenovirus-mediated gene delivery by use of an oligopeptide with dual binding specificity. Hum Gene Ther 1999;10: 2577–86.
29. De Jong JC, Wermenbol AG, Verweij-Uijterwaal MW, Slaterus KW, Wertheim-van Dillen GP, van Doornum GJ, et al. Adenoviruses from human immunodeficiency virus-infected individuals, including two strains that represent new candidate serotypes Ad50 and Ad51 of species B1 and D, respectively. J Clin Microbiol 1999;37:3940–5.
30. Muruve DA, Barnes MJ, Stillman IE, Libermann TA. Adenoviral gene therapy leads to rapid induction of multiple chemokines and acute neutrophil-dependent hepatic injury in vivo. Hum Gene Ther 1999;10:965–76.
31. Huang MR, Olsson M, Kallin A, Pettersson U, Totterman TH. Efficient adenovirus-mediated gene transduction of normal and leukemic hematopoietic cells. Gene Ther 1997;4:1093–9.
32. Haddada H, Lopez M, Martinache C, Ragot T, Abina MA, Perricaudet M. Efficient adenovirus-mediated gene transfer into human blood monocyte-derived macrophages. Biochem Biophys Res Commun 1993;195:1174–83.

ARTHRITIS & RHEUMATISM
Vol. 44, No. 3, March 2001, pp 578–584

Osteopontin

An Intrinsic Inhibitor of Inflammation in Cartilage

Mukundan G. Attur,[1] Mandar N. Dave,[1] Steven Stuchin,[1] Aaron J. Kowalski,[2] German Steiner,[3] Steven B. Abramson,[4] David T. Denhardt,[2] and Ashok R. Amin[4]

Objective. **To identify extracellular and intraarticular matrix components that are differentially expressed in normal and osteoarthritis (OA)–affected cartilage and to investigate their functions with respect to regulation of mediators of inflammation.**

Methods. **Differential-display reverse transcriptase–polymerase chain reaction (RT-PCR) analysis of a pool of messenger RNA (mRNA) from 10 human OA cartilage samples and 5 normal cartilage samples was performed using arbitrary primers. Confirmatory analysis of the up-regulated transcripts of fibronectin (FN) and osteopontin (OPN) was performed by RT-PCR of individual RNA samples from a separate set of donors. The effect of recombinant OPN (or anti-OPN antiserum) on chondrocyte function was examined by analyzing the spontaneous or interleukin-1 (IL-1)–induced release of nitric oxide (NO) and prostaglandin E_2 (PGE_2) from human OA-affected cartilage under ex vivo conditions.**

Results. **Up-regulation (300–700%) of FN and OPN mRNA was observed in human OA-affected cartilage as compared with normal cartilage. Functional analysis of the role of OPN in OA cartilage showed that 1) Addition of 1 μg/ml (20 n*M*) of recombinant OPN to human OA-affected cartilage under ex vivo conditions inhibited spontaneous and IL-1β–induced NO and PGE_2 production, and 2) neutralization of intraarticular OPN with anti-OPN antiserum augmented NO production.**

Conclusion. **The data indicate that one of the functions of intraarticular OPN, which is overexpressed in OA cartilage, is to act as an innate inhibitor of IL-1, NO, and PGE_2 production. These findings suggest that the production of pleiotropic mediators of inflammation that influence cartilage homeostasis, such as NO and PGE_2, is regulated by the interaction of chondrocytes with differentially expressed proteins within the extracellular matrix.**

Historically, osteoarthritis (OA) has been considered a "noninflammatory" disease, due to the absence of infiltrating neutrophils and the lack of characteristic signs of inflammation such as redness and swelling with heat and pain (*rubor et tumor cum colore et dolor*). However, studies from this and other laboratories have shown that OA articular cartilage, in contrast to normal cartilage, is characterized by the superinduction of proinflammatory genes (which include nitric oxide synthase [NOS], cyclooxygenase 2 [COX-2], interleukin-1β [IL-1β], IL-6, and IL-8) and corresponding gene products (1–4). It is now accepted that the excessive, spontaneous production of these cytokines and mediators of inflammation plays a significant role in the molecular pathogenesis of OA, contributing to a highly catabolic state, chondrocyte apoptosis, and the resultant progressive degeneration of articular cartilage (1–8). Among these, NO and prostaglandin E_2 (PGE_2) have detrimental effects on cartilage homeostasis (for review, see refs. 3, 5, and 9). This localized "molecular inflammation," which is driven by activated chondrocytes within avascular and aneural articular cartilage, is not typically reflected by clinical signs of inflammation. However,

Drs. Abramson and Amin's work was supported by a grant from the National Arthritis Foundation. Dr. Denhardt's work was supported by NIH grants AR-44434 and ES-06897.

[1]Mukundan G. Attur, PhD, Mandar N. Dave, PhD, Steven Stuchin, MD: Hospital for Joint Diseases, New York, New York; [2]Aaron J. Kowalski, PhD, David T. Denhardt, PhD: Rutgers University, Piscataway, New Jersey; [3]German Steiner, MD: New York University Medical Center, New York, New York; [4]Steven B. Abramson, MD, Ashok R. Amin, PhD: Hospital for Joint Diseases and New York University Medical Center, New York, New York.

Address correspondence and reprint requests to Ashok R. Amin, PhD, Department of Medicine and Rheumatology, Rheumatology Research Laboratory, Room 1600, Hospital for Joint Diseases, 301 East 17th Street, New York, NY 10003.

Submitted for publication March 27, 2000; accepted in revised form November 8, 2000.

elucidation of the initiation and regulation of these processes has the potential to reveal novel molecular targets for future therapeutic intervention in OA.

The synthesis and degradation of cartilage matrix is regulated by chondrocytes via mechanisms that depend, in part, upon the interaction of chondrocytes with the extracellular matrix (ECM) proteins. These include collagens, proteoglycans, and noncollagen proteins (10). It is increasingly recognized that there is specific induction and repression of chondrocyte gene expression, controlled through cellular contact with ECM proteins (fibronectin [FN], osteopontin [OPN], collagen, and proteoglycans) in the pericellular environment surrounding the chondrocytes (chondron), which control cartilage homeostasis.

Receptors for ECM components are integrins, a family of cell surface glycoproteins (11–14). Ligands for integrins on chondrocytes are often large ECM proteins such as collagen, laminin, and FN, and soluble proteins such as vitronectin and OPN. Recently, Tavella et al studied the expression of both FN and laminin and related integrin receptors in chondrocyte differentiation (15). Previous studies have shown that addition of FN fragments or recombinant extra domain A (EDA) region of FN in cartilage up-regulated inflammatory mediators and induced chondrolysis via the ligation of the chondrocyte $\alpha5\beta1$ integrin (12,14,16,17). OPN binds to various receptors including integrins (e.g., $\alpha v\beta3$ and CD44) and induces cellular chemotaxis in neutrophils, but, unlike hyaluronate, OPN does not induce homotypic aggregation (18). Margerie et al have demonstrated expression of OPN in human OA chondrocytes; the expression of OPN was down-regulated by IL-1 in vitro (19).

Although several studies have indicated that various ligands bind to chondrocytes via their integrins, the outcome of these interactions with respect to "outside-in" and "inside-out" signaling function is elusive in spite of the literature available in this field with respect to other cell types (11). We therefore utilized differential-display analysis of messenger RNA (mRNA) from normal and OA-affected cartilage to identify abnormal expression of intraarticular matrix components produced by chondrocytes. The functions of one of these matrix components in OA cartilage, OPN, was investigated with respect to regulation of mediators of inflammation.

MATERIALS AND METHODS

Procurement of human cartilage. Cartilage slices were obtained from the knees of patients with advanced OA (age 50–70 years) who were undergoing knee replacement surgery. Patients had not taken nonsteroidal antiinflammatory drugs for at least 2 weeks prior to surgery. Nonarthritic knee cartilage was obtained from patients with fractures or from patients undergoing amputation due to trauma. The use of discarded human cartilage was approved by appropriate institutional review boards, and informed consent was obtained.

Histologic analysis of cartilage. Histologic evaluation was performed on sagittal sections of normal and OA-affected cartilage from the medial femoral condyle and tibial plateau. Following dissection, specimens were fixed in 10% buffered formalin and embedded in paraffin. Sections (6μ) were stained with Safranin O as previously described (20).

RNA extraction from cartilage. Total RNA from OA cartilage and normal cartilage was extracted by the guanidine thiocyanate–phenol/chloroform extraction method, with minor modifications. The cartilage was milled into fine powder and extracted with 4*M* guanidine thiocyanate, 25 m*M* sodium citrate, 0.5% sodium dodecyl sarcosine, and 0.1*M* 2-mercaptoethanol. The aqueous phase was layered onto a cesium trifluoroacetate gradient for ultracentrifugation (24,000 revolutions per minute/24 hours), and the RNA was extracted. Total RNA obtained by this method showed a 260:280 ratio of 1.8:2.0. The integrity of the RNA was also confirmed using a 1% formaldehyde agarose gel.

Differential display of mRNA. Differential-display reverse transcriptase–polymerase chain reaction (DDRT-PCR) of complementary DNA (cDNA) from a pool of 5 normal and 10 OA-affected cartilage samples was performed using 0.1 μg total RNA (21). Briefly, the cDNA were synthesized using total RNA and oligo(dT) and amplified using arbitrary primers as described previously (19). The DDRT-PCR–amplified ^{32}P-labeled cDNA fragments were separated on a 6% sequencing gel. The differentially expressed cDNA were isolated and purified from the gels and cloned in TA cloning vector (Invitrogen, Carlsbad, CA). The cDNA was cloned and sequenced on an automatic DNA Sequencer (Protein DNA Technology Center, Rockefeller University, New York, NY).

Sequence analysis. Sequence searches for the cDNA clones were performed with the BLAST program.

OA explant assay. Knee articular cartilage from the OA patients was cut into 3-mm discs, and 4–6 discs were placed (in triplicate or quadruplicate) in a 24-well plate containing 2 ml Ham's F-12 medium and 0.1% human serum albumin in the presence or absence of OPN and anti-OPN antiserum (1,2).

RT-PCR analysis of OPN and FN. Total RNA (1 μg) isolated from OA and normal cartilage (2) was used for cDNA synthesis by RT-PCR (Gibco BRL, Grand Island, NY). The sense primer 5′-GGACTCCATTGACTCGAACG-3′ and antisense primer 5′-TAATCTGGACTGCTTGTGGC-3′ were used for mRNA amplification of OPN, the sense primer 5′-GCGCCTGGTCACCAGGGCTGC-3′ and antisense primer 5′-GGATCTCGCTCCTGGAAGATC-3′ were used for amplification of GAPDH, and the sense primer 5′-AATTACCACAACCCCTACAAAC-3′ and antisense primer 5′-CAACTCTGCAACATCTTCCTC-3′ were used for amplification of FN. All of the amplified products were subjected to sequence analysis as described above.

Expression and purification of OPN. Human OPN was expressed in human embryonic kidney cells as described by

Hwang et al (22). It was purified from conditioned medium by ion-exchange chromatography on a DEAE-Sepharose fast flow column, followed by elution from a sodium dodecyl sulfate–polyacrylamide gel. OPN purified by this method was >98% pure (22). The purified protein was not cytotoxic to cells and had no detectable endotoxin activity according to the *Limulus* assay. OPN at 5 μg/ml has no effect on the cell viability of bovine chondrocytes in vitro as assayed by trypan blue dye exclusion.

Preparation of anti-OPN antiserum. Polyclonal OPN antiserum was prepared as described by Harlow and Lane (23). Briefly, OPN was injected intraperitoneally into female OPN knockout mice. The rationale was to generate highly specific antibodies that recognize epitopes conserved between species as well as all those present on mouse OPN itself (24,25). The anti-OPN antiserum, but not pre-bleed serum (or normal mouse serum), identified recombinant OPN and its degraded products by Western blot analysis (26).

Recombinant histidine-tagged human OPN (~20 μg; synthesized in *Escherichia coli* and purified on a nickel chelating column) in 250 μl phosphate buffered saline was mixed with 250 μl Freund's complete adjuvant and injected intraperitoneally. After 2 weeks and after 5 weeks, the mice were boosted with an equal amount of protein in Freund's incomplete adjuvant. Ten days later, the mice were anesthetized and bled retroorbitally. Serum was collected, aliquoted, and stored at −70°C.

Nitrite and PGE_2 analysis. The stable NO metabolite, nitrite, was measured in conditioned medium by modified Griess reaction (27). PGE_2 was estimated by radioimmunoassay as previously described (2).

Semiquantitation of PCR products. Quantitation of PCR products was performed with a personal densitometer (SI; Molecular Dynamics, Sunnyvale, CA) using Quantimage 5 software, after normalization of the FN and OPN with GAPDH.

Statistical analysis. Data were expressed as the mean ± SD, and statistical analyses were performed using GraphPad Software (version 1.14). Significance of the data was determined by Student's *t*-test or by nonparametric testing (Mann-Whitney U test or Wilcoxon's signed rank test).

RESULTS

Differential display of mRNA in normal and OA-affected cartilage. We have recently standardized methods to perform differential display of mRNA of novel matrix metalloproteinases (e.g., tumor necrosis factor α convertase) expressed in human OA and normal cartilage, by using degenerate oligonucleotides to conserved motifs to amplify cDNA from RNA (28). We have also performed differential display of mRNA from normal and OA cartilage mRNA using arbitrary primers and the Gene Hunter kit (29) as described in Materials and Methods.

Cartilage from the superficial layer was scraped and utilized for RNA extraction. Representative samples of normal and OA cartilage that were used for the extraction of total RNA are shown in Figure 1. DDRT-PCR was performed from a pool of RNA obtained from 5 normal and 10 OA cartilage samples. Approximately 80 differentially expressed cDNA clones were sequenced and examined using a BLAST search. Among these sequences, 2 cDNAs coding for the ECM proteins FN and OPN were found to be up-regulated in human OA cartilage as compared with normal cartilage in the first screen.

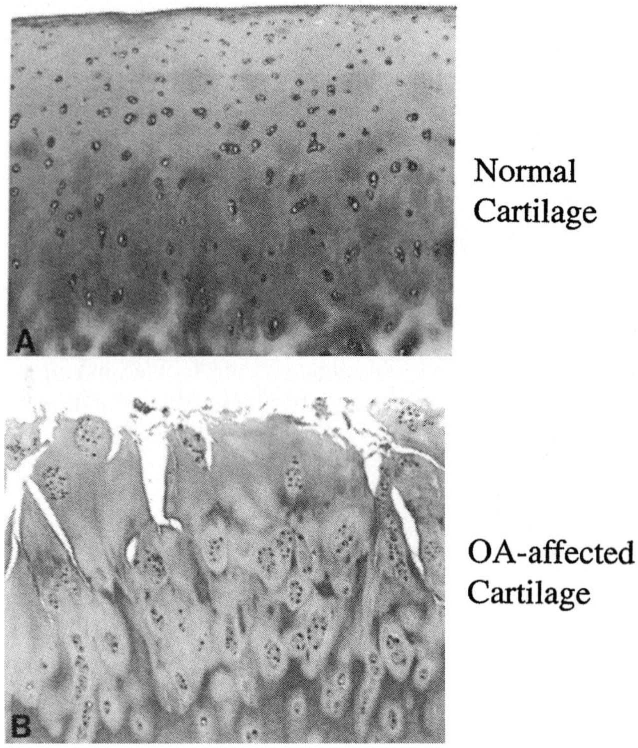

Figure 1. Histologic analysis of normal cartilage (**A**) and osteoarthritis (OA)–affected cartilage (**B**). Cartilage samples from human knees were sectioned and stained as described in Materials and Methods. Results are representative of several samples used in this study. (Original magnification × 70.)

To verify the up-regulation of FN and OPN mRNA in human OA cartilage, we assessed the expression of FN mRNA in RNA obtained from 4 OA and 2 normal cartilage samples, by RT-PCR using specific primers designed from the cDNA sequences obtained in the first screen. RT-PCR analysis showed ~300% up-regulation of FN mRNA in all 4 OA cartilage samples analyzed (Figure 2). We also analyzed OPN mRNA levels in 5 different OA and 5 normal cartilage samples by RT-PCR using specific primers. All 5 OA samples showed an average increase of OPN mRNA of ~700%

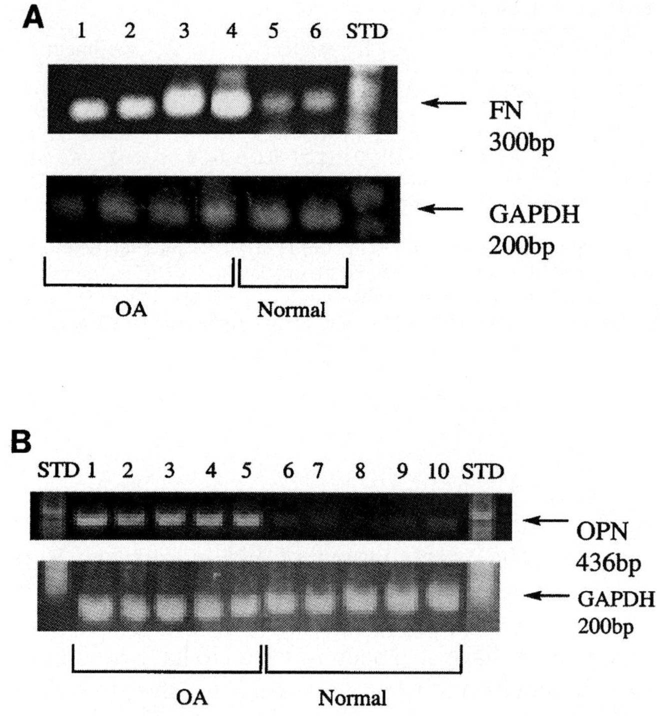

Figure 2. Up-regulation of fibronectin (FN) and osteopontin (OPN) mRNA in human osteoarthritis (OA)–affected cartilage. Normal and OA-affected cartilage samples were obtained from different individuals and total RNA was extracted without releasing the cells from the cartilage, as described in ref. 2. **A,** Equal amounts of total RNA (100 ng) from 4 OA and 2 normal cartilage samples were analyzed for expression of FN mRNA by reverse transcriptase–polymerase chain reaction (RT-PCR) using specific FN primers (25–28 cycles). **B,** Equal amounts of total RNA (100 ng) from 5 OA patients and 5 normal subjects were subjected to RT-PCR analysis (25–28 cycles) using specific OPN primers as described in Materials and Methods. GAPDH in all of the samples was also amplified by RT-PCR in the same preparations. STD = molecular weight standards. Results are representative of 2 similar experiments.

as compared with normal cartilage (Figure 2). These results confirm the enhanced expression of FN and OPN mRNA isolated from human OA cartilage as compared with normal cartilage. Attempts to quantitate OPN protein (by Western blot and enzyme-linked immunosorbent assay) in conditioned medium (under ex vivo conditions) or cartilage (by Western blot) were unsuccessful because of the apparent low amount of intact OPN protein (<1 μg/ml) and/or the susceptibility of OPN to proteases, as previously described for serum OPN (30).

Regulation of NO by OPN. In view of the multifunctional properties of FN and OPN (31,32) and the chondrolytic/proinflammatory activity of FN fragments in cartilage (13,33), we tested the hypothesis that up-regulated OPN may regulate inflammatory mediators known to be spontaneously released under ex vivo conditions in human OA cartilage. Addition of 1 μg/ml (20 n*M*) of recombinant OPN inhibited the spontaneous production of NO in human OA cartilage (Figure 3). These results suggest that OPN is able to suppress the spontaneous production of NO that had been induced in vivo and detected in cartilage organ cultures ex vivo. These findings further indicate that OPN is a negative innate modulator of NO production and can significantly decrease the accumulation of NO in human OA-affected cartilage.

We also examined the role of endogenous up-regulated OPN in human OA cartilage with respect to NO production, by adding anti-OPN antiserum. Addition of anti-OPN antiserum (but not normal murine serum) significantly augmented the spontaneous production of NO in human OA cartilage (Figure 3). These results further confirm the role of endogenous (intra-articular) OPN in chondrocyte function.

Regulation of PGE_2 production by OPN. We have previously reported superinduction of COX-2 and spontaneous production of PGE_2 (under ex vivo conditions) in human OA cartilage. Competitive NOS inhibitors, such as N^G-monomethyl-L-arginine monoacetate (L-NMMA), augment production of PGE_2 in human OA cartilage (2). In view of these observations, we assumed that the inhibition of NO production by endog-

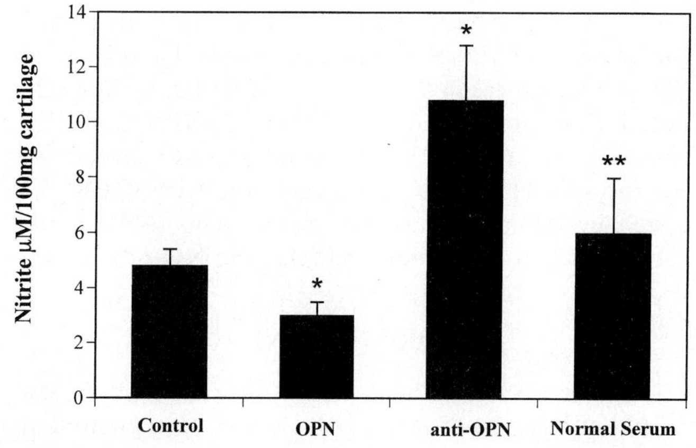

Figure 3. Regulation of nitric oxide in human osteoarthritis (OA)–affected cartilage by osteopontin (OPN) and anti-OPN antiserum. OA-affected knee cartilage was incubated in 2 ml Ham's F-12 medium in the presence of 1 μg/ml OPN or 1:500-diluted anti-OPN antiserum (and normal mouse serum), in triplicate. Values are the mean and SD amounts of nitrite released (μM/100 mg cartilage) (n = 3) at the end of the 72 hours. Results are representative of 2 similar experiments. * = $P \leq 0.01$ versus control; ** = $P \leq 0.5$ versus control.

Table 1. Effect of OPN on spontaneous and IL-1–induced NO and PGE_2 production in human OA*

	Experiment 1		Experiment 2		Experiment 3		Experiment 4		Experiment 5	
	Nitrite	PGE_2	Nitrite	PGE_2	Nitrite	PGE_2	Nitrite	PGE_2	Nitrite	PGE_2
Uninduced	4.2 ± 0.6	56.7 ± 2.7	18.5 ± 3.2	39.9 ± 2.0	8.0 ± 2.1	38.2 ± 1.7	2.1 ± 1.0	16.9 ± 0.9	<0.1	ND
+OPN (1 μg/ml)	0.3 ± 0.1†	8.0 ± 1.0†	9.6 ± 4.6‡	13.6 ± 2.5	3.2 ± 2.2†	2.5 ± 0.2†	0.4 ± 0.01‡	9.6 ± 0.5‡	ND	ND
+IL-1β (1 ng/ml)	17.1 ± 5.8	78.3 ± 4.6	22.1 ± 4.3	155.5 ± 12.0	26.8 ± 8.4	108.1 ± 14.0	14.1 ± 3.6	119.4 ± 1.5	4.1 ± 0.2	ND
+IL-1β + OPN	17.0 ± 3.4	11.8 ± 0.3§	28.7 ± 3.5	169.4 ± 7.9	20.9 ± 3.1¶	41.7 ± 1.2§	9.5 ± 2.0§	102.7 ± 3.5¶	1.4 ± 0.4§	ND

* Osteoarthritis (OA) cartilage from 5 different patients (experiments 1–5) was incubated in organ cultures in 2 ml Ham's F-12 medium with 0.1% human serum albumin for 3 days. Levels of nitric oxide (NO) (measured as nitrite, μM/100 mg cartilage) and prostaglandin E_2 (PGE_2; ng/ml/100 mg cartilage) were determined at the end of 72 hours. In experiments 1 and 2, osteopontin (OPN) and interleukin-1β (IL-1β) were added simultaneously, whereas in experiments 3–5, cultures were preincubated with OPN for 2 hours before addition of IL-1β. Data are expressed as the mean ± SD nitrite and PGE_2 accumulated (n = 3). ND = not done.
† $P \leq 0.001$ versus uninduced cultures.
‡ $P \leq 0.01$ versus uninduced cultures.
§ $P \leq 0.001$ versus cultures treated with IL-1 alone.
¶ $P \leq 0.01$ versus cultures treated with IL-1 alone.

enous OPN may cause up-regulation of PGE_2 production. We therefore tested the effect of recombinant OPN on NO and PGE_2 production. Table 1 shows that spontaneous production of NO and that of PGE_2 were both significantly inhibited by OPN in human OA cartilage. These results suggest that OPN (unlike L-NMMA) may not directly inhibit NOS activity, but may be inhibiting an "upstream" stimulus common to both NO and PGE_2 in cartilage.

Since spontaneous production of NO and PGE_2 is known to be induced in an autocrine manner by IL-1 in OA cartilage (4), we examined the influence of OPN on IL-1–induced production of those inflammation mediators in OA cartilage organ cultures. The addition of IL-1β augmented NO and PGE_2 production in OA cartilage, as shown in Table 1. OPN (1 μg/ml) significantly inhibited the production of both NO and PGE_2 in the organ cultures in the presence of IL-1β. It should be noted that simultaneous addition of OPN and IL-1 (experiments 1 and 2) did not inhibit NO production significantly. However, preincubation with OPN followed by addition of IL-1β (experiments 3–5) significantly blocked IL-1–induced PGE_2 and NO production.

DISCUSSION

The results of the present study demonstrate that 1) FN mRNA and OPN mRNA are up-regulated in human OA cartilage, 2) OPN production by chondrocytes inhibits both NO and PGE_2 production, and 3) preincubation with OPN inhibits IL-1β–induced NO and PGE_2 production in human OA-affected cartilage.

FN has previously been reported to be up-regulated in advanced rheumatoid arthritis and OA cartilage, synovial tissue, and synovial fluid (34). Our studies confirm these observations with regard to OA cartilage. The up-regulation of FN in cartilage is of enormous significance because proteolytic fragments of FN and recombinant proteins representing the EDA region of FN have also been reported to have proinflammatory activity and to promote cartilage chondrolysis in vitro (12,14).

OPN is secreted by various cell types, including activated T cells, macrophages, osteoblasts, and chondrocytes (35). Expression of OPN during chondrocyte maturation is one of the key events involved in cartilage-to-bone transitions in fracture repair (36). In embryonic growth plates, OPN was shown to be expressed in bone-forming cells and hypertrophic chondrocytes (37). In this study, we demonstrated that OPN, which is one of the hypertrophic chondrocyte-specific markers, is over-expressed in OA cartilage versus normal cartilage. These findings suggest that human OA chondrocytes express differentiation markers that resemble those identified in the epithelial growth plate chondrocytes (37). Additionally, OPN in the cartilage matrix inhibits PGE_2 synthesis. It is tempting to speculate that PGE_2 may be involved in chondrocyte differentiation, as observed in bone cells (38).

In distinction to FN fragments, which bind to α5β1 integrin and thereby up-regulate production of inflammation mediators (33), our data indicate that OPN is an endogenous inhibitor of the production of inflammation mediators in cartilage. FN and OPN may have opposing effects on the regulation of inflammatory mediators. This is similar to findings in several inflammatory conditions in which both pro- and antiinflammatory mediators are induced simultaneously (e.g., IL-1 and IL-1 receptor antagonist/IL-1 receptor II) (39). This hypothesis was further strengthened by our recent observation that specific monoclonal antibodies to FN and OPN receptors $\alpha 5\beta 1$ or $\alpha v\beta 3$ mimic the agonist functions of FN fragments and OPN, respectively, in what appears to be a yin/yang regulation of chondrocyte function via integrin signaling pathways (17). One of these monoclonal antibodies (LM609), which competitively inhibits the binding of OPN (17,40) to $\alpha v\beta 3$ (antagonist) and simultaneously mimics the function of OPN (agonist) (17) with respect to inhibition of inflammation mediators, may have therapeutic potential in some forms of arthritis, including OA. Several observations suggest that chondrocytes are the main sources of inflammatory mediators in OA joints (3,5,6), and this inflammatory response may be regulated in situ by abnormally expressed ECM proteins, including FN (41) and OPN.

In summary, the results of these studies further strengthen the hypothesis that the specific induction and repression of chondrocyte gene expression in OA has the potential to modify the course of disease progression. In particular, our findings suggest that differentially expressed ECM proteins in the pericellular environment surrounding the chondrocyte (chondron) act via a complex array of cell surface receptors on chondrocytes to regulate cartilage homeostasis.

Addendum. While this manuscript was in review, 2 articles that also describe the differential expression and regulation of OPN in OA were published (42,43).

ACKNOWLEDGMENTS

We thank Una Yearwood and Andrea L. Barrett for preparation of the manuscript. Some of the normal cartilage samples were provided by NDRI (Philadelphia, PA).

REFERENCES

1. Amin AR, di Cesare P, Vyas P, Attur MG, Tzeng E, Billiar TR, et al. The expression and regulation of nitric oxide synthase in human osteoarthritis-affected chondrocytes: evidence for up-regulated neuronal nitric oxide synthase. J Exp Med 1995;182:2097–102.
2. Amin AR, Attur MG, Patel RN, Thakker GD, Marshall PJ, Rediske J, et al. Superinduction of cyclooxygenase-2 activity in human osteoarthritis-affected cartilage: influence of nitric oxide. J Clin Invest 1997;99:1231–7.
3. Amin AR, Attur MG, Abramson SB. Regulation of nitric oxide and inflammatory mediators in human osteoarthritis-affected cartilage: implication for pharmacological intervention. In: Rubanyi GM, editor. The pathophysiology & clinical applications of nitric oxide. Newark (NJ): Harwood Academic Publishers; 1999. p. 397–413.
4. Attur MG, Patel IR, Patel RN, Abramson SB, Amin AR. Autocrine production of IL-1β by human osteoarthritis-affected cartilage and differential regulation of endogenous nitric oxide, IL-6, prostaglandin E_2 and IL-8. Proc Assoc Am Physicians 1998;110: 1–8.
5. Amin AR, Abramson SB. The role of nitric oxide in articular cartilage breakdown in osteoarthritis. Curr Opin Rheumatol 1998; 10:263–8.
6. Melchiorri C, Meliconi R, Frizziero L, Silvestri T, Pulsatelli L, Mazzetti I, et al. Enhanced and coordinated in vivo expression of inflammatory cytokines and nitric oxide synthase by chondrocytes from patients with osteoarthritis. Arthritis Rheum 1998;41: 2165–74.
7. Moos V, Fickert S, Muller B, Weber U, Sieper J, Bloom L, et al. Immunohistological analysis of cytokine expression in human osteoarthritic and healthy cartilage. J Rheumatol 1999;26:870–9.
8. Pelletier JP, Jovanovic D, Fernandes JC, Manning P, Connor JR, Currie MG, et al. Reduced progression of experimental osteoarthritis in vivo by selective inhibition of inducible nitric oxide synthase. Arthritis Rheum 1998;41:1275–86.
9. Amin AR, Dave MN, Attur MG, Abramson SB. COX-2, NO and cartilage damage and repair. Curr Rheumatol Rep 2000;2:447–53.
10. Heinegard D, Oldberg A. Structure and biology of cartilage and bone matrix noncollagenous macromolecules. FASEB J 1989;3: 2042–51.
11. Aplin AE, Howe A, Alahari SK, Juliano RL. Signal transduction and signal modulation by cell adhesion receptors: the role of integrins, cadherins, immunoglobulin-cell adhesion molecules, and selectins. Pharmacol Rev 1998;50:197–263.
12. Homandberg GA, Hui F, Wen C, Purple C, Bewsey K, Koepp H, et al. Fibronectin-fragment-induced cartilage chondrolysis is associated with release of catabolic cytokines. Biochem J 1997;321: 751–7.
13. Homandberg GA, Wen C, Hui F. Cartilage damaging activities of fibronectin fragments derived from cartilage and synovial fluid. Osteoarthritis Cartilage 1998;6:231–44.
14. Saito S, Yamaji N, Yasunaga K, Saito T, Matsumoto S, Katoh M, et al. The fibronectin extra domain A activates matrix metalloproteinase gene expression by an interleukin-1-dependent mechanism. J Biol Chem 1999;274:30756–63.
15. Tavella S, Bellese G, Castagnola P, Martin I, Piccini D, Doliana R, et al. Regulated expression of fibronectin, laminin and related integrin receptors during the early chondrocyte differentiation. J Cell Sci 1997;110:2261–70.
16. Arner EC, Tortorella MD. Signal transduction through chondrocyte integrin receptors induces matrix metalloproteinase synthesis and synergizes with interleukin-1. Arthritis Rheum 1995;38: 1304–14.
17. Attur MG, Dave MN, Clancy RM, Patel IR, Abramson SB, Amin AR. Functional genomic analysis in arthritis-affected cartilage: yin-yang regulation of inflammatory mediators by $\alpha_5\beta_1$ and $\alpha_v\beta_3$ integrins. J Immunol 2000;164:2684–91.
18. Weber GF, Ashkar S, Glimcher MJ, Cantor H. Receptor-ligand interaction between CD44 and osteopontin (Eta-1). Science 1996; 271:509–12.
19. Margerie D, Flechtenmacher J, Buttner FH, Karbowski A, Puhl W, Schleyerbach R, et al. Complexity of IL-1beta induced gene expression pattern in human articular chondrocytes. Osteoarthritis Cartilage 1997;5:129–38.
20. Fernandes J, Tardif G, Martel-Pelletier J, Lascau-Coman V, Dupuis M, Moldovan F, et al. In vivo transfer of interleukin-1 receptor antagonist gene in osteoarthritic rabbit knee joints: prevention of osteoarthritis progression. Am J Pathol 1999;154: 1159–69.
21. Hu SI, Carozza M, Klein M, Nantermet P, Luk D, Crowl RM. Human HtrA, an evolutionarily conserved serine protease identified as a differentially expressed gene product in osteoarthritic cartilage. J Biol Chem 1998;273:34406–12.
22. Hwang S-M, Lopez CA, Heck DE, Gardner CR, Laskin DL, Laskin JD, et al. Osteopontin inhibits induction of nitric oxide

synthase gene expression by inflammatory mediators in mouse kidney epithelial cells. J Biol Chem 1994;269:711–5.
23. Harlow E, Lane D. Antibodies: a laboratory manual. Cold Spring Harbor (NY): Cold Spring Harbor Laboratory Press; 1988.
24. Declerck PJ, Carmeliet P, Verstreken M, De CF, Collen D. Generation of monoclonal antibodies against autologous proteins in gene-inactivated mice. J Biol Chem 1995;270:8397–400.
25. Zanusso G, Liu D, Ferrari S, Hegyi I, Yin X, Aguzzi A, et al. Prion protein expression in different species: analysis with a panel of new mAbs. Proc Natl Acad Sci U S A 1998;95:8812–6.
26. Feng B, Rollo EE, Denhardt DT. Osteopontin (OPN) may facilitate metastasis by protecting cells from macrophages NO-mediated cytotoxicity: evidence from cell lines down-regulated for OPN expression by a targeted ribozyme. Clin Exp Metastasis 1995;13:453–62.
27. Gilliam MB, Sherman MP, Griscavage JM, Ignarro LJ. A spectrophotometric assay for nitrate using NADPH oxidation by Aspergillus nitrate reductase. Anal Biochem 1993;212:359–65.
28. Patel IR, Attur MG, Patel RN, Stuchin SA, Abagyan RA, Abramson SB, et al. TNF-α convertase from human arthritis-affected cartilage: isolation of cDNA by differential display, expression of the active enzyme, and regulation of TNF-α. J Immunol 1998;160: 4570–9.
29. Liang P, Pardee AB. Differential display of eukaryotic messenger RNA by means of the polymerase chain reaction. Science 1992; 257:967–71.
30. Fujisaki S. A study on development of enzyme immunoassay of human osteopontin: molecular fragility of serum osteopontin. Hokkaido Igaku Zasshi 2000;75:45–52.
31. Johansson S, Svineng G, Wennerberg K, Armulik A, Lohikangas L. Fibronectin-integrin interactions. Front Biosci 1997;2:d126–46.
32. Oates AJ, Barraclough R, Rudland PS. The role of osteopontin in tumorigenesis and metastasis. Invasion Metastasis 1997;17: 1–15.
33. Yonezawa I, Kato K, Yagita H, Yamauchi Y, Okumura K. VLA-5-mediated interaction with fibronectin induces cytokine production by human chondrocytes. Biochem Biophys Res Commun 1996;219:261–5.
34. Dutu A, Vlaicu-Rus V, Bolosiu HD, Parasca I, Cristea A. Fibronectin in plasma and synovial fluid of patients with rheumatic diseases. Med Interne 1986;24:61–8.
35. Denhardt DT, Noda M. Osteopontin expression and function: role in bone remodeling. J Cell Biochem Suppl 1998;30–31:92–102.
36. Nakase T, Sugimoto M, Sato M, Kaneko M, Tomita T, Sugamoto K, et al. Switch of osteonectin and osteopontin mRNA expression in the process of cartilage-to-bone transition during fracture repair. Acta Histochem 1998;100:287–95.
37. McKee MD, Glimcher MJ, Nanci A. High-resolution immunolocalization of osteopontin and osteocalcin in bone and cartilage during endochondral ossification in the chicken tibia. Anat Rec 1992;234:479–92.
38. Kawaguchi H, Pilbeam CC, Harrison JR, Raisz LG. The role of prostaglandins in the regulation of bone metabolism. Clin Orthop 1995;313:36–46.
39. Dinarello CA. Interleukin-1, interleukin-1 receptors and interleukin-1 receptor antagonist. Int Rev Immunol 1998;16:457–99.
40. Miyauchi A, Alvarez J, Greenfield EM, Teti A, Grano M, Colucci S, et al. Binding of osteopontin to the osteoclast integrin $\alpha v \beta 3$. Osteoporos Int 1993;3 Suppl 1:132–5.
41. Homandberg GA. Potential regulation of cartilage metabolism in osteoarthritis by fibronectin fragments. Front Biosci 1999;4: D713–30.
42. Petrow PK, Hummel KM, Schedel J, Franz JK, Klein CL, Müller-Ladner U, et al. Expression of osteopontin messenger RNA and protein in rheumatoid arthritis: effects of osteopontin on the release of collagenase 1 from articular chondrocytes and synovial fibroblasts. Arthritis Rheum 2000;43:1597–1605.
43. Pullig O, Weseloh G, Gauer S, Swoboda B. Osteopontin is expressed by adult human osteoarthritic chondrocytes: protein and mRNA analysis of normal and osteoarthritic cartilage. Matrix Biol 2000;19:245–55.

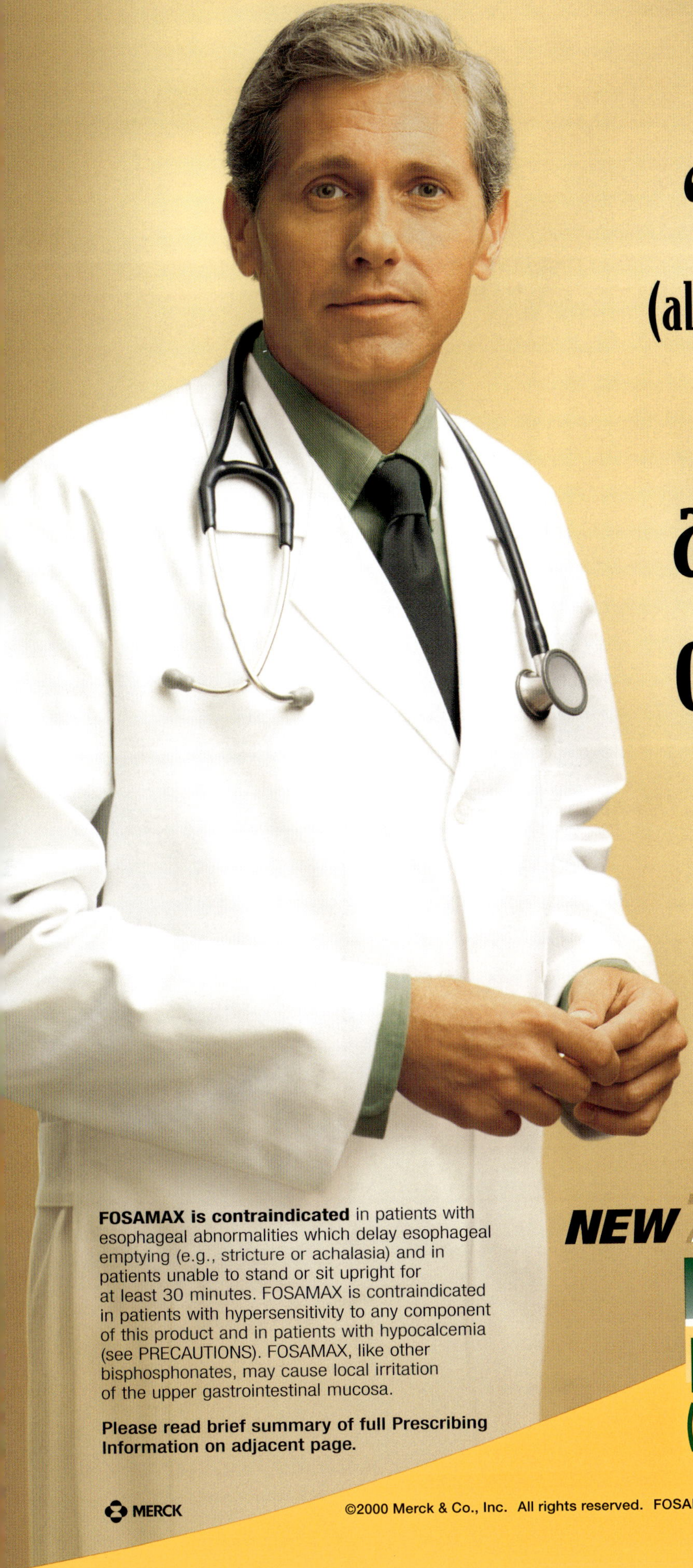

FOSAMAX®(alendronate sodium tablets) BRIEF SUMMARY OF PRESCRIBING INFORMATION

CONTRAINDICATIONS

- Abnormalities of the esophagus which delay esophageal emptying such as stricture or achalasia
- Inability to stand or sit upright for at least 30 minutes
- Hypersensitivity to any component of this product
- Hypocalcemia (see PRECAUTIONS, *General*)

WARNINGS

FOSAMAX, like other bisphosphonates, may cause local irritation of the upper gastrointestinal mucosa. Esophageal adverse experiences, such as esophagitis, esophageal ulcers and esophageal erosions, occasionally with bleeding and rarely followed by esophageal stricture, have been reported in patients receiving treatment with FOSAMAX. In some cases these have been severe and required hospitalization. Physicians should therefore be alert to any signs or symptoms signaling a possible esophageal reaction and patients should be instructed to discontinue FOSAMAX and seek medical attention if they develop dysphagia, odynophagia, retrosternal pain, or new or worsening heartburn. The risk of severe esophageal adverse experiences appears to be greater in patients who lie down after taking FOSAMAX and/or who fail to swallow it with a full glass (6–8 oz) of water, and/or who continue to take FOSAMAX after developing symptoms suggestive of esophageal irritation. Therefore, it is very important that the full dosing instructions are provided to, and understood by, the patient (see DOSAGE AND ADMINISTRATION). In patients who cannot comply with dosing instructions due to mental disability, therapy with FOSAMAX should be used under appropriate supervision. Because of possible irritant effects of FOSAMAX on the upper gastrointestinal mucosa and a potential for worsening of the underlying disease, caution should be used when FOSAMAX is given to patients with active upper gastrointestinal problems (such as dysphagia, esophageal diseases, gastritis, duodenitis, or ulcers). There have been post-marketing reports of gastric and duodenal ulcers, some severe and with complications, although no increased risk was observed in controlled clinical trials.

PRECAUTIONS

General

Causes of osteoporosis other than estrogen deficiency, aging, and glucocorticoid use should be considered. Hypocalcemia must be corrected before initiating therapy with FOSAMAX (see CONTRAINDICATIONS). Other disturbances of mineral metabolism (such as vitamin D deficiency) should also be effectively treated. Presumably due to the effects of FOSAMAX on increasing bone mineral, small, asymptomatic decreases in serum calcium and phosphate may occur, especially in patients with Paget's disease, in whom the pretreatment rate of bone turnover may be greatly elevated and in patients receiving glucocorticoids, in whom calcium absorption may be decreased. Ensuring adequate calcium and vitamin D intake is especially important in patients with Paget's disease of bone and in patients receiving glucocorticoids.

Renal insufficiency

FOSAMAX is not recommended for patients with renal insufficiency (creatinine clearance <35 mL/min). (See DOSAGE AND ADMINISTRATION.)

Glucocorticoid-induced osteoporosis

The risk versus benefit of FOSAMAX for treatment at daily dosages of glucocorticoids less than 7.5 mg of prednisone or equivalent has not been established (see INDICATIONS AND USAGE). Before initiating treatment, the hormonal status of both men and women should be ascertained and appropriate replacement considered. A bone mineral density measurement should be made at the initiation of therapy and repeated after 6 to 12 months of combined FOSAMAX and glucocorticoid treatment. The efficacy of FOSAMAX for the treatment of glucocorticoid-induced osteoporosis has been shown in patients with a median bone mineral density which was 1.2 standard deviations below the mean for healthy young adults. The efficacy of FOSAMAX has been established in studies of two years' duration. The greatest increase in bone mineral density occurred in the first year with maintenance or smaller gains during the second year. Efficacy of FOSAMAX beyond two years has not been studied. The efficacy of FOSAMAX in respect to fracture prevention has been demonstrated for vertebral fractures. However, this finding was based on very few fractures that occurred primarily in postmenopausal women. The efficacy for prevention of non-vertebral fractures has not been demonstrated.

Information for Patients

General

Physicians should instruct their patients to read the patient package insert before starting therapy with FOSAMAX and to reread it each time the prescription is renewed. Patients should be instructed to take supplemental calcium and vitamin D, if daily dietary intake is inadequate. Weight-bearing exercise should be considered along with the modification of certain behavioral factors, such as cigarette smoking and/or excessive alcohol consumption, if these factors exist.

Dosing Instructions

Patients should be instructed that the expected benefits of FOSAMAX may only be obtained when each tablet is swallowed with plain water the first thing upon arising for the day at least 30 minutes before the first food, beverage, or medication of the day. Even dosing with orange juice or coffee has been shown to markedly reduce the absorption of FOSAMAX (see CLINICAL PHARMACOLOGY, *Pharmacokinetics, Absorption*). To facilitate delivery to the stomach and thus reduce the potential for esophageal irritation patients should be instructed to swallow FOSAMAX with a full glass of water (6–8 oz) and not to lie down for at least 30 minutes and until after their first food of the day. Patients should not chew or suck on the tablet because of a potential for oropharyngeal ulceration. Patients should be specifically instructed not to take FOSAMAX at bedtime or before arising for the day. Patients should be informed that failure to follow these instructions may increase their risk of esophageal problems. Patients should be instructed that if they develop symptoms of esophageal disease (such as difficulty or pain upon swallowing, retrosternal pain or new or worsening heartburn) they should stop taking FOSAMAX and consult their physician. Patients should be instructed that if they miss a dose of once weekly FOSAMAX, they should take one tablet on the morning after they remember. They should not take two tablets on the same day but should return to taking one tablet once a week, as originally scheduled on their chosen day.

Drug Interactions (also see CLINICAL PHARMACOLOGY, *Pharmacokinetics, Drug Interactions*)

Estrogen/hormone replacement therapy (HRT)

Concomitant use of HRT (estrogen ± progestin) and FOSAMAX was assessed in two clinical studies of one or two years' duration in postmenopausal osteoporotic women. In these studies, the safety and tolerability profile of the combination was consistent with those of the individual treatments; however, the degree of suppression of bone turnover (as assessed by mineralizing surface) was significantly greater with the combination than with either component alone. The long-term effects of combined FOSAMAX and HRT on fracture occurrence have not been studied (see CLINICAL PHARMACOLOGY, *Clinical Studies, Concomitant use with estrogen/hormone replacement therapy (HRT)* and ADVERSE REACTIONS, *Clinical Studies, Concomitant use with estrogen/hormone replacement therapy*).

Calcium Supplements/Antacids

It is likely that calcium supplements, antacids, and some oral medications will interfere with absorption of FOSAMAX. Therefore, patients must wait at least one-half hour after taking FOSAMAX before taking any other oral medications.

Aspirin

In clinical studies, the incidence of upper gastrointestinal adverse events was increased in patients receiving concomitant therapy with daily doses of FOSAMAX greater than 10 mg and aspirin-containing products.

Nonsteroidal Anti-inflammatory Drugs (NSAIDs)

FOSAMAX may be administered to patients taking NSAIDs. In a 3-year, controlled, clinical study (n=2027) during which a majority of patients received concomitant NSAIDs, the incidence of upper gastrointestinal adverse events was similar in patients taking FOSAMAX 5 or 10 mg/day compared to those taking placebo. However, since NSAID use is associated with gastrointestinal irritation, caution should be used during concomitant use with FOSAMAX.

Pregnancy

Pregnancy Category C:

Reproduction studies in rats showed decreased postimplantation survival at 2 mg/kg/day and decreased body weight gain in normal pups at 1 mg/kg/day. Sites of incomplete fetal ossification were statistically significantly increased in rats beginning at 10 mg/kg/day in vertebral (cervical, thoracic, and lumbar), skull, and sternebral bones. The above doses ranged from 0.26 times (1 mg/kg) to 2.6 times (10 mg/kg) a maximum recommended daily dose of 40 mg (Paget's disease) based on surface area, mg/m^2. No similar fetal effects were seen when pregnant rabbits were treated at doses up to 35 mg/kg/day (10.3 times a 40 mg human daily dose based on surface area, mg/m^2). Both total and ionized calcium decreased in pregnant rats at 15 mg/kg/day (3.9 times the 40 human daily dose based on surface area, mg/m^2) resulting in delays and failures of delivery. Protracted parturition due to maternal hypocalcemia occurred in rats at doses as low as 0.5 mg/kg/day (0.13 times a 40 mg human daily dose based on surface area, mg/m^2) when rats were treated from before mating through gestation. Maternotoxicity (late pregnancy deaths) occurred in the female rats treated with 15 mg/kg/day for varying periods of time ranging from treatment only during pre-mating to treatment only during early, middle, or late gestation; these deaths were lessened but not eliminated by cessation of treatment. Calcium supplementation either in the drinking water or by minipump could not ameliorate the hypocalcemia or prevent maternal and neonatal deaths due to delays in delivery; calcium supplementation IV prevented maternal, but not fetal deaths. There are no studies in pregnant women. FOSAMAX should be used during pregnancy only if the potential benefit justifies the potential risk to the mother and fetus.

Nursing Mothers

It is not known whether alendronate is excreted in human milk. Because many drugs are excreted in human milk, caution should be exercised when FOSAMAX is administered to nursing women.

Pediatric Use

Safety and effectiveness in pediatric patients have not been established.

Use in the Elderly

Of the patients receiving FOSAMAX in the United States and Multinational osteoporosis treatment studies in women, the osteoporosis study in men, glucocorticoid-induced osteoporosis studies, and Paget's disease studies (see CLINICAL PHARMACOLOGY, *Clinical Studies*), 45%, 50%, 37%, and 70%, respectively, were 65 years of age or over. No overall differences in efficacy or safety were observed between these patients and younger patients but greater sensitivity of some older individuals cannot be ruled out.

ADVERSE REACTIONS

Clinical Studies

In clinical studies of up to five years in duration adverse experiences associated with FOSAMAX usually were mild, and generally did not require discontinuation of therapy. FOSAMAX has been evaluated for safety in approximately 8000 postmenopausal women in clinical studies.

Treatment of osteoporosis

Postmenopausal women

In two identically designed, three-year, placebo-controlled, double-blind, multicenter studies (United States and Multinational; n=994), discontinuation of therapy due to any clinical adverse experience occurred in 4.1% of 196 patients treated with FOSAMAX 10 mg/day and 6.0% of 397 patients treated with placebo. In the Fracture Intervention Trial (n=6459), discontinuation of therapy due to any clinical adverse experience occurred in 9.1% of 3236 patients treated with FOSAMAX 5 mg/day for 2 years and 10 mg/day for either one or two additional years and 10.1% of 3223 patients treated with placebo. Discontinuations due to upper gastrointestinal adverse experiences were: FOSAMAX, 3.2%; placebo, 2.7%. In these study populations, 49-54% had a history of gastrointestinal disorders at baseline and 54-89% used nonsteroidal anti-inflammatory drugs or aspirin at some time during the studies. Adverse experiences from these studies considered by the investigators as possibly, probably, or definitely drug related in ≥1% of patients treated with either FOSAMAX or placebo are presented in the following table.

Osteoporosis Treatment Studies in Postmenopausal Women–Adverse Experiences Considered Possibly, Probably, or Definitely Drug Related by the Investigators and Reported in ≥1% of Patients

	United States/Multinational Studies		Fracture Intervention Trial	
	FOSAMAX* % (n=196)	Placebo % (n=397)	FOSAMAX** % (n=3236)	Placebo % (n=3223)
Gastrointestinal				
abdominal pain	6.6	4.8	1.5	1.5
nausea	3.6	4.0	1.1	1.5
dyspepsia	3.6	3.5	1.1	1.2
constipation	3.1	1.8	0.0	0.2
diarrhea	3.1	1.8	0.6	0.3
flatulence	2.6	0.5	0.2	0.3
acid regurgitation	2.0	4.3	1.1	0.9
esophageal ulcer	1.5	0.0	0.1	0.1
vomiting	1.0	1.5	0.2	0.3
dysphagia	1.0	0.0	0.1	0.1
abdominal distension	1.0	0.8	0.0	0.0
gastritis	0.5	1.3	0.6	0.7
Musculoskeletal				
musculoskeletal (bone, muscle or joint) pain	4.1	2.5	0.4	0.3
muscle cramp	0.0	1.0	0.2	0.1
Nervous System/Psychiatric				
headache	2.6	1.5	0.2	0.2
dizziness	0.0	1.0	0.0	0.1
Special Senses				
taste perversion	0.5	1.0	0.1	0.0

*10 mg/day for three years **5 mg/day for 2 years and 10 mg/day for either 1 or 2 additional years

Rarely, rash and erythema have occurred.

One patient treated with FOSAMAX (10 mg/day) who had a history of peptic ulcer disease and gastrectomy and who was taking concomitant aspirin developed an anastomotic ulcer with mild hemorrhage, which was considered drug related. Aspirin and FOSAMAX were discontinued and the patient recovered.

The adverse experience profile was similar for the 401 patients treated with either 5 or 20 mg doses of FOSAMAX in the United States and Multinational studies. The adverse experience profile for the 296 patients who received continued treatment with either 5 or 10 mg doses of FOSAMAX in the two-year extension of these studies (treatment years 4 and 5) was similar to that observed during the three-year placebo-controlled period. During the extension period, of the 151 patients treated with FOSAMAX 10 mg/day, the proportion of patients who discontinued therapy due to any clinical adverse experience was similar to that during the first three years of the study.

In a one-year, double-blind multicenter study, the overall safety and tolerability profiles of once weekly FOSAMAX 70 mg and FOSAMAX 10 mg daily were similar. The adverse experiences were considered by investigators as possibly, probably, or definitely drug related in ≥1% of patients treated with either FOSAMAX 70 mg once weekly (n=519), or FOSAMAX 10 mg daily (n=370), respectively, were: *Gastrointestinal*: abdominal pain (3.7%; 3.0%), dyspepsia (2.7%; 2.2%), acid regurgitation (1.9%; 2.4%), nausea (1.9%; 2.4%), abdominal distension (1.0%; 1.4%), constipation (0.8%; 1.6%), flatulence (0.4%; 1.6%), gastritis (0.2%; 1.1%), gastric ulcer (0.0%; 1.1%); *Musculoskeletal:* musculoskeletal (bone, muscle, joint) pain (2.9%; 3.2%), muscle cramp (0.2%; 1.1%).

Men

In a two-year, placebo-controlled, double-blind multicenter study, discontinuation of therapy due to any clinical adverse experience occurred in 2.7% of men treated with FOSAMAX 10 mg/day and 10.5% of men treated with placebo. The adverse experiences considered by investigators as possibly, probably, or definitely drug related in ≥2% of patients treated with either FOSAMAX 10 mg/day (n=146), or placebo (n=95), respectively, were: *Gastrointestinal:* acid regurgitation (4.1%; 3.2%), flatulence (4.1%; 1.1%), dyspepsia (3.4%; 0.0%), abdominal pain (2.1%; 1.1%), nausea (2.1%; 0.0%).

Prevention of osteoporosis in postmenopausal women

The safety of FOSAMAX 5 mg/day in postmenopausal women 40-60 years of age has been evaluated in three double-blind, placebo-controlled studies involving over 1,400 patients randomized to receive FOSAMAX for either two or three years. In these studies the overall safety profiles of FOSAMAX 5 mg/day and placebo were similar. Discontinuation of therapy due to any clinical adverse experience occurred in 7.5% of 642 patients treated with FOSAMAX 5 mg/day and 5.7% of 648 patients treated with placebo.

In a one-year, double-blind multicenter study, the overall safety and tolerability profiles of once weekly FOSAMAX 35 mg and FOSAMAX 5 mg daily were similar.

The adverse experiences from these studies considered by the investigators as possibly, probably, or definitely drug related in ≥1% of patients treated with either once weekly FOSAMAX 35 mg, FOSAMAX 5mg/day or placebo are presented in the following table.

Osteoporosis Prevention Studies in Postmenopausal Women–Adverse Experiences Considered Possibly, Probably, or Definitely Drug Related by the Investigators and Reported in ≥1% of Patients

	Two/Three-Year Studies		One-Year Study	
	FOSAMAX 5 mg/day % (n=642)	Placebo % (n=648)	FOSAMAX 5 mg/day % (n=361)	Once-Weekly FOSAMAX 35 mg % (n=362)
Gastrointestinal				
dyspepsia	1.9	1.4	2.2	1.7
abdominal pain	1.7	3.4	4.2	2.2
acid regurgitation	1.4	2.5	4.2	4.7
nausea	1.4	1.4	2.5	1.4
diarrhea	1.1	1.7	1.1	0.6
constipation	0.9	0.5	1.7	0.3
abdominal distension	0.2	0.3	1.4	1.1
Musculoskeletal				
musculoskeletal (bone, muscle or joint) pain	0.8	0.9	1.9	2.2

Concomitant use with estrogen/hormone replacement therapy

In two studies (of one and two years' duration) of postmenopausal osteoporotic women (total: n=853), the safety and tolerability profile of combined treatment with FOSAMAX 10 mg once daily and estrogen ± progestin (n=354) was consistent with those of the individual treatments.

Treatments of glucocorticoid-induced osteoporosis

In two one-year, placebo-controlled, double-blind multicenter studies, in patients receiving glucocorticoid treatment, the overall safety and tolerability profiles of FOSAMAX 5 and 10 mg/day were generally similar to that of placebo. The adverse experiences considered by the investigators as possibly, probably, or definitely drug related in ≥1% of patients treated with either FOSAMAX 10 mg/day (n=157), FOSAMAX 5 mg/day (n=161), or placebo (n=159), respectively, were: *Gastrointestinal:* abdominal pain (3.2%; 1.9%; 0.0%), acid regurgitation (2.5%; 1.9%; 1.3%), constipation (1.3%; 0.6%; 0.0%), melena (1.3%; 0.0%; 0.0%), nausea (0.6%; 1.2%; 0.6%), diarrhea (0.0%; 0.0%; 1.3%), *Nervous System/Psychiatric*: headache (0.6%; 0.0%; 1.3%).

The overall safety and tolerability profile in the glucocorticoid-induced osteoporosis population that continued therapy for the second year of the studies (FOSAMAX: n=147) was consistent with that observed in the first year.

Paget's disease of bone

In clinical studies (osteoporosis and Paget's disease), adverse experiences reported in 175 patients taking FOSAMAX 40 mg/day for 3-12 months were similar to those in postmenopausal women treated with FOSAMAX 10 mg/day. However, there was an apparent increased incidence of upper gastrointestinal adverse experiences in patients taking FOSAMAX 40 mg/day (17.7% FOSAMAX vs. 10.2% placebo). One case of esophagitis and two cases of gastritis resulted in discontinuation of treatment. Additionally, musculoskeletal (bone, muscle, or joint) pain, which has been described in patients with Paget's disease treated with other bisphosphonates, was considered by the investigators as possibly, probably, or definitely drug related in approximately 6% of patients treated with FOSAMAX 40 mg/day vs. approximately 1% of patients treated with placebo, but rarely resulted in discontinuation of therapy. Discontinuation of therapy due to any clinical adverse experience occurred in 6.4% of patients with Paget's disease treated with FOSAMAX 40 mg/day and 2.4% of patients treated with placebo.

Laboratory Test Findings

In double-blind, multicenter, controlled studies, asymptomatic, mild, and transient decreases in serum calcium and phosphate were observed in approximately 18% and 10%, respectively, of patients taking FOSAMAX versus approximately 12% and 3% of those taking placebo. However, the incidences of decreases in serum calcium to <8.0 mg/dL (2.0 mM) and serum phosphate to ≤2.0 mg/dL (0.65 mM) were similar in both treatment groups.

Post-Marketing Experience

The following adverse reactions have been reported in post-marketing use: *Body as a Whole*: hypersensitivity reactions including urticaria and rarely angioedema. *Gastrointestinal:* esophagitis, esophageal erosions, esophageal ulcers, rarely esophageal stricture, and oropharyngeal ulceration. Gastric or duodenal ulcers, some severe and with complications have also been reported (see WARNINGS, PRECAUTIONS, and *Information for Patients*, and DOSAGE AND ADMINISTRATION). *Skin:* rash (occasionally with photosensitivity). *Special Senses:* rarely uveitis.

For more detailed information, consult your Merck representative or see the full Prescribing Information.

MERCK

007129(1)(017)-FOS Printed in USA Minimum 10% Recycled Paper

ARTHRITIS & RHEUMATISM
Vol. 44, No. 3, March 2001, pp 585–594

Matrix Metalloproteinase and Proinflammatory Cytokine Production by Chondrocytes of Human Osteoarthritic Cartilage

Associations With Degenerative Changes

Lynne C. Tetlow, Daman J. Adlam, and David E. Woolley

Objective. **To examine by immunohistochemistry the relative distributions of 6 matrix metalloproteinases (MMPs 1, 2, 3, 8, 9, and 13) and the 2 proinflammatory cytokines interleukin-1β (IL-1β) and tumor necrosis factor α (TNFα) in osteoarthritic (OA) cartilage compared with normal, age-matched articular cartilage.**

Methods. **Articular cartilage samples were obtained from the tibial plateau of OA knees removed at arthroplasty and from normal, nonarthritic, knees obtained at autopsy. Specimens were promptly fixed in Carnoy's fixative, processed, embedded in paraffin, sectioned, and examined by immunohistochemistry for MMP and cytokine production. In addition, human articular chondrocytes (HAC) were treated in vitro with either IL-1β, TNFα, or phorbol myristate acetate (PMA) to assess their potential to produce each of the MMPs, as determined by Western blotting and gelatin zymography.**

Results. **Immunodetection of the collagenases (MMPs 1, 8, and 13) and stromelysin 1 (MMP-3) was demonstrated in a proportion of chondrocytes in the superficial zone of almost all of the OA specimens that had degenerative matrix changes. The gelatinases (MMPs 2 and 9) were also demonstrated by immunohistochemistry but were not so prominent. IL-1β– and TNFα-positive chondrocytes were also observed in a proportion of cells in the superficial zones of OA specimens. Much less immunostaining for MMPs and cytokines was observed in the deep zone of all OA specimens, where the cartilage matrix and chondrocyte morphology appeared normal. In contrast, full-thickness normal cartilage specimens showed virtually no immunostaining for these MMPs or cytokines. Confirmation that chondrocytes can produce these 6 MMPs was obtained from HAC cultures treated with either IL-1β, TNFα, or PMA; conditioned medium from *activated* HAC contained all the MMPs demonstrated by immunohistochemistry. Dual immunolocalization studies of OA cartilage specimens demonstrated the coexpression of IL-1 with MMP-8 by individual chondrocytes in situ.**

Conclusion. **These results indicate that the superficial zone of OA cartilage specimens, which is characterized by fibrillations, chondrocyte clusters, and degenerative matrix changes, contains a variable proportion of cells that immunostain for IL-1β, TNFα, and 6 different MMPs. These observations support the concept that cytokine–MMP associations reflect a modified chondrocyte phenotype and an intrinsic process of cartilage degradation in OA.**

Osteoarthritis (OA) is the most prevalent disease of articular joints and is the major cause of disability in the elderly (1). Degeneration and loss of articular cartilage are characteristic features of OA. The appearance of fibrillations, matrix depletion, cell clusters, and changes in matrix composition reflect the aberrant behavior of resident chondrocytes (2). Although biomechanical factors are strongly implicated, at present it is unclear which stimuli regulate the hyperactive pheno-

Supported by the Arthritis Research Campaign and the Teaching Company Scheme: Biogenesis Ltd., Poole, UK.

Lynne C. Tetlow, BSc, PhD, Daman J. Adlam, BSc, MSc, David E. Woolley, PhD, DSc: The University of Manchester, Manchester, UK.

Address correspondence and reprint requests to Lynne C. Tetlow, BSc, PhD, University Department of Medicine, Manchester Royal Infirmary, Oxford Road, Manchester M13 9WL, UK.

Submitted for publication June 26, 2000; accepted in revised form October 13, 2000.

type of OA chondrocytes, including their ability to express cartilage-degrading proteinases.

The matrix metalloproteinases (MMPs) are considered important for the chondrolytic processes that contribute to the degenerative changes in OA cartilage (3–5). Recent studies have identified the messenger RNA (mRNA) for some MMPs, such as MMP-1, MMP-3, MMP-9, and MMP-13, in human OA cartilage (5,6), and others have reported specific MMP proteins and collagenase-mediated type II collagen degradation products (7–9). There is now a consensus that these enzymes contribute to intrinsic chondrocyte-mediated degenerative changes of the cartilage matrix in OA, but as yet, the relative importance of each proteinase and the factors responsible for their expression remain uncertain.

Many factors are implicated in the complex regulation of MMP production by chondrocytes, including their response to proinflammatory cytokines, such as interleukin-1 (IL-1) or tumor necrosis factor (TNF) (6,10–13). There is much evidence from animal and in vitro studies to support the role of MMPs in cartilage damage (14–16), but direct evidence of their relative expressions and MMP-inducing cytokines in human OA cartilage remains unresolved.

Herein we report the comparative immunohistochemical distributions of 6 MMPs, the collagenases 1, 2, and 3 (MMPs 1, 8, and 13, respectively), the gelatinases A and B (MMPs 2 and 9, respectively), and stromelysin 1 (MMP-3), together with those for IL-1β and TNFα, in specimens of articular cartilage from the tibial plateau of OA knees representing 3 grades of clinical severity and compare the findings with those in samples of age-matched normal cartilage. In vitro experiments have demonstrated the potential of human articular chondrocytes to elaborate each of these MMPs in response to stimulation by IL-1β, TNFα, or phorbol myristate acetate (PMA). In addition, we demonstrate the dual production of a specific cytokine and MMP by the same chondrocytes in situ, especially in locations showing severe degenerative changes.

PATIENTS AND METHODS

Tissue specimens and histologic assessment. Tissues from OA knees (n = 34) removed at the time of joint replacement surgery were placed in Hanks' balanced salt solution (HBSS) and transferred to the laboratory, where specimens of cartilage were sampled from the tibial plateau within 60 minutes of operation. Age-matched normal cartilage samples from subjects who had no history of arthritis were obtained from early autopsy cases (n = 6) and were processed in parallel with the OA cartilage specimens for comparative studies.

Table 1. Histologic grading of osteoarthritic changes in human knee cartilage*

Grade	Histologic features (acid toluidine blue staining)
0	Normal matrix and chondrocyte morphology
1	Uneven cartilage surface, with loss of metachromasia around enlarged chondrocytes of the superficial zone; no fibrillations or chondrocyte clusters
2	Some surface erosion; fibrillations and small chondrocyte clusters in the superficial zone; decreased metachromasia extending to the deep zone
3	Deeper surface erosions, with fibrillations extending into the deep zone; large number of chondrocyte clusters containing several cells; major degenerative changes and loss of metachromasia in the cartilage matrix

* Adapted, with permission, from studies described in references 5, 11, and 17.

All cartilage samples were fixed in Carnoy's fixative for 2 hours at 20°C, dehydrated in alcohol, processed, and embedded in paraffin. Cartilage tissue sections (5 μm) from the different specimens were initially stained with acidified toluidine blue to determine histologic grading. Two cartilage zones were identified, as previously defined and illustrated (2,9): one a "superficial zone," which included the upper midzone area beneath the articular surface, and the other a "deep zone," which included the lower midzone. These 2 zones represent approximately 25% and 75%, respectively, of the full cartilage thickness.

Each specimen was examined by 2 independent assessors (LCT and DEW) and graded as 0, 1, 2, or 3 (Table 1) according to a system adapted from previous studies of clinical grading (5,11,17). Seventeen specimens representative of each grade were selected for an immunologic study of MMP and cytokine distributions. The specimens were derived from patients in the age range 49–78 years (mean age 70 years).

Antibodies. Sheep polyclonal antibodies to MMPs 1, 2, 3, 9, and 13 were either prepared in-house or by The Binding Site (Birmingham, UK). Each was checked for monospecificity, including immunoadsorption with purified antigens, as previously described (18,19). Goat polyclonal antibodies to IL-1β and TNFα were purchased from R&D Systems (Abingdon, UK), and mouse monoclonal antibody to MMP-8 was purchased from Calbiochem (Nottingham, UK).

Immunolocalization of MMPs 1, 2, 3, 9, and 13. Tissue sections were first incubated for 30 minutes with 10% (volume/volume) donkey serum in Tris buffered saline (TBS). Sheep polyclonal antibodies to each of the MMPs 1, 2, 3, 9, and 13 were used at predetermined dilutions of 1:500, 1:500, 1:750, 1:500, and 1:1,000, respectively, in TBS and applied to the sections for 2 hours at 20°C; after which the sections were washed 3 times for 10 minutes in TBS. Biotinylated donkey anti-sheep IgG (Sigma, Poole, UK) was diluted 1:300 in TBS and applied to the sections for 45 minutes at 20°C. After further washing, alkaline phosphatase (AP)–conjugated avidin–biotin complex (ABC; Dako, Cambridge, UK) was applied and developed using New Fuchsin. Tissue sections were lightly counterstained with either toluidine blue or Harris' hematoxylin and mounted in Histomount permanent mountant (National Diagnostics, Hull, UK).

Immunolocalization of MMP-8. Tissue sections were preincubated for 30 minutes with 10% (v/v) rabbit serum in TBS followed by incubation for 2 hours at 20°C with mouse monoclonal antibody to MMP-8 (Calbiochem) diluted to 10 μg/ml. After 3 10-minute washes in TBS, sections were incubated with biotinylated rabbit anti-mouse IgG diluted 1:300 in TBS for 45 minutes at 20°C. After further washing, AP-conjugated ABC was diluted as described by the supplier and applied to the sections for 45 minutes at 20°C. After TBS washing, the AP was developed and the sections counterstained.

Immunolocalization of cytokines IL-1β and TNFα. Tissue sections were pretreated with 10% (v/v) normal rabbit serum in TBS for 30 minutes at 20°C. Goat polyclonal antibodies to human IL-1β or TNFα (R&D Systems) were diluted in TBS to give a final IgG concentration of 10 μg/ml and applied to the sections for 2 hours at 20°C. After 3 10-minute washes in TBS, biotinylated rabbit anti-goat IgG (Dako) diluted 1:200 in TBS was applied for 45 minutes at 20°C. After further washing, AP-conjugated ABC was applied for 45 minutes at 20°C and developed with New Fuchsin. Sections were then counterstained and mounted.

Dual immunolocalization of IL-1β and MMP-8. To examine the possible coproduction of IL-1β and MMP-8 by the same chondrocytes, dual localization studies were performed. Tissue sections were immunostained for IL-1β as described above, but substituting fast red for New Fuchsin in the development of the AP. Microscopic fields of the section showing IL-1β–stained chondrocytes were photographed, after which the red stain was removed by washing for ~1 hour in 95% ethanol. Following rehydration in TBS the sections were immunostained for MMP-8 using the antibody described above, but using horseradish peroxidase (HRP)–conjugated rabbit anti-mouse IgG (diluted 1:100; Dako) as the detection system. The HRP was developed using 3, 3′-diaminobenzidine tetrahydrochloride in TBS (Sigma) to give a brown color, indicating the presence of MMP-8. Carefully matched fields were photographed for comparative analysis of IL-1β and MMP-8. Control incubations using nonimmune immunoglobulins were carried out as described above, and were consistently negative.

All tissue sections were photographed using a Zeiss Photomicroscope III (Zeiss, Wetzlar, Germany) and Ektachrome 160T tungsten film (Eastman Kodak, Rochester, NY).

Human articular chondrocytes (HAC). HAC were prepared as previously described (20). Briefly, slices of full-thickness articular cartilage from the nonarthritic joints of subjects undergoing lower limb amputation were diced into ~2-mm^3 fragments and incubated with 10 ml of 1 mg/ml hyaluronidase in HBSS in a shaking water-bath at 37°C for 15 minutes. The liquid was decanted, and 10 ml of 0.25% (weight/volume) trypsin in HBSS was added to the tissue. After 30 minutes, the liquid was decanted, and 10 ml of 5 mg/ml bacterial collagenase in Dulbecco's modified Eagle's medium (DMEM) + 5% (v/v) FCS was added. After overnight incubation in a shaking water-bath at 37°C, the resulting cell suspension was filtered through sterile gauze, flushed through with a further 10 ml of DMEM, and centrifuged at 2,000 revolutions per minute for 10 minutes. The chondrocyte pellet was resuspended in DMEM + 20% FCS and seeded into a 25-cm^2 flask. After 24 hours, the medium was changed, and the chondrocytes were subsequently grown in DMEM + 10% FCS.

Chondrocytes were grown to confluence and, after trypsinization, re-seeded at first passage into 12-well culture dishes. After forming confluent monolayers, triplicate wells were incubated with 1 of the following 4 treatments: DMEM + 0.2% (w/v) lactalbumin hydrolysate (LH); DMEM + 0.2% LH + 0.1 ng/ml of IL-1β; DMEM + 0.2% LH + 20 ng/ml of TNFα; or DMEM + 0.2% LH + 25 ng/ml of PMA. Conditioned medium was harvested after 48 hours and examined for MMPs 1, 3, 8, and 13 by Western blotting, and for MMPs 2 and 9 by gelatin zymography.

Western blotting. Western blotting was carried out as previously described (19). Briefly, samples were separated by sodium dodecyl sulfate–polyacrylamide gel electrophoresis (SDS-PAGE) under dithiothreitol reducing conditions and were electrotransferred to an Immobilon-P membrane (Millipore, Watford, UK). The primary antibodies used were as described for the immunohistochemistry but at 10-fold greater dilutions for MMPs 1, 3, 8, and 13, respectively. HRP-conjugated rabbit anti-sheep and rabbit anti-mouse secondary antibodies (Dako) were diluted 1:1,000 before use, these being developed using the chemiluminescent peroxidase substrate SuperSignal CL (Novagen, Madison, WI) and detected by exposure to Kodak X-Omat film (Sigma).

Gelatin zymography. Samples were separated by SDS-PAGE on 7.5% (w/v) gels, containing gelatin at 1 mg/ml, under nonreducing conditions. The gels were washed twice for 30 minutes each in 2.5% (v/v) Triton X-100 in H_2O and incubated for 16 hours at 37°C in 50 m*M* Tris HCl, pH 7.5, containing 5 m*M* $CaCl_2$, 0.1% (v/v) Triton X-100, and 0.02% (w/v) NaN_3. Gels were stained with Coomassie brilliant blue R250 in 50% methanol and 10% acetic acid solution, and gelatinolytic activity was detected by negative staining. Western blots and gelatin zymograms were scanned using a Bio-Rad GS-700 imaging densitometer (Bio-Rad, Hertfordshire, UK) with molecular analysis software.

RESULTS

The immunodistributions of MMPs 1, 2, 3, 8, 9, and 13 were examined in specimens of OA and nonarthritic, normal cartilage. The specimens provided examples that were representative of OA grades 1, 2, and 3, for comparison with age-matched normal articular cartilage, graded as 0. The 3 collagenases (MMPs 1, 8, and 13) were detected in the superficial zones of almost all OA specimens (Figures 1A, B and C), but to variable extents. In most cases, the collagenase immunostaining was intracellular and restricted to the chondrocytic lacunae; extracellular staining was more evident for MMP-13.

MMP-3 was observed in the superficial zones of all but 1 of the specimens, again showing microfocal

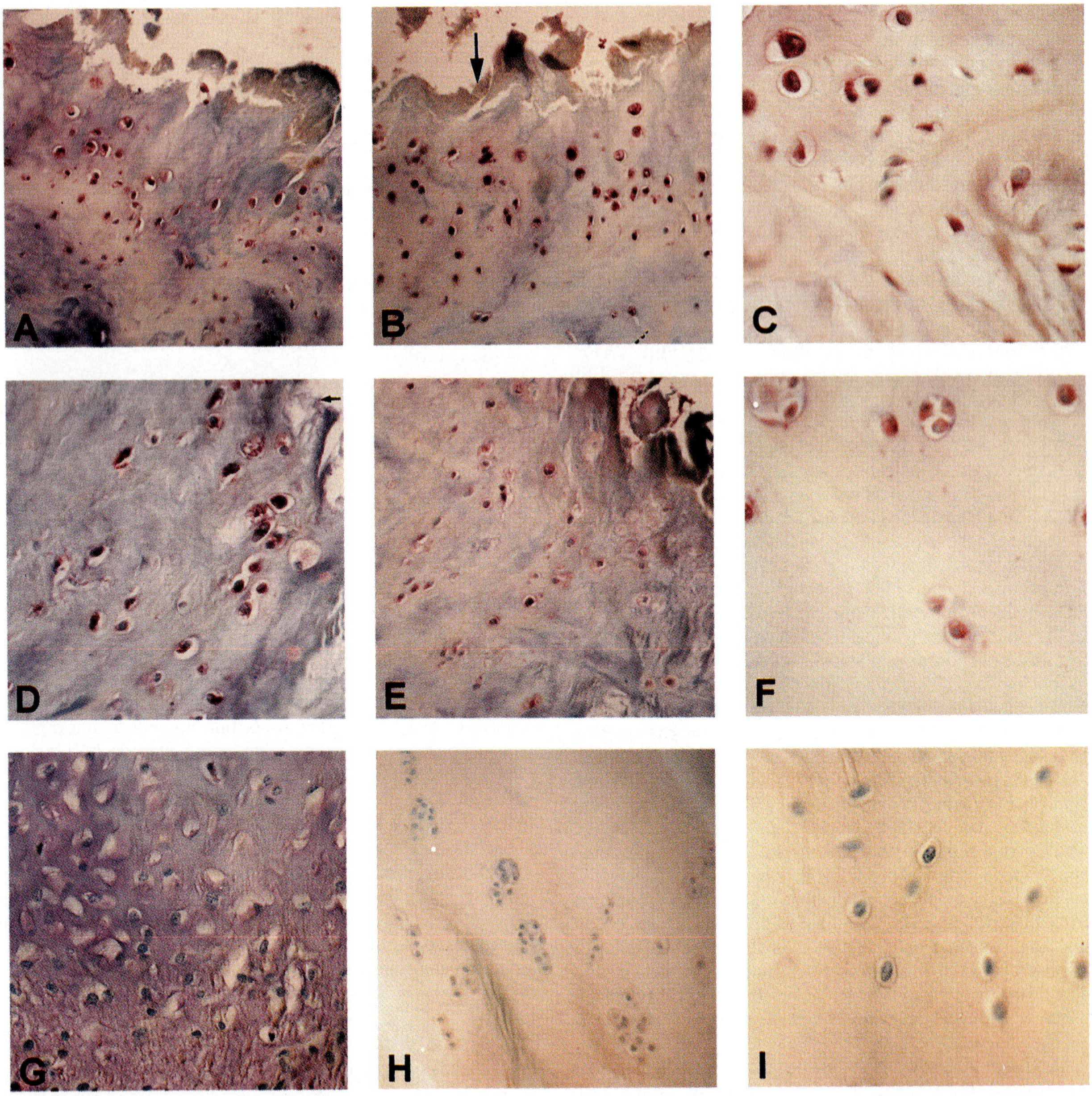

Figure 1. Immunolocalization of matrix metalloproteinases (MMPs) 1, 2, 3, 8, 9, and 13 in osteoarthritic (OA) cartilage. **A,** MMP-1 in OA cartilage specimen 699/3, grade 2. Positive cells stained red. **B,** MMP-8 in OA cartilage specimen 699/3, grade 2. Note prominent staining of chondrocytes in the superficial zone near the articular surface **(arrow)**. **C,** High-power view of chondrocytes stained for MMP-13 in the superficial zone of OA cartilage specimen 667/1, grade 1. Note the positive staining of the chondrocytic cytoplasm and extracellular staining around the edges of lacunae. **D,** MMP-3 in the superficial zone of OA cartilage specimen 697/3, grade 2. Note the presence of both positive and negative cells. **Arrow** shows articular surface. **E,** MMP-9 in the superficial zone of OA cartilage specimen 699/3, grade 2. Both positive and negative cells are present. **F,** MMP-2 in the superficial zone of OA cartilage specimen 635/3, grade 2. Note the intracellular staining. **G,** OA cartilage specimen 804/2, grade 3, treated with nonimmune sheep IgG as a negative control for the primary antibodies to MMPs 1, 2, 3, 9, and 13 shown in **A**, **C**, **D**, **E**, and **F**. **H,** OA cartilage specimen 707/3, grade 3, treated with nonimmune mouse IgG as a negative control for the MMP-8 shown in **B**. **I,** High-power view of OA cartilage specimen 792/5, grade 2, treated with nonimmune sheep IgG as a negative control for MMPs 1, 2, 3, 9, and 13. Cartilage sections were weakly counterstained with either toluidine blue (**A**, **B**, **D**, **E**, and **G**) or Harris' hematoxylin (**C**, **F**, **H**, and **I**). (Original magnification × 160 in **A**, **B**, **E**, and **H**; × 400 in **C**, **F**, and **I**; × 250 in **D** and **G**.)

Table 2. Frequency and distribution of MMPs 1, 8, 13, 2, 9, and 3 (collagenases 1, 2, and 3, gelatinases A and B, and stromelysin 1, respectively) in OA cartilage of varying disease progression*

		Superficial zone						Deep zone					
Specimen	Grade	MMP-1	MMP-8	MMP-13	MMP-2	MMP-9	MMP-3	MMP-1	MMP-8	MMP-13	MMP-2	MMP-9	MMP-3
OA													
698/2	3	++	+++	++++	+	–	++	+	++	+++	–	–	+
771/1	3	+	++	ND	ND	+	++	+	+	ND	ND	–	–
707/3	3	+++	+++	++	ND	+	++	++	++	+	ND	++	++
805/2	3	++++	+++	++	ND	+	+++	++	+	–	ND	–	++
635/3	2	++	+++	+++	++	ND	+	–	++	+++	+	ND	–
697/3	2	++	+++	++	++	+++	+++	+	+++	++	++	++	++
699/3	2	+++	+++	++++	++	++	++	++	+	+	–	–	–
792/5	2	+	++	ND	ND	–	+	–	–	ND	ND	–	–
794/2	2	+	++	+	ND	+	–	–	–	–	ND	–	–
667/1	1	++	++	+++	–	–	+	–	–	++	–	–	–
692/9	1	+	+++	++	+	–	+	+	+++	++	+	–	–
804/2	1	++	+++	ND	ND	+	++	+	+++	ND	ND	–	–
Normal													
NC/98/1	0	–	–	–	–	–	–	–	–	–	ND	–	–
NC/98/3	0	+	+	–	–	–	–/+	–	–	–/+	–	–	–
NC/98/6	0	–	–	–/+	–	–	–	–	–	–	–	–	–
NC/98/8	0	–	–/+	–	–	–	–/+	–	–	–	–	ND	–
NC/99/2	0	–	–	–	–	–	–	–	–	–	–	–	–

* Values are the percentage of total chondrocytes in each zone that stained positive for antigen: – = none, + = <10%; ++ = 10–40%; +++ = 40–80%, and ++++ = >80%; ND = not done. See Table 1 for an explanation of the histologic grading system. Statistical analyses (by Student's *t*-test) for comparisons between the osteoarthritic (OA; grades 1, 2, and 3) and normal cartilage specimens showed significant differences for all 6 matrix metalloproteinases (MMPs): $P = 0.0001$ for MMP-1, $P = 0.0000001$ for MMP-8, $P = 0.00001$ for MMP-13, $P = 0.0067$ for MMP-2, $P = 0.026$ for MMP-9, and $P = 0.0007$ for MMP-3. In addition, comparisons between the superficial and deep zones of OA cartilage showed the following values: $P = 0.005$ for MMP-1, $P = 0.006$ for MMP-8, $P = 0.06$ for MMP-13, $P = 0.19$ for MMP-2, $P = 0.085$ for MMP-9, and $P = 0.003$ for MMP-3; only those for MMPs 1, 8, and 3 were significant.

distributions with only a proportion of chondrocytes appearing positive (Figure 1D). Immunolocalization of the 2 gelatinases (MMP-2 and MMP-9) was not as prominent as that for the other 4 MMPs and, when observed, was limited to small groups of chondrocytes with rather weak staining (Figures 1E and F). Control tissue sections from OA grade 3 cartilage treated with nonimmune sheep IgG in place of the primary antibody consistently gave negative results (Figures 1G, H, and I).

An assessment of the frequency and distribution of these MMPs in each specimen is shown in Table 2 and compared with age-matched normal articular cartilage. Immunostaining for MMPs 1, 3, 8, and 13 was most prominent in the superficial zone of OA grades 2 and 3, especially associated with areas of matrix depletion, fibrillations, chondrocyte clusters, and loss of metachromasia. By contrast, the MMP immunostaining was much reduced or absent from the deep zone of these specimens, which apart from a few cell clusters, showed apparently normal hyaline cartilage and chondrocyte morphology. All the OA specimens showed a greater frequency and distribution of each MMP compared with normal articular cartilage specimens.

Since many MMPs are reported to be up-regulated by the proinflammatory cytokines IL-1 and TNF, the distribution of these 2 potential MMP-induction factors was also examined by immunohistochemistry. Both IL-1β and TNFα were localized to a proportion of chondrocytes in the superficial zone of specimens showing grade 2 or 3 features, the numbers of IL-1β+ and TNFα+ cells usually reflecting a range of ~5–40% total cells. Single chondrocytes as well as those contributing to cell clusters were shown to be positive for IL-1β or TNFα, in contrast to the scarce cytokine distributions observed for cells in the deep zones (Figure 2).

Fewer cells were stained for the 2 cytokines in grade 1 specimens. No cytokine immunostaining was observed in the normal cartilage specimens (Table 3). Such observations suggested an autocrine expression of both cytokines by chondrocytes in regions of OA cartilage showing degenerative changes.

The demonstration of 6 different MMPs in OA cartilage specimens, albeit with interspecimen variation and no regular pattern apart from prominent

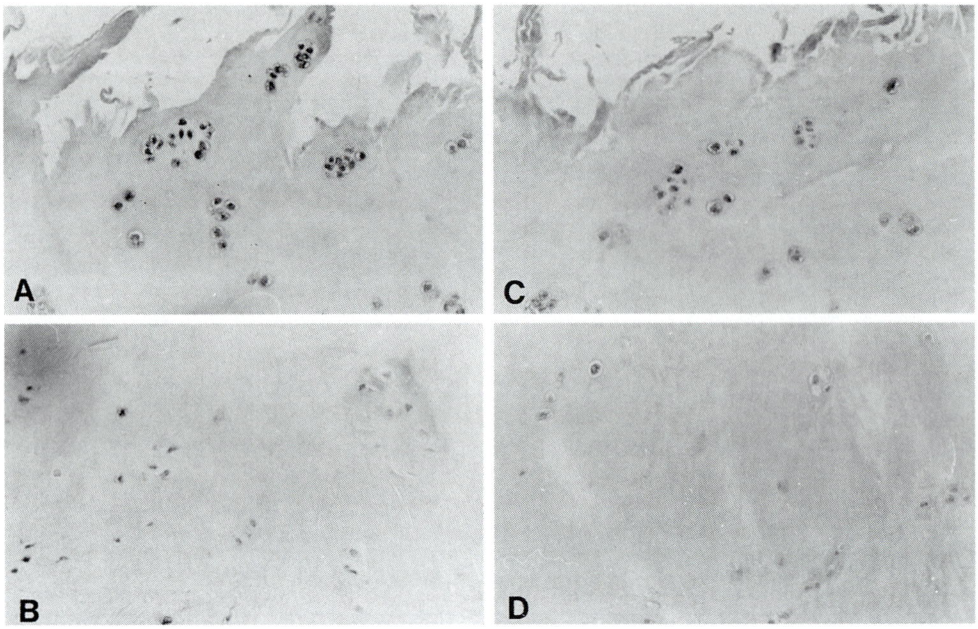

Figure 2. Immunolocalization of interleukin-1β (IL-1β) and tumor necrosis factor α (TNFα) in the superficial and deep zones of osteoarthritic (OA) cartilage. **A,** IL-1β in the superficial zone of OA cartilage grade 3. Note that most of the chondrocytes in the characteristic OA clusters are positively stained (black). **B,** IL-1β in the deep zone of the same specimen shown in **A.** Note the smaller proportion of chondrocytes stained for IL-1β. **C,** TNFα in the superficial zone of OA cartilage grade 2. A proportion of cells in the chondrocytic clusters are positively stained. **D,** TNFα in the deep zone of the same specimen shown in **C.** Note that the majority of cells are negative. Negative controls were consistently obtained using either nonimmune rabbit IgG or immunoadsorbed primary antibodies. (Original magnification × 160.)

collagenase expression in the superficial zone, was subsequently supported by the production of each MMP by human chondrocytes in vitro, especially after "activation" by IL-1β or TNFα. Conditioned culture media derived from HAC cultures treated with the MMP-inducing agents IL-1β, TNFα, or PMA showed that activated cells produced MMPs 1, 3, 8, and 13, as shown by Western blotting. Gelatin zymography showed the release of MMP-2 and MMP-9, the latter following PMA stimulation (Figure 3). The results presented in Figure 3 were typical of those produced by 3 different HAC cultures, indicating that IL-1β activation was generally more effective than TNFα or PMA for MMP induction, and thus suggesting discoordinate regulatory pathways for specific MMPs. Thus, chondrocytes in vitro have shown their potential to produce these 6 MMPs when "activated," an observation in contrast to those in HAC cultures which received no stimulatory treatments and appeared to be restricted to constitutive MMP-2 production.

Table 3. Frequency and distribution of the cytokines IL-1β and TNFα in osteoarthritic cartilage of varying disease progression*

		Superficial zone		Deep zone	
Specimen	Grade	IL-1β	TNFα	IL-1β	TNFα
OA					
771/3	3	++	++	+	–
707/3	3	++	++	–	–
805/2	3	+++	++	–	+
635/3	2	+	–	–	–
699/3	2	+	+	–	–
667/1	1	+	–	–	–
692/9	1	–	–	–	–
Normal					
NC/98/3	0	–	–	–	–
NC/98/6	0	+	–	–	–
NC/99/2	0	–	–	–	–

* Values are the percentage of total chondrocytes in each zone that stained positive for antigen: – = none; + = <10%; ++ = 10–40%; and +++ = 40–80%. See Table 1 for an explanation of the histologic grading system. IL-1β = interleukin-1β; TNFα = tumor necrosis factor α.

Dual immunolocalization studies demonstrated that some chondrocytes of OA cartilage specimens were immunostained for both IL-1β and MMP-8, indicating that these proteins were coexpressed by the same cell

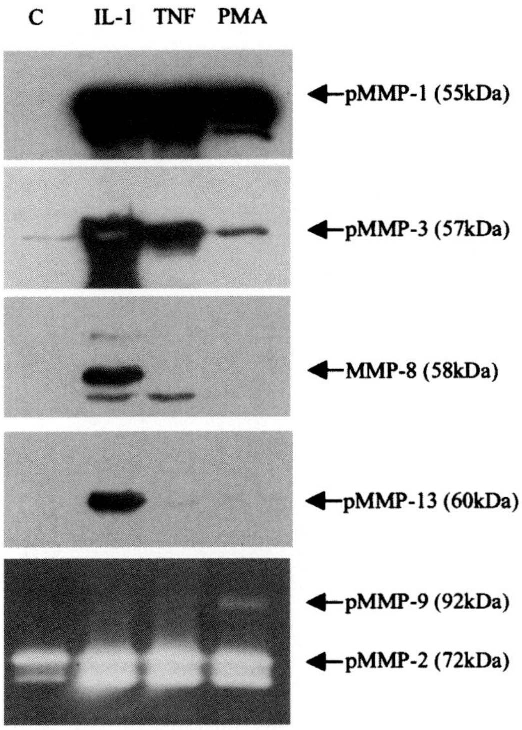

Figure 3. Western blot demonstrating the production and release of matrix metalloproteinases (MMPs) 1, 3, 8, 13 and gelatin zymography demonstrating the production and release of MMPs 2 and 9 by stimulated human articular chondrocytes in vitro. The results are from 1 human articular chondrocyte culture. Lane 1, Control (C) conditioned medium; lane 2, conditioned medium + interleukin-1β (IL-1; 0.1 ng/ml); lane 3, conditioned medium + tumor necrosis factor α (TNF; 20 ng/ml); lane 4, conditioned medium + phorbol myristate acetate (PMA; 25 ng/ml).

(Figure 4). By contrast, other chondrocytes within the same location were negative for both antigens (Figures 4A and B). Such observations of behavioral heterogeneity indicate a modified chondrocyte phenotype that may not be restricted to IL-1β and MMP-8, but further work is needed to examine the coproduction of other MMPs with IL-1β– or TNFα-positive chondrocytes.

DISCUSSION

Cartilage degradation and loss are the major features of OA; degenerative changes include fibrillations, chondrocyte proliferation into cell clusters, and matrix disruption. Recent studies have implicated the up-regulation of several matrix-degrading metalloproteinases in OA cartilage (7,8,21), as well as a role for the plasminogen activator–plasmin system and specific inhibitors of both groups of proteinases, such as the tissue inhibitors of metalloproteinases and plasminogen activator inhibitors (9,22,23). Several reports have proposed that chondrocyte production of MMPs in OA cartilage reflects a local synthesis which varies with the extent of cartilage degeneration (for review, see refs. 6, 7, 8, 24, and 25). However, the mechanisms which regulate MMP expression, the relative importance of individual MMPs, and their distributions in situ remain uncertain. The major aims of the present study were to examine the MMP and cytokine phenotypes of chondrocytes in human OA cartilage specimens and to determine whether these were related to the progressive degenerative changes of OA. To this end, we adopted a simplified grading system for OA cartilage specimens based on that described in other recent studies (5,11,17).

There have been numerous reports from immunohistochemical and in situ hybridization studies of several MMP and plasminogen activator enzymes in OA cartilage derived from humans and from various animal species, many of which identify enzyme distributions, but have not always been in agreement. One explanation for this may relate to differences in the relatively short-term experimental OA models in animals compared with the different cartilage locations, joints, and clinical gradings of human OA specimens (compare with refs. 4, 7, and 11). Other studies have used isolated chondrocytes in vitro or cartilage explant cultures to examine the production of mRNA and/or protein for various MMPs and cytokines to compare OA and normal chondrocyte phenotypes (4,10,24,26,27). Such studies have provided important data, but it is likely that some of the parameters that were measured represent the response of a minority of chondrocytes within any experiment, in accord with the heterogeneity of chondrocyte phenotype within zones of normal cartilage, as demonstrated by earlier studies (28).

Even within the present study, the MMP and cytokine profiles of OA chondrocytes showed variations within specimens of the same grade. Only occasionally was the extent of immunostaining in the deep zone similar to that of the superficial zone, this being limited to 3 of 9 specimens for MMPs 8 and 13 (compare with ref. 30). Thus, not every specimen conforms to an expected pattern, although in general it is concluded that each of the 6 MMPs showed greater expression by chondrocytes of the superficial zone, where degenerative changes were more prominent. Such findings are largely consistent with the data reported by Walter et al (25) who reported a greater immunoreaction and direct correlation for MMP-1, MMP-3, and urokinase plasmin-

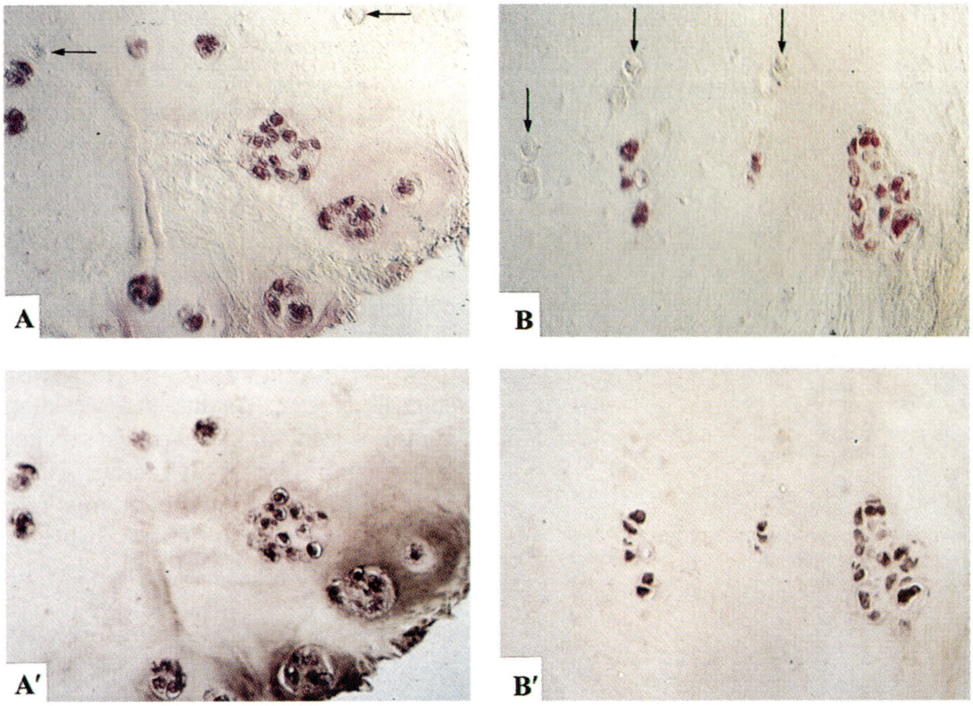

Figure 4. Dual immunolocalization of interleukin-1β (IL-1β) and matrix metalloproteinase 8 (MMP-8) in osteoarthritic (OA) cartilage. **A** and **B,** IL-1β (red stain) in OA cartilage grade 2 near the articular surface **(A)** and in a chondrocyte cluster deeper within the superficial zone **(B)**. Note IL-1β–positive and IL-1β–negative chondrocytes **(arrows)** in both fields. **A′** and **B′**, MMP-8 (brown stain) in the same sections as in **A** and **B**, respectively. Note both MMP-8–positive and MMP-8–negative cells, which correspond to those in **A** and **B**. (Original magnification × 180.)

ogen activator in chondrocytes of the superficial zones of OA cartilage with more advanced degradation.

Of the 3 collagenases, MMPs 1, 8 and 13, the latter has assumed greater importance in OA because of its preferential ability to degrade type II collagen (4,29). Several studies have identified MMP-13 in human OA cartilage, either its mRNA or enzyme protein, but reports on its frequency of expression and distribution within human cartilage illustrate variable findings (4,7,30). Recent evidence derived from the action of the selective collagenase inhibitor RS102,481 on collagen degradation in explanted bovine articular cartilage reported that MMP-1 and MMP-8 were probably not involved in type II collagen degradation (27). While we have no evidence as to whether any of the immunodetected MMPs of the present study are in an active, precursor, or complexed form, it is evident that all 3 collagenases are elaborated in situ, supporting the possibility that each makes some contribution to the processes of cartilage breakdown in human OA (see ref. 31).

A variety of cytokines are reportedly involved in cartilage breakdown, with OA chondrocytes being capable of synthesizing TNFα, IL-1β, IL-6, and others (4,10,32,33). The proinflammatory cytokines IL-1 and TNF up-regulate MMP synthesis by chondrocytes under both normal and pathologic conditions (4,13,34,35). Several studies have implicated the measurable levels of TNFα and IL-1β in the synovial fluids of normal and diseased joints as a contributory factor for MMP expression by chondrocytes (36,37). Previous work has shown that human chondrocytes in situ can produce their own IL-1 and TNF (1,38,39); observations suggest that local chondrocyte synthesis of these cytokines may represent an alternative or even prime source for MMP induction within OA cartilage. This is supported in the present studies by dual immunolocalization showing the coexpression of IL-1β and MMP-8 within the same chondrocytes of OA cartilage, possibly suggesting a local autocrine function for IL-1. TNFα plays a pivotal role in the induction of a proinflammatory cytokine cascade (40) and induces chondrocytes to increase receptor expression for other cytokines (6). It therefore seems likely that those OA chondrocytes shown to be TNFα+ and IL-1β+ may assume an autocrine function, possibly inducing changes in cytokine receptor expression and increased IL-6 and transforming growth factor α production, as described for isolated chondrocytes by Shlopov et al (6), but these have yet to be examined in situ.

The realization that OA cartilage specimens show microenvironmental variations in MMP and cytokine expression despite similar histologic grading probably reflects the recognized intermittent nature of active and quiescent phases of disease progression in OA.

The in vitro observations reported herein show that chondrocyte "activation" appears to be necessary for the local elaboration of specific MMPs. The demonstration of chondrocytes producing IL-1β and TNFα within the superficial zones of OA cartilage and the expression of 6 different MMPs in similar locations support the concept that cytokine–MMP associations contribute to what appears to be an intrinsic process of cartilage degeneration by resident chondrocytes. These findings add weight to the many earlier ex vivo studies on chondrocytes or cartilage explants, or localization studies of human OA cartilage, which have emphasized the importance of different MMPs, their induction by proinflammatory cytokines, and their associations with localized sites of cartilage matrix degradation (6,27,41).

ACKNOWLEDGMENTS

We thank consultant orthopedic surgeons T. Dunningham (Tameside Hospital, Manchester, UK) and M. Morris (Devonshire Royal Hospital, Buxton, UK) for the supply of joint tissues and Professor A. J. Freemont for help with the supply of normal cartilage. We also extend our thanks to Roddy McColl and Mark Jotham (Medical Illustration Unit, Manchester Royal Infirmary) for help with preparation of the color figures.

REFERENCES

1. Howell DS, Pelletier J-P. Etiopathogenesis of osteoarthritis. In: McCarty DJ, Koopman WJ, editors. Arthritis and allied conditions: a textbook of rheumatology. Vol. 2. 12th ed. Philadelphia: Lea & Febiger; 1993; p. 1723–34.
2. Poole AR. Cartilage in health and disease. In: Koopman WJ, editor. Arthritis and allied conditions: a textbook of rheumatology. 13th ed. Baltimore: Williams and Wilkins; 1997. p. 279–333.
3. Woessner JF Jr, Gunja-Smith Z. Role of metalloproteinases in human osteoarthritis. J Rheumatol 1991;18:99–101.
4. Shlopov BV, Lie W-R, Mainardi CL, Cole AA, Chubinskaya S, Hasty KA. Osteoarthritic lesions: involvement of three different collagenases. Arthritis Rheum 1997;40:2065–74.
5. Freemont AJ, Hampson V, Tilman R, Goupille P, Taiwo Y, Hoyland JA. Gene expression of matrix metalloproteinase 1, 3, and 9 by chondrocytes in osteoarthritic human knee articular cartilage is zone and grade specific. Ann Rheum Dis 1997;56: 542–9.
6. Shlopov BV, Gumanovskaya ML, Hasty KA. Autocrine regulation of collagenase 3 (matrix metalloproteinase 13) during osteoarthritis. Arthritis Rheum 2000;43:195–205.
7. Freemont AJ, Byers RJ, Taiwo YO, Hoyland JA. In situ zymographic localisation of type II collagen degrading activity in osteoarthritic human cartilage. Ann Rheum Dis 1999;58:357–65.
8. Billinghurst RC, Dahlberg L, Ionescu M, Reiner A, Bourne R, Rorabeck C, et al. Enhanced cleavage of type II collagen by collagenases in osteoarthritic cartilage. J Clin Invest 1997;99: 1534–45.
9. Poole AR, Alini M, Hollander AH. Cellular biology of cartilage degradation. In: Henderson B, Edwards JCW, Pettipher ER, editors. Mechanisms and models in rheumatoid arthritis. London: Academic Press; 1995. p. 163–203.
10. Borden P, Solymar D, Sucharczuk A, Lindman B, Cannon P, Heller R. Cytokine control of interstitial collagenase and collagenase-3 gene expression in human chondrocytes. J Biol Chem 1996;271:23577–81.
11. Kammermann JR, Kincaid SA, Rumph PF, Baird DK, Visco DM. Tumour necrosis factor-alpha (TNF-alpha) in canine osteoarthritis: immunolocalization of TNF-alpha, stromelysin and TNF receptors in canine osteoarthritic cartilage. Osteoarthritis Cartilage 1996;4:23–34.
12. MacNaul NK, Chartrain N. Lark M, Tocci MJ, Hutchinson NI. Discoordinate expression of stromelysin, collagenase and tissue inhibitor of metalloproteinases-1 in rheumatoid human synovial fibroblasts: synergistic effects of interleukin-1 and tumour necrosis factor-alpha on stromelysin expression. J Biol Chem 1990;265: 17238–45.
13. Lotz M, Blanco FJ, von Kempis J, Dudler J, Maier R, Villiger PM, et al. Cytokine regulation of chondrocyte functions. J Rheumatol Suppl 1995;43:104–8.
14. Pelletier J-P, DiBattista JA, Raynaud JP, Wilhelm S, Martel-Pelletier J. The in vivo effects of intraarticular corticosteroid injection on cartilage lesions, stromelysin, interleukin-1, and oncogene protein synthesis in experimental osteoarthritis. Lab Invest 1995;72:578–86.
15. Van de Loo FAJ, Joosten LAB, van Lent PLEM, Arntz OJ, van den Berg WB. Role of interleukin-1, tumor necrosis factor α and interleukin-6 in cartilage proteoglycan metabolism and destruction: effect of in situ blocking in murine antigen- and zymosan-induced arthritis. Arthritis Rheum 1995;38:164–72.
16. Martel-Pelletier J, McCollum R, Fujimoto N, Obata K, Cloutier JM, Pelletier J-P. Excess of metalloproteinase over tissue inhibitor of metalloproteinases may contribute to cartilage degradation in osteoarthritis and rheumatoid arthritis. Lab Invest 1994;70:807–15.
17. Van der Sluijs JA, Geesink RGT, van der Linden AJ, Bulstra SK, Kuyer R, Drukker J. The reliability of the Mankin score for osteoarthritis. J Orthop Res 1992;10:58–61.
18. Lees M, Taylor DJ, Woolley DE. Mast cell proteinases activate precursor forms of collagenase (pMMP-1) and stromelysin (pMMP-3) but not gelatinases A and B (pMMP-2 and pMMP-9). Eur J Biochem 1994;223:171–7.
19. Tetlow LC, Lees M, Ogata Y, Nagase H, Woolley DE. Differential expression of gelatinase B (MMP-9) and stromelysin-1 (MMP-3) by rheumatoid synovial cells in vitro and in vivo. Rheumatol Int 1993;13:53–9.
20. Meats JE, McGuire MK, Russell RGG. Human synovium releases a factor which stimulates chondrocyte production of PGE and plasminogen activator. Nature 1980;286:891–2.
21. Mehraban F, Kuo S-Y, Riera H, Chang C, Moskowitz RW. Prostromelysin and procollagenase genes are differentially upregulated in chondrocytes from the knees of rabbits with experimental osteoarthritis. Arthritis Rheum 1994;37:1189–97.
22. Cawston TE. Proteinases and connective tissue breakdown. In: Henderson B, Edwards JCW, Pettipher ER, editors. Mechanisms

and models in rheumatoid arthritis. London: Academic Press; 1995. p. 333–59.
23. Martel-Pelletier J, Faure M-P, McCollum R, Mineau F, Cloutier JM, Pelletier JP. Plasmin, plasminogen activators and inhibitor in human osteoarthritic cartilage. J Rheumatol 1991;18:1863–71.
24. Dahlberg L, Billinghurst RC, Manner P, Nelson F, Webb G, Ionescu M, et al. Selective enhancement of collagenase-mediated cleavage of resident type II collagen in cultured osteoarthritic cartilage and arrest with a synthetic inhibitor that spares collagenase 1 (matrix metalloproteinase 1). Arthritis Rheum 2000;43: 673–82.
25. Walter H, Kawashima A, Nebelung W, Neumann W, Roessner A. Immunohistochemical analysis of several proteolytic enzymes as parameters of cartilage degradation. Pathol Res Pract 1998;194: 73–81.
26. Bottomley KM, Borkakoti N, Bradshaw D, Brown PA, Broadhurst MJ, Budd JM, et al. Inhibition of bovine nasal cartilage degradation by selective matrix metalloproteinase inhibitors. Biochem J 1997;323:483–8.
27. Billinghurst RC, Wu W, Ionescu M, Reiner A, Dahlberg L, Chen J, et al. Comparison of the degradation of type II collagen and proteoglycan in nasal and articular cartilages induced by interleukin-1 and the selective inhibition of type II collagen cleavage by collagenase. Arthritis Rheum 2000;43:664–72.
28. Aydelotte MB, Kuettner KE. Heterogeneity of articular chondrocytes and cartilage matrix. In: Woessner JF Jr, Howell DS, editors. Joint cartilage degradation, basic and clinical aspects. New York: Marcel Dekker; 1993. p. 37–65.
29. Mitchell PG, Magna HA, Reeves LM, Lopresti-Morrow LL, Yocum Sa, Roesner PJ, et al. Cloning, expression and type II collagenolytic activity of matrix metalloproteinase-13 from human osteoarthritic cartilage. J Clin Invest 1996;97:761–8.
30. Moldovan F, Pelletier J-P, Hambor J, Cloutier J-M, Martel-Pelletier J. Collagenase-3 (matrix metalloproteinase 13) is preferentially localized in the deep layer of human arthritic cartilage in situ: in vitro mimicking effect by transforming growth factor α. Arthritis Rheum 1997;40:1653–61.
31. Fernandes JC, Martel-Pelletier J, Lascau-Coman V, Moldovan F, Jovanovic D, Raynaud JP, et al. Collagenase-1 and collagenase-3 synthesis in normal and early experimental osteoarthritic canine cartilage: an immunohistochemical study. J Rheumatol 1998;25: 1585–94.
32. Brinckerhoff CE. Regulation of metalloproteinase gene expression: implications for osteoarthritis. Crit Rev Eukaryot Gene Expr 1992;2:145–64.
33. Shinmei M, Masuda K, Kikuchi T, Shimomura Y, Okada Y. Production of cytokines by chondrocytes and its role in proteoglycan degradation. J Rheumatol 1991;18 Suppl 27:89–91.
34. Arend WP, Dayer J-M. Inhibition of the production and effects of interleukin-1 and tumor necrosis factor α in rheumatoid arthritis. Arthritis Rheum 1995;38:151–60.
35. Krane SM. Mechanisms of tissue destruction in rheumatoid arthritis. In: McCarty DJ, Koopman WJ. Arthritis and allied conditions: a textbook of rheumatology. Vol. 1. 12th ed. Philadelphia: Lea & Febiger; 1993. p. 763–80.
36. Chubinskaya S, Huch K, Mikecz K, Szabo C, Hasty K, Kuettner K, et al. Chondrocyte matrix metalloproteinase-8: up-regulation of neutrophil collagenase by interleukin-1β in human cartilage from knee and ankle joints. Lab Invest 1996;74:232–40.
37. Hrycaj P, Stratz T, Kovac C, Mennet P, Muller W. Microheterogeneity of acute phase proteins in patients with clinically active and clinically non-active osteoarthritis. Clin Rheumatol 1995;14: 434–40.
38. Chu CQ, Field M, Allard S, Abney E, Feldmann M, Maini RN. Detection of cytokines at the cartilage pannus junction in patients with rheumatoid arthritis: implications for the role of cytokines in cartilage destruction and repair. Br J Rheumatol 1992;32:653–61.
39. Tetlow LC, Woolley DE. Mast cells, cytokines, and matrix metalloproteinases at the rheumatoid lesion: dual immunolocalisation studies. Ann Rheum Dis 1995;54:896–903.
40. Brennan FM, Maini RN, Feldmann M. TNFα—a pivotal role in rheumatoid arthritis? Br J Rheumatol 1992;31:293–8.
41. Ohta S, Imai K, Yamashita K, Matsumoto T, Azumano I, Okada Y. Expression of matrix metalloproteinase 7 (matrilysin) in human osteoarthritic cartilage. Lab Invest 1998;78:79–87.

ARTHRITIS & RHEUMATISM
Vol. 44, No. 3, March 2001, pp 595–607

Peroxisome Proliferator–Activated Receptor γ Activators Inhibit Interleukin-1β–Induced Nitric Oxide and Matrix Metalloproteinase 13 Production in Human Chondrocytes

Hassan Fahmi,[1] John A. Di Battista,[1] Jean-Pierre Pelletier,[1] François Mineau,[1] Pierre Ranger,[2] and Johanne Martel-Pelletier[1]

Objective. **To determine the effects of peroxisome proliferator–activated receptor γ (PPARγ) agonists on interleukin-1 (IL-1) induction of nitric oxide (NO) and matrix metalloproteinase 13 (MMP-13) in human chondrocytes.**

Methods. **PPARγ expression and synthesis in human chondrocytes were determined by reverse transcriptase–polymerase chain reaction (RT-PCR) and immunohistochemistry, respectively. Chondrocytes were cultured with IL-1β, tumor necrosis factor α (TNFα), and IL-17 in the presence or absence of PPARγ agonists, and NO and MMP-13 synthesis and expression levels were measured. Transient transfection experiments were performed with the 7-kb inducible NO synthase (iNOS) and 1.6-kb MMP-13 human promoters, as well as with the PPARγ expression vector and the activator protein 1 (AP-1) and nuclear factor κB (NF-κB) reporter constructs.**

Results. **RT-PCR and immunohistochemical analysis revealed that human chondrocytes expressed and produced PPARγ. Treatment of chondrocytes with PPARγ ligands BRL 49653 and 15-deoxy-$\Delta^{12,14}$-prostaglandin J_2 (15d-PGJ_2), but not with PPARα ligand Wy 14643, decreased IL-1β–induced NO and MMP-13 production in a dose-dependent manner. In addition, both iNOS and MMP-13 messenger RNA were inhibited in the presence of 15d-PGJ_2. The inhibitory effect of PPARγ activation was not restricted to IL-1β, since TNFα- and IL-17–induced NO and MMP-13 production were also inhibited by 15d-PGJ_2. In transient transfection experiments, we showed that a constitutively active form of mitogen-activated protein kinase kinase kinase 1 (ΔMEKK-1) induced the MMP-13 and iNOS human promoter activity. This process was reduced by 15d-PGJ_2 and further inhibited by cotransfection with a PPARγ expression vector. Similarly, in a PPARγ-dependent manner, 15d-PGJ_2 inhibited ΔMEKK-1–induced AP-1– and NF-κB–luciferase reporter plasmid activation.**

Conclusion. **The findings of this study demonstrate that PPARγ agonists inhibit IL-1β induction of both NO and MMP-13 in human chondrocytes. The inhibition occurs at least at the transcriptional level through a PPARγ-dependent pathway, probably by interfering with the activation of AP-1 and NF-κB.**

Interleukin-1β (IL-1β) and tumor necrosis factor α (TNFα) are important mediators of inflammation and play a pivotal role in rheumatic diseases such as rheumatoid arthritis (RA) and osteoarthritis (OA). Indeed, in animal models, intraarticular injections of IL-1β or TNFα reproduce the major pathologies of these diseases (1,2). One mechanism through which these cytokines exert their effects is by inducing connective tissue cells, including chondrocytes and synoviocytes, to produce nitric oxide (NO) and matrix metalloproteinases (MMPs) (3–5).

In RA or OA patients, increased levels of nitrite/nitrate have been observed in the synovial fluid and serum (6). In addition, arthritis cartilage and synovium under ex vivo conditions spontaneously release NO in quantities sufficient to cause cartilage damage (4). These findings are supported by recent studies, in which we and others have shown that the in vivo selective inhibition of

[1]Hassan Fahmi, PhD, John A. Di Battista, PhD, Jean-Pierre Pelletier, MD, François Mineau, BSc, Johanne Martel-Pelletier, PhD: Hôpital Notre-Dame, Montreal, Quebec, Canada; [2]Pierre Ranger, MD: Hôpital Sacré-Coeur, Montreal, Quebec, Canada.

Address correspondence and reprint requests to Johanne Martel-Pelletier, PhD, Unité de recherche en arthrose, Centre hospitalier de l'Université de Montréal, Hôpital Notre-Dame, 1560 rue Sherbrooke est, Montreal, Quebec H2L 4M1, Canada.

Submitted for publication August 16, 2000; accepted in revised form November 9, 2000.

inducible NO synthase (iNOS) reduced the symptoms of inflammation as well as the biochemical abnormalities of affected joint tissues (7–9). NO contributes to cartilage degradation in several ways: 1) by inhibiting the synthesis of anabolic macromolecules, such as collagen and proteoglycan; 2) by inhibiting the production of IL-1 receptor antagonist; and 3) by enhancing MMP activity and inducing chondrocyte apoptosis (10–12). An MMP that may be of particular interest in the degradation of cartilage in pathologic conditions is collagenase 3 (MMP-13). MMP-13 has been found to be elevated in both RA and OA joint tissues and, more particularly, in articular cartilage (13,14). This enzyme cleaves the native collagen and is 5–10-fold more active on type II collagen than are MMP-1 and MMP-8, other collagenases also present in this tissue (14,15).

The peroxisome proliferator–activated receptors (PPARs) are ligand-activated transcription factors belonging to the nuclear receptor family (16). To date, 3 different PPARs—PPARα, PPARβ/δ, and PPARγ—have been identified and cloned in mammalian cells and were first shown to play a critical role in lipid and glucose homeostasis (16,17). Synthetic compounds that induce peroxisome proliferation in rodents, including Wy 14643, have been shown to specifically bind to and activate PPARα (18), while the synthetic antidiabetic thiazolidinediones and the natural prostaglandin 15-deoxy-$\Delta^{12,14}$-prostaglandin J_2 (15d-PGJ_2) are ligands for PPARγ (19,20). Although adipose tissue has been recognized as a principal site of expression of PPARγ, it is expressed at lower levels in many other tissues and cell types, including cells of the monocyte/macrophage lineage, neutrophils, and T lymphocytes (21–24). Although PPARγ expression has recently been shown in rat chondrocytes, in addition to some effects of PPARγ ligands (25), its presence and role have not been demonstrated in human chondrocytes.

Recent studies in different cell types suggest that PPARγ ligands may be important antiinflammatory agents (21,22,26–28). These studies showed that 15d-PGJ_2 and BRL 49653, potent PPARγ activators, inhibit the production of various inflammatory mediators, including TNFα, IL-1β, IL-6, IL-8, monocyte chemoattractant protein 1 (MCP-1), NO, and gelatinase 92 kd or MMP-9. We therefore investigated the expression of PPARγ in human chondrocytes and its role in IL-1β–induced NO and MMP-13 production.

We report that 15d-PGJ_2 inhibits NO and MMP-13 production at the transcriptional level in human chondrocytes. Using transient transfection experiments, we also show that 15d-PGJ_2 inhibits mitogen-activated protein kinase kinase kinase 1 (MAPKK kinase 1, or MEKK-1)–induced MMP-13 and iNOS promoter activation in a PPARγ-dependent manner, probably by interfering with the activation of activator protein 1 (AP-1) and nuclear factor κB (NF-κB). The PPARγ signaling pathway may present a novel target for therapeutic intervention in rheumatic diseases.

MATERIALS AND METHODS

Chemicals. Recombinant human IL-1β (rHuIL-1β) was obtained from Genzyme (Cambridge, MA), rHuTNFα was generously provided by Knoll Pharmaceutical (Markham, Ontario, Canada), and rHuIL-17 came from R&D Systems (Minneapolis, MN). The 15d-PGJ_2 and Wy 14643 were purchased from Cayman Chemical (Ann Arbor, MI). BRL 49653 was from American Radiolabeled Chemicals (St. Louis, MO). All other chemicals were purchased from either Sigma-Aldrich Canada (Oakville, Ontario, Canada) or Gibco BRL–Life Technologies (Burlington, Ontario, Canada).

Specimen selection. Normal cartilage (femoral condyles) was obtained from patients who had undergone hip replacement due to fracture (Moore hip arthroplasty). The cartilage was obtained under aseptic conditions, processed as previously described, and dissected from the underlying bone (29). To ensure that only normal tissue was used, cartilage specimens were examined thoroughly, both macroscopically and microscopically. Only those specimens with neither lesions nor alterations were processed further.

Chondrocyte culture. Chondrocytes were released from cartilage by sequential enzymatic digestion as previously described (29). Briefly, this consisted of 2 mg/ml pronase for 1 hour followed by 1 mg/ml collagenase (type IV; Sigma-Aldrich Canada) for 6 hours at 37°C in Dulbecco's modified Eagle's medium (DMEM; Gibco BRL–Life Technologies) and antibiotics (100 units/ml penicillin, 100 μg/ml streptomycin; Gibco BRL–Life Technologies). The digested tissue was briefly centrifuged and the pellet was washed. The isolated chondrocytes were seeded at high density in tissue culture flasks and cultured in DMEM supplemented with 10% heat-inactivated fetal calf serum (FCS; Hyclone, Logan, UT) and antibiotics at 37°C in a humidified atmosphere of 5% CO_2/95% air. At confluence, the chondrocytes were detached and passaged once, then seeded at high density and allowed to grow in DMEM supplemented as above. The culture medium was changed every second day, and 24 hours before the experiment the cells were incubated in fresh medium containing 0.5% FCS. Only first-passaged chondrocytes were used.

Immunohistochemistry. Cartilage specimens were processed for immunohistochemistry as previously described (30). Briefly, specimens were fixed in TissuFix #2 (Laboratoire Gilles Chaput, Montreal, Quebec, Canada) and embedded in paraffin. Five-micrometer sections of paraffin-embedded specimens were deparaffinized in toluene, hydrated in a graded series of ethanol, and preincubated with chondroitinase ABC (0.25 units/ml in phosphate buffered saline [PBS; Sigma-Aldrich Canada]) for 60 minutes at 37°C, then heated at 65°C for 20 minutes in 10 m*M* sodium citrate buffer (pH 6.0), and finally overlaid with the PPARγ antibody (final concentration

1 μg/ml) for 18 hours at 4°C in a humidified chamber. The antibody was a polyclonal goat anti-human PPARγ peptide (sc-1984; Santa Cruz Biotechnology, Santa Cruz, CA) and did not cross-react with either PPARα or PPARβ. Each slide was washed 3 times in PBS (pH 7.4) and stained using the avidin–biotin complex method (Vectastain ABC kit; Vector, Burlingame, CA). The color was developed with diaminobenzidine (Dako Diagnostics, Mississauga, Ontario, Canada). Slides were further counterstained with nuclear fast red (Trevigen, Gaithersburg, MD).

To determine specificity of staining, 3 controls were used: 1) adsorbed immune serum (for 1 hour at 37°C) with 20-fold molar excess of the specific peptide (N-20, sc-1984); 2) omission of the primary antibody; and 3) substitution of the primary antibody with nonimmune isotype IgG (Nordic, Tilburg, The Netherlands) following the same experimental protocol. The evaluation of chondrocytes staining positive was performed using our previously published method (30). For each specimen, 6 microscopic fields were examined under 40× magnification. The total number of chondrocytes and the number of chondrocytes staining positive were evaluated, and results were determined by the percentage of chondrocytes staining positive (cell score).

RNA extraction and reverse transcriptase–polymerase chain reaction (RT-PCR). Total RNA from cultured chondrocytes was isolated with the use of TRIzol (Gibco BRL–Life Technologies). RT-PCR assays were carried out with the DNA thermal cycler 480 (Perkin Elmer, Foster City, CA).

Two micrograms of total RNA were reverse transcribed into complementary DNA (cDNA) with 2 units/μl RT (Moloney murine leukemia virus; Gibco BRL–Life Technologies) at 42°C for 30 minutes in the standard buffer. Amplification of the cDNA encoding PPARγ or GAPDH was performed using the reverse-transcribed mixture as a template with the following specific oligonucleotide primers: PPARγ sense 5′-TCTCTCCGTAATGGAAGACC-3′ and antisense 5′-GCATTATGAGACATCCCCAC-3′, and GAPDH sense 5′-ACCACAGTCCATGCCATCAC-3′ and antisense 5′-TCCACCACCCTGTTGCTGTA-3′. The expected sizes of PCR products for PPARγ and GAPDH were 474 bp and 452 bp, respectively. Controls for RT-PCR amplifications were included. The PCR mixtures were incubated at 95°C for 1 minute, followed by 35 cycles each at 94°C for 30 seconds and 60°C for 1 minute, with a final elongation step at 60°C for 8 minutes. PCR product (10 μl/50 μl) reactions were separated on a 1.8% agarose gel and stained with ethidium bromide.

Plasmids and transient transfections. The PPAR-responsive element (PPRE)–luciferase construct containing 3 PPREs cloned upstream of the thymidine kinase promoter ($PPRE_3$-Tk-Luc) was generously provided by Dr. C. K. Glass (University of California, San Diego) (22). For construction of the pMMP-13-1.6-Luc plasmid, the 1.6-kb promoter region cloned into pCRII (31) was liberated as an *Nsi* fragment filled with *Klenow*, digested with *Kpn* I, and inserted into the *Kpn* I/*Sma* sites of pGL3-basic vector (Promega, Madison, WI). The luciferase reporter construct piNOS-7kb-Luc, containing the human iNOS promoter, was a gift from Dr. R. A. Shapiro (University of Pittsburgh, Pittsburgh, PA) (32). The human pSG5-PPARγ expression vector was donated by Dr. S. A. Kliewer (Glaxo Wellcome, Research Triangle Park, NC) (33). The pAP1-luciferase plasmid containing 7 AP-1 consensus sequences (pAP-1-Luc), the pNF-κB-luciferase plasmid containing 5 NF-κB consensus sequences (pNF-κB-Luc), and the pFC-MEKK1 plasmid encoding amino acids 360–672 of MEKK-1 were obtained from Stratagene (La Jolla, CA). A β-galactosidase reporter vector under the control of SV40 promoter (pSV40-β-galactosidase) were from Promega.

Chondrocytes were transiently transfected using the calcium phosphate/DNA coprecipitation method with 5 μg of luciferase reporter plasmid and 0.5 μg of pSV40-β-galactosidase (as a control of transfection efficiency), followed 4 hours later by a 15% glycerol shock for 1 minute. After washing, the cells were allowed to recover in DMEM containing 10% FCS for 24 hours. After this period, fresh DMEM containing 0.5% FCS was added, and the chondrocytes were treated with 15d-PGJ_2 (0–10 μM) or BRL 49653 (0–100 μM) for 18 hours. Cotransfection experiments with the promoters pFC-MEKK1 and pSG5-PPARγ were performed in HeLa cells at 50–60% confluency using Lipofectamine (Gibco BRL–Life Technologies) according to the manufacturer's protocol. Briefly, cells were incubated with liposomes for 5 hours, washed with DMEM, and incubated in fresh medium with vehicle or with increasing concentrations of 15d-PGJ_2 (0–10 μM) for another 24 hours. Luciferase activity was determined in cellular extracts (Luciferase Assay System; Promega) and normalized to β-galactosidase content, which was quantitated by a specific enzyme-linked immunosorbent assay (ELISA; Roche Diagnostics, Laval, Quebec, Canada).

MMP-13 and NO determinations. MMP-13 protein levels were quantitated in conditioned media of cultured chondrocytes by a specific ELISA (Amersham Pharmacia Biotech, Baie d'Urfé, Quebec, Canada). The nitrite level, used as an indicator of NO production, was determined with the Griess assay as previously described (34). All assays were performed in duplicate.

Northern blot analysis. Total RNA was resolved on 1.2% formaldehyde–agarose gels and transferred electrophoretically to nylon membranes (Hybond-N; Amersham Pharmacia Biotech) in a 10 mM sodium acetate buffer (pH 7.8), 20 mM Tris, and 0.5 mM EDTA overnight at 4°C. The RNA was crosslinked to the membranes by exposure to ultraviolet light. After prehybridization for 24 hours, hybridization was carried out at 42°C for cDNA human iNOS probe and at 68°C for RNA human MMP-13 and RNA GAPDH probes.

The iNOS cDNA probe (3.4 kb), which spanned the whole coding region of the gene, was generously provided by Dr. A. Amin (Hospital for Joint Diseases, New York, NY). The RNA MMP-13 probe consisted of the total coding sequence (1.4 kb) as well as 490 bp of the 3′-untranslated region (14). The probes were labeled with digoxigenin-11UTP (DIG-11-UTP; Boehringer Mannheim, Laval, Quebec, Canada) according to the manufacturer's specifications. Detection was carried out by chemiluminescence with the CDP-*Star* substrate (Boehringer Mannheim) and exposure to X-AR5 film (Eastman Kodak, Rochester, NY). After the first hybridization, the membranes were stripped and rehybridized with a DIG-labeled probe–specific GAPDH. The autoradiographs were scanned using the ChemiImager 4000 imaging system (Alpha Innotech, San Leandro, CA), and the messenger RNA (mRNA) values were calculated as the relative expression of

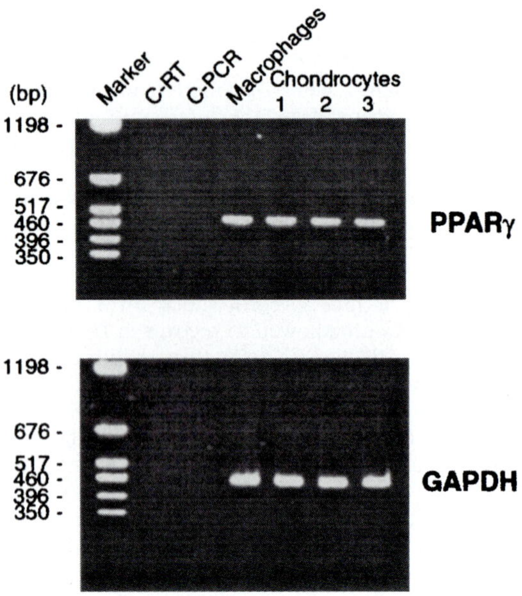

Figure 1. Expression of peroxisome proliferator–activated receptor γ (PPARγ) messenger RNA by articular chondrocytes. Shown are results of reverse transcriptase–polymerase chain reaction (RT-PCR) of total RNA from monocyte-derived macrophages (positive control) and 3 different human chondrocyte preparations. RT-PCR was performed using PPARγ- and GAPDH-specific primers. PCR products were resolved on a 1.8% agarose gel. C-RT and C-PCR are negative controls for the RT and PCR reactions, respectively. The size of the MW marker is indicated in bp.

MMP-13 and iNOS normalized to GAPDH mRNA and expressed as a percentage of the control, which was assigned a value of 100.

Statistical analysis. All results were calculated as the mean ± SEM of independent donors. Statistics were analyzed using Student's 2-tailed *t*-test. *P* values less than 0.05 were considered significant.

RESULTS

PPARγ mRNA and protein expressed by human chondrocytes. To investigate the expression of PPARγ in chondrocytes, we performed an RT-PCR analysis using specific primers on RNA from human articular cartilage chondrocytes. In 3 different chondrocyte populations derived from different donors, PPARγ mRNA was detected as a single band with the predicted size (474 bp) (Figure 1). Human monocyte–derived macrophages were used as a positive control. Two negative control experiments were also carried out in which the RT-PCR reaction was performed either without the cDNA or without the RT; these reactions yielded no PCR product.

To determine whether PPARγ protein was produced in vivo by chondrocytes, we performed immunohistochemistry studies of normal human cartilage with the use of a specific PPARγ antibody. As shown in Figure 2, positive chondrocyte staining appeared in the superficial and upper intermediate layers of the cartilage, with a mean ± SEM cell score of 21.6 ± 1.2% (n = 9 experiments). Adsorption of anti-PPARγ antibody with the peptide antigen abrogated staining (Figure 2C), indicating the specificity of the immunostaining.

Transcriptional activity of PPARγ in cultured chondrocytes. To determine whether the PPARγ receptor is functional as a transcriptional activator in human chondrocytes, cells (n = 3 experiments) were transiently transfected with a reporter construct containing 3 copies of a consensus PPRE cloned upstream of luciferase ($PPRE_3$-Tk-Luc), together with a pSV40-β-galactosidase plasmid. Cells were subsequently treated with increasing concentrations of PPARγ ligands 15d-PGJ_2 and BRL 49653. Luciferase activity was assayed and normalized to the β-galactosidase activity.

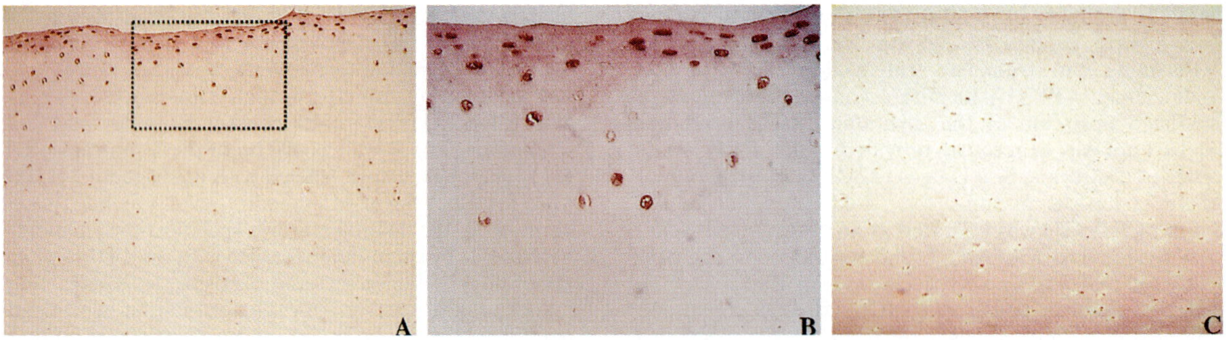

Figure 2. Expression of peroxisome proliferator–activated receptor γ (PPARγ) in human cartilage. Shown is PPARγ immunostaining in representative sections of normal human cartilage. **A,** PPARγ-specific staining found almost exclusively in the superficial zone of cartilage. **B,** Higher-magnification view of the area indicated within the dotted rectangle in **A. C,** Cartilage incubated with a 20-fold molar excess of the blocking PPARγ peptide, showing only background staining. (Original magnification × 100 in **A** and **C**; × 250 in **B.**)

As shown in Figure 3, the $PPRE_3$-Tk-Luc construct alone exhibited luciferase activity 3-fold that of the control empty basic vector. Treatment of transfected chondrocytes (n = 3 experiments) with both PPARγ ligands revealed a dose-dependent increase in the normalized activity, with a maximal 3.3-fold increase at 10 μM 15d-PGJ_2 and a maximal 3.8-fold increase at 100 μM BRL 49653. These data strongly suggest the presence of inducible PPARγ-dependent transcriptional responses in chondrocytes.

Reduction of cytokine-induced NO and MMP-13 production by PPARγ ligands. To determine whether PPAR activation could affect chondrocyte function, we investigated the effect of PPAR ligands on iNOS activity. Cultured chondrocytes (n = 4 experiments) were stimulated with IL-1β (100 pg/ml) in the presence of vehicle (control) or increasing concentrations of PPARα (Wy 14643) or PPARγ ligands (15d-PGJ_2 or BRL 49653). In preliminary experiments, cells were either preincubated with PPARγ agonists for 2 hours before IL-1β stimulation (for 18 hours) or coincubated with both IL-1β and PPARγ ligands for 18 hours. Data showed identical patterns of inhibition; therefore, the latter treatment conditions were chosen for further assays. Inducible NOS activity was monitored by measuring the levels of the nitrite/nitrate in the conditioned medium.

As shown in Figure 4A, 15d-PGJ_2 and BRL 49653 reduced IL-1β–induced NO production by chondrocytes in a dose-dependent manner. The 50% inhibition concentration (IC_{50}) values were 1 μM and 20 μM, respectively. In contrast, no effect was observed with the PPARα-specific activator Wy 14643. To further characterize the effect of PPAR ligands on chondrocytes, we examined the effect of PPAR activation on MMP-13 induction. Figure 4B shows that PPARγ ligands prevented the IL-1β–induced production of MMP-13 in a dose-dependent manner. The IC_{50} values were 2 μM for 15d-PGJ_2 and 30 μM for BRL 49653. In contrast, the PPARα-specific ligand Wy 14643 did not affect IL-1β–induced MMP-13 production. These observations suggest that PPARγ represents a novel regulatory pathway targeting IL-1β signaling in chondrocytes.

Since TNFα and IL-17 are also involved in the degradation of cartilage through induction of NO and MMPs, we assessed their effects for 18 hours with optimal concentrations of TNFα (5 μg/ml), IL-17 (50 ng/ml), and IL-1β (100 pg/ml) as comparators, in the presence of vehicle or of 10 μM 15d-PGJ_2. Interestingly, 10 μM 15d-PGJ_2 completely inhibited TNFα- and IL-17–induced NO and MMP-13 production

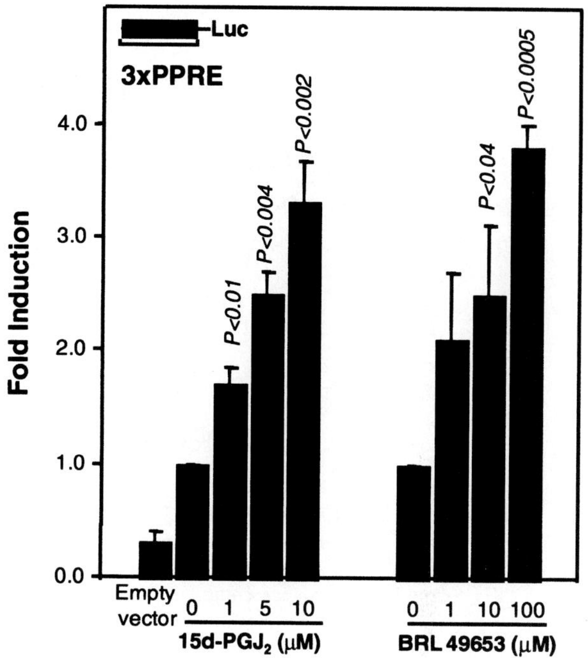

Figure 3. Activation of endogenous peroxisome proliferator–activated receptor γ (PPARγ) in human chondrocytes by PPARγ ligands 15-deoxy-$\Delta^{12,14}$-prostaglandin J_2 (15d-PGJ_2) and BRL 49653. Chondrocytes were transiently transfected with a reporter construct containing 3 copies of a consensus PPAR-responsive element (3×PPRE) placed upstream from the thymidine kinase–luciferase reporter (Tk-Luc) along with the internal control pSV40-β-galactosidase. Cells were incubated for 18 hours in the presence or absence (control) of increasing concentrations of 15d-PGJ_2 or BRL 49653. Luciferase activity normalized to β-galactosidase activity is expressed as fold induction, considering 1 as the luciferase activity of unstimulated transfected cells. Results represent the mean ± SEM of 3 independent experiments. *P* values indicate the significance of the differences from the basal value.

(Figures 5A and B), indicating that the effect of 15d-PGJ_2 was not restricted to IL-1β and that 15d-PGJ_2 might target common pathways leading to NO and MMP-13 production. It could be argued that the effects of 15d-PGJ_2 might have been due to a general toxicity; however, the trypan blue exclusion assay and the MTT salt assay showed that treatment of chondrocytes with 15d-PGJ_2 at concentrations that completely inhibited NO and MMP-13 were not cytotoxic (data not shown). Thus, the effect of 15d-PGJ_2 was probably due to the inhibition of a specific pathway involved in NO and MMP-13 production.

Inhibition of IL-1β–induced iNOS and MMP-13 expression by 15d-PGJ_2. To determine at which level 15d-PGJ_2 regulates iNOS and MMP-13, we examined its effect on induction of their mRNA (n = 3 experiments).

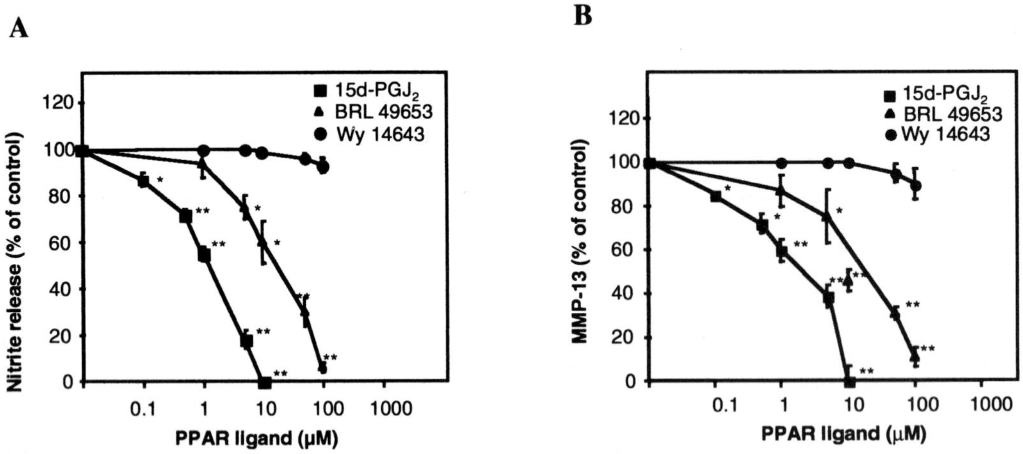

Figure 4. Inhibition by PPARγ ligands of interleukin-1β (IL-1β)–induced nitric oxide (NO) and matrix metalloproteinase 13 (MMP-13) production by human chondrocytes. Chondrocytes were incubated for 18 hours with IL-1β (100 pg/ml) in the presence or absence (control) of increasing concentrations of 15d-PGJ_2, BRL 49653, or Wy 14643. Production of **A,** NO and **B,** MMP-13 was determined in the conditioned medium. Values are expressed as the percentage of control, which was assigned a value of 100. Results represent the mean ± SEM of 4 independent experiments. $* = P < 0.01$; $** = P < 0.001$, versus absence of PPAR agonist. See Figure 3 for other definitions.

Chondrocytes were stimulated with IL-1β (100 pg/ml) in the presence of vehicle or of increasing concentrations (0–10 μM) of 15d-PGJ_2 for 18 hours, and Northern blot analysis was then performed. Results showed an undetectable level of both iNOS and MMP-13 mRNA in unstimulated cells, while higher levels were noted in the presence of IL-1β (Figure 6A). This induction was inhibited in a dose-related manner by 15d-PGJ_2, with significant inhibition at 1 μM and complete abolition at 10 μM (IC_{50} = 5 μM) (Figure 6B). As expected, no change in iNOS and MMP-13 mRNA expression was found with Wy 14643 at 100 μM.

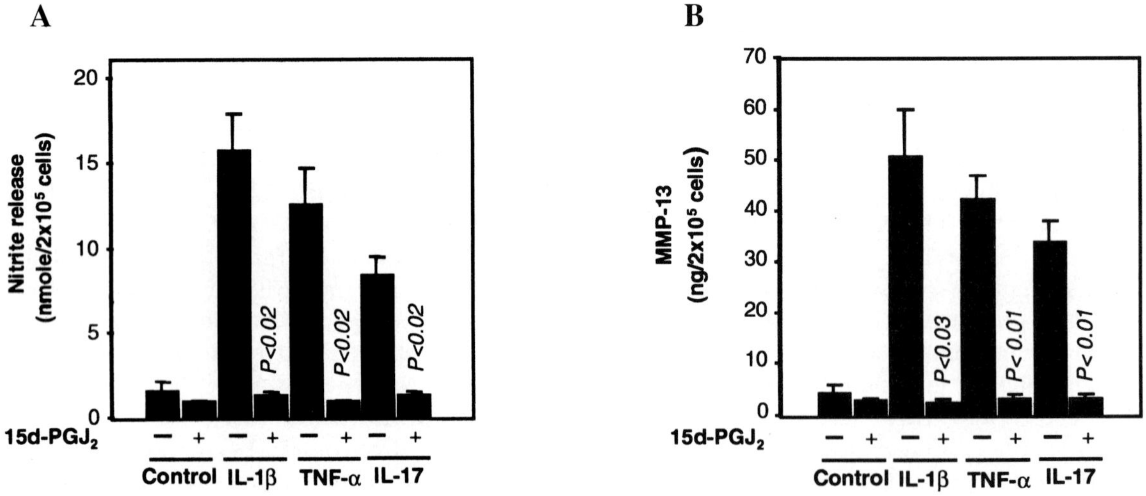

Figure 5. Inhibition by 15-deoxy-$\Delta^{12,14}$-prostaglandin J_2 (15d-PGJ_2) of tumor necrosis factor α (TNF-α)– and IL-17–induced NO and MMP-13 production by human chondrocytes. Chondrocytes were incubated for 18 hours with IL-1β (100 pg/ml), TNF-α (5 μg/ml), or IL-17 (50 ng/ml) in the presence or absence (control) of 15d-PGJ_2 (10 μM). **A,** NO levels and **B,** MMP-13 levels in the conditioned medium were determined. Results represent the mean ± SEM of 3 independent experiments. *P* values indicate the significance of the differences from the autologous control. See Figure 4 for other definitions.

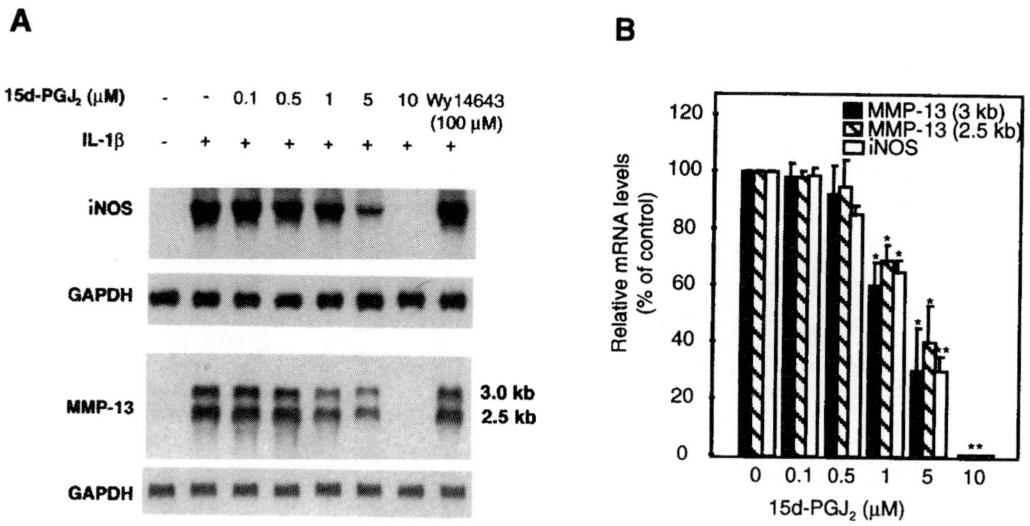

Figure 6. Inhibition by 15-deoxy-$\Delta^{12,14}$-prostaglandin J_2 (15d-PGJ_2) of IL-1β–mediated induction of inducible NO synthase (iNOS) and MMP-13 mRNA in chondrocytes. Chondrocytes were incubated for 18 hours with IL-1β (100 pg/ml) in the presence or absence (control) of increasing concentrations of 15d-PGJ_2 or 100 μM Wy 14643. **A,** Representative Northern blot autoradiograph. **B,** Relative levels of iNOS and MMP-13 mRNA expression, determined by densitometric analysis of the autoradiographic bands and normalized to the GAPDH housekeeping gene signal. Results represent the mean ± SEM of 3 independent experiments. $* = P < 0.01$; $** = P < 0.001$, versus absence of 15d-PGJ_2. See Figure 4 for other definitions.

PPARγ-dependent attenuation of activation of 7-kb iNOS and 1.6-kb MMP-13 promoters by 15d-PGJ_2. Although our understanding is incomplete regarding the intracellular events occurring after receptor occupancy by IL-1β and TNFα, recent reports indicate that exposure of cells to these cytokines leads to activation of MEKK-1 (35,36). Furthermore, MEKK-1 has been shown to potently activate signaling pathways also activated by both cytokines, namely, the NF-κB (36), c-Jun N-terminal kinase/stress-activated protein kinase 1 (JNK/SAPK-1) (37,38), extracellular signal–regulated kinase (38), and p38 MAPK (39) pathways.

The latter result suggests that 15d-PGJ_2 may be acting at the transcriptional level, given the inhibition of IL-1β–induced iNOS and MMP-13 mRNA expression. To gain insight into the mechanism mediating this inhibition, we examined the effect of 15d-PGJ_2 on the activation of iNOS and MMP-13 promoter–luciferase reporter plasmids by cotransfection with a constitutively active MEKK-1 expression vector. To assess the PPARγ-dependent effects of 15d-PGJ_2, experiments were further performed on PPARγ-negative cells. HeLa cells were used for this purpose, since they do not express PPARγ (22). Since these cells do not respond to cytokines such as IL-1β, the experiments were performed with the transient expression of an active (N-terminally truncated) form of MEKK-1 (ΔMEKK-1).

Data showed that cells transfected with the constitutively active MEKK-1 expression vector induced both promoters (iNOS and MMP-13) to a significant extent (n = 3 experiments) (Figure 7). 15d-PGJ_2 decreased the activity of both promoters, and cotransfection with a human PPARγ expression vector further enhanced the inhibitory effect of the eicosanoid (Figures 7A and B). Similar experiments were performed with IL-1β–stimulated chondrocytes transfected with the MMP-13 promoter and without the PPARγ expression vector, and similar data were obtained. However, the inhibitory effect of 15d-PGJ_2 was not affected when cotransfecting with a human PPARγ expression vector, probably because chondrocytes express enough endogenous PPARγ to mediate the effect of 15d-PGJ_2 (data not shown). These results clearly indicate that the inhibition of iNOS and MMP-13 transcription by 15d-PGJ_2 takes place, at least in part, at the transcriptional level and is mediated by PPARγ.

PPARγ-dependent inhibition of AP-1– and NF-κB–mediated transcriptional activities by 15d-PGJ_2. The transcription factors AP-1 and NF-κB are believed to mediate the induction of a host of target genes by

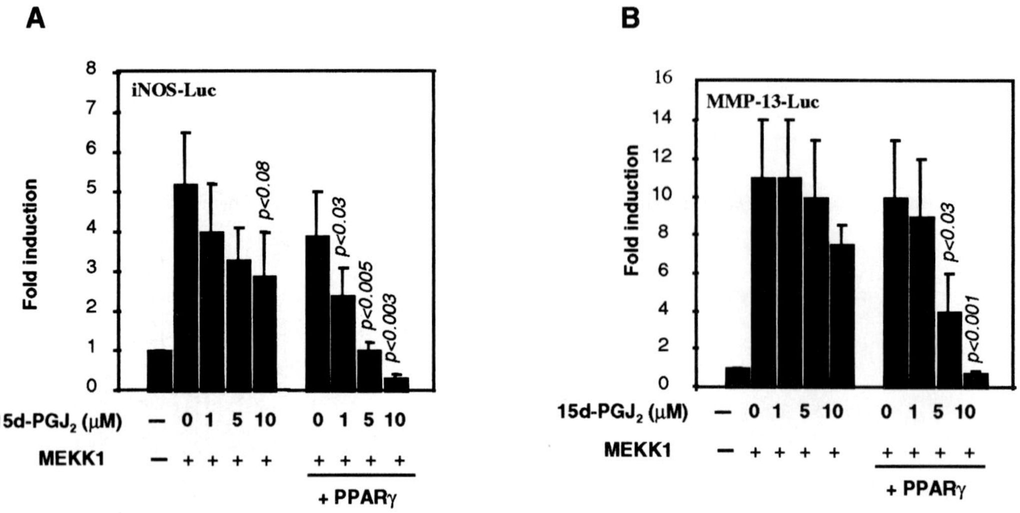

Figure 7. PPARγ-dependent inhibition by 15d-PGJ_2 of mitogen-activated protein kinase kinase kinase 1 (MEKK1)–induced activation of 1.6-kb MMP-13 and 7-kb iNOS promoters. HeLa cells were transiently cotransfected with 1 μg of either piNOS-7kb-Luc (iNOS-Luc) (**A**) or pMMP-13-1.6-Luc (MMP-13-Luc) (**B**) together with 50 ng of pFC-MEKK1 and 50 ng of pSV40-β-galactosidase in the absence or presence of 50 ng of human pSG5-PPARγ. The total amount of the DNA was kept constant by supplementation with pSG5. Cells were incubated in the presence or absence (control) of increasing concentrations of 15d-PGJ_2 and were harvested 24 hours later. Luciferase activities were determined and normalized to β-galactosidase measured in the same sample. Results are expressed as fold induction, considering 1 as the luciferase activity of unstimulated transfected cells, and represent the mean ± SEM of 3 independent experiments. *P* values indicate the significance of the differences from autologous basal values. See Figures 3, 4, and 6 for other definitions.

IL-1β and TNFα. Indeed, NF-κB plays a critical role in iNOS inducibility, while AP-1 controls MMP-13 expression to a large extent (31,32,40–42). However, MEKK-1 is a strong inducer of both AP-1 and NF-κB pathways. We therefore examined the influence of PPARγ on the transcriptional activation of the chimeric gene constructs, pNF-κB-Luc and pAP-1-Luc. pNF-κB-Luc reporter plasmid contains 5 copies of the NF-κB response element, and pAP-1-Luc reporter plasmid contains 7 copies of the AP-1 response element. We found that cotransfection with the constitutively active MEKK-1 expression vector resulted in a high induction of luciferase activity in cells transfected with either pNF-κB-Luc or pAP-1-Luc (n = 3 experiments) (Figures 8A and B). In the presence of 15d-PGJ_2, the activity of both reporter plasmids was diminished and completely blocked by cotransfection with a human PPARγ expression vector. These results suggest that 15d-PGJ_2 may decrease iNOS and MMP-13 transcription by interfering with the NF-κB and AP-1 signaling pathways.

DISCUSSION

Recently, several lines of evidence have suggested that PPAR ligands not only regulate lipid and glucose homeostasis, but may also mitigate the inflammatory processes. First, the effects of several clinically important nonsteroidal antiinflammatory drugs (e.g., indomethacin, ibuprofen, and fenoprofen) have recently been shown to be mediated not only by inhibition of cyclooxygenase (COX), but also through activation of PPARγ (43). Second, it has been shown that polyunsaturated fatty acids such as those found in fish oil activate PPARγ (44) and ameliorate inflammatory symptoms in Crohn's disease and RA (45,46). Third, resolution of inflammation was severely delayed in PPARα knockout mice following challenge with either arachidonic acid or its derivative, leukotriene B_4 (47). Finally, in vitro studies have shown that treatment with natural and synthetic PPARγ ligands inhibits the production of a number of inflammatory mediators in several cell types, including monocytes (21), macrophages (22,26,27), and a colonic epithelial cell line (28). Since chondrocytes are key players in arthritis through the elaboration of multiple proinflammatory mediators such as NO, prostaglandins, and MMPs, the role of PPARγ in the activation of these cells by IL-1β was investigated.

By RT-PCR and immunohistochemical analysis, we showed that PPARγ is expressed in human articular

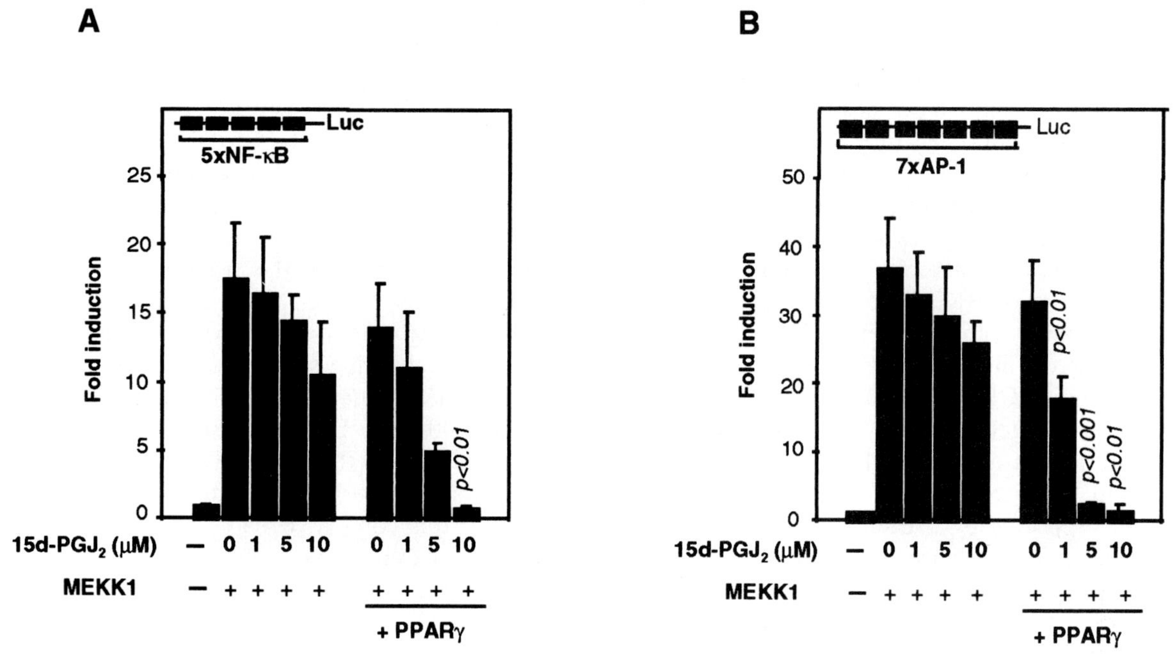

Figure 8. PPARγ-dependent inhibition by 15d-PGJ_2 of MEKK1-induced activation of the activator protein 1 (AP-1) and nuclear factor κB (NF-κB) luciferase reporter plasmids (pAP-1-Luc and pNF-κB-Luc, respectively). HeLa cells were transiently cotransfected with 1 μg of either **A,** pNF-κB-Luc, containing 5 copies of the consensus NF-κB response element (5×NF-κB), or **B,** pAP-1-Luc, containing 7 copies of the consensus AP-1 response element (7×AP-1), together with 50 ng of pFC-MEKK1 and 50 ng of pSV40-β-galactosidase, in the absence or presence of 50 ng of human pSG5-PPARγ. Cells were incubated in the presence or absence (control) of increasing concentrations of 15d-PGJ_2 and were harvested 24 hours later. Luciferase activities were determined and normalized to β-galactosidase measured in the same sample. Results are expressed as fold induction, considering 1 as the luciferase activity of unstimulated transfected cells, and represent the mean ± SEM of 3 independent experiments. *P* values indicate the significance of the differences from autologous basal values. See Figures 3 and 7 for other definitions.

chondrocytes at the mRNA and protein levels. While our study was in progress, Bordji et al described PPARγ expression in rat chondrocytes and showed that PPARγ mRNA is down-regulated by IL-1 (25). In the transcriptional study, two PPARγ ligands, 15d-PGJ_2 and BRL 49653, were added to chondrocytes transfected with a PPRE reporter plasmid. These reagents significantly increased the transcriptional activity of PPRE. Taken together, these results suggest that PPARγ is present and functional in human articular chondrocytes.

To investigate the involvement of PPARγ in chondrocyte function, we tested the ability of various PPAR ligands to modulate the production of NO and MMP-13 production. Our results showed that 15d-PGJ_2 and BRL 49653 inhibit IL-1β–stimulated NO and MMP-13 release into the culture medium in a dose-dependent manner. In contrast, the selective PPARα agonist, Wy 14643, did not affect NO and MMP-13 production. These findings contrast with previous data showing that ligands for PPARα, but not for PPARγ, inhibit inflammatory responses in vascular smooth cells (48). Although the reasons for this difference are unclear, the effects of these ligands may be tissue specific. The absence of an effect of PPARα ligands in chondrocytes may also be due either to a low level of PPARα in this tissue or to the lack of its transcriptional regulation on these genes.

Although 15d-PGJ_2 and BRL 49653 activated $PPRE_3$-Tk-Luc to the same extent, the PPARγ ligand BRL 49653, known to be more selective, showed a much weaker inhibitory effect on NO and MMP-13 production (IC_{50} of 20 μM and 30 μM, respectively) than did 15d-PGJ_2 (IC_{50} of 1 μM and 2 μM, respectively). This difference in the potency of PPARγ ligands to inhibit chondrocyte responses is comparable with that observed in other cell types (22,26,28) and is in marked contrast to their relative binding affinities for PPARγ. Indeed, the inhibition of NO and MMP-13 production by 15d-PGJ_2 occurs in a concentration range (1–10 μM) that is consistent with its dissociation constant (K_d) for PPARγ.

However, elevated concentrations of BRL 49653, much higher than its K_d for PPARγ, are required to accomplish the same effect. Although the reasons for this difference are not known, one can postulate that cellular metabolism of these compounds may affect their relative efficacy as ligands.

Our results are consistent with other reports showing that inhibition of NO and proinflammatory cytokine production by macrophages requires a much higher concentration of BRL 49653 than of 15d-PGJ_2 (22). Similarly, in a colon cancer cell line, Caco-2, 15d-PGJ_2 was also a more potent inhibitor of IL-1β–induced IL-8 and MCP-1 expression than was BRL 49653 (28). Taken together, these data, as well as our findings, suggest that additional PPARγ-independent pathways might also be involved in 15d-PGJ_2 effects. This is further supported by a recent study showing that 15d-PGJ_2 inhibits iNOS expression and its promoter activity in neuronal cells. However, troglitazone, another selective PPARγ ligand, did not mimic the 15d-PGJ_2 effect (49). Furthermore, both compounds were unable to stimulate the activity of PPAR-dependent promoters in these cells.

MEKK-1, situated upstream in the functional hierarchy of the MAP kinase family, is activated by IL-1β and TNFα (35,36). MEKK-1 has been shown to stimulate the kinase activity of inhibitor of NF-κB kinase α (IκKα) and IκKβ (36,50), which results in the phosphorylation of inhibitor of NF-κB (IκB), targeting IκB's degradation by the ubiquitin–proteasome pathway. IκB degradation leads to the release of NF-κB complexes, which can migrate to the nucleus, bind to DNA, and regulate transcription (51). Other cascades triggered by IL-1β and TNFα are the JNK/SAPK and p38 MAPK pathways. MEKK-1 has also been shown to be implicated in these pathways by activation of MAPK kinase 4 (also called SAPK/extracellular signal–regulated kinase kinase 1 and JNK kinase 1), which in turn activates JNK/SAPK and p38 MAPK (37–39). Activated JNK and p38 MAPK phosphorylate their substrates c-Jun and activating transcription factor 2, which are involved in the regulation of AP-1 activity (52). Thus MEKK-1, a kinase activated by IL-1β and TNFα, is a critical coordinate regulator of NF-κB and AP-1 pathways.

Experiments to determine the level at which PPARγ activation affected iNOS and MMP-13 expression showed that 15d-PGJ_2 suppressed IL-1β–stimulated iNOS and MMP-13 mRNA induction in human chondrocytes in a dose-dependent manner. To further evaluate whether the effect of 15d-PGJ_2 was mediated through PPARγ, transient transfection experiments were performed on HeLa cells, which do not express PPARγ (22). We showed a complete reduction in MEKK-1–induced iNOS and MMP-13 promoter activity by 15d-PGJ_2 in the presence of PPARγ, indicating that the inhibitory action of 15d-PGJ_2 takes place through PPARγ. Although the present data cannot exclude the possibility that 15d-PGJ_2 may also destabilize the MMP-13 and iNOS mRNA, the effects of 15d-PGJ_2 appear likely to be at the transcriptional level. Functional analysis of the MMP-13 and iNOS promoter regions, using deletional analysis or selective base mutation of the binding sequence, revealed that the inducibility of these genes was mediated by AP-1 and NF-κB sites (32,40–42). In transient cotransfection experiments, we showed that 15d-PGJ_2 inhibits the activities of these transcription factors induced by MEKK-1.

In this context, it has been reported that treatment of peritoneal macrophages with 15d-PGJ_2 or several synthetic PPARγ ligands inhibited interferon-γ–induced iNOS expression and suppressed the induction of gelatinase B and scavenger receptor A gene transcription in response to phorbol ester stimulation. Using minimal promoters containing binding sites for AP-1, NF-κB, and signal transducer and activator of transcription, which play a critical role in the activation of these gene promoters, those investigators showed that PPARγ activators inhibit 12-0-tetradecanoylphorbol-13-acetate–induced AP-1 as well as lipopolysaccharide-induced NF-κB activation (22). Taken together, these results suggest that 15d-PGJ_2 inhibits gene expression, at least in part, by antagonizing the activities of the transcription factors AP-1 and NF-κB.

Transcription factor–dependent gene expression involves a growing family of proteins, termed transcriptional coactivators, that most likely function by facilitating or bridging the sequence-specific activators to the basal transcription machinery and altering chromatin. Cyclic AMP–responsive element–binding protein binding protein and its structural homolog p300, along with steroid receptor coactivator 1, were shown to be essential for the activation of transcription by a large number of regulated transcription factors, including AP-1 and NF-κB (53–56). Since PPARγ has also been shown to interact with these coactivators (57), it is tempting to speculate that PPARγ exerts its inhibitory effects by titrating AP-1 and NF-κB coactivators. Furthermore, PPARγ may also antagonize AP-1 and NF-κB activity through protein–protein or protein–DNA interactions involving PPARγ itself. However, given the complexity of PPARγ expression and activity regulation, the possible involvement of other mechanisms leading to the down-regulation of AP-1 and NF-κB activity cannot be ruled out.

It has been shown that 15d-PGJ_2 is formed from PGD_2 in vivo, and PGD_2 can readily be converted to J_2 prostaglandins in the presence of plasma (58,59). PGD_2 is among the most abundantly produced prostaglandins in synovial fluid and is produced by synovial fibroblasts and synovial mast cells upon stimulation (60,61). Therefore, PGD_2 derivatives may reach a functionally significant level in the synovial fluid and act as a negative feedback loop for inflammation control. Indeed, while our study was in progress, it was shown that inflammation resolution in carrageenin-induced pleurisy in rats was associated with an increase in COX-2 expression and in PGJ_2 and PGD_2 production, as well as with a decrease in PGE_2 production. It was also shown that NS-398, a selective COX-2 inhibitor, exacerbates inflammation, a phenomenon attenuated following PGD_2 and 15d-PGJ_2 administration (62). Su et al (28) reported that troglitazone and BRL 49653 significantly inhibited intestinal inflammation in an animal model of acute colitis. Taken together, these data suggest that PPARγ ligands have antiinflammatory properties in vivo.

In summary, our study demonstrates that PPARγ is present and functionally active in human chondrocytes. We find that PPARγ ligands inhibit IL-1β–induced production of NO and MMP-13. The inhibition of iNOS and MMP-13 induction was PPARγ dependent and occurred at the transcriptional level, probably through repression of NF-κB and AP-1 signaling. In view of the crucial role that proinflammatory cytokines play in rheumatic diseases, our data provide strong evidence that the PPARγ system may represent a therapeutic target in these pathologies. Inhibitors of proinflammatory cytokine synthesis, signal transduction, and action, such as PPARγ ligands, would be of immense value in the management of these debilitating diseases. Furthermore, the centrality of proinflammatory cytokine signaling, NF-κB, and AP-1 in the biology of many immune cell types makes the PPARγ pathway extremely interesting.

ACKNOWLEDGMENTS

The authors thank Dr. C. K. Glass (University of California, San Diego) for kindly providing us with $PPRE_3$-Tk-Luc, Dr. S. A. Kliewer (Glaxo Wellcome, Research Triangle Park, NC) for the PPARγ expression vector, Dr. R. A. Shapiro (University of Pittsburgh, Pittsburgh, PA) for the iNOS promoter construct, and Dr. A. Amin (Hospital for Joint Diseases, New York, NY) for the iNOS cDNA. We are also grateful to Kayghobad Kiansa, François-Cyril Jolicoeur, Viorica Lascau-Coman, and ChangShang Geng for their technical expertise, and to Shirley McCarthy for her assistance in manuscript preparation.

REFERENCES

1. Cooper WO, Fava RA, Gates CA, Cremer MA, Townes AS. Acceleration of onset of collagen-induced arthritis by intra-articular injection of tumour necrosis factor or transforming growth factor-beta. Clin Exp Immunol 1992;89:244–50.
2. Henderson B, Pettipher ER. Arthritogenic actions of recombinant IL-1 and tumour necrosis factor alpha in the rabbit: evidence for synergistic interactions between cytokines in vivo. Clin Exp Immunol 1989;75:306–10.
3. Pelletier JP, Martel-Pelletier J, Howell DS. Etiopathogenesis of osteoarthritis. In: Koopman WJ, editor. Arthritis and allied conditions: a textbook of rheumatology. 13th ed. Baltimore: Williams & Wilkins; 1997. p. 1969–84.
4. Sakurai H, Kohsaka H, Liu MF, Higashiyama H, Hirata Y, Kanno K, et al. Nitric oxide production and inducible nitric oxide synthase expression in inflammatory arthritides. J Clin Invest 1995;96: 2357–63.
5. Burger D, Rezzonico R, Li J-M, Modoux C, Pierce RA, Welgus HG, et al. Imbalance between interstitial collagenase and tissue inhibitor of metalloproteinases 1 in synoviocytes and fibroblasts upon direct contact with stimulated T lymphocytes: involvement of membrane-associated cytokines. Arthritis Rheum 1998;41: 1748–59.
6. Farrell AJ, Blake DR, Palmer RM, Moncada S. Increased concentrations of nitrite in synovial fluid and serum samples suggest increased nitric oxide synthesis in rheumatic diseases. Ann Rheum Dis 1992;51:1219–22.
7. Pelletier J, Jovanovic D, Fernandes JC, Manning P, Connor JR, Currie MG, et al. Reduction in the structural changes of experimental osteoarthritis by a nitric oxide inhibitor. Osteoarthritis Cartilage 1999;7:416–8.
8. Pelletier JP, Lascau-Coman V, Jovanovic D, Fernandes JC, Manning P, Connor JR, et al. Selective inhibition of inducible nitric oxide synthase in experimental osteoarthritis is associated with reduction in tissue levels of catabolic factors. J Rheumatol 1999; 26:2002–14.
9. Connor JR, Manning PT, Settle SL, Moore WM, Jerome GM, Webber RK, et al. Suppression of adjuvant-induced arthritis by selective inhibition of inducible nitric oxide synthase. Eur J Pharmacol 1995;273:15–24.
10. Clancy RM, Amin AR, Abramson SB. The role of nitric oxide in inflammation and immunity. Arthritis Rheum 1998;41:1141–51.
11. Lotz M, Hashimoto S, Kuhn K. Mechanisms of chondrocyte apoptosis. Osteoarthritis Cartilage 1999;7:389–91.
12. Pelletier JP, Mineau F, Ranger P, Tardif G, Martel-Pelletier J. The increased synthesis of inducible nitric oxide inhibits IL-1ra synthesis by human articular chondrocytes: possible role in osteoarthritic cartilage degradation. Osteoarthritis Cartilage 1996;4: 77–84.
13. Stahle-Backdahl M, Sandstedt B, Bruce K, Lindahl A, Jimenez MG, Vega JA, et al. Collagenase-3 (MMP-13) is expressed during human fetal ossification and re-expressed in postnatal bone remodeling and in rheumatoid arthritis. Lab Invest 1997;76:717–28.
14. Reboul P, Pelletier JP, Tardif G, Cloutier JM, Martel-Pelletier J. The new collagenase, collagenase-3, is expressed and synthesized by human chondrocytes but not by synoviocytes: a role in osteoarthritis. J Clin Invest 1996;97:2011–9.
15. Knauper V, Lopez-Otin C, Smith B, Knight G, Murphy G. Biochemical characterization of human collagenase-3. J Biol Chem 1996;271:1544–50.
16. Lemberger T, Desvergne B, Wahli W. Peroxisome proliferator-

activated receptors: a nuclear receptor signaling pathway in lipid physiology. Annu Rev Cell Dev Biol 1996;12:335–63.
17. Spiegelman BM. PPAR-gamma: adipogenic regulator and thiazolidinedione receptor. Diabetes 1998;47:507–14.
18. Krey G, Braissant O, L'Horset F, Kalkhoven E, Perroud M, Parker MG, et al. Fatty acids, eicosanoids, and hypolipidemic agents identified as ligands of peroxisome proliferator-activated receptors by coactivator-dependent receptor ligand assay. Mol Endocrinol 1997;11:779–91.
19. Kliewer SA, Lenhard JM, Willson TM, Patel I, Morris DC, Lehmann JM. A prostaglandin J2 metabolite binds peroxisome proliferator-activated receptor gamma and promotes adipocyte differentiation. Cell 1995;83:813–9.
20. Lehmann JM, Moore LB, Smith-Oliver TA, Wilkison WO, Willson TM, Kliewer SA. An antidiabetic thiazolidinedione is a high affinity ligand for peroxisome proliferator-activated receptor gamma (PPAR gamma). J Biol Chem 1995;270:12953–6.
21. Jiang C, Ting AT, Seed B. PPAR-gamma agonists inhibit production of monocyte inflammatory cytokines. Nature 1998;391:82–6.
22. Ricote M, Li AC, Willson TM, Kelly CJ, Glass CK. The peroxisome proliferator-activated receptor-gamma is a negative regulator of macrophage activation. Nature 1998;391:79–82.
23. Greene ME, Blumberg B, McBride OW, Yi HF, Kronquist K, Kwan K, et al. Isolation of the human peroxisome proliferator activated receptor gamma cDNA: expression in hematopoietic cells and chromosomal mapping. Gene Expr 1995;4:281–99.
24. Clark RB, Bishop-Bailey D, Estrada-Hernandez T, Hla T, Puddington L, Padula SJ. The nuclear receptor PPARγ and immunoregulation: PPAR γ mediates inhibition of helper T cell responses. J Immunol 2000;164:1364–71.
25. Bordji K, Grillasca JP, Gouze JN, Magdalou J, Schohn H, Keller JM, et al. Evidence for the presence of peroxisome proliferator-activated receptor (PPAR) alpha and gamma and retinoid Z receptor in cartilage: PPARgamma activation modulates the effects of interleukin-1beta on rat chondrocytes. J Biol Chem 2000;275:12243–50.
26. Colville-Nash PR, Qureshi SS, Willis D, Willoughby DA. Inhibition of inducible nitric oxide synthase by peroxisome proliferator-activated receptor agonists: correlation with induction of heme oxygenase 1. J Immunol 1998;161:978–84.
27. Marx N, Sukhova G, Murphy C, Libby P, Plutzky J. Macrophages in human atheroma contain PPARgamma: differentiation-dependent peroxisomal proliferator-activated receptor gamma (PPARgamma) expression and reduction of MMP-9 activity through PPARgamma activation in mononuclear phagocytes in vitro. Am J Pathol 1998;153:17–23.
28. Su CG, Wen X, Bailey ST, Jiang W, Rangwala SM, Keilbaugh SA, et al. A novel therapy for colitis utilizing PPAR-γ ligands to inhibit the epithelial inflammatory response. J Clin Invest 1999;104:383–9.
29. Martel-Pelletier J, Mineau F, Jovanovic D, di Battista JA, Pelletier J-P. Mitogen-activated protein kinase and nuclear factor κB together regulate interleukin-17–induced nitric oxide production in human osteoarthritic chondrocytes: possible role of transactivating factor mitogen–activated protein kinase–activated protein kinase (MAPKAPK). Arthritis Rheum 1999;42:2399–409.
30. Moldovan F, Pelletier J-P, Hambor J, Cloutier J-M, Martel-Pelletier J. Collagenase-3 (matrix metalloprotease 13) is preferentially localized in the deep layer of human arthritic cartilage in situ: in vitro mimicking effect by transforming growth factor β. Arthritis Rheum 1997;40:1653–61.
31. Tardif G, Pelletier JP, Dupuis M, Hambor JE, Martel-Pelletier J. Cloning, sequencing and characterization of the 5′-flanking region of the human collagenase-3 gene. Biochem J 1997;323:13–6.
32. De Vera ME, Shapiro RA, Nussler AK, Mudgett JS, Simmons RL, Morris SM Jr, et al. Transcriptional regulation of human inducible nitric oxide synthase (NOS2) gene by cytokines: initial analysis of the human NOS2 promoter. Proc Natl Acad Sci U S A 1996;93:1054–9.
33. Kliewer SA, Sundseth SS, Jones SA, Brown PJ, Wisely GB, Koble CS, et al. Fatty acids and eicosanoids regulate gene expression through direct interactions with peroxisome proliferator-activated receptors alpha and gamma. Proc Natl Acad Sci U S A 1997;94:4318–23.
34. Green LC, Wagner DA, Glogowski J, Skipper PL, Wishnok JS, Tannenbaum SR. Analysis of nitrate, nitrite, and [15N]nitrate in biological fluids. Anal Biochem 1982;126:131–8.
35. Baud V, Liu ZG, Bennett B, Suzuki N, Xia Y, Karin M. Signaling by proinflammatory cytokines: oligomerization of TRAF2 and TRAF6 is sufficient for JNK and IKK activation and target gene induction via an amino-terminal effector domain. Genes Dev 1999;13:1297–308.
36. Nemoto S, DiDonato JA, Lin A. Coordinate regulation of IκB kinases by mitogen-activated protein kinase kinase kinase 1 and NF-κB-inducing kinase. Mol Cell Biol 1998;18:7336–43.
37. Yan M, Dai T, Deak JC, Kyriakis JM, Zon LI, Woodgett JR, et al. Activation of stress-activated protein kinase by MEKK1 phosphorylation of its activator SEK1. Nature 1994;372:798–800.
38. Yujiri T, Sather S, Fanger GR, Johnson GL. Role of MEKK1 in cell survival and activation of JNK and ERK pathways defined by targeted gene disruption. Science 1998;282:1911–4.
39. Lin A, Minden A, Martinetto H, Claret FX, Lange-Carter C, Mercurio F, et al. Identification of a dual specificity kinase that activates the Jun kinases and p38-Mpk2. Science 1995;268:286–90.
40. Taylor BS, de Vera ME, Ganster RW, Wang Q, Shapiro RA, Morris SM Jr, et al. Multiple NF-kappaB enhancer elements regulate cytokine induction of the human inducible nitric oxide synthase gene. J Biol Chem 1998;273:15148–56.
41. Pendas AM, Balbin M, Llano E, Jimenez MG, Lopez-Otin C. Structural analysis and promoter characterization of the human collagenase-3 gene (MMP13). Genomics 1997;40:222–33.
42. Uria JA, Jimenez MG, Balbin M, Freije JMP, Lopez-Otin C. Differential effects of transforming growth factor-beta on the expression of collagenase-1 and collagenase-3 in human fibroblasts. J Biol Chem 1998;273:9769–77.
43. Lehmann JM, Lenhard JM, Oliver BB, Ringold GM, Kliewer SA. Peroxisome proliferator-activated receptors alpha and gamma are activated by indomethacin and other non-steroidal anti-inflammatory drugs. J Biol Chem 1997;272:3406–10.
44. Yu K, Bayona W, Kallen CB, Harding HP, Ravera CP, McMahon G, et al. Differential activation of peroxisome proliferator-activated receptors by eicosanoids. J Biol Chem 1995;270:23975–83.
45. Belluzzi A, Brignola C, Campieri M, Pera A, Boschi S, Miglioli M. Effect of an enteric-coated fish-oil preparation on relapses in Crohn's disease. N Engl J Med 1996;334:1557–60.
46. Lau CS, Morley KD, Belch JJ. Effects of fish oil supplementation on non-steroidal anti-inflammatory drug requirement in patients with mild rheumatoid arthritis—a double-blind placebo controlled study. Br J Rheumatol 1993;32:982–9.
47. Devchand PR, Keller H, Peters JM, Vazquez M, Gonzalez FJ, Wahli W. The PPARα-leukotriene B4 pathway to inflammation control. Nature 1996;384:39–43.
48. Staels B, Koenig W, Habib A, Merval R, Lebret M, Torra IP, et al. Activation of human aortic smooth-muscle cells is inhibited by PPARα but not by PPARγ activators. Nature 1998;393:790–3.
49. Petrova TV, Akama KT, van Eldik LJ. Cyclopentenone prostaglandins suppress activation of microglia: down-regulation of inducible nitric-oxide synthase by 15-deoxy-Δ12,14-prostaglandin J2. Proc Natl Acad Sci U S A 1999;96:4668–73.
50. Nakano H, Shindo M, Sakon S, Nishinaka S, Mihara M, Yagita H, et al. Differential regulation of IkappaB kinase alpha and beta by two upstream kinases, NF-kappaB-inducing kinase and mitogen-activated protein kinase/ERK kinase kinase-1. Proc Natl Acad Sci U S A 1998;95:3537–42.

51. Baldwin AS Jr. The NF-kappa B and I kappa B proteins: new discoveries and insights. Annu Rev Immunol 1996;14:649–83.
52. Karin M, Liu Zg, Zandi E. AP-1 function and regulation. Curr Opin Cell Biol 1997;9:240–6.
53. Kamei Y, Xu L, Heinzel T, Torchia J, Kurokawa R, Gloss B, et al. A CBP integrator complex mediates transcriptional activation and AP-1 inhibition by nuclear receptors. Cell 1996;85:403–14.
54. Lee SK, Kim HJ, Na SY, Kim TS, Choi HS, Im SY, et al. Steroid receptor coactivator-1 coactivates activating protein-1-mediated transactivations through interaction with the c-Jun and c-Fos subunits. J Biol Chem 1998;273:16651–4.
55. Gerritsen ME, Williams AJ, Neish AS, Moore S, Shi Y, Collins T. CREB-binding protein/p300 are transcriptional coactivators of p65. Proc Natl Acad Sci U S A 1997;94:2927–32.
56. Na SY, Lee SK, Han SJ, Choi HS, Im SY, Lee JW. Steroid receptor coactivator-1 interacts with the p50 subunit and coactivates nuclear factor kappaB-mediated transactivations. J Biol Chem 1998;273:10831–4.
57. Gelman L, Fruchart JC, Auwerx J. An update on the mechanisms of action of the peroxisome proliferator-activated receptors (PPARs) and their roles in inflammation and cancer. Cell Mol Life Sci 1999;55:932–43.
58. Hirata Y, Hayashi H, Ito S, Kikawa Y, Ishibashi M, Sudo M, et al. Occurrence of 9-deoxy-delta 9,delta 12-13,14-dihydroprostaglandin D2 in human urine. J Biol Chem 1988;263:16619–25.
59. Kikawa Y, Narumiya S, Fukushima M, Wakatsuka H, Hayaishi O. 9-deoxy-delta 9, delta 12-13,14-dihydroprostaglandin D2, a metabolite of prostaglandin D2 formed in human plasma. Proc Natl Acad Sci U S A 1984;81:1317–21.
60. Pietila P, Moilanen E, Seppala E, Nissila M, Lepisto P, Laitinen O, et al. Differences in the production of arachidonic acid metabolites between healthy and rheumatic synovial fibroblasts in vitro: a preliminary study. Scand J Rheumatol 1984;13:243–6.
61. De Paulis A, Ciccarelli A, Marinò I, de Crescenzo G, Marinò D, Marone G. Human synovial mast cells. II. Heterogeneity of the pharmacologic effects of antiinflammatory and immunosuppressive drugs. Arthritis Rheum 1997;40:469–78.
62. Gilroy DW, Colville-Nash PR, Willis D, Chivers J, Paul-Clark MJ, Willoughby DA. Inducible cyclooxygenase may have anti-inflammatory properties. Nat Med 1999;5:698–701.

ARTHRITIS & RHEUMATISM
Vol. 44, No. 3, March 2001, pp 608–617

Cyclic Tensile Strain Suppresses Catabolic Effects of Interleukin-1β in Fibrochondrocytes From the Temporomandibular Joint

Sudha Agarwal,[1] Ping Long,[1] Robert Gassner,[2] Nicholas P. Piesco,[1] and Michael J. Buckley[1]

Objective. **To discern the effects of continuous passive motion on inflamed temporomandibular joints (TMJ).**

Methods. **The effects of continuous passive motion on TMJ were simulated by exposing primary cultures of rabbit TMJ fibrochondrocyte monolayers to cyclic tensile strain (CTS) in the presence of recombinant human interleukin-1β (rHuIL-1β) in vitro. The messenger RNA (mRNA) induction of rHuIL-1β response elements was examined by semiquantitative reverse transcriptase–polymerase chain reaction. The synthesis of nitric oxide was examined by Griess reaction, and the synthesis of prostaglandin E_2 (PGE_2) was examined by radioimmunoassay. The synthesis of proteins was examined by Western blot analysis of the cell extracts, and synthesis of proteoglycans via incorporation of ^{35}S-sodium sulfate in the culture medium.**

Results. **Exposure of TMJ fibrochondrocytes to rHuIL-1β resulted in the induction of inducible nitric oxide synthase (iNOS) and cyclooxygenase 2 (COX-2), which were paralleled by NO and PGE_2 production. Additionally, IL-1β induced significant levels of collagenase (matrix metalloproteinase 1 [MMP-1]) within 4 hours, and this was sustained over a period of 48 hours. Concomitant application of CTS abrogated the catabolic effects of IL-1β on TMJ chondrocytes by inhibiting iNOS, COX-2, and MMP-1 mRNA production and NO, PGE_2, and MMP-1 synthesis. CTS also counteracted cartilage degradation by augmenting expression of mRNA for tissue inhibitor of metalloproteinases 2 that is inhibited by rHuIL-1β. In parallel, CTS also counteracted rHuIL-1β–induced suppression of proteoglycan synthesis. Nevertheless, the presence of an inflammatory signal was a prerequisite for the observed CTS actions, because fibrochondrocytes, when exposed to CTS alone, did not exhibit any of the effects described above.**

Conclusion. **CTS acts as an effective antagonist of rHuIL-1β by potentially diminishing its catabolic actions on TMJ fibrochondrocytes. Furthermore, CTS actions appear to involve disruption/regulation of signal transduction cascade of rHuIL-1β upstream of mRNA transcription.**

Temporomandibular joint (TMJ) disorders are debilitating and result in progressive degeneration of articular cartilage, the disk, and/or the subchondral bone, leading to disharmonious function of the entire masticatory apparatus (1–4). As a heterogeneous group of diseases, TMJ disorders are commonly diagnosed as arthritic conditions resulting from trauma or infections (3–5). Analysis of synovial fluid from inflamed TMJ has revealed the presence of elevated levels of cytokines and other inflammatory mediators (6–10). Proinflammatory cytokines are produced by chondrocytes, cells that line the joint cavity, and cells of the immune system that have migrated into the subsynovial space (6–10). Among the proinflammatory cytokines, local production of interleukin-1 (IL-1) appears to be directly responsible for the destruction of cartilage (6–8,10). IL-1 induces catabolic responses in chondrocytes by stimulating expression of proteases, including stromelysin, collagenase, and tissue plasminogen activator. Chondrocytes stimulated with IL-1β have been found to produce massive amounts of inducible nitric oxide synthase

Supported by grants from the Oral and Maxillofacial Surgery Foundation, the NIH (grant R-15-DE-12976), and Central Medical Research Funds, University of Pittsburgh.

[1]Sudha Agarwal, PhD, Ping Long, MD, Nicholas P. Piesco, MD, Michael J. Buckley, DMD, MS: University of Pittsburgh, Pittsburgh, Pennsylvania; [2]Robert Gassner, DMD, MD: Maxillofaziale Chirurgie, Innsbruck, Austria.

Address correspondence and reprint requests to Michael J. Buckley, DMD, MS, Department of Oral and Maxillofacial Surgery, 2 South UPMC Montefiore Hospital, University of Pittsburgh, 3471 Fifth Avenue, Pittsburgh, PA 15213.

Submitted for publication July 3, 2000; accepted in revised form October 23, 2000.

(iNOS) and NO, potent mediators of the destructive effects of IL-1. NO induces the synthesis of tissue-destructive enzymes and inhibits matrix synthesis (11–17). IL-1 is also a potent inducer of cyclooxygenase 2 (COX-2) and prostaglandin E_2 (PGE_2) synthesis (18–20). IL-1 also suppresses α1(II) procollagen messenger RNA (mRNA) expression and proteoglycan synthesis. Collectively, IL-1β–induced inhibition of matrix synthesis and the induction of proteases result in cartilage resorption and pathology of the TMJ disorder (18–24).

Interestingly, physical therapies such as continuous passive motion (CPM) exert reparative effects on diseased or inflamed TMJ (25–28), as well as in postsurgical rehabilitation of TMJ. The beneficial effects of CPM are mainly attributed to the increased circulation and the removal of inflammatory exudates from synovial fluids (29). Whether CPM also acts directly on chondrocytes is not yet discerned. Since inflammatory cytokines such as IL-1β play a major role in both the initiation and the progression of cartilage destruction, we hypothesized that CPM actions may involve suppression of proinflammatory pathways. To test this hypothesis in vitro, we examined the effects of equibiaxial cyclic tensile strain (CTS) on primary cultures of chondrocytes from rabbit TMJ in the presence of recombinant human IL-1β (rHuIL-1β), to mimic effects of CPM in vivo in arthritic TMJ disorders.

MATERIALS AND METHODS

Animals and materials. New Zealand white rabbits weighing 6–7 lb were obtained from Myrtle's Rabbitry (Thompson Station, TN). Materials were obtained from the following suppliers: tissue culture media, sera, and antibiotics from Gibco (Grand Island, NY); crude clostridial collagenase from Worthington (Freehold, NJ); Luminol, Reflection autoradiographic film, ^{35}sodium sulfate (1 Ci/mmole), and PGE_2 radioimmunoassay (RIA) kit from NEN (Boston, MA); rHuIL-1β from Genentech (La Jolla, CA); pronectine-coated Bioflex II culture plates from Flexcell (Hillsborough, NC); primers for polymerase chain reaction (PCR) synthesized by Bio-Synthesis (Lewisville, TX); molecular biology reagents from Perkin-Elmer (Norwalk, CT); antibodies from Santa Cruz Biotechnology (Santa Cruz, CA); and all other reagents from Sigma (St. Louis, MO).

Isolation of chondrocytes from TMJ. Cartilage from the disk of TMJ was aseptically excised from the disk and condyles of TMJ, and the fibrochondrocytes were isolated by sequential enzymatic treatment with 0.2% trypsin and 0.2% clostridial collagenase (30). TMJ chondrocytes were then washed and resuspended in TCM (Ham's F-12, 10% fetal calf serum, penicillin [100 units/ml]/streptomycin [10 μg/ml]), and plated at a rate of 2×10^5/2 ml TCM in 6-well Bioflex culture plates and cultured for 8 days at 37°C in a CO_2 incubator (30). The cultures reached 90% confluence in 6–8 days. In primary cultures, these fibrochondrocytes retain their differentiated phenotype and express mRNA for aggrecan, biglycan, transforming growth factor β1 (TGFβ1), and type II collagen (Figure 1A), as well as synthesize chondroitin sulfate proteoglycans (Figure 1D), aggrecan, and type II collagen (Figure 1B) (31,32). Since fibrocartilage lacks blood, nerve, and lymphatics, these cultures are highly unlikely to be contaminated by other cell types. Also, such fibrochondrocytes respond to IL-1β in a manner similar to that of articular cartilage explants (33). Trypan blue exclusion confirmed >99% viability of cells in culture.

Chondrocyte activation and exposure to equibiaxial strain. Primary fibrochondrocyte cultures that were 6–8 days old and 90% confluent were grown on Bioflex plates, washed twice with TCM, and subjected to equibiaxial strain (30) in a Flexercell unit (Flexcell). The equibiaxial strain applied was at a rate of 3 cycles/minute (0.05 Hz), i.e., 10 seconds of a maximum of 6% equibiaxial strain followed by 10 seconds of relaxation per cycle (180 cycles/hour), providing reproducible suppression of IL-1β–induced iNOS mRNA expression and NO production. The strain was calculated as follows: circumferential strain = 2π (change in radius)/2π (original radius) = (change in radius)/(original radius) = radial strain. In this system, the membrane of each well of the Bioflex plate is strained on a loading post to apply equibiaxial strain on the membrane. The cells cultured on the membrane are thus subjected to the equibiaxial strain equivalent to that applied to the membrane. The chondrocytes growing on the Bioflex plates were divided into 4 groups: untreated and unstrained control cells, cells treated with CTS alone, cells treated with rHuIL-1β (1 ng/ml) alone, and cells treated with CTS and rHuIL-1β (1 ng/ml). The cells were subjected to CTS at the time of addition of rHuIL-1β in most of the experiments.

Reverse transcriptase–PCR (RT-PCR). The fibrochondrocytes on the Bioflex membrane growing above the loading posts were carefully scraped and subjected to RNA extraction with an RNA extraction kit (Qiagen, Santa Clara, CA). A total of 0.5 μg of RNA was mixed with 1 μg oligo-dT (12–18 oligomer) in reverse transcription buffer and incubated for 10 minutes at room temperature. Thereafter, the reaction mixture was cooled on ice and incubated with 200 units of Moloney murine leukemia virus reverse transcriptase for 60 minutes at 37°C. The complementary DNA thus obtained was amplified with 0.1 μg of specific primers in a reaction mixture containing 200 μM dNTP and 0.1 units of *Taq* polymerase in PCR buffer. PCR was performed in a DNA thermal cycler (Perkin-Elmer) for 30 cycles of 40 seconds at 94°C, 40 seconds at 62°C, and 60 seconds at 720°C. The sequence of sense and antisense rabbit primers used was as follows: GAPDH (293 bp) sense 5′-TCACCATCTTCCAGGAGCGA-3′, antisense 5′CAC-AATGCCGAAGTGGTCGT′; iNOS (243 bp) sense 5′-CGCCC-TTCCGCAGTTTCT-3′, antisense 5′-TCCAGGAGGACAT-GCAGCAC-3′; matrix metalloproteinase 3 (MMP-3) (322 bp) sense 5′TCAGTTCGTCCTCACTCCAG, antisense 5′-TTG-GTCCACCTGTCATCTTC; tissue inhibitor of metalloproteinases 1 (TIMP-1) (326 bp) sense 5′-GCAACTCCGACCT-TGTCATC-3′, antisense 5′-AGCGTAGGTCTTGGTGAA GC-3′, TIMP-2 (414 bp) sense 5′-GTAGTGATCAGGGCC-AAG-3′, antisense 5′-TTCTCTGTGACCCAGTCCAT-3′; biglycan (406 bp) sense 5′-GATGGCCTGAAGCTCAA-3′, antisense 5′-GGTTTTTGAAGAGGCTG-3′; COX-2 (282 bp) sense 5′-TCAGCCACGCAGCAAATCCT-3′, antisense 5′-GTCATCTGGATGTCAGCACG-3′ (34); aggrecan (350 bp) sense 5′-CTACCTTGGAGGTCGTGGTGA-3′, antisense 5′-GTGCACGTACACGGTCCTGA-3′; type I collagen $\alpha 1$ (526 bp) sense 5′-TCAACGGTGCTCCTGGTGAAG-3′, antisense 5′-GGACCTTGGCTACCCTGAGAA-3′; and type II collagen (414 bp) sense 5′-TCAACAACCAGATCGAGAGCA-3′, antisense 5′-AGGTGAACCTGCTGTTGCCCT-3′ (provided by Dr. M. Heidaran, Orquest, Mountain View, CA).

Quantitative RT-PCR (RT-QCPCR). Heterologous competitor DNA for aggrecan or iNOS was constructed by PCR using a *Bam* HI–*Eco* RI fragment of v-erbB gene as a template and a PCR MIMIC construction kit (Clontech, Palo Alto, CA), as described earlier (30). The equimolar concentrations of the gene products were estimated by densitometric analysis of ethidium bromide–stained DNA in each lane (Optimus software; Media Cybernetics, Silver Spring, MD), and results were expressed as the mean number of mRNA molecules synthesized per μg of RNA.

Proteoglycan synthesis. Total proteoglycan synthesis was measured by incorporation of Na_2-$^{35}SO_4$ into chondroitin sulfate proteoglycans during the last 8 hours of the experiment. Subsequently, culture supernatants were extracted with 0.5*M* NaOH and the incorporated precursor was separated by size exclusion chromatography using a Pharmacia (Piscataway, NJ) PD-10 column. The ^{35}S incorporation in proteoglycans was measured by scintillation counting (30).

Nitrite determination. NO production was determined as the nitrite concentration in culture medium, by use of a spectrophotometric assay based on the Griess reaction (30).

PGE_2 measurements. PGE_2 was measured in the culture supernatants of chondrocytes at various time intervals by RIA, according to the protocol recommended by the manufacturer (NEN).

Western blot analysis. Since measurable protein synthesis is apparent 8 hours after activation of cells, we selected 8 hours as the first time point at which to assess protein synthesis. Furthermore, because the effects of rHuIL-1β are sustained, we examined the effects of CTS on rHuIL-1β–induced protein synthesis 48 hours after activation of cells with rHuIL-1β. Protein synthesis in 50 μg of protein extracts was assessed by Western blot analysis (30), using goat anti–MMP-1 or anti–TIMP-2 as primary antibodies, rabbit anti-goat–horseradish peroxidase (HRP) as second antibody, and luminol as a chemiluminescent HRP substrate. The semiquantitative assessment of the luminescence in each band was performed by exposing the blots to Reflection autoradiographic film, followed by densitometric analysis of the luminescent bands using a camera equipped with a computer and Optimus software (Media Cybernetics).

Statistical analysis. Experiments were performed at least 3 times, and data are presented as the mean ± SEM. Each incubation condition was performed in triplicate, and replicates were averaged. The significance of differences between mean values was determined by Student's *t*-test.

RESULTS

TMJ cells express chondrocytic phenotype. Cells from the cartilage typically synthesize type II collagen and proteins associated with proteoglycan synthesis. However, cells from the TMJ fibrocartilage are special in nature and produce type I collagen, type II collagen, and proteoglycans. Ascertainment of the fibrochondrocyte-like phenotype of cells from TMJ showed that these cells exhibited constitutive expression of aggrecan, biglycan, TGFβ1, type I collagen, and type II collagen mRNA (Figure 1A). Additionally, these cells showed the presence of aggrecan and biglycan by immunofluorescence using anti-aggrecan and biglycan immunoglobulins as primary antibodies (Santa Cruz Biotechnology) (Figures 1B and C), and proteoglycan synthesis as observed by incorporation of Na_2-$^{35}SO_4$ into chondroitin sulfate proteoglycans (Figure 1D).

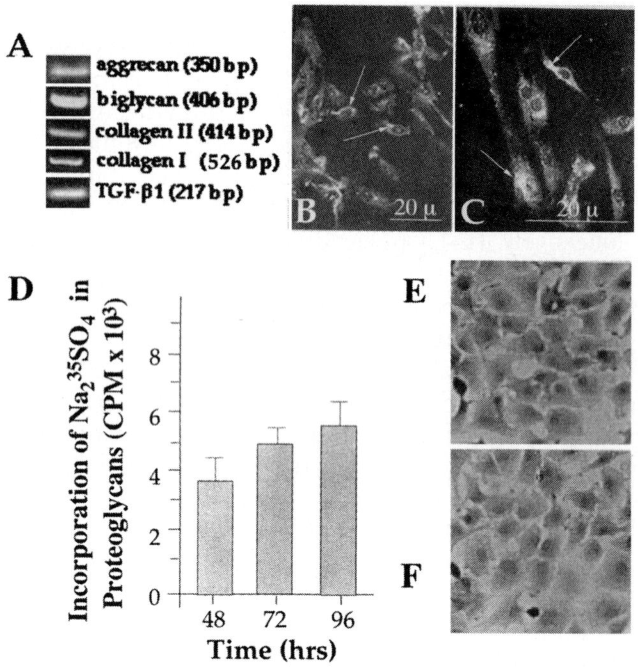

Figure 1. Phenotypic characteristics of rabbit temporomandibular joint (TMJ) fibrochondrocytes. **A,** Rabbit fibrochondrocytes exhibiting the presence of aggrecan, biglycan, type I collagen, type II collagen, and transforming growth factor β1 (TGF-β1)–specific mRNA, as assessed by reverse transcriptase–polymerase chain reaction. **B** and **C**, Rabbit TMJ disk chondrocytes showing the presence of aggrecan **(B)** and biglycan **(C)** by immunofluorescence (indicated by **arrows**). **D,** Presence of proteoglycans in TMJ disk chondrocytes as assessed by incorporation of $Na_2{}^{35}SO_4$ into chondroitin sulfate proteoglycans during the last 8 hours of the incubation. The proteoglycans were measured in a total of 2×10^6 cells in triplicate as described in Materials and Methods. Bars represent the mean and SEM of triplicate values. **E** and **F**, Morphology of fibrochondrocytes without treatment **(E)** and following exposure to cyclic tensile strain for 24 hours **(F)**.

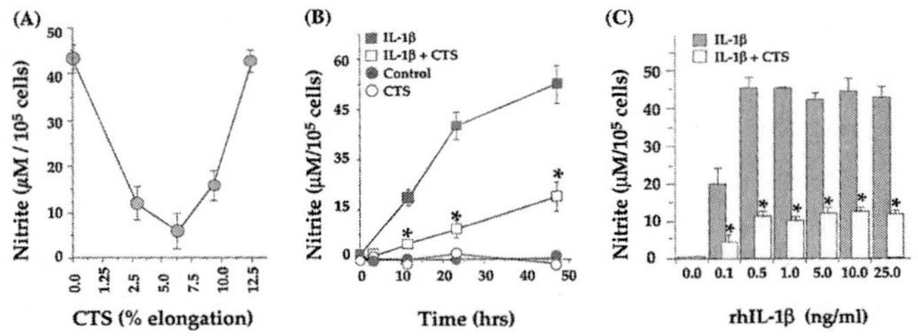

Figure 2. **A,** Effect of various magnitudes of equibiaxial cyclic tensile strain (CTS) on recombinant human interleukin-1β(rhIL-1β)–induced production of nitric oxide (NO) in temporomandibular joint (TMJ) fibrochondrocytes. TMJ chondrocytes were incubated with rHuIL-1β (1 ng/ml) and simultaneously exposed to 0%, 3%, 6%, 9%, or 12% CTS for 24 hours. **B,** Time-dependent inhibition of rhIL-1β–induced production of NO by CTS. TMJ condylar chondrocytes were untreated, or were exposed to 6% CTS, to 1 ng/ml rhIL-1β, or to rhIL-1β and CTS for 4, 12, 24, or 48 hours. **C,** Effect of CTS on production of NO in response to various concentrations of rhIL-1β. Chondrocytes were treated with 0, 0,1, 0.5, 1, 5, 10, or 25 ng/ml of rHuIL-1β for 24 hours with or without simultaneous exposure to 6% CTS for 24 hours. Accumulation of NO in the culture supernatant was assessed by Griess reaction. Data represent the mean and SEM of triplicate values in all experiments. $* = P < 0.05$ as compared with cells treated with IL-1β alone.

CTS suppresses IL-1β–dependent NO production. IL-1β initiates cartilage catabolism through transcriptional activation of multiple genes (7–14), including iNOS. Therefore, NO production initially was used as a marker to evaluate the effects of CTS on TMJ fibrochondrocytes. To evaluate the effects of CTS on rHuIL-1β actions, TMJ fibrochondrocytes were exposed to various magnitudes of equibiaxial CTS (3%, 6%, 9%, or 12% equibiaxial strain) in the presence or absence of rHuIL-1β (1 ng/ml). Fibrochondrocytes treated with rHuIL-1β alone exhibited high levels of iNOS mRNA, whereas cells treated simultaneously with rHuIL-1β and CTS for 4 hours or 24 hours exhibited a significant inhibition of NO production ($P \leq 0.05$) at 3%, 6%, and 9% elongation (Figure 2A); 12% elongation was ineffective in this respect. Since 6% CTS inhibited NO production optimally, in the rest of the experiments 6% CTS was used to examine its antiinflammatory effects on fibrochondrocytes. In these experiments, neither untreated control cells nor cells subjected to strain alone expressed iNOS mRNA. Morphologically, fibrochondrocytes subjected to CTS exhibited minimal cell deformation, compared with unstrained control cells (Figure 1E). Similarly, neither negligible cell detachment (<0.1%), as assessed by counting of nonadherent cells in the wells, nor cell death, as assessed by DNA fragmentation, was observed (data not shown).

Similar to articular chondrocytes, rHuIL-1β induces sustained NO production in fibrochondrocytes (30). Therefore, we determined whether the effects of CTS were paralleled in inhibiting the rHuIL-1β–dependent NO production in a sustained manner. As shown in Figure 2B, NO production increased rapidly after 12 hours of rHuIL-1β exposure, and this continued over a period of 48 hours. Interestingly, CTS consistently inhibited rHuIL-1β–induced NO production. Nevertheless, CTS alone did not induce NO production.

We next examined whether CTS inhibits rHuIL-1β–dependent NO production at higher concentrations of rHuIL-1β. TMJ chondrocytes were treated with 0, 0.5, 1, 10, or 25 ng/ml of rHuIL-1β for 24 hours, and the NO production was measured in the culture supernatants. As is apparent in Figure 2C, increasing the concentration of rHuIL-1β resulted in an increase in NO production between 0.1 and 1 ng/ml of rHuIL-1β, but higher concentrations of rHuIL-1β did not significantly elevate NO production. CTS (6% strain) suppressed rHuIL-1β–induced NO induction significantly ($P \leq 0.05$) at all concentrations of rHuIL-1β tested.

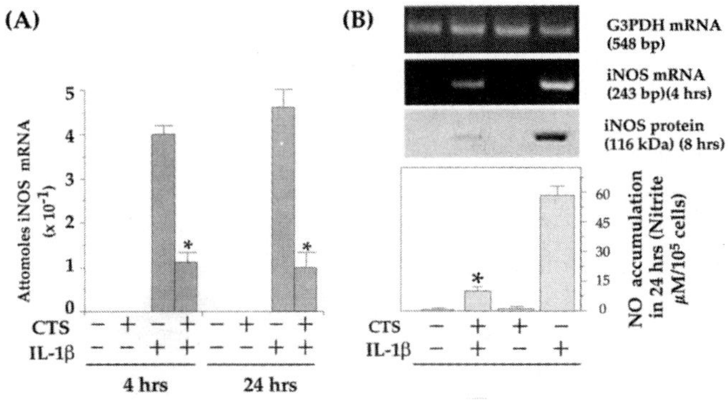

Figure 3. CTS-mediated inhibition of recombinant human IL-1β (rHuIL-1β)–dependent inducible nitric oxide synthase (iNOS) expression and production of NO in TMJ fibrochondrocytes. **A,** Quantitative reverse transcriptase–polymerase chain reaction (RT-QCPCR) analysis of iNOS mRNA expression, showing inhibition of IL-1β (1 ng/ml)–induced mRNA production by CTS in TMJ fibrochondrocytes. **B,** Parallel experiments showing CTS-mediated inhibition of rHuIL-1β–induced iNOS mRNA synthesis, iNOS protein synthesis, and total accumulation of NO in culture supernatants of the TMJ fibrochondrocytes. Control cells and those treated with CTS alone did not exhibit iNOS gene products in RT-QCPCR, iNOS protein in Western blot analysis, or production of NO in culture supernatants. Results represent the mean and SEM in 1 of 3 separate experiments, showing similar data. $* = P < 0.05$ as compared with cells treated with IL-1β alone. See Figure 2 for other definitions.

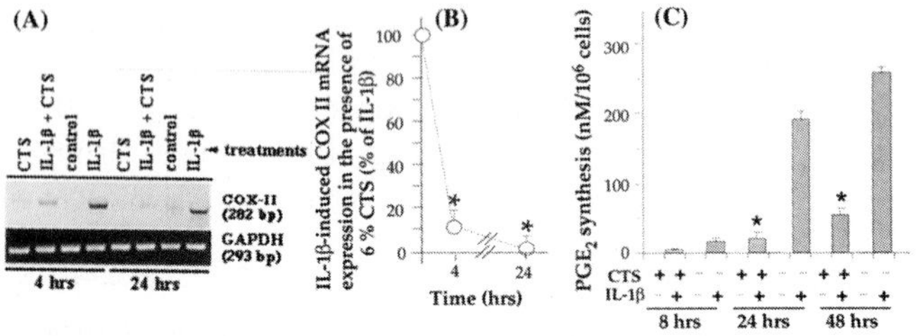

Figure 4. Inhibition of recombinant human IL-1β (rHuIL-1β)–dependent cyclooxygenase 2 (COX-II) mRNA expression and prostaglandin E_2 (PGE_2) synthesis by CTS in TMJ fibrochondrocytes. **A,** COX-II mRNA expression in chondrocytes either untreated or subjected to 1 ng/ml rHuIL-1β, 6% CTS, or rHuIL-1β and CTS for 4 or 24 hours, showing a marked inhibition of IL-1β–dependent mRNA expression of COX-II. **B,** Inhibition of COX-II mRNA expression by 6% CTS in the presence of IL-1β as compared with cells treated with IL-1β alone. **C,** PGE_2 synthesis in chondrocytes subjected to treatment regimens described in **A** for 8, 24, or 48 hours. PGE_2 synthesis was measured in the culture supernatants by radioimmunoassay. Data in **A** represent 1 of 3 separate experiments. Data in **B** and **C** represent means and SEM of triplicate values. $* = P < 0.05$ as compared with cells treated with IL-1β alone. See Figure 2 for other definitions.

CTS-mediated suppression of IL-1β–dependent NO production via inhibition of iNOS mRNA induction and iNOS synthesis. Since CTS abrogated IL-1β–induced NO production, we next examined whether this inhibition is due to the inhibition of iNOS mRNA induction. As evidenced by the data shown in Figure 3A, CTS significantly suppressed rHuIL-1β–induced iNOS mRNA expression as assessed by RT-QCPCR. Furthermore, the CTS-mediated abrogation of rHuIL-1β–induced iNOS mRNA expression was paralleled by decreased iNOS synthesis (Figure 3B). Fibrochondrocytes subjected to CTS alone, or untreated control cells, exhibited neither iNOS mRNA nor protein synthesis.

CTS suppresses IL-1β–dependent induction of COX-2 mRNA and PGE_2 synthesis. Another important proinflammatory molecule that is markedly up-regulated following IL-1β–dependent activation of chondrocytes is PGE_2, synthesized by COX-2 (18,35). To examine whether the physiologic consequences of CTS action also involve inhibition of rHuIL-1β–dependent COX-2 mRNA expression and PGE_2 production, we subjected TMJ fibrochondrocytes to rHuIL-1β and CTS simultaneously or individually for either 4 or 24 hours. As is apparent in Figure 4A, CTS significantly suppressed IL-1β–induced COX-2 mRNA expression. The semiquantitative measurement of the PCR products for COX-2 revealed 82% and 96% inhibition of COX-2 mRNA expression at 4 hours and 24 hours, respectively ($P \leq 0.01$). The inhibition of COX-2 mRNA induction by CTS was paralleled by 88% and 81% inhibition of rHuIL-1β–dependent PGE_2 production after 24 and 48 hours, respectively (Figure 4B). Unactivated control TMJ fibrochondrocytes or those exposed to CTS alone did not express COX-2 mRNA or PGE_2 production.

CTS suppresses IL-1β–dependent induction of collagenase (MMP-1). Previous studies have demonstrated that besides other MMP, induction of MMP-1 in response to IL-1β plays a critical role during cartilage degradation in inflammatory joint disease (23,36–40). Therefore, to be effective in controlling catabolic effects of rHuIL-1β, CTS actions must include suppression of collagenase production. Exposure of TMJ fibrochondrocytes to rHuIL-1β induced significant amounts of MMP-1. As expected, cells subjected to rHuIL-1β and CTS exhibited a marked (98% during the first 4 hours and 83% after 24 hours) inhibition of MMP-1 mRNA expression (Figure 5A). More important, the reduction in MMP-1 mRNA expression was reflected in the inhibition of MMP-1 synthesis as assessed by Western blot analysis, showing a 92% inhibition during the first 8 hours and 87% after 24 hours (Figure 5B). As observed above, untreated control cells, or cells treated with CTS alone, did not exhibit expression of MMP-1 mRNA.

CTS abrogates IL-1β–dependent inhibition of TIMP mRNA expression. For enhanced cartilage degradation, IL-1β not only activates metalloproteinases, but also inhibits TIMP production (41–43). This results in prolonged enzymatic activity of metalloproteinases (32–35). Therefore, to examine whether CTS also abrogates

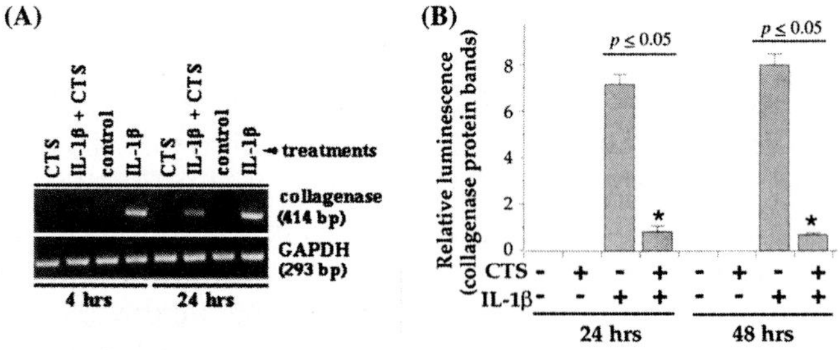

Figure 5. Effect of CTS on recombinant human IL-1β (rHuIL-1β)–dependent collagenase mRNA expression and synthesis in TMJ fibrochondrocytes. **A,** Expression of collagenase mRNA in chondrocytes either untreated or subjected to rHuIL-1β, CTS, or rHuIL-1β and CTS for 4 or 24 hours. **B,** Collagenase synthesis by fibrochondrocytes subjected to treatment regimens described in **A** for 24 or 48 hours. Collagenase synthesis was measured as the relative intensity of each band in Western blot analysis. Data in **A** represent 1 of 3 separate experiments. Data in **B** represent means and SEM of triplicate values. See Figure 2 for other definitions.

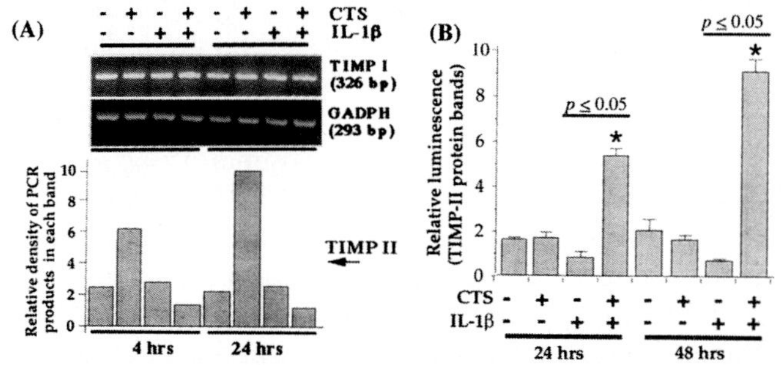

Figure 6. Effect of CTS on recombinant human IL-1β (rHuIL-1β)–dependent inhibition of tissue inhibitor of metalloproteinases (TIMP) mRNA expression. **A,** Expression of mRNA for TIMP I and TIMP II in TMJ chondrocytes either untreated or exposed to 1 ng/ml rHuIL-1β, 6% CTS, or rHuIL-1β and CTS. The mRNA expression was assessed by reverse transcriptase–polymerase chain reaction using 1 μg RNA from cells in each group. Amplification of GAPDH mRNA was used to ensure equal input in all lanes. **B,** TIMP II synthesis in cells subjected to treatment regimens described in **A.** Data in **A** represent 1 of 3 separate experiments. Data in **B** represent means and SEM of triplicate values. See Figure 2 for other definitions.

rHuIL-1β–induced suppression of mRNA for TIMP (TIMP-1 and TIMP-2), TMJ chondrocytes were exposed to CTS in the presence or absence of rHuIL-1β. The densitometric analysis of the PCR products for TIMP-1 revealed that exposure to rHuIL-1β does not inhibit TIMP-1 mRNA expression significantly after either 4 or 24 hours of exposure (Figure 6). However, treatment of chondrocytes with rHuIL-1β (1 ng/ml) resulted in a consistent inhibition of the constitutive expression of TIMP-2 mRNA. More important, coexposure of chondrocytes to rHuIL-1β and CTS resulted in hyperinduction of TIMP-2 mRNA, i.e., a 3 ± 0.44–fold increase in TIMP-2 mRNA was observed during the first 4 hours and a 6.2 ± 2.1–fold increase was observed after 24 hours compared with untreated control cells ($P < 0.05$). CTS alone did not affect TIMP-2 mRNA expression, demonstrating that CTS acted on TMJ fibrochondrocytes solely in an rHuIL-1β–dependent manner.

CTS abrogates the rHuIL-1β–dependent inhibition of proteoglycan synthesis in chondrocytes. A hallmark of cartilage degradation in inflamed joints is the inhibition of proteoglycan synthesis, which is attributed to the actions of IL-1β (18,44,45). Therefore, we next examined whether CTS abrogates rHuIL-1β–dependent inhibition of proteoglycan synthesis. TMJ fibrochondrocytes were exposed to rHuIL-1β, CTS, or rHuIL-1β and CTS for 24, 48, or 72 hours and pulsed with TCM containing Na_2-$^{35}SO_4$ during the last 8 hours of incubation. The incorporation of $^{35}SO_4$ into proteoglycans was used as an indicator of rHuIL-1β and/or CTS responses.

Quantitative assessment of CTS-mediated abrogation of rHuIL-1β–dependent inhibition of proteoglycan synthesis showed that CTS alone down-regulated proteoglycan synthesis by a mean ± SEM of 11 ± 2%, 14 ± 3%, and 9 ± 3% at 24, 48, and 72 hours, respectively. Likewise, exposure of cells to rHuIL-1β alone resulted in a 69 ± 4.4%, 62 ± 3.6%, and 57 ± 5.6% reduction in $^{35}SO_4$ incorporation in proteoglycans at 24, 48, and 72 hours, respectively. However, application of CTS almost completely abrogated rHuIL-1β–dependent inhibition of proteoglycan synthesis at all time points (Figure 7).

DISCUSSION

The data presented here provide support for a critical role of CTS on TMJ fibrochondrocytes in the modulation of proinflammatory actions of rHuIL-1β, the major inflammatory agent implicated in the etiology of TMJ disorders and other arthritic diseases (12,17,19,23,36). Rehabilitation of postoperative TMJ by

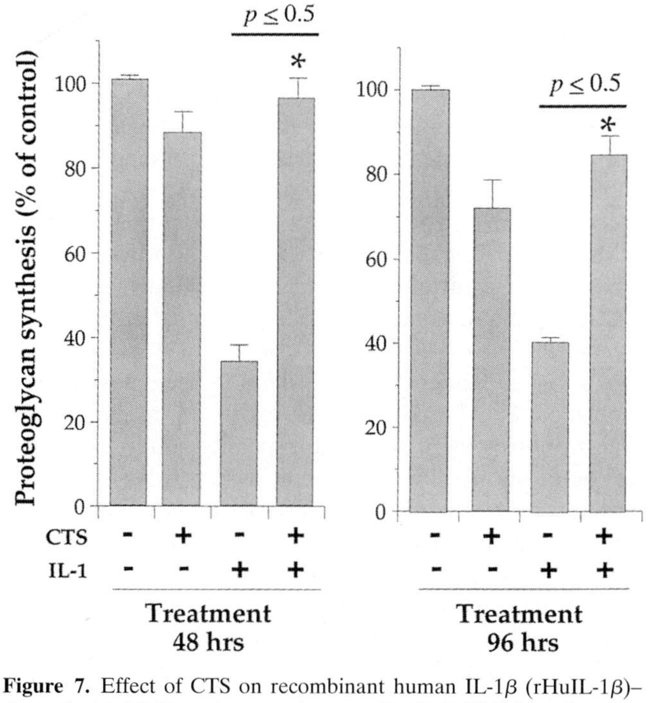

Figure 7. Effect of CTS on recombinant human IL-1β (rHuIL-1β)–dependent inhibition of proteoglycan synthesis in TMJ fibrochondrocytes. Chondrocytes were either untreated or exposed to 1 ng/ml rHuIL-1β, 6% CTS, or rHuIL-1β and CTS for 48 or 96 hours. Total proteoglycans were assessed by incorporation of Na_2-$^{35}SO_4$ during the last 8 hours of incubation followed by extraction of glycosaminoglycans with 0.5*M* NaOH and separated on PD-10 size exclusion chromatography columns. Data represent means and SEM of triplicate values in 1 of 3 separate experiments. See Figure 2 for other definitions.

continuous passive motion has been shown to augment speedier and more physiologically sound recovery in TMJ disorder patients (25–30,46). To delineate the mechanisms of continuous passive motion–mediated reparative actions, we have developed an in vitro model system. In this system, the equibiaxial CTS closely mimicks the effects of continuous passive motion in vivo because cartilage exposed to continuous passive motion is subjected to tensile strain on the superficial layers (46); chondrocytes residing in the superficial layers of cartilage are exposed to inflammatory mediators in inflamed joints; and the chondrocytes in the superficial layers of cartilage are the cells most responsive to rHuIL-1β that take part in cartilage destruction (18,48,49). Thus, this in vitro system, while closely simulating the in vivo effects of continuous passive motion on inflamed or rehabilitating joints, also provided defined parameters to examine the biochemical signals generated by CTS in TMJ chondrocytes.

We have shown that fibrochondrocytes phenotypically are distinct from articular chondrocytes, because these cells synthesize type I collagen in addition to chondrocyte-associated proteins such as type II collagen and proteoglycans. The synthesis of type I collagen by these cells is not surprising since disk cartilage synthesized by fibrochondrocytes does contain type I collagen. However, fibrochondrocytes, similar to articular chondrocytes, synthesize proinflammatory proteins such as iNOS, COX-2, and MMP-1 in response to rHuIL-1β.

Similar to articular chondrocytes, rHuIL-1β also exerts catabolic effects on TMJ fibrochondrocytes via induction of multiple proteins that mediate cartilage degradation. We have observed that application of low intensities of CTS (3–9%) consistently suppresses rHuIL-1β–dependent NO production, whereas higher intensity CTS (12.5%) fails to exert antiinflammatory effects. Interestingly, continuous passive motion therapy has been shown to yield beneficial effects in some patients, but not in all. These observations, together with our present results, tempt us to speculate that the magnitude of strain exerted on the inflamed joints may be a critical determinant of the therapeutic effects of continuous passive motion. At present it is difficult to relate the magnitude of CTS exerted on chondrocytes in vitro to the magnitude of strain experienced by chondrocytes of the TMJ disk by various regimens of continuous passive motion in vivo. Nevertheless, the understanding of the effects of various magnitudes of CTS on TMJ chondrocytes in vitro may provide leads to understand the basis for the success or failure of continuous passive motion therapy in vivo. Additionally, we have used cyclic strain at 0.05 Hz to examine the antiinflammatory actions of CTS; whether CTS also exerts antiinflammatory effects at lower or higher frequencies is yet to be determined.

With regard to the antiinflammatory actions of CTS, the data suggest that 6% CTS suppresses rHuIL-1β actions over a wide range of concentrations, encompassing those frequently found in inflamed synovial fluids (6,7). This emphasizes the potential of CTS in antagonizing the effects of rHuIL-1β and is of considerable clinical relevance regarding the treatment of inflamed joints. CTS is effective in inhibiting rHuIL-1β actions at between 3% and 10% equibiaxial strain, although 6% CTS exerts maximal inhibition of the proinflammatory responses of rHuIL-1β in vitro. Therefore, we have examined the effects of 6% CTS on the proinflammatory responses of rHuIL-1β in TMJ disk fibrochondrocytes.

CTS, by reducing the mRNA abundance of 2 pivotal proinflammatory enzymes, iNOS and COX-2, suppresses their inflammatory products, NO and PGE_2. Both NO and PGE_2 have been implicated in mediating IL-1β–induced reduction of proteoglycan synthesis (35,45). Interestingly, the presence of an inflammatory signal was a prerequisite for the observed CTS actions, since CTS (6%) alone failed to induce a response. This supports earlier reports suggesting that the low magnitude of CTS alone is not sufficient to induce synthesis of proinflammatory mediators (50). Thus, our studies point to the importance of the magnitude of CTS in its actions, i.e., low magnitude of CTS exerts antiinflammatory actions, while it is not sufficient to induce proinflammatory responses by itself. Nevertheless, as reported by others (51–53), we have also observed that a high magnitude of CTS induces iNOS and COX-2 expression in chondrocytes. High magnitude of CTS is also associated with proteoglycan degradation, which, in turn, is regulated by intracellular levels of both NO and PGE_2 (18,43,51,53,54), as well as via induction of IL-1 synthesis (51).

During cartilage degradation, cytokines such as rHuIL-1β induce extracellular matrix breakdown as well as inhibition of its synthesis. For example, chronic inflammation induces sustained collagenase production as well as inhibition of type II collagen synthesis (17,19,23,56,57). Therefore, for effective control of cartilage catabolism, prolonged suppression of collagenase production and concurrent increase in collagen synthesis is essential. In fact, our data show that CTS inhibits cartilage catabolism effectively by way of inducing prolonged suppression of rHuIL-1β–dependent collagenase synthesis via inhibition of its mRNA expression. Interestingly, application of CTS alone did not exert any effects on collagenase synthesis, which is not surprising since continuous passive motion on healthy joints has not been shown to induce cartilage degradation (51–53,58).

IL-1β has been shown to down-regulate synthesis of TIMP-2, which may facilitate increased collagen breakdown during inflammation (40–43), whereas application of TIMP-1 and TIMP-2 has been shown to inhibit IL-1β–induced collagen degradation in cartilage (41–43). Therefore, examination of the effects of CTS on the rHuIL-1β–mediated inhibition of TIMP-1 and TIMP-2 was essential to fully understand the consequences of CTS application on chondrocytes. We have observed that CTS actions indeed involve abrogation of rHuIL-1β–induced inhibition of TIMP-2 mRNA expression in parallel to inhibition of collagenase production. Furthermore, in the presence of rHuIL-1β, CTS caused hyperinduction of TIMP-2 mRNA expression, amounting to 3.2-fold and 5.6-fold increases in 4 and 24 hours, respectively. Whether all of the TIMP-2 induced by CTS is in its active form is as yet not clear. TIMP-2 blocks collagenase activity effectively at less than an equimolar ratio. This suggests that the increased production of TIMP-2 by CTS for prolonged periods may act as an effective mechanism to reduce metalloproteinase-mediated extracellular matrix degradation. Nevertheless, the presence of an inflammatory signal, such as rHuIL-1β, was essential to induce TIMP-2 mRNA expression, and exposure of chondrocytes to CTS alone was not sufficient for its induction. Interestingly, we did not observe significant down-regulation of TIMP-1 by rHuIL-1β (41,42) or its up-regulation in TMJ chondrocytes by CTS alone, or following coapplication of IL-1β and CTS.

A characteristic feature of arthritic diseases is breakdown of cartilage via degradation of chondroitin sulfate proteoglycans and inhibition of their synthesis. Our data demonstrate that CTS is effective in revoking IL-1β–dependent inhibition of proteoglycan synthesis, thus providing evidence that CTS not only antagonizes rHuIL-1β–induced proinflammatory responses, but also augments proteoglycan synthesis. Since NO inhibits sulfation of proteoglycans (47,48), it is also possible that CTS negates the effects of rHuIL-1β–dependent suppression of proteoglycan synthesis via both up-regulation of proteoglycan synthesis and inhibition of NO production, which in turn results in increased chondroitin sulfate proteoglycan synthesis. Interestingly, while continuous passive motion has been widely used for postoperative rehabilitation of TMJ patients, a number of reports have shown that its application is not always beneficial (51–53,55,58). It has been shown that a high magnitude of CTS initiates collagen degradation via induction of collagenase synthesis (50), suggesting that the magnitude of mechanical strain may be a critical determinant in the success or failure of continuous passive motion therapy. For example, the failure of continuous passive motion therapy may be due to the high magnitude of mechanical load, whereas its beneficial effects may be associated with physiologic/low magnitudes of mechanical strain in vivo, which has been shown to be reparative in nature.

In summary, our results clearly demonstrate that low magnitude of CTS is an effective antagonist of IL-1β actions and may therefore play a significant role in the repair of cartilage via inhibition of proinflammatory responses. CTS actions on TMJ fibrochondrocytes involve transcriptional regulation of multiple genes activated by IL-1β. CTS appears to disrupt/down-regulate 1 or more critical step(s) in the signal transduction cascade of IL-1β upstream of mRNA synthesis that not only result in the inhibition of inflammatory responses of TMJ chondrocytes, but also aid in their repair. Nonetheless, these actions depend on the presence of IL-1β; in the absence of IL-1β, CTS of low magnitude is ineffective in inducing reparative responses. In this regard, actions of CTS on chondrocytes appear to be strikingly comparable with those of the therapeutic agents that are currently being used to minimize cartilage degradation, such as anti–IL-1 immunoglobulins, IL-1 receptor antagonist, or metalloproteinase inhibitors (17,63–65). However, while these therapies reduce the catabolic actions of IL-1, CTS appears to initiate reparative activity in chondrocytes as well. Whether CTS specifically inhibits rHuIL-1β actions or can counteract actions of other inflammatory mediators such as tumor necrosis factor α or microbial lipopolysaccharides found in inflamed synovial joints (63,67) is yet to be determined.

ACKNOWLEDGMENT

The authors are indebted to Dr. Mohammed Heidaran, Orquest, Mountain View, CA, for providing sequences to rabbit primers for aggrecan and type II collagen.

REFERENCES

1. Kopp S. Degenerative and inflammatory temporomandibular joint disorders: clinical perspectives. In: Sessle BJ, Bryant PS, Dionne RA, editors. Progress in pain research and management. Vol 4.

Temporomandibular disorders and related pain conditions. Seattle (WA): ISAP Press; 1995. p. 119–32.
2. Albani S, Carson DA. Etiology and pathogenesis of rheumatoid arthritis. In: Koopman WJ, editor. Arthritis and allied health conditions: a textbook of rheumatology. Vol 1. Baltimore (MD): Williams & Wilkins; 1997; p. 979–91.
3. Mahan PE, Alling CC. Temporomandibular joint anatomy, function, and pathofunction. In: Mahan PE, Alling CC III, editors. Facial pain. Philadelphia: Lea & Febiger; 1991. p. 197–216.
4. Zarb GA, Carlsson GE. Osteoarthrosis/osteoarthritis. In: Zarb GA, Carlsson GE, Sessle BJ, Mohl ND, editors. Temporomandibular joint and masticatory muscle disorders. Copenhagen: Munksgaard; 1994. p. 298–327.
5. Israel HA, Diamond BE, Saed-Nejad F, Ratcliffe A. Correlation between arthroscopic diagnosis of osteoarthritis and synovitis of the human temporomandibular joint and keratan sulfate levels in the synovial fluid. J Oral Maxillofac Surg 1997;55:210–7.
6. Alstergren P, Kopp S, Theodorsson E. Synovial fluid sampling from the temporo-mandibular joint: sample quality criteria and levels of interleukin-1 beta and serotonin. Acta Odontol Scand 1999;57:16–22.
7. Alstergren P, Ernberg M, Kvarnstrom M, Kopp S. Interleukin-1beta in synovial fluid from the arthritic temporomandibular joint and its relation to pain, mobility, and anterior open bite. J Oral Maxillofac Surg 1998;56:1059–65.
8. Kubota E, Kubota T, Matsumoto J, Shibata T, Murakami KI. Synovial fluid cytokines and proteinases as markers of temporomandibular joint disease. J Oral Maxillofac Surg 1998;56:192–8.
9. Murakami KI, Shibata T, Kubota E, Maeda H. Intra-articular levels of prostaglandin E2, hyaluronic acid, and chondroitin-4 and -6 sulfates in the temporomandibular joint synovial fluid of patients with internal derangement. J Oral Maxillofac Surg 1998; 56:199–203.
10. Nordahl S, Alstergren P, Eliasson S, Kopp S. Interleukin-1beta in plasma and synovial fluid in relation to radiographic changes in arthritic temporomandibular joints. Eur J Oral Sci 1998;106: 559–63.
11. Tanaka S, Hamanishi C, Kikuchi H, Fukuda K. Factors related to degradation of articular cartilage in osteoarthritis: a review. Semin Arthritis Rheum 1998;27:392–9.
12. Evans CH, Watkins SC, Stefanovic-Racic M. Nitric oxide and cartilage metabolism. Methods Enzymol 1996;269:75–88.
13. Lotz M, Blanco FJ, von Kempis J, Dudler J, Maier R, Villiger PM, et al. Cytokine regulation of chondrocyte functions. J Rheumatol Suppl 1995;43:104–8.
14. Ratcliffe A, Israel HA, Saed-Nejad F, Diamond B. Proteoglycans in the synovial fluid of the temporomandibular joint as an indicator of changes in cartilage metabolism during primary and secondary osteoarthritis. J Oral Maxillofac Surg 1998;56:204–8.
15. Sakurai H, Kohsaka H, Liu MF, Higashiyama H, Hirata Y, Kanno K, et al. Nitric oxide production and inducible nitric oxide synthase expression in inflammatory arthritides. J Clin Invest 1995;96: 2357–63.
16. Van Lent P, van de Loo FA, Holthuysen AE, van den Bersselaar LA, Vermeer LA, van den Berg WB. Major role for interleukin-1 but not TNF in early cartilage damage in immune complex arthritis in mice. J Rheumatol 1995;22:2250–8.
17. Flugge LA, Miller-Deist LA, Petillo PA. Towards a molecular understanding of arthritis. Chem Biol 1999;6:157–69.
18. Fukuda K, Ohtani K, Dan H, Tanaka S. IL-1 inhibits keratan sulfate production by rabbit chondrocytes: possible role of prostaglandin E2. Inflamm Res 1995;44:178–83.
19. Dubois RN, Abramson SB, Crofford L, Gupta RA, Simon LS, van de Putte LB, et al. Cyclooxygenase in biology and disease. FASEB J 1998;12:1063–73.
20. Manfield L, Jang D, Murrell AC. Nitric oxide enhances cyclooxygenase activity in articular cartilage. Inflamm Res 1996;45:254–8.
21. Van de Loo FA, Arntz OJ, Otterness IG, van den Berg WB. Protection against cartilage proteoglycan synthesis inhibition by anti-interleukin-1 antibodies in experimental arthritis. J Rheumatol 1995;19:348–54.
22. Taskiran D, Stefanovic-Racic M, Georgescu H, Evans CH. Nitric oxide mediates suppression of cartilage proteoglycan synthesis by IL-1. Biochem Biophys Res Commun 1994;200:142–9.
23. Murrell GAC, Jang D, Williams RJ. Nitric oxide activates metalloprotease in articular cartilage. Biochem Biophys Res Commun 1995;206:15–21.
24. Stefanovic-Racic M, Stadler J, Evans CH. Nitric oxide and arthritis. Arthritis Rheum 1993;36:1036–44.
25. McCarty WL, Darnell MW. Rehabilitation of the temporomandibular joint through the application of motion. Cranio 1993;11: 298–306.
26. Kim HK, Kerr RG, Cruz TF, Salter RB. Effects of continuous passive motion and immobilization on synovitis and cartilage degradation in antigen induced arthritis. J Rheumatol 1995;22: 1714–21.
27. Salter RB. The physiologic basis of continuous passive motion for articular cartilage healing and regeneration. Hand Clin 1994;10: 211–8.
28. Williams JM, Moran M, Thonar E, Salter RB. Continuous passive motion stimulates repair of rabbit knee articular cartilage after matrix proteoglycan loss. Clin Orthop 1994;304:252–9.
29. Von Schroeder HP, Coutts RD, Billings J, Mai MT, Aratow M. The changes in intramuscular pressure and femoral vein flow with continuous passive motion, pneumatic compressive stockings, and leg manipulations. Clin Orthop 1991;266:218–26.
30. Gassner R, Buckley MJ, Georgescu H, Studer R, Stefanovich-Racic M, Piesco NP, et al. Cyclic tensile stress exerts anti-inflammatory actions on chondrocytes by inhibiting inducible nitric oxide synthase. J Immunol 1999;163:2187–94.
31. Fedewa MM, Oegema TR, Schwartz MH, MacLeod A, Lewis JL. Chondrocytes in cellular culture produce a mechanically functional tissue. J Orthop Res 1998;16:227–35.
32. Yu H, Grynpas M, Kandel RL. Composition of cartilagenous tissue with mineralized and non-mineralized zones formed in vitro. Biomaterials 1997;18:1425–33.
33. Hart DA, Boykiw R, Sciore P, Reno C. Complex alterations in gene expression occur in the knee ligaments of the skeletally mature multiparous rabbit during pregnancy. Biochim Biophys Acta 1998;1397:331–41.
34. Morisset S, Patry C, Lora M, de Brum-Fernandes AJ. Regulation of cyclooxygenase-2 expression in bovine chondrocytes in culture by interleukin-1α, tumor necrosis factor-α, glucocorticoids, and 17β-estradiol. J Rheumatol 1998;25:1146–53.
35. Evans CH. The role of proteinases in cartilage destruction. Agents Actions Suppl 1991;32:135–52.
36. Lotz M, Blanco FJ, von Kempis J, Dudler J, Maier R, Villiger PM, et al. Cytokine regulation of chondrocyte functions. J Rheumatol Suppl 1995;43:104–8.
37. Saito S, Katoh M, Masumoto M, Matsumoto S, Masuho Y. Involvement of MMP-1 and MMP-3 in collagen degradation induced by IL-1 in rabbit cartilage explant culture. Life Sci 1998;62:359–65.
38. Borden P, Solymar D, Sucharczuk A, Lindman B, Cannon P, Heller RA. Cytokine control of interstitial collagenase and collagenase-3 gene expression in human chondrocytes. J Biol Chem 1996;271:23577–81.
39. Kozaci LD, Buttle DJ, Hollander AP. Degradation of type II collagen, but not proteoglycan, correlates with matrix metalloproteinase activity in cartilage explant cultures. Arthritis Rheum 1997;40:164–74.
40. Cawston T, Billington C, Cleaver C, Elliott S, Hui W, Koshy P, et al. The regulation of MMPs and TIMPs in cartilage turnover. Ann N Y Acad Sci 1999;878:120–9.

41. Shingu M, Nagai Y, Isayama T, Naono T, Nobunaga M, Nagai Y. The effects of cytokines on metalloproteinase inhibitors (TIMP) and collagenase production by human chondrocytes and TIMP production by synovial cells and endothelial cells. Clin Exp Immunol 1993;94:145–9.
42. Ellis AJ, Curry VA, Powell EK, Cawston TE. The prevention of collagen breakdown in bovine nasal cartilage by TIMP, TIMP-2 and a low molecular weight synthetic inhibitor. Biochem Biophys Res Commun 1994;201:94–101.
43. Van de Loo FA, Arntz OJ, Otterness IG, van den Berg WB. Protection against cartilage proteoglycan synthesis inhibition by antiinterleukin 1 antibodies in experimental arthritis. J Rheumatol 1992;19:348–56.
44. Taskiran D, Stefanovic-Racic M, Georgescu H, Evans C. Nitric oxide mediates suppression of cartilage proteoglycan synthesis by interleukin-1. Biochem Biophys Res Commun 1994;200:142–8.
45. Kim HK, Kerr RG, Cruz TF, Salter RB. Effects of continuous passive motion and immobilization on synovitis and cartilage degradation in antigen induced arthritis. J Rheumatol 1995;22: 1714–21.
46. Häuselmann HJ, Flechtenmacher J, Michal L, Thonar EJ-MA, Shinmei M, Kuettner KE, et al. The superficial layer of human articular cartilage is more susceptible to interleukin-1–induced damage than the deeper layers. Arthritis Rheum 1996;39:478–88.
47. Hickery MS, Bayliss MT. Interleukin-1 induced nitric oxide inhibits sulphation of glycosaminoglycan chains in human articular chondrocytes. Biochim Biophys Acta 1998;1425:282–90.
48. Hayashi T, Abe E, Yamate T, Taguchi Y, Jasin HE. Nitric oxide production by superficial and deep articular chondrocytes. Arthritis Rheum 1997;40:261–9.
49. Chen J, Akyuz U, Xu L, Pidaparti RM. Stress analysis of the human temporomandibular joint. Med Eng Phys 1998;20:565–72.
50. Fujisawa T, Hattori T, Takahashi K, Kuboki T, Yamashita A, Takigawa M. Cyclic mechanical stress induces extracellular matrix degradation in cultured chondrocytes via gene expression of matrix metalloproteinases and interleukin-1. J Biochem (Tokyo) 1999;125:966–75.
51. Klein-Nulend J, Burger EH, Semeins CM, Raisz LG, Pilbeam CC. Pulsating fluid flow stimulates prostaglandin release and inducible prostaglandin G/H synthase mRNA expression in primary mouse bone cells. J Bone Miner Res 1997;12:45–51.
52. Klein-Nulend J, Semeins CM, Ajubi NE, Nijweide PJ, Burger EH. Pulsating fluid flow increases nitric oxide (NO) synthesis by osteocytes but not periosteal fibroblasts—correlation with prostaglandin upregulation. Biochem Biophys Res Commun 1995;217: 640–8.
53. Israel HA, Syrop SB. The important role of motion in the rehabilitation of patients with mandibular hypomobility: a review of the literature. Cranio 1997;15:74–83.
54. Management of temporomandibular disorders: National Institutes of Health Technology Assessment Conference Statement. J Am Dent Assoc 1996;127:1595–606.
55. Chandrasekhar S, Harvey AK, Higginbotham JD, Horton WE. Interleukin-1-induced suppression of type II collagen gene transcription involves DNA regulatory elements. Exp Cell Res 1990; 191:105–14.
56. Goldring MB, Fukuo K, Birkhead JR, Dudek E, Sandell LJ. Transcriptional suppression by interleukin-1 and interferongamma of type II collagen gene expression in human chondrocytes. J Cell Biochem 1994;54:85–99.
57. Pitsillides AA, Rawlinson SC, Suswillo RF, Bourrin S, Zaman G, Lanyon LE. Mechanical strain-induced NO production by bone cells: a possible role in adaptive bone (re)modeling? FASEB J 1995;9:1614–22.
58. Bandara G, Georgescu HI, Lin CW, Evans CH. Synovial activation of chondrocytes: evidence for complex cytokine interactions. Agents Actions 1991;34:285–8.
59. Martel-Pelletier J, McCollum R, DiBattista J, Faure M-P, Chin JA, Fournier S, et al. The interleukin-1 receptor in normal and osteoarthritic human articular chondrocytes: identification as the type I receptor and analysis of binding kinetics and biologic function. Arthritis Rheum 1992;35:530–40.
60. Dinarello CA. Biologic basis for interleukin-1 in disease. Blood 1996;87:2095–147.
61. Lane NE, Williams RJ III, Schurman DJ, Smith RL. Inhibition of interleukin 1 induced chondrocyte protease activity by a corticosteroid and a nonsteroidal antiinflammatory drug. J Rheumatol 1992;19:135–9.
62. Joosten LAB, Helsen MMA, van de Loo FAJ, van den Berg WB. Anticytokine treatment of established type II collagen–induced arthritis in DBA/1 mice: a comparative study using anti-TNFα, anti–IL-1α/β, and IL-1Ra. Arthritis Rheum 1996;39:797–809.
63. Spirito S, Doughty J, O'Byrne E, Ganu V, Goldberg RL. Metalloprotease inhibitors halt collagen breakdown in IL-1 induced bovine nasal cartilage cultures. Inflamm Res 1995;44(Suppl 2): S131–2.
64. Evans CH, Ghivizzani SC, Robbins PD. Blocking cytokines with genes. J Leukoc Biol 1998;64:55–61.
65. Van den Berg WB. Lessons for joint destruction from animal models. Curr Opin Rheumatol 1997;9:221–8.

ARTHRITIS & RHEUMATISM
Vol. 44, No. 3, March 2001, pp 618–625

The Fcγ Receptor IIIA-158F Allele Is a Major Risk Factor for the Development of Lupus Nephritis Among Caucasians but Not Non-Caucasians

Victoria A. Seligman,[1] Charlyn Suarez,[2] Raymond Lum,[1] Sven E. Inda,[2] Doris Lin,[1] Hongzhe Li,[2] Jean L. Olson,[1] Michael F. Seldin,[2] and Lindsey A. Criswell[1]

Objective. **To determine whether inheritance of Fcγ receptor (FcγR) alleles conferring lower affinity for IgG binding increases the risk of developing lupus nephritis.**

Methods. **We compared the frequency of low-affinity alleles of two FcγR polymorphisms (FcγRIIA and FcγRIIIA) among 235 patients with systemic lupus erythematosus (SLE) and proven nephritis (nephritis patients) and among 352 SLE patients with no evidence of renal disease (non-nephritis control subjects). The ethnic distribution of patients in the study was 49% Caucasian, 20% Hispanic, 17% Asian/Pacific Islander, 12% African American, and 2% from other ethnic groups. All patients were genotyped for the FcγRIIA-131R/H and FcγRIIIA-158V/F polymorphisms. We used contingency table analysis to compare allele and genotype distributions for nephritis patients and non-nephritis control subjects, including ethnic-specific strata. Multivariate logistic regression analyses included sex and disease duration as covariates.**

Results. **Univariate and multivariate analyses demonstrated a striking association between the low-affinity FcγRIIIA-158F allele and FF genotype and the risk of nephritis among Caucasians, but not among non-Caucasians (multivariate odds ratio [OR] 2.6 for Caucasians with FF genotype), (P = 0.0017). This association was even stronger among Caucasians with severe nephritis (OR 4.4, $P < 0.0001$). In contrast, inheritance of the low-affinity FcγRIIA-131R allele (and RR genotype) was not associated with an increased risk of lupus nephritis among any of the ethnic groups examined.**

Conclusion. **The FcγRIIIA-158F allele is a major risk factor for the development of lupus nephritis among Caucasians, but not among non-Caucasians. These results suggest that ethnic variation is critical in defining the specific genetic factors underlying the pathogenesis of SLE, and they have important prognostic and therapeutic implications as well.**

Systemic lupus erythematosus (SLE) is a complex systemic illness, the expression of which is influenced by multiple genetic and environmental factors (1–5). The identification of genetic risk factors for specific disease manifestations such as lupus nephritis is an area of intense current interest. Since immune complex deposition plays a pivotal role in the initiation of tissue damage in SLE, polymorphisms affecting Fcγ receptor (FcγR) function are implicated in disease pathogenesis, particularly that of glomerulonephritis.

Elimination of immune complexes follows binding of phagocytic cells via receptors to Fc portions of immunoglobulins or to attached complement components. There are 3 classes of receptors for the Fc portion of IgG: FcγRI, FcγRII, and FcγRIII. Effective clearance of immune complexes depends upon optimal functioning of these receptors and is influenced by genetic polymorphisms. For example, the FcγRIIA-131R and 131H alleles, which differ by a single amino acid at residue 131, have markedly different binding properties (6–8). Indeed, FcγRIIA-131H is the only human FcγR

Supported by grants from the NIH (AR-44804) and the Arthritis Foundation. This study was carried out in part in the General Clinical Research Center, Moffitt Hospital, University of California, San Francisco, with funds provided by the National Center for Research Resources (5-M01-RR-00079), USPHS.

[1]Victoria A. Seligman, MD, Raymond Lum, MPH, Doris Lin, BS, Jean L. Olson, MD, Lindsey A. Criswell, MD, MPH: Rosalind Russell Medical Research Center for Arthritis, University of California, San Francisco; [2]Charlyn Suarez, BS, Sven E. Inda, BS, Hongzhe Li, PhD, Michael F. Seldin, MD, PhD: University of California, Davis.

Address correspondence and reprint requests to Lindsey A. Criswell, MD, MPH, Division of Rheumatology, 374 Parnassus Avenue, Box 0500, San Francisco, CA 94143-0500.

Submitted for publication July 25, 2000; accepted in revised form October 23, 2000.

that recognizes IgG2 efficiently, while 131R binds human IgG2 poorly. Since IgG2 deposition is believed to play an important role in the pathogenesis of glomerulonephritis in human SLE, this differential binding capacity may have great clinical significance.

Polymorphisms of other FcγR classes likewise affect receptor affinity for IgG and have been examined in relationship to SLE. For example, the FcγRIIIA-158F/V polymorphism has been studied recently for its potential influence on disease expression, since the 158F isoform binds IgG1 and IgG3 with lower affinity than does the 158V isoform (9,10).

Results of previous studies examining FcγRIIA polymorphisms in SLE patients have been discordant. Some studies suggest a protective role for FcγRIIA-131H in lupus nephritis (11–13). However, other studies fail to demonstrate such an association (14–18). Data are limited regarding the FcγRIIIA-158F/V polymorphism in SLE. The two studies of predominantly Caucasian patients (9,10) demonstrated an association of FcγRIIIA-158F with SLE. A small study of Korean patients suggested an association with lupus nephritis (15). In contrast, no association was observed among the single sample of African American patients, including those with lupus nephritis, that has been studied (14). There are a number of possible explanations for the discrepancies in results of studies examining FcγRIIA and FcγRIIIA polymorphisms in SLE. For example, false-positive associations may arise due to small sample sizes, and variation in clinical characteristics of the study subjects may lead to disparate results. Importantly, some of these discrepancies may also relate to ethnic heterogeneity (i.e., variation in genetic associations according to ethnic background).

The goal of the current study was to examine the FcγRIIA-131R/H and FcγRIIIA-158F/V polymorphisms among an ethnically diverse cohort of SLE patients. Specifically, due to the role of immune complex deposition in SLE nephritis, we sought to determine whether either of the low-affinity alleles (FcγRIIA-131R or FcγRIIIA-158F) was associated with the development of SLE nephritis. The large size and ethnic diversity of our study group provided a unique opportunity to increase current understanding of the role of these polymorphisms in SLE.

PATIENTS AND METHODS

Patients and control subjects. We studied a total of 587 SLE patients, including 235 with proven nephritis (nephritis patients) and 352 SLE patients with no evidence of renal involvement (non-nephritis control). Informed consent was obtained from all patients, and the study was approved by the institutional review board at the University of California, San Francisco (UCSF). Patients were participants in the UCSF Lupus Genetics Project and were recruited from UCSF Arthritis Clinics and private rheumatology practices in northern California, as well as by nationwide outreach. All patients fulfilled the American College of Rheumatology (ACR) revised criteria for SLE (19,20). Ethnic background was determined based on the ancestries of each patient's 4 grandparents.

Definition of nephritis. The classification of nephritis was based upon review of patient questionnaires and medical records. Patients were designated as having nephritis if they met the ACR criteria for lupus nephritis (19) or if they had evidence of lupus nephritis (i.e., immune complex deposition) obtained at renal biopsy. The ACR criteria for lupus nephritis require evidence of persistent proteinuria (i.e., >0.5 gm/24 hours or +3 if only urine dipstick used) or active sediment (i.e., cellular casts: red cell, granular, tubular, or mixed).

We also used a more severe definition of nephritis in sensitivity analyses (see Statistical analysis). Specifically, only nephritis patients who had developed end-stage renal disease (ESRD) or who had proliferative lesions on renal biopsy were included in these sensitivity analyses.

A renal biopsy was performed on 189 of the nephritis patients. Original biopsy reports were available for review in the case of 118 patients and were evaluated in conjunction with one of the coauthors (JLO), a renal pathologist. Histopathologic findings were classified according to World Health Organization criteria (21). Based on an extensive review of medical records, clinical manifestations of nephritis were recorded, including proteinuria, active urinary sediment, hematuria, elevated creatinine, and ESRD.

Sample preparation and DNA marker analysis. DNA templates for polymerase chain reaction (PCR)–based genotyping were prepared from buccal cell brushings as previously described (22). The FcγRIIA-131R/H polymorphism was analyzed using a single-base extension (SBE) method (23) in which fluorescent-tagged dideoxynucleotides were utilized to distinguish between A and G bases at nucleotide position 519. These bases correspond to the H131 and R131 codon polymorphisms, respectively. Briefly, a 10-μl PCR reaction containing 0.5 units of *Taq* DNA polymerase (Qiagen, Valencia, CA); 2 μl of Q solution (Qiagen), 0.25 m*M* each of dATP, dCTP, dGTP, and dTTP, 1 μ*M* of each primer (forward 5′-GAG-AAA-CCA-TCA-TGC-TGA-GGT-GCC-ACA-GCT-G-3′; reverse 5′-GCC-CAA-TTT-TGC-TGC-TAT-GGG-C-3′), and 0.4 ng of DNA template was performed by initially denaturing the mixture at 95°C for 8 minutes, followed by 35 cycles of 95°C for 1 minute, 65°C for 1.5 minutes, and 72°C for 1 minute, and then an 8-minute final extension at 72°C.

The SBE reaction mixture included 5 μl of the PCR product (206 bp) and 5 μl of a mixture containing 0.1 μl of 1.0 μ*M* rhodamine-X (ROX)–ddUTP, 0.1 μl of 1.0 μ*M* 6-carboxy fluorescein (FAM)–ddCTP, 0.1 μl of 5.0 μ*M* ddGTP, 0.1 μl of 5.0 μ*M* ddATP, 0.1 μl of 10.0 μ*M* oligo-5′-ATG-GAG-AAG-GTG-GGA-TCC-AAA-3′, 0.5 μl of 0.32 units/μl Thermo Sequenase (Amersham Pharmacia Biotech, Piscataway, NJ), and 2 μl of 5× Sequenase buffer. The reaction was performed

Table 1. Characteristics of systemic lupus erythematosus patients with and without nephritis

Characteristic	Nephritis patients (n = 235)	Non-nephritis control (n = 352)	P*
Sex, no. (%)			
Women	200 (85.1)	329 (93.5)	0.0015
Men	35 (14.9)	23 (6.5)	
Ethnicity, no. (%)			
Caucasian	78 (33.2)	208 (59.1)	<0.00001
Hispanic	56 (23.8)	60 (17.0)	
Asian/Pacific Islander	60 (25.5)	41 (11.6)	
African American	35 (14.9)	36 (10.2)	
Other	6 (2.6)	7 (2.0)	
Age at SLE diagnosis, mean ± SD years	25.9 ± 11.2	34.6 ± 11.7	<0.0001
Disease duration, mean ± SD years	12.6 ± 8.3	6.9 ± 6.4	<0.00001

* By chi-square test for categorical variables; by Student's *t*-test for continuous variables.

in a GeneAmp PCR System 9700 (PE Applied Biosystems, Foster City, CA) using an initial denaturation of 1 minute at 96°C, followed by 30 cycles of 96°C for 30 seconds, 55°C for 30 seconds, and 60°C for 4 minutes. The resulting SBE product was then electrophoresed on a 12% polyacrylamide gel and imaged using a fluorescence scanner (FMBIO II; Hitachi Genetic Systems, Alameda, CA). Homozygotes had either a red (A base) or a green (G base) band, while heterozygotes had both band colors. The integrity and fidelity of this assay and those described below for FcγRIIIA were confirmed by sequence analysis of a subset of samples, including several from individuals of each genotype.

The FcγRIIIA-158F/V polymorphism was analyzed as described by Koene et al (9). Briefly, 1 μ*M* of each primer (forward 5′-ATA-TTT-ACA-GAA-TGG-CAC-AGG-3′; reverse 5′-GAC-TTG-GTA-CCC-AGG-TTG-AA-3′), 0.1 μl of Advantage cDNA Polymerase mix (Clontech, Palo Alto, CA), 0.25 m*M* each of dATP, dCTP, dGTP, and dTTP, and 0.4 ng of DNA template were combined in a 10-μl PCR reaction mixture. The PCR conditions were 9 minutes of denaturation at 95°C, followed by 36 cycles of 1 minute denaturation at 95°C, 1.5 minutes of primer annealing at 56°C, and 1.5 minutes of extension at 72°C, and then an 8-minute final extension at 72°C.

A nested PCR was then performed using 2 μl of the first PCR product, 1 μ*M* of each second set of primers (forward 5′-ATC-AGA-TTC-GAT-CCT-ACT-TCT-GCA-GGG-GGC-AT-3′; reverse 5′-ACG-TGC-TGA-GCT-TGA-GTG-ATG-GTG-ATG-TTC-AC-3′), 0.1 μl of Advantage cDNA Polymerase mix, and 0.25 m*M* each of dATP, dCTP, dGTP, and dTTP. The nested PCR conditions were 4 minutes of denaturation at 95°C, followed by 36 cycles of 95°C for 1 minute, 56°C for 1.5 minutes, and 72°C for 1.5 minutes, and then an 8-minute final extension at 72°C. Eight microliters of the resulting product from the nested PCR was then digested overnight with 1 μl of 10,000 units/ml *Nla* III (New England Biolabs, Beverly, MA) and loaded on a 12% polyacrylamide gel. The gel was stained with SybrGold (Molecular Probes, Eugene, OR) to detect the bands, and a Nucleovision gel imager (NucleoTech, San Carlos, CA) was used to capture the gel image.

Statistical analysis. Demographic and clinical characteristics of nephritis patients and non-nephritis control were compared using the chi-square test (for categorical variables) and Student's *t*-test (for continuous variables). Contingency table analysis using the chi-square test was used to compare allele and genotype distributions for nephritis patients and non-nephritis control subjects, including ethnic-specific strata.

Multivariate logistic regression was used to examine the association between the FcγRIIIA-158FF genotype (homozygote for low-affinity allele) and the risk of nephritis, adjusting for sex and disease duration (0–3 years, 4–7 years,

Table 2. Renal characteristics of systemic lupus erythematosus patients with nephritis*

Characteristic	Caucasian (n = 78)	Hispanic (n = 56)	Asian/Pacific Islander (n = 60)	African American (n = 35)	Total† (n = 235)
Nephrotic-range proteinuria, no. (%)	46 (59.0)	29 (51.8)	37 (61.7)	19 (54.3)	134 (57.0)
ESRD, no. (%)	32 (41.0)	23 (41.1)	20 (33.3)	8 (22.9)	85 (36.2)
Underwent renal biopsy, no. (%)	68 (87.2)	43 (76.8)	47 (78.3)	25 (71.4)	189 (80.4)
Biopsy report reviewed, no. (%)	45 (57.7)	23 (41.1)	28 (46.7)	18 (51.4)	118 (50.2)
Biopsy findings, no.					
Mesangial	2	2	3	2	9 (3.8)
FPLN	4	2	4	0	12 (5.1)
DPLN	23	15	14	4	59 (25.1)
Membranous‡	8	3	5	4	20 (8.5)
Mixed membranous and proliferative§	13	6	8	6	33 (14.0)
Sclerotic	2	2	1	0	5 (2.1)
Other	1	2	0	2	5 (2.1)

* ESRD = end-stage renal disease; FPLN = focal proliferative lupus nephritis (World Health Organization [WHO] class III); DPLN = diffuse proliferative lupus nephritis (WHO class IV).
† Totals include patients of other ethnicity.
‡ WHO classes V_A and V_B.
§ WHO classes V_C and V_D.

Table 3. FcγRIIA-131R/H allele and genotype distribution among systemic lupus erythematosus patients with and without nephritis*

Ethnic group, nephritis status	Allele distribution				Genotype distribution				
	H	R	OR†	*P*‡	HH	HR	RR	OR§	*P*‡
All patients									
Patients	207	225	1.13	0.32	38	131	47	1.14	0.57
Control	285	351			50	185	83		
Caucasian									
Patients	69	83	0.99	0.95	10	49	17	0.86	0.69
Control	170	202			28	114	44		
Non-Caucasian¶									
Patients	138	142	1.26	0.18	28	82	30	1.25	0.48
Control	115	149			22	71	39		
Hispanic									
Patients	43	53	1.22	0.49	7	29	12	0.77	0.62
Control	44	66			10	24	21		
Asian/Pacific Islander									
Patients	59	55	1.13	0.68	11	37	9	1.36	0.58
Control	39	41			6	27	7		
African American									
Patients	30	30	1.30	0.48	9	12	9	1.79	0.33
Control	27	35			6	15	10		

* Except where otherwise indicated, values are the number of patients. FcγRIIA = Fcγ receptor IIA; OR = odds ratio.
† Risk of nephritis associated with the FcγRIIA-131R allele.
‡ By 2 × 2 chi-square test.
§ Risk of nephritis for individuals with the FcγRIIA-131RR genotype compared with individuals with the other genotypes (HR and HH).
¶ Includes Hispanic, Asian/Pacific Islander, African American, and patients of other ethnicity.

8–14 years, and ≥15 years). Based on the results of contingency table analysis, logistic regressions were performed: 1) with the addition of a genotype/ethnicity interaction term, and 2) among ethnic-specific strata.

Multivariate conditional logistic regression was used for a matched-pairs analysis in which each nephritis patient was matched with a non-nephritis control subject for sex and ethnicity. When more than one appropriate matched control subject was available, the subject with the longest duration of disease was chosen. Genotype was modeled as the presence versus the absence of the FcγRIIIA-158FF genotype, and disease duration was included as a covariate, as described above. Two hundred six matched pairs were included in these analyses.

Sensitivity analyses were performed in which the logistic regression analyses were repeated using a more severe definition of nephritis, as described above.

All statistical analyses were performed on a SUN OS 5.7 platform (Sun Microsystems, Palo Alto, CA) using SAS, version 8 (24).

RESULTS

Ninety percent of the patients were women. The ethnic distribution of patients was 49% Caucasian, 20% Hispanic, 17% Asian/Pacific Islander, 12% African American, and 2% from other ethnic groups. Table 1 summarizes selected demographic and clinical characteristics of the 235 nephritis patients and 352 non-nephritis control subjects. All of these characteristics differed significantly between the two groups.

The renal characteristics of the nephritis patients are shown in Table 2. Fifty-seven percent of nephritis patients had evidence of nephrotic-range proteinuria, 36.2% developed ESRD, and 80.4% underwent renal biopsy. The most common renal pathologic finding was diffuse proliferative lupus nephritis, which was found in 25.1% of all renal biopsy samples.

Allele and genotype distributions for the FcγRIIA and FcγRIIIA polymorphisms are summarized in Tables 3 and 4, respectively. The first row of each table shows the results for all patients. Results are shown separately for Caucasians and non-Caucasians (all other ethnic groups combined) and for the largest non-Caucasian ethnic groups. The odds ratios (ORs) indicate the association of the low-affinity allele (R for FcγRIIA, F for FcγRIIIA) or the homozygous genotype (RR or FF) with the risk of developing nephritis. These data reveal striking associations of both the FcγRIIIA low-affinity allele (F) and the homozygous genotype (FF) with the risk of nephritis among Caucasians, but not

Table 4. FcγRIIIA-158F/V allele and genotype distribution among SLE patients with and without nephritis*

Ethnic group, nephritis status	Allele distribution				Genotype distribution				
	F	V	OR†	*P*‡	FF	FV	VV	OR§	*P*‡
All patients									
Patients	290	176	1.31	0.03	97	96	40	1.59	0.009
Control	388	308			108	172	68		
Caucasian									
Patients	104	52	1.91	0.0009	37	30	11	2.49	0.0008
Control	212	202			55	102	50		
Non-Caucasian¶									
Patients	186	124	0.90	0.55	60	66	29	1.05	0.84
Control	176	106			53	70	18		
Hispanic									
Patients	65	45	0.59	0.06	25	15	15	0.75	0.45
Control	81	33			30	21	6		
Asian/Pacific Islander									
Patients	73	45	1.27	0.41	22	29	8	1.44	0.41
Control	46	36			12	22	7		
African American									
Patients	41	29	1.20	0.60	11	19	5	1.90	0.25
Control	39	33			7	25	4		

* Except where otherwise indicated, values are the number of patients. See Table 3 for definitions.
† Risk of nephritis associated with the FcγRIIIA-158F allele.
‡ By 2 × 2 chi-square test.
§ Risk of nephritis for individuals with the FcγRIIIA-158FF genotype compared with individuals with the other genotypes (FV and VV).
¶ Includes Hispanic, Asian/Pacific Islander, African American, and patients of other ethnicity.

among non-Caucasians. We found no evidence of an association of the FcγRIIA-131R allele or the RR genotype with the risk of nephritis among any of the ethnic groups examined.

Next, we used multivariate logistic regression to further examine the association between the FcγRIIIA-FF genotype and the risk of nephritis, since this method allowed us to account for other differences (e.g., sex) between nephritis patients and non-nephritis control subjects that might explain the association. This method also allowed us to adjust for differences in disease duration at the time of study entry (since this might have led to misclassification of patients with recent diagnoses as non-nephritis control subjects). We accounted for the ethnic differences revealed in our contingency table analyses as described above (see Statistical analysis). These analyses confirmed the results of our contingency table analyses (see Table 5). Indeed, the ethnic-specific regressions revealed a slightly greater association between the FF genotype and the risk of nephritis among Caucasians (OR 2.6, $P = 0.0017$) and no evidence of an association among non-Caucasians (OR 0.9, $P = 0.66$).

Results for Hispanic, Asian/Pacific Islander, and African American groups also failed to demonstrate a significant association between the FF genotype and the risk of nephritis (data not shown). This interaction between genotype and ethnicity was confirmed by the logistic regression analysis that specifically modeled such an interaction ($P = 0.009$ for interaction term). The covariates of sex and disease duration were also significantly associated with nephritis in our multivariate analyses. However, the results of our matched-pairs analysis supported our regression findings (data not shown) and further suggested that other differences between the nephritis patients and non-nephritis control subjects did not explain our results.

Table 6 shows the results of our sensitivity analyses in which we used a more severe definition of nephritis. Specifically, only nephritis patients who had developed ESRD or who had proliferative lesions on renal biopsy were included in these analyses. These results revealed even more striking associations between inheritance of the FcγRIIIA-158FF genotype and the risk of nephritis among Caucasians (OR 4.4, $P < 0.0001$) and still showed no evidence of a similar association among non-Caucasians (OR 1.0, $P = 0.86$). Results for Hispanic, Asian/Pacific Islander, and African American groups also failed to demonstrate a significant association between the FcγRIIIA-158FF genotype and the risk of severe nephritis (data not shown).

Table 5. Multivariate logistic regression results for association of FcγRIIIA-158FF genotype with risk of lupus nephritis*

Ethnic group	OR (95% CI)†	*P*
Caucasian	2.6 (1.4–4.8)	0.0017
Non-Caucasian	0.9 (0.5–1.5)	0.66

* Covariates include sex and disease duration. 95% CI = 95% confidence interval (see Table 3 for other definitions).
† Risk of nephritis for individuals with the FcγRIIIA-158FF genotype compared with individuals with the other genotypes (FV and VV).

Table 6. Multivariate logistic regression results for the sensitivity analysis*

Ethnic group	OR (95% CI)†	*P*
Caucasian	4.4 (2.2–9.0)	<0.0001
Non-Caucasian	1.0 (0.5–1.7)	0.86

* This analysis was restricted to patients with severe nephritis (see text for details). Covariates include sex and disease duration. 95% CI = 95% confidence interval (see Table 3 for other definitions).
† Risk of severe nephritis for individuals with the FcγRIIIA-158FF genotype compared with individuals with the other genotypes (FV and VV).

DISCUSSION

The results of this study provide strong support for the hypothesis that inheritance of FcγR polymorphisms has a substantial impact on the risk of lupus nephritis for particular ethnic subgroups. Specifically, we demonstrated a striking association between inheritance of the FcγRIIIA-158F allele (and FF genotype) and the risk of nephritis among Caucasians. The association was stronger still in the case of severe nephritis. Several lines of evidence lend biologic support to these findings, including differential allelic binding properties and the pivotal role of immune complex deposition in lupus nephritis, particularly severe lupus nephritis (25–27). We also found compelling evidence of ethnic heterogeneity, since non-Caucasians who had inherited this particular allele were not at increased risk of nephritis.

These results may explain discrepancies among findings of previous studies of FcγRIIIA-158F/V in SLE. The two studies of predominantly Caucasian patients (9,10) demonstrated an association of FcγRIIIA-158F with SLE, although only one reported an association with nephritis. These studies provided only limited data about the risk of nephritis, however, due to incomplete descriptions of renal characteristics and/or inclusion of relatively few nephritis patients. The single study of African American SLE patients (14) failed to demonstrate an association with FcγRIIIA-158F, even for those with nephritis. In contrast to findings of the current study, one previous study suggested an association between FcγRIIIA-158F and lupus nephritis in a non-Caucasian group, specifically, Koreans (15). Since Koreans represented a very small proportion of patients in the current study, the results are not comparable. Moreover, the small sample size of the Korean study raises the possibility of a false-positive result.

In contrast to the results for FcγRIIIA, we found no evidence that the FcγRIIA-131R/H polymorphism influences the risk of nephritis among any of the ethnic groups examined. Results of previous studies examining this polymorphism in SLE patients have been discordant. Salmon et al (11) found a striking decrease in 131H/H homozygotes ($P = 0.003$) and FcγRIIA-131H allelic frequency ($P = 0.0008$) among 103 African American lupus nephritis patients compared with 100 non-SLE control subjects, suggesting a protective role for FcγRIIA-131H in lupus nephritis. In contrast, Oh et al (14) were unable to reproduce this finding in another sample of 66 African American SLE patients compared with 69 African American non-SLE control subjects when examining specific manifestations of renal disease.

Song et al (12) demonstrated a lower 131H allele frequency among Korean SLE patients, particularly those with nephritis. However, another study of Korean SLE patients (15), which included 79 lupus nephritis patients and 97 disease-free control subjects, did not confirm this finding. Among Caucasian SLE patients, the FcγRIIA-131RR genotype was associated with nephritis in a Dutch group (13), but not among Caucasians of other ancestries (16). Skewing of FcγRIIA-131R has not been substantiated by other investigators evaluating African Caribbean and Chinese lupus nephritis patients (16–18). There are potential problems with these studies, including relatively small sample sizes, lack of an SLE non-nephritis control group, and population admixture. Moreover, some of these studies focused on ethnic groups that were not well represented in the current study (e.g., African Americans of Caribbean ancestry and Koreans), and their findings are therefore not comparable.

In view of the genetic complexity of SLE (1,4,5), the striking ethnic heterogeneity we observed was not unexpected. Although a thorough examination of this finding is beyond the scope of the current study, it is of interest to consider potential causes. One possibility relates to epistasis (i.e., gene–gene interaction), since it is conceivable that the impact of FcγRIIIA-158F on the risk of nephritis is influenced by another gene that differs in allelic frequency between Caucasians and non-Caucasians. Alternatively, the observed association with FcγRIIIA may be due to linkage disequilibrium with another polymorphism(s) in close proximity that is primarily responsible for the association with nephritis. However, the growing body of literature from both animal and human studies (15,28,29) provides strong support for FcγRIIIA as an independent SLE candidate gene. Finally, the Caucasian and non-Caucasian patients examined in the present study may differ in other important characteristics that we failed to account for in our analysis.

Several characteristics of the current study, including the large size and ethnic diversity of the study sample, the availability of detailed renal characteristics, and the use of powerful multivariate methods, enhance the validity of these results and underscore the important contribution of this study. However, there are a number of limitations that warrant discussion. First, although the total number of patients examined was substantial, the relatively smaller size of individual non-Caucasian groups limited our power to examine these groups separately. Moreover, the specific ancestries of our ethnic groups may not be representative of other samples. For example, our Hispanic patients were of predominantly Mexican ancestry and were therefore not representative of all Hispanic patients (e.g., those of Puerto Rican descent).

Other design characteristics also imposed limitations. For example, these patients were not followed up prospectively from the time of their SLE diagnosis. As a result, there was variation in the amount and type of information available concerning individual patients. To compensate for this design feature, we obtained all medical records available for each patient since the time of diagnosis. For many patients, this required collection of medical records from several physicians. We also collected extensive information from patients via questionnaire to ensure that we were not missing important data relevant to their SLE diagnoses or the presence of renal involvement.

Additionally, because some patients had relatively short disease durations prior to their inclusion in the current study, it is possible that some patients who would ultimately develop renal disease were misclassified as non-nephritis control. However, to the extent that such misclassification biased our study, the bias should have been a conservative one. Furthermore, the inclusion of disease duration as a covariate in our multivariate analyses did not significantly alter the association observed between FcγRIIIA polymorphism and the risk of nephritis.

In summary, we have demonstrated that inheritance of the FcγRIIIA-158F allele (and FF genotype) has a striking influence on the risk of nephritis among Caucasian SLE patients. Similar results were not observed among non-Caucasians with SLE. In contrast, inheritance of FcγRIIA-131R/H alleles did not influence the risk of nephritis among any of the ethnic groups examined. These findings are of great significance for SLE patients, their physicians, and investigators. First, these results may provide a powerful tool to assist physicians with prognostic determinations early in the course of disease. Second, this information highlights the potential value of FcγR-directed therapies (30). Ultimately, therapeutic interventions may become available for use in patients once they have developed nephritis, or earlier, in an attempt to prevent this devastating disease manifestation. There are a number of important areas for future investigation. These include confirmation of the results for specific non-Caucasian ethnic groups and examination of ethnic groups not represented in the current study. Greater understanding of the ethnic heterogeneity we observed will also require examination of extended haplotypes in the region of FcγRIIIA in an ethnically diverse sample. Finally, as other genetic risk factors for nephritis are identified, these should be examined in conjunction with FcγRIIIA to identify important gene–gene interactions.

ACKNOWLEDGMENTS

The authors wish to thank the patients who participated in this study, their physicians, the UCSF Lupus Genetics Project staff, and the Greater Sacramento Chapter of the Lupus Foundation of America.

REFERENCES

1. Hochberg MC. The application of genetic epidemiology to systemic lupus erythematosus. J Rheumatol 1987;14:867–9.
2. Deapen D, Escalante A, Weinrib L, Horwitz D, Bachman B, Roy-Burman P, et al. A revised estimate of twin concordance in systemic lupus erythematosus. Arthritis Rheum 1992;35:311–8.
3. Lander ES, Schork NJ. Genetic dissection of complex traits. Science 1994;265:2037–48.
4. Tan FK, Arnett FC. The genetics of lupus. Curr Opin Rheumatol 1998;10:399–408.
5. Criswell LA, Amos CI. Update on genetic risk factors for systemic lupus erythematosus and rheumatoid arthritis. Curr Opin Rheum 2000;2:85–90.
6. Norris CF, Pricop L, Millard SS, Taylor SM, Surrey S, Schwartz E, et al. A naturally occurring mutation in FcgRIIA: a Q to K127 change confers unique IgG binding properties to the R131 allelic form of the receptor. Blood 1998;91:656–62.
7. Kimberly RP, Salmon JE, Edberg JC. Receptors for immunoglobulin G: molecular diversity and implications for disease. Arthritis Rheum 1995;38:306–14.
8. Rascu A, Repp R, Westerdaal NA, Kalden JR, van de Winkel JG. Clinical relevance of Fcγ receptor polymorphisms. Ann N Y Acad Sci 1997;815:282–95.
9. Koene HR, Kleijer M, Algra J, Roos D, von dem Borne A, de Haas M. FcγRIIIA-158V/F polymorphism influences the binding of IgG by natural killer cell FcγRIIIA independently of the FcgRIIIA-48L/R/H phenotype. Blood 1997;90:1109–14.
10. Wu J, Edberg JC, Redecha PB, Bansal V, Guyre PM, Coleman K, et al. A novel polymorphism of FcγRIIIa (CD16) alters receptor function and predisposes to autoimmune disease. J Clin Invest 1997;100:1059–70.
11. Salmon JE, Millard S, Schacter LA, Arnett FC, Ginzler EM, Gourley MF, et al. FcγRIIA alleles are heritable risk factors for lupus nephritis in African Americans. J Clin Invest 1996;97: 1348–54.
12. Song YW, Han C-W, Kang S-W, Baek H-J, Lee E-B, Shin C-H, et al. Abnormal distribution of Fcγ receptor type IIa polymorphisms in Korean patients with systemic lupus erythematosus. Arthritis Rheum 1998;41:421–6.
13. Duits AJ, Bootsma H, Derksen RHWM, Spronk PE, Kater L, Kallenberg CGM, et al. Skewed distribution of IgG Fc receptor IIa (CD32) polymorphism is associated with renal disease in systemic lupus erythematosus patients. Arthritis Rheum 1995;38:1832–6.
14. Oh M, Petri MA, Kim NA, Sullivan KE. Frequency of the FcγRIIIA-158F allele in African American patients with systemic lupus erythematosus. J Rheumatol 1999;26:1486–9.
15. Salmon JE, Ng S, Yoo D-H, Kim T-H, Kim SY, Song GG. Altered distribution of Fcγ receptor IIIA alleles in a cohort of Korean patients with lupus nephritis. Arthritis Rheum 1999;42:818–23.
16. Botto M, Theodoridis E, Thompson EM, Beynon HL, Briggs D, Isenberg DA, et al. FcγRIIa polymorphism in systemic lupus erythematosus (SLE): no association with disease. Clin Exp Immunol 1996;104:264–8.
17. Koene HR, Kleijer M, Swaak AJG, Sullivan KE, Bijl M, Petri MA, et al. The FcγRIIIA-158F allele is a risk factor for systemic lupus erythematosus. Arthritis Rheum 1998;41:1813–8.
18. Yap SN, Phipps ME, Manivasagar M, Tan SY, Bosco JJ. Human Fcγ receptor IIA (FcγRIIA) genotyping and association with systemic lupus erythematosus (SLE) in Chinese and Malays in Malaysia. Lupus 1999;8:305–10.
19. Tan EM, Cohen AS, Fries JF, Masi AT, McShane DJ, Rothfield NF, et al. The 1982 revised criteria for the classification of systemic lupus erythematosus. Arthritis Rheum 1982;25:1271–7.
20. Hochberg MC. Updating the American College of Rheumatology revised criteria for the classification of systemic lupus erythematosus [letter]. Arthritis Rheum 1997;40:1725.
21. Churg J, Sobin LH. Renal disease: classification and atlas of glomerular disease. Tokyo: Igaku-Shoin; 1982.
22. Bali D, Gourley IS, Kostyu DD, Goel N, Bruce I, Bell A, et al. Genetic analysis of multiplex rheumatoid arthritis families. Genes Immun 1999;1:28–36.
23. Lindblad-Toh K, Winchester E, Daly MJ, Wang DG, Hirschhorn JN, Laviolette JP, et al. Large-scale discovery and genotyping of single-nucleotide polymorphisms in the mouse. Nat Genet 2000; 4:381–6.
24. SAS. 8th ed. Cary (NC): SAS Institute, Inc.; 1999.
25. Whiting-O'Keefe Q, Henke JE, Shearn MA, Hopper J Jr, Biava CG, Epstein WV. The information content from renal biopsy in systemic lupus erythematosus: stepwise linear regression analysis. Ann Intern Med 1982;96:718–23.
26. Tateno S, Kobayashi Y, Shigematsu H, Hiki Y. Study of lupus

nephritis: its classification and significance of subendothelial deposits. QJM 1983;52:311–31.
27. Esdaile JM, Federgreen W, Quintal H, Suissa S, Hayslett JP, Kashgarian M. Predictors of one year outcome in lupus nephritis: the importance of renal biopsy. QJM 1991;295:907–18.
28. Lehrnbecher T, Foster CB, Zhu S, Leitman SF, Goldin LR, Huppi K, et al. Variant genotypes of the low-affinity Fcγ receptors in two control populations and a review of low-affinity Fcγ receptor polymorphisms in control and disease populations. Blood 1999;94: 4220–32.
29. Clynes R, Dumitru C, Ravetch JV. Uncoupling of immune complex formation and kidney damage in autoimmune glomerulonephritis. Science 1998;279:1052–4.
30. Deo YM, Graziano RF, Repp R, van de Winkel JGJ. Clinical significance of IgG Fc receptors and FcγR-directed immunotherapies. Immunol Today 1997;18:127–35.

ARTHRITIS & RHEUMATISM
Vol. 44, No. 3, March 2001, pp 626–637

Immunoglobulin V_κ Light Chain Gene Analysis in Patients With Sjögren's Syndrome

Claudia Heimbächer,[1] Arne Hansen,[1] Axel Pruss,[1] Annett Jacobi,[1] Karin Reiter,[1] Peter E. Lipsky,[2] and Thomas Dörner[1]

Objective. **Patients with Sjögren's syndrome (SS) have characteristic lymphocytic infiltration of the salivary glands with a previously reported predominance of V_κ-bearing B cells and produce a variety of autoantibodies, indicating that there is a humoral autoimmune component in this syndrome. This study was undertaken to determine whether there are primary deviations of immunoglobulin V gene usage, differences in somatic hypermutation, defects of selection, or indications for perturbances of B cell maturation in SS.**

Methods. **Individual peripheral B cells from patients with SS were analyzed for their Ig V gene usage, and the findings were compared with results in normal controls.**

Results. **Molecular differences, as reflected by findings in the nonproductive V_κ repertoire of the patients, were identified by an enhanced usage of $J_\kappa2$ gene segments and a lack of mutational targeting toward RGYW/WRCY sequences compared with controls. A greater usage of $V_\kappa1$ family members and a reduced frequency of $V_\kappa3$ gene segments in the productive repertoire suggested differences in selection, possibly driven by antigen. Overall positive selection for mutations, especially for replacements in the complementarity-determining region and for mutations in RGYW/WRCY, similar to that found in controls, was detected.**

Conclusion. **Disturbances of strictly regulated B cell maturation, during early B cell development as indicated by prominent $J_\kappa2$ gene usage and during germinal center reactions as indicated by a lack of targeting of the hypermutation mechanism, might contribute to the emergence of autoimmunity in SS.**

Sjögren's syndrome (SS) is a chronic inflammatory disease of the lacrimal and salivary glands with subsequent development of keratoconjunctivitis sicca and xerostomia. Although the cause of the disease is unknown, histopathologic findings suggest an essential role of lymphocytic infiltrates, including plasma cells, located within germinal center–like structures. Autoantibodies directed against the autoantigens Ro/SSA and La/SSB, as well as rheumatoid factor, are detected in high titers in the sera of ~80–95% of SS patients (1), indicating that there is a humoral autoimmune component in this syndrome. Whereas glandular tissue destruction has been shown to be mediated by activated CD4+ T cells that home into the lacrimal gland, a broad variety of other clinical manifestations is observed in these patients, the etiologies of which are unknown. Notably, a 44-fold increased risk for the development of lymphoid malignancy, almost exclusively of B cell origin, has been documented, and this emphasizes the intimate role of activated B cells in this autoimmune disease (2), although it is not known whether B cell activation is a primary cause or a secondary manifestation of SS.

Structures resembling germinal centers have been observed in the salivary glands of patients with SS (3,4), but it is not known whether the microenvironment of these cell clusters is sufficient for the induction of a germinal center response. Recent reports (4–6) described mutated rearranged V genes from B cells within cell clusters obtained from the salivary glands of SS patients; these findings were interpreted as being an indication of an antigen-driven immune response, as was

Supported by grants Do491/4-1 and 5-1 from the Deutsche Forschungsgemeinschaft.

[1]Claudia Heimbächer, MD, Arne Hansen, MD, Axel Pruss, MD, Annett Jacobi, MD, Karin Reiter, MD, Thomas Dörner, MD: University Hospital Charite, Berlin, Germany; [2]Peter E. Lipsky, MD: National Institutes of Health, Bethesda, Maryland.

Address correspondence and reprint requests to Thomas Dörner, MD, Department of Medicine/Rheumatology and Clinical Immunology, University Hospital Charite, Schumannstr. 20/21, 10098 Berlin, Germany.

Submitted for publication May 2, 2000; accepted in revised form November 8, 2000.

previously reported with regard to the synovial membrane in rheumatoid arthritis (7).

Specifically, one study (4) identified clonally related but different V gene rearrangements obtained from different clusters of B cells in the salivary infiltrates, and the investigators concluded that there was no major V gene preference in the 2 patients analyzed. Moreover, the ratios of replacement to silent (R:S) mutations in the V_H and V_L gene rearrangements were significantly lower than expected, and this was interpreted as an indication for selection against R mutations in both complementarity-determining regions (CDRs) and framework regions (FRs). A second study (5) analyzed V_H–D–J_H gene transcripts from lip and lymph node biopsy specimens from 2 other SS patients. The data also provided evidence for polyclonal diversification of the B cell response as evidenced by the detection of a broad variety of V gene rearrangements, although indications for clonal expansion were also found in both the lip and the lymph node samples. Consistent with the findings of the other study (4), the R:S ratio in the V_H rearrangements found was lower than expected in both the CDRs and the FRs. A third study (3) identified expanded monotypic plasma cell populations in the infiltrates of the salivary glands, which altered the κ:λ ratio to $\geq$3 in SS patients older than 43 years.

Most previous studies analyzing Ig gene rearrangements in SS focused exclusively on V genes isolated from B cells within the affected organ, i.e., the salivary glands. Since the development of B cells is governed by strict regulation of positive and negative selection at certain developmental stages of early B cell ontogeny, there remains a possibility that these influences might be disturbed in autoimmune conditions, such as SS, as either a cause or an effect of the disease. Striking abnormalities in the B cell repertoire in another autoimmune disease, systemic lupus erythematosus (SLE), have been reported (8,9). Furthermore, abnormalities in the distribution of mutations in SLE have been identified (10,11), but the role of somatic hypermutation in generating autoimmunity in SS has not been addressed.

To examine the possible roles of abnormalities in repertoire generation or somatic hypermutation in the B cell abnormalities in SS, individual peripheral B cells from patients with this condition were analyzed in the present study, by comparing nonproductive and productive V_κ gene rearrangements obtained by polymerase chain reaction (PCR) amplification of genomic DNA from individual B cells. Analysis of the nonproductive repertoire is especially important in assessing the immediate impact of recombination and somatic hypermutation, since the nonproductive rearrangements do not encode a protein, and therefore B cells expressing these rearrangements are not directly influenced by selection. In contrast, the distribution of B cells can be influenced by positive and negative selection at various stages of maturation and differentiation, based on the nature of the productive V_κ–J_κ rearrangement and the resultant expressed Ig molecule. The results demonstrate that a molecularly determined preference for $J_\kappa2$ usage, abnormal hypermutation, and aberrant selection distinguishes the peripheral V_κ gene repertoire in SS from that in normal subjects and suggest that a unique set of abnormalities characterizes the B cell repertoire in SS.

PATIENTS AND METHODS

Patients. Peripheral B cells from 3 patients fulfilling the revised criteria for classification of SS (12) were analyzed. All patients were female and exhibited typical histology of the minor salivary glands (focus score >1). Two patients (patient 1 [age 76 years, disease duration 9 years] and patient 2 [age 56 years, disease duration 2 years]) expressed high-titer anti–52-kd Ro/SSA and anti-La/SSB antibodies, whereas 1 patient (patient 3 [age 54 years, disease duration 4 years]) had only anti–52-kd Ro/SSA antibodies. All patients had hyperimmunoglobulinemia and were rheumatoid factor positive. None of the patients analyzed had a monoclonal gammopathy. Patient 1 had recurrent parotid gland enlargements in 1998 but no indications of non-Hodgkin's lymphoma by histologic examination. Patients 1 and 2 did not have extraglandular organ manifestations besides leukopenia (patient 1 with 3.6 gigaparticles/μl) and Raynaud's phenomenon (patients 2 and 3), whereas patient 3 exhibited vasculitic changes of the skin. Otherwise, the patients did not differ in any of the characteristics of SS. In terms of treatment, all patients received artificial tear drops, and patients 2 and 3 received artificial saliva. At the time of analysis, patients 1 and 2 were taking 5 mg prednisolone/day and patient 3 was receiving 7.5 mg prednisolone/day and 200 mg hydroxychloroquine/day.

Preparation of peripheral blood mononuclear cells, fluorescence-activated cell sorting of individual B cells, and the method of PCR amplification of V_κ–J_κ gene rearrangements have been reported in detail previously (13). For patients 1 and 2, 184 individual peripheral B cells were analyzed, whereas 92 individual peripheral B cells were analyzed from patient 3.

Controls. Recently reported V_κ–J_κ rearrangements from 2 healthy normal donors (ages 26 years old and 45 years old) (13) were used for comparison. Both the nonproductive and the productive repertoires of these 2 donors exhibited a comparable usage of V_κ and J_κ gene elements.

Determination of *Taq* polymerase fidelity and the frequency of potential sequence errors. The PCR error rate for this analysis has been documented to be ~1×10^{-4} mutations/basepair (14,15). Thus, few if any of the nucleotide changes encountered in this analysis can be ascribed to amplification errors.

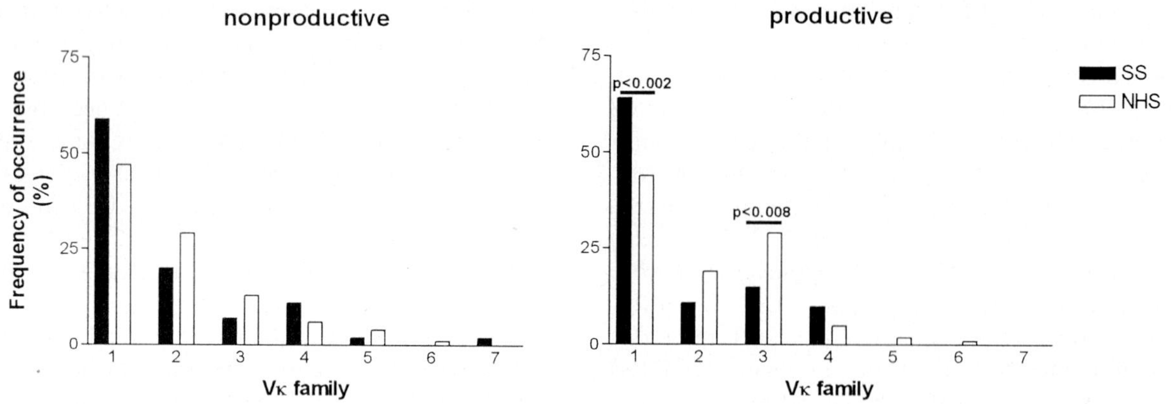

Figure 1. Distribution of Vκ gene families in peripheral B cells in the nonproductive and productive repertoires from patients with Sjögren's syndrome (SS) compared with normal controls (normal human subjects; NHS). The usage of Vκ1 family members in the productive repertoire was significantly more frequent in the SS patients compared with controls, whereas Vκ3 gene segments in the productive repertoire were found significantly less frequently in the SS patients than in controls.

Statistical analysis. Sequences were analyzed by Fisher's exact test to compare the differences in the distribution of particular gene segments, CDR3 lengths, and exonuclease and terminal deoxynucleotidyl transferase (TdT) activity. The chi-square test was used to compare the mutational frequencies between the nonproductive and productive V_κ rearrangements of the patients with SS and the controls. P values less than or equal to 0.05 were considered to be significant.

RESULTS

Seventy-nine V_κ–J_κ gene rearrangements were obtained from patient 1 (40 nonproductive and 39 productive), 28 V_κ–J_κ gene rearrangements from patient 2 (10 nonproductive and 18 productive), and 30 V_κ–J_κ rearrangements from patient 3 (6 nonproductive and 24 productive). Of note, there were no statistically significant differences between these patients with regard to V_κ and J_κ gene usage, CDR3 length, or mutational frequencies in the nonproductive or productive repertoire; therefore, the distributions were combined and analyzed as a group. This included a total of 81 productive and 56 nonproductive rearrangements.

V_κ gene family usage in SS. No significant differences in the distribution of V_κ families in the nonproductive rearrangements of the patients with SS, in comparison with the normal controls, were noted (Figure 1). In the productive repertoire, the $V_\kappa 1$ family was found significantly more frequently in the patients (52 of 81; 64%) compared with the normal controls (142 of 321; 44%) (P = 0.0018), whereas $V_\kappa 3$ family members were detected less frequently in the patients (12 of 81; 15%) than in the normal donors (94 of 321; 29%) (P = 0.0074). The remaining V_κ families did not differ signif-

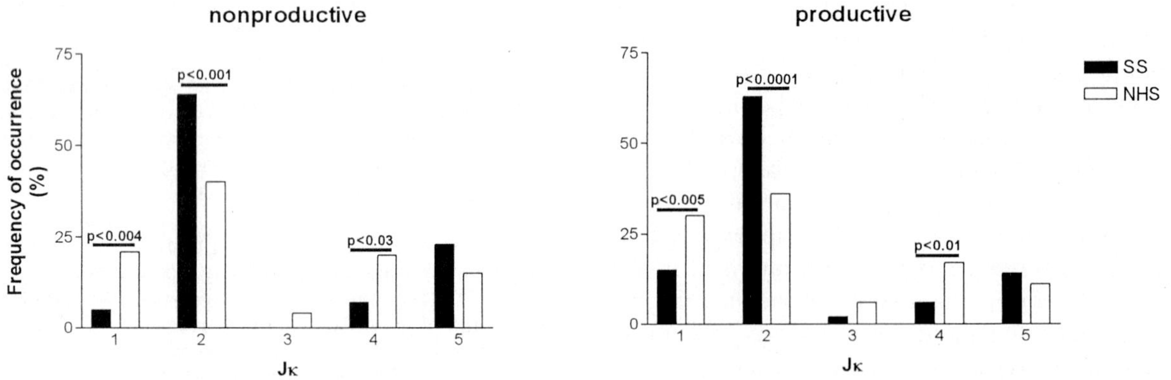

Figure 2. Distribution of Jκ genes in peripheral B cells in the nonproductive and productive repertoires from patients with SS compared with normal controls. See Figure 1 for definitions.

icantly, although members of the $V_\kappa5$ and $V_\kappa6$ families were not detected in the productive gene repertoire of the SS patients.

J_κ gene usage in SS. In the productive repertoire of the patients with SS, all 5 J_κ elements were found, whereas no V_κ rearrangement using $J_\kappa3$ was detected in the nonproductive gene repertoire (Figure 2). In the nonproductive repertoire, $J_\kappa2$ segments were significantly more frequent in patients with SS (36 of 56; 64%) than in controls (92 of 232; 40%) ($P < 0.001$), and $J_\kappa1$ (3 of 56; 5%) and $J_\kappa4$ (4 of 56; 7%) occurred significantly less frequently in patients than in controls (50 of 232; 22% and 46 of 232; 20%, respectively) ($P = 0.0036$ and $P = 0.0292$, respectively). Productive V_κ rearrangements used $J_\kappa2$ gene segments significantly more frequently in the patients than in the controls ($P < 0.0001$) (Figure 2). This was accounted for by a significantly greater usage of $J_\kappa1$ ($P < 0.005$) and $J_\kappa4$ ($P = 0.0093$) in the controls than in the patients.

Distribution of individual V_κ genes in peripheral B cells from patients with SS. The next analysis assessed the distribution of individual V_κ genes in patients with SS versus controls (Table 1). Only a few differences were detected between individual V_κ gene usage in the nonproductive and productive repertoires of the patients with SS. Thus, the O14/O4 genes were found significantly more frequently in the nonproductive repertoire (9%) than in the productive repertoire (1%) of the patients with SS ($P = 0.0416$). Moreover, the pseudogene A18 was found significantly more often in the nonproductive repertoire (7% versus 0%) ($P = 0.0262$). When the usage of particular V_κ gene segments was analyzed, L12 was found to be significantly overrepresented in the nonproductive repertoire of the patients compared with the controls (9% versus 3%) ($P = 0.042$).

When the productive repertoires of the patients and controls were compared, L12 was also detected significantly more often in the patients (17% versus 8%) ($P = 0.0209$). In contrast, A27 was found less often in the productive repertoire of the patients than in that of the controls (5% versus 14%) ($P = 0.0228$). Although A17 appeared to be less frequent in the patients (1% versus 7%), the difference was not significant ($P = 0.0595$). Some genes detected in the normal controls (L11, L10 or L25, L4, L1, A26/A10, A21, A2, A4, L16, L20, L23, and L25) were not found in the V_κ gene repertoire of patients with SS (data not shown).

Comparison of the usage of the J_κ proximal and J_κ distal cassettes. The V_κ locus is divided into a proximal and a distal cassette. To gain insight into the frequency of usage of individual V_κ genes based on their location in the chromosome (Table 2) and their rearrangement with specific J_κ segments, we analyzed the usage of proximal and distal V_κ genes in the productive and nonproductive V_κ repertoires of the patients. Of note, nonproductive V_κ rearrangements used V_κ genes J_κ distal to A18 significantly more frequently in comparison with the productive repertoire (52% versus 30%) ($P < 0.02$). Comparison of the patients and controls as shown in Tables 1 and 2 demonstrated a similarly increased usage of V genes proximal to A18 in the productive compared with the nonproductive repertoire in both groups (patients 48% in the nonproductive versus 70% in the productive repertoire [Table 2]; controls 52% in the nonproductive versus 72% in the productive repertoire). This was accounted for by a

Table 1. Distribution of rearranged V_κ genes in peripheral B cells from patients with Sjögren's syndrome (SS) and from normal controls*

		Nonproductive		Productive	
V_κ gene†	V_κ gene family	SS patients (n = 56)	Controls (n = 232)	SS patients (n = 81)	Controls (n = 321)‡
B3	$V_\kappa4$	6 (11)	14 (6)	8 (10)	17 (5)
B2	$V_\kappa5$	1 (2)	10 (4)	0	6 (2)
B1 (ψ)	$V_\kappa7$	1 (2)	0	0	0
L12	$V_\kappa1$	5 (9)§	6 (3)	14 (17)¶	26 (8)
L9	$V_\kappa1$	1 (2)	8 (3)	3 (4)	7 (2)
L8	$V_\kappa1$	1 (2)	1 (1)	3 (4)	6 (2)
L6	$V_\kappa3$	0	9 (4)	4 (5)	20 (6)
L5/L19a	$V_\kappa1$	1 (2)	2 (1)	3 (4)	9 (3)
L2	$V_\kappa3$	3 (5)	6 (3)	4 (5)	23 (7)
A30	$V_\kappa1$	3 (5)	9 (4)	5 (6)	13 (4)
A27	$V_\kappa3$	1 (2)	12 (5)	4 (5)#	46 (14)
A23	$V_\kappa2$	1 (2)	4 (2)	2 (2)	4 (1)
A20	$V_\kappa1$	1 (2)	9 (4)	1 (1)	7 (2)
A19/A3	$V_\kappa2$	1 (2)	13 (6)	5 (6)	28 (9)
A18 (ψ)	$V_\kappa2$	4 (7)**	14 (6)	0	0
A17	$V_\kappa2$	3 (5)	16 (7)	1 (1)	22 (7)
O18/O8	$V_\kappa1$	6 (11)	18 (8)	4 (5)	20 (6)
O14/O4	$V_\kappa1$	5 (9)††	8 (3)	1 (1)	6 (2)
O12/O2	$V_\kappa1$	6 (11)	20 (9)	13 (16)	34 (11)
O11/O1	$V_\kappa2$	1 (2)	4 (2)	0	1 (1)
A1	$V_\kappa2$	0	4 (2)	1 (1)	1 (1)
L15	$V_\kappa1$	1 (2)	2 (1)	0	0
L19	$V_\kappa1$	1 (2)	2 (1)	2 (2)	3 (1)
L24	$V_\kappa1$	1 (2)	4 (2)	2 (2)	3 (1)
LFVK431	$V_\kappa1$	1 (2)	0	1 (1)	0
DPK14	$V_\kappa2$	1 (2)	0	0	0

* Values are the number (%).
† V_κ genes are arranged in order from J-proximal to J-distal. The locations of 3 V_κ genes (2 LFVK431 and 1 DPK14) have not been identified (24).
‡ Data on V_κ gene usage in normal controls have been published elsewhere (13).
§ $P = 0.042$ versus controls.
¶ $P = 0.0209$ versus controls.
# $P = 0.0228$ versus controls.
** $P = 0.0262$ versus productive repertoire of SS patients.
†† $P = 0.0416$ versus productive repertoire of SS patients.

Table 2. Comparison of V_κ genes J_κ proximal or distal to A18 rearranged to J_κ1–4 or J_κ5 gene elements in patients with Sjögren's syndrome*

	Nonproductive†		Productive†	
	Proximal	Distal	Proximal	Distal
J_κ1–4	22‡	20	49	20
J_κ5	4	8	7	4
Total	26 (48)§	28 (52)	56 (70)¶	24 (30)

* Values are the number (%).
† Two V_κ genes of the nonproductive repertoire (DPK14 and LFVK431) and 1 V_κ gene of the productive repertoire (LFVK431) have not been assigned to the distal or proximal V_κ cassette (24).
‡ $P < 0.02$ versus J_κ1–4 using V_κ genes of the proximal cassette in the productive repertoire.
§ $P < 0.02$ versus usage of V_κ genes of the proximal cassettes in the productive repertoire.
¶ $P < 0.02$ versus usage of V_κ genes of the distal cassette in the productive repertoire.

reduced usage of V genes distal to A18 in the productive compared with the nonproductive repertoire by both the patients and the controls. The increased frequency of V_κ genes proximal to A18 by productive rearrangements was significant in both the patients ($P < 0.02$) and the controls ($P < 0.001$). Notably, there was no preferential usage of the V_κ distal J_κ5 element by rearrangements using J_κ distal V_κ genes in either controls (data not shown) or SS patients (Table 2).

CDR3 length. The most unique characteristic of each V–D–J gene rearrangement is the composition of CDR3. Therefore, further analysis was undertaken to compare the length of the CDR3 and the imprints of exonuclease and TdT activity on productive and nonproductive V_κ–J_κ rearrangements in the patients and controls. In general, there were no major differences between the patients and the controls with regard to CDR3 length in either repertoire (Table 3). In the nonproductive repertoire of the patients, however, 13% of the amplified V_κ rearrangements had a length of 26 bp, whereas CDR3 of this length was not found in controls ($P < 0.0001$). Overall, 77% of the rearrangements of the patients used a CDR3 length between 25 and 29 nucleotides, whereas in controls, 59% of the nonproductive V_κ rearrangements exhibited this CDR3 length.

Similarly, no significant differences between the patients and the controls were observed with regard to CDR3 length in the productive V_κ repertoire. Fifty-nine percent of the V_κ rearrangements of the patients had a CDR3 length of 27 nucleotides, and 23% contained a CDR3 length of 30 or 33 nucleotides. Only 17% of V_κ rearrangements obtained from the patients exhibited a CDR3 length of less than 18, 21, or 24 nucleotides. In normal controls, 66% of all productive V_κ gene rearrangements used a CDR3 length of 27 nucleotides, and only 13% had a shorter CDR3 length.

Exonuclease activity in V_κ rearrangements in individual B cells of the patients with SS versus controls. The imprint of exonuclease activity on the V_κ gene rearrangements of the patients was detected frequently (Tables 4 and 5). There was evidence of extreme exonuclease activity in the patients, manifested by 2 examples of the removal of 9 nucleotides in 2 V_κ rearrangements in the productive V_κ repertoire ($P = 0.0402$) (Table 4). Notably, exonuclease activity was significantly more frequent in the patients' productive V_κ repertoire (85%) compared with that in the nonproductive repertoire (71%) ($P < 0.05$). In addition, removal of 3 nucleotides was significantly more frequent in the productive V_κ repertoire of the SS patients (35%) than in the nonproductive V_κ rearrangements (13%) ($P = 0.0049$). Between 1 and 9 nucleotides were removed in the patients' V_κ repertoire, whereas 1–22 nucleotides were removed in the normal repertoire.

Table 3. Complementarity-determining region 3 length of V_κ–J_κ gene rearrangements obtained from individual B cells of patients with Sjögren's syndrome (SS) and from normal controls*

	Nonproductive		Productive	
No. of nucleotides	SS patients (n = 56)	Controls† (n = 232)	SS patients (n = 81)	Controls† (n = 321)
≤13	0	9 (4)		
14	1 (2)	1 (1)		
15			0	2 (1)
17	0	2 (1)		
18			1 (1)	3 (1)
19		3 (1)		
20	1 (2)	4 (2)		
21	0	2 (1)‡	4 (5)	7 (2)
22	0	7 (3)		
23	2 (4)	12 (5)		
24	1 (2)‡	21 (9)	9 (11)	29 (9)
25	7 (13)	25 (11)		
26	7 (13)§	0		
27	2 (4)	6 (3)‡	48 (59)	211 (66)
28	15 (27)	45 (19)		
29	11 (20)	61 (26)		
30	2 (4)‡	2 (1)‡	18 (22)	60 (19)
31	4 (7)	15 (6)		
32	2 (4)	11 (5)		
33	0	1 (1)‡	1 (1)	7 (2)
34	0	3 (1)		
35	0	2 (1)		
36	1 (2)	0	0	2 (1)

* Values are the number (%). No patients or controls had rearrangements of 16 nucleutides in either the nonproductive or the productive repertoire.
† Data on V_κ gene usage in normal controls have been published elsewhere (13).
‡ Includes pseudogenes.
§ $P < 0.0001$ versus controls.

Table 4. 5′ exonuclease activity on rearranged V_κ–J_κ genes from peripheral B cells of patients with Sjögren's syndrome (SS) and from normal controls*

No. of nucleotides removed	Nonproductive		Productive	
	SS patients (n = 56)	Controls (n = 232)	SS patients (n = 81)	Controls (n = 321)
0	16 (29)	43 (18)	12 (15)	49 (15)
1	12 (21)	32 (14)	12 (15)	52 (16)
2	11 (20)	33 (14)	10 (12)	36 (11)
3	7 (13)†	50 (22)	28 (35)	118 (37)
4	5 (9)	26 (11)	9 (11)	22 (7)
5	2 (4)	15 (6)	5 (6)	25 (8)
6	2 (4)	8 (3)	2 (2)	5 (2)
7	0	3 (1)	1 (1)	6 (2)
8	1 (2)	9 (4)	0	6 (2)
9	0	1 (1)	2 (2)‡	0
≥10–22	0	12 (5)	0	2 (<1)

* Values are the number (%).
† $P = 0.0049$ versus productive repertoire of SS patients.
‡ $P < 0.0402$ versus controls.

Evidence of exonuclease activity exerted on the J_κ gene segments was also detected frequently (Table 5). Again, this was more frequent in the patients' productive compared with their nonproductive repertoire (89% versus 73%) ($P < 0.01$). Removal of 1 nucleotide was found significantly more frequently in the productive than in the nonproductive V_κ gene repertoire (41% versus 18%) ($P < 0.005$).

Table 5. 3′ exonuclease activity on rearranged V_κ–J_κ genes from peripheral B cells of patients with Sjögren's syndrome (SS) and from normal controls*

No. of nucleotides removed	Nonproductive		Productive	
	SS patients (n = 56)	Controls (n = 232)	SS patients (n = 81)	Controls (n = 321)
0	15 (27)†	61 (26)	9 (11)‡	81 (25)
1	10 (18)§	53 (23)	33 (41)¶	88 (27)
2	6 (11)	19 (8)	15 (19)	45 (14)
3	4 (7)	27 (12)	7 (9)	32 (10)
4	7 (13)	30 (13)	4 (5)	33 (10)
5	9 (16)#	13 (7)	8 (10)	26 (8)
6	4 (7)	6 (3)	4 (5)**	2 (1)
7	1 (2)	2 (1)	1 (1)	9 (3)
8	0	8 (3)	0	2 (1)
9	0	2 (1)	0	2 (1)
10	0	4 (2)	0	1 (<1)
≥11–26	0	7 (3)		

* Values are the number (%).
† $P = 0.0226$ versus productive repertoire of SS patients.
‡ $P < 0.006$ versus controls.
§ $P = 0.005$ versus productive repertoire of SS patients.
¶ $P < 0.01$ versus controls.
# $P < 0.008$ versus controls.
** $P < 0.004$ versus controls.

Table 6. Terminal deoxynucleotidyl transferase activity on rearranged V_κ–J_κ genes from patients with Sjögren's syndrome (SS) and from normal controls*

No. of nucleotides	Nonproductive		Productive	
	SS patients (n = 56)	Controls (n = 232)	SS patients (n = 81)	Controls (n = 321)
0	22 (39)	72 (31)	40 (49)	138 (43)
1	7 (13)	42 (18)	17 (21)	61 (19)
2	15 (27)	48 (20)	12 (15)	50 (16)
3	7 (13)	29 (13)	7 (9)	38 (12)
4	4 (7)	17 (7)	4 (5)	16 (5)
5	1 (2)	12 (5)	0	9 (3)
6	0	6 (3)	0	3 (1)
7	0	2 (1)	0	2 (1)
8	0	1 (1)	1 (1)	2 (1)
≥9–15	0	3 (2)	0	2 (2)

* Values are the number (%).

Identification of the imprint of TdT activity in V_κ rearrangements in individual B cells of patients with SS versus controls. As seen in Table 6, 39% of the nonproductive rearrangements in the SS patients showed no evidence of TdT activity, whereas the remaining 61% exhibited TdT activity resulting in the addition of 1–5 nucleotides. Among the productive rearrangements in the patients, 49% had no imprint of TdT activity and 51% had 1–4 added nucleotides. Although nonproductive and productive V_κ rearrangements of controls had a greater range of added nucleotides, there was no significant difference between the controls and the patients with regard to the imprint of TdT activity.

Mutational analysis. *Frequency of mutated V_κ gene rearrangements.* It should be noted that 30.0% (patient 2), 32.5% (patient 1), and 66.7% (patient 3) of the nonproductive V_κ genes contained mutations. As a group, 20 of 56 (35.7%) of the nonproductively rearranged V_κ gene segments from the patients contained mutations, in comparison with 24% of those obtained from normal subjects (13). Among the productive V_κ repertoires, 51.3% (patient 2), 66.7% (patient 1), and 88.9% (patient 3) were mutated, for a total of 64.2% (52 of 81). Among the productive V_κ gene rearrangements of normal subjects, 41% contained mutations (13).

R:S ratio. Because of the significant differences in the mutational frequencies of the nonproductive and productive V_κ gene repertoires obtained from peripheral B cells of patients with SS (Table 7), further analysis was performed to address the nature of these mutations in more detail (Table 8). In the SS patients, no significant difference between the nonproductive and productive V_κ repertoires in terms of the R:S ratios within the FRs was observed (3.3 versus 2.7) ($P = 0.695$).

Table 7. Comparison of the mutational frequencies between V_κ gene rearrangements using J_κ1–4 and J_κ5 in patients with Sjögren's syndrome

	Nonproductive			Productive		
	No. of mutations	Total bp	Mutational frequency, %	No. of mutations	Total bp	Mutational frequency, %
J_κ1–4	57	10,562	0.54*†	189	17,017	1.11
J_κ5	7	3,303	0.21‡	26	2,578	1.00
Total	64	13,865	0.46*	215	19,595	1.10

* $P < 0.0001$ versus productive repertoire.
† $P = 0.0227$ versus V_κ rearrangements using J_κ5 in the nonproductive repertoire.
‡ $P < 0.0005$ versus productive repertoire.

However, the R:S ratio was significantly increased in the CDRs of productive compared with nonproductive rearrangements (4.0 versus 1.4) ($P < 0.01$). Analysis of specific V regions did not demonstrate significant differences in the R:S ratio between the nonproductive and productive repertoire of the patients. The same analysis identified significant differences in the R:S ratios in FR2 and FR3 of normal subjects (Table 8), consistent with an abnormality in the deletion of rearrangements with FR mutations.

Nature of mutations. As shown in Figure 3, G mutations in the patients with SS (46.9%) were significantly more frequent than A mutations and C mutations (14.1% and 12.5%, respectively) ($P < 0.001$ for both), but not significantly more frequent than T mutations (26.6%), in the nonproductive V_κ repertoire. In the productive V_κ repertoire, G mutations (30.7%) were found significantly more often than T mutations (19.5%) ($P < 0.008$), whereas A mutations (24.2%) and C mutations (25.6%) did not differ significantly. Comparison of the mutational frequency of individual nucleotides between the nonproductive and productive V_κ repertoire of SS patients demonstrated significant differences in G mutations ($P < 0.02$) and C mutations ($P < 0.03$).

Mutational analysis of V_κ gene rearrangements using J_κ5 and J_κ1–4 gene segments. The mutational frequency of V_κ rearrangements using J_κ1–4 and J_κ5 segments was also analyzed (Table 7). In the nonproductive repertoire, V_κ gene rearrangements using J_κ5 contained significantly fewer mutations than V_κ rearrangements using J_κ1–4 (mutational frequency 0.21% versus 0.54%) ($P = 0.0227$). Of note, no difference in the mutational frequency of productively rearranged V_κ genes was found when V_κ rearrangements using J_κ1–4 and those using J_κ5 were compared.

Mutational targeting in the SS patients: analysis of mutations in RGYW and WRCY motifs. Previous analyses identified the RGYW (purine, G, pyridine, A/T) motif on both DNA strands as a major target of the mutational machinery (16–18) in both V_H and V_L gene rearrangements obtained from normal subjects. As a result, a great proportion of mutations has been identified within RGYW and its countermotif, WRCY. We performed further analyses to determine the role of these motifs in mutations of the nonproductive and productive gene rearrangements in the V_κ genes from the SS patients. In the nonproductive repertoire, 12 of 64 mutations

Table 8. Comparison of the ratio of replacement to silent mutations (R:S ratio) of V_κ gene rearrangements from B cells of patients with Sjögren's syndrome (SS) and normal controls*

	SS patients							Controls		
	Nonproductive			Productive						
	R	S	R:S ratio	R	S	R:S ratio	P†	Nonproductive, R:S ratio	Productive, R:S ratio	P†
FR1	3	0	ND	7	0	ND	NS	–	–	–
CDR1	6	3	2.0	40	9	4.4	NS	3.4	4.7	NS
FR2	7	2	3.5	14	8	1.8	NS	4.2	1.3	<0.002
CDR2	4	2	2.0	25	5	5.0	NS	3.6	5.4	NS
FR3	13	5	2.6	44	16	2.8	NS	2.6	1.4	<0.03
CDR3	10	9	1.1	36	11	3.3	NS	5.7	5	NS
FR	23	7	3.3	65	24	2.7	NS	3.0 (109/36)	1.4 (195/144)	<0.035
CDR	20	14	1.4	101	25	4.0	<0.01	4.2 (79/19)	4.9 (345/70)	<0.001
Total genes	43	21	2.0	166	49	3.4	NS	3.2 (188/58)	2.5 (540/214)	<0.001

* FR = framework region; ND = not defined; NS = not significant; CDR = complementarity-determining region.
† Comparison of the R:S ratio in the nonproductive versus the productive repertoire within the particular V regions, by chi-square test.

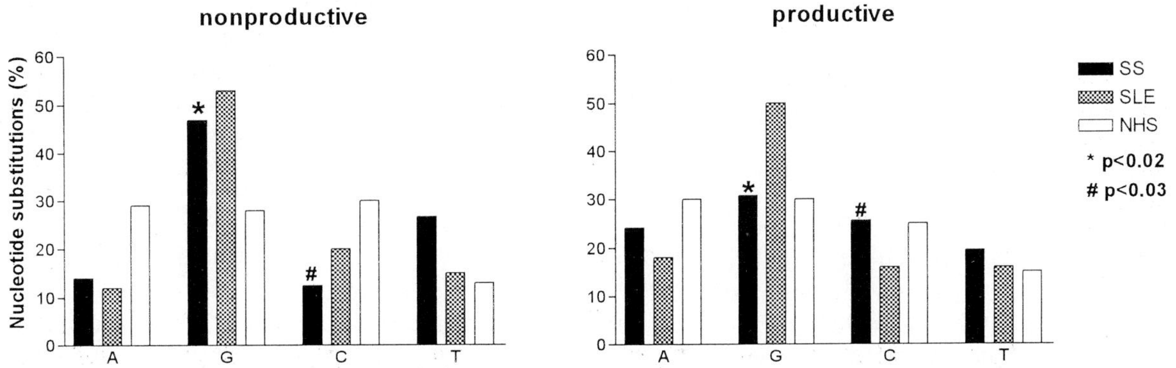

Figure 3. Analysis of nucleotide substitutions in nonproductive and productive V_κ gene rearrangements in patients with SS compared with those found in a patient with systemic lupus erythematosus (SLE) and in normal controls. Significant differences in the frequency of G and C mutations in the nonproductive versus the productive V_κ gene repertoire were found. See Figure 1 for other definitions.

(18.8%) were part of RGYW and 1 of 64 mutations (1.6%) were found within the inverse repeat of RGYW, WRCY. Altogether, 13 of 64 mutations (20.3%) were located within these motifs in the nonproductive repertoire. In the productive repertoire, 56 of 215 mutations (26.0%) were included within RGYW and 18 of 215 mutations (8.4%) occurred within WRCY sequences. Thus, 74 of 215 mutations (34.4%) were found within these consensus sequences in the productive repertoire.

Comparison with the expected percentage of mutations in randomly selected quartet sequences (23.6%) indicated no targeting of RGYW/WRCY sequences in the nonproductive repertoire (20.4%). In the productive repertoire, the frequency of mutations in RGYW/WRCY motifs (34.4%) significantly exceeded the expected percentage ($P < 0.001$) and the percentage found in the nonproductive repertoire ($P < 0.035$).

When the mutational patterns within individual RGYW motifs were compared with their specific inverse repeats (Figure 4), significant differences were detected in the patients with SS. As a reference, mutations in specific RGYW and their inverse repeats were comparable in normal subjects (16–18). There was a difference in the mutational frequency of RGYW and WRCY sequences in the nonproductive repertoire (4.1% versus 0.5%) ($P < 0.012$) and the productive repertoire (8.8% versus 4.0%) ($P < 0.002$) of the SS patients that has not been found in controls. In the nonproductive repertoire, mutations of GGCT (6.3%) were significantly more frequent than mutations of its inverse repeat, AGCC

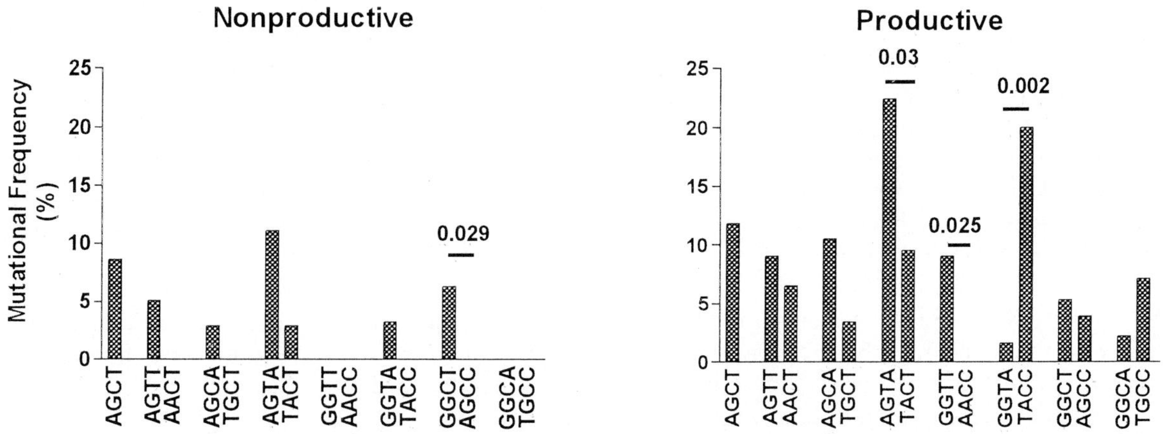

Figure 4. Mutational frequency of RGYW sequences and their inverse repeats, WRCY, in the nonproductive and productive V_κ gene repertoires of peripheral B cells from patients with Sjögren's syndrome.

(0%) ($P = 0.029$). The frequencies of RGYW mutations (8.8%) and WRCY mutations (4.1%) were increased when the productive repertoire was compared with the nonproductive repertoire ($P < 0.01$ and $P < 0.012$, respectively). In the productive repertoire, mutations of TACC (20.0%) were found significantly more frequently than mutations of its inverse repeat, GGTA (1.6%) ($P = 0.002$). A similar difference was observed between mutations of GGTT (9.0%) and mutations of AACC (0%) ($P = 0.025$), as well as between mutations of AGTA (22.4%) and mutations of TACT (9.5%) ($P = 0.03$). It should be noted that the significant increase of mutations noted when the nonproductive and productive repertoires were compared coincided with a significant increase of mutations in RGYW/WRCY motifs.

DISCUSSION

This study investigated whether patients with SS, known to have hyperimmunoglobulinemia and to produce a variety of autoantibodies, have molecular abnormalities or differences in selective influences on the generation of the V_κ light chain repertoire. Use of the single-cell PCR methodology (13,19) made it possible to amplify genomic DNA of Ig gene rearrangements from peripheral B cells and thereby to avoid biases inherent in analyzing cell lines or complementary DNA libraries (19). Since genomic DNA was used as a template, productive as well as nonproductive V_κ rearrangements could be amplified, sequenced, and analyzed. Analysis of the nonproductive repertoire is especially important for assessment of the immediate impact of molecular processes, such as recombination, somatic hypermutation, and receptor editing (8,9,13,19), since the nonproductive rearrangements do not encode an expressed Ig molecule and therefore do not influence selection of B cells expressing these Ig gene rearrangements. In contrast, the distribution of B cells and their productive Ig gene rearrangements can be affected by a variety of selective influences during development and subsequent antigenic stimulation because of the nature of the expressed μ or light chain (20). Based on these assumptions, the present study yielded new insights about both molecular and selective influences that govern the Ig repertoire in SS.

The similarity between the patients and the controls in terms of V_κ gene usage by the nonproductive gene repertoire indicated that there were no major molecular differences in the influences controlling V_κ–J_κ rearrangements in SS patients. In the productive repertoire, a significantly higher usage of $V_\kappa1$ family members ($P < 0.002$) and less frequent usage of $V_\kappa3$ genes ($P < 0.008$) indicated that after recombination, influences of negative and positive selection might have led to this difference from normal. A previous analysis of a patient with SLE (8) also revealed no differences in the frequency of particular V_κ gene families used in the nonproductive repertoire. Notably, no significant differences in V_κ family gene usage were found between the 3 patients with SS in the present study and the previously analyzed SLE patient (8). Overrepresentation of $V_\kappa1$ family members, especially in the productive repertoire, and a decreased frequency of $V_\kappa3$ family members were common findings in the SS patients and the SLE patient and suggested a characteristic bias in patients with autoimmune diseases.

This study also identified some differences in the usage of individual V_κ gene segments between SS patients and normal donors, in both the nonproductive repertoire (V_κ gene L12) and the productive repertoire (L12 and A27). Notably, the V_κ genes O04/O14 exhibited a significant reduction from the nonproductive repertoire (9%) to the productive repertoire (1%), consistent with negative selection. Moreover, rearrangements of A30/$J_\kappa2$, previously identified as a light chain binding to double-stranded DNA (21) and rearranged preferentially in SLE (8,21), were not found in the 3 SS patients. This latter finding implies that preferential rearrangements that occur in SLE are absent in SS whereas negative selection of an autoantibody encoding rearrangement is intact in SS, and is consistent with the absence of anti-DNA antibodies in the latter disease.

A variety of differences between the patients and controls in terms of J_κ gene segment usage became apparent. Thus, $J_\kappa2$ segments were used in the patients' nonproductive repertoires in 64% of rearrangements, in comparison with 40% found in controls ($P < 0.001$). Moreover, $J_\kappa1$ genes and $J_\kappa4$ segments were used significantly less often by nonproductive rearrangements in the patients ($P < 0.004$ and $P < 0.03$, respectively). In addition, $J_\kappa5$ genes were found in 23% of the patients' nonproductive repertoire, whereas these genes were found in 15% of the nonproductively rearranged V_κ–J_κ genes of controls. These findings suggest that $J_\kappa2$ is preferentially used by the SS patients, likely by molecular processes that are not under selective pressure since the frequency of $J_\kappa2$ was comparable in the productive repertoire (63%). This enhanced frequency was accounted for by a decrease in the frequency of $J_\kappa1$ and $J_\kappa4$ elements.

Although an enhanced frequency of V_κ genes distal to A18 in the nonproductive repertoire, as well as a lower mutational frequency of rearrangements using $J_\kappa 5$ (0.21%), in contrast to those using $J_\kappa 1$–4 (0.54%) ($P < 0.03$), suggested that receptor editing might have been used more frequently in SS patients, the similar usage of $J_\kappa 5$ in the nonproductive and productive V_κ repertoires of the SS patients (23% and 15%, respectively) did not indicate that there is an increased usage of secondary rearrangements. A comparable increased usage of V genes proximal to A18 in the productive compared with the nonproductive repertoire was observed in the SS patients (48% in the nonproductive and 70% in the productive repertoire) and the normal subjects (52% in the nonproductive and 72% in the productive repertoire). This increased frequency of V_κ genes proximal to A18 by productive rearrangements was significant ($P < 0.02$ in patients; $P < 0.001$ in controls). This constellation was found in all SS patients and controls and was independent of their age. Although the biologic relevance of this phenomenon is not clear, it further supports the notion that the overall V_κ gene usage in SS is very similar to that in normal individuals and is not excessively subjected to receptor editing.

Analysis of J_κ gene usage in the productive repertoire of the patients and controls identified a higher usage of $J_\kappa 2$ in the patients ($P < 0.0001$), whereas $J_\kappa 1$ ($P < 0.005$) and $J_\kappa 4$ ($P < 0.01$) were detected significantly less frequently in the patients' V_κ–J_κ repertoire. Since the frequency of $J_\kappa 2$ was the same in the nonproductive and productive repertoires of patients and exceeded the frequency of usage in controls ($P < 0.001$), it appears that the higher usage of this gene segment in SS is related to a molecular abnormality and not a selective influence. Similar findings of higher $J_\kappa 2$ usage have been reported to occur in patients with SLE (21), but have not been previously reported for SS. The differences of J_κ gene usage in the repertoire of patients with SS suggest the presence of influences exerted on the CDR3, since these gene elements encode a considerable part 3′ of this V region, although dramatic differences between patients and controls in regard to the length, 3′ and 5′ exonuclease activity, and TdT activity were not observed.

There appeared to be major differences between the mutational activity of patients with SS and that of normal subjects. The mutational frequency found in V_κ rearrangements from patients was increased in the nonproductive compared with the productive repertoire (0.46% versus 1.10%) ($P < 0.0001$). A similar constellation, consistent with positive selection of mutations into the productive V_κ gene repertoire, has been identified in normal subjects (13,17). Overall, the mutational frequencies found in the nonproductive repertoire (0.48%) and the productive repertoire (1.08%) in controls were similar. In contrast, the mutational frequencies of V_κ rearrangements in a patient with SLE (10) were significantly higher in the nonproductive repertoire (3.7%) than in the productive repertoire (2.8%) ($P < 0.003$). These data indicate that the degree of mutational activity was much more striking in the patient with SLE than in patients with SS or normal subjects. Since mutational frequency is likely to reflect the degree of B cell activity, this suggests that there is a major difference in the amount of B cell activity between SLE and SS.

Comparison of the frequency of mutated V_κ gene rearrangements from the peripheral blood revealed some notable findings. This frequency was 30–67% for the nonproductively rearranged genes and 51–89% for productively rearranged genes from SS patients, compared with 24% and 41%, respectively, from normal controls (13,17). The presence of a normal mutational frequency but an increased percentage of mutated rearrangements suggests abnormal mutational activity. In a previous analysis of an untreated SLE patient, 82% of the nonproductive and 75% of the productive V_κ repertoire harbored mutations (10). These data are consistent with the conclusion that the acquisition of mutations, and therefore, B cell memory, is enhanced in SS patients compared with normal subjects, but is not as greatly enhanced as in SLE. Whether this results from a hierarchic antigen-dependent B cell activation or, alternatively, from a diminished activation threshold in autoimmune conditions or from defects in apoptosis requires further investigation.

Mutations of individual nucleotides revealed additional differences. The frequency of A mutations was significantly lower in patients with SS (14.1% in the nonproductive repertoire, 24.2% in the productive repertoire) than in controls (29% and 30%, respectively). A constellation similar to that found in our SS patients was detected in a patient with SLE, with 12% mutated A basepairs in the nonproductive and 18% in the productive repertoire (10). In addition, G mutations were most frequent in the patients with SS (46.9% in the nonproductive and 30.7% in the productive repertoire) and in the previously reported patient with SLE (53% in the nonproductive and 50% in the productive repertoire) (10), whereas the frequency of these mutations was 28% and 30%, respectively, in controls (17).

Results were similar for mutations of T and C in the patients with SS (Figure 3). Although the mutational frequencies were different, the nature of basepair exchanges was also almost identical in the patients with SS and the SLE patient (10). These findings make it unlikely that the disturbances are related to the degree of mutations rather than to intrinsic differences in the mutational mechanism compared with normal subjects. Since defects in apoptosis among patients with SS and SLE have been reported (for review, see ref. 22), it is possible that this common characteristic might be responsible for the disturbances observed in these patients with autoimmune disease.

Whereas there was almost no evidence of differences in mutational frequency in the SS patients versus the controls, the overall targeting of mutations to RGYW motifs on both DNA strands, as clearly identified in controls (16–18), could not be identified in patients with SS. In a previous study, mutations of RGYW/WRCY motifs accounted for 36.7%, 50.6%, and 38.1% of all mutations in nonproductive V_H, V_κ, and V_λ rearrangements, respectively, in normal subjects, a significantly higher percentage than expected (23). The difference in RGYW/WRCY targeting in SS was emphasized by the lack of comparable mutations in individual RGYW motifs and their inverse WRCY repeats. Based on these differences in the markedly targeted RGYW/WRCY mutations identified in controls, nonspecific mutations are strikingly more frequent in SS. This might be a result of disturbed mismatch repair involved in mutations (25–29) that could be introduced during enhanced B cell proliferation. Since the introduction of targeted mutations appears to be related to activation by T cells with germinal centers, the present results suggest that most mutations in SS resulted from non–T cell–dependent activation. Alternatively, the germinal center–like structures in the salivary glands harboring the central inflammatory process are not able to provide an environment for a classic germinal center reaction facilitating rounds of proliferation with hypermutational and selection steps.

Consistent with positive selection of mutations from the nonproductive into the productive repertoire, RGYW/WRCY mutations were positively selected, as previously identified in normal subjects. Of note, however, the self-complementary sequence AGCT, frequently found as a highly targeted motif in normal subjects, was not mutated at the expected frequency. A possible explanation might relate to disturbed targeting of mutations without an overarching compensation by positive selection. As reported earlier with regard to the patient with SLE (10), a significant difference in the mutational frequency of AGTA/TACT and GGTA/TACC was detected in the nonproductive V_κ repertoire, indicating general perturbances of the mutational machinery or disturbed selection in systemic autoimmunity. The differences of mutations found between the complementary AGTA/TACT, GGTA/TACC, and GGTT/AACC sequences in the productive repertoire of the SS patients could also be the result of primary differences in mutational targeting. Previously, AGTT/AACT and GGCA/TGCC were identified to have significant different mutational frequencies in the patient with SLE (10). The conclusion from the current mutational analysis, that the pattern of mutations is disturbed in SS, is consistent with the findings of Manheimer-Lory et al, who reported an altered pattern of somatic mutations in the lupus-specific autoantibodies of the V_H idiotype F4+ (11). Whether these patients also had SS is not known.

The present findings are consistent with the conclusion that the SS patients exhibited differences in mutational targeting, but overall positive selection of these mutations. Whether these different mutational imprints are the result of a disturbed action of the mutational machinery or of defects in apoptosis permitting accumulation of abnormally targeted mutations not seen in normal subjects requires further elucidation.

ACKNOWLEDGMENTS

The authors are grateful to Toralf Kaiser and Gudrun Steinhauser for their technical assistance.

REFERENCES

1. Harley JB, Dickey WD. Sjögren's syndrome. In: Bigazzi PE, Reichlin M, editors. Systemic autoimmunity (Immunological series, Vol 54). New York: Dekker; 1991. p. 247–74.
2. Kassan SS, Thomas TL, Moutsopoulos HM, Hoover R, Kimberly RP, Budman DR, et al. Increased risk of lymphoma in sicca syndrome. Ann Intern Med 1978;89:888–92.
3. Bodeutsch C, de Wilde PC, Kater L, van den Hoogen FH, Hene RJ, van Houwelingen JC, et al. Monotypic plasma cells in labial salivary glands of patients with Sjögren's syndrome: prognosticator for systemic lymphoproliferative disease. J Clin Pathol 1993;46: 123–8.
4. Stott DI, Hiepe F, Hummel M, Steinhauser G, Berek C. Antigen-driven clonal proliferation of B cells within the target tissue of an autoimmune disease: the salivary glands of patients with Sjögren's syndrome. J Clin Invest 1998;1102:938–46.
5. Gellrich S, Rutz S, Borkowski A, Golembowski S, Gromnica-Ihle E, Sterry W, et al. Analysis of V_H–D–J_H gene transcripts in B cells infiltrating the salivary glands and lymph node tissues of patients with Sjögren's syndrome. Arthritis Rheum 1999;42:240–7.
6. Suzuki H, Takemura H, Suzuki M, Sekine Y, Kashiwagi H. Molecular cloning of antiSS-A/Ro 60-kDa peptide Fab fragments from infiltrating salivary gland lymphocytes of a patient with Sjögren's syndrome. Biochem Biophys Res Commun 1997;232: 101–6.
7. Schröder AE, Greiner A, Seyfert C, Berek C. Differentiation of B cells in the nonlymphoid tissue of the synovial membrane of

patients with rheumatoid arthritis. Proc Natl Acad Sci U S A 1996;93:221–5.
8. Dörner T, Foster SJ, Farner NL, Lipsky PE. Immunoglobulin kappa chain receptor editing in systemic lupus erythematosus. J Clin Invest 1998;102:688–94.
9. Dörner T, Farner NL, Lipsky PE. Immunoglobulin lambda and heavy chain gene usage in early untreated systemic lupus erythematosus suggests intensive B cell stimulation. J Immunol 1999;163: 1027–36.
10. Dörner T, Heimbächer C, Farner NL, Lipsky PE. Enhanced mutational activity of Vκ gene rearrangements in systemic lupus erythematosus. Clin Immunol 1999;92:188–96.
11. Manheimer-Lory AJ, Zandman-Goddard G, Davidson A, Aranow C, Diamond B. Lupus-specific antibodies reveal an altered pattern of somatic mutation. J Clin Invest 1997;100:2538–46.
12. Vitali C, Moutsopoulos HM, Bombardieri S. The European Community Study Group on diagnostic criteria for Sjögren's syndrome: sensitivity and specificity of tests for ocular and oral involvement in Sjögren's syndrome. Ann Rheum Dis 1994;53: 637–47.
13. Foster SJ, Brezinschek HP, Brezinschek RI, Lipsky PE. Molecular mechanisms and selective influences that shape the kappa gene repertoire of IgM+ B cells. J Clin Invest 1997;99:1614–27.
14. Dörner T, Brezinschek HP, Foster SJ, Brezinschek RI, Farner NL, Lipsky PE. Delineation of selective influences shaping the mutated expressed human immunoglobulin heavy chain repertoire. J Immunol 1998;160:2831–41.
15. Farner NL, Dörner T, Lipsky PE. Molecular mechanisms and selection influences the generation of the human VλJλ repertoire. J Immunol 1999;162:2137–45.
16. Dörner T, Foster SF, Farner NL, Lipsky PE. Targeting of somatic hypermutation. Eur J Immunol 1998;28:3384–96.
17. Foster SF, Dörner T, Lipsky PE. Targeting and subsequent selection of somatic hypermutations in the human Vκ repertoire. Eur J Immunol 1999;29:3122–32.
18. Honson NL, Dörner T, Lipsky PE. Targeting and selection of mutations in human VλJλ, gene rearrangements. Eur J Immunol 2000;30:1597–1605.
19. Brezinschek H-P, Brezinschek RI, Lipsky PE. Analysis of the heavy chain repertoire of human peripheral B cells using single-cell polymerase chain reaction. J Immunol 1995;155:190–201.
20. Rajewsky K. Burnet's unhappy hybrid. Nature 1998;394:624–5.
21. Suzuki N, Harada T, Mihara S, Sakane T. Characterization of a germline encoding cationic anti-DNA antibody and role of receptor editing for development of the autoantibody in patients with systemic lupus erythematosus. J Clin Invest 1996;98:1843–50.
22. Wallace DJ, Linker-Israeli M. It's not the same old lupus or Sjögren's any more: one hundred new insights, approaches, and options since 1990. Curr Opin Rheumatol 1999;11:321–5.
23. Dörner T, Farner NL, Lipsky PE. Mutational analysis of rearranged Ig V genes suggests two mechanisms of somatic hypermutation. Immunologist 1999;7:153–62.
24. Barbie V, Lefranc M-P. The human immunoglobulin kappa variable (IGKV) genes and joining (IGKJ) segments. Exp Clin Immunogenet 1998;15:171–83.
25. Rada C, Ehrenstein MR, Neuberger MS, Milstein C. Hot spot focusing of somatic hypermutation in MSH2-deficient mice suggests two stages of mutational targeting. Immunity 1998;9:135–41.
26. Winter DB, Phung QH, Umar A, Baker SM, Tarone RE, Tanaka K, et al. Altered spectra of hypermutation in antibodies from mice deficient for the DNA mismatch repair protein PMS2. Proc Natl Acad Sci U S A 1998;95:6953–8.
27. Phung QH, Winter DB, Alrefai R, Gearhart PJ. Hypermutation in Ig V genes from mice deficient in the MLH1 mismatch repair protein. J Immunol 1999;162:3121–4.
28. Frey S, Bertocci B, Delbos F, Quint L, Weill JC, Reynaud CA. Mismatch repair deficiency interferes with the accumulation of mutations in chronically stimulated B cells and not with the hypermutation process. Immunity 1998;9:127–34.
29. Park K, Kim J, Kim HS, Shin HS. Isolated human germinal center centroblasts have an intact mismatch repair system. J Immunol 1998;161:6128–32.

ARTHRITIS & RHEUMATISM
Vol. 44, No. 3, March 2001, pp 638–646

Polymorphisms of the *Ro52* Gene Associated With Anti–Ro 52-kd Autoantibodies in Patients With Primary Sjögren's Syndrome

Britt Nakken, Roland Jonsson, and Anne Isine Bolstad

Objective. **To screen for the *Ro52* gene encoding the 52-kd Ro autoantigen for possible mutations and polymorphisms associated with primary Sjögren's syndrome (SS).**

Methods. **The restriction enzyme fragment–single-strand conformation polymorphism method was used to search for mutations and polymorphisms in the *Ro52* gene in 97 patients with primary SS and 72 healthy control subjects. The results were verified by automated DNA sequencing and natural or amplification-created restriction site tests.**

Results. **A single-nucleotide polymorphism (SNP) was discovered in intron 3 (137 bp upstream of exon 4). The C/T genotype was significantly more prevalent among patients who were positive for anti–Ro 52-kd (20 of 38) than among healthy controls (9 of 72) (P = 0.00003); significant differences were not seen in patients who were negative for anti–Ro 52-kd. Furthermore, the frequency of the T allele in this position among groups of anti–Ro 52-kd–positive patients, anti–Ro 52-kd–negative patients, and control subjects was significantly increased in the patients who were positive for anti–Ro 52-kd compared with the controls.**

Conclusion. **We present the results of a complete screening for the *Ro52* gene in patients with primary SS and the results of an association study. An SNP in intron 3 was found to be strongly associated with the presence of anti–Ro 52-kd autoantibodies in primary SS. This finding is interesting in light of the fact that an alternative messenger RNA is made by deleting exon 4, which encodes a putative leucine zipper domain, to generate a shorter version of the Ro 52-kd protein.**

Supported by European Union Biomed II contracts (BMH4 CT96-0595 and BMH4 CT98-3489), by the Research Council of Norway (project 115563/320), and by the Norske Kvinners Sanitetsforening.

Britt Nakken, MS, Roland Jonsson, DDS, PhD, Anne Isine Bolstad, DDS, PhD: University of Bergen, and Haukeland University Hospital, Bergen, Norway.

Address correspondence and reprint requests to Britt Nakken, MS, Broegelmann Research Laboratory, Armauer Hansen Building, Haukeland University Hospital, N-5021 Bergen, Norway.

Submitted for publication May 1, 2000; accepted in revised form October 13, 2000.

Sjögren's syndrome (SS) is a systemic autoimmune disease characterized by chronic inflammation in the exocrine glands that possibly leads to mucosal and conjunctival dryness. Lymphocytic infiltration causes characteristic lesions in the salivary glands. The disease is referred to as primary SS when it occurs alone and as secondary SS when it occurs together with other connective tissue diseases. Most of the infiltrating lymphocytes are CD4+ T cells; ~20% are B cells (1). The etiology of primary SS is unknown, and genetic, infectious, and hormonal factors have all been suggested as causes (2). Most probably, several genetic and nongenetic factors cooperate to create the clinical picture recognized as primary SS.

A common characteristic in primary SS is the production of autoantibodies directed against RNP complexes composed of the Ro/SSA proteins (Ro 52 kd or Ro 60 kd) and human cytoplasmic (hY) RNA (3,4). The antigenicity of these particles is localized to the protein component (5). Anti-Ro/SSA and anti-La/SSB autoantibodies have been associated with a variety of clinical manifestations, suggesting a pathogenic role in these diseases (6–8). Whether these autoantibodies are primary pathogenic factors or develop as a result of disease activity is not clear. Detection of cells producing anti–Ro 52-kd and anti–Ro 60-kd in the salivary glands of SS patients has recently been reported (7). A strong correlation between the numbers of autoantibody-producing cells in salivary glands and the levels of autoantibodies in serum has been demonstrated (7,9, 10). For Ro 52-kd, no function has yet been assigned, but the presence of the zinc finger and leucine zipper motifs in its amino acid sequence suggest that it interacts with nucleic acids. Recently, it was shown that Ro 52-kd binds DNA in vitro, but the biologic significance of this is unknown (11,12).

The *Ro52* gene has been mapped by in situ hybridization to the end of the short arm of human chromosome 11 (13), and the *Ro52* gene has been characterized by 2 groups of investigators, who gave somewhat different results (14,15). Tsugu et al (15) identified 6 exons and a putative promoter region containing a TATA box, while Chan et al (14) found an additional exon upstream of these 6 exons that was already characterized, but they did not describe any of the promoter area. According to Chan et al, the complete gene for the full-length Ro 52-kd protein spans 10 kb of DNA and is composed of 7 exons (14). Exon 1 contains only the 5′-untranslated sequence, while the translation initiation codon is located 3 kb downstream in exon 2, which also encodes 3 zinc-finger motifs. Exon 4 encodes amino acids 168–285, including a coiled coil/leucine-zipper motif. Exon 7 is the longest and contains the human ret-finger protein–like domain and the 3′-untranslated region (UTR). A complementary DNA (cDNA) clone, p52-2, was isolated that encoded the product of an alternatively spliced messenger RNA (mRNA) derived from the deletion of exon 4, resulting in a smaller protein (Ro52β) (14). This protein has a predicted molecular weight of 45 kd and is antigenic. In neonatal lupus with congenital heart block, anti-Ro/SSA antibodies directed against the Ro52β isoform have been demonstrated (14,16). The expression of Ro 52-kd varies during embryonic development. Interestingly, a recent study showed that the time of peak expression of Ro52β in the human fetal heart coincides with the time of development of heart conduction disturbances due to neonatal lupus, suggesting a possible pathogenic role of this isoform (16).

A restriction fragment length polymorphism (RFLP) located upstream of exon 2 of the *Ro52* gene has been shown to be strongly associated with systemic lupus erythematosus (SLE) in African Americans ($P <$ 0.0005) (13). A higher disease frequency and more severe forms of the disease were noted in this ethnic group. The RFLP was detected by the restriction enzyme *Bgl* II and was later shown to be a single nucleotide substitution (15). The polymorphism was not associated with anti–Ro 52-kd autoantibodies, but rather, with the disease as a whole. It was of particular interest to examine the presence of this polymorphism in a group of Caucasian patients with primary SS to explore the possibility of this association extending to other ethnic groups as well as the possibility of a related disease.

The aim of the present study was to screen the candidate gene *Ro52* for possible mutations and polymorphisms and explore a possible association with primary SS and the presence of anti–Ro 52-kd autoantibodies.

PATIENTS AND METHODS

Patients and controls. Ninety-seven patients with primary SS who were followed up by the clinical services at the Department of Rheumatology, Haukeland University Hospital, participated in this study. The control subjects were 72 healthy sex-matched blood donors from the same area.

Biopsy tissues from the minor submucosal salivary glands of the lower lip were available from 59 patients and were subjected to histopathologic evaluation according to the method of Greenspan et al (17). In this group, 78% of the patients had a focus score ≥1. For inclusion in the study, the mean focus score was 2.4 and ranged from 1 to 10. The Ouchterlony immunodiffusion method (Immunoconcepts, Sacramento, CA) was used to test for antibodies against the specific extractable antigens Ro/SSA in all patients. Results were given as positive or negative.

The mean age of the patients at time of study was 57.2 years and ranged from 26 years to 81 years. The patients fulfilled the European Community classification criteria for primary SS (18). The study was approved by the Committee of Ethics at the University of Bergen.

Polymerase chain reaction (PCR). DNA extraction was performed using the QIAamp Blood Midi kit (Qiagen, Hilden, Germany) or using the Genepure 341 nucleic acid purification system (Applied Biosystems, Foster City, CA) following the recommended procedure for this equipment. The amount of DNA was measured using an ultraviolet (UV) spectrophotometer at $A_{260/280}$, and the quality of DNA was checked by agarose gel (0.8%) electrophoresis. Primers were designed which encompassed exons and flanking intron boundaries of *Ro52* (Table 1).

PCR was performed in a 50-μl reaction volume consisting of 5 μl of 10× SuperTaq buffer (HT Biotechnology, Cambridge, UK), 50 ng of genomic DNA, 12.5 pmoles of each primer, 0.25 m*M* of each dNTP, 1.5–2.5 m*M* $MgCl_2$, 1.25 units of AmpliTaq DNA polymerase (Perkin Elmer, Emeryville, CA), and 0.1 μl of α^{32}P-dCTP (3,000 Ci/nmole). The cycling conditions were as follows: an initial denaturation step at 94°C for 5 minutes, then 35 cycles at 94°C for 30 seconds, 55–65°C for 30 seconds, and 72°C for 30 seconds. All programs ended with a final extension step at 72°C for 10 minutes and storage at 4°C.

The Perkin Elmer GeneAmp System 2400 or 9700 thermal cyclers were used for PCR. The primers *Bgl* F (forward 5′-CAT-CCC-TTG-TCA-GAT-GGA-TAG-3′) and *Bgl* B (reverse 5′-GGA-TAT-CCA-CAT-GCA-GAA-G 3′) were designed for a PCR-based test for the *Bgl* II polymorphism reported to be associated with SLE in African Americans (13). Restriction enzyme digestion with *Bgl* II (New England Biolabs, Beverly, MA) was performed according to the manufacturer's specifications, and the samples were subjected to electrophoresis on 3% NuSieve agarose gels (FMC BioProducts

Table 1. Primers and PCR products used for REF-SSCP analysis, DNA sequencing, ACRS, and RE tests*

Exon, primer sequence†	Primer position‡	PCR product size (bp)	REF-SSCP enzymes	Enzymes used for RE testing
Exon 1				
A: 5′-AAC-TCT-GAC-TTC-TCT-TCT-CAG-CC-3′	4420–4442	339	*Sty* I	*Hinf* I
B: 5′-AGC-TGG-TCT-TGG-GTT-GAG-G-3′	4758–4740			
Exon 2				
A: 5′-CGT-CAG-ATG-ATG-TGA-TTC-CTC-CAG-3′	7567–7590	705	*Taq* I	*Nde* I
B: 5′-AAC-GAA-GCA-CTC-ACC-AGG-TGT-C-3′	8271–8250		*Fnu* 4HI	
Exon 3				
A: 5′-ACC-TCT-GGA-TTG-GAG-GGG-TTA-G-3′	8298–8390	425	*Fok* I	
B: 5′-AGC-TGG-TTT-CTG-GAG-AGT-GAG-ACG-3′	8722–8690			
Exon 3				
Ex3RsaI: 5′-CTA-TTA-CTT-GGT-TTG-CAT-GGG-GTA-3′	8441–8462	282	–	*Rsa* I
B: 5′-AGC-TGG-TTT-CTG-GAG-AGT-GAG-ACG-3′	8722–8699			
Exon 4				
A: 5′-TCA-CTG-TCC-CAG-AAA-CCT-CAA-CC-3′	9500–9522	515	*Ban* I	*Hinf* I
B: 5′-AAA-TGG-CAG-TTC-CAG-ATA-GCT-CTG-3′	10004–9522		*Bfa* I	
Exon 4				
Ex4RsaI: 5′-TGT-GTG-TGT-GTG-TGT-GTG-CGC-GCG-TGT-A-3′	9543–9570	472	–	*Rsa* I
B: 5′-AAA-TGG-CAG-TTC-CAG-ATA-GCT-CTG-3′	10004–9991			
Exon 5				
A: 5′-TGG-GCT-TCT-GGT-TAC-CTC-AC-3′	11047–11066	321	*Bsu* 36I	*Hph* I
B: 5′-GGG-AAA-ACT-TCA-GTG-CAT-GTA-CTT-C-3′	11367–11343			
Exon 6				
A: 5′-ACC-CAC-TCC-TGG-AGA-CTT-GAA-CAC-3′	11835–11858	399	*Sau* 3AI	
B: 5′-TGG-TCC-TGA-CCT-CTG-AAG-AAA-CC-3′	12234–12211			
Exon 7				
A: 5′-CTG-ATG-GTC-ATT-TCC-TCA-CAC-3′	12247–12267	847	*Ban* I	*Xmn* I
B: 5′-GAC-TTC-CCT-GCT-AAA-GCT-CG-3′	13093–13074		*Hae* III	
C: 5′-ACT-CTG-TGC-GCA-GGA-AGG-3′	12604–12621			
D: 5′-CCA-CAA-CCA-AAT-TGT-CCA-GAA-GC-3′	12671–12649			

* PCR = polymerase chain reaction; REF-SSCP = restriction enzyme fragment–single-strand conformation polymorphism; ACRS = amplification-created restriction sites; RE = restriction enzyme.
† A = forward sequence; B = reverse sequence. Ex3RsaI and Ex4RsaI primers were used for analysis of ACRS. The 7C and 7D primers were used for sequencing of exon 7.
‡ Position in the gene according to GenBank accession no. UO1882.

Europe, Vallenbaek Strand, Denmark). Positive controls (PCR products with nonpolymorphic *Bgl* II sites) were included in the restriction enzyme digestions to test the activity of the enzyme (results not shown).

Restriction enzyme fragment–single-strand conformation polymorphism (REF-SSCP) technique. Suitable restriction enzymes that produced fragments that did not exceed 350 bp were chosen. The radioactively labeled PCR products were digested with different restriction enzymes (Table 1). The labeled and cleaved DNA fragments were mixed with an equal volume of formamide loading dye (95% formamide, 20 m*M* EDTA, 0.05% bromphenol blue, and 0.05% xylene cyanol). Samples were denatured for 2 minutes at 94°C, cooled to 4°C to enable conformations, and then 4 μl of the samples was loaded on 6% polyacrylamide gels (49:1 acrylamide:bis and 1× Tris–borate–EDTA [TBE]). Electrophoresis was performed for 2–4 hours at 50W and 4°C in 1× TBE running buffer. Gels were transferred to 3-mm Whatman paper, dried, and autoradiographed with Hyperfilm-MP (Boehringer Mannheim, Mannheim, Germany) for 1–3 days.

DNA sequencing. Two or 3 samples from patients and controls who had shown REF-SSCP band shifts were selected for DNA sequencing. Every sample showing a unique mobility band shift was subjected to analysis by DNA sequencing. PCR products were purified using the QIAquick PCR Purification kit (Qiagen, San Francisco, CA) according to the manufacturer's instructions. Purified PCR products were subjected to DNA sequencing using the ABI Prism Big Dye Terminator Cycle Sequencing kit (PE Applied Biosystems, Foster City, CA). Sequencing primers were either the same as those utilized in PCR amplification or they were designed specifically when necessary (Table 1). Sequence reactions were purified using Sephadex G-150 columns, dried in a DNA SpeedVac (DNA 110; Savant, Holbrook, NY), and resolved in 4 μl of loading buffer (PE Applied Biosystems). Both sense and antisense DNA strands were sequenced.

Conformation of results by natural or amplification-created restriction site (ACRS) testing. Restriction enzyme digestion of PCR-amplified fragments containing either natural or ACRS was performed (19,20) (Table 1). New primers were designed to introduce a missense nucleotide during PCR whenever the mutation was not encompassed by a natural restriction enzyme. All restriction enzyme digestions were performed in 20-μl volumes using 5 units of restriction enzyme and were incubated according to the manufacturer's instructions (New England Biolabs). The resulting fragments were

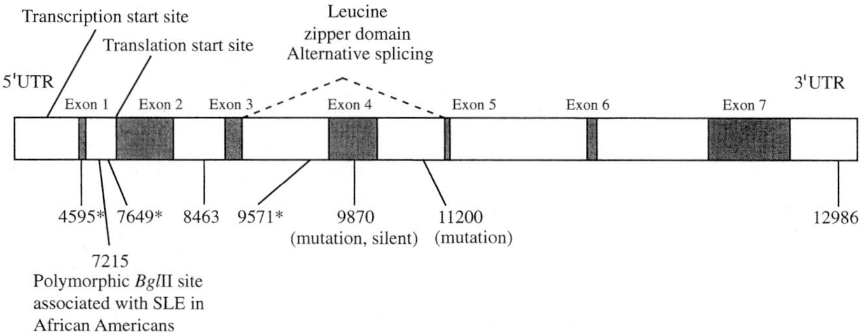

Figure 1. The *Ro52* gene. Major features of the gene are shown, together with the localization of mutations and polymorphic sites. The nucleotide numbers refer to GenBank accession no. UO1882. Asterisks indicate polymorphisms found at significantly increased frequencies in anti–Ro 52-kd–positive patients with primary Sjögren's syndrome, as compared with controls. The intron distances are not drawn proportionally. UTR = untranslated region; SLE = systemic lupus erythematosus.

analyzed on 3% NuSieve gels (FMC BioProducts Europe) containing ethidium bromide. The resulting DNA fragments were visualized by UV light.

Detection of anti–Ro 52-kd antibodies by enzyme-linked immunosorbent assay (ELISA). Patient sera were tested for the presence of anti–Ro 52-kd, anti–Ro 60-kd, and anti-La autoantibodies of the IgG isotype by ELISA. Analyses of anti–Ro 60-kd and anti-La were performed as previously described (21). For the analysis of anti–Ro 52-kd autoantibodies, high-binding Costar enzyme immunoassay/radioimmunoassay plates (Costar, Cambridge, MA) were used, and the analyses were performed in duplicate. Recombinant Ro 52-kd protein was diluted in phosphate buffered saline (PBS) to a concentration of 8 μg/ml, and the plates were coated by adding 50 μl of the dilution to each well, followed by overnight incubation at 4°C. The recombinant Ro 52-kd antigen was a kind gift from Dr. Marie Wahren-Herlenius (Karolinska Institute, Stockholm, Sweden) (22). Plates were then washed 3 times using PBS containing 0.05% Tween 20 (PBST; Merck-Schuchardt, Hohenbrunn, Germany). Nonspecific binding of antibodies was blocked with 75 μl of 5% skim milk powder (Oxoid, Basingstoke, UK) in PBST in room temperature for 1 hour.

Patient sera were diluted 1:3,000 in 5% skim milk/PBST, 50 μl of diluted sera was added to each well, wells were incubated at room temperature for 2 hours, and the plates were washed 4 times in PBST. Fifty microliters of horseradish peroxidase–conjugated goat anti-human IgG (γ-chain specific) antibody (diluted 1:8,000 in 5% skim milk/PBST; Southern Biotechnology, Birmingham, AL) was added to each well. Wells were incubated for 1 hour at room temperature, and then the plates were washed 4 times with PBST. Fifty microliters of 1,2-phenylenediamine dihydrochloride (diluted 1:7,000 in 5% skim milk/PBST; Dako, Glostrup, Denmark) was added to each well, and wells were incubated for 22 minutes at room temperature.

To stop the reaction, 50 μl of 1*M* H_2SO_4 was added to each well, and the optical density (OD) was read at 490 nm using an Emax precision microplate reader (SOFTmax Macintosh; Molecular Devices, Sunnyvale, CA). Sera were considered positive when the relative unit values exceeded 3 SD above the mean values obtained in controls. The healthy controls all had very low reactivity against the Ro 52-kd protein (OD <0.05).

Statistical analysis. Pearson's chi-square test or Fisher's exact test was used for statistical analyses. We performed multiple tests in this study, but the Bonferroni correction was not used since tests for these polymorphisms located in the same gene are not independent. *P* values less than 0.05 were considered to be statistically significant.

RESULTS

Measurement of anti–Ro 52-kd autoantibodies in primary SS patients by ELISA. Sera from 97 patients with primary SS and 31 healthy blood donors were analyzed for the presence of anti–Ro 52-kd and anti–Ro 60-kd by ELISA. Sera from 84 patients were tested for anti-La autoantibodies of the IgG isotype by ELISA. Anti–Ro 52-kd antibodies were detected in 38 of the 97 patients with primary SS (39%) and in none of the control sera; 65% of the patients were positive for anti–Ro 60-kd and 25% were positive for anti-La.

Screening of the *Ro52* gene for mutations/polymorphisms using REF-SSCP techniques. REF-SSCP analyses were carried out on 70 primary SS patients and 10 healthy control subjects. Samples showing mobility shifts were subjected to automated DNA sequencing to reveal the nature of the mutation/polymorphism. Restriction enzyme–based tests were designed to screen 97 primary SS patients and 72 control subjects. Naturally occurring restriction enzyme sites were utilized whenever possible. If a restriction enzyme site was not available at the place of the genetic variation, ACRS tests were designed. Polymorphisms were

Table 2. Distribution of genotypes among the anti–Ro 52-kd–positive and anti–Ro 52-kd–negative patients with primary SS and the control subjects

		Genotype frequency, no. (%)				
		Primary SS patients (n = 97)			*P*†	
Location (position)*	Nucleotide change	Anti–Ro 52-kd–positive (n = 38)	Anti–Ro 52-kd–negative (n = 59)	Control subjects (n = 72)	Anti–Ro 52-kd–positive vs. controls	Anti–Ro 52-kd–negative vs. controls
5′-UTR	C/C	23 (60.5)	45 (76.3)	60 (83.3)		
(4595)	C/T	13 (34.2)	12 (20.3)	10 (13.9)	0.029	0.59
	T/T	2 (5.3)	2 (3.4)	2 (2.8)		
Intron 1	A/A	22 (57.9)	45 (76.3)	58 (80.5)		
(7649)	A/G	13 (34.2)	12 (20.3)	12 (16.7)	0.038	0.84
	G/G	3 (7.9)	2 (3.4)	2 (2.8)		
Intron 2	C/C	32 (84.2)	49 (83.0)	63 (87.5)		
(8463)	C/G	6 (15.8)	9 (15.3)	9 (12.5)	0.63	0.48
	G/G	0 (0.0)	1 (1.7)	0 (0.0)		
Intron 3	C/C	17 (44.7)	44 (74.6)	61 (84.7)		
(9571)	C/T	20 (52.6)	13 (22.0)	9 (12.5)	0.00003	0.33
	T/T	1 (2.6)	2 (3.4)	2 (2.8)		
Exon 4	C/C	38 (100.0)	57 (96.6)	72 (100.0)		
(9870)	C/T	0 (0.0)	2 (3.4)	0 (0.0)	ND	0.20‡
Intron 4	C/C	36 (94.7)	59 (100.0)	72 (100.0)		
(11200)	C/T	2 (5.3)	0 (0.0)	0 (0.0)	0.117‡	ND
3′-UTR	C/C	27 (71.1)	50 (84.7)	63 (87.5)		
(12986)	C/A	11 (28.9)	9 (15.3)	9 (12.5)	0.033	0.65

* Position in the gene according to GenBank accession no. UO1882. UTR = untranslated region.
† Comparison between anti–Ro 52-kd–positive and anti–Ro 52-kd–negative patients with primary Sjögren's syndrome (SS) gave a *P* value of 0.008 for the intron 3 polymorphism. No other comparisons of polymorphisms in these two groups reached statistical significance. ND = not done.
‡ By Fisher's exact test.

detected in the 5′-UTR, intron 1, intron 2, intron 3, and in the 3′-UTR, whereas mutations were detected in exon 4 and intron 4 (Figure 1).

Case–control–based association study. The genotype and allele frequencies of the detected polymorphisms were analyzed in relation to anti–Ro 52-kd antibody production (Tables 2 and 3). Nucleotides were numbered according to Chan et al (14) (GenBank accession no. UO1882), unless stated otherwise.

The polymorphisms that were found in exon 1 (which contains only the 5′-UTR) (14) and intron 1 (position 7649) were linked, and therefore gave similar genotype and allele frequencies (Table 2). A statistically significant association between both of these polymorphisms and the presence of anti–Ro 52-kd antibodies was noted ($P = 0.029$ and $P = 0.038$, respectively). Interestingly, the polymorphism at position 7649 is located in a proposed TATA box (15). A C/G polymorphism was detected in intron 2 at position 8463, but genotype frequencies did not give significant differences among the anti–Ro 52-kd–positive or anti–Ro 52-kd–negative primary SS patients versus the control group. A C/T polymorphism was detected 137 bp upstream of exon 4 (in intron 3) at position 9571. The C/T genotype was present among anti–Ro 52-kd–positive patients (52.6%) at a significantly higher frequency than in the controls (12.5%) ($P = 0.00003$). This difference was not observed between anti–Ro 52-kd–negative patients and the controls.

A silent mutation was found in exon 4 at position 9870; heterozygosity (C/T) for this mutation was found in 2 patients with primary SS but in none of the controls. A single-base mutation was also found in intron 4 at position 11200; the C/T genotype was found in 2 patients with primary SS and in none of the controls. A C/A polymorphism was detected in the 3′-UTR at position 12986. The genotype distribution between the primary SS patients and the controls was as follows: homozygosity for the C allele was found in 71.1% of anti–Ro 52-kd–positive primary SS patients and in 87.5% of the controls ($P = 0.033$) (Table 2). No significant difference could be observed for homozygosity of the C allele between anti–Ro 52-kd–negative patients and the controls. Furthermore, comparison between anti–Ro 52-kd–positive and anti–Ro 52-kd–negative patients gave a *P* value of 0.008 for the intron

Table 3. Allele frequencies among anti–Ro 52-kd–positive and anti–Ro 52-kd–negative patients with primary SS and the control subjects

		Allele frequency, no. (%)			*P*†	
		Primary SS patients (n = 97)				
Location (position)*	Nucleotide change	Anti–Ro 52-kd–positive (n = 38)	Anti–Ro 52-kd–negative (n = 59)	Control subjects (n = 72)	Anti–Ro 52-kd–positive vs. controls	Anti–Ro 52-kd–negative vs. controls
5′-UTR	C	59 (77.6)	102 (86.4)	130 (90.3)		
(4595)	T	17 (22.4)	16 (13.6)	14 (9.7)	0.01	0.33
Intron 1	A	57 (75.0)	102 (86.4)	128 (88.9)		
(7649)	G	19 (25.0)	16 (13.6)	16 (11.1)	0.007	0.55
Intron 2	C	70 (92.1)	107 (90.7)	135 (93.8)		
(8463)	G	6 (7.9)	11 (9.3)	9 (6.3)	0.65	0.35
Intron 3	C	54 (71.1)	101 (85.6)	131 (91.0)		
(9571)	T	22 (28.9)	17 (14.4)	13 (9.0)	0.00012	0.17
Exon 4	C	76 (100.0)	116 (98.3)	144 (100.0)		
(9870)	T	0 (0.0)	2 (1.7)	0 (0.0)	ND	0.20‡
Intron 4	C	74 (97.4)	118 (100.0)	144 (100.0)		
(11200)	T	2 (2.6)	0 (0.0)	0 (0.0)	0.12‡	ND
3′-UTR	C	65 (85.5)	109 (92.4)	135 (93.8)		
(12986)	A	11 (14.5)	9 (7.6)	9 (6.3)	0.04	0.66

* Position in the gene according to GenBank accession no. UO1882.
† Comparison between anti–Ro 52-kd–positive and anti–Ro 52-kd–negative patients with primary Sjögren's syndrome (SS) gave a *P* value of 0.013 and 0.02 for the intron 3 polymorphism and the intron 1 polymorphism, respectively. No other comparisons of polymorphisms between these two groups reached statistical significance. ND = not done.
‡ By Fisher's exact test.

3 polymorphism, and no other polymorphisms reached statistical significance.

Allele frequencies of the different polymorphic sites are shown in Table 3. The allele frequencies of the polymorphism at position 8463 (intron 2) and the mutation at position 11200 did not reach statistical significance between anti–Ro 52-kd–positive primary SS patients and controls. The linked polymorphisms at positions 4595 (5′-UTR) and 7649 (intron 1) gave *P* values of 0.01 and 0.007, respectively, when anti–Ro 52-kd–positive patients were compared with the controls. The frequency of the C allele at position 4595 was 77.6% of anti–Ro 52-kd–positive patients, 86.4% of anti–Ro 52-kd–negative patients, and 90.3% of controls, whereas the A allele at position 7649 was present in similar frequencies: 75.0%, 86.4%, and 88.9%, respectively.

The T allele of the polymorphism at position 9571 (intron 3) gave a highly statistically significant association with the anti–Ro 52-kd–positive patients compared with the control subjects ($P = 0.00012$). The allele frequencies of the C/A polymorphism at position 12986 located in the 3′-UTR gave a statistically significant association between anti–Ro 52-kd–positive patients and the controls ($P = 0.04$), while statistical significance was not reached in comparisons of the anti–Ro 52-kd–negative patients and the controls ($P = 0.66$).

When anti–Ro 52-kd–positive and anti–Ro 52-kd–negative primary SS patients were compared, *P* values of 0.013 and 0.02 for the intron 3 polymorphism and the intron 1 polymorphism, respectively, were found. No other polymorphisms reached statistical significance.

Association between *Ro52* polymorphisms and the presence of anti–Ro 60-kd and anti-La. To investigate the possible associations between the *Ro52* polymorphisms and the presence of anti–Ro 60-kd and anti-La autoantibodies, we analyzed genotype and allele frequencies in relation to the presence of anti–Ro 60-kd and anti-La autoantibodies (data not shown). An association between the intron 3 polymorphism and the presence of anti–Ro 60-kd autoantibodies ($P = 0.004$) was detected. The same association was evident for the genotype frequencies: the C/T genotype of the intron 3 polymorphism was significantly associated with the presence of anti–Ro 60-kd autoantibodies ($P = 0.004$). No statistical significant difference was detected in comparisons of anti–Ro 60-kd–positive and anti–Ro 60-kd–negative patients.

With regard to correlations between the polymorphisms and the presence of anti-La autoantibodies, we found the genotype frequency of the intron 3 polymorphism to be associated with anti-La ($P = 0.007$). In addition, the 3′-UTR polymorphism gave a highly statistically significant result ($P = 0.0005$). The T allele of the 5′-UTR polymorphism and the G allele of the intron 1 polymorphism (in linkage disequilibrium) were associated with the presence of anti-La ($P = 0.003$ and $P = 0.001$, respectively). Moreover, the 3′-UTR polymorphism was associated with the presence of anti-La ($P = 0.001$). There was a statistically significant difference in the allele frequencies in the anti-La–positive and anti-La–negative patient groups for the intron 1 and 3′-UTR polymorphisms ($P = 0.02$ and $P = 0.001$, respectively). A statistically significant difference between these patient groups was also noted for comparison of the genotype frequency of the 3′-UTR polymorphism ($P = 0.0006$).

Screening for an SLE-associated *Bgl* II polymorphism. A total of 70 patients with primary SS and 72 healthy controls were screened for the *Bgl* II polymorphism. No genetic variation was evident among either the primary SS patients or the control subjects. These results were confirmed by DNA sequencing of several samples (data not shown).

DISCUSSION

Sjögren's syndrome is a systemic autoimmune disease in which lymphocyte infiltration causes characteristic lesions of the exocrine glands, which possibly leads to dry eyes and dry mouth. Autoimmune diseases aggregate in families, and family and animal studies indicate that genetic susceptibility confers a significant risk for primary SS (23–26). Characteristic of primary SS are autoantibodies to Ro/SSA (Ro 52-kd and Ro 60-kd) and La/SSB, and several studies have suggested a pathogenic role for these autoantibodies. To date, it is not known what triggers and perpetuates the production of these autoantibodies.

In the present study, we present the results of a complete screen of the *Ro52* gene in patients with primary SS and in healthy control subjects, as well as the results of an association study. We report the finding of 2 single-nucleotide polymorphisms (SNPs) that were linked and associated with anti–Ro 52-kd autoantibodies. Interestingly, the SNP in intron 1 (position 7649) is located in a putative TATA box identified by Tsugu et al (15). However, it is difficult to evaluate the biologic significance of this finding because of the conflicting results of gene characterization studies (14,15) and the lack of information about the true promoter region. Moreover, an SNP located 137 bp upstream of exon 4 was identified which was strongly associated with the presence of anti–Ro 52-kd autoantibodies. When comparisons between the primary SS patients who were positive and those who were negative for anti–Ro 52-kd were performed, a statistically significant difference in genotype frequencies ($P = 0.008$) was detected. This statistically significant difference was also evident when allele frequencies were compared ($P = 0.013$).

The possible association(s) between the detected *Ro52* polymorphisms and the presence of autoantibodies to Ro 60-kd and La was also investigated. An association between the intron 3 polymorphism and anti–Ro 60-kd ($P = 0.004$) was noted. This association may result from the presence of both anti–Ro 60-kd and anti–Ro 52-kd in these patients. This polymorphism is also statistically significant when primary SS patients and controls are compared ($P = 0.005$) (results not shown). However, the strongest association is evident with the presence of anti–Ro 52-kd. Regarding the comparison between *Ro52* polymorphisms and the presence of anti-La, we detected associations with the 5′-UTR, intron 1, intron 3, and 3′-UTR polymorphisms ($P = 0.015$, $P = 0.01$, $P = 0.007$, and $P = 0.0005$, respectively) for the genotype frequencies (results not shown). The co-occurrence of anti–Ro 52-kd and anti-La correlated to a high degree in our primary SS cohort (data not shown), and this is most likely the explanation for the observed association of *Ro52* polymorphisms with the presence of anti-La. In conclusion, we believe that the primary association between the intron 3 polymorphism is with the presence of anti–Ro 52-kd.

The localization of the intron 3 polymorphism is upstream of an alternatively spliced exon encoding a leucine-zipper domain, producing a shorter version of the protein (Ro52β). It is tempting to speculate that this polymorphism is located in a putative binding site for a factor involved in alternative splicing. However, the functional significance of this polymorphism is difficult to evaluate, since the regulation of alternative splicing is poorly understood. Further studies should examine whether this polymorphism has an effect on production of the Ro52β version of the protein and whether this isoform has an altered localization and/or function in the cell that could influence the development of autoantibodies to this protein.

Several reports have stated that under a variety of conditions that lead to cell stress, altered localizations for the Ro/SSA and La/SSB autoantigens have been observed (27,28). These effects, provoked by UV irradiation, apoptotic stimuli, and viral infections, have been most extensively studied for La/SSB. However, accumulation of Ro/SSA proteins in apoptotic blebs near the cell surface have been demonstrated (29). Such changes, especially those observed after viral infection and during apoptosis, are of particular interest for the initiation of autoimmunity to these antigens. Surface expression of Ro/SSA provides a possible explanation of how an autoantigen can be recognized by the immune system and accessed by autoantibodies. Thus, abnormal expression or localization of Ro/SSA is a hypothesis for the development of autoimmune reactions to this antigen.

Alternatively spliced forms of nuclear autoantigens are already known for La/SSB, which is another autoantibody target in primary SS (30). Tröster et al (31) described the isolation of an alternative transcript of the *La* gene from a cDNA library derived from a patient with primary SS. The identified mRNA is transcribed from an alternative promoter within intron 1 and represents the result of an alternative splicing event. The different mRNA isoforms were found to be expressed in salivary gland tissue from patients with primary SS (32). Further studies identified several cDNA that harbored frame-shift mutations in exon 7 of the *La* gene, resulting in a shorter version of the protein, which localized to the cytoplasm (33). The C-terminal region of La/SSB is known to contain one of the major autoepitopes of this protein, and these findings could be important in triggering the autoimmune response against La/SSB (33).

An RFLP located upstream of exon 2 in the *Ro52* gene has previously been shown to be strongly associated with SLE in African Americans ($P < 0.0005$) (13). This polymorphism was not associated with anti–Ro 52-kd autoantibodies but, rather, with the disease as a whole. However, our Caucasian patients with primary SS did not have the polymorphism, and subsequently, a *Bgl* II site could not be found in this position. We therefore suggest that the significance of this polymorphism does not extend to primary SS or to other ethnic groups, a conclusion supported by Frank et al (13).

Association studies are case–control studies based on comparison between unrelated affected and unaffected persons (34). An allele is said to be associated with a trait if it occurs at a significantly higher frequency among affected subjects compared with controls. A positive association occurs if the allele is involved in pathogenesis. It can also occur if the allele is in linkage disequilibrium with the allele that is involved in pathogenesis. If this is the case, the disease-causing allele should be found either upstream or downstream of that particular allele. We have undertaken a complete screening for mutations and polymorphisms in the coding regions of *Ro52*, including the intron/exon boundaries. Therefore, we would argue that it is highly unlikely that there are other polymorphisms in linkage disequilibrium in the coding region of *Ro52* of the patients included in our analyses. Still, there is the possibility that a polymorphism in the upstream regulatory region is in linkage disequilibrium with the C/T polymorphism at position 9571. Furthermore, there is also the possibility that a polymorphism in linkage disequilibrium can be found in nearby genes. Another possibility is that association can arise as a result of population admixture, giving false-positive results. To prevent this latter possibility, we chose as controls persons from the same ethnic group who were living in the same region of Norway as the patients.

In conclusion, we report the findings of our complete screening of the *Ro52* gene in patients with primary SS and in healthy control subjects. Polymorphisms were detected in the 5′-UTR, intron 1, intron 2, intron 3, and 3′-UTR, while mutations were detected in exon 4 and intron 4. Only the intron 3 polymorphism was strongly associated with the presence of anti–Ro 52-kd autoantibodies in primary SS patients. The polymorphism is associated more with the anti–Ro 52-kd autoantibodies than the disease itself. The importance of this polymorphism in the pathogenesis of primary SS is not known. Further studies are needed to investigate whether this polymorphism will influence the level of the alternatively spliced product Ro52 and whether it is present in anti–Ro 52-kd–positive patients who have diseases other than primary SS.

ACKNOWLEDGMENTS

The authors gratefully acknowledge the expert technical assistance of Turid Tynning, Anna Wargelius, and Solrun Steine. We also thank Professor Hans-Jacob Haga and his colleagues at the Section of Rheumatology, Institute of Medicine, Haukeland University Hospital, for allowing us to study their patients.

REFERENCES

1. Jonsson R, Haga H-J, Gordon T. Sjögren's syndrome. In: Koopman W, editor. Arthritis and allied conditions: a textbook of rheumatology. 14th ed. Philadelphia (PA): Lippincott, Williams & Wilkins; 2000. p. 1826–49.
2. Isenberg DA, Hrosfall AC. Autoimmune diseases: focus on Sjögren's syndrome. Oxford (UK): Bios Scientific Publishers; 1994.
3. Harley JB, Alexander EL, Bias WB, Fox OF, Provost TT, Reichlin M, et al. Anti-Ro (SS-A) and anti–La (SS-B) in patients with Sjögren's syndrome. Arthritis Rheum 1986;29:196–206.
4. Harley JB, Scofield RH, Reichlin M. Anti-Ro in Sjögren's syn-

drome and systemic lupus erythematosus. Rheum Dis Clin North Am 1992;18:337–58.
5. Slobbe RL, Pruijn GJ, van Venrooij WJ. Ro (SS-A) and La (SS-B) ribonucleoprotein complexes: structure, function and antigenicity. Ann Med Interne (Paris) 1991;142:592–600.
6. Ben-Chetrit E, Fischel R, Rubinow A. Anti-SSA/Ro and anti-SSB/La antibodies in serum and saliva of patients with Sjögren's syndrome. Clin Rheumatol 1993;12:471–4.
7. Tengnér P, Halse A-K, Haga H-J, Jonsson R, Wahren-Herlenius M. Detection of anti-Ro/SSA and anti-La/SSB autoantibody–producing cells in salivary glands from patients with Sjögren's syndrome. Arthritis Rheum 1998;41:2238–48.
8. Wahren M, Tengnér P, Gunnarsson I, Lundberg I, Hedfors E, Ringertz NR, et al. Ro/SS-A and La/SS-B antibody level variation in patients with Sjögren's syndrome and systemic lupus erythematosus. J Autoimmun 1998;11:29–38.
9. Halse A-K, Harley JB, Kroneld U, Jonsson R. Ro/SS-A-reactive B lymphocytes in salivary glands and peripheral blood of patients with Sjögren's syndrome. Clin Exp Immunol 1999;115:203–7.
10. Halse A-K, Wahren-Herlenius M, Jonsson R. Ro/SS-A- and La/SS-B-reactive B lymphocytes in peripheral blood of patients with Sjögren's syndrome. Clin Exp Immunol 1999;115:208–13.
11. Frank MB, McCubbin VR, Heldermon C. Expression and DNA binding of the human 52 kDa Ro/SSA autoantigen. Biochem J 1995;305:359–62.
12. Frank MB. Characterization of DNA binding properties and sequence specificity of the human 52 kDa Ro/SS-A (Ro52) zinc finger protein. Biochem Biophys Res Commun 1999;259:665–70.
13. Frank MB, Itoh K, Fujisaku A, Pontarotti P, Mattei MG, Neas BR. The mapping of the human 52-kD Ro/SSA autoantigen gene to human chromosome 11, and its polymorphisms. Am J Hum Genet 1993;52:183–91.
14. Chan EK, Di Donato F, Hamel JC, Tseng CE, Buyon JP. 52-kD SS-A/Ro: genomic structure and identification of an alternatively spliced transcript encoding a novel leucine zipper-minus autoantigen expressed in fetal and adult heart. J Exp Med 1995;182: 983–92.
15. Tsugu H, Horowitz R, Gibson N, Frank MB. The location of a disease-associated polymorphism and genomic structure of the human 52-kDa Ro/SSA locus (SSA1). Genomics 1994;24:541–8.
16. Buyon JP, Tseng C-E, Di Donato F, Rashbaum W, Morris A, Chan EKL. Cardiac expression of 52β, an alternative transcript of the congenital heart block–associated 52-kd SS-A/Ro autoantigen, is maximal during fetal development. Arthritis Rheum 1997;40: 655–60.
17. Greenspan JS, Daniels TE, Talal N, Sylvester RA. The histopathology of Sjögren's syndrome in labial salivary gland biopsies. Oral Surg Oral Med Oral Pathol Oral Radiol Endod 1974;37: 217–29.
18. Vitali C, Bombardieri S, Moutsopoulos HM, Balestrieri G, Bencivelli W, Bernstein RM, et al. Preliminary criteria for the classification of Sjögren's syndrome: results of a prospective concerted action supported by the European Community. Arthritis Rheum 1993;36:340–7.
19. Eiken HG, Odland E, Boman H, Skjelkvale L, Engebretsen LF, Apold J. Application of natural and amplification created restriction sites for the diagnosis of PKU mutations. Nucleic Acids Res 1991;19:1427–30.
20. Eiken H, Knappskog PM, Apold J. Restriction enzyme-based assays for complete genotyping of phenylketonuria patients. Dev Brain Dysfunct 1993;6:53–9.
21. Halse A-K, Marthinussen MC, Wahren-Herlenius M, Jonsson R. Isotype distribution of anti-Ro/SS-A and anti-La/SS-B antibodies in plasma and saliva of patients with Sjögren's syndrome. Scand J Rheumatol 2000;29:13–9.
22. Wahren M, Skarstein K, Blange I, Pettersson I, Jonsson R. MRL/lpr mice produce anti-Ro 52,000 MW antibodies: detection, analysis of specificity and site of production. Immunology 1994; 83:9–15.
23. Arnett FC, Bias WB, Reveille JD. Genetic studies in Sjögren's syndrome and systemic lupus erythematosus. J Autoimmun 1989; 2:403–13.
24. Arnett FC, Goldstein R, Duvic M, Reveille JD. Major histocompatibility complex genes in systemic lupus erythematosus, Sjögren's syndrome, and polymyositis. Am J Med 1988;85:38–41.
25. Reveille JD, Wilson RW, Provost TT, Bias WB, Arnett FC. Primary Sjögren's syndrome and other autoimmune diseases in families: prevalence and immunogenetic studies in six kindreds. Ann Intern Med 1984;101:748–56.
26. Reveille JD, Arnett FC. The immunogenetics of Sjögren's syndrome. Rheum Dis Clin North Am 1992;18:539–50.
27. LeFeber WP, Norris DA, Ryan SR, Huff JC, Lee LA, Kubo M, et al. Ultraviolet light induces binding of antibodies to selected nuclear antigens on cultured human keratinocytes. J Clin Invest 1984;74:1545–51.
28. Golan TD, Elkon KB, Gharavi AE, Krueger JG. Enhanced membrane binding of autoantibodies to cultured keratinocytes of systemic lupus erythematosus patients after ultraviolet B/ultraviolet A irradiation. J Clin Invest 1992;90:1067–76.
29. Casciola-Rosen LA, Anhalt G, Rosen A. Autoantigens targeted in systemic lupus erythematosus are clustered in two populations of surface structures on apoptotic keratinocytes. J Exp Med 1994; 179:1317–30.
30. Tan EM. Antinuclear antibodies: diagnostic markers for autoimmune diseases and probes for cell biology. Adv Immunol 1989;44:93–151.
31. Tröster H, Metzger TE, Semsei I, Schwemmle M, Winterpacht A, Zabel B, et al. One gene, two transcripts: isolation of an alternative transcript encoding for the autoantigen La/SS-B from a cDNA library of a patient with primary Sjögren's syndrome. J Exp Med 1994;180:2059–67.
32. Bachmann M, Hilker M, Grolz D, Tellmann G, Hake U, Kater L, et al. Different La/SS-B mRNA isoforms are expressed in salivary gland tissue of patients with primary Sjögren's syndrome. J Autoimmun 1996;9:757–66.
33. Bachmann M, Tröster H, Bartsch H, Grolz D. A frame shift mutation in a hot spot region of the nuclear autoantigen La (SS-B). J Autoimmun 1996;9:747–56.
34. Lander ES, Schork NJ. Genetic dissection of complex traits. Science 1994;265:2037–48.

ARTHRITIS & RHEUMATISM
Vol. 44, No. 3, March 2001, pp 647–652

Long-Term Outcome of Mothers of Children With Isolated Heart Block in Finland

Heikki Julkunen[1] and Marianne Eronen[2]

Objective. To study the long-term outcome of mothers of children with isolated heart block in a defined population.

Methods. We reviewed the Finnish hospital registries for patients born between 1950 and 1999 who had been diagnosed as having isolated heart block before the age of 15 years. We identified 101 children with isolated congenital heart block (CHB) and 55 with isolated heart block detected after the newborn period. Eighty-three (91%) of the 91 mothers of children with CHB and 48 (87%) of the 55 mothers of children with heart block detected after the newborn period were studied according to a protocol defining clinical characteristics (mean 9.9 years, range 0–49 years, and mean 22.9 years, range 4–47 years after the index delivery, respectively). Maternal survival was compared with survival in an age-matched population of normal Finnish women.

Results. Before the index delivery, 29 (37%) of the 78 surviving mothers of children with CHB had a self-reported clinical diagnosis of a chronic autoimmune disease, and 55 (71%) had had symptoms, signs, or abnormal laboratory findings suggesting an underlying subclinical disease. Of the 23 mothers who were completely asymptomatic before the index delivery, 10 (13% of the surviving mothers) remained so after a mean followup of 9.6 years (range 0–21 years). In mothers of children with CHB, clinical characteristics different from those of healthy mothers were photosensitivity, fatigue, dry eyes, and dry mouth. Forty-eight (58%) of these 83 mothers developed an autoimmune disease during followup. The most common diagnosis was primary Sjögren's syndrome (22 definite, 11 probable), followed by systemic lupus erythematosus (SLE). The standardized mortality ratio of mothers of children with CHB was 5.1, and 3 of the 5 deaths were associated with SLE. Mothers of children with heart block detected after the newborn period had similar symptoms and signs of autoimmune diseases as the healthy controls, and their standardized mortality ratio was 1.9.

Conclusion. Primary Sjögren's syndrome, either definite or subclinical, is the predominant autoimmune disorder in mothers of children with CHB. Mothers of children with isolated heart block detected after the newborn period do not, as a group, have clinical features suggestive of autoimmune diseases.

Congenital heart block (CHB), that is, heart block existing at or dating from birth, may be associated with major intracardiac malformations or, most commonly, is an isolated finding in a structurally normal heart of an otherwise healthy baby. Isolated CHB (CHB in this report) is caused by maternal antibodies to SSA and/or SSB and is considered a part of the neonatal lupus erythematosus syndrome, which also includes mild, and usually transient, cutaneous, hepatic, and hematologic abnormalities (1). Neonatal lupus was so termed because the cutaneous lesions of the affected newborn children resembled those of systemic lupus erythematosus (SLE) (2).

The association of CHB with maternal SLE was originally described in the 1950s (3), and since that time, the common belief was that most mothers of children with CHB had SLE (4), a potentially serious connective tissue disease with a poor prognosis. Other diseases that have also been associated with CHB are rheumatoid arthritis (RA) and primary Sjögren's syndrome (SS) (4,5). Studies conducted in the 1980s and 1990s have found that many mothers of children with CHB do not have a well-defined disease, but only mild symptoms suggesting an underlying autoimmune disorder, and that some mothers may be totally asymptomatic (4,6–9).

Supported by a grant from the Helsinki University Hospital Research Foundation.

[1]Heikki Julkunen, MD: Peijas Hospital, Vantaa, Finland; [2]Marianne Eronen, MD: Helsinki University Hospital, Helsinki, Finland.

Address correspondence and reprint requests to Heikki Julkunen, MD, Department of Internal Medicine, Peijas Hospital, 01400 Vantaa, Finland.

Submitted for publication June 16, 2000; accepted in revised form October 13, 2000.

The cause of isolated heart block detected after the newborn period may be myocarditis, rheumatic heart disease, cardiac tumor, Lyme disease, Marfan's syndrome, or Ehlers-Danlos syndrome (10). It is also plausible that heart block detected after the newborn period actually dates from birth and is associated with antibodies to SSA and/or SSB. CHB may be incomplete or intermittent and thus escape detection during pregnancy or the postpartum period (11). It has also been reported that lesser degrees of heart block can progress to third-degree heart block after birth (12). Therefore, it is possible that mothers of children with heart block detected after the newborn period may have clinical features characteristic of autoimmune diseases.

There are only a few recent studies on the outcome of mothers of children with isolated heart block (4–9). In those studies, the number of mothers has been rather low (4–7), the followup has been short (5,6,8), referral bias has been strong (8), or objective tests to diagnose SS have seldom been performed (4,6,8,9). Furthermore, no study has evaluated the survival of these mothers.

In the present population-based study, we examined the long-term outcome of a large group of mothers who had given birth in Finland to a child with isolated heart block (both congenital and detected after the newborn period) between 1950 and 1999.

PATIENTS AND METHODS

Children with isolated heart block. One of us, a pediatric cardiologist (ME), sought to identify all patients who had been diagnosed as having isolated heart block before the age of 15 years and who were born in Finland between 1950 and 1999 (13). Patients were identified from the hospital discharge registries and the pacemaker insertion registries of all 5 university central hospitals in Finland (Helsinki, Turku, Tampere, Kuopio, and Oulu).

The obstetric case records of the mothers and the hospital records of the neonates, children, and adults were reviewed to verify the time of detection of heart block and to demonstrate associated structural abnormalities. Patients were included in the study only if the heart block was second degree or third degree, was diagnosed before the age of 15 years, and there were no intracardiac anatomic malformations considered to be causally related to heart block (13).

Children whose heart block had been diagnosed by ultrasound examination during pregnancy or by electrocardiogram immediately after birth were defined as having isolated CHB. All others had isolated heart block detected after the newborn period.

Mothers of children with isolated heart block. The mothers of children (and adults) with isolated heart block were identified and contacted personally by mail and/or by telephone. Data on demographics, reproductive history, hospital admissions and followup visits to specialists and/or general practitioners, a self-reported diagnosis, and initial and cumulative symptoms and signs of different autoimmune diseases were collected from each mother according to a protocol that consisted of 39 items. The initial clinical feature in the mothers was defined as the first symptom, sign, or abnormal laboratory value that was clearly attributable to an underlying autoimmune disorder.

After obtaining permission from the Ministry of Health, the medical records of the mothers who were seen at different hospitals and/or health care centers in Finland were requested and examined. The diagnoses were made by using the common classification criteria for rheumatic and connective tissue diseases (the American College of Rheumatology [formerly, the American Rheumatism Association] criteria for SLE and RA, and the European Community criteria for SS [14–16]). The time of diagnosis was defined as the earliest time at which the patient fulfilled the criteria. For other autoimmune diseases, the diagnoses were made according to clinical findings.

Of the mothers who had died, the cause of death was verified by examining the hospital case records and/or the certificate of death, which was obtained from the Central Statistical Office of Finland.

The rheumatologist who was responsible for collecting and analyzing the clinical data of the mothers (HJ) was blinded to whether the index child had isolated CHB or isolated heart block diagnosed after the newborn period.

Healthy controls. Healthy controls were 89 parous women without a previously diagnosed chronic autoimmune disease who were staff of the Helsinki University Hospital.

Statistical analysis. Comparisons between groups were calculated using Fisher's exact test. We used the Bonferroni correction for multiple comparisons. Survival of the affected mothers was compared with normal survival of all age-matched Finnish women (life tables published in 1984 by the Central Statistical Office of Finland). In the calculations, the zero point was the mother's age at the birth of her first child with isolated heart block, and the end point was the time point when this study was performed or death.

RESULTS

Findings in mothers of children with isolated CHB. We identified 101 offspring with isolated CHB. There were 2 pairs of twins who were concordant for CHB, and 8 mothers each had 2 children with CHB. Of the 91 mothers who had given birth to at least 1 child with CHB, 2 could not be identified, 2 were not contacted, 3 refused participation in the study, and clinical data from 1 were incomplete. The final population, therefore, consisted of 83 mothers of children with CHB.

The mean ± SD age of these 83 mothers at the time of the study was 39.8 ± 9.0 years (range 26–75 years) and they were studied for a mean ± SD of 9.9 ± 9.0 years (range 0–49 years) after the index delivery.

Before the birth of their first child with CHB, 29

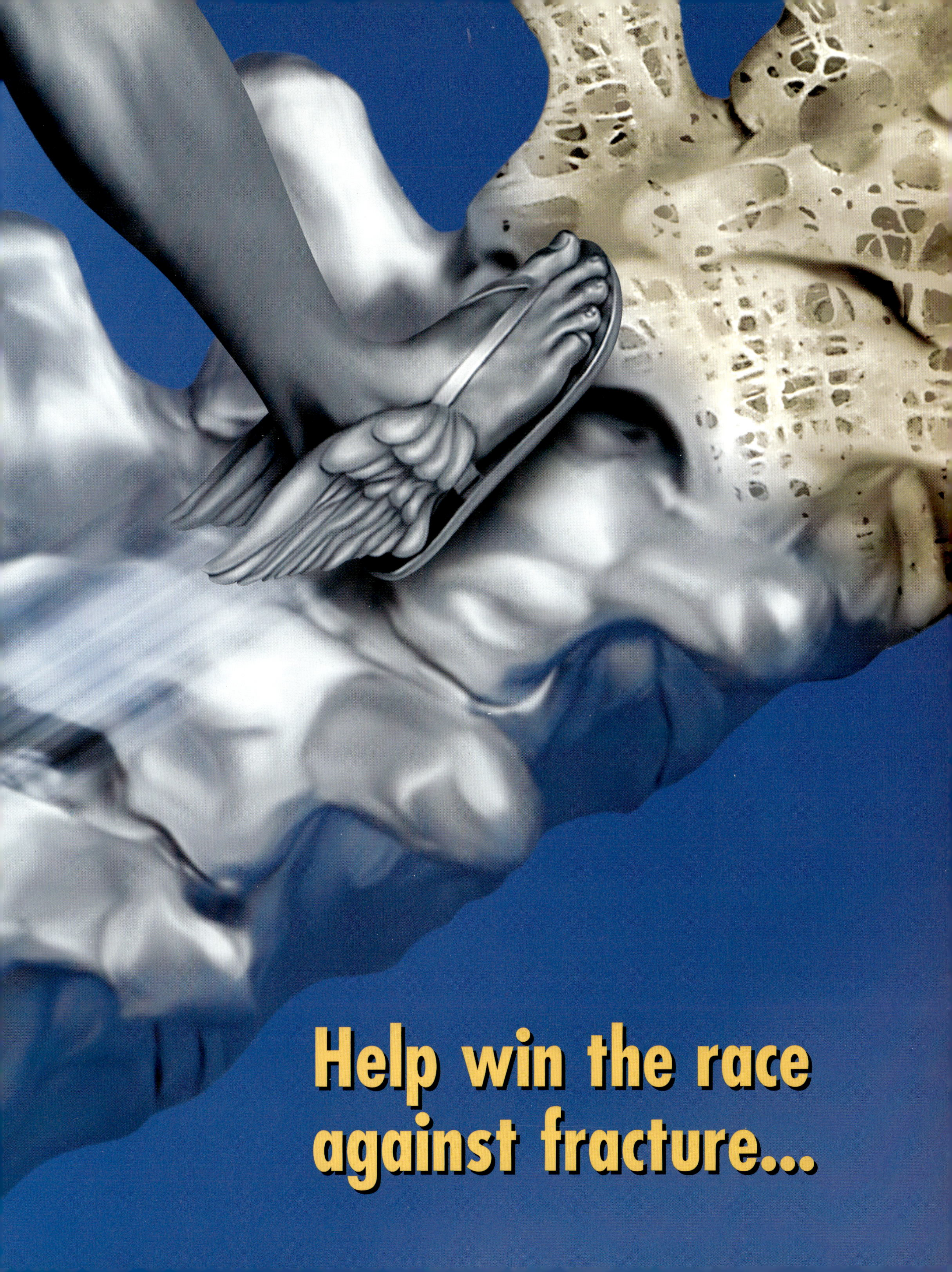
Help win the race
against fracture...

Actonel® 5 mg Efficacy you expect.

(risedronate sodium tablets)

Rapid and sustained fracture protection

Rapid—the only therapy proven to significantly reduce vertebral fractures in just 1 year[1-3]

Up to 65% reduction in vertebral fractures in postmenopausal osteoporosis[2]

Control 6.4%, Actonel 2.4%

$p<0.001$ vs control. Three-year clinical study in 2458 postmenopausal women. All patients received 1000 mg/d calcium and, if baseline levels were low, 500 IU/d vitamin D. Vertebral fractures were confirmed radiographically; some were associated with symptoms.

Sustained fracture protection in postmenopausal osteoporosis over 3 years[1-3]

Up to 49% reduction in vertebral fractures in postmenopausal osteoporosis[3]

Control 29.0%, Actonel 18.1%

$p<0.001$ vs control. Three-year clinical study in 1226 postmenopausal women. All patients received 1000 mg/d calcium and, if baseline levels were low, 500 IU/d vitamin D. Vertebral fractures were confirmed radiographically; some were associated with symptoms.

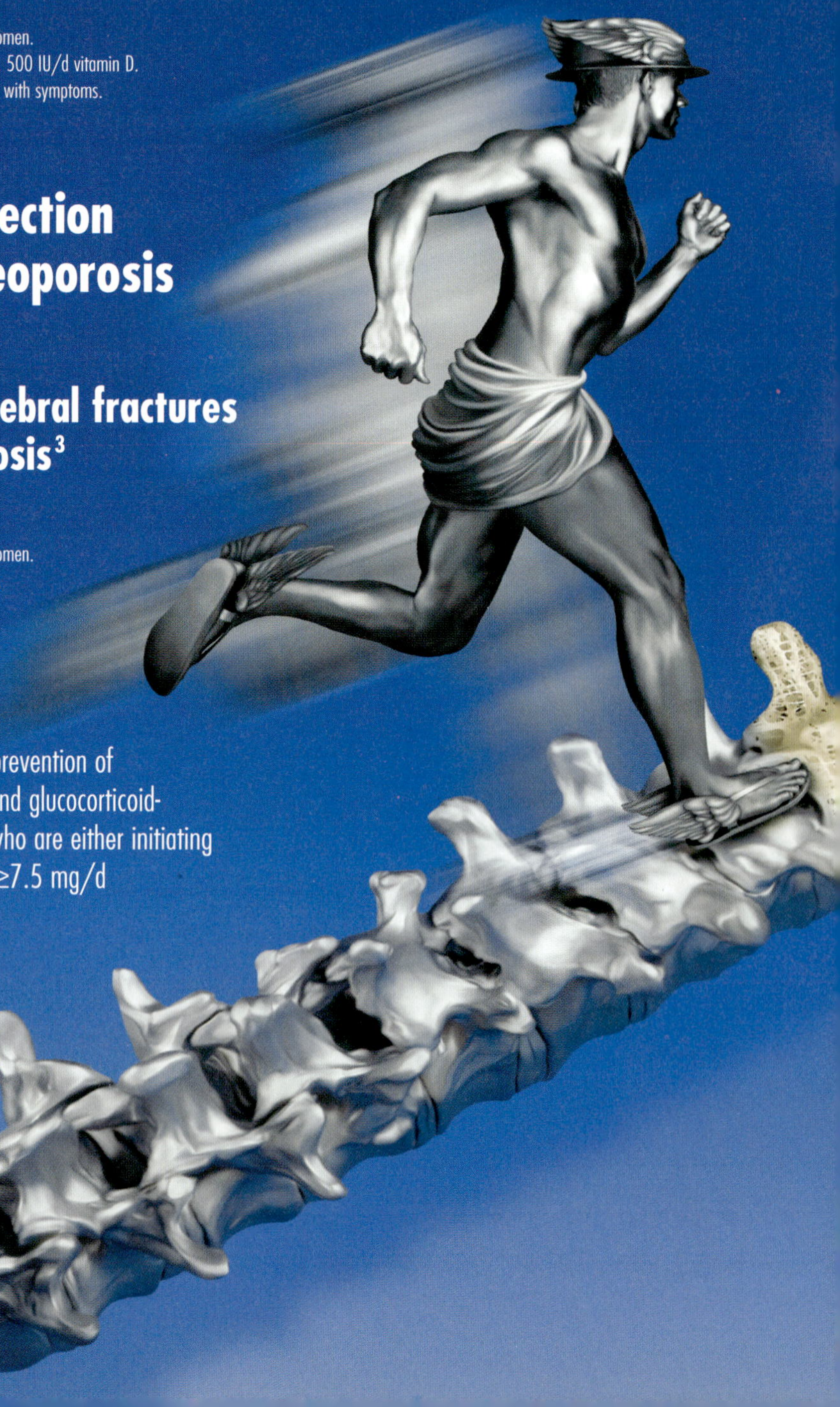

Actonel 5 mg is indicated for the treatment and prevention of postmenopausal osteoporosis (PMO) in women and glucocorticoid-induced osteoporosis (GIO) in men and women who are either initiating or continuing systemic glucocorticoid treatment (≥7.5 mg/d prednisone or equivalent) for chronic diseases.

ACTONEL® (risedronate sodium tablets)
Brief Summary: See package insert for full prescribing information.

INDICATIONS AND USAGE

Postmenopausal Osteoporosis: ACTONEL is indicated for the treatment and prevention of osteoporosis in postmenopausal women.

Treatment of Osteoporosis: In postmenopausal women with osteoporosis, ACTONEL increases BMD and reduces the incidence of vertebral fractures and a composite endpoint of nonvertebral osteoporosis-related fractures (see CLINICAL STUDIES). Osteoporosis may be confirmed by the presence or history of osteoporotic fracture, or by the finding of low bone mass (for example, at least 2 SD below the premenopausal mean).

Prevention of Osteoporosis: ACTONEL may be considered in postmenopausal women who are at risk of developing osteoporosis and for whom the desired clinical outcome is to maintain bone mass and to reduce the risk of fracture.

Factors such as family history of osteoporosis, previous fracture, smoking, BMD (at least 1 SD below the premenopausal mean), high bone turnover, thin body frame, Caucasian or Asian race, and early menopause are associated with an increased risk of developing osteoporosis and fractures. The presence of these risk factors may be important when considering the use of ACTONEL for prevention of osteoporosis.

Glucocorticoid-Induced Osteoporosis: ACTONEL is indicated for the prevention and treatment of glucocorticoid-induced osteoporosis in men and women who are either initiating or continuing systemic glucocorticoid treatment (daily dosage equivalent to 7.5 mg or greater of prednisone) for chronic diseases. Patients treated with glucocorticoids should receive adequate amounts of calcium and vitamin D.

Paget's Disease: ACTONEL is indicated for treatment of Paget's disease of bone (osteitis deformans).

Treatment is indicated in patients with Paget's disease of bone (1) who have a level of serum alkaline phosphatase (SAP) at least two times the upper limit of normal, or (2) who are symptomatic, or (3) who are at risk for future complications from their disease, to induce remission (normalization of serum alkaline phosphatase).

CONTRAINDICATIONS

- Hypocalcemia (See PRECAUTIONS, General)
- Known hypersensitivity to any component of this product
- Inability to stand or sit upright for at least 30 minutes

WARNINGS: Bisphosphonates may cause upper gastrointestinal disorders such as dysphagia, esophagitis, and esophageal or gastric ulcer (see PRECAUTIONS).

PRECAUTIONS

General: Hypocalcemia and other disturbances of bone and mineral metabolism should be effectively treated before starting ACTONEL therapy. Adequate intake of calcium and vitamin D is important in all patients, especially in patients with Paget's disease in whom bone turnover is significantly elevated. ACTONEL is not recommended for use in patients with severe renal impairment (creatinine clearance < 30 mL/min).

Bisphosphonates have been associated with gastrointestinal disorders such as dysphagia, esophagitis, and esophageal or gastric ulcers. This association has been reported for bisphosphonates in postmarketing experience, but has not been found in most pre-approval clinical trials, including those conducted with ACTONEL. Patients should be advised that taking the medication according to the instructions is important to minimize the risk of these events. They should take ACTONEL with sufficient plain water (6 to 8 oz) to facilitate delivery to the stomach, and should not lie down for 30 minutes after taking the drug.

Glucocorticoid-Induced Osteoporosis: The risk versus benefit of ACTONEL for the prevention and treatment of glucocorticoid-induced osteoporosis at daily doses of glucocorticoids < 7.5 mg of prednisone or equivalent has not been established. Before initiating treatment, the hormonal status of both men and women should be ascertained and appropriate replacement considered.

The efficacy of ACTONEL has been established in studies of 1-year's duration. The efficacy of ACTONEL beyond 1 year has not been studied.

Information for Patients: The patient should be informed to pay particular attention to the dosing instructions as clinical benefits may be compromised by failure to take the drug according to instructions. Specifically, ACTONEL should be taken at least 30 minutes before the first food or drink of the day other than water.

To facilitate delivery to the stomach, and thus reduce the potential for esophageal irritation, patients should take ACTONEL while in an upright position (sitting or standing) with a full glass of plain water (6 to 8 oz). Patients should not lie down for 30 minutes after taking the medication (see PRECAUTIONS, General). Patients should not chew or suck on the tablet because of a potential for oropharyngeal irritation.

Patients should be instructed that if they develop symptoms of esophageal disease (such as difficulty or pain upon swallowing, retrosternal pain or severe persistent or worsening heartburn) they should consult their physician before continuing ACTONEL.

Patients should receive supplemental calcium and vitamin D if dietary intake is inadequate (see PRECAUTIONS, General). Calcium supplements or calcium-, aluminum-, and magnesium-containing medications may interfere with the absorption of ACTONEL and should be taken at a different time of the day, as with food.

Weight-bearing exercise should be considered along with the modification of certain behavioral factors, such as excessive cigarette smoking, and/or alcohol consumption, if these factors exist.

Physicians should instruct their patients to read the Patient Information before starting therapy with ACTONEL 5 mg and to re-read it each time the prescription is renewed.

Drug Interactions: No specific drug-drug interaction studies were performed. Risedronate is not metabolized and does not induce or inhibit hepatic microsomal drug-metabolizing enzymes (Cytochrome P450).

Calcium Supplements/Antacids: Co-administration of ACTONEL and calcium, antacids, or oral medications containing divalent cations will interfere with the absorption of ACTONEL.

Hormone Replacement Therapy: One study of about 500 early postmenopausal women has been conducted to date in which treatment with ACTONEL (5 mg/day) plus estrogen replacement therapy was compared with estrogen replacement therapy alone. Exposure to study drugs was approximately 12 to 18 months and the primary endpoint was change in BMD. If considered appropriate, ACTONEL may be used concomitantly with hormone replacement therapy.

Aspirin/Nonsteroidal Anti-Inflammatory Drugs (NSAIDs): Of over 5700 patients enrolled in the ACTONEL Phase 3 osteoporosis studies, aspirin use was reported by 31% of patients, 24% of whom were regular users (3 or more days per week). Forty-eight percent of patients reported NSAID use, 21% of whom were regular users. Among regular aspirin or NSAID users, the incidence of upper gastrointestinal adverse experiences in ACTONEL-treated patients (24.5%) was similar to that in placebo-treated patients (24.8%).

H_2 Blockers and Proton Pump Inhibitors (PPIs): Of over 5700 patients enrolled in the ACTONEL Phase 3 osteoporosis studies, 21% used H_2 blockers and/or PPIs. Among these patients, the incidence of upper gastrointestinal adverse experiences in the ACTONEL-treated patients was similar to that in placebo-treated patients.

Drug/Laboratory Test Interactions: Bisphosphonates are known to interfere with the use of bone-imaging agents. Specific studies with ACTONEL have not been performed.

Carcinogenesis, Mutagenesis, Impairment of Fertility:

Carcinogenesis: In a 104-week carcinogenicity study, rats were administered daily oral doses up to 24 mg/kg/day (approximately 7.7 times the maximum recommended human daily dose of 30 mg based on surface area, mg/m²). There were no significant drug-induced tumor findings in male or female rats. The high dose male group of 24 mg/kg/day was terminated early in the study (Week 93) due to excessive toxicity, and data from this group were not included in the statistical evaluation of the study results. In an 80-week carcinogenicity study, mice were administered daily oral doses up to 32 mg/kg/day (approximately 6.4 times the 30 mg/day human dose based on surface area, mg/m²). There were no significant drug-induced tumor findings in male or female mice.

Mutagenesis: Risedronate did not exhibit genetic toxicity in the following assays: *In vitro* bacterial mutagenesis in *Salmonella* and *E. coli* (Ames assay), mammalian cell mutagenesis in CHO/HGPRT assay, unscheduled DNA synthesis in rat hepatocytes and an assessment of chromosomal aberrations *in vivo* in rat bone marrow. Risedronate was positive in a chromosomal aberration assay in CHO cells at highly cytotoxic concentrations (> 675 mcg/mL, survival of 6% to 7%). When the assay was repeated at doses exhibiting appropriate cell survival (29%), there was no evidence of chromosomal damage.

Impairment of Fertility: In female rats, ovulation was inhibited at an oral dose of 16 mg/kg/day (approximately 5.2 times the 30 mg/day human dose based on surface area, mg/m²). Decreased implantation was noted in female rats treated with doses ≥ 7 mg/kg/day (approximately 2.3 times the 30 mg/day human dose based on surface area, mg/m²). In male rats, testicular and epididymal atrophy and inflammation were noted at 40 mg/kg/day (approximately 13 times the 30 mg/day human dose based on surface area, mg/m²). Testicular atrophy was also noted in male rats after 13 weeks of treatment at oral doses of 16 mg/kg/day (approximately 5.2 times the 30 mg/day human dose based on surface area, mg/m²). There was moderate-to-severe spermatid maturation block after 13 weeks in male dogs at an oral dose of 8 mg/kg/day (approximately 8 times the 30 mg/day human dose based on surface area, mg/m²). These findings tended to increase in severity with increased dose and exposure time.

Pregnancy: Pregnancy Category C: Survival of neonates was decreased in rats treated during gestation with oral doses ≥ 16 mg/kg/day (approximately 5.2 times the 30 mg/day human dose based on surface area, mg/m²). Body weight was decreased in neonates from dams treated with 80 mg/kg (approximately 26 times the 30 mg/day human dose based on surface area, mg/m²). In rats treated during gestation, the number of fetuses exhibiting incomplete ossification of sternebrae or skull was statistically significantly increased at 7.1 mg/kg/day (approximately 2.3 times the 30 mg/day human dose based on surface area, mg/m²). Both incomplete ossification and unossified sternebrae were increased in rats treated with oral doses ≥ 16 mg/kg/day (approximately 5.2 times the 30 mg/day human dose based on surface area, mg/m²). A low incidence of cleft palate was observed in fetuses from female rats treated with oral doses ≥ 3.2 mg/kg/day (approximately 1 time the 30 mg/day human dose based on surface area, mg/m²). The relevance of this finding to human use of ACTONEL is unclear. No significant fetal ossification effects were seen in rabbits treated with oral doses up to 10 mg/kg/day during gestation (approximately 6.7 times the 30 mg/day human dose based on surface area, mg/m²). However, in rabbits treated with 10 mg/kg/day, 1 of 14 litters were aborted and 1 of 14 litters were delivered prematurely.

Similar to other bisphosphonates, treatment during mating and gestation with doses as low as 3.2 mg/kg/day (approximately 1 time the 30 mg/day human dose based on surface area, mg/m²) has resulted in periparturient hypocalcemia and mortality in pregnant rats allowed to deliver.

There are no adequate and well-controlled studies of ACTONEL in pregnant women. ACTONEL should be used during pregnancy only if the potential benefit justifies the potential risk to the mother and fetus.

Nursing Women: Risedronate was detected in feeding pups exposed to lactating rats for a 24-hour period post-dosing, indicating a small degree of lacteal transfer. It is not known whether risedronate is excreted in human milk. Because many drugs are excreted in human milk and because of the potential for serious adverse reactions in nursing infants from bisphosphonates, a decision should be made whether to discontinue nursing or to discontinue the drug, taking into account the importance of the drug to the mother.

Pediatric Use: Safety and effectiveness in pediatric patients have not been established.

Geriatric Use: Of the patients receiving ACTONEL in postmenopausal osteoporosis studies (see CLINICAL STUDIES), 43% were between 65 and 75 years of age, and 20% were over 75. The corresponding proportions were 26% and 11% in glucocorticoid-induced osteoporosis trials, and 40% and 26% in Paget's disease trials. No overall differences in efficacy or safety were observed between these patients and younger patients.

Use in Men: Safety and effectiveness have been demonstrated in clinical studies in men receiving ACTONEL both for Paget's disease and for treatment and prevention of glucocorticoid-induced osteoporosis. However, the safety and effectiveness in men for osteoporosis due to other causes have not been established.

ADVERSE REACTIONS

Osteoporosis: ACTONEL has been studied in over 5700 patients enrolled in the Phase 3 glucocorticoid-induced osteoporosis clinical trials and in postmenopausal osteoporosis trials of up to 3 years duration. The overall adverse event profile of ACTONEL 5 mg in these studies was similar to that of placebo. Most adverse events were either mild or moderate and did not lead to discontinuation from the study. The incidence of serious adverse events in the placebo group was 24.9% and in the ACTONEL 5 mg group was 26.3%. The percentage of patients who withdrew from the study due to adverse events was 14.4% and 13.5% for the placebo and ACTONEL 5 mg groups, respectively. Table 1 lists adverse events from the Phase 3 osteoporosis trials reported in ≥ 2% of patients and in more ACTONEL-treated patients than placebo-treated patients. Adverse events are shown without attribution of causality.

Table 5
Adverse Events Occurring at a Frequency ≥ 2% and in More ACTONEL-Treated Patients than Placebo-Treated Patients Combined Phase 3 Osteoporosis Trials

Body System	Placebo % (N = 1914)	ACTONEL 5 mg % (N = 1916)
Body as a Whole		
Infection	29.7	29.9
Back Pain	23.6	26.1
Pain	13.1	13.6
Abdominal Pain	9.4	11.6
Neck Pain	4.5	5.3
Asthenia	4.3	5.1
Chest Pain	4.9	5.0
Neoplasm	3.0	3.3
Hernia	2.5	2.9
Cardiovascular		
Hypertension	9.0	10.0
Cardiovascular Disorder	1.7	2.5
Angina Pectoris	2.4	2.5
Digestive		
Nausea	10.7	10.9
Diarrhea	9.6	10.6
Flatulence	4.2	4.6
Gastritis	2.3	2.5
Gastrointestinal Disorder	2.1	2.3
Rectal Disorder	1.9	2.2
Tooth Disorder	2.0	2.1
Hemic and Lymphatic		
Ecchymosis	4.0	4.3
Anemia	1.9	2.4
Musculoskeletal		
Arthralgia	21.1	23.7
Joint Disorder	5.4	6.8
Myalgia	6.3	6.6
Bone Pain	4.3	4.6
Bone Disorder	3.2	4.0
Leg Cramps	2.6	3.5
Bursitis	2.9	3.0
Tendon Disorder	2.5	3.0
Nervous		
Depression	6.2	6.8
Dizziness	5.4	6.4
Insomnia	4.5	4.7
Anxiety	3.0	4.3
Neuralgia	3.5	3.8
Vertigo	3.2	3.3
Hypertonia	2.1	2.2
Paresthesia	1.8	2.1
Respiratory		
Pharyngitis	5.0	5.8
Rhinitis	5.0	5.7
Dyspnea	3.2	3.8
Pneumonia	2.6	3.1
Skin and Appendages		
Rash	7.2	7.7
Pruritus	2.2	3.0
Skin Carcinoma	1.8	2.0
Special Senses		
Cataract	5.4	5.9
Conjunctivitis	2.8	3.1
Otitis Media	2.4	2.5
Urogenital		
Urinary Tract Infection	9.7	10.9
Cystitis	3.5	4.1

Duodenitis and glossitis have been reported uncommonly (0.1% to 1%). There have been rare reports (< 0.1%) of abnormal liver function tests.

Laboratory Test Findings: Asymptomatic and small decreases were observed in serum calcium and phosphorus levels. Overall, mean decreases of 0.8% in serum calcium and of 2.7% in phosphorus were observed at 6 months in patients receiving ACTONEL. Throughout the Phase 3 studies, serum calcium levels below 8 mg/dL were observed in 18 patients, 9 (0.5%) in each treatment arm (ACTONEL and placebo). Serum phosphorus levels below 2 mg/dL were observed in 14 patients, 11 (0.6%) treated with ACTONEL and 3 (0.2%) treated with placebo.

Endoscopic Findings: ACTONEL clinical studies enrolled over 5700 patients, many with pre-existing gastrointestinal disease and concomitant use of NSAIDs or aspirin. Investigators were encouraged to perform endoscopies in any patients with moderate-to-severe gastrointestinal complaints while maintaining the blind. These endoscopies were ultimately performed on equal numbers of patients between the treated and placebo groups [75 (14.5%) placebo; 75 (11.9%) ACTONEL]. Across treatment groups, the percentage of patients with normal esophageal, gastric, and duodenal mucosa on endoscopy was similar (20% placebo, 21% ACTONEL). The number of patients who withdrew from the studies due to the event prompting endoscopy was similar across treatment groups. Positive findings on endoscopy were also generally comparable across treatment groups. There was a higher number of reports of mild duodenitis in the ACTONEL group, however there were more duodenal ulcers in the placebo group. Clinically important findings (perforations, ulcers, or bleeding) among this symptomatic population were similar between groups (51% placebo; 39% ACTONEL).

Paget's Disease: ACTONEL has been studied in 392 patients with Paget's disease of bone. As in trials of ACTONEL for other indications, the adverse experiences reported in the Paget's disease trials have generally been mild or moderate, have not required discontinuation of treatment, and have not appeared to be related to patient age, gender, or race.

In a double-blind, active-controlled study, the adverse event profile was similar for ACTONEL and Didronel: 6.6% (4/61) of patients treated with ACTONEL 30 mg/day for 2 months discontinued treatment due to adverse events, compared with 8.2% (5/61) of patients treated with Didronel 400 mg/day for 6 months.

Table 6
Adverse Events Reported in ≥ 2% of ACTONEL-Treated Patients* in Phase 3 Paget's Disease Trials

Body System	30 mg/day x 2 months ACTONEL % (N = 61)	400 mg/day x 6 months Didronel % (N = 61)
Body as a Whole		
Flu Syndrome	9.8	1.6
Chest Pain	6.6	3.3
Asthenia	4.9	0
Neoplasm	3.3	1.6
Gastrointestinal		
Diarrhea	19.7	14.8
Abdominal Pain	11.5	8.2
Nausea	9.8	9.8
Constipation	6.6	8.2
Belching	3.3	1.6
Colitis	3.3	3.3
Metabolic & Nutritional		
Peripheral Edema	8.2	6.6
Musculoskeletal		
Arthralgia	32.8	29.5
Bone Pain	4.9	4.9
Leg Cramps	3.3	3.3
Myasthenia	3.3	0
Nervous		
Headache	18.0	16.4
Dizziness	6.6	4.9
Respiratory		
Bronchitis	3.3	4.9
Sinusitis	4.9	1.6
Skin		
Rash	11.5	8.2
Special Senses		
Amblyopia	3.3	3.3
Tinnitus	3.3	3.3
Dry Eye	3.3	0

*Considered to be possibly or probably causally related in at least one patient

Three patients that received ACTONEL 30 mg/day experienced acute iritis in one supportive study. All three patients recovered from their events; however, in one of these patients, the event recurred during ACTONEL treatment and again during treatment with pamidronate. All patients were effectively treated with topical steroids.

OVERDOSAGE

Decreases in serum calcium and phosphorus following substantial overdose may be expected in some patients. Signs and symptoms of hypocalcemia may also occur in some of these patients. Milk or antacids containing calcium should be given to bind ACTONEL and reduce absorption of the drug.

In cases of substantial overdose, gastric lavage may be considered to remove unabsorbed drug. Standard procedures that are effective for treating hypocalcemia, including the administration of calcium intravenously, would be expected to restore physiologic amounts of ionized calcium and to relieve signs and symptoms of hypocalcemia.

Lethality after single oral doses was seen in female rats at 903 mg/kg and male rats at 1703 mg/kg. The minimum lethal dose in mice and rabbits was 4000 mg/kg and 1000 mg/kg. These values represent 320 to 620 times the 30-mg human dose based on surface area (mg/m²).

DOSAGE AND ADMINISTRATION

ACTONEL should be taken once per day at least 30 minutes before the first food or drink of the day other than water.

To facilitate delivery to the stomach, ACTONEL should be swallowed while the patient is in an upright position and with a full glass of plain water (6 to 8 oz). Patients should not lie down for 30 minutes after taking the medication (see PRECAUTIONS, General).

Patients should receive supplemental calcium and vitamin D if dietary intake is inadequate (see PRECAUTIONS, General). Calcium supplements and calcium-, aluminum-, and magnesium-containing medications may interfere with the absorption of ACTONEL and should be taken at a different time of the day. ACTONEL is not recommended for use in patients with severe renal impairment (creatinine clearance < 30 mL/min). No dosage adjustment is necessary in patients with a creatinine clearance ≥ 30 mL/min or in the elderly.

Treatment and Prevention of Postmenopausal Osteoporosis/Glucocorticoid-Induced Osteoporosis (see INDICATIONS AND USAGE): The recommended regimen is 5 mg orally daily.

Paget's Disease (see INDICATIONS AND USAGE): The recommended treatment regimen is 30 mg once daily for 2 months. Retreatment may be considered (following post-treatment observation of at least 2 months) if relapse occurs, or if treatment fails to normalize serum alkaline phosphatase. For retreatment, the dose and duration of therapy are the same as for initial treatment. No data are available on more than one course of retreatment.

Store at controlled room temperature 20°-25°C (68°-77°F) [See USP].

Mfg. and Dist. by:
Procter & Gamble Pharmaceuticals, TM Owner
Cincinnati, Ohio 45202
Mkt. with:
Aventis Pharmaceuticals Inc.
(formerly Hoechst Marion Roussel, Inc.)
Kansas City, Missouri 64137
AUGUST 2000

5 mg Actonel.
(risedronate sodium tablets)

References: 1. Actonel [package insert]. Cincinnati, Ohio: Procter & Gamble; 2000. **2.** Harris ST, Watts NB, Genant HK, et al. Effects of risedronate treatment on vertebral and nonvertebral fractures in women with postmenopausal osteoporosis: a randomized controlled trial. *JAMA.* 1999;282(14):1344-1352. **3.** Reginster J-Y, Minne HW, Sorensen OH, et al. Randomised trial of the effects of risedronate on vertebral fractures in women with established postmenopausal osteoporosis. *Osteoporos Int.* 2000;11:83-91. **4.** Data on file, Procter & Gamble, Cincinnati, Ohio.

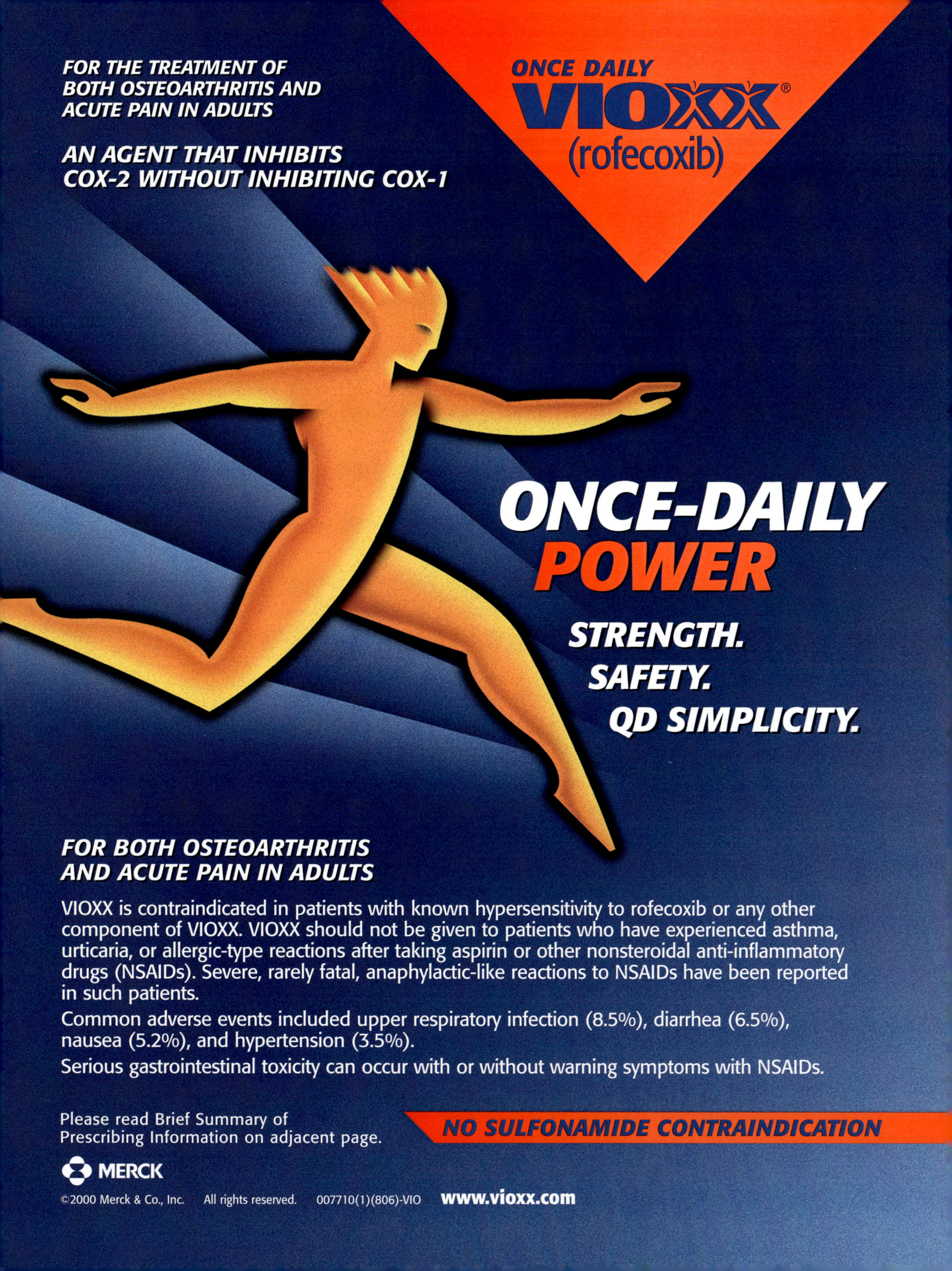

FOR THE TREATMENT OF BOTH OSTEOARTHRITIS AND ACUTE PAIN IN ADULTS
AN AGENT THAT INHIBITS COX-2 WITHOUT INHIBITING COX-1
ONCE DAILY
VIOXX®
(rofecoxib)
ONCE-DAILY
POWER
STRENGTH.
SAFETY.
QD SIMPLICITY.
FOR BOTH OSTEOARTHRITIS AND ACUTE PAIN IN ADULTS
VIOXX is contraindicated in patients with known hypersensitivity to rofecoxib or any other component of VIOXX. VIOXX should not be given to patients who have experienced asthma, urticaria, or allergic-type reactions after taking aspirin or other nonsteroidal anti-inflammatory drugs (NSAIDs). Severe, rarely fatal, anaphylactic-like reactions to NSAIDs have been reported in such patients.
Common adverse events included upper respiratory infection (8.5%), diarrhea (6.5%), nausea (5.2%), and hypertension (3.5%).
Serious gastrointestinal toxicity can occur with or without warning symptoms with NSAIDs.
Please read Brief Summary of Prescribing Information on adjacent page.
NO SULFONAMIDE CONTRAINDICATION
MERCK
©2000 Merck & Co., Inc. All rights reserved. 007710(1)(806)-VIO
www.vioxx.com

VIOXX® (rofecoxib tablets and oral suspension)

Brief Summary of Prescribing Information

INDICATIONS AND USAGE: VIOXX is indicated for: relief of the signs and symptoms of osteoarthritis (OA); management of acute pain in adults; treatment of primary dysmenorrhea.

CONTRAINDICATIONS: VIOXX is contraindicated in patients with known hypersensitivity to rofecoxib or any other component of VIOXX.

VIOXX should not be given to patients who have experienced asthma, urticaria, or allergic-type reactions after taking aspirin or other nonsteroidal anti-inflammatory drugs (NSAIDs). Severe, rarely fatal, anaphylactic-like reactions to NSAIDs have been reported in such patients (see WARNINGS, *Anaphylactoid Reactions* and PRECAUTIONS, *Preexisting Asthma*).

WARNINGS: *Gastrointestinal (GI) Effects—Risk of GI Ulceration, Bleeding, and Perforation:* Serious GI toxicity, such as bleeding, ulceration, and perforation of the stomach, small intestine, or large intestine, can occur at any time, with or without warning symptoms, in patients treated with NSAIDs. Minor upper GI problems, such as dyspepsia, are common and may also occur at any time during NSAID therapy. Therefore, physicians and patients should remain alert for ulceration and bleeding, even in the absence of previous GI tract symptoms. Patients should be informed about the signs and/or symptoms of serious GI toxicity and the steps to take if they occur. The utility of periodic laboratory monitoring has not been demonstrated, nor has it been adequately assessed. Only 1 in 5 patients who develop a serious upper GI adverse event on NSAID therapy is symptomatic. It has been demonstrated that upper GI ulcers, gross bleeding, or perforation caused by NSAIDs, appear to occur in approximately 1% of patients treated for 3–6 months, and in about 2%–4% of patients treated for 1 year. These trends continue thus, increasing the likelihood of developing a serious GI event at some time during the course of therapy. However, even short-term therapy is not without risk.

It is unclear, at the present time, how the above rates apply to VIOXX. Among 3,357 patients who received VIOXX in controlled clinical trials of 6 weeks to 1 year in duration (most were enrolled in 6-month or longer studies) at a daily dose of 12.5 mg to 50 mg, a total of 4 patients experienced a serious upper GI event, using protocol-derived criteria. Two patients experienced an upper GI bleed within 3 months (at Days 62 and 87, respectively) (0.06%). One additional patient experienced an obstruction within 6 months (Day 130) and the remaining patient developed an upper GI bleed within 12 months (Day 322) (0.12%). Approximately 23% of these 3,357 patients were in studies that required them to be ulcer free at study entry. It is unclear if this study population is representative of the general population. Prospective, long-term studies required to compare the incidence of serious, clinically significant upper GI adverse events in patients taking VIOXX vs comparator NSAID products have not been performed.

NSAIDs should be prescribed with extreme caution in patients with a prior history of ulcer disease or GI bleeding. Most spontaneous reports of fatal GI events are in elderly or debilitated patients and therefore special care should be taken in treating this population. **To minimize the potential risk for an adverse GI event, the lowest effective dose should be used for the shortest possible duration.** For high-risk patients, alternate therapies that do not involve NSAIDs should be considered.

Studies have shown that patients with a *prior history of peptic ulcer disease and/or GI bleeding* and who use NSAIDs, have a greater than 10-fold higher risk for developing a GI bleed than patients with neither of these risk factors. In addition to a past history of ulcer disease, pharmacoepidemiologic studies have identified several other cotherapies or comorbid conditions that may increase the risk for GI bleeding, such as: treatment with oral corticosteroids, treatment with anticoagulants, longer duration of NSAID therapy, smoking, alcoholism, older age, and poor general health status.

Anaphylactoid Reactions: As with NSAIDs in general, anaphylactoid reactions have occurred in patients without known prior exposure to VIOXX. In postmarketing experience, rare cases of anaphylactoid reactions and angioedema have been reported in patients receiving VIOXX. VIOXX should not be given to patients with the aspirin triad. This symptom complex typically occurs in asthmatic patients who experience rhinitis with or without nasal polyps, or who exhibit severe, potentially fatal bronchospasm after taking aspirin or other NSAIDs (see CONTRAINDICATIONS and PRECAUTIONS, *Preexisting Asthma*). Emergency help should be sought in cases where an anaphylactoid reaction occurs.

Advanced Renal Disease: No safety information is available regarding the use of VIOXX in patients with advanced kidney disease. Therefore, treatment with VIOXX is not recommended in these patients. If VIOXX therapy must be initiated, close monitoring of the patient's kidney function is advisable (see PRECAUTIONS, *Renal Effects*).

Pregnancy: In late pregnancy, VIOXX should be avoided because it may cause premature closure of the ductus arteriosus.

PRECAUTIONS: *General:* VIOXX cannot be expected to substitute for corticosteroids or to treat corticosteroid insufficiency. Abrupt discontinuation of corticosteroids may lead to exacerbation of corticosteroid-responsive illness. Patients on prolonged corticosteroid therapy should have their therapy tapered slowly if a decision is made to discontinue corticosteroids.

The pharmacologic activity of VIOXX in reducing inflammation, and possibly fever, may diminish the utility of these diagnostic signs in detecting infectious complications of presumed noninfectious, painful conditions.

Hepatic Effects: Borderline elevations of 1 or more liver tests may occur in up to 15% of patients taking NSAIDs, and notable elevations of ALT or AST (~3 or more times the upper limit of normal) have been reported in approximately 1% of patients in clinical trials with NSAIDs. These laboratory abnormalities may progress, may remain unchanged, or may be transient with continuing therapy. Rare cases of severe hepatic reactions, including jaundice and fatal fulminant hepatitis, liver necrosis, and hepatic failure (some with fatal outcome) have been reported with NSAIDs. In controlled clinical trials of VIOXX, the incidence of borderline elevations of liver tests at doses of 12.5 mg and 25 mg daily was comparable to the incidence observed with ibuprofen and lower than that observed with diclofenac. In placebo-controlled trials, approximately 0.5% of patients taking rofecoxib (12.5 mg or 25 mg q.d.) and 0.1% of patients taking placebo had notable elevations of ALT or AST.

A patient with symptoms and/or signs suggesting liver dysfunction, or in whom an abnormal liver test has occurred, should be monitored carefully for evidence of the development of a more severe hepatic reaction while on therapy with VIOXX. Use of VIOXX is not recommended in patients with moderate or severe hepatic insufficiency. If clinical signs and symptoms consistent with liver disease develop, or if systemic manifestations occur (e.g., eosinophilia, rash, etc.), VIOXX should be discontinued.

Renal Effects: Long-term administration of NSAIDs has resulted in renal papillary necrosis and other renal injury. Renal toxicity has also been seen in patients in whom renal prostaglandins have a compensatory role in the maintenance of renal perfusion. In these patients, administration of an NSAID may cause a dose-dependent reduction in prostaglandin formation and, secondarily, in renal blood flow, which may precipitate overt renal decompensation. Patients at greatest risk of this reaction are those with impaired renal function, heart failure, liver dysfunction, those taking diuretics and angiotensin-converting enzyme (ACE) inhibitors, and the elderly. Discontinuation of NSAID therapy is usually followed by recovery to the pretreatment state. Clinical trials with VIOXX at daily doses of 12.5 mg and 25 mg have shown renal effects (e.g., hypertension, edema) similar to those observed with comparator NSAIDs; these occur with an increased frequency with chronic use of VIOXX at doses above the 12.5-mg to 25-mg range (see ADVERSE REACTIONS). Caution should be used when initiating treatment with VIOXX in patients with considerable dehydration. It is advisable to rehydrate patients first and then start therapy with VIOXX. Caution is also recommended in patients with preexisting kidney disease (see WARNINGS, *Advanced Renal Disease*).

Hematologic Effects: Anemia is sometimes seen in patients receiving VIOXX. In placebo-controlled trials, there were no significant differences observed between VIOXX and placebo in clinical reports of anemia. Patients on long-term treatment with VIOXX should have their hemoglobin or hematocrit checked if they exhibit any signs or symptoms of anemia or blood loss. VIOXX does not generally affect platelet counts, prothrombin time, or partial thromboplastin time, and does not inhibit platelet aggregation at indicated dosages.

Fluid Retention and Edema: Fluid retention and edema have been observed in some patients taking VIOXX® (rofecoxib tablets and oral suspension) (see ADVERSE REACTIONS). VIOXX should be used with caution and should be introduced at the lowest recommended dose in patients with fluid retention, hypertension, or heart failure.

Preexisting Asthma: Patients with asthma may have aspirin-sensitive asthma. The use of aspirin in patients with aspirin-sensitive asthma has been associated with severe bronchospasm, which can be fatal. Since cross-reactivity, including bronchospasm, between aspirin and other NSAIDs has been reported in such aspirin-sensitive patients, VIOXX should not be administered to patients with this form of aspirin sensitivity and should be used with caution in patients with preexisting asthma.

Information for Patients: VIOXX can cause discomfort and, rarely, more serious side effects, such as GI bleeding, which may result in hospitalization and even fatal outcomes. Although serious GI tract ulcerations and bleeding can occur without warning symptoms, patients should be alert for the signs and symptoms of ulcerations and bleeding, and should ask for medical advice when observing any indicative signs or symptoms. Patients should be apprised of the importance of this follow-up (see WARNINGS, *Gastrointestinal (GI) Effects—Risk of GI Ulceration, Bleeding, and Perforation)*.

Patients should promptly report signs or symptoms of GI ulceration or bleeding, skin rash, unexplained weight gain, or edema to their physicians.

Patients should be informed of the warning signs and symptoms of hepatotoxicity (e.g., nausea, fatigue, lethargy, pruritus, jaundice, right upper quadrant tenderness, and "flu-like" symptoms). If these occur, patients should be instructed to stop therapy and seek immediate medical therapy.

Patients should also be instructed to seek immediate emergency help in the case of an anaphylactoid reaction (see WARNINGS).

In late pregnancy, VIOXX should be avoided because it may cause premature closure of the ductus arteriosus.

Laboratory Tests: Because serious GI tract ulcerations and bleeding can occur without warning symptoms, physicians should monitor for signs or symptoms of GI bleeding.

Drug Interactions: ACE Inhibitors: Reports suggest that NSAIDs may diminish the antihypertensive effect of ACE inhibitors. In patients with mild to moderate hypertension, administration of 25 mg daily of VIOXX with the ACE inhibitor benazepril, 10 to 40 mg for 4 weeks, was associated with an average increase in mean arterial pressure of about 3 mmHg compared to ACE inhibitor alone. This interaction should be given consideration in patients taking VIOXX concomitantly with ACE inhibitors. *Aspirin:* Concomitant administration of low-dose aspirin with VIOXX may result in an increased rate of GI ulceration or other complications, compared to use of VIOXX alone. At steady state, VIOXX 50 mg once daily had no effect on the antiplatelet activity of low-dose (81 mg once daily) aspirin, as assessed by ex vivo platelet aggregation and serum TXB_2 generation in clotting blood. VIOXX is not a substitute for aspirin for cardiovascular prophylaxis. *Cimetidine:* Coadministration with high doses of cimetidine (800 mg twice daily) increased the C_{max} of rofecoxib by 21%, the $AUC_{0\text{-}120hr}$ by 23%, and the $t_{1/2}$ by 15%. These small changes are not clinically significant and no dose adjustment is necessary. *Digoxin:* Rofecoxib 75 mg once daily for 11 days does not alter the plasma concentration profile or renal elimination of digoxin after a single 0.5-mg oral dose. *Furosemide:* Clinical studies, as well as postmarketing observations, have shown that NSAIDs can reduce the natriuretic effect of furosemide and thiazides in some patients. This response has been attributed to inhibition of renal prostaglandin synthesis. *Ketoconazole:* Ketoconazole 400 mg daily did not have any clinically important effect on the pharmacokinetics of rofecoxib. *Lithium:* NSAIDs have produced an elevation of plasma lithium levels and a reduction in renal lithium clearance. In postmarketing experience, there have been reports of increases in plasma lithium levels. Thus, when VIOXX and lithium are administered concurrently, subjects should be observed carefully for signs of lithium toxicity. *Methotrexate:* VIOXX 75 mg administered once daily for 10 days increased plasma concentrations by 23%, as measured by $AUC_{0\text{-}24hr}$ in patients receiving methotrexate 7.5 mg to 15 mg/week for rheumatoid arthritis. An equivalent magnitude of reduction in methotrexate renal clearance was observed. At 24 hours postdose, a similar proportion of patients treated with methotrexate alone (94%) and subsequently treated with methotrexate coadministered with 75 mg of rofecoxib (88%) had methotrexate plasma concentrations below the measurable limit (5 ng/mL). The effects of the recommended doses for OA (12.5 mg and 25 mg) of VIOXX on plasma methotrexate levels are unknown. Standard monitoring of methotrexate-related toxicity should be continued if VIOXX and methotrexate are administered concomitantly. *Oral Contraceptives:* Rofecoxib did not have any clinically important effect on the pharmacokinetics of ethinyl estradiol and norethindrone. *Prednisone/Prednisolone:* Rofecoxib did not have any clinically important effect on the pharmacokinetics of prednisone or prednisolone. *Rifampin:* Coadministration of VIOXX with rifampin 600 mg daily, a potent inducer of hepatic metabolism, produced an approximate 50% decrease in rofecoxib plasma concentrations. Therefore, a starting daily dose of 25 mg of VIOXX should be considered for the treatment of OA when VIOXX is coadministered with potent inducers of hepatic metabolism. *Warfarin:* Anticoagulant activity should be monitored, particularly in the first few days after initiating or changing VIOXX therapy in patients receiving warfarin or similar agents, since these patients are at an increased risk of bleeding complications. In single- and multiple-dose studies in healthy subjects receiving both warfarin and rofecoxib, prothrombin time (measured as INR) was increased by approximately 8% to 11%. In postmarketing experience, bleeding events have been reported, predominantly in the elderly, in association with increases in prothrombin time in patients receiving VIOXX concurrently with warfarin.

Carcinogenesis, Mutagenesis, Impairment of Fertility: Rofecoxib was not carcinogenic in mice given oral doses up to 30 mg/kg (male) and 60 mg/kg (female) (~5- and 2-fold the human exposure at 25 mg and 50 mg daily based on $AUC_{0\text{-}24}$) and in male and female rats given oral doses up to 8 mg/kg (~6- and 2-fold the human exposure at 25 mg and 50 mg daily based on $AUC_{0\text{-}24}$) for 2 years. Rofecoxib was not mutagenic in an Ames test or in a V-79 mammalian cell mutagenesis assay, nor clastogenic in a chromosome aberration assay in Chinese hamster ovary (CHO) cells, in an in vitro and an in vivo alkaline elution assay, or in an in vivo chromosomal aberration test in mouse bone marrow. Rofecoxib did not impair male fertility in rats at oral doses up to 100 mg/kg (~20- and 7-fold human exposure at 25 mg and 50 mg daily based on $AUC_{0\text{-}24}$) and rofecoxib had no effect on fertility in female rats at doses up to 30 mg/kg (~19- and 7-fold human exposure at 25 mg and 50 mg daily based on $AUC_{0\text{-}24}$).

Pregnancy: Teratogenic Effects: Pregnancy Category C. Rofecoxib was not teratogenic in rats at dosages up to 50 mg/kg/day (~28- and 10-fold human exposure at 25 mg and 50 mg daily based on $AUC_{0\text{-}24}$). There was a slight, nonstatistically significant increase in the overall incidence of vertebral malformations only in the rabbit at doses of 50 mg/kg/day (~1- or <1-fold human exposure at 25 mg and 50 mg daily based on $AUC_{0\text{-}24}$). There are no studies in pregnant women. VIOXX should be used during pregnancy only if the potential benefit justifies the potential risk to the fetus.

Nonteratogenic Effects: Rofecoxib produced periimplantation and postimplantation losses and reduced embryo/fetal survival in rats and rabbits at oral doses ≥10 and ≥75 mg/kg/day, respectively (~9- and 3-fold [rats] and 2- and <1-fold [rabbits] human exposure based on $AUC_{0\text{-}24}$ at 25 mg and 50 mg daily). These changes are expected with inhibition of prostaglandin synthesis and are not the result of permanent alteration of female reproductive function. There was an increase in the incidence of postnatal pup mortality in rats at ≥5 mg/kg/day (~5- and 2-fold human exposure at 25 mg and 50 mg daily based on $AUC_{0\text{-}24}$). In studies in pregnant rats administered single doses of rofecoxib, there was a treatment-related decrease in the diameter of the ductus arteriosus at all doses used (3–300 mg/kg: 3 mg/kg is ~2- and <1-fold human exposure at 25 mg or 50 mg daily based on $AUC_{0\text{-}24}$). As with other drugs known to inhibit prostaglandin synthesis, use of VIOXX during the third trimester of pregnancy should be avoided.

Labor and Delivery: Rofecoxib produced no evidence of significantly delayed labor or parturition in females at doses 15 mg/kg in rats (~10- and 3-fold human exposure as measured by the $AUC_{0\text{-}24}$ at 25 mg and 50 mg). The effects of VIOXX on labor and delivery in pregnant women are unknown. Merck & Co., Inc., maintains a registry to monitor the pregnancy outcomes of women exposed to VIOXX while pregnant. Healthcare providers are encouraged to report any prenatal exposure to VIOXX by calling the Pregnancy Registry at 1-800-986-8999.

Nursing Mothers: Rofecoxib is excreted in the milk of lactating rats at concentrations similar to those in plasma. There was an increase in pup mortality and a decrease in pup body weight following exposure of pups to milk from dams administered VIOXX® (rofecoxib tablets and oral suspension) during lactation. The dose tested represents an approximate 18- and 6-fold human exposure at 25 mg and 50 mg daily based on $AUC_{0\text{-}24}$. It is not known whether this drug is excreted in human milk. Because many drugs are excreted in human milk and because of the potential for serious adverse reactions in nursing infants from VIOXX, a decision should be made whether to discontinue nursing or to discontinue the drug, taking into account the importance of the drug to the mother.

Pediatric Use: Safety and effectiveness in pediatric patients below the age of 18 years have not been evaluated.

Geriatric Use: Of the patients who received VIOXX in OA clinical trials, 1,455 were 65 years of age or older (this included 460 who were 75 years or older). No substantial differences in safety and effectiveness were observed between these subjects and younger subjects. Greater sensitivity of some older individuals cannot be ruled out. Dosage adjustment in the elderly is not necessary; however, therapy with VIOXX should be initiated at the lowest recommended dose. In 1 of these studies (a 6-week, double-blind, randomized clinical trial), VIOXX 12.5 mg or 25 mg once daily was administered to 174 OA patients ≥80 years of age. The safety profile in this elderly population was similar to that of younger patients treated with VIOXX.

ADVERSE REACTIONS: *OA:* Approximately 3,600 patients with OA were treated with VIOXX; approximately 1,400 patients received VIOXX for 6 months or longer, and approximately 800 patients for 1 year or longer. The following paragraph lists all adverse events, regardless of causality, occurring in at least 2% of patients receiving VIOXX in 9 controlled studies of 6 weeks' to 6 months' duration conducted in patients with OA at the therapeutically recommended doses (12.5 mg and 25 mg), which included a placebo and/or positive control group.

Clinical adverse experiences occurring in ≥2.0% of patients treated with VIOXX vs placebo, ibuprofen 2400 mg, or diclofenac 150 mg: *Body as a Whole/Site Unspecified:* abdominal pain, 3.4% (vs 4.1%, placebo; 4.6%, ibuprofen; 5.8%, diclofenac); asthenia/fatigue, 2.2% (vs 1.0%; 2.0%; 2.6%); dizziness, 3.0% (vs 2.2%; 2.7%; 3.4%); influenza-like disease, 2.9% (vs 3.1%; 1.5%; 3.2%); lower extremity edema, 3.7% (vs 1.1%; 3.8%; 3.4%); upper respiratory infection, 8.5% (vs 7.8%; 5.8%; 8.2%). *Cardiovascular System:* hypertension, 3.5% (vs 1.3%; 3.0%; 1.6%). *Digestive System:* diarrhea, 6.5% (vs 6.8%; 7.1%; 10.6%); dyspepsia, 3.5% (vs 2.7%; 4.7%; 4.0%); epigastric discomfort, 3.8% (vs 2.8%; 9.2%; 5.4%); heartburn, 4.2% (vs 3.6%; 5.2%; 4.6%); nausea, 5.2% (vs 2.9%; 7.1%; 7.4%). *Eyes, Ears, Nose, and Throat:* sinusitis, 2.7% (vs 2.0%; 1.8%; 2.4%). *Musculoskeletal System:* back pain, 2.5% (vs 1.9%; 1.4%; 2.8%). *Nervous System:* headache, 4.7% (vs 7.5%; 6.1%; 8.0%). *Respiratory System:* bronchitis, 2.0% (vs 0.8%; 1.4%; 3.2%). *Urogenital System:* urinary tract infection, 2.8% (vs 2.7%; 2.5%; 3.6%).

The general safety profile of VIOXX 50 mg q.d. in OA clinical trials of up to 6 months (476 patients) was similar to that of VIOXX at the recommended OA doses of 12.5 mg and 25 mg q.d., except for a higher incidence of GI symptoms (abdominal pain, epigastric pain, heartburn, nausea, and vomiting), lower extremity edema (6.3%), and hypertension (8.2%).

In the OA studies, the following spontaneous adverse events occurred in >0.1% to 1.9% of patients treated with VIOXX, regardless of causality:

Body as a Whole: abdominal distension, abdominal tenderness, abscess, chest pain, chills, contusion, cyst, diaphragmatic hernia, fever, fluid retention, flushing, fungal infection, infection, laceration, pain, pelvic pain, peripheral edema, postoperative pain, syncope, trauma, upper extremity edema, viral syndrome. *Cardiovascular System:* angina pectoris, atrial fibrillation, bradycardia, hematoma, irregular heartbeat, palpitation, premature ventricular contraction, tachycardia, venous insufficiency. *Digestive System:* acid reflux, aphthous stomatitis, constipation, dental caries, dental pain, digestive gas symptoms, dry mouth, duodenal disorder, dysgeusia, esophagitis, flatulence, gastric disorder, gastritis, gastroenteritis, hematochezia, hemorrhoids, infectious gastroenteritis, oral infection, oral lesion, oral ulcer, vomiting. *Eyes, Ears, Nose, and Throat:* allergic rhinitis, blurred vision, cerumen impaction, conjunctivitis, dry throat, epistaxis, laryngitis, nasal congestion, nasal secretion, ophthalmic injection, otic pain, otitis, otitis media, pharyngitis, tinnitus, tonsillitis. *Immune System:* allergy, hypersensitivity, insect bite reaction. *Metabolism and Nutrition:* appetite change, hypercholesterolemia, weight gain. *Musculoskeletal System:* ankle sprain, arm pain, arthralgia, back strain, bursitis, cartilage trauma, joint swelling, muscular cramp, muscular disorder, muscular weakness, musculoskeletal pain, musculoskeletal stiffness, myalgia, osteoarthritis, tendinitis, traumatic arthropathy, wrist fracture. *Nervous System:* hypesthesia, insomnia, median nerve neuropathy, migraine, muscular spasm, paresthesia, sciatica, somnolence, vertigo. *Psychiatric:* anxiety, depression, mental acuity decreased. *Respiratory System:* asthma, cough, dyspnea, pneumonia, pulmonary congestion, respiratory infection. *Skin and Skin Appendages:* abrasion, alopecia, atopic dermatitis, basal cell carcinoma, blister, cellulitis, contact dermatitis, herpes simplex, herpes zoster, nail unit disorder, perspiration, pruritus, rash, skin erythema, urticaria, xerosis. *Urogenital System:* breast mass, cystitis, dysuria, menopausal symptoms, menstrual disorder, nocturia, urinary retention, vaginitis.

The following serious adverse events have been reported rarely (estimated <0.1%) in patients taking VIOXX, regardless of causality. Cases reported only in the postmarketing experience are indicated in italics.

Cardiovascular: cerebrovascular accident, congestive heart failure, deep venous thrombosis, myocardial infarction, pulmonary embolism, transient ischemic attack, unstable angina. *GI:* cholecystitis, colitis, colonic malignant neoplasm, *duodenal perforation*, duodenal ulcer, *esophageal ulcer, gastric perforation, gastric ulcer*, GI bleeding, *hepatitis,* intestinal obstruction, *jaundice,* pancreatitis. *Hemic and Lymphatic: agranulocytosis, leukopenia,* lymphoma, *thrombocytopenia. Immune System: anaphylactoid reaction, angioedema. Nervous System: aseptic meningitis. Psychiatric: confusion, hallucinations. Skin and Skin Appendages: severe skin reactions, including Stevens-Johnson syndrome. Urogenital System: acute renal failure,* breast malignant neoplasm, *interstitial nepphritis*, prostatic malignant neoplasm, urolithiasis, *worsening chronic renal failure.*

In 1-year controlled clinical trials and in extension studies for up to 86 weeks (~800 patients treated with VIOXX for 1 year or longer), the adverse-experience profile was qualitatively similar to that observed in studies of shorter duration.

Analgesia, Including Primary Dysmenorrhea: Approximately 1,000 patients were treated with VIOXX in analgesia studies. All patients in postdental surgery pain studies received only a single dose of study medication. Patients in primary dysmenorrhea studies may have taken up to 3 daily doses of VIOXX, and those in the postorthopedic surgery pain study were prescribed 5 daily doses of VIOXX.

The adverse-experience profile in the analgesia studies was generally similar to those reported in the OA studies. The following additional adverse experience, which occurred at an incidence of ≥2% of patients treated with VIOXX, was observed in the postdental pain surgery studies: postdental extraction alveolitis (dry socket).

In 110 patients treated with VIOXX (average age ~65 years) in the postorthopedic surgery pain study, the most commonly reported adverse experiences were constipation, fever, and nausea.

DOSAGE AND ADMINISTRATION: VIOXX is administered orally. The lowest dose of VIOXX should be sought for each patient.

OA: The recommended starting dose of VIOXX is 12.5 mg once daily. Some patients may receive additional benefit by increasing the dose to 25 mg once daily. The maximum recommended daily dose is 25 mg.

Management of Acute Pain and Treatment of Primary Dysmenorrhea: The recommended initial dose of VIOXX is 50 mg once daily. Subsequent doses should be 50 mg once daily as needed. Use of VIOXX for more than 5 days in management of pain has not been studied.

VIOXX Tablets may be taken with or without food.

Oral Suspension: VIOXX Oral Suspension 12.5 mg/5 mL or 25 mg/5 mL may be substituted for VIOXX Tablets 12.5 mg or 25 mg, respectively, in any of the above indications. Shake before using.

For more detailed information, consult your Merck representative and read the full Prescribing Information.

MERCK

Table 1. Cumulative clinical characteristics common to chronic rheumatic autoimmune diseases in mothers of children with isolated congenital heart block (CHB), in mothers of children with isolated heart block detected after the newborn period, and in healthy mothers*

	Mothers of children with isolated CHB (n = 81)†‡	Mothers of children with isolated heart block detected after the newborn period (n = 41)§	Healthy mothers (n = 89)
Malar rash	5 (6)	0 (0)	1 (1)
Discoid rash	1 (1)	0 (0)	0 (0)
Photosensitivity	29 (36)	6 (15)	2 (2)
Oral ulcers	1 (1)	0 (0)	2 (2)
Arthritis	7 (9)	2 (5)	3 (3)
Serositis	1 (1)	0 (0)	0 (0)
Nephritis	1 (1)	0 (0)	2 (2)
Seizures/psychosis	2 (2)	0 (0)	0 (0)
Fatigue	41/78 (52)	14 (34)	13 (15)
Raynaud's phenomenon	14/78 (18)	7 (17)	10 (11)
Dry eyes	38/78 (49)	4 (10)	6 (7)
Dry mouth	43/78 (55)	7 (17)	8 (10)

* Values are the number (%) of subjects. Fatigue was defined as a subjective feeling of unusual tiredness for >3 months. Dry eyes and dry mouth were defined as present if any of the answers to the 3 validated questions predictive of eye and oral involvement, respectively, were positive. Only P values less than 0.05 are given. The Bonferroni correction for multiple comparisons yielded a P value of 0.0042.
† $P = 0.02$ for photosensitivity and $P < 0.0001$ for dry eyes and mouth, versus mothers of children with isolated heart block detected after the newborn period.
‡ $P < 0.0001$ for photosensitivity, fatigue, dry eyes, and dry mouth, versus healthy mothers.
§ $P = 0.02$ for photosensitivity and fatigue, versus healthy mothers.

(37%) of the 78 living mothers had a self-reported diagnosis of a chronic autoimmune disease (mean ± SD duration 7.3 ± 6.5 years, range 0–28 years). Fifty-five mothers (71%) had had symptoms, signs, or abnormal laboratory findings clearly suggesting an underlying autoimmune disorder before the index delivery (mean ± SD 9.7 ± 5.6 years, range 1–31 years). Common initial symptoms were arthralgia, arthritis, dry mouth, swelling of the parotid glands, dry eyes, fatigue, and/or photosensitivity; rare symptoms were cutaneous lupus and fever. Rare initial clinical signs and/or abnormal laboratory findings were an unexplained high erythrocyte sedimentation rate, thyrotoxicosis, hyperglobulinemic purpura, pernicious anemia, and rheumatoid factor.

Mothers of children with isolated CHB had photosensitivity, fatigue, dry eyes, and dry mouth significantly more often than the healthy control subjects (Table 1). No other differences were statistically significant. Dry eyes and dry mouth were already common in affected mothers before the index delivery (in 32% and 36% of the mothers, respectively).

Twenty-three (29%) of the 78 mothers who were still living had been completely asymptomatic before the index delivery, and 10 (13%) of them remained so after a mean followup of 9.6 years (range 0–21 years).

Fifteen (18%) of all 83 mothers had developed signs and symptoms that met the criteria for a chronic rheumatic disease or had another medically documented autoimmune disease a mean ± SD of 6.8 ± 5.9 years (range 0–21 years) before the index delivery (Table 2); by a mean of 9.9 years after the index delivery, 33 (40%) of the mothers had met the criteria. The most common diagnosis was primary SS followed by SLE, both of which were often associated with other autoimmune disorders (Table 2).

Of the 83 mothers studied, 5 had died during the followup period. Two mothers not known to have an autoimmune disease died of myocardial infarction and pancreatic carcinoma, respectively. One mother who satisfied the criteria for SLE 20 years after the index delivery died of a myocardial infarction. One mother died of liver cirrhosis mainly caused by alcohol consumption; she had satisfied the criteria for SLE 12 years after the index delivery. One mother died of a fatal arrhythmia associated with pericarditis at the age of 27 years. Mothers of children with CHB had a standardized mortality ratio of 5.1 (95% confidence interval 1.6–11.8).

Findings in mothers of children with isolated heart block detected after the newborn period. We identified 55 offspring with isolated heart block detected after the newborn period. Of the 55 mothers, 1 could not

Table 2. Chronic autoimmune diseases diagnosed and number of ACR criteria for SLE and EC criteria for SS fulfilled in 83 mothers during followup after the birth of their first child with isolated congenital heart block*

Autoimmune disease	No. of mothers	Occurrence before/after index delivery	Mean no. of ACR or EC criteria fulfilled (range) SLE	SS	Diagnoses of associated autoimmune diseases (no. of patients)
Definite primary SS	22	5/17	2.1 (0–3)	4.4 (4–6)	Pernicious anemia (1), autoimmune hypothyroidism (2)†
Probable primary SS	11	4/7	1.5 (0–3)	3 (3)	Ulcerative colitis (1), autoimmune hypothyroidism (2)
SLE	9	3/6	5.1 (4–6)	2.0 (0–6)	Definite secondary SS (1), probable secondary SS (2)
Rheumatoid arthritis	1	0/1	2	2	–
Autoimmune hypothyroidism	3	1/2	1.3 (1–2)	0.7 (0–2)	–
Graves' disease	1	1/0	2	1	–
Sarcoidosis	1	1/0	0	1	–
No autoimmune disease	35	–	1.0 (0–3)	1.0 (0–2)	–

* The mean ± SD followup period was 9.9 ± 9.0 years (range 0–49 years). In mothers who had 2 autoimmune diseases, the primary diagnoses were systemic lupus erythematosus (SLE) and rheumatoid arthritis, the secondary diagnosis was primary Sjögren's syndrome (SS), and other diagnoses were tertiary. ACR = American College of Rheumatology; EC = European Community.
† One patient had both pernicious anemia and autoimmune hypothyroidism.

be identified and 6 refused participation in the study. Clinical data were available from 48 mothers, 41 of whom were still living.

The mean ± SD age of the 48 mothers at the time of the study was 53.4 ± 14.4 years (range 28–84 years). The mothers were studied a mean ± SD of 22.9 years ± 12.5 years (range 4–47 years) after the index delivery.

Before the index delivery, 2 of the 48 mothers had a medically documented diagnosis of an autoimmune disease (sarcoidosis and ulcerative colitis, respectively). One mother was diagnosed as having primary biliary cirrhosis 16 years after the index delivery.

Cumulative clinical characteristics common to chronic rheumatic autoimmune diseases were not significantly different in the 41 living mothers of children with isolated heart block detected after the newborn period compared with the healthy controls (Table 1). Mothers of children who were diagnosed as having isolated heart block after birth but before the age of 12 months were no more likely than the mothers of children who were diagnosed as having heart block after the age of 12 months to satisfy at least 1 criterion for SLE or SS (5 of 14 versus 7 of 27; *P* not significant).

Of all 54 mothers who were identified and studied, 7 had died during the followup. None of the deaths was related to an autoimmune disease. The standardized mortality ratio of these women was 1.9 (95% confidence interval 0.8–3.9).

DISCUSSION

In a nationwide study, we identified the majority of all children who had been born in Finland and had been diagnosed as having isolated heart block between 1950 and 1999. We could also clinically characterize practically all of the mothers of these children. Thus, our study is of an unselected and sufficiently large population to draw more definitive conclusions about the long-term outcome of mothers who have a child with isolated heart block, either congenital or detected after the newborn period.

We found that the common symptoms in mothers of children with CHB were photosensitivity, fatigue, dry eyes, and dry mouth. These symptoms are typical of primary SS, and it was also the most common autoimmune disease for which the criteria were fulfilled during the followup of the study in these mothers. In previous studies, the number of mothers with primary SS has been low (4,6,8,9), and it is obviously due to lack of objective tests for diagnosing keratoconjunctivitis sicca and xerostomia.

The finding that primary SS is the predominant autoimmune disease in mothers of children with CHB is not surprising considering the high prevalence of primary SS in the adult female population and the high titers of antibodies to SSA and/or SSB in these patients compared with those in patients with SLE or other autoimmune diseases (17–19).

Except for photosensitivity, specific clinical characteristics of SLE were uncommon in the mothers of children with CHB. Nine (11%) of the 83 mothers who were studied satisfied the criteria for SLE. Serious manifestations of the disease were rare; only 1 mother had nephritis (mesangial glomerulonephritis), none had central nervous system lupus, and 3 had definite or probable secondary SS. Active full-blown SLE was practically nonexistent. Our study therefore suggests that only a few mothers of children with CHB have SLE, and if they have it, the clinical picture is generally mild and overlaps with symptoms of SS.

Somewhat different findings have been reported by Waltuck and Buyon (8). In their study, 19 of 57 mothers of children with CHB had SLE; 4 of the 19 had nephritis and 1 had central nervous system disease. The explanation for the differences may be that in the Waltuck study, mothers of children with CHB were recruited from different centers including the Lupus Foundation of the United States.

Uncommon autoimmune diseases in our study population of mothers of children with CHB were Graves' disease and Hashimoto thyroiditis, both of which are known to be associated with SS (20). One mother each had sarcoidosis, ulcerative colitis, and erosive RA, and all these mothers had clinical characteristics of SS and/or SLE. Other uncommon diseases reported previously in mothers of children with CHB have been linear scleroderma, ankylosing spondylitis (9), and mixed connective tissue disease (21).

In our study, 58% of the mothers of children with CHB had developed a definitive autoimmune disease by a mean of 10 years after the index delivery, and almost all had symptoms and/or signs suggestive of a subclinical disease. These results are in considerable agreement with recent studies reporting that one-third to two-thirds of mothers of children with CHB have or will later develop a connective tissue disease (8,9). We speculate that the number may be even higher than two-thirds if affected mothers are followed up long enough (decades) and if all objective tests for diagnosing primary SS are performed.

Mortality in the mothers after the birth of the first child with CHB was somewhat higher than that in the normal population. This could be explained by chance, since the number of deaths was low. Another explanation is that mothers of children with CHB who are diagnosed as having SLE may have a poor prognosis. Three of all 5 deaths in our study occurred in patients with SLE; 1 death was directly related to the disease and 2 were indirectly related.

Mothers of children with heart block detected after the newborn period did not have, as a group, clinical characteristics clearly suggesting an underlying chronic autoimmune disease, and none of them was diagnosed as having a rheumatic disease. However, some of these mothers, especially those whose children were diagnosed as having isolated heart block before the age of 12 months, had clinical characteristics compatible with a subclinical primary SS or SLE. It is possible that, in these cases, the heart block was congenital but had escaped detection during pregnancy. Late detection of CHB may have been a problem previously, but nowadays, practically all cases are diagnosed by fetal ultrasound examinations during pregnancy.

In conclusion, we show that 10 years after the index delivery, more than half of the mothers of children with CHB have developed an autoimmune disease and that the most common diagnosis is primary SS. We also show that practically all of the mothers have subclinical features typical of SS and many have subclinical features typical of SLE. Mothers of children with isolated heart block detected after the newborn period do not, as a group, have clinical characteristics suggestive of autoimmune diseases.

ACKNOWLEDGMENT

We thank Seppo Sarna, PhD, for statistical advice.

REFERENCES

1. Tseng CE, Buyon JP. Neonatal lupus syndromes. Rheum Dis Clin North Am 1997;23:31–54.
2. McCuistion CH, Schoch EP. Possible discoid lupus erythematosus in a newborn infant: report of a case with subsequent development of acute systemic lupus erythematosus in the mother. Arch Dermatol Syph 1954;70:782–5.
3. Hogg GR. Congenital, acute lupus erythematosus associated with subendocardial fibroelastosis. Am J Clin Pathol 1957;28:648–54.
4. Brucato A, Franceschini F, Gasparini M, DeJuli E, Ferraro G, Quinzanini M, et al. Isolated congenital heart block: long-term outcome of mothers, maternal antibody specificity and immunogenetic background. J Rheumatol 1995;22:533–40.
5. Hansen BU, Manthorpe T, Manthorpe R, Marsal K. Isolated complete congenital heart block in offspring of mothers with primary Sjögren's syndrome. Scand J Rheumatol 1989;18:227–30.
6. McCune AB, Weston WL, Lee LA. Maternal and fetal outcome in neonatal lupus erythematosus. Ann Intern Med 1987;106:518–23.
7. Julkunen H, Kurki P, Kaaja R, Heikkilä R, Immonen I, Chan EKL, et al. Isolated congenital heart block: long-term outcome of mothers and characterization of the immune response to SS-A/Ro and SS-B/La. Arthritis Rheum 1993;36:1588–98.
8. Waltuck J, Buyon JP. Auto-antibody-associated congenital heart block: outcome of mothers and children. Ann Intern Med 1994; 120:544–51.
9. Press J, Uziel Y, Laxer RM, Luy L, Hamilton RM, Silverman ED. Long-term outcome of mothers of children with congenital heart block. Am J Med 1996;100:328–32.
10. Bharati S, Lev M. Pathology of atrioventricular block. Cardiol Clin 1984;2:741–51.
11. McCarron DP, Hellman DB, Traill TA, Watson RM. Neonatal lupus erythematosus syndrome: late detection of isolated heart block. J Rheumatol 1993;20:1212–4.
12. Geggel RL, Tucker L, Szer I. Postnatal progression from second- to third-degree heart block in neonatal lupus erythematosus syndrome. J Pediatr 1998;113:1049–52.
13. Eronen M, Siren MK, Ekblad H, Tikanoja T, Julkunen H, Paavilainen T. Short and long-term outcome of the children with

isolated complete heart block diagnosed in utero or as a newborn. Pediatrics 2000;106:86–91.
14. Tan EM, Cohen AS, Fries JF, Masi AT, McShane DJ, Rothfield NF, et al. The 1982 revised criteria for the classification of systemic lupus erythematosus. Arthritis Rheum 1982;25:1271–7.
15. Arnett FC, Edworthy SM, Bloch DA, McShane DJ, Fries JF, Cooper NS, et al. The American Rheumatism Association 1987 revised criteria for the classification of rheumatoid arthritis. Arthritis Rheum 1988;31:315–24.
16. Vitali C, Bombardieri S, Moutsopoulos HM, Balestrieri G, Bencivelli W, Bernstein RM, et al. Preliminary criteria for the classification of Sjögren's syndrome: results of a prospective concerted action supported by the European Community. Arthritis Rheum 1993;36:340–7.
17. Youinou P, Adler Y, Muller S, Lamour A, Baron D, Humbel RL. Anti-Ro(SSA) and anti-La(SSB) antibodies in autoimmune rheumatic diseases. Clin Rev Allergy 1994;12:253–74.
18. Julkunen H, Siren MK, Kaaja R, Kurki P, Friman C, Koskimies S. Maternal HLA antigens and antibodies to SS-A/Ro and SS-B/La: comparison with systemic lupus erythematosus and primary Sjögren's syndrome. Br J Rheumatol 1995;34:901–7.
19. Thomas E, Hay EM, Hajeer A, Silman AJ. Sjögren's syndrome: a community-based study of prevalence and impact. Br J Rheumatol 1998;37:1069–76.
20. Perez B, Kraus A, Lopez G, Cifuentes M, Alarcón-Segovia D. Autoimmune thyroid disease in primary Sjögren's syndrome. Am J Med 1995;99:480–4.
21. Nolan RJ, Shulman ST, Victorica BE. Congenital complete heart block associated with maternal mixed connective tissue disease. J Pediatr 1979;95:420–2.

ARTHRITIS & RHEUMATISM
Vol. 44, No. 3, March 2001, pp 653–661

The Disability Index of the Health Assessment Questionnaire Is a Predictor and Correlate of Outcome in the High-Dose Versus Low-Dose Penicillamine in Systemic Sclerosis Trial

Philip J. Clements,[1] Weng Kee Wong,[2] Eric L. Hurwitz,[2] Daniel E. Furst,[3] Maureen Mayes,[4] Barbara White,[5] Fredrick Wigley,[6] Michael Weisman,[7] Walter Barr,[8] Larry Moreland,[9] Thomas A. Medsger, Jr.,[10] Virginia Steen,[11] Richard W. Martin,[12] David Collier,[13] Arthur Weinstein,[14] Edward Lally,[15] John Varga,[16] Steven R. Weiner,[1] Brian Andrews,[17] Micha Abeles,[18] and James R. Seibold[19]

Objective. **To explore the clinical implications of a score of ≥1.0 on the Disability Index of the Health Assessment Questionnaire (HAQ DI) at the first patient visit, and to examine the implications of improvement in HAQ DI score over 2 years in a cohort of systemic sclerosis (SSc) patients with diffuse cutaneous scleroderma.**

Methods. **SSc skin and visceral involvement was assessed in 134 SSc patients with diffuse scleroderma (mean ± SD disease duration of 10 ± 4 months) when they entered a multicenter drug trial and again 2 years later. Mortality and the occurrence of scleroderma renal crisis were assessed for a mean ± SD of 4.0 ± 1.1 years. Logistic and linear regression analyses were used to examine the relationship of the baseline HAQ DI score to morbidity, mortality, and visceral involvement, as well as the relationship of changes in the HAQ DI score to changes in physical examination, laboratory, and functional variables over 2 years.**

Results. **A baseline HAQ DI score of ≥1.0 was predictive of mortality (odds ratio 3.22, 95% confidence interval 1.097–9.468) over 4 years. Multivariate linear regression demonstrated that a model which included the erythrocyte sedimentation rate at baseline (P = 0.005) and changes at 2 years in the swollen joint count (P = 0.002), total skin score (P = 0.005), and white blood cell count (P = 0.005) best explained the change in HAQ DI score over 2 years (R^2 = 0.528). The HAQ DI score and total skin score at baseline were highly correlated (correlation coefficient 0.368), as were changes in the HAQ DI score and the total skin score over 2 years (correlation coefficient 0.492). Although the HAQ DI score was heavily influenced by hand dysfunction at baseline and at 2 years, improvement (reduction) in the HAQ DI score over 2 years was related to factors other than hand dysfunction.**

Conclusion. **A baseline HAQ DI score of ≥1.0 predicted mortality over 4 years. Improvement in the**

Supported in part by grants from the Scleroderma Federation, United Scleroderma Foundation, FDA Orphan Drug Program, and Arthritis Foundation, CRC grants M01-RR-00865 and M01-RR-00827, and bequests from the estates of Winifred Krause, Morris Goldsmith, and Takako Ito.

[1]Philip J. Clements, MD, MPH, Steven R. Weiner, MD: UCLA School of Medicine, Los Angeles, California; [2]Weng Kee Wong, PhD, Eric L. Hurwitz, PhD: UCLA School of Public Health, Los Angeles, California; [3]Daniel E. Furst, MD: Virginia Mason Research Center, Seattle, Washington; [4]Maureen Mayes, MD, MPH: Wayne State University, Hutzel Hospital, Detroit, Michigan; [5]Barbara White, MD: University of Maryland School of Medicine, Baltimore; [6]Fredrick Wigley, MD: The Johns Hopkins University, Baltimore, Maryland; [7]Michael Weisman, MD: Cedars–Sinai Medical Center, Los Angeles, California; [8]Walter Barr, MD: Northwestern University Medical School, Chicago, Illinois; [9]Larry Moreland, MD: The University of Alabama at Birmingham; [10]Thomas A. Medsger, Jr., MD: University of Pittsburgh School of Medicine, Pittsburgh, Pennsylvania; [11]Virginia Steen, MD: Georgetown University Medical Center, Washington, DC; [12]Richard W. Martin, MD: Michigan State University College of Human Medicine, Grand Rapids; [13]David Collier, MD: University of Colorado Health Sciences Center, Denver; [14]Arthur Weinstein, MD: The George Washington University Medical Center, Washington, DC; [15]Edward Lally, MD: Brown University School of Medicine, Roger Williams General Hospital, Providence, Rhode Island; [16]John Varga, MD: University of Illinois, Chicago; [17]Brian Andrews, MD, PhD: University of California, Irvine; [18]Micha Abeles, MD: University of Connecticut Health Center, Farmington; [19]James R. Seibold, MD: UMDNJ–Robert Wood Johnson Medical School, New Brunswick, New Jersey.

Address correspondence and reprint requests to Philip J. Clements, MD, MPH, UCLA Medicine–Rheumatology, 32-59 Rehabilitation Center, Box 951670, Los Angeles, CA 90095-1670.

Submitted for publication July 13, 2000; accepted in revised form November 9, 2000.

HAQ DI score in these patients with diffuse scleroderma was associated with improvement in skin thickening, hand function, oral aperture, lung function, signs of arthritis, serum creatinine level, and the investigator's global assessment of improvement. The HAQ DI is a self-administered questionnaire that SSc patients can complete easily and rapidly and that gives the practicing physician important information about prognosis, patient status, and changes in disease course over time.

Systemic sclerosis (SSc) is a disorder characterized by overproduction and deposition of collagen in the skin and visceral organs, abnormalities of the microcirculation, and autoimmunity (1,2). Although it is well known that the disorder can be disabling, the degree of functional impairment has only recently been quantified using the Disability Index of the Health Assessment Questionnaire (HAQ DI) (3–9). We recently reported that moderate-to-severe functional impairment (HAQ DI score of ≥1.0) was already present within 18 months of SSc onset in 53% of 134 patients with diffuse cutaneous scleroderma (diffuse scleroderma) (3). This observation corroborates the findings of Poole, Steen, and others (4–9) who have also shown that moderate-to-severe functional impairment is frequent in SSc, especially in patients with diffuse scleroderma.

Recently, Steen and Medsger reported on the course of the HAQ DI score over a mean of 4 years in SSc patients followed up at the University of Pittsburgh (5). Their results showed that patients with diffuse scleroderma who ultimately died not only had higher first-visit HAQ DI scores than those of surviving patients with diffuse scleroderma, but also had a significant increase (worsening) in mean HAQ DI score prior to their deaths. Their analysis also showed that changes in the skin score were highly correlated with changes in the HAQ DI score (correlation coefficient 0.683) over 4 years. Few other published studies have addressed the issue of how functional impairment changes over time in patients with SSc, how these changes correlate with physical and laboratory changes, and what these changes imply regarding future morbidity or mortality.

In this study, we tested whether baseline data (derived from 134 SSc patients with diffuse scleroderma as they entered a randomized controlled trial of high-dose versus low-dose penicillamine for SSc) predicted survival over a 4-year period, and whether the courses of the HAQ DI score and the skin score were correlated in patients with diffuse scleroderma over 2 years of observation. More importantly, our present analysis explored changes in functional impairment in the subset of 68 SSc patients who completed the 2-year trial, as well as how these changes correlated with other physical and laboratory parameters.

What patients consider an "important symptomatic difference" in functional level has been quantified in 2 studies using the HAQ DI (10,11). In both studies, the average patient with rheumatoid arthritis (RA) concluded that if her or his HAQ DI score was lower by ≥0.2 units than another patient's HAQ DI score, this difference would be enough for the first patient to say that she or he was at least "somewhat better" than the other patient. In the present study, we tested whether an improvement of ≥0.2 units in the HAQ DI score in SSc patients with diffuse scleroderma correlated with changes in other physical and laboratory parameters over 2 years of study.

PATIENTS AND METHODS

Patients. To be eligible to enter the low-dose versus high-dose penicillamine in early SSc trial, patients had to meet American College of Rheumatology (formerly, the American Rheumatism Association) criteria for SSc, have diffuse cutaneous scleroderma (cutaneous induration proximal to, as well as distal to, the elbow and/or knee, with or without facial skin thickening), and have a disease duration of ≤18 months from the onset of the first SSc manifestation (other than Raynaud's phenomenon) (12,13). All patients signed a consent form approved by the Institutional Review Board at each center. The details and results of the high-dose versus low-dose penicillamine drug trial have been published elsewhere (14).

Patients were excluded if they had only limited cutaneous scleroderma (cutaneous induration distal to, but not proximal to, the knees and elbows) or only one of the localized forms of scleroderma, or if they met any of the following criteria or had any of the following conditions: age <18 or >75 years, pregnancy, presence of another well-defined rheumatic disease, severe organ involvement as defined previously (14), another chronic debilitating illness (e.g., cancer), history of a chronic blood dyscrasia, occurrence of scleroderma renal crisis (SRC) within the preceding 2 months, or intractable congestive heart failure. If patients required treatment with corticosteroids, the dose had to be stable at ≤10 mg/day prednisone (or equivalent) for at least 1 month prior to entry. D-penicillamine, azathioprine, cyclophosphamide, methotrexate, chlorambucil, potassium aminobenzoate, colchicine, or captopril had to have been discontinued for >1 month prior to entry.

Diagnostic tests. At baseline and every 6 months thereafter for up to 2 years, skin thickness was quantified using the modified Rodnan skin thickness score (total skin score) technique (3,14–16). Hand spread, fist closure, and vertical interlabial distance (oral aperture) were measured as previously described (3,14,16).

Organ system function was assessed at baseline and yearly thereafter for up to 2 years, as previously described (3,14,16). Assessments included pulmonary function tests (diffusing capacity for carbon monoxide [DL_{CO}; percent of predicted] and forced vital capacity [FVC; recorded in milliliters as well as percent of predicted]), posteroanterior chest radiograph; tests of 24-hour urine for creatinine clearance and protein level; serum creatine kinase (CK) level (recorded as the percent of the upper limit of normal); manual muscle testing; joint tenderness and swelling (each assessed in 8 joints [elbows, wrists, metacarpophalangeal joints, and knees; scored on a 0–1 scale] as well as the number of tender or swollen joints summed to give joint tenderness and joint swelling counts); presence and number of contractures of the elbows, wrists, and knees bilaterally, presence of palpable tendon friction rubs of the elbows, wrists, hands, knees, ankles, and other areas; serum creatinine level; and routine urinalysis.

Patients also performed self assessments of their functional capacity by completing the 20-item HAQ DI (3). In this instrument, the 20 items (each assessed on a 0–3 scale) were divided into 8 domains; the highest scores in each of the 8 domains were summed and divided by 8 to derive the HAQ DI score (range 0–3).

Assessment of organ system involvement. Involvement of the lung, kidney, muscle, joint, and heart were defined as previously described (3,14,16).

Change scores. Since complete data were only available for patients who finished the 2-year trial, calculation of change scores was possible only for those 68 patients. Change scores for these variables were derived by calculating the difference between the baseline and the 2-year values. Linear regression was employed in the analysis of normally distributed continuous or ordinal values. Logistic regression was used in the analysis of binary outcome variables. For calculating logistic regression, change scores were dichotomized as "improved" or "not improved" ("no change" was always considered "not improved") based on whether the change was above or below zero (no change).

Outcomes. Five outcomes of interest were studied. One outcome, change in HAQ DI score, was continuous. The other 4 outcomes (mortality, SRC, improvement in HAQ DI score, and global improvement) were dichotomous. The occurrence of mortality and SRC were assessed for a mean ± SD of 4.0 ± 1.1 years after entry. Improved HAQ DI was defined as a decrease in the HAQ DI score of ≥0.2 units at 24 months compared with the value at entry. At 2 years, the physician examiners made a global assessment of each SSc patient's disease course as improved, worsened, or unchanged compared with disease status at entry (using a 7-point Likert scale), as previously described (16). Because this ordinal outcome was not normally distributed (the data were heavily skewed toward improvement), the global assessment of a patient's disease course over 2 years was dichotomized as "improved" if the investigator assessed the patient's course as any grade of improved, and "not improved" if the patient's course was assessed as unchanged or as any grade of worsened.

Because 1 patient was lost to followup, data needed for the prediction of mortality and SRC were available for only 133 patients. Because change score data were available for only the 68 patients who completed (received medication for the duration of) the 2-year study, the correlations of change in HAQ DI, improved HAQ DI, and global assessment with explanatory variables were possible only for this subset of 68 patients.

Statistical analysis. All of the statistical analyses were performed using Stata (Stata Corporation, College Station, TX) and SAS (SAS Institute, Cary, NC) software. All continuous data are reported as the mean ± SD, unless otherwise specified. Group means were compared using Student's *t*-test (2-tailed, unpaired). Clinical subsets were developed based on dichotomous variables (occurring naturally or when continuous variables were made dichotomous by division above or below a cut point, usually the median). Since the data were frequently not normally distributed, Spearman (rather than Pearson) correlation coefficients were calculated. Spearman correlation coefficients were calculated with mortality, SRC, improved HAQ DI, and global improvement as binary outcome variables, and with change in HAQ DI as a continuous outcome variable. Other variables served as independent or explanatory variables (continuous where available, dichotomous otherwise).

Crude odds ratios (ORs) and 95% confidence intervals (95% CIs) were estimated using univariate logistic regression, with the outcome variable and the explanatory variables as dichotomous variables. Only variables with P values of <0.05 by chi-square testing during univariate analysis were selected for further multivariate logistic regression. Separate logistic models were built for each outcome variable (i.e., mortality, SRC, improved HAQ DI, and global improvement). Independent variables of interest were entered as dichotomous explanatory variables into each backward stepwise multivariate logistic model. Adjusted ORs and 95% CIs were used to model associations of multiple potential predictors with each outcome. R^2 was the measure of how well the regression explained the outcome (17). The effect of explanatory variables on mortality and SRC was also analyzed by life-table (Kaplan-Meier method) and Cox proportional hazards methods.

For change in HAQ DI, linear regression was used. The effect of explanatory variables on change in HAQ DI was analyzed by univariate and backward stepwise multivariate linear regression (using variables which had P values of ≤ 0.05 on univariate regression). R^2 was the measure of the proportion of variance in each outcome that was explained by the regression model.

RESULTS

Patient characteristics at baseline (n = 133 patients). The details of the randomized controlled trial of high-dose (1,000 mg/day) versus low-dose (125 mg/every other day) penicillamine for the diffuse scleroderma variant of SSc have been published elsewhere (14). In summary, the courses of the 3 major outcomes in the drug trial were similar in the 2 dosage groups. Skin thickness scores improved to similar degrees in both groups over the 2 years of the study, while the number of patients who died or experienced renal crisis were similar in the 2 groups followed up for a mean ± SD of 4.0 ± 1.1 years. Since 1 patient was lost to followup, the data for the remaining 133 patients were pooled for this analysis. During the followup period of 4.0 ± 1.1 years, 18 patients developed renal crisis and 20 patients died.

The demographic and baseline disease-related characteristics of the original 134 patients studied (104 women and 30 men) have been described in detail

Table 1. Baseline variables that correlated with or predicted mortality (n = 133 patients)*

Variable	Correlations: Coefficient†	Correlations: P	Univariate logistic regression: OR	95% CI	P	Group at risk	Kaplan-Meier: Log rank P	Wilcoxon P
Heart involvement	0.256	0.003	4.23	1.532–11.668	0.005	Heart involved	0.001	0.001
Lung involvement	0.220	0.012	4.07	1.280–12.954	0.017	Lung involved	0.008	0.001
Total skin score	0.214	0.014	3.59	1.227–10.548	0.020	Total skin score ≥20	0.018	0.034
Joint contractures	0.148	0.0907	3.59	1.130–11.425	0.030	Contractures	0.016	0.011
FVC, % of predicted	−0.233	0.008	3.46	1.178–10.173	0.024	FVC <85% of predicted	0.020	0.002
Hematocrit, %	−0.262	0.002	3.34	1.136–9.814	0.028	Men with hematocrit of <41.6% Women with hematocrit of <38.6%	0.018	0.002
ESR, mm/hour	0.267	0.003	3.33	1.121–9.870	0.030	ESR ≥20 mm/hour	0.018	0.002
HAQ DI score	0.266	0.002	3.22	1.097–9.468	0.033	HAQ DI score ≥1.0	0.034	0.011
Oral aperture, mm	−0.251	0.004	3.18	1.071–9.421	0.037	Oral aperture ≤45 mm	0.028	0.012
DLco, % of predicted	−0.233	0.008	3.00	1.075–8.375	0.036	DLco <76% of predicted	0.045	0.039
Platelets/mm^3	0.119	0.176	1.09	0.412–2.891	0.176	≥330,000 platelets/mm^3	0.019	0.013

* OR = odds ratio; 95% CI = 95% confidence interval; FVC = forced vital capacity; ESR = erythrocyte sedimention rate; HAQ DI = Disability Index of the Health Assessment Questionnaire; DLco = diffusing capacity for carbon monoxide.
† For positive correlations, higher (more abnormal) values at baseline predict greater risk of mortality. For negative correlations, lower (more abnormal) values at baseline predict greater risk of mortality.

elsewhere (3,14). Briefly, their age was 43.7 ± 12.4 years (mean ± SD), their modified Rodnan skin thickness score was 21.0 ± 8.0, their duration of SSc prior to entry was 10 ± 4 months, and their HAQ DI score was 1.04 ± 0.67. Tendon friction rubs were noted in 37% of patients, large joint contractures in 56%, joint involvement in 38%, muscle involvement in 16%, renal involvement in 25% (no patient had experienced SRC prior to entry), heart involvement in 20%, and lung involvement in 54%. Thirty percent of patients were taking prednisone at a dosage of 7.5 ± 2.5 mg/day.

Baseline predictors of outcome (n = 133 patients). *Mortality.* During 4.0 ± 1.1 years of followup, 20 patients died (15%) of the 133 for whom the outcome was known.

Table 2. Frequency of dichotomous variables at baseline, proportion and frequency of patients who improved, and proportion and frequency of patients who developed new-onset involvement over 2 years*

Variable	Baseline, no. (%) of patients: HAQ DI improved (n = 33)	HAQ DI not improved (n = 35)	P‡	Patients abnormal at baseline who improved, proportion (%): HAQ DI improved	HAQ DI not improved	P‡	Patients at risk who had new onset of involvement, proportion (%)†: HAQ DI improved	HAQ DI not improved	P‡
Female	23 (70)	28 (80)	0.340	–	–	–	–	–	–
Prednisone use	8 (24)	7 (20)	0.673	–	–	–	–	–	–
Digital tip ulcer	4 (12)	7 (20)	0.378	3/4 (75)	2/5 (40)	0.242	1/29 (3)	6/28 (21)	0.436
Non–digital tip ulcer	7 (21)	7 (20)	0.902	6/7 (86)	2/6 (33)	0.103	0/26 (0)	6/28 (21)	0.013§
Proximal muscle weakness	2 (6)	1 (3)	0.520	2/2 (100)	1/1 (100)	1.000	1/31 (3)	3/34 (9)	0.314
Tendon rub	12 (36)	9 (26)	0.342	5/6 (83)	4/6 (67)	1.000	3/21 (14)	3/26 (12)	0.839
Contractures	19 (58)	13 (37)	0.092	9/19 (47)	5/13 (38)	0.725	7/14 (50)	7/22 (32)	0.280
Joint involvement	14 (42)	14 (40)	0.839	8/13 (62)	7/14 (50)	0.704	2/19 (11)	5/21 (24)	0.283
Muscle involvement	3 (9)	3 (9)	0.938	1/1 (100)	2/3 (67)	1.000	1/30 (3)	5/32 (16)	0.084
Renal involvement	7 (21)	10 (29)	0.484	4/7 (57)	7/10 (70)	0.644	3/26 (12)	6/25 (24)	0.264
Heart involvement	8 (24)	2 (6)	0.031§	6/8 (75)	1/2 (50)	1.000	2/25 (8)	6/33 (18)	0.273
Lung involvement	17 (52)	18 (51)	0.994	7/17 (41)	10/18 (56)	0.505	1/16 (6)	6/17 (35)	0.041§
Swollen joints	11 (33)	8 (23)	0.336	10/11 (91)	6/8 (75)	0.546	0/22 (0)	4/27 (15)	0.058

* HAQ DI = Disability Index of the Health Assessment Questionnaire.
† Proportions are the number of patients with new onset of involvement/number of patients at risk (i.e., without that involvement at baseline).
‡ By Fisher's exact test.
§ $P < 0.05$, by chi-square test.

Table 3. Baseline and change score variables (continuous) in the 68 systemic sclerosis patients who completed the 2-year study, classified according to improvement in HAQ DI score*

	Baseline			Change scores at 2 years		
Variable	HAQ DI improved (n = 33)†	HAQ DI not improved (n = 35)‡	*P*	HAQ DI improved (n = 33)†	HAQ DI not improved (n = 35)‡	*P*
Demographic						
Age, years	43.3 ± 14.4	45.1 ± 11.9	0.581	–	–	–
History						
Duration of Raynaud's phenomenon at entry, days	712 ± 1,481	957 ± 1,841	0.550	–	–	–
Physical examination						
Total skin score, 0–51	21.5 ± 7.7	18.8 ± 9.1	0.199	−9.2 ± 7.4	−2.7 ± 10.0	0.004§
HAQ DI score, 0–3	1.13 ± 0.60	0.85 ± 0.54	0.050§	−0.61 ± 0.35	0.28 ± 0.39	0.000§
Maximum oral aperture, mm	46.1 ± 11.3	50.2 ± 9.6	0.116	4.7 ± 7.2	−0.7 ± 8.6	0.008§
Right hand spread, mm	177.3 ± 24.5	183.7 ± 33.8	0.384	−3.3 ± 15.7	−7.1 ± 19.2	0.384
Right fist closure, mm	29.3 ± 18.4	20.2 ± 22.7	0.000§	−12.3 ± 16.2	3.8 ± 18.1	0.000§
Tender joint count, 0–8	1.6 ± 2.2	1.6 ± 2.3	1.000	−0.9 ± 1.9	0.0 ± 2.7	0.032§
Swollen joint count, 0–8	1.0 ± 1.6	0.5 ± 1.0	0.130	−0.9 ± 1.5	0.0 ± 1.8	0.032§
Laboratory						
Hematocrit, %	39.2 ± 3.1	40.4 ± 3.3	0.133	0.6 ± 2.8	−0.5 ± 2.9	0.123
White blood cells, $\times 1{,}000/mm^3$	8.3 ± 2.1	8.4 ± 2.5	0.861	−1.5 ± 1.8	−0.6 ± 2.2	0.075
Platelets, $\times 1{,}000/mm^3$	344 ± 98	326 ± 95	0.291	−63 ± 69	−56 ± 88	0.721
ESR, mm/hour	26.3 ± 15.8	17.3 ± 11.1	0.009§	−5.0 ± 14.1	−1.8 ± 10.1	0.291
Creatine kinase, % of upper limit of normal	86.1 ± 203.8	80.6 ± 94.3	0.008§	−0.7 ± 34.7	−19.3 ± 78.7	0.224
DLco, % of predicted	73.3 ± 16.1	78.2 ± 19.0	0.264	3.1 ± 20.9	−6.3 ± 16.7	0.047§
FVC, % of predicted	83.2 ± 21.4	85.7 ± 16.0	0.591	10.2 ± 13.5	−0.2 ± 11.2	0.001§
Creatinine clearance, ml/minute	95.4 ± 33.2	88.5 ± 30.5	0.382	−7.4 ± 30.9	−5.8 ± 37.6	0.851
Serum creatinine, mg/dl	0.9 ± 0.2	0.9 ± 0.2	1.000	0.0 ± 0.2	−0.1 ± 0.2	0.047§

* Except where indicated otherwise, values are the mean ± SD. See Table 1 for definitions.
† Patients whose HAQ DI score improved by ≥0.2 units from the baseline value.
‡ Patients whose HAQ DI score did not improve by ≥0.2 units from the baseline value.
§ $P \leq 0.05$, by 2-tailed unpaired *t*-test.

Using Spearman correlations, univariate logistic regression, and life-table methods, 11 potential predictors of mortality were found at baseline (Table 1), including HAQ DI score (univariate OR 3.22, 95% CI 1.097–9.468). Since FVC and DLco were included in the composite lung involvement parameter, and since lung involvement had a stronger relationship with mortality than FVC or DLco alone, only the composite lung involvement parameter was explored further in multivariate logistic regression. Backward stepwise multivariate logistic regression suggested that of the remaining 9 potential predictors, lung involvement (multivariate OR 6.09, 95% CI 1.613–23.073) and total skin score of ≥20 (multivariate OR 3.69, 95% CI 1.169–11.670) together contributed the most to predicting mortality ($R^2 = 0.139$). The addition of other variables did not appreciably increase the R^2. Although the HAQ DI score was a significant predictor of mortality in univariate regression, it did not contribute significantly in multivariate regression.

SRC and other visceral involvements. At baseline, no patient had ever had an episode of SRC. The HAQ DI score did not correlate with the presence of heart, lung, or renal involvement at baseline. During 4.0 ± 1.1 years of followup, 18 of the 133 patients at risk (14%) developed SRC. The baseline HAQ DI score predicted neither SRC over 4 years nor new-onset heart or lung involvement over 2 years.

Patient characteristics over 2 years (n = 68 patients). Sixty-six patients withdrew before completing the full 2 years of the study. Two-year data were complete, therefore, only for the 68 patients who completed the 2-year study (completers). Improvement in completers was noted in a number of clinical and laboratory variables. The modified Rodnan skin thickness score decreased by 5.9 ± 9.4 units, the HAQ DI score by 0.17 ± 0.59 units, the tender joint count by 0.4 ± 2.4 units, and fist closure by 3.8 ± 18.9 mm, while FVC (percent of predicted) increased by 4.8 ± 13.4 percentage points and hand spread by 5.3 ± 17.6 mm. Over 2 years of followup, new onset of heart involvement occurred in 8 of 58 patients at risk (14%), while new onset of lung involvement occurred in 7 of 33 patients at risk (21%) (Table 2).

The HAQ DI score decreased (improved) by ≥0.2 units compared with the baseline value in 33 patients, and these patients were considered to be "HAQ DI improved" (Tables 2 and 3). The other 35 patients did not show such an improvement and were considered to be "HAQ DI not improved." In HAQ DI–

Table 4. Baseline and 2-year change variables that correlated with change in HAQ DI over the same 2-year period*

	Correlation		Linear regression		
	Coefficient†	*P*	R^2	*P*	Association with improved HAQ DI‡
Change variable					
Total skin score	0.492	0.000	0.246	0.000	Decreased skin score
Right fist closure	0.524	0.000	0.240	0.000	Tighter fist
Oral aperture	−0.452	0.000	0.194	0.000	Greater oral aperture
WBC count	0.445	0.000	0.186	0.000	Decreased WBC count
Joint swelling	0.334	0.006	0.137	0.001	Fewer swollen joints
FVC	−0.384	0.002	0.113	0.007	Increased FVC
Right hand spread	−0.217	0.082	0.108	0.008	Increased hand spread
Tender joints	0.276	0.024	0.101	0.009	Fewer tender joints
Contractures	0.255	0.039	0.072	0.029	Fewer contractures
Tendon rubs	0.205	0.097	0.068	0.033	Fewer tendon rubs
Skin ulcers	0.242	0.050	0.064	0.041	Fewer skin ulcers
Baseline variable					
ESR	−0.299	0.016	0.148	0.002	Higher ESR
HAQ DI score	−0.252	0.040	0.126	0.003	Higher HAQ DI score
Swollen joints	−0.237	0.053	0.109	0.006	More swollen joints
Total skin score	−0.309	0.011	0.068	0.034	Higher total skin score
Right hand spread	0.254	0.039	0.065	0.039	Decreased hand spread
Hematocrit	0.224	0.069	0.061	0.043	Lower hematocrit level

* WBC count = white blood cell count (see Table 1 for other definitions).
† For positive correlations, higher values show stronger relationship with change in HAQ DI. For negative correlations, lower values show stronger relationship with change in HAQ DI.
‡ For change variables, the direction of the change is shown. For baseline variables, the baseline level is shown.

improved patients, baseline values for the HAQ DI, fist closure, erythrocyte sedimentation rate (ESR), and CK were higher (more abnormal), and heart involvement more frequent, than in the HAQ DI–not improved group (P = 0.000 to P = 0.050) (Tables 2 and 3). Otherwise, baseline characteristics were similar in the 2 groups.

At 2 years, HAQ DI–improved patients showed significantly more improvement than HAQ DI–not improved patients in total skin score, HAQ DI score, oral aperture, tender and swollen joint counts, fist closure, DLco (percent of predicted), FVC (percent of predicted), and serum creatinine level (P = 0.000 to P = 0.047) (Table 3). Also, HAQ DI–not improved patients were more likely to have developed new onset of non–digital tip cutaneous ulcers and new-onset lung involvement at 2 years than were HAQ DI–improved patients (P = 0.013 and P = 0.041, respectively) (Table 2). Therefore, these data support the conclusion that improvement in the HAQ DI score was associated with improvement in multiple other important aspects of disease involvement, including skin thickness, hand function, and oral aperture, as well as lung, kidney, and joint involvement.

Correlates of outcome over 2 years (n = 68 patients). *HAQ DI.* The baseline and change variables which were related to changes in HAQ DI scores (by Spearman correlation coefficient and univariate regression R^2) are shown in Table 4. When these relationships were analyzed by backward stepwise multiple linear regression, 1 baseline variable and 3 change variables together explained 53% of the variance of the change in HAQ DI (R^2 = 0.528). These were ESR at baseline (P = 0.005) and changes in the swollen joint count (P = 0.002), total skin score (P = 0.005), and white blood cell count (P = 0.005). The addition of other variables did not increase the R^2 appreciably.

Improvement in HAQ DI. No baseline variable predicted improved the HAQ DI at 24 months in the 68 patients who completed the trial.

Global improvement. Of the 68 patients who completed the 2-year trial, 50 were judged to have "improved" the globally. Using Spearman correlations and univariate logistic regression, the absence of large joint contractures (multivariate OR 4.46, 95% CI 1.230–16.136) and the presence of higher hematocrit levels (defined as ≥41.6% in men and ≥38.6% in women) (multivariate OR 4.11, 95% CI 1.131–14.950) at baseline were the only variables that together best explained global improvement (R^2 = 0.157). Addition of other variables did not improve the prediction.

Conversely, 10 change variables correlated with global improvement (Table 5). Two of the change variables (change in total skin score and change in HAQ DI) had exceptionally strong associations with global improvement. When analyzed in multivariate logistic regression, improvement in the total skin score (multivariate OR 18.91, 95% CI 3.058–116.981) and improvement in the HAQ DI (multivariate OR 17.96, 95% CI 2.890–111.550) were the only 2 variables that indepen-

Table 5. Change over 2 years in variables that correlated with or were associated with physician's (MD) global assessment of "improved" over the same 2-year period*

Change in variable	Correlation		Univariate logistic regression			
	Coefficient†	*P*	OR	95% CI	*P*	Change associated with MD global assessment of "improved"
Total skin score	−0.685	0.000	24.62	5.475–110.711	0.000	Improved skin score
HAQ DI score	−0.581	0.000	22.15	4.469–109.463	0.000	Improved HAQ DI score
Right fist closure	−0.434	0.000	4.20	1.181–14.937	0.027	Tighter fist
Oral aperture	0.437	0.000	3.89	1.212–12.460	0.022	Increased aperture
WBC count	−0.403	0.001	6.16	1.617–23.463	0.008	Decreased WBC count
Contractures	−0.460	0.000	5.62	0.677–46.685	0.110	Fewer contractures
Right hand spread	0.359	0.003	3.22	0.817–12.677	0.095	Greater hand spread
Skin ulcers	−0.302	0.008	2.60	0.297–22.868	0.388	Fewer ulcers
FVC	0.264	0.035	1.90	0.611–5.887	0.268	Increased FVC
Tender joints	−0.264	0.030	0.92	0.249–3.381	0.896	Fewer tender joints

* WBC count = white blood cell count (see Table 1 for other definitions).
† For positive correlations, higher values predict an MD global assessment of "improved." For negative correlations, lower values predict an MD global assessment of "improved."

dently contributed to the model (R^2 = 0.445). Addition of other variables did not improve the prediction.

Correlates of HAQ DI score at baseline and at 2 years in completers (n = 68 patients). We were concerned that the relationship of the baseline HAQ DI score with variables in the 68 completers might be different from the relationship we found previously in the 134 patients of the initial cohort. Using stepwise logistic regression in these 68 patients, we found that the oral aperture and hand spread at baseline (Table 6) best explained the model (R^2 = 0.374). No other variables remained in the model.

We also examined the relationship of other explanatory variables to the HAQ DI score at 2 years in the completers (Table 6). We recalculated medians for continuous variables at 2 years in these 68 patients. We then converted continuous variables to binary variables (using cut points at or near the median) while maintaining naturally occurring dichotomous variables as binary variables. Stepwise multivariate logistic regression showed that a model including oral aperture, hand spread, tender joints, and fist closure together best explained the relationship (R^2 = 0.586).

Relationship between HAQ DI score and total skin score. The HAQ DI score and total skin score at baseline were highly correlated (correlation coefficient of 0.368, *P* = 0.000) (3), as were the courses of the HAQ DI score and total skin score over the 2-year study period (correlation coefficient 0.4918, *P* = 0.000). We explored this relationship further by comparing the courses of change in HAQ DI and its 8 components in patients whose skin score decreased by ≥25% over 2 years (skin improved) with those courses in patients whose skin score did not improve by ≥25% over the 2 years (skin not improved). While no baseline differences were found (Table 7), there were significantly greater improvements over 2 years in the arising, walking, hygiene, and reaching components of the HAQ DI in skin-improved patients compared with skin–not-improved patients (Table 7). Conversely, there were no differences between skin-improved and skin–not-improved patients in the courses of the dressing, eating, gripping, or activity components of the HAQ DI over 2 years.

DISCUSSION

Although the level of functional impairment in SSc has now been documented in several reports (3–9), few published studies have documented how function in SSc changes over time. Steen and Medsger recently reported their analysis of HAQ DIs that were completed annually by 1,250 SSc patients attending the University of Pittsburgh Scleroderma Clinic over a mean of 4.0 years (5). Their major findings were that HAQ DI scores in diffuse scleroderma correlated directly with skin

Table 6. Variables that had a significant (*P* < 0.05) relationship to HAQ DI at baseline and at 2 years by stepwise multivariate logistic regression in the 68 patients who completed the 2-year study*

Variables	OR	95% CI	*P*
At baseline			
Oral aperture	6.882	1.955–24.233	0.003
Hand spread	5.820	1.784–18.993	0.004
At 2 years			
Oral aperture	9.681	1.724–54.353	0.010
Hand spread	10.785	1.952–59.586	0.006
Tender joints	21.208	2.757–163.108	0.003
Fist closure	10.347	1.769–60.513	0.010

* See Table 1 for definitions.

Table 7. Baseline and change score values at 2 years for the 8 component scores of the HAQ DI (ordinal) in the 68 systemic sclerosis patients who completed the 2-year study, classified according to improvement in final skin score*

	Baseline values			Change score values at 2 years		
HAQ DI variable	Skin improved (n = 42)†	Skin not improved (n = 26)‡	*P*	Skin improved (n = 42)†	Skin not improved (n = 26)‡	*P*
Dressing	0.857 ± 0.718	0.923 ± 0.744	0.718	−0.146 ± 0.823	0.154 ± 1.008	0.187
Arising	0.881 ± 0.633	0.654 ± 0.689	0.169	−0.463 ± 0.552	0.038 ± 0.824	0.009§
Eating	1.048 ± 0.764	1.154 ± 1.047	0.631	−0.073 ± 0.848	−0.154 ± 0.849	0.726
Walking	0.667 ± 0.570	0.692 ± 0.549	0.856	−0.220 ± 0.652	0.192 ± 0.849	0.029§
Hygiene	1.190 ± 1.042	1.038 ± 1.076	0.566	−0.293 ± 0.716	0.423 ± 0.809	0.001§
Reaching	1.071 ± 0.808	1.115 ± 0.864	0.833	−0.463 ± 0.977	0.077 ± 1.093	0.039§
Gripping	0.881 ± 0.633	1.192 ± 0.895	0.129	−0.244 ± 0.734	−0.231 ± 0.951	0.950
Activity	1.119 ± 0.803	1.385 ± 0.852	0.200	−0.390 ± 0.703	−0.077 ± 1.017	0.176
Overall	0.964 ± 0.550	1.019 ± 0.649	0.710	−0.287 ± 0.486	−0.053 ± 0.664	0.019§

* Values are the mean ± SD. HAQ DI = Disability Index of the Health Assessment Questionnaire.
† Patients whose final skin score decreased by ≥25% of the baseline value.
‡ Patients whose final skin score did not decrease by ≥25% of the baseline value.

involvement, scleroderma heart and kidney disease, tendon friction rubs, finger contractures, and proximal muscle weakness at entry; over time, changes in HAQ DI scores correlated with changes in total skin scores and was a good predictor of survival.

Our recently published analysis of the relationship of baseline HAQ DI score to other physical and laboratory parameters at entry (3) and our present analysis of changes in HAQ DI over time confirm several of Steen and Medsger's findings relative to the relationship of HAQ DI to other variables. We found that the HAQ DI score was directly correlated with skin and joint involvement, scleroderma heart disease, tendon friction rubs, hand contractures, and proximal muscle weakness at entry. Also, changes in the HAQ DI were highly correlated with changes in skin score over 2 years (correlation coefficient 0.4918).

We also found that the HAQ DI score was predictive of survival. We realize, however, that this relationship between functional status and mortality is not unique to SSc; such a relationship has been noted previously in RA, in general medical patients, and in congestive heart failure (18–20). In the present study, when we further explored the relationship of the HAQ DI score and other variables to the prediction of survival using multivariate logistic regression, we found that a combination of lung involvement and total skin score of ≥20 at baseline was superior to the HAQ DI score (alone or in combination) as a predictor of survival.

More importantly, we explored the relationship of changes in HAQ DI scores to changes in other physical examination and laboratory variables over time in the cohort of 68 patients who completed the 2-year study. The question of what represents a meaningful change or difference in HAQ DI from the patient's point of view has been addressed and answered in 2 recent cross-sectional studies of RA patients (10,11). Both studies reported that a difference in HAQ DI score of ≥0.2 units was judged by patients to be symptomatically important (10,11). Although no similar study in SSc patients has been reported, we have assumed for this analysis that SSc patients would have rated themselves in a similar manner.

The HAQ DI score decreased by ≥0.2 units in 33 of the 68 completers, and they might therefore have rated themselves at least "somewhat better" (an important symptomatic difference) over the study period. Our analysis showed that patients whose HAQ DI score decreased by ≥0.2 units (HAQ DI–improved patients) also showed greater improvements in numerous other physical examination and laboratory parameters than did the HAQ DI–not improved patients (Tables 2 and 3). These improvements included skin involvement (total skin score), joint involvement (tender and swollen joint counts, tendon friction rubs), oral aperture, lung involvement (DLco, FVC), serum creatinine level, and hand function (fist closure).

We queried physician investigators about how each of their patients fared over the 2-year study period (physician's global assessment). In multivariate logistic regression, only 2 variables remained as independent contributors to the physician's global assessment: change in total skin score (multivariate OR 18.91) and change in HAQ DI score (multivariate OR 17.96), with R^2 = 0.445. This suggests that the physician's assessment of the patient's course is greatly influenced by improvements in skin thickening and in function.

In our recent analysis of HAQ DI scores at baseline (3), we hypothesized that the major factors that determine the HAQ DI score early in the disease course might not be those that influence the HAQ DI later in time. At 2 years, we found that hand function was still a very important influence on the HAQ DI score. We also found, however, that the improvements in HAQ DI recorded in skin-improved patients over 2 years were attributable primarily to the arising, walking, hygiene, and reaching components of the HAQ DI and not to the dressing, eating, gripping, or activity components. In reviewing the 20 questions that make up the HAQ DI, we noted that only 2 of the 9 questions that ask about arising, walking, hygiene, and reaching are directly related to hand function, while 8 of the 11 questions that ask about dressing, eating, gripping, or activity are directly related to hand function. This suggests that although the total HAQ DI score (at baseline and at 2 years) was heavily influenced by hand function, the improvement in function that occurred over 2 years was largely related to improvement in factors other than hand dysfunction (i.e., possible improvements in large joint flexibility, muscle strength, joint pain, and energy level).

In summary, our analyses further elucidate the performance characteristics and clinical usefulness of the HAQ DI in SSc patients with recent-onset diffuse scleroderma (3,5,14). Although our data cannot specifically address how severe heart, lung, or kidney involvement might have affected the HAQ DI score, the HAQ DI appears to have several attributes which are useful in the clinical management of SSc patients with early diffuse scleroderma. The HAQ DI can be used to document functional impairment at a given point in time (i.e., the initial visit) and how it changes over time. Baseline HAQ DI scores of $\geq$1.0 predict a greater risk of mortality. Improvement (decline) in the HAQ DI score suggests that a number of other SSc physical and laboratory involvements are probably improving as well. Finally, our data suggest that the assessment of patient function using the HAQ DI (a self-administered questionnaire that SSc patients can easily complete in less than 5 minutes), coupled with physician assessment of the total skin score (16), provides the practicing physician with important information about prognosis, patient status, and changes in disease course over time in SSc patients with early diffuse scleroderma.

REFERENCES

1. Medsger TA Jr. Systemic sclerosis (scleroderma): clinical aspects. In: Koopman WJ, editor. Arthritis and allied conditions: a textbook of rheumatology. Baltimore: Williams & Wilkins; 1997. p. 1433–64.
2. Seibold JR. Scleroderma. In: Kelley WN, Harris ED, Ruddy S, Sledge CB, editors. Textbook of rheumatology. Philadelphia: WB Saunders; 1997. p. 1133–62.
3. Clements PJ, Wong WK, Hurwitz EL, Furst DE, Mayes M, White B, et al. Correlates of the Disability Index of the Health Assessment Questionnaire: a measure of functional impairment in systemic sclerosis. Arthritis Rheum 1999;42:2372–80.
4. Poole JL, Steen VD. The use of the Health Assessment Questionnaire (HAQ) to determine physical disability in systemic sclerosis. Arthritis Care Res 1991;4:27–31.
5. Steen VD, Medsger TA Jr. The value of the Health Assessment Questionnaire and special patient-generated scales to demonstrate change in systemic sclerosis patients over time. Arthritis Rheum 1997;40:1984–91.
6. Moser DK, Clements PJ, Brecht M-L, Weiner SR. Predictors of psychosocial adjustment in systemic sclerosis: the influence of formal education level, functional ability, hardiness, uncertainty, and social support. Arthritis Rheum 1993;36:1398–405.
7. Roca RP, Wigley FM, White B. Depressive symptoms associated with scleroderma. Arthritis Rheum 1996;39:1035–40.
8. Merkel PA, Martin RW, Herlyn K. Health status measurements in patients with Raynaud's phenomenon and scleroderma [abstract]. Arthritis Rheum 1997;40:S255.
9. Callahan LF, Smith WJ, Pincus T. Self-report questionnaires in five rheumatic diseases: comparisons of health status constructs and associations with formal education level. Arthritis Care Res 1989;2:122–31.
10. Redelmeier DA, Lorig K. Assessing the clinical importance of symptomatic improvement: an illustration in rheumatology. Arch Intern Med 1993;153:1337–42.
11. Wells GA, Tugwell P, Kraag GR, Baker PR, Groh J, Redelmeier DA. Minimum important difference between patients with rheumatoid arthritis: the patient's perspective. J Rheumatol 1993;20:557–60.
12. Medsger TA Jr, Steen VD. Classification, prognosis. In: Clements PJ, Furst DE, editors. Systemic sclerosis. Baltimore: Williams and Wilkins; 1996. p. 51–64.
13. Subcommittee for Scleroderma Criteria of the American Rheumatism Association Diagnostic and Therapeutic Criteria Committee. Preliminary criteria for the classification of systemic sclerosis (scleroderma). Arthritis Rheum 1980;23:581–90.
14. Clements PJ, Furst DE, Wong W-K, Mayes M, White B, Wigley F, et al. High-dose versus low-dose D-penicillamine in early diffuse systemic sclerosis: analysis of a two-year, double-blind, randomized, controlled clinical trial. Arthritis Rheum 1999;42:1194–203.
15. Clements P, Lachenbruch P, Seibold JR, White B, Weiner S, Martin RW, et al. Inter and intraobserver variability of total skin thickness score (modified Rodnan TSS) in systemic sclerosis. J Rheumatol 1995;22:1281–5.
16. Clements PJ, Hurwitz EL, Wong WK, Seibold JR, Mayes M, White B, et al. Skin thickness score is a predictor and correlate of outcome in systemic sclerosis: high-dose versus low-dose penicillamine trial. Arthritis Rheum 2000;43:2445–54.
17. Nagelkerke NJD. A note on a generalized definition of the coefficient of determination. Biometrika 1991;78:691–2.
18. Pincus T, Brooks RH, Callahan LF. Prediction of long-term mortality in patients with rheumatoid arthritis according to simple questionnaire and joint count measures. Ann Intern Med 1994;120:26–34.
19. Inouye SK, Peduzzi PN, Robison JT, Hughes JS, Horwitz RI. Concato J. Importance of functional measures in predicting mortality among older hospitalized patients. JAMA 1998;279:1187–93.
20. Edwards BS, Rodeheffer RJ. Prognostic features in patients with congestive heart failure and selection criteria for cardiac transplantation. Mayo Clin Proc 1992;67:485–92.

ARTHRITIS & RHEUMATISM
Vol. 44, No. 3, March 2001, pp 662–665

Cytochrome P2 Polymorphisms and Susceptibility to Scleroderma Following Exposure to Organic Solvents

A. Povey,[1] M. J. Guppy,[1] M. Wood,[1] C. Knight,[2] C. M. Black,[2] and A. J. Silman[1]

Objective. **To determine whether there are specific cytochrome P450 (CYP2) alleles that increase susceptibility to scleroderma in individuals who have been exposed to organic solvents.**

Methods. **CYP alleles at 2 loci, 2E1 and 2C19, were compared in 7 patients who had developed scleroderma after exposure to solvents versus 71 patients with scleroderma without solvent exposure ("sporadic" disease) and 106 population controls.**

Results. **The 2E1*3 allele was found in 2 of the 7 patients who had been exposed to organic solvents, with a greater frequency than occurred in either the disease controls or the population controls (odds ratio [95% confidence interval] 9.1 [1.5–59.1] and 10.2 [1.8–62.2], respectively). All 7 patients with solvent exposure carried the 2C19EM genotype, compared with 89% of patients with sporadic scleroderma.**

Conclusion. **Our results suggest that alleles at CYP loci may be involved in increasing susceptibility to scleroderma among subjects who have been exposed to organic solvents.**

Scleroderma is found predominantly in females (1,2), and cases occurring in males of working age are relatively infrequent in most populations (3). Despite this, a number of occupational exposures have been linked to the development of the disease, most particularly, exposure to a wide variety of organic solvents, including trichlorethylene and trichloroethane. Many of these observations come from case reports (4–7), but more recent case–control studies have confirmed that there is an increased likelihood of exposure to solvents in scleroderma cases compared with controls (8,9).

However, exposure to organic solvents is fairly frequent in many occupational groups, and, given the rarity of scleroderma, it is likely that there are genetic susceptibility factors that might occur relatively infrequently in normal populations, which increase the likelihood of disease development in the setting of solvent exposure. A model for this comes from studies of individuals with vinyl chloride disease, a disorder related to scleroderma. Individuals with HLA–DR7 were found to be more likely to develop this disease than individuals without that allele (10). Polymorphisms within the cytochrome P450(CYP) genes are another target for genetic investigation. These genes are important in encoding for enzymes that metabolize a number of external agents, including organic solvents and drugs. Specific genes of interest include CYP2E1, which is important in metabolizing organic solvents (11), and CYP2C19, which is the major S-mephenytoin 4-hydroxylase (12). Furthermore, individuals who are poor hydroxylators of this drug are at an increased risk of developing scleroderma (13). We therefore examined the hypothesis that there are certain genetic susceptibility factors encoded within the CYP system that increase the likelihood of development of scleroderma after exposure to organic solvents.

PATIENTS AND METHODS

Subjects and study design. This was a case–control study with 2 referent groups. Cases were individuals with scleroderma who had developed the disease while working in a job in which they were exposed daily to organic solvents. The 2 control groups were a group of patients with "sporadic" scleroderma (no history of solvent exposure) and a group of population controls. Exposure to organic solvents in the cases was by self-report. Seven such cases (mean age 49) were ascertained, all of whom were male; 6 had diffuse disease and 1 had limited disease. The controls with sporadic scleroderma had all completed an occupational history questionnaire. This questionnaire, used in a previous investigation (9), asked

Supported by the UK Arthritis Research Campaign and the Cancer Research Campaign.

[1]A. Povey, PhD, M. J. Guppy, PhD, M. Wood, MSc, A. J. Silman, MD: University of Manchester, Manchester, UK; [2]C. Knight, MSc, C. M. Black, MD: Royal Free Hospital, London, UK.

Address correspondence and reprint requests to A. J. Silman, MD, ARC Epidemiology Unit, Stopford Building, University of Manchester, Oxford Road, Manchester M13 9PT, UK.

Submitted for publication February 23, 2000; accepted in revised form October 23, 2000.

Table 1. Association between CYP2 alleles and solvent-induced scleroderma: comparison with findings in patients with sporadic disease*

	Solvent-induced scleroderma (n = 7)	Sporadic scleroderma (n = 71)	Odds ratio (95% confidence interval)	*P*†
CYP2E				
2E1*3				
Present	2 (28.6)	3 (4.2)	9.1 (1.5–59.1)	
Absent	5 (71.4)	68 (95.8)		
2E1*4				
Present	2 (28.6)	8 (11.3)	3.2 (0.3–17.0)	
Absent	5 (71.4)	63 (88.7)		
CYP2C19 genotype				
EM	7 (100)	63 (88.7)		0.45
PM	0 (0)	8 (11.3)		

* Values are the number (%).
† By Fisher's exact test.

subjects to list all occupations prior to symptom onset and to indicate whether the job involved exposure to any organic solvents on a daily basis. A total of 71 patients who had no evidence of exposure to solvents in occupational settings were identified: 42 had diffuse disease, 20 had limited disease, and 9 had a mixed pattern of cutaneous involvement. The population control group consisted of 106 healthy individuals recruited from population samples from various other studies.

Genotyping. DNA was extracted from whole blood, and polymorphisms in the transcription regulation region (2E1*3) and intron 6 (2E1*4) of the CYP2E1 gene, and in exon 5 of the 2C19 gene (2C19*2), were identified after polymerase chain reaction amplification by digestion with *Pst 1/Rsa* 1, *Dra* 1, and *Sma* 1, respectively (14–16). Successful genotyping was carried out for all samples except for the 2E1*4 allele and the 2C19 gene in 1 population control.

Analysis. The percentage of individuals in each group carrying (a) the 2E1*3 allele and (b) the 2E1*4 allele was compared with the percentage not carrying those alleles, by calculating the odds ratios and 95% confidence intervals. The frequency of individuals in each group with the EM genotype was compared with the frequency carrying the PM genotype at the 2C19 locus, using Fisher's exact test.

RESULTS

Comparisons between the solvent-exposed cases and the sporadic disease controls are shown in Table 1. Despite the small number of solvent-exposed cases, there was a statistically significant association between the presence of the 2E1*3 allele and solvent exposure. There was also a trend, though nonsignificant, of increased carriage of the 2E1*4 allele. Comparisons between the solvent-exposed cases and the population controls are shown in Table 2. The results were very similar to those found in the comparison with the disease control group, with a significantly increased association

Table 2. Association between CYP2 alleles and solvent-induced scleroderma: comparison with findings in population controls*

	Solvent-induced scleroderma (n = 7)	Population controls (n = 106)	Odds ratio (95% confidence interval)	*P*†
CYP2E				
2E1*3				
Present	2 (28.6)	4 (3.8)	10.2 (1.8–62.2)	
Absent	5 (71.4)	102 (96.2)		
2E1*4‡				
Present	2 (28.6)	17 (16.2)	2.1 (0.2–10.2)	
Absent	5 (71.4)	88 (83.8)		
CYP2C19 genotype‡				
EM	7 (100)	99 (94.3)		0.67
PM	0 (0)	6 (5.7)		

* Values are the number (%).
† By Fisher's exact test.
‡ Data not available for 1 population control.

with the 2E1*3 allele and a nonsignificant increase in the frequency of the 2E1*4 allele. Interestingly, all 7 solvent-exposed cases carried the EM genotype at the 2C19 locus, whereas 8 patients with sporadic disease and 6 population controls were negative for that genotype. These differences were not significant ($P = 0.45$ versus patients with sporadic disease; $P = 0.67$ versus controls, by Fisher's exact test).

DISCUSSION

In this study investigating the possibility that genetically determined impaired metabolism of organic solvents might be linked to the development of scleroderma, we found an association with the 2E1*3 allele, but not with the 2E1*4 allele or the 2C19 genotype. Increased risk of developing solvent-induced chronic toxic encephalopathy has been associated with the glutathione S transferase M1-null genotype (17). To our knowledge, however, there have been few studies linking polymorphisms within the CYP2E1 gene to disease susceptibility resulting from exposure to organic solvents, although liver expression of CYP2E1 is associated with metabolism of solvents (e.g., benzene [18]). Associations between CYP2E1 polymorphisms and alcohol-induced diseases and cancer have been studied (19–22). The *Dra* 1 site, located in intron 6 (2E1*4 allele), has no known functional significance but may be associated with alcoholic liver disease in some, but not all, populations (20,23). The *Pst* 1/*Rsa* 1 restriction sites, located in the transcription regulation region (2E1*3 allele) of CYP2E1, are, however, associated with increased gene expression (14), and there is an association between the 2E1*3 allele and alcoholic liver disease (24). The genetic polymorphism identified by *Sma* 1 in exon 5 of the 2C19 gene (2C19*2) has been shown to be a genetic defect leading to the poor-metabolizer phenotype that is associated with increased scleroderma risk (12,13).

The most important limitation of our findings is clearly the very small number of solvent-exposed cases studied. It is always hazardous, when studying patients with a disease who have been exposed to solvents, to conclude that there is a cause-and-effect relationship between the solvent exposure and the disease. We chose to restrict consideration of cases to those who had obvious occupational exposure and had developed the disease while still working in the given occupation. Given the nature of the exposure (i.e., occupations in which few women work), all of our subjects were male. It is obviously important to replicate these findings in a larger group of subjects. Our control subjects had no exposure to solvents either as far as they could recall or as would be expected based on job title. We did not attempt to validate the self-reported exposures by reference back to occupational records. This would have enhanced the quality of the exposure data but was ruled out for medicolegal reasons. Any misclassification of solvent exposure by the cases or controls, however, would have made it more difficult to have observed a difference. The nature of employment by most of these individuals was such that exposure to many different solvents had occurred, and, particularly given the small numbers, we did not attempt within this analysis to separate out whether there are differences in susceptibility in relation to specific solvents.

It does seem likely that genetic factors are involved in increasing the susceptibility to scleroderma in the context of exposure to putative environmental agents, such as solvents. This is based mainly on the observation that in most patients who have developed scleroderma after solvent exposure this exposure was not substantially different, either in amount or in nature, from exposure in individuals who did not develop scleroderma (4–9). Interestingly, the influences of HLA alleles on scleroderma susceptibility are generally weak, although they might mediate disease expression in the related vinyl chloride disease (10). It is perhaps biologically more plausible that the genetic handling of solvents is more closely linked to the development of disease in the small subset of patients whose disease has an environmental component.

In conclusion, this small study demonstrates the possibility that there are specific genotypes, linked to impaired metabolism of organic solvents, that increase susceptibility to scleroderma. The results require replication in a larger group.

REFERENCES

1. Mayes M. Scleroderma epidemiology. Rheum Dis Clin North Am 1996;22:751–64.
2. Fresko I, Soy M, Hamuryudan V, Yurdakul S, Yavuz Ş, Tümer Z, et al. Genetic anticipation in Behcet's syndrome. Ann Rheum Dis 1998;57:45–8.
3. Steen VD, Oddis CV, Conte CG, Janoski J, Casterline GZ, Medsger TA Jr. Incidence of systemic sclerosis in Allegheny County, Pennsylvania: a twenty-year study of hospital-diagnosed cases, 1963–1982. Arthritis Rheum 1997;40:441–5.
4. Walder BK. Do solvents cause scleroderma? Int J Dermatol 1983;22:157–8.
5. Czirjak L, Katalin D, Schlammadinger J, Surányi P, Tamási L, Szegedi GY. Progressive systemic sclerosis occurring in patients exposed to chemicals. Int J Dermatol 1987;26:374–8.
6. Lockey JE, Kelly CR, Cannon GW, Colby TV, Aldrich V, Livingston GK. Progressive systemic sclerosis associated with exposure to trichloroethylene. J Occup Med 1987;29:493–6.

7. Garcia-Zamalloa AM, Ojeda E, Gonzalez-Beneitez C, Goni J, Garrido A. Systemic sclerosis and organic solvents: early diagnosis in industry [letter]. Ann Rheum Dis 1994;54:618.
8. Bovenzi M, Barbone F, Betta A, Tommasini M, Versini W. Scleroderma and occupational exposure. Scand J Work Environ Health 1995;21:289–92.
9. Silman AJ, Jones S. What is the contribution of occupational environmental factors to the occurrence of scleroderma in men? Ann Rheum Dis 1992;51:1322–4.
10. Black C, Pereira S, McWhirter A, Welsh K, Laurent R. Genetic susceptibility to scleroderma-like syndrome in symptomatic and asymptomatic workers exposed to vinyl chloride. J Rheumatol 1986;13:1059–62.
11. Lieber CS. Cytochrome p-4502E1: its physiological and pathological role. Physiol Rev 1997;77:517–44.
12. Goldstein JA, Faletto MB, Romkes SM, Sullivan T, Kitareewan S, Raucy JL, et al. Evidence that CYP2C19 is the major (S)-mephenytoin 4′-hydroxylase in humans. Biochemistry 1994;33:1743–52.
13. May DG, Black CM, Olsen NJ, Csuka ME, Tanner SB, Bellino L, et al. Scleroderma is associated with differences in individual routes of drug metabolism: a study with dapsone, debrisoquin and mephenytoin. Clin Pharmacol Ther 1990;49:286–95.
14. Hayashi S-I, Watanabe J, Kawajiri K. Genetic polymorphisms in the 5′-flanking region change transcription regulation of the human cytochrome p450IIE1 gene. J Biochem 1991;110:559–65.
15. Kato S, Shields PG, Caporaso NE, Sugimura H, Trivers H, Tucker GE, et al. Analysis of cytochrome p4502E1 genetic polymorphisms in relation to human lung cancer. Cancer Epidemiol Biomarkers Prev 1994;3:515–8.
16. De Morais SMF, Wilkinson GR, Blaisdell J, Nakamura K, Meyer UA, Goldstein JA. The major genetic defect responsible for the polymorphism of S-mephenytoin metabolism in humans. J Biol Chem 1994;269:15419–22.
17. Soderkvist P, Ahmadi A, Akerback A, Axelson A, Flodin U. Glutathione S-transferase M1 null genotype as a risk modifier for solvent-induced chronic toxic encephalopathy. Scand J Work Environ Health 1996;22:360–3.
18. Nedelcheva V, Gut I, Soucek P, Tichavsha P, Tynkova B, Mraz L, et al. Metabolism of benzene in human liver microsomes: individual variations in relation to CYP2E1 expression. Arch Toxicol 1999;73:33–40.
19. D'Errico A, Malats N, Vineis P, Boffetta P. Review of studies on selected metabolic polymorphisms and cancer. In: Vineis P, Malats N, Land M, d'Errico A, Caporaso N, Cuzick N, et al, editors. Metabolic polymorphisms and susceptibility to cancer. Lyon: IARC Scientific Publications; 1999. p. 323–93.
20. Ingelman-Sundberg M, Johansson I, Yin H, Terelius Y, Eliasson E, Clot P, et al. Ethanol-inducible cytochrome P4502E1: genetic polymorphism, regulation and possible role in the etiology of alcohol induced liver disease. Alcohol 1993;10:447–52.
21. Itoga S, Nomura F, Harada F, Tsutsumi M, Takase S, Nakai T. Mutations in the exons and exon-intron junction regions of human cytochrome P-4502E1 gene and alcoholism. Alcohol Clin Exp Res 1999;23 Suppl 4:13S–16S.
22. Marsh JC, Chowdry J, Parry-Jones N, Ellis SW, Muir KR, Gordon-Smith EC, et al. Study of the association between cytochromes p450 2D6 and 2E1 genotypes and the risk of drug and chemical induced idiosyncratic aplastic anaemia. Br J Haematol 1999;104:266–70.
23. Savolainen VT, Pajarinen VT, Perola M, Penttila A, Karhunen PJ. Polymorphism in the cytochrome P450 2E1 gene and the risk of alcoholic liver disease. J Hepatol 1997;26:55–61.
24. Grove J, Brown AS, Daly AK, Bassendine MF, James OF, Day CP. The Rsa1 polymorphism of CYP2E1 and susceptibility to alcoholic liver disease in Caucasians: effect on age of presentation and dependence on alcohol dehydrogenase genotype. Pharmacogenetics 1998;8:335–42.

ARTHRITIS & RHEUMATISM
Vol. 44, No. 3, March 2001, pp 666–675

Long-Term Followup of Polyarteritis Nodosa, Microscopic Polyangiitis, and Churg-Strauss Syndrome

Analysis of Four Prospective Trials Including 278 Patients

Martine Gayraud,[1] Loïc Guillevin,[1] Philippe le Toumelin,[1] Pascal Cohen,[1] François Lhote,[2] Philippe Casassus,[1] Bernard Jarrousse,[1] and the French Vasculitis Study Group

Objective. **To determine the long-term outcome of patients with polyarteritis nodosa (PAN), microscopic polyangiitis (MPA), and Churg-Strauss syndrome (CSS), to compare the long-term outcome with the overall French population, to evaluate the impact on outcome of the type of vasculitis, prognostic factors, and treatments administered at diagnosis, and to analyze treatment side effects and sequelae.**

Methods. **Data from PAN, MPA, and CSS patients (n = 278) who were enrolled between 1980 and 1993 were collected in 1996 and 1997 and analyzed. Two prognostic scoring systems, the Five-Factors Score (FFS) and the Birmingham Vasculitis Activity Score (BVAS), were used to evaluate all patients at the time of diagnosis.**

Results. **The mean ($\pm$SD) followup of the entire population was 88.3 $\pm$ 51.9 months (range 3 days to 192 months). Of the 85 deaths recorded, at least 41 were due to progressive vasculitis or its consequences. Death rates reflected disease severity, as assessed by the FFS ($P = 0.004$) and the BVAS ($P < 0.0002$), and the 2 scores were correlated (r = 0.69). Relapses, rarer in hepatitis B virus (HBV)–related PAN (7.9%) than in MPA (34.5%) ($P = 0.004$), occurred in 56 patients (20.1%) and did not reflect disease severity. Survival curves were similar for the subpopulation of 215 patients with CSS, MPA, and non–HBV-related PAN who were given first-line corticosteroids (CS) with or without cyclophosphamide (CYC). However, CS with CYC therapy significantly prolonged survival for patients with FFS scores $\geq$2 ($P = 0.041$). Relapse rates were similar regardless of the treatment regimen; only patients treated with CS alone had uncontrolled disease. CYC was associated with a greater frequency of side effects ($P < 0.00001$).**

Conclusion. **Rates of mortality due to PAN (related or unrelated to HBV), MPA, and CSS reflected disease severity and were higher than the mortality rate in the general population ($P < 0.0004$). Rates of relapse, more common in MPA than HBV-related PAN patients, did not reflect disease severity. Survival rates were better among the more severely ill patients who had received first-line CYC. Based on these findings, we recommend that the intensity of the initial treatment be consistent with the severity of the disease. The use of the FFS and BVAS scores improved the ability to evaluate the therapeutic response.**

At the beginning of the 1950s, the prognosis of systemic vasculitis dramatically improved with the introduction of corticosteroids (CS), increasing the 5-year survival rate from 13% without treatment to 48–57% (1). Patients with renal disease had a poorer prognosis (1–5). For vasculitides refractory to CS, Fauci et al (6) demonstrated that cyclophosphamide (CYC) further improved the prognosis. However, for polyarteritis nodosa (PAN), when CYC or other cytotoxic agents were given in combination with CS at the time of diagnosis, an

Supported by grants from the Institut National de la Santé et de la Recherche Médicale (INSERM), the Caisse Nationale d'Assurance Maladie des Travailleurs Salariés (CNAMTS), and the Association pour la Recherche sur les Angéites Nécrosantes (ARAN).

[1]Martine Gayraud, MD (current address: Institut Mutualiste Montsouris, Paris, France), Loïc Guillevin, MD, Philippe le Toumelin, MD, Pascal Cohen, MD, Philippe Casassus, MD, Bernard Jarrousse, MD: Hôpital Avicenne, Bobigny, France; [2]François Lhote, MD: Hôpital Delafontaine, St. Denis, France.

Address correspondence and reprint requests to Loïc Guillevin, MD, Department of Internal Medicine, Hôpital Avicenne, 125 rue de Stalingrad, 93009 Bobigny Cedex, France.

Submitted for publication March 16, 2000; accepted in revised form October 23, 2000.

advantage in terms of survival had not been demonstrated, except in 1 retrospective study (7). In a prospective study on the treatment of PAN, microscopic polyangiitis (MPA), and Churg-Strauss syndrome (CSS) conducted by the French Vasculitis Study Group (8), no survival advantage was demonstrated when CYC was given in combination with CS as first-line therapy.

The objectives of the present study were as follows: 1) to determine the long-term outcome of patients and to compare it with the overall French population; 2) to evaluate the impact, in terms of morbidity and mortality, of the type of vasculitis, the prognostic factors, and the treatments administered at the time of diagnosis; and 3) to analyze the number and severity of treatment side effects and sequelae.

PATIENTS AND METHODS

Study population and study design. The 278 patients were enrolled from 1980 through 1993 in general or university hospitals participating in the French Vasculitis Study Group (see Acknowledgments for names of the investigators). Data concerning the patients were prospectively recorded in a computerized database. All patients, except 5, were randomized to 1 of 4 consecutive, prospective, multicenter therapeutic trials. Five patients had received treatment before a definitive diagnosis had been made; they were treated according to the protocol but were not randomized. These trials have been described in detail previously (8–12), and the protocols are briefly summarized below.

Protocol 1. For 68 patients who had PAN associated or not associated with hepatitis B virus (HBV) markers, MPA, or CSS (August 1980 through December 1983) (8), CS and plasma exchanges were prescribed for all patients, 31 of whom were subsequently randomized to receive CYC (2 mg/kg/day) for 1 year.

Protocol 2. For 71 patients who had PAN without HBV infection, MPA, or CSS (December 1983 through December 1988) (9), CS was prescribed for every patient and plasma exchanges were administered in a randomized manner (mean of 11 plasma exchanges for each of 32 patients).

Protocol 3. Patients who had PAN without HBV infection, MPA, or CSS (January 1989 through August 1993) were categorized into 2 subgroups: those with factors of poor prognosis (Five-Factors Score [FFS] ≥1; see explanation below) and those with factors of good prognosis. The 62 patients with poor prognostic factors were treated with CS and a monthly pulse of CYC for 1 year; after randomization, 34 received 9 plasma exchanges (3/week) (10). The 25 patients with good prognostic factors (FFS 0) were treated with CS and, after randomization, received oral CYC (n = 15) or monthly pulses of CYC (n = 10) for 1 year.

Protocol 4. For 47 patients with PAN with HBV markers (beginning in 1983) (11), treatment consisted of a combination of 2 weeks of CS followed by an antiviral agent, vidarabine (n = 39), until 1987, then interferon-alfa (n = 8) and plasma exchanges. In the case of relapse, treatment was adapted to the severity of the symptoms: CS, CYC, or other immunosuppressive agents.

Five patients were not randomized because they had been treated before a definitive diagnosis had been established. They all received CS, and 4 of them received oral CYC.

The CS regimen in protocols 1, 2, and 3 was the same. Prednisone was prescribed at a dosage of 1 mg/kg/day for 1 month, decreased by 2.5 mg every 10 days for 1 month, then decreased by 2.5 mg each week until a level equal to half the initial dose was reached. This dosage was maintained for 3 weeks, further decreased by 2.5 mg every week until patients were taking 20 mg/day, and then decreased by 1 mg every week.

Among the entire group of 278 patients, 122 received CYC as initial therapy: 50 orally and 72 via intravenous pulses. Ten patients (3 in protocol 1, 6 in protocol 2, 1 in protocol 4) received CYC therapy because of uncontrolled disease or relapse.

When our studies were initiated, the vasculitides were classified according to the Fauci classification system (13). Patients with vasculitis of the PAN group, which comprised PAN, CSS, and overlap vasculitis, were included. Diagnoses were based on histologic and/or angiographic features and, for 4 patients, on clinical criteria.

Patients have been reclassified according to the American College of Rheumatology criteria for CSS (14) and PAN (15). In addition, classic PAN and MPA were diagnosed according to the Chapel Hill Consensus Conference nomenclature (16) and our own recommendations for the diagnosis of MPA (17). Nevertheless, we cannot exclude the possibility that a few patients might have been misclassified between the PAN and MPA groups because of the limitations inherent in all classification systems (18).

Evaluation criteria. Two scores were applied to evaluate disease activity at the time of diagnosis. The 5 factors that comprise the FFS (19) are the following: classes of serum creatinine levels (≤1.58 mg/dl and >1.58 mg/dl) and proteinuria (≤1 gm/day and >1 gm/day), presence of severe gastrointestinal (GI) tract involvement, cardiomyopathy, and/or central nervous system involvement. The presence of each factor is accorded 1 point, and the score is defined as follows: 0 represents no factors present, 1 represents 1 factor present, 2 represents ≥2 factors present.

We also applied the Birmingham Vasculitis Activity Score (BVAS) (20) to test its ability to correlate with prognosis and to compare it with the FFS. The BVAS is a clinical index of disease activity based on symptoms and signs in 9 categories: systemic signs; skin; mucous membranes and eyes; ear, nose, and throat (ENT); chest; heart and vessels; GI tract; kidney; and nervous system. Maximum points were accorded to each category; the maximum score is 63. Disease features were scored only when they were attributable to active vasculitis. We used the BVAS in its first presentation form; modified forms of the BVAS have been published subsequently and can be used at successive steps of the disease (21). Our patients were evaluated according to 4 arbitrarily defined BVAS categories: scores of ≤10, 10 to ≤20, 20 to ≤30, and >30.

Uncontrolled vasculitis was defined as the occurrence of new manifestations or aggravation of manifestations already present despite treatment for the disease. Relapses were defined as recurrence of signs or new symptoms after an initial

Table 1. Demographics and vasculitis scores of the 278 patients with CSS, MPA, and PAN

Parameter	CSS (n = 64)	MPA (n = 58)	Non–HBV-related PAN (n = 93)	HBV-related PAN (n = 63)
Sex, no. females/no. males	35/29	28/30	46/47	22/41
Mean age, years	51.1	59.5	53.4	51.9
FFS, mean ± SD*	0.75 ± 0.9	1.86 ± 1.3	0.72 ± 1	0.95 ± 1
BVAS, mean ± SD†	22.1 ± 6.3	23.4 ± 8.4	15.1 ± 6.4	18.6 ± 7.3
Deaths, no. (%)‡	20 (31.3)	22 (37.9)	22 (23.7)	21 (33.3)
Deaths due to vasculitis, no.	4	7	5	6
Patients with relapses, no. (%)§	13 (20.3)	20 (34.5)	18 (19.4)	5 (7.9)

* Differences in the Five-Factors Score (FFS) between the group with microscopic polyangiitis (MPA) and the other 3 groups were significant ($P < 0.001$). No significant differences were noted between the groups with Churg-Strauss syndrome (CSS), non–hepatitis B virus (HBV)–related polyarteritis nodosa (PAN), and HBV-related PAN.
† Differences in the Birmingham Vasculitis Activity Score (BVAS) between the group with non–HBV-related PAN and the other 3 groups were significant ($P < 0.001$). No significant differences were noted between the groups with CSS, MPA, and HBV-related PAN.
‡ Death rates were comparable among the 4 groups.
§ Relapse rates differed significantly among the 4 groups ($P = 0.004$).

remission had been achieved; early relapses were those that occurred <12 months after the beginning of remission.

To gather information concerning the long-term survival of the patients, a questionnaire was sent to the hospital physician who had included the patients in the study and/or to their treating practitioner. The following questions were asked: 1) Is the patient dead or alive? 2) If the patient is dead, what was the cause of death? 3) Had the patient suffered a relapse(s) since inclusion in the study? If yes, what were the characteristics, date, and treatment of the relapse(s)? 4) Is the patient still receiving treatment for the vasculitis? 5) Did the patient experience treatment side effects? Answers were collected from January 1, 1996 to December 31, 1997. The end point was December 31, 1997. When the information was not obtained at the time of the inquiry or if the patient had not been seen by the physician who included the patient in the trial, the treating physician was contacted by mail or phone. When the patient was lost to followup, his or her demographic data were obtained from the French death registry, in which every French citizen's date and place of birth and of death are recorded; for ethical reasons, the cause of death is not reported.

Antineutrophil cytoplasmic antibodies (ANCA) had been sought in 118 of the 278 patients (42.4%). The technique that was used followed the recommendations of the European ANCA Assay Standardization Group (22).

Statistical analysis. Statistical analyses were carried out using SAS version 6.12 (SAS Institute, Cary, NC). The baseline characteristics of the study patients were expressed as percentages for categorical variables and as means for continuous variables. For univariate analysis, the chi-square test was used for categorical variables and Student's *t*-test for continuous variables. We used Spearman's correlation coefficient to determine the relationship between 2 continuous variables. Analysis of variance was performed for multiple comparisons of means and with the Bonferroni conversion for differences between means.

To compare our cohort with the general population, we used a model constructed according to the stochastic Monte Carlo method (23), which matched our control cohort of 278 persons according to year of study entry, age at study entry, sex, and duration of followup. A computerized program was designed with Visual Basic. Expected survival probabilities were calculated year-by-year on the basis of probabilities published by the Institut National de la Statistique et des Etudes Economiques (demographic data in France) (24). Survival curves were constructed according to the Kaplan-Meier method (25) using the log-rank test (26) or adjusted to prognostic factors and using the SAS Proc Lifetest, and using the log-rank test or the Cox model (27) adjusted to the prognostic factors using the SAS PROC PHREG. Survival curves were used to compare the clinical forms (CSS, MPA, PAN related or not related to HBV). These curves were plotted according to the 3 FFS classes and 4 BVAS classes described above. The survival curves evaluating the impact of CYC considered only 215 patients because those with HBV-related PAN were treated differently. The side effects were compared according to whether the patients received CYC or not. For all the statistical analyses, $P < 0.05$ was considered significant.

RESULTS

Demographics. Two hundred seventy-eight patients with a mean ± SD age of 53.8 ± 15.1 years at the time of diagnosis were included in the study; 54.3% were men and 45.7% were women. Regardless of the disease, no difference was noted between male and female patients in terms of clinical symptoms and causes of death. Of this total group, 64 had CSS, 58 had MPA, 93 had non–HBV-related PAN, and 63 had HBV-related PAN. Two hundred sixty-two of the patients (94.2%) were European Caucasians, 10 were born in North Africa, 3 were born in Asia, and 3 were black (2 Caribbean and 1 African). The patients were treated in different centers in France (see Acknowledgments). Nine patients were lost to followup after a mean of 82.3 months. The mean ± SD followup of the entire series of patients was 88.3 ± 51.9 months (range 3 days to 192 months).

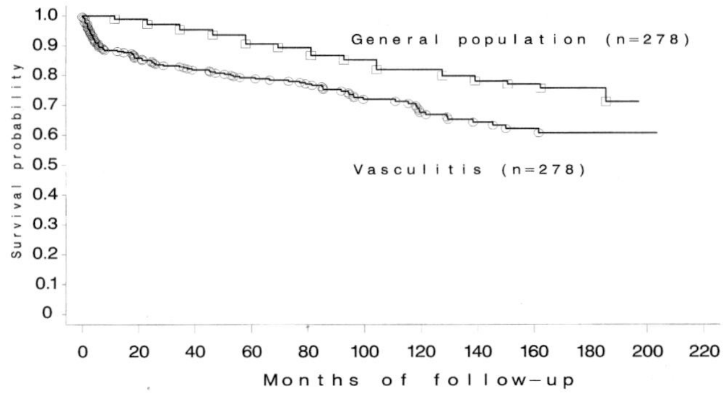

Figure 1. Survival of vasculitis patients (Churg-Strauss syndrome, microscopic polyangiitis, and polyarteritis nodosa with and without hepatitis B virus markers; n = 278) as compared with the general population of France ($P < 0.0004$).

The sex ratio, mean age, mean FFS and BVAS scores, deaths, and relapses for the different clinical forms of vasculitis are shown in Table 1. For the 64 patients with CSS, the ENT and chest manifestations accounted, respectively, for 3.52 ± 1.6 and 2.6 ± 1.1 BVAS points (mean ± SD). The mean BVAS, excluding ENT and chest signs (with the exception of hemorrhagic alveolitis), was 16 ± 6.4.

ANCA were sought in 118 of the 278 patients and were positive by immunofluorescence assay in 40 (14 of 30 CSS patients, 19 of 30 MPA, 7 of 35 non–HBV-related PAN, and 0 of 23 in HBV-related PAN).

Outcome. As shown by the Kaplan-Meier survival curves (Figure 1), the overall death rate of the study patients exceeded that of the general population of France, regardless of their age ($P < 0.0004$). A sharp drop in survival was observed within the first 18 months of followup. Afterwards, the curves tended to be parallel.

The mean ± SD FFS score for the entire cohort was 1 ± 1.13. The numbers of patients in each FFS group were 126 for an FFS of 0, 60 for an FFS of 1, 63 for an FFS of 2, 20 for an FFS of 3, 7 for an FFS of 4, and 2 for an FFS of 5. The mean ± SD BVAS score for the entire group was 19.1 ± 7.8, which was distributed as follows: 32 for a BVAS of ≤10, 130 for a BVAS of 10 to ≤20, 91 for a BVAS of 20 to ≤30, and 25 for a BVAS of >30.

Mortality was significantly associated with disease severity, as assessed by the FFS ($P = 0.004$) (Figure 2A) and the BVAS ($P < 0.0002$) (Figure 2B). Despite a tendency toward increased mortality in the MPA patients, no statistically significant difference was observed among the 4 clinical forms of vasculitis (Table 1 and Figure 3). Nevertheless, we observed more deaths during the followup of the MPA patients. Patients in this

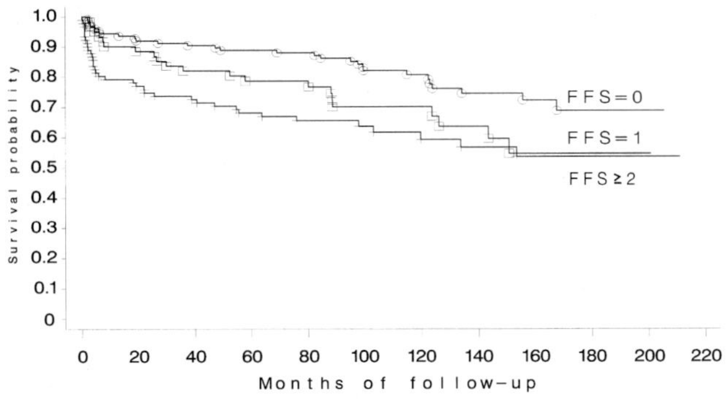

A

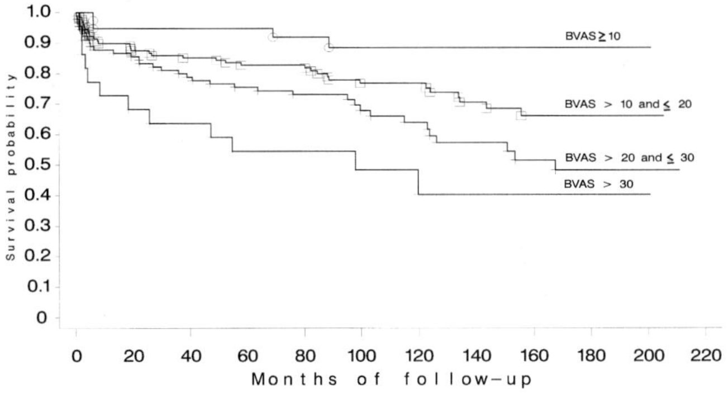

B

Figure 2. Survival of vasculitis patients (Churg-Strauss syndrome, microscopic polyangiitis, and polyarteritis nodosa with and without hepatitis B virus markers; n = 278) as a function of **A,** their Five-Factors Scores (FFS) ($P = 0.004$) and **B,** their Birmingham Vasculitis Activity Scores (BVAS) ($P < 0.0002$).

group were older at the time of diagnosis, 2 of them experienced severe relapses (108 and 120 months, respectively, after the diagnosis of vasculitis), and 2 CS-

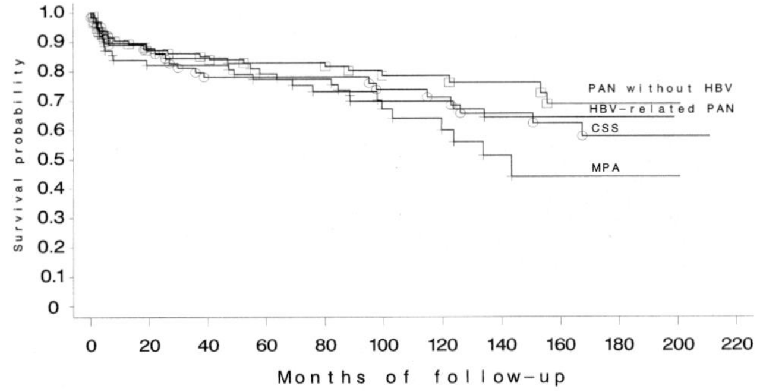

Figure 3. Survival of vasculitis patients (Churg-Strauss syndrome [CSS], microscopic polyangiitis [MPA], and polyarteritis nodosa [PAN] with and without hepatitis B virus [HBV] markers; n = 278) as a function of the type of vasculitis, adjusted to the Five-Factors Score ($P = 0.53$) and to the Birmingham Vasculitis Activity Score ($P = 0.79$).

dependent patients developed sepsis due to severe immunosuppression. A correlation was established between the FFS and BVAS scores (r = 0.69, $P < 0.01$) (Figure 4).

Relapses. Fifty-six patients (20.1%) experienced 84 relapses. No relationship was observed between the initial disease severity and the occurrence of relapse (mean ± SD FFS 0.94 ± 1.1 and BVAS 18.8 ± 8 in the group with relapses and FFS 1.05 ± 1.1 and BVAS 19 ± 7.8 in the group without). The first relapse occurred a mean ± SD of 31.6 ± 26.9 months after the initiation of first-line therapy. Treatment with cytotoxic agents did not prevent relapses: among the 215 patients treated with CS and CYC for CSS, MPA, or non–HBV-related PAN, 23.4% experienced a relapse, compared with 24.2% among those treated with CS alone. The time to relapse for the group treated with CYC and CS was 33.6 ± 20.8 months, and the time to relapse or uncontrolled disease for those treated with CS alone was 26.9 ± 24 months. It should be noted that the 6 patients whose disease became uncontrollable before the end of this initial treatment, between the sixth and eighth months, had received CS alone. No patient receiving CS and CYC had uncontrolled disease during the treatment period.

The number of relapses differed according to the type of vasculitis: 5 (7.9%) of the 63 patients with HBV-related PAN, 18 (19.4%) of the 93 patients with non–HBV-related PAN, 13 (20.3%) of the 64 CSS patients, and 20 (34.5%) of the 58 MPA patients experienced at least 1 relapse ($P = 0.004$ for the comparison of relapses versus no relapses among the 4 groups, by chi-square test with 3 degrees of freedom). The time to the first relapse was comparable for all the vasculitides: 24.6 ± 18 months in CSS, 37 ± 26 months in MPA, 29.4 ± 20.5 months in non–HBV-related PAN, and 36.6 ± 60.1 months in HBV-related PAN.

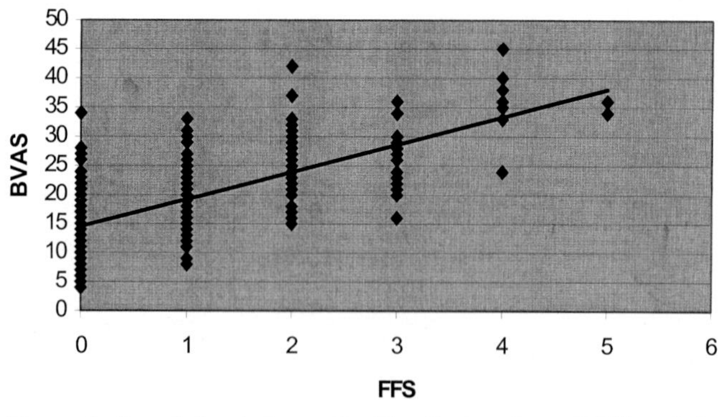

Figure 4. Correlation between the Five-Factors Score (FFS) and the Birmingham Vasculitis Activity Score (BVAS) in 278 patients with vasculitis (Churg-Strauss syndrome, microscopic polyangiitis, and polyarteritis nodosa with and without hepatitis B virus markers) (r = 0.69, $P < 0.01$).

Table 2. Causes of the 85 deaths of the vasculitis patients

Cause of death	No. (%) of patients
Progressive vasculitis	22 (25.9)
Bowel infarction	10
Cardiac failure	5
Multivisceral involvement	3
Renal failure	3
Stroke	1
Infectious side effects of treatment	11 (12.9)
Bacterial pneumonia	5
Septicemia	6
Sudden deaths	9 (10.6)
Heart disease	8 (9.4)
Cancer	13 (15.3)
Pulmonary embolism	3 (3.5)
Chronic respiratory disease	3 (3.5)
Fulminant viral hepatitis	2 (2.4)
Miscellaneous	14 (16.5)

Deaths. The causes of the 85 deaths that were recorded are shown in Table 2. Four sudden deaths of unknown cause were noted during the first 6 months after the start of treatment and were considered to be related to the disease. Three patients died of heart-related conditions (sequelae of specific cardiomyopathy in 2, hypertensive heart disease in 1). Two occurrences of pulmonary emboli were observed during the first 4 months of treatment. Thirteen patients died of cancers that developed in the following sites: lung (n = 3), throat (n = 2), GI tract (2 colon, 1 stomach), liver (n = 1), prostate (n = 1), lymphatic system (n = 2), unknown (n = 1). These patients were older than the rest of the study patients at the time of study inclusion (60.3 ± 10 years); their mean ± SD duration of followup was 71.9 ± 57.6 months. One patient developed breast carcinoma but died of cardiac failure secondary to cardiomyopathy that was specifically associated with CSS.

Two patients were treated for malignancies during followup. One had bladder cancer secondary to CYC therapy, and the other had uterine cancer considered to be independent of the vasculitis and its treatment. Both are still alive and in remission of both the vasculitis and the malignancy. The patient who had uterine cancer also developed thrombotic thrombocytopenic purpura 16 years after HBV-related PAN; the condition was attributed to the radiotherapy that had been used to treat the cancer.

Among the total of 15 patients who developed

Table 3. Patient characteristics and vasculitis scores, according to outcome*

Parameter	Study population (n = 278)	Survivors (n = 193)	Deaths: Overall (n = 85)	Deaths: Uncontrolled vasculitis (n = 22)	Deaths: Sepsis (n = 11)
Age, years	53.6 ± 15.5	51.3 ± 15.3	58.9 ± 13.6	52.1 ± 16.2	63.5 ± 9.2
FFS	1 ± 1.1	0.9 ± 1	1.3 ± 1.2	2.3 ± 1.3	1.5 ± 1.1
BVAS	19.1 ± 7.7	17.9 ± 7.5	21.9 ± 7.6	25.2 ± 9.2	22.1 ± 6.3
Followup, months	88.5 ± 51.7	106 ± 42.5	49 ± 42.5	26.6 ± 40.4	17.9†

* The patients' age, Five-Factors Score (FFS), and Birmingham Vasculities Activity Score (BVAS) were recorded at diagnosis. Values are the mean ± SD.
† The SD is not reported because 9 of the 11 deaths occurred before 4 months and the other 2 occurred at 10 years and 11 years, respectively.

cancers, 7 received CS plus CYC, and 8 received CS alone. One of the 2 lymphoma patients received CYC.

Forty-one patients died as a consequence of their vasculitis or its treatment: 22 died of uncontrolled vasculitis, 11 of treatment side effects (sepsis), 6 of early sudden death, and 2 of sequelae of cardiomyopathy, representing 14.7% of the total population and 48.2% of all the deaths (Table 3). Eighteen of the 22 patients who died of uncontrolled vasculitis had poor prognostic factors. The mean followup of this group was 39 ± 17.4 months. Thirty (73.2%) of the 41 deaths due to the disease or its consequences occurred during the first 18 months after starting treatment.

Influence of treatment. Survival was comparable for the 215 patients receiving either CS or CS plus CYC (Figure 5). When these patients were stratified according to FFS, those with scores ≥2 who received CYC (n = 91) benefited from significantly prolonged survival ($P = 0.044$). No difference was observed between the overall population and those with an FFS score of 0 or 1 ($P = 0.46$ and $P = 0.31$, respectively). Stratification according to the BVAS failed to reveal a difference in survival. Nevertheless, among the 25 patients for whom the BVAS was >30, a tendency toward significance was observed in favor of CYC ($P = 0.069$). Fifteen of the 22 patients who died of severe vasculitis had been treated with CS alone.

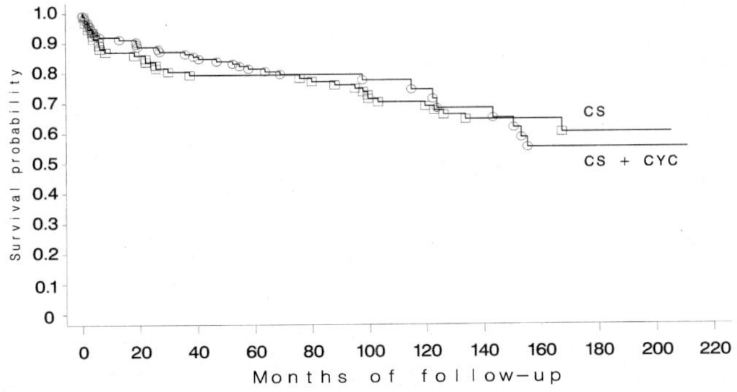

Figure 5. Survival of patients with vasculitis (Churg-Strauss syndrome, microscopic polyangiitis, and polyarteritis nodosa without hepatitis B virus markers; n = 215) as a function of treatment with corticosteroids (CS) versus CS plus cyclophosphamide (CYC) as first-line therapy (P not significant).

Treatment side effects. Only moderate and severe side effects were recorded; mild side effects were not taken into account because they were not always reported. One hundred seventy-five treatment side effects (Table 4) were reported in 93 of the 278 patients; 79 of the 93 patients (84.9%) had received CYC. The distribution of side effects among the protocols and forms of diseases were as follows: 41% in protocol 1, 9.8% in protocol 2, 64.2% in protocol 3, and none in protocol 4 (only mild effects due to antiviral agents); 37.5% of the CSS patients, 58.6% of MPA, 29% of non–HBV-related PAN, and 7.9% of HBV-related PAN. Among the 185 patients who did not experience side effects, only 53 (28.6%) had received CYC ($P < 0.0001$). The mean ± SD ages of the patients with and without side effects were, respectively, 56.5 ± 12.7 years and 52.4 ± 15.5 years.

Infectious diseases and osteoporotic fractures were the 2 major events, respectively, in 13.3% and 8.6% of the entire study population. In protocol 3, in which all patients received CS and CYC, infections occurred in 28.6% (mean ± SD age 61.8 ± 10 years), and osteoporotic fractures occurred in 19% of the whole group and in 35% of the women in the group. The 11 patients who died of sepsis had taken CYC (6 oral doses and 5 intravenous pulse doses) and were older than the other patients in the series (63.5 years versus 53.6 years). Side effects were observed in 59% of patients receiving oral CYC and in 62% of those receiving pulse doses.

Sequelae were noted in 58 patients. The main

Table 4. Distribution of side effects as a function of treatment with CS with and without CYC*

Side effect	No. of events (n = 175)	No. of patients with side effects: Total (n = 93)	No. of patients with side effects: No. taking CYC (n = 79)
Infections	40	37	31
Bacterial pneumonia	8		
Acute bronchitis	6		
Tuberculosis	3		
Pneumocystis carinii pneumonia	1		
Sinusitis	2		
Septicemia	4		
Urinary tract infections	2		
Herpes zoster infections	5		
Osteomyelitis, arthritis	2		
Furunculosis	2		
Aspergillosis, candidiasis, cryptococcosis	5		
Osteoporotic fractures	26	24	14
Vertebra	23		
Femur	3		
Amenorrhea	5	5	5
Alopecia	6	6	6
Hemorrhagic cystitis	7	7	7
Neutropenia	9	9	9
Cushing's disease	24	24	19
Weight gain	9	9	3
Diabetes	8	8	5
Hypertension	11	11	9
Depression	7	7	4
GI symptoms	5	5	5
Acne	5	5	3
Thrombosis	4	4	2
Cataract	3	3	2
Osteonecrosis	3	3	2
Cholestasis	2	2	1
Bladder cancer	1	1	1

* Some patients experienced more than 1 side effect; therefore, the sum of each of the 2 last columns is higher than the number of patients indicated at the top of the column. CS = corticosteroids; CYC = cyclophosphamide; GI = gastrointestinal.

sequelae were end-stage renal failure necessitating hemodialysis (n = 8; 2 of whom subsequently received renal allografts), moderate renal insufficiency (n = 7), peripheral neuropathy (n = 10), congestive heart failure (n = 5), hypertension (n = 4), chronic respiratory disease (n = 5), hemiplegia (n = 1), visual impairment (n = 1), amputation (n = 2), marked weight gain (n = 2), pain from vertebral fractures (n = 11), and inability to get out of bed (n = 2).

DISCUSSION

Several studies (6–12) have demonstrated an overall improvement in the prognosis of vasculitis and, recently, scores predicting the prognosis have been devised (19). However, to date, the impact of therapeutic strategies on subgroups of vasculitides according to the prognostic factors and the occurrence of long-term side effects has not been evaluated. We demonstrated in the present study that the overall mortality was significantly higher than that observed in the general population of France, despite the improvement in treatments. Deaths usually occurred early, within the first 18 months of followup. Later, survival curves tended to be parallel despite the occurrence of late relapses. Survival reflected the initial disease severity (Figures 2A and B), and in our opinion prognostic scores should be used in clinical trials to guide the initial treatment choice as a function of disease severity in the individual patient.

We observed a few discrepancies between the BVAS and the FFS. Although the scores were correlated (r = 0.69), for CSS the BVAS (20) overestimated the disease severity (Table 1) as a consequence of the points attributed to ENT involvement and chest involvement, despite the fact that neither maxillary sinusitis nor asthma has ever been demonstrated to be a factor of poor prognosis in CSS (19). Based on these data, the FFS was easier to use and better adapted for comparing the initial severity of the different types of vasculitides. However, the BVAS is a more precise measurement of the dissemination of the disease and could be used to evaluate followup (21), which is not the case for the FFS. The 2 scores are therefore complementary and are useful for decision-making and treatment followup.

In our opinion, deaths due to vasculitis or its complications did not reflect the type of vasculitis but, rather, the extent of organ involvement, e.g., kidney, GI

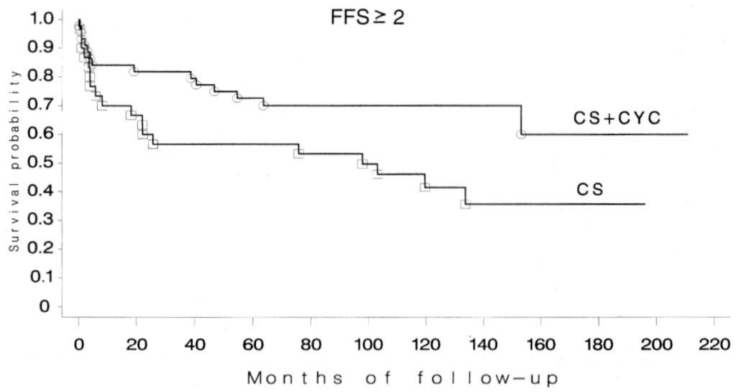

Figure 6. Survival of patients with vasculitis (Churg-Strauss syndrome, microscopic polyangiitis, and polyarteritis nodosa without hepatitis B virus markers and Five-Factors Scores [FFS] of ≥2; n = 91) as a function of treatment with corticosteroids (CS) versus CS plus cyclophosphamide (CYC) as first-line therapy (P = 0.044).

tract, or heart, or the patient's age at the time of diagnosis (in terms of treatment-related sepsis). The increased, but not significant, number of late deaths of MPA patients was partly due to more severe disease (with kidney involvement in nearly all patients), to their tendency to relapse more frequently (and thus require more treatments, which are potentially responsible for a higher number of side effects), and to their older age at study entry. Considering the entire cohort of patients, we did not observe that patients receiving CS plus CYC had better outcomes. Careful analysis of survival stratified according to prognostic factors showed that CS plus CYC significantly prolonged the survival of the more severely ill patients, who had FFS scores ≥ 2 ($P = 0.044$). A tendency toward prolonged survival was also observed for patients who received CYC and had BVAS scores >30.

Also, 15 patients taking CS alone died of uncontrolled disease. We found that CYC in combination with CS did not prevent the occurrence of the first relapse, which seemed more often to be related to the type of vasculitis and its spontaneous tendency to relapse than to the first-line therapy prescribed. Nevertheless, only patients who were being treated with CS alone had uncontrolled disease.

The causes of death in a previous French cohort of 149 patients (for the years 1958–1983) (4) were nearly identical to those seen in the present group, except for sepsis, which was lower in the present study (26.5% versus 12.9%, respectively), and can be attributed to the improved management of infections.

Side effects were frequent, being reported in at least 33.5% of the patients. Infectious events were strongly associated with the combination of CS and CYC, were more frequent in patients older than 65 years, and were responsible for 11 deaths. The increased frequency of infections in patients taking the combination of CS and CYC has previously been reported (2,28). In a few of our patients, the vasculitis was controlled by this combination, but the treatment was responsible for infection-related deaths. Although no difference was observed between oral and pulse administration of CYC, hematuria was predominantly observed with the oral form (6 of 7 cases).

Despite recommendations to prescribe calcium and vitamin D supplements to all patients, we observed a high frequency of osteoporotic fractures, higher than that which would be expected in the general population of France (annual incidence of femoral fractures 170/100,000 females, 62/100,000 males; no data concerning vertebral fractures are available) (29). Bone demineralization can be explained by the prolonged and high-dose CS regimen given in these prospective trials, the mean age of the patients at the time of diagnosis, and the high number of menopausal women without hormone replacement therapy and/or women with CYC-induced amenorrhea. Indeed, a lower CS dose, close to that used in National Institutes of Health and European trials (30), is prescribed in the ongoing trials in an attempt to lower the frequency of osteoporosis. We also recommend preventing osteoporosis in different manners: hormone replacement therapy for menopausal women, and/or calcium, vitamin D, and bisphosphonates.

In our patients, malignancies were not clearly attributable to CYC, except for 1 case of bladder cancer. Those who developed cancer were older at the time of the diagnosis of vasculitis, the mean interval between the two diagnoses was rather long, and 5 of them had risk factors (smokers and/or heavy drinkers). Comparison of the frequencies of cancers in this series with those of the general population is difficult because there is no exhaustive registry of cancers in France. They are recorded in some districts of France and extrapolated to the entire population (31). Nevertheless, the incidence of lymphomas was higher than that of the general population.

It has been reported that, in Wegener's granulomatosis, long-term treatment with CYC was the cause of a dramatically increased number of bladder cancers, with a long latency period between the first exposure and the diagnosis of cancer (32–35). The presence of microscopic hematuria is an independent risk factor for the development of cancer. Although the total CYC dose and the duration of therapy were not clearly associated with the development of cancers, most of them occurred in patients who had received a cumulative dose that exceeded 100 gm (32). In our patients, the duration of CYC treatment did not exceed 12 months, and, since 1987, pulses have been predominantly prescribed, thereby lowering the total dose, with the systematic use of hydration and mesna. The relatively short duration of CYC therapy compared with that in Wegener's granulomatosis and the use of pulses to lower the total CYC dose could explain the low number of bladder cancers observed in our patients.

Based on the results of these studies, our group has undertaken new trials that aim to specify the indications for CYC and other immunosuppressive agents and to lower the CYC dose in patients with severe vasculitis. We also intend to establish a strategy adapted to the type of vasculitis, its severity, and its predicted (according to the FFS) outcome.

ACKNOWLEDGMENTS

This research was conducted with the help of The Société Nationale Française de Médecine Interne (SNFMI). The following investigators participated in the study: M. Alcalay and P. Roblot (Poitiers); P. Amarenco, J. Cabane, P. Cacoub, J. Cadranel, B. Christoforov, P. Deblois, G. Deray, P. Druet, P. Even, M. Gayraud, P. Godeau, M. Krulik, F. Lioté, D. Molle, P. Pasquier, J. C. Piette, J. M. Visy, B. Wechsler, and J. M. Ziza (Paris); K. S. Ang, G. Dien, and P. Simon (St. Brieuc); P. Arlet, P. Bayle, P. Carles, O. Pourrat, and S. Ollier (Toulouse); P. Babinet and F. Lhote (St. Denis); J. Baillet, J. P. Ducroix, A. Fournier, R. Madkassi and S. Smaïl (Amiens); G. Baralis (Arles); J. Barrier and J. Y. Grolleau (Nantes); P. Bironne and J. Glowinski (Gonesse); J. P. Bouchon (Ivry); E. Bercoff, O. Deshayes, B. Desrumeaux, X. Le Loët, and B. Pinel (Rouen); P. Canton and M. Maignan (Nancy); J. P. Cassuto, P. Dujardin, J. G. Fuzibet and J. F. Quaranta (Nice); B. Coevoet (St. Quentin); P. Casassus, P. Cohen, D. Daupleix, P. Dreyfus, L. Guillevin, B. Jarrousse, P. Le Toumelin, and J. N. Hugues (Bobigny); G. Desproges-Gotteron, F. Liozon, R. Treves, and E. Vidal (Limoges); J. F. Desson (Caen); P. Doumovo (Eaubonne); Y. Echard (Montfermeil); A. Fischer (Evry); J. L. Debru, A. Franco, B. Imbert, and P. Micoud (Grenoble); B. Godeau, A. Schaeffer, J. C. Roujeau, and A. Sobel (Créteil); G. Janin (Mâcon); J. Jouquan (Brest); M. Kerjean (St. Malo); M. Imler (Strasbourg); S. Lassoued (Cahors); J. Mallecourt (Dreux); J. Maupetit (Libourne); O. Maurisset (La Roche-sur-Yon); P. Mornet (St. Germain-en-Laye); M. Mougeot Martin (Creil); J. Ninet, J. Pasquier, C. Trépo, and D. Vital-Durand (Lyon); O. Patey (Villeneuve St. Georges); A. M. Piette (Suresnes); M. Pointud (Montluçon); F. Rossi (Vendôme); H. Rousset (St. Etienne); M. Ruel (Senlis); M. Sigal Nahum (Argenteuil); and P. Veyssier (Compiègne). The coordinating center is at the Department of Internal Medicine, Hôpital Avicenne, Assistance Publique des Hôpitaux de Paris, Université Paris-Nord, Bobigny, France.

REFERENCES

1. Frohnert PP, Sheps SG. Long-term follow-up study of periarteritis nodosa. Am J Med 1967;43:8–14.
2. Bradley JD, Brandt KD, Katz BP. Infectious complications of cyclophosphamide treatment for vasculitis. Arthritis Rheum 1989; 32:45–53.
3. Cohen RD, Conn DL, Ilstrup DM. Clinical features, prognosis and response to treatment in polyarteritis. Mayo Clin Proc 1980;55: 146–55.
4. Cacoub P, Le Thi Huong D, Guillevin L, Godeau P. Les causes de mortalité au cours des vascularites systémiques du groupe de la périartérite noueuse: analyse d'une série de 165 malades. Ann Med Interne (Paris) 1988;139:381–90.
5. Exley AR, Carruthers DM, Luqmani RA, Kitas GD, Gordon C, Janssen BA, et al. Damage occurs early in systemic vasculitis and is an index of outcome. QJM 1997;90:391–9.
6. Fauci AS, Katz P, Haynes BF, Wolff SM. Cyclophosphamide therapy of severe necrotizing vasculitis. N Engl J Med 1979;301:235–8.
7. Leib ES, Restivo C, Paulus HE. Immunosuppressive and corticosteroid therapy of polyarteritis nodosa. Am J Med 1979;67:941–7.
8. Guillevin L, Jarrousse B, Lok C, Lhote F, Jaïs JP, Le Thi Huong Du D, et al, and the Cooperative Study Group for Polyarteritis Nodosa. Longterm follow-up after treatment of polyarteritis nodosa and Churg-Strauss angiitis with comparison of steroids, plasma exchange and cyclophosphamide to steroids and plasma exchange: a prospective randomized trial of 71 patients. J Rheumatol 1991;18:567–74.
9. Guillevin L, Fain O, Lhote F, Jarrousse B, Le Thi Huong D, Bussel A, et al. Lack of superiority of steroids plus plasma exchange to steroids alone in the treatment of polyarteritis nodosa and Churg-Strauss syndrome: a prospective, randomized trial in 78 patients. Arthritis Rheum 1992;35:208–15.
10. Guillevin L, Lhote F, Cohen P, Jarrousse B, Lortholary O, Généreau T, et al. Corticosteroids plus pulse cyclophosphamide and plasma exchanges versus corticosteroids plus pulse cyclophosphamide alone in the treatment of polyarteritis nodosa and Churg-Strauss syndrome patients with factors predicting poor prognosis: a prospective, randomized trial in sixty-two patients. Arthritis Rheum 1995;38:1638–45.
11. Guillevin L, Lhote F, Cohen P, Sauvaget F, Jarrousse B, Lortholary O, et al. Polyarteritis nodosa related to hepatitis B virus: a prospective study with long-term observation of 41 patients. Medicine (Baltimore) 1995;74:238–53.
12. Gayraud M, Guillevin L, Cohen P, Lhote F, Cacoub P, Deblois P. Treatment of good-prognosis polyarteritis nodosa and Churg-Strauss syndrome: comparison of steroids and oral or pulse cyclophosphamide in 25 patients. Br J Rheumatol 1997;36:1290–7.
13. Fauci AS, Haynes BF, Katz P. The spectrum of vasculitis: clinical, pathologic, immunologic and therapeutic considerations. Ann Intern Med 1978;89:660–76.
14. Masi AT, Hunder GG, Lie JT, Michel BA, Bloch DA, Arend WP, et al. The American College of Rheumatology 1990 criteria for the classification of Churg-Strauss syndrome (allergic granulomatosis and angiitis). Arthritis Rheum 1990;33:1094–100.
15. Lightfoot RW Jr, Michel BA, Bloch DA, Hunder GG, Zvaifler NJ, McShane DJ, et al. The American College of Rheumatology 1990 criteria for the classification of polyarteritis nodosa. Arthritis Rheum 1990;33:1088–93.
16. Jennette JC, Falk RJ, Andrassy K, Bacon PA, Churg J, Gross WL, et al. Nomenclature of systemic vasculitides: proposal of an international consensus conference. Arthritis Rheum 1994;37:187–92.
17. Guillevin L, Durand-Gasselin B, Cevallos R, Gayraud M, Lhote F, Callard P, et al. Microscopic polyangiitis: clinical and laboratory findings in eighty-five patients. Arthritis Rheum 1999;42:421–30.
18. Rao JK, Allen NB, Pincus T. Limitations of the 1990 American College of Rheumatology classification criteria in the diagnosis of vasculitis. Ann Intern Med 1998;129:345–52.
19. Guillevin L, Lhote F, Gayraud M, Cohen P, Jarrousse B, Lortholary O, et al. Prognostic factors in polyarteritis nodosa and Churg-Strauss syndrome: a prospective study in 342 patients. Medicine (Baltimore) 1996;75:17–28.
20. Luqmani RA, Bacon PA, Moots RJ, Janssen BA, Pall A, Emery P, et al. Birmingham Vasculitis Activity Score (BVAS) in systemic necrotizing vasculitis. QJM 1994;87:671–8.
21. Luqmani RA, Exley AR, Kitas GD, Bacon PA. Disease assessment and management of the vasculitides. Baillieres Clin Rheumatol 1997;11:422–47.
22. Hagen EC, Daha MR, Hermans J, Andrassy K, Csernok E, Gaskin G, et al. Diagnostic value of standardized assays for anti-neutrophil cytoplasmic antibodies in idiopathic systemic vasculitis: EC/BCR Project for ANCA Assay Standardization. Kidney Int 1998;53:743–53.
23. Mueller ME. Some continuous Monte Carlo methods for the Dirichlet problem. Ann Math Stat 1956;27:569–89.
24. Kerjosse R, Tamby I. La situation démographique en France en 1994: mouvement de la population. INSEE (Institut National de la Statistique et des Etudes Economiques); 1995. Internal Report 129–45.
25. Kaplan E, Meier P. Non parametric estimation for incomplete information. J Am Stat Assoc 1958;53:457–81.
26. Peto R, Pike MC. Conservatism of the approximation (O-E)2-E in the logrank test for survival data or tumor incidence data. Biometrics 1973;29:579–84.

27. Cox DR. Regression models and lifetable. J R Stat Soc B 1972;34:187–200.
28. Sen RP, Walsh TE, Fisher W, Brock N. Pulmonary complications of combination therapy with cyclophosphamide and prednisone. Chest 1991;99:143–6.
29. Baudoin C. Epidémiologie présente et future des ostéoporoses. Rev Prat 1995;45:1089–95.
30. Gross WL. New concept in treatment protocols for severe systemic vasculitis. Curr Opin Rheumatol 1999;11:41–6.
31. Réseau Français des Registres de Cancers FRANCIM, 37 allée Jules Guesde, 31073 Toulouse, France.
32. Stillwell TJ, Benson RC Jr, DeRemee RA, McDonald TJ, Weiland LH. Cyclophosphamide-induced bladder toxicity in Wegener's granulomatosis. Arthritis Rheum 1988;31:465–70.
33. Stillwell TJ, Benson RC. Cyclophosphamide-induced hemorrhagic cystitis: a review of 100 patients. Cancer 1988;61:451–7.
34. Hoffman GS, Kerr GS, Leavitt RY, Hallahan CW, Lebovics RS, Travis WD, et al. Wegener's granulomatosis: an analysis of 158 patients. Ann Intern Med 1992;116:488–98.
35. Talar-Williams C, Hijazi YM, Walther MM, Lineham WM, Hallahan CW, Lubensky I, et al. Cyclophosphamide-induced cystitis and bladder cancer in patients with Wegener's granulomatosis. Ann Intern Med 1996;124:477–84.

ARTHRITIS & RHEUMATISM
Vol. 44, No. 3, March 2001, pp 676–681

Invasiveness of Synovial Fibroblasts Is Regulated by p53 in the SCID Mouse In Vivo Model of Cartilage Invasion

Thomas Pap,[1] Karlfried R. Aupperle,[2] Steffen Gay,[1] Gary S. Firestein,[2] and Renate E. Gay[1]

Objective. **In vitro data suggest that the tumor suppressor p53 is critically involved in the regulation of proliferation and apoptosis in fibroblast-like synoviocytes (FLS). Based on evidence that abnormalities in p53 expression and function are found in rheumatoid arthritis (RA), we analyzed whether inhibition of p53 using gene transfer with the human papilloma virus type 18 (HPV-18) E6 protein results in an increased cellularity and invasiveness of synovial fibroblasts in vivo.**

Methods. **RA and normal FLS were transduced with a pLXSN-based construct encoding for the HPV-18 E6 protein or with the pLXSN vector alone. After selection with G418, FLS were coimplanted with normal human cartilage under the renal capsule of SCID mice. Parental, nontransduced cells were used as additional controls. After 60 days, the implants were removed, and FLS invasion into the cartilage, perichondrocytic degradation, and cellularity were assessed.**

Results. **Nontransduced and mock-transduced RA FLS exhibited characteristic invasion into the cartilage (mean ± SEM scores 2.2 ± 0.3 and 2.4 ± 0.2, respectively). Invasion was increased significantly in the E6-transduced RA FLS (mean score 3.1 ± 0.3; $P <$ 0.05). Inhibition of p53 also resulted in an increase in cellularity. Parental and mock-transduced normal FLS did not exhibit significant invasion (mean score 1.5 ± 0.1 and 1.4 ± 0.3, respectively), but transduction with E6 resulted in clear invasiveness (mean score 2.4 ± 0.4) as well as increased cellularity.**

Conclusion. **The data suggest that inhibition of endogenous p53 leads to increased invasiveness and cellularity of RA FLS and may also transform normal FLS to cells that display an aggressive, RA FLS–like behavior. Therefore, abnormalities such as somatic mutations in the p53 tumor suppressor may contribute to synovial hyperplasia and invasion in RA.**

Being a key regulator of cell proliferation and death (1), the tumor suppressor p53 is critically involved in preventing cellular transformation and ensuring normal tissue homeostasis. Specific functions of p53 are related to the maintenance of DNA integrity through the initiation of repair mechanisms and the transcriptional activation of cell cycle–related genes. Consequently, alterations in p53 expression and function have been observed in a variety of human malignancies (2,3) and are associated with cell proliferation, impaired apoptosis, and invasiveness (4,5).

In rheumatoid arthritis (RA), the progressive destruction of articular cartilage by an inflamed and hyperplastic synovial membrane is a key feature of disease. Within this membrane, activated fibroblast-like synoviocytes (FLS) contribute significantly to cartilage degradation. Although the exact mechanisms that lead to the activation of RA FLS as well as to their subsequent proliferation and invasion into the extracellular matrix remain elusive, alterations in tumor suppressor p53 have been implicated in the pathogenesis of disease. Interestingly, overexpression of p53 protein in the lining layer of the RA synovium (6–8) contrasts with the low rate of apoptosis in RA FLS at sites of invasion (9).

In their searches for possible alterations in the structure and function of p53 in the rheumatoid synovium, Firestein et al and, later, Rème et al demonstrated the presence of somatic mutations in the p53 gene in RA (10,11). In addition, Han et al showed that at least 2 of

Supported in part by grants from the NIH (5P50-AR-44850-02 and R01-AR-45347-03) and from the Swiss National Science Foundation (NFP-37; 4037-55152). Dr. Aupperle's work was supported by the Arthritis Foundation.
[1]Thomas Pap, MD, Steffen Gay, MD, Renate E. Gay, MD: University Hospital, Zurich, Switzerland; [2]Karlfried R. Aupperle, MD, Gary S. Firestein, MD: University of California, La Jolla.
Address correspondence and reprint requests to Renate Gay, MD, World Health Organization Collaborating Center for Molecular Biology and Novel Therapeutic Strategies for Rheumatic Diseases, Department of Rheumatology, University Hospital, Gloriastrasse 25, CH-8091 Zurich, Switzerland.
Submitted for publication May 12, 2000; accepted in revised form November 8, 2000.

the p53 mutants identified in RA are dominant negative and suppress endogenous p53 function (12). The most recent in vitro data further suggest that p53 is a key regulator of FLS proliferation and invasiveness (13). Therefore, it has been hypothesized that alterations in p53 may be associated with the aggressive behavior of RA FLS.

In the present studies, we sought to answer the question of whether inhibition of endogenous p53 results in increased cellularity and aggressiveness of FLS under in vivo conditions. In this context, transfer of the human papillomavirus type 18 (HPV-18) E6 protein has been demonstrated to effectively inhibit the transcription activity of p53 in FLS (13). Specifically, the E6 protein inhibits the activation of gene transcription by p53 through binding to the p53 protein (14) as well as by activating the ubiquitin protease system (15,16). Using retroviral gene transfer with the HPV-18 E6 gene to RA and normal FLS, we found that inhibition of wild-type p53 not only increases the proliferation and invasiveness of RA FLS, but also transforms normal synovial fibroblasts (normal FLS) to cells that display an aggressive, RA FLS–like behavior.

PATIENTS AND METHODS

Isolation of FLS. Synovial tissue was obtained from 2 patients with RA who met the 1987 revised criteria of the American College of Rheumatology (formerly, the American Rheumatism Association) for the disease (17). Normal synovial tissue was obtained at autopsy from an individual with no history of arthritis. The tissue specimens were minced and digested enzymatically (1 mg/ml of type VIII collagenase; Sigma, St. Louis, MO) in serum-free medium (RPMI 1640; Life Technologies, Grand Island, NY) for 1 hour at 37°C. The released cells were grown in Dulbecco's modified Eagle's medium (Life Technologies) with 10% fetal calf serum (Gemini Biological Products, Calabasas, CA) in a humidified atmosphere containing 5% CO_2.

After allowing the cells to adhere overnight, nonadherent cells were removed, and the adherent cells were grown further over 4–5 passages. Cells were screened for p53 mutations immediately after establishing the cell cultures (second passage) and were found to contain >95% wild-type p53 messenger RNA, as described previously (13). These cell lines (2 RA and 1 normal) were selected for study. These lines have been extensively characterized and described in a previous publication (13).

Transduction of FLS. A retroviral construct was used to transduce the RA and normal FLS. In this construct, the HPV-18 E6 gene (E6+*neo*) was cloned into the pLXSN vector, which has been described previously (18). The empty vector (*neo*) was used as a control. RA and normal FLS that contained wild-type p53 were incubated with the retrovirus supernatant (either E6+*neo* or *neo* alone) for 48 hours. Subsequently, the medium was replaced with fresh medium, and cells were selected with G418 (0.25 mg/ml; Gibco BRL, Life Technologies, Basel, Switzerland). For the SCID mouse experiments, E6-transduced FLS, mock (pLXSN)–transduced FLS, and the parental, nontransduced cells were used.

SCID mouse coimplantation experiments. Two-week-old, female SCID mice were provided by Charles River (Sulzfeld, Germany) and were kept permanently under germ-free conditions. Normal human articular cartilage was obtained from patients undergoing joint replacement surgery for severe trauma at the Department of Surgery, University Hospital, Zurich, Switzerland. Implantation of FLS together with normal human cartilage was performed as described previously (19). Briefly, after trypsinization, washing, and centrifugation, 10^5 cells were resuspended in 100 μl of sterile culture medium and inserted into the cavity of an inert sponge (Gelfoam; Pharmacia & Upjohn, Dübendorf, Switzerland) together with a 1-mm^3 piece of the articular cartilage.

Mice were anesthetized intraperitoneally with 0.014 mg/gm of Xylocaine (lidocaine hydrochloride; Astra Pharmaceutica, Dietikon, Switzerland) and 0.09 mg/gm of Ketalar (ketamine hydrochloride; Parke-Davis, Baar, Switzerland) in an isotonic solution, and a 1-cm incision was made on the left flank. The left kidney was exteriorized, and following a small incision, the implant was placed under the renal capsule. The peritoneal layer and the skin were closed using 5-0 Prolene suture material. After 60 days, mice were killed and the implants removed. Tissue preparation included fixation in 4% buffered formalin and paraffin embedding according to standard procedures. All experiments were performed in duplicate, using a total of 18 mice.

Invasion score. Following hematoxylin and eosin staining of the sections, histologic evaluation was performed using semiquantitative scores for invasion and perichondrocytic cartilage degradation, as described previously (19). For the invasion score, the depth of invasion was assessed by estimating the number of cell layers invaded, and the scores were defined as follows: 0 = no or minimal invasion, 1 = visible invasion (2–5 cell depths), 2 = invasion (6–10 cell depths), 3 = deep invasion (>10 cell depths), and 4 = overall deep invasion reshaping the cartilage surface. Perichondrocytic cartilage degradation was scored as follows: 0 = no degradation, with sharp halo, 1 = visible degradation (≤1 diameter of the chondrocyte), 2 = substantial degradation (1–2 diameters of the chondrocyte), 3 = major degradation (>2 diameters of the chondrocyte). The sections were evaluated by 2 experienced scientists (TP and SG) in a blinded manner.

Cellularity of FLS. The number of cells at sites of cartilage degradation was counted in 4 randomly selected high-power fields (hpf; 400× magnification). For comparability of the data, a proportion of two-thirds of the cartilage tissue and one-third of the implanted fibroblasts was chosen when selecting the hpf.

Statistical analysis. For statistical analysis, the means and SEM were calculated. Differences between groups were tested for statistical difference using the Mann-Whitney U test. Differences were considered statistically significant at $P < 0.05$.

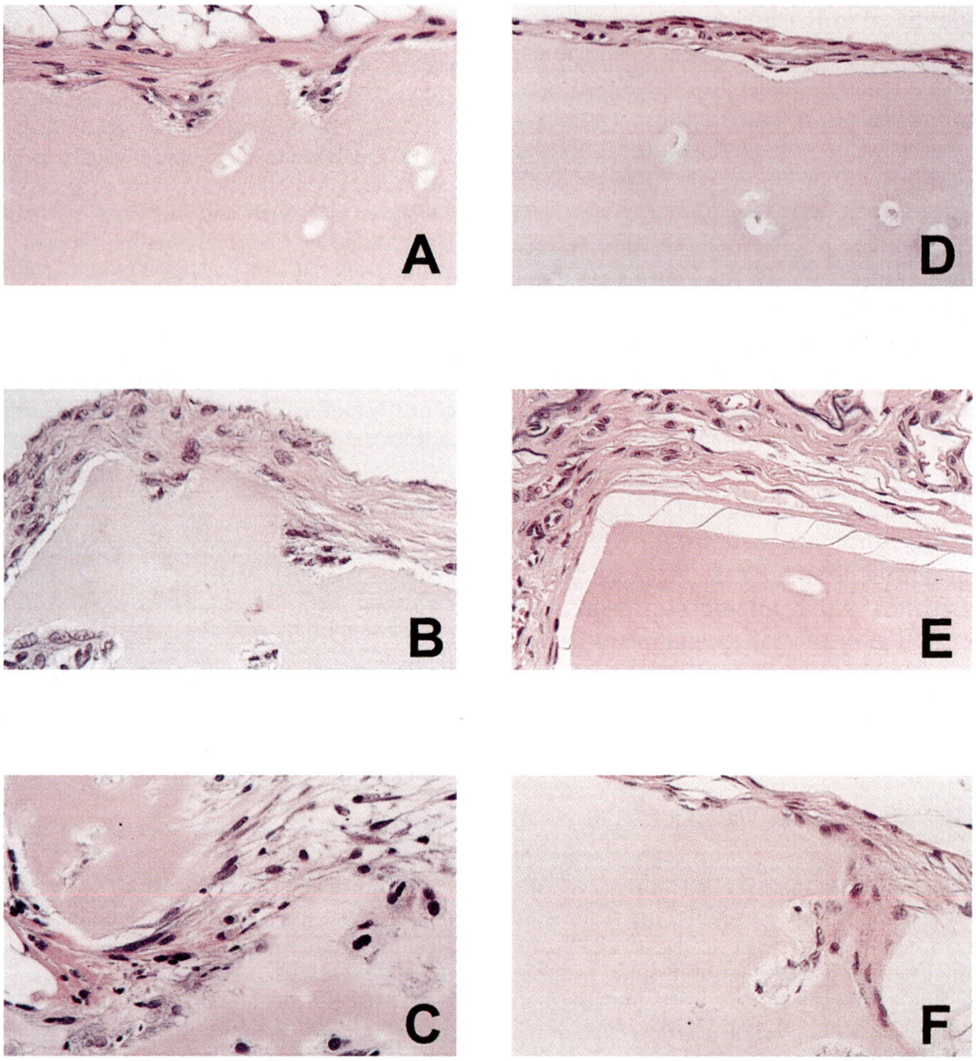

Figure 1. Invasion of fibroblast-like synoviocytes (FLS) into the coimplanted cartilage in the SCID mouse model of rheumatoid arthritis (RA). Parental, nontransduced (**A**) as well as mock-transduced (**B**) RA FLS showed a clear invasion that was enhanced by transducing these cells with the human papillomavirus type 18 (HPV-18) E6 gene (**C**). Parental (**D**) and mock-transduced (**E**) normal FLS did not show significant invasion into the cartilage, but transduction with the HPV-18 E6 gene caused a clear RA FLS–like invasiveness (**F**). (Original magnification × 400 in **A**, **B**, and **F**; × 630 in **C**; × 200 in **D** and **E**.)

RESULTS

Invasiveness of FLS. As shown in Figure 1A, a clear invasion of the parental, nontransduced RA FLS into the coimplanted cartilage was observed. The mean ± SEM invasion score of all RA FLS was 2.2 ± 0.3, with only minor differences between the cell cultures. In contrast, parental, nontransduced normal FLS did not exhibit marked invasion (Figure 1D). At sites of cartilage fissures, a few normal FLS grew into the cartilage matrix, resulting in an overall invasion score of 1.5 ± 0.1. Notably, nontransduced normal FLS did not attach as firmly to the coimplanted cartilage as the RA FLS. Thus, a partial detachment of the cartilage from the fibroblasts was seen at the time of tissue processing. Transduction of RA FLS and normal FLS with the mock pLXSN (*neo* alone) vector did not change their invasive behavior (mean ± SEM scores 2.4 ± 0.2 and 1.4 ± 0.3, respectively). The differences between RA FLS and nontransduced normal FLS are shown in Figures 1B and E; the scores were significantly different ($P < 0.05$).

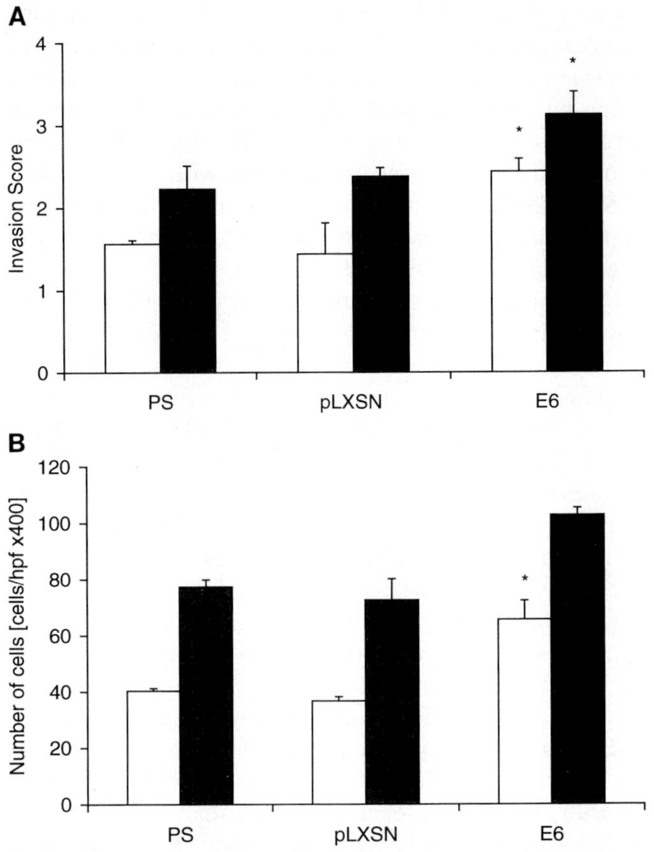

Figure 2. Comparison of the invasion scores (**A**) and the cellularity (**B**) of parental, nontransduced FLS (PS), mock-transduced (pLXSN) FLS, and HPV-18 E6 gene–transduced (E6) FLS from normal (open bars) and RA (solid bars) synovium. $*$ = $P < 0.05$ versus PS and versus pLXSN. hpf = high-power field (see Figure 1 for other definitions).

Transduction of RA FLS with the HPV-18 E6 gene resulted in a significantly higher invasiveness, with the invasion score increasing to 3.1 ± 0.3 ($P < 0.05$ versus parental, nontransduced FLS and versus pLXSN mock-transduced FLS). As can be seen in Figure 1C, E6-transduced RA FLS deeply invaded the coimplanted cartilage, reshaping the cartilage surface. An intriguing finding is that normal FLS that had been transduced with E6 also exhibited a clear invasion (Figure 1F). E6-transduced normal FLS invaded the coimplanted cartilage to a similar degree as the parental and mock-transduced RA FLS (mean ± SEM invasion score 2.4 ± 0.4). A comparison of the invasion scores is shown in Figure 2A.

Perichondrocytic degradation. Comparison of the perichondrocytic degradation revealed significant differences between the parental, nontransduced RA FLS and the normal FLS, as previously described (mean ± SEM score 1.8 ± 0.2 versus 0.7 ± 0.1; $P <$ 0.05). As with the mock vector, transduction with the HPV-18 E6 gene had no significant effects on the perichondrocytic matrix degradation (data not shown).

Cellularity. Although the same number of cells were implanted in all experiments, transduction with the E6 gene had a significant impact on the on the number of cells invading the cartilage (Figure 2B). Basal cellularity was higher in the RA FLS than in the nontransduced FLS (mean ± SEM 77 ± 3 versus 40 ± 2 cells/hpf), and transduction of either cell type with the mock vector did not result in any appreciable changes (73 ± 7 versus 37 ± 3 cells/hpf). However, inhibition of p53 resulted in a marked increase in the number and density of the cells, both in RA FLS and normal FLS implants. In the E6-transduced RA FLS, the number of cells increased to a mean of 102 ± 3 per hpf ($P = 0.07$), whereas the number of cells reached a mean of 65 ± 6 per hpf ($P < 0.05$) in the E6-transduced normal FLS.

DISCUSSION

Several lines of evidence suggest that synovial fibroblasts in the lining layer of the inflamed and hypertrophic synovium are involved in the progressive destruction of articular cartilage in RA. Apart from showing morphologic alterations, RA FLS display features of activation that distinguish them from normal and osteoarthritis synovial fibroblasts. These involve the up-regulation of proto-oncogenes as well as the pathologic expression of adhesion molecules and matrix-degrading enzymes. In addition, recent data indicate that alterations in apoptosis represent a major consequence of cellular activation in RA FLS. Although DNA strand breaks appear to be common in the RA synovium (6), only a few cells exhibit morphologic evidence of completed apoptosis (9). In addition, recent data have shown the up-regulation of antiapoptotic molecules, such as sentrin, in RA FLS (20). However, the question of how the impaired apoptosis in RA FLS is linked to the aggressive behavior of these cells at a molecular level has not yet been answered.

Recently, the p53 tumor suppressor gene has been implicated as a key regulator of cellular activation. Not only do mutations of p53 increase the invasiveness and metastatic properties of several cancers, but alterations in the p53 gene also affect apoptosis. Therefore, the observation that somatic mutations of p53 are also found in RA synovial fibroblasts is of particular interest. Although relevant mutations appear to be present in only a subset of patients with RA (21), a dominant-negative effect on the wild-type p53 has been reported (12). It has been suggested that environmental factors, such as nitric oxide, result in somatic mutations in regulatory genes, such as p53, which in turn, enhance the activated state of RA FLS. Interestingly, p53 has been shown to be a universal sensor of genotoxic stress (22), and recent in vitro data have strengthened this idea by demonstrating that p53 regulates cell proliferation, apoptosis, and degradation of the cartilage-like matrix (13).

In this study, we investigated whether inhibition of p53 affects the behavior of RA and normal FLS under in vivo conditions. For this purpose, the SCID mouse coimplantation model of RA was used. In this model, FLS are implanted together with normal human cartilage under the renal capsule of SCID mice and maintained for 60 days. Since these mice lack a functional immune system, the implants are not rejected, thus allowing for the investigation of cartilage destruction by the implanted FLS (19). The feasibility of the SCID mouse model for studying the specific properties of FLS in the absence of human inflammatory cells as well as for analyzing the effect of gene transfer approaches has been shown in several studies (23–25). For the inhibition of p53, we used a gene transfer approach that has been shown to be highly effective (13).

In our experiments, transduction of FLS with the HPV-18 E6 gene resulted in a significantly increased invasiveness into the coimplanted cartilage. This is consistent with previous data from studies of different malignancies that have linked the loss of p53 function to the invasiveness of tumors (5,26,27). Nontransduced RA FLS exhibited significant invasion in the absence of relevant p53 mutations, and the invasiveness was comparable to that seen in previous studies (19,24). Although p53-mutated RA FLS were not tested in our study, one could speculate that mutations as described in some studies (10–12) would enhance the destructive potential of these cells. However, this would be critically dependent on the effects such mutations have on the activation and action of p53. Specifically, one could anticipate that mutations exerting dominant-negative effects (12) would result in a more invasive phenotype.

Our method for detecting p53 mutations in the synoviocytes cannot exclude the possibility that a small subset (<5%) of cells have mutations and account for the increased invasiveness of RA FLS in this model. Our data may therefore also indicate that p53-independent pathways contribute significantly to the basal activation of RA FLS. On the other hand, it is of interest that inhibition of p53 through gene transfer with the E6 gene not only increased the invasiveness of RA FLS, but also transformed normal FLS into exhibiting an aggressive behavior. Notably, the grade of invasion resembled that of the parental and mock-transduced RA FLS, and the implants containing E6-transduced normal FLS were nearly indistinguishable from those with parental RA FLS at histologic examination. The invasiveness of the E6-transduced normal FLS, however, did not reach the level of the E6-transduced RA FLS.

This leads to the conclusion that inhibition of p53 may be sufficient for turning normal synovial cells into aggressive cells, but it may constitute only part of the mechanism of cellular activation in RA. Rather, it can be hypothesized that the pattern of cellular changes differ within the RA synovium. While initial events may not include the inactivation of p53, environmental factors, such as cytokine-mediated increases in nitric oxide, may become a major trigger at later stages of disease. Such mutations would then not only enhance the activation in already altered RA FLS, but also potentially transform normal cells. This could provide an explanation for the diversity of findings related to the activated phenotype of cells seen in some studies. It may be speculated that inhibition of p53 could result in an aggressive behavior by other, nonsynovial fibroblasts as well. However, whether or not such changes would lead to an invasive destruction of articular cartilage cannot be answered at this point.

Inhibition of p53 through the E6 protein also had significant effects on the cellularity at sites of cartilage destruction. This was seen both in RA and normal FLS, with the effects, again, being more pronounced in the RA FLS. The question of whether this is caused primarily by an increase in cell growth or by altered apoptosis is difficult to assess from these experiments. Although in vitro data suggest that p53 controls both proliferation and programmed cell death, several studies have demonstrated a low rate of proliferation among synovial fibroblasts in vivo (28,29). In contrast, growing evidence suggests that altered apoptosis contributes to the synovial hyperplasia in RA. In the context of the present data, the finding of increased expression of sentrin in RA FLS is of interest (20). Recent data suggest that UBC9, a member of the ubiquitin conjugation enzyme family that conjugates sentrin, also interacts with p53 (30,31). Therefore, it appears that the loss of p53 function may also be associated with alterations in the sentrin pathway, which prevents cells from undergoing apoptosis.

In summary, p53 appears to constitute a key regulator of the invasive potential and growth in synovial fibroblasts. Dominant-negative mutations in the p53 gene that are caused by environmental factors in the inflamed synovium, therefore, may contribute to the pathogenesis of RA by enhancing the destructive potential of altered RA FLS, extending the lifespan of these cells and inducing transformation in normal FLS.

ACKNOWLEDGMENTS

The authors wish to thank Elvira Walder-Jeisy and Ferenc Pataky for their technical assistance.

REFERENCES

1. Lane DP. Cancer: p53, guardian of the genome. Nature 1992;358: 15–6.
2. Hollstein M, Sidransky D, Vogelstein B, Harris CC. p53 mutations in human cancers. Science 1991;253:49–53.
3. Bártek J, Bártková J, Vojtesek B, Stasková Z, Lukás J, Rejthar A, et al. Aberrant expression of the p53 oncoprotein is a common feature of a wide spectrum of human malignancies. Oncogene 1991;6:1699–703.
4. Hsiao M, Low J, Dorn E, Ku D, Pattengale P, Yeargin J, et al. Gain-of-function mutations of the p53 gene induce lymphohematopoietic metastatic potential and tissue invasiveness. Am J Pathol 1994;145:702–14.
5. Marchetti A, Buttitta F, Pellegrini S, Campani D, Diella F, Cecchetti D, et al. p53 mutations and histological type of invasive breast carcinoma. Cancer Res 1993;53:4665–9.
6. Firestein GS, Yeo M, Zvaifler NJ. Apoptosis in rheumatoid arthritis synovium. J Clin Invest 1995;96:1631–8.
7. Firestein GS, Nguyen K, Aupperle KR, Yeo M, Boyle DL, Zvaifler NJ. Apoptosis in rheumatoid arthritis: p53 overexpression in rheumatoid arthritis synovium. Am J Pathol 1996;149:2143–51.
8. Nakajima T, Aono H, Hasunuma T, Yamamoto K, Shirai T, Hirohata K, et al. Apoptosis and functional Fas antigen in rheumatoid arthritis synoviocytes. Arthritis Rheum 1995;38: 485–91.
9. Matsumoto S, Müller-Ladner U, Gay RE, Nishioka K, Gay S. Ultrastructural demonstration of apoptosis, Fas and Bcl-2 expression of rheumatoid synovial fibroblasts. J Rheumatol 1996;23: 1345–52.
10. Firestein GS, Echeverri F, Yeo M, Zvaifler NJ, Green DR. Somatic mutations in the p53 tumor suppressor gene in rheumatoid arthritis synovium. Proc Natl Acad Sci U S A 1997;94: 10895–900.
11. Rème T, Travaglio A, Gueydon E, Adla L, Jorgensen C, Sany J. Mutations of the p53 tumour suppressor gene in erosive rheumatoid synovial tissue. Clin Exp Immunol 1998;111:353–8.
12. Han Z, Boyle DL, Shi Y, Green DR, Firestein GS. Dominant-negative p53 mutations in rheumatoid arthritis. Arthritis Rheum 1999;42:1088–92.
13. Aupperle KR, Boyle DL, Hendrix M, Seftor EA, Zvaifler NJ, Barbosa M, et al. Regulation of synoviocyte proliferation, apoptosis, and invasion by the p53 tumor suppressor gene. Am J Pathol 1998;152:1091–8.
14. Pim D, Storey A, Thomas M, Massimi P, Banks L. Mutational analysis of HPV-18 E6 identifies domains required for p53 degradation in vitro, abolition of p53 transactivation in vivo and immortalisation of primary BMK cells. Oncogene 1994;9:1869–76.
15. Band V, de Caprio JA, Delmolino L, Kulesa V, Sager R. Loss of p53 protein in human papillomavirus type 16 E6-immortalized human mammary epithelial cells. J Virol 1991;65:6671–6.
16. Scheffner M, Werness BA, Huibregtse JM, Levine AJ, Howley PM. The E6 oncoprotein encoded by human papillomavirus types 16 and 18 promotes the degradation of p53. Cell 1990;63:1129–36.
17. Arnett FC, Edworthy SM, Bloch DA, McShane DJ, Fries JF, Cooper NS, et al. The American Rheumatism Association 1987 revised criteria for the classification of rheumatoid arthritis. Arthritis Rheum 1988;31:315–24.
18. Miller AD, Bender MA, Harris EA, Kaleko M, Gelinas RE. Design of retrovirus vectors for transfer and expression of the human beta-globin gene. J Virol 1988;62:4337–45.
19. Müller-Ladner U, Kriegsmann J, Franklin BN, Matsumoto S, Geiler T, Gay RE, et al. Synovial fibroblasts of patients with rheumatoid arthritis attach to and invade normal human cartilage when engrafted into SCID mice. Am J Pathol 1996;149:1607–15.
20. Franz JK, Pap T, Hummel KM, Nawrath M, Aicher WK, Shigeyama Y, et al. Expression of sentrin, a novel antiapoptotic molecule, at sites of synovial invasion in rheumatoid arthritis. Arthritis Rheum 2000;43:599–607.
21. Kullmann F, Judex M, Neudecker I, Lechner S, Jüsten HP, Green DR, et al. Analysis of the p53 tumor suppressor gene in rheumatoid arthritis synovial fibroblasts. Arthritis Rheum 1999;42: 1594–600.
22. Liu ZG, Baskaran R, Lea-Chou ET, Wood LD, Chen Y, Karin M, et al. Three distinct signalling responses by murine fibroblasts to genotoxic stress. Nature 1996;384:273–6.
23. Jorgensen C, Gay S. Gene therapy in osteoarticular diseases: where are we? Immunol Today 1998;19:387–91.
24. Müller-Ladner U, Roberts CR, Franklin BN, Gay RE, Robbins PD, Evans CH, et al. Human IL-1Ra gene transfer into human synovial fibroblasts is chondroprotective. J Immunol 1997;158: 3492–8.
25. Müller-Ladner U, Evans CH, Franklin BN, Roberts CR, Gay RE, Robbins PD, et al. Gene transfer of cytokine inhibitors into human synovial fibroblasts in the SCID mouse model. Arthritis Rheum 1999;42:490–7.
26. Campbell C, Quinn AG, Ro YS, Angus B, Rees JL. p53 mutations are common and early events that precede tumor invasion in squamous cell neoplasia of the skin. J Invest Dermatol 1993;100: 746–8.
27. Kovach JS, Hartmann A, Blaszyk H, Cunningham J, Schaid D, Sommer SS. Mutation detection by highly sensitive methods indicates that p53 gene mutations in breast cancer can have important prognostic value. Proc Natl Acad Sci U S A 1996;93: 1093–6.
28. Aicher WK, Heer AH, Trabandt A, Bridges SLJ, Schroeder HWJ, Stransky G, et al. Overexpression of zinc-finger transcription factor Z-225/Egr-1 in synoviocytes from rheumatoid arthritis patients. J Immunol 1994;152:5940–8.
29. Nykänen P, Bergroth V, Raunio P, Nordström D, Konttinen YT. Phenotypic characterization of ^{3}H-thymidine incorporating cells in rheumatoid arthritis synovial membrane. Rheumatol Int 1986;6: 269–71.
30. Liu Q, Jin C, Liao X, Shen Z, Chen DJ, Chen Y. The binding interface between an E2 (UBC9) and a ubiquitin homologue (UBL1). J Biol Chem 1999;274:16979–87.
31. Shen Z, Pardington-Purtymun PE, Comeaux JC, Moyzis RK, Chen DJ. Associations of UBE2I with RAD52, UBL1, p53, and RAD51 proteins in a yeast two-hybrid system. Genomics 1996;37: 183–6.

ARTHRITIS & RHEUMATISM
Vol. 44, No. 3, March 2001, pp 682–692

Variations in Susceptibility to Proteoglycan-Induced Arthritis and Spondylitis Among C3H Substrains of Mice

Evidence of Genetically Acquired Resistance to Autoimmune Disease

Tibor T. Glant,[1] Tamás Bárdos,[1] Csaba Vermes,[2] Raman Chandrasekaran,[1] Juan C. Valdéz,[1] Jeffrey M. Otto,[1] David Gerard,[1] Sonja Velins,[1] György Lovász,[2] Jian Zhang,[1] Katalin Mikecz,[1] and Alison Finnegan[1]

Objective. **To identify and screen the level of arthritis susceptibility in C3H murine strains known to be resistant to proteoglycan (aggrecan)–induced arthritis, and to measure and correlate various immunologic and inflammatory parameters with susceptibility to either arthritis or spondylitis in various C3H substrains.**

Methods. **Mice of 10 C3H substrains (subcolonies) were immunized with cartilage proteoglycan (aggrecan) for induction of arthritis. Animals were assessed for clinical symptoms, and the peripheral joints and spine were studied by histologic methods. Proteoglycan-specific T cell responses (T cell proliferation and production of interleukin-2 [IL-2], interferon-γ, and IL-4) and the B cell response to lipopolysaccharide (LPS) were measured in spleen cell cultures. Serum levels of heteroantibodies and autoantibodies as well as various cytokines (IL-6, IL-10, IL-12, and tumor necrosis factor α) and soluble CD44 were determined by enzyme-linked immunosorbent assay.**

Results. **Immunization with cartilage proteoglycan induced severe arthritis in the C3H/HeJCr substrain (95–100% incidence), whereas the original parent mice of the C3H/HeJ colony were resistant to proteoglycan (aggrecan)–induced arthritis. Furthermore, the progressive polyarthritis that is characteristic in susceptible C3H/HeJCr mice was accompanied by progressive inflammation around the spine. In subsequent experiments, 10 different C3H colonies with largely identical genetic backgrounds (all originating from the National Institutes of Health or Jackson Laboratory) exhibited extreme differences in susceptibility. Although none of the laboratory findings, including LPS hyporesponsiveness, immunologic parameters, and inflammatory markers, showed a correlation with susceptibility or resistance in the C3H/HeJCr and C3H/HeJ substrains, respectively, significant differences were found when all arthritic C3H mice were compared with all nonarthritic animals, regardless of their substrain origin.**

Conclusion. **Because many of the C3H substrains lost arthritis susceptibility or acquired resistance, our results suggest that a preferred site for a mutation(s) in a gene(s) in a relatively upstream position of the inflammatory cascade is present. This is the first autoimmune model that exhibits extreme differences in arthritis susceptibility in the same murine strain, and is therefore a valuable tool for identification of arthritis-susceptible (or arthritis-suppressive) genes.**

Immunization of BALB/c mice with deglycosylated human or canine cartilage proteoglycan (PG) induces progressive polyarthritis (1–5). To date, no other mouse strain or other laboratory animal species, such as rat, hamster, guinea pig, rabbit, and dog, have

Supported by NIH grants AR-40310 and AR-45652.

[1]Tibor T. Glant, MD, PhD, Tamás Bárdos, MD, Raman Chandrasekaran, PhD, Juan C. Valdéz, PhD, Jeffrey M. Otto, PhD, David Gerard, BS, Sonja Velins, MS, Jian Zhang, MD, Katalin Mikecz, MD, PhD, Alison Finnegan, PhD: Rush University at Rush–Presbyterian–St. Luke's Medical Center, Chicago, Illinois; [2]Csaba Vermes, MD, György Lovász, MD: University of Medicine, Pécs, Hungary.

Address correspondence and reprint requests to Tibor T. Glant, MD, PhD, Department of Orthopedic Surgery, Rush–Presbyterian–St. Luke's Medical Center, 1653 West Congress Parkway, Chicago, IL 60612.

Submitted for publication July 27, 2000; accepted in revised form October 23, 2000.

been found to be susceptible to PG (aggrecan)–induced arthritis (PGIA). Cartilage PGs from other species (e.g., sheep or bovine) are either nonarthritogenic or induce only a very mild, transient synovitis in susceptible BALB/c mice (2,6). PGIA has many similarities to rheumatoid arthritis, as indicated by clinical assessments and histopathologic studies (1,3,7). During the course of arthritis, progressively more joints are affected, and repeated inflammatory episodes result in complete deterioration of the articular cartilage and bone erosion with severe deformations of the peripheral joints (1,2,8,9). Arthritis development is based on cross-reactive immune responses between the immunizing heterologous and autologous (mouse) PGs (2,5,7,10).

Recently, genome scan studies were performed to identify susceptibility-conferring loci in PGIA (11–14). For these studies, mice were obtained from the National Cancer Institute (NCI; Frederick, MD) instead of the Jackson (Bar Harbor, ME) or Charles River (Wilmington, MA) Laboratories, from which mice had been purchased for previous experiments (3,7,8). PGIA-susceptible BALB/c female mice were mated with either major histocompatibility complex (MHC)–matched ($H\text{-}2^d$) DBA/2 male mice or MHC-unmatched C57BL/6, C3H, and DBA/1 male mice ($H\text{-}2^b$, $H\text{-}2^k$, and $H\text{-}2^q$, respectively). Depending on the parent strains, 10–28% of the F_2 hybrid mice developed PGIA, as described earlier (2,3,13,14). However, the incidence of PGIA in (BALB/c × C3H [NCI])F_2 hybrids was 54%. Since BALB/c mice of the NCI colony have been used in previous studies (7), the C3H/HeJCr background may be responsible for the high arthritis incidence in (BALB/c × C3H)F_2 hybrids. To confirm the findings in our earlier studies (3,7,8,13) and reproduce current observations (12,14), we immunized C3H mice of different colonies. We were intrigued to find that while the C3H/HeJ colony (from Jackson Laboratory) was essentially resistant to arthritis, the C3H/HeJCr colony (from NCI) was 95–100% susceptible.

The finding of a new strain whose PGIA susceptibility and histopathology are comparable with those in BALB/c mice, and especially the unique observation that 2 C3H sublines/colonies with the same genetic origin exhibit extreme differences in disease susceptibility, initiated a series of studies that are summarized herein. Arthritis-susceptible and -resistant C3H mice can provide a powerful tool for identification of disease-associated genes in a largely identical genetic background. We believe that a very few genes, or gene clusters, govern the critical traits that confer either susceptibility or resistance to arthritis in C3H mice. Herein we describe the newly discovered phenomenon of PGIA in C3H mice and compare different C3H colonies with respect to their disease susceptibility as well as various markers of PG immunity and inflammation. The first genome scan using F_2 hybrids of susceptible C3H/HeJCr and resistant C57BL/6 strains has already identified 4 new quantitative trait loci (*Pgia* 12–15) associated with arthritis susceptibility (12).

MATERIALS AND METHODS

Sources and preparation of cartilage PG (aggrecan). PG from human fetal (27–30 weeks gestation), human adult (26–72 years old), canine (3–12 years old), and bovine (16–18 months of age) articular cartilage was prepared as previously described (5,7,15). Human cartilage samples were obtained from autopsy material within 2–8 hours after death through either the Cooperative Human Tissue Network (Columbus, OH) or the Comprehensive Cancer Center (Birmingham, AL), or were collected from osteoarthritic knee joints removed during joint replacement surgeries. All procedures involving human samples were approved by the Institutional Review Board at Rush–Presbyterian–St. Luke's Medical Center. Bovine articular cartilage was obtained from a local slaughterhouse, canine cartilage was collected from the knee joints of dogs used for surgery training of medical students, and mouse cartilage was obtained from the knee joints of 5–7-day-old BALB/c mice. PG samples were digested with protease-free chondroitinase ABC (Seikagaku America, Rockville, MD) and endo-β-galactosidase (7) to remove glycosaminoglycan side chains, which can interfere with the immune responses to cartilage PG (2,3,5).

Animals and immunization of mice with cartilage PGs. Female BALB/c and C3H mice from various colonies as well as BALB.B and BALB.K congenic mice (all serum antivirus antibody free), weighing 17–18 gm, were purchased from different vendors (listed in Table 3) and maintained in standard (non–germ-free) conditions in the same room. Several sets of experiments were performed and all animals of the different groups and/or colonies were treated identically. Typically, we coordinated all animal arrivals from different vendors within 1 week, and then mice were left for acclimatization for 10–14 days prior to the immunization as approved by the Institutional Animal Care and Use Committee (IACUC). Mice were injected intraperitoneally with 100 μg of cartilage PGs (measured as protein) using a standard immunization method described elsewhere (2,4,7).

Mice were injected intraperitoneally on days 0, 7, 28, and 49. The first and fourth injections were given in Freund's complete adjuvant and the second and third injections were in Freund's incomplete adjuvant. The development of PGIA requires a relatively long period of time and the earliest onset can be noted after the third antigen injection (Table 1). In each comparative study described in this report, mice were injected simultaneously, maintained under identical conditions, and killed at the same time point (as indicated in the Tables and Figures). Based on the IACUC regulation, representative serum samples were tested at the Charles River Laboratory

Table 1. Arthritis susceptibility and immune responses to human cartilage proteoglycan*

	Incidence of arthritis, no./total (%)	Arthritic animals: Highest cumulative score	Arthritic animals: Onset, days	All immunized animals: T cell response (by CTLL-2 assay), SI	All immunized animals: Antibody response, arbitrary units: Hetero-	All immunized animals: Antibody response, arbitrary units: Auto-
NCI-BALB/c	20/21 (95)	9.4 ± 3.9	42 ± 11	1.76 ± 0.58	1.08 ± 0.52	0.96 ± 0.38
NCI-C3H/HeJCr	36/38 (95)	9.3 ± 4.5	63 ± 11†	3.34 ± 1.28‡	3.32 ± 2.35‡	1.99 ± 0.76†
Jackson-C3H/HeJ	3/28 (11)	0.7 ± 1.4‡	89 ± 19‡	3.78 ± 1.13‡	3.10 ± 0.26‡	1.89 ± 0.56†

* Except where otherwise indicated, values are the mean ± SD. Animals were immunized simultaneously with deglycosylated human cartilage proteoglycan in adjuvant. A total of 5 antigen injections were given at 3-week intervals. The highest (maximum) cumulative acute arthritis score measured at any time point of the experiment was used for calculation. Cytotoxic lymphoid line 2 (CTLL-2) assay using spleen cells was performed on week 14 (end of experiment, 2 weeks after the fifth antigen injection). SI = stimulation index; NCI = National Cancer Institute.
† $P < 0.05$ versus control BALB/c mice.
‡ $P < 0.01$ versus control BALB/c mice.

every sixth week for serum antibodies of pathogenic viruses and bacteria.

Clinical and histologic assessments of arthritis. The limbs of all mice were examined daily and abnormalities due to arthritic changes in the joints were documented as described previously (1,4,5). The appearance of joint swelling was recorded as the time (day) of onset of arthritis. The other recorded clinical parameter was joint swelling (ranging from 0 to 4 for each paw), which was expressed as the cumulative acute arthritis score of the 4 limbs of each animal (4,5,16). Thus, maximum swelling in all 4 paws resulted in an arthritis score of 16. Animals were assessed by the same person (either TTG or TB) over the entire experiment, and the observer was blinded to the previous score. For standard histopathologic assessments of arthritis, the paws were fixed, decalcified, embedded in paraffin, sectioned, and stained as described elsewhere (1,7). Sections from other joints (knee, hip, elbow, sacroiliac), the spine, and nonskeletal organs (trachea, lung, ear, eyes, kidney) were examined for microscopic abnormalities.

Measurements of anti-PG immune responses (T cell responses and antibodies), cytokines, and soluble CD44 (sCD44). Antigen (PG)–specific interleukin-2 (IL-2) production was measured by cytotoxic lymphoid line 2 (CTLL-2) bioassay on day 2, and T cell proliferation was determined by direct ^{3}H-thymidine incorporation on day 5 (5,7,10). Splenic lymphocytes (3×10^5 cells/well) were cultured in the absence or presence of PG antigens (100 μg protein/ml) used for immunization. The assays were performed using quadruplicate samples in 96-well plates in the presence of 1.5% fetal calf serum in Dulbecco's modified Eagle's medium as described previously (5,10,17), and 16-hour ^{3}H-thymidine incorporation was measured in both CTLL-2 and lymphocyte proliferation assays. The stimulation index was calculated by dividing the counts per minute in antigen-stimulated cultures by the cpm in nonstimulated cultures.

Serum antibodies were measured by enzyme-linked immunosorbent assay (ELISA) using either the immunizing antigen or native (intact) mouse cartilage PG immobilized in Nunc Maxisorp (Nunc International, Hanover Park, IL) microtitration plates (18). For PG-specific IgG isotype assays, peroxidase-labeled goat anti-mouse IgG1 or IgG2a (Zymed Laboratories, San Francisco, CA) was employed. In each case, results were calculated in arbitrary units, which was the ratio of the serum dilution of the standard (pooled serum from arthritic BALB/c mice; n = 62) to that of the test sample at the same optical density.

Interferon-γ (IFNγ) was determined in the conditioned media of human cartilage PG-stimulated and nonstimulated spleen cell cultures on day 3, and IL-4 was measured in 5-day-old cultures by capture ELISAs (PharMingen, San Diego, CA) (19). IFNγ and IL-4 levels in PG-stimulated cultures were calculated for 1×10^6 cells. Serum IL-1 levels were determined by D10S bioassay using human recombinant IL-1β standard (R&D Systems, Minneapolis, MN) as previously described (13). All other cytokines (tumor necrosis factor α [TNFα], IL-6, IL-10, IL-12) and sCD44 (as a marker of inflammation) were determined by capture ELISAs. Cytokine assay reagents were purchased from PharMingen, and the sCD44 assay was developed in our laboratory (20).

Assays for lipopolysaccharide (LPS) sensitivity. Spleen cells were stimulated with 2 different serotypes of *Escherichia coli* LPS (0127.B8 and 055.B5; both from Sigma, St. Louis, MO) at dilutions ranging from 0.1 to 100 μg/ml. Cells in control wells were stimulated with phorbol myristate acetate (PMA; 50–500 ng/ml) or concanavalin A (1.25–10.0 μg/ml). Sixteen-hour ^{3}H-thymidine incorporation was measured at 36-hour time points, and the results of incorporated radioactivity were expressed as the ratio of cpm of LPS-stimulated cultures to that of nonstimulated cultures. In addition, peritoneal macrophages after 48-hour adherence were stimulated similarly with LPS (0.1–10.0 μg/ml) or with 250 ng/ml PMA, and TNFα production in the macrophages was measured in 24-hour conditioned media by ELISA.

Statistical analysis. Results were analyzed using a two-factor repeated-measures multivariate analysis of variance, and the Pillai's trace criterion was employed to calculate multivariate significance. The Mann-Whitney and Wilcoxon tests and paired Kruskal-Wallis tests were used for intergroup comparisons, with Bonferroni correction. For determination of correlation coefficients, Spearman's rho test was used. All

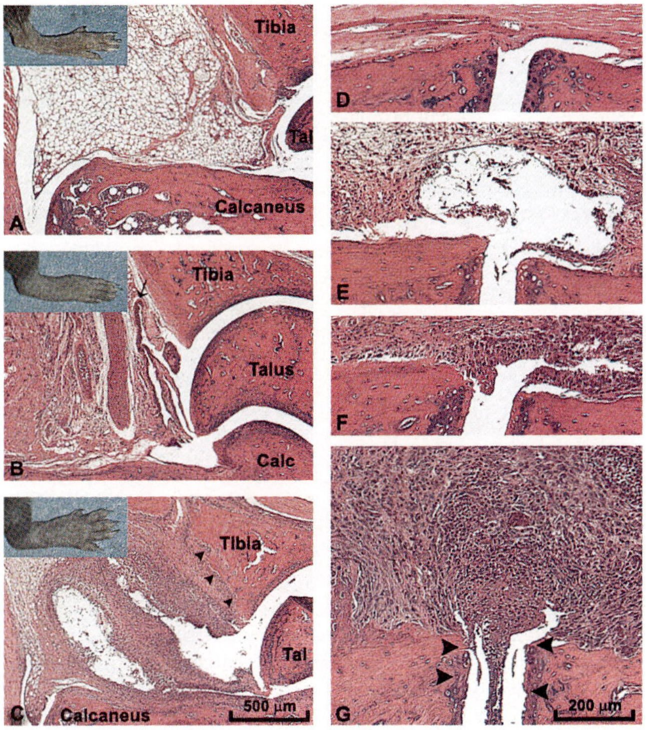

Figure 1. Histopathologic findings in the peripheral joints of resistant C3H/HeJ (**A** and **D**) and susceptible C3H/HeJCr (**B, C,** and **E–G**) mice immunized with cartilage proteoglycan. Ankle joints are shown on the left and tarsal joints on the right. Inserts in **A–C** depict the paws from which the ankle joints were taken. **A** and **D** show normal (noninflamed) joints, **B** and **E** demonstrate early/weak inflammatory reactions in joints with an acute arthritis score of 2, and **C, F,** and **G** are representative of severely inflamed joints (with a score of 4). **Arrowheads** point to bone and cartilage erosions. Calc = calcaneus; Tal = talus. (Stained with hematoxylin and eosin; original magnification × 10 in **A–C;** × 25 in **D–G.**)

statistical analyses were performed using SPSS/PC, version 7.5, statistical software (SPSS, Chicago, IL).

RESULTS

Arthritis susceptibility of C3H mice. Earlier studies concluded that only BALB/c mice were susceptible to PGIA (2,3,13). Susceptibility completely disappeared in the F_1 hybrids of all BALB/c combinations with PGIA-resistant mouse strains (2), whereas it returned in ~15% of the intercross F_2 hybrids (13). An unexpectedly high incidence of PGIA (54%) found in (BALB/c × C3H/HeJCr [NCI])F_2 hybrids (12) compelled us to compare PGIA susceptibility in C3H/HeJ (Jackson Laboratory) and C3H/HeJCr (NCI) mice. Control BALB/c mice exhibited the "usual" response with respect to immune reactions, susceptibility, and severity of PGIA, as previously described (1,2,5,7). Consistent with earlier findings (2,3,13), the Jackson C3H/HeJ mice were resistant to arthritis. In contrast, 95% of the NCI C3H/HeJCr mice developed PGIA (Table 1). Although both C3H sublines were high responders to PG immunization, no significant differences were found in antigen-specific autoantibody or heteroantibody production or in T cell responses between

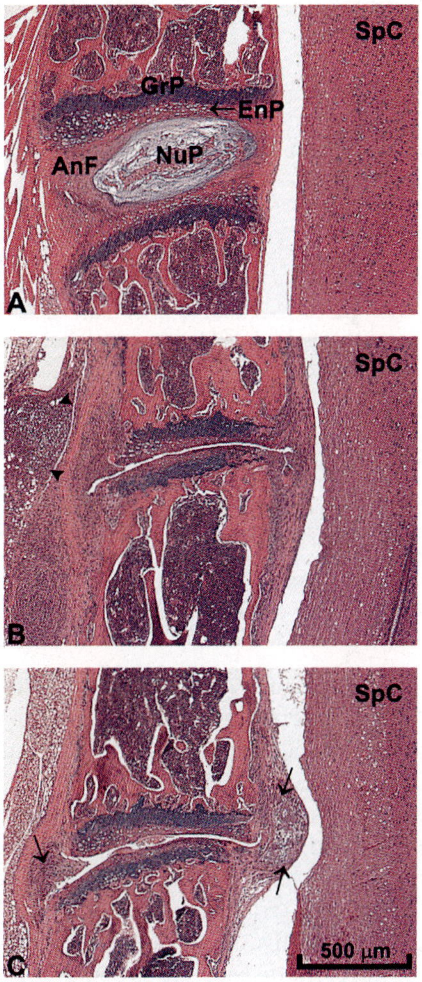

Figure 2. Histopathologic findings in the spine (intervertebral discs) of a C3H/HeJCr mouse. Three intervertebral discs and neighboring vertebra bodies of the lower cervical/upper thoracic region of the same animal are shown. **A,** Morphologically intact (normal C5–C6) intervertebral disc and vertebral bodies. **B,** Completely resorbed intervertebral disc surrounded by an acute inflammatory reaction **(arrowheads)**. In an area 3 discs distal to that shown in **B,** the intervertebral disc is also resorbed and the margins of vertebra bodies are fused **(C)**. This newly formed chondrophyte-like tissue **(arrows)** causes the compression of the spinal cord (SpC). NuP = nucleus pulposus; AnF = annulus fibrosus; EnP = end plate; GrP = growth plate. (Stained with hematoxylin and eosin; original magnification × 10.)

Table 2. Immune responses to cartilage proteoglycans in susceptible BALB/c and C3H/HeJCr strains*

	Incidence of arthritis, no./total (%)	Arthritic animals: Onset, days	Arthritic animals: Highest cumulative score	All immunized animals: T cell response (by CTLL-2 assay), SI†	All immunized animals: Serum antibody response, arbitrary units: Hetero-	All immunized animals: Serum antibody response, arbitrary units: Auto-
BALB/c (Charles River Laboratories, Kingston colony K51, NY)						
HFPG (Chase)	8/8 (100)	49 ± 12	9.5 ± 4.2	2.9 ± 1.4	1.1 ± 0.1	0.97 ± 0.12
HAC (Chase only)	1/8 (12.5)	63	2.0	1.9 ± 1.1	2.8 ± 0.2	0.36 ± 0.13
HAC (Chase + Eβg)	8/8 (100)	52 ± 18	7.9 ± 3.5	2.1 ± 0.8	2.2 ± 0.3	1.01 ± 0.26
DAC (Chase)	8/8 (100)	61 ± 7	9.1 ± 3.5	2.9 ± 0.3	1.8 ± 0.4	0.98 ± 0.18
BAC (Chase)	0/8 (0)	NA	NA	1.8 ± 0.9	1.7 ± 0.3	1.16 ± 0.19
H/B-CII	0/16 (0)	NA	NA	ND	0.8 ± 0.2‡	ND
C3H/HeJCr (National Cancer Institute, Kingston colony, NY)						
HFPG (Chase)	12/12 (100)	62 ± 12	9.2 ± 4.2	2.8 ± 0.9	2.8 ± 0.6	2.11 ± 0.21
HAC (Chase only)	5/12 (42)	84 ± 14	2.7 ± 1.2	3.0 ± 0.7	5.4 ± 2.2	1.92 ± 0.36
HAC (Chase + Eβg)	15/16 (94)	58 ± 9	7.6 ± 1.4	3.2 ± 1.7	4.1 ± 1.9	2.03 ± 0.18
DAC (Chase)	6/18 (33)	75 ± 16	4.5 ± 0.7	3.6 ± 1.5	5.2 ± 0.7	1.65 ± 0.27
BAC (Chase)	7/18 (39)	86 ± 15	3.2 ± 0.9	3.9 ± 1.8	4.9 ± 0.9	0.92 ± 0.18
H/B-CII	0/24 (0)	NA	NA	ND	1.1 ± 0.2‡	ND

* Except where otherwise indicated, values are the mean ± SD. All mice were immunized and tests performed simultaneously. All cartilage proteoglycans were digested with chondroitinase ABC (Chase) and, when indicated, with endo-β-galactosidase (Eβg), to remove chondroitin sulfate and keratan sulfate side chains. Animals were immunized by standard protocols, except that mice that remained nonarthritic 3 weeks after the fourth antigen injection received a fifth injection of the same antigen in Freund's complete adjuvant. Animals were killed on weeks 13–14 of the experiment. The cumulative score shows the maximum score of acute arthritic animals measured at any time during the experiment. Immunization with type II collagen from human or bovine cartilage showed the same results, and was thus combined (H/B-CII). Phosphate buffered saline and adjuvant controls were negative for all parameters in both groups (data not shown). Source of antigen: HFPG = human fetal cartilage proteoglycan; HAC = human adult articular cartilage (proteoglycan); DAC = dog articular cartilage (proteoglycan); BAC = bovine articular cartilage (proteoglycan). NA = not applicable (no arthritis detected); ND = not determined (see Table 1 for other definitions).

† Immunization antigens (100 μg protein/ml) were used for the CTLL-2 (interleukin-2) assays.

‡ Arbitrary units of anti–type II collagen were calculated in a similar manner as that for anti-proteoglycan, using pooled arthritic sera of mice with collagen-induced arthritis.

the arthritis-susceptible and -resistant C3H sublines (Table 1). These observations indicate that the (auto)immune responses of the 2 C3H sublines were independent of their susceptibility to PGIA.

Histopathologic findings in the peripheral joints. Animals were killed on week 14 of immunization and the paws, spine, and other organs, including the hip and sacroiliac joints, ribs, trachea/lung, ears, eyes, and kidneys, were examined histologically. At this time point, a full range of different disease states could be observed in the various joints of the arthritic animals. Joints of clinically negative (noninflamed) paws were also found to be negative histologically (Figures 1A and D), and nonskeletal tissues showed normal morphology in all C3H mice (data not shown).

As in BALB/c mice, the first clinical symptoms of PGIA (paw swelling and redness) in C3H/HeJCr mice were associated with early mononuclear leukocyte infiltration and tissue edema, accompanied and/or followed by polymorphonuclear cell accumulation in the joint cavities (Figures 1B and E). In joints with more advanced arthritis, there was a progressive proliferation of synovial macrophage- and fibroblast-like cells, which was still accompanied by both lymphocyte and polymorphonuclear cell infiltration (Figures 1F and G). Joints in the subacute phase became deformed and this was accompanied by massive cartilage (Figure 1G) and bone (Figures 1C and G) erosions.

Histopathologic findings in the spine. Along with the routine histopathologic screening of various organs and joints, we frequently noted inflammatory reactions around the intervertebral discs of the spine in C3H/HeJCr mice. Almost all mice of the susceptible C3H/HeJCr colony exhibited spondylitis that was localized in 1 or several intervertebral discs (Figure 2), irrespective of the severity of peripheral arthritis. In contrast, no inflammation was found around the spine tissues of any of the resistant C3H/HeJ mice. Similar to that described in the peripheral joints (Figure 1), there were large individual variations in spine involvement, and fre-

Table 3. List and origin of C3H substrains, showing both congenic and inbred mice*

Strains/colonies	Vendor	Year established (generation)	Origin and major known characteristics of the current substrain (ref.)
1. **C3H/HeJCr†‡**	NCI	1967 (unk)	From the Jackson Laboratory as C3H/HeJ (Heston, 1947); carries point mutation(s) in *Tlr-4* (*Lps*) gene (responsible for LPS sensitivity); MTV+ and the strain carries the *rd/rd* gene.
2. C3H/HeNCrlBR	CRL	1974 (unk)	From the NIH as C3H/HeN (21).
3. **C3H/HeOuJ**	Jackson	1981 (F_{93})	Subline; established from C3H/HeJ (1952) before the *Tlr-4* mutation occurred and returned to the Jackson Laboratory from Outzen et al in 1981 (22,23); homozygous for normal *Lps* allele; F_{144} was in 1995.
4. **C3HeB/FeJ**	Jackson	1950 (F_3)	Subline selected for MTV resistance; established by Hummel et al in 1948 by transferring fertilized egg of C3H/HeJ to C57BL/6 and then maintained by the Jackson Laboratory from 1950 (23,24); F_{166} generation was in 1995.
5. C3H/HeNCr-MTV+	NCI	1998 (unk)	Subline from the NIH; annually tested for 14 genetic markers and reciprocal skin graft; MTV+.§
6. C3H/HeNCr-MTV−	NCI	1998 (unk)	Subline from NIH (MTV−); Cesarian-derived C3H/HeN newborns were suckled by a C57BL/6 MTV− foster mother.§
7. C3H/HeNHsd	Harlan	1978 (unk)	From the NIH (MTV−).
8. C3H/HeNTac	Taconic	1987 (F_{147})	From the NIH (MTV−).
9. C3H/BiDACr	NCI	1985 (unk)	Established by Clide J. Dawe at the NCI from a C3H/Bi (Bittner, 1931) subline; highly susceptible to MTV infection but resistant to MTV provirus.§
10. **C3H/HeJ†‡**	Jackson	1947 (F_{48})	LPS hyporesponsive due to Lps^d mutation in the cytoplasmic domain of *Tlr-4* (21,23); MTV+ and carries the *rd/rd* gene as the parent C3H/HeJ line (group 1); F_{223} generation was in 1995.
11. BALB.B-UK	Harlan		Congenic; parent lines: Jackson's BALB/cJ × C57BL/10Sn (25).
12. BALB.K-UK‡	Harlan		Congenic; parent lines: Jackson's BALB/cJ × AKR (26).
13. BALB/c†‡	CRL or NCI		Both sublines have BALB/cAnN origin received from the NIH; NIH from Andover (An) in 1951.

* Note that the C3H/HeJ, C3H/HeJCr, C3H/HeOuJ, and C3HeB/FeJ sublines (all shown in boldface) have a common origin. These lines were established before (groups 3 and 4) or after (group 1) the mutation occurred in the *Tlr-4* gene. Vendors include the National Cancer Institute (NCI; Frederick, MD), Charles River Laboratory (CRL; Kingston colonies; Wilmington, MA), Jackson Laboratory (Bar Harbor, ME), Harlan-Sprague Dawley (Indianapolis, IN; UK indicates that congenic mice were purchased from Harlan UK Limited, Blackthorn, England), and Taconic Laboratory Animals (Germantown, NY). unk = generation number is unknown; *Tlr-4* = toll-like receptor 4; LPS = lipopolysaccharide; MTV+/− = highly susceptible/resistant to mammary tumor virus infection; *rd/rd* = retinal degeneration; NIH = National Institutes of Health.
† Colonies used in repeated experiments (see Tables 1 and 2).
‡ A colony used in the companion study (12) or in earlier studies for proteoglycan-induced arthritis (2,3,13).
§ Information was collected from the references listed in the review by Beck et al (27) and from additional references (23,28,29). Additional information was obtained from C. Reeder at NCI, from the technical services of animal laboratories, and through the Web site http://www.informatics.jax.org.

quently, intervertebral discs of the same animal showed various stages of inflammation, cartilage, and bone resorption, with or without osteophyte formation (Figure 2). Typically, 3–5 weeks after the onset of arthritis in the peripheral joints, 1 or 2 intervertebral discs of the lower cervical/upper thoracic region, and frequently in the lumbar region, showed resorption of the annulus fibrosus and nucleus pulposus due to a massive inflammation around the disc (Figure 2B), and the immediate proximal or distal discs were either intact (Figure 2A) or completely resorbed (Figure 2C).

Recognition and arthritogenicity of cartilage PGs in C3H mice. Fetal, newborn, and adult cartilage PGs of 11 species were tested for arthritis induction, and only human and canine PGs induced arthritis in BALB/c mice (1–3,6). Since BALB/c and C3H strains carry different MHC haplotypes (H-2^d and H-2^k, respectively), we hypothesized that the epitope recognition and arthritogenicity of cartilage PGs might be different in the 2 mouse strains. Therefore, susceptible BALB/c and C3H/HeJCr mice (both from the Kingston colonies of the NCI) were immunized with different cartilage PGs, and the incidence of PGIA, antibody production, and T cell responses using various PGs were compared.

As expected, human fetal and adult cartilage PGs, depleted of glycosaminoglycans, induced arthritis with 100% incidence in both BALB/c and C3H/HeJCr mice. Although the incidence and severity of PGIA were highly comparable in BALB/c and C3H/HeJCr mice, the C3H mice demonstrated significantly higher T cell responses and serum antibody levels, with significantly delayed disease onset (Tables 1 and 2). Unlike in BALB/c mice (2,5), partially deglycosylated (keratan sulfate–containing) human adult or bovine cartilage PGs

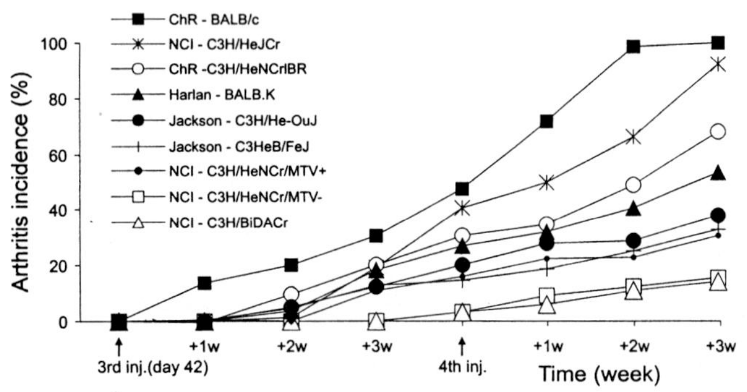

Figure 3. Progression of acute inflammation in various murine (sub-) strains after the third antigen (proteoglycan) injection (inj.). Animals were immunized identically with deglycosylated human cartilage proteoglycan. The incidence of arthritis in the immunized groups is shown on a weekly timescale. Standard deviation is omitted for clarity, and results for the negative congenic BALB.B mice and groups with a cumulative acute arthritis score <1.0 (C3H colonies from Harlan and Taconic, and Jackson Laboratory's C3H/HeJ mice) are not shown. ChR = Charles River Laboratory; NCI = National Cancer Institute; MTV = mammary tumor virus.

did induce arthritis in C3H mice. However, arthritis induced by immunization with canine PG resulted in significantly lower incidence (33%; $P < 0.01$) in C3H/HeJCr mice than in BALB/c mice (Table 2). These observations suggest that beyond a partially different pattern of epitope recognition, other genetic factors may control the onset and incidence of PGIA in susceptible BALB/c and C3H mice.

Comparative studies on different C3H sublines and colonies. To determine whether there was a distinct pattern of PGIA susceptibility in the 2 C3H/HeJ sublines (Table 1), C3H mice of 10 different colonies, purchased from 5 different vendors (Table 3), were identically immunized with deglycosylated human cartilage PG. Inbred BALB/c (PGIA-susceptible) and congenic BALB.B and BALB.K strains served as controls. Approximately 40% of BALB/c mice developed arthritis soon after the third PG injection, and 100% after the fourth injection (Figure 3). At each time point of immunization, C3H sublines showed a lower incidence of arthritis (Figure 3) and less severe disease (data not shown) than did BALB/c mice.

The differences among C3H colonies became evident after the fourth injection: mice from 3 colonies (the Harlan and Taconic C3H/HeN and the Jackson Laboratory C3H/HeJ mice) were essentially resistant, while 2 substrains (the NCI C3H/HeNCr-MTV− and NCI C3H/BiDACr mice) exhibited low arthritis scores, but slightly higher disease incidence (Figure 4A). Importantly, mice of 5 C3H colonies (groups 1–5 in Table 3 and Figure 4) demonstrated high arthritis susceptibility and severity that was comparable with that seen in BALB/c mice (groups 1–5 versus group 13 in Figure 4A). Most of the BALB.K mice (70% [44 of 63]; group 12 in Figure 4A) developed arthritis with a relatively low arthritis score (mean ± SD 1.8 ± 1.9), but none of the 29 immunized animals of the BALB.B strain (group 11 in Figure 4A) showed any symptoms of inflammation. These results demonstrate a mixed pattern of resistance and susceptibility to PGIA in various C3H sublines.

Antigen-specific in vitro T cell responses and production of cytokines, as well as serum levels of anti-PG antibodies, proinflammatory cytokines, and sCD44 (used as an inflammation marker) were examined in the 10 C3H substrains/colonies and in the control groups (Figures 4B and C). All animals were killed 4 weeks after the fourth injection, and the various immune and inflammatory parameters were measured simultaneously. Finally, animals were grouped according to disease status, i.e., in the order of descending clinical score (Figure 4A), and the results were reanalyzed for correlations. Comparisons among the 10 different C3H substrains demonstrated positive correlations between antigen-specific IL-2 production (by CTLL-2 assay) and T cell proliferation ($P < 0.0$, $\sigma = 0.449$), between T cell responses (by CTLL-2 assay and proliferation) and sCD44 levels ($P < 0.001$, $\sigma = 0.492$–0.565), and, except for the C3H/BiDACr subline, between the heteroantibody (immunizing) and autoantibody (mouse) anti-PG (both IgG1 and IgG2a) levels ($P < 0.02$–0.001, $\sigma = 0.246$–0.627).

Although the C3H substrains exhibited differences in PG-specific antibody production as well as in T cell responses and cytokine levels (Figures 4B and C), we were unable to detect a consistent correlation between any of the measured parameters and arthritis susceptibility. However, IL-4 levels in PG-stimulated T cell cultures were significantly lower in the 5 most susceptible C3H colonies (groups 1–5) than in the rest of the C3H mice (Figure 4C), but this did not correlate with the production of IFNγ (Figure 4C) measured in the same culture media. In addition, serum IL-6 and sCD44 levels were significantly higher in the 5 most PGIA-susceptible sublines than in the other 5 groups of C3H mice (Figure 4C), but neither the serum IL-10 nor the serum IL-12 levels showed a similar correlation (data not shown).

Because neither susceptibility in the C3H/HeJCr mice nor resistance to PGIA in the C3H/HeJ subline showed an evident correlation with the disease-related markers (group 1 versus group 10 in Figure 4), addi-

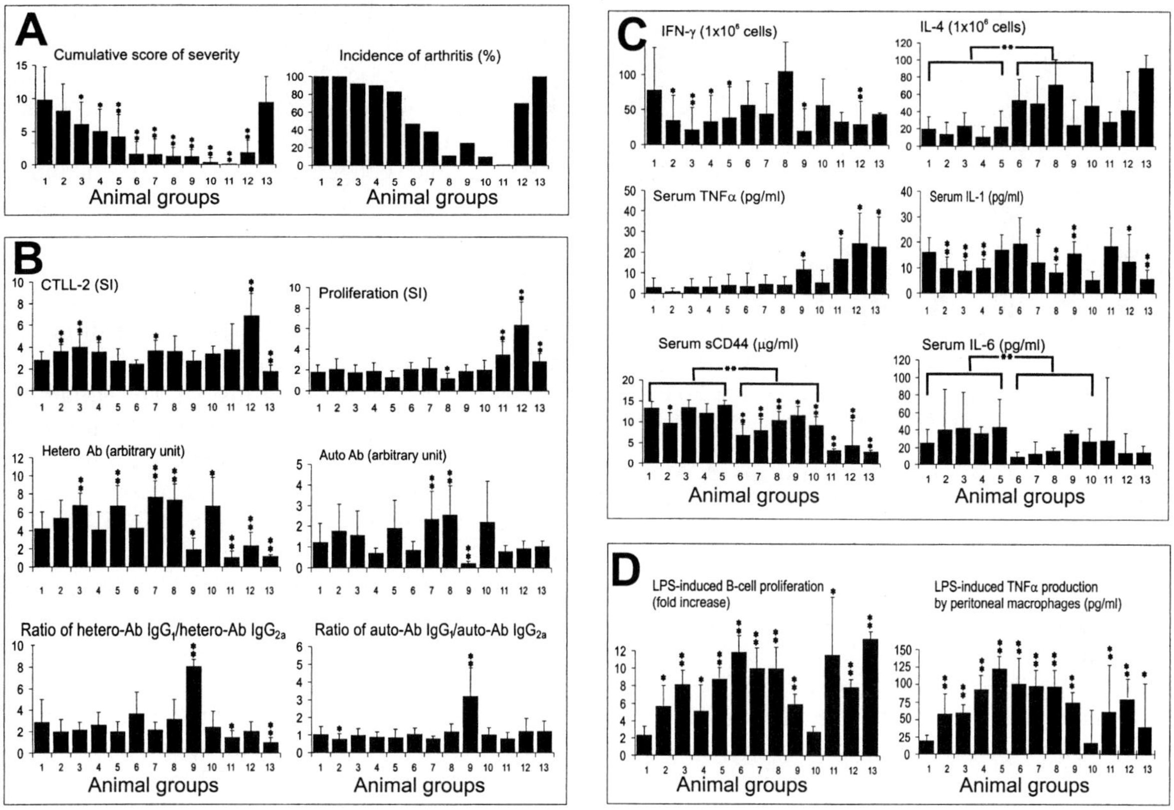

Figure 4. Comparative analysis of 10 C3H substrains, control BALB/c mice, and BALB.B and BALB.K congenic mice after immunization with deglycosylated human cartilage proteoglycan. Animals were killed 4 weeks after the fourth antigen injection. Data on all immunized animals are shown. C3H colonies (groups 1–10) are organized in order of descending cumulative (clinical) score followed by the BALB.B (group 11), BALB.K (group 12), and BALB/c (group 13) control groups **(A)** (corresponding numbers are shown in Table 3). T and B cell responses **(B)** and inflammatory marker/cytokine levels **(C)** were determined in the same groups of mice. **D,** Lipopolysaccharide (LPS)–induced B cell proliferation and tumor necrosis factor α (TNFα) production by peritoneal macrophages were also examined. Significant differences between the National Cancer Institute's C3H/HeJCr mice (group 1) and all other strains (n = 14–30 animals/group) and, if applicable, the differences between the first set of 5 and second set of 5 C3H strains are shown (indicated with horizontal bars). $* = P < 0.05$ and $** = P < 0.01$. Bars show the mean and SD. CTLL-2 = cytotoxic lymphoid line 2; SI = stimulation index; Ab = antibodies; IFN-γ = interferon-γ; IL-4 = interleukin-4; sCD44 = soluble CD44.

tional analyses were performed on arthritic and nonarthritic animals. Unexpectedly, arthritic C3H mice (n = 164) showed significantly lower ($P < 0.05$) antigen (human PG)–specific T cell proliferation rates than did the nonarthritic mice (n = 78). Th2-dependent IL-4 production and Th2-supported IgG1 levels (both hetero- and autoantibodies) were lower in arthritic than in nonarthritic animals (Figure 5). Serum levels of IL-1 ($P < 0.05$), IL-6 ($P < 0.01$), and sCD44 ($P < 0.01$) were significantly higher in arthritic than in nonarthritic C3H mice (Figure 5).

Comparison of LPS sensitivity and arthritis susceptibility in C3H mice. C3H mice of different colonies differ in their sensitivity to LPS. The Jackson Laboratory's C3H/HeJ mice are hyporesponsive, whereas sublines coded with C3H/HeN (National Institutes of Health [NIH] origin) are highly sensitive to LPS stimulation (30–32). It is believed that a point mutation, or mutations, occurred at the *Lps* locus in C3H/HeJ mice, which was recently identified as toll-like receptor 4 (*Tlr-4*) (33–35). This gene is responsible for LPS-induced B cell proliferation and TNFα production by macrophages (32,34,36,37).

To detect a potential correlation between LPS sensitivity and arthritis susceptibility, spleen cells of each colony (Table 3) were cultured in the presence or absence of LPS, and B cell proliferation was determined by ^{3}H-thymidine incorporation. As shown in Figure 4D,

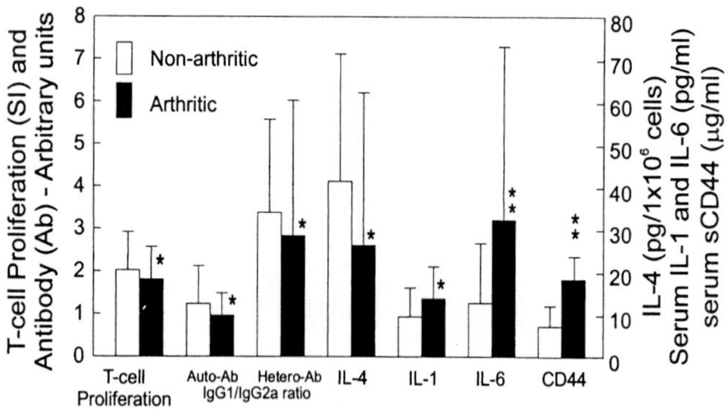

Figure 5. Comparative analysis of various immunologic and inflammatory parameters in all arthritic versus nonarthritic animals of the 10 C3H substrains 4 weeks after the fourth antigen (proteoglycan) injection. Only statistically significant differences are shown. Bars show the mean and SD. * = $P < 0.05$ and ** = $P < 0.01$ versus nonarthritic mice. See Figure 4 for definitions.

there was a 2.5–6-fold difference in LPS-induced cell proliferation among C3H sublines, but the responses of arthritis-susceptible C3H/HeJCr (NCI) and resistant C3H/HeJ (Jackson Laboratory) mice to LPS stimulation were identical. LPS-induced TNFα production by peritoneal macrophages was also highly comparable (low in the C3H/HeJ-related colonies and high in the C3H/HeN-related colonies), but no correlation was found between TNFα production and arthritis susceptibility in the different C3H sublines (Figure 4D). Furthermore, there was no correlation between serum TNFα levels (Figure 4C) and the in vitro TNFα production measured in conditioned media of LPS-stimulated peritoneal macrophages (Figure 4D).

DISCUSSION

To identify disease-responsible loci in PGIA, genome scan studies were carried out using F_2 intercross hybrids of the only known PGIA-susceptible BALB/c strain and either MHC-matched (DBA/2) or MHC-unmatched (C57BL/6, C3H, and DBA/1) PGIA-resistant strains (7,11–14). In contrast to a "standard" 15% ratio of F_2 susceptibility to PGIA, more than 50% of the hybrid mice from the BALB/c × C3H/HeJCr intercross developed arthritis (12). This unexpected observation compelled us to repeat earlier experiments (2,3,13) in anticipation of finding the C3H/HeJCr strain that is susceptible to PGIA. Indeed, while the previously used C3H/HeJ mice from the Jackson Laboratory were essentially resistant (<10% incidence and very low inflammation score), C3H/HeJCr mice from the NCI used for the genome-wide screening study (12) demonstrated 95–100% incidence of PGIA. Because of this extreme difference between the C3H/HeJ and C3H/HeJCr sublines, we compared 10 different C3H colonies for arthritis susceptibility, along with highly susceptible BALB/c and congenic BALB.B (H-2^b) and BALB.K (H-2^k) strains. PGIA could be induced in a few colonies of C3H mice as well as in the BALB/c and BALB.K strains.

An important observation was the massive inflammation around the intervertebral discs in arthritic C3H mice, resulting in resorption of the disc and the development of vertebral fusion. The inflammatory reaction, characterized by a predominantly lymphocytic infiltration around the intervertebral disc (Figure 2B), suggests that an immune attack occurred against spine tissue components, most likely against PG, which is a dominant component in the nucleus pulposus and cartilaginous end and growth plates of vertebral bodies. Spondylitis with complete resorption of the intervertebral disc and fusion of the neighboring vertebra has been described, to date, in BALB/c mice only (1,8). However, there are a number of questions to be resolved, such as the following: How does the spondylitis correlate with arthritis in peripheral joints? Why are only a few discs attacked/resorbed when neighboring intervertebral discs remain intact? Most importantly, how is the spine involvement (either in BALB/c or C3H mice) related to human ankylosing spondylitis? It is also unclear whether PGs of the nucleus pulposus and cartilage plates of vertebra are the target antigens in spondylitis; if so, why do nonarticular cartilages (e.g., in the ear or trachea) remain intact in arthritic animals? We have collected all spine tissues of all mice involved in this and corresponding studies (11–13), with the goal of describing the cascade of inflammatory events around the spine. To this end, PGIA accompanied by spondylitis in C3H mice may provide a novel autoimmune and unique genetic model that demonstrates striking similarities to human ankylosing spondylitis.

C3H is one of the most frequently used murine strains. The first founder C3H colony was generated in 1920 when a female Bagg albino (a founder of the BALB/c strain) was mated with a DBA male (the latter was the founder of DBA/1 and DBA/2 strains [29,38]). After a few generations, the "C3H" strain was noted for a high incidence of developing mammary tumor (24,39). The Jackson Laboratory received breeding pairs at the F_{48} generation from W. E. Heston (He) (39,40) in 1947, and established an inbred C3H/HeJ colony (Table 3). The NIH generated a similar colony in 1951 (C3H/

HeN). Essentially, all available C3H sublines originated from these 2 founder colonies and were maintained as inbred strains. A common feature of all C3H mice is that they carry the *rd/rd* (retinal degeneration) gene leading to blindness by 3–4 months of age (41), and most C3H sublines exhibit susceptibility to both mammary tumor (39,42) and hepatoma (40). A known mutation in the *Lps* receptor genes occurred between 1960 and 1967 in the original C3H/HeJ colony maintained by the Jackson Laboratory (30,31). This *Lps* gene has been identified recently as the *Tlr-4* on chromosome 4, which is responsible for LPS-mediated signaling in B cells, macrophages, and fibroblasts (36,37,43).

The B cell response to LPS stimulation is normal in all NIH-derived C3H/HeN colonies and in all C3H/HeJ-derived sublines that had been separated from the founder colony prior to the occurrence of the point mutation in the *Tlr4* gene (23). Because a normal response (versus hyporesponsiveness) to LPS by B cells and macrophages is one of the most prominent differences among C3H colonies, we tested the general B cell response to LPS (measured as proliferation) as well as the TNFα production by LPS-stimulated macrophages in the 10 C3H sublines (Figure 4D). Although dramatic differences were measured by both assays in the different C3H sublines, the most PGIA-susceptible C3H/HeJCr (NCI) mice and the most arthritis-resistant C3H/HeJ (Jackson Laboratory) mice were equally hyporesponsive to LPS stimulation. Since the NCI received the C3H/HeJCr founders from the Jackson Laboratory in 1967, the *Tlr-4* mutation was probably already present at that time. However, additional mutations in the genome and/or genetic contamination within any of the 2 colonies may have occurred, resulting in NCI's C3H/HeJCr mice being susceptible or Jackson Laboratory's C3H/HeJ mice being resistant to PGIA.

Although BALB/c and C3H mice differ in haplotype, as discussed above, the 2 strains share a common heritage, since the founder mother of both strains was the same (29). Thus, this common heritage suggests that some non-MHC genes that had already existed in the founder mother could have conferred arthritis susceptibility to both the BALB/c and the C3H strains of mice. Assuming that no genetic contamination occurred in the inbred C3H colonies maintained by the different vendors, we can hypothesize that additional mutations in the genome caused the variations in PGIA susceptibility in C3H mice. This seems to be very similar to the genetic alterations responsible for differences in susceptibility to mammary tumors and hepatoma, or the differences in LPS sensitivity reported in different colonies/sublines of the C3H strain (27). Since several C3H sublines (from either the Jackson Laboratory or the NIH) lost their PGIA susceptibility (Figure 4), we speculate that a mutation or mutations occurred in an "autoimmune suppressor" gene or gene clusters (11). Such a mutation might result in the loss of control over a "cascade" of either arthritis-permissive or -promoting genes.

Although it is a challenging idea to find such a gene mutation, alternatively it is possible that the arthritis susceptibility is a result of an imbalanced (patho)physiologic network, and very-far-upstream events (e.g., genetic mutations) might have much less importance than the local (micro)environmental components in the joint or in the perivertebral soft tissue. Nonetheless, the high variation in arthritis susceptibility among C3H substrains is of special interest. Using C3H mice will make it possible to identify disease (arthritis)–associated candidate genes on the same MHC background. The first study in this direction is summarized in our corresponding report (12).

ACKNOWLEDGMENTS

We thank Edit Buzás, MD, PhD, Cory Holgren, and Ann Mikhail for technical help, Dr. Susan Shott for advice in statistical analyses, our colleagues of the Departments of Immunology and Biochemistry for thoughtful discussions and critical reviewing of the manuscript, and for information received from the technical services of Harlan-Sprague Dawley, Taconic, Charles River Laboratory, and Clarence Reeder at the NCI.

REFERENCES

1. Glant TT, Mikecz K, Arzoumanian A, Poole AR. Proteoglycan-induced arthritis in BALB/c mice: clinical features and histopathology. Arthritis Rheum 1987;30:201–12.
2. Mikecz K, Glant TT, Poole AR. Immunity to cartilage proteoglycans in BALB/c mice with progressive polyarthritis and ankylosing spondylitis induced by injection of human cartilage proteoglycan. Arthritis Rheum 1987;30:306–18.
3. Glant TT, Mikecz K, Thonar EJ-MA, Kuettner KE. Immune responses to cartilage proteoglycans in inflammatory animal models and human diseases. In: Woessner JF, Howell DS, editors. Cartilage degradation: basic and clinical aspects. New York: Marcel Dekker; 1992. p. 435–73.
4. Mikecz K, Brennan FR, Kim JH, Glant TT. Anti-CD44 treatment abrogates tissue edema and leukocyte infiltration in murine arthritis. Nat Med 1995;1:558–63.
5. Glant TT, Buzás EI, Finnegan A, Negroiu G, Cs-Szabó G, Mikecz K. Critical role of glycosaminoglycan side chains of cartilage proteoglycan (aggrecan) in antigen recognition and presentation. J Immunol 1998;160:3812–9.
6. Glant TT, Fülöp C, Cs-Szabó G, Buzás EI, Ragasa DR, Mikecz K. Mapping of arthritogenic/autoimmune epitopes of cartilage aggrecans in proteoglycan-induced arthritis. Scand J Rheumatol 1995; 24:43–9.
7. Glant TT, Cs-Szabó G, Nagase H, Jacobs JJ, Mikecz K. Progres-

sive polyarthritis induced in BALB/c mice by aggrecan from normal and osteoarthritic human cartilage. Arthritis Rheum 1998; 41:1007–18.
8. Mikecz K, Glant TT, Buzás E, Poole AR. Proteoglycan-induced polyarthritis and spondylitis adoptively transferred to naive (nonimmunized) BALB/c mice. Arthritis Rheum 1990;33:866–76.
9. Singer II, Kawka DW, Bayne EK, Donatelli SA, Weidner JR, Williams HA, et al. VDIPEN, a metalloproteinase-generated neoepitope, is induced and immunolocalized in articular cartilage during inflammatory arthritis. J Clin Invest 1995;95:2178–86.
10. Buzás E, Mikecz K, Brennan FR, Glant TT. Mediators of autopathogenic effector cells in proteoglycan-induced arthritic and clinically asymptomatic BALB/c mice. Cell Immunol 1994;158: 292–304.
11. Otto JM, Bárdos T, Adarichev V, Valdez JC, Mikecz K, Finnegan A, et al. A combined autoimmune model of arthritis reveals novel, and shared and independent binary and quantitative trait loci. J Immunol 2001; in press.
12. Otto JM, Chandrasekaran R, Vermes C, Mikecz K, Finnegan A, Rickert SE, et al. A genome scan using a novel genetic cross identifies new susceptibility loci and traits in a mouse model of rheumatoid arthritis. J Immunol 2000;165:5278–86.
13. Otto JM, Cs-Szabó G, Gallagher J, Velins S, Mikecz K, Buzás EI, et al. Identification of multiple loci linked to inflammation and autoantibody production by a genome scan of a murine model of rheumatoid arthritis. Arthritis Rheum 1999;42:2524–31.
14. Otto JM, Mikecz K, Finnegan A, Buzas EI, Cs-Szabo G, Enders JT, et al. A genome scan in a murine model of rheumatoid arthritis localizes loci associated with different traits and genetic backgrounds [abstract]. Arthritis Rheum 1999;42:S233.
15. Glant TT, Mikecz K, Poole AR. Monoclonal antibodies to different protein-related epitopes of human articular cartilage proteoglycans. Biochem J 1986;234:31–41.
16. Buzás EI, Brennan FR, Mikecz K, Garzó M, Negroiu G, Holló K, et al. A proteoglycan (aggrecan)-specific T cell hybridoma induces arthritis in BALB/c mice. J Immunol 1995;155:2679–87.
17. Hakeda Y, Shiokawa M, Mano H, Kameda T, Raisz LG, Kumegawa M. Prostaglandin $F_{2\alpha}$ stimulates tyrosine phosphorylation and mitogen-activated protein kinase in osteoblastic MC3T3-E1 cells via protein kinase C activation. Endocrinology 1997;138: 1821–8.
18. Holló K, Glant TT, Garzó M, Finnegan A, Mikecz K, Buzás EI. Complex pattern of Th1 and Th2 activation with a preferential increase of autoreactive Th1 cells in BALB/c mice with proteoglycan (aggrecan)-induced arthritis. Clin Exp Immunol 2000;120: 167–73.
19. Finnegan A, Mikecz K, Tao P, Glant TT. Proteoglycan (aggrecan)-induced arthritis in BALB/c mice is a Th1-type disease regulated by Th2 cytokines. J Immunol 1999;163:5383–90.
20. Mikecz K, Dennis K, Shi M, Kim JH. Modulation of hyaluronan receptor (CD44) function in vivo in a murine model of rheumatoid arthritis. Arthritis Rheum 1999;42:659–68.
21. Glode LM, Rosenstreich DL. Genetic control of B cell activation by bacterial lipopolysaccharide is mediated by multiple distinct genes or alleles. J Immunol 1976;117:2061–6.
22. Outzen HC, Corrow D, Schultz LD. Attenuation of exogenous murine mammary tumor virus virulence in the C3H/HeJ mouse substrain bearing the Lps mutation. J Natl Cancer Inst 1985;75: 917–23.
23. Handbook on genetically standardized JAX mice. 5th ed. Bar Harbor (ME): Jackson Laboratories; 1997.
24. Hummel KP, Richardson RL, Fekete E. Anatomy. In: Green EL, editor. Biology of the laboratory mouse. New York: McGraw-Hill; 1966. p. 247–307.
25. Freedman HA, Lilly F. Properties of cell lines derived from tumors induced by friend virus in BALB/c BALB/c-*H-2*^{b} mice. J Exp Med 1975;142:212–23.
26. Shearer GM, Schmitt-Verhulst A-M, Pettinelli CB, Miller MW, Gilheany PE. H-2-linked genetic control of murine T-cell-mediated lympholysis to autologous cells modified with low concentrations of trinitrobenzene sulfonate. J Exp Med 1979;149:1407–23.
27. Beck JA, Lloyd S, Hafezparast M, Lennon-Pierce M, Eppig JT, Festing MFW, et al. Genealogies of mouse inbred strains. Nat Genet 2000;24:23–5.
28. Stasiuk LM, Abehsira-Amar O, Fournier C. Collagen-induced arthritis in DBA/1 mice: cytokine gene activation following immunization with type II collagen. Cell Immunol 1996;173:269–75.
29. Festing MFW. Inbred strains of mice. Mouse Genome 1996;94: 523–677.
30. Watson J, Riblet R. Genetic control of responses to bacterial lipopolysaccharides in mice. I. Evidence for a single gene that influences mitogenic and immunogenic responses to lipopolysaccharides. J Exp Med 1974;140:1147–61.
31. Coutinho A, Möller G, Gronowicz E. Genetical control of B-cell responses. IV. Inheritance of the unresponsiveness to lipopolysaccharides. J Exp Med 1975;142:253–8.
32. Rosenstreich DL, Glode LM. Difference in B cell mitogen responsiveness between closely related strains of mice. J Immunol 1975;115:777–80.
33. Wong PM, Chugn SW, Sultzer BM. Genes, receptors, signals and responses to lipopolysaccharide endotoxin. Scand J Immunol 2000;51:123–7.
34. Vogel SN, Johnson D, Perera PY, Medvedev A, Larivière L, Qureshi ST. Functional characterization of the effect of the C3H/HeJ defect mice that lack an Lpsn gene: in vivo evidence for a dominant negative mutation. J Immunol 1999;162:5666–70.
35. Takeuchi O, Takeda K, Hoshino K, Adachi O, Ogawa T, Akira S. Cellular responses to bacterial cell wall components are mediated through MyD88-dependent signaling cascades. Int Immunol 2000; 12:113–7.
36. Qureshi ST, Gros P, Malo D. The Lps locus: genetic regulation of host responses to bacterial lipopolysaccharide. Inflamm Res 1999; 48:613–20.
37. Hoshino K, Takeuchi O, Kawai T, Sanjo H, Ogawa T, Takeda Y, et al. Toll-like receptor 4 (TLR-4)-deficient mice are hyporesponsive to lipopolysaccharide: evidence for TLR4 as the Lps gene product. J Immunol 1999;162:3749–52.
38. Staats J. The laboratory mouse. In: Green EL, editor. Biology of the laboratory mouse. New York: McGraw-Hill; 1996. p. 1–9.
39. Heston WE, Parks WP. Mammary tumor virus and host genome in the transmission and causation of mammary tumors in mice. Can J Genet Cytol 1975;17:493–502.
40. Heston WE, Vlahakis G. Factors in the causation of spontaneous hepatomas in mice. J Natl Cancer Inst 1966;37:839–43.
41. Nagy ZM, Misanin JR. Visual perception in the retinal degenerate C3H mouse. J Comp Physiol Psychol 1970;72:306–10.
42. Heston WE. Genetics of neoplasia. In Burdette WJ, editor. Methodology in mammalian genetics. San Francisco: Holden-Day; 1963. p. 247–68.
43. Du X, Poltorak A, Silva M, Beutler B. Analysis of Tlr4-mediated LPS signal transduction in macrophages by mutational modification of the receptor. Blood Cells Mol Dis 1999;25:328–38.

ARTHRITIS & RHEUMATISM
Vol. 44, No. 3, March 2001, pp 693–702

Elevated Proapoptotic Bax and Caspase 3 Activation in the NOD.*scid* Model of Sjögren's Syndrome

Reiji Masago,[1] Sonomi Aiba-Masago,[1] Norman Talal,[2] Fabio Jimenez Zuluaga,[1] Ibtisam Al-Hashimi,[3] Michael Moody,[3] C. Allen Lau,[4] Ammon B. Peck,[5] Jason Brayer,[5] Michael G. Humphreys-Beher,[5] and Howard Dang[1]

Objective. **Salivary gland epithelial cells in patients with Sjögren's syndrome (SS) and in NOD and NOD.*scid* mice express Fas and Fas ligand, and these cells die from apoptosis. To elucidate the intracellular molecular mechanisms responsible for this salivary gland epithelial cell apoptosis, expression of the Bcl-2 family of proteins (Bcl-2, Bcl-x_L, Bax) and caspase (caspases 3 and 8) was studied in young (ages 8–10 weeks) and old (ages 17–28 weeks) NOD and NOD.*scid* mice.**

Methods. **Sections of frozen salivary gland tissue were obtained from NOD and NOD.*scid* mice and from the lip biopsy material of SS patients. Immunohistochemistry or Western blot analysis was performed to assess the apoptotic-associated proteins.**

Results. **Levels of Bax and caspase 3 were elevated in the epithelial cells of glands from old NOD mice, but not in those from young NOD mice. In contrast, epithelial cells from both young and old NOD.*scid* mice exhibited strong expression of Bax and caspase 3. Western blot analysis showed that the activated form of caspase 3 was increased 2–5-fold in the glands from old NOD, old NOD.*scid*, and young NOD.*scid* mice compared with those from young NOD mice. Caspase 3 was also significantly elevated ($P < 0.01$) in SS patients whose focus scores were grade 3 or 4. In the SS patients' biopsy tissue and in the mouse glands, cells with fragmented DNA were positive for caspase 3.**

Conclusion. **These results demonstrate that salivary gland epithelial cells in NOD and NOD.*scid* mice overexpress the proapoptotic molecules Bax and caspase 3. Bax could be the gene responsible for initiation of caspase activation, epithelial cell destruction, and lymphocyte glandular localization in SS.**

Sjögren's syndrome (SS) is an autoimmune rheumatic disease characterized by lymphocyte infiltration of exocrine glands (e.g., salivary and lacrimal glands) that leads to glandular dysfunction as well as oral and ocular dryness. SS exocrine epithelial cells undergo apoptosis, which is initiated by Fas (1–5) or granzyme A (6,7). An accelerated and inappropriate epithelial cell death may initiate the autoimmune attack against the salivary glands (8–10). In the NOD mouse model of SS (11), we have shown that the submandibular gland acinar epithelial cells undergo apoptosis (12). Furthermore, since acinar epithelial cell apoptosis is also present in the congenic immunodeficient NOD strain (NOD.*scid*), it is likely that a low level of apoptosis occurs in the absence of lymphocytes (10).

Apoptosis is a highly regulated biologic process in cell physiology and pathology. Proteins from the Bcl-2 family act as important regulators of apoptosis by conferring to the cell either resistance or sensitivity to apoptotic signals (13). The molecules Bcl-2 and Bcl-x_L confer resistance, whereas Bax is proapoptotic. Since these molecules form dimers with one another (14), the relative levels of Bcl-2, Bcl-x_L, and Bax are important in determining a cell's eventual fate in the life cycle.

Supported by grants from The RKG Foundation (Austin, Texas) and the NIH (NIDCR, DE-12203).

[1]Reiji Masago, MD, Sonomi Aiba-Masago, MD, Fabio Jimenez Zuluaga, Howard Dang, PhD: The University of Texas Health Science Center, San Antonio; [2]Norman Talal, MD: Columbia University College of Physicians & Surgeons, New York, New York; [3]Ibtisam Al-Hashimi, PhD, Michael Moody, MD: Baylor College of Dentistry, Dallas, Texas; [4]C. Allen Lau, PhD: Harcourt Brace Educational Measurement, San Antonio, Texas; [5]Ammon B. Peck, MD, Jason Brayer, Michael G. Humphreys-Beher, PhD: University of Florida, Gainesville.

Drs. Masago and Aiba-Masago contributed equally to this work.

Address correspondence and reprint requests to Howard Dang, PhD, Department of Medicine, Division of Clinical Immunology, Mail Code 7874, 7703 Floyd Curl Drive, San Antonio, TX 78229-3900.

Submitted for publication February 25, 2000; accepted in revised form October 13, 2000.

Enzymes—in particular, the cysteine proteases called caspases—cause the destruction that is characteristic of apoptosis. Fas signaling leads to the activation of the initiator caspase, caspase 8, which in turn activates effector caspases, such as caspase 3. Caspase 3 plays a major role in apoptosis by cleaving proteins that are essential for cell survival, such as actin, poly (ADP-ribose) polymerase (PARP), and focal adhesion kinase. Caspase 3 also activates an endonuclease, called CAD, that leads to DNA fragmentation, which is a hallmark of apoptosis. Bcl-2 and Bcl-x_L regulate the activation of caspase 3 by maintaining mitochondrial membrane integrity and preventing the cleavage of caspase 3 from its proenzyme state (15,16). Bax has the opposite effect by altering the mitochondrial outer membrane permeability and allowing the release of proapoptotic molecules (e.g., cytochrome c) (17,18).

We and others have reported abnormal expression of Bcl-2 family members in lip biopsy tissue from the salivary glands of patients with SS (1,3,19). In particular, the epithelial acinar cells display increased Bax levels, which is associated with apoptosis. In contrast, the lymphocytes show increased levels of Bcl-2, which no doubt plays a role in the lymphomagenesis characteristic of SS (20).

Studies were performed in NOD and NOD.*scid* mice to further elucidate the molecular mechanism responsible for salivary gland epithelial cell apoptosis. The data show that salivary gland epithelial cells in NOD and NOD.*scid* mice overexpress the proapoptotic molecules Bax and caspase 3, as do those in SS patients. Since this is true even in the absence of lymphocytes, these results suggests that Bax in epithelial cells may trigger the apoptotic death that leads to lymphocyte invasion and glandular destruction in SS.

PATIENTS AND METHODS

Animals and tissue preparation. NOD, NOD.*scid*, and BALB/c mice at 8 and 18 weeks of age (young and old groups, respectively) were obtained from the University of Florida (Gainesville, FL) specific pathogen–free environment mouse breeding facilities. Penetrance of salivary abnormalities is 100% in NOD and NOD.*scid* mice. In NOD mice, salivary and lacrimal gland lymphocytic infiltrates begin at 10–12 weeks and lose secretory function by 15 weeks of age. The epithelial cell pathology in both NOD and NOD.*scid* mice, which is characterized by decreased amylase and epidermal growth factor synthesis along with aberrant parotid secretory protein expression and processing, begins at 8–10 weeks of age.

The submandibular glands were removed and immediately frozen in a dry-ice/isopentane bath or fixed in 10% buffered formalin. Frozen tissues were stored at −80°C. Fixed tissues were embedded in paraffin.

Biopsy material from SS patients (21) was obtained from the Salivary Dysfunction Clinic (Baylor College of Dentistry, Dallas, TX) and embedded in paraffin. SS biopsy samples were graded for disease severity on a scale of 1–4, according to the method of Chisholm and Mason (22). Formalin-fixed normal salivary glands were obtained from The National Disease Research Interchange (Philadelphia, PA).

Antibody reagents. For immunohistochemistry, goat polyclonal antibody to caspase 8 (Mch5 p20, T-16) and rabbit polyclonal antibody to Bcl-2 (N-19), Bcl-x_L (H-62), Bax (Δ21), and caspase 3 (CPP32, H-277) were purchased from Santa Cruz Biotechnology (Santa Cruz, CA). Rabbit polyclonal antibody to the activated form of caspase 3 (PharMingen, San Diego, CA) was also used for immunohistochemistry. Rat monoclonal antibody to Bcl-2 (4c11; Santa Cruz Biotechnology) and goat polyclonal antibody to PARP (A-20; Santa Cruz Biotechnology) were used for Western blot analysis. Rabbit polyclonal antibodies to caspase 3 and Bax were purchased from PharMingen and utilized for Western blot analysis.

Immunohistochemistry. Frozen sections (4 μm) were air dried, fixed in 4% paraformaldehyde for 10 minutes, and washed in Tris buffered saline (with 0.05% Tween 20, pH 7.6). Paraffin-embedded tissue sections were deparaffinized with xylene, rehydrated in sequential ethanol/H_2O baths of descending ethanol concentrations, and subjected to microwave fixation (15 minutes) in 10 m*M* citrate buffer. Endogenous peroxidase was quenched with 0.3% H_2O_2 in methanol for 10 minutes. Nonspecific binding was inhibited by 1% (weight/volume) bovine serum albumin (BSA) for 30 minutes at room temperature. Primary antibodies (1:40 volume/volume) were added to the slides in blocking 1% (w/v) BSA solution and incubated for 30 minutes at room temperature. Tissue sections were incubated for 30 minutes at room temperature with a peroxidase-conjugated secondary antibody (1:100 v/v) in blocking buffer. After washing, tissue sections were incubated for 5 minutes at room temperature with biotinyl tyramide (1:50 v/v) in 50 m*M* Tris HCl (0.01% H_2O_2, pH 8) followed by a 30-minute incubation with alkaline phosphatase–conjugated streptavidin (1:100 v/v) in blocking buffer.

Color development was achieved by incubation for 10 minutes at room temperature with Vector Red (Vector Laboratories, Burlingame, CA) with 5 m*M* levamisole in 100 m*M* Tris HCl (pH 8.3). The counterstain was 1% methyl green.

Paraffin-embedded or frozen tissue sections were double-stained for DNA fragmentation (i.e., apoptosis) and caspase 3 or Bax expression. Apoptosis was assessed using ApopTag (Intergen, Purchase, NY). Diaminobenzidine was used to visualize fragmented DNA. Thereafter, sections were stained for either caspase 3 or Bax as described above. BCIP/nitroblue tetrazolium (paraffin-embedded sections) or Vector Red (frozen sections) was used as the substrate to detect the expression of these 2 molecules. The counterstain was 1% methyl green or hematoxylin.

Slides were photographed with a light microscope (Olympus BX40) equipped with a 35-mm camera (Olympus PM40) with Elite chrome 100 ASA film (Eastman Kodak, Rochester, NY).

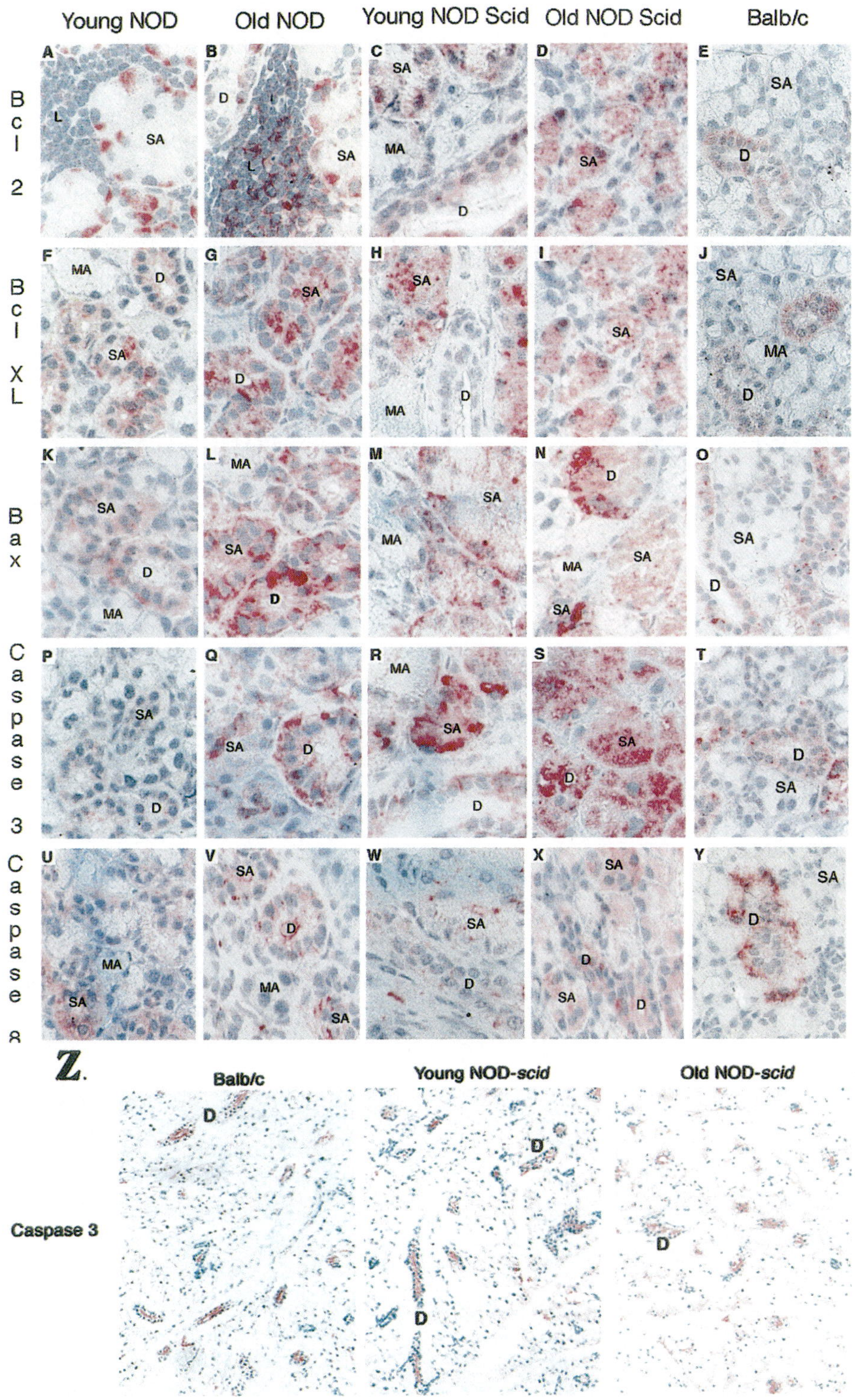

Figure 1. Immunohistochemical staining for Bcl-2 family members (Bcl-2, Bcl-x_L, Bax) and caspases 3 and 8. Submandibular glands from NOD and NOD.*scid* mice were stained with antibodies to Bcl-2 (**A–E**), Bcl-x_L (**F–J**), Bax (**K–O**), caspase 3 (**P–T**, and **Z**), and caspase 8 (**U–Y**). The substrate was Vector Red and slides were counterstained with hematoxylin. Acinar and ductal (**D**) cells from old NOD and NOD.*scid* mice (young and old) stained stronger for Bax and caspase 3 compared with cells from young NOD and BALB/c mice. Note that the mucous acinar cells (**MA**) stained weakly for all protein markers compared with the serous acinar cells (**SA**). (Original magnification × 400 in **A–Y**; × 200 in **Z**.)

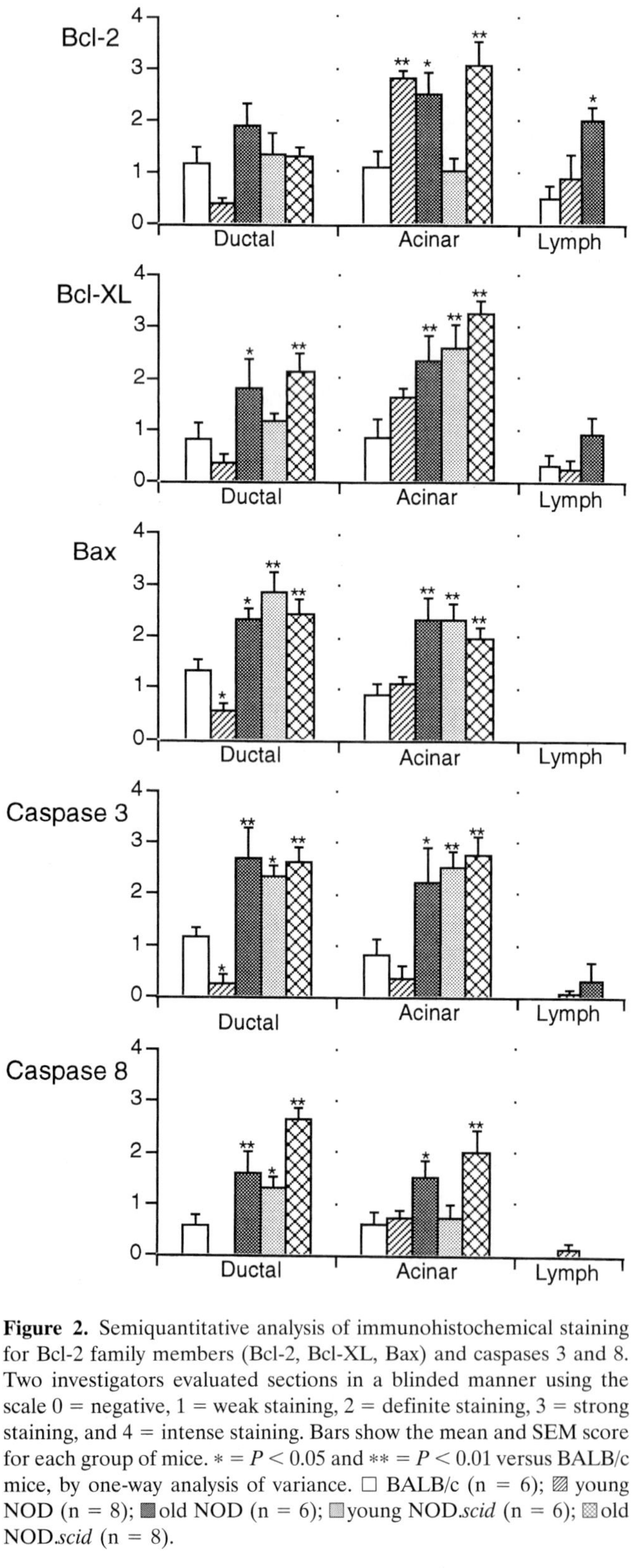

Figure 2. Semiquantitative analysis of immunohistochemical staining for Bcl-2 family members (Bcl-2, Bcl-XL, Bax) and caspases 3 and 8. Two investigators evaluated sections in a blinded manner using the scale 0 = negative, 1 = weak staining, 2 = definite staining, 3 = strong staining, and 4 = intense staining. Bars show the mean and SEM score for each group of mice. * = $P < 0.05$ and ** = $P < 0.01$ versus BALB/c mice, by one-way analysis of variance. □ BALB/c (n = 6); ▨ young NOD (n = 8); ■ old NOD (n = 6); □ young NOD.*scid* (n = 6); ▩ old NOD.*scid* (n = 8).

Western blotting. Frozen tissues were dissected into small pieces using a clean sterile razor blade and thawed in lysis buffer (10 m*M* Tris HCl [pH 7.5], 10 m*M* NaH_2PO_4/Na_2HPO_4, 130 m*M* NaCl, 1% Triton X-100, 10 m*M* inorganic sodium pyrophosphate). Samples were homogenized by ultrasonication and centrifuged at 14,000*g* for 20 minutes at 4°C. The supernatant was mixed with an equal volume of sample buffer (1*M* Tris HCl [pH 6.8] containing 10% sodium dodecyl sulfate [SDS], 10% glycerol, 10% β-mercaptoethanol, and 1% bromphenol blue). Proteins were denatured by boiling for 5 minutes. Protein concentration was determined by the Bradford method (Bio-Rad protein assay kit; Bio-Rad, Hercules, CA).

Aliquots containing 50 μg of total protein were separated on 15% SDS–polyacrylamide gels and blotted to polyvinylidene difluoride membranes (Bio-Rad). Nonspecific binding was blocked by incubating membranes with 0.5% (v/v) Tween 20/0.05*M* Tris buffered saline (TBS) containing 3% (w/v) nonfat dry milk for 1 hour at room temperature. Membranes were incubated for another 1 hour with the first antibody (1:1,000 v/v). After washing with 0.5% (v/v) Tween/TBS, membranes were incubated for 1 hour with biotinylated secondary antibody (1:1,000 v/v) in blocking buffer, and subsequently washed with 0.5% (v/v) Tween/TBS for 10 minutes at room temperature with peroxidase-conjugated streptavidin (1:1,000 v/v). After several washes, membranes were incubated for 10 minutes at room temperature with biotinyl tyramide (1:1,000 v/v) in 50 m*M* Tris HCl, pH 8.3, with 0.01% H_2O_2, washed, and incubated for 30 minutes at room temperature with alkaline phosphatase–conjugated streptavidin (1:1,000 v/v). Immun-Star Chemiluminescence Protein Detection System (Bio-Rad) was used for detection on XAR film (Eastman Kodak).

Quantification and statistical analysis. Semiquantitative analysis was used to measure levels of expression. The intensity of immunohistochemical staining was subjectively evaluated by 2 individuals in a blinded manner on a 5-point ranking scale as follows: 0 = negative, 1 = weak staining, 2 = definite staining, 3 = strong staining, and 4 = intense staining. One-way analysis of variance (ANOVA) or Kruskal-Wallis test was used to perform statistical comparisons.

RESULTS

Distribution of Bcl-2 family members (Bcl-2, Bcl-x_L, Bax). Submandibular glands from young (ages 8–10 weeks) and old (ages 17–28 weeks) NOD, NOD.*scid*, and BALB/c mice were stained for expression of the Bcl-2 family of proteins (Bcl-2, Bcl-x_L, Bax) and caspases 3 and 8 (Figures 1 and 2). The proapoptotic oncogene Bax was significantly elevated in both the ductal and acinar cells of old NOD mice and NOD.*scid* (young and old) mice compared with those from BALB/c mice. Acinar cells from young NOD mice, however, had normal levels of Bax.

Bcl-2 and Bcl-x_L were significantly elevated in the acinar cells of NOD and NOD.*scid* mice compared with

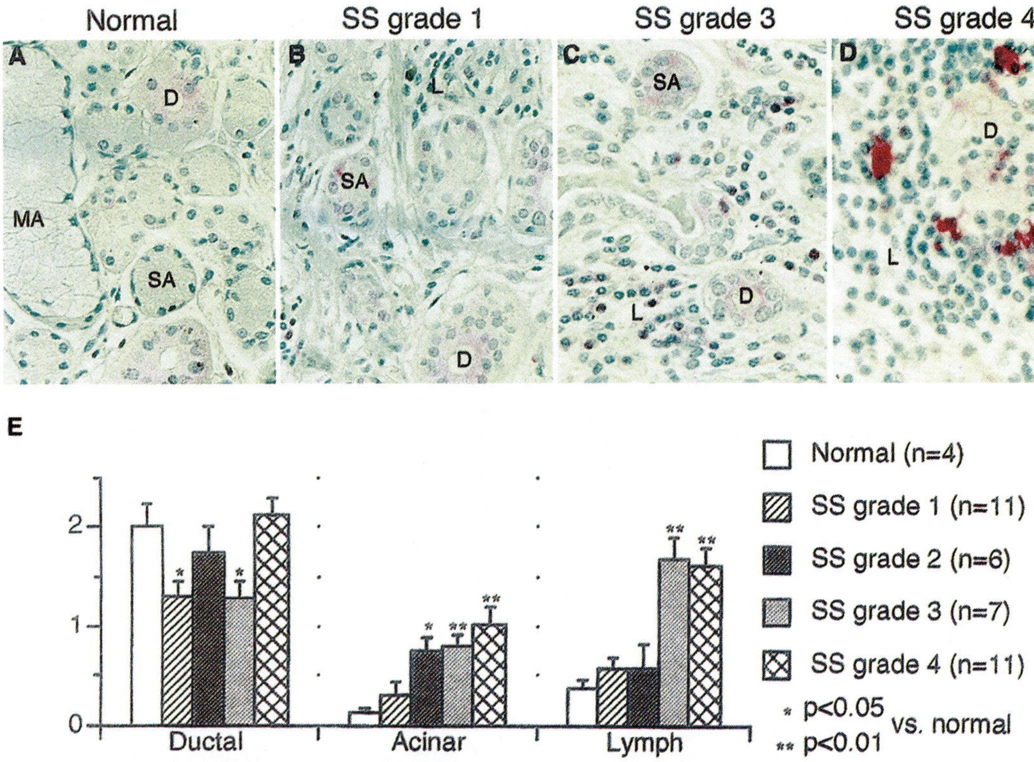

Figure 3. Caspase 3 expression in Sjögren's syndrome (SS) salivary glands compared with that in normal salivary glands. Note that only ductal (**D**) staining was observed in normal salivary glands (**A**), whereas both ductal and serous acinar (**SA**) **cells and lymphocytes** (**L**) were positive for caspase 3 in the SS glands (**B–D**) (original magnification × 400). Bars in **E** show the mean and SEM score for each group of subjects. One-way analysis of variance was used for comparisons between groups.

submandibular acinar cells of BALB/c mice; however, the NOD and NOD.*scid* glands from young mice displayed normal expression of Bcl-x_L and Bcl-2, respectively. There was no significant difference in Bcl-2 expression among the ductal cells of either of the NOD strains compared with the expression in similar cells from BALB/c mice.

Lymphocytes were positive for Bcl-2 and Bcl-x_L in both young and old NOD mice, but negative for Bax. This is consistent with our previous finding that few of the infiltrating lymphocytes in the NOD submandibular gland are apoptotic (12).

Distribution of caspases 3 and 8. The Bcl-2 family regulates caspase activity in many types of cells. Therefore, staining for caspase 8 and caspase 3 was performed to determine the relationship of the Bcl-2 family and caspases in cells of the salivary gland. The initiator caspase, caspase 8, was elevated in the acinar cells of old NOD mice and old NOD.*scid* mice, while younger mice had caspase 8 levels comparable with those in BALB/c mice. The executioner caspase, caspase 3, was significantly elevated in the acinar cells of NOD.*scid* mice of both age groups and old NOD mice. This expression of caspase 3 correlated with the expression of Bax.

Defects in SS cells. We have reported that Bax expression is elevated in the salivary acinar cells of SS patients (19). To show that these observations in NOD mice reflect the characteristics of the human disease, SS biopsy samples were stained for caspase 3 (Figure 3). In glands from subjects with no known salivary dysfunction, only the ductal cells stained for caspase 3. Both the ductal and acinar cells in SS salivary glands expressed caspase 3. There was a significant difference in acinar staining between the SS and normal glands ($P < 0.05$, by Kruskal-Wallis test). ANOVA showed that the significant difference in acinar staining was found in SS biopsy

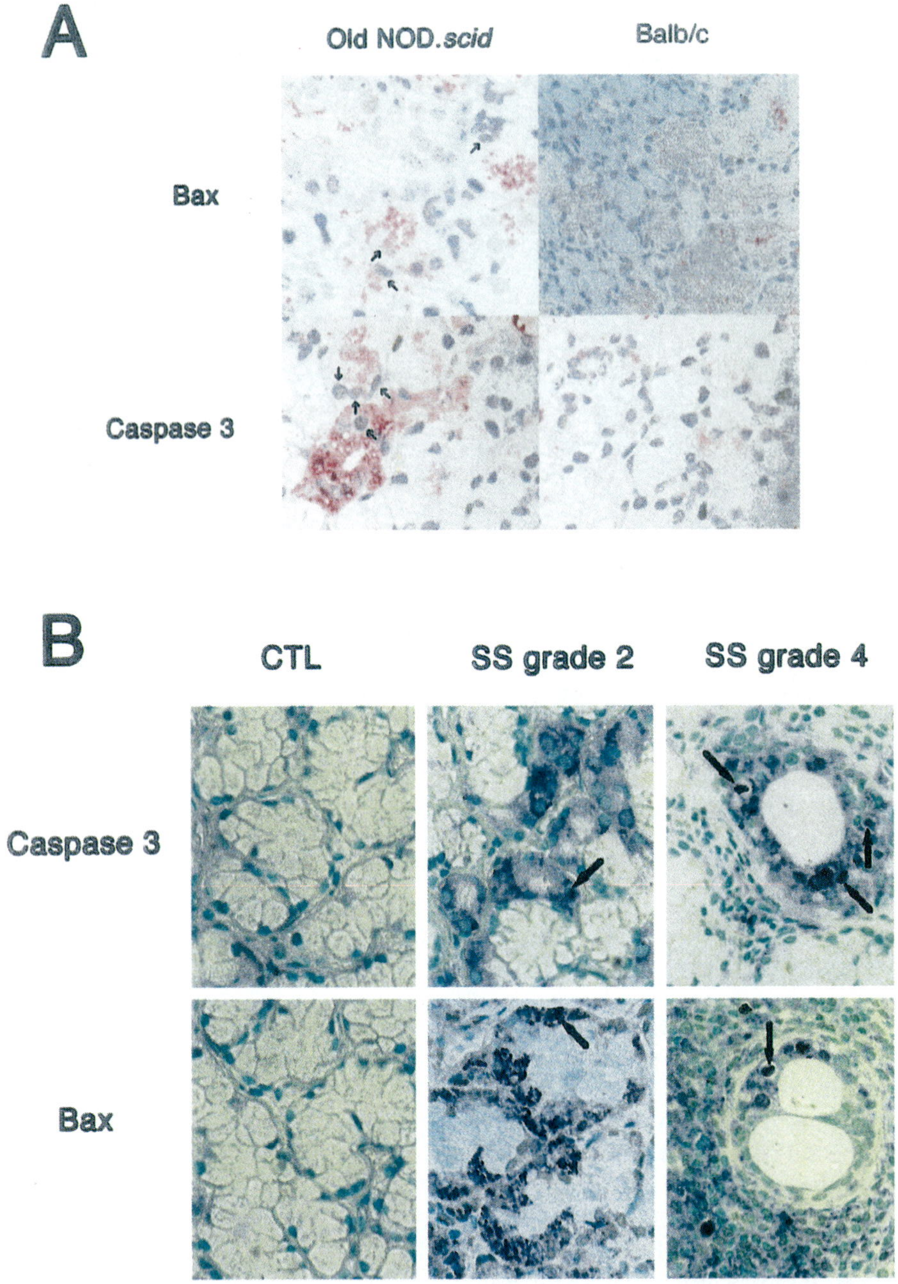

Figure 4. Expression of caspase 3 and Bax in apoptotic and nonapoptotic cells. Tissue sections from salivary glands were double-stained for fragmented DNA (by TUNEL assay) and caspase 3 or Bax. Frozen sections were obtained from old NOD.*scid* mice and age-matched BALB/c mice **(A)**, while normal (CTL) and Sjögren's syndrome (SS) sections **(B)** were derived from paraffin-embedded human tissues. Both apoptotic **(arrows)** and nonapoptotic ductal cells expressed caspase 3 and Bax. Note the condensed nuclei of apoptotic cells. (Original magnification × 400.)

samples with a focus score of >2. Caspase 3 was also significantly increased in SS lymphocytes infiltrating the gland.

Tissue sections were stained for DNA fragmentation (i.e., by TUNEL assay) followed by staining for either caspase 3 or Bax (Figure 4). Caspase 3 and Bax were observed in both apoptotic and nonapoptotic cells. All of the apoptotic cells stained positive for caspase 3

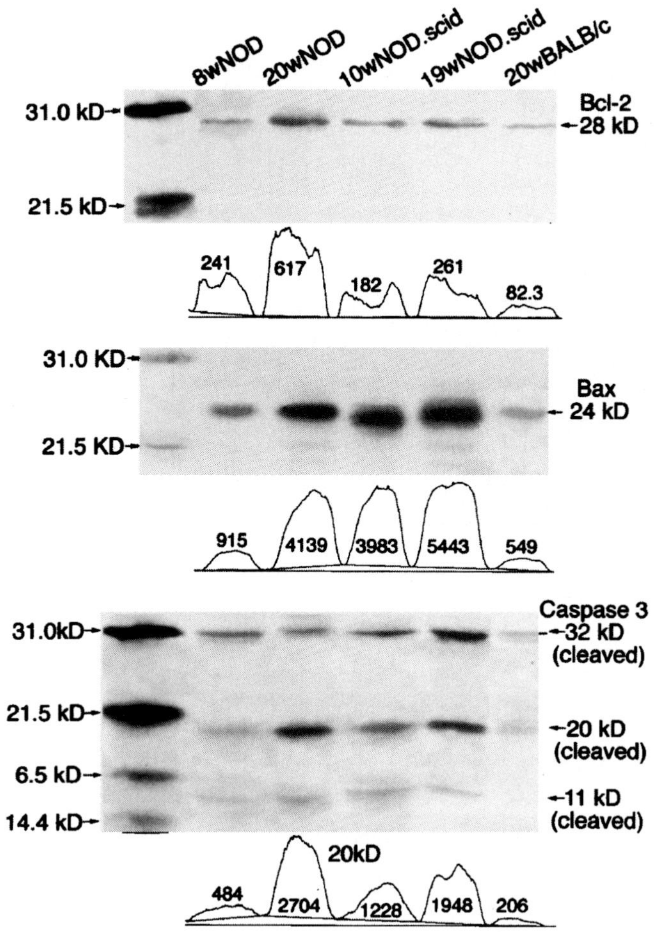

Figure 5. Western blotting for Bcl-2, Bax, and caspase 3. Aliquots of total protein (50 μg) from submandibular glands were separated by gel electrophoresis and transferred to polyvinylidene difluoride membranes. Chemiluminescence was used to reveal specific bands, and the intensity of the bands was quantified with the use of NIH Image. Numbers represent arbitrary units.

and Bax. Similar observations were made in tissues from old NOD.*scid* mice. This suggests that the expression of these gene products precedes DNA fragmentation.

Western blot analysis. Lysates from mouse submandibular tissue were subjected to Western blot analysis for Bcl-2, Bax, and caspase 3 (Figure 5). Given the heterogenous nature of the tissue lysates, there was good agreement between the immunohistochemical staining results and the findings on Western blot. There were no large differences among the strains with regard to Bcl-2 expression. Bax was elevated >4-fold in old NOD mice and was also elevated in NOD.*scid* mice of both age groups. Similarly, caspase 3 expression was increased in these 3 groups of mice. Moreover, caspase 3 was found in its activated state by the appearance of the 20-kd fragment. There was more activated caspase 3 in tissues from older mice compared with tissues from the younger mice of both NOD strains.

Localization of activated caspase 3. A specific antibody for the activated form of caspase 3 was used for immunohistochemical analysis (Figure 6). Although salivary ductal and acinar cells from old NOD and NOD.*scid* mice stained positive for caspase 3 (as shown in Figure 1), only activated caspase 3 was found in the serous acinar cells. In contrast, salivary acinar cells from young NOD mice and BALB/c mice stained weakly for this enzyme form. Ductal cells and lymphocytes in all groups were found to be negative for activated caspase 3.

DISCUSSION

NOD and NOD.*scid* mice develop salivary dysfunction with age. In the NOD mouse, lymphocytic infiltrates are seen in the salivary and lacrimal glands between 18 and 20 weeks of age. Although lacking a mature immune system, the NOD.*scid* mouse shows alterations in salivary protein composition and epithelial cell apoptosis. The exocrine glands in both strains have acinar cells that undergo apoptosis. These features in the NOD and NOD.*scid* mice are similar to features seen in the exocrine glands of patients with SS (19). The present study demonstrates that proapoptotic molecules (i.e., Bax and caspases) are elevated in the epithelial cells of these 2 strains. The finding of elevated levels of Bax and the caspases in the absence of lymphocytes points once again to an intrinsic apoptotic defect in the epithelial cells.

Bax is a proapoptotic member of the Bcl-2 family that regulates cell death (23). Bax can form ion-conducting channels in planar lipid bilayers that may be the biochemical mechanism through which it exerts its effects on the mitochondria (17). Mice deficient in Bax develop hematopoietic malignancies (24) and are resistant to neuronal cell death in vitro (25). We report herein that the levels of Bax are elevated in the acinar salivary cells in the NOD and NOD.*scid* model of SS. We and other investigators have observed a possible role for Bax in the initiation of epithelial cell apoptosis in biopsy tissue from SS patients (1,19). Recently, it was shown that retinal cells of diabetic patients have elevated levels of Bax (26). Overexpression of Bax has also been reported in other diseases. Increased staining for Bax in the muscles of patients with myopathies has been reported (27,28). Moreover, abnormally high Bax expres-

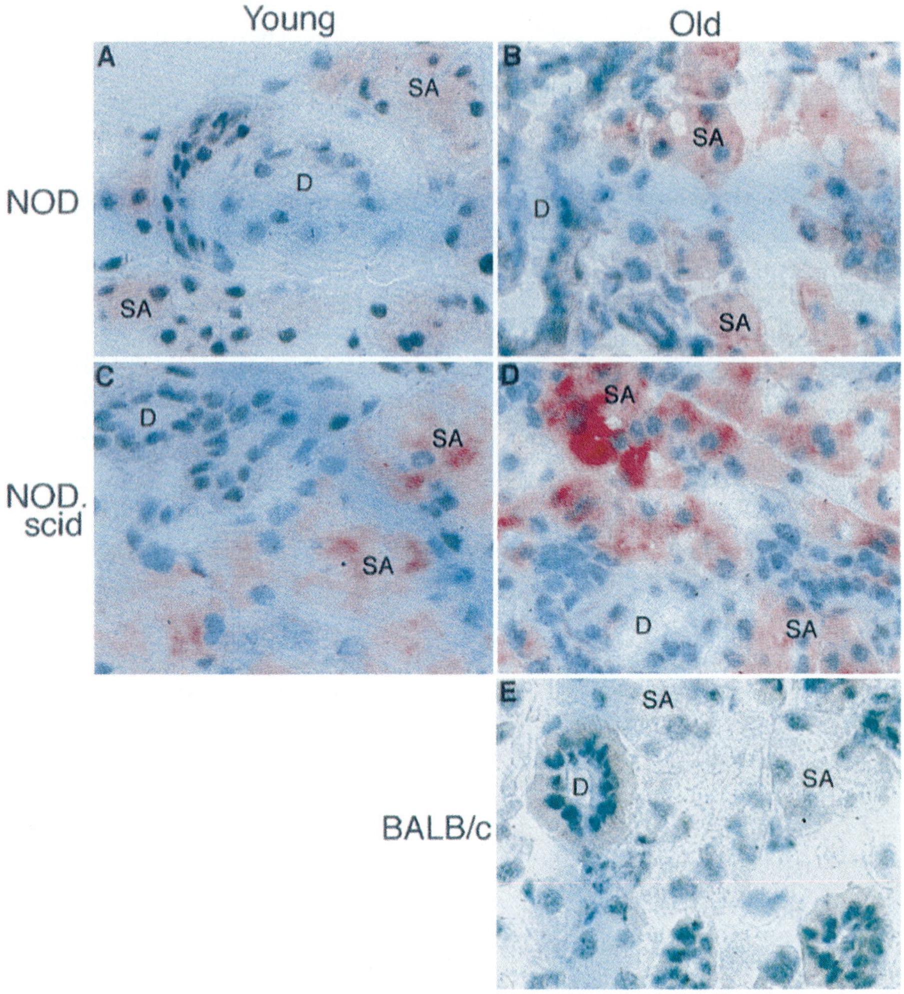

Figure 6. Immunohistochemical analysis of activated caspase 3. Submandibular glands from NOD and NOD.*scid* mice were stained with specific antibodies to activated caspase 3. The substrate was Vector Red and slides were counterstained with methyl green. Serous acinar (**SA**) cells from old NOD and NOD.*scid* mice (young and old) stained stronger for caspase 3 compared with cells from young NOD and BALB/c mice. Note that lymphocytes and ductal (**D**) cells stained weakly or were negative for this enzyme. (Original magnification × 400.)

sion may be important in the cell loss leading to glomerulosclerosis (29). Bax may also contribute to tissue destruction in the synovium of patients with rheumatoid arthritis (30).

The Bcl-2 family controls caspase activation by regulating the release of caspase activators such as cytochrome c, ATP, and Apaf-1 from the mitochondria (16,31). Caspase 3 is an important effector caspase that predominates in many apoptotic pathways, including the Fas and granzyme pathways. Inhibition of caspase activation may hold therapeutic potential. In the mouse model of Huntington's disease, the intracerebroventricular administration of a caspase inhibitor delays disease progression and mortality (32). The baculoviral protein p35 has caspase inhibitory properties. This protein, when specifically expressed in the retina, has been associated with retention of vision in a *Drosophila* model of retinal degeneration (33). Finally, the systemic administration of a peptidic caspase inhibitor prevented Fas-mediated liver damage in mice (34).

Our studies to date suggest a 2-stage model for SS in which initial epithelial apoptosis in NOD and NOD.*scid* mice occurs first and leads to lymphocyte infiltration and gland destruction (10,12). The first stage could be caused by abnormal expression of proapoptotic molecules.

The products of apoptotic cells can generate immunogenic autoantigens that initiate the autoimmune process (35,36). Apoptotic cells have membrane blebs containing nucleoproteins that are targets for autoantibodies (37). Mice immunized with syngeneic apoptotic thymocytes develop autoantibodies commonly seen in autoimmune rheumatic diseases (38). It is interesting to note that α-fodrin, which is cleaved by caspases and calpain during apoptosis, induces SS-like salivary lesions in mice after immunization (39). We believe that the abnormal expression of Bax results in caspase activation, leading to protein degradation and release of autoantigens. These autoantigens drive the autoimmune response and recruit lymphocytes to the exocrine glands. Once there, the lymphocytes cause further damage, eventually resulting in the clinical presentation of secretory dysfunction. Indeed, the presence of lymphocytes may be protective early in the disease in NOD mice. Certain cytokines (e.g., interferons and interleukin-10), produced by activated T cells, may protect cells from apoptosis (40–42). However, as the inflammatory process progresses, other cytokines may shift the balance from survival to apoptosis.

REFERENCES

1. Polihronis M, Tapinos NI, Theocharis SE, Economou A, Kittas C, Moutsopoulos HM. Modes of epithelial cell death and repair in Sjogren's syndrome (SS). Clin Exp Immunol 1998;114:485–90.
2. Kong L, Ogawa N, Nakabayashi T, Liu GT, D'Souza E, McGuff HS, et al. Fas and Fas ligand expression in salivary glands of patients with primary Sjögren's syndrome. Arthritis Rheum 1997; 40:87–97.
3. Manganelli P, Quaini F, Andreoli AM, Lagrasta C, Pilato FP, Zuccarelli A, et al. Quantitative analysis of apoptosis and bcl-2 in Sjogren's syndrome. J Rheumatol 1997;24:1552–7.
4. Matsumura R, Umemiya K, Kagami M, Tomioka H, Tanabe E, Sugiyama T, et al. Glandular and extraglandular expression of the Fas-Fas ligand and apoptosis in patients with Sjogren's syndrome. Clin Exp Rheumatol 1998;16:561–8.
5. Matsumura R, Kagami M, Tomioka H, Tanabe E, Sugiyama T, Sueishi M, et al. Expression of ductal Fas antigen in sialoadenitis of Sjogren's syndrome. Clin Exp Rheumatol 1996;14:309–11.
6. Tsubota K, Saito I, Miyasaka N. Granzyme A and perforin expressed in the lacrimal glands of patients with Sjogren's syndrome. Am J Ophthalmol 1994;117:120–1.
7. Alpert S, Kang H-I, Weissman I, Fox RI. Expression of granzyme A in salivary gland biopsies from patients with primary Sjögren's syndrome. Arthritis Rheum 1994;37:1046–54.
8. El Kaissouni J, Bene MC, Faure GC. Investigation of activation markers demonstrates significant overexpression of the secretory component on salivary gland epithelial cells in Sjogren's syndrome. Clin Immunol Immunopathol 1996;79:236–43.
9. Moutsopoulos HM. Sjogren's syndrome: autoimmune epithelitis. Clin Immunol Immunopathol 1994;72:162–5.
10. Humphreys-Beher MG, Peck AB, Dang H, Talal N. The role of apoptosis in the initiation of the autoimmune response in Sjogren's syndrome. Clin Exp Immunol 1999;116:383–7.
11. Robinson CP, Yamachika S, Bounous DI, Brayer J, Jonsson R, Holmdahl R, et al. A novel NOD-derived murine model of primary Sjögren's syndrome. Arthritis Rheum 1998;41:150–6.
12. Kong L, Robinson CP, Peck AB, Vela-Roch N, Sakata KM, Dang H, et al. Inappropriate apoptosis of salivary and lacrimal gland epithelium of immunodeficient NOD-scid mice. Clin Exp Rheumatol 1998;16:675–81.
13. Reed JC. Bcl-2 family proteins. Oncogene 1998;17:3225–36.
14. Sato T, Hanada M, Bodrug S, Irie S, Iwama N, Boise LH, et al. Interactions among members of the Bcl-2 protein family analyzed with a yeast two-hybrid system. Proc Natl Acad Sci U S A 1994;91:9238–43.
15. Susin SA, Zamzami N, Castedo M, Hirsch T, Marchetti P, Macho A, et al. Bcl-2 inhibits the mitochondrial release of an apoptogenic protease. J Exp Med 1996;184:1331–41.
16. Kroemer G. The proto-oncogene Bcl-2 and its role in regulating apoptosis. Nat Med 1997;3:614–20.
17. Basanez G, Nechushtan A, Drozhinin O, Chanturiya A, Choe E, Tutt S, et al. Bax, but not Bcl-xL, decreases the lifetime of planar phospholipid bilayer membranes at subnanomolar concentrations. Proc Natl Acad Sci U S A 1999;96:5492–7.
18. Shimizu S, Narita M, Tsujimoto Y. Bcl-2 family proteins regulate the release of apoptogenic cytochrome c by the mitochondrial channel VDAC. Nature 1999;399:483–7.
19. Kong L, Ogawa N, McGuff HS, Nakabayashi T, Sakata K-M, Masago R, et al. Bcl-2 family expression in salivary glands from patients with primary Sjögren's syndrome: involvement of bax in salivary gland destruction. Clin Immunol Immunopathol 1998;88: 133–41.
20. Talal N, Bunim JJ. The development of malignant lymphoma in the course of Sjogren's syndrome. Am J Med 1964;36:529–40.
21. Vitali C, Bombardieri S, Moutsopoulos HM, Balestrieri G, Bencivelli W, Bernstein R, et al. Preliminary criteria for the classification of Sjögren's Syndrome: results of a prospective concerted action supported by the European Community. Arthritis Rheum 1993;36:340–7.
22. Chisholm DM, Mason DK. Labial salivary gland biopsy in Sjögren's disease. J Clin Pathol 1968;21:656–60.
23. Brady HJ, Gil-Gomez G. Bax: the pro-apoptotic Bcl-2 family member, Bax. Int J Biochem Cell Biol 1998;30:647–50.
24. Meijerink JPP, Mensink EJBM, Wang K, Sedlak TW, Slöetjes AW, de Witte T, et al. Hematopoietic malignancies demonstrate loss-of-function mutations of BAX. Blood 1998;91:2991–7.
25. Deckwerth TL, Elliott JL, Knudson CM, Johnson EM Jr, Snider WD, Korsmeyer SJ. BAX is required for neuronal death after trophic factor deprivation and during development. Neuron 1996; 17:401–11.
26. Podesta F, Romeo G, Liu WH, Krajewski S, Reed JC, Gerhardinger C, et al. Bax is increased in the retina of diabetic subjects and is associated with pericyte apoptosis in vivo and in vitro. Am J Pathol 2000;156:1025–32.
27. Tews DS, Goebel HH, Meineck HM. DNA-fragmentation and apoptosis-related proteins of muscle cells in motor neuron disorders. Acta Neurol Scand 1997;96:380–6.
28. Olive M, Ferrer I. Bcl-2 and Bax protein expression in human myopathies. J Neurol Sci 1999;164:76–81.
29. Yoshimura A, Uda S, Inui K, Nemoto T, Sugenoya Y, Sharif S, et al. Expression of bcl-2 and bax in glomerular disease. Nephrol Dial Transplant 1999;14 Suppl 1:55–7.
30. Sioud M, Mellbye O, Førre Ø. Analysis of the NF-kappa B p65 subunit, Fas antigen, Fas ligand and Bcl-2-related proteins in the synovium of RA and polyarticular JRA. Clin Exp Rheumatol 1998;16:125–34.

31. Nuñez G, Benedict MA, Hu Y, Inohara N. Caspases: the proteases of the apoptotic pathway. Oncogene 1998;17:3237–45.
32. Ona VO, Li M, Vonsattel JP, Andrews LJ, Khan SQ, Chung WM, et al. Inhibition of caspase-1 slows disease progression in a mouse model of Huntington's disease. Nature 1999;399:263–7.
33. Davidson FF, Steller H. Blocking apoptosis prevents blindness in Drosophila retinal degeneration mutants. Nature 1998;391: 587–91.
34. Rodriguez I, Matsuura K, Ody C, Nagata S, Vassalli P. Systemic injection of a tripeptide inhibits the intracellular activation of CPP32-like proteases in vivo and fully protects mice against Fas-mediated fulminant liver destruction and death. J Exp Med 1996;184:2067–72.
35. Tan EM. Autoimmunity and apoptosis. J Exp Med 1994;179: 1083–6.
36. Ogawa N, Dang H, Talal N. Apoptosis and autoimmunity. J Autoimmun 1995;8:1–20.
37. Casciola-Rosen LA, Anhalt G, Rosen A. Autoantigens targeted in systemic lupus erythematosus are clustered in two populations of surface structures on apoptotic keratinocytes. J Exp Med 1994; 179:1317–30.
38. Mevorach D, Zhou JL, Song X, Elkon KB. Systemic exposure to irradiated apoptotic cells induces autoantibody production. J Exp Med 1998;188:387–92.
39. Haneji N, Nakamura T, Takio K, Yanagi K, Higashiyama H, Saito I, et al. Identification of α-fodrin as a candidate autoantigen in primary Sjögren's syndrome. Science 1997;276:604–7.
40. Karsen A, Yee E, Kaushansky K, Harlan JM. Cloning of a human bcl-2 homologue: inflammatory cytokines induce human A1 in cultured endothelial cells. Blood 1996;87:3089–96.
41. Horie T, Dobashi K, Iizuka K, Yoshii A, Shimizu Y, Nakazawa T, et al. Interferon-gamma rescues TNF-alpha induced apoptosis mediated by up-regulation of TNFR2 on EoL-1 cells. Exp Hematol 1999;27:512–9.
42. Rivera DL, Olister SM, Liu X, Thompson JH, Zhang XJ, Pennline K, et al. Interleukin-10 attenuates experimental fetal growth restriction and demise. FASEB J 1998;12:189–97.

ARTHRITIS & RHEUMATISM
Vol. 44, No. 3, March 2001, pp 703–711

Cysteine Protease Activity Is Up-Regulated in Inflamed Ankle Joints of Rats With Adjuvant-Induced Arthritis and Decreases With In Vivo Administration of a Vinyl Sulfone Cysteine Protease Inhibitor

Sandra L. Biroc,[1] Steffen Gay,[2] Klaus Hummel,[3] Catherine Magill,[4] James T. Palmer,[4] Donna R. Spencer,[5] Susan Sa,[6] Jeffrey L. Klaus,[7] Beat A. Michel,[2] David Rasnick,[8] and Renate E. Gay[2]

Objective. **Cysteine proteases are postulated to play a role in tissue destruction in the joints of animals with arthritis. The purpose of the present study was to confirm the concept that cysteine proteases are enzymes involved in the pathology of rheumatoid arthritis (RA).**

Methods. **Arthritis was induced in Lewis rats by adjuvant injection (adjuvant-induced arthritis [AIA] model) and scored for inflammation. At necropsy, the rear paws were either fixed in formalin and assigned a histologic score (based on synovial cell proliferation, cartilage erosion, bone erosion, and fibroproliferative pannus) or frozen, cryosectioned, and assayed for enzyme activity either by in situ cytochemical staining with a post-azo-coupling method using a chromogenic substrate (Z-arg-arg-MNA) or by a novel assay placing the tissue section directly in a cuvette using the fluorogenic substrate Z-arg-arg-AMC.**

Results. **Enzymatic activity, measured either in frozen sections in situ or in the cuvette assay, was positively correlated with joint destruction (r = 0.7) and inflammation (r = 0.8). Activity was not inhibited significantly by Pefabloc (a serine protease inhibitor), EDTA (a metalloprotease inhibitor), or pepstatin A (an aspartyl protease inhibitor) but was inhibited by E-64 and vinyl sulfone irreversible inhibitors of cysteine proteases. The effect of one of the vinyl sulfone cysteine protease inhibitors, Mu-Leu-HomoPhe-vinylsulfone, was tested in vivo by dietary administration at 2.2 mg/kg/day in the AIA model; this resulted in a significant decrease in inflammation and in the amount of cysteine protease activity measured in the joint tissue.**

Conclusion. **Cysteine protease activity levels increase in the diseased state and may be an important target for designing small molecule inhibitors to reduce the inflammation and tissue destruction associated with RA.**

[1]Sandra L. Biroc, PhD: Berlex Biosciences, Richmond, California; [2]Steffen Gay, MD, Beat A. Michel, MD, Renate E. Gay, MD: University Hospital, Zurich, Switzerland; [3]Klaus Hummel, MD: University Hospital Gottingen, Gottingen, Germany; [4]Catherine Magill, PhD, James T. Palmer, PhD: Axys Pharmaceuticals, Inc., South San Francisco, California; [5]Donna R. Spencer, MS: AP Cells, Menlo Park, California; [6]Susan Sa, BS: LabVelocity, San Francisco, California; [7]Jeffrey L. Klaus, BS: Abbott Laboratories, Abbott Park, Illinois; [8]David Rasnick, PhD: University of California, Berkeley.

Address correspondence and reprint requests to Catherine Magill, PhD, Axys Pharmaceuticals, Inc., Department of Pharmacology and Cell Biology, 180 Kimball Way, South San Francisco, CA 94080.

Submitted for publication June 7, 2000; accepted in revised form November 9, 2000.

Rheumatoid arthritis (RA) is a systemic disease characterized by chronic joint inflammation and destruction of articular cartilage and periarticular bone. Common therapeutic approaches have resulted in reducing symptoms of inflammation, i.e., pain and swelling, but not in diminishing joint destruction. Proteases are prime culprits in tissue wasting diseases and, as such, represent a target for drug discovery efforts for small molecule inhibitors.

Cysteine proteases are 1 of 4 major classes of proteolytic enzymes that are characterized by the presence of a cysteine residue at their active site. They are mainly localized within lysosomes but are also found to be secreted into the extracellular milieu (1). It is important to demonstrate not only that protein levels, messenger RNA (mRNA) levels, and inactive forms of the enzyme are up-regulated but also that actual enzymatic activity is up-regulated and that the increase is concomitant with disease severity. It is not known whether the enzymatic activity increases concurrently with protein levels.

There is a wealth of evidence pointing to up-regulation of cysteine proteases, especially cathepsins B, L, S, and K, in disease processes (2). Increased levels of cysteine proteases have been implicated in tissue- and bone-degrading diseases such as arthritis (3) and osteoporosis (4,5). Cysteine proteases are present in increased quantities in the synovial fluid of patients with RA (6,7). Increased levels of cathepsins B and L are found in the joint tissue of animals with experimentally induced RA (8–11) as well as in the synovium of patients with RA (10). Furthermore, inhibitors of cathepsin B have been shown to decrease the severity of joint inflammation and reduce joint destruction in adjuvant-induced arthritis (AIA) in rats (12–14).

In this study, a method for demonstrating increased levels of cysteine proteases in frozen tissue sections (8,15,16) was modified to quantitate enzyme activity. These values were compared with the degree of inflammation and of tissue destruction. One of the cysteine protease inhibitors used in the in vitro assay was tested in vivo, mixed with the food and fed to the animals for the duration of the AIA trial. The results indicate that there is a strong positive correlation between the amount of cysteine protease enzyme activity and the severity of arthritic lesions and that oral administration of an inhibitor of cysteine proteases reduces the severity of inflammation and tissue destruction in the AIA model of RA.

MATERIALS AND METHODS

AIA in rats. Female Lewis/SsN rats (5 weeks old; Charles River, Wilmington, MA) were housed in standard cages and fed powdered 4% rat chow (Harlan Teklad, Madison, WI) and water ad libitum. All procedures were in accordance with the Institutional Animal Care and Use policies at the University of Alabama at Birmingham, where the in-life portion of this study was conducted. To provide mild analgesia, acetaminophen (3 mg/ml) was administered in the drinking water at an estimated dosage of 110–300 mg/kg/day. It should be noted that acetaminophen has antiinflammatory properties and may have had some effect on the outcome of the study. On day 0, 70 rats were injected intradermally, at the base of the tail, with 0.1 ml of heat-inactivated *Mycobacterium butyricum* (Difco, Becton Dickinson, Franklin Lakes, NJ) in light mineral oil (6 mg/100 μl). Body weight and articular inflammation were determined at weekly intervals. Rear paw edema (swelling) was scored as follows: 0 = no edema, 1 = slight edema of the digital joints, 2 = edema of the digital joints and foot pads, 3 = gross edema of the entire foot pad below the ankle, and 4 = gross edema of the entire foot pad including the ankle or elbow joint. For erythema (redness), the scoring was as follows: 0 = normal, 1 = pink, 2 = red, 3 = violet, and 4 = deep violaceous. On day 34, the animals were killed by CO_2 asphyxia.

Joint histology. The left hind paw from each animal was fixed and prepared for scoring of tissue destruction; the right paw was snap frozen for enzyme activity measurements. Cryopreservation was accomplished by removing the ankle, submerging it in a 50:50 mixture of OCT TissueTek (Fisher Scientific, Hampton, NH) and water, and then plunging it into a beaker of supercooled hexane (in a dry ice/ethanol bath). Specimens were stored at −80°C. Morphology of the joint tissue was assessed by first fixing the tissue in 10% neutral buffered formalin, decalcifying (Fisher Chelating Agent [0.003*M* EDTA, 1.35*N* hydrochloric acid]; Fisher Scientific), embedding in paraffin (58°C, 3 times for 45 minutes each time), and staining the 5-μm sections with hematoxylin and eosin. Two sections of each joint were evaluated by 2 independent investigators (SG and REG), who were blinded to the treatment information. Total joint histopathologic scores were calculated by determining the severity or extent of (a) synovial proliferation, (b) cartilage erosion, (c) bone erosion, and (d) fibroproliferative pannus, each on a scale of 0–3 where 0 = normal, 1 = mild, 2 = moderate, and 3 = severe. The scores from the 2 investigators were summed and used as the score for the joint.

In situ enzyme activity. In situ enzyme activity was measured by the method of van Noorden et al (8). Paw joints were collected at the time the rats were killed and were snap frozen. Without any prior fixation or decalcification, the specimens were cryosectioned into 10-μm slices, using a Jung CM 3000 cryostat (Leica, Deerfield, IL) and a tungsten carbide D-profile knife, and the slices collected onto clear tape (Scotch, 1″, type 600). The samples were first incubated for 45 minutes at 37°C with the substrate solution, consisting of 3.2 m*M* Z-arg-arg-MNA (Bachem Bioscience, Philadelphia, PA) in 100 m*M* potassium phosphate buffer, pH 6.0, to which was added 10% polyvinyl alcohol (Sigma, St. Louis, MO), 10 m*M* dithiothreitol (DTT), 2.7 m*M* L-cysteine, and 1.3 m*M* EDTA. The samples were then placed in *N*-ethylmaleimide (Sigma) at 125 mg/ml in potassium phosphate buffer, pH 8, for 1 minute at room temperature and then at 55°C for another 5 minutes. They were then soaked in Fast Blue B solution (FBB; Sigma) (prepared from 21 mg FBB dissolved in 1 ml dimethylformamide [Baxter, McGraw Park, IL] and then added to 100 ml potassium phosphate buffer, pH 8.0) for 30 minutes at room temperature. Finally, the slides were placed into 0.1*M* cupric sulfate solution (Sigma) for 15 minutes at room temperature.

After a short rinse with 0.9% saline, the samples were mounted in Aquamount (Fisher Scientific) and immediately viewed under a microscope with 4× and 10× objectives, and the intensity of the developing red color was scored on a scale of 0–4. Pictures were taken using 64 Tungsten or Daylight color slide film (Sigma) or captured as a 640 × 480 digital image using an Optronics DEI 750 3 chip camera (Technical Instruments, San Francisco, CA) on a Leitz/Wild M3Z dissecting microscope with a 0.63× reducing lens on the C-mount. Adjacent sections were fixed in formalin and stained briefly in hematoxylin for location of major morphologic landmarks. Also, adjacent sections were treated with 10 μM cysteine protease inhibitor in the initial reaction mixture.

Cuvette enzyme activity. Cysteine protease enzyme activity was measured in frozen tissue sections by a novel method. The ankle was cryosectioned using a Leica cryostat and a tungsten carbide D-profile knife at a cutting angle of 10°, as suggested by Johnstone (15). The tape with adhering tissue slice was placed into a test tube to which was added 2 ml reaction buffer (50 m*M* sodium phosphate buffer, pH 6.0; 2.5 m*M* EDTA, 3.0 m*M* DTT) and 0.005 ml substrate solution (10 m*M* Z-arg-arg-AMC [Sigma] in dimethyl formamide [DMF]). The tube was incubated for 10 minutes at 30°C, then the reaction was stopped with the addition of 0.3 ml 1.7% trifluoroacetic acid in acetonitrile (Baxter). The fluorescence intensity was read on a fluorimeter (Applied Biosystems, Foster City, CA) at excitation 380 nm and emission 450 nm. To obtain the activity per cross-sectional area of tissue, an adjacent section was stained with hematoxylin, mounted as above, placed on a light box, and the shape traced onto clear x-ray film. The shapes were cut out from the film and weighed. The weights were compared with a standard curve of weight versus square centimeter. The number for the cross-sectional area obtained from the standard curve was divided into the fluorescence intensity value, which represents total enzyme activity normalized to the size of the tissue sample.

Substrate/inhibitor profile. To better characterize the cuvette assay, various substrates and inhibitors were tested. Both Z-val-val-arg-AMC and Z-phe-arg-AMC (synthesized by one of the authors [JLK]) were used as substrates at 5 μM for 3 minutes at 30°C. The inhibitors, Pefabloc (1 m*M*; Pierce, Rockford, IL), EDTA (12.5 m*M*; Sigma), pepstatin A (1 μM, Sigma), and E-64 (10 μM, Sigma), were added to buffer and tissue section 10 minutes before the addition of substrate. Irreversible cysteine protease inhibitors, Mu-Phe-HomoPhe-vinylsulfone, Mu-Leu-HomoPhe-vinylsulfone (LHVS), Mu-3,5-diiodo-Tyr-HomoPhe-vinylsulfone, and Mu-2-naphthylalanine-HomoPhe-vinylsulfone-2-Naphthyl, were synthesized according to a method previously described by us (17). They were dissolved in DMF at a concentration of 10 m*M*, and were added to the reaction mixture at a final concentration of 10 μM, 10 minutes before the addition of substrate.

In vivo administration of LHVS to arthritic rats. Two separate studies were performed to determine if a vinyl sulfone cysteine protease inhibitor, LHVS, would reduce the signs of inflammation, the evidence of joint destruction, or the measured enzyme activity in the affected ankle joints. In the first study, 10 animals were injected with adjuvant on day 0 as above. Five rats were fed powdered Harlan Teklad (4%) rat chow. The remaining 5 rats were given the same food (from day 2 to day 28), which had been powdered in a blender with the test article mixed into the food at a level of 30 mg/1 kg of food. This converts to 2.2 mg of LHVS/kg body weight/day assuming an average daily food intake of 18 gm/200-gm rat. The dosage of 2.2 mg/kg/day was determined in a preliminary dose-ranging study using 100, 30, and 10 mg LHVS per kg food. The actual food intake for each animal was not monitored. The food was replenished daily. The rats were killed on day 29. In the second study, there were 3 treatment groups (n = 10 in each). One group received adjuvant and normal food (disease control), another received adjuvant and LHVS in the food at 2.2 mg/kg/day, and the third received saline injection instead of adjuvant injection and normal food (saline control). LHVS-treated food was administered from day 2 to day 28, and all animals were killed on day 32. No obvious acute or long-term drug-related toxicity was observed over the dosing period.

Statistical analysis. Data were analyzed by Sigma-Plot or Kaleidagraph, and r values obtained by linear regression least squares analysis. Statistical analyses were performed on Statview using analysis of variance and the Bonferroni-Dunnett post hoc test. *P* values less than 0.05 were considered significant.

RESULTS

Increased cysteine protease activity in the joints of arthritic rats. To demonstrate that cysteine proteases are up-regulated in inflamed joint tissue from rats in which arthritis has been induced by a single injection of adjuvant, 85 animals were tested, 10 of which received no adjuvant at all and served as the noninflamed saline controls. Frozen tissue sections were tested for in situ enzyme activity by the post-azo-coupling procedure, using Z-arg-arg-MNA as the substrate. In nearly all of the inflamed joints, there was a marked increase in colored product, whereas, in the tissue sections from the control joints, very little or no color was seen (Figure 1). This increase in enzyme activity is due either to the increased amount of cysteine proteases or to an increase in the activation of enzyme in the diseased state. The histochemical enzyme activity staining could be completely abolished by the addition of cysteine protease inhibitors (at 10 μM) to the reaction medium 10 minutes before adding substrate solution (results not shown). The in situ reaction was scored qualitatively by assigning a relative score of 0–4 for the intensity of red color.

To quantitate this observed increase in enzyme activity, a novel cuvette assay was developed. The tissue section adhering to the clear tape was placed into a tube with reaction buffer and fluorogenic substrate. The resulting increase in fluorescence was both linear and quantitative over a 10-minute period at 30°C (data not shown). Thus, an end point assay was adopted to screen joint tissue from ~80 animals. The mean ± SD value in nondiseased (saline control) rat ankles and diseased ankles was 186 ± 34 fluorescent units (n = 10) and 481 ± 247 fluorescent units (n = 70), respectively. Although there was great variation in the values obtained from individual animals, on average, tissue from adjuvant-injected rats had greater enzyme activity than tissue from control animals.

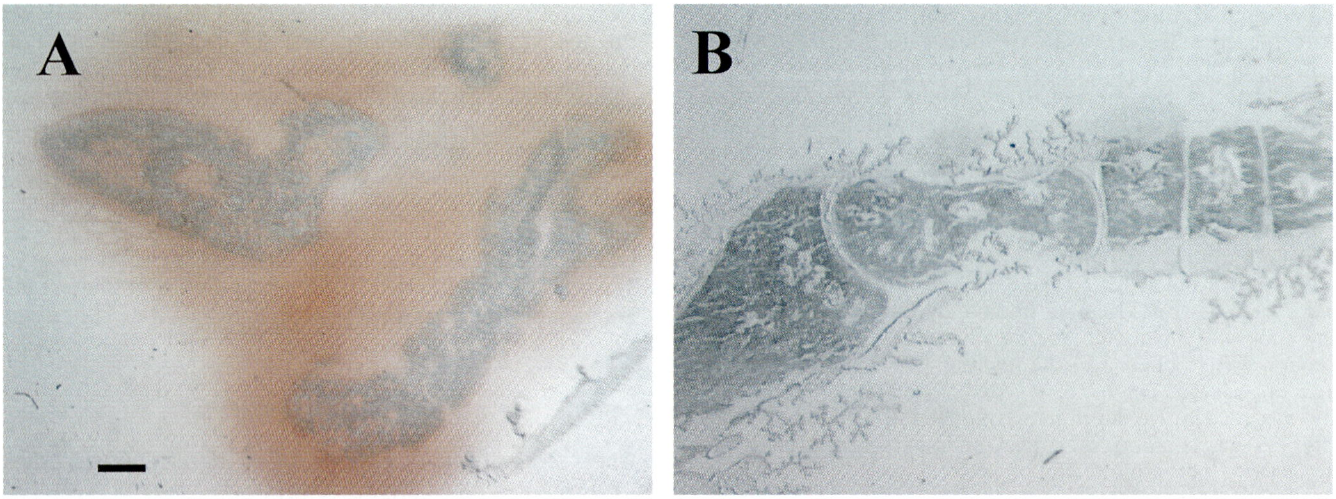

Figure 1. In situ cysteine protease enzyme activity in frozen tissue sections from the ankles of arthritic and normal rats. Ankle joints from arthritic rats and from normal rats were snap frozen and cryosectioned, and tissue sections were stained for cysteine protease activity. **A,** Arthritic rat (inflammation score 19 [scale 0–24], tissue destruction score 6 [scale 0–12], in situ enzyme score 4 [scale 0–4], cuvette assay score 636 fluorescent units [scale 0–1,000]). **B,** Normal rat (inflammation score 0, tissue destruction score 0, in situ enzyme score 0.25, cuvette assay score 234 fluorescent units). Even though enzyme staining is diffuse and cannot be localized to a particular compartment, cysteine protease activity is dramatically increased in the arthritic ankle compared with the normal ankle. An adjacent tissue section from the arthritic rat was treated with 10 μM Mu-Leu-HomoPhe-vinylsulfone, and, when stained for cysteine protease activity, produced no signal (results not shown). **Bar** = 1 mm.

Positive correlation of enzyme activity with inflammation and severity of tissue destruction. The scores for inflammation and tissue destruction were correlated with the quantitative values for enzyme activity. The weekly measurements of paw swelling and redness were added together for a score of inflammation on a total scale of 0–24 (3 weekly values summed). A general histologic score (0–12 scale) representing the severity of tissue destruction, obtained by summing individual scores for synovial cell proliferation, fibroproliferative pannus, bone erosion, and cartilage erosion, was also assigned. The results are shown in Figure 2. Enzymatic activity in frozen sections in situ (scored on a scale of 0–4) was positively correlated (by linear least-squares analysis) with joint destruction ($r = 0.70$) and inflammation ($r = 0.82$). Enzymatic activity measured by cleavage of Z-arg-arg-AMC was also positively correlated with joint destruction ($r = 0.75$) and inflammation ($r = 0.86$).

Cathepsin B–like activity measured by tissue section cuvette assay. To rule out the possibility that the cuvette assay was measuring another class of protease, several inhibitors and several substrates were tested in the cuvette end point assay with adjacent frozen sections from 1 severely arthritic ankle. The results are shown in Table 1. The tissue slices were tested with Z-arg-arg-AMC (a substrate selective for cathepsin B), Z-phe-arg-AMC (a substrate with broad-range specificity for cathepsins B, L, S, and K), and Z-val-val-arg-AMC (a substrate for cathepsins B, L, S, and K but with a preference for cathepsin S). Adjacent sections of the same rat ankle gave values of 861 fluorescent units after 10 minutes for Z-arg-arg-AMC, 968 fluorescent units after 3 minutes for Z-phe-arg-AMC, and 590 fluorescent units after 3 minutes for Z-val-val-arg-AMC (assayed at 30°C). The reaction was linear for the duration of the assay for all 3 substrates. To test whether known cysteine protease inhibitors indeed inhibit the tissue enzymes, several inhibitors were tested with the 3 substrates in the cuvette end point assay. In all cases, the cysteine protease inhibitors decreased the enzyme activity by 83–97% compared with the noninhibited control value.

The substrates used can also serve as substrates for other proteases. Certainly metalloproteases are present in great quantity in the inflamed joint (18–20). Serine proteases and aspartyl proteases may also be present. To rule out the possibility that serine proteases, metalloproteases, or aspartyl proteases interfere positively with the activity measurement, selective inhibitors for these classes of proteases were also tested (Table 1). Using concentrations known to inhibit the respective enzymes, Pefabloc (a serine protease inhibitor), EDTA (a metalloprotease inhibitor) and pepstatin A (an aspartyl protease inhibitor) were each added to the reaction

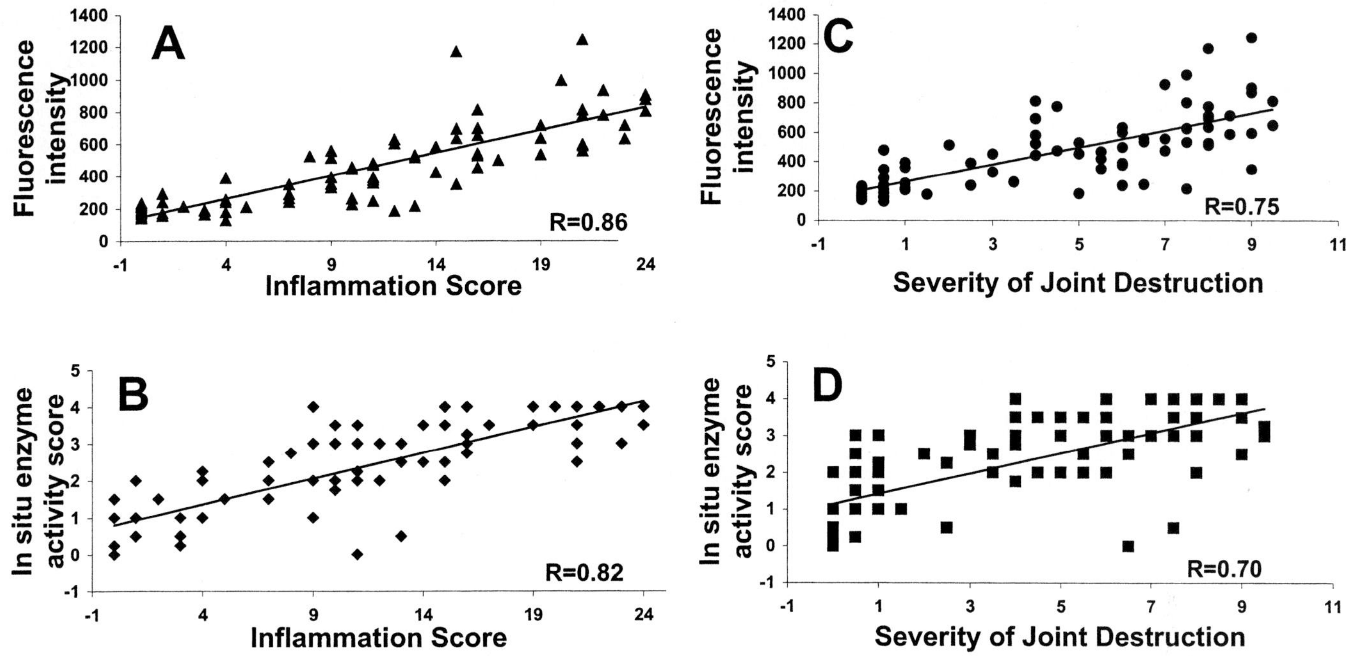

Figure 2. Correlations between cysteine protease activity and inflammation or tissue destruction. The scores from individual animals are plotted pairwise and compared by linear regression least squares analysis. The score for inflammation was plotted against enzyme activity by cuvette assay (**A**) and in situ cytochemical assay (**B**). Likewise, the degree of tissue destruction (summed histologic score for bone erosion, cartilage erosion, fibroproliferative pannus, and synovial cell proliferation) was plotted against enzyme activity by cuvette assay (**C**) and in situ cytochemical assay (**D**). In all 4 cases, the correlation values (>0.7) indicate good correlation between enzyme activity and degree of inflammation or tissue destruction.

mixture 10 minutes before addition of substrate. None of these significantly inhibited the reaction. However, known inhibitors of cysteine protease activity (E-64 and several irreversible vinyl sulfones) greatly inhibited the enzyme activity of the tissue slices. Taken together, these data suggest that the enzymatic activity is primarily from cysteine proteases that are of the cathepsin B–like family.

Reduction of disease severity in AIA rats fed LHVS. Since inhibitors of cysteine protease decreased the enzyme activity in the in vitro enzyme assay, it was reasonable to suggest that cysteine protease inhibitors

Table 1. Inhibition of endogenous, up-regulated enzyme activity in frozen tissue sections of arthritic joints, as determined by the cuvette assay*

Compound	Inhibition specificity	Concentration	Inhibition as % of uninhibited control activity		
			Z-arg-arg-AMC†	Z-phe-arg-AMC‡	Z-val-val-arg-AMC§
Mu-Phe-Hph-VSPh¶	Cysteine proteases, irreversible	10 μM	94	96	85
Mu-Leu-Hph-VSPh¶	Cysteine proteases, irreversible	10 μM	97	96	86
Mu-Tyr(I_2)-Hph-VSPh¶	Cysteine proteases, irreversible	10 μM	95	95	83
Mu-Na2-Hph-VS2-Nap¶	Cysteine proteases, irreversible	10 μM	94	94	85
E-64	Cysteine proteases, irreversible	10 μM	97	95	86
EDTA	Metalloproteases	12.5 mM	26	0	7
Pefabloc	Serine proteases	1 mM	19	13	17
Pepstatin A	Aspartyl proteases	1 μM	1	1	4

* A cuvette assay was performed, in duplicate, on adjacent tissue sections from an individual rat ankle as described in Materials and Methods. Inhibition, as a percent of uninhibited control, was determined using substrates with varying specificity for cathepsins B, L, S, or K.
† Z-arg-arg-AMC is a substrate specific for cathepsin B.
‡ Z-phe-arg-AMC is a substrate for cathepsins B, L, S, and K.
§ Z-val-val-arg-AMC is a substrate with a preference for cathepsin S.
¶ The vinyl sulfones inhibit cathepsins B, L, S, and K with varying degrees of selectivity.

Table 2. Histologic and inflammation scores in animals treated with Mu-Leu-HomoPhe-vinylsulfone (LHVS)*

Treatment group	Histologic score†					Inflammation score‡		
	SCP	CE	BE	FPP	Sum	Edema	Erythema	Sum
Adjuvant	2.1 ± 0.82	1.3 ± 1.03	4.0 ± 0.79	1.8 ± 1.037	9.2 ± 1.94	8.6 ± 1.94	1.0 ± 1.0	9.6 ± 2.5
LHVS	1.4 ± 0.74	0.23 ± 0.27	2.7 ± 1.44	1.3 ± 1.5	5.6 ± 3.34	6.00 ± 3.67	2.8 ± 2.16	8.8 ± 5.4
P§	0.195	0.051	0.115	0.56	0.070	0.199	0.13	0.77

* Animals were fed normal food (adjuvant; n = 5) or food mixed with vinyl sulfone to deliver 2.2 mg/kg/day (LHVS; n = 5) from day 2 to day 28 after adjuvant injection. Values are the mean ± SD.
† Paraffin-embedded/hematoxylin and eosin–stained tissue sections were scored for the degree of synovial cell proliferation (SCP), cartilage erosion (CE), bone erosion (BE), and fibroproliferative pannus (FPP), each on a scale of 0–3, for a total possible summed score of 12.
‡ In-life measurements of inflammation are the sum of edema (scale 0–4) and erythema (scale 0–4) for 3 weeks, for a total possible summed score of 24.
§ Treatment group versus adjuvant-injected control group, by Bonferroni-Dunnett post hoc test for significance.

might decrease enzyme activity in vivo in the joints of rats with induced polyarthritis. In a pilot study with 5 animals per treatment group, LHVS was administered in the food of 1 group of arthritic rats for 4 weeks. Table 2 shows the inflammation scores and histologic scores for joint destruction. Inflammation was decreased by ~10%

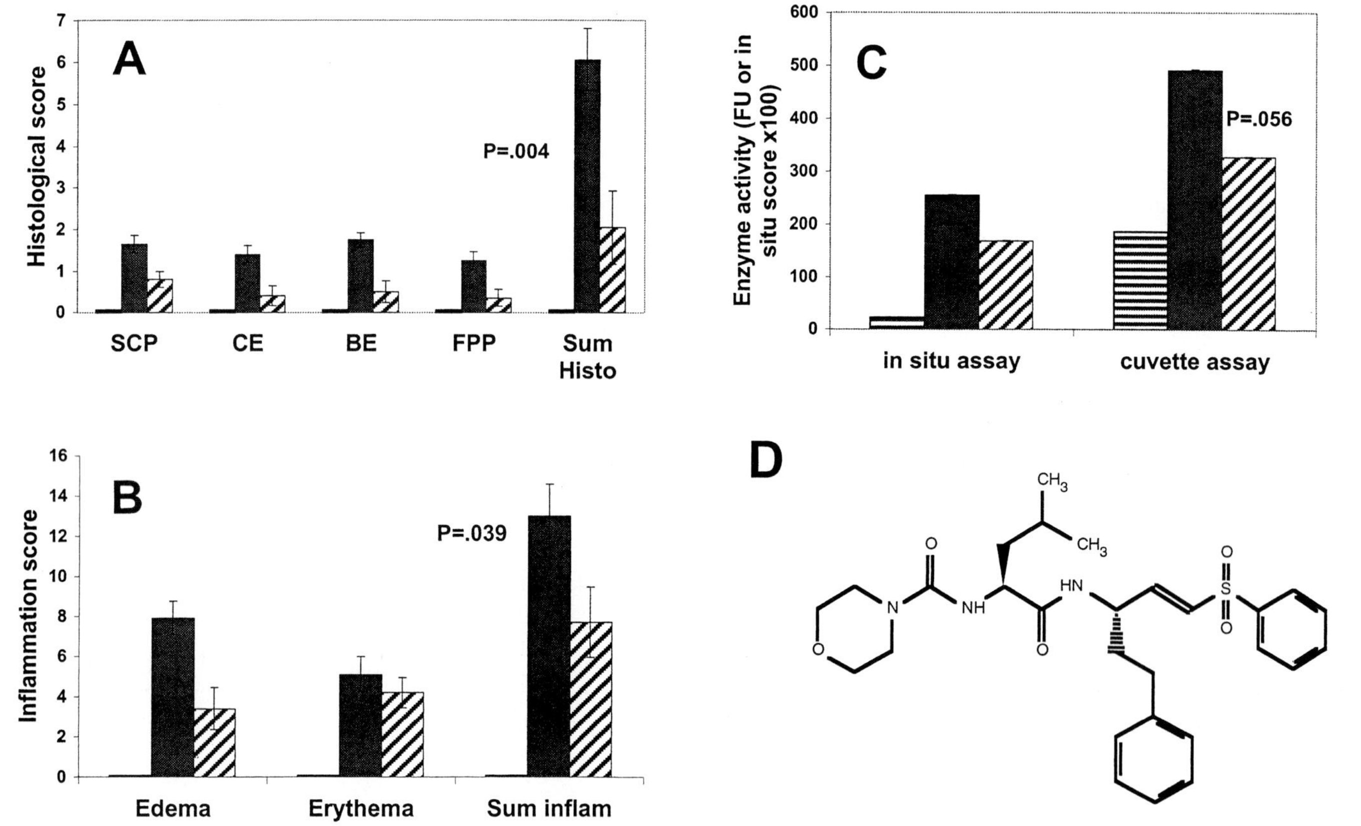

Figure 3. Effects of oral administration of Mu-Leu-HomoPhe-vinylsulfone (LHVS) in the adjuvant-induced arthritis model. **A,** Joint destruction, assessed by scoring paraffin-embedded/hematoxylin and eosin–stained tissue sections for degree of synovial cell proliferation (SCP), cartilage erosion (CE), bone erosion (BE), and fibroproliferative pannus (FPP), each on a scale of 0–3, for a total possible summed score (Sum Histo) of 12. **B,** Clinical inflammation, assessed by scoring swelling (edema) and redness (erythema), 3 weekly values, each on a scale of 0–4, for a total possible summed score (Sum inflam) of 24. LHVS-treated animals showed statistically significant decreases in the total summed score for histologic features and inflammation. **C,** Enzyme activity, measured either by in situ staining or by the fluorogenic cuvette assay (in fluorescent units [FU]), showing a decrease in animals treated with the cysteine protease inhibitor. ▤ = nondisease (saline-treated) controls; ■ = disease (adjuvant-injected) controls; ▨ = disease rats treated with LHVS. Values are the mean ± SEM of 10 animals. **D,** Chemical structure of LHVS.

and joint destruction decreased by ~40% in the animals treated with LHVS; however, neither of these decreases was statistically significant. When the total histologic score was broken down into the 4 individual components, cartilage erosion showed the greatest decrease.

Since the results of the pilot study did not reach statistical significance, a second study was initiated, with 10 animals in each treatment group and a nonarthritic saline control group added. LHVS was administered in the food at 2.2 mg/kg/day for 4 weeks after adjuvant injection. The total histologic score for joint destruction (Figure 3A) was decreased by 66% (from a mean ± SD of 6.05 ± 2.35 to 2.05 ± 2.77 in control adjuvant-injected rats and LHVS-treated adjuvant-injected rats, respectively; $P = 0.004$), with dramatic decreases in cartilage erosion and bone erosion. Likewise, the scores for inflammation (Figure 3B) showed a dramatic decrease with LHVS treatment. There was a concomitant decrease in cysteine protease enzyme activity in the frozen ankle tissue as measured by the in situ enzyme staining assay or by the fluorogenic substrate cuvette assay (Figure 3C). Thus, dietary administration of an irreversible vinyl sulfone inhibitor of cysteine proteases resulted in a statistically significant reduction in the severity of clinical signs of the disease in this model of RA.

DISCUSSION

In this study, the up-regulation of cysteine proteases in the arthritic ankle joints of rats with AIA correlates positively with the severity of joint destruction and with measurements of the degree of inflammation. Other investigators have previously shown that proteases in general are increased in the inflamed joint (10,21). Cathepsins are lysosomal enzymes that contribute to the normal process of cellular turnover by digesting intracellular proteins. However, if overexpressed or misrouted to the extracellular compartment, they may give rise to a pathologic condition, contributing to tissue destruction. In addition, mislocalized cathepsins may proteolytically activate other tissue-destructive enzymes, e.g., converting the precursor form of a matrix metalloprotease (MMP), tissue collagenase or elastase, to the active form (22). Thus, the correlation between increased cysteine protease activity and markers of the disease is an important observation.

Two different methods were used to measure the increased enzyme activity in frozen slices of arthritic joints: in situ staining and a cuvette assay. The tissue staining, post-azo-coupling method developed by van Noorden and Vogels (9) unfortunately allows for diffusion of the colored product, so localization can be assigned only to general regions and quantitated by assigning a visual score. Using this method, it was found that cysteine protease activity increased with disease severity.

The second method, a novel cuvette assay of frozen tissue slices, allows better quantitation of the observed increase in enzyme activity. The advantage of this new technique is that it provides a numeric value for comparison with the visual localization information obtained from the adjacent in situ–stained sections. The comparisons can be expanded to include additional adjacent sections immunostained for localization of the protein (which may not have enzymatic activity) or sections stained by in situ hybridization for localization of cathepsin mRNAs. However, both pre- and proforms of the enzyme will be recognized by immunostaining techniques but will not be enzymatically active. Using our methods, the enzyme activity is still inhibitable because LHVS added directly, either to the tissue section or to the cuvette, at 10 μM, greatly reduced the enzyme activity values. A distinct disadvantage is that tissue preservation of these frozen sections is not nearly good enough to enable the kind of in-depth morphologic analysis that was performed on the paraffin-embedded sections.

Cathepsins B, L, S, and K are members of the papain family of cysteine proteases. Even though several cathepsins are present in the inflamed joint (7,23), cathepsin B appears to be the primary cysteine protease measured in the in situ and cuvette assays. Herein the presence of cathepsin B or B-like activity was confirmed by substrate profile analysis. Z-phe-arg-AMC is a substrate for all cathepsins, and Z-val-val-arg-AMC also serves as a substrate for all cathepsins (with a preference for cathepsin S), but Z-arg-arg-AMC is selective for cathepsin B. Since the frozen joint tissue reacted well with Z-arg-arg-AMC, it can be concluded that cathepsin B activity is present in the joint. Another piece of evidence pointing to cathepsin B is the fact that cystatins, extracellular endogenous cysteine protease inhibitors, inhibit most other cysteine proteases but not cathepsin B (24). Since extracellular and intracellular compartments may be allowed to mix in this assay, cathepsin B might be the dominant activity, because all other cysteine proteases are inhibited by cystatins. This is not to say that cathepsin B is the only cysteine protease present but that the assay used here is likely measuring primarily cathepsin B activity.

As can be seen in Figure 2, there is a definite correlation between enzyme activity and joint inflammation and destruction, with r values in the range of 0.7–0.8. However, the correlation for joint destruction (0.7) was not quite as good as that for inflammation (0.8). There are several possible reasons for this discrepancy. The most likely is that the inflammation score is obtained from both joints in all animals, whereas the tissue destruction is from 1 joint only; therefore the difference may be due to simple sampling error.

Oral administration of LHVS showed efficacy in this animal arthritis model, reducing the signs of inflammation and tissue destruction, but the mechanism of action is not known. The AIA model is a complex one involving first an immune response, then an inflammatory phase affecting diarthroidal joints, and finally a tissue destruction phase in which cartilage and bone are degraded. LHVS could be acting in any 1, or all 3, of these phases. It is possible that the irreversible cysteine protease inhibitor enters the periarticular space from the circulation and directly inhibits the cysteine proteases present in the synovial fluid. The fact that enzyme activity in the joint tissue decreases concomitantly with the decrease in inflammation and joint destruction would support this view. However, there may be other explanations for the target and mechanism of action of LHVS.

Instead of acting locally, at the joint, LHVS may be acting systemically by disrupting class II major histocompatibility complex antigen presentation. LHVS preferentially inhibits cathepsin S, which is implicated in class II–restricted antigen presentation (25). This lipid-soluble inhibitor acts in vivo and in vitro, by entering the splenocyte and interfering with degradation of the invariant chain and thus antigen presentation (26). Therefore, it is possible that inhibition of cathepsin S in antigen-presenting cells is a contributor to the efficacy seen in this model. Alternatively, cathepsin K may be the relevant target of LHVS. Since cathepsin K is known to be involved in the process of bone resorption, LHVS may be acting by preventing the destruction of bone tissue. Finally, all cysteine proteases may act "upstream" by converting the pro- form of an enzyme, such as MMPs (known contributors to joint tissue destruction) (19,27,28), to the active form. Thus, LHVS may be acting by any one of several mechanisms and with several different targets to show efficacy in this animal model.

In summary, our data show that papain-like cysteine protease activity correlates well with the destructive events in the inflamed joint and that an irreversible cysteine protease inhibitor, administered orally in vivo in the AIA model, inhibits inflammation and joint destruction. Thus, this family of cysteine proteases may be a good target for structure-based RA drug design.

ACKNOWLEDGMENTS

We wish to thank Barry Franklin for expert technical assistance. We are also grateful to Dr. Tineke Meijers for instruction on cryosectioning and enzyme staining of the tissue sections.

REFERENCES

1. Reddy VY, Zhang Q-Y, Weiss SJ. Pericellular mobilization of the tissue-destructive cysteine proteinases, cathepsins B, L, and S, by human monocyte derived macrophages. Proc Natl Acad Sci U S A 1995;92:3849–53.
2. Muller-Ladner U, Gay RE, Gay S. Cysteine proteinases in arthritis and inflammation. Perspect Drug Discovery Design 1996;97–8.
3. Page AE, Hayman AE, Andersson LMB, Chambers TJ, Warburton MJ. Degradation of bone matrix proteins by osteoclast cathepsins. Int J Biochem 1993;25:545–50.
4. Brömme D, Okamoto K. Human cathepsin O2 (Cat K) a novel cysteine protease highly expressed in osteoclastomas and ovary: molecular cloning sequencing and tissue distribution. Biol Chem Hoppe Seyler 1995;376:379–84.
5. Brömme D, Okamoto K, Wang BB, Biroc S. Human cathepsin O2 (Cat K), a matrix protein-degrading cysteine protease expressed in osteoclasts: functional expression of human cathepsin O2 in Spodoptera frugiperda and characterization of the enzyme. J Biol Chem 1996;271:2126–32.
6. Gabrijelcic D, Annan-Prah A, Rodic B, Rozman B, Cotic V, Turk V. Determination of cathepsin B and H in sera and synovial fluids of patients with different joint diseases. J Clin Chem Clin Biochem 1990;28:149–153.
7. Lenarcic B, Gabrijelcic D, Rozman B, Drobnic-Kosorok M, Turk V. Human cathepsin B and cysteine proteinase inhibitors (CPIs) in inflammatory and metabolic joint disease. Biol Chem Hoppe Seyler 1988;369:257–61.
8. Van Noorden CJF, Smith RE, Rasnick D. Cysteine proteinase activity in arthritic rat knee joints and the effects of a selective systemic inhibitor, Z-phe-ala-CH2F. J Rheumatol 1988;15: 1525–35.
9. Van Noorden CJF, Vogels IMC. Enzyme histochemical reactions in unfixed and undecalcified cryostat sections of mouse knee joints with special reference to arthritic lesions. Histochemistry 1986;86: 127–33.
10. Trabandt A, Gay RE, Fassbender H-G, Gay S. Cathepsin B in synovial cells at the site of joint destruction in rheumatoid arthritis. Arthritis Rheum 1991;34:1444–51.
11. Trabandt A, Aicher WK, Gay RE, Sukhatme VP, Nilson-Hamilton M, Hamilton RT, et al. Expression of the collagenolytic and ras-induced cysteine proteinase cathepsin L and proliferation-associated oncogenes in synovial cells of MRL/l mice and patients with rheumatoid arthritis (RA). Matrix 1990;10:349–61.
12. Esser RE, Watts LM, Angelo RA, Thornburg SP, Prior JJ, Palmer JT. The effect of fluoromethyl ketone inhibitors of cathepsin B on adjuvant induced arthritis. J Rheumatol 1993;20:1176–83.
13. Esser RE, Angelo RA, Murphey MD, Watts LM, Thornburg LP, Palmer JT, et al. Cysteine proteinase inhibitors decrease articular cartilage and bone destruction in chronic inflammatory arthritis. Arthritis Rheum 1994;37:236–47.
14. Ahmed NK, Martin LA, Watts LM. Peptidyl fluoromethyl ketones

as inhibitors of cathepsin B: implication for the treatment of rheumatoid arthritis. Biochem Pharmacol 1992;44:1201–7.
15. Johnstone JJA. The routine sectioning of undecalcified bone for cytochemical studies. Histochem J 1979;11:359–65.
16. McElroy HH, Shih M-S, Parfitt AM. Producing frozen sections of calcified bone. Biotech Histochem 1993;68:50–5.
17. Palmer JT, Rasnick D, Klaus JL, Brömme D. Vinyl sulfones as mechanism-based cysteine protease inhibitors. J Med Chem 1995; 38:3193–6.
18. Matrisian LM. Metalloproteinases and their inhibitors in matrix remodeling. Trends Genet 1990;6:121–5.
19. Conway JG, Wakefield JA, Brown RH, Marron BE, Sekut L, Stimpson SA, et al. Inhibition of cartilage and bone destruction in adjuvant arthritis in the rat by a matrix metalloproteinase inhibitor. J Exp Med 1995;182:449–57.
20. Keyszer GM, Heer AH, Kriegsmann J, Geiler T, Trabandt A, Keyszer M, et al. Comparative analysis of cathepsin L, cathepsin D, and collagenase messenger RNA expression in synovial tissues of patients with rheumatoid arthritis and osteoarthritis, by in situ hybridization. Arthritis Rheum 1995;38:976–84.
21. Meijers MHM, Koopdonk-Kool J, Meacock SCR, van Noorden CJF. Cysteine proteinase activity in the development of arthritis in an adjuvant model of the rat. Agents Actions 1993;39:C219–21.
22. Yan S, Sameni M, Sloane BF. Cathepsin B and human tumor progression. Biol Chem 1998;379:113–23.
23. Maciewicz RA, Etherington DJ. Enzyme immunoassay for cathepsins B & L in synovial fluids from patients with arthritis. Biochem Soc Trans 1988;16:812–3.
24. Barrett AJ. The cystatins: a diverse superfamily of cysteine peptidase inhibitors. Biomed Biochim Acta 1986;45:1363–74.
25. Riese RJ, Wolf PR, Bromme D, Natkin LR, Villadangos JA, Ploegh HL, et al. Essential role for cathepsin S in MHC class II-associated invariant chain processing and peptide loading. Immunity 1996;4:357–66.
26. Riese RJ, Mitchell RN, Villadangos JA, Karp ER, DeSanctis GT, Ploegh HL, et al. Cathepsin S activity regulates antigen presentation and immunity. J Clin Invest 1998;101:2351–63.
27. Van Meurs JB, van Lent PL, van de Loo AA, Holthuysen AE, Bayne EK, Singer II, et al. Increased vulnerability of postarthritic cartilage to a second arthritic insult: accelerated MMP activity in a flare up of arthritis. Ann Rheum Dis 1999;58:350–6.
28. Van Meurs J, van Lent P, Stoop R, Holthuysen A, Singer I, Bayne E, et al. Cleavage of aggrecan at the Asn^{341}–Phe^{342} site coincides with the initiation of collagen damage in murine antigen-induced arthritis: a pivotal role for stromelysin 1 in matrix metalloproteinase activity. Arthritis Rheum 1999;42:2074–84.

ARTHRITIS & RHEUMATISM
Vol. 44, No. 3, March 2001, pp 712–722

Activation of a Fibroblast-Specific Enhancer of the Proα2(I) Collagen Gene in Tight-Skin Mice

Christopher P. Denton,[1] Bing Zheng,[1] Xu Shiwen,[2] Zhaoping Zhang,[1] George Bou-Gharios,[1] Heidi Eberspaecher,[1] Carol M. Black,[2] and Benoit de Crombrugghe[1]

Objective. **Reporter transgenes were introduced into the type 1 tight-skin (*Tsk1*/+) mouse model of scleroderma to test the hypothesis that fibroblast-specific genetic programs are activated in fibrosis.**

Methods. **Transgenes harboring upstream fragments of the 5′ flanking region of the mouse proα2(I) collagen gene (*Col1a2*), linked to a 400-bp minimal *Col1a2* promoter driving an *Escherichia coli* β-galactosidase (*LacZ*) reporter gene, were introduced into *Tsk1*/+ mice by breeding. Expression of these transgenes, which function as lineage-specific markers of fibroblast differentiation, was compared between the *Tsk-LacZ* mice and non-*Tsk* littermates. Responsiveness of these constructs to the profibrotic cytokine, transforming growth factor β1 (TGFβ1), was investigated by transient transfection of reporter constructs in tissue-culture cells.**

Results. **There was significant activation of reporter genes harboring the upstream enhancer in *Tsk1*/+ mice starting from 1 week of age. This was maximal at 6 weeks old (mean ± SD 237 ± 24% of non-*Tsk* controls; $P = 0.001$). Recombinant TGFβ1 significantly activated reporter genes regulated by the upstream enhancer in transient transfection, and *Tsk-LacZ* fibroblasts showed elevated *LacZ* expression in tissue culture.**

Conclusion. **These data suggest that activating signals in *Tsk1*/+ mice may act via fibroblast-specific regulatory elements within the murine *Col1a2* gene. Although TGFβ has been implicated in the pathogenesis of fibrosis, and reporter genes regulated by the upstream enhancer appear to be TGFβ responsive in vitro, our results suggest that fibroblast-specific pathways may also be involved.**

Dermal and visceral fibrosis is a pathologic hallmark of the connective tissue disease, scleroderma (systemic sclerosis). It coexists with immunologic perturbation and vascular dysfunction (1), both of which may contribute to the development of fibrosis by activating connective tissue fibroblasts (2). These cells deposit increased extracellular matrix within the skin and certain internal organs, including the lungs, heart, and gastrointestinal tract (3). Fibroblasts cultured from lesional skin or lung in scleroderma show increased levels of transcription of extracellular matrix genes including type I collagen (4–6). That these properties persist over several passages in tissue culture provides support for the view that although initial activating signals may originate from other cell types, the fibroblast is a critical effector cell in this disease.

The type 1 tight-skin (*Tsk1*/+) mouse, originally described by Green et al in 1976 (7), demonstrates features of established scleroderma, including the development of dermal fibrosis, with associated up-regulation of type I collagen messenger RNA (mRNA) levels on Northern blot analysis (8) and in situ hybridization (9). Fibroblasts from *Tsk1*/+ mice show increased extracellular matrix gene expression in tissue culture, reminiscent of scleroderma cells. The genetic defect responsible for the *Tsk1*/+ strain has been identified as an in-frame reduplication of exons 17–40 within the fibrillin-1 gene (10). This gene encodes a larger-than-normal protein, which appears to be incorporated into microfibrils, although the mechanism by which this leads to the

Supported by NIH Specialized Center of Research in Scleroderma grant P-50-AR-44888, and by The Wellcome Trust and The Arthritis Research Campaign (UK).

[1]Christopher P. Denton, PhD, MRCP, Bing Zheng, MSc, Zhaoping Zhang, MS, George Bou-Gharios, PhD, Heidi Eberspaecher, MS, Benoit de Crombrugghe, MD: University of Texas, Houston; [2]Xu Shiwen, PhD, Carol M. Black, MD, FRCP: University College London, London, UK.

Address correspondence and reprint requests to Christopher P. Denton, PhD, MRCP, Centre for Rheumatology, Royal Free and University College Medical School, Royal Free Campus, Rowland Hill Street, London NW3 2PF, UK.

Submitted for publication September 15, 2000; accepted in revised form November 20, 2000.

development of a characteristic tight-skin phenotype is uncertain (11). The *Tsk1/+* mouse strain provides an experimental system in which to investigate the regulation of collagen gene expression in vivo, and represents one of the best-characterized animal models for human scleroderma.

The use of transgenic mice has led to substantial progress toward understanding collagen gene regulation. Expression patterns of reporter transgenes controlled by different promoter constructs from mouse collagen genes suggests a modular arrangement of regulatory elements, with certain critical sequences directing expression of collagen genes to specific mesenchymal cell types at the appropriate time in embryonic development (12). Reporter transgenes regulated by such *cis*-acting sequences therefore function as differentiation markers for mesenchymal cell lineages and have helped to define osteoblast (13) and chondrocyte (14) differentiation pathways. Previous studies from this laboratory have identified a fibroblast-specific transcriptional enhancer located in the far-upstream region of the murine proα2(I) collagen (*Col1a2*) gene (15). A 6-kb sequence (−19.5 kb to −13.5 kb upstream of the transcription start site) was shown to endow high-level fibroblast-specific expression to reporter genes linked to endogenous and heterologous (16) minimal promoters in transgenic mouse embryos. Additional recent studies by our group have identified a homologous enhancer element in the human *COL1A2* gene, suggesting that fibroblast-specific regulatory pathways may be conserved between human and murine cells (17).

The precise molecular mechanisms underlying increased extracellular matrix gene expression in scleroderma remain incompletely understood, although regulatory elements in the proximal promoter that interact with the transcription factor Sp1 and NF1 (18), and also sequences within the first intron of the proα1(I) collagen (*COL1A1*) gene (19), have been implicated. We hypothesize that the same regulatory elements that direct high-level collagen gene expression in embryonic development are also important for activation of these genes postnatally in pathologic conditions such as fibrosis. If so, then lineage-specific regulatory elements within the far-upstream region of the *Col1a2* gene may be targets for activation, and fibroblast-specific or fibroblast-enriched transcription factors may be present at greater levels, or in more active forms, in fibrosis. Defining these pathways may provide logical targets for therapeutic modulation (20).

In the present study, we have investigated activation of reporter genes regulated by fibroblast-specific enhancer sequences from the *Col1a2* gene in tight-skin mice, and examined whether pathways acting on these might be selectively activated in fibrosis. Our experiments show, for the first time, that lineage-specific transcriptional regulators are targets for activation in this murine model system. Since similar regulatory processes appear to operate in the human *COL1A2* gene, these pathways may also be activated in human fibrotic conditions such as scleroderma.

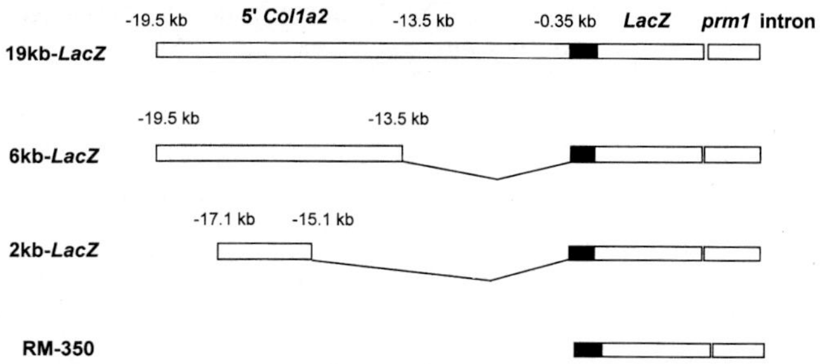

Figure 1. Transgene constructions harboring far-upstream enhancer elements of the mouse or human proα2(I) collagen gene. Three constructs incorporating far-upstream sequences of the mouse proα2(I) collagen (*Col1a2*) gene were introduced into type 1 tight-skin mice. The 19kb-*LacZ* construct includes the region between −19.5 kb upstream of the transcription start site and +54 bp of the *Col1a2* gene. Construction of the 6kb-*LacZ* (similar to pGB19.5/13.5 [see ref. 15]) eliminates sequences between −13.5 kb and −350 bp, and 2kb-*LacZ* incorporates 2 kb of the upstream region linked to a minimal 400-bp promoter. RM-350 includes only the *Col1a2* minimal promoter.

MATERIALS AND METHODS

Plasmids incorporating mouse *Col1a2* gene sequences. The far-upstream region of the mouse *Col1a2* gene was subcloned from a cosmid clone and a lambda phage clone, as described previously (15). Constructions containing 4 different portions of the *Col1a2* gene were generated, as shown in Figure 1. Intermediate constructions were subcloned into pBluescript or into a modified pBluescript containing a *Bgl* II site, depending on the restriction sites used for cloning. The −19.5 to −13.5 kb fragment cloned between *Bam* H1 and *Bgl* II of modified pBluescript was excised by *Xho* 1 and *Not* 1 and subcloned into the expression vector pRM350 (to produce the construct, 6kb-*LacZ*). The pRM350 vector incorporates a minimal (−350 bp to +54 bp) *Col1a2* promoter (15) driving an *Escherichia coli* β-galactosidase gene (*LacZ*) fused to the splice sites, intron, and polyadenylation signal of the mouse protamine 1 gene (21). A full-length 19.5-kb construct (19kb-*LacZ*) was assembled by introduction of the 6-kb *Bgl* II–*Bgl* II fragment (−19.5 kb to −13.5 kb) into a plasmid harboring the −13.5 kb to +54 bp fragment of the *Col1a2* gene. A central 2-kb fragment of the −19.5 kb to −13.5 kb fragment, between 2 *Eco* R1 sites at −17.1 kb to −15.1 kb, was blunted by *Klenow* and subcloned into the blunted *Xho* 1 site of pRM350, to produce the construction, 2kb-*LacZ*.

Table 1. Transgenic mouse lines harboring far-upstream sequences of the mouse proα2(I) collagen gene crossed with type 1 tight-skin (*Tsk1*/+)

Designation	Enhancer sequence	Copy number	*LacZ* expression, mean ± SEM RLU/DNA*	Staining intensity	Time to maximum staining, hours
19kb-*LacZ*	−19.5 kb upstream of transcription start site	2	648 ± 141	++++	8
6kb-*LacZ*-1	−19.5 kb to −13.5 kb	2	651 ± 18	+++++	6
6kb-*LacZ*-2	−19.5 kb to −13.5 kb	1	358 ± 39	++++	8
6kb-*LacZ*-3	−19.5 kb to −13.5 kb	3	248 ± 9	+++	16
2kb-*LacZ*	−17.1 kb to −15.1 kb	2	256 ± 84	+++	16

* RLU = relative luminescence units.

Generation of transgenic mice. Plasmids were digested with *Sac II* and *Nru I* and transgene constructs were gel purified. Transgenic mice were generated by pronuclear injection of transgene constructions into fertilized B6D2F2 oocytes as described previously (22). Injected eggs were transferred into CD1 foster mothers. All animal procedures were performed in accordance with local ethical practice guidelines and approved by the M. D. Anderson Cancer Center Institutional Review Board.

To identify transgenic mice, genomic DNA was extracted from the tails of 10-day-old mice and genotyping was performed by polymerase chain reaction (PCR) for *LacZ*, using sequence-specific primers (5′-CGGATAAACGGAACT-GGAAA-3′ and 5′-TAATCACGACTCGCTGTATC-3′) to yield a 500-bp product. Amplification was undertaken by 35 cycles of annealing for 60 seconds at 58°C, Mg^{++} 2.6 m*M*, and extension for 60 seconds at 72°C. For the genotyping of the embryos, genomic DNA was isolated from placenta.

A novel PCR was used for confirmation of the *Tsk1* genotype in *LacZ-Tsk* progeny, since coat color could not be used, unlike that in the *Tsk1*/+ line. The fibrillin-1 mutation associated with the *Tsk1* phenotype causes duplication of exons 17–40, with an in-frame fusion of intron 40 and intron 16 (10). Using an upstream primer (5′-ACCGTTGGC-AACTATACCTG-3′) in exon 40 and a downstream one (5′-TCCTGGTAACATAGGAAAGC-3′) complementary to the sequence of intron 16 of the fibrillin-1 gene, a unique 250-bp product is obtained for mice harboring the fibrillin-1 mutation (35 cycles of 60 seconds of annealing at Mg^{++} 1.5 m*M* at 57°C, and 45 seconds of extension). The mutant, but not wild-type, fibrillin-1 gene binds these primers to amplify the intervening sequence. Direct palpation of interscapular skin could determine the tight-skin phenotype from 10 days old and was invariably present in mice that were positive for the mutation by PCR.

Transgene copy number was estimated by Southern blot (12) of genomic tail DNA using a 3-kb *Bam* H1 probe from the *LacZ* gene. Mice from each 6kb-*LacZ* line or from the 19kb-*LacZ* and the 2kb-*LacZ* lines were assessed, comparing signal intensity with that of genomic DNA containing a single copy of the *LacZ* gene per genome (*ROSA*26-*LacZ* mouse line [23]). For the construct 6kb-*LacZ,* 3 lines were generated and these were designated 6kb-*LacZ*-1, 2, and 3. Details of the expression level and copy number for the transgenic lines generated for this study are summarized in Table 1.

Introduction of reporter transgenes into tight-skin mice. Reporter transgenes were established in tight-skin mice by mating *Tsk1*/+ with transgenic mice. For 6kb-*LacZ*-1, a female mouse homozygous for the transgene was mated with a male *Tsk1*/+. For the other reporter lines, heterozygous female transgenic mice were mated with *Tsk1*/+ males. Progeny were genotyped at 10 days old and nontransgenic littermates were killed. Transgenic pups were weaned at 19 days old, and the responses in *Tsk-LacZ* and non–*Tsk-LacZ* littermates were compared.

X-gal staining. Whole mouse embryos or dissected skin fragments were fixed for 60 minutes (0.1*M* sodium phosphate, pH 7.3, 5 m*M* EGTA, pH 8.0, 2 m*M* magnesium chloride, 0.2% glutaraldehyde, 0.3% formaldehyde), rinsed for 90 minutes, and stained with X-gal (5-bromo-4-chloro-3-indoyl β-D-galactopyranoside) staining solution (1 mg/ml) at room temperature, as described previously (24). Tissue was processed through increasing concentrations of ethanol and stored in 80% ethanol at −20°C. For histologic examination, tissues were dehydrated and embedded in paraffin wax, and 7-μm sections were cut and counterstained with eosin.

Measurement of β-galactosidase activity in tissue extracts. Biopsy samples (5 mm × 5 mm) of shaved areas of skin from the upper back of *Tsk* and non-*Tsk* littermates for each of the transgenic mice were obtained with the mice placed under anesthesia. Fresh tissue was homogenized for 90 seconds and centrifuged at 3,000*g* for 5 minutes, and the β-galactosidase activity in the tissue extract was measured by Galacto-Light chemiluminescence assay, according to the manufacturer's instructions (Tropix, Bedford, MA). In brief, 20 μl of extract supernatant was added to 100 μl reaction buffer/Galacton substrate mixture, and luminescence was measured (in relative luminescence units) after a 30-minute incubation. Wild-type control tissue extract included in each assay confirmed negligible background β-galactosidase activity (data not shown). Biopsy tissue wet weight or DNA content of the tissue extract was used for standardization of raw data for comparison of *LacZ* activity between mice. DNA concentration was measured by fluorometry using the Hoechst 3358 fluorochrome in a dedicated filter fluorometer (Hoefer TKO 100; Pharmacia, San Francisco, CA). The concentration of DNA was compared with DNA standards (Sigma, St. Louis, MO) in each assay (25).

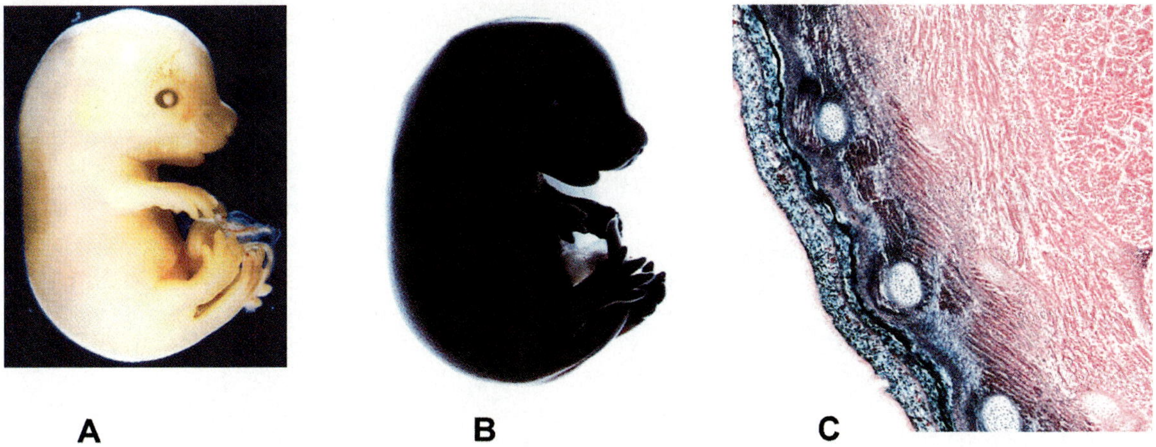

Figure 2. A 2-kb fragment of the far-upstream region directs high-level reporter gene expression. A representative founder embryo (15.5 days postconception) harboring *LacZ* under the control of a proα2(I) collagen minimal promoter (RM350; −350 bp to +54 bp) showed very weak X-gal staining in the skin over the snout and upper limbs and in the parietal region of the developing skull (**A**). In contrast, the 2-kb fragment (−17.1 kb to −15.1 kb) linked to this minimal promoter directed strong *LacZ* expression in the skin (**B**). Histologic findings from the embryo harboring the 2-kb enhancer fragment were identical to those from the strong-staining 6-kb and 19-kb reporter lines (**C**).

Northern hybridization. Mice were killed by cervical dislocation, and full-thickness samples of skin from the upper back of *Tsk* (n = 3) or non-*Tsk* (n = 3) littermates from the 6kb-*LacZ* line 1 or from the upper back of control wild-type (n = 2) and *Tsk* (n = 1) mice were obtained. The tissue was homogenized on ice in guanidium isothiocyanate lysis buffer and homogenates were stored at −80°C until used. Total RNA was isolated from shaved skin taken from the upper back, using RNEasy spin columns (Qiagen, Chatsworth, CA) according to the manufacturer's protocol. Northern blot analysis was performed using a random primer–labeled 321-bp *Eco* R1–*Hind* III mouse *Col1a1* probe and a 200-bp *Pst* 1–*Eco* R1 *Col1a2* probe, as previously described (26).

Culture of fibroblasts from transgenic mice. To extend the data obtained from analysis of skin biopsy samples from transgenic mice, dermal fibroblasts were cultured from 10-day-old pups. This allowed expression of the reporter transgene to be examined in tissue culture, and allowed the effect of exogenous transforming growth factor β1 (TGFβ1) on transgene expression level to be examined, to assess whether the increased expression of *LacZ* observed in *Tsk-LacZ* fibroblasts may result from increased TGFβ1 activity. Briefly, 1-cm skin samples were finely chopped and fibroblasts grown by explant culture. Fibroblasts were maintained in Dulbecco's modified Eagle's medium (Gibco BRL, Grand Island, NY) supplemented with 10% fetal calf serum (Gibco), 100 units/ml penicillin, and 100 mg/ml streptomycin, and cultured in a humidified atmosphere of 5% CO_2 in air. At confluence, cells were trypsinized and passaged. For experiments, fibroblasts were used at the first or second passage.

Transfection of reporter constructs and assessment of TGFβ1 responsiveness. To examine whether TGFβ ligands might be responsible for the greater expression of reporter transgenes, the effect of exogenous TGFβ1 was examined in tissue-culture cells. Primary cultures of dermal fibroblasts were established from 10-day-old wild-type transgenic (6kb-*LacZ*) mice or *Tsk-LacZ* littermates. Transient transfection was used to assess TGFβ1 responsiveness of the *Col1a2* promoter constructs, as shown in Figure 1. Test constructs and control plasmids (herpes simplex virus thymidine–kinase–renilla luciferase) were mixed and transfected with LipofectAMINE PLUS (Life Technologies, Rockville, MD), according to the manufacturer's protocol. Reporter gene expression was determined using the Galactolight assay kit (Tropix) or the Dual-Luciferase Reporter Assay System (Promega, Madison, WI). Raw data were corrected for transfection efficiency and DNA concentrations were standardized (0.4 mg DNA per tissue-culture well) using empty vector. Initial experiments using control fibroblasts transiently transfected with the plasminogen activator inhibitor 1 (*PAI-1*)–luciferase plasmid (27) confirmed a concentration-dependent response to recombinant human TGFβ1 (R&D Systems, Minneapolis, MN), with maximum activation using a final concentration of 10 ng/ml and incubation of 12–16 hours. Subsequent experiments were performed under these conditions using fibroblasts cultured from transgenic mice or NIH-3T3 fibroblasts (CRL-1658; American Type Culture Collection, Rockville, MD) transiently transfected with the 3 *Col1a2*-promoter reporter plasmids. For each experiment, transfection was performed when the cell layer was 60–70% confluent in a 24-well tissue-culture plate.

RESULTS

Earlier studies demonstrated that reporter genes under the control of a far-upstream enhancer of the mouse *Col1a2* gene are expressed at high levels in a variety of embryonic mesenchymal cells, especially in fibroblasts of the dermis, fascia, and internal organs (15). Our initial experiments using *LacZ* reporter lines incorporating far-upstream enhancer sequences con-

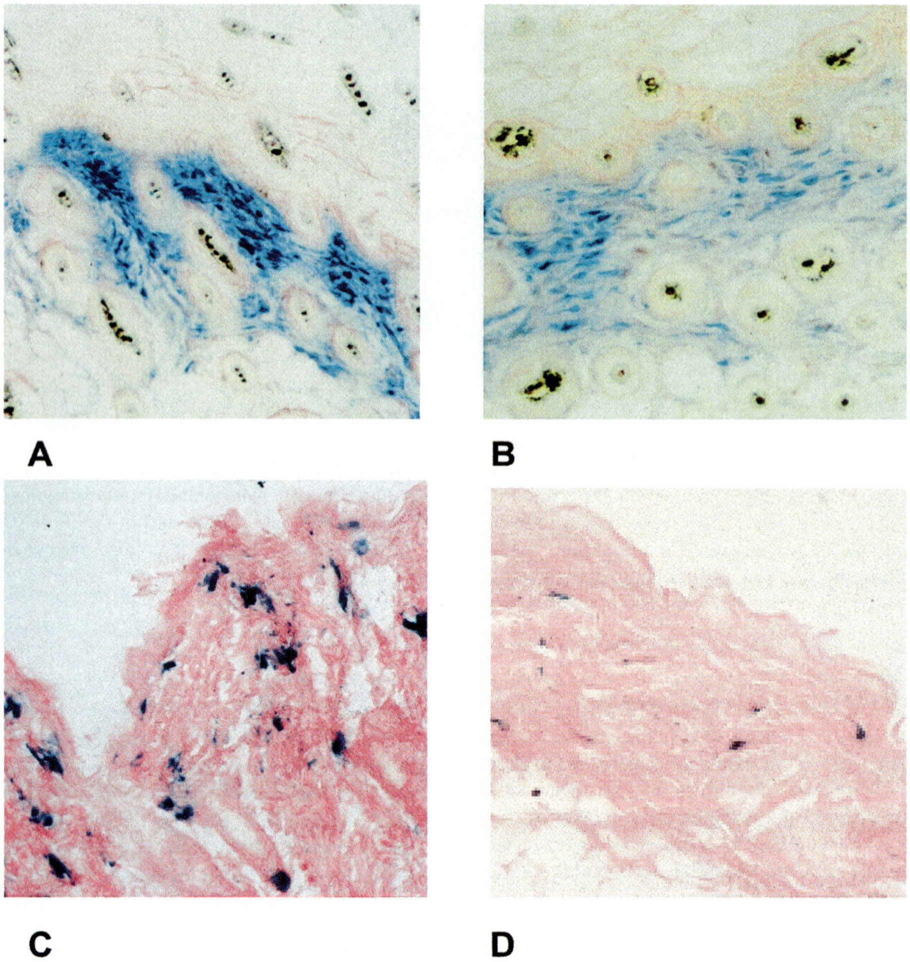

Figure 3. Increased expression of *LacZ* in the skin of tight-skin (*Tsk*)–transgenic mice compared with non-*Tsk* littermates. At 4 weeks old, tight-skin mice harboring 6kb-*LacZ* reporter transgenes showed more intense X-gal staining in the dermis (**A**) than did non-*Tsk* transgenic littermates (**B**). The staining at 12 weeks old remained stronger in *Tsk* mice (**C**) than in non-*Tsk* mice (**D**).

firmed a similar expression pattern postnatally, which persisted into adulthood. With the use of X-gal staining of whole-mount F1 or F2 embryos, we compared the expression levels in founders for each transgene. The 6kb-*LacZ* lines (1,2, and 3) all showed expression in the dermis, both macroscopically and histologically. Expression levels varied between lines.

The maximum intensity of X-gal staining and the time taken to reach maximal staining intensity in embryos (15.5 days postconception), together with the results of quantitation of *LacZ* expression in skin extracts of 4-week-old mice are shown in Table 1. These data considerably extend previous characterizations of the minimal enhancer sequence, by delineating enhancer activity to a relatively short 2-kb fragment (−17.1 kb to −15.1 kb). Experiments examining a series of transgenic founder embryos confirmed that this 2-kb sequence directed strong *LacZ* expression in dermal fibroblasts in ~80% of transgenic founders, with some mice demonstrating a very high level of expression that was comparable with that observed in the high-expressing 6kb-*LacZ* and 19kb-*LacZ* lines (Figure 2). In contrast, as previously reported, expression of reporter genes linked to only a minimal *Col1a2* promoter (−350 bp to +54 bp) in the absence of far-upstream elements was very weak in embryos (28) and was not detectable in the skin of mice postnatally, either by X-gal staining or by biochemical assay.

Introduction of the 6-kb reporter transgene into *Tsk-1*/+ mice was consistently associated with increased

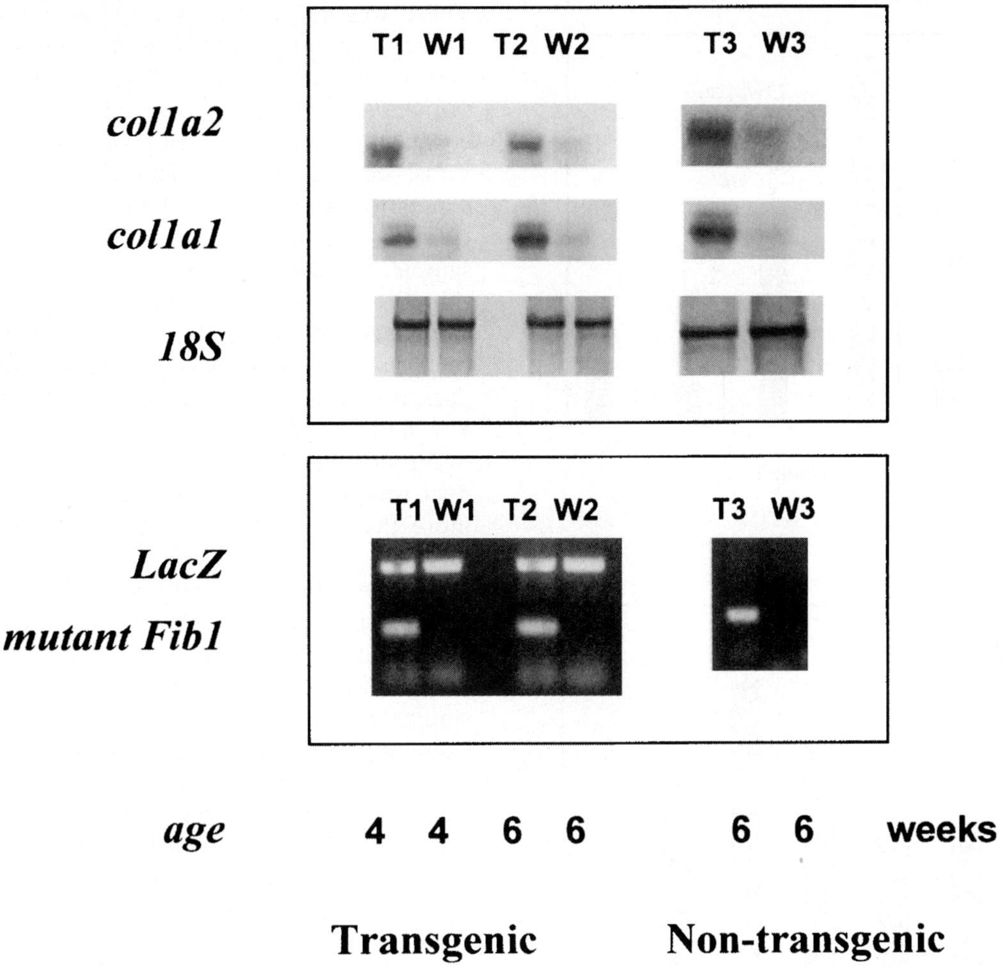

Figure 4. Up-regulation of endogenous proα1(I) and proα2(I) collagen genes (*col1a1* and *col1a2*, respectively) in transgenic mice harboring the type 1 tight-skin (*Tsk1*) mutant fibrillin-1 (Fib1) gene. Upper panel shows Northern hybridization of total RNA (5 μg per lane) extracted from skin homogenates of *Tsk*-6kb-*LacZ* mice (T1 = 4 weeks old, T2 = 6 weeks old) and non-*Tsk* 6kb-*LacZ* littermates (W1 and W2). T3 and W3 are nontransgenic *Tsk* or non-*Tsk* littermates (age 6 weeks). Bands of 18S RNA confirm equal loading of lanes. Blots were probed for *col1a2* and *col1a1* as described in Materials and Methods. The lower panel shows polymerase chain reaction genotyping of genomic DNA isolated from these mice, and demonstrates the transgene and mutant fibrillin-1 gene.

expression of the *LacZ* reporter gene in skin. This was apparent macroscopically when biopsy samples taken from *Tsk* and non-*Tsk* transgenic progeny were compared for 3 independently derived 6kb-*LacZ* lines after overnight X-gal staining (data not shown), and was confirmed by histologic examination. This difference was present from 4 weeks of age (Figures 3A and B) and was particularly obvious in areas of thickened interscapular skin, which are a hallmark of this mutant strain (Figures 3C and D).

The tight-skin phenotype did not appear to be modified by introduction of the *LacZ* reporter construct. Thus, in addition to the typical macroscopic and histologic features, there was up-regulation of *Col1a1* and *Col1a2* mRNA species (Figure 4) in *Tsk*-transgenic mice. This is consistent with the findings in previous reports (29) and suggests that any changes in genetic background that occurred with introduction of the *Tsk* mutation into transgenic mice was not significant. Furthermore, it shows that 6kb-*LacZ* reporter transgene expression reflects the activity of the endogenous type I collagen genes. Levels of type I collagen mRNA in wild-type mice were similar for transgenic and nontransgenic wild-type littermates, confirming that the reporter

A

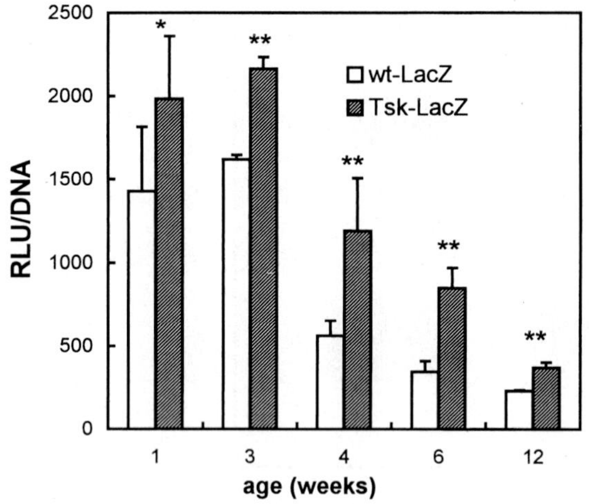

B

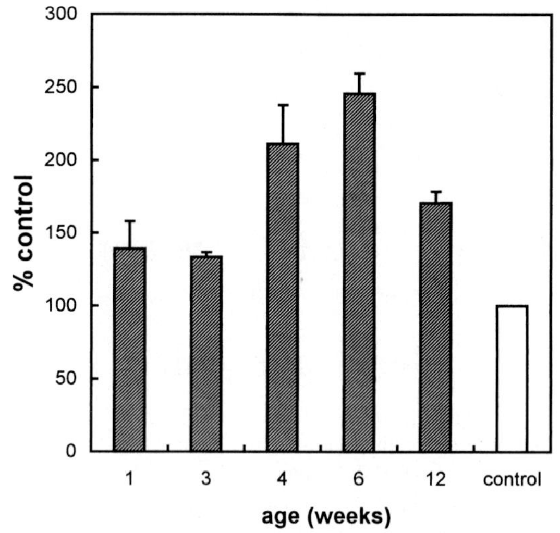

Figure 5. Increased reporter transgene expression in tight-skin (*Tsk*)–transgenic mice. Activity of β-galactosidase was assessed in skin homogenates from mice harboring the 6kb-*LacZ* transgene between ages 1 week and 12 weeks, and the results are corrected for DNA concentration of tissue extracts (**A**) or expressed as a percentage of the non-*Tsk* littermates (**B**). Three pairs of mice were examined at each time point and bars show the mean and SEM. $* = P < 0.05$ and $** = P < 0.01$, by Student's paired *t*-test. RLU = relative luminescence units; wt-LacZ = wild-type *LacZ*.

transgene does not alter the expression level of the endogenous *Col1a2* gene.

Direct measurement of β-galactosidase activity in skin extracts provided valuable additional information. The results of longitudinal studies of transgene expression in the 6kb-*LacZ* lines are summarized in Figure 5. There was consistently greater activity in the *Tsk1*/+ mice than in non-*Tsk* mice at time points between 7 days and 12 weeks old ($P < 0.05$ at all time points, by Student's *t*-test). The measured β-galactosidase activity corresponded with intensity of dermal X-gal staining. Thus, in both non-*Tsk* and *Tsk*-transgenic mice, the expression level decreased with time in adult mice. To correct for differences in the cellularity of each biopsy sample, raw data were adjusted for the DNA content of skin *LacZ*-expression homogenates. In fact, these data were very similar to those obtained following correction for the size of each biopsy sample (by wet weight of skin; data not shown), suggesting that differences between *Tsk* and non-*Tsk* *LacZ* expression were not due to differences in cell number. Activation of *LacZ* in *Tsk* mice was greatest between 4 and 6 weeks of age, at levels more than 2-fold greater than those in non-*Tsk* littermates.

The 19kb-*LacZ* and 2kb-*LacZ* lines also demonstrated significantly greater transgene expression in *Tsk*-transgenic mice than in non–*Tsk*-transgenic littermates. For the non–*Tsk*-19-kb line, β-galactosidase activity was similar to that of the strongest of the 3 6-kb lines examined (Table 1), but there was greater enhancement of transgene activation in *Tsk*-6kb-*LacZ* mice compared with *Tsk*-19kb-*LacZ* mice (Figure 6). Strong transactivation via the 6-kb enhancer suggests that this region contains sites that respond to activating factors in the *Tsk1*/+ mice, and the qualitatively similar effect observed using the central 2-kb *Eco* R1–*Eco* R1 fragment appears to delineate these responsive elements to the central portion of the 6-kb fragment. This 2-kb region includes 3 hypersensitive sites present in the chromatin of fibroblasts, but not in non–type I collagen–producing cells (15), and regions of sequence conservation between the mouse and human enhancer element (17). Overall, these data suggest that lineage-specific enhancer elements in the far-upstream region of the mouse *Col1a2* gene are involved in transactivation of genes in this mouse model of fibrosis.

Previous studies of several TGFβ-responsive promoters, including those of the *COL1A2* and the *PAI-1* genes (27), have shown that the nucleotide sequence, GACACA, within the proximal promoter interacts with Smad3/Smad4 complexes, which are crucial downstream mediators of TGFβ signaling, and that this motif underlies TGFβ responsiveness (30). Sequence analysis of the far-upstream enhancer of the *Col1a2* gene identified a number of Smad3 consensus binding sites in the 6kb-*LacZ* reporter transgene (at around −19.3, −16.8, −16.7, and −15.6 kb upstream of the transcription start

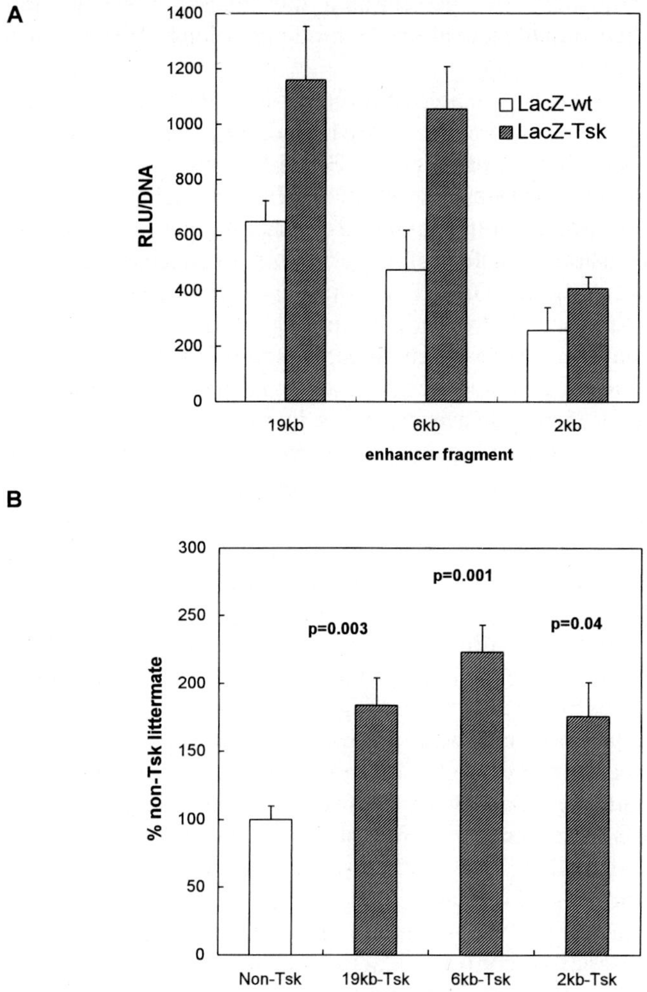

Figure 6. Transactivation of the *LacZ* reporter gene under the control of different enhancer constructions. Activation of reporter gene expression was examined in type 1 tight-skin (*Tsk1*/+) mice for the 19-kb (−19.5 kb to −350 bp), 6-kb (−19.5 kb to −13.6 kb), and 2-kb (−17.1 kb to −15.1 kb) flanking sequences linked to a minimal (−350 bp to +54 bp) endogenous *Col1a2* promoter (**A**). Bars show the mean and SEM results of a series of 3 independent experiments using the transgenic lines described in Table 1, and the relative activation via these sequences (expressed as a percentage of the non-*Tsk* littermates) is also shown (**B**). *P* values are by Student's paired *t*-test. RLU = relative luminescence units; LacZ-wt = wild-type *LacZ*.

site), as well as 1 consensus sequence at −252 bp in the minimal promoter (Figure 7A). Three of these motifs lay within the minimal 2-kb enhancer fragment, and suggest that Smad3/Smad4 complexes may interact with these transgene constructs.

Transient transfection experiments confirmed the responsiveness of dermal fibroblasts to TGFβ1. Thus, the *PAI-1*–luciferase construct demonstrated an ~6-fold induction by TGFβ1 in dermal fibroblasts cultured from neonatal mice. In contrast, NIH-3T3 fibroblasts showed a consistent 2-fold induction under similar experimental conditions (data not shown). The minimal promoter (RM350) construct showed consistent modest induction by TGFβ1 to ~140% (±4 SD) of basal activity in transfected NIH-3T3 cells, but there was much greater induction of *LacZ* when the minimal promoter was linked to elements of the upstream enhancer. Thus,

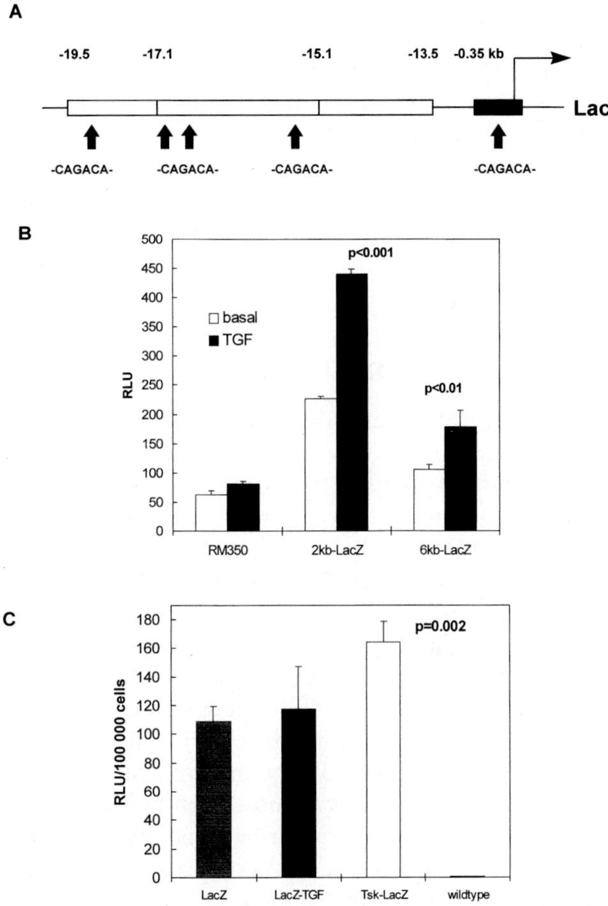

Figure 7. In vitro responsiveness of reporter transgenes to transforming growth factor β1 (TGFβ1). Sequence analysis of the far-upstream enhancer indicated consensus binding sites for Smad3 in the 6kb-*LacZ* reporter transgene (**A**). NIH-3T3 fibroblasts transiently transfected with 3 different reporter constructs (2kb-*LacZ*, 6kb-*LacZ*, and RM350) were treated with recombinant TGFβ1. Constructs harboring the upstream enhancer sequences showed greater responsiveness (**B**). Primary cultures of dermal fibroblasts were established from 10-day-old wild-type transgenic (6kb-*LacZ*) mice or tight-skin (*Tsk*)–*LacZ* littermates. Transgenic-*Tsk* fibroblasts showed significantly greater *LacZ* expression than did cells from a non-*Tsk* littermate, consistent with the findings using skin homogenates (**C**). Bars show the mean and SEM relative luminescence units (RLU).

for the 2kb-*LacZ* construct, TGFβ1 induced expression to 194% (±9 SD), and for the 6kb-*LacZ* construct, to 170% (±29 SD) of basal activity (Figure 7B). Levels of expression, when corrected for transfection efficiency, were also higher than those observed for the minimal promoter, suggesting that some of the enhancer activity observed in vivo may also be demonstrated in vitro, although these experiments do not address whether this is cell-type specific. Overall, these data strongly suggest that sequences within the far-upstream enhancer are responsive to TGFβ1 in vitro.

Consistent with the results from skin homogenates, dermal fibroblasts cultured from neonatal transgenic mice also showed high-level *LacZ* expression, and levels of expression in *Tsk-LacZ* fibroblasts were significantly elevated compared with those in littermate controls (Figure 7C). However, there was no significant induction of *LacZ* expression after pretreatment of these transgenic cells with TGFβ1, suggesting that these pathways may already be maximally activated in these cells.

DISCUSSION

These experiments demonstrate the usefulness of transgenic methods for better understanding gene regulation in mutant mouse strains. The type 1 tight-skin mouse was originally characterized as a spontaneously arising mutant strain that developed thickening of the interscapular skin together with more subtle skeletal abnormalities including increased bone length (7). Despite one contradictory report (31), analysis of the tight-skin phenotype in interspecific backcross experiments mapped it to the fibrillin-1 locus on chromosome 2, and Siracusa et al (10) identified an in-frame partial duplication of the fibrillin-1 gene in tight-skin mice. This mutation is designated *Tsk1*. Subsequently it was shown that the mutant gene is transcribed and that increased type I collagen mRNA levels correlate with mRNA levels for the mutant protein (32).

More recently it has been confirmed that the mutant protein is secreted and incorporated into extracellular matrix in vitro, forming abnormal microfibrils (33). The mechanism by which this mutant protein induces a tight-skin phenotype is less clear. Fibrillin-1 has domains that are homologous to those of latent TGFβ binding protein type 1 and has been shown to bind to TGFβ family members (34). TGFβ is a potent profibrotic cytokine and has been implicated in the development of a number of fibrotic disorders including scleroderma (35). It is possible that abnormal fibrillin-1 molecules are incorporated into microfibrils and alter their stability and ability to bind and release TGFβ family members (36).

It is plausible that the far-upstream elements may directly respond to TGFβ1, and sequence analysis has identified a number of Smad-binding consensus sequences within the enhancer. Interestingly, 3 of these are located in the smaller 2-kb transgene. Our data from transient transfection experiments do suggest that there is functional TGFβ1 responsiveness for these transgene constructs, but do not completely exclude the possibility that the upstream enhancer element is acting by amplification of responses mediated via previously described TGFβ1-responsive elements in the proximal promoter of the *Col1a2* gene, which include a Smad3-binding consensus sequence at −259 bp upstream of the transcription start site.

Despite these in vitro data we were unable to induce transgene expression in fibroblasts cultured from infant transgenic mice. This suggests that TGFβ1-responsive pathways are already maximally activated in these cells. It appears, therefore, that specific fibroblastic pathways are regulating trangene expression in these cells and that these pathways are up-regulated in *Tsk* mice. Interestingly, dermal fibroblasts cultured from *Tsk*-transgenic mice showed sustained activation of *LacZ* expression above the levels observed for non-*Tsk* littermates. This further suggests that as with systemic sclerosis fibroblasts, the transcriptional activation of these cells is sustained, at least temporarily, in the absence of continuing activating stimuli.

The present study provides support for the concept that highly controlled cell or tissue-specific regulatory mechanisms governing temporal and spatial expression of genes in embryonic development are also important in postnatal regulation and may be recruited in pathologic states such as fibrosis. Although our data suggest that far-upstream regulatory enhancer elements respond directly to transactivating signals in *Tsk1*/+ mice, they do not exclude the possibility that these effects may also be mediated via proximal elements within the 400-bp minimal promoter, and perhaps amplified by the upstream enhancer. However, greater activation of the −19.5 kb to −13.5 kb fragment in *Tsk1*/+ mice, compared with the full-length 19.5-kb transgene, in lines which show similar levels of β-galactosidase activity in non-*Tsk* mice, together with the undetectable (by X-gal staining or biochemical assay) postnatal expression levels of *LacZ* linked only to this minimal promoter, indicate an important in vivo role for the far-upstream elements. Conversely, the lower level of transactivation for the 2-kb construction is consistent with the possible existence of additional response elements within the 6-kb fragment that are outside the −17.1 kb to −15.1 kb region. A modular arrangement of regulatory elements has previously been postulated for a number of genes, including the proximal promoter of the mouse *Col1a1* gene, with some sequences that regulate cell-specific expression and others that control the level of expression (13).

Although our data confirm that the far-upstream enhancer contained elements that are activated postnatally, the level of transgene expression in the skin appears to decline markedly up to 12 weeks of age. This is reminiscent of previous studies examining expression of type I collagen genes in *Tsk* mice by in situ hybridization (9). The apparent decrease may reflect the rate of normal connective tissue turnover in the adult dermis, with relatively few cells actively synthesizing collagen. It also probably reflects changes that occur in tissue architecture, since the neonatal dermis is highly cellular, compared with the mature adult dermis which consists mainly of collagen-rich extracellular matrix. It should be noted, however, that correction of *LacZ* expression for tissue weight gave very similar results to those observed when expressing activity in terms of DNA concentration (a surrogate for cell number), so that changes in cell number do not explain the differences observed between the *Tsk1/+* and wild-type skin, even if they contribute to the apparent reduction in transgene activity in mature mice.

Increased *LacZ* activity in the skin of *Tsk1/+* transgenic mice, compared with non–*Tsk*-transgenic littermates, implies either an increased proportion of *LacZ*-expressing cells or that *Tsk* fibroblasts express *LacZ* more strongly. The histologic features of X-gal–stained tissue suggest that both processes may be relevant. Thus, there is stronger *LacZ* expression at 4 weeks, with X-gal staining fairly uniformly distributed within the dermis. However, by 12 weeks, the main difference between *Tsk1/+* and non-*Tsk* mice appears to be an increased number of cells expressing *LacZ.* It has been shown that skin fibroblasts are phenotypically heterogeneous in terms of collagen production (37), adhesion molecule expression (38), and proliferation rate (39). It is possible that there are greater proportions of high-level collagen–producing cells in *Tsk1/+* mice and that this is the basis for the skin pathology.

For the 3 6kb-*LacZ* reporter genes harboring the same construction, the effect of position and copy number of the transgene expression could be examined. Although high-level–, medium-level–, and low-level–expressing lines all showed an ~2-fold increase in *LacZ* expression in *Tsk-LacZ* progeny at 6 weeks old, levels of *LacZ* expression varied between lines. This appears to be predominantly due to position effect, since even single copies of the transgene could produce high-level skin expression. It should be noted that a relatively high proportion of transgenic founders expressed the reporter gene for all constructs (more than 50%). This may reflect preferential integration into open chromatin, or alternatively, that the upstream regulatory elements are able to modify chromatin at the integration site, similar to that observed with some locus control regions of other genes (40).

In addition to the presence of a far-upstream fibroblast-specific enhancer in the murine *Col1a2* gene, our own data have demonstrated a region of sequence and functional similarity in the upstream region of the human *COL1A2* gene. In addition, hypersensitive sites in chromatin for the upstream region of the mouse *Col1a1* gene have recently been described (41). This suggests that upstream regulatory elements may exist in a number of extracellular matrix genes, and that these may be targets for activation by similar cell-specific, or cell-enriched, transactivating factors. Further definition of such elements should help to better understand the molecular pathology of fibrotic disorders, and also provide insight into genetic factors influencing the severity of or susceptibility to these diseases. Elucidating upregulatable fibroblast-specific *cis*-acting elements should facilitate identification of the transactivating factors involved in fibrosis and may eventually make possible targeted genetic therapies for some of the most intractable human diseases.

REFERENCES

1. Kahaleh MB, LeRoy EC. Autoimmunity and vascular involvement in systemic sclerosis (SSc). Autoimmunity 1999;31:195–214.
2. Varga J, Jimenez SA. Modulation of collagen gene expression: its relation to fibrosis in systemic sclerosis and other disorders. Ann Intern Med 1995;122:60–2.
3. Clements PJ. Systemic sclerosis (scleroderma) and related disorders: clinical aspects. Baillieres Best Pract Res Clin Rheumatol 2000;14:1–16.
4. Kahari VM, Vuorio T, Nanto-Salonen K, Vuorio E. Increased type I collagen mRNA levels in cultured scleroderma fibroblasts. Biochim Biophys Acta 1984;781:183–6.
5. Jimenez SA, Feldman G, Bashey RI, Bienkowski R, Rosenbloom J. Co-ordinate increase in the expression of type I and type III collagen genes in progressive systemic sclerosis fibroblasts. Biochem J 1986;237:837–43.
6. Shi-Wen X, Denton CP, McWhirter A, Bou-Gharios G, Abraham DJ, du Bois RM, et al. Scleroderma lung fibroblasts exhibit elevated and dysregulated type I collagen biosynthesis. Arthritis Rheum 1997;40:1237–44.

7. Green, MC, Sweet HO, Bunker LE. Tight-skin, a new mutation of the mouse causing excessive growth of connective tissue and skeleton. Am J Pathol 1976;82:493–512.
8. Jimenez SA, Williams CJ, Myers JC, Bashey RI. Increased collagen biosynthesis and increased expression of type I and type III procollagen genes in tight skin (TSK) mouse fibroblasts. J Biol Chem 1986;261:657–62.
9. Pablos JL, Everett ET, Harley R, LeRoy EC, Norris JS. Transforming growth factor-beta 1 and collagen gene expression during postnatal skin development and fibrosis in the tight-skin mouse. Lab Invest 1995;72:670–8.
10. Siracusa LD, McGrath R, Ma Q, Moskow JJ, Manne J, Christner PJ, et al. A tandem duplication within the fibrillin 1 gene is associated with the mouse tight skin mutation. Genome Res 1996;6:300–13.
11. Saito S, Nishimura H, Brumeanu TD, Casares S, Stan AC, Honjo T, et al. Characterization of mutated protein encoded by partially duplicated fibrillin-1 gene in tight skin (TSK) mice. Mol Immunol 1999;36:169–76.
12. Rossert J, Eberspaecher H, de Crombrugghe B. Separate cis-acting DNA elements of the mouse pro-alpha 1(I) collagen promoter direct expression of reporter genes to different type I collagen-producing cells in transgenic mice. J Cell Biol 1995;129: 1421–32.
13. Rossert JA, Chen SS, Eberspaecher H, Smith CN, de Crombrugghe B. Identification of a minimal sequence of the mouse pro-alpha 1(I) collagen promoter that confers high-level osteoblast expression in transgenic mice and that binds a protein selectively present in osteoblasts. Proc Natl Acad Sci U S A 1996;93:1027–31.
14. Lefebvre V, Zhou G, Mukhopadhyay K, Smith CN, Zhang Z, Eberspaecher H, et al. An 18-base-pair sequence in the mouse proalpha1(II) collagen gene is sufficient for expression in cartilage and binds nuclear proteins that are selectively expressed in chondrocytes. Mol Cell Biol 1996;16:4512–23.
15. Bou-Gharios G, Garrett LA, Rossert J, Niederreither K, Eberspaecher H, Smith C, et al. A potent far-upstream enhancer in the mouse pro-alpha 2(I) collagen gene regulates expression of reporter genes in transgenic mice. J Cell Biol 1996;134:1333–44.
16. Rabe C, Denton CP, de Crombrugghe B. Transcriptional regulation of type-I collagen genes. In: Ooyama T, editor. Extracellular matrix-cell interactions. Tokyo: Japan Scientific Society Press; 1998. p. 217–34.
17. Denton CP, Zheng B, Rabe C, Bou-Gharios G, Zhang Z, Black CM, et al. Identification of highly conserved fibroblast-specific regulatory elements involved in type I collagen gene activation [abstract]. Clin Sci 1999;97:14.
18. Hitraya EG, Varga J, Artlett CM, Jiménez SA. Identification of elements in the promoter region of the α1(I) procollagen gene involved in its up-regulated expression in systemic sclerosis. Arthritis Rheum 1998;41:2048–58.
19. Hitraya EG, Jiménez SA. Transcriptional activation of the α1(I) procollagen gene in systemic sclerosis dermal fibroblasts: role of intronic sequences. Arthritis Rheum 1996;39:1347–54.
20. Denton CP, Black CM, Korn JH, de Crombrugghe B. Systemic sclerosis: current pathogenetic concepts and future prospects for targeted therapy. Lancet 1996;347:1453–8.
21. Schmidt A, Rossi P, de Crombrugghe B. Transcriptional control of the mouse alpha 2(I) collagen gene: functional deletion analysis of the promoter and evidence for cell-specific expression. Mol Cell Biol 1986;6:347–54.
22. Hogan B, Costantini F, Lacy E. Manipulating the mouse embryo: a laboratory manual. Cold Spring Harbor (NY): Cold Spring Harbor Press; 1980.
23. Soriano P. Generalized LacZ expression with the ROSA26 Cre reporter strain. Nat Genet 1999;21:70–1.
24. Mercer EH, Hoyle GW, Kapur RP, Brinster RL, Palmiter RD. The dopamine beta-hydroxylase gene promoter directs expression of E coli LacZ to sympathetic and other neurons in adult transgenic mice. Neuron 1991;7:703–16.
25. Labarca C, Paigen K. A simple, rapid and sensitive DNA assay procedure. Anal Biochem 1980;102:344–52.
26. Niederreither K, D'Souza R, Metsaranta M, Eberspaecher H, Toman PD, Vuorio E, et al. Coordinate patterns of expression of type I and III collagens during mouse development. Matrix Biol 1995;14:705–13.
27. Van Waarde MA, van Assen AJ, Kampinga HH, Konings AW, Vujaskovic Z. Quantification of transforming growth factor-beta in biological material using cells transfected with a plasminogen activator inhibitor-1 promoter-luciferase construct. Anal Biochem 1997;247:45–51.
28. Frazier K, Williams S, Kothapalli D, Klapper H, Grotendorst GR. Stimulation of fibroblast cell growth, matrix production, and granulation tissue formation by connective tissue growth factor. J Invest Dermatol 1996;107:404–11.
29. Goldberg H, Helakoski T, Garrett LA, Karsenty G, Pellegrino A, Lozano G, et al. Tissue-specific expression of the mouse alpha 2(I) collagen promoter: studies in transgenic mice and in tissue culture cells. J Biol Chem 1992;267:19622–30.
30. Chen SJ, Yuan W, Lo S, Trojanowska M, Varga J. Interaction of Smad3 with a proximal Smad-binding element of the human alpha2(I) procollagen gene promoter required for transcriptional activation by TGF-beta. J Cell Physiol 2000;183:381–92.
31. Doute RC, Clark SH. Tight-skin (Tsk) maps on mouse chromosome 2 within the region of linkage homology with human chromosome 15. Genomics 1994;22:223–5.
32. Yufit T, Christner P, Siracusa LD, McGrath R, Jimenez SA. A mutation in the fibrillin gene influences the expression of several genes encoding extracellular matrix proteins in Tsk1 mouse embryonic cell lines [abstract]. Arthritis Rheum 1997;40:S334.
33. Kielty CM, Raghunath M, Siracusa LD, Sherratt MJ, Peters R, Shuttleworth CA, et al. The tight skin mouse: demonstration of mutant fibrillin-1 production and assembly into abnormal microfibrils. J Cell Biol 1998;140:1159–66.
34. Sinha S, Nevett C, Shuttleworth CA, Kielty CM. Cellular and extracellular biology of the latent transforming growth factor-beta binding proteins. Matrix Biol 1998;17:529–45.
35. Cotton SA, Herrick AL, Jayson MI, Freemont AJ. TGF beta—a role in systemic sclerosis? J Pathol 1998;184:4–6.
36. Raghunath M, Unsold C, Kubitscheck U, Bruckner-Tuderman L, Peters R, Meuli M. The cutaneous microfibrillar apparatus contains latent transforming growth factor-beta binding protein-1 (LTBP-1) and is a repository for latent TGF-β1. J Invest Dermatol 1998;111:559–64.
37. Jelaska A, Arakawa M, Broketa G, Korn JH. Heterogeneity of collagen synthesis in normal and systemic sclerosis skin fibroblasts: increased proportion of high collagen–producing cells in systemic sclerosis fibroblasts. Arthritis Rheum 1996;39:1338–46.
38. Needleman BW. Increased expression of intercellular adhesion molecule 1 on the fibroblasts of scleroderma patients. Arthritis Rheum 1990;33:1847–51.
39. Feldman SR, Trojanowska M, Smith EA, Leroy EC. Differential responses of human papillary and reticular fibroblasts to growth factors. Am J Med Sci 1993;305:203–7.
40. Ellis J, Tan-Un KC, Harper A, Michalovich D, Yannoutsos N, Philipsen S, et al. A dominant chromatin-opening activity in 5′ hypersensitive site 3 of the human beta-globin locus control region. EMBO J 1996;15:562–8.
41. Salimi-Tari P, Cheung M, Safar CA, Tracy JT, Tran I, Harbers K, et al. Molecular cloning and chromatin structure analysis of the murine alpha1(I) collagen gene domain. Gene 1997;198:61–72.

ARTHRITIS & RHEUMATISM
Vol. 44, No. 3, March 2001, pp 723–727

Development of the Tight-Skin Phenotype in Immune-Deficient Mice

Tatjana D. Dodig, Kristine T. Mack, Deborah F. Cassarino, and Stephen H. Clark

Objective. **To determine if cutaneous thickening, a major phenotypic feature of the tight-skin (Tsk) mutation, could develop in an immune-deficient mouse.**

Methods. **Experimental crosses among different strains of mice were conducted to create mice that were genetically Tsk/+, and that were also homozgyous for a mutation at the Prkdc^{scid} locus and thus lacked mature T and B lymphocytes. Skin samples prepared from experimental and control genotypic groups of mice were evaluated for skin thickness.**

Results. **The data showed that the Tsk/+ mice developed the Tsk phenotype in the absence of a functional immune system.**

Conclusion. **Mature T and B cells are not required for the development of the cutaneous thickening in mice carrying the Tsk mutation.**

The tight-skin (Tsk) mutation was first described by Green et al (1) as a spontaneous mutation in the mouse that causes excessive growth of connective tissue, which maps to chromosome 2 approximately 2 cM distal to the pallid locus. The fully viable heterozygotes (Tsk/+ mice) are recognizable at 7 days of age by a tightness in the skin, and by 2 months of age, there is a pronounced thickening of the skin that is particularly apparent in the dorsum and interscapular regions. Homozygotes (Tsk/Tsk mice) die in utero at 7–8 days of development. The skin of Tsk/+ mice is thicker and stiffer than the skin of normal siblings and is associated with increased cellularity, largely comprising fibroblasts, and excessive collagen accumulation and glycosaminoglycans (2–5). This phenotype parallels the abnormalities observed in scleroderma, in which both collagens and glycosaminoglycans are elevated, and thus this murine mutation serves as an important animal model for the human connective tissue disease (for review, see refs 6–8). In addition to the cutaneous hyperplasia, the Tsk defect has an impact on several internal organs. Tsk/+ mice have enlarged hearts and display a lung phenotype that resembles human emphysema (9).

Recently, the Tsk defect has been associated with a tandem duplication of the fibrillin 1 gene (*Fbn1*) (10,11). The duplicated *Fbn1* gene produces a larger messenger RNA chain encoding an abnormal fibrillin molecule. Most recently, Kielty et al (12) described the synthesis and secretion of mutant fibrillin molecules into the extracellular matrix of Tsk dermal fibroblasts. However, how this abnormal peptide drives various cellular and molecular events leading to the global dysregulation of connective tissue metabolism is not yet understood.

In addition to alterations in extracellular matrix macromolecule biosynthesis, several studies have pointed to an autoimmune component for the Tsk phenotype, including the presence of antinuclear antibodies, one of which is anti–topoisomerase I, an autoantibody specific to scleroderma (13–17). Anti–RNA polymerase I autoantibodies have also been detected in Tsk sera (18). Further involvement of the immune system was suggested by the adoptive transfer of tight-skin fibrosis and the production of autoantibodies in normal (+/+) mice by transplanting Tsk immunocompetent cells (19,20). The experiments of Wallace et al (17) utilizing targeted disruptions of the CD4 and CD8 gene loci indicated an important role of CD4+ T cells in the development of Tsk cutaneous fibrosis and CD8+ T cells for the production of antitopoisomerase. Finally, a report by Kasturi et al (21) showed full development of

Supported in part by a grant from the Department of Veterans Affairs.

Tatjana D. Dodig, MD, Kristine T. Mack, BS, Deborah F. Cassarino, BS, Stephen H. Clark, PhD: Veterans Affairs Connecticut Healthcare System, Newington, Connecticut, and University of Connecticut Health Center, Farmington.

Address correspondence and reprint requests to Stephen H. Clark, PhD, Department of Genetics and Developmental Biology, University of Connecticut Health Center, 263 Farmington Avenue, Farmington, CT 06030.

Submitted for publication August 16, 1999; accepted in revised form November 9, 2000.

the Tsk cutaneous hyperplasia in Ig knockout mice that were devoid of mature B cells and immunoglobins.

In the present report, we describe the results of experiments to determine if the Tsk phenotype could develop in a mouse in the absence of a functional immune system. We observed that Tsk mice that are deficient in both B and T cell function ($Prkdc^{scid}$/$Prkdc^{scid}$) develop cutaneous thickening that is indistinguishable from that in Tsk mice with a fully functional immune system. Our observations are consistent with the recent findings of Siracusa et al (22), who demonstrated the development of skin tightness in Tsk mice homozygous for a knockout of the recombination-activating gene 2 and thus lacking mature T and B lymphocytes.

MATERIALS AND METHODS

Mouse strains. C57BL/6-Tsk/pa+, C57BL/6-pa+/pa+, and BALB/cByJSmn-$Prkdc^{scid}$/J mice were purchased from The Jackson Laboratory (Bar Harbor, ME). We maintained the C57BL/6-Tsk/pa+ mice in an American Association for Accreditation of Laboratory Animal Care–accredited facility by brother–sister matings with C57BL/6-pa+/pa+. Tsk/+ genotypes are easily distinguished from those of normal mice by physical examination. Mice homozygous for the mutant $Prkdc^{scid}$ allele have a severely compromised immune system due to a failure in B and T lymphocyte maturation (23). In this study, the immune-deficient phenotype was confirmed by the absence of circulating antibodies in the sera of homozygous mutant mice. All procedures involving mice were conducted using protocols that were reviewed and approved by the Institutional Animal Care and Use Committee.

Experimental matings. In the P_1 cross, the C57BL/6-Tsk/pa+ males were mated to BALB/cByJSmn-$Prkdc^{scid}$/J females. Males with a Tsk phenotype were identified among the F_1 progeny by tightness of the skin in the interscapular region. These F_1 males were backcrossed to BALB/cByJSmn-$Prkdc^{scid}$/J females. Among the progeny of these matings, 4 genotypes were anticipated, of which 2 were Tsk genotypes (Tsk/+;$Prkdc^{scid}$/$Prkdc^{+}$ and Tsk/+;$Prkdc^{scid}$/$Prkdc^{scid}$) and 2 were normal genotypes (+/+;$Prkdc^{scid}$/$Prkdc^{+}$ and +/+;$Prkdc^{scid}$/$Prkdc^{scid}$). The 4 genotypes were identified utilizing simple sequence-length polymorphic loci that mapped close to the Tsk locus on chromosome 2, D2MIT30, and the $Prkdc^{scid}$ locus on chromosome 16, D16MIT34. Polymorphisms for both of these loci had been identified between the parental inbred lines C57BL/6 and BALB/c. Genotyping was conducted by a polymerase chain reaction (PCR) analysis of DNA extracted from tail biopsy samples.

Serum samples from these mice were evaluated for circulating antibodies. Any mice that were genotyped with the homozygous $Prkdc^{scid}$ mutation, as determined by the D16MIT34 marker, and yet displayed circulating antibodies were discarded from the study without further analysis, since these mice either represented crossovers between the $Prkdc^{scid}$ mutant allele and the D16MIT34 marker or, alternatively, were "leaky" for the $Prkdc^{scid}$ phenotype. Furthermore, had the Tsk phenotype failed to develop in an immune-deficient mouse ($Prkdc^{scid}$/$Prkdc^{scid}$), a second marker flanking the other side on the Tsk locus would have been tested to confirm the Tsk genotype.

PCR genotyping. DNA was extracted from tail biopsy samples collected from N_2 mice. Simple sequence-length polymorphisms were used in order to genotype the mice. Primer pairs for the 2 markers used in this study, D2MIT30 and D16MIT34, were purchased from Research Genetics (Huntsville, AL). A PCR amplification reaction of tail genomic DNA was done using an MJ Research (Watertown, MA) PT-100 thermal cycler, with reaction conditions for the 2 markers provided by Research Genetics. The products from 10-μl PCR reactions, labeled with a trace amount of α^{32}P-dCTP, were electrophoresed on a 6% polyacrylamide/50% urea denaturing gel. The gel was then exposed to film and visualized by autoradiography. The PCR products for the C57BL/6 and BALB/cByJSmn alleles had the following sizes: D2MIT30, B6 320 and BALB/c 136 bp, and for D16MIT34, B6 138 bp and BALB/c 110 bp. In the genotyping of N_2 progeny, the D2MIT30 locus served as a marker for the Tsk mutation, while the D16MIT34 locus provided a marker for the $Prkdc^{scid}$ mutation.

Assessment of antibody levels by enzyme-linked immunosorbent assay (ELISA). To assess potential leakiness of the $Prkdc^{scid}$ mutant phenotype, the levels of circulating antibodies in the serum samples collected from N_2 mice were assayed by using an ELISA. Rajan et al (24) have successfully used this assay to detect possible leakiness of the $Prkdc^{scid}$ mutant phenotype. Briefly, microtiter wells were coated with a rat anti-mouse κ light-chain antibody that was at a concentration of 1 μg/ml, and the wells were then washed with phosphate buffered saline (PBS) containing 0.02% Tween 20. Blocking solution, consisting of 1% bovine serum albumin (BSA) in PBS, was added to the wells, which were then washed again with 0.02% Tween/PBS. Various dilutions of serum samples in 100-μl volumes were added to the wells. Serial dilutions were done on the sera.

Serum samples from Tsk/pa+ mice served as positive controls, while serum from a young $Prkdc^{scid}$/$Prkdc^{scid}$ mouse served as a negative control. Our experimental sera were derived from all the N_2 progeny. The wells were washed again with 0.02% Tween 20/PBS. A second antibody, an alkaline phosphatase–conjugated goat anti-mouse Ig heavy- and light-chain–specific antiserum, was applied to the wells. After more washes with 0.02% Tween 20/PBS, an alkaline phosphatase colorimetric substrate, *p*-nitrophenyl phosphate disodium, was added, which then caused a color to develop. The ELISA plate was read at an optical density of 410 nm. Although there is some assay-to-assay variability with this method, at a serum dilution of 1:1,000, normal mice displayed an optical density of $>$0.450 nm, whereas serum samples from $Prkdc^{scid}$/$Prkdc^{scid}$ mice displayed an optical density of $<$0.1 nm, and often $\ll$0.1 nm.

Histology. The interscapular region of the mouse was shaved, and a piece of skin that included the epidermis to the muscle layer was excised from the body. Samples were placed in 10% neutral buffered formalin at room temperature overnight. The following day, the samples were washed in running tap water and then kept in 70% ethanol. Samples were

Table 1. Genotype and phenotype analyses of progeny of the mating of Tsk/+; $Prkdc^{scid}/Prkdc^{+}$ males to BALB/cByJSmn-$Prkdc^{scid}$/J females

Genotype	No. of mice	Phenotype	D2MIT30 genotype	D16MIT34 genotype	Circulating antibodies
Tsk/+; $Prkdc^{scid}/Prkdc^{scid}$	11	Tight skin	B6/BALB/c	BALB/c/BALB/c	No
Tsk/+; $Prkdc^{scid}/Prkdc^{+}$	24	Tight skin	B6/BALB/c	B6/BALB/c	Yes
+/+; $Prkdc^{scid}/Prkdc^{scid}$	16	Normal	BALB/c/BALB/c	BALB/c/BALB/c	No
+/+; $Prkdc^{scid}/Prkdc^{+}$	33	Normal	BALB/c/BALB/c	B6/BALB/c	Yes

processed through a series of dehydration steps, cleared with xylene, and embedded in paraffin. Skin samples were sectioned and stained with Harris' hematoxylin and eosin.

Skin measurements. Sections of skin were measured for the width of the subcutaneous fibrous layer, using a light microscope equipped with a computer analyzer. Twenty independent measurements of both the dermis and hypodermis were taken from each skin section. For these measurements, the dermis is defined as the tissue beneath the epidermis extending to the adipose layer, and the hypodermis is the fibrous band between the adipose tissue and underlying muscle. All skin measurements are reported in millimeters.

Statistical tests conducted on these skin-thickness data included a calculation of the standard error of the mean and *t*-tests for comparisons between Tsk and normal genotypes.

RESULTS

Table 1 presents the results of the genotyping analysis conducted on the progeny of the mating of Tsk/+; $Prkdc^{scid}/Prkdc^{+}$ males to BALB/cByJSmn-$Prkdc^{scid}$/J females. The $Prkdc^{scid}$ phenotype and lack of "leakiness" was confirmed by the absence of circulating antibodies in $Prkdc^{scid}/Prkdc^{scid}$ mice and by their presence in control mice. The anticipated 1:1 ratio of $Prkdc^{scid}/Prkdc^{scid}$ homozygotes to $Prkdc^{scid}$/Prkdc+ heterozygotes was not observed; however, reduction in the $Prkdc^{scid}/Prkdc^{scid}$ genotypes is not correlated with the presence of the Tsk mutant allele. Tsk/+ genotypes were readily distinguished from those of normal mice by physical examination, which revealed a tightness of the skin in the interscapular region. The Tsk physical phenotype was indistinguishable between $Prkdc^{scid}/Prkdc^{scid}$ homozygotes and $Prkdc^{scid}/Prkdc^{+}$ heterozygotes.

Figure 1 presents the results of measurements of the subcutaneous fibrous layer conducted on histologic preparations of skin samples isolated from Tsk and normal mice. As with the Tsk physical phenotype assessed by manual examination, cutaneous thickening in Tsk mice determined by histologic evaluation was indistinguishable between $Prkdc^{scid}/Prkdc^{scid}$ homozygotes and $Prkdc^{scid}/Prkdc^{+}$ heterozygotes. The total dermal thickness of the skin samples from Tsk genotypes was greater than that in samples collected from normal mice. This cutaneous thickening was largely due to an increased thickness in the hypodermal layer.

Statistical analyses (*t*-test) were performed on the thickness data. These analyses did not reveal any statistically significant differences between Tsk genotypes with and without a functional immune system (Tsk/+; $Prkdc^{scid}/Prkdc^{+}$ compared with Tsk/+; $Prkdc^{scid}/Prkdc^{scid}$). Also, the absence of functional immune cells in normal mice did not alter the skin thickness, since no statistically significant difference in skin thickness was observed when measurements were compared between +/+; $Prkdc^{scid}/Prkdc^{+}$ and +/+; $Prkdc^{scid}/Prkdc^{scid}$ genotypes. In contrast, statistical analyses comparing the skin thickness in mice with the Tsk and normal genotypes did reveal significant differences in skin-thickness measurements. The Tsk mice with a functional immune system (Tsk/+; $Prkdc^{scid}/Prkdc^{+}$) had a total thickness (hypodermis + dermis) as well as a hypodermis thickness that was statistically significantly greater than that in normal mice (+/+; $Prkdc^{scid}/Prkdc^{+}$) ($P = 0.010$ for total-thickness comparisons and $P = 0.000$ for hypodermis comparisons). Also, similar results were observed in Tsk and normal mice without a functional immune system;

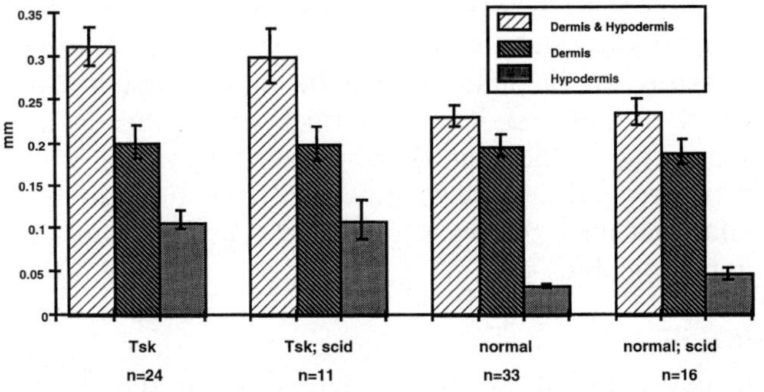

Figure 1. Thickness of the dermis and hypodermis of skin samples isolated from Tsk/+ and +/+ mice with and without a functional immune system. The different genotypes are as follows: Tsk = Tsk/+; $Prkdc^{scid}/Prkdc^{+}$, Tsk; scid = Tsk/+; $Prkdc^{scid}/Prkdc^{scid}$, normal = +/+; $Prkdc^{scid}/Prkdc^{+}$, and normal; scid = +/+; $Prkdc^{scid}/Prkdc^{scid}$. Bars show the mean ± SEM.

statistically significant differences in skin-thickness measurements between Tsk/+; $Prkdc^{scid}/Prkdc^{scid}$ and +/+; $Prkdc^{scid}/Prkdc^{scid}$ genotypes were observed for total skin thickness (hypodermis and dermis) ($P = 0.046$) and hypodermis ($P = 0.000$).

DISCUSSION

In this study, the role of the immune system in the development of cutaneous thickening in Tsk mice was assessed. These experiments were conducted because several reports have indicated an autoimmune component for the Tsk phenotype, including the presence of antinuclear antibodies as well as the adoptive transfer of tight-skin fibrosis and the production of autoantibodies in normal mice by transplanting Tsk/+ immunocompetent cells. In the present experiments, the development of the Tsk skin phenotype was examined in mice that lacked functional T and B cells as a result of a mutation at the Prkdc locus. Although histology experiments were not performed to examine the immune system in $Prkdc^{scid}/Prkdc^{scid}$ mice, all $Prkdc^{scid}/Prkdc^{scid}$ mice used in the present study lacked circulating antibodies in their sera. Tsk mice that were also homozygous for the $Prkdc^{scid}$ mutation ($Prkdc^{scid}/Prkdc^{scid}$) developed excessive cutaneous thickening that was indistinguishable from that observed in Tsk mice that were heterozygous for the $Prkdc^{scid}$ mutation ($Prkdc^{scid}/Prkdc^{+}$).

Concordant with this observation, statistically significant differences were observed in comparisons of hypodermis and total-skin (hypodermis + dermis) thickness measurements between Tsk/+ and +/+ genotypes. These data are consistent with those in the recent report by Siracusa et al (22) that showed the full development of the Tsk phenotype in mice lacking mature T and B lymphocytes. The present report and the observations by Siracusa et al (22) indicate that the immune system is not the cause of the Tsk skin thickening. This is also supported by the findings of Kasturi et al (21), which demonstrated the development of Tsk fibrosis in Ig knockout mice that were devoid of mature B cells and immunoglobins.

In aggregate, the results of these studies indicate that the autoimmune component of the Tsk phenotype is not required for the development of the dermal thickening observed in Tsk mice. It is possible that the fibrotic process itself may stimulate an autoimmune response. Although this type of stimulating mechanism in Tsk mice is unknown, it may involve the excessive production/turnover of extracellular matrix macromolecules. This prospect is supported by the fact that the Tsk cutaneous phenotype develops in young mice, while autoantibodies are detected in older animals (13), as well as by the observation of elevated levels of collagen-degrading enzymes in the skin of Tsk mice (6).

REFERENCES

1. Green MC, Sweet HO, Bunker LE. Tight-skin, a new mutation of the mouse causing excessive growth of connective tissue and skeleton. Am J Pathol 1976;82:493–512.
2. Menton DN, Hess RA, Lichenstein JR, Eisen AZ. The structure and tensile properties of the skin of tight-skin (TSK) mutant mice. J Invest Dermatol 1978;70:4–10.
3. Menton DN, Hess RA. The ultrastructure of collagen in the dermis of tight-skin (TSK) mutant mice. J Invest Dermatol 1980;74:139–47.
4. Jimenez SA, Millan A, Bashey RI. Scleroderma-like alterations in collagen metabolism occurring in the TSK (tight skin) mouse. Arthritis Rheum 1984;27:180–5.
5. Ross SC, Osborn TG, Dorner RW, Zuckner J. Glycosaminoglycan content in skin of the tight-skin mouse. Arthritis Rheum 1983;26: 653–7.
6. Jimenez SA, Bashey RI, Williams CJ, Millan AH. The tight skin (TSK) mouse as an experimental model of scleroderma. In: Greenwald RA, Diamond HS, editors. CRC handbook of animal models for the rheumatic diseases. Boca Raton (FL): CRC Press; 1988. p. 169–93.
7. Bocchieri MH, Jimenez SA. Animal models of fibrosis. Rheum Dis Clin North Am 1990;16:153–67.
8. Jimenez SA, Christner P. Animal models of systemic sclerosis. Clin Dermatol 1994;12:425–36.
9. Gardi C, Martorana PA, de Santi MM, van Even P, Lungarella G. A biochemical and morphological investigation of the early development of genetic emphysema in tight-skin mice. Exp Mol Pathol 1989;50:398–410.
10. Siracusa LD, McGrath R, Ma Q, Moslow JJ, Manne J, Christner PJ, et al. A tandem duplication of the fibrillin 1 gene is associated with the mouse tight skin mutation. Genome Res 1996;6:300–13.
11. Bona CA, Murai C, Casares S, Kasturi K, Nishimura H, Honjo T, et al. Structure of the mutant fibrillin-1 gene in the tight skin (TSK) mouse. DNA Res 1997;4:267–71.
12. Kielty CM, Raghunath M, Siracusa LD, Sherratt MJ, Peters R, Shuttleworth CA, et al. The tight skin mouse: demonstration of mutant fibrillin-1 production and assembly into abnormal microfibrils. J Cell Biol 1998;140:1159–66.
13. Bocchieri MH, Henriksen PD, Kasturi KN, Muryoi T, Bona CA, Jimenez SA. Evidence for autoimmunity in the tight skin mouse model of systemic sclerosis. Arthritis Rheum 1991;34:599–605.
14. Muryoi T, Kasturi KN, Kafina MJ, Saitoh Y, Usuba O, Perlish JS, et al. Self reactive repertoire of tight skin mouse: immunochemical and molecular characterization of anti-topoisomerase I autoantibodies. Autoimmunity 1991;9:109–17.
15. Muryoi T, Andre-Schwartz J, Saitoh Y, Daian C, Hall B, Dimitriu-Bona A, et al. Self-reactive repertoire of tight skin (TSK/+) mouse: immunochemical and molecular characterization of anti-cellular autoantibodies. Cell Immunol 1992;144:43–54.
16. Bona C, Rothfield N. Autoantibodies in scleroderma and tight skin mice. Curr Opin Immunol 1994;6:931–7.
17. Wallace VA, Kondo S, Kono T, Xing Z, Timms E, Furlonger C, et al. A role for CD4+ T cells in the pathogenesis of skin fibrosis in tight skin mice. Eur J Immunol 1994;24:1463–6.
18. Shibata S, Muryo T, Saitoh Y, Brumeanu T-D, Bona C, Kasturi KN. Immunochemical and molecular characterization of anti-

RNA polymerase I autoantibodies produced by tight skin mouse. J Clin Invest 1993;92:984–92.
19. Walker M, Harley R, Maize J, DeLustro F, LeRoy EC. Mast cells and their degranulation in the Tsk mouse model of scleroderma. Proc Soc Exp Biol Med 1985;180:323–8.
20. Phelps RG, Daian C, Shibata S, Fleischmajer R, Bona CA. Induction of skin fibrosis and autoantibodies by infusion of immunocompetent cells from tight skin mice into C57BL/6 Pa/Pa mice. J Autoimmun 1993;6:701–18.
21. Kasturi KN, Hatakeyama A, Murai C, Gordon R, Phelps RG, Bona CA. B-cell deficiency does not abrogate development of cutaneous hyperplasia in mice inheriting the defective fibrillin-1 gene. J Autoimmun 1997;10:505–17.
22. Siracusa LD, McGrath R, Fisher JK, Jimenez SA. The mouse tight skin (Tsk) phenotype is not dependent on the presence of mature T and B lymphocytes. Mamm Genome 1998;9:907–9.
23. Bosma MJ, Carroll AM. The scid mouse mutant: definition, characterization and potential uses. Annu Rev Immunol 1991;9: 323–50.
24. Rajan TV, Schultz LD, Yates J, Greiner DL. B lymphocytes are not required for murine resistance to the human filarial parasite, Brugia malayi. J Parasitol 1995;81:490–3.

ARTHRITIS & RHEUMATISM
Vol. 44, No. 3, March 2001, pp 728–734

CONCISE COMMUNICATIONS

Prolonged remission without treatment after autologous stem cell transplantation for refractory childhood systemic lupus erythematosus

Improved care and drug treatment have considerably decreased morbidity and mortality in childhood systemic lupus erythematosus (SLE), although renal failure, infections, and drug-related toxicity remain major concerns. In recent years, potent immunosuppressive drug regimens have been introduced to control the disease (1). Nevertheless, a small proportion of children have not responded to these drugs or have developed severe side effects. Autologous stem cell transplantation (ASCT) has recently been described as a possible treatment for severe chronic autoimmune diseases that have been refractory to conventional therapy (2,3). This was based on several case reports that described prolonged remission of autoimmune disease in patients who were treated with bone marrow transplantation for a malignancy (4). Regression of adjuvant-induced arthritis was observed in rats after total-body irradiation (TBI) and autologous bone marrow transplantation (5,6). The rationale of this therapy is to suppress the immune system maximally and then "rescue" the patient from prolonged or persistent aplasia by infusing autologous stem cells. Between 1994 and 1999, more than 20 cases of adult SLE patients treated with ASCT have been reported (7,8), and participants in several workshops have proposed inclusion criteria for this experimental treatment.

Herein we present the first report of ASCT in children with SLE. ASCT was administered to 2 children, both of whom were steroid dependent but experienced severe side effects from the steroids. They were treated with high-dose cyclophosphamide (CYC), which induced strong immunosuppression but little immunoablation. We added low-dose TBI to their regimens based on the finding, in an animal arthritis model, that this induces a very profound depletion of T memory cells (6). T cell depletion of the graft was performed to avoid reinfusion of putative autoreactive T cells. We hypothesize that immune reconstitution in the absence of mature T memory cells in a patient with aplasia may induce tolerance to unknown autoantigens responsible for the disease.

The protocol was approved by our institutional research board. Written informed consent was obtained. Clinical details on the patients are shown in Table 1.

Patient 1, a 14-year-old girl, presented at the age of 10 with fever, Raynaud's phenomenon, malar rash, sunlight hypersensitivity, vasculitic skin lesions on her fingers and toes, and polyarthritis. A few months later she developed hemorrhagic pneumonitis, glomerulonephritis (World Health Organization [WHO] class IV), and pancytopenia. She was treated for 6 months with pulse CYC, which was stopped because of severe hemorrhagic cystitis. In the following years, azathioprine (AZA) and hydroxychloroquine (HCQ) were added to her treatment regimen. Tapering of the prednisone to <1 mg/kg/day resulted repeatedly in exacerbations of her SLE, with vasculitic lesions in the fingers, malar rash, fever, malaise, and a concomitant decrease in complement levels and increase in the anti–double-stranded DNA (anti-dsDNA) titer.

Patient 2, a 14-year-old boy, was diagnosed with SLE at the age of 9, presenting with Coombs-positive hemolytic anemia, polyarthritis, lymphadenopathy, and malar rash. A few months later, he lost vision in his right eye due to vasculitis. In the following years, he developed glomerulonephritis (WHO class IV) that remained active despite treatment with steroids (both pulse methylprednisolone and oral maintenance therapy), pulse CYC, AZA, and HCQ. He developed severe pericarditis that responded well to steroids. Tapering of steroids to <0.75 mg/kg/day resulted in flares of the pericarditis, fatigue, and/or hypocomplementemia.

Hemopoietic stem cells were obtained by conventional bone marrow aspiration under general anesthesia without priming. In patient 1, the graft was purged by 2 cycles of T cell depletion with CD2 and CD3 antibodies, yielding a suspension with a CD34+ count of 0.55×10^6/kg and a T cell count of 0.5×10^4/kg (9). During this period, a new method of cell separation using the Clinimacs column (Miltenyi Biotec, Bergisch-Gladbach, Germany) coated with an anti-CD34 monoclonal antibody was introduced into our clinic, yielding an even more profound cell depletion. Bone marrow obtained from the second patient was processed by this positive CD34+ selection, resulting in 1.2×10^6/kg CD34+ cells and 1.3×10^4/kg T cells.

The conditioning regimen included 4 days of antithymocyte globulin (rabbit ATG; IMTIX, Pasteur-Merieux, France) at a dosage of 5 mg/kg from day -9 to day -6, CYC at a dosage of 50 mg/kg/day from day -5 to day -2, and low-dose TBI (4 Gy, single fraction) on day -1. On day 0, the frozen stem cell suspension was thawed and infused. HCQ and tolmetin were stopped before ASCT. Prednisone treatment was continued throughout the procedure and was slowly tapered after 2–6 months. During conditioning and the aplastic period, the patients were hospitalized in private rooms at our transplant unit for 6–8 weeks.

The patients were monitored at 3-month intervals. Clinical evaluation of SLE activity after ASCT was done with the SLE Disease Activity Index (SLEDAI) (10). The prednisone dosage was adjusted in accordance with the actual disease activity and laboratory values. White blood cell and differential cell counts were performed by hemocytometry. Lymphocyte subsets were determined using fluorescein isothiocyanate– or phycoerythrin-conjugated antibodies to CD3 (T lymphocytes), CD4 (T helper lymphocytes), CD8 (T cytotoxic/suppressor lymphocytes), CD20 (B lymphocytes), CD45RA (naive T cells), CD45RO (memory T cells), or CD16/CD57 (natural killer cells) (all from Becton Dickinson, San Jose, CA). Cells were analyzed by flow cytometry on a Calibur fluorescence-activated cell sorter (Becton Dickinson). In vitro lymphocyte function was assessed by the proliferative response to activation with mitogens, recall antigens, or allogeneic cells. Hemolytic complement activity (CH50) was determined on sensitized sheep red blood cells and expressed as a percentage of the activity in normal human serum. Complement components C1q, C3, and C4 were determined by radial immunodiffusion (Behring, Marburg, Germany). Antinuclear antibodies were determined by indirect immunofluorescence on HEp-2 cells; anti-dsDNA antibodies were determined by

Table 1. Characteristics of the patients before, during, and after ASCT*

	Before ASCT		During ASCT		After ASCT	
	Patient 1	Patient 2	Patient 1	Patient 2	Patient 1	Patient 2
Specific clinical problems	Pneumonitis, glomerulonephritis, cyclophosphamide-related cystitis	Retinal vasculitis, glomerulonephritis despite cyclophosphamide, recurrent pericarditis, avascular necrosis of the tibial head	ATG-related fever, RSV pneumonia	ATG-related fever, enterovirus-associated pericarditis	VZV (skin), no vasculitis	Mild sinobronchitis, no pericarditis, no vasculitis
SLEDAI score	20	27	ND	ND	0	8
Laboratory values						
Hemoglobin, mmoles/liter	6–8	5–6.7			8–9	4.6–7.4
Lymphocytes/μl	120–500	90–400	Neutrophil count >500/ml after 22 days	Neutrophil count >500/ml after 30 days	500–1,500	250–1,500
Platelets, $\times 10^6$/liter	250–350	240–400	>20,000 after 17 days	>20,000 after 24 days	180–320	150–250
Creatinine, μmoles/liter	50–60	45–56			50–60	46–63
Urinalysis	Erythrocytes, and protein positive	Erythrocytes, and protein positive			Normal	Normal
Complement (CH50), %	30–50	39–66			>100	45–161
ANA titer	1:200–1:1,600	1:40–1:400	ND	ND	1:40	Negative
DsDNA (Farr assay), IU/mL	52–750	47–120	ND	ND	Negative	Negative
Lymphocyte proliferation in vitro	Normal	Normal	ND	ND	Normal after 7 months	Normal after 11 months
Treatment						
Prednisone, mg/day	20–50	30–60	15	30	Stopped 6 months after ASCT	Stopped 3 months after ASCT
Azathioprine, mg/day	75	75	–	–	–	–
Cyclophosphamide, mg/m^2/month	750, 6 times	750, 9 times	–	–	–	–
Hydroxychloroquine, mg/day	200	200	–	–	During summer	–
Tolectin (NSAID), mg/day	1,200		–	–	–	200
IV gamma globulin, gm/kg/3 weeks	0.4	–	0.4	–	Stopped 12 months after ASCT	–
Growth, cm	2 in last 3 years	5 in last 3 years			8 in last year	6 in last year
Months of followup					18	12

*ASCT = autologous stem cell transplantation; ATG = antithymocyte globulin; RSV = respiratory syncytial virus; VZV = varicella zoster virus; SLEDAI = Systemic Lupus Erythematosus Disease Activity Index; ND = not determined; ANA = antinuclear antibody; dsDNA = double-stranded DNA; NSAID = nonsteroidal antiinflammatory drug; IV = intravenous.

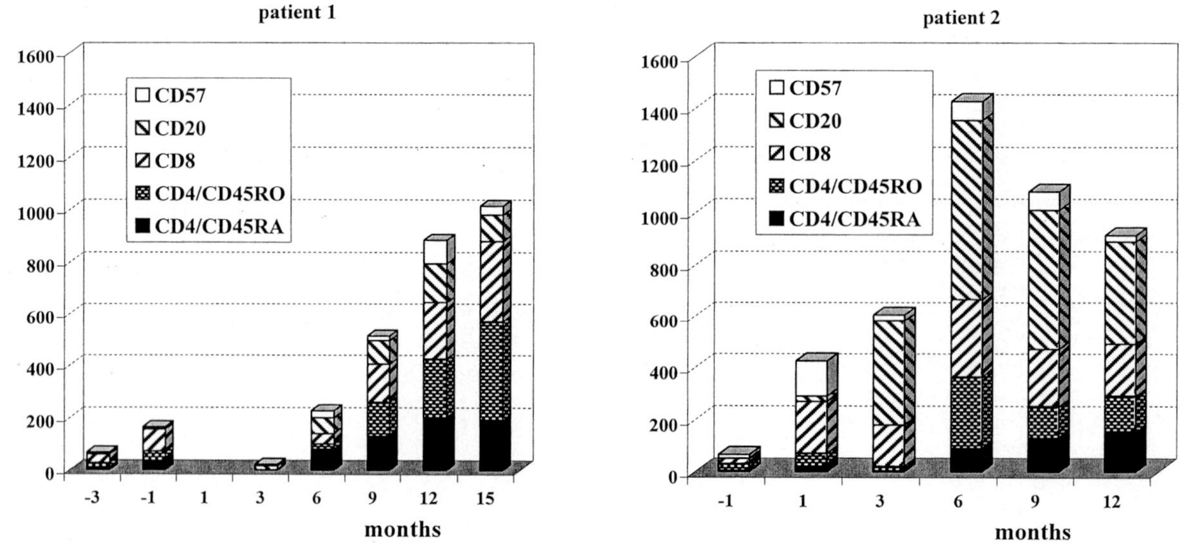

Figure 1. Immune reconstitution in patients 1 and 2, after autologous stem cell transplantation (ASCT). All values are the number of cells/μl. Before ASCT, the number of CD4 cells was only 50–100/μl, illustrating the immunocompromised state. After ASCT, a gradual increase in all T cell subsets was seen. Only 12–15 months after ASCT, the number of CD4 cells (CD45RO and CD45RA together) was >500/μl in patient 1 and 290/μl in patient 2.

the Farr assay. Renal function was monitored by determination of the serum creatinine level, examination of urinary sediment, and screening for proteinuria at each visit.

The conditioning regimen was reasonably well tolerated, although both patients experienced fever, chills, and hypotension after the first ATG dose. After ASCT, their total lymphocyte counts rose to 1,000/μl after 6–12 months. Immunologic reconstitution has been slow in both patients. In patient 1, the CD4 count increased to >500/μl only 12–15 months after ASCT (Figure 1). Eleven months after ASCT, the CD4 count in patient 2 is only 290/μl. Serum immunoglobulins from both patients were within the normal range, with normal antibody responses to recall antigens 8–11 months after ASCT.

Both patients showed a remarkable and persistent decrease in SLE activity after ASCT (Table 1). At present, patients 1 and 2 have been in complete remission without immunosuppressive medication for 12 months and 9 months, respectively, with SLEDAI scores of 0 and 8, respectively (the score of 8 in patient 2 is due to permanent vasculitic lesions of the retina). The ASCT was well tolerated apart from well-known ATG-related side effects and viral infections. Complete clinical treatment-free remission was induced by this experimental treatment, but a longer observation time is necessary to determine whether ASCT can lead to a definite cure. The findings in our 2 patients are consistent with the results of ASCT in adult SLE patients, reported to the European Group for Bone and Marrow Transplantation (EBMT) Working Party for Autoimmune Diseases (7,8).

With regard to the application of ASCT for severe autoimmune disease, several issues arise. First, is ASCT needed, or can similar results be obtained by conventional therapy? (1,11,12). The results of other studies, especially those reported by Brodsky et al (11,12), show prolonged remission after high-dose CYC, given at the same dosage we used in this study. It is not clear whether T cell depletion of the marrow is crucial to the process of the transplant, or whether an intensive but nonmyeloablative regimen without stem cell support would be just as effective. A major concern is that autoreactive T cells will be reinfused with the autograft. In most cases reported to date, T cell depletion of the autograft was performed, because in one of the earliest studies, early relapses after non–T cell–depleted ASCT were noted in a series of 5 patients with a malignant disorder and coincidental SLE (13). In our opinion, only randomized trials with prolonged followup can show differences between high-dose CYC, with and that without stem cell support. For this purpose, protocols are presently being developed. Recently, a joint EBMT/Autologous Blood and Marrow Transplant Registry form for clinical followup after ASCT for SLE was developed. Use of this form will enable accurate evaluation of the clinical response.

We did not perform mobilization of bone marrow progenitor cells with CYC and granulocyte–colony-stimulating factor (G-CSF) because G-CSF has been associated with reactivation of rheumatoid arthritis and SLE and development of leukocytoclastic vasculitis (14,15). Graft manipulation by either negative CD2/CD3 or positive CD34 selection resulted in a prolonged CD4 lymphopenia in both patients for whom this has been reported (14,15), with the risk of opportunistic infections, comparable with the lymphopenia after ASCT observed in patients with juvenile idiopathic arthritis (JIA) (2,16).

In the first 200 adults and children who have had ASCT for autoimmune disease, the reported transplant-related mortality is 5–10%, comparable with the transplant-related mortality of ASCT for non-Hodgkin's lymphoma (17).

A serious complication observed in JIA after ASCT is virus-associated hemophagocytic syndrome or macrophage activation syndrome (16). Though very rare, this has been observed in SLE. Therefore, SLE patients who have undergone ASCT must also be considered at risk for this complication. A 10% rate of transplant-related mortality can be acceptable only if it is counterbalanced by significant drug toxicity from conventional treatment or markedly impaired quality of life. The preliminary results of ASCT for JIA, as well as the cases reported here, do indicate a marked improvement in the quality of life. Several European and American workshops have addressed the issue of inclusion criteria for this putative new treatment. ASCT must be performed only for the most severely affected patients with SLE. For adults, inclusion criteria have been developed, and these include CYC-resistant class III or IV glomerulonephritis, uncontrollable vasculitis (lungs, brain, heart) or transfusion-dependent cytopenias (7,8). Similar criteria have been proposed for children (workshops in Utrecht, the Netherlands, May 1998, and Worcester, Massachusetts, September 1999).

N. M. Wulffraat, MD
E. A. M. Sanders, MD
S. S. M. Kamphuis, MD
G. T. Rijkers, MD
W. Kuis, MD
M. Lilien, MD
I. C. M. Slaper-Cortenbach, MD
University Medical Centre Utrecht
Utrecht, The Netherlands

1. Lehman TJ, Onel K. Intermittent intravenous cyclophosphamide arrests the progression of the renal chronicity index in childhood systemic lupus erythematosus. J Pediatr 2000;136:243–7.
2. Wulffraat NM, van Royen A, Bierings M, Vossen JM, Kuis W. Autologous haemopoietic stem cell transplantation in four patients with refractory juvenile chronic arthritis. Lancet 1999;353:550–3.
3. Tyndall A, Gratwohl A. Blood and marrow stem cell transplants in auto-immune disease: a consensus report written on behalf of the European League against Rheumatism (EULAR) and the European Group for Blood and Marrow Transplantation (EBMT). Bone Marrow Transplant 1997;19:643–5.
4. Lowenthal RM, Cohen ML, Atkinson K, Biggs JC. Apparent cure of rheumatoid arthritis by bone marrow transplantation. J Rheumatol 1993;20:137–40.
5. Van Bekkum DW. Effectiveness and risks of total body irradiation for conditioning in the treatment of autoimmune disease with autologous bone marrow transplantation. Rheumatology (Oxford) 1999;38:757–61.
6. Van Bekkum DW. Conditioning regimens for the treatment of experimental arthritis with autologous bone marrow transplantation. Bone Marrow Transplant 2000;25:357–64.
7. Tyndall A, Gratwohl A. Immune ablation and stem-cell therapy in autoimmune disease: clinical experience. Arthritis Res 2000;2:276–80.
8. Traynor AE, Schroeder J, Rosa RM, Cheng D, Stefka J, Mujais S, et al. Treatment of severe systemic lupus erythematosus with high-dose chemotherapy and haemopoietic stem-cell transplantation: a phase I study. Lancet 2000;356:701–7.
9. Slaper-Cortenbach ICM, Wijngaarden-duBois MJGJ, de Vries-van Rossen A, Borst HPE, van der Lelie H, van Heugten HG, et al. The depletion of T cells from haematopoietic stem cell transplants. Rheumatology (Oxford) 1999;38:751–4.
10. Bombardier C, Gladman DD, Urowitz MB, Caron D, Chang CH, and the Committee on Prognosis Studies in SLE. Derivation of the SLEDAI: a disease activity index for lupus patients. Arthritis Rheum 1992;35:630–40.
11. Brodsky RA, Petri M, Smith BD, Seifter EJ, Spivak JL, Styler M, et al. Immunoablative high-dose cyclophosphamide without stem-cell rescue for refractory, severe autoimmune disease. Ann Intern Med 1998;129:1031–5.
12. Brodsky RA, Petri M, Jones RJ. Hematopoietic stem cell transplantation for systemic lupus erythematosus. Rheum Dis Clin North Am 2000;26:377–87.
13. Euler HH, Marmont AM, Bacigalupo A, Fastenrath S, Dreger P, Hoffknecht M, et al. Early recurrence or persistence of autoimmune diseases after unmanipulated autologous stem cell transplantation. Blood 1996;88:3621–5.
14. Farhey YD, Herman JH. Vasculitis complicating granulocyte colony stimulating factor treatment of leucopenia and infection in Felty's syndrome. J Rheumatol 1995;22:1179–82.
15. Euler HH, Harten P, Zenner RA, Schwab AM. Recombinant human granulocyte colony stimulating factor in patients with SLE neutropenia and associated infections. J Rheumatol 1997;24:2153–7.
16. Wulffraat NM, Kamphuis SSM, Brinkman D, ten Cate R, Kuis W. Autologous hemopoietic stem cell transplantation in 12 cases with refractory juvenile idiopathic arthritis. Osteol Bull 2000;5:62–5.
17. Tyndall A, Fassas A, Passweg J, Ruiz de Elvira C, Attal M, Brooks P, et al. Autologous hemopoietic stem cell transplants for autoimmune disease: feasibility and transplant related mortality. Bone Marrow Transplant 1999;24:729–34.

Up-regulated expression of transforming growth factor β receptors in dermal fibroblasts in skin sections from patients with localized scleroderma

Localized scleroderma is a connective tissue disorder limited to the skin and subcutaneous tissue, often involving the muscular tissues beneath the cutaneous lesions. The absence of Raynaud's phenomenon, of acrosclerosis, and of involvement of internal organs differentiates it from systemic sclerosis (SSc). However, the 2 diseases may share similar pathogenetic processes, since abnormal collagen metabolism (1) and autoimmunity (2) are considered to be fundamental characteristics of both. Elevated collagen synthesis by skin fibroblasts derived from involved lesions, which has been demonstrated in an in vitro culture system (1), is one of the common characteristics of the 2 conditions and may be closely related to their pathogenesis.

Transforming growth factor β (TGFβ) has gained attention as an important factor in the pathogenesis of fibrosis (3). TGFβ causes the deposition of extracellular matrix (ECM) by simultaneously stimulating skin fibroblasts to increase the production of ECM proteins such as collagen, fibronectin, or proteoglycan, to decrease the production of matrix-degrading proteases, to increase the production of inhibitors of these proteases, and to modulate the expression of integrins (4). Increased expression of TGFβ has been noted in skin biopsy specimens from patients with sclerotic skin disorders, including SSc and localized scleroderma (5). It is suspected that the TGFβ signaling pathway plays an important role in fibrosis.

There are 3 isotypes of receptors for TGFβ, referred to as types I, II, and III, among which types I and II receptors are involved in the TGFβ signaling pathway (6). The TGFβ type II receptor (TGFβRII) binds TGFβ, and then TGFβRI is re-

Table 1. Characteristics of the patients with localized scleroderma and the normal controls, and results of in situ hybridization and immunohistochemical staining*

				In situ hybridization						Immunohistochemical staining			
			Disease duration,	Type I receptor			Type II receptor			Type I receptor		Type II receptor	
Subject	Age/sex	Diagnosis	years	Epidermis	Fibroblasts	No.	Epidermis	Fibroblasts	No.	Epidermis	Fibroblasts	Epidermis	Fibroblasts
Patients													
1	20/F	Morphea	1	+++	++	>30	+++	++	10–20	+++	++	++	+
2	65/M	Generalized morphea	0.5	+++	+++	>30	+++	++	>30	+++	+++	++	++
3	10/F	Linear scleroderma	5	++	+	10–20	+++	+++	>30	+	++	+	+
4	43/F	Morphea	1	+++	+++	>30	+++	++	10–20	+++	++	+	+
5	24/F	Linear scleroderma	1	++	+++	>30	+++	+++	>30	++	+++	+++	++
Controls													
1	43/M			++	+	0–1	++	+	1–5	++	++	++	+
2	30/M			++	−	0	+	−	0	++	+	++	+
3	20/F			+	−	0	+	−	0	++	−	++	−
4	22/F			++	+	0–1	++	+	1–5	++	++	+	−
5	45/F			++	−	0	++	+	0–1	+	−	+	−
6	43/F			++	−	0	++	−	0	+++	+	+	−

* Localized scleroderma included morphea. Skin sections from patients were obtained from affected areas. Staining intensity was graded as − = none, + = slight staining, +++ = strong staining, and ++ = staining between + and +++. No. = approximate number of positively stained fibroblasts in a 200× magnified area.

cruited to form a heteromeric complex. TGFβRII transphosphorylates the glycine/serine-rich domain of TGFβRI kinase (6). The complex can directly act as a transcriptional activator and can indirectly regulate gene transcription by interacting with transcriptional factors (7). Overexpression of TGFβRI and TGFβRII in cultured dermal fibroblasts derived from skin biopsy specimens from patients with SSc has been demonstrated by Northern blot analysis in an in vitro system (8). To examine their expression in localized scleroderma, we performed immunohistochemical staining and in situ hybridization studies of skin sections of patients with localized scleroderma.

Skin biopsy specimens were obtained from 6 normal controls and from 5 patients with localized scleroderma (including morphea) (Table 1). All of the patients with localized scleroderma were diagnosed by clinical appearance and histologic findings, and none of them had any other collagen disease, including SSc. All patient biopsy specimens were obtained from affected skin at the time of diagnosis. All samples were fixed in neutral buffered formalin, embedded in paraffin, and prepared for hematoxylin and eosin staining. On hematoxylin and eosin examination, all patients with localized scleroderma demonstrated histologic evidence of sclerosis, with perivascular and perifollicular lymphocytic infiltration in the dermis. The dermal collagen bundles were packed and thickened, and the dermal–epidermal junctions were flattened. Dermal sclerosis extended into the subjacent adipose tissues.

Formalin-fixed, paraffin-embedded skin tissue samples were investigated using the nonradioactive in situ hybridization technique with digoxigenin (DIG)–labeled RNA probes, with slight modification as described previously (9). Briefly, paraffin-embedded sections were cut to a thickness of 5 μm, mounted on silane-coated slides, deparaffinized, and treated with 0.2*M* HCl for 15 minutes, followed by 1.5 mg/ml proteinase K digestion for 15 minutes at 37°C. The sections were postfixed with 4% paraformaldehyde in phosphate buffered saline (PBS) for 30 minutes and treated with PBS containing 2 mg/ml glycine twice, for 15 minutes each time. After rinsing with PBS, the samples were soaked twice in standard saline–sodium citrate buffer (SSC) with 50% formamide and subjected to hybridization.

A 2,300-bp fragment from TGFβRI complementary DNA (cDNA; kindly provided by Dr. P. ten Dijke, Ludwig Institute for Cancer Research, Uppsala, Sweden) (8) and a 4,000-bp fragment from TGFβRII cDNA (kindly provided by Dr. R. A. Weinberg, Whitehead Institute for Biochemical Research, Cambridge, MA) (8) were subcloned into the SPT18 phagemid (Roche Diagnostics, Indianapolis, IN) and pcDNA 3.1 (Invitrogen, San Diego, CA) and used to make probes. The sense probes and antisense probes for TGFβRI and TGFβRII were labeled with DIG-11–UTP using a DIG RNA-labeling kit (Roche Diagnostics). The labeled RNA probes (final concentration 1 μg/ml) in a mixture containing 50% formamide, 10% dextran sulfate, 1× Denhardt's solution, 100 μg/ml transfer RNA, 5× SSC, 0.25% sodium dodecyl sulfate, 1 m*M* EDTA, and 50 m*M* NaH_2PO_4 were placed on the slides and covered with a coverslip. Hybridization was performed in a humidified chamber for 18 hours at 45°C, after which the specimens were washed in 2× SSC with 50% formamide at 50°C. Unhybridized probes were digested in 2.5 μg/ml RNase A, 500 m*M* NaCl, 1 m*M* EDTA, and 10 m*M* Tris HCl (pH 8.0) for 15 minutes at 37°C. The slides were then washed for 15 minutes in 2× SSC and for 15 minutes in 0.2× SSC, twice at 50°C. After post-hybridization washing, DIG-labeled probes were visualized as described in the DIG nucleic acid detection kit protocol (Roche Diagnostics). We used the following grading system: + = slight staining, +++ = strong staining, and ++ = staining between + and +++. The approximate number of stained cells in a 200× magnified area was counted.

Immunohistochemical staining on paraffin-embedded

sections was performed using a Vectastain ABC kit (Vector, Burlingame, CA) according to the manufacturer's recommendations. Five micrometer–thick sections were mounted on APES-coated slides, deparaffinized with xylene, and rehydrated through a graded series of ethyl alcohol and PBS. The sections were then incubated with antibodies against TGFβRI and TGFβRII (Santa Cruz Biotechnology, Santa Cruz, CA) and diluted 1:500 in PBS overnight at 4°C. The immunoreactivity was visualized with diaminobenzidine. The sections were then counterstained with hematoxylin. Staining was graded using the same scoring system as described above.

In normal skin, TGFβRI messenger RNA (mRNA) and TGFβRII mRNA were expressed strongly in the follicles and the sebaceous glands, moderately in the epidermis and blood vessels, and slightly in spindle-shaped cells. The distributions of TGFβRI mRNA and TGFβ-RII mRNA were roughly the same, especially when staining was stronger. In the skin sections from patients with localized scleroderma, TGFβRI mRNA and TGFβRII mRNA were expressed strongly in follicles, sebaceous glands, and spindle-shaped cells between collagen bundles and moderately in the epidermis and blood vessels (Table 1). Tissue sections from patients with localized scleroderma had increased numbers of spindle-shaped cells with strong expression of TGFβRI and TGFβRII mRNA. At higher magnification, these spindle-shaped cells appeared to be fibroblasts morphologically. Furthermore, prominent expression of both TGFβRI mRNA and TGFβRII mRNA was observed on round cells around the vessels. With hematoxylin counterstaining, these round cells appeared to be lymphocytes. There was no staining or coloration after in situ hybridization, except for basal pigmentation in the epidermis in the tissue sections from normal skin or from localized scleroderma skin studied using TGFβRI and TGFβRII sense probes.

By immunohistochemical staining, expression of TGFβRI protein and TGFβRII protein in normal skin sections was found to be strong in the follicles and the sebaceous glands, moderate in the epidermis and the blood vessels, and slight in the spindle-shaped cells between collagen bundles. Skin sections from patients with localized scleroderma showed strong expression of TGFβRI and TGFβRII proteins in the follicles, the sebaceous glands, and the round cells around the vessels, and moderate expression in the epidermis, blood vessels, and spindle-shaped cells between collagen bundles, by immunohistochemical staining (Table 1). The distribution of expression of TGFβRI protein and of TGFβRII protein was similar, especially where staining was stronger. The results of immunohistochemical staining were similar to those of in situ hybridization, though the findings were not perfectly identical due to differences in the sensitivity of these methods.

TGFβ is presently recognized as a central mediator in various fibrotic diseases, including SSc and localized scleroderma (3). It principally affects human skin fibroblasts as a stimulator of ECM production, leading to excessive ECM deposition. TGFβ can increase expression of collagen types I, III, VI, VII, and X, fibronectin, and proteoglycans (10). Stimulation of ECM production by TGFβ is further enhanced by its inhibitory effect on matrix degradation via decreasing synthesis of proteases and increasing levels of protease inhibitors (10). An important mechanism for regulating the cellular response to cytokines and hormones resides at the level of receptor expression. Modulation of the levels of TGFβRI and TGFβRII expression may play an important role in both the mechanism of wound healing and the pathogenesis of various fibrogenic disorders. Several types of cells, including immune, endothelial, and mesenchymal cells, are thought to be sources of TGFβ in fibrotic lesions, and sustained production of TGFβ in the lesion may be maintained by the establishment of an autocrine cytokine loop (11).

In this study, we demonstrated elevated levels of expression of both TGFβRI and TGFβRII mRNA in skin sections from patients with localized scleroderma in comparison with normal control skin sections, in spite of the small number and heterogeneity of the patients investigated and the semiquantitative nature of the methods. In an in vitro analysis, the elevated expression of mRNA for these receptors was correlated with elevated $\alpha 2(1)$ collagen mRNA levels (8). These results suggest that overtransduction of the TGFβ signaling pathway and overexpression of these receptors may induce overexpression of the ECM, including collagen (8).

In immunohistochemical studies, staining was also detected in epidermal cells, adnexal tissues, vascular cells, and fibroblasts with distribution quite similar to that found for expression of TGFβRI and TGFβRII mRNA. Furthermore, the up-regulated expression of TGFβRI and TGFβRII proteins in localized scleroderma was also demonstrated in immunohistochemical studies. The sensitivity of in situ hybridization for TGFβRI and TGFβRII exceeded that of immunohistochemical staining. Thus, it is more accurate to evaluate overexpression of TGFβRI and TGFβRII by in situ hybridization than by immunohistochemical staining using available antibodies.

In conclusion, TGFβRI and TGFβRII are up-regulated in dermal fibroblasts in the affected skin of patients with localized scleroderma. Autocrine TGFβ signaling due to the overexpression of both TGFβRI and TGFβRII in dermal fibroblasts may be involved in the pathogenesis of dermal fibrosis in this disease.

Masahide Kubo, MD, PhD
Hironobu Ihn, MD, PhD
Kenichi Yamane, MD
Kunihiko Tamaki, MD, PhD
University of Tokyo
Tokyo, Japan

1. LeRoy EC. Increased collagen synthesis by scleroderma fibroblasts in vitro: a possible defect in the regulation or activation of the scleroderma fibroblast. J Clin Invest 1974;54:880–9.
2. Falanga V, Medsger TA Jr, Reichlin M, Rodnan GP. Linear scleroderma: clinical spectrum, prognosis, and laboratory abnormalities. Ann Intern Med 1986;104:849–57.
3. LeRoy EC, Smith EA, Kahaleh MB, Trojanowska M, Silver RM. A strategy for determining the pathogenesis of systemic sclerosis: is transforming growth factor β the answer? Arthritis Rheum 1989;32:817–25.
4. Border WA, Noble NA. Transforming growth factor β in tissue fibrosis. N Engl J Med 1994;331:1286–92.
5. Higley H, Persichitte K, Chu S, Waegell W, Vancheeswaran R, Black C. Immunocytochemical localization and serologic detection of transforming growth factor $\beta 1$: association with type I procollagen and inflammatory cell markers in diffuse and limited systemic sclerosis, morphea, and Raynaud's phenomenon. Arthritis Rheum 1994;37:278–88.

6. Wrana JL, Atissano L, Weiser R, Ventura F, Massague J. Mechanism of activation of the TGF-β receptor. Nature 1994;370:341–7.
7. Dennler S, Itoh S, Vivien D, ten Dijke P, Huet S, Gauthier JM. Direct binding of Smad3 and Smad4 to critical TGF beta-inducible elements in the promoter of human plasminogen activator inhibitor-type 1 gene. EMBO J 1998;17:3091–100.
8. Kawakami T, Ihn H, Xu W, Smith E, LeRoy EC, Trojanowska M. Increased expression of TGF-β receptors by scleroderma fibroblasts: evidence for contribution of autocrine TGF-β signaling to scleroderma phenotype. J Invest Dermatol 1998;110:47–51.
9. Igarashi A, Nashiro K, Kikuchi K, Sato S, Ihn H, Grotenddorst GR, et al. Significant correlation between connective tissue growth factor gene expression and skin sclerosis in tissue sections from patients with systemic sclerosis. J Invest Dermatol 1995;105:280–4.
10. Massagúe J. The transforming growth factor-β family. Annu Rev Cell Biol 1990;6:597–641.
11. Assonian RK, Fleurdelys BE, Stevenson HC, Miller PJ, Madtes DK, Ranines EW, et al. Expression and secretion of type β transforming growth factor by activated human macrophages. Proc Natl Acad Sci U S A 1987;84:6020–4.

ARTHRITIS & RHEUMATISM
Vol. 44, No. 3, March 2001, pp 735–738

LETTERS

Updating the American College of Rheumatology preliminary classification criteria for systemic sclerosis: addition of severe nailfold capillaroscopy abnormalities markedly increases the sensitivity for limited scleroderma

To the Editor:

We read with interest the article by Poormoghim et al (1), in which they note that some patients with systemic sclerosis (SSc) have disease that does not satisfy the American College of Rheumatology (ACR; formerly, the American Rheumatism Association) preliminary classification criteria for definite SSc (2). Poormoghim and colleagues suggest that the ACR classification criteria for SSc should be revised to more adequately incorporate such patients (1). We concur with their view and wish to share data showing our approach to this issue.

The ACR classification criteria for SSc were not designed for diagnostic purposes but rather with the intent "to establish a standard for definite disease in order to permit comparison of groups of patients from different centers" (2). However, these criteria are perceived as diagnostic criteria (3) and thus are often used by clinicians to diagnose SSc. Yet, like Medsger (4) and others, we have observed that the ACR criteria paradoxically exclude certain patients who have been diagnosed by experienced clinicians as having definite SSc. Therefore, we wished to evaluate the potential diagnostic value of ACR criteria in our SSc cohort. Furthermore, given that the ACR criteria were published 20 years ago, we wanted to determine whether addition of more recently described SSc features, such as nailfold capillary microscopy (NCM) features, could increase their sensitivity.

Between 1984 and 1999, 259 consecutive French Canadian patients at the Connective Tissue Diseases Clinics, Notre-Dame Hospital (5,6) were diagnosed by expert clinicians (DC, J-RG, FJ, AR, ER, J-LS) as having definite SSc. The clinical diagnosis of SSc was made without awareness of NCM or anticentromere antibody (ACA) test results. Patients were evaluated at first visit with a standard clinical, visceral extension, and NCM protocol encompassing 215 variables computerized into an Access database. They were categorized into 3 SSc subsets according to a slightly modified version of the definitions described by Barnett et al (7), based on extent of sclerodermatous skin involvement: diffuse (must include trunk involvement; 29 patients), intermediate (must include upper extremities proximal to metacarpophalangeal [MCP] joints without trunk involvement; 78 patients), and limited (sclerodactyly only, plus Raynaud's phenomenon [RP]; 152 patients). Patients with overlap syndrome features were not included in this classification. Patients were further classified as fulfilling the ACR 1980 preliminary criteria for SSc (ACR+) or not (ACR−), based on the presence or absence of the major criterion, i.e., sclerodermatous skin involvement proximal to MCP joints (including facial skin thickening), or 2 or more of the minor criteria: 1) sclerodactyly, 2) digital pitting scars or loss of substance of the distal finger pad, and 3) bibasilar pulmonary fibrosis (2).

NCM was performed as previously described (6,8). All digits of both hands were examined with an SR stereomicroscope (Carl Zeiss, Montreal, Quebec, Canada) at 8–50× magnification using a cool source of illumination, and the following were recorded: degree of capillary dilatation (0 = normal; 1 = borderline [<2× normal diameter]; 2 = definitely dilated [≥2× but ≤4× normal diameter]; 3 = extremely dilated [>4× normal diameter]) and avascular areas (A = no capillary loss; B = rare avascular areas; C = moderate capillary loss; D = extensive capillary loss). The capillary origin of clinically visible telangiectasias of the hands was confirmed by NCM. In our patient population, the specificity of grade 2 or 3 capillary dilatations for SSc ranges from 95.6% to 100%, as determined in studies using controls with primary RP (n = 507), systemic lupus erythematosus (SLE; n = 27), and rheumatoid arthritis (RA; n = 20). All of the SLE and RA controls were selected because they had RP. In studies using the same controls, the specificity of grade C or D avascular areas for SSc ranges from 93.1% to 100%.

As expected, all patients (100%) in the diffuse and intermediate SSc subsets were ACR+. However, in the limited SSc subset, only 51 patients (33.6%) were ACR+. Thus, 101 patients (66.4%) diagnosed by expert clinicians as having limited SSc could not be classified as having SSc according to the ACR 1980 criteria. No significant differences were observed between the limited SSc ACR+ and limited SSc ACR− groups in the proportion of women (92% versus 84.1%, respectively), age at SSc onset (mean ± SD 38.4 ± 14.3 years versus 41.2 ± 13.6 years), age at first evaluation (mean ± SD 50.5 ± 12.5 years versus 51 ± 11.3 years), or frequency of clinically visible capillary telangiectasias of the hands, face, lips, or tongue (62.7% versus 50.4%), capillary dilatations of grades 0 and 1 (30.6% versus 34.7%), or of grades 2 and 3 (69.4% versus 65.2%), and presence of ACA (56.8% versus 50%).

In contrast, several clinical variables were significantly more common in the limited SSc ACR+ group: digital pitting scars (86.2% versus 0%; $P < 0.001$), pulmonary fibrosis (11.7% versus 0%; $P < 0.01$), esophageal involvement (62.7% versus 34.6%; $P < 0.01$), and calcinosis (45.1% versus 20.8%; $P < 0.01$). More severe capillary loss was also significantly more common in the limited SSc ACR+ versus the limited SSc ACR− group: 20.4% versus 45.2% for grade A or B avascular areas, and 79.6% versus 54.7% for grade C or D avascular areas ($P < 0.05$).

To determine whether the sensitivity of the ACR criteria for limited SSc could be improved, we computed the sensitivities generated by addition of single clinical variables as novel minor criteria, selected because their frequency was equal or greater in the limited SSc ACR+ group. Figure 1 is a regression tree showing the best improvement in sensitivity. Introduction of grade 2 or 3 dilated capillaries improved the sensitivity from 33.4% to 74.3%. The sensitivity further improved to 82.9% by adding grade C or D avascular areas, and to 88.8% with clinically visible capillary telangiectasias. Finally, the presence of ACA increased the sensitivity to 91.5%.

Due to the exclusion of a large number of patients with limited SSc, accounting for 39% of our SSc cohort, the

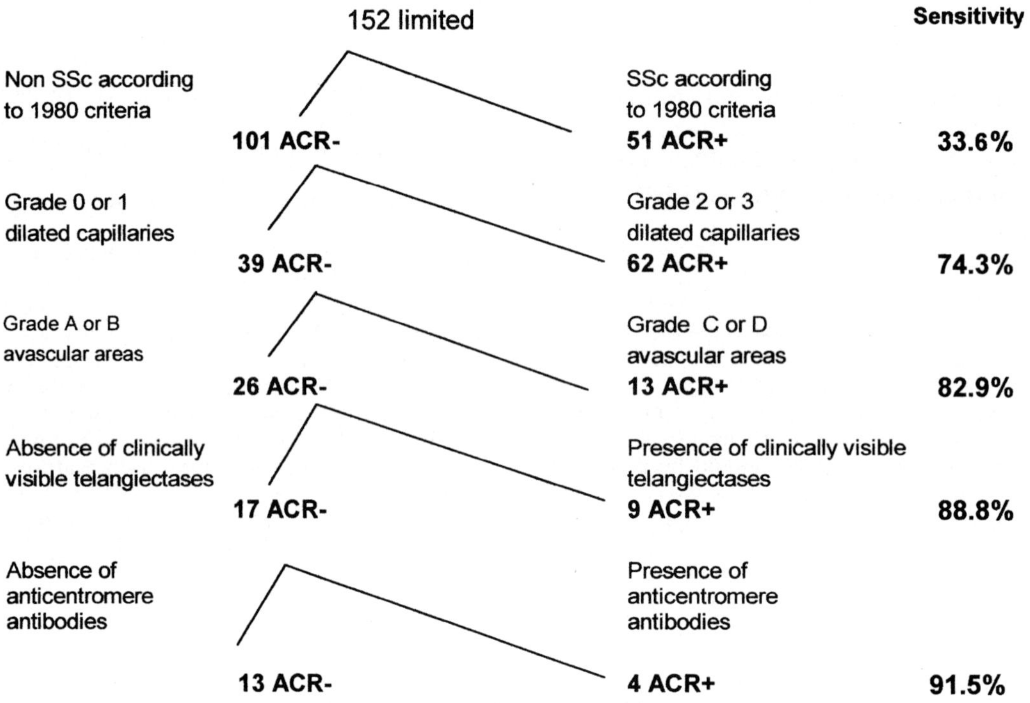

Figure 1. Regression tree showing the sensitivity of possible minor criteria additions to the American College of Rheumatology (ACR; formerly, the American Rheumatism Association) criteria for systemic sclerosis (SSc), as applied to patients with limited SSc at first evaluation. Patients (n = 152) were diagnosed as having limited SSc by expert clinicians. All patients had Raynaud's phenomenon plus the 1980 minor criterion of sclerodactyly. Patients with 2 minor criteria, i.e., sclerodactyly plus 1 of these novel criteria, are designated ACR+. Patients with sclerodactyly as the only minor criterion are designated ACR−.

sensitivity of the ACR criteria is low. Our data support the view of Poormoghim et al (1) and previous findings by Medsger (4) emphasizing the need to revise the ACR criteria to more adequately incorporate patients with limited SSc. These results suggest that the diagnostic sensitivity of ACR criteria may be markedly improved by addition of simple clinical variables, including NCM abnormalities and ACA positivity, as novel minor criteria. These variables were not included in the original ACR criteria, because they were described after publication of the criteria. They should be evaluated in a multicenter trial aimed at revising the 1980 criteria.

Supported by Sclérodermie Québec.

Lilian Scussel Lonzetti, MD
France Joyal, MD, FRCPC
Jean-Pierre Raynauld, MD, FRCPC
André Roussin, MD, FRCPC
Jean-Richard Goulet, MD, FRCPC
Éric Rich, MD, FRCPC
Denis Choquette, MD, FRCPC
Yves Raymond, PhD
Jean-Luc Senécal, MD, FRCPC
Notre-Dame Hospital
Centre Hospitalier de l'Université de Montréal
Montreal, Quebec, Canada

1. Poormoghim H, Lucas M, Fertig N, Medsger TA Jr. Systemic sclerosis sine scleroderma: demographic, clinical, and serologic features and survival in forty-eight patients. Arthritis Rheum 2000; 43:444–51.
2. Subcommittee for Scleroderma Criteria of the American Rheumatism Association Diagnostic and Therapeutic Criteria Committee. Preliminary criteria for the classification of systemic sclerosis (scleroderma). Arthritis Rheum 1980;23:581–90.
3. Wigley FM. Systemic sclerosis: clinical features. In: Klippel JH, Dieppe PA, editors. Rheumatology. Philadelphia: Mosby; 1998. p. 7.9.1–13.
4. Medsger TA Jr. Comment on scleroderma criteria cooperative study. In: Black CM, Myers AR, editors. Current topics in rheumatology: systemic sclerosis (scleroderma). New York: Gower; 1985. p. 16–7.
5. Weiner ES, Earnshaw WC, Senécal JL, Bordwell B, Johnson P, Rothfield NF. Clinical associations of anticentromere antibodies and antibodies to topoisomerase I: a study of 355 patients. Arthritis Rheum 1988;31:378–85.
6. Joyal F, Choquette D, Roussin A, Senécal JL. Evaluation of the severity of systemic sclerosis by nailfold capillary microscopy in 112 patients. Angiology 1992;43:203–10.
7. Barnett AJ, Miller MH, Littlejohn GO. A survival study of patients with scleroderma diagnosed over 30 years (1953–1983): the value of a simple cutaneous classification in the early stages of the disease. J Rheumatol 1988;15:276–83.
8. Maricq HR. Widefield capillary microscopy: technique and rating scale of abnormalities seen in scleroderma and related disorders. Arthritis Rheum 1981;24:1159–65.

Possible role of antiidiotypes in the loss of anti–topoisomerase I antibodies: comment on the article by Kuwana et al

To the Editor:

We read with great interest the article by Kuwana et al (1) reporting on a subset of anti–topoisomerase I antibody (anti–topo I)–positive patients with systemic sclerosis who lost this autoantibody during their disease course, independent of immunosuppressive treatment. These patients, referred to as group 1, had a favorable clinical outcome compared with patients who were persistently positive for this autoantibody (group 2). Topo I reactivity of group 1 patients' circulating lymphocytes, isolated from an antibody-negative blood sample, was intermediate between that observed with healthy donors and that with group 2 patients. Kuwana et al attribute the disappearance of anti–topo I to a loss of antigenic stimulation of topo I–reactive lymphocytes, rather than to their elimination.

We would like to propose an alternative theory to account for the disappearance of anti–topo I in these patients, based on antiidiotypic regulation of another disease-specific autoantibody, antiribosomal P. These antibodies are detected by conventional assays only in patients who have systemic lupus erythematosus (SLE) or overlap diseases with SLE (2). Interestingly, we identified these antibodies in all healthy individuals' sera after treatment with immobilized ribosomal P protein (3,4). Antiidiotypic antibodies, which are displaced by this treatment, mask antiribosomal P antibodies, thereby preventing their detection by conventional assays (5). SLE patients who persistently lack antiribosomal P antibodies also have masking antiidiotypes, whereas those who are persistently positive for antiribosomal P antibodies have absent or dysfunctional antiidiotypes (5). We also identified a subset of antiribosomal P antibody–positive patients (n = 7) who lost these antibodies during their disease course. Covert antiribosomal P antibodies and their antiidiotypes were recoverable from their sera when overt antiribosomal P antibodies were not demonstrable. Thus, we hypothesize that antiidiotypes contribute to the disappearance of antiribosomal P antibodies in these patients.

We would like Kuwana and colleagues to consider the possibility that antiidiotypes to anti–topo I fulfill a similar role in topo I–specific autoimmunity. These antibodies could prevent the serologic detection and in vitro production of anti–topo I in healthy individuals and account for their loss in group 1 patients. Regulatory antiidiotypes could be responsible for the delayed antigen-specific T lymphocyte proliferation and decreased T lymphocyte precursor numbers in healthy individuals and group 1 patients. If this scenario is accurate, then anti–topo I autoantibodies would join the growing list of autoantibodies that are regulated by antiidiotypes, e.g., anti-DNA, antimitochondrial antibodies, and a variety of organ-specific autoantibodies (6).

Haraldine A. Stafford, PhD, MD
University of Oklahoma Health Sciences Center
Oklahoma Medical Research Foundation
and Department of Veterans Affairs
Zi-Jian Pan, MD
Camille J. Anderson, MS
Oklahoma Medical Research Foundation
Oklahoma City, OK

1. Kuwana M, Kaburaki J, Mimori T, Kawakami Y, Tojo T. Longitudinal analysis of autoantibody response to topoisomerase I in systemic sclerosis. Arthritis Rheum 2000;43:1074–84.
2. Elkon KB, Bonfa E, Brot N. Antiribosomal antibodies in systemic lupus erythematosus. Rheum Dis Clin North Am 1992;18:377–90.
3. Stafford HA, Anderson CJ, Reichlin M. Unmasking of antiribosomal P autoantibodies in healthy individuals. J Immunol 1995;155:2754–61.
4. Anderson CJ, Neas BR, Pan Z, Taylor-Albert E, Reichlin M, Stafford HA. The presence of masked antiribosomal P autoantibodies in healthy children. Arthritis Rheum 1998;41:33–40.
5. Pan Z, Anderson CJ, Stafford HA. Anti-idiotypic antibodies prevent the serologic detection of anti-ribosomal P autoantibodies in healthy adults. J Clin Invest 1998;102:215–22.
6. Stafford HA, Reichlin M. Dysregulation of the idiotype network in autoimmune diseases. In: Paul S, editor. Contemporary immunology: autoimmune reactions. Totowa, NJ: Humana Press; 1999. p. 157–76.

Reply

To the Editor:

We thank Dr. Stafford and colleagues for their valuable comments on our study of longitudinal anti–topo I responses in patients with systemic sclerosis (SSc). We attributed the disappearance of serum anti–topo I in the group 1 patients to a loss of antigenic stimulation that activates topo I–reactive T and B cells. Dr. Stafford and coworkers propose possible alternative explanations.

Stafford et al raise 2 different points. First, they suggest a possible interpretation of the negative serum anti–topo I findings in group 1 patients, i.e., that covert anti–topo I is still present in sera, but antiidiotypes prevent their detection of conventional serologic assays. Unfortunately, we have not examined "masked" anti-topo I after treatment of group 1 sera with immobilized topo I, and there is no reported study examining antiidiotypes to anti–topo I in sera from SSc patients or healthy individuals. However, analysis of anti–topo I idiotypes by Vazquez-Abad et al showed the presence of both cross-reactive and private idiotypes (1). In addition, the majority of anti–topo I–positive SSc sera contain heterogeneous antibodies directed against several distinct epitopes, including continuous and conformational epitopes (2,3). These findings strongly suggest that anti–topo I in SSc sera are heterogeneous in terms of idiotypic expression and antigenic specificity. Therefore, it is unlikely that induction of antibodies to 1 or a few idiotypes alone prevents the serologic detection of the entire range of anti–topo I antibodies, although multiple types of antiidiotypes to antiribosomal P have been shown to exist in some individuals (4).

Stafford and colleagues also suggest an alternative theory to account for the disappearance of anti–topo I, i.e., that autoreactive T and B cell responses to topo I are suppressed by antiidiotypic regulation, rather than a loss of antigenic stimulation. In this regard, it has been shown that antiidiotypes suppress antibody production from B cells by crosslinking B cell receptors (5,6). In addition, we have reported that topo I–specific B cells are acting not only as anti–topo I–producing cells but also as efficient antigen-presenting cells that activate topo I–reactive CD4+ T cells (7). Therefore, antiidiotypes may inhibit antigen uptake by blocking the antigen-binding site of B cell receptors, resulting in insufficient presentation of "cryptic" epitopes to topo I–reactive CD4+ T cells. The delayed kinetics of antigen-induced T cell proliferation and the decreased T cell precursor frequencies in group 1 patients after loss of anti–topo I could be explained by this regulatory action of antiidiotypes. On the other hand, we recently identified CD8+ T cells that specifically killed topo I–specific CD4+ T cells in SSc patients with anti–topo I, probably by recognition of the unique determinants on the T cell receptor. It is believed that immune tolerance to the variable regions in the T cell receptors and immunoglobulins that determine antigen binding specificity does not develop, since during the neonatal period these unique binding regions are present at levels that are too low to induce tolerance. Individual T cell receptors and immunoglobulins are therefore immunogenic by virtue of these unique sequences, and immune responses to these idiotypes are capable of influencing the outcome of an immune response.

Taken together, these observations indicate that further studies examining immune responses to the idiotypes of both T cell receptors and immunoglobulins are necessary to understand mechanisms regulating autoantibody responses in patients with autoimmune diseases.

Masataka Kuwana, MD
Keio University School of Medicine
Junichi Kaburaki, MD
Tokyo Electric Power Company Hospital
Tokyo, Japan

1. Vazquez-Abad D, Pascual V, Zanetti M, Rothfield NF. Analysis of human antitopoisomerase I idiotypes. J Clin Invest 1993;93: 1301–13.
2. Kuwana M, Kaburaki J, Mimori T, Tojo T, Homma M. Autoantigenic epitopes on DNA topoisomerase I: clinical and immunogenetic associations in systemic sclerosis. Arthritis Rheum 1993;36: 1406–13.
3. Kuwana M, Kaburaki J, Medsger TA Jr, Wright TM. An immunodominant epitope on DNA topoisomerase I is conformational in nature: heterogeneity in its recognition by systemic sclerosis sera. Arthritis Rheum 1999;42:1179–88.
4. Pan Z, Anderson CJ, Stafford HA. Anti-idiotypic antibodies prevent the serologic detection of anti-ribosomal P autoantibodies in healthy adults. J Clin Invest 1998;102:215–22.
5. Rajewsky K, Takemori T. Genetics, expression, and function of idiotypes. Annu Rev Immunol 1983;1:569–607.
6. Geha RS. Idiotypic-anti-idiotypic interactions in man. Am J Dis Child 1985;139:417–20.
7. Kuwana M, Medsger TA Jr, Wright TM. T–B cell collaboration is essential for the autoantibody response to DNA topoisomerase I in systemic sclerosis. J Immunol 1995;155:2703–14.

RHEUMATOLOGIST
Suburb of Pittsburgh, Pennsylvania

Excellent opportunity for well qualified BC/BE Rheumatologist to join 2 other Rheumatologists in a well established practice, physician owned and directed. The practice is associated with 3 community hospitals and has 2 office locations that include laboratory, X-rays, Bone Mineral Density, approximately 90% Rheumatology and 10% Internal Medicine. The position will also entail teaching duties in an Internal Medicine Residency program. Offering a competitive salary, attractive fringe benefits, and an opportunity for partnership. (Preferably without Visa problems) Please fax or send CV with cover letter to:

Denise Brakeall / 500 Naysmith Road
North Versailles, PA 15137 / Fax: (412) 673-6223

South Florida

BC/BE Rheumatologist to join well established 5 MD, 100% Rheumatology practice. The practice is affiliated with 3 community hospitals and has 3 office locations with modern facilities that include a laboratory, DEXA, x-ray, and clinical research site. Exceptional candidate will enjoy a competitive salary package with fringe benefits that include a 401K plan. Our practice, is located in beautiful Boca Raton with excellent schools and quality of life. Please fax or mail CV to:

Rheumatology Associates
1050 NW 15th Street, Suite 212A
Boca Raton, FL 33486
Attn: Leslie Smiciklas / Fax: 561-361-6818

Park Nicollet

Rheumatologist

We are a dynamic 5 person group in a large, nationally recognized, multispecialty clinic in Minneapolis. Our interests include the full range of rheumatologic practice, as well as an extremely active osteoporosis program. Clinical research activities abound in many areas including osteoporosis and traditional rheumatologic arenas. These activities are supported by a reaseach staff who serve under the auspices of an affiliated research foundation. Opportunities exist for university affiliation. We enjoy an excellent referral base, excellent salary and benefits, enviable collegiality, and the lifestyle and amenities, including wide ranging cultural offerings, major sporting events, and easy access to beautiful lakes and country during all 4 seasons, of one of America's greatest cities.

Please send CV to Missy Fisher, Manager Clinician Recruitment, Park Nicollet Health Services, 3800 Park Nicollet Blvd. - 7N, Minneapolis, MN 55416; fax (952) 993-2819; email: fishem@parknicollet.com. For more information, call Missy Fisher (952) 993-6025 or (888) 437-5004.

KAISER PERMANENTE

A Great History. A Greater Future.

What has 50 years of medical excellence brought our professionals at The Permanente Medical Group Inc.? A longstanding reputation for progress that not only offers them the stability they need for a fulfilling career, but also the freedom to explore innovative ideas on the horizon. We currently have an exceptional opportunity in Northern California.

RHEUMATOLOGY
San Francisco Bay Area

For more information, please contact Mazie Blanks, Physician Recruiter, Physician Recruitment Services, Dept A159, 1814 Franklin Street, 4th Floor, Oakland, CA 94612; Phone: (800) 777-4912; Fax: (510) 873-5006. Email: Mazie.Blanks@kp.org.

KAISER PERMANENTE®

www.kp.org/ca • EEO/AA Employer

SOUTH CAROLINA

Graduating fellows and experienced Rheumatologists are invited to call **Dr. Chermol at (800) 866-6045** to discuss an exceptional private practice opportunity with an established, successful, board certified Rheumatologist. Located between two major cities and the mountains and the beach; excellent family environment; new office; modern hospital. Not a J-1 visa site.

RHEUMATOLOGIST

The VA Western New York Healthcare System has an immediate opening for a full-time staff Rheumatologist at the Buffalo Medical Center. The selected candidate will work in the Rheumatology clinic providing treatment to veterans on an outpatient basis; perform consults for inpatients on an as-needed basis; provide clinical instruction to medical students, residents and fellows; and participate in an active research program. The selected candidate will also receive a faculty appointment at the affiliated Department of Medicine, SUNY at Buffalo School of Medicine. Must be BC/BE in Rheumatology. Candidates interested in investigative careers highly desirable. Salary based on experience. Please respond with CV and three (3) letters of reference to: **Human Resources Management Office, VA Western New York Healthcare System, 3495 Bailey Avenue, Buffalo, NY 14215. Fax: (716) 862-3281. E-mail: hrms.buffalo@med.va.gov.** *Equal Opportunity Employer.*

Enbrel® etanercept

BRIEF SUMMARY

See package insert for full Prescribing Information.

INDICATIONS AND USAGE

ENBREL is indicated for reducing signs and symptoms and delaying structural damage in patients with moderately to severely active rheumatoid arthritis. ENBREL can be used in combination with methotrexate in patients who do not respond adequately to methotrexate alone.

ENBREL is indicated for reducing signs and symptoms of moderately to severely active polyarticular-course juvenile rheumatoid arthritis in patients who have had an inadequate response to one or more DMARDs.

CONTRAINDICATIONS

ENBREL should not be administered to patients with sepsis or with known hypersensitivity to ENBREL or any of its components.

WARNINGS

IN POSTMARKETING REPORTS, SERIOUS INFECTIONS AND SEPSIS, INCLUDING FATALITIES, HAVE BEEN REPORTED WITH THE USE OF ENBREL. MANY OF THESE SERIOUS EVENTS HAVE OCCURRED IN PATIENTS WITH UNDERLYING DISEASES THAT IN ADDITION TO THEIR RHEUMATOID ARTHRITIS COULD PREDISPOSE THEM TO INFECTIONS. PATIENTS WHO DEVELOP A NEW INFECTION WHILE UNDERGOING TREATMENT WITH ENBREL SHOULD BE MONITORED CLOSELY. ADMINISTRATION OF ENBREL SHOULD BE DISCONTINUED IF A PATIENT DEVELOPS A SERIOUS INFECTION OR SEPSIS. TREATMENT WITH ENBREL SHOULD NOT BE INITIATED IN PATIENTS WITH ACTIVE INFECTIONS INCLUDING CHRONIC OR LOCALIZED INFECTIONS. PHYSICIANS SHOULD EXERCISE CAUTION WHEN CONSIDERING THE USE OF ENBREL IN PATIENTS WITH A HISTORY OF RECURRING INFECTIONS OR WITH UNDERLYING CONDITIONS WHICH MAY PREDISPOSE PATIENTS TO INFECTIONS, SUCH AS ADVANCED OR POORLY CONTROLLED DIABETES (see **PRECAUTIONS, ADVERSE REACTIONS, Infections**).

Neurologic Events- Rare cases of central nervous system demyelinating disorders have been described in spontaneous adverse event reports (see **ADVERSE REACTIONS**). The causal relationship to ENBREL therapy remains unclear. However, while no clinical trials have been performed evaluating ENBREL therapy in multiple sclerosis, other TNF antagonists administered to patients with multiple sclerosis have been associated with increases in disease activity. Prescribers should exercise caution in considering the use of ENBREL in patients with preexisting or recent onset of central nervous system demyelinating disorders. **Hematologic Events**- Rare reports of pancytopenia, including aplastic anemia, some with a fatal outcome, have been reported in patients with rheumatoid arthritis treated with ENBREL (see **ADVERSE REACTIONS**). The causal relationship to ENBREL therapy remains unclear. Although no high risk group has been identified, caution should be exercised in patients being treated with ENBREL who have a previous history of significant hematologic abnormalities. All patients should be advised that if they develop signs and symptoms suggestive of blood dyscrasias or infection (e.g., persistent fever, bruising, bleeding, pallor) while on ENBREL, they should seek immediate medical attention. If significant hematologic abnormalities are confirmed, consideration should be given to discontinuation of ENBREL therapy.

PRECAUTIONS: General-Allergic reactions associated with administration of ENBREL during clinical trials have been reported in <2% of patients. If an anaphylactic reaction or other serious allergic reaction occurs, administration of ENBREL should be discontinued immediately and appropriate therapy initiated. **Information to Patients**-If a patient or caregiver is to self-administer ENBREL, he/she should be instructed in injection techniques and how to measure the correct dose to help ensure the proper administration of ENBREL (see **How to Use ENBREL, Instructions for Preparing and Giving an Injection**). The first injection should be performed under the supervision of a qualified health care professional. The patient's or caregiver's ability to self-inject subcutaneously should be assessed. A puncture-resistant container for disposal of needles and syringes should be used. Patients and caregivers should be instructed in the technique as well as proper syringe and needle disposal, and be cautioned against reuse of these items. **Immunosuppression**-The possibility exists for anti-TNF therapies, including ENBREL, to affect host defenses against infections and malignancies since TNF mediates inflammation and modulates cellular immune responses. In a study of 49 patients with RA treated with ENBREL, there was no evidence of depression of delayed-type hypersensitivity, depression of immunoglobulin levels, or change in enumeration of effector cell populations. The impact of treatment with ENBREL on the development and course of malignancies, as well as active and/or chronic infections is not fully understood (see **WARNINGS, ADVERSE REACTIONS, Infections** and **Malignancies**). The safety and efficacy of ENBREL in patients with immunosuppression have not been evaluated. **Immunizations**-No data are available on the effects of vaccination in patients receiving ENBREL. Live vaccines should not be given concurrently with ENBREL. No data are available on the secondary transmission of infection by live vaccines in patients receiving ENBREL (see **PRECAUTIONS, Immunosuppression**). It is recommended that JRA patients, if possible, be brought up to date with all immunizations in agreement with current immunization guidelines prior to initiating ENBREL therapy. Two JRA patients developed varicella infection and signs and symptoms of aseptic meningitis, which resolved without sequelae. Patients with a significant exposure to varicella virus should temporarily discontinue ENBREL therapy and be considered for prophylactic treatment with Varicella Zoster Immune Globulin. **Autoantibody Formation**-Treatment with ENBREL may result in the formation of autoimmune antibodies (see **ADVERSE REACTIONS, Autoantibodies**). **Drug Interactions**-Specific drug interaction studies have not been conducted with ENBREL. **Carcinogenesis, Mutagenesis, and Impairment of Fertility**-Long-term animal studies have not been conducted to evaluate the carcinogenic potential of ENBREL or its effect on fertility. Mutagenesis studies were conducted in vitro and in vivo, and no evidence of mutagenic activity was observed. **Pregnancy (Category B)**-Developmental toxicity studies have been performed in rats and rabbits at doses ranging from 60- to 100-fold higher than the human dose and have revealed no evidence of harm to the fetus due to ENBREL. There are, however, no studies in pregnant women. Because animal reproduction studies are not always predictive of human response, this drug should be used during pregnancy only if clearly needed. **Nursing Mothers**-It is not known whether ENBREL is excreted in human milk or absorbed systemically after ingestion. Because many drugs and immunoglobulins are excreted in human milk, and because of the potential for serious adverse reactions in nursing infants from ENBREL, a decision should be made whether to discontinue nursing or to discontinue the drug. **Geriatric Use**-A total of 197 RA patients ages 65 years or older have been studied in clinical trials. No overall differences in safety or effectiveness were observed between these patients and younger patients. Because there is a higher incidence of infections in the elderly population in general, caution should be used in treating the elderly. **Pediatric Use**-ENBREL is indicated for treatment of polyarticular-course juvenile rheumatoid arthritis in patients who have had an inadequate response to one or more DMARDs. For issues relevant to pediatric patients, in addition to other sections of the label, see also **PRECAUTIONS, Immunizations,** and **ADVERSE REACTIONS, Adverse Reactions in Pediatric Patients.** ENBREL has not been studied in children <4 years of age.

ADVERSE REACTIONS: ENBREL has been studied in 1197 patients with RA, followed for up to 36 months. The proportion of patients who discontinued treatment due to adverse events was approximately 4% in both ENBREL and placebo-treated patients. **Injection Site Reactions**-In controlled trials, 37% of patients treated with ENBREL developed injection site reactions. All injection site reactions were described as mild to moderate (erythema and/or itching, pain, or swelling) and generally did not necessitate drug discontinuation. Injection site reactions generally occurred in the first month and subsequently decreased in frequency. The mean duration of injection site reactions was 3 to 5 days. Seven percent of patients experienced redness at a previous injection site when subsequent injections were given. In post-marketing experience, injection site bleeding and bruising have also been observed in conjunction with ENBREL therapy. **Infections**-In controlled trials, there were no differences in rates of infection among patients treated with ENBREL and those treated with placebo or MTX. The most common type of infection was upper respiratory infection, which occurred in 16% of placebo-treated patients and 29% of patients treated with ENBREL. When the longer observation of patients on ENBREL was accounted for, the event rate was similar in both groups. In placebo-controlled trials in DMARD-refractory RA, no increase in the incidence of serious infections was observed (approximately 1% in both placebo and ENBREL-treated groups). The rates of infections for the ENBREL arm in Study III were similar. In all clinical trials in RA, 50 of 1197 subjects exposed to ENBREL for up to 36 months experienced serious infections, including pyelonephritis, bronchitis, septic arthritis, abdominal abscess, cellulitis, osteomyelitis, wound infection, pneumonia, foot abscess, leg ulcer, diarrhea, sinusitis, and sepsis. Serious infections, including sepsis and death, have also been reported during post-marketing use of ENBREL. Some have occurred within a few weeks after initiating treatment with ENBREL. Many of the patients had underlying conditions (e.g., diabetes, congestive heart failure, history of active or chronic infections) in addition to their rheumatoid arthritis (see **WARNINGS**). Data from a sepsis clinical trial not specifically in patients with RA suggest that ENBREL treatment may increase mortality in patients with established sepsis. **Malignancies**-Seventeen malignancies of various types were observed in 1197 RA patients treated in clinical trials with ENBREL for up to 36 months. The observed rates and incidences were similar to those expected for the population studied. **Autoantibodies**-Patients had serum samples tested for autoantibodies at multiple timepoints. In Studies I and II, the percentage of patients evaluated for antinuclear antibodies (ANA), the percentage of patients who developed new positive ANA (≥1:40) was higher in patients treated with ENBREL (11%) than in placebo-treated patients (5%). The percentage of patients who developed new positive anti-double-stranded DNA antibodies was also higher by radioimmunoassay (15% of patients treated with ENBREL compared to 4% of placebo-treated patients) and by crithidia lucilae assay (3% of patients treated with ENBREL compared to none of placebo-treated patients). The proportion of patients treated with ENBREL who developed anticardiolipin antibodies was similarly increased compared to placebo-treated patients. In Study III, no pattern of increased autoantibody development was seen in ENBREL patients compared to MTX patients. No patients in placebo- and active-controlled trials developed clinical signs suggestive of a lupus-like syndrome. The impact of long-term treatment with ENBREL on the development of autoimmune diseases is unknown. **Other Adverse Reactions**-The following table summarizes events reported in at least 3% of all patients with higher incidence in patients treated with ENBREL compared to controls in placebo-controlled RA trials (including the combination methotrexate trial), and relevant events from Study III.

Percent of RA Patients Reporting Adverse Events in Controlled Clinical Trials*

	Placebo Controlled		Active Controlled (Study III)	
	Percent of patients		Percent of patients	
Event	Placebo† (n=152)	ENBREL (n=349)	MTX (n=217)	ENBREL (n=415)
Injection site reaction	10	37	7	34
Infection	32	35	72	64
Non-upper respiratory infection**	32	38	60	51
Upper respiratory infection**	16	29	39	31
Headache	13	17	27	24
Nausea	10	9	29	15
Rhinitis	8	12	14	16
Dizziness	5	7	11	8
Pharyngitis	5	7	9	6
Cough	3	6	6	5
Asthenia	3	5	12	11
Abdominal pain	3	5	10	10
Rash	3	5	23	14
Peripheral edema	3	2	4	8
Respiratory disorder	1	5	NA	NA
Dyspepsia	1	4	10	11
Sinusitis	2	3	3	5
Vomiting	–	3	8	5
Mouth ulcer	1	2	14	6
Alopecia	1	1	12	6
Pneumonitis ("MTX lung")	–	–	2	0

* *Includes data from the 6-month study in which patients received concurrent MTX therapy.*

† *The duration of exposure for patients receiving placebo was less than the ENBREL-treated patients.*

** *Includes data from two of the three placebo-controlled trials.*

Among patients with rheumatoid arthritis treated in placebo-controlled trials, serious adverse events occurred at a frequency of 4% in 349 patients treated with ENBREL compared to 5% of 152 placebo-treated patients. In Study III, serious adverse events occurred at a frequency of 6% in 415 patients treated with ENBREL compared to 8% of 217 MTX-treated patients. Among patients with RA in placebo-controlled, active-controlled, and open-label trials of ENBREL, malignancies (see **ADVERSE REACTIONS, Malignancies**) and infections (see **ADVERSE REACTIONS, Infections**) were the most common serious adverse events observed. Other infrequent serious adverse events observed included heart failure, myocardial infarction, myocardial ischemia, cerebral ischemia, hypertension, hypotension, cholecystitis, pancreatitis, gastrointestinal hemorrhage, bursitis, depression, dyspnea, deep vein thrombosis, pulmonary embolism, membranous glomerulonephropathy, polymyositis, and thrombophlebitis.

Adverse Reaction Information from Spontaneous Reports-Adverse events have been reported during post-approval use of ENBREL. Because these events are reported voluntarily from a population of uncertain size, it is not always possible to reliably estimate their frequency or establish a causal relationship to ENBREL exposure.

In post-marketing experience, patients being treated for RA have reported developing additional manifestations of RA while receiving ENBREL therapy. There are uncommon reports of joint pain, generalized pain, fatigue, and dry mouth. There have also been rare reports of patients developing pulmonary disease, ocular inflammation, anorexia, cutaneous vasculitis, subcutaneous nodules, and dry eyes.

Additional adverse events are listed by body system below:

Body as a whole:	fever, flu syndrome, angioedema, weight gain
Cardiovascular:	chest pain, vasodilation (flushing)
Digestive:	diarrhea, altered sense of taste
Hematologic/Lymphatic:	adenopathy, anemia, leukopenia, thrombocytopenia, pancytopenia, aplastic anemia (see **WARNINGS**)
Nervous:	stroke, paresthesias, seizures and central nervous system events suggestive of multiple sclerosis or isolated demyelinating condition such as transverse myelitis or optic neuritis (see **PRECAUTIONS**)
Respiratory:	dyspnea, worsening of prior lung disorder
Skin:	urticaria, pruritis

Adverse Reactions in Pediatric Patients-In general, the adverse events in pediatric patients were similar in frequency and type as those seen in adult patients. Differences from adults and other special considerations are discussed in the following paragraphs.

Severe adverse reactions reported in 69 JRA patients ages 4 to 17 years included varicella (see also **PRECAUTIONS, Immunizations**), gastroenteritis, depression/personality disorder, cutaneous ulcer, esophagitis/gastritis, group A streptococcal septic shock, type I diabetes mellitus, and soft tissue and post-operative wound infection.

Forty-three of 69 (62%) children with JRA experienced an infection while receiving ENBREL during 3 months of study (part 1 open-label), and the frequency and severity of infections was similar in 58 patients completing 12 months of open-label extension therapy. The types of infections reported in JRA patients were generally mild and consistent with those commonly seen in outpatient pediatric populations.

The following adverse events were reported more commonly in 69 JRA patients receiving 3 months of ENBREL compared to the 349 adult RA patients in placebo-controlled trials. These included headache (19% of patients, 1.7 events per patient year), nausea (9%, 1.0 events per patient year), abdominal pain (19%, 0.74 events per patient year), and vomiting (13%, 0.74 events per patient year).

In post-marketing experience, very rare cases of cutaneous vasculitis in children with JRA have been reported. A causal relationship to ENBREL therapy for this condition has not been established.

OVERDOSAGE: The maximum tolerated dose of ENBREL has not been established in humans. Toxicology studies have been performed in monkeys at doses up to 30 times the human dose with no evidence of dose-limiting toxicities. No dose-limiting toxicities have been observed during clinical trials of ENBREL. Single IV doses up to 60 mg/m² have been administered to healthy volunteers in an endotoxemia study without evidence of dose-limiting toxicities. The highest dose level evaluated in RA patients has been a single IV loading dose of 32 mg/m² followed by SC doses of 16 mg/m² (~25 mg) administered twice weekly. In one RA trial, one patient mistakenly self-administered 62 mg ENBREL SC twice weekly for 3 weeks without experiencing adverse effects.

RX only

This Brief Summary is based on document 0311-06, issued 10/00.

Manufactured by:
Immunex Corporation
Seattle, Washington 98101
U.S. License Number 1132

Marketed by Immunex Corporation and Wyeth-Ayerst Pharmaceuticals

IMMUNEX® WYETH-AYERST LABORATORIES

Immunex U.S. Patent Numbers: 5,395,760; 5,605,690; 5,945,397; Re. 36,755
For more information, please call 1-888-436-2735.

61697-00